Brief Contents

Fundamentals of Nursing

THE ART AND SCIENCE OF NURSING CARE

Fundamentals of Nursing

THE ART AND SCIENCE OF NURSING CARE

Seventh Edition

Carol R. Taylor, PhD, MSN, RN
Center for Clinical Bioethics
Professor of Nursing
Georgetown University
Washington, DC

Carol Lillis, MSN, RN
Faculty Emerita, Assistant to the Provost
Delaware County Community College
Media, Pennsylvania

Priscilla LeMone, DSN, RN, FAAN
Associate Professor Emerita, Sinclair School of Nursing
University of Missouri
Columbia, Missouri
Adjunct Associate Professor, College of Nursing
The Ohio State University
Columbus, Ohio

Pamela Lynn, MSN, RN
Instructor
School of Nursing
Gwynedd-Mercy College
Gwynedd Valley, Pennsylvania

Wolters Kluwer | Lippincott Williams & Wilkins
Health
Philadelphia • Baltimore • New York • London
Buenos Aires • Hong Kong • Sydney • Tokyo

Executive Acquisitions Editor: Carrie Brandon
Senior Product Manager: Betsy Gentzler
Editorial Assistants: Shawn Loht, Amanda Jordan
Design Coordinator: Holly Reid McLaughlin
Illustration Coordinator: Brett MacNaughton
Manufacturing Coordinator: Karin Duffield
Prepress Vendor: Aptara, Inc.

7th Edition

Library of Congress Cataloging-in-Publication Data

Fundamentals of nursing : the art and science of nursing care / Carol R.
    Taylor . . . [et al.]. – 7th ed.
        p. ; cm.
    Includes bibliographical references and index.
        ISBN 978-0-7817-9383-4 (alk. paper)
    1. Nursing. I. Taylor, Carol, CSFN.
    [DNLM: 1. Nursing Care. 2. Nursing Process. WY 100.1]
    RT41.T396 2011
    610.73–dc22

                                2010030027

LWW.com

To Bob, my husband and best friend, who makes life a joy!
—CAROL TAYLOR

To my husband, Jack: Your support and sense of humor have made everything possible.
—CAROL LILLIS

I dedicate this book to all the students who will become the nurses of tomorrow and to all the students I have taught, who are the nurses of today.
—PRISCILLA LEMONE

To John, Jenn, and Anna: The best support system anyone could ask for.
—PAM LYNN

Contributors and Reviewers

CONTRIBUTORS

Lynn Burbank, MSN, RN, CPNP
Learning Resource Coordinator
Dixon School of Nursing
Abington Memorial Hospital
Abington, Pennsylvania
> CHAPTER 29: MEDICATIONS

Kerry H. Cheever, PhD, RN
Professor and Chairperson, St. Luke's
    School of Nursing at Moravian College
Assistant Vice President, St. Luke's
    Hospital & Health Network
Bethlehem, Pennsylvania
> PICO IN PRACTICE: ASKING CLINICAL
>   QUESTIONS

Joanne O'Brien, RN, MSN
Associate Professor
Delaware County Community College
Media, Pennsylvania
> CONCEPT MAPS

Christine E. Smith, MSN, RN, CNOR
Perioperative Clinical Nurse Specialist
Lucile Packard Children's Hospital at
    Stanford
Palo Alto, California
> CHAPTER 30: PERIOPERATIVE NURSING

REVIEWERS

Robin Abrams, RN, MS, CDE
Nursing Faculty
Alvin Community College
Alvin, Texas

Faisal Aboul-Enein, DrPH, MSN,
    MPH, NP
Clinical Assistant Professor
Texas Women's University
Houston, Texas

Lavonne M. Adams, PhD, RN, CCRN
Associate Professor of Nursing
Texas Christian University, Harris College
    of Nursing & Health Sciences
Fort Worth, Texas

Gerry Ehrmann Altmiller, EdD, MSN,
    APRN
Assistant Professor
La Salle University, School of Nursing and
    Health Sciences
Philadelphia, Pennsylvania

Jane G. Anderson, MSN, RN, BC, GCNS
Instructor, Undergraduate Program,
    College of Nursing
Medical University of South Carolina
Charleston, South Carolina

Lyda Arévalo-Flechas, PhD, MSN, RN
Assistant Professor
JAHF Claire M. Fagin Fellow
University of Texas Health Science Center
    at San Antonio, School of Nursing
San Antonio, Texas

Lisa Ayers, RN, MSN, CNE
Assistant Professor
Harper College
Palatine, Illinois

Helen Ballestas, PhD, RN, CRRN
Assistant Professor of Nursing
Adelphi University
Garden City, New York

Judith Bateman, RN, MSN
Assistant Professor
Coordinator, CNA Program
Black Hawk College
Moline, Illinois

Joyce Bates, RN, MSN
Assistant Professor
Fairmont State University
Fairmont, West Virginia

Cynthia Bechtel, PhD(c), RN, CEN,
    CNE, EMT-I
Assistant Professor
Nursing Coordinator, MSN Program
Framingham State College
Framingham, Massachusetts

Jennifer Beck, PhD, RN, CNE
Associate Professor of Nursing
Our Lady of the Lake College
Baton Rouge, Louisiana

Kathy Becker, RN, MSN Med
Associate Professor
St. Louis Community College, Forest
    Park
St. Louis, Missouri

Diana R. Beckner, RN, MSN, CS, FNP
Nursing Instructor
Lincoln Memorial University
Harrogate, Tennessee

Amy Bigham, MSN, APRN, BC
Instructor
University of Alabama, Capstone College
    of Nursing
Tuscaloosa, Alabama

Mary Bjorklund, RN, MSN, CPN
Professor, Associate Degree Nursing
Lonestar College—Kingwood
Kingwood, Texas

Kathleen Blust, MSN, RN, BC
Professor of Nursing
Collin College
McKinney, Texas

Joanne Bonesteel, MS, RN
Nursing Faculty
Excelsior College School of Nursing
Albany, New York

Connie J. Booth, RN, MSN
Professor
Des Moines Area Community College
Boone, Iowa

Dana M. Botz, RN, MSN
Nursing Instructor
North Hennepin Community College
Brooklyn Park, MN

Ethel Bratt, RN, BScN
Nursing Instructor
Saskatchewan Institute of Applied Science
    and Technology
Regina, Saskatchewan

Nell Britton, MSN, RN, CNE
Nursing Division New Student Coordinator/
    Nursing Instructor
Trident Technical College
Charleston, South Carolina

Anna Bruch
Nursing Faculty
Illinois Valley Community College
Oglesby, Illinois

Beverly Bryant, RN, MSN
Instructor
Athens Technical College
Athens, Georgia

Donna Bumpus, RN, MSN
Assistant Professor of Nursing
Lamar University
Beaumont, Texas

Deborah Burton, RN, MSN
Instructor
San Bernardino Valley College
San Bernardino, California

Cecelia Carew, RN(BC), MA, CNE,
    CCRN, CPAN, CEN, LNC
Associate Professor
Bronx Community College
Bronx, New York

Julie Calvery Carman, MS, APN, FNP-BC
Family Nurse Practitioner
Van Buren Family Medical Clinic
Van Buren, Arkansas

Dr. Veronica Clarke-Tasker, PhD, RN, MBA, MPH
Professor of Nursing
Howard University, College of Pharmacy, Nursing & Allied Health Sciences
Washington, DC

Sandra Cleveland, MSN, RN
Assistant Professor
University of Detroit—Mercy
Detroit, Michigan

Nancy Cohen, MSN, RN, CGRN, CNE
Nursing Instructor 1
University of Pittsburgh Medical Center (UPMC), Shadyside School of Nursing
Pittsburgh, Pennsylvania

Annie Collins, RN, MSN
Assistant Professor of Nursing
Washburn University
Topeka, Kansas

John F. Conklin, RN, MSN, PhD
Assistant Professor of Nursing and Department Chair
State University of New York (SUNY) at Canton
Canton, New York

Marnie Connelly
Professor, Practical Nursing
Algonquin College
Ottawa, Ontario, Canada

Susan Cristofori, RN, MSN
Professor
St. Clair County Community College
Port Huron, Michigan

Becky Daniels, RN, MSN, CPNP
Faculty, Associate's Degree Program
Holmes Community College, Ridgeland Campus
Ridgeland, Mississippi

Ann Denney, MSN, RN
Assistant Professor of Nursing
Thomas More College
Crestview Hills, Kentucky

Maddie Diedo, RN, BSN, MSN
Nursing Faculty
Wayne County Community College District
Detroit, Michigan

Evelyn Dogbey, PhD, APRN, BC
Assistant Professor of Nursing
Temple University
Philadelphia, Pennsylvania

Kris Thomas Dreifuerst
Nursing Faculty
University of Wisconsin, Oshkosh
Oshkosh, Wisconsin

Kathleen M. Reilly Dolin, RN, MSN, DNP
Associate Professor of Nursing
Northampton Community College
Bethlehem, Pennsylvania

Linda Dolphus, MSN, RN, BSN
Nursing Faculty
Wayne County Community College District
Detroit, Michigan

Michelle Dorin, BS, ADN, BSN, PhD
Assistant Professor of Nursing
Texas Women's University
Dallas, Texas

Denise Edinger, RN, MS
Assistant Chairperson
Level II Coordinator
Laboure College
Dorchester, Massachusetts

Maureen Eisenstein, RN, MS
Nursing Instructor
Signature-Healthcare, Brockton Hospital School of Nursing
Brockton, Massachusetts

Kim Everett, MSN, RN
Assistant Professor of Nursing
Southern Arkansas University
Magnolia, Arkansas

Carol Fanutti, EdD, RN, CNE
Professor
Director of Nursing
Trocaire College
Buffalo, New York

Carla Ferguson, RN, MSN, CNE
Associate Professor
Oakton Community College
Des Plaines, Illinois

Ruth Fiedler, EdD, PMHCNS-BC, CNE
Assistant Professor
Rush University
Chicago, Illinois

Cynthia Figueroa-Haas, PhD, ANP-BC
Clinical Assistant Professor
ANP Track Coordinator
Department of Adult & Elderly Nursing
University of Florida
Gainesville, Florida

Karen Flanigan, RN, MS
Nursing Faculty
Chandler-Gilbert Community College
Mesa, Arizona

Jacqueline Frock, MSN, RN
Professor of Nursing
Oklahoma City Community College
Oklahoma City, Oklahoma

Sally Gaines, MSN, RN
Nursing Instructor
Amarillo College
Amarillo, Texas

Linda Garcia
Faculty—Health, Physical Education, and Nursing
Bucks County Community College
Newtown, Pennsylvania

Michelle Gardner
Albany College of Pharmacy
Albany, New York

Patricia Gautreaux, MSN, M.Ed., RN
Nursing Instructor
University of Southern Mississippi
Hattiesburg, Mississippi

Mary Gers, MSN, CNS, RNC
Associate Professor
Director of Simulation and Technology
Northern Kentucky University
Highland Heights, Kentucky

Carol Girocco, MSN, RN
Professor, Associate Degree of Nursing
Lonestar College—Montgomery
Conroe, Texas

Carolyn Godfrey, RN, MSN
Associate Professor, Nursing
St. Louis Community College, Forest Park
St. Louis, Missouri

Ramesh Upadhyaya, RN, CRRN, MSN, MBA
Clinical Instructor
University of North Carolina, Greensboro
Greensboro, North Carolina

Jeanne Ann Van Fossan, RN, MSN, NP
Professor, Nursing
West Virginia Northern Community College
Weirton, West Virginia

Barbara Vickers, RN, MS, CCRN
Nursing Professor
Erie Community College
State University of New York (SUNY)
Buffalo, New York

Susan Waltz, RN, DNP
Professor—School of Health Sciences
Ivy Tech Community College of Indiana
Columbus, Indiana

Marsha Wamsley, RN, MS
Professor of Nursing
Sinclair Community College
Dayton, Ohio

Andrea Weber, MSN, RN
Associate Professor
St. Louis Community College, Forest Park
St. Louis, Missouri

Mary Welhaven, BS, MSN, PhD
Professor, Nursing
Winona State University
Winona, Minnesota

Julie Wells-Tsiatsos, MSN, RN
Nursing Instructor
St. Elizabeth College of Nursing
Utica, New York

Kathleen S. Wilson, RN, MSN
Nursing Professor
Houston Community College
Houston, Texas

Becky Wolff, RN, MSN
Assistant Professor of Nursing
University of South Dakota, Vermillion
Vermillion, South Dakota

Donna Woshinsky, RN, MSN, CNE
Associate Professor of Nursing
Springfield Technical Community College
Springfield, Massachusetts

Robert Wyatt, MSN, RN
Assistant Professor of Nursing
Jackson State Community College
Jackson, Tennessee

Yin Xu, PhD, MSN, RN
Assistant Professor
University of Cincinnati
Cincinnati, Ohio

Joanne M. Yastik, MSN, RN
Assistant Professor of Nursing
University of Detroit Mercy
Detroit, Michigan

Jean Yockey, RN, MSN, CNE
Assistant Professor
University of South Dakota, Vermillion
Vermillion, South Dakota

Preface

Today's competitive, market-driven healthcare environment is challenging the very nature of professional nursing practice. *Fundamentals of Nursing: The Art and Science of Nursing Care,* seventh edition, promotes nursing as an evolving art and science, directed to human health and well-being. It challenges students to cultivate the blended skills they will need to serve patients and the public well. Our aim is to prepare nurses who combine the highest level of scientific knowledge and technologic skill with responsible, caring practice. We want to challenge students to identify and master the cognitive and technical skills as well as the interpersonal and ethical/legal skills they will need to effectively nurse the patients in their care. We refuse to allow accountability and caring relationships to become relics of a bygone era.

Those new to nursing can quickly become overwhelmed by the demands placed on the nurse's knowledge, technical competence, interpersonal skills, and commitment. Therefore, much care has once again gone into the selection of both the content in this edition and the manner of its presentation. We strive to capture the unique essence of both the art and science of nursing, distilling what the person beginning the study and practice of nursing needs to know. We invite students to identify with the profession, to share in its pride, and to respond to today's challenges competently, enthusiastically, and accountably.

LEARNING EXPERIENCE

This text and the entire Taylor Suite have been created with the student's experience in mind. Care has been taken to appeal to all learning styles. The student-friendly writing style ensures that students will comprehend and retain information. The updated art program and strong features enhance understanding of important concepts. Free video clips clearly demonstrate and reinforce important skill steps; as students watch and listen to the videos, comprehension increases. In addition, each element of the Taylor Suite, which is described later in the preface, coordinates to provide a consistent and cohesive learning experience.

ORGANIZATION

Fundamentals of Nursing: The Art and Science of Nursing Care, seventh edition, is organized into eight units. Ideally, the text is followed sequentially, but every effort has been made to respect the differing needs of diverse curricula and students. Thus, each chapter stands on its own merit and may be read independently of others.

Unit I, Foundations of Nursing Practice

Unit I opens with a description of contemporary nursing. Successive chapters introduce content foundational to nursing practice: cultural diversity; health and illness; health of the individual, family, and community; theory, research, and evidence-based practice; values, ethics, and advocacy; and legal implications.

Unit II, Community-Based Settings for Patient Care

Unit II introduces the multiple settings in which nursing is practiced and prepares students to ensure continuity of care in what could be a fragmented healthcare system. Chapters address the variety of community-based healthcare settings; continuity of care as the patient enters a healthcare facility, is transferred within the facility, and is discharged into another setting within the community; and care provided within the home.

Unit III, The Nursing Process

Unit III offers a detailed, step-by-step guide to each component of the nursing process. Practical guidelines and examples are included in each chapter. Separate chapters address the nursing process as a whole, nursing's blended skills, critical thinking, assessing, diagnosing, outcome identification and planning, implementing, and evaluating. A chapter on documentation, reporting, conferring, and using informatics highlights these nursing responsibilities. New NANDA International and NIC/NOC content has been added along with a stronger emphasis on clinical decision making.

Unit IV, Promoting Health Across the Life Span

Unit IV provides the basis for understanding growth and development across the life span and acknowledges nursing's differing requirements arising from the various developmental stages and abilities to meet developmental tasks.

Unit V, Roles Basic to Nursing Care

Unit V describes major roles in which nurses function as they interact holistically with patients. Chapters focus on the communicator, teacher and counselor, and leader and manager roles of the nurse as caregiver.

Unit VI, Actions Basic to Nursing Care

Unit VI introduces the foundational skills used by nurses: measuring vital signs, assessing health, promoting safety, maintaining asepsis, incorporating complementary and alternative therapies, administering medication, and caring for surgical patients.

Unit VII, Promoting Healthy Physiologic Responses

Unit VII explores the nurse's role in helping patients meet basic physiologic needs: hygiene, skin integrity and wound care, activity, rest and sleep, comfort, nutrition, urinary elimination, bowel elimination, oxygenation, and fluid, electrolyte, and acid–base balance. In each chapter, guidelines are included for assessing and diagnosing unhealthy responses and for planning, implementing, and evaluating appropriate care strategies. Chapters conclude with a *Nursing Plan of Care* illustrating the use of the nursing process and nursing's blended skills to resolve selected nursing diagnoses.

Unit VIII, Promoting Healthy Psychosocial Responses

Unit VIII uses the same format as Unit VII to focus on the psychosocial needs of patients: self-concept; stress and adaptation; loss, grief, and dying; sensory functioning; sexuality; and spirituality.

THEMES

In this edition, we capitalize on the strengths of the first six editions and address new priorities. The following themes are interwoven throughout the text to provide a broad knowledge base of nursing essentials while emphasizing holistic care.

Emphasis on Partnering With Patients, Family, and Professional Caregivers

From the very first edition of this text, students were encouraged to actively partner with patients and their family caregivers in designing and implementing care. Those familiar with early editions of this text may remember that we initially used the term *client* rather than *patient* to highlight the active role that most individuals prefer to play in directing their healthcare. Today, we have witnessed the healthcare "industry" transform patients to "customers," who buy healthcare (if they are able) as a commodity in the marketplace. We do not believe that a "customer-orientation" serves patients or nurses well. One of our students shared her belief that she owes less to a "customer" and even to a "client" than she does to a "patient." We, therefore, have chosen to reclaim the term *patient*—in its most positive sense—to designate the recipient of nursing care.

Careful attention is paid to directing students to identify, value, and develop the interpersonal skills that will allow them to effectively partner with patients, family, and professional caregivers. The National Patient Safety Foundation (NPSF) Universal Patient Compact now offers principles for partnership between healthcare provider and patient. This will set a tone for successful practice.

Efforts have been made to highlight nursing strategies for actively engaging patients, family caregivers, and the public in the development of health goals and strategies to achieve these goals. Patients may be individuals, families, or communities. Care has been taken to communicate that both nurses and patients may be male or female and that they come from every racial and ethnic background and socioeconomic group. Whenever possible, we have tried to avoid male/female distinctions in personal pronouns.

Integrated Nursing Process

After the nursing process is introduced in Unit III, it provides the organizational framework for successive chapters. Chapters in Units VII and VIII, which deal with physiologic and psychosocial responses, begin with a succinct background discussion of the concept, followed by identification of factors that influence how different individuals respond to these needs. Steps in the nursing process are used to describe related nursing responsibilities. Throughout these chapters, students will find numerous practical examples of how to conduct focused assessments, develop and write diagnostic statements, identify goals and outcomes, and select, implement, and evaluate appropriate nursing interventions. These examples will reinforce the student's mastery of nursing process skills. Most chapters in Units VII and VIII conclude with a *Nursing Plan of Care* that illustrates each step of the nursing process and a sample documentation of nursing assessment or intervention. In addition, concept maps demonstrating the nursing process are included in several chapters.

Assessing

Common elements of both a comprehensive and problem-focused nursing assessment are presented; sample interview questions are included within *Focused Assessment Guides,* and specific physical assessment techniques are described. Students will learn the what, why, when, and how of assessment.

Diagnosing

NANDA International-approved nursing diagnoses related to the human need being discussed are identified. *Examples* *of NANDA Nursing Diagnoses* boxes illustrate the relationship between related factors and the problem statement, and provide sample-defining characteristics.*

Outcome Identification and Planning

Expected outcomes are suggested based on patient health problems and strengths within Unit III: The Nursing Process and *Nursing Plans of Care.* Nursing Outcomes Classification (NOC) is also discussed within Unit III. Sample nursing outcomes have been added in this edition to the *Examples of Nursing Interventions and Nursing Outcomes Classifications (NIC/NOC)* boxes.

Implementing

Nursing interventions are clearly explained and are illustrated when appropriate. *Skills* have been streamlined to facilitate mastery and appear at the end of the chapters for easy reference. A sufficient variety of nursing interventions is provided to foster the development of a repertoire of nursing actions that makes practicing the art of nursing possible. *Examples of Nursing Interventions and Nursing Outcomes Classifications (NIC/NOC)* boxes provide a sampling of potential nursing interventions for specific topics.

Evaluating

Criteria for evaluating the effectiveness of the plan of care are suggested.

Nursing as an Art and Science

Nursing, as a science, is characterized by a growing body of knowledge that links technical and interpersonal interventions to desired patient outcomes; as an art, nursing demands of its practitioners sufficient competency to creatively design individualized strategies to assist patients to reach personal health goals. A unique spirit of caring always must prevail.

Health Orientation

A health rather than an illness orientation provides a framework for presentation of content. *Promoting Health* boxes highlight assessment checkpoints for specific components of

*Material related to nursing diagnoses from *Nursing Diagnoses—Definitions and Classification 2009–2011*. Copyright (c) 2009, 2007, 2005, 2003, 2001, 1998, 1996, 1994 by NANDA International. Used by arrangement with Wiley-Blackwell Publishing, a company of John Wiley & Sons, Inc. In order to make safe and effective judgments using NANDA-I nursing diagnoses, it is essential that nurses refer to the definitions and defining characteristics of the diagnoses listed in this work.

high-level health and include suggestions for designing a self-care prescription. These boxes serve as a self-care model for the learner and an invaluable aid to the individual who is developing the role of patient healthcare educator. *Teaching Tips* boxes also focus on health and wellness by providing health topics and teaching strategies.

Aims of Nursing

Learners are gradually introduced to the theory and blended skills that will enable them to work successfully with patients to promote health, prevent illness, restore health, and facilitate coping with altered functioning. Early attention to these broad aims of nursing will prepare learners to meet the needs of patients in diverse healthcare settings.

Basic Human Needs

Common to all people and essential to health and survival are basic human needs. The clinical chapters in Unit VII, Promoting Healthy Physiologic Responses, and Unit VIII, Promoting Healthy Psychosocial Responses, prepare the learner to assist patients and family members in meeting these needs. Learners are encouraged to explore human responses to health and illness as indicators of how well an individual is functioning to meet basic human needs.

Holistic Care Across the Life Span

A holistic orientation to basic human needs exists across the life span. This orientation is emphasized through information about growth and development in Unit IV, Promoting Health Across the Life Span; through developmental considerations and related tables and displays in Unit VII, Promoting Healthy Physiologic Responses, and in Unit VIII, Promoting Healthy Psychosocial Responses; through age considerations in many *Skills;* and through the diverse ages and needs of patients represented in numerous features. Wherever appropriate, cultural considerations are included.

Attention to Special Needs of the Older Person

Because the age of the population is increasing, nurses encounter growing numbers of older patients in all practice settings. *Chapter 20, The Aging Adult,* the *Focus on the Older Adult* boxes, and general considerations for the older patient that appear within the text aim to sensitize students to the special nursing needs of this population. Readers of the seventh edition will find expanded information related to dementia, depression, and delirium; a discussion of cascade iatrogenics; the Fulmer SPICES tool used to identify common problems that lead to negative outcomes in older adults; the Hendrich II Fall Risk Model; and the American Geriatrics Society Position Statement on Restraint Use. The textbook has been reviewed by a gerontology consultant to ensure the material complies with guidelines for addressing the needs of older adults.

Critical Thinking

Critical thinking content is emphasized in *Chapter 11, Blended Skills and Critical Thinking Throughout the Nursing Process* and in the Nursing Process chapters that follow. The *Reflective Practice* boxes, *Focused Critical Thinking Guides,* and *Developing Critical Thinking Skills* material in each chapter challenge students to use new knowledge and experience to "think through" learning exercises designed to demonstrate how critical thinking can change outcomes.

Personal Accounts

We have invited students, patients, and family caregivers to share their experiences. Boxes entitled *Through the Eyes of a Student, Through the Eyes of a Patient,* and *Through the Eyes of a Family Caregiver* speak eloquently of nursing's power to "make a difference." The *Reflective Practice* boxes are written by students and are designed to engage readers in real-life scenarios encountered by their peers. These personal accounts will evoke smiles, pride, and empathy, and they will unite nurse caregivers in their struggles to perfect their caregiving skills as they make a difference in the lives of others.

Nursing Skills

Skills are presented in a concise, straightforward, and simplified format that is intended to facilitate competent performance of nursing skills. A scientific rationale accompanies each nursing action, and many color photographs and illustrations further reinforce mastery. Special considerations, including modifications and age and home care considerations, are given where appropriate. Unexpected outcomes and associated interventions are included to help students think critically about the skills they are performing. In this edition, we have added documentation guidelines and samples to help students learn what and how to document when performing skills.

Guidelines for Nursing Care provide a quick reference for additional nursing actions. Free video clips and interactive exercises on the Student Resource DVD-ROM facilitate understanding. A companion skills textbook, a skills video series, and new skills handbook are part of the Taylor Suite. Available as separate purchases, these products expand upon

the skills provided in this *Fundamentals* text and, additionally, address numerous basic, intermediate, and advanced skills. One unique benefit of the Taylor Suite products is that skill instruction is consistent in all products; this consistency is especially helpful for beginning students.

Broad Scope of Nursing Practice

Fundamentals of Nursing: The Art and Science of Nursing Care, seventh edition, is written to encompass fundamental skills in a laboratory as well as in actual clinical settings where nurses care for both well and ill patients. To acquaint students of nursing with many exciting career options in nursing, numerous examples are given to illustrate nurses interacting with patients of all ages and backgrounds and in traditional and nontraditional settings.

Focus on Community and Expanded Nursing Roles

Patients today spend fewer days in the hospital, are frequently transferred both within the hospital and between healthcare institutions and home, and need to rely on rapidly proliferating community-based healthcare resources. Content, photos, and illustrations throughout the text highlight both traditional and innovative nursing roles in institutional and community-based practice settings. This text encourages students to dream about new ways nurses can serve the public by creatively responding to health needs and problems.

Focus on Safety

New content highlights today's emphasis on patient safety, including expanded safety information related to children, adolescents, and older adults. The Institute of Medicine Safety content, 2010 Joint Commission National Patient Safety Goals and Sentinel Event Statistics are highlighted, and new information is provided on healthcare-associated infections (HAIs). Safe Patient Handling and Movement Practices, based on guidelines from VISN 8 Patient Safety Center, 2006, 2007, and 2009 are included in this edition.

Research as a Strength to Practice

Content on research and evidence-based practice has been updated and is included in Unit I for increased emphasis early in the learning experience. A new feature, *PICO in Practice: Asking Clinical Questions,* encourages readers to delve into research to solve a clinical question using the PICO format and guidelines. Updated *Research in Nursing: Bridging the Gap to Evidence-Based Practice* boxes, appearing throughout the book, promote the value of research and apply its relevance to nursing practice. Students are challenged to become informed participants in, or consumers of, clinical research. To that end, students can explore additional research in nursing journal articles provided for each chapter on thePoint (http://thePoint.lww.com/Taylor7e).

Up-to-Date Clinical Information

Revisions in each clinical chapter will help educators and students remain current. Sample new content includes:

- Increased emphasis on research, evidence-based practice, and nursing management
- Expanded emphasis on complementary and alternative therapies
- Joint Commission 2010 National Patient Safety Goals
- Expanded information on healthcare-associated infections (HAIs), including Centers for Medicare and Medicaid Services' refusal to reimburse hospitals for 8 preventable HAIs, the Institute for Healthcare Improvement's promotion of use of carebundles or evidence-based protocols that reduce incidence of catheter-related infections and ventilator-associated pneumonia, and the impact of staffing issues on HAIs.
- Safe Patient Handling and Movement Practices, including discussion of current research related to identifying high-risk lifting and movement activities for caregivers and promotion of a safe working environment
- SBAR communication to improve patient "hand-offs" from one professional caregiver to another.
- Updated ANA Standards of Practice, ICN Definition of Nursing, and Healthy People 2010
- New delegation decision tree
- 2010 Recommended Immunization Schedule
- New information on child maltreatment
- Discussion of aggressive interpersonal behavior between healthcare personnel and horizontal violence (nurse-to-nurse hostility)
- Ask Me 3 Tool to enhance health literacy included in new *Promoting Health Literacy* feature
- New Quality Standards and Indicators for Magnet Recognition Program
- Increased cultural competence content
- Updated content on pressure ulcer staging, based on the National Pressure Ulcer Advisory Panel, 2007
- New information about traumatic brain injuries (e.g., concussions) in children
- Discussion of teenage abuse of prescribed drugs and over-the-counter medications
- Updated information on electronic medical records, new information technologies, and privacy considerations
- Conscience objections

Self-Assessment Guides

Fundamentals of Nursing has always encouraged students to be independent learners. Checklists throughout the text (e.g., blended skills assessment, use of nursing process, health assessments) allow students to evaluate their personal strengths and limitations and develop related learning goals.

RECURRING FEATURES
Chapter Opening Features

- **Patient Scenarios.** Chapter openers present three "patients" with photos and a short description of their cases. To reinforce learning and engage the reader, the three "patients" are mentioned throughout the chapter to support clinical examples from the text.
- **Learning Objectives and Key Terms.** By beginning each chapter with the learning objectives, we are offering a valuable learning checklist to assess mastery of essential content. Students can use these objectives as a basis for learning outlines or self-testing, or the instructor may use them for evaluating student knowledge and abilities. The key terms for each chapter also appear in the beginning of the chapter. When these terms are defined in the chapter, they are in bold type for clarity. A Glossary appears at the back of the book for easy review of these terms.

In-Text Features

- **Reflective Practice Boxes** are written by students to describe a challenge to their blended skills: cognitive, technical, interpersonal, or ethical/legal. Students identify possible courses of action and *the criteria they would use to identify a successful outcome,* and then describe what they learned after reflecting on their response. The readers are asked if they think they would respond in the same way; what this tells them about themselves and the adequacy of their blended skills; and whether the criteria for a successful outcome were appropriate.
- **Nursing Process Demonstrations.** This text continues to set the standard for practical demonstrations of each step of the nursing process. As they read through clinical chapters, students see multiple examples of assessment questions and skills, diagnostic statements, plans of care, documented nursing interventions, evaluative statements, and discharge and teaching plans. For visual learners, these tools greatly facilitate mastery of the complex behaviors students must master quickly when beginning clinical experiences.

- **Case scenario extracts** provide real-world examples and lend significance to conceptual content. These extracts refer back to the chapter-opening patient scenarios for a cohesive learning experience.
- **Concept maps** walk students through the nursing process for selected case study patients.
- **Nursing Skills** show both actions and rationales and highlight special considerations. Unexpected outcomes and associated interventions plus special considerations are included. *New* to this edition is the inclusion of documentation guidelines and samples.
- **Guidelines for Nursing Care** boxes outline important points to remember in practice.
- **Watch and Learn** icons direct students to free video clips that show students how to perform a skill.
- **Practice and Learn** icons direct students to free activities that allow students to apply skills to patient care.
- **Through the Eyes of a Student, Through the Eyes of a Patient,** and **Through the Eyes of a Family Caregiver** offer personal anecdotes from different perspectives in order to help students relate to their patients.
- **Promoting Health** boxes highlight assessment checkpoints for various health and wellness issues and include suggestions for patient and self-care.
- **New! Nursing Advocacy in Action** boxes present scenarios and challenge readers to begin to identify what a student nurse, newly graduated nurse, and experienced nurse can do to advocate for vulnerable individuals. Students are urged to identify what needs to change at the level of individuals, practice settings, and society to prevent the recurrence of injustice.
- **New! Promoting Health Literacy** boxes help readers identify patients/families at risk for poor health outcomes related to low health literacy. In each scenario, nurses instruct patients to ask: *What is the main problem? What do they need to do? Why is it important for them to do this?*
- **New! PICO in Practice: Asking Clinical Questions** boxes demonstrate how to do a systematic search for and critical appraisal of the most relevant evidence to answer a burning clinical question by following the PICO model.
- **Research in Nursing: Bridging the Gap to Evidence-Based Practice** boxes highlight recent findings in nursing care.
- **Examples of NANDA Nursing Diagnoses** and **Examples of Nursing Interventions and Nursing Outcomes Classifications (NIC/NOC)** boxes highlight nursing diagnoses and nursing interventions and outcomes for quick and easy reference. The inclusion of nursing outcomes in these boxes is new to this edition.
- **Focused Assessment Guides** provide sample interview questions to foster independent learning.
- **Focused Critical Thinking Guides** help students follow the step-by-step critical thinking process and develop critical thinking skills.
- **Teaching Tips** boxes provide patient teaching tips for nurse–patient communication.
- **Focus on the Older Adult** boxes emphasize gerontologic care.
- **Nursing Plans of Care with Patient Case Studies** conclude clinical chapters. The patient case study is often derived from the chapter opener cases. Students will find concrete examples of each step of the nursing process, as well as related examples of documentation. The diagnoses that are worked up in these studies illustrate common health problems and the wide variety of independent and collaborative interventions nurses manage in different practice settings.
- **A vibrant, modern art program** uses illustrations and photos to enhance students' understanding. Hundreds of new photos have been added to this edition.

Chapter Ending Features

- **Developing Critical Thinking Skills** sections provide exercises that challenge students to synthesize, rather than just reiterate, the information they have learned. By thinking through various scenarios to a final outcome, students will begin to see how their decisions influence end results.
- **Practicing for NCLEX** exercises in *every chapter* will assist students who are attempting to improve their objective test-taking skills. Students who want additional practice with NCLEX-type questions will find the student study guide useful.
- **Taylor Suite Resources** lists at the end of every chapter outline which products in the Taylor Suite relate to the chapter topic and help students coordinate their studying.
- **Bibliographies** at the end of each chapter help make students aware of the variety of resources for information on nursing and give additional reference materials for instructors or students.

TEACHING/LEARNING PACKAGE

To facilitate mastery of this text's foundational content, a comprehensive teaching/learning package has been developed to assist faculty and students.

Resources for Instructors

Tools to assist you with teaching your course are available upon adoption of this text on thePoint at http://thePoint.lww.com/Taylor7e. Many of these tools are also included on the Instructor's Resource DVD-ROM.

- An **E-Book** on thePoint gives you access to the book's full text and images online.
- The **Test Generator** lets you put together exclusive new tests from a bank containing hundreds of questions to help you in assessing your students' understanding of the material. Test questions link to chapter learning objectives. This test generator comes with a bank of more than 1,250 questions.
- An extensive collection of materials is provided for each book chapter:
  - **Pre-Lecture Quizzes** (and answers) are quick, knowledge-based assessments that allow you to check students' reading.
  - **PowerPoint Presentations** provide an easy way for you to integrate the textbook with your students' classroom experience, either via slide shows or handouts. Multiple-choice and true/false questions are integrated into the presentations to promote class participation and allow you to use i-clicker technology.
  - **Guided Lecture Notes** walk you through the chapters, objective by objective, and provide you with corresponding PowerPoint slide numbers.
  - **Discussion Topics** (and suggested answers) can be used as conversation starters or in online discussion boards.
  - **Assignments** (and suggested answers) include group, written, clinical, and Web assignments.
  - **New! Case Studies** with related questions (and suggested answers) give students an opportunity to apply their knowledge to a client case similar to one they might encounter in practice.
- An **Image Bank** lets you use the photographs and illustrations from this textbook in your PowerPoint slides or as you see fit in your course.
- A sample **Syllabus** provides guidance for structuring your nursing fundamentals course.
- **Journal Articles,** updated for the new edition, offer access to current research available in Lippincott Williams & Wilkins journals.
- Adaptable **Skill Checklists** walk through skills step by step and can be used to help you evaluate your students' mastery of skills.
- **New! Master Checklist for Skills Competency** provides a list of all skills in the book to help you track your students' progress in achieving skill competency.

Contact your sales representative or check out LWW.com/Nursing for more details and ordering information.

Resources for Students

An exciting set of free resources is available to help students review material and become even more familiar with vital concepts. Students can access all these resources on thePoint at http://thePoint.lww.com/Taylor7e using the codes printed in the front of their textbooks. Many of these resources are also available on the DVD-ROM bound in this textbook.

- An **E-Book** on thePoint allows access to the book's full text and images online.
- **NCLEX-Style Review Questions** for each chapter help students review important concepts and practice for NCLEX. Over 900 questions are included.
- **New! Taylor's Fundamentals of Nursing Q&A iPhone Application** allows you to create and complete personalized NCLEX practice quizzes from the book's NCLEX-Style Student Review Questions—all from your iPhone.
- **Multimedia Resources** appeal to a variety of learning styles. Icons in the text direct readers to relevant resources:
  - **Watch & Learn Video Clips** from *Taylor's Video Guide to Clinical Nursing Skills* reinforce skills from the textbook and appeal to visual and auditory learners.
  - **Practice & Learn Activities** present case scenarios and offer interactive exercises and questions to help students apply what they have learned.
  - **Concepts in Action Animations** bring physiologic and pathophysiologic concepts to life and enhance student comprehension.
- A **Spanish–English Audio Glossary** provides helpful terms and phrases for communicating with patients who speak Spanish.
- **Journal Articles** offer access to current research available in Lippincott Williams & Wilkins journals.
- **Dosage Calculation Quizzes** provide opportunities for students to practice math skills and calculating drug dosages.

TAYLOR SUITE OF PRODUCTS

From traditional texts to video and interactive products, the Taylor Fundamentals suite is tailored to fit every learning style. This integrated suite of products offers students a seamless learning experience you won't find anywhere else. The following products accompany *Fundamentals of*

Nursing: The Art and Science of Nursing Care, seventh edition:

- ***Study Guide for Fundamentals of Nursing: The Art and Science of Nursing Care,* 7th Edition,** by Carol Taylor, Carol Lillis, Priscilla LeMone, Pamela Lynn, and Marilee LeBon. This guide reinforces the Taylor Fundamentals suite by offering exercises and study review tools to enhance the learning process. It also includes hundreds of NCLEX-style questions in both multiple choice and the alternate format.
- ***Skill Checklists for Fundamentals of Nursing: The Art and Science of Nursing Care,* 7th Edition,** by Carol Taylor, Carol Lillis, Priscilla LeMone, Pamela Lynn, and Marilee LeBon. The checklists are designed to accompany the comprehensive fundamentals textbook and promote proper technique while increasing confidence.
- *Taylor's Clinical Nursing Skills,* **3rd Edition,** by Pamela Lynn, MSN, RN. This text covers all of the *Skills* and *Guidelines for Nursing Care* identified in *Fundamentals of Nursing,* as well as additional skills, at the basic, intermediate, and advanced levels. Each Skill follows the nursing process format. Features include Fundamentals Review displays, which reinforce important concepts; Skill Variations, which present alternate techniques; Documentation Guidelines and Samples; Unexpected Situations and Associated Interventions; and Special Considerations. A new feature for the third edition, Evidence for Practice, highlights available best practice guidelines and/or research-based evidence to support the skills as available.

- **New!** *Taylor's Handbook of Clinical Nursing Skills* by Pamela Lynn, MSN, RN. This brand new offering in the Taylor Suite provides streamlined skills consistent with those in *Taylor's Clinical Nursing Skills*, 3rd Edition. Presented for quick reference or on-the-go review, skills are organized alphabetically by key word.
- *Taylor's Video Guide to Clinical Nursing Skills,* **2nd Edition.** From reinforcing fundamental nursing skills to troubleshooting clinical problems on the fly, this dynamic video series follows nursing students and their instructors as they perform and discuss a range of essential nursing procedures. The second edition of these videos is updated with tons of brand new footage to reflect the most current best practice, to address changes in medication administration and equipment, and to include even more skills. Ideal as a stand-alone learning tool or as a companion to this book, these videos parallel the text and are organized into topical modules for easy reference. Schools can purchase the videos on enhanced DVD or for video streaming. Student versions of the videos are available on enhanced DVD or online through thePoint.

Contact your sales representative, visit your college bookstore, or check out LWW.com/Nursing for more details and ordering information.

Carol Taylor, PhD, MSN, RN
Carol Lillis, MSN, RN
Priscilla LeMone, DSN, RN, FAAN
Pamela Lynn, MSN, RN

Letter to the Student

Dear Student,

Congratulations on choosing an exciting and rewarding profession! All of us who have been part of the writing of this text welcome you warmly to our profession and prize our role as your guides to excellent practice. We have tried in this text to present in a readable and enjoyable format the scientific and technical knowledge you will need to design safe and effective nursing care. But we want to do more than prepare you intellectually and technically. You will also find narratives that will teach you valuable interpersonal skills and content specifically designed to prepare you to meet the ethical and legal challenges in today's practice. So take a deep breath and dig in. Your patients are counting on you and so are we!

Carol Taylor

Carol Lillis

Priscilla LeMone

Pamela Lynn

How to Use *Fundamentals of Nursing*

New Features—Taylor Made

READ ALL ABOUT IT!

Check out the brand-new features in the seventh edition! Read the **PICO in Practice: Asking Clinical Questions** boxes to think about how you can formulate questions and apply evidence-based answers to your practice.

PICO IN PRACTICE
Asking Clinical Questions

Scenario: You are a staff nurse newly hired to a general medicine unit. Your assigned preceptor calls in sick one day. Another seasoned nurse assigned to the unit, Donna, agrees to serve as your substitute preceptor for that shift. One of your assigned patients must have a nasogastric tube placed. You ask Donna to observe you perform this procedure and

- COMPARISON: Removal of gloves only without hand hygiene
- OUTCOME: Lower rates of hospital-associated infections on the unit

PICO Question: Among direct-care gloved nurses who have not soiled their hands, is performing hand hygiene

NURSING ADVOCACY IN ACTION

Patient Scenario

Ms. Samol is a 38-year-old patient in the medical intensive care unit who is dying of AIDS-related complications. Since being diagnosed with AIDS, she has refused to inform her husband and family of her AIDS status. She even has an advance directive, which for-

Reflect on the **Nursing Advocacy in Action** boxes to consider how you might advocate for vulnerable patient populations.

Promoting Health Literacy boxes demonstrate how you might help your patients improve their knowledge and health literacy to improve outcomes.

Promoting Health Literacy
IN PATIENTS WITH HYPERTENSION

Patient Scenario

Harry Miller, 66, went to his primary healthcare provider for his annual health assessment. He had gained 15 pounds in the past year. When the office nurse took his blood pressure, it was 166/92 mm Hg. The nurse took Mr. Miller's blood pressure again and then repeated it later

is important to control his high blood pressure to prevent serious risks, such as heart attack and stroke. Urge Mr. Miller and his wife to talk to a dietitian about a nutritious diet that would help him to lose weight; contains recommended servings of fiber, fruits, and vegetables; and contains less salt. Explain the action of the prescribed medication importance of taking medication to

STUDY ON THE GO!

Download a new iPhone app designed to help you study for your course anytime, anywhere! **Taylor's Fundamentals of Nursing Q&A** app lets you complete personalized practice quizzes from this book's accompanying NCLEX-Style Review Questions—all from your iPhone.

LOOK AHEAD!

Before reading the chapter content, read the **Learning Objectives.** These roadmaps help you understand what is important and why. Review the **Key Terms** lists to become familiar with new vocabulary presented throughout the narrative.

FOLLOW THE STORY LINES!

Get to know your patients by reading the chapter opening **Case Scenarios.** In-text references to Case Scenarios throughout the chapter allow you to consider how the chapter content applies to care of real patients.

LUCIUS EVERLY

Lucius, who has a history of diabetes and circulatory problems, underwent abdominal surgery several days ago and is in the critical care unit. He is slouched down in bed; his abdominal dressing is moist, and only part of the tape securing the dressing is adhering to the skin. His level of consciousness

---

REFLECTIVE PRACTICE
Challenge to Ethical and Legal Skills

I had a tough clinical 2 weeks ago while caring for Lucius Everly, a critical care postop patient with a history of diabetes and circulation problems. The nurse I was working with had floated to the unit on this day, but I didn't know that at the time. Mr. Everly appeared to be neglected by other caregivers, and because he was not communicating and had a decreased level of consciousness, he could not express his needs. I saw that he needed bathing, wound care, repositioning in bed, and some additional attention. While in the room, the nurse spoke about Mr. Everly as though he was deaf. In my opinion, the nurse did not respect his inability to communicate. I became frustrated because she did not share my sense of concern for him. I became irritated when I asked what we could do to care for the poor circulation to his feet. . . .lized that he was developing a pre. . . . . . .'s heel.

Read **Reflective Practice** boxes and discover how other nursing students confront challenging situations related to the Case Scenarios. After reading these boxes, consider how you would respond to similar situations.

DEVELOP CRITICAL THINKING SKILLS!

Learn how critical thinking can change patient outcomes. Like nursing care, critical thinking follows a process. Study the **Focused Critical Thinking Guides** to gain skill in working through the step-by-step critical thinking process.

FOCUSED CRITICAL THINKING GUIDE • 32-1

Wound Care: Promoting Acceptance of Changes in Body Image

During both clinical days in 1 week, you (a female student) have been assigned to care for a middle-aged woman who has had a breast removed because of cancer. The patient, Mrs. Nola, is an attractive woman who is usually cheerful and eager to get better and return home. However, on both days, she turned her head away and would not look at the incision when her dressing was

Time constraints: Some decision about wound care must be made before her discharge the next day.

3. Address Potential Problems

There are several potential obstacles to critical thinking in this situation. As a student, you want to exhibit safe, knowledgeable care, and the importance of teaching for . . . . . . .an emp. . . . .

Challenge yourself! Use the new knowledge you've gained to "think through" learning exercises presented in **Developing Critical Thinking Skills.**

MASTER NURSING PROCESS!

Throughout the clinical chapters, follow the step-by-step organization of the Nursing Process to understand nursing responsibilities. Review the sample interview questions within **Focused Assessment Guides** to strengthen your assessment skills.

FOCUSED ASSESSMENT GUIDE • 32-1

SKIN INTEGRITY

Factors to Assess	Questions and Approaches
Appearance of skin	• Do you have any skin areas that are discolored? • Do some areas of skin on your body feel warmer or colder than others? • Describe the moisture in your skin: is it damp, dry, oily? • Have you noticed that your skin seems to be thinner? Where? • Have you noticed any swelling in your feet, ankles, or fingers?

Examples of NANDA Nursing Diagnoses

Patient With a Wound or Pressure Ulcer

Nursing Diagnoses	Related Factors	Sample Defining Characteristics
Impaired Skin Integrity	Any condition that alters the dermis and/or epidermis, such as a surgical incision or traumatic wound; moisture, physical immobilization	• Presence of intentional or unintentional wound • Presence of a pressure ulcer

Discover how to develop and write diagnostic statements in **Examples of NANDA Nursing Diagnoses.**

Learn to select, implement, and evaluate appropriate nursing interventions and outcomes in **Examples of Nursing Interventions and Nursing Outcomes Classifications (NIC/NOC)** boxes.

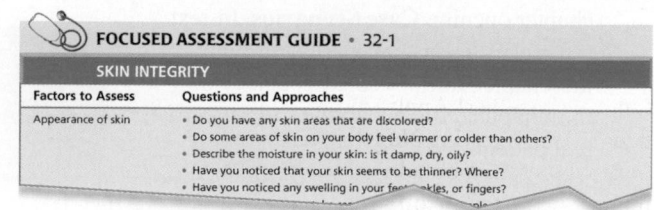

Examples of Nursing Interventions and Nursing Outcomes Classifications (NIC/NOC)

Risk for Impaired Skin Integrity

Nursing Interventions	Nursing Outcomes
• Bedrest Care • Incision Site Care • Wound Care • Pressure Management	• Wound Healing: Primary Intention • Immobility Consequences: Physiological • Tissue Integrity: Skin and Mucous Membranes

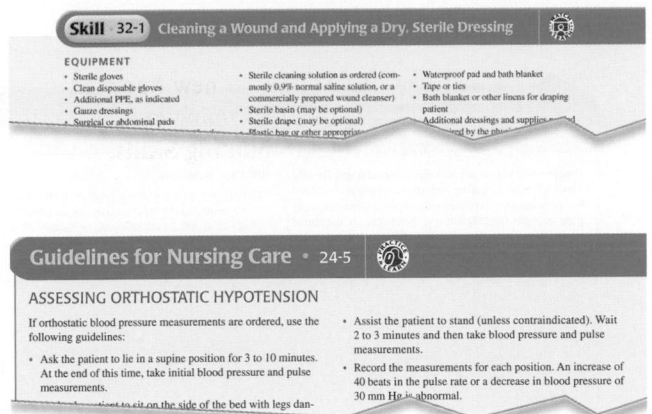

Carefully follow the concise, straightforward, and simplified format of the nursing **Skills** and **Guidelines for Nursing Care** to gain competence in performing nursing skills. Many skills and guidelines have free accompanying video clips, indicated by the **Watch & Learn** icon, or free accompanying activities, indicated by the **Practice & Learn** icon.

Put it all together! Apply chapter content to clinical practice through studying **Nursing Plan of Care** boxes. These boxes represent a broad range of the health problems you might encounter in different settings. The patient case study introduces a specific case, and the related Care Plan follows through the interventions. Each step of the nursing process is covered, and related documentation is included.

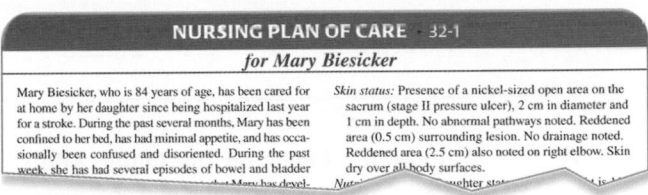

NURSING PLAN OF CARE · 32-1

for Mary Biesicker

Mary Biesicker, who is 84 years of age, has been cared for at home by her daughter since being hospitalized last year for a stroke. During the past several months, Mary has been confined to her bed, has had minimal appetite, and has occasionally been confused and disoriented. During the past week, she has had several episodes of bowel and bladder...

Skin status: Presence of a nickel-sized open area on the sacrum (stage II pressure ulcer), 2 cm in diameter and 1 cm in depth. No abnormal pathways noted. Reddened area (0.5 cm) surrounding lesion. No drainage noted. Reddened area (2.5 cm) also noted on right elbow. Skin dry over all body surfaces.

In addition, several clinical chapters include **Concept Maps** that walk you through the nursing process for one of the case study patients.

Lucius Everly, who has a history of diabetes and circulatory problems, underwent abdominal surgery several days ago and is now in the critical care unit. When you enter, he is slouched down in bed. Assessment reveals that his abdominal dressing is moist, and only part of the tape securing the dressing is adhering to the skin. His level of consciousness is decreased, and he responds only to moderate touch and pain. With repositioning, he moans. Further assessment reveals the beginning of a pressure ulcer on his heel. He is NPO and has a central intravenous catheter in place for administration of total parenteral nutrition (TPN). An indwelling catheter is in place to accurately measure intake and output. He is currently afebrile but has been prescribed antibiotics prophylactically.

Priority 1	Priority 2	Priority 3
Risk for Infection related to surgical incision and invasive therapy **Supporting Data:** • Abdominal surgical incision with moist dressing • Pressure ulcer on heel • Weakened defenses from chronic illness, such as diabetes and circulatory problems • Central venous catheter • Indwelling urinary catheter • Afebrile • IV antibiotics prescribed	**Impaired Skin Integrity related to surgical incision and parenteral therapy** **Supporting Data:** • Abdominal surgical incision • Moist dressings, loosely secured • History of factors impeding healing (diabetes and circulatory problems) • Central venous catheter • NPO receiving TPN	**Impaired Tissue Integrity related to altered mobility and chronic illness** **Supporting Data:** • Decreased level of consciousness • Unable to turn independently • Pressure ulcer on heel • History of circulatory problems and diabetes
Outcome: Patient will remain afebrile with absence of redness or purulent drainage at surgical site. Urine will remain clear.	**Outcome:** Patient will demonstrate signs of a healing incision, absence of skin irritation, absence of IV infiltration, and will maintain optimal nutrition	**Outcome:** Patient will demonstrate signs of healing in pressure ulcer on heel; no further skin breakdown will occur.
Nursing Interventions: • Maintain aseptic technique with dressing change, parenteral therapy, and indwelling urinary catheter • Use proper handwashing technique • Dispose of soiled dressings appropriately • Change dressing as needed • Note appearance of pressure ulcer, incision, and IV insertion sites • Monitor characteristics of urine • Monitor temperature every 4 hours	**Nursing Interventions:** • Change abdominal dressing daily and as needed to prevent saturated dressings • Inspect surgical incision for signs of healing • Cleanse surgical incision • Use Montgomery straps to secure dressing and prevent skin irritation from tape • Use transparent dressing to cover central venous catheter insertion site to allow inspection of insertion site • Inspect insertion site frequently and administer TPN as prescribed to meet nutritional needs and promote healing	**Nursing Interventions:** • Inspect skin, noting areas that are reddened • Use Braden scale to assess risk for pressure ulcer • Turn and reposition patient at least every 2 hours, using padded devices • Use linen to assist in position change to decrease shearing force • Apply heel protectors • Avoid pressure on heels by placing pillow under calves when patient in supine position • Cover pressure ulcer on heel with appropriate protective dressing • Consider consult with wound care specialist
Evaluation: Lucius is afebrile. His urine is clear. No drainage is noted from pressure ulcer. His surgical incision is draining serosanguineous material. Continue interventions.	**Evaluation:** Surgical dressings have been changed as needed to minimize moisture against skin. Pink granulation tissue is noted at the surgical incision. Nutrition has been maintained as noted by stable weight and a preabumin level within normal limits. Parenteral therapy maintained without signs of infiltration.	**Evaluation:** Lucius has been consistently turned every 2 hours; healthy granulation tissue is noted in wound bed.

- - - - - Relationship ■ Assessment ■ Nursing Diagnosis ■ Outcome Identification ■ Interventions ■ Evaluation

Concept map displaying the nursing process for Lucius Everly.

PROMOTE HEALTH!

Learn not only to treat illness but also to promote the health and wellness of your patients. Check out the **Promoting Health** boxes, which include assessment checkpoints for specific health and wellness topics and suggestions for designing a self-care prescription. Use the Promoting Health boxes for yourself as well as your patients. After all, it is important to take care of yourself and serve as a role model for your patients.

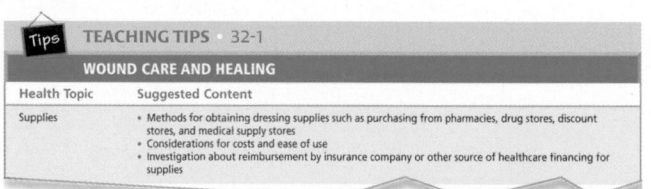

Review the teaching strategies presented in **Teaching Tips** boxes to develop your role as patient educator.

Study the **Focus on the Older Adult** boxes, which provide general considerations for older patients and address their special nursing needs.

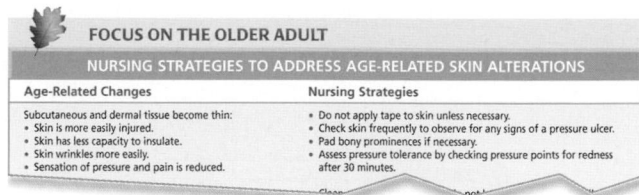

GAIN NEW INSIGHTS!

Read **Through the Eyes of a Patient/Family Caregiver/ Student** to gain insight into nursing care from various perspectives. These real-life stories demonstrate how nursing can make a difference in the lives of patients and their families.

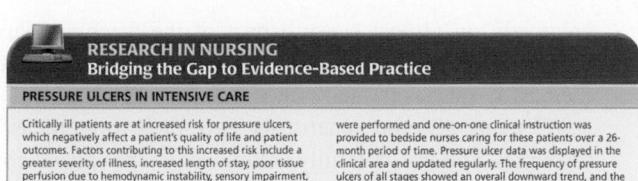

RESEARCH IN NURSING
Bridging the Gap to Evidence-Based Practice

PRESSURE ULCERS IN INTENSIVE CARE

Critically ill patients are at increased risk for pressure ulcers, which negatively affect a patient's quality of life and patient outcomes. Factors contributing to this increased risk include a greater severity of illness, increased length of stay, poor tissue perfusion due to hemodynamic instability, sensory impairment, and poor nutritional status. Facilities usually have policies and protocols in place, as well as products and procedures, address-ing pressure ulcer prevention and treatment. These policies and

were performed and one-on-one clinical instruction was provided to bedside nurses caring for these patients over a 26-month period of time. Pressure ulcer data was displayed in the clinical area and updated regularly. The frequency of pressure ulcers of all stages showed an overall downward trend, and the prevalence decreased from 50% to 8%. The appropriate alloca-tion of pressure-relieving devices increased from 75% up to 95% to 100%. The origin of the ulcer (community or hospital acquired) ...

Gain insight into the "why" behind nursing care. Consider **Research in Nursing: Bridging the Gap to Evidence-Based Practice** boxes to discover recent findings in nursing care and relate their relevance to nursing practice.

PREPARE FOR NCLEX!

Start preparing for NCLEX right from the beginning of your nursing education. Familiarize yourself with the multiple-choice format of test taking. Multiple-choice questions presented in **Practicing for NCLEX** test your knowledge of basic through complex concepts.

● **Practicing for NCLEX**

1. A nurse assesses an oral temperature for a patient as 38.5°C (101.3°F). What term would the nurse use to report this temperature?
   a. Fever
   b. Hypothermia
   c. Hypertension
   d. Afebrile

COORDINATE YOUR STUDY PLAN!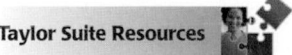
Taylor Suite Resources

Look for the **Taylor Suite Resources** listed at the end of every chapter to see what other parts of the Taylor Suite can help you learn, review, and apply knowledge and skills related to the chapter.

Acknowledgments

This revision is the work of many talented and committed people, and we wish to gratefully acknowledge the assistance of all who have contributed in any way to the completion of this project. Our first debt of gratitude is to all the nurse educators and students who have adopted the text and shared with us their experiences in using the teaching and learning package. We are deeply grateful for their revision suggestions and trust they will enhance the learning experiences of others.

The work of this revision was capably facilitated by our Senior Product Manager, Betsy Gentzler. She worked tirelessly behind the scenes to make sure that a superb, state of the art product was delivered on time! Our very special thanks to her and to Jean Rodenberger, Executive Acquisitions Editor for their hard work and guidance throughout the project. Thank you to the members of the Creative Services department, who brought a fresh look to the entire Taylor Suite of products: Holly Reid McLaughlin, Design Coordinator; and Brett MacNaughton, Illustration Coordinator. The Instructional Services Consultants also deserve special thanks for their focus on our products to provide curriculum guidance, instructional design, technology support, and training. We also want to thank Marilee LeBon who works creatively on almost every aspect of the teaching/learning package to ensure that faculty and students alike are getting the best resources to facilitate learning.

We thank all who generously gave their time, ideas, and resources, and we gratefully acknowledge the special contributions of the following:

- Rick Brady, Joe Mitchell, Ken Kasper, Barbara Proud, Gates Rhodes, and Kathy Sloane, photographers
- Marie Clark, who developed the math problems and solutions in the "Medications" chapter
- Kathleen Lucente, RN, MT, CIC, Infection Control Manager at Paoli Hospital, Paoli, Pennsylvania, for advising and updating us on changing infection-control protocols.

We gratefully acknowledge the influence of our mentors and teachers who have influenced our thoughts and writing; each person we have been privileged to care for as nurses; our students, who continually challenge us to find more effective means to teach nursing; our professional colleagues; and perhaps most important, our families and friends, whose love sustained us through the long hours of research and writing.

Expanded Contents

FOUNDATIONS OF NURSING PRACTICE

Nursing is both an art and a science. It is a profession that uses specialized knowledge and skills to promote wellness and to provide care for people in both health and illness in a variety of practice settings. Unit I introduces concepts that provide the foundation for nursing practice by defining nursing as a whole. Chapters in this unit introduce the profession of nursing; cultural diversity; health and illness; basic needs and health of individuals, their families, and the community; theory, research, and evidence-based nursing practice; and ethical and legal implications for nursing practice.

Historical perspectives, educational preparation, professional organizations, and guidelines for professional nursing practice serve as a base for understanding what nursing is and how it is organized. The diverse society in which nurses care for others mandates the ability to provide culturally competent care. An understanding of basic human needs and the individualized definitions of wellness and illness prepare the nurse to integrate the human dimensions—the physical, intellectual, emotional, sociocultural, spiritual, and environmental aspects of each person—into nursing care to promote wellness, prevent illness, restore health, and facilitate coping with altered function or death. Knowledge of the varied methods of care delivery is necessary in today's complex healthcare system.

Nursing theories and nursing research provide a foundation for evidence-based nursing practice, defining the rationale for nursing actions and offering a focus for nursing care. An understanding of the influence of values on human behavior and of the ethical dimensions of nursing practice is essential to responsible and accountable patient care. Finally, sensitivity to the legal implications of professional nursing practice is imperative in today's culture.

Unit I explores the foundations for nursing practice from both the perspective of the nurse and a holistic understanding of the patient. Students of nursing are introduced to a challenging and rewarding profession and are provided with a knowledge base to ground the development of caregiving skills and professional relationships and behaviors.

" *Basic to any philosophy of nursing seems to be these three concepts: (1) reverence for the gift of life; (2) respect for the dignity, worth, autonomy, and individuality of each human being; (3) resolution to act dynamically in relation to one's beliefs.*"

ERNESTINE WIEDENBACH (1900–1996) • *a faculty member at Yale University School of Nursing, where she developed her model of nursing from years of experience in various nursing positions*

1 Introduction to Nursing

ROBERTO PECORINI

Roberto is a 38-year-old man diagnosed with metastatic colon cancer. Having undergone radiation treatments and chemotherapy, he is extremely weak and malnourished. He is receiving intravenous fluids via a central venous catheter. He has two pressure ulcers on his sacrum, each approximately 1½″ in diameter, requiring wound care. He also has a colostomy that he cannot care for independently.

MICHELLE FINE

Michelle, a 19-year-old first-time mother who was discharged with her healthy 7-lb 8-oz baby girl 2 days ago, calls the nursery. She reports, "My baby isn't taking to my breast and she hasn't had any real feeding for 24 hours."

ALBERT ROWLINGS

Albert, a 62-year-old male who is at risk for heart disease, is being taught about lifestyle modifications, such as diet and exercise. He states, "Just save your breath. Why should I bother about all that? I'd be better off dead than living like I am now, anyway!"

What is nursing? Consider the following examples of who nurses are and what they do:

- Delton Nix, RN, graduated from an associate degree nursing program 3 years ago. He is now working full-time as a staff nurse in a hospital medical unit while attending school part-time toward a baccalaureate degree in nursing; his goal is to become a nurse anesthetist.
- Jeiping Wu, RN, MSN, FNP, specializes as an advanced practice family nurse practitioner. She has an independent practice in a rural primary health clinic.
- Samuel Cohen, LPN, decided to follow his life's dream to become a nurse after 20 years as a postal worker. After examining all his options and goals, he completed a practical nursing program and is now a member of an emergency ambulance crew in a large city.
- Amy Orlando, RN, BSN, graduated 2 years ago and recently began a new job in an urban community health service.
- Roxanne McDaniel, RN, PhD, with a doctorate in nursing, teaches and conducts research at a large university.

These examples show how difficult it is to describe nursing simply. If everyone in your class were asked to complete the sentence, "Nursing is . . . ," there would be many different responses because each person would answer based on his or her own personal experience and knowledge of nursing at that time. As you progress toward graduation and as you practice nursing after graduation, your own definition will reflect changes as you learn about and experience nursing.

Nursing is a profession focused on assisting individuals, families, and communities to attain, recover, and maintain optimum health and function from birth to old age. Nursing care involves any number of activities, from carrying out complicated technical procedures to something as seemingly simple as holding a hand. Nursing is a blend of science and art. The science of nursing is the knowledge base for the care that is given, and the art of nursing is the skilled application of that knowledge to help others reach maximum health and quality of life.

This chapter introduces you to nursing, including a brief history of nursing from its beginnings to the present, and provides the definitions and aims of nursing. In examining nursing as a profession, educational preparation, professional organizations, and guidelines for professional nursing practice are discussed to help you better understand what nursing is and how it is organized. (For an example demonstrating the importance of licensure to nursing practice and responsibilities, see the accompanying Reflective Practice box.) Because nursing is a part of an ever-changing society, current trends in nursing also are discussed.

HISTORIC PERSPECTIVES ON NURSING

Caregivers for those who were ill or injured have always been a part of history. The roles, settings, and responsibilities, however, have changed over time, as is summarized in the following section.

Development of Nursing from Early Civilizations to the 16th Century

Most early civilizations believed that illness had supernatural causes. The theory of animism attempted to explain the cause of mysterious changes in bodily functions. This theory was based on the belief that everything in nature was alive with invisible forces and endowed with power. Good spirits brought health; evil spirits brought sickness and death. In providing treatment, the roles of the physician and the nurse were separate and distinct. The physician was the medicine man who treated disease by chanting, inspiring fear, or opening the skull to release evil spirits (Dolan, Fitzpatrick, & Herrmann, 1983). The nurse usually was the mother who cared for her family during sickness by providing physical care and herbal remedies. This nurturing and caring role of the nurse has continued to the present.

As civilizations grew, temples became the centers of medical care because of the belief that illness was caused by sin and the gods' displeasure (i.e., disease literally means "disease"). Priests were highly regarded as physicians, but neither human life nor women were valued by society. In some

REFLECTIVE PRACTICE

Challenge to Ethical and Legal Skills

During nursing school, I was working as a nurse's aide on a busy oncology unit. It was here that I met Roberto Pecorini, a 38-year-old man diagnosed with metastatic colon cancer. He had undergone radiation treatments and chemotherapy and was extremely weak and malnourished. He was receiving numerous intravenous fluids via a central venous catheter. In addition, he had developed two pressure ulcers on his sacrum, each approximately 1½" in diameter, that required wound care. He also had a colostomy that he could not care for independently.

Although the staff was very helpful, the orientation I received to the unit was brief because they were very short staffed. During one occasion, shortly after I had been oriented to the floor, I was working a night shift and was the only nurse's aide on the unit. The nurses I was working with asked me to care for Mr. Pecorini, including performing several tasks and skills with which I was unfamiliar. In addition to my lack of familiarity with skills such as changing central line dressings and performing blood draws and wound care, I was not licensed to perform these tasks. I felt uncomfortable performing these skills on my own. However, the nurses were extremely busy and I wanted to help them as much as possible. If I performed these skills on my own, I could be putting the patient at risk. Moreover, I could be threatening the license of the nurses.

Thinking Outside the Box: Possible Courses of Action

- Perform the tasks requested despite the fact that I had little experience with them.
- Inform the nurses that I did not feel comfortable completing these skills on my own and ask that they assign me other tasks within my scope of duty.
- Ask the nurses to be present when I performed these tasks so that they could observe my skills and intervene if necessary.

- Refrain from performing these tasks and alert the nurse manager the following day that I was assigned to tasks outside my scope of duty.

Evaluating a Good Outcome: How Do I Define Success?

- The patient received safe, comprehensive care without being placed at risk.
- I performed tasks and skills within my scope of practice.
- The nurses understood my job duties and properly delegated the necessary tasks.

- The nurses' licensure was not put in jeopardy.
- I felt comfortable and competent in my job performance.

Personal Learning: Here's to the Future!

Since I felt uncomfortable in performing the duties assigned to me by the nurses, I confronted them and told them that I had recently been oriented to the floor and did not have experience with these skills. Although somewhat surprised that I didn't have the experience, they understood, not wanting me to do anything I felt uncomfortable with. The nurses were used to having an LPN as a night aide, and the LPN's scope of practice was broader than mine. Throughout the night, I observed the nurses performing the skills and tasks, with the nurses walking me through several of the skills that I was allowed to perform but in which I did not feel proficient.

In the morning, we spoke with the nurse manager, who realized the need for clarifying the job duties of the nurse's aides and the appropriate delegation of tasks. I feel that I made the right decision in speaking to the nurses because patient safety could have been compromised by my inexperience. The nurses' licensure also could have been put at risk. As a result of our conversation with the nurse manager, the orientation for new nurse's aides was reorganized, helping greatly to define the scope of duties for the aides.

Colleen Kilcullen, Georgetown University

Reflection

How do you think you would respond in a similar situation? Why? What does this tell you about yourself and about the adequacy of your skills for professional practice? Can you think of other ways to respond? How was the nursing student's action ethical? Legal? Please explain. What other skills (cognitive, interpersonal, technical, ethical/legal) would you need to respond well in this situation? Do you agree with the criteria to evaluate a successful outcome? Based on the nursing student's personal learning, were the criteria met? Please explain why or why not.

societies, the nurse was viewed as a slave, carrying out menial tasks based on the orders of the priest–physician. During the same period, the ancient Hebrews developed rules through the Ten Commandments and the Mosaic Health Code for ethical human relationships, mental health, and disease control. Nurses cared for sick people in the home and the community and also practiced as nurse–midwives (Dolan et al., 1983).

In the early Christian period, nursing began to have a formal and more clearly defined role. Led by the idea that love and caring for others were important, women called deaconesses made the first organized visits to sick people, and members of male religious orders gave nursing care and buried the dead. Both male and female nursing orders were founded during the Crusades (11th to 13th centuries). Hospitals were built for the enormous number of pilgrims needing healthcare, and nursing became a respected vocation. Although the early Middle Ages ended in chaos, nursing had developed purpose, direction, and leadership.

At the beginning of the 16th century, many Western societies changed from having a religious orientation to emphasizing warfare, exploration, and expansion of knowledge. Many monasteries and convents closed, leading to a tremendous shortage of people to care for the sick. To meet this need, women who had committed crimes were recruited into nursing in lieu of serving jail sentences. In addition to having a poor reputation, nurses received low pay and worked long hours in unfavorable conditions.

Florence Nightingale and the Birth of Modern Nursing

From the middle of the 18th century to the 19th century, social reforms changed the roles of nurses and of women in general. It was during this time that nursing as we now know it began, based on many of the beliefs of Florence Nightingale. Born in 1820 to a wealthy family, she grew up in England, was well educated, and traveled extensively. Despite strong opposition from her family, Nightingale began training as a nurse at the age of 31. The outbreak of the Crimean War and a request by the British to organize nursing care for a military hospital in Turkey gave Nightingale an opportunity for achievement (Kalisch & Kalisch, 2004). As she successfully overcame enormous difficulties, Nightingale challenged prejudices against women and elevated the status of all nurses. After the war, she returned to England, where she established a training school for nurses and wrote books about healthcare and nursing education. Florence Nightingale's contributions include:

- Identifying the personal needs of the patient and the role of the nurse in meeting those needs
- Establishing standards for hospital management
- Establishing a respected occupation for women
- Establishing nursing education
- Recognizing the two components of nursing: health and illness
- Believing that nursing is separate and distinct from medicine
- Recognizing that nutrition is important to health
- Instituting occupational and recreational therapy for sick people
- Stressing the need for continuing education for nurses
- Maintaining accurate records, recognized as the beginnings of nursing research

Florence Nightingale elevated the status of nursing to a respected occupation, improved the quality of nursing care, and founded modern nursing education. Florence Nightingale, other historically important nurses, and images of early nursing can be seen in Figure 1-1. People important to the development of nursing are listed in Table 1-1. Foundational documents for nursing are discussed in Box 1-1.

Development of Nursing from the 19th to 21st Centuries

Both the work of Florence Nightingale and the care provided for battle casualties during the Civil War focused attention on the need for educated nurses in the United States. Schools of nursing, founded in connection with hospitals, were established on the beliefs of Nightingale, but the training they provided was based more on apprenticeship than on educational principles. Hospitals saw an economic advantage in having their own schools, and most hospital schools were organized to provide more easily controlled and less expensive staff for the hospital. This resulted in a lack of clear guidelines separating nursing service and nursing education. As students and as graduates, female nurses were under the control of male hospital administrators and physicians. The lack of educational standards, the male dominance in healthcare, and the pervading Victorian belief that women depended on men combined to contribute to several decades of slow progress toward professionalism in nursing (Kalisch & Kalisch, 2004).

World War II had an enormous effect on nursing. For the first time, large numbers of women worked outside the home. They became more independent and assertive. These changes in women and in society led to an increased emphasis on education. The war itself had created a need for more nurses and resulted in a knowledge explosion in medicine and technology, which broadened the role of nurses. After World War II, efforts were directed at upgrading nursing education. Schools of nursing were based on educational objectives and were increasingly developed in university and college settings, leading to degrees in nursing for men, women, and minorities.

Nursing has broadened in all areas, including practice in a wide variety of healthcare settings, the development of a specific body of knowledge, the conduct and publication of nursing research, and recognition of the role of nursing in promoting health. Increased emphasis on nursing knowledge as the base for evidence-based practice has led to the growth of nursing as a professional discipline.

DEFINITIONS OF NURSING

The word *nurse* originated from the Latin word *nutrix,* meaning "to nourish." Most definitions of **nursing** describe the nurse as a person who nourishes, fosters, and protects and who is prepared to take care of sick, injured, and aged people. With the expanding roles and functions of the nurse in today's society, however, any one definition may be too limited.

The International Council of Nurses (2002) captures much of what nursing means in its definition:

Nursing encompasses autonomous and collaborative care of individuals of all ages, families, groups, and communities, sick or well and in all settings. Nursing includes the promotion of health, prevention of illness, and the care of ill, disabled, and dying people. Advocacy, promotion of a safe environment, research, participation in shaping health policy and in patient and health systems management, and education are also key nursing roles.

Clara Barton, founder of the American Red Cross in 1882

Florence Nightingale, initiator of major reforms in healthcare and nursing training in England

Vassar training camp classroom, 1918

Isabel Hampton Robb, outstanding leader in nursing and nursing education

Mary Mahoney, America's first African American nurse to graduate from a school of nursing

Philadelphia General Hospital nurse, late 1800s

Post-WWII nursing school poster

FIGURE 1-1. Images of nurses spanning more than 100 years of service. *(Courtesy of the Center for the Study of the History of Nursing, University of Pennsylvania.)*

The American Nurses Association (ANA) describes the values and social responsibility of nursing, provides a definition and scope of practice for nursing, discusses nursing's knowledge base, and describes the methods by which nursing is regulated within its Nursing's Social Policy Statement (2003). Within the definition, nurses focus on human experiences and responses to birth, health, illness, and death within the context of individuals, families, groups, and communities. The knowledge base for nursing practice includes diagnosis, interventions, and evaluation of outcomes from an established plan of care. In addition, the nurse integrates objective data with knowledge gained from an understanding of the patient's or group's subjective experience, applies scientific knowledge in the nursing process, and provides a caring relationship that facilitates health and healing.

The central focus in all definitions of nursing is the patient (the person receiving care) and includes the physical, emotional, social, and spiritual dimensions of that person. Nursing is no longer considered to be concerned primarily with illness care. Nursing's concepts and definitions have expanded to include the prevention of illness and the promotion and maintenance of health for individuals, families, and communities.

AIMS OF NURSING

Four broad aims of nursing practice can be identified in the definitions of nursing:

1. To promote health
2. To prevent illness
3. To restore health
4. To facilitate coping with disability or death

TABLE • 1-1	PEOPLE IMPORTANT TO THE DEVELOPMENT OF NURSING IN NORTH AMERICA
Person	**Contribution**
19th Century	
Florence Nightingale	Defined nursing as both an art and a science, differentiated nursing from medicine, created free-standing nursing education; published books about nursing and healthcare; is regarded as the founder of modern nursing (see text for further information)
Clara Barton	Volunteered to care for wounds and feed Union soldiers during the Civil War; served as the supervisor of nurses for the Army of the James, organizing hospitals and nurses; established the Red Cross in the United States in 1882
Dorothea Dix	Served as superintendent of the Female Nurses of the Army during the Civil War; was given the authority and the responsibility for recruiting and equipping a corps of army nurses; was a pioneering crusader for the reform of the treatment of the mentally ill
Mary Ann Bickerdyke	Organized diet kitchens, laundries, and an ambulance service and supervised nursing staff during the Civil War
Louise Schuyler	A nurse during the Civil War; returned to New York and organized the New York Charities Aid Association to improve care of the sick in Bellevue Hospital; recommended standards for nursing education
Linda Richards	Graduated in 1873 from the New England Hospital for Women and Children in Boston, Massachusetts, as the first trained nurse in the United States; became the night superintendent of Bellevue Hospital in 1874 and began the practice of keeping records and writing orders
Jane Addams	Provided social services within a neighborhood setting; a leader for women's rights; recipient of the 1931 Nobel Peace prize
Lillian Wald	Established a neighborhood nursing service for the sick poor of the Lower East Side in New York City; the founder of public health nursing
Mary Elizabeth Mahoney	Graduated from the New England Hospital for Women and Children in 1879 as America's first African American nurse
Harriet Tubman	A nurse and an abolitionist; active in the underground railroad movement before joining the Union Army during the Civil War
Nora Gertrude Livingston	Established a training program for nurses at the Montreal General Hospital (the first 3-year program in North America)
Mary Agnes Snively	Director of the nursing school at Toronto General Hospital and one of the founders of the Canadian Nurses Association
Sojourner Truth	Provided nursing care to soldiers during the Civil War and worked for the women's movement
Isabel Hampton Robb	A leader in nursing and nursing education; organized the nursing school at Johns Hopkins Hospital; initiated policies that included limiting the number of hours in a day's work and wrote a textbook to help student learning; the first president of the Nurses Associated Alumnae of the United States and Canada (which later became the American Nurses Association)
20th Century	
Mary Adelaide Nutting	Became the first professor of nursing in the world as a faculty member of Teachers' College, Columbia University; with Lavinia Dock, published the four-volume *History of Nursing*
Elizabeth Smellie	A member of the original Victorian Order of Nurses for Canada (a group who provided public health nursing); organized the Canadian Women's Army Corps during World War II
Lavinia Dock	A nursing leader and women's rights activist; instrumental in the Constitutional amendment giving women the right to vote
Mary Breckenridge	Established the Frontier Nursing Service and one of the first midwifery schools in the United States
Margaret Sanger	Founder of Planned Parenthood

To meet these aims, the nurse uses knowledge, skills, and critical thinking to give care in a variety of traditional and expanding nursing roles. See Box 1-2 for examples. Nurses use four essential competencies: *cognitive, technical, interpersonal,* and *ethical/legal skills* to provide safe and knowledgeable care.

Cognitively skilled nurses think about the nature of things sufficiently to "make sense" of their world and to grasp con-

ceptually what is necessary to achieve valued goals. Cognitively skilled nurses are able to accomplish the following:

- Offer a scientific rationale for the patient's plan of care (sciences include nursing and medical science, as well as basic sciences, such as chemistry, microbiology, anatomy, physiology, psychology, sociology, and anthropology)

Box 1-1   TIMELINE OF THE DEVELOPMENT OF FOUNDATIONAL NURSING DOCUMENTS

1859	Florence Nightingale publishes *Notes on Nursing: What It Is and What It Is Not.*
1896	The Nurses' Associated Alumnae of the United States and Canada is founded. Later to become the American Nurses Association (ANA), its first purpose is to establish and maintain a code of ethics.
1940	A "Tentative Code" is published in *American Journal of Nursing,* although never formally adopted.
1950	*Code for Professional Nurses,* in the form of 17 provisions that are a substantive revision of the "Tentative Code" of 1940, is unanimously accepted by the ANA House of Delegates.
1952	*Nursing Research* publishes its premiere issue.
1956	*Code for Professional Nurses* is amended.
1960	*Code for Professional Nurses* is revised.
1968	*Code for Professional Nurses* is substantively revised, condensing the 17 provisions of the code into 10 provisions.
1973	ANA publishes its first *Standards of Nursing Practice.*
1976	*Code for Nurses With Interpretive Statements,* a modification of the provision and interpretive statements, is published as 11 provisions.
1980	ANA publishes *Nursing: A Social Policy Statement.*
1985	The National Institutes of Health organizes the Center for Nursing Research.
	ANA publishes *Titling for Licensure.*
	Code for Nurses with Interpretive Statements retains the provisions of the 1976 version and includes revised interpretive statements.
	The ANA House of Delegates forms a task force to formally document the scope of practice for nursing.
1987	ANA publishes *The Scope of Nursing Practice.*
1990	The ANA House of Delegates forms a task force to revise the 1973 *Standards of Nursing Practice.*
1991	ANA publishes *Standards of Clinical Nursing Practice.*
1995	ANA publishes *Nursing's Social Policy Statement.*
	The Congress of Nursing Practice directs the Committee on Nursing Practice Standards and Guidelines to establish a process for periodic review and revision of nursing standards.
1996	ANA publishes *Scope and Standards of Advanced Practice Registered Nursing.*
1998	ANA publishes *Standards of Clinical Nursing Practice,* 2nd ed. (also known as *Clinical Standards*).
2001	*Code of Ethics With Interpretive Statements* is accepted by the ANA House of Delegates.
	ANA publishes *Bill of Rights for Registered Nurses.*
2002	ANA publishes *Nursing's Agenda for the Future: A Call to the Nation.*
2003	ANA publishes *Nursing's Social Policy Statement,* 2nd ed.
	ANA publishes *Nursing: Scope and Standards of Practice.*

Source: American Nurses Association (ANA). (2003). *Nursing: Scope and standards of practice.* Washington DC: Nursebooks.org. © 2001 By American Nurses Association, Reprinted with permission. All rights reserved.

- Select those nursing interventions that are most likely to yield the desired outcomes
- Use critical thinking to solve problems creatively

Technically skilled nurses manipulate equipment skillfully to produce a desired outcome or result. Technical competence involves everything from manual dexterity and good eye–hand coordination to an ability to troubleshoot when equipment malfunctions, based on an understanding of the technical workings of the equipment. Technically skilled nurses are able to accomplish the following:

- Use technical equipment with sufficient competence and ease to achieve goals with minimal distress to participants involved
- Creatively adapt equipment and technical procedures to the needs of individual patients in diverse circumstances

Interpersonally skilled nurses establish and maintain caring relationships that facilitate the achievement of valued goals while simultaneously affirming the worth of those in the relationship. Nurses skilled in interpersonal relations are able to accomplish the following:

- Use interactions with patients, their significant others, and colleagues to affirm their worth
- Elicit the personal strengths and abilities of patients and their significant others to achieve valued health goals
- Provide the healthcare team with knowledge about the patient's valued goals and expectations
- Work collaboratively with other members of the healthcare team as a respected and credible colleague to reach valued goals

Ethically and legally skilled nurses conduct themselves in a manner consistent with their personal moral code and

Box 1-2   HOW CAN YOU BE A NURSE?

How can you be a nurse? How can you bear to watch children suffer?
Wait until you've rocked and soothed a suffering child into peaceful sleep, and you feel the child's relief washing over you like a blessing. Then you won't need to ask.

Photo by Joe Mitchell.

How can you be a nurse? How can you bear to care for frustrating, confused Alzheimer's patients?
Wait until you've devised a combination of strategies that provide exercise and permit safe wandering, and you see a lift, almost a spring, in a patient's shuffling gait. You'll feel the lightness of Baryshnikov in your own step that day.

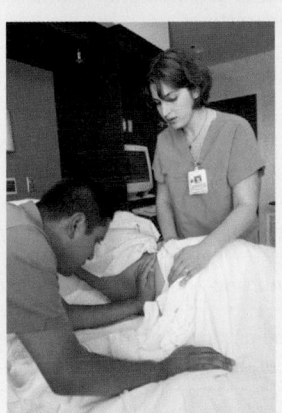

Photo by Joe Mitchell.

How can you be a nurse? So many of your patients are so old, so sick, these days. How can you bear the thought that, in the end, your care may make no difference?
Wait until you've used your hands and eyes and voice to dispel terror, to show a helpless person that his life is respected, that he has dignity. Your caring helps him care about himself . . .

Photo © Barbara Proud.

How can you be a nurse? How can you bear the sound of babies crying?
Wait until your combination of vigilance, bulldog advocacy, and gentle handling has given a preemie's lungs the time they needed to develop, and you hear his first lusty cry. You'll laugh out loud!

Photo by Joe Mitchell.

So you keep choosing to be a nurse. You have days of frustration, nights of despair, terrible angers. Your highs and lows are peaks and chasms, not hills and valleys. The defeats come more than often enough to keep you humble: the problems you can't untangle, the lives that seep away too fast, the meanings that elude your understanding. But you keep working at it, learning from it, knowing the next peak lies ahead.

Mary Mallison
Editorial, April 1987
American Journal of Nursing

professional role responsibilities. Nurses skilled in ethical/legal competence are able to accomplish the following:

- Be trusted to act in ways that advance the interests of patients
- Be accountable for their practice to themselves, the patients they serve, the caregiving team, and society
- Act as effective patient advocates
- Mediate ethical conflicts among the patient, significant others, the healthcare team, and other interested parties
- Practice nursing faithful to the tenets of professional codes of ethics and appropriate standards of practice
- Use legal safeguards that reduce the risk of litigation

The primary role of the nurse as caregiver is given shape and substance by the interrelated roles of communicator, teacher, counselor, leader, researcher, advocate, and collaborator. These roles are described in Table 1-2 and are fully discussed in Unit V. The nurse carries out these roles in many different settings, with care increasingly provided in the home and in the community. Examples of settings for care are listed in Box 1-3 and are fully described in Chapters 8 and 10.

➤ Recall Roberto Pecorini, the 38-year-old patient with metastatic cancer. When providing care for Mr. Pecorini, the nurse assumes the role of caregiver, maintaining the patient's safety throughout, and explaining to the patient all interventions being performed, thereby educating the patient. ∎

| Box 1-3 | EXAMPLES OF SETTINGS FOR NURSING CARE |

Hospitals
Ambulatory surgery centers
Emergency helicopter services
Clinics
Homes
Educational programs
Public health offices
Doctors' offices
Industry
Long-term care facilities
Mobile healthcare units
Schools
Offices
Hospice
Mental health facilities
State health programs
Skilled-care facilities
Churches
Prisons

Promoting Health

Health is a state of optimal functioning or well-being. As defined by the World Health Organization, one's health includes physical, social, and mental components and is not merely the absence of disease or infirmity. Health is often a subjective state—a person may be medically diagnosed with an illness but still consider himself or herself healthy. Wellness, a term that is often associated with health, is an active

TABLE • 1-2	NURSING ROLES IN ALL SETTINGS
Role	**Function**
Caregiver	The provision of care to patients that combines both the art and the science of nursing in meeting physical, emotional, intellectual, sociocultural, and spiritual needs. As a caregiver, the nurse integrates the roles of communicator, teacher, counselor, leader, researcher, advocate, and collaborator to promote wellness through activities that prevent illness, restore health, and facilitate coping with disability or death. The role of caregiver is the primary role of the nurse.
Communicator	The use of effective interpersonal and therapeutic communication skills to establish and maintain helping relationships with patients of all ages in a wide variety of healthcare settings
Teacher/Educator	The use of communication skills to assess, implement, and evaluate individualized teaching plans to meet learning needs of patients and their families
Counselor	The use of therapeutic interpersonal communication skills to provide information, make appropriate referrals, and facilitate the patient's problem-solving and decision-making skills
Leader	The assertive, self-confident practice of nursing when providing care, effecting change, and functioning with groups
Researcher	The participation in or conduct of research to increase knowledge in nursing and improve patient care
Advocate	The protection of human or legal rights and the securing of care for all patients based on the belief that patients have the right to make informed decisions about their own health and lives
Collaborator	The effective use of skills in organization, communication, and advocacy to facilitate the functions of all members of the healthcare team as they provide patient care

state of being healthy by living a lifestyle that promotes good physical, mental, and emotional health. Models of health and wellness are described in Chapter 3.

Health is an essential part of each of the other aims of nursing. Nurses promote health by identifying, analyzing, and maximizing each patient's own individual strengths as components of preventing illness, restoring health, and facilitating coping with disability or death.

> *When teaching Mr. Rowlings, the patient described at the beginning of the chapter with risk factors for heart disease, the nurse would focus the teaching plan to rely on the patient's strengths. Although his statements reflect a reluctance to learn and change, emphasizing the patient's strengths would help the patient feel more in control of his health, and thus, hopefully, spur him to make the necessary changes.* ■

Health promotion is motivated by the desire to increase a person's well-being and health potential (Pender, Murdaugh, & Parsons, 2006). A person's level of health is affected by many different interrelated factors that either promote health or increase the risk for illness. These factors include genetic inheritance, cognitive abilities, educational level, race and ethnicity, culture, age and gender, developmental level, lifestyle, environment, and socioeconomic status. A level of health or wellness is also strongly influenced by what is termed "health literacy." Health literacy, defined by the U.S. Department of Health and Human Services in the document *Healthy People 2010,* is the ability of patients to obtain, process, and understand the basic information needed to make appropriate decisions about health. Examples of ways nurses can promote health literacy are included throughout this text.

Healthy People 2010 also establishes health promotion guidelines for the nation as a whole. The guidelines are focused on meeting two overarching goals: (1) to increase quality and years of healthy life, and (2) to eliminate health disparities. The guidelines contain 10 Leading Health Indicators, which are being used to measure the health of the nation over 10 years. The Leading Health Indicators, listed in Box 1-4, reflect the major health concerns in the United States at the beginning of

---

| Box 1-4 | **HEALTHY PEOPLE 2010: LEADING HEALTH INDICATORS** |

- Physical Activity
- Overweight and Obesity
- Tobacco Use
- Substance Abuse
- Responsible Sexual Behavior
- Mental Health
- Injury and Violence
- Environmental Quality
- Immunization
- Access to Healthcare

U.S. Department of Health and Human Services, Office of Disease Prevention and Health Promotion. (2000). *Healthy people 2010.* Washington, DC: U.S. Department of Health and Human Services.

---

the 21st century. They were selected on the basis of their ability to motivate action, availability to measure progress, and importance as public health issues.

Health promotion is the framework for nursing activities. The nurse considers the patient's self-awareness, health awareness, and use of resources while providing care. Through knowledge and skill, the nurse accomplishes the following:

- Facilitates decisions about lifestyle that enhance quality of life and encourage acceptance of responsibility for one's own health
- Increases health awareness by assisting in the understanding that health is more than just not being ill, and by teaching that certain behaviors and factors can contribute to or diminish health
- Teaches self-care activities to maximize achievement of goals that are realistic and attainable; serves as a role model
- Encourages health promotion by providing information and referrals

Preventing Illness

The objectives of illness-prevention activities are to reduce the risk for illness, to promote good health habits, and to maintain optimal functioning. The motivation for illness prevention is to avoid or achieve early detection of illness or to maintain function within the constraints of an illness (Pender et al., 2006). Nurses prevent illness primarily by teaching and by personal example. Such activities include the following:

- Educational programs in areas such as prenatal care for pregnant women, smoking-cessation programs, and stress-reduction seminars
- Community programs and resources that encourage healthy lifestyles, such as aerobic exercise classes, "swimnastics," and physical fitness programs
- Literature, television, radio, or Internet information on a healthy diet, regular exercise, and the importance of good health habits
- Health assessments in institutions, clinics, and community settings that identify areas of strength and risks for illness

> *Think back to Albert Rowlings, the 62-year-old man at risk for heart disease who was described at the beginning of the chapter. The nurse participates in illness prevention, thus promoting healthier behavior by addressing his resistance to change and teaching him lifestyle modifications necessary to reduce his risk for developing heart disease.* ■

Restoring Health

Activities to restore health encompass those traditionally considered to be the nurse's responsibility. These focus on the individual with an illness and range from early detection of a disease to rehabilitation and teaching during recovery. Such activities include the following:

- Performing assessments that detect an illness (e.g., taking blood pressure, measuring blood sugars)

- Referring questions and abnormal findings to other healthcare providers as appropriate
- Providing direct care of the person who is ill by such measures as giving physical care, administering medications, and carrying out procedures and treatments
- Collaborating with other healthcare providers in providing care
- Planning, teaching, and carrying out rehabilitation for illnesses such as heart attacks, arthritis, and strokes
- Working in mental health and chemical-dependency programs

Facilitating Coping With Disability and Death

Although the major goals of healthcare are promoting, maintaining, and restoring health, these goals cannot always be met. Nurses also facilitate patient and family coping with altered function, life crisis, and death. Altered function decreases an individual's ability to carry out activities of daily living and expected roles. Nurses facilitate an optimal level of function through maximizing the person's strengths and potentials, through teaching, and through referral to community support systems. Nurses provide care to both patients and families during end-of-life care, and they do so in hospitals, long-term care facilities, and homes. Nurses are active in hospice programs, which assist patients and their families in preparing for death and in living as comfortably as possible until death occurs.

NURSING AS A PROFESSIONAL DISCIPLINE

As definitions of nursing have expanded to describe more clearly the roles and actions of nurses, increased attention has been given to nursing as a professional discipline. Nursing uses existing and new knowledge to solve problems creatively and meet human needs within ever-changing boundaries. Nursing is recognized increasingly as a **profession** based on the following defining criteria:

- Well-defined body of specific and unique knowledge
- Strong service orientation
- Recognized authority by a professional group
- Code of ethics
- Professional organization that sets standards
- Ongoing research
- Autonomy

Nursing involves specialized skills and application of knowledge based on an education that has both theoretical and clinical practice components. Nursing is guided by standards set forth by professional organizations and an established code of ethics. Nursing focuses on human responses to actual or potential health problems and is increasingly focused on wellness, an area of caring that encompasses nursing's unique knowledge and abilities. Nursing is increasingly recognized as scholarly, with academic qualifications, research, and publications specific to the profession that are accepted and respected widely. In addition, nursing interventions are focused on evidence-based practice, which is practice based on research and not intuition.

Nursing has evolved through history from a technical service to a person-centered process that maximizes potential in all human dimensions. This has been an active development process, using lessons from the past to gain knowledge for practice in the present and in the future.

EDUCATIONAL PREPARATION FOR NURSING PRACTICE

Educational preparation for nursing practice involves several different types of programs that lead to **licensure,** or the legal authority to practice as a nursing professional. Students may choose to enter a practical nursing program and become a licensed practical nurse (LPN), or they may enter a diploma, an associate degree, or a baccalaureate program to be licensed as a registered nurse (RN). State laws in the United States recognize both the LPN and the RN as credentials to practice nursing. Increasingly, various levels of nursing education are providing programs for educational advancement. For example, the LPN can complete an associate degree and become an RN, and the RN prepared at the diploma or associate degree level can attain a bachelor of science in nursing (BSN) degree. There are also programs that provide RN-to-master's degrees as well as BSN and master's degree-to-PhD. Graduate programs in nursing provide master's and doctoral degrees.

Educational preparation for the nurse has become a major issue in nursing; the multiple methods of preparation are confusing to employers, consumers of healthcare services, and nurses themselves. Nursing organizations are working hard to answer questions such as "What is technical nursing?" and "What is professional nursing?" as well as "Should graduates of different programs take the same licensing examination and have the same title?" These questions are likely to be resolved during your nursing career. The following sections discuss current education for LPNs and RNs, as well as graduate nursing education, continuing education for nurses, and in-service education.

Practical and Vocational Nursing Education

Practical (also labeled vocational) nursing programs were established to teach graduates to give bedside nursing care to patients. Schools for practical nursing programs are located in varied settings, such as high schools, technical or vocational schools, community colleges, and independent agencies. Most programs are 1 year in length, divided into one-third classroom hours and two-thirds clinical laboratory hours. On completion of the program, graduates can take the National Council Licensure Examination-Practical Nurse (NCLEX-PN) for licensure as an LPN. LPNs work under the direction of a physician or RN to give direct care to patients, focusing on meeting healthcare needs in hospitals, nursing homes, and home health agencies.

Registered Nursing Education

Three types of educational programs lead to licensure as an RN: (1) diploma, (2) associate degree, and (3) baccalaureate programs. Graduates of all three programs take the NCLEX-RN examination. Although it is a national examination, it is administered by, and the nurse is licensed in, the state in which the examination is taken and passed. *It is illegal to practice nursing unless one has a license verifying completion of an accredited (by state) program in nursing and has passed the licensing examination.* Nurses gain legal rights to practice nursing in another state by applying to that state's board of nursing and receiving reciprocal licensure. Table 1-3 summarizes the types of education for RNs. A more in-depth discussion of licensure is included later in this chapter under Nurse Practice Acts and Licensure.

Diploma in Nursing

Many nurses practicing in the United States today received their basic nursing education in a 3-year, hospital-based diploma school of nursing (Ellis & Hartley, 2007). The first schools of nursing established to educate nurses were diploma programs, and until the 1960s, they were the major source of graduates. In recent years, the number of diploma programs has decreased greatly.

Graduates of diploma programs have a sound foundation in the biologic and social sciences, with a strong emphasis on clinical experience in direct patient care. Graduates work in acute, long-term, and ambulatory healthcare facilities (Ellis & Hartley, 2007).

Associate Degree in Nursing

Most associate degree in nursing (ADN) programs are in community or junior colleges. These 2-year educational programs attract more men, more minorities, and more nontraditional students than do the other types of programs. Associate degree education prepares nurses to give care to patients in various settings, including hospitals, long-term care facilities, and home healthcare settings. Graduates are technically skilled and well prepared to carry out nursing roles and functions. As defined by the National League for Nursing (NLN), competencies of the ADN on entry into

TABLE • 1-3	SUMMARY OF TYPES OF EDUCATIONAL PROGRAMS FOR REGISTERED NURSES (RNs)		
	Diploma	**Associate Degree**	**Baccalaureate**
Location	Hospital	Community college	Senior college or university
Length	24–36 mo	2 academic or calendar years	4 academic years
Course work	Biologic science Physical science Nursing theory Nursing practice	Basic sciences Social sciences General education Nursing theory Nursing practice	Basic sciences General education Social sciences Nursing theory Nursing practice Nursing research Community health Management
Clinical component	Both hospital and community settings	Both hospital and community settings	A variety of settings in which healthcare and nursing care are provided
Further education opportunity	If affiliated with a college, may transfer some credit toward a bachelor of science in nursing (BSN) degree	Credits often apply toward a bachelor of science in nursing (BSN) degree	Base for advanced education at the master's and doctoral levels
Competencies on graduation	Plans and gives direct care to patients in structured settings Works with other members of the healthcare team to plan and provide care to ill patients	Plans and gives direct care to patients in structured settings Works with other members of the healthcare team to plan and provide care to ill patients	Plans and gives direct care to individual patients, groups, and communities Directs other members of the healthcare team in planning and providing care to ill and well patients in a variety of settings; assumes beginning leadership roles; provides comprehensive healthcare, including health promotion, illness prevention, and rehabilitative, educational, and health counseling

practice encompass the roles of provider of care, manager of care, and member of the discipline of nursing.

Baccalaureate in Nursing

The first baccalaureate nursing programs were established in the United States in the early 1900s. The number of programs and the number of enrolling students, however, did not increase markedly until the 1960s. Most graduates receive a bachelor of science in nursing (BSN).

Recommendations by national nursing organizations that the entry level for professional practice be at the baccalaureate level have resulted in increased numbers of these programs. Although BSN nurses practice in a wide variety of settings, the 4-year degree is required for many administrative, managerial, and community health positions.

In BSN programs, the major in nursing is built on a general education base, with concentration on nursing at the upper level. Students acquire knowledge of theory and practice related to nursing and other disciplines, provide nursing care to individuals and groups, work with members of the healthcare team, use research to improve practice, and have a foundation for graduate study. Nurses who graduate from a diploma or associate degree program and wish to complete requirements for a BSN may choose to enroll in an on-campus, online, or external degree RN-to-BSN program. In addition, there are accelerated BSN programs for people who already have a degree in another area.

Graduate Education in Nursing

The two levels of graduate education in nursing are the master's and doctoral degrees. A master's degree prepares advanced practice nurses to function in educational settings, in managerial roles, as clinical specialists, and in various advanced practice areas, such as nurse–midwives and nurse practitioners (Table 1-4). Many master's graduates gain national certification in their specialty area, for example, as family nurse practitioners (FNPs). Nurses with doctoral degrees meet requirements for academic advancement and organizational management. They also are prepared to carry out research necessary to advance nursing theory and practice.

Continuing Education

The ANA defines continuing education as those professional development experiences designed to enrich the nurse's contribution to health. Colleges, hospitals, voluntary agencies, and private groups offer formal continuing education through

TABLE • 1-4 EXPANDED EDUCATIONAL AND CAREER ROLES OF NURSES	
Title	**Description**
Clinical nurse specialist (e.g., enterostomal therapist, geriatrics, infection control, medical–surgical, maternal–child, oncology, quality assurance, nursing process)	A nurse with an advanced degree, education, or experience who is considered to be an expert in a specialized area of nursing; carries out direct patient care; consultation; teaching of patients, families, and staff; and research
Nurse practitioner	A nurse with an advanced degree, certified for a special area or age of patient care; works in a variety of healthcare settings or in independent practice to make health assessments and deliver primary care
Nurse anesthetist	A nurse who completes a course of study in an anesthesia school; carries out preoperative visits and assessments; administers and monitors anesthesia during surgery; and evaluates postoperative status of patients
Nurse–midwife	A nurse who completes a program in midwifery; provides prenatal and postnatal care; and delivers babies for women with uncomplicated pregnancies
Nurse educator	A nurse, usually with an advanced degree, who teaches in educational or clinical settings; teaches theoretical knowledge and clinical skills; conducts research
Nurse administrator	A nurse who functions at various levels of management in healthcare settings; is responsible for the management and administration of resources and personnel involved in giving patient care
Nurse researcher	A nurse with an advanced degree who conducts research relevant to the definition and improvement of nursing practice and education
Nurse entrepreneur	A nurse, usually with an advanced degree, who may manage a clinic or health-related business, conduct research, provide education, or serve as an adviser or consultant to institutions, political agencies, or businesses

courses, seminars, and workshops. In some states, continuing education is required for an RN to maintain licensure.

In-Service Education

Many hospitals and healthcare agencies provide education and training for employees of their institution or organization, called in-service education. This is designed to increase the knowledge and skills of the nursing staff. Programs may involve learning, for example, a specific nursing skill or how to use new equipment.

PROFESSIONAL NURSING ORGANIZATIONS

One of the criteria of a profession is having a professional organization that sets standards for practice and education. Nursing's professional organizations are concerned with current issues in nursing and healthcare, and influence healthcare policy and legislation. The benefits of belonging to a professional nursing organization include networking with colleagues, having a voice in legislation affecting nursing, and keeping current with trends and issues in nursing.

International Nursing Organization

The International Council of Nurses (ICN), founded in 1899, was the first international organization of professional women. By sharing a commitment to maintaining high standards of nursing service and nursing education and by promoting ethics, the ICN provides a way for national nursing organizations to work together.

National Nursing Organizations

Professional nursing organizations in the United States include the American Nurses Association (ANA), the National League for Nursing (NLN), and the American Association of Colleges in Nursing (AACN). The National Student Nurses' Association (NSNA) prepares students to participate in professional nursing organizations.

ANA

The ANA is the professional organization for RNs in the United States. Founded in the late 1800s, its membership is comprised of the state nurses' associations to which individual nurses belong. Its primary mission is to be involved in public education, clinical nursing standards, and lobbying state and federal lawmakers to advance the profession of nursing. The ANA addresses ethics, public policy, and the economic and general welfare of nurses. Publications of the ANA include *American Nurse Today, The American Nurse, Foundations of Nursing,* and *Capitol Update.*

NLN

The NLN is an organization open to all people interested in nursing, including nurses, nonnurses, and agencies. Estab-

lished in 1952, its objective is to foster the development and improvement of all nursing services and nursing education. The NLN conducts one of the largest professional testing services in the United States, including pre-entrance testing for potential students and achievement testing to measure student progress. It also serves as the primary source of research data about nursing education, conducting annual surveys of schools and new RNs. The organization also provides voluntary accreditation for educational programs in nursing.

AACN

The AACN is the national voice for baccalaureate and higher degree nursing education programs. The organization's goals focus on establishing quality educational standards, influencing the nursing profession to improve healthcare, and promoting public support of baccalaureate and graduate education, research, and nursing practice. National accreditation for collegiate nursing programs is provided (based on meeting standards) through the AACN by the Commission on Collegiate Nursing Education (CCNE).

NSNA

Established in 1952 with the assistance of the ANA and the NLN, the NSNA is the national organization for students enrolled in nursing education programs. Through voluntary participation, students practice self-governance, advocate for student and patient rights, and take collective, responsible action on social and political issues.

Specialty Practice and Special Interest Nursing Organizations

A wide variety of specialty practice and special interest nursing organizations are available to nurses. These organizations provide information on specific areas of nursing, often have publications in the specialty area, and may be involved in certification activities. Examples of these organizations are listed in Box 1-5.

Box 1-5 **EXAMPLES OF US SPECIALTY PRACTICE AND SPECIAL INTEREST NURSING ORGANIZATIONS**

- American Academy of Nurse Practitioners
- American Assembly for Men in Nursing
- American Association for the History of Nursing
- American Association of Nurse Attorneys
- American Holistic Nurses' Association
- Association of Nurses in AIDS Care
- Dermatology Nurses Association
- Hospice Nurses Association
- Oncology Nurses Society
- Sigma Theta Tau International
- Transcultural Nursing Society

GUIDELINES FOR NURSING PRACTICE

Nursing controls and guarantees its practice through standards of practice, nurse practice acts and licensure, and the use of the nursing process. Each of these will guide your nursing education as a student and how you practice after graduation.

Standards of Nursing Practice

The ANA's 2003 *Nursing: Scope and Standards of Practice* defines activities that are specific and unique to nursing. **Standards** allow nurses to carry out professional roles, serving as protection for the nurse, the patient, and the institution where healthcare is given. Each nurse is accountable for his or her own quality of practice and is responsible for the use of these standards to ensure knowledgeable, safe, and comprehensive nursing care. The 2003 ANA standards outlined in Box 1-6 apply to the practice of professional nursing for all RNs, in all settings.

Nurse Practice Acts and Licensure

Nurse practice acts are laws established in each state in the United States to regulate the practice of nursing. They are broadly worded and vary among states, but all of them have certain elements in common, such as the following:

- Protect the public by defining the legal scope of nursing practice, excluding untrained or unlicensed people from practicing nursing
- Create a state board of nursing or regulatory body having the authority to make and enforce rules and regulations concerning the nursing profession

- Define important terms and activities in nursing, including legal requirements and titles for RNs and LPNs
- Establish criteria for the education and licensure of nurses

The board of nursing for each state has the legal authority to allow graduates of approved schools of nursing to take the licensing examination. Those who successfully meet the requirements for licensure are then given a license to practice nursing in the state. The license, which must be renewed at specified intervals, is valid during the life of the holder and is registered in the state. Many states have a requirement for a specified number of continuing education units (CEUs) to renew and maintain licensure. There are two ways in which nurses can practice in a state other than in the one they were originally licensed. One is by **reciprocity,** which allows a nurse to apply for and be endorsed as a registered nurse by another state. There are also 23 states that are members of the Nurse Licensure Compact, allowing a nurse who is licensed and permanently lives in one of the member states to practice in the other member states without additional licensure (National Council of State Boards of Nursing, 2008). The license and the right to practice nursing can be denied, revoked, or suspended for professional misconduct (e.g., incompetence, negligence, chemical impairment, or criminal actions).

As nursing roles continue to expand and issues in nursing are resolved, revised nurse practice acts will reflect those changes. All nurses must be knowledgeable about the specific nurse practice act for the state in which they practice.

Nursing Process

The **nursing process** is another of the major guidelines for nursing practice. Nurses implement their roles through the

---

> **Box 1-6** ANA STANDARDS OF NURSING PRACTICE

Standards of Practice
- Assessment: The nurse collects comprehensive data pertinent to the patient's health or the situation.
- Diagnosis: The nurse analyzes the assessment data to determine the diagnoses or issues.
- Outcomes Identification: The nurse identifies expected outcomes for a plan individualized to the patient or the situation.
- Planning: The nurse develops a plan that prescribes strategies and alternatives to attain expected outcomes.
- Implementation: The nurse implements the identified plan, coordinates care delivery, employs strategies to promote health and a safe environment (the APRN* also provides consultation and uses prescriptive authority and treatment).
- Evaluation: The nurse evaluates progress toward attainment of outcomes.

Standards of Professional Performance
- Quality of Practice: The nurse systematically enhances the quality and effectiveness of nursing practice.
- Practice Evaluation: The nurse evaluates one's own practice in relation to professional practice standards and guidelines, relevant statutes, rules, and regulations.
- Education: The nurse attains knowledge and competency that reflects current nursing practice.
- Collegiality: The nurse interacts with and contributes to the professional development of peers and colleagues.
- Collaboration: The nurse collaborates with patient, family, and others in the conduct of nursing practice.
- Ethics: The nurse integrates ethical provisions in all areas of practice.
- Research: The nurse integrates research findings into practice.
- Resource Utilization: The nurse considers factors related to safety, effectiveness, cost, and impact on practice in the planning and delivery of nursing services.
- Leadership: The nurse provides leadership in the profession and the professional practice setting.

*APRN = Advanced Practice Registered Nurse

American Nurses Association (ANA). (2003). *Nursing: Scope and standards of practice: Professional development.* Washington, DC: Author. Reproduced with permission of the American Nurses Association.

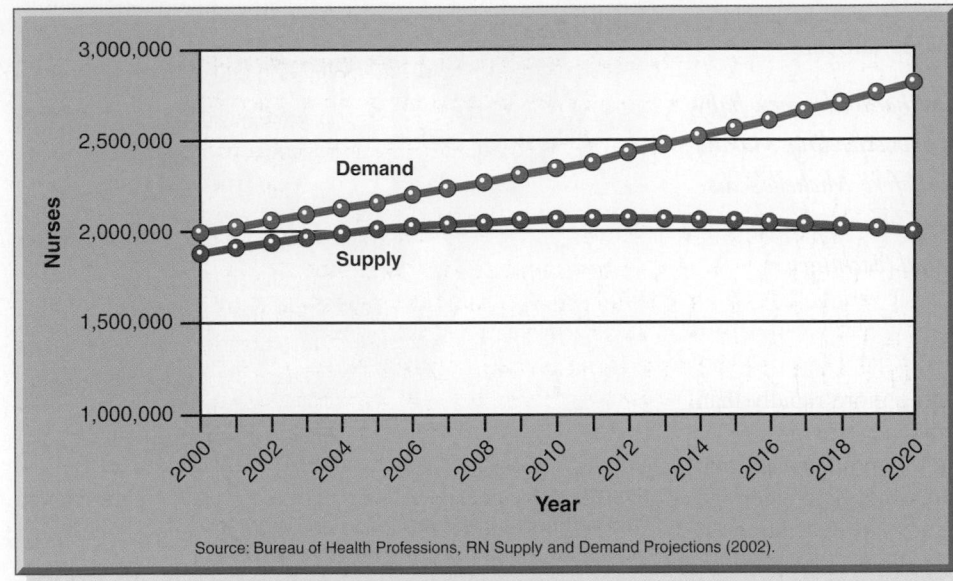

FIGURE 1-2. National supply and demand projection for FTE registered nurses: 2000 to 2020. (Source: Bureau of Health Professions [2002]. *Projected supply, demand, and shortages of registered nurses: 2000–2020*).

nursing process, which integrates both the art and the science of nursing—that is, the nursing process is nursing made visible.

The nursing process is used by the nurse to identify the patient's healthcare needs and strengths, to establish and carry out a plan of care to meet those needs, and to evaluate the effectiveness of the plan to meet established outcomes. The nursing process allows nurses to use critical thinking when providing care that is individualized and holistic, and to define those areas of care that are within the domain of nursing. Critical thinking and the nursing process are fully described in Unit III.

CURRENT TRENDS IN NURSING

Nursing changes continually in response to the needs and resources of society as a whole. It also changes in response to factors such as definitions of nursing, the aims of nursing, the educational preparation for nursing, and expanded practice roles. The trends discussed in the following text are currently affecting nursing education and practice. These trends and many others provide the background for nursing in this century. As nurses continue to define their own practice, the special and distinctive role of nursing in caring for others will become increasingly recognized in society.

Nursing Shortage

Registered nurses are the largest group of healthcare providers in the United States, numbering nearly 2.9 million, with 2.4 million employed in nursing (American Nurses Association, 2006). However, various forces are in effect to decrease that number. The nursing workforce is aging, as are the faculty needed to educate nursing students. Although more men and more minorities are entering

nursing, their numbers are not high enough to compensate for those retiring. By 2020, a shortage of nurses will put the nursing workforce in critical condition, as illustrated in Figure 1-2. This reduction in the workforce continues to occur at the same time as the population is aging and developing chronic illnesses and disabilities that require skilled nursing care.

Evidence-Based Practice

Although nurses have conducted and published research since the 1950s, only recently has the importance of using scientific evidence to develop guidelines for nursing care been recognized. By identifying and analyzing the best available scientific evidence, nurses are steadily developing further guidelines for clinical practice that are useful nationally and internationally. Additional information about evidence-based practice is provided in Chapter 5.

Community-Based Nursing

Healthcare is increasingly provided in community-based settings such as clinics, outpatient settings, and homes. These are discussed in Unit II. The impetus for this change has largely been the implementation of a system of managed care to control and monitor healthcare services to minimize costs.

Decreased Length of Hospital Stay

Though patients who require in-hospital care are more acutely ill or injured than in the past, their length of stay in the hospital has decreased. This trend affects nursing in several ways. Nurses employed in hospital settings must have the knowledge and skills to provide often-complex care to very ill patients. In the home, nurses may find themselves providing much the same type of care, as well as teaching patients and their families how to provide self-care.

> *Recall Michelle Fine, the young mother with a new baby who calls the nursery for help with breastfeeding. Making a referral for home care follow-up before Michelle's discharge from the hospital would have been appropriate to offer support, guidance, and additional teaching.* ∎

Aging Population

The older adult population is expanding more rapidly than any other age group, with the greatest increase in those older than 75 years of age. This population trend means that patients in all healthcare settings increasingly are older and require teaching and nursing interventions designed to meet needs different from those of younger patients. Older healthcare consumers are also demanding more disease-prevention interventions, new building designs to meet their housing needs, and a focus on communities of care. Nursing will continually need to research health issues related to the oldest old, ethnically diverse populations, quality of life, and innovative systems of care.

Increase in Chronic Health Conditions

Chronic health conditions, such as heart disease, cancer, respiratory disease, and acquired immunodeficiency syndrome (AIDS), are major health problems in our society. As the population ages, it has been projected that by the year 2030, nearly 171 million people will have a chronic health condition, with half of that number having more than one chronic disease (Robert Wood Johnson Foundation, 2009). Meeting the healthcare needs of so many people will be more difficult for society, particularly for those who live in poverty, are homeless, are mentally ill, or are of different cultures.

Culturally Competent Care and Complementary Therapies

The importance of culturally competent care and the use of alternative or complementary therapies to treat illnesses are recognized as crucial to providing holistic, individualized care. Nurses must become more culturally aware as our society becomes increasingly global.

Independent Nursing Practice

Advanced practice nurses, such as nurse practitioners and nurse–midwives, are increasingly establishing independent practices in which they diagnose and treat illnesses, promote health, provide well-women care, and deliver babies (Fig. 1-3). Depending on state certification requirements, they may also practice in collaboration with a physician. There are over 200,000 advanced practice nurses providing primary healthcare services and establishing the need for

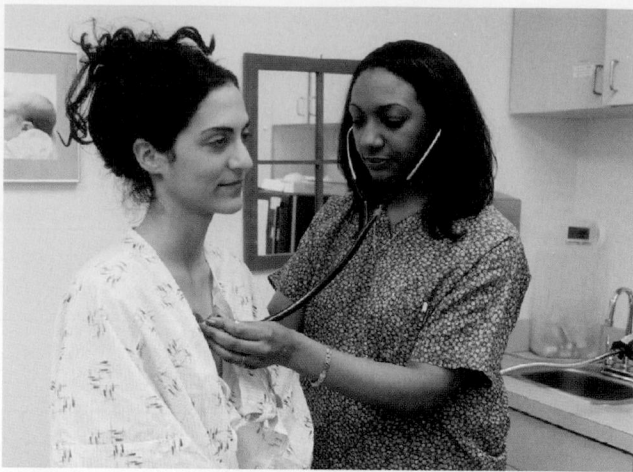

FIGURE 1-3. Growing numbers of women's health centers staffed with certified nurse practitioners and nurse–midwives provide affordable health maintenance care.

increased use of such nurses in the future (American Nurses Association, 2007).

● Developing Critical Thinking Skills

1. Consider the roles and functions of professional nursing (see Table 1-2). Interview several nurses in different settings to see how much value they attach to these roles and how much time they are able to devote to them.

2. Describe how a nurse would meet the aims of nursing as described in this chapter (promoting health, preventing illness, restoring health, and facilitating coping) when caring for the following patients:
   • A single mother who has just delivered her first child and is scheduled to be discharged 12 hours after delivery
   • An 82-year-old woman who wants to begin an exercise program
   • A 32-year-old man dying of AIDS at home

As you consider these situations, try to identify factors that either promote or inhibit the fulfilling of these aims.

● Practicing for NCLEX

1. Which phrase best describes the science of nursing?
   a. The skilled application of knowledge
   b. The knowledge base for care
   c. Hands-on care, such as giving a bath
   d. Respect for each individual patient

2. Which nurse in history is credited with establishing nursing education?
   a. Clara Barton
   b. Lillian Wald
   c. Lavinia Dock
   d. Florence Nightingale

3. What historic event in the 20th century led to an increased emphasis on nursing and broadened the role of nurses?
   a. Religious reform
   b. Crimean War
   c. World War II
   d. Vietnam War

4. Which of the following phrases describes one of the purposes of the ANA's Nursing's Social Policy Statement?
   a. To describe the nurse as a dependent caregiver
   b. To provide standards for nursing educational programs
   c. To regulate nursing research
   d. To describe nursing's values and social responsibility

5. A school nurse is teaching a class of junior-high students about the effects of smoking. This educational program will meet which of the aims of nursing?
   a. Promoting health
   b. Preventing illness
   c. Restoring health
   d. Facilitating coping with disability or death

6. Which of the following nursing degrees prepares a nurse for advanced practice as a clinical specialist or nurse practitioner?
   a. LPN
   b. ADN
   c. BSN
   d. Master's

7. Which nursing organization was the first international organization of professional women?
   a. ICN
   b. ANA
   c. NLN
   d. NSNA

8. What is the purpose of the ANA's Scope and Standards of Practice?
   a. To describe the ethical responsibility of nurses
   b. To define the activities that are special and unique to nursing
   c. To establish nursing as an independent and free-standing profession
   d. To regulate the practice of nursing

9. What type of authority regulates the practice of nursing?
   a. International standards and codes
   b. Federal guidelines and regulations
   c. State nurse practice acts
   d. Institutional policies

10. Who are the largest group of healthcare providers in the United States?
    a. Registered nurses
    b. Physicians
    c. Physical therapists
    d. Social workers

● Answers With Rationale

1. **b.** The science of nursing is the knowledge base for care that is provided. In contrast, the skilled application of that knowledge is the art of nursing.

2. **d.** Florence Nightingale established nursing education.

3. **c.** During World War II, large numbers of women worked outside the home. There was an increased emphasis on education and a knowledge explosion in medicine and technology, broadening the roles of nurses.

4. **d.** The Nursing's Social Policy Statement describes the values and social responsibility of nursing.

5. **b.** Educational programs can reduce the risk of illness by teaching good health habits.

6. **d.** A master's degree prepares advanced practice nurses.

7. **a.** The ICN, founded in 1899, was the first international organization of professional women.

8. **b.** The ANA's Scope and Standards of Practice define the activities of nurses that are specific and unique to nursing.

9. **c.** Nurse practice acts are established in each state to regulate the practice of nursing.

10. **a.** Registered nurses are the largest group of healthcare providers in the United States.

Taylor Suite Resources

The Taylor Suite offers these additional resources to enhance learning and facilitate understanding of this chapter:

- thePoint online resource, http://thepoint.lww.com/Taylor7E
- Student DVD included with the book
- Study Guide for Taylor's Fundamentals of Nursing

BIBLIOGRAPHY

American Nurses Association (ANA). (2003). *Nursing: Scope and standards of practice: Professional development.* Washington, DC: Author.

American Nurses Association (ANA). (2005). *Core issues.* Washington, DC: Author.

American Nurses Association (ANA). (2009). *Considering nursing?* Available http://www.nursingworld.org/EspeciallyForYou/StudentNurses.aspx

Blais, K., Hayes, J., & Kozier, B. (2005). *Professional nursing practice: Concepts and perspectives* (5th ed.). Upper Saddle River, NJ: Pearson Prentice Hall.

Buerhaus, P. (2007). Dealing with reality: Confronting the global nursing shortage. *Reflections on Nursing Leadership, Fourth Quarter,* 6 p.

D'Antonio, P. (2004). Women, nursing, and baccalaureate education in 20th century America. *Journal of Nursing Scholarship, 36*(4), 379–384.

D'Antonio, P. (2006). History for a practice profession. *Nursing Inquiry, 13*(4), 242–248.

Dolan, J. A., Fitzpatrick, M. L., & Herrmann, E. K. (1983). *Nursing in society: A historical perspective.* Philadelphia: W. B. Saunders.

Donley, R., Sr. (2005). Challenges for nursing in the 21st century. *Nursing Economics, 23*(6), 312–318.

Ellis, J., & Hartley, C. (2007). *Nursing in today's world: Challenges, issues, trends* (9th ed.). Philadelphia: Lippincott Williams & Wilkins.

Fairman, J. (2008). Context and contingency in the history of post World War II nursing scholarship in the United States. *Journal of Nursing Scholarship, 40*(1), 4–11.

International Council of Nurses. (2002). *The ICN definition of nursing.* Geneva: Imprimeries Populaires.

Kalisch, P. A., & Kalisch, B. J. (2004). *American nursing: A history.* Philadelphia: Lippincott Williams & Wilkins.

Lauridsen, B. (2005). Stepping stones on which today's nursing was built. *Nursing BC, 37*(2), 5.

National Council of State Boards of Nursing. (2008). Nurse licensure compact administration, Participating states in the NLC. Available at https://www.ncsbn.org/158.htm

Nightingale, F. (1992). *Notes on nursing: What it is and what it is not.* (Commemorative ed.). Philadelphia: J. B. Lippincott.

Pender, N. J., Murdaugh, C., & Parsons, M. A. (2006). *Health promotion in nursing practice* (5th ed.). Upper Saddle River, NJ: Prentice Hall.

Price-Spratlen, L., & Mahoney, M. (2006). February, Black History Month: A time to review nursing's past, present, and future. *Washington Nurse, 36*(1), 12–13.

Robert Wood Johnson Foundation. (2009). *The chronic care model.* Available at http://www.improvingchroniccare.org/index.php?p=The_Chronic_Care_Model&s=2.

Smeltzer, C. H., Vlasses, F. R., & Robinson, C. R. (2005). A look back . . . "If we only had a nurse" . . . historical view of a nurse shortage. *Journal of Nursing Care Quality, 20*(2), 190–192.

Stanley, D. (2007). Lights in the shadows: Florence Nightingale and others who made their mark. *Contemporary Nurse, 24*(1), 45–51.

U.S. Department of Health and Human Services, Office of Disease Prevention and Health Promotion. (2000). *Healthy people 2010.* Washington, DC: U.S. Department of Health and Human Services.

U.S. Department of Labor. Bureau of Labor Statistics. (2008). Occupational Outlook Handbook, 2008–2009 Edition. Registered Nurses. Available at http://www.bls.gov/oco/ocos083.htm

Wall, B. M. (2008). Celebrating nursing history. *American Journal of Nursing, 108*(6), 26–29.

West, R. A., Griffith, G. P., & Iphofen, R. (2007). A historical perspective on the nursing shortage. *MEDSURG Nursing, 16*(2), 124–130.

Cultural Diversity 2

DANIELLE DORVALL

Danielle is an immigrant from Haiti who has been in the United States for approximately 8 months. She recently had surgical repair of a fractured femur and is now confined to bed in skeletal traction. She asks that a Haitian folk healer from her neighborhood be allowed to come to the hospital to help heal her broken leg.

KHALIFA ABDUL HAKIM

Khalifa, the husband of a Muslim patient, requests that only female healthcare practitioners care for his wife. In the Muslim culture, it is deemed immodest for the body of a married woman to be seen by any male other than her husband.

JANICE GOLDBERG

Janice, a 23-year-old woman of Jewish ancestry, comes to the women's health clinic for a routine examination. During the visit, she asks, "I've been dating this man who also is Jewish, and we're thinking about getting married and having children. But I've heard about a hereditary disorder called Tay-Sachs disease that occurs in Jews. Should I be concerned?"

LEARNING OBJECTIVES

After completing the chapter, you will be able to accomplish the following:

1. Explain concepts of cultural diversity.
2. Describe influences that affect culturally competent healthcare.
3. Discuss examples of diversity in health and illness care, including culturally based traditional care.
4. Practice cultural competence when assessing and providing nursing care for patients from diverse cultural groups.
5. Discuss factors in the healthcare system and in nursing that facilitate or impede culturally competent nursing care.

KEY TERMS

cultural assimilation
cultural blindness
cultural diversity
cultural imposition
culture
culture conflict
culture shock
ethnicity
ethnocentrism
personal space
race
stereotyping
subculture

Our society is made up of people from many diverse backgrounds. The definition of **cultural diversity** includes, but is not limited to, people of varying cultures, racial and ethnic origin, religion, language, physical size, gender, sexual orientation, age, disability, socioeconomic status, occupational status, and geographic location. The essential knowledge and skills of understanding cultural diversity and providing culturally competent care have become essential components of nursing practice. (For an example, see the accompanying Reflective Practice display). This chapter focuses on the concepts of cultural diversity and discusses their influence on nursing care.

CONCEPTS OF CULTURAL DIVERSITY

Cultural diversity, including culture, ethnicity, and race, is an integral component of both health and illness because of the cultural values and beliefs we learn in our families and communities, as well as the need to know physiological characteristics common to certain populations that influence health. To be able to provide culturally competent care to people from diverse backgrounds, nurses must be sensitive to these factors. It is also vital to remember that each indi-

vidual may be a member of multiple cultural, ethnic, and racial groups at one time. Therefore, different cultural values may guide an individual in different situations based on what is most important to them at the time.

Culture

Culture may be defined as a shared system of beliefs, values, and behavioral expectations that provides social structure for daily living. Culture defines roles and interactions with others as well as within families and communities, and is apparent in the attitudes and institutions unique to particular groups (Andrews & Boyle, 2008). The characteristics of culture include the following:

- Culture guides what is acceptable behavior for people in a specific group. It is shared by, and provides an identity for, all members of the same cultural group.
- Culture is learned by each new generation through both formal and informal life experiences. Language is the primary means of transmitting culture.
- The practices of a particular culture often arise because of the group's social and physical environment.
- Cultural practices and beliefs may evolve over time, but they mainly remain constant as long as they satisfy a group's needs.
- Culture influences the way people of a group view themselves, have expectations, and behave in response to certain situations. Because a culture is made up of individuals, there are differences both within cultures and among cultures.

> Recall Mr. Hakim, the Muslim man described in the Reflective Practice display. The nurse's knowledge of his culture and beliefs would be important in ensuring culturally appropriate care as well as staffing needs. The nurse would need to understand actions and behaviors that would be acceptable to Mr. Hakim and his wife. ■

Within most cultures are **subcultures.** A subculture is a large group of people who are members of an even larger cultural group, but who have certain ethnic, occupational, or physical characteristics that are not common to the larger culture. For example, nursing is a subculture of the larger healthcare system culture, and teenagers and older adults are often regarded as subcultures of the general population in the United States.

Societies include both dominant culture groups and minority culture groups. A dominant group is the group that has the most ability to control the values and sanctions of the society. It usually is (but does not have to be) the largest group in a society. Minority groups usually have some physical or cultural characteristic (such as race, religious beliefs, or occupation) that identifies the people within it as different from the dominant group.

When a minority group lives within a dominant group, many of their members may lose the cultural characteristics that once made them different, and their values may be

REFLECTIVE PRACTICE

Challenge to Intellectual Skills

I had thought that I'd pretty much gotten used to all sorts of questions from patients about why a guy like me would go into nursing. Today, however, I was surprised when Khalifa Abdul Hakim, the husband of a newly admitted patient, demanded that I leave his wife's room immediately. Stepping into the corridor with me, he explained that he and his family were Muslim and that in their culture it was deemed immodest for the body of a married woman to be seen by any male other than her husband. He asked me to make sure that his wife's chart made it clear that there were to be no male nurses. He also asked about female physicians. Since we were short-staffed and all trying to cover for one another to get through the day, I wasn't sure that I could make that promise, especially since our unit has three or four male nurses. I wasn't clear if this was just a personal preference, a religious or cultural matter or both, or if this mattered at all. I have to admit that I had absolutely no clue as to how to respond. I remembered classes about the importance of culturally appropriate care, but didn't remember ever learning about how to respond to requests such as this one. I also wasn't sure if the hospital had a policy about these types of requests.

Thinking Outside the Box: Possible Courses of Action

- Find someone to swap patients with me and forget about having to deal with the situation (probably the simplest response).
- Use the opportunity to research the Muslim culture and talk with the patient's male family members about what is important to them. Since our Muslim patient population seems to be growing, suggest an in-service program on this topic for everyone.

- Explain to Mr. Hakim that his wife is in a U.S. hospital, and that while here, they should observe U.S. customs, meaning she may have male nurses or other male healthcare practitioners.
- Check the hospital's policy on these sorts of requests and then follow it.

Evaluating a Good Outcome: How Do I Define Success?

- I need to know enough to do whatever is necessary to ensure the patient's health and well-being as well as respect the integrity of all participants involved within the scope of my responsibilities.

- The patient and her family feel sufficiently comfortable in our environment (culturally appropriate care) for healing to be maximized.
- I know more at the end of the experience than I when I started.

Personal Learning: Here's to the Future!

I was pretty surprised when two of the older, more experienced nurses said they had never encountered such a request, and that they didn't know if the hospital had a policy on these sorts of matters. Luckily, one of them referred me to our patient-relations person, and she came right up to the unit. I had never met her before, but I was impressed with her knowledge and her strong commitment to patient advocacy. She showed me the hospital policy that obligates all workers to respect the beliefs and values of patients unless this entails compro-

mising their own integrity or the safety of other persons. She said that we will be seeing more Muslim patients because of a new influx into our community and recommended a Web site to get more information. I have to admit that I haven't checked it out yet, but I did talk some with the patient's family and have a better understanding of why these things matter to them. I'm thinking of trying to cultivate the attitude that each patient and family could be an important learning opportunity for me if I'm open to what they have to teach!

Reflection

How do you think you would respond in a similar situation? Why? What does this tell you about yourself and about the adequacy of your skills for professional practice? Can you think of other ways to respond? What type of information would you need to respond in a different manner? Imagine if the nurse had been female. Would this situation have arisen? Explain why or why not. What other skills (cognitive, interpersonal, technical, ethical/legal) would you need to respond well in this situation? Do you agree with the criteria to evaluate a successful outcome? Did the nursing student meet the criteria?

replaced by the values of the dominant culture. This process is called **cultural assimilation** or acculturation. For example, when people immigrate and encounter a new dominant culture, as they go to work, go to school, and learn the dominant language, they often move closer to the dominant culture. The process and the rate of assimilation are individualized.

Mutual cultural assimilation also does occur, with some characteristics of both groups being traded. For example,

many Hispanic immigrants to the United States learn to speak English, and many Americans learn to cook and enjoy traditional Hispanic foods. In this way, we gain from the many cultures with which we live. Although we seldom think about it, the clothes we wear, the foods we eat, the music we enjoy, many of the words we use, and the leisure activities we practice are all characteristics in which we have become acculturated.

Another possibility is **culture shock,** or the feelings a person experiences when placed in a different culture perceived as strange. Culture shock may result in psychological discomfort or disturbances, as the patterns of behavior a person found acceptable and effective in his or her own culture may not be adequate or even acceptable in the new one. The person may then feel foolish, fearful, incompetent, inadequate, or humiliated. These feelings eventually can lead to frustration, anxiety, and loss of self-esteem.

Ethnicity

Ethnicity is a sense of identification with a collective cultural group, largely based on the group's common heritage. One belongs to a specific ethnic group or groups either through birth or through adoption of characteristics of that group. People within an ethnic group generally share unique cultural and social beliefs and behavior patterns, including language and dialect, religious practices, literature, folklore, music, political interests, food preferences, and employment patterns. Ethnicity largely develops through day-to-day life with family and friends within the community.

Race

Although the term ethnicity often is used interchangeably with **race,** these terms are not the same. Racial categories are typically based on specific physical characteristics such as skin pigmentation, body stature, facial features, and hair texture. Because of the significant blending of physical characteristics through the centuries, however, race is becoming harder to define using the simple classifications once used, and physical characteristics are not considered a reliable way to determine an individual's race. Federal standards for race classification provide five categories including American Indian or Alaska Native, Asian, Black or African American, Native Hawaiian or Other Pacific Islander, and White,

and provide the opportunity for an individual to identify themselves in multiple categories.

Factors Inhibiting Sensitivity to Diversity

A variety of factors may affect sensitivity to others. When one assumes that all members of a culture, ethnic group, or race act alike, **stereotyping** is at work. Stereotyping may be positive or negative. Negative stereotyping includes racism, ageism, and sexism. These are beliefs that certain races, an age group, or one gender is inherently superior to others, leading to discrimination against those considered inferior (Fig. 2-1).

Also affecting cultural sensitivity are **cultural imposition,** which is the belief that everyone should conform to your own belief system, and **cultural blindness,** which occurs when one ignores differences and proceeds as though they do not exist. This has been true of the healthcare system, especially in regard to what are considered nontraditional methods of care. **Culture conflict** occurs when people become aware of cultural differences, feel threatened, and respond by ridiculing the beliefs and traditions of others to make themselves feel more secure about their own values (Andrews & Boyle, 2008).

CULTURAL INFLUENCES ON HEALTHCARE

The United States is multicultural, multiethnic, and multiracial. Therefore, nurses must be aware of, and sensitive to, the needs of a culturally diverse patient population. In most situations, a person interprets the behaviors of another person in terms of her or his own familiar culture. This process usually is multidirectional; for example, in a healthcare setting, the patient evaluates the attitudes and actions of the healthcare provider at the same time the healthcare provider interprets the behavior of the patient. Remember that what may seem reasonable and important to a patient may seem ridiculous and irrelevant to a nurse. The reverse is also true; practices a nurse

FIGURE 2-1. Identifying one's own prejudices is the first step toward eliminating them. Think about the assumptions you make about the people in these images. (Left to right, First photo © Christopher Briscoe, Science Source/Photo Researchers; Third photo © Renee Lynn, Science Source/Photo Researchers; Fourth photo © Ken Cavanagh, Science Source/Photo Researcher)

perceives as logical and effective may seem senseless or even dangerous to a patient.

> *Consider Danielle Dorvall, described at the beginning of the chapter. She might view skeletal traction as worthless, while the nurse may view her request for a folk healer in the same way. The nurse needs to be aware of these possible attitudes and beliefs to ensure maximum effective care while still meeting the patient's cultural needs.* ■

The following sections present an overview of general considerations in providing culturally competent care.

Physiologic Variations

Various studies have shown that certain racial and ethnic groups are more prone to developing specific diseases and conditions. For example, a hereditary disorder, Tay-Sachs disease, is associated with individuals of Eastern European Jewish descent. Although the incidence of this disorder has declined over the years due to improved and earlier testing, it is still a concern. Use knowledge of these individualized risk factors when interviewing a patient to complete a health history. Table 2-1 provides examples of diseases that are more often diagnosed in specific populations.

TABLE • 2-1	EXAMPLES OF COMMON HEALTH PROBLEMS IN SPECIFIC POPULATIONS
Population	**Common Health Problems**
American Indians and Alaska Natives	Heart disease Cirrhosis of the liver Diabetes mellitus Fetal alcohol syndrome
African Americans	Hypertension Stroke Sickle cell anemia Lactose intolerance Keloids
Asian/Pacific Islanders	Hypertension Cancer of the liver Lactose intolerance Thalassemia
Hispanics	Diabetes mellitus Lactose intolerance
Whites	Breast cancer Heart disease Hypertension Diabetes mellitus Obesity

> *Recall Janice Goldberg, the young woman described at the beginning of the chapter? Knowledge of the Tay-Sachs disorder and screening and early detection methods would be important for the nurse to use as a foundation when counseling and teaching Janice.* ■

Reactions to Pain

Healthcare researchers have discovered that many of the expressions and behaviors exhibited by people in pain are culturally prescribed. Some cultures allow and even encourage the open expression of emotions experienced by a person in pain, whereas other cultures frown on the open and free expression of emotions.

The main issue for nurses in this area of cultural expression is their attitude toward the "ideal patient." Nurses often assume that a patient who does not complain of pain is not having pain. Therefore, a patient who deals with pain quietly and stoically may have their pain-reduction needs ignored. To avoid this, be sensitive to other signals of discomfort, such as holding or applying pressure to the painful area, self-restriction of activities that intensify the pain, and uncontrollable, spontaneous expressions of discomfort, such as facial grimacing and moaning. You also should not consider patients who freely express their discomfort as constant complainers whose requests for pain relief seem excessive. Pain is a warning from the body that something is wrong. Pain is what the patient says it is, and every complaint of pain should be assessed carefully.

Nursing care for the patient in pain is always individualized (see Chapter 35), but important culture-sensitive considerations include the following:

- Recognize that culture is an important component of individuality and that each person holds (and has the right to hold) various beliefs about pain.
- Respect the patient's right to respond to pain in whatever manner is culturally and individually appropriate.
- Never stereotype a patient's perceptions or responses to pain based on the person's culture.

Mental Health

Most mental health norms are based on research and observations made of white, middle-class people. Many ethnic groups have their own norms or acceptable patterns of behavior for psychological well-being and normal psychological reactions to certain situations. For example, many Hispanic people deal with problems within the family and would view it as inappropriate to tell problems to a stranger. Traditional Chinese people often consider mental illness a stigma; therefore, seeking psychiatric help would be a disgrace to the family. In times of high stress or anxiety, some Puerto Ricans may demonstrate a hyperkinetic seizure activity known as *ataques*. This behavior is a culturally accepted reaction. Be aware of these variations and accept them as culturally appropriate.

Gender Roles

In many cultures, the man is the dominant figure and generally makes decisions for all family members. For example, if approval for medical care is needed, the man gives it regardless of which family member is involved. In male-dominant cultures, women are usually passive. On the other hand, in many African American and Caucasian families, the woman is often dominant.

Knowing who is the dominant member of the family is important when planning nursing care. For example, if the dominant member is ill and can no longer make decisions, the whole family may be anxious and confused. If a non-dominant family member is ill, he or she may require help in verbalizing needs, particularly if they differ from those the dominant member perceives as being important.

> ➤ *Think back to Mr. Hakim, the Muslim man concerned about his wife's care providers being male. Because Mr. Hakim, and not his wife, was the person who made the request about no male care providers, the nurse would interpret this as indicating that Mr. Hakim is the dominant family member.* ■

Language (Linguistics) and Communication

When people from another part of the world move to the United States, they may speak their own language fluently but have difficulty speaking English. This is especially true for the women or older adults in the family if they do not work outside the home, or for people who live in proximity to others who speak their primary language. Assimilation is likewise slower for people who stay at home, especially if they live in communities of their ethnic and cultural background. Children usually assimilate more rapidly and learn the language of the dominant culture quickly because they leave home each day to go to school, making new friends in the dominant culture. Wage earners also tend to learn a new language more quickly through the work setting. Language acquisition is thus tied to necessity and assimilation rather than to degree of difficulty.

Because the United States has such a diverse population, with many languages spoken, communication problems can arise during healthcare activities. This problem is not unique to non–English-speaking patients; even in different regions of the country, certain dialects or word meanings can cause differences in understanding. Consider how difficult it must be to describe symptoms or give a personal health history when you do not understand the questions being asked. In addition, patients may forget English words or revert to their more familiar language when experiencing the stress of an injury, illness, or pain.

Nurses who work in a geographic area with a high population of residents who speak a language other than English should learn pertinent words and phrases in that language. See the accompanying Through the Eyes of a Student account. Many agencies also have a qualified interpreter, or one can be found in the community. To avoid misinterpretation of

Through the Eyes of a Student

I was doing my maternity rotation and was assigned to labor and delivery. I was assigned a woman who spoke no English—she and her husband were from Central America and had been in the United States for only 2 months.

When I arrived at 7 am, the night nurse was giving a report about my patient to the day nurse. The night nurse was frantic—no one understood the couple, all efforts to locate a translator had come up empty, and, quite frankly, she had no idea exactly what condition this woman was in.

I quickly began to think back on my 2 years of Spanish. Could I be of any help to this couple? I wondered. Would I remember enough to communicate with them about giving birth? Then I decided that any little bit of communication at this point was better than none, so I spoke up. I told both nurses that I spoke some Spanish and asked if I could be of any help. The night nurse literally hugged me!

I began by telling the expectant couple that I was a nursing student and that I spoke some Spanish. We exchanged introductions and then I asked the woman some assessment questions. Nothing I said was complicated—all of my sentences were short and simple, but who needed more than that?

Then the couple asked me some questions. They had heard about "cutting open the stomach" to deliver a baby. I naturally assumed that they meant a cesarean delivery. They looked so afraid but I had to be honest. They wanted to know how it was done and why. The words I could not remember or did not know I acted out. They looked so relieved when I was finished.

The man said that they thought all babies were born this way in our country. He said that they had never heard of this procedure until coming to the United States. No wonder they were so frightened!

The doctor came in, examined the woman, and said she was fully dilated. The doctor asked if I could teach a crash course in Lamaze breathing to the woman. She also asked me if I would stay throughout the delivery because she would need assistance in translating directions to the woman. Of course, I said yes.

The woman was terrified. I told her that it was normal to be afraid and that I would be with her during the delivery. She took my hand and whispered, "Muchas gracias." I never felt more useful than I did at that moment.

—*A. Kelly Gaylor*
Holy Family College, Philadelphia

questions and answers, it is important to use an interpreter who understands the healthcare system. Sometimes a family member or friend can translate for the nurse, but such a person may be protective and not the most reliable means of transferring information. Nurses may find themselves talking in a louder tone of voice to a patient who does not understand what they are saying; remember that this is a communication problem, not a hearing problem.

One of the most culturally variable forms of nonverbal communication is eye contact. Although the following examples are not true of all members of a group, they are given to provide general guidelines for consideration. The American dominant culture emphasizes eye contact while speaking, but other cultures regard this behavior in different ways. For example, direct eye contact may be considered impolite or aggressive by Asians, Native Americans, Indochinese, Arabs, and Appalachians; these groups of people tend to avert their eyes while speaking with another. Hispanics may look downward in deference to age, gender, social position, economic status, and authority. Muslim–Arab women indicate modesty by avoiding eye contact with men, and Hasidic Jewish men tend to avoid direct eye contact with women (Andrews & Boyle, 2008).

When caring for culturally and ethnically diverse patients, it is it important to perform a transcultural assessment of communication (adapted from Andrews & Boyle, 2008):

• What language does the patient speak during usual activities of daily living?
• How well does the patient speak and write in English?
• Does the patient need an interpreter? Are family members or friends available? Are there people the patient would not want to serve as an interpreter?
• How does the patient prefer to be addressed?
• What cultural values and beliefs of the patient may change your techniques of communication and care (such as eye contact, space, or social taboos)?
• How does the patient's nonverbal behavior affect the responses of members of the healthcare team?
• What are the cultural characteristics of the patient's communications with others?

Chapter 21 provides additional information on communicating with non–English-speaking patients.

Orientation to Space and Time

Personal space is the area around a person regarded as part of the person. This area, individualized to each person and to different cultures and ethnic groups, is the area into which others should not intrude during personal interactions. If others do not consider a person's personal space, that person may become uncomfortable or even angry. When providing nursing care that involves physical contact, you should know the patient's cultural personal space preferences. For example, people of Arabic and African origin commonly sit and stand close to one another when talking, whereas people of Asian and European descent are more comfortable with some distance between themselves and others.

Many people and almost all institutions in the United States value promptness and punctuality. When arriving for an appointment, doing a job, or carrying out an activity, being on time and getting the job done promptly are viewed as important. This is not true in some other cultures. For example, in some South Asian cultures, being late is considered a sign of respect. In addition, while some cultures are future-oriented (including activities that promote future good health), other cultures are more concerned with the present or the past. Understanding the patient's orientation to time is important as you communicate, for example, the need to be on time for appointments for healthcare procedures and when taking medications.

Food and Nutrition

Food preferences and how foods are prepared often are related culturally. Certain food groups serve as staples of the diet based on culture and remain so even when members of that culture are living in a different country.

Patients in a hospital or long-term care setting often do not have much choice of foods. This means that people with cultural food preferences may not be able to select appealing foods and thus may be at risk for inadequate nutrition. When assessing the cause of decreased appetite in patients, try to determine whether the problem may be related to culture. It may be possible for family or friends to bring in foods that satisfy the patient's nutritional needs while still meeting dietary restrictions. Dietary teaching must be individualized according to cultural values about the social significance and sharing of food. A culturally sensitive assessment of nutrition is provided in Box 2-1.

Box 2-1   CULTURALLY SENSITIVE NUTRITION ASSESSMENT

1. Which foods are considered edible and which are not?
   • In France, corn is considered an animal feed, whereas corn is a commonly eaten vegetable in the United States.
   • Religious beliefs prohibit some Jewish, Muslim, and Seventh-Day Adventist patients from eating pork.
   • Patients who follow a vegetarian diet do not eat pork, beef, or chicken.
2. What times and types of food are considered meals?
   • Anglo-Americans typically eat three meals a day, with foods such as bacon and eggs or cereal for breakfast, sandwiches and soup for lunch, and meat with potatoes and vegetables for dinner.
   • Vietnamese may eat soup for every meal.
   • Beans are a staple for meals among Mexican people.
   • People from Middle Eastern countries often eat cheese and olives for breakfast.
   • Native American and Latin American people usually eat two meals a day.
   • Rural southern African Americans may eat large amounts of food on weekends and less food at meals during the week.
   • Holy days or religious holidays influence food choices for almost all cultures.

Family Support

In many cultural and ethnic groups, people have large, extended families and consider the needs of any family member to be equal to or greater than their own. They may be unwilling to share private information about family members with those outside the family (including healthcare providers). Other cultural groups have great respect for the elders in the family and would never consider institutional care for them. Including the family in planning care for any patient is a major component in nursing care to meet individualized needs, especially if those needs can be met only through consideration of all members of the family.

Socioeconomic Factors

Low income is a major problem in the United States, and is often described as having created a culture of poverty. A report from the U.S. Census Bureau (2008) noted that an estimated 13% of the U.S. population had income below the poverty threshold. Of that population, the lowest income was found in African Americans, American Indians, and Alaska Natives. There has been much debate about how to define poverty. In terms of economics, a person or family whose income falls below the poverty line is considered poor. The U.S. Census Bureau defines poverty by using a set of money/income guidelines that vary by family size and composition. If the family's total income is less than that family's threshold, all members of the family are considered poor. Others have stated that poverty is a relative term that reflects a judgment on the basis of community standards. Such standards vary at different times and in different places; what is judged poverty in one community might be regarded as wealth in another (Spector, 2009). No matter how poverty is defined, it is an increasingly devastating epidemic, fueled by real estate foreclosures and credit debt that has evolved into a culture of its own. At highest risk are children, older people, families headed by single mothers, and future generations of those now living in poverty. The amount of money a person or family has affects how they meet their basic needs and maintain their health. Poverty leads to other problems such as lack of health insurance, care of infants and children, and homelessness. All these areas are of concern to nursing.

The feminization of poverty threatens to increase the number of people who are living at poverty level. The number of female-headed households is increasing as a result of divorce, abandonment, unmarried motherhood, and changes in abortion laws. Because it is now common in many households that two incomes are required for economic survival, a single woman supporting a household is at a financial disadvantage. The number of single-parent families headed by women is associated closely with the increasing number of children living in poverty and the number of homeless families with children.

The increasing population of older people has also raised problems associated with poverty. Many older people live on fixed incomes that often do not keep up with inflation, and many (particularly widows) are on the borderline of poverty or have already slipped below the poverty level. Socioeconomic status often differs by the cultural group of the older adult. For example, Pacific/Asian, African American, Native American, and Hispanic elders generally have lower incomes than do elders in the Anglo-American majority population. The work history of the cultural group, especially those who have worked all their lives as agricultural workers, often means an individual has no Social Security or Medicare benefits.

In some cases, the culture of poverty is passed from generation to generation. This appears to be especially true in such groups as migrant farm workers, families living on welfare, and people who live in isolated areas of Appalachia. Poverty cultures have the following characteristics:

- Feelings of despair, resignation, and fatalism
- Day-to-day attitude toward life, with no hope for the future
- Unemployment and need for financial or government aid
- Unstable family structure, possibly characterized by abusiveness and abandonment
- Decline in self-respect and retreat from community involvement

Poverty has long been a barrier to adequate healthcare. It prevents many people from consistently meeting their basic human needs. The lack of affordable or adequate housing is a problem experienced frequently by poor people. When low-income housing is available, it sometimes lacks such necessities as running water, heat, and electricity. To stretch their available money and to pool resources, many poor people live in crowded conditions, with several families living together in one household.

Research has demonstrated that crowded living conditions foster depersonalization, correlate with higher crime rates, and lead to psychological problems such as schizophrenia, alienation, and feelings of worthlessness (Spector, 2009). Such conditions also contribute to an increased incidence of disease and illness because of the proximity of people, the sharing of utensils and belongings, poor sanitation, and poor health habits. The health effects of such conditions include a higher incidence and severity of illness in poor people than in people of higher income groups.

Accessing healthcare facilities frequently requires transportation, which many times is neither affordable nor available to poor people. Their access to health insurance also is frequently limited, and they often must choose between purchasing food and purchasing healthcare. Those in upper-income groups tend to live longer and to experience less disability than those in lower-income groups. Other barriers to healthcare include isolation, language or communication difficulties, seasonal occupations, migration patterns, depersonalization, and institutional prejudice (Spector, 2009).

CULTURAL INFLUENCES ON HEALTH AND ILLNESS

People's values and beliefs about health, illness, and care for an illness develop as a direct result of cultural and ethnic influences. For example, in some groups, illnesses are classified as natural or unnatural. "Natural illnesses" are caused by dangerous agents, such as cold air or impurities in the air, water, or food. "Unnatural illnesses" are punishments for failing to follow God's rules, resulting in evil forces or witchcraft causing physical or mental health problems.

In some cultures, the power to heal is thought to be a gift from God bestowed on certain people. People in these cultures believe that these folk or traditional healers know what is wrong with them through divine intervention and experience. A patient used to traditional healers may think healthcare providers are incompetent because they have to ask many questions before they can treat an illness. Traditional healers speak the patient's language, often are more accessible, and are usually more understanding of the patient's cultural and personal needs.

> *Think back to Danielle Dorvall, the immigrant from Haiti asking for a folk healer. The use of a folk healer, as appropriate, demonstrates respect for and an understanding of the patient's cultural beliefs.* ∎

People from different cultures may also have different beliefs about the best way to treat an illness or disease. For example, herbs are a common method of treatment in many cultures. In fact, many medications used today have a basis in herbs or other plant sources that have been used for centuries to cure illnesses. If a patient traditionally drinks an herbal tea to alleviate symptoms of an illness, there is no reason both the herbal tea and prescribed medications cannot be used, as long as the tea is safe to drink and the ingredients do not interfere with or exaggerate the action of the medication.

Other types of traditional therapies include the use of cutaneous stimulation, Therapeutic Touch, acupuncture, and acupressure. Cutaneous stimulation by massage, vibration, heat, cold, or nerve stimulation reduces the intensity of the sensation of pain. Therapeutic Touch is an intentional act that involves an energy transfer from the healer to the patient to stimulate the patient's own healing potential. Acupuncture, long used in China, is a method of preventing, diagnosing, and treating pain and disease by inserting special needles into the body at specified locations. Acupressure involves a deep-pressure massage of appropriate points of the body.

CULTURALLY COMPETENT NURSING CARE

Providing culturally competent nursing care means that care is planned and implemented in a way that is sensitive to the needs of individuals, families, and groups from diverse populations within society. The nurse who recognizes and respects cultural diversity will be better equipped to exhibit cultural sensitivity and provide nursing care that accepts the significance of cultural factors in health and illness. See Examples of NANDA Nursing Diagnoses.

The healthcare system is itself a culture with customs, rules, values, and a language of its own, with nursing as its largest subculture. As you progress through your education, you will be acculturated into the culture of the healthcare system and will develop values related to health and healthcare. Box 2-2 lists some common cultural norms of the healthcare system.

Although nursing as a whole is actively recruiting more diverse members, many nurses are members of, and have the same value systems as, the dominant middle-class culture in the United States. When a nurse with a particular set of cultural values about health interacts with a patient who has his or her own set of cultural values about health, the following factors affect this interaction:

- The cultural background of each participant
- The expectations and beliefs of each about healthcare
- The cultural context of the encounter (e.g., hospital, clinic, home)
- The degree of agreement between the two persons' sets of beliefs and values (Andrews & Boyle, 2008)

Examples of NANDA Nursing Diagnoses
Cultural Diversity

The following nursing diagnoses are examples of those that might be appropriate for providing culturally competent care:

- Impaired Verbal Communication related to inability to speak English and interpreter unavailable
- Social Isolation related to recent move away from neighborhood and friends of same ethnic group
- Impaired Parenting related to use of culturally based discipline considered inappropriate or abusive by current country of residence
- Spiritual Distress related to inability to take part in significant culturally based rituals regularly

- Readiness for Enhanced Family Process related to request for information about child care
- Ineffective Management of Therapeutic Regimen (Individual) related to mistrust of traditional healthcare personnel
- Situational Low Self-Esteem related to language difficulties and inability to secure employment
- Powerlessness related to inability to make healthcare providers understand the importance of dietary and social values and beliefs

Box 2-2   CULTURAL NORMS OF THE HEALTHCARE SYSTEM

Beliefs
- Standardized definitions of health and illness
- Omnipotence of technology

Practices
- Maintenance of health and prevention of illness
- Annual physical examinations and diagnostic procedures

Habits
- Documentation
- Frequent use of jargon
- Use of a systematic approach and problem-solving methodology

Likes
- Promptness
- Neatness and organization
- Compliance

Dislikes
- Tardiness
- Disorderliness and disorganization

Customs
- Professional deference and adherence to the pecking order found in autocratic and bureaucratic systems
- Use of certain procedures attending birth and death

Box 2-3   ASSURING CULTURAL COMPETENCE IN HEALTHCARE

- Ensure that all patients/consumers receive from all staff members effective, understandable, and respectful care that is provided in a manner compatible with their cultural health beliefs and practices and preferred language.
- Implement strategies to recruit, retain, and promote at all levels of the organization a diverse staff and leadership that are representative of the demographic characteristics of the service area.
- Ensure that staff at all levels and across all disciplines receive ongoing education and training in culturally and linguistically appropriate service delivery.
- Offer and provide language assistance services, including bilingual staff and interpreter services, at no cost to each patient/consumer with limited English proficiency at all points of contact, in a timely manner during all hours of operation.
- Make available easily understood patient-related materials and post signs in the language of the commonly encountered groups and/or groups represented in the service area.
- Ensure that data on the individual patient's/consumer's race, ethnicity, and spoken and written language are collected in health records, integrated into the organization's management information systems, and periodically updated.
- Maintain a current demographic, cultural, and epidemiological profile of the community, as well as a needs assessment to accurately plan for and implement services that respond to the cultural and linguistic characteristics of the service area.

Data from The Office of Minority Health, Public Health Service, U.S. Department of Health and Human Services. (2001, December). *Assuring cultural competence in health care: Recommendations for national standards and an outcomes-focused research agenda. Federal Register, 65*(247), 80865–80879.

Nursing care can become complicated when the patient and the nurse have distinctly different cultural norms. Cultural imposition in healthcare is the tendency for health personnel to impose their beliefs, practices, and values on people of other cultures. Closely related to cultural imposition is **ethnocentrism,** the belief that one's own ideas, beliefs, and practices are the best, are superior, or are most preferred to those of others. When health professionals assume that they have the right to make choices and decisions for patients, patients may respond in the same way that minority cultures often respond to such an attitude by the dominant culture: by becoming passive, resistive, angry, or resistant to treatment.

Unless the nurse is willing to examine carefully and clarify his or her own attitudes and values and to be sensitive to others who are "different," the use of cultural concepts to provide care will be unsuccessful. The nurse's role is to understand the patient's needs and to adapt care to meet those needs. A careful merging of modern and traditional cultural beliefs is a necessary prerequisite for safe, considerate, and successful nursing care of all patients.

National standards issued by the Office of Minority Health (2001) were developed in response to the need to ensure that all people entering the healthcare system be provided equitable and effective treatment in a culturally and linguistically appropriate manner. Examples of these standards are provided in Box 2-3.

Cultural Assessment

When caring for patients who are from a different culture, it is important to first ask a patient how they want to be treated based on their values and beliefs. An effective way to identify specific factors that influence a patient's behavior is to perform a cultural assessment. The primary informant should be the patient, if possible. If the patient is not able to respond to the questions, a family member or a friend can be consulted. A useful tool for this is the Andrews and Boyle Transcultural Nursing Assessment Guide (2008), part of which is included in Box 2-4.

You can also anticipate a patient's cultural needs by obtaining this information through research before initiating contact with the patient. Remember, however, that information about any culture is general, and that it must be individualized for the specific patient once the actual interaction begins.

Guidelines for Nursing Care

Transcultural nursing care has been both developed as a specialty and established as a formal area of practice as the result of theory development by Dr. Madeleine M. Leininger, a nurse–anthropologist. Her Theory of Cultural Care Diversity and Universality (1991) provides the foundation for providing

Box 2-4 TRANSCULTURAL ASSESSMENT: HEALTH-RELATED BELIEFS AND PRACTICES

1. To what cause(s) does the patient attribute illness and disease (e.g., divine wrath, imbalance in hot/cold or yin/yang, punishment for moral transgressions, hex, soul loss, pathogenic organism)?
2. What are the patient's cultural beliefs about the ideal body size and shape? What is the patient's self-image compared to the ideal?
3. What name does the patient give to his or her health-related condition?
4. What does the patient believe promotes health (eating certain foods; wearing amulets to bring good luck; sleep; rest; good nutrition; reducing stress; exercise; prayer; rituals to ancestors, saints, or intermediate deities)?
5. What is the patient's religious affiliation (e.g., Judaism, Islam, Pentecostalism, West African voodooism, Seventh-Day Adventism, Catholicism, Mormonism)? How actively involved in the practice of this religion is the patient?
6. Does the patient rely on cultural healers (e.g., curandero, shaman, spiritualist, priest, minister, monk)? Who

determines when the patient is sick and when the patient is healthy? Who influences the choice/type of healer and treatment that should be sought?
7. In what types of cultural healing practices does the patient engage (use of herbal remedies, potions, massage; wearing of talismans, copper bracelets, or charms to discourage evil spirits; healing rituals, incantations, prayers)?
8. How are biomedical/scientific healthcare providers perceived? How does the patient and his or her family perceive nurses? What are the expectations of nurses and nursing care?
9. What comprises appropriate "sick role" behavior? Who determines what symptoms constitute disease/illness? Who decides when the patient is no longer sick? Who cares for the patient at home?
10. How does the patient's cultural group view mental disorders? Are there differences in acceptable behaviors for physical versus psychological illnesses?

Adapted from Andrews, M., & Boyle, J. (2008). *Transcultural concepts in nursing care* (5th ed.). Philadelphia: Lippincott Williams & Wilkins.

culturally competent care for patients of all ages, as well as to families, groups, and communities. A nurse who is culturally competent has the knowledge and skills to adapt nursing care to cultural similarities and differences (see the accompanying Research in Nursing box). Cultural competence

takes time. It involves developing awareness, acquiring knowledge, and practicing skills. Box 2-5 lists information about selected diverse cultures to illustrate similarities and differences. It is important to remember that these are only general guidelines and that each patient must be considered

(continued text on page 36)

RESEARCH IN NURSING
Bridging the Gap to Evidence-Based Practice

NURSING CARE OF ARAB MUSLIMS IN THE UNITED STATES

The Arab Muslim population is an increasing minority population in the United States. This population is at increased risk for several diseases and faces many barriers to accessing the American healthcare system. Some of those barriers, such as modesty, gender preference in healthcare providers, and misconceptions about the cause of illness, arise out of their cultural beliefs and practices. This review of the literature provides important information for nurses caring for this population.

Related Research

Yosef, A. R. O. (2008). Health beliefs, practice, and priorities for health care of Arab Muslims in the United States. *Journal of Transcultural Nursing, 19*(3), 284–291.

Cultural factors that arise from religious beliefs and practices have the potential to affect health. Islam is a way of life, providing guidance for carrying out daily activities and practicing a healthy lifestyle. Muslims believe that God created humans and gave them their bodies as gifts to be cared for through general hygiene, diet, and exercise. However, there are also Islam tenets that might hinder health promotion, including the reluctance of Muslim women to expose their bodies or reveal their health problems to male healthcare providers. In addition, the American healthcare system is more complex than those in Arab countries, and language barriers, cultural misconceptions, and

perceptions of disrespect toward Arabs are other examples of obstacles in seeking care. As a result, although the Arab Muslim population is at increased risk for heart disease, diabetes, and cancer, they may lack the knowledge or skills to prevent, detect, and treat these diseases.

Relevance to Nursing Practice

Nurses must incorporate knowledge of the health-related effects of the practice of Islam on Arab Muslims in health promotion activities. Selected examples include:

- The Islamic religion does not allow the use of healthcare professionals of the opposite gender unless it is impossible to locate one of the same gender.
- Some Muslims might not participate in health promotion activities because they believe God has preordained their life.
- Issues such as safe sex and family planning cannot be discussed with Arab teenagers because no sexual relations are accepted before marriage.
- Abortion is prohibited, unless the mother's life is threatened by the pregnancy.
- Giving intravenous fluids leads Muslims to break their fast.
- Organ transplantation is allowed only in the case of saving a patient's life.

For additional research, visit the Point.

Box 2-5   CULTURAL FACTORS THAT AFFECT NURSING CARE

White Middle Class

Family
- Nuclear family is highly valued.
- Elderly family members may live in a nursing home when they can no longer care for themselves.

Folk and Traditional Healthcare
- Self-diagnosis of illnesses
- Use of over-the-counter drugs (especially vitamins and analgesics)
- Dieting (especially fad diets)
- Extensive use of exercise and exercise facilities

Values and Beliefs
- Youth is valued over age
- Cleanliness
- Orderliness
- Attractiveness
- Individualism
- Achievement
- Punctuality

Nursing Considerations
- Careful assessment of client's use of over-the-counter medications (observe for signs and symptoms of toxic medication levels, especially fat-soluble vitamins)
- Nutritional assessments of dietary habits

African American

Family
- Close and supportive extended-family relationships
- Strong kinship ties with nonblood relatives from church or organizational and social groups
- Family unity, loyalty, and cooperation are important.
- Usually matriarchal

Folk and Traditional Healthcare
- Varies extensively and may include spiritualists, herb doctors, root doctors, conjurers, skilled elder family members, voodoo, faith healing

Values and Beliefs
- Present oriented
- Members of the African American clergy are highly respected in the black community.
- Frequently highly religious

Nursing Considerations
- Many African American families may still use various folk healing practices and home remedies for treating particular illnesses.
- Special care may be necessary for the hair and skin.
- Special consideration should be given to the sometimes extensive and frequently informal support networks of patients (i.e., religious and community group members who offer assistance in a time of need).

Asian
(Beliefs and practices vary, but most Asian cultures share some characteristics.)

Family
- Welfare of the family is valued above the person.
- Extended families are common.
- A person's lineage (ancestors) is respected.
- Sharing among family members is expected.

Folk and Traditional Healthcare
- Theoretical basis is in Taoism, which seeks a balance in all things.
- Good health is achieved through the proper balance of yin (feminine, negative, dark, cold) and yang (masculine, positive, light, warm).
- An imbalance in energy is caused by an improper diet or strong emotions.
- Diseases and foods are classified as hot or cold, and a proper balance between them will promote wellness (e.g., treat a cold disease with hot foods).
- Many Asian healthcare systems use herbs, diet, and the application of hot or cold therapy. Also, many Asians believe that there are points on the body that are located on the meridians or energy pathways. If the energy flow is out of balance, treatment of the pathways may be necessary to restore the energy equilibrium.
  Acumassage—Technique of manipulating points along the energy pathways
  Acupressure—Technique for compressing the energy pathway points
  Acupuncture—Technique by which fine needles are inserted into the body at energy pathway points

Values and Beliefs
- Strong sense of self-respect and self-control
- High respect for age
- Respect for authority
- Respect for hard work
- Praise of self or others is considered poor manners
- Strong emphasis on harmony and the avoidance of conflict

Nursing Considerations
- Some members of Asian cultures may be upset by the drawing of blood for laboratory tests. They consider blood to be the body's life force, and some do not believe that it can be regenerated.
- Some members believe that it is best to die with the body intact, so they may refuse surgery except in dire circumstances.
- Members of many Asian cultures seldom complain about what is bothering them. Therefore, the nurse must carefully assess the patient for pain or discomfort by observing for nonverbal signs of discomfort, such as facial grimacing or wincing and holding of the painful area.
- Some Asians consider it polite to give a person the responses the person is expecting. Therefore, misinformation may be transmitted to the questioner in an effort, on the client's part, to be respectful.
- Some members may move from physician to physician in an attempt to be cured of an illness, but to avoid insulting or embarrassing a physician, they will not inform him or her that they are going to another physician. This can result in confusion, inaccuracies, and overmedication.
- Some Asians may refuse to have diagnostic studies done because they believe that a skilled and competent physician can diagnose an illness solely through a physical examination.
- Some members may have a difficult time understanding the importance of taking a regimen of medications because many of their folk treatments involve the ingestion of one dose of herbal mixtures.
- Dietary counseling may be necessary if the patient is on a salt-restricted diet because many Asian foods have a high salt content related to the use of soy sauce.

Box 2-5 CULTURAL FACTORS THAT AFFECT NURSING CARE *(continued)*

Hispanic

Family
- Familial role is important.
- *Compadrazgo:* special bond between a child's parents and his or her grandparents
- Family is the primary unit of society.

Folk and Traditional Healthcare
- *Curanderas(os):* folk healers who base treatments on humoral pathology—basic functions of the body are controlled by four body fluids or "humors":
  Blood—hot and wet
  Yellow bile—hot and dry
  Black bile—cold and dry
  Phlegm—cold and wet
- The secret of good health is to balance hot and cold within the body; therefore, most foods, beverages, herbs, and medications are classified as hot (*caliente*) or cold (*fresco, frio*) (a cold disease will be cured with a hot treatment).

Values and Beliefs
- Respect is given according to age (older) and sex (male).
- Roman Catholic Church may be very influential.
- God gives health and allows illness for a reason; therefore, may perceive illness as a punishment from God. An illness of this type can be cured through atonement and forgiveness.

Nursing Considerations
- It may be difficult to convince an asymptomatic patient that he or she is ill.
- Special diet considerations are necessary if the patient believes in the hot/cold theory of treating illnesses.
- Diet counseling may be necessary at times, because many members have a normal diet that is high in starch.

Puerto Rican
(Since the Jones Act of 1917, all Puerto Ricans are American citizens.)

Family
- *Compadrazgo*—same as in Hispanic culture

Folk and Traditional Healthcare
- Similar to that of other Spanish-speaking cultures

Values and Beliefs
- Place a high value on safeguarding against group pressure to violate a person's integrity (may be difficult for Puerto Ricans to accept teamwork)
- Close-mouthed about personal and family affairs (psychotherapy may be difficult to achieve at times because of this belief)
- Proper consideration should be given to cultural rituals, such as shaking hands and standing up to greet and say goodbye to people.
- Time is a relative phenomenon; little attention is given to the exact time of day.
- *Ataques*—culturally acceptable reaction to situations of extreme stress, characterized by hyperkinetic seizure activity

Nursing Considerations
- It may be difficult to teach Puerto Rican patients to follow time-oriented actions (e.g., taking medications, keeping appointments).

Native American
(Each tribe's beliefs and practices vary to some degree.)

Family
- Families are large and extended.
- Grandparents are official and symbolic leaders and decision makers.
- A child's namesake may become the same as another parent to the child.

Folk and Traditional Healthcare
- Medicine men (*shaman*) are heavily used.
- Heavy use of herbs and psychological treatments, ceremonies, fasting, meditation, heat, and massages

Values and Beliefs
- Present oriented. Taught to live in the present and not to be concerned about the future. This time consciousness emphasizes finishing current business before doing something else.
- High respect for age
- Great value is placed on working together and sharing resources.
- Failure to achieve a personal goal frequently is believed to be the result of competition.
- High respect is given to a person who gives to others. The accumulation of money and goods often is frowned on.
- Some Native Americans practice the Peyotist religion, in which the consumption of peyote, an intoxicating drug derived from mescal cacti, is part of the service. Peyote is legal if used for this purpose. It is classified as a hallucinogenic drug.

Nursing Considerations
- The family is expected to be part of the nursing care plan.
- Note taking often is taboo. It is considered an insult to the speaker because the listener is not paying full attention to the conversation. Good memory skills often are required by the nurse.
- Indirect eye contact is acceptable and sometimes preferred.
- It often is considered rude or impolite to indicate that a conversation has not been heard.
- A low tone of voice often is considered respectful.
- A Native American patient may expect the caregiver to deduce the problem through instinct and not through asking many questions and history taking. If this is the case, it may help to use declarative sentences rather than direct questioning.

Hawaiian

Family
- Familial role is important.
- *Ohana*, or extended families, are jointly involved in childrearing.
- Hierarchy of family structure—each gender and age have specific duties
- Closely knit families in small, isolated communities

Folk and Traditional Healthcare
- *Kahuna La'au Lapa'nu* is the ancient Hawaiian medical practitioner.
- View patient's illness as part of the whole.
- Relationships among the physical, psychological, and spiritual
- Emphasis on preventive medicine
- Treatment uses more than 300 medicinal plants and minerals

(continued)

Box 2-5 CULTURAL FACTORS THAT AFFECT NURSING CARE *(continued)*

Values and Beliefs
- Aloha: a deep love, respect, and affection between people and the land
- Christian God replaced the myriad of Hawaiian gods.
- Lifestyle more revered than compliance with healthcare issues
- Present oriented, less initiative and drive rather than direction and achievement
- Death seen as part of life and not feared

Nursing Considerations
- Many Hawaiians may still use folk healing practices and home remedies.
- Special consideration given to the extensive family network during hospitalization
- Acceptance from healthcare practitioners of current health practices and lifestyle

Appalachian
Family
- Intense interpersonal relations
- Family is cohesive, and several generations often live close to each other.
- Elderly are respected as providers.
- Tend to live in rural, isolated areas

Folk and Traditional Healthcare
- "Granny" woman, or folk healer, provides care and may be consulted even if receiving traditional care.
- Various herbs, such as foxglove and yellow root, are used for common illnesses such as malaise, chest discomfort, heart problems, and upper respiratory infections.
- Elderly may have had only limited contact with healthcare providers and be skeptical of modern healthcare.

Values and Beliefs
- Independence and self-determination
- Isolation is accepted as a way of life.
- Person oriented
- May be fatalistic about losses and death
- Belief in a divine existence rather than attending a particular church

Nursing Considerations
- Treat each person with regard for personal dignity.
- Allow family members to remain with patient as support system.
- Acceptance from healthcare providers of current health practices and lifestyle
- Allow patients to make decisions about care.

a unique individual. What is true of one person may not be true of another, even if they are from the same cultural background.

When providing care to different people from different cultures, it is important to use past experiences as a guide, but never as the answer to all cultural solutions. Learn from your mistakes and do not repeat them. All nurses make mistakes at some time when caring for culturally different patients. Inadvertent mistakes are just that, but repeated mistakes are careless and disrespectful; they will adversely affect your interaction with patients and coworkers. The following sections provide additional guidelines that are useful in providing appropriate nursing care.

Develop Cultural Self-Awareness

Before you can provide culturally competent care to patients from diverse backgrounds, it is important to become aware of the role of cultural influences in your own life. Objectively examine your own beliefs, values, practices, and family experiences. As you become more sensitive to the importance of these factors, you will also become more sensitive to cultural influences in others' lives. Identify your biases. How do they affect your feelings about others? How could they affect your nursing care of others? Box 2-6 lists a cultural self-assessment that will help you gain the insight necessary to overcome ethnocentric tendencies and stereotypic behaviors.

Develop Cultural Knowledge

Learn as much as possible about the belief system and practices of people in your community and of patients in the area

in which you work. Practice techniques of observation and listening to acquire knowledge of the beliefs and values of patients for whom you are caring. Some people, especially those of minority cultures, may have been belittled and subjected to ridicule and may be hesitant to discuss their beliefs and practices. Approach this topic with patients carefully. If you are motivated by sincerity, respect, and concern, your attitude will convey this, and most patients will respond positively. On the other hand, if you are motivated by curiosity and have a condescending attitude, most patients will respond negatively.

Accommodate Cultural Practices in Healthcare

Incorporate factors from the patient's cultural background into healthcare whenever possible and when the practices are not considered harmful to health. To ignore or contradict the patient's background may result in the patient refusing care or failing to follow prescribed therapy. Modify care to include traditional practices and practitioners as much as possible, and be an advocate for patients from diverse cultural groups.

Accommodate the cultural dietary practices of patients as much as possible. Dietary departments in many hospitals and long-term care facilities can supply patients with meals that are consistent with special dietary practices. Families may be encouraged to bring food from home for patients with particular preferences when this practice does not violate policy. Teaching patients and families about therapeutic diets can also be done within the framework of particular cultural practices.

Box 2-6   HOW DO YOU RELATE TO VARIOUS GROUPS OF PEOPLE IN SOCIETY?

Described below are different levels of response you might have toward a person.

Levels of Response
1. Greet: I can greet this person warmly and welcome him or her sincerely.
2. Accept: I can honestly accept this person as he or she is and be comfortable enough to listen to his or her problems.
3. Help: I can genuinely try to help this person with his or her problems.
4. Background: I have the background of knowledge and/or experience to be able to help this person.

5. Advocate: I can honestly be an advocate for this person.

Instructions
The following is a list of individuals. Read down the list and place a checkmark next to anyone you could not greet, accept, help, use your background, or advocate for. Try to respond honestly, not as you think would be socially or professionally desirable. Your answers are only for your personal use in clarifying your initial reactions to different people.

Individual	Level of Response				
	1	**2**	**3**	**4**	**5**
	Greet	*Accept*	*Help*	*Background*	*Advocate*
1. Haitian	☐	☐	☐	☐	☐
2. Child abuser	☐	☐	☐	☐	☐
3. Jewish person	☐	☐	☐	☐	☐
4. Person with hemophilia	☐	☐	☐	☐	☐
5. Neo-Nazi	☐	☐	☐	☐	☐
6. Mexican American	☐	☐	☐	☐	☐
7. IV drug user	☐	☐	☐	☐	☐
8. Senile, elderly person	☐	☐	☐	☐	☐
9. Prostitute	☐	☐	☐	☐	☐
10. Jehovah's Witness	☐	☐	☐	☐	☐
11. Gay/lesbian	☐	☐	☐	☐	☐
12. Person with AIDS	☐	☐	☐	☐	☐
13. Black American	☐	☐	☐	☐	☐
14. Amputee	☐	☐	☐	☐	☐
15. Klu Klux Klansman	☐	☐	☐	☐	☐
16. Alcoholic	☐	☐	☐	☐	☐
17. Person with cancer	☐	☐	☐	☐	☐
18. Hispanic	☐	☐	☐	☐	☐
19. Amish person	☐	☐	☐	☐	☐
20. Atheist	☐	☐	☐	☐	☐

Adapted from the Association for the Care of Children's Health, 7910 Woodmont Avenue, Suite 300, Bethesda, MD 20814, from Randall-David, E. L. (1989). *Strategies for working with culturally diverse communities and clients*, pp. 7–9.

Respect Culturally Based Family Roles

Take into consideration the cultural role of the family member who makes most of the important decisions. In some cultures, it is the husband or father, whereas in others, it is the grandmother or another respected elder. To disregard this fact or to proceed with nursing care that is not approved by this person can result in conflict or in disregard for what has been taught. Be careful to involve this person in the nursing care planning.

Avoid Mandating Change

Keep in mind that health practices are part of the overall culture and that changing them may have widespread implica-

tions for the person. You need to provide the necessary support and reinforcement for the patient if a change in a health practice with a cultural basis is considered necessary.

Do not force the patient to participate in care that conflicts with his or her values. If the patient is forced to accept it, the care may become harmful because resulting feelings of guilt and alienation from a religious or cultural group are likely to threaten the patient's well-being.

Seek Cultural Assistance

Seek assistance of a respected family member, member of the clergy, or traditional healer, as indicated, so that the patient is more likely to accept healthcare services. Acknowledging the role of the person's traditional healer can be an important way of building trust. If invited, folk medicine practitioners can work closely with professional health practitioners in the interest of the patient and family. Such efforts promote mutual understanding, respect, and cooperation.

● Developing Critical Thinking Skills

1. Analyze the following situations, identifying potential sources of cultural imposition:
   • A young Ethiopian woman with terminal breast cancer requests that all treatment decisions be made by her uncle, who is the family elder. Her primary nurse is an active feminist.
   • A Native American woman refuses a life-saving amputation of her leg because she believes it is essential to enter the next world "whole."

2. Interview family members or friends who have recently received healthcare, such as for a health screening, diagnostic testing, emergency care, routine checkup, office/clinic visit, or hospitalization. What aspects of the healthcare culture were most distressing to them? What factors were most helpful? Do their answers vary according to the setting for care? If so, why do you think they felt as they did?

● Practicing for NCLEX

1. Which of the following phrases best defines culture?
   a. A dominant group within a society
   b. A shared system of beliefs, values, and behaviors
   c. One's values are replaced by the values of the dominant culture
   d. Categories are based on specific physical characteristics

2. Minority groups living within a dominant culture may lose the cultural characteristics that made them different. What is this process called?
   a. Cultural diversity
   b. Cultural imposition
   c. Cultural assimilation
   d. Ethnocentrism

3. Which of the following terms is defined as the sense of identification with a collective cultural group?
   a. Ethnicity
   b. Race
   c. Cultural acquisition
   d. Culture shock

4. A nurse states, "That woman is 78 years old—too old to learn how to change a dressing." What is the nurse demonstrating?
   a. Cultural imposition
   b. Clustering
   c. Cultural competency
   d. Stereotyping

5. A young Hispanic mother comes to the local clinic because her baby is sick. She speaks only Spanish and the nurse speaks only English. What should the nurse do?
   a. Use short words and talk more loudly
   b. Ask an interpreter for help
   c. Explain why care can't be provided
   d. Provide instructions in writing

6. A nurse is interviewing a newly admitted patient. Which question would be considered culturally sensitive?
   a. "Do you think you will be able to eat the food we have here?"
   b. "Do you understand that we can't prepare special meals?"
   c. "What types of food do you eat for meals?"
   d. "Why can't you just eat our food while you are here?"

7. What group is the largest subculture of the healthcare system?
   a. Nurses
   b. Physicians
   c. Social workers
   d. Physical therapists

8. A nurse states, "I know I am cleaner than most of my patients." What does this statement indicate?
   a. Cultural assimilation
   b. Racism
   c. Ethnocentrism
   d. Stereotyping

9. A nurse wants to acquire knowledge of a specific culture. What could be done first?
   a. Talk to coworkers
   b. Review literature
   c. Talk to family members of the patient
   d. Ask others with more experience for help

10. Although all of the following are important to culturally competent nursing care, which one is most basic?
    a. Learning another language
    b. Having significant information
    c. Treating each person as an individual
    d. Recognizing the importance of family

● Answers With Rationale

1. *b.* Culture may be defined as a shared system of beliefs, values, and behavioral expectations that provide social structure for daily living.

2. *c.* When minority groups live within a dominant group, many members lose the cultural characteristics that once made them different.

3. *a.* Ethnicity is the sense of identification with a collective cultural group, largely based on the group's common heritage.

4. *d.* Stereotyping is assuming that all members of a group are alike.

5. *b.* Many agencies have a qualified interpreter who understands the healthcare system and can reliably provide assistance.

6. *c.* Asking patients what types of foods they eat for meals is culturally sensitive.

7. *a.* Nurses are the largest subculture of the healthcare system.

8. *c.* Ethnocentrism occurs when one believes that one's own ideas and practices are superior to those of others.

9. *b.* Reviewing the literature about a specific culture can provide the nurse with a starting point for information about cultural values, dietary practices, family lines of authority, and health and illness beliefs and practices.

10. *c.* In all aspects of nursing, it is important to treat each patient as an individual. This is also true in providing culturally competent care.

Taylor Suite Resources

The Taylor Suite offers these additional resources to enhance learning and facilitate understanding of this chapter:

- thePoint online resource, http://thepoint.lww.com/Taylor7E
- Student DVD included with the book
- Study Guide for Taylor's Fundamentals of Nursing

BIBLIOGRAPHY

Andrews, M. M., & Boyle, J. S. (2008). *Transcultural concepts in nursing care* (5th ed.). Philadelphia: Lippincott Williams & Wilkins.

Bigshaw, A., & Semega, J. (2008). *Income, earnings, and poverty data from the 2007 American Community Survey.* Washington, DC: U.S. Government Printing Office.

Blackford, J. (2005). Equity in care for people of culturally and linguistically diverse backgrounds. *Australian Nursing Journal, 13*(2), 29–31.

Broome, B., & McGuinness, T. (2007). A CRASH course in cultural competence for nurses. *Urologic Nursing, 27*(4), 292–295, 304.

Browne, K. (2005). Ethnographic interviewing as a technique to increase cultural competence in health care. *Nursingmatters, 16*(7), 4, 14.

DeRosa, N., & Kochurka, K. (2006). Implement culturally competent healthcare in your workplace. *Nursing Management, 37*(10), 18, 20, 22.

Del Vecchio, P., & Fricks, L. (2007). Cultural competency and recovery within diverse populations. *Psychiatric Rehabilitation Journal, 31*(1), 49–53.

Eggenberger, S., Grassley, J., & Restrepo, E. (2006). Culturally competent nursing care for families listening to the voices of Mexican-American women. *The Online Journal of Issues in Nursing, 11*(3).

Hall, L., Callister, L. C., Berry, J. A., & Matsumura, G. (2007). Meanings of menopause: Cultural influences on perception and management of menopause. *Journal of Holistic Nursing, 25*(2), 106–118.

Henderson, G., & Primeaux, M. (1981). *Transcultural health care.* Menlo Park, CA: Addison-Wesley.

Leininger, M. M. (1991). *Culture care diversity and universality: A theory of nursing.* New York: John Wiley & Sons.

Miller, E. (2005). Embracing diversity to overcome health disparities. *Rehabilitation Nursing, 30*(4), 122, 139.

Mold, F., Fitzpatrick, J., & Roberts, J. (2005). Caring for minority ethnic older people in nursing care homes. *British Journal of Nursing, 14*(11), 601–606.

Muñoz, C., & Hilgenberg, C. (2005). Ethnopharmacology: Understanding how ethnicity can affect drug response is essential to providing culturally competent care. *American Journal of Nursing, 105*(8), 40–49.

Murray, R., Zentner, J., & Yakimo, R. (2009). *Health promotion strategies through the life span* (8th ed.). Upper Saddle River, NJ: Prentice Hall Health.

Office of Minority Health, Public Health Service, U.S. Department of Health and Human Services. (2001). *National standards for culturally and linguistically appropriate services (CLAS) in health care.* Washington, DC: Office of Minority Health.

Pullen, R. L. (2007). Tips for communicating with a patient from another culture. *Nursing, 37*(10), 48–49.

Resnick, L. K. (2008). The meaning of health among midlife Russian-speaking women. *Journal of Nursing Scholarship, 40*(3), 248–253.

Spector, R. (2009). *Cultural diversity in health and illness* (7th ed.). Upper Saddle River, NJ: Prentice Hall.

U.S. Census Bureau News. (2008). An older and more diverse nation by mid-century. Available at http://www.census.gov/Press-Release/www/releases/archives/population/012496.html.

U.S. Census Bureau, Housing and Household Economic Statistics Division. (2008). *Income, earnings, and poverty data from the 2007 American community survey.* Washington, DC: U.S. Government Printing Office.

Wilson, P., Wright, K., & Isbell, M. T. (2008). *Left behind: Black America; A neglected priority in the global AIDS epidemic.* Los Angeles, CA: Black AIDS Institute.

Yosef, A. R. O. (2008). Health beliefs, practice, and priorities for health care of Arab Muslims in the United States: Implications for care. *Journal of Transcultural Nursing, 19*(3), 284–291.

3 Health and Illness

RUTH JACOBI

Ruth is a 62-year-old woman who was hospitalized after a "mini-stroke." She has now returned to her pre-event level of functioning and is being prepared for discharge. She states, "I know that I have an increased risk for a major stroke, so I want to do everything possible to stay as active and as healthy as I possibly can."

SARA GELBART

Sara, a college freshman, is encouraged to visit the student health center by her roommate because she rarely visits the dining hall for meals, runs 5 to 8 miles a day, and has recently lost a significant amount of weight. Sara states, "I'm plenty healthy, just a bit 'nuts' about being fit!"

DANIEL STERNMAN

Daniel is a 27-year-old man with history of schizophrenia. He comes to the mental health clinic, loudly demanding relief from the voices who are telling him to hurt himself. Mr. Sternman is well known by the clinic staff. His medical record reveals that he has had numerous visits to the clinic and that he has difficulty interacting and dealing with various staff members.

After completing the chapter, you will be able to accomplish the following:

1. Describe concepts and models of health, wellness, and illness.

2. Compare and contrast acute illness and chronic illness.

3. Explain how the human dimensions, basic human needs, and self-concept influence health and illness.

4. Summarize the role of the nurse in promoting health and preventing illness.

5. Explain the levels of preventive care.

KEY TERMS

acute illness	illness
chronic illness	morbidity
disease	mortality
exacerbation	remission
health	risk factor
health promotion	wellness
holistic care	

The primary objectives of the nurse as caregiver are to promote health, to prevent illness, to restore health, and to facilitate coping with illness, disability, or death. These objectives focus care on maximizing the health of patients of all ages, in all settings, and in both health and illness. Health is more than just the absence of illness; it is an active process in which an individual moves toward his or her maximum potential. It also has different definitions for different individuals. (See the accompanying Reflective Practice box for an example.) To give **holistic care,** care that addresses the many dimensions that comprise the whole individual, the nurse must understand and respect each person's own definition of health and responses to illness and should be familiar with models of health and illness. The nurse's knowledge of health and illness is even more important because of today's focus on health promotion and advocacy, the continuing trend toward care being provided in the home and community, the increasing numbers of older adults, and the growing incidence of chronic illnesses.

CONCEPTS OF HEALTH AND WELLNESS

Meguni Kuni, 4 years old, was born with cystic fibrosis. Although she requires ongoing treatment for this illness, she is now an active member of her preschool class, takes gymnastics lessons, and wants to be a doctor when she grows up.

Shondra Cole, 34 years old, is married and has two school-aged children. She has chronic rheumatoid arthritis and is in a wheelchair. Shondra takes care of her house and family and uses a specially designed car to get to her part-time job. Samuel Cohen is 67 years old. He was diagnosed with type 2 diabetes and high blood pressure last year and takes medications for both health problems. Samuel is retired but volunteers 3 days a week in a local hospital as a transport technician. Would Meguni, Shondra, and Samuel be described as healthy? Although they each have a physical condition that might lead them to define themselves as being ill, they are all productive members of their society and would say they are healthy.

Health

A classic definition of **health** is that health is a state of complete physical, mental, and social well-being, not merely the absence of disease or infirmity (World Health Organization, 1974). The health of the public is measured more globally by **morbidity,** how frequently a disease occurs and **mortality,** numbers of deaths. On a personal level, however, most individuals define health according to how they feel ("I feel really sick"), the absence or presence of symptoms of illness ("I have a terrible pain in my stomach"), or their ability to carry out activities of daily living ("I felt so much better that I got up and cooked supper"). See the accompanying Through the Eyes of a Student.

Each person defines health in terms of his or her own values and beliefs. The family, culture, community, and society in which one lives also influence one's personal perception of health.

> *Think back to Sara Gelbart, the college freshman who rarely eats and runs several miles almost daily. According to her statement, she considers herself to be healthy. However, her roommate is concerned because of what she views as excessive exercise and Sara's poor nutrition. The nurse needs to investigate each person's views a bit further to determine exactly what each believes to be healthy. Doing so provides a foundation on which to develop an appropriate plan of care.* ■

Health, as defined by each person, integrates all the human dimensions—the physical, intellectual, emotional, sociocultural, spiritual, and environmental aspects of the whole person. The nurse giving holistic nursing care must equally consider all these interrelated and interdependent dimensions of the whole person (Fig. 3-1).

Wellness

Wellness, a term often used interchangeably with health, is an active state of being healthy by living a lifestyle that promotes good physical, mental, and emotional health. Dunn (1980) described his model of high-level wellness as functioning to one's maximum potential while maintaining balance and a purposeful direction in the environment. Dunn differentiated "wellness" from "good health," believing that good health is a passive state wherein the person is not ill. Wellness is a more

REFLECTIVE PRACTICE
Challenge to Intellectual Skills

My first college roommate, Sara Gelbart, seemed the ideal roommate when I first met her. A good student, she was thoughtful, outgoing, and fun. By October, however, I was really worried about her. I noticed that she rarely wanted to come to the dining hall with our group of friends. When she did come, she just seemed to pick at her food. She also spent a lot of time at the athletic center, running 5 to 8 miles almost daily. I wasn't surprised when she started losing significant amounts of weight. What worried me was her lack of willingness to talk about her nutritional habits and health. She told me that she was plenty healthy, just a bit "nuts" about being fit! She also kidded that I'd be healthier if I worked out more often with her. While she was certainly right about that, I was worried that she had a serious eating disorder and wasn't sure what I could do to help. She politely told me to "mind my own business" when I asked her if she had ever spoken with anyone about her health and eating.

Thinking Outside the Box: Possible Courses of Action

- Respect Sara's wishes and simply try to be a good friend without continuing to confront her about her nutritional status.
- Tell Sara I am concerned that she has a serious eating disorder, and then plan the next steps with her, fully respecting her right to seek or refuse professional help.
- Tell Sara that if she fails to get professional help, I will contact her parents or a counselor at school.

Evaluating a Good Outcome: How Do I Define Success?

- Sara gets whatever help she needs to address her eating problems and regain health.
- Sara's right to make her own decisions is respected.
- My obligations as a friend are fulfilled.
- My beginning ability to identify and correctly respond to health problems affirms my choice for nursing.

Personal Learning: Here's to the Future!

Unfortunately, I did not intervene because (1) I failed to recognize how serious a problem this would become, and (2) I wasn't sure what I could do after Sara refused my initial offers of help. Sara dropped out of school at the end of our freshman year and she has not returned my calls, so I'm not sure how she is doing. I've read more about eating disorders, and I now know how important it is to get professional help early. I learned too late that Sara had been in treatment for anorexia during high school and that the pressures of college life had led to a relapse. I think I valued her friendship more than I valued getting her the help that she needed to address a serious health problem.

Reflection

How do you think you would respond in a similar situation? Why? What does this tell you about yourself and about the adequacy of your skills for professional practice? What pressures of college life might have affected the nursing student's actions? Sara's actions? Please explain. How did the nursing student view health and illness? How did Sara view it? Can you think of other ways to respond? How might the student's and Sara's developmental level affected their responses? What other skills (cognitive, interpersonal, technical, ethical/legal) would you need to respond well in this situation? Do you agree with the criteria to evaluate a successful outcome? Are there any other criteria that could been used? Please explain.

active state, regardless of one's level of health. Dunn also defined processes that help a person know who and what he or she is. These processes, which are a part of each individual's perception of his or her own wellness state, are being (recognizing self as separate and individual), belonging (being part of a whole), becoming (growing and developing), and befitting (making personal choices to befit the self for the future). Dunn's model encourages the nurse to care for the total person, with regard for all factors affecting the person's state of being while striving to reach maximum potential.

CONCEPTS OF ILLNESS AND DISEASE

Disease is a medical term, meaning that there is a pathologic change in the structure or function of the body or mind. Box 3-1 lists examples of causes of disease. An **illness** is the response of the person to a disease; it is an abnormal process in which the person's level of functioning is changed when compared with a previous level. This response is unique for each person and is influenced by self-perceptions, others' perceptions, the effects of changes in body structure and function, the effects of those changes on roles and relationships, and cultural and spiritual values and beliefs. A disease is traditionally diagnosed and treated by a physician (although nurses with advanced educations are increasingly doing so), while nurses focus on the person with an illness. However, the two terms are often used interchangeably. It is important for nurses to remember that a person may have an illness or injury but still achieve maximum functioning and quality of life and consider themselves to be healthy.

Through the Eyes of a Student

Carrie was a 17-year-old brunette who attended my high school, dated my best friend Ricky, and participated in many of the same clubs and activities as me. By looking at her, I never would have guessed anything was wrong. However, once I got to know her, I learned that she was diagnosed with cancer and that the disease had spread through her heart and lungs. The situation, as doctors continually told her, did not look promising. Yet, she never once let that slow her down, and she lived each day to the fullest. It was almost 1 year ago I watched this friend pass away from bone cancer. However, until the days before her last breath, in my eyes she was a happy and healthy girl. She never once let the disease get the best of her, and she fought for life every second of every day. Her constant optimism and determined smile touched and moved so many others. So you ask me, was Carrie healthy?

Health to me is a state of mind, not the physical condition of a person's body. Carrie, in my opinion, was the definition of healthy; she was happy, she lived her life to the fullest, and she continually inspired others to embrace life. The dictionary may state that health is the absence of a disease; however, for me it is the way a person thinks and reacts to life. A person's health con-

sists of being able to work to the best of her capability, look out for herself, and her ability to respond to life enthusiastically. In my eyes, a person like Carrie can be physically unwell, but in terms of living, is healthy. Perhaps this is where health and wellness differ in that, to me, health means the person's entire state of being and is decided by the individual, whereas wellness refers more to the physical condition of a person and is determined more readily by society. The words illness and disease also correspond with these words. I believe that illness, like health, is a matter of thinking, while disease is a medical term that relates to physical condition and wellness. All of these states are constantly changing, and I have probably experienced the best and worst of all of them. However, as I embark on this new and exciting journey of college, I consider myself extremely healthy. I am living each day to the fullest, trying to impact other people's lives, and am filled with optimism. This all may change shortly, but as I look back on Carrie's life and the effect she has had on me, I will always try to live my life in a healthy and grateful way.

—Molly Proskine
Georgetown University

Classifications of Illness

Illnesses are classified as either acute or chronic. A person may have an acute illness, a chronic illness, or both at the same time; for example, an adult with diabetes (a chronic illness) may also have appendicitis (an acute illness).

Acute Illness and Illness Behaviors

An **acute illness** usually has a rapid onset of symptoms and lasts only a relatively short time. Although some acute ill-

nesses are life threatening, with self-treatment and use of over-the-counter medications simple acute illnesses, such as the common cold or diarrhea, do not usually require medical treatment. If medical care is required, a specific treatment with medications (e.g., antibiotics for pneumonia) or surgical procedures (e.g., an appendectomy for appendicitis) usually return the person to normal functioning.

When a person becomes acutely ill, certain illness behaviors may occur in identifiable stages (Suchman, 1965). These behaviors are the way people cope with alterations in function caused by the disease. They are unique to the individual and are influenced by age, gender, family values, economic status, culture, educational level, and mental status.

There is no specific timetable for the stages-of-illness behaviors, which may occur rapidly or slowly. Nursing roles throughout the stages remain constant. In all stages, the nurse accepts the patient as an individual, gives nursing care based on prioritized needs, and facilitates recovery

FIGURE 3-1. The human dimensions. All of these interdependent parts compose the whole person.

Box 3-1   CAUSES OF DISEASES

- Inherited genetic defects
- Developmental defects resulting from exposure to such factors as virus or chemicals during pregnancy
- Biologic agents or toxins
- Physical agents such as temperature, chemicals, and radiation
- Generalized tissue responses to injury or irritation
- Physiologic and emotional reactions to stress
- Excessive or insufficient production of body secretions (hormones, enzymes, and so forth)

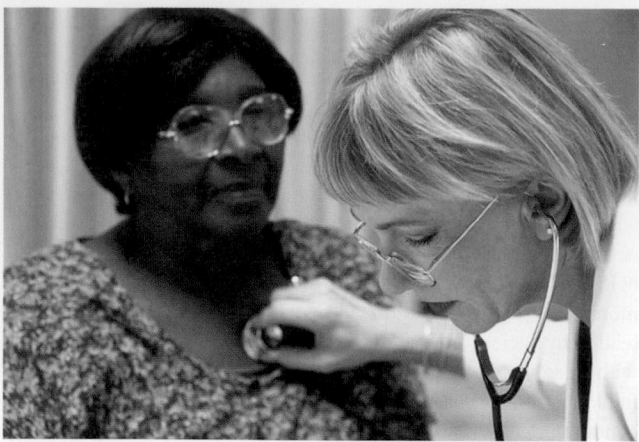

FIGURE 3-2. The nurse is assessing the patient as a basis for teaching healthy heart behaviors.

through physical care, emotional support, and health education (Fig. 3-2).

STAGE 1: EXPERIENCING SYMPTOMS

How do people define themselves as "sick"? The first indication of an illness usually is recognizing one or more symptoms that are incompatible with one's personal definition of health. Although pain is the most significant symptom indicating illness, other common symptoms include a rash, fever, bleeding, or a cough. If the symptoms last for a short time or are relieved by self-care, the person usually takes no further action. If the symptoms continue, however, the person enters the next stage.

STAGE 2: ASSUMING THE SICK ROLE

The person now defines himself or herself as being sick, seeks validation of this experience from others, gives up normal activities, and assumes a "sick role." At this stage, most people focus on their symptoms and bodily functions. Depending on individual health beliefs and practices, the person may choose to do nothing, may buy over-the-counter medications to relieve symptoms, or may seek out a healthcare provider for diagnosis and treatment. In our society, an illness becomes legitimate when a healthcare provider diagnoses it and prescribes treatment. When help from the healthcare provider is sought, the person becomes a patient and enters the next stage.

➤ *Recall Daniel Sternman, the young man with schizophrenia. His arrival at the mental health clinic indicates that he is seeking help from a healthcare provider. The nurse would interpret this behavior as signaling his assumption of the sick role.* ■

STAGE 3: ASSUMING A DEPENDENT ROLE

This stage is characterized by the patient's decision to accept the diagnosis and follow the prescribed treatment plan. The person conforms to the opinions of others, often requires assistance in carrying out activities of daily living,

and needs emotional support through acceptance, approval, physical closeness, and protection.

If the disease is serious (such as a heart attack or stroke), the patient may enter the hospital for treatment. If the symptoms can be managed by the patient or family alone or with the assistance of home care providers, the patient is cared for at home. To facilitate adherence to the treatment plan, the patient needs effective relationships with caregivers, knowledge about the illness, and an individualized plan of care. The patient's responses to care depend on a variety of factors, including the seriousness of the illness, the patient's degree of fear about the disease, the loss of roles, the support of others, and previous experiences with illness care. The patient is expected by both caregivers and family to get well and resume normal roles.

STAGE 4: ACHIEVING RECOVERY AND REHABILITATION

Recovery and rehabilitation might begin in the hospital and conclude at home, or may be totally concluded at a rehabilitation center or at home. Most patients complete this final stage of illness behavior at home. In this stage, the person gives up the dependent role and resumes normal activities and responsibilities. If the plan of care includes health education, the individual may return to health at a higher level of functioning and health than before the illness.

➤ *Remember Ruth Jacobi, the woman being prepared for discharge after a mini-stroke. The patient's stated desire to be as active and as healthy as she possibly can reflects her desire to give up the dependent role. The nurse would use this knowledge as a basis for the patient's teaching plan, thereby fostering a return to health, possibly at a level higher than before the patient's mini-stroke.* ■

Chronic Illness

Chronic illness is a broad term that encompasses many different physical and mental alterations in health, with one or more of the following characteristics:

- It is a permanent change.
- It causes, or is caused by, irreversible alterations in normal anatomy and physiology.
- It requires special patient education for rehabilitation.
- It requires a long period of care or support.

Chronic illnesses usually have a slow onset and many have periods of **remission** (when the disease is present, but the person does not experience symptoms) and **exacerbation** (the symptoms of the disease reappear). Examples of common chronic illnesses are heart disease, diabetes mellitus, lung diseases, and arthritis.

➤ *Recall Daniel Sternman, the young man with schizophrenia. The nurse would integrate knowledge of this disorder, understanding that it is a chronic illness that can be controlled with treatment. The patient's arrival at the clinic with reports of hearing voices would indicate to the nurse that symptoms of the disorder have reappeared, necessitating treatment.* ■

Chronic illnesses are the leading health problem in the world, with the yearly cost of chronic illness in the United States estimated to be $1 trillion (Sobering statistics, 2008). This makes the health promotion and illness prevention activities discussed later in this chapter even more vital to nursing care. Current trends that result in an increase in chronic illnesses include growing numbers of older adults, lifestyle choices (such as smoking and drug use), environmental factors (increasing air and water pollution), and the AIDS epidemic. Nursing care of more patients with chronic illnesses will be required in the future. Although not all people with a chronic illness require care, all who are chronically ill must accept certain conditions of life to be able to live with the illness on a day-to-day basis for the rest of their lives. People with a chronic illness often grieve over losses or changes in physical structure and function, worry about finances, status, roles, and dignity, and must face the possibility of an earlier death. Of the 10 leading causes of death in the United States, seven are the result of chronic illnesses (heart disease, cancer, stroke, respiratory disease, diabetes, Alzheimer's disease, and kidney disease) (National Center for Health Statistics, 2008).

To successfully adapt to a chronic illness, the individual must learn to live as normally as possible and maintain a positive self-concept and sense of hope, despite symptoms and treatments that may make an individual feel different from others. Activities of daily living, relationships, and self-care activities must often be modified, and it is important that the person maintain a feeling of being in control of his or her own life and the prescribed treatments.

Nurses care for individuals of all ages with chronic illnesses, and provide that care in all types of settings, including homes, hospitals, clinics, long-term care facilities, and institutions. Regardless of the age of the patient or the effects and demands of the illness or the setting, the nurse must make every effort to promote health for patients with chronic illness, with a focus of care that emphasizes what is possible rather than what can no longer be.

Effects of Illness on the Family

Most nursing care is given to patients with some form of support system, usually family members. When an illness occurs, roles change for both the patient and the family. For example, a chronic illness creates stress for the patient and family because it might require lifelong alterations in roles or lifestyle, frequent hospitalizations, economic problems, and decreased social interactions among family members. The responses of family members to an illness are also individualized. Some family members want to be with the patient all the time, while others might avoid visiting. Parents of a sick child often react with blame, overprotection, and severe anxiety, and family members of patients requiring intensive care often feel alone and frightened. In both cases, they might also feel guilty and imagine the worst possible outcome. See Chapter 4 for more information.

FACTORS AFFECTING HEALTH AND ILLNESS

Many factors influence a person's health status, health beliefs, and health practices. These factors may be internal or external to the individual and may or may not be under the person's conscious control. To plan and provide holistic care, the nurse must understand how these factors influence behavior in both healthy and ill patients.

Basic Human Needs

A basic human need is something that is essential to the emotional and physiologic health and survival of humans. A person whose needs are met may be considered to be healthy, and a person who has one or more unmet needs is at an increased risk for illness. (Basic human needs are discussed in detail in Chapter 4).

The Human Dimensions

The factors influencing a person's health–illness status, health beliefs, and health practices relate to the person's human dimensions (refer back to Fig. 3-1). Each dimension interrelates with each of the others, and influences the behaviors of the person in health and in illness. Nursing assessments of strengths and weaknesses in each dimension are used to develop a plan of care that is individualized and holistic. The nursing process, used to plan, implement, and evaluate plans of care, is discussed in Unit III.

Physical Dimension

The physical dimension includes genetic inheritance, age, developmental level, race, and gender. These components strongly influence the person's health status and health practices. As examples, inherited genetic disorders include Down syndrome, hemophilia, cystic fibrosis, and color blindness; the toddler is at greater risk for drowning, and the adolescent and young adult male are at greater risk for automobile crashes from excessive speed; there are specific racial traits for disease, including sickle cell anemia, hypertension, and stroke; a young woman who has a mother and grandmother with breast cancer is more likely to have an annual clinical breast examination and mammogram.

Emotional Dimension

How the mind affects body function and responds to body conditions also influences health. Long-term stress affects body systems, and anxiety affects health habits; conversely, calm acceptance and relaxation can actually change body responses to illness. As examples of the negative effects of emotions, a student always has diarrhea before examinations and an adolescent with poor self-esteem begins to experiment with drugs. The positive effects of emotions include reducing surgical pain with relaxation techniques and reducing blood pressure with biofeedback skills.

> *Knowledge of the emotional dimension would be important when planning care for Sara Gelbart, the college freshman described at the beginning of the chapter. The nurse would need to examine how she responds to stress and anxiety.* ■

Intellectual Dimension

The intellectual dimension encompasses cognitive abilities, educational background, and past experiences. These influence responses to teaching about health and reactions to nursing care during illness. They also play a major role in health behaviors. Examples of situations involving this dimension include a young college student with diabetes who follows a diabetic diet but continues to drink beer and eat pizza with friends several times a week, and a middle-aged man who quits taking his high-blood-pressure medication after developing unpleasant side effects.

Environmental Dimension

The environment has many influences on health and illness. Housing, sanitation, climate, and pollution of air, food, and water are elements in the environmental dimension. A few examples of environmental causes of illness are deaths in older adults from inadequate heating and cooling, increased incidence of asthma and respiratory problems in large cities with smog, and increased incidence of skin cancer in people who live in hot, sunny areas of the world.

Sociocultural Dimension

Health practices and beliefs are strongly influenced by a person's economic level, lifestyle, family, and culture. In general, low-income groups are less likely to seek medical care to prevent illness, and high-income groups are more prone to stress-related habits and illness. The family and the culture to which a person belongs influence the person's patterns of living and values about health and illness; such patterns are often unalterable. All of these factors are involved in personal care, patterns of eating, lifestyle habits, and emotional stability. Examples of other sociocultural situations that influence health and illness are an adolescent who sees nothing wrong with smoking or drinking because her parents smoke and drink, parents of a sick infant who do not seek medical care because they have no health insurance, a single parent (abused as a child) who in turn physically abuses her own small son, and a person of Asian descent who uses herbal remedies and acupuncture to treat an illness.

Spiritual Dimension

Spiritual beliefs and values are important components of a person's health and illness behaviors (see Chapter 46). It is important that nurses respect these values and understand their importance for the individual patient. Examples of the influences of the spiritual dimension on healthcare include the Roman Catholic requirement of baptism for both live births and stillborn babies; Kosher dietary laws, prohibiting the intake of pork and shellfish, practiced by Orthodox and Conservative Jews; and opposition to blood transfusion common to Jehovah's Witnesses.

Self-Concept

Another variable influencing health and illness is a person's self-concept (see Chapter 41), which incorporates both how the person feels about self (self-esteem) and the way he or she perceives his or her physical self (body image). Self-concept has both physical and emotional aspects and is an important factor in the way the individual reacts to stress and illness, follows self-care health practices, and relates to others.

> *Consider Sara Gelbart, the college freshman with a suspected eating disorder. Although she has lost a significant amount of weight, she states that she is healthy, but just "nuts" about being fit. Her self-concept is most likely one of being overweight. Subsequently, she rarely eats. In contrast, a person who is overweight may feel that nothing will change the way he or she looks and refuse to follow a diet and exercise program.* ■

A person's self-concept results from a variety of past experiences, interpersonal interactions, physical and cultural influences, and education. It includes perceptions of one's own strengths and weaknesses. Illness can alter a person's self-concept as it affects roles, independence, and relationships with important others.

Risk Factors for Illness or Injury

A **risk factor** is something that increases a person's chances for illness or injury. Like other components of health and illness, risk factors are often interrelated. Risk factors may be further defined as modifiable (able to be changed, such as quitting smoking) or nonmodifiable (unable to be changed, such as a family history of cancer). As the number of risk factors increases, so does the possibility of illness. For example, an overweight executive, under pressure to increase sales, smokes and drinks alcohol in excess. These factors, combined with a family history of heart disease, place this person at higher risk for illness. The six general types of risk factors are described in Table 3-1. Risk factors for each developmental level across the life span are included in Unit II, and cultural influences on health are discussed in Chapter 2.

HEALTH PROMOTION AND ILLNESS PREVENTION

Health promotion is the behavior of an individual that is motivated by a personal desire to increase well-being and

TABLE • 3-1	MAJOR AREAS OF RISK FACTORS
Risk Factor	**Examples**
Age	School-aged children are at high risk for communicable diseases. After menopause, women are more likely to develop cardiovascular disease.
Genetic factors	A family history of cancer or diabetes predisposes a person to developing the disease.
Physiologic factors	Obesity increases the possibility of heart disease. Pregnancy places increased risk on both the mother and the developing fetus.
Health habits	Smoking increases the probability of lung cancer. Poor nutrition can lead to a variety of health problems.
Lifestyle	Multiple sexual relationships increase the risk for sexually transmitted infections (e.g., gonorrhea or acquired immunodeficiency syndrome). Events that increase stress (e.g., divorce, retirement, work-related pressure) may precipitate accidents or illness.
Environment	Working and living environments (such as hazardous materials and poor sanitation) may contribute to disease.

health potential. In contrast, illness/disease prevention is behavior motivated by a desire to avoid or detect disease, or to maintain functioning within the constraints of illness or disability (Pender, Murdaugh, & Parsons, 2006). Health promotion and illness prevention activities have traditionally been described as occurring on primary, secondary, and tertiary levels (Leavell & Clark, 1965). Definitions and examples of nursing activities for each level are discussed below and are illustrated in Table 3-2.

Primary Health Promotion and Illness Prevention

Primary health promotion and illness prevention is directed toward promoting health and preventing the development of disease processes or injury. Nursing activities at the primary level may focus on individuals or groups. Examples of primary-level activities are immunization clinics, family planning services, providing poison-control information, and accident-prevention education. Other nursing interventions include teaching about a healthy diet, the importance of regular exercise, safety in industry and farms, using seat belts, and safer sex practices.

Health-risk assessments are an important part of primary health promotion and preventive care. A health-risk assess-

ment is an assessment of the total person. The resulting "picture" of the individual indicates areas of risk for disease or injury as well as areas that support health. A variety of formats are used to perform the assessment, but all of them take a broad approach to health, focusing on lifestyle and behaviors. Box 3-2 contains an example of a health-style self-test that is completed by the patient. As you work with patients to provide care, use this self-test to help your patients assess their state of health and health risks, and learn a new health style through recommended lifestyle practices that support health.

Secondary Health Promotion and Illness Prevention

Secondary health promotion and illness prevention focuses on screening for early detection of disease with prompt diagnosis and treatment of those found. The goals of secondary preventive care are to identify an illness, reverse or reduce the severity of the disease or provide a cure, and thereby return the individual to maximum health, as quickly as possible. Examples of nursing activities at this level are assessing children for normal growth and development and encouraging regular medical, dental, and vision examination. Other activities include screenings (e.g., blood pressure, cholesterol, and

TABLE • 3-2	EXAMPLES OF NURSING ACTIVITIES BY LEVEL OF HEALTH PROMOTION AND PREVENTIVE CARE
Level	**Topic**
Primary	Weight loss Diet Exercise Smoking cessation Alcohol consumption Drugs Farm safety Seat belts and child safety seats Immunizations Water treatment Safer sex practices Parenting
Secondary	Screenings (Blood pressure, cholesterol, glaucoma, HIV, skin cancer) Pap smears Mammograms Testicular examinations Family counseling
Tertiary	Medications Medical therapy Surgical treatment Rehabilitation Physical therapy Occupational therapy Job training

Box 3-2   A HEALTH-STYLE SELF-TEST

All of us want good health, but many of us do not know how to be as healthy as possible. Health experts now describe *lifestyle* as one of the most important factors affecting health. In fact, it is estimated that as many as 7 of the 10 leading causes of death could be reduced through common-sense changes in lifestyle. That's what this brief test, developed by the Public Health Service, is all about. Its purpose is simply to tell you how well you are doing to stay healthy. The behaviors covered in the test are recommended for most Americans. Some of them may not apply to people with certain chronic diseases or disabilities, or to pregnant women. Such people may require special instructions from their physicians.

Cigarette Smoking

If you never smoke, enter a score of 10 for this section and go to the next section on Alcohol and Drugs.

almost always / sometimes / almost never

2 1 0   1. I avoid smoking cigarettes.
2 1 0   2. I smoke only low-tar and nicotine cigarettes *or* I smoke a pipe or cigars.

Smoking score: _____

Alcohol and Drugs

4 1 0   1. I avoid drinking alcoholic beverages *or* I drink no more than one or two drinks a day.
2 1 0   2. I avoid using alcohol or other drugs (especially illegal drugs) as a way of handling stressful situations or the problems in my life.
2 1 0   3. I am careful not to drink alcohol when taking certain medicines (eg, medicine for sleeping, pain, colds, and allergies), or when pregnant.
2 1 0   4. I read and follow the label directions when using prescribed and over-the-counter drugs.

Alcohol and drugs score: _____

Eating Habits

4 1 0   1. I eat a variety of foods each day, such as fruits and vegetables, whole-grain breads and cereals, lean meats, dairy products, dry peas and beans, and nuts and seeds.
2 1 0   2. I limit the amount of fat, saturated fat, and cholesterol I eat (including fat on meats, eggs, butter, cream, shortenings, and organ meats such as liver).
2 1 0   3. I limit the amount of salt I eat by cooking with only small amounts, not adding salt at the table, and avoiding salty snacks.
2 1 0   4. I avoid eating too much sugar (especially frequent snacks of sticky candy or soft drinks).

Eating habits score: _____

Exercise and Fitness

3 1 0   1. I maintain a desired weight, avoiding overweight and underweight.
3 1 0   2. I do vigorous exercises for 15 to 30 minutes at least three times a week (examples include running, swimming, brisk walking).
2 1 0   3. I do exercises that enhance my muscle tone for 15 to 30 minutes at least three times a week (examples include yoga and calisthenics).
2 1 0   4. I use part of my leisure time participating in individual, family, or team activities that increase my level of fitness (such as gardening, bowling, golf, and baseball).

Exercise/fitness score: _____

Stress Control

2 1 0   1. I have a job or do other work that I enjoy.
2 1 0   2. I find it easy to relax and express my feelings freely.
2 1 0   3. I recognize early, and prepare for, events or situations likely to be stressful for me.
2 1 0   4. I have close friends, relatives, or others whom I can talk to about personal matters and call on for help when needed.
2 1 0   5. I participate in group activities (such as church and community organizations) or hobbies that I enjoy.

Stress control score: _____

Safety

2 1 0   1. I wear a seat belt while riding in a car.
2 1 0   2. I avoid driving while under the influence of alcohol and other drugs.
2 1 0   3. I obey traffic rules and the speed limit when driving.
2 1 0   4. I am careful when using potentially harmful products or substances (such as household cleaners, poisons, and electrical devices).
2 1 0   5. I avoid smoking in bed.

Safety score: _____

What Your Scores Mean to You

Scores of 9 and 10

Excellent! Your answers show that you are aware of the importance of this area to your health. More important, you are putting your knowledge to work for you by practicing good health habits. As long as you continue to do so, this area should not pose a serious health risk. It's likely that you are setting an example for your family and friends to follow. Because you got a very high test score on this part of the test, you may want to consider other areas where your scores indicate room for improvement.

Scores of 6 to 8

Your health practices in this area are good, but there is room for improvement. Look again at the items you answered with "Sometimes" or "Almost never." What changes can you make to improve your score? Even a small change can often help you achieve better health.

Scores of 3 to 5

Your health risks are showing! Would you like more information about the risks you are facing and about why it is important for you to change these behaviors? Perhaps you need help in deciding how to make the changes you desire. In either case, help is available.

(continued)

Box 3-2   **A HEALTH-STYLE SELF-TEST**   *(continued)*

Scores of 0 to 2
Obviously, you were concerned enough about your health to take the test, but your answers show that you may be taking serious and unnecessary risks with your health. Perhaps you are unaware of the risks and what to do about them. You can easily get the information and help you need to improve, if you wish. The next step is up to you.

SUGGESTED SELF-CARE BEHAVIORS
Start by asking yourself a few frank questions: *Am I really doing all I can to be as healthy as possible? What steps can I take to feel better? Am I willing to begin now?* If you scored low in one or more sections of the test, decide what changes you want to make for improvement. You might pick that aspect of your lifestyle where you feel you have the best chance for success and tackle that one first. Once you have improved your score there, go on to other areas.

Lifestyle practices that promote health include:

- Sleeping regularly, 7 to 8 hours per night
- Eating regular meals, which include recommended food groups
- Maintaining ideal body weight
- Having a regular schedule of exercise
- Using alcohol in moderation, if at all
- Not smoking
- Maintaining positive mental health and self-concept
- Practicing safer sex
- Wearing seatbelts, using car seats for children, and wearing bicycle helmets

- Having recommended screenings and checkups by your medical and dental healthcare providers

If you already have tried to change your health habits (to stop smoking or exercise regularly, for example), don't be discouraged if you haven't yet succeeded. The difficulty you have encountered may be due to influences you've never really thought about—such as advertising—or to a lack of support and encouragement. Understanding these influences is an important step toward changing the way they affect you.

There's help available. In addition to personal actions you can take on your own, there are community programs and groups (such as the YMCA or the local chapter of the American Heart Association) that can assist you and your family to make the changes you want to make. If you want to know more about these groups or about health risks, contact your local health department or the National Health Information Clearinghouse. There's a lot you can do to stay healthy or to improve your health—and there are organizations that can help you. Start a new "health-style" today!

For assistance in locating specific information on these and other health topics, write to the National Health Information Clearinghouse:

National Health Information Clearinghouse
P.O. Box 1133
Washington, DC 20013

(Adapted with permission of the National Health Information Clearinghouse.)

skin cancer), recommending gynecologic examinations and mammograms for women as age-appropriate, and teaching testicular self-examination to men. Direct nursing care interventions at the secondary level include administering medications and caring for wounds.

Tertiary Health Promotion and Illness Prevention

Tertiary health promotion and disease prevention begins after an illness is diagnosed and treated to reduce disability and to help rehabilitate patients to a maximum level of functioning. Nursing activities on a tertiary level include teaching a patient with diabetes how to recognize and prevent complications, using physical therapy to prevent contractures in a patient who has had a stroke or spinal cord injury, and referring a woman to a support group after removal of a breast because of cancer. Nurses are important in monitoring the responses of the patient to the prescribed therapy and in providing services to patients to facilitate recovery or improve quality of life while living with the effects of an illness or injury.

> *Think back to Sara Gelbart, the college freshman with a suspected eating disorder. The nurse would use tertiary preventive care by referring the patient to an eating disorders support group. For Ruth Jacobi, the woman being*

discharged after a mini-stroke, tertiary preventive care would include educating her about the warning signs and symptoms of a major stroke and about measures to reduce her risk. ■

MODELS OF HEALTH PROMOTION AND ILLNESS PREVENTION

Models of why and how individuals carry out behaviors to promote health and prevent illness are useful in helping healthcare providers understand health-related behaviors and adapt care to people from diverse economic and cultural backgrounds. This knowledge can be used to overcome barriers to health from disparities in care resulting from such factors as the increasing number of people without health insurance, a predicted upward trend in minority populations, and a lack of accessible and essential healthcare services for low-income and rural populations.

The Health Belief Model

Free or low-cost screens and health information are available in most areas to help in the early detection of disease and to educate people about healthy living. Why, then, don't more people take advantage of these services or change their lifestyles? This question can be answered with the widely used health belief model, which describes health behaviors.

The health belief model (Rosenstock, 1974) is concerned with what people perceive, or believe, to be true about themselves in relation to their health. This model is based on three components of individual perceptions of threat of a disease: (1) perceived susceptibility to a disease, (2) perceived seriousness of a disease, and (3) perceived benefits of action.

Perceived susceptibility to a disease is the belief that one either will or will not contract a disease. It ranges from being afraid of contracting a disease to completely denying that certain behaviors will result in illness. For example, one person who smokes cigarettes may believe he or she is at danger for lung cancer and may stop smoking, while another person may believe smoking poses no serious threat and continues to smoke.

Perceived seriousness of a disease concerns the perception of the threat to health posed by the disease and its effect on the person's lifestyle. This component is related to how much the person knows about the disease and can result in a change in health behavior. If a person who smokes believes that lung cancer can lead to physical disability or death and would, therefore, affect his or her ability to work and care for the family, the person is more likely to stop smoking.

Perceived benefits of action is concerned with how effective the individual believes measures will be in preventing illness. This factor is influenced by the person's conviction that carrying out a recommended action will prevent or modify the disease and by the person's perception of the cost and unpleasant effects of performing the health behavior (compared with not taking any action). For example, the person may believe that stopping smoking will prevent future breathing problems and that the initial withdrawal symptoms can be overcome; therefore, the person may stop smoking.

Modifying factors for one's health beliefs include demographic variables (such as age and gender), sociopsychological variables (such as personality and peer group pressure), and structural variables (such as knowledge and prior contact with the disease). These factors interact to influence the perceived benefits of preventive action minus the perceived barriers to preventive action. Cues to action are also modifying factors and are provided by activities such as others' advice, mass-media campaigns, literature, appointment-reminder telephone calls or postcards, and illness of a significant other. The likelihood of taking a recommended preventive health action is thus a composite of individual perceptions and modifying factors.

The health belief model is useful when teaching individuals about health and illness. You can assess the patient's related beliefs and mutually structure goals to help realistically meet health needs. Teaching and health promotion activities are ineffective, however, unless the patient believes they are important and necessary.

> *Consider Ruth Jacobi, the woman being discharged after a mini-stroke. The patient indicates that she is positively motivated to achieve health, providing the nurse with valuable information about the patient's health beliefs. Together, the nurse and patient can determine realistic goals. The nurse, then, could use this model to develop the patient's teaching plan, including information about the underlying disease process, risk factors for stroke, and ways to reduce the patient's risk for a major stroke.* ■

The Health Promotion Model

The health promotion model (Pender, Murdaugh, & Parsons, 2006) was developed to illustrate how people interact with their environment as they pursue health. The model incorporates individual characteristics and experiences and behavior-specific knowledge and beliefs, to motivate health-promoting behavior. The components of the model can be used to design and provide nursing interventions to promote health for individuals, families, and communities.

Individual characteristics and experiences can be useful in predicting if an individual will incorporate and use health-related behaviors. If a behavior has been used before and becomes a habit, it is more likely to be used again. Personal biologic, psychological, and sociocultural factors, including age, gender, strength, self-esteem, perceived health status, definition of health, acculturation, and socioeconomic status are all predictive of a given health-related habit. For example, the person who has high self-esteem, defines self as healthy, and has an adequate income might be less likely to use alcohol or tobacco and more likely to follow a healthy diet and take part in regular exercise. Conversely, a person with low self-esteem, a fatalistic attitude toward health, and a low socioeconomic base might be more likely to have poor nutrition, never exercise, and use addictive substances.

Behavior-specific knowledge, beliefs, and relationships are considered to be major motivators for engaging in health-promoting behaviors. These include the belief that there will be a positive outcome from a specific health behavior, that one has the skill and competence to engage in health behaviors, and that one is affected by the interpersonal influences of others (especially family, peers, and healthcare providers). Situational influences, such as no-smoking policies, also influence health behaviors. Barriers to action, which include perceptions of unavailability, inconvenience, expense, difficulty, or time, usually result in avoidance of a behavior.

A health-related behavior is initiated by committing to a plan of action, accompanied by developing associated strategies to perform the valued behavior. Failure to sustain the behavior may result from competing demands. For example, a person may begin a low-fat diet but "give in" to the convenience of fast foods. Health-related behavior is the outcome of the model and is directed toward attaining positive health outcomes and experiences throughout the life span.

The Health–Illness Continuum

The health–illness continuum is one way to measure a person's level of health. This model views health as a constantly changing state, with high-level wellness and death being on

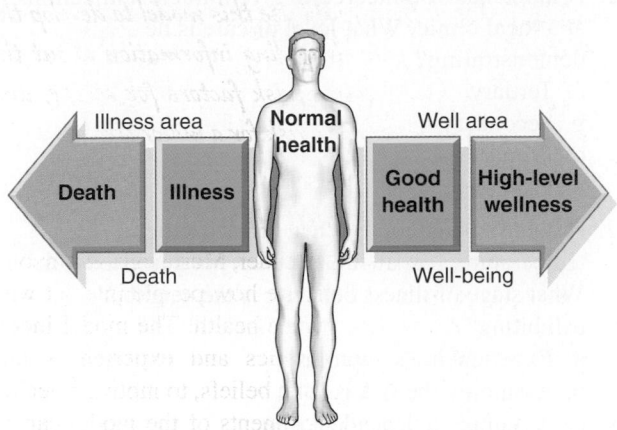

FIGURE 3-3. The health–illness continuum.

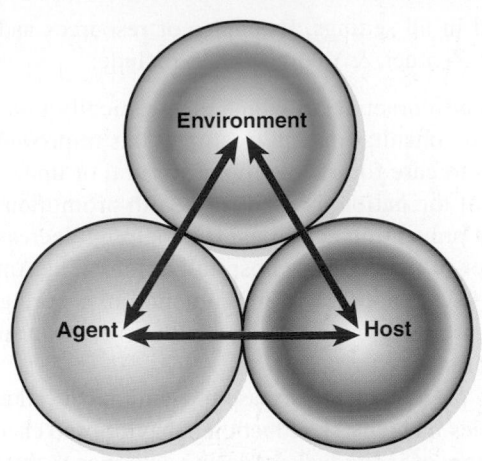

FIGURE 3-4. The agent–host–environment triangle.

opposite ends of a graduated scale, or continuum (Fig. 3-3). This continuum illustrates the ever-changing state of health as a person adapts to changes in the internal and external environments to maintain a state of well-being. For example, a patient with cancer may view himself or herself at different points on the continuum at any given time, depending on how well the patient believes he or she is functioning with the illness.

> *Think back to Sara Gelbart, the college freshman described in the Reflective Practice display. The nurse could apply the health–illness continuum model when assessing this patient, recognizing that the stressors of college life have resulted in a shift along the continuum for this patient away from high-level wellness.* ∎

The Agent–Host–Environment Model

The agent–host–environment model of health and illness, developed by Leavell and Clark (1965), is useful for examining the causes of disease in an individual. An agent is an environmental factor or stressor that must be present or absent for an illness to occur. For example, the factor may be bacteria or a virus, a chemical substance, or a form of radiation whose presence, excessive presence, or absence (such as in a vitamin-deficiency disease) is necessary for an illness. A host is a living organism capable of being infected or affected by an agent. The host reaction is influenced by family history, age, and health habits. The environment includes all the factors external to the host that make illness more or less likely. The factors can include any that influence health, including physical, social, biologic, and cultural factors. For example, a person who has poor nutritional habits and gets little sleep is at increased risk for infection during an outbreak of influenza. If that person also is immune deficient (as in AIDS), the risk is even greater. The triangle in Figure 3-4 illustrates how each of the agent–host–environment factors affects and is affected by the others. These factors are constantly interacting, and a combination of factors may increase the risk of illness. When the factors are balanced, health is maintained; when they are out of balance, disease occurs. Thus, health is an ever-changing state.

NURSING CARE TO PROMOTE HEALTH AND PREVENT ILLNESS

The current focus on health promotion and illness prevention at local, state, national, and global levels is important to nursing. Chapter 1 provides information about *Healthy People 2010*, a national agenda to promote health. Nursing interventions to promote health in the community are discussed in Chapters 4 and 8. Chapters 19 and 20 discuss recommended screenings, immunizations, and safety practices across the life span.

Nurses must take care of their own health to be able to give effective nursing care to others. Good personal health not only enables nurses to practice more efficiently, but also enables them to serve as role models for patients and families. Nurses can help patients acquire new health behaviors by modeling the very behaviors they are trying to promote. It is difficult for nurses to be sincerely attentive to the needs of patients when their own needs are not being met. Because no one is perfectly healthy all of the time, it is important that nurses who are preparing for professional practice spend time getting to know themselves. From this self-knowledge should come a commitment to actively pursue holistic health. To help you increase your self-knowledge, you should go back and complete the health-style self-test in Box 3-2.

The Promoting Health boxes highlighted throughout this text may be useful to you, as well as to your patients. Use these guides to assess and identify both strengths and risks for alterations in health. The guides can also serve as a basis for teaching self-care to patients.

As we move further into the 21st century, resources for healthcare practices for self and others and maintaining knowledge of healthcare trends can help in promoting health and serving as an advocate for patients and families of all ages and in all settings. Examples of resources and trends (Murray, Zentner, & Yakimo, 2009) include:

- Telehealth practice, in which electronically transmitted clinical consultation and treatment has improved access to care for people living in rural or underserved areas of the nation, is used for health promotion and illness prevention activities. It is helping decrease the number of unnecessary hospitalizations. The American Nurses Association was instrumental in securing Medicare repayment for telehealth services in specific rural areas.
- Health promotion and disease prevention education and activities include risk reduction behaviors and changing behaviors of individuals; tailoring activities to the unique health risk environment, age, and gender of the individual patient.
- Industries and other work settings increasingly have programs for employees that emphasize stress reduction, exercise, smoking cessation, and weight guidance.
- Health promotion sites are now found in a wide variety of locations, including university campuses, retirement centers, day schools, churches, community centers, grocery stores, and senior nutrition sites.
- Healthcare services must be given in nontraditional sites to provide screening and education to people who are, for example, homeless, migrant workers, and carnival workers.

● Developing Critical Thinking Skills

1. Identify a family in which someone has a chronic illness. Interview as many of the other family members as possible, and discuss the effect of the illness on them. What do you observe about the effects of the illness in relation to the patient's age, type of illness (e.g., AIDS versus cancer), gender, and family role?

2. List the six human dimensions described in this chapter, and identify your personal strengths and weaknesses in each area. For example, you may have inherited a genetic tendency toward being overweight (a weakness), but have controlled your weight through nutrition and exercise (a strength). After considering your strengths and weaknesses, develop a personal plan for health promotion.

● Practicing for NCLEX

1. Of the following statements, which is most true of health and illness?
   a. Health and illness are the same for all people.
   b. Health and illness are individually defined by each person.
   c. People with acute illnesses are actually healthy.
   d. People with chronic illnesses have poor health beliefs.

2. A nurse has volunteered to give influenza injections at a local clinic. What level of care is he demonstrating?
   a. Tertiary
   b. Secondary
   c. Primary
   d. Promotive

3. A nurse's neighbor tells her, "I have a high temperature, feel awful, and I am not going to work." What stage of illness behavior is the neighbor exhibiting?
   a. Experiencing symptoms
   b. Assuming the sick role
   c. Assuming a dependent role
   d. Achieving recovery and rehabilitation

4. A nurse is caring for a patient with heart failure, a chronic illness. Which of the following characteristics is not a part of chronic illness?
   a. Permanent change in body structure or function
   b. Self-treatment that relieves symptoms
   c. Long period of treatment and care
   d. Often has remissions and exacerbations

5. The agent–host–environment model of health and illness is based on what concept?
   a. Risk factors
   b. Infectious diseases
   c. Behaviors to promote health
   d. Stages of illness

6. When providing health promotion classes, a nurse uses concepts from models of health. What do both the health–illness continuum and the high-level wellness models demonstrate?
   a. Illness as a fixed point in time
   b. The importance of family
   c. Wellness as a passive state
   d. Health as a constantly changing state

7. Following the birth of his first child and after reading about the long-term effects of nicotine, John decides to stop smoking. This behavior change is most likely based on John's perceptions of all but one of the following. Which one is **not** true?
   a. His susceptibility to lung cancer
   b. How serious lung cancer would be
   c. What benefits his stopping smoking will have
   d. Personal choice and economic factors

8. Of the following clinic patients, which one is most likely to have annual breast examinations and mammograms based on the physical human dimension?
   a. Jane, because her best friend had a benign breast lump removed
   b. Sarah, who lives in a low-income neighborhood
   c. Tricia, who has a family history of breast cancer
   d. Nancy, because her family encourages regular physical examinations

9. A nurse is asked to teach a group of young adults a healthy lifestyle. One young man says, "I stopped eating fast foods to lose weight." What model of health or illness explains this behavior?
   a. Health–illness continuum
   b. Agent–host–environment model
   c. Health promotion model
   d. Health belief model

10. A nurse follows the guidelines for a healthy lifestyle. How can this promote health in others?
    a. By being a role model for healthy behaviors
    b. By not requiring sick days from work
    c. By never exposing others to any type of illness
    d. By spending less money on food

Answers With Rationale

1. *b.* Each person defines health and illness individually, based on a number of factors.

2. *c.* Giving influenza injections is an example of primary health promotion and illness prevention.

3. *b.* When people assume the sick role, they define themselves as ill, seek validation of this experience from others, and give up normal activities.

4. *b.* Acute illnesses are often self-treated to relieve symptoms.

5. *a.* The interaction of the agent–host–environment creates risk factors that increase the probability of disease.

6. *d.* Both these models view health as a dynamic (constantly changing state).

7. *d.* Responses *a, b,* and *c* are components of the health belief model.

8. *c.* A family history of breast cancer is a major risk factor.

9. *c.* The health promotion model illustrates how health-related behaviors and beliefs promote health.

10. *a.* Good personal health enables the nurse to serve as a role model for patients and families.

Taylor Suite Resources

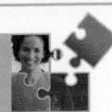

The Taylor Suite offers these additional resources to enhance learning and facilitate understanding of this chapter:

- thePoint online resource, http://thepoint.lww.com/Taylor7E
- Student DVD included with the book
- Study Guide for Taylor's Fundamentals of Nursing

BIBLIOGRAPHY

Condon, M., & Welker-Hood, K. (2007). Environment, health, and safety. *American Nurse Today, 2*(6), 56.

Delgado, C. (2007). Sense of coherence, spirituality, stress, and quality of life in chronic illness. *Journal of Nursing Scholarship, 39*(3), 229–234.

Dunn, H. (1980). *High-level wellness.* Thorofare, NJ: Slack, Inc.

Edelman, C., & Mandle, C. (2006). *Health promotion throughout the life span* (5th ed.). St. Louis, MO: Mosby.

How to lower your health risks, at any age. (2008). *Consumer Reports on Health, 20*(8), 1, 45.

Leavell, H., & Clark, E. G. (1965). *Preventive medicine for the doctor in the community* (3rd ed.). New York: McGraw Hill.

Mason, D. (2005). The state of the science: Focus on chronic illness. *American Journal of Nursing, 105*(2), 27–28.

Murray, R. B., Zentner, J. P., & Yakimo, R. (2009). *Health promotion strategies through the lifespan* (8th ed.). Upper Saddle River, NJ: Pearson Prentice Hall.

National Center for Health Statistics. (2008). Deaths—leading causes. Available at http://www.cdc.gov/nchs/FASTATS/lcod.htm

Pender, N., Murdaugh, C., & Parsons, M. (2006). *Health promotion in nursing practice* (6th ed.). Upper Saddle River, NJ: Pearson Prentice Hall.

Rosenstock, I. (1974). Historical origin of the health belief model. *Health Education Monographs, 2,* 334.

Sheer, B. (2007). Nursing and the impact of worldwide poverty. *Topics in Advanced Practice Nursing eJournal, 7*(3). Available at http://www.medscape.com/viewarticle/564102

Sobering statistics. (2008). *American Journal of Nursing, 108*(1), 22.

Stanhope, M., & Lancaster, J. (2006). *Foundations of nursing in the community.* (2nd ed.). St. Louis: Mosby.

Suchman, E. (1965). Stages of illness and medical care. *Journal of Health and Human Behavior, 6,* 114.

U.S. Department of Health and Human Services. (2000). *Healthy people 2010.* Washington, DC: Author.

World Health Organization. (1974). *Constitution of the World Health Organization: Chronicle of the World Health Organization.* Geneva: Author.

4 Health of the Individual, Family, and Community

ROLANDA SIMPKINS

Rolanda, a sexually active 16-year-old girl, comes to the clinic seeking information about contraception. She states, "My mother would 'kill me' if she knew I was asking about this."

SAMUEL KAPLAN

Samuel is the 80-year-old husband of a 76-year-old woman who was diagnosed with Alzheimer's disease 1 year ago. Visibly tearful, he states, "I don't think that I can continue to care for my wife at home anymore. But how can I even consider putting her in a nursing home?"

CARLOTTA RIOS

Carlotta is a 17-year-old girl who was brought to the mental health–psychiatric unit because of attempted suicide. She does not speak English very well and lives with her sister because of the recent death of her mother. Further assessment reveals possible verbal abuse by her sister and a desire to "disappear" and not return to her sister's home.

After completing the chapter, you will be able to accomplish the following:

1. Describe each level of Maslow's hierarchy of basic human needs.

2. Explain nursing care necessary to meet needs for each level of Maslow's hierarchy.

3. Discuss family concepts, including family roles, structures, functions, developmental stages, tasks, and health risk factors.

4. Identify aspects of the community that affect individual and family health.

5. Describe nursing interventions to promote and maintain health of the individual as a member of a family and as a member of a community.

KEY TERMS

basic human needs	nuclear family
blended family	physiologic needs
community	safety and security needs
extended family	
family	self-actualization needs
love and belonging needs	self-esteem needs

Humans are complex organisms, influenced by and responsive to both the internal and external environments. Our behaviors, our feelings about ourselves and others, our values, and the priorities we set for ourselves all relate to our physiologic and psychosocial needs. These needs are common to all people, and meeting these needs is essential to the health and survival of all people; hence, they are labeled **basic human needs.** Basic human needs can be met or unmet in a variety of ways. A person can meet some needs independently, but most needs require relationships and interactions with others for partial or complete fulfillment. Satisfying one's needs often depends on the social and physical environment, especially one's family and community.

Holistic nursing care, which is based on considering all the dimensions that affect how the patient's basic human needs are met in health and in illness, allows the nurse to provide individualized and health-oriented care. This chapter discusses how basic human needs, the family, and the community environment affect the health of the individual. (For an example, see the accompanying Reflective Practice box.)

THE INDIVIDUAL'S BASIC HUMAN NEEDS

In nursing, we consider both the physical and psychosocial needs of each individual patient. Abraham Maslow (1968) developed a hierarchy of basic human needs (Fig. 4-1) that can be used to consider which needs of a person are the most important at any given time. Certain needs are more basic or essential than others and must be at least minimally met before other needs can be considered.

Maslow's hierarchy is useful for understanding the relationships of basic human needs and for establishing priorities of care. The hierarchy is based on the theory that something is a basic need if it has the following characteristics:

- Its absence results in illness.
- Its presence helps prevent illness or signals health.
- Meeting it restores health.
- It is preferred over other satisfactions when unmet.
- One feels something is missing when the need is unmet.
- One feels satisfaction when the need is met.

Maslow arranged the hierarchy to show that certain needs are more basic than others. Although all people have all the needs all the time, people generally strive to meet certain of the needs (at least to a minimal level) before attending to other needs. The five levels of needs, with physiologic being the most basic, are as follows:

Level 1: Physiologic needs
Level 2: Safety and security needs
Level 3: Love and belonging needs
Level 4: Self-esteem needs
Level 5: Self-actualization needs

Nursing care is often directed toward meeting unmet or threatened needs. Maslow's hierarchy provides a framework for nursing assessment and for understanding the needs of patients at all levels, so that interventions to meet priority needs become a part of the plan of care. Many of the nursing interventions that you learn as you progress through your education are aimed at meeting patients' basic human needs. The following sections describe each level of need in more detail.

Physiologic Needs

Physiologic needs—oxygen, water, food, temperature, elimination, sexuality, physical activity, and rest—must be met at least minimally to maintain life. These needs are the most basic in the hierarchy of needs, are the most essential to life and, therefore, have the highest priority. Most healthy children and adults meet their physiologic needs through self-care, but meeting physiologic needs is often a major part of the nursing care plan for young, old, disabled, and ill people who require assistance in meeting them.

Oxygen is the most essential of all needs because all body cells require oxygen for survival. Oxygenation of body cells is carried out primarily by the respiratory and cardiovascular systems, and any alteration in their structure or function can result in an increased need for oxygen. This need may be acute (such as when cardiopulmonary resuscitation is

REFLECTIVE PRACTICE

Challenge to Ethical and Legal Skills

Junior year was full of excitement and new experiences. I was both nervous and excited about our mental health clinical rotation. Although the staff was very helpful and cooperative in providing as great an experience as they could, I found this clinical rotation to be difficult. I was going to be speaking with patients who had mental-health problems and developing nurse–patient relationships that were different from the ones that I had been exposed to in the past. To tell the truth, I was fearful. I was afraid I would say the wrong thing, causing the person to react, possibly injuring himself or others.

One patient really made an impression on me—Carlotta Rios, a 17-year-old girl who was brought to the unit because of attempted suicide. She did not speak English very well and lived with her sister because her mother had recently passed away. The nurses asked me to speak with her because I spoke Spanish.

When talking with her, I found out that Carlotta did not like living with her sister because the sister verbally abused her, always putting her down and constantly reminding Carlotta that the only reason she was here was because of her sister. Carlotta reported that her sister constantly told her about all of the sacrifices that she was making just so that Carlotta could be with her. According to Carlotta, her sister said that Carlotta did not appreciate everything that her sister was doing. The sister constantly reminded Carlotta of everything she bought for her, making sure to keep a record so that Carlotta would pay her back. Carlotta said that she was not happy and figured that the only way she would stop feeling bad and that her sister would be happy again would be if Carlotta disappeared. Carlotta no longer wanted to exist.

Talking with Carlotta further, I found out that she did not want to return home, which currently was her sister's home. Unfortunately, this was a problem because legally she was not considered an adult. Therefore, Carlotta's sister would have to be contacted. Yet, it seemed that Carlotta's current family and living situation was not the safest. At the same time, it also seemed to be the cause of Carlotta's desperate attempt to take her life. If she chose not to return to her sister's house, Carlotta would be taken to court in handcuffs and placed in a foster home. Although this placement would only be until she turned 18 years old, which was at the end of the month, it also meant that once she was 18 years old, she would be on her own. It was apparent that she was not ready for such a drastic change.

Thinking Outside the Box: Possible Courses of Action

- Call her sister and have her pick her up, because she is legally responsible for the patient.
- Gain the trust of the patient by speaking to her as an adult and informing her of all the options, ultimately assisting her with carrying them out.
- Call someone with whom she felt comfortable to provide support and also to hear the options available; in this way, the patient would have the opinion of someone she knew and trusted before she made a decision on which course of action to take.

Evaluating a Good Outcome: How Do I Define Success?

- Patient's safety is ensured.
- Patient benefits from the course of action decided on.
- The patient's human dignity is respected.
- No violations of the American Nurses Association's Code of Ethics occur.
- Patient makes the most appropriate decision, resulting in the best outcome for her.
- The ethical and legal obligations for myself and those of the hospital are met.

Personal Learning: Here's to the Future!

I figured the best way to approach this situation was to develop a trusting relationship. So, after getting Carlotta up, we went to a brighter, better-lit room, where we had breakfast. I started by asking simple questions, eventually progressing to those that pertained to why she was in the hospital. Throughout our talks, I reinforced that her sister was considered the person legally responsible for Carlotta, explaining that if Carlotta decided not to call home, she would be taken in handcuffs to court, where she then would be placed in a foster home. I told her that this would only be until she turned 18 years old; upon turning 18, she then would be on her own. After listening to all of her options, she decided that she would call her sister to let her know where she was. She also told her sister that she would be staying with a best friend until she had figured things out. For Carlotta, this was the best decision to make because she felt safest. As a result of informing her sister, Carlotta would not have to go to court. Subsequently, any upset or disruption for her sister would be minimized, further adding to Carlotta's feelings of being safe. The priority for Carlotta was a safe environment. We were able to establish a trusting relationship and work together toward this end.

Stephanie Cuellar, Georgetown University

Reflection

How do you think you would respond in a similar situation? Why? What does this tell you about yourself and about the adequacy of your skills for professional practice? Can you think of other ways to respond? How might the death of Carlotta's mother have impacted her "desire to disappear"? What family risk factors were evident here? Were they addressed in this scenario? If so, how; if not, then how could they be? What community resources might have been helpful for Carlotta? How were the nursing student's actions legal? Ethical? Please explain. What other skills (cognitive, interpersonal, technical, ethical/legal) would you need to respond well in this situation? Do you agree with the criteria to evaluate a successful outcome? Were the stated criteria met? Why or why not?

FIGURE 4-1. Maslow's hierarchy of basic human needs.

needed) or chronic (requiring special positioning, treatments, and teaching). Nurses evaluate patients' oxygen needs by assessing skin color, vital signs, anxiety levels, responses to activity, restlessness, and mental responsiveness.

A balance between the intake and elimination of fluids is essential to life. Healthy people drink fluids to satisfy thirst, and they maintain fluid balance through various physiologic processes. Either dehydration or edema (the collection of fluid in body tissues) evidences changes in the water balance of the body. Dehydration occurs from conditions such as severe diarrhea or vomiting, whereas causes of edema include diseases of the cardiovascular or renal system and trauma. Measuring intake and output, testing the resiliency of the skin, checking the condition of the skin and mucous membranes, and weighing the patient help assess water balance.

Food is a physiologic need, with balance maintained through digestive and metabolic processes. The need for food is manifested through hunger. Insufficient nutrient intake results in nutrient and electrolyte imbalances and weight loss. A component of the digestive processes that is also a physiologic need is elimination. Waste products are eliminated from the body through the skin, lungs, kidneys, and intestines. Nutritional status is assessed with a variety of indicators, including weight, muscle mass, strength, and laboratory values.

The human body functions best within a narrow range of temperatures, usually considered as plus or minus 98.6°F (37°C). Homeostatic mechanisms and adaptive responses, such as shivering, maintain this temperature. Nurses assess body temperature as a vital sign (discussed in Chapter 24).

Sexuality is an integral component of each individual and may be affected by physical and emotional illnesses. Sexual practices are dependent on a variety of factors, such as a per-

son's age, sociocultural background, self-esteem, and level of health. There is increasing awareness in healthcare that the consideration of sexuality is a vital part of holistic care.

➤ *Recall Rolanda Simpkins, the 16-year-old girl described at the beginning of the chapter requesting information about contraception. The nurse would use knowledge about Rolanda's sexuality and sexual practices in helping to determine the most appropriate method of contraception for her.* ■

Physical activity and rest are also basic physiologic needs. Physical activity is primarily accomplished by intact and functioning neuromuscular and skeletal systems. Rest and sleep allow time for the body to rejuvenate and be free of stress. Individual requirements for rest and sleep vary widely, but the effects of deprivation have been well documented as significant. Factors that influence sleep are age, environment, exercise, stress, and drug use.

➤ *Think back to Samuel Kaplan, the older man caring for his wife with Alzheimer's disease at home. The nurse would assess the effect of providing this care on his activity, rest, and sleep patterns, thereby developing an appropriate plan of care for Mr. Kaplan to ensure that his needs are met.* ■

Safety and Security Needs

Safety and security needs come next in priority and involve both physical and emotional components. Physical safety and security means being protected from potential or actual harm. Nurses carry out a wide variety of activities to meet patients' physical safety needs, such as the following:

- Using proper hand hygiene and sterile techniques to prevent infection
- Using electrical equipment properly
- Administering medications knowledgeably
- Using skill when moving and ambulating patients
- Teaching parents about household chemicals that are dangerous to children

Emotional safety and security involves trusting others and being free of fear, anxiety, and apprehension. Patients entering the healthcare system often fear the unknown and may have significant emotional security needs. Nurses can help meet such needs by encouraging spiritual practices that are a source of strength and support, by allowing as much independent decision making and control as possible, and by carefully explaining new and unfamiliar procedures and treatments.

➤ *Remember Carlotta Rios, the adolescent described in the Reflective Practice display? The nurse fosters the development of a trusting relationship to promote emotional safety and security. Doing so would assist Carlotta in her decision-making process about going home.* ■

Love and Belonging Needs

All humans have a basic need for love and belonging. After physiologic and safety and security needs, this is the next priority and is often called a higher-level need. **Love and belonging needs** include the understanding and acceptance of others in both giving and receiving love, and the feeling of belonging to families, peers, friends, a neighborhood, and a community.

People who believe that their love and belonging needs are unmet often feel lonely and isolated. They may withdraw physically and emotionally, or they may become overly demanding and critical. Often, these behaviors are a signal that the person has unmet love and belonging needs. Nurses should always consider love and belonging needs when developing a plan of care (Fig. 4-2). Some nursing interventions to help meet this need are as follows:

- Including family and friends in the care of the patient
- Establishing a nurse–patient relationship based on mutual understanding and trust (by demonstrating caring, encouraging communication, and respecting privacy)
- Referring patients to specific support groups (such as a cancer support group or Alcoholics Anonymous)

> *Think back to Samuel Kaplan, the man caring for his wife with Alzheimer's disease. The nurse could refer Mr. Kaplan to a support group for caregivers of patients with Alzheimer's disease to help in meeting Mr. Kaplan's needs for love and belonging.* ■

Self-Esteem Needs

The next highest priority on the hierarchy is **self-esteem needs,** which include the need for a person to feel good about himself or herself, to feel pride and a sense of accomplishment, and to believe that others also respect and appreciate those accomplishments. Positive self-esteem facilitates the individual's confidence and independence.

FIGURE 4-2. By providing time for the mother and newborn to bond, the nurse is helping to fulfill the need for love and belonging of both mother and child.

Many factors affect self-esteem. When a person's role changes (e.g., through a job change or through the death of a spouse), self-esteem can be seriously altered because the person's responsibilities and relationships have also changed. Other changes that may affect self-esteem include a change in body image, such as the loss of a breast, an injury, or a growth spurt during puberty. Nurses must remember that the person's perception of the change—rather than the actual change itself—is what affects that individual's self-esteem.

Nurses can help meet patients' self-esteem needs by respecting their values and beliefs, encouraging patients to set attainable goals, and facilitating support from family or significant others. These actions promote a sense of worth and self-acceptance.

Self-Actualization Needs

The highest level on the hierarchy of needs is **self-actualization needs,** which include the need for individuals to reach their full potential through development of their unique capabilities. In general, each lower level of need must be met to some degree before this need can be satisfied. The process of self-actualization is one that continues throughout life. Maslow lists the following qualities that indicate achievement of one's potential:

- Acceptance of self and others as they are
- Focus of interest on problems outside oneself
- Ability to be objective
- Feelings of happiness and affection for others
- Respect for all people
- Ability to discriminate between good and evil
- Creativity as a guideline for solving problems and pursuing interests

To help meet patients' self-actualization needs, the nurse focuses on the person's strengths and possibilities rather than on problems. Nursing interventions are aimed at providing a sense of direction and hope and providing teaching that is aimed at maximizing potentials.

> *Recall Carlotta Rios, the 17-year-old who had attempted suicide. By focusing on her strengths as well as providing her with a sense of direction through decision making, the nurse helps to meet Carlotta's self-actualization needs.* ■

Applying Maslow's Theory

Nurses can apply Maslow's hierarchy of basic needs in the assessment, planning, implementation, and evaluation of patient care. The hierarchy can be used with patients at any age, in all settings where care is provided, and in both health and illness. It helps the nurse identify unmet needs as they become healthcare needs. The hierarchy of basic needs allows the nurse to locate the patient on the health–illness continuum and to incorporate the human dimensions and health models into meeting needs (Table 4-1).

	Basic Human Need	Examples
Physical dimension	Physiologic needs	Breathing Circulation Temperature Intake of food and fluids Elimination of wastes Movement
Environmental dimension	Safety and security needs	Housing Community/ neighborhood Climate
Sociocultural dimension	Love and belonging needs	Relationships with others Communications with others Support systems Being part of a community Feeling loved by others
Emotional dimension	Self-esteem needs	Fear Sadness Loneliness Happiness Accepting self
Intellectual and spiritual dimensions	Self-actualization needs	Thinking Learning Decision making Values Beliefs Fulfillment Helping others

TABLE • 4-1 THE HUMAN DIMENSIONS AND BASIC HUMAN NEEDS

As the nurse identifies and carries out interventions to help meet patients' needs, it is important to remember that this is only a framework or guideline and that, in actuality, each individual sets priorities for meeting needs on levels most important to that person. Additionally, basic human needs are interrelated and may require nursing actions at more than one level at a given time. For example, in caring for a person coming into the emergency department with a heart attack, the nurse's immediate concern is the patient's physiologic needs (i.e., oxygen and pain relief). At the same time, however, safety needs (e.g., following proper precautions with oxygen use and ensuring the person does not fall off the examining table) and love and belonging needs (e.g., letting a family member stay with the person, if possible) are still major considerations. You will learn how nurses meet basic human needs throughout the rest of this book.

THE FAMILY

Almost every person is a member of a number of groups, such as friends, colleagues at work, or members of a church

or school class. Each of these groups involves a specific part of the person's life and is important to the person. Only one group, however, is concerned with all parts of a person's life and with meeting his or her basic human needs to promote health. That group is the family.

A **family** can be defined simply as any group of people who live together and are emotionally bonded. Families exist in all sizes and configurations and are essential to the health and survival of the individual family members, as well as to society as a whole. The family is a buffer between the needs of the individual member and the demands and expectations of society. The role of the family is to help meet the basic human needs of its members while also meeting the needs of society (Friedman, Bowden, & Jones, 2003).

Family Structures

A family may consist of two or more people. The members of the family may be unrelated either biologically or legally, may be of the same gender, and/or may include several generations (such as grandparents raising grandchildren). Nurses must remember that there are no absolute "rights" or "wrongs" about what makes a family, and one person's values must not be imposed on another person. Respect for of all kinds of family members and relationships is essential to holistic, individualized patient care.

Nuclear Family

The **nuclear family,** also called the traditional family, is composed of two parents and their children. The parents might be heterosexual or homosexual, are often married or in a committed relationship, and all members of the family live in the same house until the children leave home as young adults. The nuclear family may be composed of biologic parents and children, adoptive parents and children, surrogate parents and children, or stepparents and children.

In the classic nuclear family, the father was the family member who went to work, providing economic security, whereas the mother stayed at home, providing physical and emotional safety and security. This family group usually lived in close geographic proximity to relatives, such as aunts, uncles, and grandparents, who are a part of the **extended family.** Couples without children and couples with grown children who no longer live at home are considered traditional families as well. The **blended family** is also a traditional family, formed when parents bring unrelated children from previous relationships together to form a new family.

The contemporary nuclear family still has the same basic form, but the roles of the members have changed considerably. The two major causes of this change are increased education and career opportunities for women and changes in our economy resulting in a need for additional income to maintain a desired standard of living. As a result, two-career families, in which both parents work outside the home, have become the norm. When both parents work, there is usually a blending of tasks, with both parents taking a more active role in housework and childcare as well as economic support.

With changes in family structure have come other influences on the basic human needs of family members. Considerations for the family, and for nursing care, include support systems (in our mobile society, family members may live hundreds or thousands of miles away), availability of childcare, time for leisure and recreation, struggles to meet financial commitments, and changing role models.

Single-Parent Family

Single parents may be separated, divorced, widowed, or never married. Increasing numbers of never-married men and women are choosing to become parents. It is estimated that more than one fourth of all children in North America live in single-parent families. Many single-parent families are African American and headed by women. Single parents have special problems and needs, including financial concerns and role shifts (i.e., having the roles of both parents), becoming remarried or having new relationships. These problems are important considerations when planning and implementing nursing care.

Other Family Structures

In addition to traditional and single-parent families, cohabiting adults and single adults are other family structures. Cohabiting families are individuals who choose to live together for a variety of reasons—relationships, financial need, or changing values. Cohabiting families include unmarried adults (of any age, including retired people who choose not to marry because it would impose financial hardship) living together, and communal or group marriages. Other family structures include binuclear (where divorced parents assume joint custody of children) and dyadic nuclear (in which the couple chooses not to have children).

Single adults may not be living with others, but they are part of a family of origin, usually have a social network with significant others, or may even regard a pet as family. Most single adults living alone are either young adults who achieve independence and enter the workforce or older adults who never married or are left alone after the death of a spouse.

Family Functions

Families have functions that are important in how individual family members meet their basic human needs and maintain their health. The family provides the individual with the necessary environment for development and social interactions. Families also are important to society as a whole because they provide new and socialized members for society.

The five major areas of family function are physical, economic, reproductive, affective and coping, and socialization. Physically, the family provides a safe, comfortable environment necessary for growth, development, and rest or recuperation. Economically, the family provides financial aid to family members and also helps meet monetary needs of society. The reproductive function of the family is raising children. The affective and coping function of the family involves providing emotional comfort to family members. It

also helps members to establish an identity and to maintain that identity in times of stress. Finally, through socialization, the family teaches; transmits beliefs, values, attitudes, and coping mechanisms; provides feedback; and guides problem solving (Friedman, Bowden, & Jones, 2003).

Developmental Tasks of Families

Duvall (1977) identified critical family developmental tasks and stages in the family life cycle. Duvall's theory, based on Erikson's theory of psychosocial development (described in Chapter 18), states that all families have certain basic tasks for survival and continuity and specific tasks related to the sequential stages of development throughout the life of the family. These stages and related developmental tasks are outlined in Table 4-2. If the family does meet certain developmental tasks, societal disapproval may lead to intervention by children's services, social services, police departments, welfare agencies, or health departments (Edelman & Mandle, 2010). The successful mastery of each developmental stage is important to the family's adaptation and growth through successive stages.

The Family in Health and Illness

Individuals learn healthcare activities, health beliefs, and health values in the family. In health and illness, as well as in other areas of life, the individual reflects behaviors learned from the family. When patients enter the healthcare system, they bring their own personal behaviors and needs, but they also bring (in a sense) their family too.

Friedman and associates (2003) identified the importance of family-centered nursing care, based on four rationales. First, the family is composed of interdependent members who affect one another. If some form of illness occurs in one member, all other members become a part of the illness. Second, a strong relationship exists between the family and the health status of its members; therefore, the role of the family is essential in every level of nursing care. The third rationale is that the level of health of the family and, in turn, each member, can be significantly improved through health promotion activities. Finally, illness of one family member may suggest the possibility of the same problem in other members. Through assessment and intervention, the nurse can assist in improving the health status of all family members.

Illness may precipitate a health crisis in a family. Brief changes in family tasks may occur if an illness is relatively minor, such as a viral infection in a child. If an injury or illness to a family member is serious, roles and responsibilities, as well as functions, of individual family members change. This is especially true if the illness is chronic and long-term, results in disability, or decreases time to live. Some families find it difficult to adapt to the stress of changes in financial, social, and caregiving resources, whereas other families experience renewed family closeness and stability. Regardless of how the family adapts, members of the family must constantly adjust roles and responsibilities to manage the needs of the ill family member and the family.

TABLE • 4-2	FAMILY STAGES, TASKS, HEALTH RISK FACTORS, AND NURSING INTERVENTIONS TO PROMOTE HEALTH		
Family Stage*	**Tasks**	**Risk Factors**	**Nursing Interventions/ Referrals**
Couple and family with children	Establish a mutually satisfying marriage Plan to have or not to have children Have and adjust to infant Support needs of all family members Adjust to cost of family life Adapt to needs and activity of children Cope with loss of energy and privacy Encourage and support growth and development and educational achievements	Inadequate knowledge of contraception and family Inadequate knowledge of sexual and marital roles Lack of knowledge about child safety and health Child abuse and neglect First pregnancy before age 16 Inadequate nutrition; obesity Drug and alcohol abuse Sexually transmitted diseases Rubella	Family planning clinics Prenatal classes Well-child clinics Immunization information Vision and hearing screenings Dental health information Parent support groups Communicable disease control Safety in the home, daycare, school, neighborhood, and community
Family with adolescents and young adults	Maintain open communications Support moral and ethical family values Balance teenagers' freedom with responsibility Maintain supportive home base Strengthen marital relationships	Family of origin Low socioeconomic status Family value of aggressiveness Dependence on welfare Inadequate problem-solving abilities Conflict between family members Physical or sexual abuse Use of drugs or alcohol Sexually transmitted diseases	Alcohol and drug information Accident prevention programs Sex education Nutrition support groups Mental health programs Screening for chronic illness
Family with middle-aged adults	Maintain ties with younger and older generations Prepare for retirement	Diet high in fat, sugar, salt Obesity Use of drugs or alcohol Physical inactivity Depression Exposure to environmental or work-related health risks, such as sunlight, asbestos, radiation, coal dust, and air or water pollution	Blood pressure screenings Screening for chronic illness Nutrition information Support groups (e.g., for loss, grief, smoking cessation, alcohol or drug abuse)
Family with older adults	Adjust to retirement Adjust to loss of spouse May move from family home	Increasing age with loss of physical function Chronic illness Poor nutrition Lack of exercise Depression Death of spouse Limited income Past lifestyle	Screening for chronic illness Nutrition information Exercise information Home safety information Retirement information Pharmacology information

Data from Duvall, E. (1977). *Marriage and family development* (5th ed.). Philadelphia: J. B. Lippincott; Aldous, J. (1975). *The developmental approach to family analysis.* Minneapolis: University of Minnesota Press.

*Family includes all forms: nuclear, extended, single-parent, etc.

▶ *Remember Mr. Kaplan, the 80-year-old man caring for his wife with Alzheimer's disease? Now the primary caregiver, Mr. Kaplan's role has changed. The disease and family member role changes may affect the family's ability to function. The nurse would incorporate knowledge of this when developing the most appropriate plan for Mr. Kaplan and his wife.* ■

Nursing interventions for the family in a health crisis include providing teaching that is honest, open, and respectful; using therapeutic communication skills; applying knowledge of family dynamics; and making referrals to community healthcare and financial resources to support realistic hope. In addition, it is important to involve family members in the plan of care and the implementation of care.

Family Risk Factors

Family patterns of behavior, the environment in which the family lives, and genetic factors can all place family members at risk for health problems (see the Research in Nursing box). It is important for nurses to assess these factors before developing nursing care plans. Typical questions that should be part of a family assessment include the following:

- What is the family structure?
- What is the family's socioeconomic status?
- What are the cultural backgrounds and religious affiliations of family members?
- Who cares for children if both parents work?
- What health practices are common (e.g., types of foods eaten, meal times, immunizations, bedtime, exercise)?
- What habits are common (e.g., do any family members smoke, drink to excess, or use drugs)?
- How does the family cope with stress?
- Do close friends or family members live nearby, and can they help if necessary?

> *These questions would be extremely important to ask when assessing Carlotta Rios, the adolescent described in the Reflective Practice display, and Samuel Kaplan, the older adult caring for his ill wife at home. Each patient's answers to these questions would provide the nurse with valuable*

information about determining the best way to meet each patient's needs. For Carlotta, this would include information about viable options for her living arrangements that provide physical and emotional safety. For Mr. Kaplan, answers would provide information about available sources of help so that he can continue to care for his wife at home, or if necessary, ease the transition and adjustment to moving his wife to a long-term care facility. ■

When conducting a health assessment for a family, the nurse should consider the risk factors for altered health described in Box 4-1.

Nursing Interventions to Promote Health

The role of the nurse in reducing risk factors involves activities that promote health for all family members at any level of development. Each person has his or her own definition of health, based on family beliefs and values about health and illness. Through interventions that emphasize health, the nurse assists both the individual and the family to meet their basic human needs. Examples of nursing interventions to promote health in the family are shown in Table 4-2. Nurses may carry out such activities themselves or may refer the individual or family to other healthcare providers for additional education.

RESEARCH IN NURSING
Bridging the Gap to Evidence-Based Practice

DISCLOSING GENETIC TEST RESULTS TO FAMILY MEMBERS

All humans are composed of genes, which are the basic units of heredity that direct the structure, development, and function of the human body. The international Human Genome Project, which analyzed the structure of human DNA and determined the location of all genes on chromosomes, has greatly influenced all areas of healthcare, including nursing practice. With increased knowledge of how genes affect both human growth and development and health and disease, healthcare providers will be better able to promote health and prevent illness. It is increasingly obvious that nurses must become knowledgeable of genetics to effectively integrate that knowledge into the care and counseling of patients in a variety of diverse settings.

Related Research

Hamilton, R., Bowers, B., & Williams, J. (2005). Disclosing genetic test results to family members. *Journal of Nursing Scholarship, 37*(1), 18–24.

This study was conducted to describe the experiences of family members tested for Huntington's disease or hereditary breast and ovarian cancer as they disclosed genetic test results to biological family members. The primary focus of the study was to gain an increased understanding of how people at risk understand and communicate test results, as well as the dynamics of

family relationships and communication. Most of the study participants used three processes when disclosing genetic test results: (1) they considered the effects on themselves and family members, (2) they selectively disclosed particular aspects of the information, and (3) they planned the timing of the disclosure by assessing how vulnerable and receptive to the information the family member was (e.g., based on life situations, personality, and age). Information was disclosed after deciding who could "handle it" and a desire to protect family members from harm by determining the right time for disclosure.

Relevance to Nursing Practice

Disclosing that one has had genetic testing for a hereditary disease affects not only the person tested, but also the family members. Determining what is heard when genetic test results are disclosed to family members is a part of the genetic testing process. Nurses who provide genetic counseling must consider both the perceptions of the person being tested and the ability of that person to share information with family members. Interventions to provide support for the person being tested should be based on the knowledge that the patient recognizes a responsibility to warn others but at the same time realizes that disclosure of test results will make a family disease more obvious.

For additional research, visit thePoint.

Box 4-1   RISK FACTORS FOR ALTERED FAMILY HEALTH

Lifestyle Risk Factors

- Lack of knowledge about sexual and marital roles, leading to teenage marriage and pregnancy; divorce; sexually transmitted infections; child, spouse, or elder abuse; and lack of prenatal or child care
- Alterations in nutrition—either more or less than body requirements at any age
- Chemical dependency, including the use of alcohol, drugs, and nicotine
- Inadequate dental care and hygiene
- Unsafe or unstimulating home environment

Psychosocial Risk Factors

- Inadequate childcare resources, when both parents work, for preschool and school-aged children
- Inadequate income to provide safe housing, food, clothing, and healthcare
- Conflict between family members

Environmental Risk Factors

- Lack of knowledge or finances to provide safe and clean living conditions
- Work or social pressures that cause stress
- Air, water, or food pollution

Developmental Risk Factors

- Families who have new babies, especially if support systems are unavailable
- Older people, especially those living alone or on a fixed income
- Unmarried adolescent mothers who lack personal, economic, and educational resources

Biologic Risks

- Birth defects
- Mental retardation
- Genetic predisposition to certain diseases, including cardiovascular diseases and cancer

The family is the primary educational and support structure for the individual. The family, as a social unit, provides the environment and relationships necessary for members to meet their basic human needs. Health beliefs and practices are learned within the family context and are influenced by the family's developmental level. Health promotion activities and nursing actions can reduce the risk for illness and facilitate healthy behaviors at any age within the family life cycle.

> *Consider Rolanda Simpkins, the adolescent seeking contraceptive information. The nurse would need to evaluate further Rolanda's statement that her mother would "kill her," questioning Rolanda further to determine the family's health beliefs and practices.* ∎

THE COMMUNITY

A person, as an individual and as a member of a family, is also a member of a community. The community environment affects the ability of the individual to meet basic human needs. This section discusses the relationship of the community to basic human needs, including influences on health and illness.

A **community** can be defined in a variety of ways, but the most basic definition is that a community is a specific population or group of people living in the same geographic area under similar regulations and having common values, interests, and needs. A community may be a small neighborhood in a major urban city or a large rural area encompassing a small town. Communities are formed by the characteristics of people, area, social interaction, and common familial, cultural, or ethnic heritage and ties. Within a community, people interact and share resources.

Many community factors affect the health of residents. A healthy community provides elements that enable people to maintain a high quality of life and productivity. For example, a healthy community:

- Offers access to healthcare services for all members of the community, which provide both treatment for illnesses and activities to promote health
- Has roads, schools, playgrounds and other services to meet needs of the people in the community
- Provides and maintains a safe and healthy environment

Health of the residents of a community is affected by the social support systems, the community health structure, environmental factors, and types of agencies providing assistance for those in need of shelter, housing, and food. Examples of community factors affecting health are listed in Box 4-2 and are discussed further in the following sections.

Box 4-2   EXAMPLES OF COMMUNITY FACTORS AFFECTING HEALTH

- Number and availability of healthcare institutions and services
- Housing codes
- Police and fire departments
- Nutritional services for low-income infants, mothers, school-aged children (e.g., lunch programs), and older people
- Zoning regulations separating residential and industrial areas
- Waste disposal services and locations
- Air and water pollution
- Food sanitation
- Health education services and dissemination
- Recreational opportunities
- Violent crimes or drug use

Social Support Systems

The social support systems of an individual are made up of all the people who help meet financial, personal, physical, and emotional needs. In most instances, family, friends, and neighbors provide the best social support within a community. To understand the social support systems of a community, it is important to know who and what provides support (such as family, neighbors, friends, church, and organizations).

Community Healthcare Structure

The healthcare structure of a community has a direct effect on the health of the people living within it. The size and location of the community often determine the types of services available. For example, urban residents have various means of transportation to a variety of healthcare providers, whereas rural residents might need to travel long distances for care. In addition, the county and state funding for community healthcare services also determines the type and number of healthcare institutions and agencies that are available.

Economic Resources

Financial and insurance coverage affect an individual's access to healthcare services within a community. As private health insurance costs continue to escalate, fewer citizens have it. Many part-time and unskilled jobs provide no insurance benefits at all, resulting in a substantial number of citizens who do not have any financial assistance for healthcare screenings or care for illnesses. Although this problem is being examined by state and federal policy makers, no clear solution is yet available.

Environmental Factors

The environment of the community in which an individual lives and works might have both helpful and harmful effects on health. The quality of air and water differ across communities. Large urban areas are often affected by air pollution, whereas smaller communities may be at risk for water pollution from run-off of chemical or livestock wastes. There is also increasing concern about how global warming affects health. Environmental barriers to accessing healthcare within a community include lack of transportation, distance to services, and location of the services.

Effect on Individuals and Families

The community has a strong influence on health promotion and illness-prevention activities of individuals and families in the community (Fig. 4-3). Just as there are family risk factors for the health of individual members, so are there community risk factors involving resources, economics, and services. For nursing assessments and interventions to be comprehensive and individualized, the nurse must also consider the community's influence.

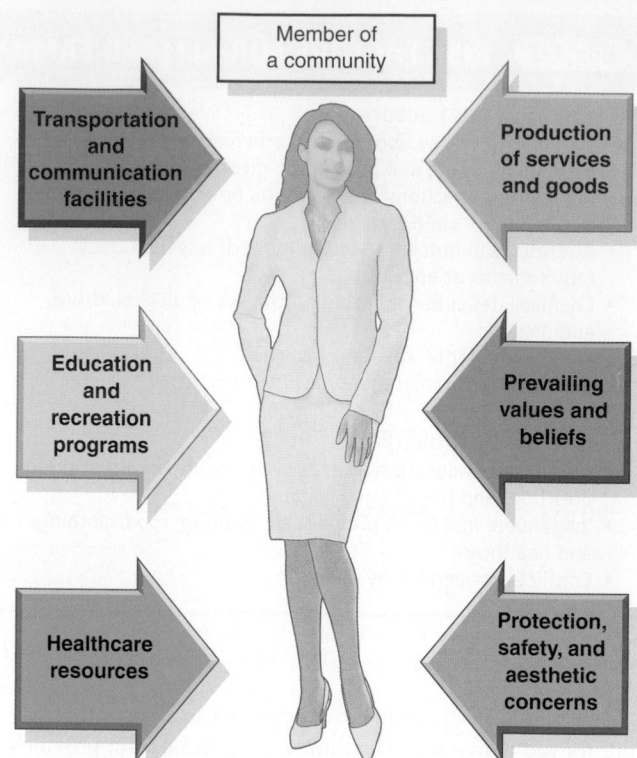

FIGURE 4-3. Many characteristics of a community influence the health of its members. This diagram shows six categories of characteristics that influence the health of a member of a community.

To illustrate how the community can affect the individual's and family's needs, consider the following examples. Maria, 20 years old, lives in an inner-city, two-room apartment with her 6-month-old baby girl. The apartment lacks adequate heat and plumbing. Maria has no family living nearby, and her husband has left her. Maria rarely leaves her apartment because she fears the street gangs and drug addicts. She has never taken her baby to a local clinic for checkups because she doesn't know how to get there.

Anne, 22 years old, lives in a small house in a rural area with her 2-year-old son. She is a single mother and works as a secretary at an insurance agency. Anne often sees her family members, who live nearby. Anne and her son have regular health assessments.

These two different examples illustrate that the community plays a major role in the health of people who live there. Maria and her baby are at much greater risk for illness than are Anne and her son. Even if the two women had identical healthcare needs, their care plans would have different interventions because of their different community environments.

Nursing in the Community

In contrast to community health nursing, which focuses on populations within a community, community-based nursing is centered on individual and family healthcare needs.

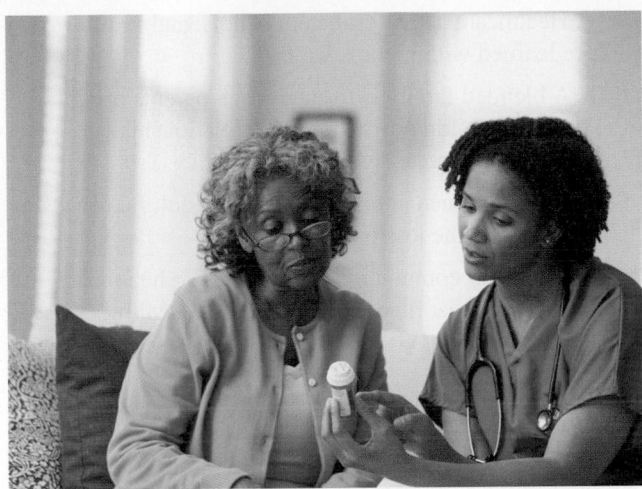

FIGURE 4-4. A nurse at work in a home healthcare setting.

The nurses practicing community-based nursing provide interventions to manage acute or chronic health problems, promote health, and facilitate self-care. The nursing care provided within a community must be culturally competent and family centered.

Nurses providing community-based care must know about the location and specialty of healthcare providers, the availability and accessibility of services and supplies, and public health services. Other factors to consider include facilities (such as daycare or long-term care), housing, and the number and type of agencies providing services.

Nurses carry out a variety of activities that involve the community, designed to promote health and prevent illness. Nurses promote health as individuals, as caregivers within institutional settings, and as community-based healthcare providers. Nurses also provide community services as volunteers in health-related activities (e.g., screenings, educational programs, and blood drives) and as role models for health practices and lifestyles. Nurses working in a variety of healthcare settings consider community influences when developing individualized nursing care plans and when making referrals to community agencies and support groups. Community-based nurses are employed in many different kinds of practice settings, including home care (Fig. 4-4), community health centers, school nursing, occupational nursing, and independent nursing practice. Community-based care is discussed in more detail in Chapter 8.

● Developing Critical Thinking Skills

1. What do you believe to be the most important basic human need that is actually or potentially unmet in the following situations?
   - A toddler falls into a swimming pool.
   - An elderly woman falls at home and is not found for 3 days.
   - A preschooler is admitted to the hospital with multiple bruises and burn marks.
   - A teenager is constantly told "you are no good" by his parents.
   - A nursing home resident says, "I never did anything right in my life."

2. Our own family experiences often affect the way we relate to the families of our patients. Describe at least two possible responses to the families described below.
   - Suspecting child abuse, a nurse asks a mother about her child's bruises. The woman says, "In our family, we believe in 'spare the rod and spoil the child.'"
   - A single woman wants to have a child and comes to a fertility clinic for information on artificial insemination.
   - Several members of a patient's large, extended family are in the patient's long-term care facility room and are trying to do everything for the patient.

● Practicing for NCLEX

1. A nurse is providing care based on Maslow's hierarchy of basic human needs. For which of the following nursing activities is this approach useful?
   a. Making accurate nursing diagnoses
   b. Establishing priorities of care
   c. Communicating concerns more concisely
   d. Integrating science into nursing care

2. Which of the following levels of basic human needs is most basic?
   a. Physiologic
   b. Safety and security
   c. Love and belonging
   d. Self-actualization

3. Of all the physiologic needs, which one is the most essential?
   a. Food
   b. Water
   c. Elimination
   d. Oxygen

4. Practicing careful hand hygiene and using sterile techniques are ways in which nurses meet which basic human need?
   a. Physiologic
   b. Safety and security
   c. Self-esteem
   d. Love and belonging

5. Of the following statements, which one is true of self-actualization?
   a. Humans are born with fully developed self-actualization.
   b. Self-actualization needs are met by having confidence and independence.

c. The self-actualization process continues throughout life.

d. Loneliness and isolation occur when self-actualization needs are unmet.

6. What is the best broad definition of a family?
   a. A father, a mother, and children
   b. A group whose members are biologically related
   c. A unit that includes aunts, uncles, and cousins
   d. A group of people who live together

7. Where do individuals learn their health beliefs and values?
   a. In the family
   b. In school
   c. From school nurses
   d. From peers

8. John and Mary, each parents of one child, are both divorced. When they marry, the family structure that is formed will be described as which of the following?
   a. Nuclear family
   b. Extended family
   c. Blended family
   d. Cohabiting family

9. Which of the following is one of the developmental tasks of the older adult family?
   a. Maintain a supportive home base
   b. Prepare for retirement
   c. Cope with loss of energy and privacy
   d. Adjust to loss of spouse

10. Which of the following is one element of a healthy community?
    a. Meets all the needs of its inhabitants
    b. Offers access to healthcare services
    c. Has mixed residential and industrial areas
    d. Is little concerned with air and water quality

● Answers With Rationale

1. *b.* Maslow's hierarchy of basic human needs is useful for establishing priorities of care.

2. *a.* Physiologic needs are the most basic and must be met at least minimally to sustain life.

3. *d.* Oxygen is the most essential of all needs because all body cells require oxygen for survival.

4. *b.* By carrying out careful hand hygiene and using sterile technique, nurses provide safety from infection.

5. *c.* Self-actualization, or reaching one's full potential, is a process that continues through life.

6. *d.* Although all the responses may be true, the best definition is a group of people who live together.

7. *a.* Healthcare activities, health beliefs, and health values are learned within one's family.

8. *c.* A blended family is formed when parents bring unrelated children from previous relationships together to form a new family.

9. *d.* A developmental task of the older adult family is adjusting to the loss of a spouse.

10. *b.* A healthy community offers access to healthcare services to treat illness and to promote health.

Taylor Suite Resources

The Taylor Suite offers these additional resources to enhance learning and facilitate understanding of this chapter:

- thePoint online resource, http://thepoint.lww.com/Taylor7E
- Student DVD included with the book
- Study Guide for Taylor's Fundamentals of Nursing

BIBLIOGRAPHY

Aldous, J. (1975). *The developmental approach to family analysis.* Minneapolis: University of Minnesota Press.

American Nurses Association (ANA). (2005). *ANA's health care agenda 2005.* Washington, DC: Author.

Boltz, M. (2007). Assessing family preferences for participation in care in hospitalized older adults. *Try This: Best Practices in Nursing Care to Older Adults, 22.* Available at http://consultgerirn.org/uploads/File/trythis/issue22.pdf

Condon, M., & Welker-Hood, K. (2007). Environment, health, and safety. *American Nurse Today, 2*(6), 56.

Duvall, E. (1977). *Marriage and family development* (5th ed.). Philadelphia: J.B. Lippincott.

Ebersole, P., Touhy, T., Hess, P., Jett, K., & Luggen, A. (2007). *Toward healthy aging: Human needs and nursing response* (7th ed.). St. Louis: Mosby.

Edelman, C., & Mandle, C. (2010). *Health promotion throughout the lifespan* (7th ed.). St. Louis: Mosby Elsevier.

Friedman, M., Bowden, V., & Jones, E. (2003). *Family nursing: Research, theory, and practice* (5th ed.). Upper Saddle River, NJ: Prentice Hall.

Hamilton, R., Bowers, B., & Williams, J. (2005). Disclosing genetic test results to family members. *Journal of Nursing Scholarship, 37*(1), 18–24.

Hoffman, E. (2008). The Maslow effect: A humanist legacy for nursing. *American Nurse Today, 3*(8), 36–37.

Jacobson, J. (2008). The top news stories of 2007 (Uninsured and underinsured Americans…). *American Journal of Nursing, 108*(1), 19.

Long, S., Liu, K., Black, K., O'Keeffe, J., & Molony, S. (2005). Getting by in the community: Lessons from frail elders. *Journal of Aging & Social Policy, 17*(1), 19–44.

Maslow, A. (1968). *Toward a psychology of being* (2nd ed.). New York: Van Nostrand–Reinhold.

Miyashita, M., Morita, T., & Hirai, K. (2008). Evaluation of end-of-life cancer care from the perspective of bereaved family members: The Japanese experience. *Journal of Clinical Oncology, 26*(23), 3845–3852.

NANDA International. (2009). *Nursing diagnoses: Definitions & classification, 2009–2011.* Oxford: Wiley-Blackwell.

O'Connor, A., & Roy, C. (2008). Electric power plant emission & public health. *American Journal of Nursing, 108*(2), 62–69.

Pender, N. J., Murdaugh, C., & Parsons, M. A. (2006). *Health promotion in nursing practice* (6th ed.). Upper Saddle River, NJ: Prentice Hall.

Snitzer, P., & Ewigman, B. (2008). Household composition and fatal unintentional injuries related to child maltreatment. *Journal of Nursing Scholarship, 40*(1), 91–97.

Stanhope, M., & Lancaster, J. (2010). *Foundations of community health nursing—community oriented practice* (3rd ed.). St. Louis: Mosby Elsevier.

U.S. Department of Health and Human Services. (2000). *Healthy people 2010.* Washington, DC: Author.

Vandall-Walker, V., Jensen, L., & Oberle, K. (2007). Nursing support for family members of critically ill adults. *Qualitative Health Research, 17*(9), 1207–1218.

Zwillich, T. (2007). Experts: Global warming affects health. WebMD Health. Available at http://www.medscape.com/viewarticle/564806

5 Theory, Research, and Evidence-Based Practice

JOE WIMMER

Joe, a first-time father of a healthy 8-lb baby girl delivered several hours ago, is visiting with his wife and new daughter. He asks, "Why is my daughter wearing that funny little cap on her head?"

CHARLOTTE HORN

Charlotte, the daughter of a 57-year-old patient being discharged with an order for intermittent nasogastric tube feedings, is being taught how to perform the procedure. During one of the teaching sessions, Charlotte asks, "How will I know that the tube is in the right place?"

MARIBELLA SANTOS

Maribella, who had just arrived back on the unit after undergoing abdominal surgery, is complaining of nausea. A while later she states, "My nausea is gone. The nurse did something with her hands and the feeling just went away."

After completing the chapter, you will be able to accomplish the following:

1. Explain the sources of, types of, and historical influences on nursing knowledge.

2. Compare and contrast systems theory, adaptation theory, and developmental theory.

3. Explain the significance of the four concepts common to all nursing theories.

4. Discuss the evolution of nursing research.

5. Compare and contrast quantitative and qualitative research methods.

6. Describe evidence-based practice in nursing, including the rationale for its use.

7. Outline the steps in implementing evidence-based practice.

8. Read and understand, on a beginning level, a published research article.

KEY TERMS

applied research
basic research
concept
conceptual framework
  or model
data
deductive reasoning
evidence-based practice
evidence-based practice
  guideline
inductive reasoning
informed consent
nursing research
nursing theory
philosophy
process
qualitative research
quantitative research
research
science
systematic review
theory

Nursing is a unique healthcare discipline in which nurses provide a service based on knowledge and skill. Nursing has two essential elements: a body of knowledge and the application of that knowledge in nursing care interventions. The body of knowledge provides the rationale for nursing interventions. There is a growing knowledge base developed specifically for nursing through theory development and research. (See the accompanying Reflective Practice display for an example.) Rationales for nursing interventions also come from many different disciplines, including anatomy, physiology, chemistry, nutrition, psychology, and sociology.

This chapter discusses the concepts of nursing knowledge, nursing theory, nursing research, and evidence-based practice as separate entities, but in fact, they are often intertwined in clinical practice.

NURSING KNOWLEDGE

Knowledge is an awareness of the reality one acquires through learning or investigation. Every individual collects, organizes, and arranges facts to build a knowledge base relevant to his or her personal reality.

Sources of Knowledge

Knowledge comes from a variety of sources and may be traditional, authoritative, or scientific.

Traditional Knowledge

Traditional knowledge is that part of nursing practice passed down from generation to generation. When questioned about the origin of such nursing practices, nurses might reply, "We've always done it this way." Changing bedclothes is an example of how traditional knowledge has affected nursing practice. It is customary in acute care settings to change a patient's bedclothes daily, whether soiled or not. There are no research data to support this, yet virtually millions of hospital beds are changed daily because this practice is accepted as a necessary component of quality patient care. Until this practice is challenged scientifically and its assumed value disproved, it will remain a traditional part of patient care.

Authoritative Knowledge

Authoritative knowledge comes from an expert and is accepted as truth based on the person's perceived expertise—for example, when a senior staff nurse teaches a new graduate nurse a more efficient method of doing a technical procedure, such as inserting an intravenous catheter. The senior nurse has gained knowledge through experience, and the new graduate nurse accepts it as truth based on the perceived authority of the experienced nurse. Authoritative knowledge generally remains unchallenged as long as the presumed authority maintains his or her perceived expertise.

Scientific Knowledge

Scientific knowledge is that knowledge arrived at through the scientific method (implying through research). New ideas are tested and measured systematically using objective criteria.

> *Think back to Maribella Santos, the woman complaining of nausea after undergoing abdominal surgery. The nurse would integrate scientific knowledge about the effects of surgery and anesthesia on the body and the side effects of pain medication to develop the postoperative plan of care.* ■

REFLECTIVE PRACTICE

Challenge to Cognitive Skills

One of the nurses, Danielle, on a surgical floor where I was assigned, took a course in Therapeutic Touch. When she returned to work, she was eager to use her new "intervention." My patient, Maribella Santos, had come back to the unit after undergoing abdominal surgery. Upon her return, she complained of nausea. Danielle used her "unruffling" technique to calm the patient, whose nausea then "disappeared." Excited, I reported this in postconference, only to learn from my instructor that Therapeutic Touch was "a lot of bunk" without scientific support.

Thinking Outside the Box: Possible Courses of Action

- Accept my instructor's dismissal of Therapeutic Touch.
- Learn more about Therapeutic Touch from my colleague Danielle and professional literature.

- Become an advocate for Therapeutic Touch if it DOES work!

Evaluating a Good Outcome: How Do I Define Success?

- Patient is not harmed by anyone using an unproven therapy.
- Patient benefits from my openness to new (potentially beneficial) therapies.

- I rely on research, not hearsay, as a basis for my clinical judgments and actions.

Personal Learning: Here's to the Future!

I was surprised to find the literature so inconclusive about the benefits of Therapeutic Touch. Obviously, its adherents claim that they can measure its efficacy. Others find these claims unsupported. Since this event happened at the beginning of my clinical rotation, I decided to observe Danielle throughout my rotation. What I saw made me a believer in this technique. Danielle was using

Therapeutic Touch as an adjuvant to other therapies and it seemed to be working. I want to learn more about this technique. My goal is to attend a workshop on Therapeutic Touch to see if it is something I can incorporate into my practice.

Katherine Figliala, Georgetown University

Reflection

How do you think you would respond in a similar situation? Why? What does this tell you about yourself and about the adequacy of your skills for professional practice? Can you think of other ways to respond? What sources of knowledge did the nursing student use? Did the nursing student use theory and research? If so, please explain how. Would you consider Therapeutic Touch to be evidence-based practice? Why or why not? How might the patient's culture have affected the response? What other skills (cognitive, interpersonal, technical, ethical/legal) would you need to respond well in this situation? Propose possible reasons for the instructor's response. Do you agree with the criteria to evaluate a successful outcome? Did the nursing student meet the criteria? Please explain your answer.

Significance of Knowledge Sources

All sources of knowledge are useful in the collective body of knowledge that constitutes the nursing profession. Although these three sources provide nursing with important contributions, each has inherent strengths and limitations. Both traditional and authoritative knowledge are practical to implement but are often based on subjective data, limiting their usefulness in a wide variety of practice settings. For this reason, nurses increasingly focus on scientific knowledge to provide care, commonly called evidence-based practice.

Types of Knowledge

Some of the types of knowledge include science, philosophy, and process.

Science

Science is observing, identifying, describing, investigating, and explaining events and occurrences that are perceived in

the world. It implies a body of knowledge. The science of nursing is the knowledge in and of nursing.

Philosophy

Philosophy is the study of wisdom, fundamental knowledge, and the processes used to develop and construct one's perceptions of life. Philosophy provides a viewpoint and implies a system of values and beliefs. Each individual develops a personal philosophy to give meaning to experiences and to guide behavior and attitudes. Personal philosophies are developed by learning from interpersonal relationships, through formal and informal educational experiences, through religion and culture, and from the environment.

Every nurse's philosophy, developed through education and practice, forms the basis for providing nursing care. Nurses demonstrate both a personal and a professional philosophy through their values and beliefs about concepts such as goodness, health, illness, accountability, and ethics. In the same way, nursing education and nursing practice settings provide education or patient care based on philosophic beliefs about humans, health, teaching and learning, and quality patient care.

Process

A **process** is a series of actions, changes, or functions intended to bring about a desired result. During a process, one takes systematic and continuous steps to meet a goal and uses both assessments and feedback to direct actions to meet the goal. A particular theory or conceptual framework directs how these actions are carried out. The delivery of nursing care within the nursing process (described in Unit III) is directed by the way specific conceptual frameworks and theories define the person (patient), the environment, health, and nursing.

Historical Influences on Nursing Knowledge

The development of nursing knowledge has been influenced by the work of Florence Nightingale and by societal changes.

Nightingale's Contributions

Nightingale influenced nursing knowledge and practice by demonstrating efficient and knowledgeable nursing care, defining nursing practice as separate and distinct from medical practice, and differentiating between health nursing and illness nursing. (See Chapter 1 for further information.)

The training of nurses was initially carried out under the direction and control of the medical profession (Kalish & Kalish, 1995). Because the conceptual and theoretical basis for nursing practice came from outside the profession, nursing struggled for years to establish its own identity and to receive recognition for its significant contributions to healthcare.

Societal Influences on Nursing Knowledge

Most early schools of nursing established in the United States were adapted from Nightingale's model. There was no planned educational curriculum; instead, knowledge was acquired from lectures by physicians and through practical experience by caring for sick people in hospitals. This service orientation for nursing education remained the strongest influence on nursing practice until the 1950s. Nursing care was carried out under the control and direction of the hospital administration and physicians practicing in that hospital. Nursing care was based on traditional ideas about following orders, as well as on common wisdom about caring for others based on either "common sense" or widely accepted scientific principles (Chinn & Kramer, 2008). As a result, nursing knowledge remained undeveloped and fragmented.

During the first half of the 20th century, a change in the structure of society resulted in changed roles for women and, in turn, for nursing. As a result of World Wars I and II, women increasingly entered the workforce, became more independent, and sought higher education. At the same time, nursing education began to focus more on education than hands-on training, and nursing research was conducted and published. As women became more independent and assertive, nursing's need for a clearly defined identity based on unique contributions to the healthcare system emerged. In the mid-20th century, the idea of nursing as a science became more generally accepted, and philosophic beliefs and a knowledge base for nursing practice began to evolve.

NURSING THEORY

A **theory** is composed of a group of concepts that describe a pattern of reality. **Concepts,** like ideas, are abstract impressions organized into symbols of reality. Concepts describe objects, properties, and events and relationships among them. A group of concepts that follows an understandable pattern makes up a **conceptual framework or model.** Concepts can be thought of as the individual bricks and boards used to build a house, with the conceptual framework being the blueprint that specifies where each brick and board should go. Theories can be tested, changed, or used to guide research or to provide a base for evaluation. They are derived through two principal methods: **deductive reasoning,** in which one examines a general idea and then considers specific actions or ideas, and **inductive reasoning,** in which the reverse process is used—one builds from specific ideas or actions to conclusions about general ideas.

Nursing theory is developed to describe nursing. Nursing theory differentiates nursing from other disciplines and activities in that it serves the purposes of describing, explaining, predicting, and controlling desired outcomes of nursing care practices. Thus, theories provide a means of testing knowledge through research and for expanding nursing's knowledge base to meet the healthcare needs of patients in an ever-changing society.

Interdisciplinary Base for Nursing Theories

Nursing theories are often based on, and influenced by, other broadly applicable processes and theories. The ideas and principles of the theories described briefly in the following sections are basic to many nursing concepts and are a part of the nursing literature. Nurses need to understand these theories and terminologies as they develop their own knowledge base in nursing.

General Systems Theory

General systems theory has been used in a wide range of disciplines since it emerged in the 1920s. Its primary theorist, Ludwig von Bertalanffy, developed the theory for universal application. This theory describes how to break whole things into parts and then to learn how the parts work together in "systems." It emphasizes relationships between the whole and the parts and describes how parts function and behave. These concepts may be applied to different kinds of systems, for example, to molecules in chemistry, cultures in sociology, organs in anatomy, and health in nursing. Key points in general systems theory are outlined in Box 5-1.

Box 5-1   KEY POINTS IN GENERAL SYSTEMS THEORY

- A system is a set of interacting elements, all contributing to the overall goal of the system. The whole system is always greater than the sum of its parts.
- Systems are hierarchical in nature and are composed of interrelated subsystems that work together in such a way that a change in one element could affect other subsystems, as well as the whole.
- Boundaries separate systems both from each other and from their environments.
- A system communicates with and reacts to its environment through factors that enter the system (input) or are transferred to the environment (output).
- An open system allows energy, matter, and information to move freely between systems and boundaries, whereas a closed system does not allow input from or output to the environment (no totally closed systems are known to exist in reality).
- To survive, open systems maintain balance through feedback.

> *Recall Maribella Santos, the woman described in the Reflective Practice display who received Therapeutic Touch? The nurse would need to integrate knowledge of systems theory, including system communication, open systems, and energy transfer to better understand the goal of this technique.* ■

Adaptation Theory

Adaptation theory defines adaptation as the adjustment of living matter to other living things and to environmental conditions. Adaptation is a continuously occurring process that effects change and involves interaction and response. Human adaptation occurs on three levels: the internal (self), the social (others), and the physical (biochemical reactions). Chapter 42 describes adaptation in relation to stress.

Developmental Theory

Developmental theory outlines the process of growth and development of humans as orderly and predictable, beginning with conception and ending with death. Although the pattern has definite stages, the progress and behaviors of an individual within each stage are unique. Heredity, temperament, emotional and physical environment, life experiences, and health status influence the growth and development of an individual.

Several theorists have made important contributions to developmental theory, but only two are mentioned here because their work is often used to develop nursing theory and to organize nursing practice. Erikson based his theory of psychosocial development on the process of socialization, emphasizing how individuals learn to interact with the world. Erikson recognized the role of social, biologic, and environmental factors in development, and defined specific tasks or conflicts that people accomplish or over-

come during what he defined as the eight stages of life. Chapters 18, 19, and 20 present more information on developmental theory.

Abraham Maslow developed his theory of human needs in terms of physical and psychosocial needs considered essential to human life, rather than by chronologic age as Erikson did. As described in Chapter 4, Maslow defined five levels of need in a hierarchy, with different needs existing simultaneously.

> *Think back to Joe Wimmer, the new father of a baby girl. When explaining about the use of the cap on the baby's head, the nurse would incorporate knowledge of Maslow's hierarchy of needs, specifically physiologic needs, and the need to minimize heat loss as a priority.* ■

As you continue in your nursing education and practice, you will learn how systems, adaptation, and developmental theories are used in planning and giving holistic care to patients. The following sections on specific nursing theories will help you better understand the knowledge base used to develop the concepts unique to nursing.

Nursing Theories

Even though nurses have difficulty agreeing on precise definitions of nursing, theory-based nursing directs nurses toward a common goal, with the ultimate outcome being improved patient care. Nursing theory provides rational and knowledgeable reasons for nursing interventions, based on descriptions of what nursing is and what nurses do. Additionally, nursing theory gives nurses the knowledge base necessary for acting and responding appropriately in nursing care situations, provides a base for discussion, and, ideally, helps resolve current nursing issues. Theory gives nurses who know and practice theory better problem-solving skills, so that nursing interventions are better organized, considered, and purposeful. Nursing theory also prepares nurses to question assumptions and values in nursing, thus further defining nursing and increasing the knowledge base.

Nursing theories identify and define interrelated concepts important in nursing and clearly state the relationships between and among these concepts. Nursing theories should be simple and general; simple terminology and broadly applicable concepts ensure their usefulness in a wide variety of nursing practice situations. Nursing theories should also increase the nursing profession's body of knowledge by generating research to guide and improve practice. Overall, nursing theory guides nursing practice by providing a knowledge base, organizing concepts, providing guidelines for practice, and identifying nursing care goals.

Nursing theories may be descriptive or prescriptive (Meleis, 2006). Descriptive theories describe a phenomenon, an event, a situation, or a relationship. They further identify the properties and components of each of these as well as the circumstances in which it occurs. Prescriptive theories address nursing interventions and the consequences of those interventions; they are designed to control, promote, and change clinical nursing practice.

The aims of nursing, described in Chapter 1, are the same for all nursing theorists, but the values, assumptions, and beliefs individualize each theory when it is applied to nursing care. Theoretical frameworks of nursing provide a focus for nursing care activities. The person receiving care is the central theme, but the way each theorist defines that person, the environment, health, and nursing gives a unique focus specific to a particular theory. The ultimate goal of each framework is holistic patient care, individualized to meet needs, promote health, and prevent or treat illness. Selected theories of nursing are outlined in Table 5-1.

Common Concepts in Nursing Theories

Four concepts common in nursing theory that influence and determine nursing practice are (1) the person (patient), (2) the environment, (3) health, and (4) nursing. Each of these concepts is usually defined and described by a nursing theorist, and although these concepts are common to all nursing theories, both the definitions and the relations among them may differ from one theory to another. Of the four concepts, the most important is that of the person. The focus of nursing, regardless of definition or theory, is the person (Fig. 5-1).

Nursing Theory in Clinical Practice

As a discipline, nursing is increasingly defining its own independent functions and contributions to healthcare. The development and use of nursing theory provide autonomy (independence and self-governance) in the practice of nursing in many ways. As nurses demonstrate that nursing care does indeed make a difference and that nursing services are valuable, the discipline becomes more independent. Having a body of knowledge specific to the discipline allows members to be viewed by others as experts; this, in turn, gives nurses authority to carry out actions. In addition, interventions carried out and based on sound rationales are trusted and respected.

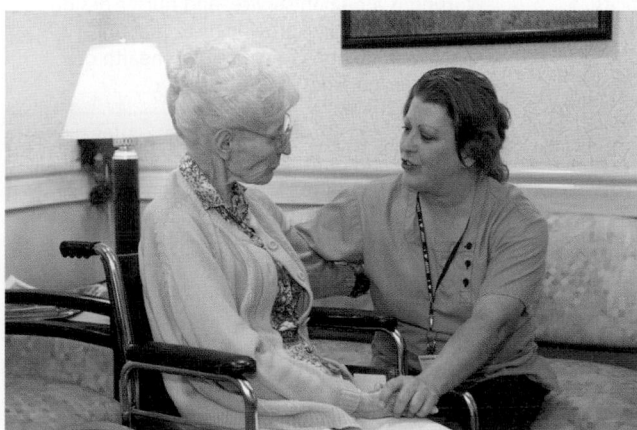

FIGURE 5-1. Four concepts common to all nursing theories are person, environment, health, and nursing. The most important concept, and the focus of nursing, is the person. *(Photo by Rick Brady.)*

Today, it has become even more necessary and important for nurses to demonstrate efficient, cost-effective, high-quality care within organized healthcare delivery systems. By practicing theory-based nursing combined with critical thinking skills, nurses are able not only to deliver care that meets those criteria but also to describe and document what it is they do. Professional nurses use theories from nursing and from the behavioral sciences to collect, organize, and classify patient data and to understand, analyze, and interpret patients' health situations. Theoretical concepts and theories guide all phases of the nursing process, including planning, implementing, and evaluating nursing care, while also describing and explaining desired responses to and outcomes of care.

The major concepts of a chosen model or theory guide each step of the nursing process. The concepts serve as categories to guide the nurse in determining what information is relevant and should be collected to make assessments and to formulate nursing diagnoses. The concepts also suggest the appropriate types of nursing interventions and patient outcomes to be included in the care plan (see Table 5-1, on the following pages, for the purpose and clinical application of selected nursing theories). It is important to realize that as the focus of nursing changes, so does the applicability of the concepts within a specific theory.

NURSING RESEARCH

Research most simply defined means to examine carefully or to search again. Research as scientific inquiry is a process that uses observable and verifiable information (**data**), collected in a systematic manner, to describe, explain, or predict events. Research is conducted to validate and refine current knowledge or to develop new knowledge. The goals of research are to develop explanations (in theories) and to find solutions to problems.

> *Consider Charlotte Horn, the daughter who is being taught how to give tube feedings and is asking about ensuring proper tube placement. The nurse would recommend the best method to use based on scientific evidence from research.* ■

Nursing research, broadly defined, encompasses both research to improve the care of people in the clinical setting and also the broader study of people and the nursing profession, including studies of education, policy development, ethics, and nursing history. Research is included as an essential component of nursing by the American Nurses Association (ANA), by the International Council of Nurses, and by nursing specialty organizations. One of the many ways to promote nursing's development of greater autonomy and strength is nursing research. Nurses, depending on their level of education, conduct or participate in research to improve their efforts to deliver high-quality, cost-efficient care. Nurses also increasingly use the findings of research to provide evidence-based nursing practice (discussed in the next section).

TABLE • 5-1   SELECTED THEORISTS AND THEORIES OF NURSING

Nursing Theorist and Date of Theory	Central Theme	Application to Clinical Practice
Florence Nightingale (1860)	Meeting the personal needs of the patient within the environment	Concern for the environment of the patient, including cleanliness, ventilation, temperature, light, diet, and noise
Hildegard Peplau (1952)	Nursing is a therapeutic, interpersonal, and goal-oriented process.	Nursing interventions are directed toward developing the patient's personality for productive personal and community living.
Virginia Henderson (1955)	The patient is an individual who requires help to reach independence.	Nursing practice is independent; autonomous nursing functions are identified, and self-help concepts are described.
Faye Abdullah (1960)	Nursing is a problem-solving art and science used to identify the nursing problems of the patients as they move toward health and cope with illness-related health needs.	The 21 nursing-care problems identified were based on research and can be used to determine patient needs and formulate nursing-focused care.
Ida Jean Orlando (1961)	The nurse reacts to the patient's verbal and nonverbal expression of needs both to understand the meaning of the distress and to know what is needed to alleviate it.	Uses the nursing process to provide solutions to problems as well as to prevent problems
Ernestine Wiedenbach (1964)	Nursing as an art; nursing is providing nurturing care to patients.	Clinical nursing includes a philosophy, a purpose, the practice, and the art. Care is directed toward a specific purpose to meet the patient's perceived healthcare needs.
Lydia E. Hall (1966)	A focus on rehabilitation, encompassing nursing's autonomy, is therapeutic use of self, treatment within the healthcare team (cure), and nurturing (care).	The major outcome of nursing care is rehabilitation and feelings of self-actualization by the patient.
Myra E. Levine (1967)	Emphasis is on the ill person in the healthcare setting; describes detailed nursing skills and actions	The patient is the center of nursing activities, with nursing care provided based on four conservation principles to help patients adapt to their environment.
Martha Rogers (1970)	Emphasis on the science and art of nursing, with the unitary human being central to the discipline of nursing	Nursing interventions are directed toward repatterning human environment fields or assisting in mobilizing inner resources.
Dorothea Orem (1971)	Self-care is a human need, self-care deficits require nursing actions.	Nursing is a human service, and nurses design interventions to provide or to manage self-care actions for sustaining health or recovering from illness or injury.
Imogene King (1971)	The patient is a personal system within a social system; the nurse and the patient experience each other and the situation, act and react, and transact.	Nursing is a process of human interactions as nurses and patients communicate to mutually set goals, and explore and agree on the means to reach those goals.
Betty Newman (1972)	Humans are in constant relationship with stressors in the environment.	The major concern for nursing is keeping the client system stable through accurately assessing the effects of environmental stressors and in assisting client adjustments required for optimal wellness.
Sr. Callista Roy (1974)	Humans are biopsychosocial beings existing within an environment. Needs are created within interrelated adaptive modes: physiological self-concept, role function, and interdependence.	Nursing interventions are required when individuals demonstrate ineffective adaptive responses.

(continued)

TABLE • 5-1 SELECTED THEORISTS AND THEORIES OF NURSING *(continued)*		
Nursing Theorist and Date of Theory	**Central Theme**	**Application to Clinical Practice**
Madeline Leininger (1978)	Caring is the central theme of nursing care, nursing knowledge, and nursing practice.	Provides the foundation of transcultural nursing care. Caring improves human conditions and life processes.
Jean Watson (1979)	Nursing is concerned with promoting and restoring health, preventing illness, and caring for the sick.	Clinical nursing care is holistic to promote humanism, health, and quality of living. Caring is universal and is practiced through interpersonal relationships.
Margaret A. Newman (1979)	Nursing interventions are purposeful, using a total-person approach to patient care to help individuals, families, and groups attain and maintain wellness.	Nursing care is directed toward reducing stress factors and adverse conditions that increase the risk for or actually affect optimal patient functions.
Dorothy E. Johnson (1980)	Nursing problems arise when there are disturbances in the system or subsystem or the level of behavioral functioning is below an optimal level.	Nursing interventions are designed to support/maintain, educate, counsel, and modify behavior.
Rosemarie Parse (1981)	The individual continually interacts with the environment and participates in maintaining health.	Health is a continual, open process (rather than an absence of illness), with nursing care planned based on the patient's perspective of health and care.
Nola Pender (1982)	The goal of nursing is the optimal health of the individual, with a focus on how individuals make healthcare decisions.	Factors significant to health-promoting behaviors include an individual's beliefs about the importance of health, the perceived benefits of, and perceived barriers to those behaviors. Participation in health-promoting behaviors is modified by one's demographic and biologic characteristics, interpersonal influences, and situational and behavioral factors.
Patricia Benner & Judith Wrubel (1989)	Nursing practice within a context of caring and skill development. Caring is a common bond of persons situated in a state of being that is essential to nursing.	A systematic description of stages of nursing practice: novice, advanced beginner, competent, proficient, and expert.

Nursing research is fundamental to the recognition of nursing as a profession. As an occupation, nursing has existed since the beginning of human history. One of the essential elements that differentiate a profession from an occupation is the existence of a unique and distinct knowledge base. The ultimate goal of expanding nursing's body of knowledge is to learn improved ways to promote and maintain health. As healthcare and illness patterns change, nursing interventions must change. Ongoing practice-based research reflects the nursing profession's commitment to meet the ever-changing demands of healthcare consumers.

➤ *Remember Joe Wimmer, the new father described at the beginning of the chapter? Before responding to Mr. Wimmer, the nurse would need knowledge of newborn heat loss and methods to minimize it. A review of the literature would provide theoretical information necessary to explain the scientific rationale for using caps on the heads of newborns to reduce heat loss.* ■

The Evolution of Nursing Research

While caring for victims of the Crimean War, Florence Nightingale kept careful and objective records. These records provided baseline data that she later used to determine which nursing interventions were most effective in treating her patients.

Although nurses have always provided care through nursing interventions and have evaluated the response of the patient, for a long time those interventions were primarily based on a philosophy of "It's always been done that way." As advances were made in technology and medical research during the 20th century, nursing leaders realized that research about the practice of nursing was necessary to meet the health needs of modern society. Increasing numbers of nurses began to conduct research and publish articles telling other nurses how to conduct nursing research.

During the 1950s and 1960s, nursing research was increasingly recognized as important. Early studies provided the basis for the development of nursing practice standards and the most effective educational preparation for registered nurses. The

American Nurses Association (ANA) sponsored a series of nursing research conferences. A focus on clinical studies to examine quality of care and the development of outcomes of care grew out of the newly developed intensive care units.

The 1970s and 1980s focused on clinical research, with published studies of clinical interventions, such as vital signs and treatment procedures. Primary patient care was a popular method of nursing care, with research investigating outcomes and quality of care. The nursing process also was studied, with research into assessment and effective nursing diagnosis of patient responses to the effects of illness. Studies of nursing education were concerned with student learning experiences and clinical evaluation methods, as well as differentiation of practice by educational preparation. In addition, models, conceptual frameworks, and theories were developed to guide nursing practice. More nurses were prepared at the doctoral level, and federal funding for nursing research increased. Journals specific to nursing research and nursing research in specialty areas were published. Of major importance was the creation of the National Center for Nursing Research (NCNR) by the ANA in 1985 with promotion to the National Institute of Nursing Research (NINR) in 1993, thereby gaining equal status with other National Institutes of Health. Further contributing to a focus on research in the clinical setting are the increased numbers of graduates from nursing master's and doctoral programs.

Methods of Conducting Nursing Research

Nursing research is conducted by quantitative and qualitative methodology. Each method is summarized here to facilitate understanding published research so that findings may be used in clinical practice.

Quantitative Research Methods

Quantitative research involves the concepts of basic and applied research. Box 5-2 provides definitions of important terms for quantitative research. **Basic research,** sometimes called pure or laboratory research, is designed to generate and

---

| Box 5-2 | IMPORTANT TERMS IN QUANTITATIVE RESEARCH |

- *Variable:* Something that varies and has different values that can be measured
- *Dependent variable:* The variable being studied, determined as a result of a study
- *Independent variable:* Causes or conditions that are manipulated or identified to determine the effects on the dependent variable
- *Hypothesis:* Statement of relationships between the independent and dependent variables that the researcher expects to find
- *Data:* Information the researcher collects from subjects in the study (expressed in numbers)
- *Instruments:* Devices used to collect and record the data, such as rating scales, pencil and paper tests, and biologic measurements. Instruments should be both reliable (produce the same results [data] on repeated use) and valid (test what they are supposed to test).

---

refine theory, and the findings are often not directly useful in practice. **Applied research,** also called practical research, is designed to directly influence or improve clinical practice.

The types of quantitative research depend on the level of current knowledge about a research problem. Table 5-2 describes the various types. The steps of quantitative research are followed carefully, although they may be designed in different ways. The basic steps of the quantitative research process are outlined and described briefly in Table 5-3.

Qualitative Research Methods

Qualitative research is a method of research conducted to gain insight by discovering meanings. It is based on the belief that reality is based on perceptions, which differ for each person and change over time. The research design follows many of the same steps as quantitative research, but differs in that the researcher primarily analyzes words rather than numbers. Table 5-4 outlines and briefly describes the methods of qualitative research.

| TABLE • 5-2 | TYPES OF QUANTITATIVE RESEARCH |

Type	Purpose
Descriptive Research	To explore and describe events in real-life situations, describing concepts and identifying relationships between and among events. Often used to generate new knowledge about topics with little or no prior research.
Correlational Research	To examine the type and degree of relationships between two or more variables. The strength of the relationship varies from a -1 (perfect negative correlation, in which one increases as the other decreases) to a $+1$ (perfect positive correlation, with both variables increasing or decreasing together).
Quasi-experimental Research	To examine cause-and-effect relationships between selected variables. Often conducted in nursing to examine the effects of nursing interventions on patient outcomes.
Experimental Research	To examine cause-and-effect relationships between variables under highly controlled conditions. These are often conducted in a laboratory setting.

TABLE • 5-3   STEPS OF THE QUANTITATIVE RESEARCH PROCESS

Step	Description
1. State the research problem.	Often stated as a question, the problem should be focused narrowly on the problem being studied. For example: "What is the optimal time for taking a rectal temperature with a digital thermometer?"
2. Define the purpose of the study.	The purpose explains "why" the problem is important and what use the findings will be.
3. Review related literature.	The literature review provides information about what is already known, provides information about concepts, and how the concepts have been measured. It also identifies gaps in knowledge that will be studied.
4. Formulate hypotheses and variables.	Hypotheses are statements about two or more concepts or variables. Variables are concepts of varying levels of abstraction that are measured, manipulated, or controlled in a study.
5. Select the research design.	The design is a carefully determined, systematic, and controlled plan for finding answers to the question of the study. This provides a "road map" for all aspects of the study, including how to collect and analyze the data.
6. Select the population and sample.	The population is the group to be studied. The sample refers to specific people or events in the population from which data will be collected.
7. Collect the data.	Sources of data may include people, literature, documents, and findings (for example, from sources such as laboratory data or measurements of vital signs). Data may be collected from interviews, questionnaires, direct measurement, or examinations (such as physical or psychological tests).
8. Analyze the data.	Statistical procedures are used to analyze the data and provide answers to the research question.
9. Communicate findings and conclusions.	Through publications and presentations, the researcher explains the results of the study and links them to the existing body of knowledge in the literature. The researcher also describes the implications of the study and suggests directions for further research.

TABLE • 5-4   QUALITATIVE RESEARCH METHODS

Method	Description
Phenomenology	The purpose of phenomenology (both a philosophy and a research method) is to describe experiences as they are lived by the subjects being studied. Analysis of data provides information about the meaning of the experience within each person's own reality (for example, the experience of health or of having a heart attack).
Grounded Theory	The basis of grounded theory methodology is the discovery of how people describe their own reality and how their beliefs are related to their actions in a social scene. The findings are grounded in the data from subjects and are used to formulate concepts and to generate a theory of the experience, supported by examples from the data (for example, coping with a seriously ill child).
Ethnography	Developed by the discipline of anthropology, ethnographic research is used to examine issues of a culture that are of interest to nursing.
Historical	Historical research examines events of the past to increase understanding of the nursing profession today. Many historical studies focus on nursing leaders, but there is increasing interest in the historical patterns of nursing practice.

Protection of the Rights of Human Subjects

Many nurses work in healthcare institutions in which patients are invited to participate in clinical research. With their focus on the overall well-being of the patient, nurses play an important role in ensuring that patient interests are not sacrificed to research interests. Nursing priorities include determining that the studies have met appropriate scientific and ethical criteria before their implementation, and protecting patient rights. Specific patient rights include **informed consent,** the patient's right to consent knowledgeably to participate in a study without coercion (knowing that this consent may be withdrawn at any time) or to refuse to participate without jeopardizing the care that he or she will receive, the right to confidentiality, and the right to be protected from harm.

Federal regulations require that institutions receiving federal funding or conducting studies of drugs or medical devices regulated by the Food and Drug Administration establish institutional review boards (IRBs). The IRBs review all studies conducted in the institution to determine the risk status of all studies and to ensure that ethical principles are followed (see Chapter 6 for full discussion of values and ethics in nursing).

Application of Research to Practice

The most common impediments to nursing research include restricted access to resources, limited time to participate in research-related activities, and lack of educational preparation needed by nurses for research. Research about nursing education, administration, and practice all affect patient care directly or indirectly. Too often, practicing nurses mistakenly think research is far removed from caring for patients at the bedside. This false impression has slowed the progress of practice-based nursing research. Yet much of what bedside nurses routinely do constitutes research. The nursing process (i.e., assessing, diagnosing, planning, implementing, and evaluating) represents the basic framework of the research process.

Unless the research findings of nurse researchers are used by practicing nurses to improve the quality of patient care, clinical nursing research is useless. Nursing students developing clinical skills must understand the scientific rationale that makes one course of action preferable to another (Fig. 5-2). Throughout this text, Research in Nursing boxes highlight current studies that have the potential to make a positive difference in nursing practice and patient outcomes.

EVIDENCE-BASED PRACTICE

Nurses make decisions about many different aspects of patient care each day. For example, questions for consideration range from "what route should I use to take an infant's temperature?" to "how can I move my patient in bed to decrease complications and promote safety?" Patient safety and health may be adversely affected unless

FIGURE 5-2. A student questions her instructor about the discrepancy between what she sees staff nurses doing to treat a wound and what her text and literature search recommend.

the most current best evidence is used to answer questions and make clinical decisions. **Evidence-based practice (EBP)** in nursing is a problem-solving approach to making clinical decisions, using the best evidence available (considered "best" because it is collected from sources such as published research, national standards and guidelines, and reviews of targeted literature). EBP blends both the science and the art of nursing so that the best patient outcomes are achieved. The information that is collected is analyzed and used to answer questions (the science of nursing), taking into consideration patient preferences and values, as well as the clinical experiences of the nurse (the art of nursing). EBP may consist of specific nursing interventions or may use guidelines established for the care of patients with certain illnesses, treatments, or surgical procedures.

Implementing EBP in clinical practice can present multiple challenges. Resistance to using EBP may arise in the current healthcare setting as a result of the nursing shortage, the acuity level of patients, nurse's skill in reading and evaluating published research, and an organizational culture that does not support change. However, to achieve desired outcomes for quality patient care and to demonstrate clinical nursing effectiveness, it is critical that nurses gain the necessary knowledge and skills to provide the best possible nursing care. The practice setting in which nurses work must support changes made based on EBP. The changes may be implemented by an individual nurse, by groups of nurses working together, or by interdisciplinary teams of healthcare providers.

Rationale for Using EBP

The impetus for EBP is based in the Institute of Medicine report (2001) *Crossing the Quality Chasm: A New Health System for the 21st century* that challenged healthcare professionals to provide care based on scientific evidence. In addition, those interested in quality and cost control want

TABLE • 5-5 **PARTS OF A RESEARCH JOURNAL ARTICLE**

Sections (in usual order)	Description
Abstract	The abstract is at the beginning of the article. It summarizes the entire article and usually provides the purpose of the study, a description of the subjects, data collection and data analysis, and a summary of important findings.
Introduction • Review of the literature • Statement of the purpose	The literature review discusses relevant studies that have been conducted in the area of this study. A statement of the specific goals or purpose of the study often follows the review.
Method • Subjects • Design • Data collection • Data analysis	The methods section provides in detail how the study was conducted, including who and how many subjects, what research design was used, what data were collected and how, and types of analysis done. There should be enough information so that the study could be replicated (repeated).
Results	The results (findings) are often presented both in words and in charts, tables, or graphs. It is important to understand what the results were and if they are meaningful.
Discussion (Conclusions)	The discussion section reports what the results mean in regard to the purpose of the study and the literature review. It may also include suggestions for further research and application to nursing education or practice, as appropriate.
References	The references are at the end of the article and include a list of articles and books used by the researcher.

evidence that the services and interventions being funded or reimbursed are effective in securing valued goals.

Until the mid 1990s, many large hospitals had research utilization departments directed by doctorally prepared nurse scientists. These departments conducted research within the hospital to answer clinical practice questions, and used the research findings to dictate practice changes. Today, few hospitals use findings from their own research to direct clinical nursing practice. As a result of recent advances in information technology, findings from published literature can be found, analyzed, and applied to answer clinically relevant questions. Key databases and search engines may be easily accessed on most work computer stations as well as home computer systems. Many research articles in journals and guidelines developed by expert panels can be downloaded to paper copies, read, evaluated, and shared with colleagues.

Therefore, the use of EBP mandates the analysis and systematic review of research findings. The first step for you as a student is to be able to read and understand a research article. To help you, the typical format of a research journal article with a description of each part is outlined in Table 5-5.

Steps in Implementing EBP

To practice EBP, nurses carry out the following 5 steps (Melnyk & Fineout-Overholt, 2005).

Step 1: Ask a question about a clinical area of interest or an intervention. There are several different methods that can be used to ask clinical questions. The most common method is the PICO format (Melnyk & Fineout-Overholt, 2002), described in Table 5-6. See the accompanying display,

TABLE • 5-6 **ASKING CLINICAL QUESTIONS IN PICO FORMAT**

Components	Considerations
P = Patient, population, or problem of interest	Need for explicit description; may include setting, limiting to subgroups (such as by age).
I = Intervention of interest	The more defined, the more focused search of the literature will be; may include exposure, treatment, patient perception, diagnostic test, or predicting factor.
C = Comparison of interest	Usually the comparison is to another treatment or the usual standard of care.
O = Outcome of interest	Specifically identifying the outcome to enable a literature search to find evidence that examined the same outcome, perhaps in different ways.

PICO IN PRACTICE
Asking Clinical Questions

Scenario: You are the director of nurses in a large long-term care facility. At the end of each 3 months, a round-table discussion is held about the prevalence of pressure ulcers (bedsores). At the latest meeting, it was noted that the prevalence was higher than it had been the previous two periods of time. A new type of mattress has been suggested by a salesman that is air-fluidized and is "more effective in preventing pressure ulcers than the foam mattress overlays now in use." However, the air-fluidized mattress is more expensive. You wonder if you should recommend buying the new mattresses for the entire facility.

- POPULATION: Adult inpatients at risk for pressure ulcers
- INTERVENTION: Air-fluidized mattress
- COMPARISON: Foam-mattress overlays
- OUTCOME: Pressure ulcer rates

PICO Question: Is the use of air-fluidized mattresses associated with lesser rates of pressure ulcers than foam-mattress overlays among adult inpatients at-risk for pressure ulcers?

Finding: From a MEDLINE search: Reddy, M., Gill, S. S., & Rochon, P. A. (2006). Preventing pressure ulcers: A systematic review. *Journal of the American Medical Association, 296*(8), 974–984.

Findings from research studies on pressure ulcer prevention do not suggest that either dynamic mattresses (e.g., dynamic air-fluidized mattresses) or static mattress overlays (e.g., foam mattress overlays) are better mattress choices that prevent pressure ulcers.

Strength of Evidence: Level I—Systematic Review

Recommendation: You decide not to purchase the more expensive air-fluidized mattresses.

(Adapted from information presented by Cheever, K. [2007]. *Integrating evidence-based practice findings into the classroom.* Philadelphia: Lippincott Williams & Wilkins.)

PICO in Practice, for a sample of the development of a clinical question using PICO and the EBP decision-making process; additional samples are found in selected chapters of this text.

Step 2: Collect the most relevant and best evidence. It is important to collect information that is regarded as the strongest level of evidence. The level for strength of evidence is numerical, with level 1 being the strongest and level 7 the lowest. The strongest ("best") evidence is pro-

vided by findings from systematic reviews, evidence-based practice guidelines, and meta-analyses. **Systematic reviews** summarize findings from multiple studies of a specific clinical practice question or topic, and recommend practice changes and future directions for research. **Evidence-based practice guidelines** synthesize information from multiple studies and recommend best practices to treat patients with a disease (e.g., hypertension), a symptom (e.g., chronic pain), or a disability (e.g., cognitive impairment); these guidelines are typically written by a panel of experts. A *meta-analysis* uses statistical analysis of the effect of a specific intervention across multiple studies, providing stronger evidence than results from a single study. If systematic reviews, EBP guidelines, and meta-analyses are not available, collect reviews of descriptive or qualitative studies or articles of original quantitative studies listed in databases such as MEDLINE and CINAHL (Cumulative Index to Nursing and Allied Health Literature). Box 5-3 provides a suggested list of resources for collecting evidence.

Step 3: Critically appraise the evidence. Ask three questions: (1) What were the results of the study? (2) Are the

Box 5-3   WEB-BASED RESOURCES FOR EVIDENCE-BASED PRACTICE

- The Cochrane Collection (http://www.cochrane.org) produces systematic reviews and other types of evidence reports. Holdings can be searched by topic or keyword.
- The Joanna Briggs Institute (http://www.joannabriggs.edu.au) produces systematic reviews, evidence summaries, and best practice series that tend to be nursing focused. Holdings can be searched by topic or keyword
- PubMed's Clinical Queries (http://www.ncbi.nlm.nih.gov/entrez/query/static/clinical.shtml) provides access to Medline and the National Library of Medicine's database of medical, nursing, and other life sciences articles, as well as evidence summaries and literature reviews.
- Center for Evidence-Based Nursing in England works with nurses to identify evidence-based practice through primary research and systematic reviews.
- Agency for Health Care Research and Quality (AHRQ), formerly the Agency of Health Care Policy and Research (AHCPR), (http://www.ahcpr.gov) has developed several clinical guidelines based on the best available evidence.
- National Guideline Clearinghouse (http://www.guidelines.gov) publishes evidence-based practice guidelines.
- CINAHL (http://www.cinahl.com) is a cumulative index of nursing and allied health literature from 1982 to present.
- MEDLINE is a cumulative index of medical, nursing, biomedical, dentistry, and allied health literature from 1966 to present.
- Specialty Organizations often have evidence-based guidelines for practice.

results valid (did the investigator measure what was intended to be measured) and reliable (were the measurements consistent across time)? (3) Will the results of the study improve patient care?

Step 4: Integrate the evidence with clinical expertise, patient preferences, and values in making a decision to change. Patients want to be involved in decision making about their care; if evidence is found to support a change but the patient does not want it, the change should not occur. If the change that is proposed cannot be applied in a practical sense, or is too costly or too risky, then the change should also not occur. For example, the most reliable method to determine if a nasogastric tube is correctly placed is by x-ray examination. However, this method of verification is costlier and more risky to the patient (i.e., through exposure to radiation) than other methods; therefore, it is not considered the preferred method in many situations.

Step 5: Evaluate the practice decision or change. The evaluation step is essential to determining if the change is effective for a particular patient or setting and if the expected outcomes resulted from the change.

It is important for nurses and the patients they care for to implement EBP in their clinical practice. "In doing so, patients, healthcare professionals, and healthcare systems will be able to place more confidence in the care that is being delivered and know the best outcomes for patients and their families are being achieved" (Melnyk & Fineout-Overholt, 2005, p. 22).

● Developing Critical Thinking Skills

1. Describe your own beliefs about the patient, the nurse, health, and what nursing is. Compare and contrast your answers with another student. How are they different, and how are they alike? How do you think such differences might influence nursing practice for each of you?

2. In preparation for your clinical assignment, you read three research articles about positioning and moving patients who are at risk for pressure ulcers (bedsores). The staff nurse responsible for the patient tells you, "Oh, I don't pay any attention to that stuff." What would you do?

● Practicing for NCLEX

1. When you ask an older student why it is necessary to change the patient's bed every day, he says, "I guess we have always done it that way." This answer is an example of which of the following?
   a. Unsubstantiated knowledge
   b. Scientific knowledge
   c. Authoritative knowledge
   d. Traditional knowledge

2. One method of developing a theory is by first examining a general idea and then considering specific actions or ideas. What is this method called?
   a. Inductive reasoning
   b. Deductive reasoning
   c. Conceptual modeling
   d. Concept development

3. When describing the term *concept* to a group of students, which word would the instructor most likely use?
   a. Fact
   b. Science
   c. Idea
   d. Truth

4. Which type of theory focuses on clinical nursing practice?
   a. Prescriptive theory
   b. Descriptive theory
   c. Developmental theory
   d. Systems theory

5. After reviewing information about the four concepts common to nursing theories, the students demonstrate understanding of the information when they identify which concept as most important?
   a. Person
   b. Environment
   c. Health
   d. Nursing

6. When conducting research, information is collected. This would be identified as which of the following?
   a. Subject
   b. Analysis
   c. Data
   d. Abstract

7. Which type of quantitative research is conducted to directly influence or improve clinical practice?
   a. Basic research
   b. Applied research
   c. Experimental research
   d. Descriptive research

8. A nurse researcher is studying the effects of exercise and sleep on blood pressure. The researcher identifies blood pressure as which type of variable?
   a. Exploratory
   b. Correlational
   c. Dependent
   d. Independent

9. Of the following types of qualitative research, which method developed in anthropology?
   a. Historical
   b. Ethnography
   c. Grounded theory
   d. Phenomenology

10. A nurse is formulating a clinical question in PICO
    format. Which of the following is represented by
    the letter P?
    a. Comparison to another similar treatment
    b. Clearly defined, focused literature review
    c. Specific identification of the desired outcome
    d. Explicit descriptions of population of interest

● Answers With Rationale

1. **d.** Traditional knowledge is the part of nursing practice
   passed down from generation to generation, often without research data to support it.

2. **b.** Moving from a general idea to specific ideas is
   deductive reasoning.

3. **c.** A concept, like an idea, is an abstract impression of
   reality.

4. **a.** Prescriptive theories address nursing interventions
   and are designed to control, promote, and change clinical nursing practice.

5. **a.** Of the four concepts, the most important is the person.

6. **c.** Data are observable and verifiable information
   collected to describe, explain, or predict events.

7. **b.** Applied research, a type of quantitative research, is
   designed to directly influence or improve clinical
   practice.

8. **c.** The dependent variable is the variable being studied
   and is determined by manipulating conditions (the
   independent variables).

9. **b.** Ethnographic research was developed by the
   discipline of anthropology and is used to examine
   issues of culture of interest to nursing.

10. **d.** The P in the PICO format represents an explicit
    description of the patient population of interest.

Taylor Suite Resources

The Taylor Suite offers these additional resources to enhance
learning and facilitate understanding of this chapter:

• thePoint online resource, http://thepoint.lww.com/Taylor7E
• Student DVD included with the book
• Study Guide for Taylor's Fundamentals of Nursing

BIBLIOGRAPHY

Alligood, M., & Marriner-Tomey, A. (2006). *Nursing theory: Utilization and application* (3rd ed.). St. Louis, MO: Mosby.

Allyn, D. (2007). Primum non nocere (first, do no harm): Prayer,
culture, and evidence-based practice. *Topics in Advanced Practice
Nursing eJournal, 7*(2). Available at http://www.medscape.com/
viewarticle/561760_print

Armola, R. R., Bourgault, A. M., Halm, M. A., Board, R. M.,
Bucher, L., Harrington, L., et al. (2009). Upgrading the
American Association of Critical Care Nurses' evidence-
leveling hierarchy. *American Journal of Critical Care,
18*(5), 405–409.

Beyea, S. (2004). Evidence-based practice in perioperative
nursing. *American Journal of Infection Control, 32*(2),
97–100.

Burns, N., & Groves, S. (2007). *Understanding nursing research:
Building an evidence-based practice* (4th ed.). Philadelphia:
Elsevier Saunders.

Chinn, P., & Kramer, M. (2008). *Integrated knowledge development
in nursing* (7th ed.). St. Louis: Mosby Elsevier.

Cronenwett, L., Sherwood, G., Barnsteiner, J., Disch, J., Johnson, J.,
Mitchell, P., et al. (2007). Quality and safety education for
nurses. *Nursing Outlook, 55*(3), 122–131.

Dale, A. (2006). Determining guiding principles for evidence-
based practice. *Nursing Standard, 20*(25), 41–46.

Dontje, K. (2007). Evidence-based practice: Understanding the
process. *Topics in Advanced Practice Nursing eJournal, 7*(4).
Available at http://medscape.com/viewarticle/567786_print

Fawcett, J. (2005). Scholarly dialogue. Influences on advancement
of nursing knowledge. *Nursing Science Quarterly, 18*(3),
227–232.

Grace, J., & Powers, B. (2009). Claiming our core: Appraising
qualitative evidence for nursing questions about human
response and meaning. *Nursing Outlook, 57*(1), 27–34.

Hockenberry, M., Wilson, D., & Barrera, P. (2006). Implementing
evidence-based nursing practice in a pediatric hospital.
Pediatric Nursing, 32(4), 371–377.

Hood, L., & Leddy, S. (2006). *Leddy & Pepper's conceptual bases
of professional nursing* (6th ed.). Philadelphia: Lippincott
Williams & Wilkins.

Institute of Medicine (IOM). (2001). *Crossing the quality chasm:
A new health system for the 21st century.* Washington, DC:
National Academy of Sciences.

Kalish, P., & Kalish, B. (1995). *The advance of American nursing*
(3rd ed.). Philadelphia: J. B. Lippincott.

Lamp, J., & Zadvinskis, I. (2008). Kangaroo care: Making the
leap to an evidence-based practice. *American Nurse Today,
3*(3), 13–15.

Marriner-Tomey, A., & Alligood, M. (2006). *Nursing theorists
and their work* (6th ed.). St. Louis, MO: Mosby.

McCutcheon, Z. (2005). Tradition, rituals, and standards: In a
realm of evidence-based nursing care. *Contemporary Nurse,
18*(3), 300–308.

McEwen, M., & Wills, E. (2007). *Theoretical basis for
nursing* (2nd ed.). Philadelphia: Lippincott Williams &
Wilkins.

Meleis, A. I. (2006). *Theoretical nursing: Development and
progress* (4th ed.). Philadelphia: Lippincott Williams &
Wilkins.

Melnyk, B., & Fineout-Overholt, E. (2005). *Evidence-based practice in nursing: A guide to best practice.* Philadelphia: Lippincott
Williams & Wilkins.

Melnyk, B., & Fineout-Overholt, E. (2002). Key steps in
evidence-based practice. Asking compelling clinical questions
and searching for the best evidence. *Pediatric Nursing, 28,*
262–263, 266.

Neuman, B., & Faucett, J. (2002). *The Neuman systems model.*
(4th ed.). Upper Saddle River, NJ: Prentice Hall.

Pipe, T., Wellik, K., Buchda, V., Hansen, C., & Martyn, D. (2005).
Implementing evidence-based nursing practice. *Urologic Nursing, 25*(5), 365–370.

Polit, D., & Beck, C. (2008). *Nursing research: Generating and
assessing evidence for nursing practice* (8th ed.). Philadelphia:
Lippincott Williams & Wilkins.

Rauen, C., Vollman, K., Arbour, R., & Chulary, M. (2008).
Challenging nursing's sacred cows. *American Nurse Today,
3*(4), 23–26.

Remshardt, M., & Flowers, D. (2007). Understanding qualitative research. *American Nurse Today, 2*(9), 20–23.

Rycroft-Malone, J., Harvey, G., Seers, K., Kitson, A., McCormack, B., & Titchen, A. (2004). An exploration of the factors that influence the implementation of evidence into practice. *Journal of Clinical Nursing, 13*(8), 913–924.

Talsma, G., Feetham, S., Heinrich, J., & Steinwachs, D. (2008). The perfect storm: Patient safety and nursing shortages within the context of health policy and evidence-based practice. *Nursing Research, 57*(1S): S15–21.

Van Achterberg, T., Schoonhoven, L., & Grol, R. (2008). Nursing implementation science: How evidence-based nursing requires evidence-based implementation. *Journal of Nursing Scholarship, 40*(4), 302–310.

Winsett, R., & Cashion, A. (2007). The nursing research process. *Nephrology Nursing Journal, 34*(6), 635–643.

6 Values, Ethics, and Advocacy

CHENGYU ZHANG

Chengyu is an alert 32-year-old man in the intensive care unit who is begging to be removed from the ventilator. He understands that it is highly unlikely that he will be able to breathe on his own without the ventilator. He writes on the communication board, "If I die, I die. I can't keep living like this."

MARISSA SANDOVAL

Marissa, a 44-year-old woman who has just recently undergone extensive surgery to treat uterine cancer, is experiencing several serious postoperative complications. She states, "I don't know why all of these things are happening. I ask the doctors. So does my family. But we get no answers. We just want to know what is happening." The nurse is surprised to observe that not only does the surgeon not answer Marissa's questions, but that he also dismisses her fears without any explanation.

WILLIAM RAINES

William, a homeless, 68-year-old indigent man diagnosed with schizophrenia, developmental delays, and uncontrolled hypertension, was admitted for control of moderately severe elevated blood pressure. A review of his medical record reveals that Mr. Raines was getting samples of medications for blood pressure treatment from the pharmaceutical representatives at the clinic, but recent policy changes stopped this practice approximately 4 weeks ago. Mr. Raines is about to be discharged with several prescriptions for medications and no way to fill them.

After completing the chapter, you will be able to accomplish the following:

1. List five common modes of value transmission.

2. Describe seven steps in the valuing process.

3. Use values clarification strategies in clinical practice.

4. Compare and contrast the principle-based and care-based approaches to bioethics.

5. Describe nursing practice that is consistent with the code of ethics for nursing.

6. Describe the purpose of the Bill of Rights for Registered Nurses.

7. Recognize ethical issues as they arise in nursing practice.

8. Use an ethical framework and decision-making process to resolve ethical problems.

9. Identify four functions of institutional ethics committees.

10. Describe three typical concerns of the nurse advocate.

KEY TERMS

advocacy	fidelity
autonomy	justice
beneficence	morals
bioethics	nonmaleficence
care-based approach	nursing ethics
clinical ethics	paternalism
code of ethics	principle-based
deontologic	approach
ethical agency	utilitarian
ethical dilemma	value
ethical distress	value system
ethics	values clarification
feminist ethics	

The unique nature of nursing places nurses both at the bedside and in groups of professionals where critical decisions are made about the best way to treat injury and illness and to solve healthcare problems. Often, the question confronting the nurse is not "How do I do this?" but, rather, "Should I do this?" The more that science and technology increase the options available to patients and healthcare professionals, the more frequently nurses will find themselves asking "We can do this, but should we, here and now, for this patient?"

"Should the professionals in the intensive care unit keep Mr. Zhang on ventilatory support?"

Nurses also are increasingly distressed by the failure of society to provide adequate care for its most vulnerable members. Nothing is more disturbing for professional nurses than seeing firsthand the consequences of unmet healthcare needs. When nurses care for patients like Mr. Raines, who lack the financial resources to obtain the medications and treatment they need, they have special advocacy obligations. A shortage of nurses further complicates the nursing work environment, creating the necessity for nurses to be skilled advocates for safety, quality care, and their own needs. Never has it been more important for nurses to grasp the ethical dimensions of professional practice and to be confident in "doing the ethically right thing simply because it's the right thing to do!" With their moral integrity on the line every day, nurses understand the need to be as skilled ethically as they are intellectually, interpersonally, and technically. Nurses who understand how patients' values and their own values shape nurse–patient interactions, and who continually develop sensitivity to the ethical dimensions of nursing practice, are best able to provide quality care and advocate for their patients. (For an example, see the accompanying display, Reflective Practice: Challenge to Ethical and Legal Skills.)

VALUES

A **value** is a belief about the worth of something, about what matters, that acts as a standard to guide one's behavior. If you think back to how you spent your last weekend, you may observe something about your own values. The amount of time, passion, and money you devote to relationships, work, study, fitness activities, leisure, and other experiences reveals something about the importance (value) you attach to these endeavors.

A **value system** is an organization of values in which each is ranked along a continuum of importance, often leading to a personal code of conduct. A person's values influence beliefs about human needs, health, and illness; the practice of health behaviors; and human responses to illness. For example, individuals who place a high value on health and personal responsibility often work hard to reach their fitness goals. Individuals who value high-risk leisure activities may attach less value to life and health. Nurses who work effectively with patients are sensitive to how a patient's values and their own values influence their interactions.

Development of Values

An individual is not born with values; rather, values are formed during a lifetime from information from the environment, family, and culture.

> *Recall Chengyu Zhang, the 32-year-old man in the intensive care unit asking to be removed from the ventilator, even if it means that he will die. The nurse can integrate knowledge of the patient's culture and family and their influence on the patient's value of independence as a key aspect in planning his care.* ■

REFLECTIVE PRACTICE

Challenge to Ethical and Legal Skills

I have faced a common ethical dilemma both as a student in the clinical area and as a nurse extern during the summers. My lack of confidence prevents me from being a patient advocate. My lack of status in the unit makes it very difficult for me to stand up to more senior, experienced staff to act as a patient advocate. However, patient advocacy is a crucial duty for any nurse. I feel that when I neglect this duty, I am being unethical because I am not fulfilling one of the most important nursing roles. An example of this dilemma occurred during one of my first weeks on the gynecologic surgical floor, where I was an extern this summer.

Mrs. Marissa Sandoval was a 44-year-old woman who had just recently undergone extensive surgery for treatment of newly diagnosed uterine cancer. She also developed several postoperative complications. Mrs. Sandoval and her family were unhappy about the lack of answers they were getting from the attending surgeon and the residents about the complications she was experiencing from the surgery. After observing the surgeon interacting with the patient and her family in her room, I could easily understand the patient's distress. In addition to the surgeon not answering any of the family's questions, he dismissed all of her legitimate fears without an explanation. I felt this was a terrible way to treat a patient and that as patient advocate, I had an ethical and professional duty to make sure the patient and her family received adequate answers.

Thinking Outside the Box: Possible Courses of Action

- Confront the surgeon, explaining the patient's anxiety and asking him to return to her room to answer the questions.
- Try to answer the patient's questions to the best of my ability.
- Pretend that the doctor was acting appropriately. Tell the patient that the doctor will return tomorrow during rounds, and that she will have the opportunity to ask questions then.
- Ask another, more experienced nurse to answer my patient's questions.
- Tell the patient not to worry so much because the doctors and nurses will take good care of her.

Evaluating a Good Outcome: How Do I Define Success?

- The patient receives satisfactory answers to her questions.
- The situation is handled in a respectful manner for all parties involved.
- The American Nurses Association's Bill of Rights is followed: "Nurses have the right to freely and openly advocate for themselves and their patients, without fear of retribution."
- No one involved in the situation suffers from a violation of integrity.
- The ANA Code of Ethics is followed: "The nurse promotes, advocates for, and strives to protect the health, safety, and rights of the patient."

Personal Learning: Here's to the Future!

In retrospect, when I examine the situation, I don't think that I handled the situation in the most ethical manner. Rather than dealing with the situation myself, I sought out the help of a more experienced nurse to answer the patient's questions to the best of her ability. Unfortunately, because of the complexity of the case, the more experienced nurse was not able to answer all of the questions adequately. I should have spoken with the surgeon and expressed my concern regarding the patient's questions going unanswered. However, I was greatly intimidated by this surgeon, and thus, I did not want to confront him. My actions demonstrate that I was compromising my role as a patient advocate. I compromised this role because of personal anxiety and lack of confidence associated with confronting the surgeon.

I do feel that I am trying to base my personal practice on a strong ethical foundation, with my personal actions reflective of this, as I hold my own actions to a high ethical standard. However, I am not a very confrontational person. This, coupled with my great insecurities about working in the hospital setting, makes it difficult for me to confront other healthcare providers when I think they are acting in an unethical manner. Therefore, while I think my personal actions have a strong ethical foundation, I have a lot of room for growth when acting in an ethical manner when needing to confront coworkers. I hope that as I grow more comfortable in the hospital setting, I will not compromise my role as a patient advocate because of my personal fears.

Elizabeth Nalli, Georgetown University

Reflection

How do you think you would respond in a similar situation? Why? What does this tell you about yourself and about the adequacy of your skills for professional practice? How might the surgeon's values have influenced his actions? Please explain. Did the student adhere to the ANA's Bill of Rights? ANA Code for Nurses? Canadian Nurses Association Code of Ethics? Explain your answer. Evaluate whether the patient's rights as stated in the American Hospital Association's Bill of Rights were respected. How did the student use or not use ethical agency? What ethical principles were involved in this situation? How did the student attempt to use these principles? Can you think of other ways to use these principles or respond? What other skills (cognitive, interpersonal, technical, ethical/legal) would you need to respond well in this situation? Do you agree with the criteria to evaluate a successful outcome? Was anyone's integrity violated? Please explain.

As children observe the actions of others, they quickly learn what has high and low value for family members. If the parents spend a good portion of each day cooking, and the family spends a long time eating and talking at the table, the children learn to value food and the good times it represents. Similarly, children learn that helpfulness is a good and respected quality if praised when helping parents, grandparents, and siblings. Common modes of value transmission include:

- Modeling
- Moralizing
- Laissez-faire
- Rewarding and punishing
- Responsible choice

Through modeling, children learn what is of high or low value by observing parents, peers, and significant others. Thus, modeling may lead to socially acceptable or unacceptable behaviors. Children whose caregivers use the moralizing mode of value transmission are taught a complete value system by parents or an institution (e.g., church or school) that allows little opportunity for them to weigh different values.

Those who use the laissez-faire approach to value transmission leave children to explore values on their own (no one set of values is presented as best for all) and to develop a personal value system. This approach often involves little or no guidance and can lead to confusion and conflict.

Through rewarding and punishing, children are rewarded for demonstrating values held by parents and punished for demonstrating unacceptable values. Finally, caregivers who follow the responsible-choice mode of value transmission encourage children to explore competing values and to weigh their consequences. Support and guidance are offered as children develop a personal value system.

Values Essential to the Professional Nurse

Professional values provide the foundation for nursing practice and guide the nurse's interactions with patients, colleagues, and the public. In 1998, the American Association of Colleges of Nursing identified five values that epitomize the caring, professional nurse. Box 6-1 lists these values and sample behaviors illustrating each of these values. Every nurse should critically examine his or her personal values to see if they match these essential professional values. For example, if I value self-promotion to the extent that I won't make the sacrifices demanded by a genuine commitment to the welfare of the patients entrusted to my care, I will never be successful as a nurse. Similarly, if I attach low value to respecting people who are different from me, I may interact with patients and colleagues in a way that is demeaning and unprofessional. It is helpful to identify nurses in your practice

---

Box 6-1 PROFESSIONAL VALUES

Altruism
Altruism is a concern for the welfare and well-being of others. In professional practice, altruism is reflected by the nurse's concern for the welfare of patients, other nurses, and other healthcare providers. Sample professional behaviors include the following:
- Demonstrates understanding of cultures, beliefs, and perspectives of others
- Advocates for patients, particularly the most vulnerable
- Takes risks on behalf of patients and colleagues
- Mentors other professionals

Autonomy
Autonomy is the right to self-determination. Professional practice reflects autonomy when the nurse respects patients' rights to make decisions about their healthcare. Sample professional behaviors include the following:
- Plans care in partnership with patients
- Honors the right of patients and families to make decisions about healthcare
- Provides information so that patients can make informed choices

Human Dignity
Human dignity is respect for the inherent worth and uniqueness of individuals and populations. In professional practice, human dignity is reflected when the nurse values and respects all patients and colleagues. Sample professional behaviors include the following:

- Provides culturally competent and sensitive care
- Protects the patient's privacy
- Preserves the confidentiality of patients and healthcare providers
- Designs care with sensitivity to individual patient needs

Integrity
Integrity is acting in accordance with an appropriate code of ethics and accepted standards of practice. Integrity is reflected in professional practice when the nurse is honest and provides care based on an ethical framework that is accepted within the profession. Sample professional behaviors include the following:
- Provides honest information to patients and the public
- Documents care accurately and honestly
- Seeks to remedy errors made by self or others
- Demonstrates accountability for own actions

Social Justice
Social justice is upholding moral, legal, and humanistic principles. This value is reflected in professional practice when the nurse works to assure equal treatment under the law and equal access to quality healthcare. Sample professional behaviors include the following:
- Supports fairness and nondiscrimination in the delivery of care
- Promotes universal access to healthcare
- Encourages legislation and policy consistent with the advancement of nursing care and healthcare

From American Association of Colleges of Nursing. (2008). *The essentials of baccalaureate education for professional nursing practice.* Washington, DC: Author.

setting who epitomize nursing's essential values and to learn from observing their behavior.

To encourage healthcare professionals to respect and accept the individuality of patients, some educators have advised that professionals be "value neutral" and "nonjudgmental" in their professional roles. Thus, the nurse has a "commitment to patients whether or not the nurse and the patients hold the same values. The nurse does not assume that her personal values are right and should not judge the patient's values as right or wrong depending on their congruence with the nurse's personal value system" (Steele & Harmon, 1983, p. 27). This kind of thinking encourages effective care for patients with values different from the nurse's. For example, a nurse who strongly believes that any premarital or extramarital sex is wrong can still offer competent and compassionate nursing care to a young woman prostitute with active herpes lesions. On the other hand, if the same patient, after receiving education, indicates that she is unconcerned about whom she might infect in future sexual encounters, the nurse has an ethical obligation to protect the patient and others from the harm the patient's values may cause.

Values Clarification

Values clarification is a process by which people come to understand their own values and value system. "It is a process of discovery and allows the person to discover through feelings and analysis of behavior what choices to make when alternatives are presented, and to identify whether or not these choices are rationally made or are the result of previous conditioning" (Steele & Harmon, 1983, p. 13). Values clarification has a beneficial application to nursing. When nurses understand the values that motivate the decisions and behaviors of patients, they can tap these values when teaching and counseling patients. For example, a man who does not value his own health and well-being may be motivated by the value he attaches to being a good father for his children to make needed lifestyle changes.

Values theorists most often describe the process of valuing as having seven steps focusing on three main activities (Raths, Simon, & Harmin, 1978):

1. Choosing
2. Prizing (treasuring)
3. Acting

When one values something, one chooses freely from alternatives after careful consideration of the consequences of each alternative. Prizing something one values involves pride, happiness, and public affirmation. Finally, the person who values something acts by combining choice into one's behavior with consistency and regularity on the value.

> *Remember Chengyu Zhang described at the beginning of the chapter? Understanding the patient's values would aid the nurse in developing an appropriate plan of care for the client based on his request to be removed from the ventilator.* ∎

Example of Values Clarification by the Nurse

If respect for human dignity is a value that characterizes your nursing practice, you choose freely to believe in the worth and uniqueness of each individual, to realize that you have other options (e.g., you could treat with dignity only those people who are most like you), and to believe that respecting each person's human dignity yields the best consequences for you and for all of society.

You also will prize your choice. For example, you especially enjoy when patients let you know they appreciate your care and when nursing colleagues and supervisors compliment you on interpersonal skills. You also prize your ability to defend this value when someone's human dignity is being ignored.

Clarifying this value of respect for human dignity will motivate you to incorporate this value into your practice. You strive to respect human dignity consistently in your personal as well as professional life.

As you become more conscious of this value, you will be sensitive to your actions that are inconsistent with it. For example, you may feel uncomfortable gossiping with other nurses during break about a patient no one likes, realizing that this behavior contradicts your basic respect for human dignity.

Clinical Applications

Box 6-2 illustrates how the steps in the valuing process can be used to help a patient with high blood pressure take charge of his health and manage his medications. Other clinical examples follow.

PATIENT PLACES LOW VALUE ON HEALTH AND HEALTH BEHAVIORS

You become frustrated when repeated attempts to teach or counsel a 26-year-old pharmaceutical salesperson meet with failure. Although hospitalized with a serious duodenal ulcer, all he can talk about is his job and meeting his sales quota.

To facilitate values clarification for this patient, first help him identify his basic life values. Ask him, "What three things are most important to you in life?" or have him rank the following behaviors in terms of how he would most likely spend an unexpected free day:

_____ Enjoy some quiet time alone (e.g., thinking, reading, listening to music)

_____ Spend time with family, friends

_____ Do something active (e.g., hiking, playing ball, swimming)

_____ Watch television

_____ Volunteer time and energy to help someone else

_____ Use time for my job

_____ Other

Discuss with the patient what these rankings suggest about his values. Determine whether his rankings would be

Box 6-2 STEPS IN THE VALUING PROCESS

Situation: Mr. Jefferson is a 49-year-old man with uncontrolled high blood pressure

Choosing
1. *Freely.* Rehospitalized for high blood pressure after abruptly stopping his antihypertensive medication, Mr. Jefferson decides from now on to take his medication as prescribed.
2. *From Alternatives.* After a teaching–learning session with a nurse, Mr. Jefferson understands he has basically three options:
   - Comply with prescribed treatment regimen
   - Refuse to take the medication but try harder to control his blood pressure through diet, exercise, and stress management
   - Refuse to take the medication and assume a "we'll see" attitude
3. *After Consideration of the Consequences.* Mr. Jefferson understands the *probable* consequences of these options:
   - Compliance with the treatment regimen will yield the best control of high blood pressure (but may cause some annoying side effects).
   - Diet, exercise, and stress management may reduce his blood pressure somewhat but did not yield sufficient control in the past.

- High blood pressure may result in serious complications such as stroke, kidney disease, or impaired vision.

Prizing
4. *With Pride and Happiness.* Mr. Jefferson states, "Now that I understand high blood pressure better and know what I can do to control it, I feel more in charge of my life—and I like that!"
5. *With Public Affirmation.* Mr. Jefferson states to his wife, "I guess I was wrong to stop taking that medicine when I blamed it for how lousy I was feeling. You can bet that won't happen again. If you ever hear me complaining about my pills, remind me to see my doctor right away."

Acting
6. *With Incorporation of the Choice Into One's Behavior.* After discharge from the hospital, Mr. Jefferson takes the medication as prescribed.
7. *With Consistency and Regularity on the Value.* Mr. Jefferson seeks to understand any new medication he is prescribed (i.e., reason for the medication, possible side effects, consequences of the noncompliance) and successfully manages the treatment regimen; he feels proud of his new knowledge and self-care abilities.

different if he were asked how he *wished* he could spend the free day versus how he would *most likely* spend it.

VALUES OF PATIENT AND FAMILY MEMBERS CONFLICT

You sense a growing tension while counseling the young parents of a child with asthma. Questioning them ("You seem uncomfortable with what I'm saying now. Is there something wrong?") reveals that the wife is a smoker and cat lover who has told her husband that even if these behaviors are hurting their child, she is unwilling to give them up.

To facilitate values clarification, suggest that both parents complete the following exercise, and then talk with them about their different responses:

Where do you stand on the following issues? (Indicate your responses in the following manner: SA, strongly agree; A, agree; D, disagree; SD, strongly disagree; U, undecided.)

_____ A parent's primary obligation is to meet the needs of his or her child.

_____ Each member of a family is entitled to pursue personal pleasures, even if these are not in the best interest of all.

_____ Pleasure is more important than health.

_____ The choices one family member makes can dramatically affect other family members (positively or negatively).

This exercise will help the parents to evaluate their basic values, explore areas of conflict, and, perhaps, move toward joint choosing, prizing, and acting on several health-promoting values.

ETHICS

Ethics is systematic inquiry into principles of right and wrong conduct, of virtue and vice, and of good and evil as they relate to conduct and human flourishing. The ability to be ethical, to make decisions, and to act in an ethically justified manner, begins in childhood and develops gradually. See Chapter 18 for a description of two popular accounts of moral development, Kohlberg's justice-based account and Gilligan's care-based account.

Many people use the term ethics when describing the systematic ethics incorporated into a code of professional conduct, such as nursing codes of ethics. The term **morals,** although similar in meaning to ethics, usually refers to personal or communal standards of right and wrong. It is important to distinguish ethics from religion, law, custom, and institutional practices. For example, the fact that an action is legal or customary does not in itself make the action ethically or morally right.

Since values are beliefs about what is important, they are intimately related to and direct ethical conduct. If I place a high value on patient safety and well-being, I am more likely to inconvenience myself to secure the patient's safety and well-being—even when this entails sacrifice—than a nurse who places less value on securing the patient's interests.

Types of Ethics

There are many types of ethics. Those of particular concern to the nurse are bioethics, clinical ethics, and nursing ethics. The *Encyclopedia of Bioethics* describes the scope of **bioethics** as encompassing a number of fields and disciplines grouped broadly under the rubric "the life sciences":

> They encompass all those perspectives that seek to understand human nature and behavior, characteristically the domain of the social sciences, and the natural world that provides the habitat of human and animal life, primarily the population and environmental sciences. Yet it is the medical and biological sciences in which bioethics found its initial impetus and in which it has seen the most intense activity.

(Callahan, 1995, p. 255)

Issues in bioethics include responsible research conduct, genetic enhancement, environmental ethics, and sustainable healthcare.

Clinical ethics is that branch of bioethics literally concerned with ethical problems "at the bedside," that is, ethical concerns that arise within the context of caring for actual patients, wherever they are found. Clinical ethics developed in response to three criticisms of bioethics.

1. The need for a contextual approach to ethical inquiry that takes more careful account of the variety of contexts in clinical care and the special needs of ill and suffering patients
2. The need to emphasize the relevance of clinical experience that draws on the knowledge available only through the intimacy of the clinician–patient relationship when doing clinical ethics
3. The need for an orientation toward service in clinical ethics that addresses ethics education, policy making to address ethical issues in patient care, ethics consultation, and clinical ethics research (Fletcher, Spencer, & Lombardo, 2005, p. 5)

Examples of issues in clinical ethics include valid consent or refusal and how one ought to respond to requests for medically futile treatment or assisted suicide.

Nursing ethics, which is a subset of bioethics, is the formal study of ethical issues that arise in the practice of nursing and of the analysis used by nurses to make ethical judgments.

As nurses assume increasing responsibility for managing care, it is critical that we are prepared to recognize the ethical dimensions of our practice and to participate competently in ethical decision making. Common ethical issues encountered by nurses in daily practice include cost-containment issues that jeopardize patient welfare, end-of-life decisions, breaches of patient confidentiality, and incompetent, unethical, or illegal practices of colleagues.

> ➤ *Recall Mr. Raines, the 68-year-old indigent, homeless man who is being discharged with several medication prescriptions. Due to policy changes, this patient is no longer able to receive his medications at the clinic free of charge. Whether healthcare is a commodity that can be bought and sold in the marketplace ("too bad, Mr. Raines, if you don't have insurance to cover your meds or money in your pocket...")*

or a social good owed everyone is a basic question in bioethics. Clinical ethics might evaluate whether or not the institution should have a policy to cover patients like Mr. Raines who are too poor to buy the treatment they need. Nursing ethics will ask about the moral obligations of the nurse case manager caring for Mr. Raines. ■

Theories of Ethics

Ethical theories or frameworks are systems of thought that attempt to explain how we ought to live and why. These theories may be broadly categorized as action-guiding theories that answer the question "What ought I to do?" or character-guiding theories that answer the question "What kind of person ought I to be?" Action-guiding theories fall into two main categories:

- **Utilitarian.** The rightness or wrongness of an action depends on the consequences of the action.
- **Deontologic.** An action is right or wrong independent of its consequences.

These distinctions are important because they form the basis of many ethical conflicts we experience in practice. For example, one nurse may believe that abortion is ethically justified in situations that result in the best consequences for the woman, child, and society (utilitarian argument). Another nurse may agree that certain abortions yield better consequences than allowing an unplanned and unwanted pregnancy to continue, but believe that the act of abortion is nonetheless ethically wrong because no consequences justify the taking of innocent life (deontologic argument).

Nurse ethicists frequently use two popular theoretical and practical approaches to "doing ethics"—the principle-based approach and the care-based approach.

Principle-Based Approach

The **principle-based approach** to ethics combines elements of both utilitarian and deontologic theories and offers specific action guides for practice. The Beauchamp and Childress principle-based approach to bioethics (2001) identifies four key principles: **autonomy, nonmaleficence, beneficence,** and **justice** (Table 6-1). Many nurses add **fidelity,** veracity, accountability, privacy, and confidentiality to this list because they play a central role in the tradition of nursing (and medical) ethics and guide the behavior of healthcare professionals toward patients and their families.

> ➤ *Recall Marissa Sandoval, the 44-year-old woman who developed complications following extensive surgery for uterine cancer? The nurse would likely feel that the surgeon and residents are not being faithful (principle of fidelity) to their responsibility to address the patient's questions and fears. Unless the nurse can effectively advocate for Marissa with the medical team, her own ability to*

TABLE • 6-1 PRINCIPLES OF BIOETHICS		
Principle	**Moral Rule**	**Implications for Nursing Practice**
Autonomy (self-determination)	Respect the rights of patients or their surrogates to make healthcare decisions.	Provide the information and support patients and families need to make the decision that is right for them; at times, this may mean collaborating with other members of the healthcare team to advocate for the patient.
Nonmaleficence	Avoid causing harm.	Seek not to inflict harm; seek to prevent harm or risk of harm whenever possible.
Beneficence	Benefit the patient, and balance benefits against risks and harms.	Commit yourself to actively promote the patient's benefit (health and well-being or good dying). Be sensitive to the fact that individuals (patients, family members, and professional caregivers) may identify benefits and harms differently. A benefit to one may be a burden to another.
Justice	Give each his or her due; act fairly.	Always seek to distribute the benefits, risks, and costs of nursing care justly. This may involve recognizing subtle instances of bias and discrimination.
Fidelity	Keep promises.	Be faithful to the promise you made to the public to be competent and to be willing to use your competence to benefit the patients entrusted to your care. Never abandon a patient entrusted to your care without first providing for the patient's needs.

be faithful to Marissa and accountable for her well-being will be compromised. ■

The principles offer general guides to action. All things being equal, we ought to act at all times in a manner that respects the autonomy of others, does not harm, does benefit others, treats others fairly, and is faithful to the promises we make to others. Rarely is this as simple as it sounds. Be sensitive to the fact that individuals (patients, family members, and professional caregivers) may identify benefits and harms differently. A benefit to one may be a burden to another.

➤ *Review the request by Mr. Zhang, the 32-year-old man described at the beginning of the chapter. Although the nurse may view the request for removal from the ventilator as harmful, most likely leading to the patient's death, the patient's view differs, that is, he does not want to be dependent on a ventilator to live. When conflict about how to apply these principles cannot be resolved, the nurse can request an ethics consult, which is described at the end of this chapter.* ■

Ethical dilemmas arise when attempted adherence to basic ethical principles results in two conflicting courses of action. There is no foolproof method for identifying which principle is most important when there is conflict between competing principles. Popularized versions of the principle-based approach to bioethics have too frequently resulted in a type of "quandary ethics" that diminishes in importance the everyday ethical concerns of nurses (Taylor, 1997), and misleadingly suggests that how ethical dilemmas are resolved is unimportant, as long as one can justify one's recommendation with recourse to a principle. Thus, many healthcare professionals equate ethics with decisions about whether to "pull the plug," ignoring the ethical challenges involved in daily decisions about what constitutes an honest day's work, how respectful we are to others, how truthful, and how compassionate.

Care-Based Approach

Dissatisfaction with the principle-based approach to bioethics led many nurses to look to care as the foundation for nursing's ethical obligations. The nurse–patient relationship is central to the **care-based approach,** which directs attention to the specific situations of individual patients viewed within the context of their life narrative. The care perspective directs that how you choose to "be" and act each time you encounter a patient or colleague is a matter of ethical significance. Ethics is not reduced to a decision to withhold or withdraw life-sustaining treatment. Characteristics of the care perspective include the following:

- Centrality of the caring relationship
- Promotion of the dignity and respect of patients as people
- Attention to the particulars of individual patients
- Cultivation of responsiveness to others and professional responsibility
- A redefinition of fundamental moral skills to include virtues like kindness, attentiveness, empathy, compassion, reliability (Taylor, 1993)

Feminist Ethics

Feminist ethics is a particular type of ethical approach popular among nurses. It aims to critique existing patterns of oppression and domination in society, especially as these affect women and the poor. There are many forms of feminist ethics and their subjects range from gender-related inequities to concern for the least well-off. Nurses working within a feminist framework promote social policy that reflects a fundamental trust in the moral agency of women and those on the margins. This trust is recognition that all persons deserve the opportunity to make legitimate choices about conditions that affect their lives and are deserving of respect whenever they exercise such agency. This approach reflects a full commitment to full personhood for marginalized persons and provides for basic human needs that are consistent with one's capacity to flourish and that honors human dignity and relationality (Holland, 2001, pp. 74–75).

An excellent example of feminist ethics is Holland's critique of human embryonic stem cell research:

> It is true that women, the poor, persons of color and marginals could benefit from the regenerative medical therapies and drug therapies heralded by hES (human embryonic stem) cell and EG (embryonic germ) cell research, but it is not at all likely that they will be the ones who do benefit. Such therapies, when they are perfected, are likely to be cost-prohibitive for all but the wealthy and the well-insured, assuming that insurance companies agree to such coverage, a big assumption in any case. The poor, who are primarily women and most persons of color, will simply be marginalized from these therapies, even as it is possible that their eggs are commercialized downstream for profit.

(Holland, 2001, p. 83)

ETHICAL CONDUCT

Nurses committed to high-quality care base their practice on professional standards of ethical conduct. The study of professional ethical behavior begins in nursing school, continues in formal and informal discussions with colleagues and peers, and culminates when nurses "try on" and adopt the behaviors of role models who practice professional nursing consistent with high ethical standards. How do nurses learn the standards for professional ethical behavior? At the very least, nurses should identify and develop the essential elements of ethical agency, cultivate the virtues of nursing, understand ethical theories that dictate and justify professional conduct, and be familiar with bioethical standards for professional nursing conduct.

Ethical Agency

It is unrealistic to assume that the simple desire to be a nurse is accompanied by the natural ability to behave in an ethical way and to do the ethically right thing because it is the right thing to do. This ability, **ethical agency,** must be cultivated in the same way that nurses cultivate the ability to do the scientifically right thing in response to a physiologic alteration. Nurses who appreciate the ethical challenges in professional practice value their ethical development sufficiently to work hard to develop these skills. Essential elements of ethical agency include:

- *Ethical sensibility:* Ability to recognize the "ethical moment" when an ethical challenge presents itself

- *Ethical responsiveness:* Ability and willingness to respond to the ethical challenge
- *Ethical reasoning and discernment:* Knowledge of and ability to use sound theoretical and practical approaches to "thinking through" ethical challenges, to ultimately decide how to respond to this particular situation after identifying and critiquing alternative courses of action; these approaches are used to inform as well as to justify moral behavior
- *Ethical accountability:* Ability and willingness to accept responsibility for one's ethical behavior and to learn from the experience of exercising ethical agency
- *Ethical character:* Cultivated dispositions that allow one to act as one believes one ought to act
- *Ethical valuing:* Valuing in a conscious and critical way that which squares with good ethical character and ethical integrity
- *Transformative ethical leadership:* Commitment and proven ability to create a culture that facilitates the exercise of ethical agency, a culture in which people do the right thing because it is the right thing to do

Box 6-3 illustrates these elements of ethical agency in action.

The Virtues of Nurses

Virtues are human excellencies, cultivated dispositions of character and conduct that motivate and enable us to be good human beings. Clinical virtues enable nurses to provide good care to patients. While there is no official list of essential virtues of nurses, the following virtues are frequently named:

- Competence
- Compassionate caring
- Subordination of self-interest to patient care
- Self-effacement
- Trustworthiness
- Conscientiousness
- Intelligence
- Practical wisdom
- Humility
- Courage
- Integrity

Since these human qualities cannot be "put on" the way one puts on a uniform or identity badge, it is important that they are part of the nurse's character, part of who the nurse is. They form an important basis of what allows patients to trust us!

Nursing Codes of Ethics

According to the American Nurses Association (2001), individuals who become nurses are expected not only to adhere to the moral norms of the profession but also to embrace them as part of what it means to be a nurse. The ethical tradition of nursing is self-reflective, enduring, and distinctive. A **code of ethics** is a set of principles that reflect the primary goals, values, and obligations of the profession.

The Code of Ethics for Nurses serves the following purposes:

- It is a succinct statement of the ethical obligations and duties of every individual who enters the nursing profession.

Box 6-3 ELEMENTS OF ETHICAL AGENCY

Situation: A 75-year-old patient with end-stage lung cancer suffers a respiratory arrest and is coded, ventilated, and admitted to the intensive care unit (ICU). When the receiving nurse reviews his chart, she discovers that upon admission, his nurse documented that he "did not want to be resuscitated" and that he wanted to prepare an advance directive specifying "no heroics." There is no do-not-resuscitate order on the chart, and the nurse can find no advance directive.

Ethical Sensibility
The ICU nurse notes the discrepancy between the patient's documented preferences and the care that he has received. She senses personal discomfort about this disregard for his wishes.

Ethical Responsiveness
The nurse can decide to ignore her discomfort and simply provide excellent technologic care, or acknowledge her discomfort and respond. She decides to talk with the attending physician about his knowledge concerning the patient's preferences and learns that the attending was unaware of the patient's documented preferences and has no personal knowledge of these. She contacts the nurse who originally admitted the patient and learns that although the patient was quite clear about his preference, no one followed up and translated this conversation into orders on his chart. She calls an ethics consult when the attending says that there is "nothing to be done now that treatment is initiated."

Ethical Reasoning and Discernment
During the ethics consult, family members agree that the patient would not be happy to find himself on a ventilator and request that he be weaned—even if this results in his death. The ethicist explains that weaning him from an ineffective treatment (the ventilator will not cure his lung cancer) that is disproportionately burdensome is an ethically justified action.

Ethical Accountability
The nurse initiated the ethics consult because she believed that she could not be an advocate for this patient and merely provide good physical care. Once she knew (or suspected) that his preferences had been ignored, she felt accountable for determining how the system had failed this patient and for remedying the problem. The nurse prides herself on being responsible and accountable; therefore, she could not "stick her head in the sand" and pretend that this was not her problem! After the ethics consult, she participates in plans to find an optimal time and conditions to wean the patient from the ventilator and makes sure that his family is present. The patient does not survive the weaning, and although they are grieving, his family members are grateful to the nurse for her care for the patient and for them.

Ethical Character
Because she had cultivated the virtues of responsibility and fidelity, the nurse's course of action was natural.

Ethical Valuing
Because she places a high value on being an effective patient advocate, the nurse was willing to confront the attending physician and initiate an ethics consult, even though these actions caused her some discomfort and the expense of time and inconvenience.

Transformative Ethical Leadership
When her colleagues asked her where she got the "guts" to follow through with this course of action, the nurse knew that the culture within the hospital had to change so that more nurses would choose to do the same thing she did without fearing negative consequences. She asks the nurse educator on her unit to explore the possibility of pursuing this theme in a future Nursing Grand Rounds and is willing to work to make this happen.

- It is the profession's nonnegotiable ethical standard.
- It is an expression of nursing's own understanding of its commitment to society.

The International Council of Nurses writes that, to achieve its purpose, The Code of Ethics for Nurses must be available to students and nurses throughout their study and work lives. They recommend that nursing students:

- Study the standards under each element of the Code.
- Reflect on what each standard means to them. Think about how they can apply ethics in their own nursing domain: practice, education, research, and management.
- Discuss the Code with coworkers and others.
- Use a specific example from experience to identify ethical dilemmas and standards of conduct as outlined in the Code. Identify how they would resolve the dilemma.
- Work in groups to clarify ethical decision making and reach a consensus on standards or ethical conflict.
- Collaborate with their national nurses' association, coworkers, and others in continuous application of ethical standards in nursing practice, education, management, and research.

Codes are effective in accomplishing their goals only to the extent that members of the profession uphold them. Code requirements may exceed legal requirements. Violations of the law subject a nurse to civil or criminal liability (see Chapter 7), and violations of the code of ethics may result in reprimands, censure, suspension, and expulsion.

Codes of ethics for nursing include the International Council of Nurses (ICN) *ICN Code of Ethics for Nurses* (adopted in 1953 and revised in 1965, 1973, 2000, and 2006) (Box 6-4); the *ANA Code for Nurses With Interpretive Statements* (adopted in 1950 and revised in 1968, 1976, 1985, and 2001) (Box 6-5); and the Canadian Nurses Association (CNA) *Code of Ethics for Registered Nurses* (adopted in 1980 and revised in 2002 and 2008) (Box 6-6).

Nursing Standards of Practice

When the American Nurses Association revised its Standards of Clinical Nursing Practice in 1991, it developed standards of professional performance as well as standards of care. Standard V of professional performance, Ethics, describes

THE ICN CODE OF ETHICS FOR NURSES

An international code of ethics for nurses was first adopted by the International Council of Nurses (ICN) in 1953. It has been revised and reaffirmed at various times since, most recently with this review and revision completed in 2005.

Preamble

Nurses have four fundamental responsibilities: to promote health, to prevent illness, to restore health, and to alleviate suffering. The need for nursing is universal.

Inherent in nursing is respect for human rights, including cultural rights, the right to life and choice, to dignity, and to be treated with respect. Nursing care is respectful of and unrestricted by considerations of age, colour, creed, culture, disability or illness, gender, sexual orientation, nationality, politics, race, or social status.

Nurses render health services to the individual, the family, and the community and co-ordinate their services with those of related groups.

The ICN Code

The *ICN Code of Ethics for Nurses* has four principal elements that outline the standards of ethical conduct.

1. Nurses and People

The nurse's primary professional responsibility is to people requiring nursing care. In providing care, the nurse promotes an environment in which the human rights, values, customs, and spiritual beliefs of the individual, family, and community are respected.

The nurse ensures that the individual receives sufficient information on which to base consent for care and related treatment.

The nurse holds in confidence personal information and uses judgement in sharing this information.

The nurse shares with society the responsibility for initiating and supporting action to meet the health and social needs of the public, in particular those of vulnerable populations.

The nurse also shares responsibility to sustain and protect the natural environment from depletion, pollution, degradation, and destruction.

2. Nurses and Practice

The nurse carries personal responsibility and accountability for nursing practice, and for maintaining competence by continual learning.

The nurse maintains a standard of personal health such that the ability to provide care is not compromised.

The nurse uses judgement regarding individual competence when accepting and delegating responsibility.

The nurse at all times maintains standards of personal conduct, which reflect well on the profession and enhance public confidence.

The nurse, in providing care, ensures that use of technology and scientific advances are compatible with the safety, dignity, and rights of people.

3. Nurses and the Profession

The nurse assumes the major role in determining and implementing acceptable standards of clinical nursing practice, management, research, and education.

The nurse is active in developing a core of research-based professional knowledge.

The nurse, acting through the professional organisation, participates in creating and maintaining safe, equitable social and economic working conditions in nursing.

4. Nurses and Co-Workers

The nurse sustains a co-operative relationship with co-workers in nursing and other fields.

The nurse takes appropriate action to safeguard individuals, families, and communities when their health is endangered by a co-worker or any other person.

the nurse's ethical obligations; the nurse's decisions and actions on behalf of patients are determined in an ethical manner. Measurement Criteria for Standard V (American Nurses Association, 2004, pp. 13–14) are:

1. The nurse's practice is guided by the Code for Nurses.
2. The nurse maintains patient confidentiality within legal and regulatory parameters.
3. The nurse acts as a patient advocate and assists patients in developing skills so they can advocate for themselves.
4. The nurse delivers care in a nonjudgmental and non-discriminatory manner that is sensitive to patient diversity.
5. The nurse delivers care in a manner that preserves or protects patient autonomy, dignity, and rights.
6. The nurse seeks available resources to help formulate ethical decisions

Remember Marissa Sandoval, the 44-year-old woman who wants answers but is not getting them? Integration of

these standards would be essential for the nurse to act professionally and ethically when obtaining the needed answers. ■

A Patient's Bill of Rights

The American Hospital Association developed *A Patient's Bill of Rights* in 1972 (revised in 2003 as *The Patient Care Partnership;* see Chapter 7, Box 7-5). The bill of rights includes the rights and responsibilities of the patient while receiving care in the hospital, which range from "the right to considerate and respectful care" to "the right to be informed of hospital policies and practices that relate to patient care, treatment and responsibilities." With care moving increasingly from the hospital to the community, nurses must be familiar with how different institutions and professional groups define patient rights and responsibilities. Other bills of rights include Pregnant Patient's Bill of Rights, Indian Patient's Bill of Rights, Nursing Home Bill of Rights, and Veterans Administration Code of Patient Concern. Each

Box 6-5 AMERICAN NURSES ASSOCIATION CODE FOR NURSES

1. The nurse, in all professional relationships, practices with compassion and respect for the inherent dignity, worth, and uniqueness of every individual, unrestricted by considerations of social or economic status, personal attributes, or the nature of health problems.
2. The nurse's primary commitment is to the patient, whether an individual, family, group, or community.
3. The nurse promotes, advocates for, and strives to protect the health, safety, and rights of the patient.
4. The nurse is responsible and accountable for individual nursing practice and determines the appropriate delegation of tasks consistent with the nurse's obligation to provide optimum patient care.
5. The nurse owes the same duties to self as to others, including the responsibility to preserve integrity, to maintain competence, and to continue personal and professional growth.
6. The nurse participates in establishing, maintaining, and improving healthcare environments and conditions of employment conducive to the provision of quality healthcare and consistent with the values of the profession through individual and collective action.
7. The nurse participates in the advancement of the profession through contributions to practice, education, administration, and knowledge development.
8. The nurse collaborates with other health professionals and with the public in promoting community, national, and international efforts to meet health needs.
9. The profession of nursing, as represented by associations and their members, is responsible for the articulating of nursing values, for maintaining the integrity of the profession and its practice, and for shaping social policy.

From *Code of Ethics for Nurses with Interpretive Statements*. © 2001 By American Nurses Association. Reprinted with permission. All rights reserved.

Box 6-6 CANADIAN NURSES ASSOCIATION CODE OF ETHICS FOR REGISTERED NURSES*

A. Nurses provide safe, compassionate, competent and ethical care.
B. Nurses work with people to enable them to attain their highest possible level of health and well-being.
C. Nurses recognize, respect, and promote a person's right to be informed and make decisions.
D. Nurses recognize and respect the intrinsic worth of each person.
E. Nurses recognize the importance of privacy and confidentiality and safeguard personal, family and community information obtained in the context of a professional relationship.
F. Nurses uphold principles of justice by safeguarding human rights, equity, and fairness and by promoting the public good.
G. Nurses are accountable for their actions and answerable for their practice.

*This represents only one element of the code—values. Nurses in all domains of practice bear the ethical responsibilities identified under each of the seven primary nursing values. These are intended to help nurses apply the code.

Reprinted with permission from Canadian Nurses Association. (2008). *Code of ethics for registered nurses*. Ottawa, Ontario: Author.

emphasizes a specific aspect of patient rights within a particular health agency and implies a code of ethics the nurse observes professionally.

> *The nurse could use knowledge of the Patient's Bill of Rights to ensure that the questions from Marissa Sandoval, the woman described at the beginning of the chapter, and those of her family, are answered.* ■

Bill of Rights for Registered Nurses

Two of the chief reasons nurses cite for the declining quality of nursing care at their facilities are inadequate staffing and decreased nurse satisfaction. Advocacy on behalf of nurses and the profession has resulted in a tangible tool, the Bill of Rights for Registered Nurses, to aid in improving workplaces and ensuring nurses' ability to provide safe, quality patient care. The Bill of Rights is intended to empower nurses by making clear what is absolutely nonnegotiable in the workplace. "The ANA and its constituent member organ-

izations will continue their longstanding work, through political and legislative activism, collective bargaining, workplace advocacy, and public education, to ensure that the basic tenets of this Bill of Rights are a reality for nurses across the country" (Wiseman, 2001).

The seven basic tenets of the Bill of Rights for Registered Nurses are (American Nurses Association, 2001, p. 1; used with permission):

1. Nurses have the right to practice in a manner that fulfills their obligations to society and to those who receive nursing care.
2. Nurses have the right to practice in environments that allow them to act in accordance with professional standards and legally authorized scopes of practice.
3. Nurses have the right to a work environment that supports and facilitates ethical practice, in accordance with the Code of Ethics for Nurses and its interpretive statements.
4. Nurses have the right to freely and openly advocate for themselves and their patients, without fear of retribution.
5. Nurses have the right to fair compensation for their work, consistent with their knowledge, experience, and professional responsibilities.
6. Nurses have the right to a work environment that is safe for themselves and their patients.
7. Nurses have the right to negotiate the conditions of their employment, either as individuals or collectively, in all practice settings.

Box 6-7   **TYPES OF ETHICAL EXPERIENCES AND SITUATIONS**

When nurses can name the type of ethical concern they are experiencing, they are better able to discuss it with colleagues and supervisors, take steps to address it at an early stage, and receive support and guidance in dealing with it. Identifying an ethical concern can often be a defining moment that allows positive outcomes to emerge from difficult experiences. There are a number of terms that can assist nurses in identifying and reflecting on their ethical experiences and discussing them with others:

- *Ethical problems* involve situations where there are conflicts between one or more values and uncertainty about the correct course of action. Ethical problems involve questions about what is right or good to do at individual, interpersonal, organizational, and even societal levels.
- *Ethical (or moral) uncertainty* occurs when a nurse feels indecision or a lack of clarity, or is unable even to know what the moral problem is, while at the same time feeling uneasy or uncomfortable.
- *Ethical dilemmas or questions* arise when there are equally compelling reasons for and against two or more possible courses of action, and where choosing one course of action means that something else is relinquished or let go. True dilemmas are infrequent in health care. More often, there are complex ethical problems with multiple courses of actions from which to choose.

- *Ethical (or moral) distress* arises when nurses know or believe they know the right thing to do, but for various reasons (including fear or circumstances beyond their control) do not or cannot take the right action or prevent a particular harm. When values and commitments are compromised in this way, nurses' identity and integrity as moral agents are affected, and they feel moral distress.
- *Ethical (or moral) residue* is what nurses experience when they seriously compromise themselves or allow themselves to be compromised. The moral residue that nurses carry forward from these kinds of situations can help them reflect on what they would do differently in similar situations in the future.
- *Ethical (or moral) disengagement* can occur if nurses begin to see the disregard of their ethical commitments as normal. A nurse may then become apathetic or disengage to the point of being unkind, noncompassionate, or even cruel to other healthcare workers and to persons receiving care.
- *Ethical violations* are actions or failures to act that breach fundamental duties to the persons receiving care or to colleagues and other healthcare providers.
- *Ethical (or moral) courage* is exercised when a nurse stands firm on a point of moral principle or a particular decision about something in the face of overwhelming fear or threat to himself or herself.

Used with permission. Canadian Nurses Association. (2008). *Code of Ethics for Registered Nurses.* 2008 Centennial Edition. Ottawa, Ontario: Author.

ETHICAL EXPERIENCE AND DECISION MAKING

Ethical experience comes in many varieties for professional nurses (Box 6-7).

Two types of ethical problems commonly faced by nurses are ethical dilemmas and ethical distress. In an ethical dilemma, two (or more) clear moral principles apply but support mutually inconsistent courses of action. **Ethical distress** occurs when the nurse knows the right thing to do but either personal or institutional factors make it difficult to follow the correct course of action. When what nurses choose to do is different than what they believe to be the ethically correct course of action, either their ethical agency is deficient or they are experiencing ethical distress—or some combination of both. Nurses need sound analytic skills and the ability to engage in ethical reasoning to resolve ethical dilemmas and ethical distress. The American Association of Critical Care Nurses has developed a helpful model to "rise above moral distress," which is illustrated in Figure 6-1 and is accessible at their Web site, www.aacn.org.

The Joint Commission mandates that all accredited agencies have a mechanism for addressing ethical problems. Nurses should be familiar with (and use) the resources within their institution. Most institutions have ethics committees (discussed later in the chapter), and many employ staff ethicists. A few have nurse ethicists. Resources for ethical decision making are highlighted in Box 6-8. Also see the

content on creating and sustaining healthy work environments in Chapter 16.

Using the Nursing Process to Make Ethical Decisions

Every nurse needs to be confident in using a process of ethical decision making. One process with which nurses are familiar and thus can use to make ethical decisions is the nursing process. Using the nursing process to make ethical decisions involves following the steps discussed below. The accompanying patient care study illustrates this five-step model of ethical decision making that is based on the nursing process (Box 6-9).

Assess the Situation (Gather Data)

Recognize and then describe the situation and contextual factors that give rise to the ethical problem. This involves the main people involved (their views and interests); the patient's overall nursing, medical, and social situation; and relevant legal, administrative, and staff considerations.

Diagnose (Identify) the Ethical Problem

Clarify that the issue is ethical in nature: (1) Is there a conflict at the personal, interpersonal, institutional, or societal level? Is there a question that arises either at the level of thought or feeling? (2) Does the question have a moral or ethical component? Why? (e.g., does it raise issues of rights,

ASK
You may be unaware of the exact nature of the problem but are feeling distress.

Ask: *"Am I feeling distressed or showing signs of suffering? Is the source of my distress work related? Am I observing symptoms of distress within my team?"*

Goal: You become aware that moral distress is present.

ACT
Prepare to Act
Prepare personally and professionally to take action.

Take Action
Implement strategies to initiate the changes you desire.

Maintain Desired Change
Anticipate and manage setbacks. Continue to implement the 4 A's to resolve moral distress.

Goal: You preserve your integrity and authenticity.

Creation of a healthy environment where critical care nurses make their optimal contributions to patients and families

AFFIRM
Affirm your distress and your commitment to take care of yourself.

Validate feelings and perceptions with others.

Affirm professional obligation to act.

Goal: You make a commitment to address moral distress.

ASSESS
Identify sources of your distress.
• Personal
• Environment
Determine the severity of your distress.
Contemplate your readiness to act.
• You recognize there is an issue but may be ambivalent about taking action to change it.
• You analyze risks and benefits.

Goal: You are ready to make an action plan.

FIGURE 6-1. The 4 A's to Rise Above Moral Distress. (From American Association of Critical Care Nurses, available at http://www.aacn.org/WD/Practice/Docs/4As_to_Rise_Above_Moral_Distress.pdf.)

moral character?) State the problem clearly. Identify your relationship to the decision. Identify time parameters. Make sure that the problem is an ethical problem as opposed to a communication or legal problem. Some suggest that whenever human dignity is being threatened, you have an ethical problem.

Plan

Identify options and explore the probable short-term and long-term consequences of each for each stakeholder. Use ethical reasoning to decide on a course of action that you can justify ethically:

• Identify your personal and professional moral positions and those of other involved individuals

• Apply pertinent ethical theories and principles
• Apply codes of conduct and ethics, professional position statements or guides as applicable
• Consider consultation with a respected and wise colleague or an institutional ethics committee
• Decide on the course of action you are best able to support

Implement Your Decision

Implement your decision and compare the outcome of your action with what you considered and hoped for in advance.

Evaluate Your Decision

What have you learned from this process that will help you in the future? How can you improve your reasoning and

Box 6-8   ETHICS RESOURCES

The following are ethics resources for healthcare professionals.

American Nurses Association Center for Ethics and Human Rights
http://www.nursingworld.org/ethics/index.htm

In September 1990, the Center for Ethics and Human Rights was established, with the following guiding objectives:

- *Promulgate* in collaboration with ANA constituents a body of knowledge, both theoretical and practical, designed to address issues in ethics and human rights at the state, national, and international level.
- *Develop and disseminate* information about and advocate for public policy to assure that ethics and human rights are addressed in healthcare.
- *Assure* that short- and long-range objectives regarding ethics and human rights will be addressed within the Association, and expressed to appropriate bodies external to the Association.

Be sure to note their policy statements.

The American Society for Bioethics and Humanities
http://www.asbh.org/

This is a professional society of more than 1500 individuals, organizations, and institutions interested in bioethics and humanities. Their website serves as a source of information for members, prospective members, and anyone interested in bioethics and humanities. There is a special interest group for nurses.

The American Society for Law, Medicine and Ethics
http://www.aslme.org/

Within this site you will find information about two nationally acclaimed peer-reviewed journals, *The Journal of Law, Medicine & Ethics* and *The American Journal of Law & Medicine*. You will be able to search for information from hundreds of articles that have been published. You will also be able to register for ASLME educational conferences and connect to relevant web links from the ASLME site.

The Medical College of Wisconsin's Center for the Study of Bioethics
http://www.mcw.edu/bioethics.htm

The Medical College of Wisconsin's Center for the Study of Bioethics is dedicated to nationally and internationally recognized innovation and excellence in:

- *Bioethics Education:* Educating healthcare professionals, researchers, policy makers, and students in bioethics
- *Bioethics Research and Scholarship:* Advancing current knowledge through research in bioethics and health policy
- *Bioethics Consultation:* Assisting ethics committees and healthcare providers in shared bioethical decision making with patients and their representatives
- *Bioethics Community Service:* Fostering greater understanding of bioethics issues locally, regionally, nationally, and internationally, through conferences, programs, and the development and dissemination of resource materials

National Reference Center for Bioethics Literature
http://bioethics.georgetown.edu/nrc/

A specialized collection of library resources concerned with contemporary biomedical issues in the fields of ethics, philosophy, medicine, nursing, science, law, religion, and the social sciences. Call for bioethics information, BIOETHICSLINE searches (computerized database), search strategies, reference help, and publication orders.

The Hastings Center
http://www.thehastingscenter.org/

The Hastings Center is an independent, nonpartisan, and nonprofit bioethics research institute, founded in 1969 to explore fundamental and emerging questions in healthcare, biotechnology, and the environment. Publishes *The Hastings Center Report*.

Centre for Applied Ethics
http://www.ethics.ubc.ca/resources/

Provides links to many ethics resources in healthcare and other disciplines

---

decision making in the future? In what ways does your institutional culture need to change to prevent similar conflicts in the future?

Ethically Relevant Considerations

Fletcher, Spencer, and Lombardo (2005) recommend attention to eight ethical considerations that have the greatest weight and relevance in the care of patients, which bridge between ethical principles, an ethics of caring, and the clinical situation (p. 12).

The Balance between Benefits and Harms in the Care of Patients

Nurses are superbly positioned to contribute to reasoning about what counts as the benefits or burdens of treatment and what are the related harms, since their relationships with patients enable them to see more than physiologic effects.

Disclosure, Informed Consent, and Shared Decision Making

There are three basic models of healthcare decision making. In the paternalistic model, clinicians acting to benefit the patient decide what ought to be done and inform the patient, and the patient's role is to comply. In the patient sovereignty model, patients or their surrogates, expressing their right to be autonomous, tell the clinician what they want, and the clinician's role is to comply. Most ethicists reject these models in their extremes and recommend a model of shared decision making, which respects and uses the preferences of the patient and the expertise and judgment of the clinician. *The object of all clinical decision making is decisions that secure the health and well-being of the patient and that honor and respect the integrity of all participants in the decision-making process.* Nurses can play an important role in ensuring that patients and their surrogates receive the information *and support they need* to make healthcare decisions that secure their interests.

Box 6-9 PATIENT CARE STUDY USING A FIVE-STEP PROCESS FOR RESOLVING ETHICAL CONFLICT

Jean Watts is a labor and delivery room nurse in a small community hospital that serves both private and clinic patients. Jean has always felt that certain members of the obstetrics–gynecology medical staff have treated these two groups of clients differently. On this particular morning, Jean is caring for a woman who is scheduled for an elective cesarean delivery. The woman (who is a clinic patient) has made it very clear that she wants to be awake for the delivery and has requested epidural or spinal anesthesia. Jean is dismayed when the anesthesiologist enters the delivery room because the anesthesiologist's success rate with epidural anesthesia is poor. The anesthesiologist unsuccessfully attempts to perform an epidural block. After waiting 20 minutes for results, the obstetrician is growing impatient and instructs the anesthesiologist to put the patient to sleep. Jean feels the rights of this patient are being violated but is unsure of what her response should be.

Step 1: Assess the Situation (Gather Data)

The patient is in stable medical condition (elective cesarean delivery, not an emergency) and has made it very clear that she wishes to be awake for the delivery. The patient is not a private paying patient of the obstetrician. The nurse believes her role is to promote and protect the patient's interests; she knows of no reason in this case why the patient's preferences should be disregarded.

The anesthesiologist has a poor success record with epidural anesthesia.

The obstetrician seems to want to complete delivery quickly. In the past, he has seemed to give more weight to following wishes of private patients, as opposed to clinic patients. He is the head of the obstetrics–gynecology department; he believes nurses should obey physicians unquestioningly.

Nurses have in the past expressed dissatisfaction with the different levels of care being provided to private and clinic patients, but no one to date has formally addressed the concern.

Step 2: Diagnose (Identify) the Ethical Problem

Jean objects to the obstetrician's intent to disregard the patient's wish to be awake for her delivery; she is aware of no good reasons justifying this course of action.

The nurse will be a participant in carrying out the decision.

The decision for this case must be made immediately; it would be helpful to plan to avoid situations like this in the future.

Step 3: Plan

a. Identify Options

The nurse can say nothing to the obstetrician and help with the delivery. If asked by the patient later why she needed to be put to sleep, the nurse can (1) tell the truth, (2) refer her to the obstetrician, (3) express sympathy that she could not be awake, or (4) say nothing. *Outcome:* The patient's wishes are disregarded; delivery occurs in record time, and the obstetrician is happy; the nurse fulfills obligation to physician and hospital but feels she has betrayed the patient's trust. *Long-term outcome:* There is a good probability the same problem will happen again.
Or

The nurse can remind the obstetrician that the patient was adamant about wanting to be awake and suggest that a differ-

ent anesthesiologist be called in. If the obstetrician agrees, the patient may get her wish and everyone is satisfied with the outcome (the nurse must still decide how to prevent recurrence of this dilemma). If the obstetrician refuses and insists that the patient be put to sleep, the nurse can (1) refuse to participate (if another nurse is unavailable or unwilling to replace her, the nurse has abandoned the patient and harm may ensue) or (2) participate and proceed as above or resolve to speak to the obstetrician in a "cool moment" after the delivery to see how to avoid this problem in the future. If the nurse does not get satisfaction with the obstetrician, then she must decide whether to move through the proper administrative channels. Depending on the institution and people involved, the nurse may be affirmed or censored for this move. *Long-term outcome:* Future patients may be helped by the nurse following through with her concerns.
Or

The nurse can say nothing and assist with this delivery, believing it to be the wisest course of action for the time being, but resolve to take the steps above to correct the perceived injustice. *Outcome:* There is no benefit for the present patient but potential benefit to future patients.

b. Think the Ethical Problem Through

Basic moral principles: The good of patients (beneficence) should be the nurse's primary concern (ANA Code of Ethics for nurses); this strongly suggests that the nurse should act, but it does not address the nurse's obligation to do so if she feels it would jeopardize her own good (job security).

Respect for persons would suggest that the patient's autonomy (right to self-determination) should be respected unless there is strong justification for not doing so.

Justice would suggest that whether a patient pays the obstetrician privately should have no bearing on the quality of care received.

Care-based ethics would obligate Jean to serve as an effective advocate for her patient, respecting the nurse's commitment to be faithful to the nurse–patient relationship.

c. Make a Decision

Jean feels from past interactions with this obstetrician that her speaking up will not influence his decision to have the patient put to sleep. She decides to speak with the obstetrician after the delivery and follow up with whatever approach is necessary to avoid recurrence.

Steps 4–5: Implement and Evaluate Your Decision

Jean will never know if speaking up would have resulted in the patient's wishes being respected. Although she is dissatisfied with the outcome of this case, she hopes to prevent this from happening to other clinic patients in the future. In this instance, a hospital committee was formed to study the problem and make recommendations. If Jean had been told to "mind her own business" unless she wanted trouble, she would have to make a decision weighing patient benefit on one hand with potential personal risk or harm on the other.

Norms of Family Life

Most patients do not present as isolated individuals. Nurses who are sensitive to how a patient's injury or illness influences family members and significant others will be better able to appreciate how this influences decisions about care and can bring this information to the interdisciplinary team.

The Relationship between Clinicians and Patients

The healing encounter is central to nursing ethics. As nurses reason ethically about what ought to be done, it is always in the context of the relationships, which hold us accountable to patients and their families, and the professional caregivers with whom we work. Much ethical distress for nurses results from the strong conviction that we owe individual patients more than present work environments allow us to deliver.

The Professional Integrity of Clinicians

While the 2001 ANA Code of Ethics for Nurses clearly states that the primary commitment of the nurse is the patient, it also states that the nurse owes the same duties to self as to others—including the responsibility to preserve integrity, to maintain competence, and to continue personal and professional growth. Nurses should think long and hard when they find themselves asked to sacrifice personal integrity to meet the needs of another.

Cost-Effectiveness and Allocation

The increasing awareness of how difficult it is to make valued and scarce health resources available to all in need has resulted in new appreciation for the moral relevance of cost-effectiveness. Nurses who are committed to patient advocacy bridge the sometimes overwhelming needs of patients and their families and the limited resources available to professional caregivers. Justice is the principle of bioethics that speaks to distributing the benefits and burdens of healthcare delivery fairly. Nurses are uniquely positioned within the interdisciplinary team to speak to what it means to give patients or patient cohorts "their due."

Issues of Cultural and/or Religious Variation

Since many conflicts about what ought to be done are rooted in different cultural or religious beliefs and values, nurses who are sensitive to the cultural and/or religious identity of patients and caregivers can help mediate these conflicts.

Considerations of Power

Differences in power underlie many of the ethical challenges encountered in clinical practice. Injury and illness create vulnerabilities in the most sophisticated consumer of healthcare and mandate vigilance on the part of the nurse and other caregivers to challenge any abuses of power by clinicians. Clinicians who believe they lack power to influence care settings and delivery may also experience ethical conflict and distress.

A Final Note About Trustworthiness

Common to all of the standards discussed above is the obligation for nurses to be competent and willing to use their competence to secure the health and well-being or good dying of the patient. Whom you choose to be on any day you arrive for practice literally has the power to influence how people are born, live, and die. When you become aware that something is interfering with patients getting the care they need, you are responsible for responding within the scope of your power and responsibility. If you cannot independently resolve the problem, you are responsible for alerting the appropriate party, who may be the attending physician, a nursing supervisor, or a medical director. While some nurses believe "the problem is out of their hands" once they notify the next person in the chain of command, the problem remains theirs until appropriate action is taken. Thus, you should know and use the chain of command and continue to refer a problem upwards until it is resolved and the patient's needs are met.

Examples of Ethical Problems

Ethical problems commonly arise between nurses and patients, nurses and physicians, nurses and other nurses, and nurses and their employing institutions. Moreover, nurses are often most conflicted when good practice seems to require acting against their personal moral convictions. As you read through the following mini-cases, try to determine how you would respond. The process of ethical decision making described above should prove helpful. Note that many ethical challenges will be addressed in other chapters, especially Chapters 43 and 45.

Nurses and Patients

Troublesome nurse–patient situations that can result in ethical problems for nurses include **paternalism** (acting for patients without their consent to secure good or prevent harm), deception, confidentiality, allocation of scarce nursing resources, advocacy, valid consent or refusal, conflicts between the patient's and nurse's values and interests, and conflicts concerning new technologies.

PATERNALISM

An alert older resident who lives in a nursing home and who is now at high risk for falls refuses to call the nurse for assistance when getting out of bed. The nurse must decide whether to obtain an order to restrain the patient. Does preventing potential harm justify violating the patient's right to autonomy and make it acceptable for the nurse to act as a "parent" and choose an action the patient does not want because the nurse believes it to be in the patient's best interest?

DECEPTION

A postoperative patient asks the student nurse, who is about to administer an intramuscular injection for pain, "Is this your first shot?" It does happen to be the student's first injection, and the student is anxious. Would the student's intent to decrease the patient's anxiety justify telling the patient, "No, I've given several before"?

CONFIDENTIALITY

A nurse asks a middle-aged woman who is crying quietly, "Would you like to share what's troubling you?" The woman tells the nurse she has no idea how she will pay for this clinic visit because she entered the country illegally 2 months ago and is trying to earn enough money to help her family back home. She begs the nurse not to tell anyone. If the nurse believes this anxiety is interfering with the patient's ability to obtain needed healthcare, would it be ethical to break the woman's confidence to obtain help for her?

ALLOCATION OF SCARCE NURSING RESOURCES

A nurse has just been pulled from your unit, leaving it understaffed. Among your patients is a 33-year-old man recovering from a heart attack who is being discharged in the morning (he tells you he still has many questions), an older patient who is close to death, and a woman with cancer who has been vomiting all day and who is in severe pain. You know you cannot meet everyone's needs well. How do you "distribute" your nursing care? (You really like the patient who is going home in the morning.)

ADVOCACY IN MARKET-DRIVEN ENVIRONMENT

A hospitalized 57-year-old woman who underwent two lengthy bowel resections has just been informed by her health plan that she has exceeded her allowable length of stay and needs to be discharged immediately. She lives alone and has no family members or friends who are able to assist with her care. You believe that she would benefit immensely from extra hospital days so that she could regain her strength and learn how to provide necessary self-care. She does not have the money to pay for more days. What do you do?

VALID CONSENT OR REFUSAL

A resident is attempting to perform a spinal tap on an adolescent who you know dislikes the resident. After one failed attempt, the adolescent tells the resident to stop. The resident asks you to administer an antianxiety medication to the patient so the resident can get the spinal tap done quickly. Should you administer the medication knowing the patient no longer consents to the procedure?

CONFLICTS BETWEEN THE PATIENT'S AND NURSE'S INTERESTS

A homeless man who is well known to the emergency room nurses arrives one night in an inebriated state looking like it has been weeks since he washed or changed clothes. He is known to have tuberculosis and hepatitis B. One nurse, who is breastfeeding her 8-month-old infant, refuses to take him as a patient, fearing she will transmit something to her baby. The other nurses tell her she must accept this assignment because it is her "duty" and none of them is willing to cover for her. Is a nurse ever justified in refusing to provide care to a patient assigned to his or her care?

CONFLICTS CONCERNING NEW TECHNOLOGIES

An infertile woman asks you what you think about in vitro fertilization. She tells you that she is "desperate to produce a child for her husband and in-laws" but also has grave reservations about the whole process. "I've read about couples who end up with seven frozen embryos, and I think that would kill me, thinking I've got seven potential kids 'on ice.'"

Nurses and Physicians

Nurse–physician situations can also result in ethical distress for nurses. Common problems include disagreements about a proposed medical regimen, conflicts regarding the scope of the nurse's role, and physician incompetence.

DISAGREEMENTS ABOUT THE PROPOSED MEDICAL REGIMEN

In the nursing home where you work, any patient who loses a significant amount of weight (more than 10% of usual body weight) is automatically subjected to an exhaustive battery of tests (including a complete gastrointestinal [GI] series) to determine whether there are any physical causes for the weight loss (e.g., a tumor). You strongly object to one patient being put through these tests because she has made it clear that she wants to die and will starve herself to death if that is the only way she can do it. The medical director insists that the patient undergo the diagnostic studies because there is a long history of patient family dissatisfaction with the facility's medical care. The director wants to avoid causing further dissatisfaction. Are you responsible for preparing the patient for these diagnostic studies and scheduling them? Are there grounds for refusing to participate?

CONFLICTS REGARDING THE SCOPE OF THE NURSE'S ROLE

A young woman needing surgery that will result in a permanent colostomy tells the nurse how afraid she is and how much she dreads depending on "the thing." The nurse is certain this patient would benefit greatly from the help of the young staff enterostomal therapist, who also has a colostomy. When this suggestion is mentioned to the surgeon, however, the surgeon tells the nurse that he does his own teaching and counseling for all his patients and does not "believe" in enterostomal therapists. He points out that the nurse's duty here is to carry out his orders. Does it fall within the scope of nursing to recommend the enterostomal therapist to the woman? Is the nurse obligated to make this recommendation to the patient?

UNPROFESSIONAL, INCOMPETENT, UNETHICAL, OR ILLEGAL PHYSICIAN PRACTICE

A nurse who works in the operating room notices that a pediatric surgeon who has been on the staff for several years and done excellent work suddenly seems not to be concentrating during surgery and to be making more mistakes than usual. Rumors have been circulating about the surgeon having a problem with cocaine abuse after his recent divorce. The parents of one pediatric patient are dissatisfied with the progress the patient is making and ask the nurse for an opinion about the surgeon. Should the nurse voice personal concerns? Is the nurse obligated to report the physician to the proper hospital authority for investigation?

Nurses and Other Nurses

Some of the most difficult ethical problems nurses encounter result from nurse–nurse interactions, which may be complicated by obligations of friendship. Problems include claims of loyalty and nurse incompetence.

CLAIMS OF LOYALTY

A nurse working the 11 p.m. to 7 a.m. shift tells the other nurse on the unit, "I just made rounds and everyone is OK. Please cover for me while I catch an hour of sleep. I had an awful day." She neglects to tell the other nurse that a report mentioned that one patient needed special monitoring. This patient dies unexpectedly while the nurse sleeps. When she wakes up and discovers what happened, she begs the other nurse, her friend, never to tell anyone she was sleeping. "That patient could have died anyway between my rounds," she says. "Besides, you're my best friend, right?"

UNPROFESSIONAL, INCOMPETENT, UNETHICAL, OR ILLEGAL NURSE PRACTICE

When you make your morning rounds, a patient tells you that one of the nurses fondled her body and made suggestive remarks during the previous night shift. You suspect that the patient may simply be trying to cause trouble, and because you like the nurse in question, you find it hard to believe the patient. What should you do?

Nurses and Institutional and Public Policy

As nurses assume increased responsibility for decision making at all levels of care, the institutional and public policy arenas offer unique dilemmas. Three current examples are short staffing, whistle-blowing, and healthcare rationing.

SHORT STAFFING AND WHISTLE-BLOWING

Restructuring has resulted in chronic understaffing on the unit where you work. You believe that patients are now at risk because there simply are not enough nurses to provide quality care. Some nurses are talking about forming a union and going on strike. Because yours is the only major hospital in a rural area, you are unsure whether striking is a morally legitimate option. Because efforts to get management involved in addressing the issues have repeatedly failed, you are also contemplating "going public" with your concerns. Your brother works for the local newspaper, and you are pretty sure he would be willing to do a story about the situation at the hospital. What do you do?

HEALTHCARE RATIONING

In the United States, as many as 43 million people are uninsured or underinsured and have limited access to healthcare. Whether each person has a "right" (is entitled) to basic healthcare continues to be the subject of debate. There are plans for rationing healthcare that could limit the options available to the elderly, the poor, the terminally ill, and those in society whom many view as having limited "social value." What moral obligation do you have to contribute to this debate? How might you ensure that your voice and the nursing viewpoint are heard?

Nurses' Personal Moral Convictions and Institutional or Professional Ethics

Nurses sometimes experience a challenge to their personal ethical integrity because what they believe ought to be done in a particular situation is forbidden by the ethics of their place of employment or profession.

BEGINNING-OF-LIFE ISSUES

You are a psychiatric mental health nurse working in a Catholic hospital whose ethical and religious directives forbid abortion and abortion counseling. You are talking with a single woman recently hospitalized with bipolar disorder who is in the first trimester of an unplanned pregnancy and who is expressing great ambivalence about continuing the pregnancy. You personally believe that your ethical obligation is to explore abortion as an option with this woman and to refer her to outside resources if she elects to abort. The charge nurse tells you that these are not appropriate options within this hospital.

END-OF-LIFE ISSUES

You are the nurse case manager for a woman with a history of breast cancer whose cancer recurred (metastasis to the spine) after she had been cancer free for 7 years. She frequently tells you when you come to visit her at home that she is unwilling to fight anymore and wants to die with some dignity while she is still in control. She begs you to get her something that will "put me gently to sleep once and for all before my pain gets worse." You believe that this is her sincere wish, not just depression speaking, and you honestly believe that she would be better off spared the last stage of her illness. Your religious beliefs, however, tell you that assisted suicide is wrong under any circumstances. How do you reconcile your desire to help this woman with your profession's ethical code and your religious conviction that what she is asking for is intrinsically wrong? For a fuller discussion of ethical issues at the end of life, see Chapter 43.

Nurses and Ethics Committees

An increasing number of healthcare institutions have developed ethics committees whose chief functions include education, policy making, case review, consultation, and, in some cases, research. Some committees focus on clinical ethics and some on organizational ethics. These committees are uniquely equipped to deal with the complexities of modern healthcare because they are multidisciplinary and provide a forum in which radically divergent views can be aired without fear of repercussion. Nurses bring an important voice to the ethics committee. When clinical issues are being reviewed, nurses can help to ensure that the technical facts are understood, that the appropriate decision makers have been identified, that the patient's medical and overall best interests have been identified, and that the course of action selected from the alternatives is justified by sound ethical principles. Nurses' strong backgrounds in interpersonal communications allow us to contribute unique knowledge about the patient and family to the discussion and to facilitate the ethics committee's group dynamics.

Nurses also play an important role in policy making. They are frequently able to identify what policies are needed to address recurring ethical concerns and to suggest needed modifications of existing policies.

ADVOCACY IN NURSING PRACTICE

Bridging vulnerable patients and the resources they need to secure health outcomes, nurses have always been strong patient advocates. **Advocacy** is the protection and support of another's rights. This role is increasingly important because of patients' changing expectations and demands, and because the public has learned that in our increasingly market-driven healthcare economy, there are no guarantees that the healthcare system will work to secure their safety and health. See the Nursing Advocacy in Action box in this and other chapters.

Nurses who value patient advocacy:

- Make sure that their loyalty to an employing institution or colleague does not compromise their primary commitment to the patient
- Give priority to the good of the individual patient rather than to the good of society in general
- Carefully evaluate the competing claims of the patient's autonomy (self-determination) and patient well-being

When respecting autonomy, the nurse respects and supports the patient's right to make decisions. Informed consent is described in Chapter 7. When promoting patient well-being, the nurse acts in the best interests of the patient. Ideally, both autonomy and patient well-being are promoted in every nurse–patient interaction; however, conflicts sometimes arise.

> ▶ *For example, when Mr. Zhang, the 32-year-old man described at the beginning of the chapter, requests to be removed from the ventilator, the principle of autonomy demands respect for his treatment preferences at the same time that the principle of nonmaleficence obligates us to prevent the harm of his likely death. Nurses sensitive to the need to promote both patient autonomy and well-being may often experience conflict, but they are more likely than other nurses to succeed in securing the patient's genuine best interests.* ■

NURSING ADVOCACY IN ACTION

Patient Scenario

Mrs. Abigail Winthur is repeatedly asking the staff in your nursing home NOT to encourage her husband to eat. Mr. Winthur, age 88, has advanced Alzheimer's disease. He seems to enjoy eating and has no difficulty swallowing, but an aide has to sit by Mr. Winthur and lift the spoon to his mouth and place his cup in his hand. If you merely put the tray in front of him, he will most likely not eat.

Mrs. Winthur reports that her husband would never want to live the way he is now and she is sure that he would refuse to eat if capable of doing so. She also states that society is going to have to decide what to do about all the people we are currently warehousing. She seems to love her husband, but she is very open about the horror of being his caregiver for 3 years. He was always a gentle man, but then suddenly he became aggressive and would just as soon hit or punch you as take your hand.

Implications for Nursing Advocacy

How will you respond if you are Mr. Winthur's nurse? Talk with your classmates and experienced nurses about the questions that follow.

- If you elect to advocate for Mr. and Mrs. Winthur, what practical steps can you take to ensure better health outcomes?
- What is it reasonable to expect of a student nurse, a graduate nurse, and an experienced nurse in this situation?
- What advocacy skills are needed to effectively respond to this challenge?

Representing Patients

Most nurses would agree that a great deal of nursing time is spent representing patients' interests or guiding patients in protecting their own rights. The nurse is often involved as an intermediary between the patient and the family, especially when the patient and family have conflicting ideas about the management of healthcare situations (Fig. 6-2). For example, a patient with terminal cancer may want to go home to die. He tells this to his nurse. The patient's family, however, tells the nurse that they cannot care for him at home. As an advocate, the nurse recognizes the rights of both the patient and his family. The nurse then works to assist them in finding a solution that benefits both the patient and them. By informing the family of the availability of home care and hospice care, the nurse gives them knowledge that may help satisfy the patient's right to a dignified death. Working alone, most people would be unable to get the financial help needed

FIGURE 6-2. The nurse acts as a patient advocate in discussing all aspects of the patient's healthcare with family members.

for such care. Nurses have the resources available to help them and can arrange referrals from other healthcare workers, such as social workers, to achieve the desired outcomes.

Nurses may also serve as intermediaries between patients and the medical profession. Nurse ethicist Patricia Murphy (1990) documented a moving account of how nurses interceded for a 43-year-old woman with amyotrophic lateral sclerosis who was on a ventilator but wished to die. The patient's primary physicians refused to help remove her from the ventilator, and more than 20 other physicians declined to accept her as a patient when they learned what she wanted to do. After unsuccessful appeals for help to the county medical society and her own attorney, the patient's visiting nurse, working with a supportive social worker, contacted her state nurses association and finally secured the assistance she needed to help the patient achieve her goal of a dignified death.

Patients with special advocacy needs include those who are uninformed concerning their rights and opportunities, those with sensory impairment, those who do not speak English well or at all, the very young and the elderly, those who are seriously ill, those who are mentally or emotionally impaired, those with physical disabilities, and those who lack adequate financial or human resources.

> *Consider Mr. Raines, the 68-year-old man described at the beginning of the chapter. Awareness of his special needs would be critical in developing his discharge plan of care.* ∎

Promoting Self-Determination

Advocacy is linked to the belief that making choices about health is a fundamental human right that promotes the individual's dignity and well-being. Ethical dilemmas may arise when people are unable or unwilling to make choices or when they are not given the opportunity to do so. Faulty communication among patients, family members, and caregivers frequently contributes to these dilemmas. Nurses have an important advocacy role in educating the public about the value of written advance directives (described in Chapter 43).

Nurses as advocates must realize that they do not make ethical decisions for their patients. Instead, they facilitate patients' decision making. Nurses interpret findings for their patients, inform them of various aspects to be considered, help them verbalize and organize their feelings, call in those people who should be involved in the decision making (e.g., family, primary nurse, physician, or clergy), and help patients assess all of their options in relation to their beliefs. In this way, nurses advocate for the right of patients to make their own decisions concerning their health. Not all individuals want to make their own treatment decisions; however, you should not violate the spirit of autonomy (self-determination) by forcing it on anyone. Nurses sometimes advocate for patients by helping them to delegate decisions to a preferred decision maker whom they trust. In addition, when claiming to be a patient advocate, nurses must be careful to clarify exactly what it is they mean by advocacy because, in most instances, this is not simply supporting patients in all of their preferences. For example, if a patient in the early stages of Alzheimer's disease, with the support of her husband, asks a nurse for help in terminating her life, the nurse would have strong ethical grounds for refusing to advocate for this particular request.

Being Politically Active

No discussion of nursing advocacy would be complete without noting nursing's continuing voice in the political arena on behalf of those least well served by the existing healthcare system, including homeless people, minorities, women, and children. As the government becomes more involved in the delivery and funding of healthcare services, and as those designing rationing plans speak seriously of age and other variables as criteria for limiting care, nurses must continue to advocate for the healthcare needs of those least empowered to do so for themselves. Nurses are a powerful block of voters whose potential for influencing healthcare legislation is just beginning to be tapped. See Chapter 7 for helpful guides to contacting your legislative representatives.

● Developing Critical Thinking Skills

1. Students choose nursing as a career because of different values. A desire to help others, a love of money, wanting a career that allows you to work anywhere at any time, a commitment to provide for your children's well-being, a love of science and technology, and respect for your parents' wishes are all values that may lead to choosing nursing as a career.
   - Interview your classmates and identify the values that brought everyone to nursing. When a classmate lists more than one value, ask him or her to rank these in order of their importance. Compare your lists.
   - Discuss which values, if any, provide the best motivation for professional nursing. Are there certain values that are incompatible with professional nursing and that ought to be grounds for rejecting candidates for professional nursing?
   - Make a judgment about how well your personal values equip you for professional nursing. Would your patients affirm your values? Are any modifications needed?

2. Make a list of all the values that might positively or negatively influence someone's ability to lose weight. Think about how you could use this knowledge when counseling obese patients.

3. Another student tells you "Who I am outside of school is no one's business and has no effect on my nursing." Do you agree? Why or why not?

4. Take any current ethical issue (assisted suicide, human cloning, how to allocate scarce organs for transplantation, everyone's right to healthcare) and poll your class to see the range of opinions among your classmates. Reflect on what it is that causes people to reach different conclusions about what is the ethically right thing to do. How might you use this knowledge as you experience ethical conflict in your professional practice?

● Practicing for NCLEX

1. Five-year-old Bobby has dietary modifications related to his diabetes. His parents want him to value good nutritional habits and they decide to deprive him of a favorite TV program when he becomes angry after they deny him foods not on his diet. This is an example of what mode of value transmission?
   a. Modeling
   b. Moralizing
   c. Laissez-faire
   d. Rewarding and punishing
   e. Responsible choice

2. Which of the following is the best professional response to a patient who tells you that she believes that "white nurses are smarter than nurses of color" and then asks if you agree?
   a. "You are right!" (The patient/customer is always right!)
   b. "What I think doesn't matter. What's important is whatever you believe." (Value neutrality)
   c. "I don't believe being smart is related to race or ethnicity." (Commitment to human dignity)

3. The American Association of Colleges of Nursing identified five values that epitomize the caring professional nurse. Which of these is best described as acting in accordance with an appropriate code of ethics and accepted standards of practice?
   a. Altruism
   b. Autonomy
   c. Human dignity
   d. Integrity
   e. Social justice

4. A professional nurse with a commitment to social justice is most apt to:
   a. Provide honest information to patients and the public
   b. Promote universal access to healthcare
   c. Plan care in partnership with patients
   d. Document care accurately and honestly

5. When an older nurse complains that nurses just aren't ethical anymore, which reply reflects the best understanding of moral development?
   a. "The ability to behave ethically must be carefully cultivated; maybe we don't value this sufficiently to pay it the attention it deserves."
   b. "I don't agree that nurses were more ethical in the past. It's a new age and the ethics are new!"
   c. "Ethics is genetically determined . . . it's like having blue or brown eyes. Maybe we're evolving out of the ethical sense you and your generation had."
   d. "No kidding! Who could be ethical in a practice setting like this!"

6. A home health nurse who performs a careful safety assessment of the home of a frail elderly patient to prevent harm to the patient is acting in accord with which of the principles of bioethics?
   a. Autonomy
   b. Beneficence
   c. Justice
   d. Fidelity
   e. Nonmaleficence

7. A professional nurse committed to the principle of autonomy would be careful to:
   a. Provide the information and support a patient needed to make decisions to advance her own interests
   b. Treat each patient fairly, trying to give everyone his or her due

c. Keep any promises made to a patient or another professional caregiver

d. Avoid causing harm to a patient

8. A friend asks you about the new Bill of Rights for nurses. What can you tell her that accurately reflects the concerns of the drafters of these rights?
   a. The Bill of Rights was drafted by nurses who care more about themselves than they do about patients.
   b. The Bill of Rights was drafted by union nurses who are always looking for a reason to strike.
   c. The Bill of Rights was drafted to empower nurses and to improve conditions in the workplace.

9. Janie wants to call an ethics consult to clarify treatment goals for a patient no longer able to speak for himself. She believes his dying is being prolonged painfully. She is troubled when the patient's doctor tells her that she'll be fired if she raises questions about his care or calls the consult. This is a good example of:
   a. Ethical uncertainty
   b. Ethical distress
   c. Ethical dilemma

10. Nurse advocates often are conflicted about respecting a patient's right to be self-determining, while at the same time wanting to do everything in their power to promote the patient's best interests. Which is the best general guideline for situations like these?
    a. Patient rules! "It's my life!"
    b. Nurse rules! "It may be your life, but in this instance you don't know enough to make the right choice!"
    c. When in conflict, weigh the benefits and risks of following each option and then choose wisely.

● Answers With Rationale

1. *d.* When rewarding and punishing are used to transmit values, children are rewarded for demonstrating values held by parents and punished for demonstrating unacceptable values.

2. *c.* While it is true that value neutrality commits nurses to care for patients whether or not the nurse and patient hold the same value, it is not true that nurses should sacrifice their moral integrity and compromise their beliefs or values to please a patient.

3. *d.* The American Association of Colleges of Nursing defines integrity as acting in accordance with an appropriate code of ethics and accepted standards of practice.

4. *b.* The American Association of Colleges of Nursing lists promoting universal access to healthcare as an example of social justice. Providing honest information and documenting care accurately and honestly are examples of integrity, and planning care in partnership with patients is an example of autonomy.

5. *a.* The ability to be ethical, to make decisions, and to act in an ethically justified manner, begins in childhood and develops gradually.

6. *e.* Nonmaleficence is defined as the obligation to prevent harm. Autonomy is respect for another's right to make decisions, beneficence obligates us to benefit the patient, justice obligates us to act fairly, and fidelity obligates us to keep our promises.

7. *a.* The principle of autonomy obligates us to provide the information and support patients and their surrogates need to make decisions that advance their interests.

8. *c.* The American Nurses Association's Bill of Rights for Registered Nurses was a result of advocacy on behalf of nurses, to aid in improving workplaces and to ensure that nurses would have what they needed to provide safe, quality patient care. It is not true that these nurses cared more for themselves than patients (*a*) nor that these were nurses looking for reasons to strike (*b*).

9. *b.* Ethical distress results from knowing the right thing to do but finding it almost impossible to execute because of institutional or other constraints (in this case, fear of losing her job). Ethical uncertainty (*a*) results from feeling troubled by a situation but not knowing if it is an ethical problem. Ethical dilemmas occur when the principles of bioethics justify two or more conflicting courses of action (*c*).

10. *c.* Neither respecting and supporting patient preferences (*a*) nor ignoring patient preferences to achieve a medical benefit (*b*) routinely trump all other considerations. When a nurse cannot do both simultaneously, she must carefully weigh the benefits and risks of each option and then choose wisely.

Taylor Suite Resources

The Taylor Suite offers these additional resources to enhance learning and facilitate understanding of this chapter:

• thePoint online resource, http://thepoint.lww.com/Taylor7E
• Student DVD included with the book
• Study Guide for Taylor's Fundamentals of Nursing

BIBLIOGRAPHY

American Association of Colleges of Nursing. (2008). *The essentials of baccalaureate education for professional nursing practice*. Washington, DC: Author.

American Association of Critical-Care Nurses. (n.d.). *4 A's to rise above moral distress*. Available at http://www.aacn.org/WD/Practice/Docs/4As_to_Rise_Above_Moral_Distress.pdf.

American Association of Critical-Care Nurses. (2005). *AACN standards for establishing and sustaining healthy work environments*. Available at http://www.aacn.org/WD/HWE/Content/hwehome.pcms?menu=Practice&lastmenu=American Nurses Association. (2001). *Code for nurses with interpretive statements*. Washington, DC: Author.

American Nurses Association. (n.d.). Ethics and human rights. ANA policy statements. Available at http://www.nursingworld.org/MainMenuCategories/HealthcareandPolicyIssues/ANAPositionStatements/EthicsandHumanRights.aspx.

American Nurses Association. (2003). *Nursing's social policy statement* (2nd ed.). Washington, DC: Author.

American Nurses Association. (2004). *Nursing: Scope and standards of practice.* Washington, DC: Author.

American Nurses Association's Code of Ethics Task Force. (2000). A new code of ethics for nurses. *AJN, 100*(7), 69, 71–72.

Beauchamp, T. L., & Childress, J. F. (2001). *Principles of biomedical ethics* (5th ed.). New York: Oxford University Press.

Bishop, A. H., & Scudder, J. R. (1990). *The practical, moral, and personal sense of nursing.* Albany: State University of New York Press.

Burkhardt, M. A., & Nathaniel, A. K. (2008). Ethical issues in contemporary nursing (3rd ed.). Clifton Park, New York: Thomson Delmar Learning.

Callahan, D. (1995). Bioethics. In W. T. Reich (Ed.), *Encyclopedia of bioethics* (Rev. ed., pp. 247–256). New York: Macmillan.

Canadian Nurses Association. (2008). *Code of ethics for registered nurses.* Ottawa, Ontario: Author.

Corley, M. C., Elswick, R. K., Gorman, M., & Clor, T. (2001). Development and evaluation of a moral distress scale. *Journal of Advanced Nursing, 33*(2), 250–256.

Corley, M. C., Minick, P., Elswick, R. K., & Jacobs, M. (2005). Nurse moral distress and ethical work environment. *Nursing Ethics, 12*(4), 381–390.

Crigger, N. J. (2004). Always having to say you're sorry: An ethical response to making mistakes in professional practice. *Nursing Ethics, 11*(6), 568–576.

DeWolf Bosek, M. S., & Savage, T. A. (2007). The ethical component of nursing education. Philadelphia: Lippincott, Williams & Wilkins.

Drew, M., & Garrahan, K. (2005). Whistleblower protection for nurses and other health care professionals. *Journal of Nursing Law, 10*(2), 79–87.

Fletcher, J. C., Spencer, E. M., & Lombardo, P. A. (Eds.). (2005). *Fletcher's introduction to clinical ethics* (3rd ed.). Hagerstown, MD: University Publishing Group.

Fowler, M. D. M. (Ed.). (2008). *Guide to the code of ethics for nurses: Interpretation and application.* Silver Spring, MD: American Nurses Association.

Fry, S. T., & Veatch, R. M. (2006). *Case studies in nursing ethics* (3rd ed.). Sudbury, MA: Jones and Bartlett Publishers.

Grace, P. J., & McLaughlin, M. (2005). Ethical issues. When consent isn't informed enough: What's the nurse's role when a patient has given consent but doesn't fully understand the risks? *American Journal of Nursing, 105*(4), 79, 81–84.

Grady, C., Danis, M., Soeken, K. L., O'Donnell, P., Taylor, C., Farrar, A., et al. (2008). Does ethics education influence the moral action of practicing nurses and social workers? *American Journal of Bioethics, 8*(4), 4–11.

Holland, S. (2001). Beyond the embryo: A feminist appraisal of the embryonic stem cell debate. In S. Holland, K. Lebacqz, & L. Zoloth (Eds.), *The human embryonic stem cell debate* (pp. 73–86). Cambridge, MA: A Bradford Book.

International Council of Nurses. (2000). *ICN code of ethics for nurses: Ethical concepts applied to nursing.* Geneva: Imprimeries Populaires.

Jensen, A., & Lidell, E. (2009). The influence of conscience in nursing. *Nursing Ethics, 16*(1), 31–42.

Kilpatrick, S. D., Weaver, A. J., McCullough, M. E., Puchalski, C., Larson, D. B., Hays, J. C., et al. (2005). A review of spiritual and religious measures in nursing research journals: 1995–1999. *Journal of Religion and Health, 44*(1), 55–66.

Kirschbaum, H. (1977). *Advanced values clarification.* La Jolla, CA: University Associates.

Lachman, V. D. (Ed.). (2006). *Applied ethics in nursing.* New York: Springer.

Maze, C. D. M. (2005). Registered nurses' personal rights vs. professional responsibility in caring for members of underserved and disenfranchised populations. *Journal of Clinical Nursing, 14*(5), 546–554.

Milton, C. L. (2005). Ethical issues. Symbols and ethics: Integrity and the discipline of nursing. *Nursing Science Quarterly, 18*(3), 211–214.

Morris, P. E., & Dracup, K. (2008). Time for a tool to measure moral distress. *American Journal of Critical Care, 17*(5), 398–401.

Murphy, P. (1990). Helping Joanne die with dignity: A nursing profile in courage. *Nursing, 20*(9), 44–49.

Numminen, O., van der Arend, A., & Leino-Kilpi, H. (2009). Nurse educators' and nursing students' perspectives on teaching codes of ethics. *Nursing Ethics, 16*(1), 69–82.

Penticuff, J. H., & Waldron, M. (2000). Influence of practice environment and nurse characteristics on perinatal nurses' responses to ethical dilemmas. *Nursing Research, 49*(2), 64–72.

Pinch, W. J. E., & Haddad, A. M. (2008). *Nursing and health care ethics: A legacy and a vision.* Silver Spring, MD: American Nurses Association.

Raths, L. E., Simon, S. B., & Harmin, M. (1978). *Values and teaching* (2nd ed.). Columbus, OH: Charles E. Merrill.

Redman, B., & Fry, S. T. (2000). Nurses' ethical conflicts: What is really known about them? *Nursing Ethics, 7*(4), 360–366.

Schluter, J., Winch, S., Holzhauser, K., & Henderson, A. (2008). Nurses' moral sensitivity and hospital ethics climate: A literature review. *Nursing Ethics, 15*(3), 304–321.

Steele, S. M., & Harmon, V. M. (1983). *Values clarification in nursing* (2nd ed.). Norwalk, CT: Appleton-Century-Crofts.

Storch, J. L., Rodney, P., & Starzomski, R. (Eds.). (2004). *Toward a moral horizon: Nursing ethics for leadership and practice.* Toronto, Ontario: Pearson/Prentice Hall.

Storch, J. L., & Kenny, N. (2007). Shared moral work of nurses and physicians. *Nursing Ethics, 14*(4), 478–491.

Taylor, C. (1993). Nursing ethics: The role of caring. *AWHONN's Clinical Issues in Perinatal and Women's Health Nursing, 4*(4), 552–560.

Taylor, C. (1997). Everyday nursing concerns: Unique? Trivial? Or essential to healthcare ethics? *HEC Forum, 9*(1), 68–84.

The Patient Care Partnership. (2003). Available at http://www.aha.org/aha/issues/Communicating-With-Patients/pt-care-partnership.html

U.S. General Accounting Office. (2001). *Nursing workforce: Emerging nurse shortages due to multiple factors. Report to Chairman, Subcommittee on Health, Committee on Ways and Means, House of Representatives.* (Publication No. GAO-01-944). Washington, DC: Author.

Uustal, D. B. (1978). Values clarification in nursing: Application to practice. *American Journal of Nursing, 78*(12), 2058–2063.

Volker, D. L. (2003). Is there a unique nursing ethic? *Nursing Science Quarterly, 16*, 207–211.

Wiseman, R. (2001). The ANA develops Bill of Rights for Registered Nurses. *American Journal of Nursing, 101*(11), 55, 57.

Wright, L. D. (2007). When does a nurse–patient relationship cross the line? *American Nurse Today, 2*(6), 52–53.

Zuzelo, P. R. (2007). Exploring the moral distress of registered nurses. *Nursing Ethics, 14*(3), 344–359.

7 Legal Implications of Nursing

RAMONE SCOTT

Ramone, a 66-year-old man, had surgery to repair a fractured hip earlier in the day. He just received a dose of an intravenous antibiotic that was prescribed for another patient.

MEREDITH BEDFORD

Meredith is the mother of a terminally ill child with a brain tumor who is admitted to the pediatric oncology unit for a pain management program. One morning she comes out to the nurses' station and firmly states, "I'm very unhappy with the care my son is receiving. I'm going to talk with my attorney as soon as possible to press charges against the hospital."

ELLA RODRIGUEZ

Ella, an 8-year-old girl, comes to the emergency department (ED) with a right forearm fracture. She requires diazepam (Valium) sedation for a closed reduction procedure. The protocol for administration to a child states that a physician must be present throughout the entire sedation procedure. One of the physicians has been working his 14th hour, and the ED is overflowing. He orders the nurse to begin the sedation protocol, stating that he will be back in the room in 10 minutes.

LEARNING OBJECTIVES

After completing the chapter, you will be able to accomplish the following:

1. Define law and describe its four sources.

2. Describe the professional and legal regulation of nursing practice.

3. Identify the purpose of credentialing, using as examples accreditation, licensure or registration, and certification.

4. Identify grounds for suspending or revoking a license or registration.

5. Differentiate intentional torts (assault and battery, defamation, invasion of privacy, false imprisonment, fraud) and unintentional torts (negligence).

6. Evaluate personal areas of potential liability in nursing.

7. Describe the legal procedure once a plaintiff files a complaint against a nurse for negligence.

8. Describe the roles of the nurse as defendant, fact witness, and expert witness.

9. Use appropriate legal safeguards in nursing practice.

10. Explain the purpose of incident reports.

11. Describe laws affecting nursing practice.

KEY TERMS

accreditation	fraud
assault	liability
battery	licensure
certification	litigation
common law	malpractice
credentialing	misdemeanor
crime	negligence
defamation of character	plaintiff
defendant	sentinel event
expert witness	statutory law
fact witness	tort
felony	whistle-blowing

As the roles and duties of nurses expand, so does their legal accountability. In the past, many nurses worked under the supervision of a physician, few carried liability insurance, and even if a nurse's actions were the direct cause of harm to a patient, the primary liability for the nursing action fell on the employing agency or physician. In modern practice, nurses assess and diagnose patients and plan, implement, and evaluate nursing care. Full legal responsibility and accountability for these nursing actions rest with the nurse. (See the accompanying Reflective Practice box for an example.) Nurses are increasingly the subjects of both civil and criminal negligence cases and are being brought to court to defend their practice.

Although many nurses continue to work in traditional settings like hospitals and nursing homes, more nurses are working in nontraditional community settings such as home care agencies, clinics, day-care centers, and nurse-managed health centers. Advanced practice nurses may have independent practices. It has never been more important for nurses to document their actions carefully and act in ways to prevent malpractice accusations. Nurses who wish to avoid legal conflicts need to develop trusting nurse–patient relationships (satisfied patients rarely sue), practice within the scope of their competence, and identify potential liabilities in their practice and work to prevent them.

LEGAL CONCEPTS

As you begin professional practice, it is essential to understand how the law defines the nurse's legal responsibilities and duties.

Definition of Law

A law is a standard or rule of conduct established and enforced by the government that is intended chiefly to protect the rights of the public. Public law is law in which the government is involved directly. It regulates relationships between individuals and the government, for example, describing the powers of the government. Private law, also called civil law, regulates relationships among people. Civil law includes laws relating to contracts, ownership of property, and the practice of nursing, medicine, pharmacy, and dentistry. Criminal law concerns state and federal criminal statutes, which define criminal actions such as murder, manslaughter, criminal negligence, theft, and illegal possession of drugs.

Sources of Laws

Four sources of laws exist at both the federal and state level: constitutions, statutory law, administrative law, and common law.

Constitutions

Federal and state constitutions indicate how the federal and state governments are created, and they give authority and state the principles and provisions for establishing specific laws. Although they contain relatively few laws (called constitutional laws), constitutions serve as guides to legislative bodies.

Statutory Law

A legislative body enacts **statutory law.** Statutory laws must be in keeping with both the federal constitution and the state

REFLECTIVE PRACTICE
Challenge to Ethical and Legal Skills

This past summer, I worked in the emergency department of a very reputable hospital. Overall, I felt that the department was a desirable working environment and that the relationships between physicians and nurses were very open. However, one incident occurred that I felt put the patient's safety at risk.

Ella Rodriguez, an 8-year-old girl, had come to the emergency department with a right forearm fracture. She required diazepam (Valium) sedation for a closed reduction procedure. The protocol for administration for a child states that a physician must be present throughout the entire sedation procedure. One of the physicians had been working his 14th hour, and the ED was overflowing. He ordered the nurse to begin the sedation protocol, stating that he would be back in the room in 10 minutes. The nurse taking care of the patient was a new graduate and did not feel comfortable giving the drug alone, but also did not feel comfortable speaking up to the doctor. She proceeded to go into the room and inject the first dose of diazepam (Valium), against protocol.

This nursing action completely undermined the patient's safety because she not only stated previously that she did not feel comfortable with the sedation procedure, but she also went against protocol. Although the physician was also responsible for giving the nurse orders against protocol, her obligation to herself and the patient should have been the priority, and thus, she should have refused to give the drug until the physician was in the room.

Thinking Outside The Box: Possible Courses of Action

- Hope and pray that nothing happens to the patient until the physician comes back into the room.
- Get the physician back into the room; if he refuses an invitation to be present, report this to someone in a leadership position.
- Ask the nurse why she is violating protocol.
- Seek the help of my preceptor immediately.

Evaluating a Good Outcome: How Do I Define Success?

- Patient is benefited or at the very least not harmed.
- The physician, nurse, and unit leaders accept responsibility for safely implementing protocols.
- All healthcare team members demonstrate accountability for failures to adhere to protocols.
- Patient safety is put first, even when this means challenging other members of the team.

Personal Learning: Here's to the Future!

My preceptor, the charge nurse, realized that the nurse was in the room administering the medication. Once he realized this, he immediately got the physician to go into the patient's room. After the procedure was completed successfully, he discussed the implications of both the nurse's and the doctor's actions with each of them together and separately. I did not have time to respond to this incident because the charge nurse had acted so quickly and appropriately.

Obviously, I think that the nurse should have spoken to the physician and refused to give the medication, but I can understand her feelings, especially being a new graduate. The entire situation can be very intimidating, but as nurses, our responsibility is to the patient. By not standing up for the patient and herself, the nurse put the patient in danger and herself in danger, and did nothing to change the climate of the ED. The experienced and exceptionally capable charge nurse was not afraid to stand up to the doctor. Not only did his actions put the patient's safety first, but he also demonstrated to the nurse, myself, and other nurses that it is imperative that nurses stand up for themselves and patients.

I believe that no matter what the circumstance is, nurses need to stand up for themselves and their patients, especially now, when our healthcare climate yields to nurses' voices being heard. The only way that nurses' roles and reputations will change is if we, the nurses, speak up, and speak loudly. Right now, we have a unique opportunity to change the way medicine is practiced to benefit both patients and nurses. If all nurses grab this opportunity and make something of it, we can really make a difference, but it needs to be a collective effort to be successful. Regardless of how small the problem is, it must be addressed.

Julia Strobel, Georgetown University

Reflection

How do you think you would respond in a similar situation? Why? What does this tell you about yourself and about the adequacy of your skills for professional practice? Can you think of other ways to respond? Do you think that the nurse would be able to admit that she made a mistake by not following the protocol? How was the nurse's integrity compromised? The nursing student's integrity? What legal principles were violated by not following the sedation protocol? What influence, if any, might the patient's age have had on the nurse's action? What types of leadership skills did the charge nurse demonstrate? What other skills (cognitive, interpersonal, technical, ethical/legal) would you need to respond well in this situation? Suppose the charge nurse had not intervened. What might have occurred? Do you agree with the criteria to evaluate a successful outcome? Did the nursing student meet the criteria?

constitution. Nurse Practice Acts are an example of statutory laws. These are discussed fully in the section "Professional and Legal Regulation of Nursing Practice."

Administrative Law

Executive officers (e.g., the President of the United States, state governors, or city mayors) administer agencies that, among other functions, are responsible for law enforcement. These agencies have the power to make administrative rules and regulations, in conformity with enacted law, that act as laws and are enforceable. Boards of nursing are administrative agencies at the state level. The rules and regulations they adopt are administrative laws. An example of a municipal administrative agency is the city board of health.

Common Law

The government provides for a judiciary system, which is responsible for reconciling controversies. It interprets legislation at the local, state, and national levels as it has been applied in specific instances and makes decisions concerning law enforcement. A body of law known as **common law** has evolved from these accumulated judiciary decisions. Common law is thus court-made law. Most law involving malpractice is common law.

Common law is based on the principle of *stare decisis*, or "let the decision stand." After a decision has been made in a court of law, the principle in that decision becomes the rule to follow in other similar cases. The case that first sets down the rule by decision is called a precedent. Court decisions can be changed, but only with strong justification. Common law helps prevent one set of rules from being used to judge one person and another set to judge another person in similar circumstances.

Litigation

A lawsuit is a legal action in a court. **Litigation** is the process of bringing and trying a lawsuit. The person or government bringing suit against another is called the **plaintiff.** The one being accused of a crime or tort (defined later) is called the **defendant.** The defendant is presumed innocent until proved guilty of a crime or tort.

> *Recall Meredith Bedford, the mother of the terminally ill child threatening to bring charges against the hospital. The mother would be considered the plaintiff, while those named in the lawsuit would be considered the defendants.* ■

The two levels of courts in the United States are trial courts and appellate courts. The trial court, the first-level court, hears all the evidence in a case and makes decisions based on facts, usually through a jury. The appellate court hears only cases questioning a point of law decided by the trial court. No witnesses testify at the appellate court level. The opinions of appellate judges are published and become common law.

PROFESSIONAL AND LEGAL REGULATION OF NURSING PRACTICE

Nurses who practice safely respect both the voluntary and legal controls that map the boundaries of nursing practice. Both of these controls are designed to ensure quality healthcare and to protect society from unsafe actions.

Nurse Practice Acts

Your state's Nurse Practice Act is the most important law affecting your nursing practice. Each state has a Nurse Practice Act that protects the public by broadly defining the legal scope of nursing practice. You should obtain a copy of this act from your state Board of Nursing and study it carefully. Visit the Web site of the National Council of State Boards of Nursing for more information about nurse practice acts and how to contact your State Board of Nursing (https://www.ncsbn.org/about.htm). Each nurse is expected to care for patients within defined practice limits. Practicing beyond those limits (e.g., performing an appendectomy) makes you vulnerable to charges of violating the state Nurse Practice Act.

> *Consider Ella Rodriguez, the 8-year-old with the fractured arm requiring administration of sedation based on a protocol. The nurse would need to integrate knowledge of the state's Nurse Practice Act when administering the medication, understanding the need to adhere to the protocol that requires a physician to be present throughout the administration.* ■

Nurse Practice Acts list the violations that can result in disciplinary actions against a nurse and also serve to exclude untrained or unlicensed people from practicing nursing. Table 7-1 illustrates different sources of rules affecting nursing practice, examples of issues covered, where these rules are documented, and suggestions for initiating change. Sharp (2003, p. 12) claims that gaining power and influence for nurses is easier than we think: "Simple as it seems, the written word can get us exactly what we want and what our patients need—more nurses and improved working conditions. . . . To get what we want, we have to make sure our legislators hear us loud and clear. What easier way to do this than with a letter or e-mail?" Examples of a letter and an e-mail to members of Congress to support funding for the Nurse Reinvestment Act (NRA) are provided in Box 7-1, and two students share their lobbying experiences in Through the Eyes of Students.

Standards

Voluntary standards, developed and implemented by the nursing profession itself, are not mandatory but are used as guidelines for peer review. Professional nursing organizations continually reassess the functions, standards, and qualifications of their members. These organizations are guided by their own assessment of society's need for nursing and by the public's expectations of nursing. Examples of voluntary

TABLE • 7-1	WHO MAKES NURSING PRACTICE RULES?		
Source of Practice Rules	**Examples of Issues Covered**	**Where Rules Are Documented**	**How to Initiate Change**
Federal legislation	• Medicare and Medicaid provisions related to reimbursement for nursing services	• Federal statutes	• Review documents. • Draft desired legislative changes. • Obtain support of colleagues, nursing organizations, other healthcare providers, and the public, if appropriate. • Obtain support and sponsorship from a U.S. congressperson or senator, who will introduce the bill. • Lobby for the bill's passage.
State legislation	• Scope of practice for RNs, LPNs, advanced practice nurses • Nursing educational requirements • Composition and disciplinary authority of board of nursing	• Nurse Practice Act • Medical Practice Act • Other statutes	• Review documents. • Draft desired legislative changes. • Obtain support of colleagues, nursing organizations, other healthcare providers, and the public, if appropriate. • Obtain support and sponsorship from a state legislator, who will introduce the bill. • Lobby for the bill's passage.
Board of nursing	• Delegation • Medication administration • Unprofessional conduct • Licensing	• Rules and regulations • Position statements • Declaratory rulings (as found in meeting minutes or newsletters), which may be specific to a particular setting or institution	• Review documents. • Initiate a formal query to the licensing board. • Obtain board support for change. • The board may issue a position statement or declaratory ruling or hold a formal public hearing before voting to promulgate new rules or change existing ones.
Healthcare institution	• Clinical procedures, such as wound dressing changes • Policies specific to the institution, specialty, or practice setting • Personnel and employment policies	• Unit-based policies • Institutional policies • Institutional credentialing policies	• Review institutional policies. • Follow institutional policies or the chain of command to make inquiries or propose change.

From Laskowshi-Jones, L. (1998). Reaching beyond the rules: Understanding—and influencing—your scope of practice. *Nursing, 28*(9), 45.

standards include the American Nurses Association (ANA) standards of practice (see Chapter 1), professional standards for the accreditation of education programs and service organizations, and standards for the certification of individual nurses in general and specialty areas of practice.

Legal standards, on the other hand, are developed by a legislature and are implemented by authority granted by the state to determine minimum standards for the education of nurses, to set requirements for licensure or registration, and to decide when a nurse's license may be suspended or revoked. Examples of legal standards include state Nurse Practice Acts and rules and regulations of nursing.

Credentialing

Nursing has taken several steps to ensure the competence of its practitioners, including the credentialing process.

Credentialing refers to ways in which professional competence is ensured and maintained.

Three processes are used for credentialing in nursing. The first is **accreditation,** which is the process by which an educational program is evaluated and recognized as having met certain standards. The second is **licensure,** which is the process by which a state determines that a candidate meets certain minimum requirements to practice in the profession and grants a license to do so. The third is **certification,** which is the process by which a person who has met certain criteria established by a nongovernmental association is granted recognition in a specified practice area.

Accreditation

State constitutions give states a responsibility for the public welfare. State legislative bodies have used this principle to

Box 7-1   **EXAMPLES OF A LETTER AND AN E-MAIL TO CONGRESS TO SUPPORT FUNDING FOR THE NURSE REINVESTMENT ACT (NRA)**

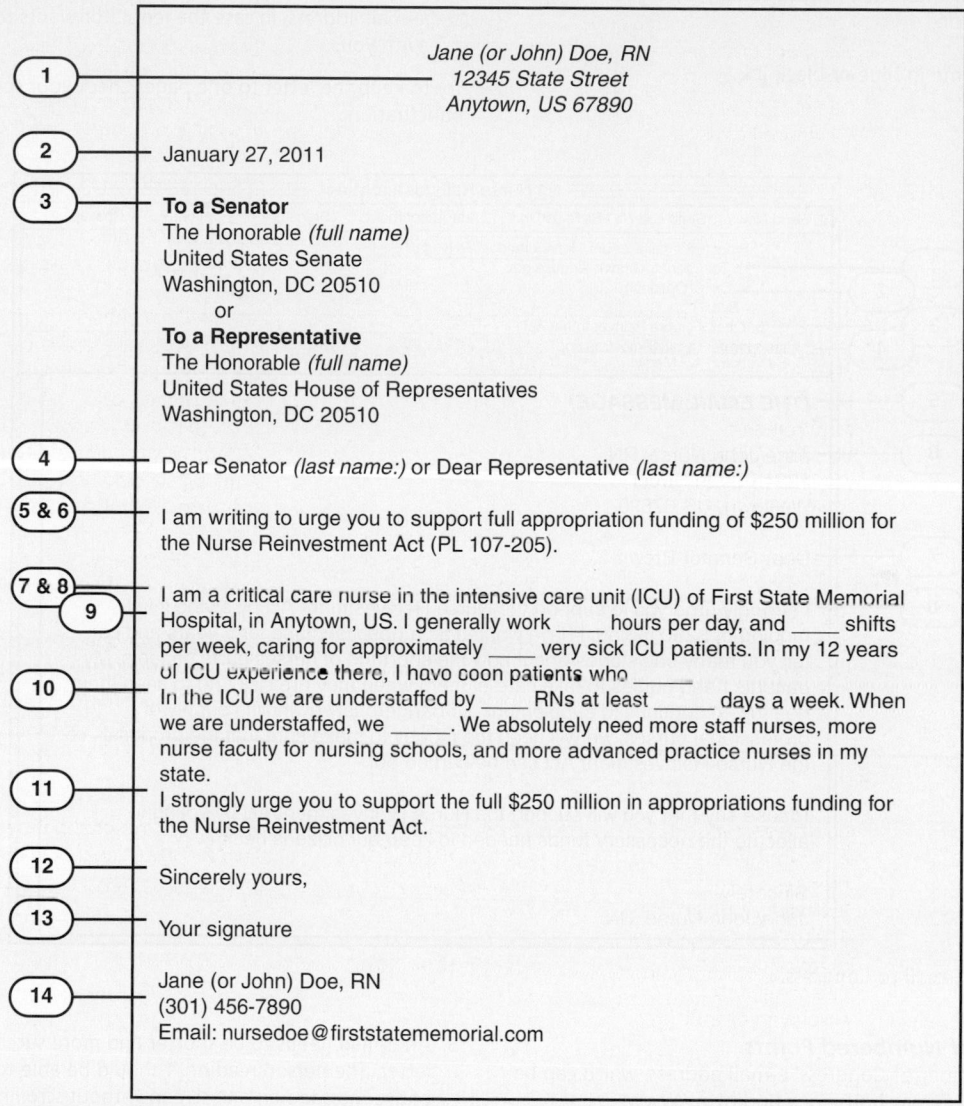

①
Jane (or John) Doe, RN
12345 State Street
Anytown, US 67890

② January 27, 2011

③ **To a Senator**
The Honorable *(full name)*
United States Senate
Washington, DC 20510
or
To a Representative
The Honorable *(full name)*
United States House of Representatives
Washington, DC 20510

④ Dear Senator *(last name:)* or Dear Representative *(last name:)*

⑤ & ⑥ I am writing to urge you to support full appropriation funding of $250 million for the Nurse Reinvestment Act (PL 107-205).

⑦ & ⑧ I am a critical care nurse in the intensive care unit (ICU) of First State Memorial
⑨ Hospital, in Anytown, US. I generally work _____ hours per day, and _____ shifts per week, caring for approximately _____ very sick ICU patients. In my 12 years of ICU experience there, I have seen patients who _____
⑩ In the ICU we are understaffed by _____ RNs at least _____ days a week. When we are understaffed, we _____. We absolutely need more staff nurses, more nurse faculty for nursing schools, and more advanced practice nurses in my state.
⑪ I strongly urge you to support the full $250 million in appropriations funding for the Nurse Reinvestment Act.

⑫ Sincerely yours,

⑬ Your signature

⑭ Jane (or John) Doe, RN
(301) 456-7890
Email: nursedoe@firststatememorial.com

Letter to Congress.

Explanation of Numbered Points

1. Use either letterhead stationery of your own, or just type your name and address (centered) at the top of the sheet.
2. Write the month, day, and year you are writing the letter.
3. Find the names of your members of Congress (two senators and one representative) at http://www.house.gov or http://www.senate.gov. Just type in your state and ZIP code, and the names will come up. Write to each member of Congress separately.
4. Use the appropriate title—either "Senator" or "Representative"—along with the member of Congress' last name in your salutation.
5. State your purpose for writing briefly and clearly in the first paragraph. If you know the specific piece of legislation, identify it accordingly as shown (PL 107-205) or make your subject clear (for example, "Nurse Reinvestment Act").
6. Talk about only one legislative issue in each letter.

7. State clearly that you are a nurse.
8. Name the city and state where you live to identify that you are a voter, live in the legislator's district, and are, therefore, eligible to vote (this may not be where you practice). Be sure that you are contacting the legislator in the place you are eligible to vote. If you decide also to contact a legislator in the place where you work—for instance, if you live in one state or district and work in another—write the letter to show the impact the legislation will have on the legislator's constituents, who are your patients.
9. Be courteous and to the point, and include key information.
10. Talk about what you know and what you do in your own words. Use specific examples from your workplace to support your position. For example, "As a result of having too few nurses, some patients suffered unnecessary complications such as . . ."

(continued)

Box 7-1 **EXAMPLES OF A LETTER AND AN E-MAIL TO CONGRESS TO SUPPORT FUNDING FOR THE NURSE REINVESTMENT ACT (NRA)** *(continued)*

11. At the end of the letter, restate exactly what you want the legislator to do.
12. Closing
13. Sign your name in blue or black ink.

14. Be sure to list all your contact information, including your e-mail address, in case the legislator wants to get in touch with you.

Try to keep the letter to one page. Check your spelling and punctuation.

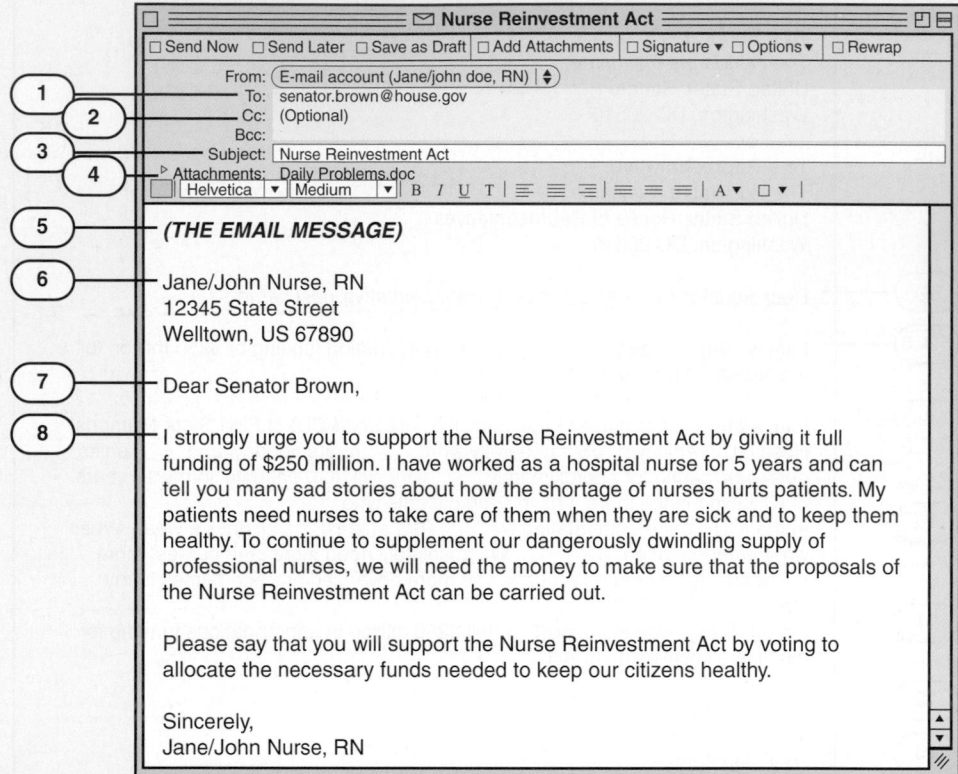

E-mail to Congress.

Explanation of Numbered Points

1. Use your member of Congress' e-mail address, which can be found at http://www.house.gov and http://www.senate.gov. Send an individual e-mail to each member of Congress separately, with only one e-mail address in the "To:" line. You may want to send an e-mail to the member who represents voters from the place where you work, if you live in a different state or district from where you work. If you do this, be sure to write the e-mail to describe the impact the legislation will have on your patients, who are the legislator's constituents.
2. You can copy this e-mail to a professional nursing organization or leave this blank. Do not copy it to another member of Congress.
3. State as clearly as possible the legislation you are addressing (e.g., nursing shortage). Although not necessary, you can use the bill number, if known.
4. If you want to attach a letter you have written that is longer and more fully explains your position, you may do so here.

5. An e-mail needs to be shorter and more succinct than a letter. The person reading it should be able to view your entire message on one screen without scrolling down. If you want to write more, attach a letter (see above).
6. Put your name and address at the top to show the legislator that you are a voter in his or her district or state.
7. The legislator's title—either "Representative" or "Senator"—and last name make up the salutation.
8. Body of the e-mail:
   • State what you want the legislator to do in the first sentence.
   • Identify yourself as a concerned nurse.
   • Tell why the legislator should do what you are asking.
   • Ask the legislator to vote for/support what you are asking.

Finally, use spell-check and reread the e-mail to make sure the message you want to get across is clear and concise.

Used with permission. Sharp, N. (Jan. 27, 2003). The "write stuff." *Nursing Spectrum, 13*(2), 12–13.

Through the Eyes of Students

I was extremely nervous to go to Capitol Hill and meet with my congressional representative; I had begun to feel so comfortable in my scrubs at the hospital that I felt out of place in a suit. I was very fortunate that Representative Christopher Shays agreed to meet with me to discuss my views on medical malpractice liability. Although the meeting was very short, Mr. Shays gave me his attention and respect and listened to my point of view and that of the ANA with political tact. He said that he appreciated my taking time to meet with him and share my views on the subject as a voter and student nurse. He found the issue to be especially important in Connecticut because our state is currently facing crises in regard to high medical malpractice insurance rates and a large number of physicians having to end their practice because of these rates. Mr. Shays shared his belief that it is critical to reform medical malpractice to provide quality, affordable healthcare. He explained his view that excessive jury awards have driven the cost of healthcare up for everyone and that he believes a noneconomic damage cap of $250,000 will help in containing healthcare costs and make insurance more affordable to Americans. I was able to reiterate the ANA's view of postponing judgment on the institution of a medical malpractice cap until an impartial commission could complete and release a report on the effect of the controversial topic, helping him to make an informed decision. I thanked Mr. Shays for his time, and he thanked me for sharing my views on the subject and wished me luck in my study of such a "noble profession." It was thrilling to talk to Mr. Shays, if only briefly, and to feel like such an important part of the legislative process. Nurses definitely have the power to impact our nation's healthcare legislation.

—Maureen McFadden
Georgetown University

I went to visit Senator Hillary Rodham Clinton's office in Washington, DC. I spoke to her legislative aide, Ann Garaghan, who handles many of the current healthcare issues. We discussed the initiative "Funding for Nursing Workforce Development."

At the meeting, I introduced myself to Ms. Garaghan, who was very pleasant and patient with me. She gave me her full attention, as I explained the initiative that I was there to advocate. Hillary Clinton is a big supporter of nurses and of healthcare in general, so she is already in favor of and advocating many of my positions. I told Ms. Garaghan that as a nursing student, I can already foresee the major problems that will arise in the future because of a lack of nurses. Nurses have such a major role in society and in many aspects of life. Without them, the aging population and the ill will not have anyone to care for them. I reiterated several of the points of the "Funding for Nursing Workforce Development" initiative and urged her to reject the funding cut related to nursing development that was approved in the House of Representatives.

Overall, I enjoyed my time on "the Hill." It was a new and interesting experience, and I realized how important it is for nurses to be advocates not only for their patients, but also for themselves. Becoming politically active and joining nursing organizations is an important step. If enough people get involved, it can make a major difference. After this experience, I know that once I become a registered nurse, I will have the confidence to contact representatives and get involved in supporting initiatives related to nursing and the advancement of healthcare.

—Gwen E. Hobson
Georgetown University

enact laws controlling occupational and professional groups. One function of these laws is to see that schools preparing practitioners maintain minimum standards of education. Nursing is one of the groups operating under state laws that promote the general welfare by determining minimum standards of education through accreditation of schools of nursing. State-approved, or accredited, educational programs in nursing include practical or vocational, associate degree, diploma, baccalaureate, and graduate programs in nursing (see Chapter 1).

Legal accreditation of a school preparing nursing personnel by the state Board of Nursing should not be confused with voluntary accreditation. The National League for Nursing Accrediting Commission (NLNAC) and the American Association of Colleges of Nursing (AACN) are voluntary agencies that accredit schools when they meet certain criteria. Most schools choose to seek this voluntary accreditation, and many prospective students prefer selecting accredited schools. Accreditation by NLNAC or AACN is not a legal requirement for a school to exist; state accreditation is a legal requirement.

Licensure

Licensure is a specialized form of credentialing based on laws passed by a state legislature. A license is a legal document that permits a person to offer to the public skills and knowledge in a particular jurisdiction, where such practice would otherwise be unlawful without a license. Licensure is discussed in Chapter 1.

According to the National Council of State Boards of Nursing, a mutual recognition model of nurse licensure exists that allows a nurse to have one license in his or her state of residency and to practice in other states (both physically and electronically) as well, subject to each state's practice law and regulation, unless otherwise restricted. This is referred to as a multistate nurse licensure model, specifically the Nurse Licensure Compact (NLC). All states that currently belong to the NLC also operate the single state licensure model for those nurses who do reside legally in a NLC state or do not qualify for multistate licensure. *You must legally reside in an NLC state to be eligible to have a multistate license.* For questions related to the multistate license or privilege to practice, please contact the Board of Nursing in your state of residence (https://www.ncsbn.org/nlc.htm).

Once earned, a license to practice is a property right and may not be revoked without due process. This includes notice of an investigation, a fair and impartial hearing, and a proper decision based on substantial evidence. Crucial to a nurse's successful defense are early legal counsel, character and expert witnesses, and thorough preparation for all proceedings.

The State Board of Nurse Examiners in the United States may revoke or suspend a nurse's license or registration for various reasons. Drug or alcohol abuse is currently the most frequent reason. Other reasons for revocation or suspension of a license or registration include fraud, deceptive practices, criminal acts, previous disciplinary action by other state boards, gross or ordinary negligence, and physical or mental impairments, including those resulting from aging.

Certification

Whereas licensure measures entry-level competence, certification validates specialty knowledge, experience, and clinical judgment. Nursing certification is offered by many U.S. professional organizations, including two primary organizations: the American Association of Critical-Care Nurses, which represents the specialty with the largest number of certified nurses, and the American Nurses Credentialing Center, a subsidiary of ANA, which began certifying nurses in 1974. The latter is the largest and most prestigious nurse credentialing organization in the United States and more than a quarter million nurses have been certified by ANCC since 1990. More than 75,000 advanced practice nurses are currently certified by ANCC (http://www.nursecredentialing.org/Certification.aspx). Although certification, which involves special testing, is voluntary, nurse specialists are increasingly becoming certified.

Certification is one means to demonstrate advanced proficiency and a commitment to ensuring competence in the context of the current U.S. healthcare crisis, with daily reports of unsafe care, rising litigation, escalating costs, and a worsening nursing shortage. A call to action was issued in 2002 in a white paper drafted by the American Association of Critical-Care Nurses and AACN Certification Corporation: "Today's critically ill patients require heightened vigilance and extraordinarily intricate care. As skilled and responsible health professionals, the 403,000 critical care nurses in the United States must acquire the specialized knowledge and skills needed to provide this care and demonstrate their competence to the public, their employers and profession. Recognizing that nurses can validate specialty competence through certification, this white paper . . . puts forth a call to action for all who can influence and will benefit from nurses' contributions to patient care."

CRIMES AND TORTS

A wrong committed against a person or his or her property may be categorized as a crime or a tort. A **crime** is a violation punishable by the state, whereas a **tort** is subject to action in a civil court with damages usually being settled with money. By its very nature, a wrong tried as a crime is considered a more serious offense, with more legal implications, than a tort.

Crime

Though there may only be one victim of a crime, criminal acts are considered to be against the public as well. In a criminal case, the government, called "the people," prosecutes the offender. When a crime is committed, the factor of intent to commit wrong is present in most cases. Nonetheless, people who break certain laws are guilty of a crime regardless of whether they intended it. For example, failure to observe the Federal Food, Drug, and Cosmetic Act may constitute a crime.

Criminal law is in most cases statutory law (e.g., federal Controlled Substance Acts and kidnapping laws or state criminal codes that define murder, manslaughter, criminal negligence, rape, fraud, illegal possession of drugs, theft, assault and battery); only infrequently is it common law. Examples of common law are informed consent and the right to refuse treatment. Crimes are further classified as misdemeanors or felonies (rape, murder). A **misdemeanor** is a less serious crime than a felony. Misdemeanors are commonly punishable with fines, imprisonment for less than 1 year, or both, or with parole. A **felony** is punishable by imprisonment in a state or federal penitentiary for more than 1 year.

Torts

Torts may be intentional or unintentional acts of wrongdoing. Some of the intentional torts for which nurses may be held liable include assault and battery, defamation of character, invasion of privacy, false imprisonment, and fraud. A person committing an intentional tort is considered to have knowledge of the permitted legal limits of his or her words or acts. Violating these limits is grounds for prosecution. For example, although there are policies that specify when a nurse may use restraints to protect an incompetent patient, restraining a competent patient to enable you to administer medications forcefully while the patient is refusing is assault and battery. Unintentional torts are referred to as negligence. A nurse who fails to initiate proper precautions to prevent patient harm (falls, skin breakdown) is subject to the charge of negligence.

An act that is a tort may also be a crime. For example, gross negligence that demonstrates the offender is guilty of complete disregard for another's life may be tried as both a civil and a criminal action. It is then prosecuted under both civil and criminal law.

Intentional Torts

ASSAULT AND BATTERY

Assault is a threat or an attempt to make bodily contact with another person without that person's consent. **Battery**

is an assault that is carried out and includes willful, angry, and violent or negligent touching of another person's body or clothes or anything attached to or held by that other person. Forcibly removing a patient's clothing, administering an injection after the patient has refused it, and pushing a patient into a chair are all examples of battery. Threatening to do any of these actions if the patient does not cooperate is assault. When a nurse needs to defend himself or herself or others from an aggressive patient, only actions necessary for self-protection or the aid of another are permitted.

Every individual has the right to be free from invasion of his or her person, and adult patients who are alert and oriented have the right to refuse any treatment. The fact that treatment is desirable does not allow the nurse or physician to proceed without the consent of the patient or to go beyond the limits to which the patient has consented (see "Informed Consent or Refusal" within "Legal Safeguards for the Nurse").

DEFAMATION

Defamation of character is an intentional tort in which one party makes derogatory remarks about another that diminish the other party's reputation. Slander is oral defamation of character; libel is written defamation. Defamation of character is grounds for an award of civil damages. Damages are awarded to the plaintiff based on the amount of harm done to the plaintiff. Nurses who make false or exaggerated statements about their patients or coworkers run the risk of being sued for slander or libel. A person charged with slander or libel may be found not liable if it can be proved that the statement was made not to injure another but for a non-malicious, justifiable purpose (e.g., proof of consent, truth, privilege, or fair comment).

INVASION OF PRIVACY

The U.S. Supreme Court has interpreted the right against invasion of privacy as inherent in the U.S. Constitution. The Fourth Amendment gives citizens the right of privacy and the right to be left alone. State courts have also been strong in protecting a patient's right to have information kept confidential. What is confidential? All information about patients is considered private or confidential, whether written on paper, saved on a computer, or spoken aloud. This includes their name and all identifiers such as address, telephone and fax numbers, Social Security number, and any other personal information. It also includes the reason the patient is sick or in the hospital, office, or clinic, the treatments he or she receives, and information about past health conditions. Protected health information may be found in the patient medical record, computer systems, telephone calls and voice mails, fax transmissions, e-mails that contain patient information, and conversations about patients between clinical staff.

Congress passed the Health Insurance Portability and Accountability Act (HIPAA) in 1996; the final regulations were published in December 2000, modified by the Bush administration, and released in August 2002. Most agencies now require workers to undergo HIPAA training and to review and sign a confidentiality agreement when hired and at each performance review. As a student in a healthcare setting, it is important for you to discuss privacy guidelines with your instructor and nurse mentors. According to HIPAA, patients have a right:

- To see and copy their health record
- To update their health record
- To get a list of the disclosures a healthcare institution has made independent of disclosures made for the purposes of treatment, payment, and healthcare operations
- To request a restriction on certain uses or disclosures
- To choose how to receive health information

If a health institution wants to release a patient's health information for purposes other than treatment, payment, and routine healthcare operations, the patient must be asked to sign an authorization. Box 17-2 in Chapter 17 gives a list of permitted disclosures of patient health information and incidental disclosures.

The doctrine of privileged communication specifies that individuals in a protected relationship, such as a doctor and patient, cannot be forced, even during legal proceedings, to reveal communication between them unless the person who benefits from the protection agrees to it. State laws determine which relationships are protected by the privilege doctrine, and not all states privilege nurse–patient communication. Disclosure of confidential information, such as inappropriately discussing a patient's problem with a third party, may be construed as invasion of privacy and may subject the nurse to liability. The nurse's intimate knowledge of the patient increases legal risk in this regard.

HIPAA includes punishments for anyone caught violating patient privacy: Those who do so for financial gain can be fined as much as $250,000 or go to jail for up to 10 years. Even accidentally breaking the rules can result in penalties—and embarrassment—for you and your organization.

Certain acts by nurses could constitute invasion of privacy, as the following examples illustrate:

- Unnecessary exposure of patients while moving them through a corridor or while caring for them in rooms they share with others
- Talking with patients in rooms that are not soundproof
- Discussing patient information with people not entitled to the information (e.g., with the patient's employer or the press)
- Pressing the patient for information not necessary for care planning
- Interacting with the patient's family in ways not authorized by the patient
- Using tape recorders, dictating machines, computers, and the like without taking precautions to ensure the patient's confidentiality (see Chapter 17 and Box 7-2).
- Preparing written or oral class assignments about patients without concealing their identity
- Carrying out research without taking proper precautions to ensure the anonymity of patients

At times, an individual's right to privacy may conflict with other rights, such as the public's right to information. When

---

Box 7-2 **PRIVACY AND CONFIDENTIALITY OF HEALTHCARE RECORDS**

Security measures that a nurse can be aware of, particularly when using computerized healthcare records, include the following:

- Authorized users of an automated information system should have individual passwords and identification codes that are changed frequently.
- Terminals, including those at the point of care, should have key locks as an additional measure to prevent unauthorized access to data.
- The computer system should "time out" when not in use for a specific period of time. The authorized user would need to reenter the password and identification code to regain access.
- Temporary employees, such as traveling nurses, should have temporary passwords assigned.
- Employees who leave the organization should have their passwords and IDs terminated.
- The system should be able to track which users viewed, deleted, or updated patient information.

- Some information, such as results of acquired immuno-deficiency syndrome testing, should not be stored on a computer.
- Computer printouts must be discarded appropriately because they may contain sensitive data about a patient.
- Your organization should have a policy regarding the use of patient data in research. Patient identifiers should be removed before the data are analyzed.
- Every nurse must be aware of the laws and statutes that protect the confidentiality of medical records. Most states have guidelines on the sharing of medical information. Your State Board of Nursing may revoke your license for serious breaches of patient confidentiality.

Protecting the privacy and confidentiality of healthcare records is the duty of every nurse (McMullen & Philipsen, 1996).

---

in doubt about disclosing confidential information, consult the nursing supervisor, ethics committee, or public relations department of the institution.

FALSE IMPRISONMENT

Unjustified retention or prevention of the movement of another person without proper consent can constitute false imprisonment. For example, only a reasonable amount of restraint should be used in circumstances that warrant it. The indiscriminate and thoughtless use of restraints on a patient can constitute false imprisonment.

A person cannot be legally forced to remain in a health agency, such as a hospital, if he or she is of sound mind, even when health practitioners believe the person should remain for additional care. Health agencies have special forms to use when a patient insists on being discharged against medical orders. The patient signs to indicate that he or she does not hold the agency responsible for any harm that may result from leaving. People who are mentally ill may be committed to a psychiatric institution for treatment without their consent (involuntary commitment) only when it can be proved that they may be harmful to themselves or others.

FRAUD

Fraud is willful and purposeful misrepresentation that could cause, or has caused, loss or harm to a person or property. Misrepresentation of a product is a common fraudulent act. A person fraudulently misrepresenting himself or herself to obtain a license to practice nursing may be prosecuted under the state's Nurse Practice Act. Also, misrepresenting the outcome of a procedure or treatment may constitute fraud.

Unintentional Torts

NEGLIGENCE AND MALPRACTICE

Negligence is defined as performing an act that a reasonably prudent person under similar circumstances would not

do or, conversely, failing to perform an act that a reasonably prudent person under similar circumstances would do. As the definition implies, an act of negligence may be an act of omission or commission. **Malpractice** is the term generally used to describe negligence by professional personnel.

ELEMENTS OF LIABILITY

Liability involves four elements that must be established to prove that malpractice or negligence has occurred: duty, breach of duty, causation, and damages. Duty refers to an obligation to use due care (what a reasonably prudent nurse would do) and is defined by the standard of care appropriate for the nurse–patient relationship. Breach of duty is the failure to meet the standard of care. Causation, the most difficult element of liability to prove, shows the failure to meet the standard of care (breach) actually caused the injury. Damages are the actual harm or injury resulting to the patient. Examples of these four elements are presented in Table 7-2.

STANDARDS OF CARE

Whether negligence has occurred depends on a standard of care—what a reasonably prudent person would or would not have done under similar circumstances. All nurses are responsible for following the standards of care for their particular areas of practice. For example, labor and delivery nurses must understand how standards for nursing practice differ from those for medical obstetric practice (according to the state's Nurse Practice Act), must be familiar with specific standards for obstetric nursing (e.g., Association of Women's Health, Obstetrics, and Neonatal Nursing [AWHONN]), and must carry out the nursing responsibilities detailed in the hospital's policies and procedures and in their job description. If hospital policy dictates an assessment of each woman in the early stages of labor every 30 minutes, nurses must adhere to this standard unless they document a reason for doing otherwise.

TABLE • 7-2 PROOF OF MALPRACTICE

An example of how a plaintiff (person bringing the lawsuit) proves that the nurse defendants are guilty of malpractice.

Element	Example
Duty	Hospital staff nurses are responsible for • Accurate assessment of patients assigned to their care • Alerting responsible healthcare professionals to changes in a patient's condition • Competent execution of safety measures for patients
Breach of duty	• Failure to note and report that an elderly patient assessed as alert on admission is exhibiting periods of confusion • Failure to execute and document use of appropriate safety measures (e.g., upper and lower bedside rails, use of restraints if necessary, assisted ambulation)
Causation	• Failure to use appropriate safety measures; this failure causes the patient to fall while attempting to get out of bed, resulting in a fractured left hip
Damages	• Fractured left hip, pain and suffering, lengthened hospital stay, and need for rehabilitation

Table 7-3 lists areas of potential liability associated with each of the ANA standards of clinical nursing practice. Nursing errors can result in serious outcomes for the patient, as these examples show. To read more about standards, see Chapters 14 and 16.

Malpractice Litigation

When a patient believes that he or she has been injured because of the negligence of a nurse or other healthcare professional and pursues legal action, one of three outcomes usually occurs:

- All parties work toward a fair settlement.
- The case is presented to a malpractice arbitration panel (in the United States).
- The case is brought to trial court.

The steps involved in malpractice litigation are as follows:

1. The basis for the claim is determined to be appropriate and timely; all elements of liability are present (duty, breach of duty, causation, and serious damages).
2. All parties named as defendants (nurses, physicians, healthcare agency), as well as insurance companies and attorneys, work toward a fair settlement.
3. The case is presented to a malpractice arbitration panel. The panel's decision is either accepted or rejected, in which case a complaint is filed in trial court.
4. The defendants contest allegations (believe there is no basis for alleging deviation from the appropriate standard of care or for proving causation and damages).
5. Pretrial discovery activities occur: review of medical records and depositions of plaintiff, defendants, and witnesses
6. Trial takes place
7. Decision or verdict is reached
8. If the verdict is not accepted by both sides, it may be appealed to an appellate court.

The nurse may be involved in legal proceedings as a defendant, a fact witness, or an expert witness. For a tangible illustration of how the legal process operates, you and your class may want to implement the malpractice lawsuit simulation developed by Jenkins and Lemak (2009).

NURSE AS DEFENDANT

A nurse who is named a defendant should work closely with an attorney while preparing the defense. The attorney representing the nurse's interests is secured by either the nurse (if carrying personal liability insurance) or the employing agency. Recommendations for the nurse defendant include the following:

- Do not discuss the case with anyone at your agency (with the exception of the risk manager), with the plaintiff, with the plaintiff's lawyer, with anyone testifying for the plaintiff, or with reporters.
- Do not alter the patient's records. Tampering with a chart is the worst mistake you can make—you may well ruin your defense.
- Cooperate fully with your attorney. Do not hide any information from him or her. Make sure you are fully prepared before you go on the witness stand.
- Be courteous on the witness stand. Do not volunteer any information.

NURSE AS FACT WITNESS

Either the defense or the prosecuting attorney may call a nurse who has knowledge of the actual incident prompting the legal case to testify as a **fact witness.** Fact witnesses, who are placed under oath, must base their testimony on only firsthand knowledge of the incident and not on assumptions. The nurse will be asked if the testimony is based on independent recollection of the incident or on documentation in the patient record. The nurse may testify, "I do not remember Ms. Jones, but I see from review of her record that I cared for her on the evenings of June 10, 13, 14, and 17." When in doubt about facts, the nurse should simply testify, "I do not remember that." New research into memory is showing that people often remember things differently from the way they were; this challenges the value of eyewitness memory. Thus, accurate documentation remains the nurse's best defense.

TABLE • 7-3 AREAS OF POTENTIAL LIABILITY FOR NURSES

Areas of Potential Liability	Examples
Standard I: Assessment The nurse collects patient health data. • Incomplete database obtained (occurs frequently when patient is too ill at admission to respond to questions) • Significant omissions or errors in recorded database • Failure to note in the patient's plan of care (and to execute) the need for more frequent nursing assessments • Failure to recognize and to report significant changes in the patient's condition	• Child too weak to be weighed on admission; chart contains no record of patient's weight; dosage of postoperative antibiotic therapy (which should be calculated on child's weight) too small to prevent infection; abscess develops • Nurse fails to detect and report observable signs that an older patient is at risk for abuse in her home from her granddaughter • Previously alert patient was exhibiting periods of confusion; found beating roommate with a hairbrush • Mother's labor is failing to progress, nurses unaware of signs of fetal distress; obstetrician not informed; irreversible cerebral damage to fetus • Healthy patient making slower than usual postanesthesia recovery; signs of developing cerebrovascular accident (slurred speech, difficulty moving extremities, falling to one side) present and unnoted
Standard II: Diagnosis The nurse analyzes the assessment data in determining diagnoses. • Failure to identify priority nursing diagnosis critical to the patient's care • Nursing diagnosis incorrectly developed and "labels" the patient negatively	• Nowhere in the resident's plan of care was it noted that the patient had a history of choking on food ("impaired swallowing") and that close supervision was indicated during meals; patient aspirated Brussels sprout and died. • Homosexual male patient without acquired immunodeficiency syndrome (AIDS) admitted for gallbladder surgery questions the few interactions he has with staff; nursing diagnosis on Kardex reads "High Risk for Violence: Directed at Others (AIDS), related to homosexuality"
Standards III and IV: Outcome Identification and Planning The nurse identifies expected outcomes individualized to the patient and develops a plan of care that prescribed interventions to attain expected outcomes. • No indication in nursing care plan that nurses were aware of and sensitive to the patient's healthcare priorities	• Obese patient with a history of impaired circulation continually refuses to ambulate after major abdominal surgery; patient dies after a massive pulmonary embolism; plan of care showed no concern or attempt to compensate for patient's lack of mobility; family states no nurse consulted them to encourage mobility
Standard V: Implementation The nurse implements the interventions identified in the plan of care. • Patient's record contains no documentation of attempts to teach appropriate self-care measures to patient and family • Nursing interventions deviate from usual standard of care (understaffing, indifference on part of nurse, inexperience of nurse, faulty or scarce equipment or resources)	• Male patient discharged from short-procedure unit on crutches; falls first day home, refracturing leg; alleges his not receiving instructions for crutch walking caused fall; patient record contains no documentation of client education • Skin breakdown on frail, older homebound patient worsens with eventual muscle deterioration; sepsis; nurses seem confused about treatment regimen for pressure ulcers; treatment is inconsistent
Standard VI: Evaluation The nurse evaluates the patient's progress toward attainment of outcomes. • No evidence in plan of care and nursing notes that nurses evaluated whether the patient achieved target goals • Patient discharged before key goals are met and without follow-up instruction	• Male patient, newly started on insulin therapy, discharged after giving himself the insulin only once, and without understanding the relationship among food, exercise, and insulin. No referral made to visiting nurse; patient readmitted after 2 weeks with dangerously low blood sugar after overdose with insulin

American Nurses Association. (2004). *Nursing scope and standards of practice.* Washington, DC: Author.

NURSING ADVOCACY IN ACTION/ADVOCATING FOR VULNERABLE POPULATIONS

Patient Scenario

Mr. Spahn is a 49-year-old attorney who suffered a cerebral bleed. He had surgery on his brain and his surgeon then informed the family that Mr. Spahn has massive, irreversible neurological damage. In short, barring an act of God or nature he will have no meaningful recovery. His wife is already suing the first hospital who saw her husband because they delayed in performing the appropriate diagnostic tests. She and her daughter complain frequently about the nursing care Mr. Spahn is receiving now, and no one wants to take care of him because they are afraid of being named in a lawsuit. Mrs. Spahn keeps a notebook in which she writes down the name of every caregiver who helps her husband. She has placed numerous calls to complain to administration about everything from the cleanliness of the room to a torn sheet. You believe that he is receiving less than optimal care because everyone is afraid of his family bringing a lawsuit.

Implications for Nursing Advocacy

How will you respond if you are Mr. Spahn's nurse? Talk with your classmates and experienced nurses about the questions that follow.

- If you elect to advocate for Mr. Spahn, what practical steps can you take to ensure better health outcomes?
- What is it reasonable to expect of a student nurse, a graduate nurse, and an experienced nurse in this situation?
- What advocacy skills are needed to effectively respond to this challenge?

NURSE AS EXPERT WITNESS

A nurse may be called by either attorney to testify as an **expert witness:** to explain to the judge and jury what happened based on the patient's record and to offer an opinion about whether the nursing care met acceptable standards. Nurse expert witnesses need a solid educational background and strong clinical experience comparable with those of the nurse defendant. The expert witness also needs an understanding of the legal aspects of nursing and malpractice liability and knowledge of the state Nurse Practice Act and the standard of nursing care where the incident occurred.

LEGAL SAFEGUARDS FOR THE NURSE

A variety of safeguards are in place in the healthcare system, both to protect nurses from exposure to legal risks while performing the duties of their role, and to ensure the practice environment is geared towards enhancing patient and personal safety. As you read the following information, consider the scenario featured in the Nursing Advocacy in Action display and the implications for nursing practice.

Informed Consent or Refusal

Every person is granted freedom from bodily contact by another person unless consent is granted. In all healthcare agencies, informed and voluntary consent is needed for admission (for routine treatment), for each specialized diagnostic procedure or medical or surgical treatment, and for any experimental treatments or procedures. The consent must be written, designated for the procedure to be performed, and signed by the patient or person legally responsible for the patient. A signed consent is not needed in an emergency if there is an immediate threat to life or health, if experts would agree that it is an emergency, and if the patient is unable to consent and a legally authorized person cannot be reached. Although some value informed consent mostly as a protection against lawsuits, the central values underlying informed consent include promoting the patient's well-being and respecting the patient's self-determination (President's Commission for the Study of Ethical Problems in Medicine and Biomedical and Behavioral Research, 1982). Elements of informed consent include disclosure, comprehension, competence, and voluntariness (Box 7-3).

Obtaining informed consent is the responsibility of the person who will perform the diagnostic or treatment procedure or the research study. Your role as a nurse is to confirm that a signed consent form is present in the patient's chart and to answer any patient questions about the consent. In some instances, you may be responsible for having a patient sign the consent form after a physician has explained the procedure, its risks and benefits, and alternative treatments

Box 7-3 CHECKLIST TO ENSURE INFORMED CONSENT

Disclosure
Patient/surrogate has been informed of the (1) nature of the procedure, (2) risks (nature of the risk, magnitude, probability that the risk will materialize) and benefits, (3) alternatives (including the option of nontreatment), and (4) fact that no outcomes can be guaranteed.

Comprehension
Patient/surrogate can correctly repeat in his or her own words that for which they are giving consent.

Competence
The patient understands the information needed to make *this* decision, is able to reason in accord with a relatively consistent set of values, and can communicate a preference.

The surrogate (if needed) meets the above criteria, knows the patient's wishes to the extent that this is possible, and is free from undue emotional stress and conflict of interests.

Voluntariness
The patient is voluntarily consenting or refusing. Care has been taken to avoid manipulative and coercive influences.

to the patient. Increasingly, nurses are part of interdisciplinary teams that meet with the patient to obtain consent for complex interventions (e.g., bone marrow transplants).

The documentation of the consent process through the use of a printed consent form should not be confused with the actual explanation given to the patient and the informed consent itself. When documenting consent, assess whether the patient understands what he or she is signing and is acting voluntarily and report to the physician any problems. Having patients describe in their own words what they understand they are consenting to is the best way to make sure they understand. Nurses often find themselves in a position in which they question the patient's understanding of the proposed procedure and its risks or the patient's ability to consent voluntarily to the procedure. Impediments include the effects of anxiety, pain, medication, depression, language barriers, and temporary or permanent states of disorientation and confusion. Unless actually obtaining consent for a nurse-prescribed and -initiated intervention, as a nurse you sign the consent form as a witness to having seen the patient sign the form, not as having obtained the consent (Fig. 7-1). Consequences of not obtaining a valid consent include the possibility of charges of battery against the nurse, the doctor,

FIGURE 7-1. Informed consent is a process. A mere signature does not guarantee each of the elements of consent: disclosure, comprehension, competence, and voluntariness.

and the healthcare agency, which has a duty to protect patients and is responsible for its employees' actions.

A patient's refusal to sign a consent should be documented, and the patient should be informed of the possible consequences of the refusal. The patient should sign a release form indicating his or her refusal to consent and releasing the nurse, physician, and agency from responsibility for outcomes of this act. This statement should be witnessed.

Contracts

A contract may be defined as the exchange of promises between two parties. The agreement may be in writing or oral, although oral contracts may be more difficult to prove. The law of contracts provides a remedy for a breach of contract so that the person who suffers from a broken contract may be compensated for any resulting loss. For a contract to be legally enforceable, it must involve real consent of the parties, a valid consideration, a lawful purpose, competent parties, and the format required by law.

Practicing nurses enter into legally valid and binding contracts with both their employers and their patients. Thus, it is important to understand and be able to fulfill the terms of a nursing agreement before giving consent. Your employment contract should specify what it is reasonable for you to expect of your employer and what the employer can expect of you. An employer that repeatedly expects you to assume supervisory responsibilities without benefit or who fires you without just cause is most likely guilty of contract violations. Similarly, you may be guilty of contract violations if you refuse to accept reasonable assignments, repeatedly fail to arrive on time for work, or are habitually unable to complete reasonable work assignments. Any action by your employer that violates a federal or state law would be the basis of a grievance, even if the employment contract permits the action. Examples include a female nurse receiving less pay for performing the same work as a male nurse, or a supervisor's failure to promote on the basis of race. When discrimination is suspected, complaints should be filed with the Equal Employment Opportunity Commission (EEOC).

Contracts with patients are often implied. There may not be a written contract specifying what is reasonable for patients to expect of nurses, but courts will uphold that an implied contract exists obligating the nurse to be competent and to provide responsible care.

> *Remember Meredith Bedford, the mother of the terminally ill child threatening to sue the hospital. The nurse would need to understand what the implied contract is between the patient (and his family) and the healthcare team.* ■

Collective Bargaining

The 2001 revision of the American Nurses Association's Code of Ethics for Nurses states that the nurse "participates in establishing, maintaining and improving health care environments and conditions of employment conducive to the provision of quality health care and consistent with the values of the profession through individual and collective action."

Although individual contracts serve many nurses adequately, an increasing number of nurses have joined other groups of workers in finding their interests better protected when contracts are negotiated for them as a group. Collective bargaining is a legal process in which representatives of organized employees negotiate with employers about such matters as wages, hours, and conditions. Arbitration, strikes, and threats of strikes may be used to enhance the terms of employment and to enforce contracts. Many nurses choose their state nurses' association, versus a trade organization, as their collective bargaining representative. Other nurses question whether collective bargaining is an appropriate role for a professional organization to play. The *Nurse's Legal Handbook* (Shaw, 2004) recommends asking the following questions before deciding whether to participate in collective bargaining:

- Will collective bargaining help my professional and economic status?
- Can I address my professional concerns through collective bargaining?
- Can I devote the time and effort that such organized activity demands?
- Can I change my working conditions as an individual, or do I need to organize with other nurses?

Competent Practice

Competent practice remains the nurse's most important and best legal safeguard (Fig. 7-2). Each nurse is responsible for

making sure that his or her educational background and clinical experience are adequate to fulfill the nursing responsibilities described in the job description. Legal safeguards include the following:

- Respecting legal boundaries of practice
- Following institutional procedures and policies
- "Owning" personal strengths and weaknesses; seeking means of growth, education, and supervised experience to ensure continued competence for new and evolving responsibilities
- Evaluating proposed assignments; refusing to accept responsibilities for which you are unprepared
- Keeping current
- Respecting patient rights and developing rapport with patients
- Keeping careful documentation
- Working within the agency to develop and support management policies

> *Think back to Ella Rodriguez, the girl with a fractured arm requiring the administration of sedation according to the agency's protocol. The nurse would need to incorporate knowledge of the legal safeguards for competent practice when preparing to administer the medication and knowledge of the unit's protocol. In addition, the nurse would need to identify personal limitations and confront the physician, stressing the need for his presence to ensure the patient's safety.* ∎

Competent practice includes developing sensitivity to common sources of patient injury, such as falls, restraints, and malfunctioning equipment, and then taking specific measures to prevent patient injury. Box 7-4 lists the most frequent allegations against nurses and related prevention tips.

Patient Education

U.S. courts affirm the patient's right to know and view patient education as the legal duty of the nurse. Standards for patient education are derived from national professional standards and from state Nurse Practice Acts as well as the local standards described in agency policies, procedure manuals, and job descriptions. Special forms for documenting the nurse's assessment of the patient's learning needs and for subsequent teaching are available in some agencies. Failure to conduct or document the assessment of learning needs and teaching may later be construed as negligence.

Determine in your practice setting what specific aspects of patient education are the responsibility of nursing. Consult your job description, and be familiar with agency policies regarding patient education and its documentation. Remember that an important aim of nursing is to assist patients in managing their own care. Discuss the nursing plan of care with patients and family members, and identify their learning needs and learning readiness. Document the teaching

FIGURE 7-2. Competent practice is the nurse's most important legal safeguard. Careful documentation is the key to competent practice.

Box 7-4 NURSING MALPRACTICE PREVENTION

Most Frequent Allegations Against Nurses and Related Prevention Tips

1. **Failure to ensure patient safety**
   - Monitor patients in a timely manner. Assess and document potential for injury. Incorporate safety needs into plan of care.
   - Clearly define criteria for use of restrictive devices. Ensure that the use of restrictive devices is consistent with agency policy. Use the least restrictive devices that will be effective in preventing injury.
   - Update knowledge on patient safety and new interventions to prevent and reduce injury.
   - Evaluate whether patients at high risk for injury are routinely being identified before injury results.

2. **Improper treatment or performance of treatment**
   - Question treatments you believe are improper. Know your agency's policy for questioning a problematic order.
   - Use proper techniques when performing procedures, and follow agency procedures.
   - Seek assistance when unsure of a new procedure. Never perform an intervention until you know what you are doing, why you are doing it, and your ongoing assessment and teaching responsibilities.
   - Update your clinical skills through continuing education classes, conferences, and workshops.

3. **Failure to monitor and report**
   - Follow physician orders regarding monitoring of patients unless changes in the patient's condition necessitate a change in the frequency of monitoring; report need for change to the physician.
   - Report any requested information or significant changes in a patient's condition. If unsure of the significance of an observed change, consult with an experienced colleague.
   - Perform appropriate and timely nursing assessments.
   - Ensure that the nurse–patient ratio is adequate.

4. **Medication errors and reactions**
   - Verify any questionable medical orders.
   - Verify patient's name before administering medication.
   - Listen to patient's objections regarding medication and investigate patient's concerns before administering the medication.
   - Refer to a drug reference for any questions about appropriate dosages, side effects, and reactions.
   - Know your agency's policies on verbal and written medication orders and on medication administration.
   - Update your knowledge of medications and new medication administration protocols.

5. **Failure to follow agency procedure**
   - Know your agency's procedures. Ensure that your orientation to new responsibilities familiarizes you with pertinent policies and procedures.
   - If you must deviate from a procedure, discuss the incident with your supervisor and decide on appropriate action.
   - Advise the appropriate person of procedures that need to be revised.

6. **Documentation**
   - Document significant information about your patients objectively and factually.
   - Know and follow the agency's documentation policies.
   - Be time-specific about the information such as when you performed actions, made observations, or performed patient assessments.
   - Document legibly when writing, spell correctly, and use only agency-approved abbreviations.
   - Be sensitive to privacy considerations when documenting on a computer.
   - Routinely evaluate the quality of documentation and update your knowledge of new documentation methodologies.

7. **Equipment use**
   - Learn how to operate equipment in a safe and appropriate manner. Never operate equipment with which you are unfamiliar.
   - Use predetermined procedures when teaching patients how to use equipment and ensure that all the nurses involved in client education are teaching the same procedures.
   - Provide home care patients with the telephone number of a 24-hour backup hospital or home care service available in case of emergency.
   - Have patients demonstrate their competence with equipment before allowing them to use it.
   - Attend orientations and in-services on the use of new or modified equipment.

8. **Adverse incidents**
   - When adverse incidents occur, complete the appropriate documentation and report the incident to the designated individual after agency policy.
   - Do not assume, voice, or record any blame for the incident.
   - Know the institutional chain of command for reporting instances when patient care is at issue.
   - Support agency loss prevention programs that identify potential liabilities, guard against patient injuries, and maximize the defense of the agency and its employee nurses.

9. **Clients with human immunodeficiency virus (HIV)**
   - Be conscious of actions that could result in a lawsuit:
     - Discrimination in treatment
     - Nosocomial (in-hospital) transmission of virus
     - Breach of confidentiality
     - Participation in testing a patient for HIV without first obtaining informed consent
   - Know and follow agency policies and procedures for the care of patients with infectious diseases.
   - Update your knowledge of HIV infection; be familiar with national standards (such as those established by the Centers for Disease Control) and pertinent state/ province laws.

Adapted in part from *American Nurse*, June 1989, p. 28.

plan as part of the nursing plan of care. Document all nursing efforts to educate the patient and family about healthcare management, and also document the patient's response. If a patient refuses health education or refers you to a family member (e.g., "Talk to my wife about my pills; she'll be giving them to me at home"), document this in the patient's record. If patient education greatly increases the patient's anxiety and the patient requests not to be given any more information, document the patient's initial response to teaching, the patient's request that it be stopped, and, if you complied, the reason for doing so.

Because a lack of time is a frequently offered reason for failing to document patient education, assess what type of patient documentation is performed routinely. If possible, develop forms or checklists that will facilitate rapid documentation. For example, preoperative checklists have greatly facilitated the recording of preoperative teaching and are often introduced as evidence in court that preoperative teaching was done. Other successful models include forms for documenting diabetic patient teaching, teaching after a myocardial infarction, and teaching postpartum and baby care to mothers. The teaching role of the nurse is discussed in Chapter 22.

Executing Physician Orders

Nurses are legally responsible for carrying out the orders of the physician in charge of a patient unless an order would lead a reasonable person to anticipate injury if it were carried out. Guidelines when executing orders follow:

1. Be familiar with the parties designated in your state's Nurse Practice Act who can legally write orders for the nurse to execute (in many states, a physician assistant cannot legally write orders for the nurse).
2. Be familiar with your institution's or agency's policy regarding physician orders.
3. Attempt to get all physicians' orders in writing. Verbal and telephone orders should be countersigned within 24 hours. Take the following steps to eliminate errors caused by telephone orders:
   a. Limit telephone orders to true emergency situations in which there is no alternative.
   b. Designate which nurses may take telephone orders (e.g., those who have more education and experience, such as primary nurses).
   c. Repeat a telephone order back to the physician for confirmation.
   d. Document the order, its time and date, the situation necessitating the order, the physician prescribing and reconfirming the order as it is read back, and your name; indicate if the order is a VO (verbal order) or TO (telephone order).
   e. When telephone extensions make this possible, have two nurses listen to a questionable telephone order, with both nurses countersigning the order. See Chapter 17 for additional guidelines on executing verbal, telephone, and fax orders.

4. Question any physician order that is:
   a. Ambiguous
   b. Contraindicated by normal practice (e.g., dose of medication that is abnormally high)
   c. Contraindicated by the patient's present condition (e.g., as a patient's present condition improves, he or she may no longer need aggressive forms of treatment)

> *Remember Ella Rodriguez, the young girl requiring a sedation protocol for closed reduction of her fracture. The nurse would understand that the child is at risk for complications if the physician is not present during the drug administration. Therefore, the nurse would need to question the physician's order to "start without him" to ensure the patient's safety.* ■

It is good practice to double-check any order that a patient questions. See Chapter 17 for another discussion of orders.

Delegating Nursing Care

Professional nurses are responsible for delegating nursing activities, but although RNs may delegate elements of care, they do not delegate the nursing process itself. As a nurse, you remain accountable for any actions you delegate. You can read about the ANA principles for delegation at the following Web site: http://www.safestaffingsaveslives.org//WhatisSafeStaffing/SafeStaffingPrinciples/PrinciplesforDelegationhtml.aspx. Chapters 15 and 23 address nursing's delegation responsibilities.

Documentation

Documentation is discussed in Chapter 17; this chapter addresses only the legal implications of documentation.

Although most nurses prefer to spend their time interacting with patients rather than writing in a patient's record, careful documentation is a crucial legal safeguard for the nurse. Documentation must be factual, accurate, complete, and entered in a timely fashion. The presumption of the law is that if something was not documented, it was not done. This includes even routine acts, such as taking vital signs, repositioning patients, and ensuring the patient's safety.

Be sure that the nursing plan of care is part of the patient's permanent record. Agencies should have flow sheets or some type of documentation form that enables you to check off routine aspects of care rapidly and completely. You should also write a comprehensive nursing note for each patient problem addressed during your time of duty. The note should include the current nature of the problem, how you intervened, the patient's response, and, when appropriate, future priorities for care. After a problem is noted, nursing documentation should demonstrate continuity of care until the problem is resolved.

A common problem reported by nurses is not knowing how to document an incident—for example, if you believe the patient needs medical attention and intervention but the responsible physicians are not responding to calls for assistance. In this case, the best legal safeguard is to document the facts of the incident, being careful not to make incriminatory statements, such as, "Anyone could see we were losing this patient rapidly" or "Once again, Dr. Jones was unavailable when her patient needed her." The note should document the time the physician was called, the time of response or lack of response, and the subsequent nursing response (e.g., nursing supervisor notified). Such a note documents that you are carefully assessing the patient, recognizing significant cues, and reporting them appropriately. The nursing supervisor should write the next note after reviewing the case and choosing a course of action. Patient noncompliance with a treatment also should be documented, along with your attempts to increase compliance.

Adequate Staffing

Understaffing is a problem that results in reduced quality of nursing care and may jeopardize patient safety. Temporary management solutions to understaffing, such as floating nurses from one unit to another or asking (or mandating) nurses to work overtime or double (back-to-back) shifts, are ineffective because they can further jeopardize patient safety. A nurse in an understaffed agency will be held to a professional standard of judgment with respect to accepting responsibility for work and for delegating nursing responsibilities to others. Thus, if a patient claims negligent care, a nurse who claims that she was overworked that evening because of an unrealistic assignment does not have adequate grounds for a legal defense. If patient injury results, the agency and nurse employee will most likely be named as codefendants. Some state nursing associations are using "protest of assignment forms" to track employer practices of routine understaffing.

Whistle-blowing

Many nurses who are frustrated with unsafe practice environments are speaking up. **Whistle-blowing** is an effort by a member or past member of an organization to deliver a warning to the public concerning a serious wrongdoing or danger created or masked by the organization (Lachman, 2008a). Nurses should understand that the decision to whistle-blow can be difficult since some nurses have been threatened with the loss of their jobs and licenses. Whistle-blower laws intended to prevent employers from taking retaliatory action against nurses, such as suspension, demotion, harassment, or discharge, for reporting improper patient care or business practices. As part of the American Nurses Association's (ANA) Nationwide State Legislative Agenda, ANA and State Nurses Associations are promoting strong whistle-blower laws on the state level that provide legal protections for nurses advocating for patients, without fear of reprisal. A number of states are now including some protections in other legislation such as safe staffing and mandatory overtime prohibition. See information about whistle-blower protection on the Nursing World Web site (http://www.nursingworld.org) to learn more.

Professional Liability Insurance

Although a nurse's best legal safeguard is always competent practice, the increasing number of malpractice claims naming nurses as defendants makes it wise for nurses to carry their own liability insurance. Nurses may obtain this insurance through the ANA and other nursing associations and other sources.

Reasons the ANA (1990) lists for purchasing a personal professional liability insurance policy are as follows:

- Protection of the nurse's best interests. If the nurse is named as a defendant in a malpractice action along with the agency, a conflict of interest could arise between the nurse and the agency. Nurses have no assurance that their best interest will be represented unless they have their own coverage, which provides their own attorney.
- Limitations of employer's coverage. Most healthcare facilities carry "claims made" insurance, which means that if the nurse is no longer working there or the facility closes, the nurse is not covered when a claim is filed.
- Care or advice given outside of work. An employer's policy covers the nurse only within the confines of the work setting.

Risk Management Programs

Hoping to reduce malpractice claims, many healthcare agencies have initiated risk management programs designed to identify, analyze, and treat risks. Elements of a comprehensive risk management program include the following:

- Safety program. The aim is to provide a safe environment in which the basic safety needs of patients, employees, and visitors are met.
- Product safety program. The aim is to ensure safe and adequate equipment; this involves ongoing equipment evaluation and maintenance.
- Quality assurance program. The aim is to provide quality healthcare to patients; this involves ongoing evaluation of all systems used in the care of the patient.

Nurses with legal questions often find risk managers a helpful resource. Many risk managers are encouraging nurses and other clinicians to report "near misses" to better identify factors contributing to errors. A "near miss" is an error that would have happened except for someone's alertness and ability to identify and prevent the error.

Incident, Variance, or Occurrence Reports

An incident report, also called a variance or occurrence report, is used by healthcare agencies to document the occurrence of anything out of the ordinary that results in, or has the potential to result in, harm to a patient, employee, or visitor (Fig. 7-3). These reports are used for quality improvement and should not be used for disciplinary action against

Medication Occurrence Information Report/PI   ADDRESSOGRAPH
Send completed form to Risk Management
This document is part of a quality improvement process
CONFIDENTIAL: Do Not PHOTOCOPY
Do Not File in Patient Record
All Sections Must Be Completed

Patient age:_____

Definition of occurrence: Any preventable event that may cause or lead to inappropriate medication use or patient harm while the medication is in the control of the healthcare professional, patient, or consumer. Such events may be related to professional practice, healthcare products, procedures and systems, including prescribing, order communication, product labeling, packaging and nomenclature; compounding; dispensing; distribution; administration; education; monitoring; and use.

Section A: Report filed by (please print): _____Title: _____Date/Time: _____
Location of event
Floor/Unit: _____Date of event: _____Time of event (24 hour): _____ ☐ Inpatient   ☐ Outpatient

Error discovered: ☐ Within same shift   ☐ Within 24 hours   ☐ Greater than 24 hours

Staff involved in initial error: ☐ Staff RN ☐ Agency RN ☐ Pharmacist ☐ NP ☐ House staff ☐ Attending MD Name: _____
Other staff also involved (i.e., perpetuated the error): ☐ Staff RN   ☐ Agency RN   ☐ Pharmacist   ☐ Physician

Staff that discovered error: ☐ Staff RN   ☐ Agency RN   ☐ Pharmacist   ☐ Physician

Physician notified? ☐ No   ☐ Yes   Date: _____Time: _____Attending: _____

Section B: Medication type: Medication(s) involved: Incident documented in medical record? ☐ Yes   ☐ No
    ☐ IV   A. _____   Patient/family aware of incident? ☐ Yes   ☐ No
    ☐ Non-IV   B. _____   *(If yes, please comment below)*

TYPE OF ERROR *(See reverse for definitions)*	**BREAKDOWN POINT** *(Where in process did the initial error occur?)*	**BREAKDOWN POINT** *(Where in process did the initial error occur?)* *(continued from the previous column)*

☐ Prescribing
☐ Omission—Total #
_____ Schedule: _____
☐ Monitoring error
☐ Wrong patient
☐ Wrong time
☐ Wrong route
☐ Wrong dose/quantity/extra dose
  • dose ordered _____
  • dose given _____
☐ Medication D/C'd, given
  • extra doses:
  _____
☐ Wrong drug
  • med ordered _____
  • med given _____
☐ Medication not ordered
  • med given _____
  • dose _____
☐ Wrong drug preparation
☐ Wrong rate of administration
☐ Given to patient with known allergy
☐ Investigational protocol not followed
☐ Other _____
	☐ Prescribing
	circle:
	• illegible handwriting
	• wrong chart/order sheet
	• incorrect order
	• incomplete order
	• other, please describe below
	☐ Order processing
	circle:
	• carbon not pulled/pulled late
	• order not transcribed
	• transcribed incorrectly
	• other, please describe below
	☐ Dispensing
	circle:
	• incorrectly entered into computer by pharmacist/not entered at all
	• wrong strength sent
	• wrong med sent
	• label incorrect/unclear
	• delay in delivery of medication
	• other, please describe below
	
	(continued next column)
		☐ Administration
		circle:
		• med given, but not charted
		• med charted, but not given
		• held med given
		• incorrect medication taken from floorstock/Pyxis and given
		• incorrect dose/rate calculation
		• pump error
		  –tubing clamped
		  –incorrect rate setting
		  –pump malfunction
		  –pump turned off
		☐ Other, please describe below
		ERROR SEVERITY/OUTCOME
		☐ **Category A:** Circumstances or events that have the capacity to cause error
		☐ **Category B:** Error occurred; medication not given
		☐ **Category C:** Medication given but did not cause patient harm
		☐ **Category D:** Resulted in the need for increased patient monitoring but no harm
		☐ **Category E:** Resulted in the need for treatment or intervention and caused temporary patient harm
		☐ **Category F:** Resulted in initial or prolonged hospitalization and caused temporary patient harm
		☐ **Category G:** Resulted in permanent patient harm
		☐ **Category H:** Resulted in a near-death event (e.g., anaphylaxis, cardiac arrest)
		☐ **Category I:** Resulted in patient death

COMMENTS/DESCRIBE EVENT (include any intervention/treatment given and outcome):
_____
_____
_____

FIGURE 7-3. Medication occurrence information report. (From Georgetown University Medical Center. Used with permission.) *(continued)*

Section C: ANALYSIS/RECOMMENDATIONS/ACTION PLAN *(Manager to complete):*

Possible causes: ☐ abbreviation ☐ calculation error ☐ communication confusing/intimidating/lacking ☐ computer order entry ☐ decimal point/leading zero missing/trailing zero ☐ equipment design ☐ facsimile order ☐ handwriting illegible ☐ inexperienced staff ☐ staffing level ☐ labeling (GUMC) confusing/incomplete/inaccurate ☐ labeling (manufacturer) confusing/incomplete/inaccurate ☐ similar name ☐ patient identification ☐ shift change ☐ floating staff ☐ poor lighting ☐ performance deficit ☐ preparation error ☐ procedure/protocol not followed ☐ reference manual confusing/inaccurate/unclear/outdated ☐ verbal order confusing/incomplete/misunderstood ☐ written order confusing/incomplete/misunderstood ☐ other _____

_____

_____

_____

Signature of Manager: _____ Date: _____

FIGURE 7-3. *(Continued)*

staff members. They are a means of identifying risks. More harm than good results from ignoring mistakes. Incident reports improve the management and treatment of patients by identifying high-risk patterns and initiating in-service programs to prevent future problems. These forms also make all the facts about an incident available to the agency in case of litigation.

The nurse responsible for a potentially or actually harmful incident or who witnesses an injury is the one who fills out the incident form. This form should contain the complete name of the person or people involved and the names of all witnesses; a complete factual account of the incident; the date, time, and place of the incident; pertinent characteristics of the person or people involved (e.g., alert, ambulatory, asleep) and of any equipment or resources being used; and any other variables believed to be important to the incident.

▶ *Think back to Ramone Scott, the patient who received the wrong medication. The nurse would document the incident, including the actions taken upon finding the error such as immediately stopping the medication, assessing the patient, and notifying the physician. In addition, the nurse would need to document continued follow-up assessments and interventions taken to ensure the patient's safety.* ■

A physician completes the incident form with documentation of the medical examination of the patient, employee, or visitor with an actual or potential injury.

In some states, incident reports may be used in court as evidence. When documenting a patient incident, be sure to include a complete account of what happened in the patient's record and also prepare the incident report. *Documentation in the patient record, however, should not include the fact that an incident report was filed.*

Sentinel Events

The Joint Commission implemented its Sentinel Event Policy in 1996 and has made revisions since that time. The Joint Commission defines a **sentinel event** as an unexpected occurrence involving death or serious physical or psychological injury, or the risk thereof. Serious injury specifically includes loss of limb or function. The phrase "or the risk thereof" includes any process variation for which a recurrence would carry a significant chance of a serious adverse outcome. Such events are called "sentinel" because they signal the need for immediate investigation and response. Accredited organizations are expected to identify and respond appropriately to all sentinel events occurring in the organization or associated with services that the organization provides, or provides for. Appropriate response includes a thorough and credible root cause analysis, implementation of improvements to reduce risk, and monitoring of the effectiveness of those improvements. Nurses play a critical role in responding to sentinel events. Doni Haas, RN, director of risk management, described in 1998 her hospital's response to a medication error that caused the death of a 7-year-old boy: "Every step in any process needs to be viewed as an opportunity for error. Opportunities for error are opportunities for improvement that must not be ignored. It does not matter how long a process has been 'the standard.' Challenge it."

Never Events

On November 15, 2006, the National Quality Forum released a newly revised list of 28 events that they termed "serious reportable events," extremely rare medical errors that should never happen to a patient. Often termed "never events," these include errors such as surgery performed on the wrong body part or on the wrong patient, leaving a foreign object inside a patient after surgery, or discharging an infant to the wrong person. By reporting and following suggested guidelines when a Never Event occurs, the likelihood of such an error happening again is greatly decreased.

There is growing consensus that hospitals should not be reimbursed for the treatment of the consequences of never events. The Leapfrog Group, a voluntary program aimed at recognizing and rewarding big leaps in healthcare safety, quality, and customer value, gives public recognition to hospitals if they agree to the following if a never event occurs within their facility:

- We will apologize to the patient and/or family affected by the never event
- We will report the event to at least one of the following agencies: The Joint Commission, as part of its Sentinel Events policy*; state reporting program for medical errors; or a Patient Safety Organization
- We agree to perform a root cause analysis, consistent with instructions from the chosen reporting agency
- We will waive all costs directly related to a serious reportable adverse event
- We will make a copy of our policy available to patients and payers upon request

See http://www.leapfroggroup.org/for_hospitals/leapfrog_hospital_quality_ and_safety_survey_copy/never_events for more on the Leapfrog Group Position Statement on Never Events.

Patient's Bill of Rights

The American Hospital Association developed "A Patient's Bill of Rights" in 1972 (revised in 1992 and 2003) (Box 7-5). Renamed "The Patient Care Partnership," it addresses the expectations, rights, and responsibilities of the patient while receiving care in the hospital and ranges from "high-quality hospital care" to "helping prepare you and your family for when you leave the hospital." With care moving increasingly from the hospital to the community, nurses must be familiar with how different institutions and professional groups define patient rights and responsibilities. Other bills of rights include the Pregnant Patient's Bill of Rights, the Indian Patient's Bill of Rights, a Nursing Home Bill of Rights, and the Veterans Administration Code of Patient Concern. Each emphasizes a specific aspect of patient rights within a particular health agency and implies a code of ethics the nurse observes professionally.

Good Samaritan Laws

Good Samaritan laws are designed to protect health practitioners when they give aid to people in emergency situations. For example, a nurse at the scene of an automobile accident may give emergency care without fear of legal suit if such care appears necessary, unless care is given in a grossly negligent manner.

Forty-eight states and the District of Columbia have Good Samaritan laws, although the laws vary considerably. Nurses are covered in some states but not in others, and in some states, only certain acts are covered. While in many states no person has a legal obligation to help another (except in employment situations), and a health practitioner, like any other person, may choose to help or to leave the scene of an emergency, other states consider helping to be mandatory for

anyone. You should refer to the specific laws in the state where you reside to learn more. Regardless, in many situations, there would appear to be an ethical responsibility to assist. When health practitioners assist a person in an emergency situation and obtaining consent for the care is impossible, they are expected to use good judgment in determining whether an emergency exists and to give care that a reasonably prudent person with a similar background and in similar circumstances would give.

STUDENT LIABILITY

As a student nurse, you are responsible for your own acts of negligence if these result in patient injury. Moreover, you are held to the same standard of care that would be used to evaluate the actions of a registered nurse. Your legal responsibilities include careful preparation for each new clinical experience and a duty to notify your clinical instructor if you feel in any way unprepared to carry out a nursing procedure. *For no reason should you attempt a clinical procedure if you are unsure of the correct steps involved.* As a student nurse, you are also responsible for being familiar with agency policies and procedures.

A hospital may also be held liable for the negligence of a student nurse enrolled in a hospital-controlled program because the student is considered an employee of the hospital. The status of students enrolled in college and university programs is less clear, as is the liability of the educational institution in which they are enrolled and the healthcare agency offering a site for clinical practice.

Nursing instructors may share responsibility for damages in the event of patient injury if an assignment called for clinical skills beyond a student's competency or the instructor failed to provide reasonable and prudent clinical supervision. Because the status of patients can change rapidly, especially in an acute care setting, notify your instructor or a staff member of any significant changes in the patient's condition, even if you are unsure of the meaning of these changes.

Most nursing programs require students to carry personal professional liability insurance. *School policies provide coverage only for clinical nursing done for educational purposes at the direction of the school.* Moreover, student nurses who work as nursing assistants or in some other healthcare role are legally permitted to offer only the services contained in their job description. Even if you feel confident with medication administration, catheter insertion, and other professional nursing acts, you risk disciplinary action if you perform these procedures outside the supervised clinical practice setting.

LAWS AFFECTING NURSING PRACTICE

Just as there are many safeguards in place to help protect nurses from the risk of legal action, there are many laws in place that govern the practice of nursing to protect both nurses and patients from harm.

*Reporting of Sentinel Events to the Joint Commission is voluntary for its accredited hospitals.

Box 7-5   THE PATIENT CARE PARTNERSHIP: UNDERSTANDING EXPECTATIONS, RIGHTS, AND RESPONSIBILITIES

When you need hospital care, your doctor and the nurses and other professionals at our hospital are committed to working with you and your family to meet your healthcare needs. Our dedicated doctors and staff serve the community in all its ethnic, religious, and economic diversity. Our goal is for you and your family to have the same care and attention we would want for our families and ourselves.

The sections below explain some of the basics about how you can expect to be treated during your hospital stay. They also cover what we will need from you to care for you better. If you have questions at any time, please ask them. Unasked or unanswered questions can add to the stress of being in the hospital. Your comfort and confidence in your care are very important to us.

What to Expect During Your Hospital Stay

- **High-quality hospital care.** Our first priority is to provide you the care you need, when you need it, with skill, compassion, and respect. Tell your caregivers if you have concerns about your care or if you have pain. You have the right to know the identity of doctors, nurses, and others involved in your care, as well as when they are students, residents, or other trainees.
- **A clean and safe environment.** Our hospital works hard to keep you safe. We use special policies and procedures to avoid mistakes in your care and keep you free from abuse or neglect. If anything unexpected and significant happens during your hospital stay, you will be told what happened and any resulting changes in your care will be discussed with you.
- **Involvement in your care.** You and your doctor often make decisions about your care before you go to the hospital. Other times, especially in emergencies, those decisions are made during your hospital stay. When they take place, making decisions should include:
  - *Discussing your medical condition and information about medically appropriate treatment choices.* To make informed decisions with your doctor, you need to understand several things:
    - The benefits and risks of each treatment
    - Whether it is experimental or part of a research study
    - What you can reasonably expect from your treatment and any long-term effects it might have on your quality of life
    - What you and your family will need to do after you leave the hospital
    - The financial consequences of using uncovered services or out-of-network providers

    Please tell your caregivers if you need more information about treatment choices.
  - *Discussing your treatment plan.* When you enter the hospital, you sign a general consent to treatment. In some cases, such as surgery or experimental treatment, you may be asked to confirm in writing that you understand what is planned and agree to it. This process protects your right to consent to or refuse a treatment. Your doctor will explain the medical consequences of refusing recommended treatment. It also protects your right to decide if you want to participate in a research study.
  - *Getting information from you.* Your caregivers need complete and correct information about your health and

coverage so that they can make good decisions about your care. That includes:
- Past illnesses, surgeries, or hospital stays
- Past allergic reactions
- Any medicines or diet supplements (such as vitamins and herbs) that you are taking
- Any network or admission requirements under your health plan

- *Understanding your health care goals and values.* You may have health care goals and values or spiritual beliefs that are important to your well-being. They will be taken into account as much as possible throughout your hospital stay. Make sure your doctor, your family, and your care team know your wishes.

- *Understanding who should make decisions when you cannot.* If you have signed a healthcare power of attorney stating who should speak for you if you become unable to make healthcare decisions for yourself, or a "living will" or "advance directive" that states your wishes about end-of-life care, give copies to your doctor, your family, and your care team. If you or your family need help making difficult decisions, counselors, chaplains, and others are available to help.

- **Protection of your privacy.** We respect the confidentiality of your relationship with your doctor and other caregivers, and the sensitive information about your health and healthcare that are part of that relationship. State and federal laws and hospital operative policies protect the privacy of your medical information. You will receive a Notice of Privacy Practices that describes the ways that we use, disclose, and safeguard patient information and that explains how you can obtain a copy of information for our records about your care.

- **Help preparing you and your family for when you leave the hospital.** Your doctor works with hospital staff and professionals in your community. You and your family also play an important role. The success of your treatment often depends on your efforts to follow medication, diet, and therapy plans. Your family may need to help care for you at home.

  You can expect us to help you identify sources of follow-up care and to let you know if our hospital has a financial interest in any referrals. As long as you agree we can share information about your care with them, we will coordinate our activities with your caregivers outside the hospital. You can also expect to receive information and, where possible, training about the self-care you will need when you go home.

- **Help with your bill and filing insurance claims.** Our staff will file claims for you with healthcare insurers or other programs, such as Medicare and Medicaid. They will also help your doctor with needed documentation. Hospital bills and insurance coverage are often confusing. If you have questions about your bill, contact our business office. If you need help understanding your insurance coverage or health plan, start with your insurance company or health benefits manager. If you do not have health coverage, we will try to help you and your family find financial help or make other arrangements. We need your help with collecting needed information and other requirements to obtain coverage or assistance.

While you are here, you will receive more detailed notices about some of the rights you have as a hospital patient and how to exercise them. We are always interested in improving. If you have questions, comments, or concerns, please contact
_____

Occupational Safety and Health

The Occupational Safety and Health Act of 1970 set legal standards in the United States in an effort to ensure safe and healthful working conditions for men and women. The act, intended to reduce work-related injuries and illnesses, has affected healthcare agencies and has increased certain responsibilities for many nurses. In December 1991, the Occupational Safety and Health Administration (OSHA) published a rule establishing safety standards for workers who may be exposed to bloodborne pathogens in the course of their employment. The following examples illustrate situations that could violate standards, if care is not taken, because of the potential threat to worker safety:

• Use of electrical equipment
• Use of isolation techniques for patients with infectious diseases and the management of contaminated equipment and supplies
• Use of radiation, such as infrared or ultraviolet radiation, sound or radio waves, and laser beams
• Use of chemicals, such as those that are toxic or flammable

The law, which continues to be updated, is specific in its applications, and fines can be severe when infractions are noted. Nurses can assist in implementing this law by promoting health and safety precautions wherever they work. Nurses employed in industrial settings have a particularly important role in conforming to the law's requirements. The U.S. Labor Department created a new Office of Occupational Health Nursing at OSHA to underscore the major role such nurses play in striving for safe and healthful workplaces.

National Practitioner Data Bank

The Health Care Quality Improvement Act of 1986 was enacted to encourage healthcare practitioners to identify and discipline practitioners who engage in unprofessional conduct and to restrict the ability of incompetent practitioners to move from state to state without disclosure of the practitioner's previous performance. When a state licenses, certifies, or registers practitioners, they become subject to the National Practitioner Data Bank requirements. The Act contains two major provisions: (1) immunity from civil damages for peer review and (2) establishment of the National Practitioner Data Bank as an information clearinghouse. Nurses may be reported to the National Practitioner Data Bank for medical malpractice payments, adverse licensure actions, or adverse professional actions.

Reporting Obligations

The unique nature of nurse–patient interactions frequently results in the nurse having knowledge that a state requires to be reported such as child abuse, rape, or a communicable disease. Legislation varies in this regard, and the nurse is responsible for knowing what needs to be reported in the local area and to what authority.

Nurses are frequently the first members of the public to detect abuse. Abuse includes physical, verbal, sexual, and emotional attack; neglect; and abandonment. Targets of abuse include infants, children, and adult men and women of all ages. Abusers are men and women of all ages, races, socioeconomic groups, and religious backgrounds. Nurses are obligated both ethically and legally to report abuse. In many states, the failure to report actual or suspected abuse is a crime in itself. Nurses are protected by law against suits from alleged abusers if they erroneously but in good faith filed a report of suspected abuse.

Controlled Substances

The United States has special laws governing the distribution and use of controlled substances (drugs with abuse potential) such as narcotics, depressants, stimulants, and hallucinogens. Drug abuse laws are specific, and violations are considered criminal acts. Nursing responsibilities for controlled substances include storing them in special locked compartments and adhering to specific documentation responsibilities.

A related problem is when nurses themselves are impaired by drugs or alcohol. The stresses involved in nursing and healthcare and the availability of controlled substances combine to make nurses prime candidates for alcohol and drug addiction problems. Startlingly, more than half of all impaired nurses began abusing during their nursing education days. In earlier days, nurses with substance abuse problems were promptly punished by firing and license suspension. Today, substance abuse is recognized as a treatable disorder, and the objective is to detect problems early and get nurses into treatment. Students should recognize their level of risk and know to seek help promptly if they suspect a personal problem or a problem on the part of a classmate or colleague. The public's trust and well-being and the well-being of the nurse are both at stake.

Discrimination and Sexual Harassment

Title VII of the Civil Rights Act of 1964 protects employees from discrimination based on race, color, religion, sex, or national origin and provides that pregnant women receive the same protection as other employees and applicants. The EEOC, which enforces Title VII, defines sexual harassment as "unwelcome sexual advances, requests for sexual favors, and other verbal or physical conduct of a sexual nature" occurring in the following circumstances:

• Submission to sexual advances is implicitly or explicitly considered a condition of employment.
• Submission to sexual advances is used as a basis for employment decisions.
• Sexual harassment interferes with job performance even if it only creates an intimidating, offensive, or hostile atmosphere. (EEOC, 1980, sections 3950.10 to 3950.11).

See Chapter 45 for a lengthier discussion of sexual harassment including a discussion of hostile environment harassment.

Health Insurance Portability and Accountability Act (HIPAA)

See earlier discussion in this chapter under the heading "Invasion of Privacy."

Restraints

The Nursing Home Reform Act of 1987 states that the nursing home resident has the right to be free from physical or chemical restraints imposed for purposes of discipline or convenience and not required to treat the resident's medical symptoms. When caring for a patient who requires restraints, be sure that you are familiar with your institution's policies and the guidelines set forth by the Joint Commission. Safe use of restraints is discussed in Chapter 26.

People With Disabilities

Noting that there are at least 43 million Americans with physical or mental disabilities and that discrimination against such individuals persists in such crucial areas as employment, housing, public accommodations, education, transportation, communication, and health services, in 1990 Congress passed the Americans With Disabilities Act (ADA). The ADA provides a broad definition of "disability"; it covers any individual who has a physical or mental impairment that substantially limits one or more major life activities or who has a record of such impairment. In addition to covering people who have impairments that have traditionally been perceived as disabilities, the ADA also specifically protects people who have communicable diseases such as AIDS or HIV infection, people who are recovering from drug or alcohol addiction, and people who are regarded as being disabled, whether or not they are in fact disabled. The ADA imposes two requirements on businesses covered by the Act. First, it prohibits such entities from discriminating against disabled people. Second, it requires covered entities to "reasonably accommodate" individuals who are protected by the Act.

Wills

State and provincial laws regulate requirements for wills. The person who makes a will is called the testator. A will describes the intentions of a testator to be carried out upon his or her death. A person who receives money or property from a will is called a beneficiary. Nurses are occasionally asked to witness a testator's signing of his or her will and should be familiar with the following guidelines:

- The witness should feel sure that the testator is of sound mind—that is, that the testator knows what he or she is doing and is free of the influence of drugs that could distort his or her thinking.
- The witness should feel sure that the testator is acting voluntarily and is not being coerced in any way concerning the terms of his or her will.

- Witnesses should watch the testator sign the will, and they should sign in the presence of each other. State law indicates how many witnesses must acknowledge the testator's signature on a will; two or three witnesses are most commonly required.
- Witnesses to the signature on a will do not need to read it, but they should be sure that the document being signed is a will and not some other type of document.
- In most states, a person who is a beneficiary in a will is disqualified from acting as a witness to the testator's signature.

Legal Issues Related to Dying and Death

Legal responsibilities for the dying or deceased patient are discussed in Chapter 43. Legal issues include advance directives, do-not-resuscitate orders, assisted suicide, direct voluntary euthanasia, organ donation, autopsy, and inquest.

● Developing Critical Thinking Skills

1. Part of nursing's collaborative responsibilities are to help other practitioners obtain informed and voluntary consent for treatment in difficult situations. How might a nurse facilitate the process of obtaining informed consent in the following situations?
   - A 15-year-old boy with cancer who is tired of therapy needs a new course of chemotherapy.
   - Vietnamese parents who speak little English are being asked to consent to surgery for their newborn.
   - An older adult who has had pain with eating for 6 months is being offered an exploratory laparotomy. She tells the surgeon, "I don't care what you do, just get rid of this pain."
   - Rehabilitation options are being considered for an elderly man who is intermittently confused.

2. You are caring for a recently hospitalized patient who had been living in a retirement community. When his daughters, who tend to be critical, come to visit, they tell you that they hope their father's care here will be better than it is in the retirement community, which they are in the process of suing. How would you respond to the daughters, and what, if anything, would you share with other nurses about this incident?

3. Recent layoffs have reduced the number of professional nurses on your unit, and you are growing increasingly concerned about safety, as well as quality issues. What would you do about your concern for your personal liability for inadequate care?

4. When you bring an antipsychotic medication to your alert nursing home resident, she refuses to take it, saying, "I don't like the way it makes me feel." When you report this to one of the nurses, she tells you that they always crush the medication and administer it in food so that the resident doesn't know what she is getting. How do you respond?

● **Practicing for NCLEX**

1. When a state attorney decides to charge a nurse with manslaughter for allegedly administering a lethal medication order, this is an example of what type of law?
   a. Public law
   b. Private law
   c. Civil law
   d. Criminal law

2. If you wanted to find a list of the violations that can result in disciplinary actions against a nurse, you should read which of the following?
   a. Nurse Practice Act
   b. Code of Ethics for Nurses
   c. Nurses' Bill of Rights
   d. *American Journal of Nursing*

Questions 3 through 7 refer to the following scenario:

"Jean," a veteran nurse, pleaded guilty to a misdemeanor negligence charge in the case of a 75-year-old woman who died after slipping into a coma during routine outpatient eye surgery at an eye surgery center. Jean admitted she failed to monitor the woman's vital signs during the procedure. The surgeon who performed the procedure called the nurse's action pure negligence, saying the patient could have been saved. The patient was a vibrant grandmother of 10 who had walked three quarters of a mile the morning of her surgery and had sung in her church choir the day before. As part of her plea arrangement, the nurse agreed to serve 6 months of probation—the first 2 months on house arrest—and surrender her nursing license.

3. Those bringing the charges against Jean are called:
   a. Appellates
   b. Defendants
   c. Plaintiffs
   d. Attorneys

4. Jean's attorney was careful to explain in her defense that Jean had specialty knowledge, experience, and clinical judgment and had met certain criteria established by a nongovernmental association, as a result of which she was granted recognition in a specified practice area. What is this sort of credential called?
   a. Accreditation
   b. Licensure
   c. Certification
   d. Board approval

5. If review of this patient's record revealed that she had never consented to the eye surgery, of which intentional tort might the surgeon have been guilty?
   a. Assault
   b. Battery
   c. Invasion of privacy
   d. False imprisonment

6. What must be established to prove that malpractice or negligence has occurred in this case?
   a. The surgeon who performed the procedure called the nurse's action pure negligence, saying the patient could have been saved.
   b. The fact that this patient should not have died—she was a vibrant grandmother of 10 who had walked three quarters of a mile the morning of her surgery and had sung in her church choir the day before.
   c. The nurse intended to harm the patient and was willfully negligent.
   d. The nurse had a duty to monitor the patient's vital signs, failed to do so, the patient died, and it was Jean's failure to do her duty that caused the patient's death.

7. When the attorney representing the patient's family calls Jean and asks to talk with her about the case so that he can better understand her actions, how should Jean respond?
   a. "I'm sorry, but I can't talk with you. You'll have to contact my attorney."
   b. Answer the attorney's questions honestly and make sure that he understands her side of the story.
   c. Appeal to the attorney's sense of compassion and try to enlist his sympathy by telling him how busy it was that morning.
   d. "Why are you doing this to me? This could ruin me!"

8. If you harm a patient by administering a medication (wrong drug, wrong dose, etc.) ordered by a physician, which of the following is true?
   a. You are not responsible, since you were merely following the doctor's orders.
   b. Only you are responsible, since you actually administered the medication.
   c. Only the physician is responsible, since he or she actually ordered the drug.
   d. Both you and the physician are responsible for your respective actions.

9. A friend tells you not to even think about carrying your own insurance because "you'll be a magnet for attorneys trying to make a buck." When you seek the advice of the American Nurses Association, you are likely to read which of the following reasons for purchasing a personal professional liability insurance policy?
   (1) Protection of the nurse's best interests
   (2) Limitations of employer's coverage
   (3) Care or advice given outside of work
   (4) Protection of the institution's best interests
      a. (1)
      b. (1) and (2)
      c. (1), (2), (3)
      d. All of the above

10. A fellow student asks you about your legal liability when you do your clinical practice. Which of the following are true?
    (1) Student nurses are responsible for their own acts of negligence if these result in patient injury.
    (2) Students nurses are held to the same standard of care that would be used to evaluate the actions of a registered nurse.
    (3) A hospital may also be held liable for the negligence of a student nurse enrolled in a hospital-controlled program because the student is considered an employee of the hospital.
    (4) Nursing instructors may share a student's responsibility for damages in the event of patient injury if the instructor failed to provide reasonable and prudent clinical supervision.
       a. (1) and (3)
       b. (2) and (4)
       c. (1), (2), (3)
       d. All of the above

Answers With Rationale

1. **d.** Criminal law concerns state and federal criminal statutes, which define criminal actions such as murder, manslaughter, criminal negligence, theft, and illegal possession of drugs.

2. **a.** Each state has a Nurse Practice Act that protects the public by broadly defining the legal scope of nursing practice. Practicing beyond those limits makes you vulnerable to charges of violating the state Nurse Practice Act. Nurse Practice Acts list the violations that can result in disciplinary actions against a nurse and also serve to exclude untrained or unlicensed people from practicing nursing.

3. **c.** The person or government bringing suit against another is called the plaintiff.

4. **c.** Certification is the process by which a person who has met certain criteria established by a non-governmental association is granted recognition in a specified practice area.

5. **b.** Assault (*a*) is a threat or an attempt to make bodily contact with another person without that person's consent. Battery (*b*) is an assault that is carried out. Every person is granted freedom from bodily contact by another person unless consent is granted.

6. **d.** Liability involves four elements that must be established to prove that malpractice or negligence has occurred: duty, breach of duty, causation, and damages. Duty refers to an obligation to use due care (what a reasonably prudent nurse would do) and is defined by the standard of care appropriate for the nurse–patient relationship. Breach of duty is the failure to meet the standard of care. Causation, the most difficult element of liability to prove, shows that the failure to meet the standard of care (breach) actually caused the injury.

Damages are the actual harm or injury resulting to the patient.

7. **a.** One of the cardinal rules for nurse defendants is: Do not discuss the case with anyone at your agency (with the exception of the risk manager), with the plaintiff, with the plaintiff's lawyer, with anyone testifying for the plaintiff, or with reporters.

8. **d.** Nurses are legally responsible for carrying out the orders of the physician in charge of a patient unless an order would lead a reasonable person to anticipate injury if it were carried out. If the nurse should have anticipated injury and did not, both the prescribing physician and the administering nurse are responsible for the harms to which they contributed.

9. **c.** The ANA (1990) lists reasons (1), (2), and (3) for purchasing a personal professional liability insurance policy.

10. **d.** All of the answers are true.

Taylor Suite Resources

The Taylor Suite offers these additional resources to enhance learning and facilitate understanding of this chapter:

- thePoint online resource, http://thepoint.lww.com/Taylor7E
- Student DVD included with the book
- Study Guide for Taylor's Fundamentals of Nursing

BIBLIOGRAPHY

Aiken, T. D. (2004). *Legal, ethical and political issues in nursing* (2nd ed.). Philadelphia: F. A. Davis.

American Association of Critical Care Nurses and AACN Certification Corporation. (2002). *Safeguarding the patient and the profession: Executive summary.* Aliso Viejo, CA: Author.

American Nurses Association. (1990). *Liability prevention and you: What nurses and employers need to know.* Washington, DC: Author.

American Nurses Association. (1994). *Guidelines on reporting incompetent, unethical or illegal practices.* Washington, DC: Author.

American Nurses Association. (2004). *Nursing scope and standards of practice.* Washington, DC: Author.

Ashley, R. C. (2002). Legal counsel. Am I legally responsible for the nursing care or advice that I provide for my neighbors and friends, or other people in a situation outside work? *Critical Care Nurse, 22*(2), 128–129.

Ashley, R. C. (2004). Legal counsel. The first element of negligence. *Critical Care Nurse, 23*(6), 81.

Ashley, R. C. (2004). Legal counsel. The fourth element of negligence. *Critical Care Nurse, 24*(4), 78–79.

Ashley, R. C. (2004). Legal counsel. The third element of negligence. *Critical Care Nurse, 24*(3), 65–66.

Ashley, R. C. (2004). Legal counsel. The second element of negligence. *Critical Care Nurse, 24*(1), 68–69.

Brous, E. A. (2007). HIPAA vs. law enforcement: A nurses' guide to managing conflicting responsibilities. *American Journal of Nursing, 107*(8): 60–63.

Brown, S. M. (1999). Good Samaritan laws: Protections and limits. *RN, 62*(11), 65–68.

Carson, W. Y. (2001). Nursing malpractice: Protect yourself. What to do when you're the subject of a board of nursing complaint. *American Journal of Nursing, 101*(12), 81.

Cary, A. (2001). Certified registered nurses: Results of the study of the certified workforce. *American Journal of Nursing, 1*(1), 44–52.

Cohen, M., Rosen, L. F., & Barbacci, M. (2008). Past, present, and future: The evolution of the nurse expert witness. *Journal of Legal Nurse Consulting, 19*(4), 3–8.

Creighton, H. (2006). *Law every nurse should know* (6th ed.). Philadelphia: W. B. Saunders.

Croke, E. M. (2003). Nurses, negligence, and malpractice: An analysis based on more than 250 cases against nurses. *American Journal of Nursing, 103*(9), 54–64.

Equal Employment Opportunity Commission. (1980). Sex discrimination guidelines. In: *EEOC rules and regulations.* Chicago: Commerce Clearing House.

Fedorka, P. (2008). The expert witness: A critical role in successful litigation. *Journal of Legal Nurse Consulting, 19*(4), 20–1, 34.

Flores, J., & Dodier, A. (2005, May 31). HIPAA: Past, present and future implications for nurses. *Online Journal of Issues in Nursing.* Vol. 10 No. 2, Manuscript 4. Available at http://www.nursingworld.org/MainMenuCategories/ANAMarketplace/ANAPeriodicals/OJIN/TableofContents/Volume102005/No2May05/tpc27_416020.aspx

Haas, D. (1998, February 27). *In memory of Ben: A case study.* Sentinel Events Alert. Joint Commission on Accreditation of Healthcare Organizations. Available at http://www.jointcommission.org/NR/rdonlyres/39B79D63-7336-48E1-B2AD-632A2906F403/0/March_April_1997_Perspectives.pdf

Iyer, P. (2004). Liability in the care of the elderly. *JOGNN: Journal of Obstetric, Gynecologic, and Neonatal Nursing, 33*(1), 124–131.

Jenkins, R. C., & Lemak, C. H. (2009). A malpractice lawsuit simulation: Critical care providers learn as participants in a mock trial. *Critical care nurse, 29*(4), 52–60.

Karlsen, K. A., Hendrix, T. J., & O'Malley, M. (2009). Medical error reporting in America: A changing landscape. *Quality Management in Health Care,* 18(1), 59–70.

Lachman, V. D. (2008a). Whistleblowers: Troublemakers or virtuous nurses? *Dermatology Nursing, 20*(5), 394–396.

Lachman, V. D. (2008b). Whistleblowing: Role of Organizational Culture in Prevention and Management. *Dermatology Nursing, 20*(5), 390–393.

LaDuke, S., & Spital, J. K. (1999). What you should expect from your attorney . . . and what your attorney expects from you. *Nursing, 29*(6), 62–64.

McMullen, P. C., & Philipsen, N. C. (1996). Confidentiality: Computer security and data protection. In B. R. Heller, M. E. Mills, & C. A. Romano (Eds.). *Information management in nursing and health care.* Springhouse, PA: Springhouse.

President's Commission for the Study of Ethical Problems in Medicine and Biomedical and Behavioral Research. (1982). *Making healthcare decisions: A report (Vol. 1).* Washington, DC: U.S. Government Printing Office.

Sharp, N. (2003). The "write stuff." *Nursing Spectrum, 13*(2), 12–13.

Shaw, M. (Ed.). (2004). *Nurse's legal handbook* (4th ed.). Springhouse, PA: Springhouse Corporation.

Smetzer, J. L. (1998). Lesson from Colorado: Beyond blaming individuals. *Nursing, 28*(5), 48–51.

Sullivan, G. H. (2003). Legally speaking. Incident reports are a must. *RN, 66*(11), 71–72, 74.

The American Association Nurses Attorneys (TAANA). (2004). TAANA position paper on expert testimony in nursing malpractice actions. *Journal of Nursing Law, 9*(4), 18–25.

Tounsel, D, III., & Reising, D. L. (2005). Whether legislation can be helpful in reducing burnout among hospital nurses: A normative analysis. *Journal of Nursing Law, 10*(2), 89–95.

Verklan, M. T. (2004). Malpractice and the neonatal intensive care nurse. *JOGNN: Journal of Obstetric, Gynecologic, and Neonatal Nursing, 33*(1), 116–123.

Westrick, S. J., & Dempski, K. (2009). *Essentials of nursing law and ethics.* Sudbury, MA: Jones and Bartlett.

Zalon, M. L., Constantino, R. E., & Andrews, K. L. (2008). The right to pain treatment: A reminder for nurses. *Dimensions of Critical Care Nursing, 27*(3), 93–101; quiz 102–103.

Weld, K. K., & Garmon, B. S. C. (2009). Concept analysis: Malpractice and modern-day nursing practice. *Nursing Forum, 44*(1), 2–10.

COMMUNITY-BASED SETTINGS FOR PATIENT CARE

Nurses care for patients (persons requiring and receiving healthcare services) in a wide variety of settings. As the healthcare environment changes, nurses are increasingly providing care to promote wellness and restore health outside the traditional hospital setting. Patients may receive healthcare services as inpatients or ambulatory outpatients in a hospital, through voluntary or public health agencies, in daycare centers and schools, in offices and clinics, in their home, or through crisis intervention centers. A healthcare team often provides care to meet physical, psychological, sociocultural, economic, and spiritual needs. Healthcare services may be financed through federal funding, health maintenance organizations, or private insurance. These factors, combined with increasing concern about healthcare provision and costs, have raised questions about cost containment, consumer rights, fragmentation of care, and changing patient populations and needs.

As patients move among healthcare settings, the nurse is most often the member of the healthcare team responsible for coordinating care and teaching so that continuity of care is maintained. Unit II provides information about the various settings in which nursing care is provided and the resources for that care. Chapter 8 discusses the healthcare system as a whole, including methods of healthcare delivery, settings and services, services for caregivers and end-of-life care, healthcare agencies, members of the interdisciplinary healthcare team, financial aspects of healthcare, and selected trends and issues. Chapter 9 provides information for the nurse in maintaining continuity of care as patients are admitted, transferred, and discharged from healthcare settings. Because more and more healthcare is provided to patients in their own homes, Chapter 10 describes the characteristics and roles of the home healthcare nurse as well as the components of a home visit. The information in this unit enables the nurse to work within the healthcare system to meet individualized patient needs and provide holistic, patient-centered care.

" . . . a realization that the call to the nurse is not only for the bedside care of the sick, but to help in seeking out the deep-lying basic causes of illness and misery, that in the future there may be less sickness to nurse and to cure."

LILLIAN WALD (1867–1940) • *a visionary humanitarian who initiated child-labor law revision, improved housing conditions in tenements, supported education for the mentally handicapped, originated public health nursing, and founded the Visiting Nurse Service at the Henry Street Settlement House, in New York City*

8 Healthcare Delivery Systems

PAUL COCHRAN

Paul is a 38-year-old man with a history of mental illness and numerous visits to mental health inpatient and outpatient facilities; he comes to the mental health clinic for follow-up. He says, "I ran out of my medications last week, but I feel fine. Do I still need to take them?"

MARGARET RITCHIE

Margaret, a 63-year-old woman, is caring at home for her 67-year-old husband who has been diagnosed with amyotrophic lateral sclerosis (ALS, or Lou Gehrig's disease). She states, "All of the help from the home care agency has been a blessing. But I need more help and some other equipment now that our insurance won't cover. Plus, now the doctor says that his condition has really worsened, and he probably has 6 months or less to live."

MARITZA CORTES

Maritza, a 37-year-old Hispanic woman, brings her daughter to the emergency department. The child is diagnosed with a strep throat and is given a starting dose of penicillin. After receiving discharge instructions, including information about possible complications, and a prescription for additional doses of penicillin, she says, "I can't afford to get the prescription filled. Exactly what are these problems and what are my son's chances for also having these same problems?"

After completing the chapter, you will be able to accomplish the following:

1. Explain managed care, case management, and primary healthcare.

2. Compare and contrast settings and agencies that provide healthcare.

3. Describe the members of the interdisciplinary healthcare team.

4. Discuss various methods of financing healthcare.

5. Discuss selected trends and issues affecting healthcare delivery.

6. Describe the role of nursing in meeting the challenges of healthcare reform.

KEY TERMS

ambulatory care	managed care
case management	Medicaid
consumer	Medicare
diagnosis-related group (DRG)	outpatient
	palliative care
hospice	primary healthcare
inpatient	respite care
long-term care	

The healthcare system is comprised of healthcare settings and services, policies, payment plans, providers, patients, families, and caregivers. This chapter introduces healthcare delivery systems, facilities and frameworks for care, members of the healthcare team, financial aspects, selected trends and issues affecting the healthcare system, and nursing's role in healthcare reform. See the accompanying Reflective Practice display for an example of care in one type of healthcare system setting.

METHODS OF HEALTHCARE DELIVERY

Different methods are used to ensure continuity of care and cost-effective care as a patient moves through the healthcare system. These methods include managed care systems, case management, and primary healthcare.

Managed Care Systems

Managed care systems are a way of providing care that is designed to control the cost while still maintaining the quality of that care. The care of the individual is carefully planned and monitored by the primary care provider, sometimes referred to as the case manager or "gatekeeper," from the initial contact to discharge from a healthcare episode. A managed care system limits the choice of care providers and may require approval for specialty care.

Planning and monitoring activities are conducted to ensure that standards are followed and costs minimized. Health maintenance organizations and insurance companies are increasingly changing to managed care systems. A form of managed care has been proposed as a national healthcare plan; in general, large "umbrella" organizations would provide all aspects of care and compete for the consumer's business. Consumers would be able to choose only among managed care organizations, not among individual healthcare providers.

Case Management

Case management is a method used to coordinate a patient's healthcare to achieve patient wellness and optimum function through advocacy, communication, and education. As defined by the Case Management Society of America, case management is an interdisciplinary process of assessing, planning, facilitating, and advocating for options to meet the healthcare needs of an individual. Case managers are often nurses who maintain continuity of care across settings for patients who are seriously ill or have chronic illnesses. In this role, the nurse monitors the care provided and ensures that appropriate referrals are made and that the plan of care is evidence-based and follows established standards.

Although there are different forms of case management, all focus on enhancing continuity of care and effectively using healthcare resources. The primary objective in many case management systems is to identify specific protocols and timetables for care and treatment in a format called a critical pathway. These written critical paths (also called clinical pathways, care maps, or anticipated recovery paths) incorporate independent and collaborative nursing interventions to reach desired patient outcomes within a specific time frame.

Nursing case management is an important method of coordinating care, controlling costs, and improving access to healthcare. The nurse case manager is responsible for these goals and may follow the patient from diagnosis of an illness to hospitalization and then back to home care. During the healthcare episode, the nurse case manager is responsible for managing the patient's interactions with the entire healthcare system. Nurses who are case managers do not give direct care; rather, they coordinate the care provided by others. In this role, nurse case managers have increased autonomy and power within the healthcare system in a variety of settings, including hospitals, long-term care facilities, and clinics.

Primary Healthcare

Primary healthcare is defined as essential healthcare based on practical, scientifically sound, and socially acceptable methods and technology, made universally accessible to individuals and families in the community through their full

REFLECTIVE PRACTICE

Challenge to Cognitive Skills

Maritza Cortes, a 37-year-old Hispanic woman, came into the emergency department (ED) this summer with her daughter who was diagnosed with strep throat using a rapid strep test. The child was given an initial dose of penicillin and was getting ready for discharge. When I entered the patient's room to give her mother the discharge instructions and the prescription for 10 more doses of penicillin, Ms. Cortes said that she could not afford the medication and probably would not be able to have the prescription filled. I told her that it is essential to fill the medication because strep throat can lead to rheumatic fever and glomerulonephritis. She then asked me to elaborate, requesting exact information about the chances of her son also developing these complications. She wanted exact numbers and did not settle for my answer of "No matter what the percentage is, the medication is still necessary." She also wanted me to elaborate on the disease processes of rheumatic fever and glomerulonephritis. Although I do know basic information about these conditions, I did not feel comfortable being the primary and sole informer.

Thinking Outside the Box: Possible Courses of Action

- Make up a percentage to tell the mother and give a partial explanation of the diseases so that she would sign the discharge papers.
- Look up the answer in books available in the ED or on the Internet.
- Try to persuade her that numbers don't matter and that the possible diseases are very severe.

- Ask the nurse to inform me or explain the information to me while we were with the patient.
- Ask the physician to inform me or provide the information to me while we were with the patient.

Evaluating a Good Outcome: How Do I Define Success?

- Ms. Cortes receives adequate information regarding the medication and the conditions that may follow strep throat.
- Ms. Cortes obtains medication and gives it to her daughter, as prescribed.

- The standards of nursing care and protocols of the hospital are maintained.
- I am able to acknowledge that I need the help of others, seeking out their help; in return, those individuals help me.

Personal Learning: Here's to the Future!

Because I was working under my preceptor's license and he had to cosign my signature, I decided that he would be the best person to go to first. My preceptor said that this situation is a common occurrence in this ED because many people come in to get checked, even though they know that they cannot afford the medication, if necessary. As a justification to themselves, patients often want to know what are the exact chances for developing complications, which will likely influence whether or not they go ahead and fill the prescription.

My preceptor and I returned to the room, where he was able to explain rheumatic fever and glomerulonephritis in detail in Spanish. Because he was able to do this at the education level of the patient's mother and be very direct and persuasive, she was no longer concerned about exact numbers. She stated that she would try to get the medication filled, and then she signed the discharge document. Unfortunately, there is no way to follow-up in these situa-

tions. I still wonder if the patient was able to get her medications.

Medical information is always changing, and what people held as standards of practice years ago differ from what we practice today. Similarly, what we hold today may be obsolete and even wrong in the years ahead. As a student, I find overwhelming the vast information that is necessary to be a competent nurse, especially in pharmacology. In this example, I should have probably been able to give the patient a comprehensive explanation of rheumatic fever and glomerulonephritis. However, I didn't feel comfortable. I do feel that I have learned a lot in the past years as a student, but I know that the knowledge I need to act as a professional nurse is much greater! While it is overwhelming and very challenging at times, I think continued learning is one reason why nursing is such a wonderful profession. I think it will never get boring.

Julia Strobel, Georgetown University

Reflection

How do you think you would respond in a similar situation? Why? What does this tell you about yourself and about the adequacy of your skills for professional practice? Can you think of other ways to respond? What, if any, effect do you think the preceptor's culture had on the situation? His gender? His position or title in the ED? Please explain your answers. Reread the preceptor's statement about this type of situation being common in the ED. Do the statements reflect culturally competent nursing? Or are the statements judgmental? Support your response. Did the nursing student seek out the most appropriate resource for information? Why or why not? What other resources could have been helpful? What other skills (cognitive, interpersonal, technical, ethical/legal) would you need to respond well in this situation? Do you agree with the criteria to evaluate a successful outcome? Did the nursing student meet the criteria? Explain your answer.

participation and at a cost the community can afford. It brings healthcare as close as possible to where people live and work.

Primary healthcare was originally conceptualized in 1978 by the World Health Organization (WHO) and the United Nations International Children's Emergency Fund (UNICEF). The concept was developed based on decreases in illness and death in member countries that were achieved by simple, local, inexpensive solutions to health problems, especially when combined with economic and social development. Further discussion led to a focus on a global health strategy called primary healthcare.

Primary *healthcare* should not be confused with primary *care*. Primary care is the delivery of healthcare services, including the initial contact and ongoing care. Included in primary care is the responsibility for referral to other providers based on patient needs. Both physicians and nurse practitioners provide primary care, which focuses on the individual patient and is directed by the provider. In contrast, primary healthcare emphasizes universal access and afford ability of healthcare, health of the whole population, and consumer involvement. However, primary care and case management can both be practiced within a primary healthcare philosophy.

HEALTHCARE SETTINGS AND SERVICES

Healthcare is provided within many different types of facilities to meet the needs of people. Figure 8-1 illustrates examples of the various settings for healthcare. When one considers that only patients who require complex surgery, who are acutely ill or seriously injured, or who are having babies are hospitalized—and then only for a minimum period of time—it is apparent that most healthcare services are provided in settings outside the hospital. Some examples of these set-tings are clinics, homes, schools, prisons, and daycare centers for children and older adults. Other healthcare settings include crisis-intervention centers, mental health centers, drug and alcohol rehabilitation programs, storefront clinics, and churches.

Some healthcare agencies provide immunizations for infants and children, screenings for sexually transmitted infections (STIs) or tuberculosis, and verification of need and voucher distribution for milk and food for women and children with low incomes through the Women, Infants, and Children (WIC) program. Healthcare facilities may also focus on patients with special needs, such as older adults or terminally ill patients. Nurses are involved in caring for patients and families in all of these agencies and in many other settings. Box 8-1 lists examples of nursing activities in different types of healthcare agencies.

Hospitals

There are approximately 5,000 community hospitals in the United States. Community hospitals are defined as short-term general, nonfederal, and special (for example orthopedic, cancer, and academic medical-center) hospitals. Each year, community hospitals admit more than 35 million people, treat nearly 118 million people in their emergency departments, and deliver over 4 million babies (American Hospital Association, 2009). The average length of hospital stay in 2008 was 4.8 days, although longer stays occur in patients who have serious infections, major trauma, mental illnesses, and cardiovascular diseases (CDC, 2008). The shorter hospital stay is the result of many factors, including improved treatment of diseases, an increased emphasis on preventive care, federal regulations, and other healthcare reimbursement policies. The shorter stay means that most hospital care is focused on the acute care needs of the patient.

FIGURE 8-1. In recent years, the number and variety of healthcare settings have increased dramatically. *(Photos © B. Proud.)*

Box 8-1 EXAMPLES OF NURSING ACTIVITIES IN VARIOUS HEALTHCARE SETTINGS

Home
- Assesses the home environment and the patient
- Develops the relationship based on mutual trust
- Plans, implements, and evaluates the plan of care
- Provides direct care
- Coordinates care of others
- Teaches patient and family
- Provides support for family members
- Makes referrals

Hospitals
- Serves as administrator or manager
- Assesses and monitors patient's health status
- Provides direct care
- Coordinates the care provided by others
- Teaches patients and families
- Plans, implements, and evaluates the plan of care
- Provides staff information
- Coordinates discharge planning to ensure continuity of care

- Provides specialized care
- Makes referrals

Ambulatory Care
- Makes assessments of health status of patients
- Assists (or is) the primary care provider
- Provides direct patient care
- Coordinates care provided by others
- Teaches patients and families
- Plans, implements, and evaluates the plan of care
- Serves as patient advocate

Long-Term Care
- Serves as administrator
- Coordinates the care provided by others
- Provides direct care
- Teaches patients and families
- Plans, implements, and evaluates the plan of care
- Makes referrals

Classification

Hospitals are classified as public or private, and as for-profit or nonprofit. Public hospitals, which are nonprofit institutions, are financed and operated by local, state, or national agencies. Patients admitted to a public hospital may not have health insurance, and services are provided at little or no cost to the patient. Tax revenue or public funds cover the cost. Private hospitals may be for-profit or nonprofit and are operated by communities, churches, corporations, and charitable organizations. Many patients cared for in private hospitals have some type of personal health insurance or healthcare plan.

Size and Services

Hospital size ranges from as few as 20 beds to large medical centers with hundreds of beds. Various services are provided, depending on the size and location of the hospital. Most hospitals provide emergency care, inpatient care, surgery, diagnostic tests, and patient education. Other hospital services might include intensive care, obstetrical care, social services, outpatient clinics and surgery, educational programs, and long-term skilled nursing care facilities. Hospitals may provide care for all types of illnesses and trauma or may specialize in the treatment of certain types of illness. Specialty hospitals, or special units in general hospitals, meet the varied needs of certain patient groups such as children and patients of all ages needing rehabilitation, cancer care, psychiatric or drug-dependency care, or patients with severe burns.

Inpatient and Outpatient Services

Hospitals provide both inpatient and outpatient services. An **inpatient** is a person who enters a hospital and stays overnight for an indeterminate time (ranging from days to months).

Hospitals also have many services for **outpatients**—those who are not hospitalized overnight but who require diagnosis or treatment. Individuals who do not require inpatient care can receive treatment, care, and education on an outpatient basis. Examples of outpatient services include surgical procedures, diagnostic tests, medications, physical therapy, counseling, and health education. A form of hospital outpatient care occurs in short-stay units, where patients having diagnostic tests or surgery enter the hospital, have the procedure, and then return to the hospital room for a brief (1 to 6 hours) recovery period before going home. Patients may also be categorized as outpatients when they are admitted, treated, and discharged within a 23-hour period of time.

Nurses' Role in Hospitals

Although the trend is changing, hospitals still employ more nurses than any other type of facility. The percentage of RNs working in hospitals is declining, but about 59% of RNs are still employed in hospitals (U.S. Department of Labor, 2008). The U.S. Department of Labor projects that the number of RNs employed in hospitals will decrease while those employed in outpatient settings, home health, and long-term care will increase. Nurses employed in hospitals have many roles. Although many nurses are direct care providers, other roles include manager of other members of the healthcare team providing patient care, administrator, nurse practitioner, clinical nurse specialist, patient educator, in-service educator, and researcher.

The Magnet Recognition Program for Excellence in Nursing is administered by the American Nurses Credentialing Center (ANCC), a subsidiary of the American Nurses Association. Magnet hospitals must meet strict requirements and standards that define the highest quality of nursing practice and patient care. A designation as a magnet hospital recognizes quality patient care, nursing excellence, and innovations in professional nursing practice (American Nurses Credentialing Center, 2009).

> *Think back to Maritza Cortes, the mother who brings her daughter to the emergency department for care. The nurse, in this situation, acts primarily in the caregiver role. However, the nurse also plays a major role as educator, using knowledge about the infection to teach the mother about possible complications and the need for continued antibiotic treatment.* ∎

Primary Care Centers

Physicians and advanced practice nurses provide primary healthcare services in offices and clinics. Services include the diagnosis and treatment of minor illnesses; performing minor surgical procedures; and providing obstetrical care, well-child care, counseling, and referrals (Fig. 8-2). Many offices have laboratory and radiographic facilities. Although some physicians are general practitioners who treat all types of illness, many physicians specialize in one type of illness or surgery. An RN working in a healthcare provider's office makes health assessments, performs technical procedures, assists the physician, and provides health education.

Advanced practice registered nurses ([APRNs] nurse practitioners, midwives, or clinical nurse specialists) work independently or collaboratively with physicians to make assessments and care for patients who require health maintenance or health promotion activities. Depending on state regulations, APRNs may have their own offices and clinics to provide primary care and treatment to patients and refer only complex health problems to a physician.

> *Recall Maritza Cortes, the mother of the child with a strep throat? When thinking about healthcare for usual childhood illnesses, one might commonly think of primary healthcare services. However, in this case, Ms. Cortes uses*

FIGURE 8-2. A nurse assesses a patient during a well-child visit at a primary care center. *(Photo by Joe Mitchell.)*

> *the emergency department. Possibly the mother thought that the child was too ill and needed to be seen immediately. In this case, the nurse would develop a teaching plan for Ms. Cortes about typical childhood illnesses. Maybe she did not know of anywhere else to obtain services. Here, the nurse could contact social services to obtain information about community clinics for Ms. Cortes. Finances on the mother's part may have led to her decision to use the emergency department. In this case, the nurse also could contact social services to arrange for financial assistance.* ∎

Ambulatory Care Centers and Clinics

Ambulatory care centers and clinics (agencies that deliver medical care on an outpatient basis) may be located in hospitals, may be a free-standing service provided by a group of healthcare providers who work together, or may be managed by an APRN. Ambulatory care centers and clinics are often located in convenient areas such as shopping malls or other community agencies. Many ambulatory care centers and clinics offer walk-in services so that appointments are unnecessary, and they are also open at times other than traditional office hours. Increasing numbers of small clinics staffed by APRNs are being established in nontraditional sites, such as drugstores and grocery stores (often called Convenient Care Clinics). These clinics have dramatically improved access to care for the uninsured or for those with other barriers to healthcare (Edmonds & Scudder, 2008).

Nurses in ambulatory care centers and clinics provide technical services (e.g., administering medications), determine the priority of care needs, and provide teaching about all aspects of care. A special type of ambulatory care center is an urgent care center, which provides walk-in care for illnesses and minor trauma. Outpatient or same-day surgical centers, discussed in Chapter 30, are another form of ambulatory care center.

Home Healthcare

Home healthcare is one of the most rapidly growing areas of the healthcare system. (See Chapter 10 for a full discussion of this type of community-based care.) Home healthcare may be provided through community health departments, visiting nurses' associations, hospital-based case managers, and home health agencies. These agencies provide many different health-related services, including skilled nursing assessment, teaching and support of patients and family members, and direct care for patients.

The importance of home healthcare is evidenced by many factors. The prospective payment system of reimbursement (diagnosis-related groups, or DRGs, discussed later) encourages early discharge from the hospital, and has created a new, acutely ill population that needs skilled care at home. Increasing numbers of older people are living longer and have multiple chronic illnesses, and with sophisticated technology, people can be kept alive and relatively comfortable in their own homes. Healthcare consumers demand that services be humane and that provisions be made for a dignified death at home.

Nurses who provide care in the home make assessments and provide physical care, administer medications, teach, and support family members. They also collaborate with other healthcare providers, such as physicians, physical therapists, occupational therapists, respiratory therapists, and social workers to plan and provide patient care.

Long-Term Care

Long-term care provides medical and nonmedical care for people with chronic illnesses or disabilities. Through a variety of services, family, and other caregivers, it assists with activities of daily living for people of any age who are physically or mentally unable to care for themselves independently. In 2007, about 9 million people over the age of 65 used long-term care services; that number is projected to increase to 12 million by 2020. Most long-term care is provided to people by family or friends; for example, 70% of older adults requiring long-term care are not in any type of facility (Medicare: Long-Term Care, 2007).

Long-term care may extend for periods ranging from days to years. Facilities that provide long-term care are often independent but may be associated with a hospital. Long-term care facilities include transitional subacute care, assisted-living facilities, intermediate and long-term care, nursing homes, retirement centers, and residential institutions for mentally and developmentally or physically disabled patients of all ages. One of the newest concepts in long-term care is called "aging in place." In this type of care, patients move to a living space, such as an apartment, while they are still physically able to care for themselves, and then have access to services that are a part of the healthcare community as needed as long as they live.

Long-term care facilities have proliferated in recent years for two reasons. First, as many patients are discharged from the hospital earlier in their recovery period, they require care that is beyond the scope of home care. These patients receive transitional, subacute care in a long-term facility. Second, as the population ages, many older adults will not have caregivers available and would be unable to carry out activities of daily living independently. However, as the services available through home healthcare increase, more people are able to remain in their own homes.

Although long-term facilities, especially nursing homes, have had a negative image in the past, much has changed. Most nursing homes focus on maintaining residents' function and independence, with concern for the living environment as well as the healthcare provided. A focus on maximizing quality of life for residents has led to surroundings that include plants and animals. Many of the overall improvements in long-term care resulted from the 1987 Omnibus Budget Reconciliation Act (OBRA), which included legislation to maintain standards of quality assurance in the nursing home industry.

FIGURE 8-3. A nurse provides care and counseling at a long-term care facility.

Because patients entering long-term care facilities require so many different levels of care, it is difficult to generalize about the services provided. Those entering convalescent centers remain only until they have recovered. In some instances, an older adult may choose to move into a retirement or assisted-living facility that provides healthcare services only when needed. Other people who enter a nursing home may require complete care as long as they live. The nurse's roles in long-term care facilities may include being a provider of direct care, supervisor, administrator, or teacher (Fig. 8-3). Because most patients are older, increasing numbers of gerontology nurse specialists are contributing their knowledge and expertise to the care of these patients. Almost all long-term care facilities require that skilled nursing care be available at all times. The care given to patients can be performed only by or under the direct supervision of a licensed nurse.

Specialized Care Centers and Settings

Specialized care centers and settings provide services for a specific population or group. They are usually located in easily accessible locations within a community.

Daycare Centers

Daycare centers have a variety of purposes. Some centers care for healthy infants and children whose parents work; some also care for children with minor illnesses. Eldercare centers and senior citizen centers provide a place for older adults to socialize and to receive care while family members work. Some daycare centers provide health-related services and care to people who do not need to be in a healthcare institution but cannot be at home alone. Such centers provide services to older people for physical rehabilitation, for people with special needs (e.g., cerebral palsy), and for chemical dependency and mental health.

Nurses who work in daycare centers administer medications and treatments, conduct health screenings, teach, and counsel.

Mental Health Centers

Mental health centers may be associated with a hospital or may provide services as an independent agency. The services provided may be crisis centered or may involve long-term counseling. Patients receive outpatient care through a variety of interventions, including individual and group counseling, medications, and assistance with independent living. Crisis intervention centers are also mental health centers. They typically provide 24-hour services and hotlines for people who are suicidal, abusing drugs or alcohol, or in abusive situations. These centers also provide information and services for victims of rape and abuse.

Nurses who work in mental health centers must have strong communication and counseling skills and must be thoroughly familiar with community resources specific to the needs of patients being served in order to make appropriate referrals.

> ➤ *Remember Paul Cochran, the patient with a mental illness who ran out of his medications? The nurse needs knowledge of local mental health centers to ensure continuity of care, including follow-up with medication regimen.* ■

Rural Health Centers

Rural health centers are often located in geographically remote areas that have few healthcare providers. Many rural health centers are run by APRNs who serve as the patient's primary health provider for the care of minor acute illnesses as well as chronic illnesses. Patients who are seriously ill or injured are given emergency care and then transported to the nearest large hospital. Nurses who practice independently usually do so in collaboration with a physician who approves protocols for care. Many rural healthcare settings and providers now have immediate access to information about diagnosis and treatment of illness through telecommunication and computers.

Schools

School nurses are often the major source of health assessment, health education, and emergency care for the nation's children. The role of the school nurse reflects changes in society itself: Children in schools today are from many different racial and ethnic groups, have varying socioeconomic backgrounds, and have more complex disabilities that require expert knowledge and skills for management during school hours. School nurses provide many different services, including maintaining immunization records, providing emergency care for physical and mental illnesses, administering prescribed medications, conducting routine health screenings (e.g., vision, hearing, scoliosis), and providing health information and education.

Industry

Many large industries have their own ambulatory care clinic, staffed primarily by nurses. Occupational health nurses in industrial clinics focus on preventing work-related injury and illness by conducting health assessments, teaching for health promotion (e.g., stopping smoking, eating sensibly, using safety equipment, exercising regularly), caring for minor accidents and illnesses, and making referrals for more serious health problems.

Homeless Shelters

Homeless shelters are usually living units, such as an apartment building or home, that provide housing for people who do not have regular shelter. The homeless are at increased risk for illness or injury because of factors such as exposure to the elements, exposure to violence, drug and alcohol addiction, poor nutrition, poor hygiene, and overcrowding. Services provided by nurses in homeless shelters include immunizing children, teaching pregnant women, treating infections and illnesses, referring for diagnosis and treatment of STIs, and providing information about maintaining health.

Rehabilitation Centers

Rehabilitation centers specialize in services for patients requiring physical or emotional rehabilitation and for treatment of chemical dependency. These centers may be either free-standing or associated with a hospital. The goal is to return patients to optimal health and to return them to the community as independent members of society. Rehabilitation centers often use a multidisciplinary team composed of physicians, nurses, physical therapists, occupational therapists, and counselors. The role of the nurse includes direct care, teaching, and counseling. The practice of rehabilitation nursing is based on a philosophy of encouraging independent self-care within the patient's capabilities.

Healthcare Services for Caregivers and End-of-Life Care

Healthcare services are provided for the caregivers of those who are chronically ill and for patients and caregivers as a part of end-of-life care. These services include respite care, hospice, and palliative care. (End-of-life care is discussed further in Chapter 43.)

Respite Care

Respite care is a type of care provided for caregivers of homebound ill, disabled, or elderly patients. The main purpose is to give the primary caregiver some time away from the responsibilities of day-to-day care. Professionals or volunteers may provide care in an adult daycare center or in the patient's home. In most instances, the care is provided by trained nursing assistants or volunteers. Professional nurses provide information about how to access respite care and may make referrals. Medicaid and most insurance providers do not cover the costs of respite care.

Hospice Services

Hospice is a program of palliative and supportive care services providing physical, psychological, social, and spiritual care for dying persons, their families, and other loved ones. There are more than 3,250 hospice agencies in the United States, with services and care reimbursed by private insurance or a Medicare hospice benefit. Services are reimbursed by Medicare for an initial 90-day period, followed by a subsequent 90-day period, and an unlimited number of 60-day periods as long as the patient continues to meet eligibility requirements. The average length of service is 71 days (Hospice Association of America, 2008). Hospice services usually begin when the patient has 6 months or less to live and ends with the family 1 year after the death of the patient. This continuation of care for the family is called bereavement care (bereavement is the time of mourning experienced after a loss).

To be eligible for hospice benefits from Medicare or Medicaid, the patient must have a serious, progressive illness with a limited life expectancy. In most cases, a family (or other) caregiver must be continuously in the home with the patient. The patient must have Medicare, waive traditional Medicare benefits for the terminal illness, and have physician certification of a terminal illness with a life expectancy of 6 months or less. In addition, the care must be provided by a Medicare-certified hospice agency or program. Hospice care under Medicare includes home care, inpatient care when needed, and a variety of services not otherwise covered by Medicare (U.S. Department of Health & Human Services, 2008). The focus is on care, not cure.

> *Think back to Margaret Ritchie, who is caring for her husband at home. The physician recently informed her of her husband's prognosis. The nurse might anticipate that hospice care would be appropriate for Mrs. Ritchie and her husband.* ■

Hospice services are provided by nurses, social workers, therapists, counselors, volunteers, and chaplains working together as an interdisciplinary team. It is provided in hospitals, long-term care facilities, hospice residences, and homes. It is projected that hospice services will grow as increasing numbers of people do not want to die in a clinical setting.

The hospice nurse combines the skills of the home care nurse with the ability to provide daily emotional support to dying patients and their families. Hospice nurses are especially skilled in pain and symptom management. Their focus is on improving quality of life, as opposed to prolonging the length of it, and on preserving dignity for the patient in death. After the death, the nurse continues to care for the patient's family during the bereavement period for up to 1 year. Nurses use this time to help families work through the grief process after their loss. (See Chapter 43 for more information).

Palliative Care

Palliative care is an area of care that has evolved out of the hospice experience, but also exists outside of hospice programs. It is not restricted to the end of life and can be used from the initial diagnoses of an incurable illness. Palliative care, which can be used in conjunction with medical treatment and in all types of healthcare settings, is focused on the relief of physical, mental, and spiritual distress. The goal of palliative care is to prevent and relieve suffering by early assessment and treatment of pain and other physical problems (such as difficulty breathing, nausea, fatigue, and problems with sleeping). As with hospice care, palliative care is provided by an interdisciplinary team.

Healthcare Agencies

Many different types of agencies provide healthcare services. This section includes discussion on voluntary agencies, religious agencies, and government agencies.

Voluntary Agencies

Community agencies are often nonprofit voluntary agencies. These agencies are financed by private donations, grants, or fundraisers (although some may charge minimal fees). Examples of volunteer agencies are Meals on Wheels, which supplies meals to older and homebound people; transportation services for older and physically disabled people; and shopping or house-cleaning services. Other nonprofit voluntary community agencies include the American Heart Association and the American Lung Association. Physicians and nurses are often active members of these organizations and provide health screenings and educational programs.

Voluntary agencies may also provide a setting for support groups. These groups provide an education and support system for patients who are adjusting to their health problems. Members of these support groups have experienced the same type of problem. By sharing experiences, members learn to solve problems when dealing with a stressful or crisis situation. Professional nurses most often provide information about and make referrals to these agencies to patients and family members. The following are examples of support groups:

- Alcoholics Anonymous—an international organization for recovering alcoholics. The purpose of this support group is to help individuals stop drinking and remain sober. Meetings are held in accessible community locations, such as churches and hospitals.
- Cancer support groups—focus on support and solving problems experienced by people diagnosed with cancer. Most cancer support group meetings are held at hospitals.
- Reach to Recovery—for women who have had a breast removed for cancer or have had breast reconstruction surgery. Among other activities, members visit women before surgery, teach exercises to prevent muscle atrophy, and provide information about prostheses and clothing.

Parish Nursing

Parish nursing is an expanding area of specialty nursing practice that emphasizes holistic healthcare, health promotion, and disease-prevention activities. It combines professional nursing practice with health ministry, emphasizing health and healing within a faith community. Parish nurses function as health educators, resource and referral aids, and facilitators of lay volunteer and support groups. Parish nurses reach out to those most vulnerable such as the elderly, those who have suffered a loss or change, single parents, and children.

Government Agencies

National, state, or local taxes finance government agencies. City and county taxes help support hospitals and public health clinics, state taxes help support state mental health hospitals, and national taxes help finance national health and welfare programs.

VETERANS ADMINISTRATION AND MILITARY AGENCIES

Veterans Administration (VA) hospitals and military hospitals all come under the umbrella of government-supported and government-operated healthcare. VA hospitals provide healthcare services to veterans, and military hospitals provide care to active members of the armed forces and their immediate families. Nursing services provided in military hospitals are the same as those in other types of hospital settings.

PUBLIC HEALTH SERVICE

The Public Health Service (PHS) is a federal health agency under the direction of the U.S. Department of Health and Human Services. The PHS is a multifaceted program with a wide range of services. It is the medical branch of the U.S. Coast Guard and the principal source of Native American healthcare through the Indian Health Services. The PHS supplies funds to health centers that provide care to migrant workers and to community agencies that supply healthcare to the poor and uninsured. The principal budget of the PHS goes to grant programs for poor and uninsured people.

The Centers for Disease Control and Prevention (CDC) in Atlanta and the National Institutes of Health (NIH) are both part of the PHS. The CDC focuses on the epidemiology, prevention, control, and treatment of communicable diseases, such as STIs. The NIH is engaged in both funding and conducting various health research activities.

The PHS also supplies healthcare professionals (e.g., nurses, physicians, dentists, pharmacists) to the U.S. Department of Justice to provide care in federal prisons. The service is also involved to some extent in some state administered drug and alcohol abuse and mental health programs. PHS activities focus on community needs whenever possible. Nurses practicing in these settings provide direct care, provide information, and serve as patient advocates within the community.

PUBLIC HEALTH AGENCIES

Public health agencies are local, state, and federal agencies that provide public health services at the local, county, state, or federal level. They are usually funded by taxes and run by elected or appointed administrators. Local agencies provide services and programs to promote health and pre-

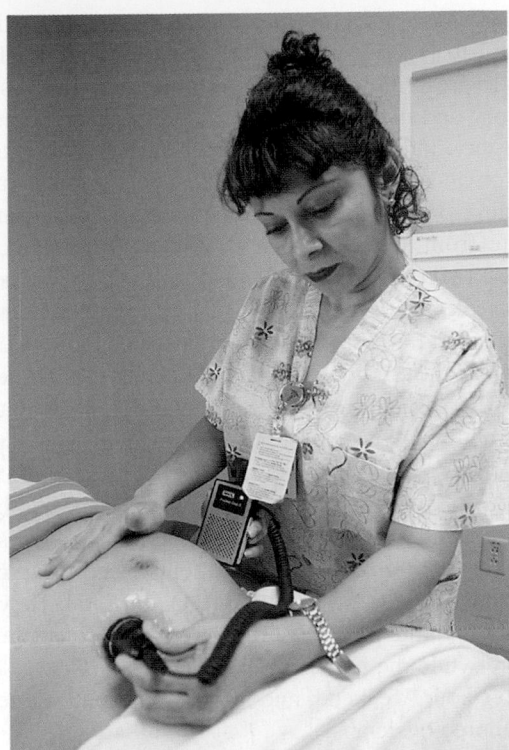

FIGURE 8-4. A nurse provides prenatal care at a public health clinic. *(Photo by Joe Mitchell.)*

vent illness, such as providing immunizations and screening for tuberculosis and STIs. Public health agencies work with state and local departments to ensure public health through activities such as inspections of restaurants and water supplies. They also provide educational programs and may provide direct care services for low-income people or people living in rural, isolated areas. Nurses who practice in public health agencies focus on prenatal care, well-child care, screening programs, education, and outreach into the community (Fig. 8-4).

INTERDISCIPLINARY CARE: THE HEALTHCARE TEAM

In any type of agency, setting, or framework, nurses with other members of the interdisciplinary healthcare team plan, provide, and evaluate patient care. For example, a nurse may request a consult with a dietitian for a patient who is not eating well or for a patient who needs to lose weight. After the dietitian talks with the patient and mutually determines a plan of care, the nurse can reinforce the plan and evaluate its effectiveness. The primary goal of each member of the healthcare team is to promote and restore health. The following sections describe members of the healthcare team (other than nurses) whom nurses work with most often.

Physician

The physician is primarily responsible for the diagnosis of illness and the medical or surgical treatment of that illness. Physicians are granted the authority to admit patients to a healthcare agency by the healthcare agency or institution itself and to practice care within that setting through such actions as prescribing medications, interpreting the results of laboratory and diagnostic tests, and performing procedures and surgery. Individuals become physicians after extensive education and clinical practice and a licensing examination. Depending on the curriculum completed, a physician may graduate from a medical school and become a Doctor of Medicine (MD) or from a college of osteopathy and become a Doctor of Osteopathy (DO). MDs and DOs have similar educations and areas of practice, but osteopathic medicine emphasizes the study of mechanical changes in tissues as a cause of illness and treatment that involves manipulation of body structures. Physicians may choose to be general practitioners or to specialize in the treatment of one type of illness or body system (such as a cardiologist) or a specific type of surgery (such as an orthopedic surgeon). Hospitalists are physicians who provide care to patients when they visit the emergency room or are admitted to the hospital. They communicate with the patient's primary care physician, but provide care while the patient is in the hospital. They also may take after-hour, weekend, and holiday calls and services for one or more physicians.

Physician Assistant

A physician assistant (PA) has completed a specific course of study and a licensing examination in preparation for providing support to the physician. The PA's responsibilities usually depend on the supervising physician and might include conducting physical examinations and suturing lacerations. In most states, nurses are not legally bound to follow a PA's orders unless a physician cosigns the orders. This is an important aspect to investigate if PAs are employed by hospitals in your area.

Physical Therapist

A physical therapist (PT) seeks to restore function or to prevent further disability in a patient after an injury or illness. PTs use various techniques to treat patients, including massage, heat, cold, water, sonar waves, exercises, and electrical stimulation. Most PTs are also educated in the use of psychological strategies to motivate patients.

Respiratory Therapist

A respiratory therapist (RT) is trained in techniques that improve pulmonary function and oxygenation. RTs may also be responsible for administering a variety of tests that measure lung function and for educating the patient about the use of various devices and machines prescribed by the physician.

Occupational Therapist

An occupational therapist (OT) assists physically challenged patients to adapt to limitations. OTs use a variety of adaptive devices and strategies to aid patients in carrying out the activities of daily living.

Speech Therapist

A speech therapist is trained to help hearing-impaired patients speak more clearly, to assist patients who have had a stroke to relearn how to speak, and to correct or modify a variety of speech disturbances in children and adults. Speech therapists also diagnose and treat swallowing problems in patients who have had a head injury or a stroke.

Dietitian

A registered dietitian (RD) manages and plans for the dietary needs of patients, based on knowledge about all aspects of nutrition. RDs can adapt specialized diets for the individual needs of patients, counsel and educate individual patients, and supervise the dietary services of an entire facility.

Pharmacist

A pharmacist, prepared at the doctoral level, is licensed to formulate and dispense medications. The pharmacist is also responsible for keeping a file of all patient medications and for informing the physician when a potential or actual medication error in prescribing has occurred, or when prescribed drugs may interact adversely. The pharmacist is an excellent resource for information related to medications for both patients and nurses.

Social Worker

A social worker counsels patients and family members and also informs them of and refers them to various community resources. Social workers are involved in many activities such as counseling, reporting suspected drug addiction or abuse, assisting with decisions about life-sustaining treatments, placing patients in long-term care facilities, and providing support to dying patients and their family members.

> *Think about Maritza Cortes, the woman who brought her daughter to the emergency department. The statement by Ms. Cortes about not having the money needed to have the prescription filled would alert the nurse to the need for consulting social service. The social worker could provide Ms. Cortes with information about available financial assistance and community resources.* ■

Unlicensed Assistive Personnel

Unlicensed assistive personnel (UAPs) help nurses provide direct care to patients. As defined by individual state boards of nursing, UAPs may have the title of certified nursing assistants, orderlies, attendants, or technicians.

FINANCIAL ASPECTS OF HEALTHCARE

Many questions have been raised about the present healthcare system. Most questions involve access to, cost of, and quality of care. These questions are debated at the local, state, and federal level, as well as by healthcare providers and consumers of healthcare services. Healthcare reform plans have been proposed at both the federal and state levels, but as of January, 2010, no one plan has been accepted. Federal legislation enacted through the 1996 Health Insurance Portability and Accountability Act has improved access to insurance for employed persons and prohibits denial of coverage for an existing illness. Increased options for health insurance for children who do not live in poverty are available. Despite these measures, the number of people without access to private insurance continues to increase.

Healthcare is very expensive, and costs continue to increase. Few citizens can afford to pay for healthcare from their own resources. The costs of most people's healthcare are covered by federally funded programs, prepaid plans, and/or private insurance.

Federally Funded Healthcare Programs

The primary federally funded healthcare programs are Medicare and Medicaid.

Medicare

The 1965 **Medicare** amendments to the Social Security Act established national and state health insurance programs for the elderly under Title 18. Within a decade, almost all citizens older than 65 years of age held Medicare insurance for hospital care, extended care, and home healthcare. Medicare coverage was increased in 1972 to include permanently disabled workers and their dependents, if they also qualified for Social Security benefits.

In 1983, Medicare converted to a prospective payment plan based on patient classification categories, called **diagnosis-related groups** (DRGs). The federal government implemented DRGs in an effort to control rising healthcare costs. The plan pays the hospital a fixed amount that is predetermined by the medical diagnosis or specific procedure rather than by the actual cost of hospitalization and care. Medicare was expanded in 1988 to include catastrophic care costs and expensive medications. In 2007, based on changes in DRGs made by the Centers for Medicare & Medicaid Services (CMS), the reimbursement to hospitals is now based on severity of illness and projected cost of care. The plan pays only the amount of money preassigned to a treatment for the diagnosis (e.g., an appendectomy); if the cost for hospitalization is greater than that assigned, the hospital must absorb the additional cost. If the cost is less than that assigned, the hospital makes a profit. In addition, Medicare will no longer reimburse hospitals for conditions that result from preventable errors and lead to increased costs. The conditions include pressure ulcers, injuries caused by falls, infections associated with indwelling urinary catheters, vascular catheter-associated infections, infections of the mediastinum after coronary artery bypass graft, air embolisms, adverse reactions to incompatible blood infusions, and sponges or instruments left inside a patient during surgery (Guadagnimo, 2007).

People who receive Medicare pay both a deductible cost and a monthly premium for full insurance coverage. Part A of Medicare, which pays most inpatient hospital costs, is paid by the federal government. Part B of Medicare, which is voluntary, is paid by a monthly premium; it covers most outpatient costs for physician visits, medications, and home health services. Because the full cost of some services is not covered by Medicare, a supplemental insurance policy offered by a private insurance company is recommended. Also, because Medicare is federally funded, benefits may change annually according to decisions related to the federal budget.

> *Remember Margaret Ritchie, the older adult woman caring for her husband at home? Most likely, she and her husband have Medicare. Medicare does pay for home healthcare services if the patient meets specific criteria. However, Medicare does not cover all equipment that may be necessary.* ∎

Medicaid

Medicaid was established in 1965 under Title 19 of the Social Security Act. Medicaid is a federally funded public assistance program for people of any age who have low incomes; for the blind, elderly, and disabled covered by supplemental security benefits; and for beneficiaries of Aid to Families With Dependent Children. The coverage depends on individual state regulations.

Current budgetary considerations are forcing state and federal agencies to trim Medicaid expenditures. The rapid growth of an aging population and an increase in the number of poor people, many of whom are women and children, are draining the Medicaid budget. In an attempt to survive, Medicaid programs are implementing changes such as reduced benefits or placing patients into managed care programs.

Group Plans

The major group plans for financing healthcare are managed care plans (such as health maintenance organizations [HMOs], preferred provider organizations [PPOs]), and private insurance. Enrollment in these plans is voluntary. An individual pays a fixed rate on a monthly or annual basis and, in turn, receives coverage for most healthcare services to maintain health and treat illness.

Because group plans such as HMOs and PPOs pay the direct costs of the healthcare services used by their subscribers, they encourage preventive healthcare to avoid the higher costs of illness and hospitalization. For the same reason, they carefully monitor the quality and quantity of the healthcare delivered to their subscribers. They also place limitations on the use of high-cost procedures and require certain guidelines to be followed when a physician recommends a costly procedure. Some people do not like these plans because they use a selective contracting approach that mandates subscribers use specific institutions and healthcare providers. Some consumers dislike not being able to control decisions about their own or their family's health.

Health Maintenance Organizations

Health maintenance organizations (HMOs) are prepaid, group-managed care plans that allow subscribers to receive all the medical services they require through a group of affiliated providers. There may be no additional out-of-pocket costs, or subscribers may pay only a small fee, called a copayment. An HMO may employ all its providers (including physicians) or may be a group of physicians in alliance who provide care as independent practitioners. In most HMOs, the patient does not have a choice about healthcare providers but receives all services from physicians who are associated with or are part of the HMO. HMOs are popular with large employers who support the concept of managed care, and they are also associated with Medicare in some states.

Preferred Provider Organizations

Preferred provider organizations (PPOs) allow a third-party payer (agencies that pay healthcare providers for services provided to individuals, such as a health insurance company) to contract with a group of healthcare providers to provide services at a lower fee in return for prompt payment and a guaranteed volume of patients and services. Although patients are encouraged to use specific providers, they may also seek care outside the panel without referral by paying additional out-of-pocket expenses. One type of PPO is called a preferred provider arrangement, in which a contract is made with an individual healthcare provider rather than with a group of providers. Similarly, a point-of-service plan encourages the use of specified physicians and services but pays a portion of expenses if referrals are made to physicians outside the organization by the patient's primary care physician.

Private Insurance

Personal healthcare can be financed by private insurance through large, nonprofit, tax-exempt organizations or through smaller, private, for-profit insurance companies. To be insured, members pay monthly premiums either by themselves or in combination with employer payments. These plans are called third-party payers because the insurance company pays all or most of the cost of care. The premiums on private insurance plans tend to be higher than those for managed care plans, but members can choose their own physician and services desired.

Long-Term Care Insurance

Increasing numbers of people are enrolling in long-term care (LTC) insurance. Some commercial insurance companies offer LTC benefits, but most LTC insurance (about 90%) is paid for by Medicaid and out-of-pocket spending. Medicare pays for only a minimal amount of LTC insurance. Promoters of LTC insurance have developed plans that cover a variety of services, such as nursing home care and home care, as well as other services that help prevent the institutionalization of older, debilitated, and chronically ill people. Adult daycare centers and respite care are also LTC services and would be covered by such benefits.

TRENDS AND ISSUES IN HEALTHCARE DELIVERY

This section discusses some current issues and trends in healthcare. In your career as a nurse, you may find that some issues are resolved, whereas other new challenges arise. It is important for you both personally and professionally to be knowledgeable about all healthcare trends affecting the healthcare delivery system (Box 8-2).

Focus on Preventive Care

Health awareness and the desire to be involved in one's own healthcare have strongly influenced the delivery of healthcare services in our society. Stress management programs, nutritional awareness, exercise and fitness programs, and antismoking and antidrug campaigns are all examples of this trend. Equally important to health are measures such as legislating the use of seat belts, promoting automobile and airplane safety, controlling smog, controlling handguns, and eliminating hazardous wastes.

Knowledgeable Consumers

A **consumer** is someone who uses a commodity or service. Healthcare consumers (patients) are increasingly knowledgeable about health, prefer to control and make decisions about their own health, and want to be active participants in planning and implementing their healthcare. Consumers of healthcare services are better educated about the services they require and the services that are available, largely because so much health information is available on the Internet. They also are concerned about access to services, the cost of those services, and the quality of the care received for services. Consumers have questioned escalating costs and the proliferation and duplication of services. Consumers have become actively involved in the administration of healthcare agencies and have helped develop standards for

---

Box 8-2 TRENDS TO WATCH IN HEALTHCARE DELIVERY

- Changing demographics
- Increasing diversity
- Technology explosion
- Globalization of economy and society
- Educated consumers
- Increasing complexity of patient care
- Costs of healthcare
- Effect of health policy and regulation
- Current nursing shortage

care, patient rights, and cost-containment measures as protection for patients when they enter a healthcare setting. A recent federal program surveys patients' experiences with nurses and doctors, while in the hospital and after leaving the hospital. Data will be used to improve and make hospitals accountable for the quality of patient care (Cipriano, 2008).

> *Remember Paul Cochran, the patient with a history of mental illness and numerous visits to inpatient and outpatient facilities? The nurse would need to obtain a thorough assessment of the patient's medications to ensure the most accurate information from which to develop a plan of care.* ∎

Cost Containment

The U.S. healthcare system has been experiencing a financial crisis. Costs have increased dramatically, and some analysts believe that cost-containment measures were implemented too late to reverse the rise in health costs. The actual short-term and long-term results of cost-containment measures remain to be seen.

Historically, payment for healthcare services encouraged the use of expensive and sometimes inappropriate or ineffective services. In the past, healthcare also focused primarily on the treatment of illnesses rather than prevention because preventive strategies were not covered by health insurance. The system of third-party reimbursement effectively insulated patients, who seldom saw the bills, from knowing the actual cost of their healthcare.

Competition among hospitals has further fueled the increase in health costs. To attract patients, hospitals have invested huge sums of money in technologically advanced equipment. As new machines and more advanced procedures have been developed and used, patients' expectations of the availability and use of those resources have also tended to increase. Supporters of cost-containment measures are encouraging hospitals to cooperate and share resources rather than compete. Other efforts at cost containment include hospital restructuring and multiple hospitals joining together as one system.

Fragmentation of Care

Expanded healthcare research has led to an upward spiral of new technology and knowledge. Because many healthcare providers can no longer keep up with all of the advances being made in all areas, specialization in smaller areas has become almost the rule rather than the exception. What does this mean for patients?

A general practitioner physician diagnoses and treats a variety of common health problems; however, a patient who requires diagnosis and treatment for a more complex problem is usually referred to a specialist physician. For example, a patient with diabetes and a heart condition may be cared for by the family physician, a cardiologist, and an endocrinologist. Hospitalized patients not only come in contact with many different healthcare providers (e.g., RNs, LPNs, nursing assistants, nurse specialists, PTs, RDs, students), but they are also frequently seen by other physician specialists who are called in on consultation or to do surgery. This can cause patients to become confused about care and treatments. This fragmentation of care can lead to a loss of continuity of care, resulting in conflicting plans of care, too much or too little medication, and higher healthcare costs.

Healthcare: A Right or a Privilege?

Two major factors influencing the provision of healthcare in the United States are the ability to pay for care and the location of facilities. Poor or uninsured people, minorities, residents of rural areas, and older people often have inadequate access to healthcare services. In the United States, millions of people have inadequate insurance or none at all. Although many people assume that everyone has a right to healthcare, consider these questions that pose ethical dilemmas for nurses who provide care, as well as for consumers of healthcare services:

- Do uninsured people who do not take care of themselves deserve the same healthcare as employed people with insurance, even if they cannot pay for it?
- Who provides funds for the healthcare needs of the unemployed and homeless?
- Is someone who pays for national television coverage to ask for an organ donation for his or her child any more deserving than someone who has been waiting months for just such a transplant?
- Are you willing to pay higher insurance premiums or taxes so that drug addicts who overdose can have intensive care?
- If 20 people need a heart transplant and only one heart is available, who decides who gets another chance at life?

These are only a few of the questions being raised, and there are no easy answers.

NURSES' ROLE IN HEALTHCARE REFORM

Changes taking place in healthcare give nurses the opportunity to help shape healthcare for the future. Projections about competencies of future healthcare practitioners, coupled with the national health promotion and disease prevention objectives outlined in the *Healthy People 2020* project (Office of Disease Prevention & Health Promotion, 2008), underscores the importance of nursing's role in improving access to care, quality of care, and cost of care.

The healthcare system in the United States has many challenges, including the rapidly increased numbers of older adults, changing expectations of healthcare consumers, rapidly expanding technologies, and an emphasis on improved quality and safety of care. To help meet these challenges, the National Academy of Sciences (2003) proposed five core competencies necessary for healthcare professionals to meet the needs of the 21st-century healthcare system. The competencies are based on communication, knowledge, technical skills, critical thinking, and values in clinical practice. These competencies are (1) to provide patient-centered care, (2) to work in interdisciplinary teams, (3) to use evidence-based practice, (4) to apply quality improvement, and (5) to use informatics.

The goals of healthcare reform focus on cost containment, improved access, and increased quality of services for all citizens. Where do nurses fit into the reform movement? First, nurses are becoming a stronger voice in protesting health-related problems in our nation. Second, nurses in greater numbers are increasing their education and becoming APRNs. As such, more nurses now provide primary healthcare services in areas and to people long neglected: the elderly, women, infants, the poor, and those living in rural areas. In addition, the focus of nursing care provided by all nurses is holistic care essential to promoting health and preventing illness. Moreover, *ANA's Health System Reform Agenda* (2008) (Box 8-3) reaffirm the association's 15 years of support for a restructured healthcare system that ensures universal access to a standard package of essential healthcare services and lays out a comprehensive strategy for achieving goals.

Nursing's Health System Reform Agenda (2008) is a strategic plan formulated by the American Nurses Association that is focused on the means to ensure safe, quality patient care and address the causes of the acute shortage of RNs, predicted to worsen in the next decade. As discussion continues about the goals of this document, the common themes for all nurses emerge: collaborating with other nurses (as individuals and as groups), developing leadership

---

> **Box 8-4** **NURSES CAN MAKE A DIFFERENCE IN HEALTHCARE POLICY AND REFORM**
>
> - Stay informed about current issues and pending legislation.
> - Write or e-mail members of Congress to support legislation to improve nursing and patient care.
> - Belong to and participate in nursing organizations.
> - Document the outcomes of nursing care and develop a database to influence healthcare costs and quality of care.
> - Be a leader in local, state, and national nursing and consumer groups.
> - Advocate for the rights of all individuals for equal, affordable, accessible, and knowledgeable healthcare.

and public communication skills, increasing collaboration with policy makers and business leaders, and communicating successes to the public. There are many ways nurses can become involved in shaping healthcare reform and healthcare policy. Selected examples are listed in Box 8-4.

The issues of who gets healthcare and who pays the bills continue to have major importance for society in the 21st century. These issues will present both challenges and opportunities for nurses of the future.

● Developing Critical Thinking Skills

1. Make a list of the different types of healthcare settings where you have received care. How many different healthcare providers did you come in contact with? How did the structure and organization of the settings differ, and how were they alike?

2. How might prenatal and well-child care differ for two women—one without health insurance and the other with a good health insurance plan? Why do you think this happens? What can nurses do?

● Practicing for NCLEX

1. A group of students are reviewing information about hospitals in preparation for a quiz the next day. Which of the following, if identified by the students as associated with a hospital, demonstrates the need for additional study?
   a. Provision of acute care
   b. Inpatient services
   c. Outpatient services
   d. Parish nursing activities

2. Which type of healthcare facility employs the largest percentage of RNs?
   a. Ambulatory care
   b. Long-term care
   c. Hospitals
   d. Physician offices

> **Box 8-3** **SELECTED ELEMENTS OF *ANA'S HEALTHCARE AGENDA***
>
> - A restructured healthcare system that enhances access to services by delivering primary healthcare in community-based settings and fosters consumer responsibility for personal health, self-care, and informed decision making in selecting healthcare services.
> - A federally defined standard package of essential healthcare services available to all citizens and residents of the United States, provided and financed through an integration of public and private plans and sources.
> - A phase-in of essential services that would include coverage of pregnant women and children and services designed specifically to assist vulnerable populations who have limited access to our nation's healthcare system.
> - Steps to reduce healthcare costs, including required use of managed care in the public plan and encouraged in the private plan, controlled growth of the healthcare system, incentives for consumers and providers to be more cost-efficient, and assuring direct access to a full range of qualified providers.
> - Case management would be required for all those with continuing healthcare needs.
> - Provision for long-term care, including public and private funding for services of short duration, public funding for extended care when needed, and emphasis on the consumers' responsibility to financially plan for their long-term care needs.

From American Nurses Association. (2008). *ANA's health system reform agenda.* Washington, DC: Author.

3. When reviewing information about the growth of healthcare services, which area would the nurse expect to find as the most rapidly growing area?
   a. Hospitals
   b. Home care
   c. Nursing homes
   d. Parish nursing

4. Which healthcare provider is a major source of health assessment and health education for children?
   a. Hospital emergency department
   b. Community center
   c. Nurse practitioner
   d. School nurse

5. A caregiver asks a nurse to explain respite care. How would the nurse respond?
   a. "A service that allows time away for caregivers"
   b. "A special service for the terminally ill and their family"
   c. "Direct care provided to individuals in nursing homes"
   d. "Living units for people without regular shelter"

6. After teaching a class about the various healthcare agencies and services, the instructor determines that the teaching was successful when the class identifies which of the following as a government agency?
   a. Alcoholics Anonymous
   b. Public Health Service
   c. Rural health center
   d. Ambulatory care center

7. Which purpose best describes managed care as a framework for healthcare?
   a. A design to control the cost of care while maintaining the quality of care
   b. Care coordination to maximize positive outcomes to contain costs
   c. The delivery of services from initial contact through ongoing care
   d. Based on a philosophy of ensuring death in comfort and dignity

8. Your newly employed friend is a part of the company's HMO. You interpret that to mean the friend
   a. Can have healthcare services from a provider of his choice
   b. Will be unable to have emergency care
   c. Receives all healthcare from providers within the organization
   d. Must pay an additional monthly premium

9. Private insurance most often is called a third-party payer, indicating which of the following?
   a. You pay no monthly premium, paying for all healthcare costs yourself.
   b. You belong to a preferred provider organization.
   c. You are at risk if your healthcare provider is not a part of the plan.
   d. You pay a monthly premium, and the insurance company pays the bills.

10. A nurse is developing a presentation for a local community group about the knowledgeable healthcare consumer. Which technology would the nurse include as having the greatest effect on this area?
    a. Television
    b. Computers
    c. Cell phones
    d. Global positioning system (GPS) devices

● Answers With Rationale

1. *d.* Hospitals are acute care providers, providing services to both inpatients and outpatients.

2. *c.* Despite a downward trend, the largest percent of RNs are employed by hospitals.

3. *b.* Home care services are the most rapidly growing area of healthcare.

4. *d.* School nurses do provide much of the health assessment and health information for the nation's children.

5. *a.* Respite care is provided to enable a primary caregiver time away from the day-to-day responsibilities of homebound patients.

6. *b.* The Public Health Service is a government agency.

7. *a.* Managed care is a way of providing care, designed to control costs while maintaining the quality of care.

8. *c.* In most HMOs, the patient does not have a choice of healthcare providers and receives all services from providers within the HMO.

9. *d.* You (and your employer, if appropriate) pay monthly premiums, and the insurance company pays all or most of the cost of care.

10. *b.* Consumers are increasingly using their home computers to access healthcare information through the Internet.

Taylor Suite Resources

The Taylor Suite offers these additional resources to enhance learning and facilitate understanding of this chapter:

- thePoint online resource, http://thepoint.lww.com/Taylor7E
- Student DVD included with the book
- Study Guide for Taylor's Fundamentals of Nursing

BIBLIOGRAPHY

American Hospital Association. (2009). Fast facts on U.S. hospitals. Available at http://www.aha.org/aha/resource-center/Statistics-and-Studies/fast-facts.html.
American Nurses Association. (2008). *ANA's health system reform agenda.* Silver Springs, MD: American Nurses Association.
American Nurses Association. (2005). *ANA's health care agenda.* Washington, DC: Author.
American Nurses Credentialing Center. (2009). *Magnet recognition program in the news.* Available http://www.nursecredentialing.org/

Bureau of Labor Statistics, U. S. Department of Labor. (2007). *Occupational outlook handbook, 2008–2009 edition: Registered nurses*. Available at http://www.bls.gov/oco/ocos083.htm

Case Management Society of America. (2008). *What is a case manager?* Available at http://www.cmsa.org/Home/CMSA/WhatisaCaseManager/tabid/224/Default.aspx

Center to Advance Palliative Care. (2009). *What is palliative care*. Available at http://www.getpalliativecare.org/whatis

Centers for Disease Control and Prevention (CDC). (2008). Hospital utilization (in non-Federal short stay hospitals). Available at http://www.cdc/gov/nchs/fastats/hospital.htm

Centers for Medicare & Medicaid Services. (2009). *Medicare information; Medicaid information*. Available at http://cms.hhs.gov.

Cipriano, P. (2008). The voice of the consumer. *American Nurse Today, 3*(3), 8.

Cohen, E., & Cesta, T. (2005). *Nursing case management: From essentials to advanced practice applications*. Philadelphia: Saunders.

Daniels, S. (2009). Advocacy and the hospital case manager. *Professional Case Management, 14*(1), 48–51.

Edmonds, M., & Scudder, L. (2008). Convenient care clinics and nurse practitioners. *Journal of Nursing Practitioners, 4*, 773–775.

Ellis, J., & Hartley, C. (2007). *Nursing in today's world: Trends, issues, and management* (9th ed.). Philadelphia: Lippincott Williams & Wilkins.

Garrett, M. (2008). Understanding Medicaid: What case managers need to know. *Professional Case Management, 13*(3), 123–126.

Guadagnino, C. (2007). Appraising CMS's new hospital reimbursement methodology. *Physician's News Digest, Inc.* Available at http://www.physiciansnews.com/spotlight/1007.html

Health & Human Services. Medicare. (2007). *Long-term care*. Available at http://www.medicare.gov/LongTermCare/static/Home.asp

Hospice Association of America. (2008). *Hospice facts & statistics*. Washington, DC: Author.

Huston, C. J. (2006). *Professional issues in nursing: Challenges & opportunities*. Philadelphia: Lippincott Williams & Wilkins.

Kurtzman, E., & Buerhaus, P. (2008). New Medicare payment rules: Danger or opportunity for nursing? *American Journal of Nursing, 108*(6), 30–35.

Lombardi, K. S. (2008, February 17). *For patients, more comfort and a bigger dose of respect. The New York Times* in the region, Hospitals 1–2.

National Academy of Sciences. (2003). *Executive summary: Health professions education. A bridge to quality*. Available at http://www.nap.edu

National Association for Home Care & Hospice. (2008). *Basic statistics about home care*. Washington, DC: Author.

Office of Disease Prevention & Health Promotion. U.S. Department of Health & Human Services. (2008). *Healthy people 2020: The road ahead*. Available at http://www.healthypeople.gov/hp2020/

Patterson, D., Wehling, B., & Mason, G. (2008). Parish nursing: Reclaiming the spiritual dimensions of care. *American Nurse Today, 3*(10), 38–40.

The National Association for Home Care & Hospice. (2008). *Basic statistics about home care*. Washington, DC: Author.

U.S. Department of Labor. Bureau of Labor Statistics. Occupational Outlook Handbook (2008). *Registered Nurses*. Available at http://www.bls.gov/oco/ocos083.htm

U.S. Department of Health and Human Services. Centers for Medicare & Medicaid Services. (2008). *Medicare hospice benefits*. (Pub. No. 02154). Baltimore, MD: Author.

Widman, M., & Lemke, S. (2008). Impact of nursing case management on an underserved population. *Home Health Care Management & Practice, 21*(1), 17–22.

White, K., Baxoli, G., Roggenkamp, S., & Gau, T. (2005). Does case management matter as a hospital cost-control strategy? *Health Care Management Review, 30*(1), 32–43.

Continuity of Care | 9

JEFF HART

Jeff is a 9-year-old with a genetic disease that includes severe mental retardation. He is transferred from the state home for children to the hospital for respiratory complications.

LAURA DEGAS

Laura, a 78-year-old woman, has been caring for her sister, Ellen, at home. She says, "She was diagnosed with Alzheimer's disease 2 years ago. This surgery to fix her broken hip has really been tough. I want to take her home, but I'm not sure if I can give her the care that she needs now."

JENNIFER LENNER

Jennifer, a 20-year-old woman diagnosed with a seizure disorder, had surgery 3 days ago. She says, "My doctor says that I'm going home today. I can't wait! My parents are coming to pick me up later this morning." Review of her medical record indicates that the attending physician had not written discharge orders.

After completing the chapter, you will be able to accomplish the following:

1. Describe the role of the nurse in ensuring continuity of care between and among healthcare settings.

2. Discuss considerations for establishing an effective nurse–patient relationship when admitting a patient to a healthcare setting.

3. Compare and contrast admission of a patient to an ambulatory care setting and a hospital setting.

4. Discuss transfer of patients within and among healthcare settings.

5. Explain how nurses use the components of discharge planning to provide continuity of care.

KEY TERMS

chart	discharge planning
community-based care	HIPAA privacy rule
continuity of care	Kardex

People enter healthcare settings and become consumers of healthcare services (patients) for many different reasons. Not all individuals have the same kinds of healthcare needs, nor are they alike as patients. Some of them will be admitted and discharged on the same day; some of them will remain in the acute care setting only as long as acute care is needed; and some will require long-term care.

Entering and leaving a healthcare setting, as well as receiving care at home, are experiences that produce anxiety for both patients and family members. The nurse is often the person who helps the patient make a smooth transition from one type of care setting to another. (See the accompanying Reflective Practice box for an example.) This chapter discusses continuity of care, community-based nursing practice, admission and discharge from a healthcare setting, transfer from one type of setting to another, and discharge planning in preparation for home healthcare. It focuses on the patient's needs and the nurse's role in providing continuity of care.

ESSENTIAL CONCEPTS

Two concepts essential to nursing care of patients within and across healthcare settings are continuity of care and community-based care. Planning for and providing individualized nursing interventions that promote health, prevent illness, and support coping with disability are critical in today's culturally diverse society. It is no longer enough only to consider the patient's needs within the hospital setting; nurses must also consider how those needs will be met as the patient makes the transition from the acute care setting to some type of long-term care or to care at home with support and services from his or her community.

▶ *Consider Laura Degas, the sister of the woman with Alzheimer's disease who had undergone a hip repair. Due to her sister's increased complexity of care, Ms. Degas is unsure if she can continue to care for her sister at home. The nurse would work with Ms. Degas to determine her needs and possibly enlist the aid of social services for assistance with a referral to home care and appropriate resources and community services.* ■

Continuity of Care

Continuity of care is a process by which healthcare providers give appropriate, uninterrupted care and facilitate the patient's transition between different settings and levels of care. Continuity of care ensures a smooth transition between ambulatory or acute care and home healthcare or other types of healthcare settings in the patient's community. Coordination helps ensure a patient-focused and individualized continuum of healthcare so that the patient may attain maximum recovery and health.

Most people are born in a hospital, thus becoming consumers of healthcare from the first day of life. Over their lifetime, most people continue to require services of some type, in a variety of healthcare settings. Although a patient's healthcare may involve many different providers and settings (discussed in Chapter 8), the nurse is often the primary person responsible for communicating the patient's needs, teaching self-care, and, in many instances, providing care. As a result, one of the primary responsibilities of the nurse as caregiver is ensuring continuity of care.

Continuity of care is essential in the current healthcare system. The emphasis on promoting health and preventing illness makes teaching individuals of all ages a crucial component of patient care. To provide continuity of care, nurses must consider teaching and referrals in the care of any person admitted to any type of healthcare setting and must also involve the patient and family in a mutual planning process. The nurse must collaborate with other members of the healthcare team in meeting the physical, psychological, sociocultural, and spiritual needs of the patient and family in all settings and at all levels of health or illness.

▶ *Think back to Jennifer Lenner, the young adult woman with a seizure disorder who had surgery. The nurse would need to collaborate with the surgeon and primary healthcare provider to ensure that all of the patient's needs are addressed. Also, since the patient lives with her parents,*

REFLECTIVE PRACTICE

Challenge to Interpersonal Skills

Last week in clinical, I was assigned to care for four patients. Although the care for the patients did not appear to be incredibly complex, this was my first time having four patients at once. Needless to say, I was slightly nervous. In report, I was told that one of the patients, Jennifer Lenner, a 20-year-old woman with a seizure disorder who had had surgery 3 days ago, was going to be discharged sometime today. Therefore, we needed to do discharge planning, as well as get her ready to go home. Although the unit nurse was very helpful, she had been feeling sick all morning and at some point needed to go down to Employee Health.

While I was completing my morning assessment of Jennifer, she told me how eager she was to get home. Her parents had been told to come to the hospital sometime in the morning to bring her home. However, when reviewing Jennifer's chart for discharge orders, I noted that no orders had been written. The nurse and I made a call to the resident to ask about Jennifer's status, because the attending physician had told her that she was going home today. The resident responded that that was not the case and that she was going to have to wait until tomorrow to go home per the order of the attending physician. The resident reported that they were concerned about postoperative complications. However, the patient was already 3 days postsurgery. In the meantime, the nurse with whom I was working had gone down to Employee Health. The charge nurse as well as my clinical instructor were still with me, but they had not been dealing with the situation the whole morning. So, I was left with two options: I could listen to what the resident said and tell the patient that the plans had changed and we were going to continue with her daily care, or I could call the attending and see if that was indeed what he had in mind for Jennifer.

Thinking Outside the Box: Possible Courses of Action

- Simply take what the resident said and continue with Jennifer's care. Although she would be very disappointed, I would just tell her that this is what her doctor wanted and there is nothing I can do.

- Look in the chart for a means of contacting the attending physician and ask him if these were the plans he had in mind for Jennifer.

Evaluating a Good Outcome: How Do I Define Success?

- The patient is first of all healthy enough to be discharged home without fear of any complications.
- The patient's interests are taken into account because she had already been told that she would be going home that day.

- I stand up and advocate for my patient when she cannot do so herself.

Personal Learning: Here's to the Future!

I paged the attending physician with the charge nurse by my side. I was very nervous because I was worried he wasn't going to want to listen to what I, a nursing student, had to say. He called back and I explained the situation to him. He replied that indeed he had intended for Jennifer to go home today, and he even thanked me for calling to

check! He sent a resident up to write discharge orders, and we took out her intravenous catheter and reviewed her discharge instructions. Jennifer was happy to go home, and I was comfortable with the fact that she was healthy enough to be sent home.

Kathryn Southerton, Georgetown University

Reflection

How do you think you would respond in a similar situation? Why? What does this tell you about yourself and about the adequacy of your skills for professional practice? How might the nursing student's patient assignment have affected the actions taken? What questions could the nursing student and/or charge nurse have posed to the resident to determine the resident's knowledge of the situation? Can you think of other ways to respond? What other skills (cognitive, interpersonal, technical, ethical/legal) would you need to respond well in this situation? How did the nursing student ensure continuity of care? Suppose the attending physician had said that the patient's discharge had to wait 1 more day. How would you respond to the situation and then inform the patient of this decision? Do you agree with the criteria to evaluate a successful outcome? Did the nursing student meet the criteria? Please explain your answer.

the nurse would need to include the parents in any discharge teaching. ■

Community-Based Care

Community-based care is healthcare provided to people who live within a defined geographic area. That geographic area might be a small neighborhood in a large urban area or a large area of rural residents. Each community is unique and is defined by the people, area, social interactions, and common ties within that community.

In contrast to community health and public health nursing (which are population based and focus on the health of the community), community-based care is centered on individual and family healthcare needs. It emphasizes the provision of comprehensive, coordinated, and continuous services for patients with acute or chronic health problems (Stanhope & Lancaster, 2008). Within a framework of community-based care, nurses help people wherever they are, including where they live, work, play, worship, and go to school.

The nurse practicing community-based care considers the continuity of the care the patient requires when moving from one level or setting of care to another, providing interventions to promote health, manage acute or chronic illnesses, and promote self-care. Community-based care is designed to meet the needs of people as they move into, between, and among different healthcare settings within the overall healthcare system.

ADMISSION TO A HEALTHCARE SETTING

As a result of increasing costs and of healthcare cost reimbursement programs that are prospective rather than retrospective (meaning that costs are predetermined for specific illnesses or treatments, including severity of illness and costs of care), hospital admissions and lengths of hospital stay have decreased. Increasing numbers of patients are having surgery, diagnostic tests, and emergency care in ambulatory care settings or on a hospital outpatient basis. Even patients who are admitted often stay for less than 24 hours, are admitted the morning of the surgery, or go home during an interim period between diagnosis and care.

All people who enter a healthcare setting take on a new role. They must add to their already established roles (e.g., spouse, parent, sibling, student) the role of patient. They also enter an environment in which they are surrounded by strangers and in which they encounter different sounds, sights, and smells.

To meet patients' healthcare needs during the admission process, nurses provide holistic care and establish the basis for how patients will respond to and evaluate the remainder of their stay. Box 9-1 describes guidelines for establishing an effective nurse–patient relationship to ensure that each patient is considered as an individual in any setting.

During admission, the nurse acts not only as a practitioner but also as an advocate concerned about the welfare of the patient and the family. The admission period corresponds to the orientation phase of the helping relationship described in Chapter 21. In addition, regulatory guidelines direct both the continuity and the quality of care. For example, the Joint Commission has established standards for admission to a hospital. These standards assert that each patient's need for nursing care related to admission should be assessed by a registered nurse; this assessment includes consideration of biophysical, psychosocial, environmental, self-care, educational, and discharge planning factors. In addition, nurses collaborate, as appropriate, with physicians and members of other clinical disciplines to make decisions regarding the patient's need for nursing care.

The HIPAA Privacy Rule

All patients entering a healthcare setting of any type (ranging from hospitals to dental offices) must sign a statement

---

Box 9-1   ESTABLISHING AN EFFECTIVE NURSE–PATIENT RELATIONSHIP ON ADMISSION

- Recognize and take steps to reduce the patient's anxiety. Anxiety is a natural reaction to the unknown, but it can be reduced by therapeutic communication, teaching, and acceptance. Some common concerns that cause anxiety are: *Will I have pain? Who will take care of my family if I die? Will strangers be looking at my body? How much will this cost? What if I can't keep my job?*
- Remember that the medical or surgical condition for which the patient is being treated is only one part of the patient's life. Other concerns include family needs, financial status, and the future.
- Communicate with the patient as an individual so that he or she can maintain his or her own identity. Ask patients how you should address them—some people prefer Mr., Mrs., Miss, or Ms. [last name]; others would rather be called by their first name. Do not call all older adults "Grandma" or "Grandpa." Do not refer to Mr. Jones, admitted to room 2218 for treatment of a ruptured appendix, as "the appendix in 2218."
- Take time to learn who the patient being admitted is, including his or her cultural and religious background. Respect the patient's values and beliefs even though they may differ from yours.
- Encourage the patient's family to participate in and make decisions about all aspects of care.

---

that they understand the protection of their medical information. A copy is given to the patient and a copy is retained with the patient's medical record. This is a requirement of the Federal Health Insurance Portability and Accountability Act of 1996 (HIPAA). The goals of the **HIPAA privacy rule** are to assure that health information is protected while allowing the flow of health information needed to provide and promote high-quality healthcare and to protect the public's health and well being (U.S. Department of Health & Human Services, 2003). Health information cannot be used and shared without a person's written permission unless the law allows it. Every healthcare provider who electronically transmits health information in connection with certain transactions is included, for example, insurance claims, questions about Medicare or other insurance eligibility, and referrals. Individual health information that would identify a person and is protected includes:

- Name and demographic information (age, address, gender)
- Past, present, or future physical or mental health or condition
- Healthcare provided to the individual
- Past, present, or future payment for the healthcare provided

This law also means, as further examples, that healthcare providers may not provide information about a patient or his/her condition to anyone without specific permission, that healthcare providers (including students) may only read the records of patients for which they are providing care, and that there can be no identifying patient information on written records used for educational or research purposes.

Admission to an Ambulatory Care Facility

Ambulatory care facilities, described in Chapter 8, are those in which the patient receives healthcare services but does not remain overnight. An individual may receive care in many different kinds of ambulatory facilities, including physician offices, clinics, hospital outpatient services, emergency rooms, and same-day surgery centers. The goal of these facilities is to provide healthcare services to patients who are able to provide self-care at home. Individuals go to ambulatory settings for health promotion, health maintenance, or medical or surgical treatment.

In most office and clinic facilities, patients enter a reception area, where they are asked to complete a short health history (unless they have already done so during a previous visit) and sign a statement acknowledging the HIPAA privacy rule. They then go to an examination room where a physical assessment (often specific to the reason for the visit) is completed. Depending on their needs, patients may be given, for example, diagnostic tests, immunizations, prescriptions for medications, or may undergo minor surgery. All patients require teaching, which should include written instructions about care at home, health promotion activities, and how to contact someone for further questions. Referrals to community agencies, support groups, or other types of healthcare settings might also be necessary.

Admission to ambulatory or same-day surgery facilities is somewhat different. Screening tests, teaching, and admission procedures are usually completed before patients enter the setting. They arrive at the setting, have the procedure, and go home when recovery is satisfactory. If patients have outpatient or short-stay surgery in the hospital setting, the regular admission procedures are completed on arrival; in most instances, screening tests and teaching are done before the day of surgery. It is the nurse's responsibility to assess what has been done and tailor the care plan to the patient's needs.

Admission to the Hospital

A scheduled admission to the hospital usually begins in the admitting office. Admitting office staff obtain information about the patient and input that information on an admission sheet. The admission sheet, which includes the information listed in Box 9-2, becomes part of the patient's permanent record.

The identification number (often included as a barcode), as well as the patient's name, physician's name, and any other information required by the particular institution is printed on an identification wristband that is placed on the patient's wrist. This wristband is an important safety component during the patient's stay because it is one of two identifiers, required by The Joint Commission national safety standards (2008), used to identify accurately a patient during

---

Box 9-2	INFORMATION COLLECTED DURING ADMISSION TO A HOSPITAL

Full name
Address
Date of birth
Name of admitting physician
Gender
Marital status
Nearest relative
Occupation and employer
Financial status for healthcare payment
Religious preference
Date and time of admission
Identification number
Admitting diagnosis

---

activities such as medication administration, blood and fluid administration, diagnostic tests, and surgery. A wristband is worn by all patients.

During the initial interview, the admitting staff provides other information about legal and ethical components of care. The patient is asked to sign forms that give consent to treatment and allow the hospital to contact healthcare insurance companies or public agencies (e.g., Medicare) for reimbursement of services. Patients are asked if they have established advance directives, such as a living will or durable power of attorney, to indicate their treatment preferences about prolonging life. If they have established advance directives, a copy becomes a part of their hospital record. If they have not, the purpose is explained and they are given a form to complete if they wish to do so. (Chapter 43 discusses advance directives and provides a sample form.) Providers must give patients a clear written explanation of how health information will be used and disclosed and a privacy statement is signed. Patients may also be asked to provide the names of family or friends to whom health status information may be given. Lastly, almost all hospitals give some form of a Patient Care Partnership (formerly titled a Patient Bill of Rights) to the patient to inform them about what to expect while in the hospital. This document, printed in several languages (e.g., English, Arabic, Spanish, Vietnamese, Chinese, Russian), includes rights to high-quality hospital care, a clean and safe environment, involvement in care, protection of privacy, help when leaving the hospital, and help with insurance claims (American Hospital Association, 2008).

After the necessary forms have been completed in the admitting office, a nurse who works in that area might complete the admission health history and physical assessment, or patients may also be taken to an assigned room for these admission procedures. Laboratory studies and x-rays, as well as the admitting office procedures, are usually completed on an outpatient basis before the day of admission. If

Guidelines for Nursing Care • 9-1

PREPARING THE ROOM FOR PATIENT ADMISSION

- Position the bed. For ambulatory patients, the bed should be in its lowest position. Place the bed in its highest position if the patient will arrive on a stretcher. Ensure that the furniture in the room is arranged to allow easy access to the bed.

- Open the bed by folding back the top bed linens (see figure).

- Assemble routine equipment and supplies. A hospital admission pack (which contains such items as a bath basin, water pitcher, drinking glass, tissues, soap, and lotion) is placed in the room. A hospital gown or pajamas should be in the room, although the patient may choose to wear his or her own pajamas or gown. Equipment for taking vital signs (i.e., stethoscope, sphygmomanometer, thermometer) and height and weight should be in the room or readily available. If laboratory work has not been done previously, a container for a clean urine specimen should be available.

- Assemble special equipment and supplies. The patient may require oxygen therapy, cardiac monitoring, or suction equipment. The nurse ensures that the equipment is functioning properly and is ready for the patient's use on arrival.

- Adjust the physical environment of the room. This may include turning on lights and setting the room temperature.

An "open" bed, ready for the patient's arrival.

---

the patient has an unscheduled admission or is going to have only a limited stay (e.g., those who are admitted the morning of a diagnostic examination and then go home later in the day), admission procedures and assessments may be completed on the unit.

Preparing the Room for Admission

The admitting office notifies the unit to which the patient is to be admitted before the patient arrives so the room can be prepared. Although the nurse might delegate most of the activities in preparing the room for an admission, it is a nursing responsibility to ensure that other personnel do them. Guidelines for Nursing Care 9-1 outlines the activities carried out in anticipation of the patient's arrival.

Admitting the Patient to the Unit

Although other members of the healthcare team may assist in the admitting procedure, the nurse is responsible for ensuring the comfort and well-being of the patient upon arrival in the unit. The patient's **chart** (a computerized or paper medical record containing information such as medical orders, assessments and care; nursing documentation of plan of care, assessments and interventions; and diagnostic/surgery results), and a **Kardex** card (a system used to provide patient information in a brief format) is completed. The nurse completes the admission assessment and documents the information on the admission database, illustrated in Figure 9-1. The sample form in Figure 9-2 illustrates typical information that is collected and documented. The information on the form is used to develop the nursing care plan for

the patient and also is used as a database for discharge planning and home care. In addition, an inventory of personal belongings and valuables is completed to ensure these are returned to the patient on discharge or transferred with the patient if he or she moves to another unit or facility. In some hospitals, a medication reconciliation form is completed on admission. This form is added to the chart; the form is checked and filled out again with each transfer and on discharge to ensure all medications have been correctly ordered or discontinued, as the patient moves through the system.

Nurses should welcome the patient to the unit in the same courteous manner that would be used in welcoming a guest

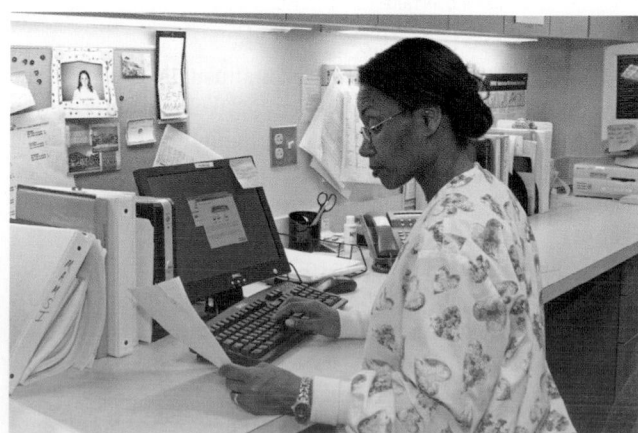

FIGURE 9-1. Documenting information in the admission database.

Example of An Admission Database

NURSING ADMISSION DATA

CURRENT MEDICATIONS, SUPPLEMENTS, NON-PRESCRIPTION DRUGS:

NAME	DOSE/FREQUENCY	LAST DOSE
Aspirin	2 prn	1 month
Maalox	prn	this Am

☐ MEDICATION TO PHARMACY ☐ MEDICATION SENT HOME

ALLERGEN: (DRUGS, FOOD, TAPES, DYES, OTHERS)

ALLERGEN	SYMPTOMS
Penicillin	rash

DATE __1-16-12__ TIME __0900__

ADMISSION   ☐ OBSERVATION

☒ AMBULATORY ☐ WHEELCHAIR ☐ STRETCHER
☐ CORRECT INDENTIFICATION BAND
ADMITTED FROM: ☒ HOME ☐ NURSING FACILITY
        ☐ EMERGENCY ROOM ☐ OTHER_____
INFORMATION GIVEN BY: ☐ FAMILY MEMBER ☐ FRIEND ☒ PATIENT
    ☐ UNABLE TO TAKE HISTORY - PATIENT UNRESPONSIVE/CONFUSED
    NOT ACCOMPANIED BY FAMILY OR FRIEND
    ☐ PREVIOUS MEDICAL RECORD

ORIENTATION TO ROOM
☒ VISITING HOURS ☒ CALL LIGHT IN REACH: ☒ EXPLAINED
☒ OPERATION OF BED AND SIDE RAILS ☒ USE OF PHONE
☒ VALUABLES SENT HOME ☐ IN SAFE ☐ IN POSSESSION
    SPECIFY _____
☒ PATIENT HANDBOOK   ☒ INTRODUCED TO ROOMMATE

MEDICAL HISTORY
ADMITTED MEDICAL DIAGNOSIS __Peptic Ulcer__

PAST HOSPITALIZATIONS AND/OR ILLNESS: (MEDICAL, SURGICAL, EMOTIONAL PROBLEMS) __1999 - Appendectomy__

WHAT IS REASON FOR ADMISSION? (PATIENT'S OWN WORDS)
"My doctor says I have An ulcer"

LEGAL GUARDIAN (NAME/PHONE)_____
CONTACT PERSON (NAME/PHONE) Mrs. Solle, 335-4001
PHYSICIAN NOTIFIED ✓   TIME 0830
PRIMARY CARE PHYSICIAN Dr. Wills

*OBJECTIVE DATA:
1. CLINICAL DATA
AGE __36__ HEIGHT __5'6"__
WEIGHT __122__ ☒ BEDSCALE ☐ STANDING APPROXIMATE
TEMP: __98.4__ PULSE: __118__ RESPIRATIONS __16__
BLOOD PRESSURE (RIGHT ARM) __120/68__ (LEFT ARM) __122/70__
    ☒ SITTING ☐ LYING
N.T./N.A. INITIALS __O.B.__

2. NUTRITIONAL/METABOLIC PATTERN
ORAL MUCOSA: ☒ HEALTHY COLOR_____
    ☐ MOIST ☐ DRY ☐ LESIONS_____
TEETH: ☒ NO PROBLEM CONDITION:_____
    ☐ DENTURES ☐ UPPER ☐ LOWER ☐ PARTIAL
    ☐ MISSING TEETH ☐ CAPS/CROWNS
☒ WELL NOURISHED ☐ OBESE ☐ EMACIATED
SKIN: ☒ TURGOR NORMAL ☐ OTHER_____
    ☒ INTACT ☐ OTHER_____
    TEMP __Warm__ COLOR __brown__ ☐ DIAPHORESIS
☐ TUBES _____

3. RESPIRATION/CIRCULATION PATTERN
BREATH SOUNDS __Clear__
LIP COLOR __pink__   ☐ USE OF ACCESSORY MUSCLES
COUGH: ☐ NON-PRODUCTIVE ☐ PRODUCTIVE SPUTUM COLOR_____
APICAL RATE __120__ RHYTHM: ☒ REGULAR ☐ IRREGULAR
ABNORMAL HEART SOUNDS NOTED __No__
NECK VEIN DISTENTION AT 45 DEGREES: ☐ PRESENT ☒ ABSENT
☐ EDEMA: LOCATION_____
RIGHT DORSALIS PEDAL PULSE: ☒ STRONG ☐ WEAK ☐ ABSENT
LEFT DORSALIS PEDAL PULSE: ☒ STRONG ☐ WEAK ☐ ABSENT
CALF TENDERNESS ☒ NO ☐ YES ☐ N/A
EXTREMITIES COLOR __brown__
    TEMP __Warm__

4. ELIMINATION PATTERN
ABDOMEN: ☒ SOFT   ☐ FIRM
    ☐ NON-TENDER ☐ TENDER
    ☐ NON-DISTENDED ☐ DISTENDED _____ Girth
☐ OSTOMIES/TUBES: TYPE_____
☐ NORMAL BOWEL SOUNDS ☐ HYPOACTIVE ☒ HYPERACTIVE ☐ ABSENT

*SUBJECTIVE DATA:
1. HEALTH PERCEPTIONS/HEALTH MANAGEMENT PATTERN
GENERAL HEALTH __Excellent__
USE OF: ☐ TOBACCO: HOW MUCH/HOW LONG? __No__
    ☐ ALCOHOL: HOW MUCH/HOW LONG? __No__
    ☐ OTHER DRUGS TYPE(s) __None__

2. NUTRITIONAL/METABOLIC PATTERN
DIET/RESTRICTIONS/SUPPLEMENTS: __Regular diet__

☐ INSTRUCTED IN DIET PREVIOUSLY BY:_____
TIME OF LAST P.O. INTAKE: __0700__
FLUID INTAKE (AMOUNT/DAY) __5-6 glasses__
WEIGHT: ☐ NO PROBLEMS
☐ GAIN_____ ☒ LOSS/HOW MUCH/HOW LONG __10 lbs / 1 month__
☒ SKIN NORMAL ☐ HEALING PROBLEMS
    ☐ COLOR CHANGE OF SKIN
    ☐ SKIN LESIONS/RASH_____

3. RESPIRATION/CIRCULATION PATTERN
HISTORY OF: ☐ COUGH ☐ SPUTUM
☐ SHORTNESS OF BREATH ☐ WITHOUT EXERCISE ☐ WITH EXERCISE

HISTORY OF: ☐ PACEMAKER ☐ RATE_____
    ☐ BLOOD CLOTS ☐ CHEST PAIN ☐ PEDAL EDEMA

☒ CHECK BOX IF DATA IS PERTINENT
*SEE NURSES NOTES FOR FURTHER NOTATIONS OR ANY CHANGES.

(Courtesy of Southeast Missouri Hospital, Cape Girardeau, Missouri.)

FIGURE 9-2. Example of an admission database. *(continued)*

Example of An Admission Database (continued)

SUBJECTIVE DATA (Cont'd) LBM_____

4.   ELIMINATION PATTERN

BOWEL HABITS: STOOLS/DAY 2   COLOR dk. brown ☒ SOFT/FORMED
           ☐ CONSTIPATION: ☐ LAXATIVE ☐ ENEMA
           ☐ DIARRHEA   ☐ INCONTINENCE

BLADDER HABITS: URINATES/DAY 5-6 ☒ NO PROBLEM ☐ SELF-CATH
           ☐ URGENCY ☐ FREQUENCY ☐ NOCTURIA
           ☐ DYSURIA ☐ HEMATURIA ☐ INCONTINENCE

**5.   SEXUALITY/REPRODUCTIVE PATTERN
    (IF APPROPRIATE)**

LAST MENSTRUAL PERIOD 1-10-12   MENSTRUAL PROBLEMS ☐ YES ☒ NO

BIRTH CONTROL MEASURES None ____ # PREGNANCIES 2

COMPLICATIONS OF PREGNANCIES None

HX VENEREAL DISEASE No

SEXUAL CONCERNS: None

6.   ACTIVITY/EXERCISE PATTERN

ENERGY LEVEL: ☐ TIRES EASILY ☐ AVERAGE ☒ HIGH/ENERGY

ABLE TO: ☒ FEED SELF ☒ BATHE SELF
        ☐ BATHE/FEED SELF WITH ASSISTANCE
        ☒ AMBULATE ☒ CLIMB STAIRS !
        ☒ CAN DO HOUSEHOLD CHORES

AIDS: ☐ CANE ☐ WALKER ☐ WHEELCHAIR ☐ OTHER ____

GAIT: ☐ STEADY ☐ UNSTEADY ☐ LIMP ☐ UNABLE TO WALK

PROTHESIS ____

7.   SLEEP/REST PATTERN

DO YOU FEEL RESTED AFTER SLEEP? ☒ YES ☐ NO ☐ NO PROBLEM

SLEEP PROBLEMS: ☐ TROUBLE FALLING ASLEEP ☐ EARLY AM WAKING
           ☐ OTHER ____

8.   COGNITIVE/PERCEPTUAL PATTERN

HEARING: ☒ NORMAL ☐ IMPAIRED ☐ LEFT EAR ☐ RIGHT EAR ☐ AID

VISION: ☐ NORMAL ☐ IMPAIRED ☒ GLASSES ☐ PROTHESIS
      ☐ FARSIGHTED ☐ NEARSIGHTED

OTHER PROBLEMS ____

COMMUNICATION: LANGUAGE SPOKEN English

UNDERSTANDS ____ UNABLE TO: ☐ READ ☐ WRITE

ABLE TO: ☒ READ ☒ WRITE ☐ LIP READ

COGNITION: ☒ NO PROBLEMS ☐ RECENT MEMORY CHANGE
         ☐ DIFFICULTY LEARNING

DISCOMFORT/PAIN: ☐ NO ☒ YES DESCRIBE Epigastric

HOW DO YOU MANAGE YOUR PAIN? Bland food, Maalox

9.   COPING/STRESS TOLERANCE PATTERN

SPECIAL CONCERNS REGARDING HOSPITALIZATION? ☐ NO ☒ YES
Care of Children

10.   SELF-PERCEPTION/SELF-CONCEPT PATTERN

CONCERNS ABOUT HOW YOUR ILLNESS AFFECTS YOU? ☐ NO ☒ YES
Concerned about health

11.   ROLE/RELATIONSHIP PATTERN

MARITAL STATUS: ☐ MARRIED ☐ SINGLE ☐ WIDOWED ☒ DIVORCED

CHILDREN (#) 2 ____ OTHER DEPENDENT(S) 0

OCCUPATION Secretary

RESIDENCY (TYPE) Apartment

WHO LIVES AT HOME WITH YOU? Children

SUPPORT SYSTEM (CLOSE FRIEND/FAMILY MEMBER) Yes

FAMILY CONCERNS ABOUT HOSPITALIZATION? Yes

12.   VALUE/BELIEF PATTERN

RELIGIOUS AFFILIATION Baptist

RELIGIOUS RESTRICTIONS 0

☐ WOULD LIKE CHAPLAIN TO VISIT (IF YES, NOTIFY CHAPLAIN)

☒ WOULD LIKE FAMILY MINISTER TO VISIT

NAME Mr. Ame ____ PHONE 314-6000

RELIGIOUS ACTIVITIES IMPORTANT TO YOU Bible

SUBJECTIVE DATA SIGNATURE P. LeMne RN ____ (Nurse)

6.   ACTIVITY/EXERCISE PATTERN

ROM: ☒ FULL ☐ OTHER ____

BALANCE AND GAIT: ☒ STEADY ☐ UNSTEADY ☐ LIMP ____

HAND GRASPS: ☒ EQUAL ☒ STRONG
           ☐ WEAKNESS/PARALYSIS ☐ RIGHT ☐ LEFT

LEG MUSCLES: ☒ EQUAL ☒ STRONG
           WEAKNESS/PARALYSIS ☐ RIGHT ☐ LEFT

8.   COGNITIVE/PERCEPTUAL PATTERN

LEVEL OF CONSCIOUSNESS: ☒ ALERT ☒ RESPONDS TO PAIN

ORIENTED TO: ☒ TIME ☒ PLACE ☒ PERSON

MOOD: ☒ CALM ☐ SAD ☐ ANGRY
        ☐ WITHDRAWN ☐ OTHER ____

PUPILS: ☒ EQUAL ☒ REACTIVE ☐ OTHER ____

COGNITION: ☒ ABLE TO FOLLOW SIMPLE COMMANDS
         ☒ RESPONDS APPROPRIATELY TO QUESTIONS
         ☐ UNABLE TO FOLLOW COMMANDS
         ☐ OTHER ____

HEARING: ☒ NORMAL ☐ OTHER ____

VISION: ☒ NORMAL ☐ OTHER ____

MANIFESTATIONS OF PAIN ____

10.   SELF-PERCEPTION/SELF-CONCEPT PATTERN

EYE CONTACT: ☒ APPROPRIATE ☐ DOWNCAST ☐ STARING

BODY POSTURE: ☒ RELAXED ☐ STOOPED ☐ RIGID

BEHAVIOR: ____ 1 ____ ② ____ 3 ____ 4 ____ 5 ____ (CIRCLE)
         RELAXED ____ NERVOUS

☐ OTHER ____

11.   ROLE/RELATIONSHIP PATTERN

BEHAVIOR: ① ____ 2 ____ 3 ____ 4 ____ 5 ____ (CIRCLE)
     PASSIVE ____ ASSERTIVE ____ AGGRESSIVE

INTERACTION WITH FAMILY/SIGNIFICANT OTHER: ☐ N/A

☒ RELAXED ☐ TENSE ☐ ANGRY ☐ WITHDRAWN ☐ OTHER ____

COMMENTS: ____

Worried about effect of
illness and possible surgery
on care of children, job,
and income. Has strong
support of family.

SIGNATURE P. LeMne, RN ____ (Nurse)

FIGURE 9-2. *(Continued)*

into one's own home. In most instances, the patient is accompanied by family members who may either remain with the patient to provide support and information or who may be asked to wait in the waiting room during the admission procedure. The nurse needs to assess the needs of the patient and family, and they should mutually agree about whether family should be present during admission.

TRANSFERRING WITHIN AND BETWEEN HEALTHCARE SETTINGS

It is common for some type of move to be made within settings as well as between settings. Examples of patient transfers within and between settings include the following:

- Within the hospital, such as from the emergency room to a hospital room, from an intensive care unit (ICU) to a hospital room (and vice versa), from one unit to another, or from one room to another room on the same unit.
- To and from acute care settings and long-term settings.
- From acute care settings to their homes.
- From ambulatory care settings to acute care settings.

When a transfer occurs, the patient must readjust to new surroundings, new roommates, new routines, and new people providing care. If the transfer is to a higher level of care, as in a move to the ICU, the patient and family experience unfamiliar sights and sounds. A transfer to a long-term facility may not be desired by the patient or family but may be necessary if family members cannot provide care at home or if no other support people are available. All of these factors cause stress and anxiety.

> *Recall Laura Degas, the woman who is not sure if she will be able to care for her sister at home. If it is determined that Ms. Degas cannot care for her sister at home, she may decide to have her sister transferred to a long-term care facility. In this case, the nurse must provide Ms. Degas with support and guidance to ease the transition and help minimize the stress and anxiety of this move.* ■

The nurse may not be responsible for the actual physical move but is responsible for ensuring that the comfort, safety, and teaching needs of the patient and family are met. Although documentation and procedures differ depending on the institution and type of transfer, patient needs are always a priority in ensuring a smooth transition and continuity of care.

Transfer Within the Hospital

When a patient is transferred within the hospital, personal belongings must be moved to the new room. Every effort must be made to ensure that belongings are not misplaced or lost. The patient's chart and Kardex card are moved to the new unit. Other hospital departments (e.g., dietary, pharmacy, physical therapy) must be notified of the transfer. If the patient is moved to the ICU, family members may need to take personal belongings home. It is helpful to have completed a personal belongings list and a valuables inventory on admission if family members are not available to take personal belongings.

When a patient is transferred to another unit, the nurse in the original area gives a verbal report about the patient to the nurse in the new area. The report should include the patient's name, age, physicians, admitting diagnosis, surgical procedure (if applicable), current condition and manifestations, allergies, medications and treatments, laboratory data, and any special equipment that will be needed to provide care. Nursing care priorities are identified, and the existence of advance directives is noted. Accurate, concise, and complete verbal communication is essential.

Transfer to a Long-Term Care Facility

When a patient is transferred from the hospital to a long-term care facility, he or she is discharged from the hospital setting, but a copy of the chart may be sent to the long-term care facility (depending on the physician's preference and the agency's protocol). The original chart, which is a legal document, remains at the hospital. All of the patient's belongings are carefully packed and sent to the facility with the patient. Prescriptions and appointment cards for return visits to the physician's office may also be sent with the patient.

In most instances, a detailed assessment and care plan is sent from the hospital to the long-term care facility. In addition, the nurse at the hospital often provides a verbal report to the nurse at the long-term care facility.

> *Remember Jeff Hart, the 9-year-old boy transferred from the state facility to the hospital due to respiratory complications. Once the child's problems have been resolved, the nurse would prepare Jeff to be transferred back to the state facility. Information about the events of the hospitalization would be documented and reported. In addition, communication between healthcare team members at the hospital and those at the state facility is essential to ensure continuity of care for Jeff.* ■

DISCHARGE FROM A HEALTHCARE SETTING

Patients are discharged from a healthcare facility when the expected outcomes of care are met and the patient or caregiver has the necessary knowledge and skills to provide care. In meeting the needs of the patient being discharged from a healthcare setting, nurses consider that the person may be expecting a change from a dependent role to a more independent (self-care) role. Although discharge is almost always a welcome event, it also can be stressful.

Discharge Planning

The purpose of planning for continuity of care, which is more commonly referred to in hospital-based settings as **discharge planning,** is to ensure that patient and family needs are consistently met as the patient moves from the acute care setting to care at home. Essential components of discharge planning include assessing the strengths and limitations of the patient, the family or support person, and the environment; implementing and coordinating the plan of care; considering individual, family, and community resources; and evaluating the effectiveness of care.

Planning for discharge actually begins on admission, when information about the patient is collected and documented. The key to successful discharge planning is an exchange of information among the patient, the caregivers, and those responsible for care while the patient is in the acute care setting and after the patient returns home. This coordination of care is usually the nurse's responsibility.

With earlier hospital discharges, patients often are still acutely ill when they go home, and many require complicated treatment and care by family members. It is no longer unusual for family members to change sterile dressings, administer tube feedings, monitor intravenous medications, manage high-technology equipment, give complete physical care, and prepare special diets. If they are unprepared or unable to carry out these interventions correctly, the patient may have an exacerbation of the illness or experience complications that could require readmission or additional treatment. The nurse must ensure that family members are taught the necessary knowledge and skills (Fig. 9-3) and that referrals are made to agencies such as home healthcare or social services to provide support and assistance during the recovery period. (Home care is discussed in Chapter 10.)

Initiating the process involves identifying which patients will need which level of discharge planning. All patients need discharge planning in general, but certain patients have more comprehensive needs for specific services. The nurse who conducts the initial nursing assessment is in the best position to determine these special needs.

FIGURE 9-3. Patients or caregivers must be taught special skills, such as medication administration, diet planning, or feeding, so that they can care for themselves when nursing services are no longer provided. *(Photo by Rick Brady.)*

> ➤ *Recall Jennifer Lenner, the young woman with a seizure disorder at risk for postoperative complications. Information about Jennifer's underlying neurologic problem would have been obtained when Jennifer was admitted. From that information, the nurse would develop a discharge plan that addresses the patient's specific postoperative risks. Since Jennifer lives with her parents, a referral for home care may or may not be appropriate, depending on further assessment of Jennifer's parents and the home situation.* ■

Patients who meet any of the following criteria need a formal discharge plan and referral to another agency:

- Lack of knowledge of the treatment plan
- Social isolation
- Recently diagnosed chronic disease
- Major surgery
- Prolonged recuperation from major surgery or illness
- Emotional or mental instability
- Complex home care regimen
- Financial difficulties
- Lack of available or appropriate referral sources
- Terminal illness

Guidelines for Discharge Planning

For a patient hospitalized with a serious illness or injury, discharge planning may be done over time; for a patient treated in an ambulatory facility, it may be completed relatively quickly. A nursing case manager or discharge planner is often responsible for discharge planning for patients in acute care settings and may follow a plan of care or a critical path established for the patient. No matter what organizing plan is used, the nurse assesses the patient's needs and identifies problems, develops goals with the patient, carries out teaching, and makes referrals. An example of discharge planning is provided in Box 9-3.

ASSESSING AND IDENTIFYING HEALTHCARE NEEDS

The first step in discharge planning involves collecting and organizing data about the patient. When assessing the patient for discharge, the nurse includes the family, if possible, because both the patient and family must be actively involved if the transition from the healthcare setting to home is to be effective. Factors to assess in discharge planning are listed in the accompanying Focused Assessment Guide 9-1. Other assessment formats may be used, depending on institutional procedures, to evaluate the patient's ability to carry out activities of daily living (e.g., bathing, dressing, toileting, transferring, continence, feeding) and instrumental activities of daily living (using the telephone, shopping, preparing food, doing housekeeping and laundry, taking medications, accessing transportation). The medical record and physician orders must also be consulted for the exact medication and treatment plan before the nursing care plan is developed.

Box 9-3   A DISCHARGE PLANNING EXAMPLE

Scenario

Mr. Smith is a 55-year-old married man, admitted to the hospital with a diagnosis of stroke. He now has left-side weakness and difficulty communicating verbally. He has had a history of high blood pressure for 10 years. If his blood pressure remains stable, Mr. Smith is to be discharged from the hospital in 3 days. He will be going home with four new medications and an indwelling urinary catheter. A low-sodium diet is prescribed.

After reviewing the medical record, the nurse interviews Mr. and Mrs. Smith. The assessment reveals that Mr. Smith has a limited ability to transfer from bed to chair. Both Mr. and Mrs. Smith are fearful of discharge. Mr. Smith believes he will be able to return to work as an accountant in 3 weeks and hates the thought of being an invalid at his age, but Mrs. Smith thinks he will never work again. They have never faced a life-threatening or disabling illness in the past. They have no strong cultural preferences for diet. They have two adult children who live out of state with their own families. Mrs. Smith has a younger sister who lives nearby. The Smiths are both college educated. They live in a suburban area in a two-story home with narrow stairs leading to the second floor's two baths and three bedrooms. They have adequate plumbing. Their doctor's office is about 1 mile away, and shopping is nearby.

Mrs. Smith is worried about managing care of the catheter and moving Mr. Smith in and out of bed. She needs instruction in the new medications and diet regimen. She is terrified that she may be unable to handle an emergency in the middle of the night. Financially, this two-income family has abruptly become a one-income family. Mr. Smith is not 65 years old and thus is not yet eligible for Medicare, although he does have disability insurance that will cover a portion of his salary.

Planning

How would the nurse coordinate this discharge plan? The physician must be consulted for diet, medication, other treatments, and home health orders. The dietitian needs to counsel the Smiths on a low-sodium diet and on creative ways to prepare low-salt meals. Physical therapy has already been initiated at the hospital and will continue through home healthcare. An occupational therapist will visit to provide teaching about strengthening exercises and assistive devices, such as a walker. The social worker has been called for financial assessment to determine exactly what services the Smiths can expect to have reimbursed by their insurance plan and how they will manage their out-of-pocket expenses.

The nurse discusses Mr. and Mrs. Smith's healthcare needs with the home health agency. A teaching plan for medications and care of the urinary catheter is implemented. Mrs. Smith demonstrates how to care for the catheter. The physical therapist teaches Mrs. Smith how to transfer Mr. Smith into and out of the bed and assures her that he will help her practice at home. Written information about high blood pressure, stroke, low-sodium diet, and prescribed medications is given to the Smiths, along with the telephone number of a local support group for people who have had strokes. Although Mrs. Smith still verbalizes concern about providing care at home, she says she feels more in control now. Mr. Smith is beginning to realize that recovery may take longer than he anticipated. At the time of discharge, the nurse tells the Smiths that someone from the hospital will call them the next day and that the home health nurse will visit them that afternoon.

Nursing diagnoses, developed from the discharge planning assessment, identify the needs of both the patient and the family. Examples of nursing diagnoses for a patient being discharged are listed in the Examples of NANDA Nursing Diagnoses box. It is important to determine whether problems are present now or are potential problems. For example, a patient with chronic respiratory problems may have assistance from a member of the family who has come to stay for 1 month, but after that, the patient will be alone at home. In this case, the problem is not an actual problem now but could become one unless planning is done to meet needs when there is no longer a family caregiver.

SETTING GOALS WITH THE PATIENT

The expected goals of the discharge plan are set mutually and must be realistic if they are to be met. If the patient is involved in establishing goals, it is more likely that the expected outcomes of the plan of care will be met. The patient may fail to follow the plan if the goals are not mutually agreed on or are not based on a complete assessment of the patient's needs. For example, the nurse or another healthcare provider may do a thorough job of teaching a patient about a special diet, but the patient may not actually follow the diet after discharge because he may not be able to afford the special food, he may not be able to get to the grocery store, or he may not have a refrigerator at home for food storage.

TEACHING

Important teaching topics about self-care at home must be covered before discharge. These topics include medications, procedures and treatments, diet, referrals, and health status.

The patient needs to understand the drug name, dosage, purpose, effects, times to be taken, and possible side effects. Information about medications should be given both verbally and in writing. Copies of the medication administration record are often given to the patient to use as a pattern for times and amounts of medications administered in the hospital. Patients often find it helpful when the nurse draws a clock face and writes the names of the medications in the correct time slots.

All steps of a procedure (e.g., dressing changes) should be demonstrated, practiced, and provided in writing. The patient or caregiver should then perform the procedure or treatment in the presence of the nurse to demonstrate his or her understanding and ability to carry out the procedure. The caregiver should know the purpose of what is being done and how to get supplies.

Teaching should clearly describe the purpose of the diet and its expected outcomes. Patients find examples of written diet plans and meals helpful. If the patient has been in the hospital, it is helpful to save menu or meal forms to use as a reference at home.

FOCUSED ASSESSMENT GUIDE • 9-1

DISCHARGE PLANNING

Factors to Assess	Questions and Approaches
Health data	Establish a database that includes age, gender, height and weight, medical diagnoses, past medical history, current health problems, surgery, and functional limitations (e.g., impaired sight or hearing, amputation, use of wheelchair or walker).
Personal data	Ask the patient: *"What language do you prefer to use?"* *"How do you feel about being discharged?"* *"What are your expectations for recovery?"* *"What do you do to help you cope with stress? Are these things helpful?"*
Caregivers	Establish the caregiver's age, gender, relationship to the patient, past experiences with this illness or treatment, values and beliefs, and cultural practices that might affect prescribed care. Ask the caregiver: *"Do you live with the patient?"* *"What are your expectations about providing care at home?"* *"What are your fears about providing care at home?"*
Environment	Assess the home, noting if there will be barriers to using prescribed assistive devices (e.g., wheelchairs or walkers), if the patient will be able to use bathroom facilities safely, and if hot water, heat, and room for supplies are available. Assess the community, noting location (such as rural or urban), whether healthcare is available and accessible, whether transportation is available, and any known environmental hazards.
Financial and support resources	Discuss expenses of prescribed care, including dressing supplies, medications, equipment, and special foods. Discuss available resources, including Medicare and Medicaid, parish nursing, and meal services to the home. Discuss, especially if the patient will be living alone, support services and resources and how they can be accessed. Include friends, church groups, and support groups specific to the patient's age and healthcare needs.

Examples of NANDA Nursing Diagnoses
Discharge from a Healthcare Setting

Nursing Diagnoses	Related Factors
Anxiety	Concern about uncertain future following radiation treatment for breast cancer
Risk for Caregiver Role Strain	Care of 75-year-old wife with dementia from Alzheimer's disease
Readiness for Enhanced Coping	Attendance at support group meetings and verbally defining stressors as manageable
Delayed Surgical Recovery	Infection of large abdominal wound and needed help to complete self-care
Effective Enhanced Therapeutic Regimen Management	Demonstrates accurate dressing change and verbalizes confidence in managing recovery and preventing complications

FIGURE 9-4. Written instructions for continuing self-care at home should be given to the patient. In addition, the nurse reviews the instructions with the patient to ensure that the patient understands.

Appointments for the first visit to a physician or agency are often made before discharge. Whether or not this is done, the patient and family members should know how to contact the providers of follow-up care and should know whom to call if they have questions or problems. This referral information takes into account the patient's economic situation, access to transportation, support systems, and home environment.

All aspects of the illness or effects of treatment should be clearly described, both verbally and in written materials. Many forms of written information are available to give to patients, ranging from printed literature (e.g., from the American Heart Association) to teaching materials developed by the healthcare facility. Written instructions are given to the patient (Fig. 9-4). The patient should be able to talk about the anticipated physical and emotional effects of the illness and also describe what will be done to achieve the highest level of health possible. All teaching should be documented in the patient's record and the discharge summary. The patient's or family member's demonstrations of care procedures must be satisfactory, and the patient and caregiver must have exposure to and practice with the equipment they will be using at home.

> *Think back to Jennifer Lenner, the young woman who is to be discharged after surgery. The nurse would include teaching about any antiseizure medications ordered, wound care or dressing changes needed secondary to the surgery, diet and activity level allowed and restricted, and follow-up with the surgeon and her regular physician.* ∎

MEETING ELIGIBILITY REQUIREMENTS FOR HOME HEALTHCARE

The physician must write an order for all home care services, and the patient must meet eligibility criteria for reimbursement for home healthcare visits. As much information as possible about the patient should be given to the home health agency. Such information includes the kind of surgery or injury, medications, the patient's physical and mental status, significant social factors (e.g., frail caregiver with health problems, or no caregiver), and the family's expected needs. Chapter 10 discusses home care in detail.

Evaluating Discharge Planning Effectiveness

Evaluating the discharge plan is crucial to ensure that the discharge planning works. Planning and referrals must be scrutinized to ensure the quality and appropriateness of services. Evaluation is ongoing, and care plans may need to be changed. A few weeks after the patient goes home, further evaluation of the discharge process is usually conducted by a telephone call, a questionnaire, or a home visit.

Leaving the Hospital Against Medical Advice

A patient sometimes decides to leave the hospital against medical advice (AMA). Although the patient is legally free to do so, this choice carries a risk for increased illness or complications. A patient who decides to leave AMA must sign a form that releases the physician and healthcare institution from any legal responsibility for his or her health status. The patient is informed of any possible risk before signing the form. The patient's signature must be witnessed, and the form becomes part of the patient's record.

● Developing Critical Thinking Skills

1. Interview a classmate or family member who has been admitted to a hospital. What were his or her concerns on admission? How did those concerns differ from those experienced on discharge?

2. Compare and contrast the needs of the following patients and their families:
   - A 2-year-old who is admitted to an ambulatory surgery center for minor surgery
   - A 34-year-old woman who is discharged home after treatment for a fractured arm in the emergency room
   - A 50-year-old woman who is returning to a clinic to learn the results of her mammogram
   - A 78-year-old man who is being transferred from the hospital to a nursing home

● Practicing for NCLEX

1. A nurse is the discharge planner at a large metropolitan hospital. What would the nurse do to ensure continuity of care as patients move from acute care to home care?
   a. Perform an admission health assessment
   b. Participate in the transfer of patients to the ICU
   c. Make referrals to appropriate agencies
   d. Maintain records of patient satisfaction with services

2. Which of the following phrases best describes the philosophy of community-based care?
   a. It considers the healthcare needs of the community as a whole.
   b. It centers on individuals and families with acute and chronic illness needs.
   c. It has a population-based focus, with an emphasis on illness prevention.
   d. It provides direction for the roles of the nurse in the acute care setting.

3. When admitting a patient to the hospital, the nurse may delegate some activities to other members of the healthcare team. Which activity would be appropriate to delegate?
   a. Collecting information for a health history
   b. Performing a physical assessment
   c. Contacting the physician for medical orders
   d. Preparing the bed and collecting needed supplies

4. Based on the Health Insurance Portability and Accountability Act (HIPAA), a patient admitted to a healthcare facility must be provided with a written explanation of:
   a. The names and addresses of responsible providers
   b. A Patient's Bill of Rights
   c. How health information will be used and disclosed
   d. How often family members or friends may visit or call

5. A patient is being transferred from the ICU to a regular hospital room. What must the ICU nurse be prepared to do as part of this transfer?
   a. Provide a verbal report to the nurse on the new unit
   b. Provide a detailed written report to the unit secretary
   c. Delegate the responsibility for providing information
   d. Make a copy of the patient's medical record

6. At what point during a hospital stay should discharge planning be initiated?
   a. After surgery and successful recovery
   b. After the patient is less anxious
   c. Immediately before discharge
   d. On admission to the acute care setting

7. Which of the following statements or questions would be appropriate in establishing a discharge plan for a patient who has had major abdominal surgery?
   a. "I'll bet you will be so glad to be home in your own bed."
   b. "What are your expectations for recovery from your surgery?"
   c. "Be sure and take your pain medications and change your dressing."
   d. "You will just be fine! Please stop worrying."

8. A patient who decides to leave the hospital against medical advice (AMA) must sign a form. What is the purpose of this form?
   a. To indicate the patient's wishes
   b. To use in the event of readmission
   c. To release the physician and hospital from legal responsibility for the patient's health status
   d. To ethically illustrate that the patient has control of his or her own care and treatment

9. What is the primary purpose of the identification bracelet worn by hospitalized patients?
   a. Safety
   b. Communication
   c. Advocacy
   d. Legality

10. The Patient Care Partnership form, given to patients on admission to the hospital, includes several specific rights during hospitalization. Which of the following is included in this form?
    a. The right to wear one's own bed clothing
    b. The right to use a personal cell phone
    c. The right to have help when leaving the hospital
    d. The right to take medications brought from home

● Answers With Rationale

1. *c.* Making appropriate referrals for patients as they move from acute care to home care is an essential component of discharge planning for continuity of care.

2. *b.* Community-based care centers on individuals and families with acute and chronic healthcare needs.

3. *d.* The nurse may delegate preparation of the bed and collection of needed supplies to unlicensed personnel but would perform the other activities listed.

4. *c.* HIPAA ensures privacy of information use and disclosure.

5. *a.* The ICU nurse gives a verbal report about the patient's condition and nursing care needs to the nurse on the new unit. This information is not given to a unit secretary, nor is it delegated to others. The medical record is transferred with the patient; a copy is not made.

6. *d.* Effective discharge planning begins on admission.

7. *b.* It is important to assess the expectations of the patient (and family) when assessing healthcare needs for discharge planning.

8. *c.* Patients who leave the hospital AMA sign a form releasing the physician and hospital from legal responsibility for their health status. This signed form becomes part of the medical record.

9. *a.* The identification bracelet is a safety measure ensuring that the correct patient is given medications, has surgery, and so forth.

10. *c.* One item on the Patient Care Partnership form is the right to have help when leaving the hospital.

Taylor Suite Resources

The Taylor Suite offers these additional resources to enhance learning and facilitate understanding of this chapter:

- thePoint online resource, http://thepoint.lww.com/Taylor7E
- Student DVD included with the book
- Study Guide for Taylor's Fundamentals of Nursing

BIBLIOGRAPHY

American Hospital Association. (2008). *The patient care partnership*. Available at http://www.aha.org/aha/issues/Communicating-With-Patients/pt-care-partnership.html

Bergstrom, J., Fraser, L., Quinn, M., & Wheeler, H. (2008). All roads lead to scheduled discharges. *Nursing, 38*(12), 61–63.

Boyd, C., Landefeld, C. S., Counsell, S., Palmer, R. M., Fortinsky, R. H., Kresevic, D., Burant, C., & Covinsky, K. E. (2008). Recovery of activities of daily living in older adults after hospitalization for acute medical illness. *Journal of the American Geriatrics Society, 56*, 2171–2179.

Carlson, E. (2008). Nurses' crucial role in preventing and documenting conditions not present on admission. *American Nurse Today, 3*(4), 20.

Coleman, E., Smith, J., Frank, J., Min, S. J., Parry, C., & Kramer, A. M. (2004). Preparing patients and caregivers to participate in care delivered across settings: The care transitions intervention. *Journal of the American Geriatrics Society, 52*(11), 1817–1825.

Davis, M., Smith, S., & Tyler, S. (2005). Improving transition and communication between acute care and long-term care: A system for better continuity of care. *Annals of Long-Term Care, 13*(5), 25–32.

Douglas, S., Daly, B., Kelley, C., O'Toole, E., & Montenegro, H. (2007). Discharge management program for chronically ill

patients. *American Journal of Critical Care Nursing, 16*, 447–457.

Getting the most from an admission interview. (2006). *Nursing, 36*(12), 31.

Graf, C. (2008). The hospital admission risk profile. *American Journal of Nursing, 108*(8), 62–72.

Jabonski, R., Utz, S., Steeves, R., & Gray, D. P. (2007). Decisions about transfer from nursing home to emergency department. *Journal of Nursing Scholarship, 39*(3), 266–272.

Mitty, E., & Flores, S. (2007). Assisted living practice: Admission assessment. *Geriatric Nursing, 28*(1), 27–30.

NANDA International. (2009). *Nursing diagnoses: Definitions & classification 2009–2011*. West Sussex, UK: Wiley-Blackwell.

Popejoy, L. (2008). Adult protective services use for older adults at the time of hospital discharge. *Journal of Nursing Scholarship, 40*(4), 326–332.

Shepperd, S., Parkes, J., McClaran, J., & Phillips, C. (2005). Discharge planning from hospital to home. The Cochrane Library (Oxford). (2): (ID #CD000313).

Stanhope, M., & Lancaster, J. (2008). *Community & public health nursing* (7th ed.). St. Louis: Mosby Elsevier.

The Joint Commission. (2008). *Pre-publication version: Standards Improvement Initiative, National Patient Safety Goals*. Available at http://www.jointcommission.org/patientsafety/nationalpatientsafetygoals/

Trossman, S. (2008). Care without gaps. *American Nurse Today, 3*(7), 40–42.

U.S. Department of Health and Human Services (USDHHS). (2003). *Health information privacy for consumers*. Available at http://www.hhs.gov/ocr/privacy/hipaa/understanding/consumers//index.html

Walker, C., Hogstel, M., & Cox, L. (2007). Hospital discharge of older adults. *American Journal of Nursing, 107*(6), 60–70.

Watts, R., Pierson, J., & Gardner, H. (2005). How do critical care nurses define the discharge planning process? *Intensive & Critical Care Nursing, 21*(1), 39–46.

10 Home Healthcare

JANE FRIEL

Jane, a single woman with end-stage breast cancer, lives with a friend who provides most of her care. She is receiving hospice care with weekly visits unless complications require additional visits.

ALPHONSE CALIFANO

Alphonse, a widower who lives alone, is receiving weekly visits from the home healthcare nurse. He has a history of diabetes, hypertension, and kidney disease.

JOEY MARSHALL

Joey, an extremely low-birth-weight baby (1,100 g), has spent 7 months in the hospital before being discharged home. His mother is caring for him, his twin (who is healthier), and their 3-year-old sister. Joey is still being fed artificially, is on a ventilator, and needs care round the clock.

After completing the chapter, you will be able to accomplish the following:

1. Discuss the components of the home healthcare system, including agencies, patients, referrals, primary caregivers, reimbursement sources, and legal considerations.

2. Explain the purposes and characteristics of hospice and palliative care.

3. Describe the qualities and roles of the home health nurse.

4. Explain the essential components of the pre-entry and entry phases of the home visit.

5. Provide rationale for the importance of documentation in home care.

KEY TERMS

advocacy	palliative care
bereavement care	referral source
home healthcare	reimbursement source
hospice	
Outcome and Assessment Information Set (OASIS)	

In the past decade, many changes have occurred in the healthcare system and in the settings where nurses provide care. A major and important change is an ever-increasing shift from hospital-based settings to community-based home healthcare. Home healthcare is one of the fastest-growing areas of healthcare today; the National Association for Home Care (NAHC) (2008) estimates that more than 83,000 providers deliver home healthcare services to 7.6 million people. (See the accompanying Reflective Practice box for an example.) In its effort to decrease costs, managed care has had a major effect on increasing the move from hospital to home care, and this trend is expected to continue.

Home healthcare is more than just illness care at home or the act of setting up a hospital bed in someone's home. As defined by the NAHC, home care is services provided for people with an acute illness, long-term health condition, permanent disability, or terminal illness who are in need of treatment or support to function effectively in the home environment. The home environment may be a private home, an apartment, a homeless shelter, a boarding house, a dormitory, an assisted-living or long-term care facility, or a group home. Care in the home environment is provided to patients of all ages.

> *Think back to Joey Marshall, the high-risk infant being discharged home with tube feedings and mechanical ventilation. Joey has both acute and chronic healthcare needs. As part of his plan of care, the nurse addresses not only Joey's needs but also those of his family to ensure holistic continuity of care.* ∎

When providing home healthcare, nurses focus on community-based care, taking into account the environmental, socioeconomic, cultural, and personal factors that affect the patient's and family's health. Nurses provide direct care, supervise other care providers, coordinate care with members of the healthcare team, advocate for the client and family, and teach family members or other caregivers how to care for the patient. The essential components of home healthcare include the patient, the family, healthcare professionals from various disciplines, and the goals of helping the patient reach maximum independence and health.

BRIEF HISTORY OF HOME HEALTHCARE NURSING

In the late 1800s, with the United States experiencing a large influx of immigrants, home nursing agencies were started in New York, Boston, and Philadelphia to meet the health needs of the rapidly growing cities. Lillian Wald and Mary Brewster opened the Henry Street Settlement House in New York City in 1893. Visiting nurses from this agency cared for poor residents living in tenements. Eventually, these providers of home healthcare became known as Visiting Nurse Associations (VNAs), which focused on providing personal care to the sick and teaching about health to families.

Before World War II, physicians often made house calls to treat the sick. During the war, physicians shifted their practice setting from the home to the hospital and office, and nurses began to provide most of the home healthcare visits. VNAs were started in most major cities throughout the country. Hospital-based home care agencies were also formed as hospitals looked for ways to expand services to their communities.

In the mid-1960s, federally financed healthcare services expanded to include the older population. The 1965 Social Security Act provided coverage for home healthcare to older persons participating in Medicare. Not long after, Medicaid home healthcare benefits were initiated. The Medicare and Medicaid programs (discussed in Chapter 8) provide the financing for most home healthcare agencies today.

There are many reasons for the expansion in home healthcare. The need for home healthcare services is increasing as the population ages. Fewer people live in the same community as their parents do; thus, home healthcare providers may be needed to care for ill parents if the children live far away. Because patients are discharged from the hospital earlier in their recovery, many will need skilled professional care after they return home. Increasingly, people are choosing to die with comfort and dignity in their own homes. In addition, third-party payers (such as insurance companies and managed care organizations) have sought a way to reduce the escalating costs of healthcare through the use of managed care programs that include home healthcare.

REFLECTIVE PRACTICE
Challenge to Technical Skills

Joey Marshall, an extremely low-birth-weight baby (1,100 g) spent 7 months in the hospital before being discharged home. His mother is now at home full time caring for him, his twin (who is healthier), and their 3-year-old sister. Joey is still being fed via tube feedings, is on a ventilator, and needs care around the clock. When I first visited Joey on the day he was discharged home, I was frightened at the sight of such a small baby surrounded by beeping machines and tubes. While this was not a new sight for Joey's mom, she seemed very uncomfortable being his primary caregiver. She said she had lots of practice taking care of him in the hospital, but nothing had prepared her for the reality of his coming home and needing help around the clock.

Thinking Outside the Box: Possible Courses of Action

- Take a "pass" on this family and tell my instructor that this family's needs exceed my capacity to care; an adult with a lot of tubes is one thing, but a BABY!
- Ask for an experienced mentor to guide me through a comprehensive family assessment and planning to

meet everyone's needs; use this as a challenge but ask for help until I feel competent and confident.
- Act like I know what I'm doing and pray I don't make mistakes!

Evaluating a Good Outcome: How Do I Define Success?

- Joey's mother develops the competence and confidence she needs to provide Joey's care at home.
- I am honest about my ability and seek help when I need it.

- I learn something from each situation that will prepare me to meet the next clinical challenge.
- I don't let my fear interfere with my learning.

Personal Learning: Here's to the Future!

I decided that options one (taking a pass) and three (acting like I knew what I was doing) weren't really options, although they seemed tempting. An experienced home health nurse who once worked in the neonatal intensive care unit (NICU) agreed to visit this family with me, and she talked me through a comprehensive assessment. I was able to use my fear to identify with how Joey's mom was feeling, and I believe I was able to make her feel

comfortable. I told her that we would learn how to do everything together! By the end of this rotation, we were both comfortable with Joey's care. I learned a valuable lesson: to seek help when I am in over my head and to relish a challenge. I hope I will remember this experience as I grow more confident so that I never forget how overwhelmed many families feel when they first bring a loved one home!

Reflection

How do you think you would respond in a similar situation? Why? What does this tell you about yourself and about the adequacy of your skills for professional practice? Can you think of other ways to respond? What technical skills were needed in this situation? What other skills (cognitive, interpersonal, technical, ethical/legal) would you need to respond well in this situation? What factors do you think may have influenced how Joey's mother was feeling? How the nursing student was feeling? Do you agree with the criteria to evaluate a successful outcome? Did the nursing student meet the criteria? Please explain why or why not.

THE HOME HEALTHCARE SYSTEM

Nurses provide home healthcare within a system that includes home health agencies, patients, referral sources, physicians or other primary caregivers, reimbursement sources, and legal considerations. The system functions best when its members communicate, cooperate, and collaborate with each other.

Types of Home Health Agencies

There are several different kinds of public and private home healthcare agencies. All home healthcare agencies are similar in that they must meet uniform standards for licensing, certification, and accreditation by state agencies and/or federal programs (such as Medicare). Home care agencies differ in the way they are organized and administered. They may

be official or public; voluntary or not for profit; private, proprietary; or institution-based. These types of agencies are described in Table 10-1.

In addition, home healthcare agencies are either certified or not certified by Medicare. An agency must be certified by Medicare to receive reimbursement for services from Medicare. Agencies that are not certified by Medicare are not certified for many reasons; for example, home care agencies that do not provide skilled nursing care (e.g., services provided by a registered nurse), are not eligible to participate in Medicare. Medicare is the largest single payer of home care services. It provides payment for services through a prospective payment plan based on an "episode of care" (usually considered a 60-day period). All patients receiving home healthcare services must have an order from their primary healthcare provider.

TABLE • 10-1	TYPES OF HOME HEALTHCARE AGENCIES
Type	**Description**
Official or public agencies	These agencies are operated by state or local governments and primarily financed by tax funds. Most offer home care and disease-prevention programs in the community.
Voluntary or private not-for-profit agencies	These agencies are supported by donations, endowments, charities (such as the United Way), and insurance reimbursements. They are governed by a board of directors, usually representing the community they serve.
Private, proprietary agencies	Most private, proprietary agencies are for-profit organizations governed by individual owners or national corporations. Their services are paid for through healthcare insurance or individual self-pay.
Institution-based agencies	These agencies operate under a parent organization, such as a hospital. The home care agency is governed by the institution, and most referrals for care come from within the institution.

Home healthcare services include high-technology pharmacy services, skilled professional services, custodial care, medical equipment services, hospice and respite services (discussed in Chapter 8), and community support services. Examples of each area, with related services, are listed in Table 10-2.

Depending on the agency and its geographic location, professional providers may include registered nurses, licensed practical/vocational nurses, nurse practitioners and clinical nurse specialists, home care aides, enterostomal therapists, mental health specialists, speech therapists, respiratory therapists, physical therapists, occupational therapists, social workers, dietitians, and a chaplain or minister. Regardless of the number of providers for home healthcare, the responsibility for care coordination (also called case management) remains with the registered nurse. The roles of various members of the home healthcare team are outlined in Table 10-3.

Patients and Caregivers

The patient in home healthcare is both the person receiving care and the person's family, who often are also the caregivers. When a patient enters the hospital, the family most often plays a minor role in actual care. Families and friends visit with the patient and sometimes stay overnight, but they are generally not involved in the direct care of the patient. Hospital staff provide personal care for the patient and

administer medications and treatments. After the patient is discharged, the responsibility for care is shifted to family caregivers, who may or may not be physically or mentally able to handle this responsibility.

Today's emphasis on home healthcare means that family caregivers must carry increased responsibilities. Patients are being discharged "quicker and sicker." Chronically ill patients may need long-term care at home that may not be covered by Medicare, and changes in Medicare funding may mean that fewer home visits will be covered. The financial burden associated with care is more than many families can afford, and home healthcare nurses must be alert for signs of such financial problems (e.g., no food in the refrigerator or kitchen cupboards). A referral for services such as Meals on Wheels may be necessary to provide adequate nutrition for the patient.

In addition to the financial burden, family members face the challenges of handling equipment, providing new types of

TABLE • 10-2	EXAMPLES OF HOME HEALTHCARE SERVICES
Area of Service	**Type of Service Provided**
High-technology pharmacy services	Intravenous therapy Home uterine monitoring Ventilator management Chemotherapy
Skilled professional/paraprofessional services	Nursing care (provided by a licensed practical nurse, a registered nurse, a clinical nurse specialist, or a nurse practitioner) Care by home health aides Personal care Physical therapy Occupational therapy Speech therapy Medical social work Respiratory therapy
Custodial services	Homemaking and housekeeping Hourly or shift coverage Live-in services Companionship
Home medical services	Providing durable medical equipment such as beds, braces, canes, crutches, wheelchairs, commodes, and oxygen
Hospice services	Pain management Physician services Spiritual support Respite care Bereavement counseling
Community support services	Meals on Wheels Transportation Friendly visitor Delivery services Emergency answering services

TABLE • 10-3	COLLABORATIVE ROLES OF MEMBERS OF THE HOME HEALTHCARE TEAM
Member	**Role**
Physician	Certifies that the patient has a health problem to receive home healthcare. Prescribes and certifies a plan of care for treatment for the patient receiving home healthcare.
Nurse	Supervises and coordinates direct care to patients and families. Teaches patient and family self-care. Conducts research to ensure cost-effectiveness and quality of care. May be an administrator of home health agency and serve as consultant to staff. Coordinates services of other healthcare providers.
Physical therapist	Provides direct care such as muscle-strengthening exercises, gait training, and massage. Teaches patient and family to promote self-care.
Occupational therapist	Evaluates the patient's functional level and teaching activities to promote self-care in activities of daily living. Assesses the home for safety and provides adaptive equipment as necessary.
Speech pathologist	Provides direct care services to patients with speech, language, or hearing needs. Teaches patient and family to facilitate speech and language ability, as well as eating and swallowing.
Social worker	Assists patient and family in dealing with the social, emotional, and environmental factors that affect their well-being. Makes referrals to appropriate community resources. Provides assistance with securing equipment and supplies and with healthcare finances.
Home health aide	Implements the plan of care designed by the nurse. Assists patients with hygiene. May carry out light housekeeping.

care to loved ones, and dealing with unfamiliar and often terrifying sounds, odors, and substances. Most caregivers are women, and many of them are older than 65 years of age. Older women may themselves have health problems or may not have the physical strength or energy to care for their husbands. Even family members who are themselves nurses may find that providing care at home is very different from providing care in the hospital. The accompanying box, Through the Eyes of the Family Caregiver, describes one such experience.

The home healthcare nurse must identify the needs of the family and caregiver. The nurse assesses whether the patient and family understand and agree with the plan of care and determines if the caregivers understand the instructions provided and are capable of providing care. The nurse can help the patient and family identify and use community resources to meet various needs. If a caregiver is becoming overwhelmed, the nurse can provide resources to relieve the stress. The nurse also supports family decisions about complex treatments or end-of-life care. The following questions may be used for discussion:

- What is most important to you?
- What do you want for your life and that of your family?
- How do you want to spend the rest of your life?
- How is this technology supporting or not supporting what you want?

Referrals

A **referral source** is a person who recommends home care services and supplies the home healthcare agency with details about the patient's needs. The referral source may be a nurse,

physician, social worker, therapist, or discharge planner. The referral may be to a home health agency, a hospice, or a community resource. Families sometimes generate their own referrals by contacting a home care agency. If the agency believes the patient qualifies for services, the agency contacts the patient's physician and requests a referral for the patient.

Orders for Home Care

Home healthcare cannot begin without an order from a primary caregiver (usually a physician, but may also be a nurse practitioner), nor can it proceed without the primary caregiver's approved treatment plan. This is a legal and reimbursement requirement. A nursing assessment visit to identify a patient's needs can be scheduled only after a referral is made and an initial set of primary caregiver's orders are received. At the nursing assessment visit, the nurse begins to formulate the plan of care and sends it to the primary caregiver for review and approval. See Box 10-1 for Medicare's required data for the plan of care. The primary caregiver's signature on the plan of care authorizes the home care agency to provide services. The plan is reviewed as necessary but at least once every 60 days.

Reimbursement Sources

A **reimbursement source** pays for home healthcare services. Although Medicare is the largest single source of reimbursement, services are also reimbursed by Medicaid, private insurance, patients or their families, and other public funding. The reimbursement source evaluates each plan of care, and only interventions identified on the plan are approved for reimbursement.

Through the Eyes of the Family Caregiver

"I'm So Glad to Have You Home, But What Do I Do Now?" (and this is just the first day. . . .)

I am a nurse and have been a nurse for 30 years. I have a diploma in nursing, a baccalaureate in nursing, a master's in counseling, and a doctorate in nursing. I have taught others how to be nurses for more than 25 years. Nothing in all my educational and practice experiences prepared me to care for the complex needs of my husband, Jacque, when he had surgery 2 years ago. Following diagnosis of metastatic thyroid cancer, a large lower thoracic spinal cord tumor (which put pressure on the spinal nerves, causing leg weakness and bladder malfunction) and the thyroid gland were removed surgically, and steel rods were implanted almost the entire length of the spine. After 30 days in the hospital for diagnosis, surgery, and recovery, Jacque came home—unable to do more than move from the bed to a chair, and with a catheter in his bladder that was attached to a drainage bag.

Before he came home, I got a hospital bed with electric controls, a bedside commode, and a bedside table. I cleared out the family room furniture, got a friend to put the television up on a table (so it could be seen from the hospital bed), and thought I was all ready to give my husband expert care. The first challenge came when he got up in a chair to eat his dinner—we had no chairs with a high enough seat or a straight enough back to allow use of the bedside table. I ran up and down stairs to look at chairs, and finally decided the antique armchair in the living room would work, and it did. Now another problem—where to hang the catheter drainage bag? And how best to move so it

didn't pull when he moved? And remember to empty the bag before he gets up!

I fixed a wonderful homecoming meal for this man I love, and he could only eat a few bites. Now back to bed and a new problem. He got out of the bed and into the chair just fine, but now he can't get out of the chair and into the bed because his legs are still so weak. What did I do wrong—it worked in the hospital. It took me 2 days to realize that I forgot to lower the bed height so Jacque wouldn't have to push up so hard to get his bottom on the bed.

Then, after finally literally hauling him back in bed, I realized that I did not know how to move him up in bed. The physical therapist had taught him how to get up in a chair, but not how to move himself up in bed (they always did it for him in the hospital). This is a 250-pound man we are talking about. I could turn him from side to side, but I couldn't physically move him up in bed and he couldn't stay where he was. After a lot of trials, we figured out that he could wiggle one side of his body at a time and slowly inch up in bed. Now, he was exhausted and in pain, and I felt totally incompetent. Thank goodness, the home health nurse is coming to visit tomorrow.

If I felt this way, how must family members feel who know nothing about caring for someone who is sick or in pain? I have such respect for all those family members who provide such wonderful care and for the nurses who provide home care that calms the fears and answers the questions.

—Priscilla LeMone

Medicare pays the cost of the first 100 home visits following a hospital stay (U.S. Department of Health & Human Services, 2009). Medicare does not reimburse visits to support general health, health promotion, or socioeconomic needs. To be approved for Medicare reimbursement, the patient must meet the criteria listed in Box 10-2.

Box 10-1   MEDICARE'S REQUIRED DATA FOR THE HOME PLAN OF CARE

- Mental status
- Types of services and equipment required
- Prognosis and rehabilitation potential
- Functional limitations
- Activities permitted
- Nutritional requirements
- Medications and treatments
- Safety measures to protect against injury
- Instructions for timely discharge

(Source: Health Care Financing Administration [1999]. *CMS manuals, Home health agency center; Participation, enrollment & certification*, Section 484.30. Available at http://www.cms.hhs.gov/center/hha.asp.)

Box 10-2   ELIGIBILITY REQUIREMENTS FOR MEDICARE REIMBURSEMENT FOR HOME HEALTH SERVICES

The home health agency must be Medicare certified, and the patient must meet the following requirements:
- Be confined to the home.
- Under the care of a physician.
- Receiving services under a plan of care established and periodically reviewed by a physician
- Be in need of skilled nursing care on an intermittent basis (provided or needed on fewer than 7 days a week or less than 8 hours of each day for periods of 21 days or less, although extensions may be possible).
- Have an intermittent need for physical therapy, speech–language therapy, or to continue occupational therapy.

Although a patient may leave home for medical treatment or short infrequent trips for nonmedical reasons (such as to the barbershop or to attend religious services), leaving the home must require considerable and taxing effort.

(Source: U. S. Department of Health and Human Services, Centers for Medicare and Medicaid Services. [2007]. *Medicare and home health. Section 1 Medicare coverage of home health care*. Available at http://www.medicare.gov/Publications/Pubs/pdf/10969.pdf)

In addition, Medicare will provide reimbursement only if the nurse teaches about a new or acute situation, assesses an acute change in the patient's condition, or performs a skilled procedure requiring the professional skill, knowledge, ability, and judgment of a licensed nurse. It is imperative to thoroughly document all nursing interventions with each home visit so that reimbursement is provided.

Legal Considerations

Legal considerations in home care involve a variety of factors, including issues of privacy and confidentiality, the patient's access to health information, the patient's freedom from reasonable restraint, informed consent, and matters of negligence and malpractice. The same codes and standards that guide all other nurses also guide nurses providing care in the home. The American Nurses Association (ANA) *Home Health Nursing Scope and Standards of Practice* (2007) are used as a basis for practice in the home. The standards address the nursing process, interdisciplinary collaboration, quality assurance, professional development, and research. Another source of guidance is the NAHC Bill of Rights. Home care agencies are required by federal law to address the concepts in the Bill of Rights with all home care patients on the initial visit. See Box 10-3 for selected examples from the Bill of Rights. Nurses can best avoid lawsuits by knowing standards of practice, providing care that is consistent with agency policies, and documenting all care fully and accurately.

HOSPICE AND PALLIATIVE CARE

Hospice is comprehensive and coordinated care for patients with limited life expectancy, provided both at home and in institutional settings. Provided by hospice agency nurses and other members of a healthcare team (usually including social workers, ministers, home health aides, and volunteers), it is based on a philosophy of dying with comfort and dignity, encompassing biomedical, psychosocial, and spiritual aspects of the dying experience. Although most hospice care is provided in the home, it may also be provided in hospitals, long-term care facilities, or other community-based settings.

There are approximately 3,500 hospice agencies in the United States, with most services and care reimbursed by a Medicare hospice benefit (National Association for Home Care & Hospice, 2008). Services are reimbursed by Medicare for an initial 90-day period, followed by a subsequent 90-day period, and an unlimited number of 60-day periods, as long as the patient continues to meet eligibility requirements. Most hospice users have care episodes of less than 6 months, but the number of long hospice episodes is increasing (MedPac, 2008). Hospice services usually begin when the patient has 6 months or less to live and end with the family 1 year after the death of the patient. This continuation of care for the family is called **bereavement care** (bereavement is the time of mourning experienced after a loss).

Palliative care is a related area of care that has evolved out of the hospice experience but is used earlier in the disease process. The goal of palliative care is to improve quality of life at the end of life by preventing and relieving suffering through early assessment and treatment of pain and other physical, psychosocial, and spiritual needs. It can be used in all healthcare settings, integrating the knowledge and skills of the patient's physician, a nurse specialist, and/or a team of specialists in palliative care. The World Health Organization's (2009) definition of palliative care encompasses the following selected components:

- Provides relief from pain and other distressing symptoms
- Affirms life and regards dying as a normal process
- Offers a support system to help patients live as actively as possible until death
- Uses a team approach to address the needs of patients and families

THE HOME HEALTHCARE NURSE

For most people, the home is a place of safety and security and has meaning and value, rooted in ownership, family relationships and memories, and independence. When healthcare is provided in the home, the nurse must remember that this setting is controlled by the patient and family. Instead of the patient coming to the nurse, the nurse goes to the patient. The nurse cannot regulate the home setting, but must adapt to the patient's environment, instead of the patient adapting to the hospital environment (Fig. 10-1). The home healthcare nurse must have the ability to blend clinical skills with flexibility.

> *Consider Alphonse Califano, the older man with several health problems. The nurse providing home care to Mr. Califano needs to adapt to his schedule. For example, the nurse might want to visit around breakfast time to evaluate his meal pattern and his diabetes. However, the*

| Box 10-3 | EXAMPLES OF RIGHTS AS A HOME HEALTHCARE PATIENT |

A home healthcare patient has the right to:
- Be fully informed of all his or her rights and responsibilities by the home health agency
- Choose care providers
- Receive reasonable continuity of care
- Receive information necessary to give informed consent before the start of any treatment or procedure
- Refuse treatment within the confines of the law and to be informed of the consequences of his or her action
- Have healthcare providers comply with advance directives in accordance with state law requirements
- Voice grievances and suggest changes in service or staff without fear of restraint or discrimination
- Be informed of what to do in the case of an emergency

(Source: These are part of a longer list of patient rights published by the National Association for Home Care & Hospice. [2009]. *Consumer information: What are my rights as a patient?* Available at http://www.nahch.org/consumer/rights.html)

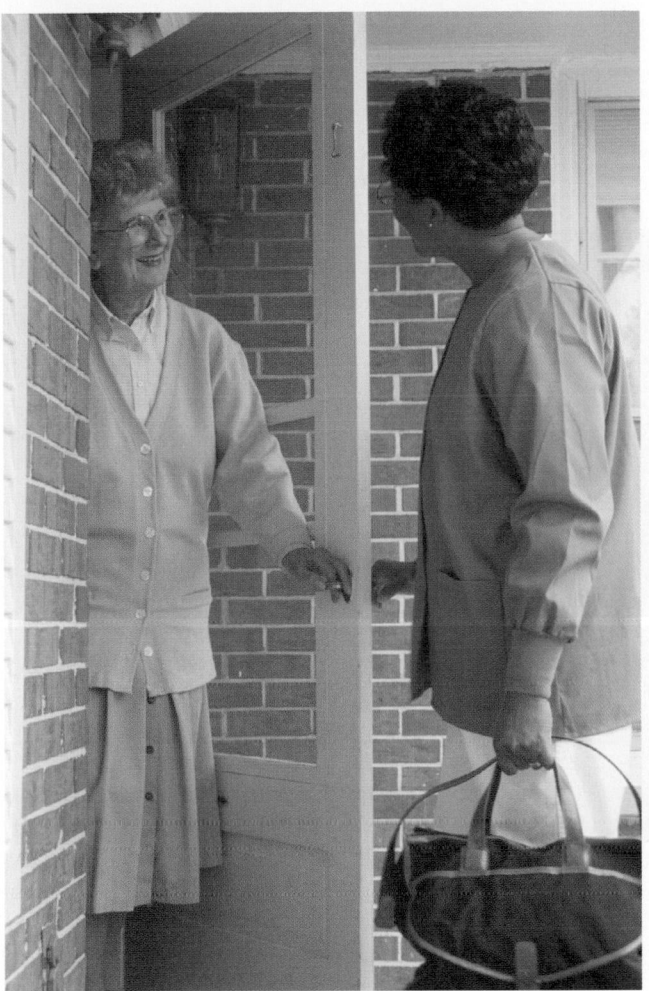

FIGURE 10-1. The nurse providing home healthcare must adapt to the patient's environment, instead of the patient adapting to the hospital or clinic environment.

patient says that he likes to take his time in the morning and doesn't want the nurse to visit until the afternoon. Even after the nurse explains the rationale for wanting to visit earlier in the day, the patient insists that the nurse visit in midafternoon. The nurse must abide by the patient's request. ■

Until about 1990, home healthcare nurses were considered generalists, but recently many home healthcare nurses have gained advanced skills to meet the growing demands of acutely ill patients being cared for at home. These specialties include enterostomal therapy, cardiac care, mental health, and maternal and child health. Specialized nursing knowledge and skills and sophisticated technology allow many patients with acute and chronic healthcare needs to be treated safely and effectively in the home.

Qualities of a Home Healthcare Nurse

Nurses choose to practice home healthcare nursing in both urban and rural settings for various reasons. Many nurses

enjoy practicing in an autonomous setting where they can use their expertise in an expanded role. Others enjoy managing their time independently and like the satisfaction they derive from patients welcoming them into their home and life. Home healthcare nurses find satisfaction in networking with community agencies to provide individualized care. The home setting also provides an opportunity for nurses to be creative in delivering care. Home healthcare nurses must possess several key qualities: they must be knowledgeable and skilled in their practice, must be able to make decisions independently, and must remain accountable.

Knowledgeable and Skilled

Nurses who provide care in the home must have the knowledge and skills needed to provide appropriate care. Both effective communication and clinical skills are essential, as shown in Figure 10-2. In fact, many home healthcare agencies require a minimum of 1 year of clinical practice as a prerequisite for employment. Physical assessment skills are necessary to identify positive and negative changes in a patient's health status. Procedures such as administering intravenous fluids, changing complex wound dressings, caring for ostomies, and providing ventilator care are often required. Home healthcare nurses have identified the following areas of knowledge as most important in home care: legal regulations, physical assessment, body mechanics, nursing diagnoses, and infection control.

Independent in Making Decisions

Nurses providing care in the home make independent decisions and assume responsibility for decision making. They are generally alone when providing care and must be able to make patient care decisions independently. The combination of a sound theoretical foundation, proficiency in clinical skills, and ability to solve problems creatively enables the nurse to make appropriate patient care decisions.

> ➤ *Think back to Jane Friel, the woman who is terminally ill with breast cancer. The nurse has been visiting once a week but would increase the frequency of visits if needed, based on the patient's condition. This situation requires the nurse to make an independent decision based on a solid foundation of knowledge about the disease and its complications.* ■

Accountable

Accountability is another important characteristic of home healthcare nurses. In a hospital, the nurse generally works a shift and reports to the next shift nurse, who then continues to care for the patient. The home healthcare nurse generally does not have a next shift to report to, but must rely on family or other caregivers to continue the care. If there is no caregiver in the home, the nurse returns to face the same issues at the next visit. The nurse is accountable to the

FIGURE 10-2. Home health nurses combine effective communication skills with a sound clinical knowledge base when caring for patients and their families.

patient, the family, and the primary healthcare provider. Home healthcare nurses must consider questions such as the following:

- Whom do I call if the patient's physician is not available?
- What should I do if a family member becomes acutely ill?
- How do I learn to perform advanced procedures?
- How do I document the patient's decisions about treatment?
- How do I ensure that other providers know about and document the plan of care?

Roles of the Home Healthcare Nurse

In addition to having caregiving skills, the nurse providing care in the home is a patient advocate, coordinator of services, and patient and family educator.

Caregiver

It is within the caregiver role that the nurse develops and implements a plan of care. Although the licensed practical nurse may assist with assessment and data collection, only a registered nurse has the legal authority to make the nursing diagnoses that structure the nursing care provided. Skilled nursing care provided by a registered nurse includes assessment, management, evaluation, administration of medications, wound care, tube feedings, catheter care, and behav-

ioral health interventions. As caregiver, the nurse delegates some aspects of care to other healthcare providers, but assumes responsibility for the care and safety of the patient. Selected examples of specific activities performed by the nurse as a caregiver include:

- Completing an in-depth assessment of the patient, family, home environment, and community services.
- Providing wound care by interventions such as changing dressings, debriding and irrigating wounds, and culturing wound drainage.
- Assessing nutritional and hydration status.
- Inserting feeding tubes and providing tube feedings.
- Administering intravenous medications, chemotherapeutic agents, and blood products.

Patient Advocate

Advocacy—the protection and support of another's rights—is an important role of the home healthcare nurse. Patients often need help understanding the complex healthcare system, handling insurance problems, or dealing with state and federal regulations affecting their care and their environment. For example, the nurse may have to convince the patient's insurance carrier of the need for continued home health services. Patients might need help understanding complex billing issues related to their care. Home healthcare nurses can often mobilize services needed to improve the patient's environment.

Coordinator of Services

The home healthcare nurse is generally the coordinator of all other healthcare providers visiting the patient and is the primary source of communication and coordination of the patient's care with the primary healthcare provider. He or she must use effective communication skills with other healthcare providers while coordinating services for the patient. The sample forms shown in Figures 10-3 and 10-4 illustrate how the home healthcare nurse coordinates services among other healthcare providers, teaches the patient's

FIGURE 10-3. Example of home health plan of care.

SKILLED NURSING VISIT NOTE

Patient _____ Samuel Smythe _____

DATE 061311   TIME 11:00–11:45

VISIT FREQUENCY   **Daily**
☐ Change   ☐ Patient informed

BP 140/86 Standing (Sitting) Lying

TEMPERATURE   98.2°

PULSE 80, regular (Apical) Radial

RESPIRATIONS 26

LUNG SOUNDS Clear

DIET/ APPETITE   1800 cal.
Taught fiber sources.

ACTIVITY LEVEL   **Weak. Transfers with 1.**

AIDE SUPERVISION   **Observed K. Jackson**

PHYSICIAN CONTACT/APPT.   **Appt. 061511**

CARE COORDINATION   **Reviewed PT program with aide.**

CONFERENCE

☐ PROGRESS NOTE

No S/S fluid retention. Wound measures 9x5x3 cm. Small amount of purulent drainage. Wound bed 70% slough, 30% granulation tissue. Wound care performed: irrigated with normal saline, covered with ABD. Surrounding skin intact. Expresses discomfort during procedure Taught use of pain med 1 hr. before procedure. Reports occasional constipation. Observed aide transfer patient. Uses safe technique. Patient satisfied with care. Can demonstrate exercises but reluctant to do alone. Taught wife how to assist.

SIGNATURE _Susan Jackson RN_

SKILLED NURSING VISIT NOTE

Patient _____ Samuel Smythe _____

DATE 091911   TIME 7:30–8:20

VISIT FREQUENCY Weekly. Aide dc'd 0913
☐ Change   ☒ Patient informed

BP 132/76 Standing (Sitting) Lying

TEMPERATURE   97.6°

PULSE 70, regular (Apical) Radial

RESPIRATIONS 22

LUNG SOUNDS Clear

DIET/ APPETITE   1800 cal. ADA
"Good appetite"

ACTIVITY LEVEL   **Ambulates 30' – walker No longer uses wheelchair.**

AIDE SUPERVISION

PHYSICIAN CONTACT/APPT.   **Appt. 092311**

CARE COORDINATION

CONFERENCE

☒ PROGRESS NOTE   091911

Venipuncture for FBS – (L) antecubital. Verbalizes routine for blood, urine testing. Still has difficulty performing finger stick. Does not get enough blood on strip for accurate reading. Demonstrated procedure for finger stick.

Blood sugar 175–225.

Feeling more comfortable about performing care.

SIGNATURE _Susan Jackson RN_

FIGURE 10-4. Example of home health nursing progress note.

caregiver to assist in or provide care, and documents the care given.

The home healthcare nurse is also responsible for coordinating community resources needed by the patient. A sound knowledge of community resources enables the nurse to provide comprehensive services to the patient. For example, the nurse must understand the role of a social worker or physical therapist to determine a need for these services. The nurse should know about available community resources, such as Meals on Wheels, the American Cancer Society, services for patients who are visually or hearing impaired, and local services for the aging. As the coordinator of care, the nurse directs the various services toward a common goal of improving the patient's health and promoting independence.

Patient and Family Educator

Nurses providing home healthcare teach patients and families about all the aspects of care in the home, including the disease process or treatment, nutrition, medications, and treatment and care of wounds. The nurse identifies learning needs; then the nurse, patient, and family mutually develop goals for teaching information necessary to promote health. Family members or other caregivers may be taught any skill that they are able and willing to perform.

The nurse provides the information necessary to keep the patient safe until the next visit, using methods that work best in the home. The goal is to increase the patient's ability to provide self-care and the caregiver's ability to care for the patient. The teaching and learning process is fully described in Chapter 22.

> ➤ *Remember Joey Marshall, the high-risk infant coming home after 7 months in the neonatal intensive care unit. In this situation, the home healthcare nurse will fill many roles; one of the major roles will be that of educator, with the goal of teaching Joey's mother so that she can ultimately care for Joey independently.* ■

THE HOME VISIT

Home healthcare patients often feel frightened, in pain, and abandoned, and family members often feel nervous about their new roles as caregivers. The home healthcare nurse must keep these concerns and needs in mind when planning and carrying out care.

The Pre-entry Phase of the Home Visit

In the referral process, the physician or discharge planner of a hospital contacts the home care agency and provides them with a brief medical history, along with indications for home health services. During this pre-entry phase, the referral nurse at the home care agency collects as much information as possible about the patient's diagnoses, surgical experience, socioeconomic status, and treatments ordered. This phase of the home care visit is called the pre-entry phase. Once assigned the case, the nurse reviews the information and calls the patient to make initial contact and schedule a visit. During this conversation, the nurse can determine whether the patient's caregiver can answer questions related to the patient's and family's needs and can also learn about the patient's cognitive abilities, orientation, and caregiver status. This information is important to the nurse planning the first visit.

In the pre-entry phase, the nurse gathers the supplies that will be needed for the first visit, such as wound care products, dressings, and educational materials. The nurse organizes and takes to the first visit a field chart to document the assessment and care provided to the patient. This chart accompanies the nurse on subsequent visits.

The nurse should evaluate safety issues before making the first home visit; this includes the safety of the neighborhood where the patient lives. The nurse may need to arrange the visit at a time when it is safe to be in that area and should always know the exact destination before arriving for the visit. In some unsafe areas, police or security officers may accompany the nurse. Other guidelines for safety include carrying a cell phone programmed with emergency numbers, making sure someone from the agency knows the nurse's itinerary, and being continuously alert to the environment.

The Entry Phase of the Home Visit

The second phase of the visit is the entry phase. In the entry phase, the nurse develops rapport with the patient and family, makes assessments, determines nursing diagnoses, establishes desired outcomes (along with the patient and family), plans and implements prescribed care, and provides teaching. The nurse must remember that he or she is a guest in the patient's home and is offering services that the patient may accept or reject. Important considerations include negotiating and honoring visit times, establishing a rapport with the patient and family, defining what nursing care will be provided, and teaching to promote independence in self-care.

The nurse must gain the trust of the patient and family and must recognize and respect their values. Accepting the patient's living conditions is necessary, even when they differ from those of the nurse. The nurse must ask permission before using the patient's home for activities such as handwashing. The nurse might believe the furniture in the patient's home or sick room needs to be rearranged to allow the use of equipment and to remove safety hazards, but the patient should give permission before any changes are made.

Nurses who provide home healthcare interventions do so based on an individualized plan of care for each patient, based initially on identifying individualized healthcare needs. In identifying the patient's needs and determining the interventions, the nurse fulfills the roles discussed earlier in the chapter.

Identifying Needs

The ability to assess patients accurately is an important skill for home care nurses. Most of the initial assessment takes place during the first home visit, although ongoing focused assessment occurs during subsequent visits. The nurse must be skilled not only in physical assessment but also in psychological, socioeconomic, environmental, spiritual, and cultural assessment. Skilled assessment allows the nurse to make appropriate diagnoses. (See Examples of NANDA Nursing Diagnoses: Home Healthcare.) In addition, the nurse must determine and provide culturally sensitive care (see Chapter 2); although important for inpatients, this is even more important in the patient's home. Family caregivers must also be considered, taking into account the various roles that each family member plays and how they contribute to the patient's health status.

Factors to consider include the following:

- What are the roles and responsibilities of family members? Who makes the decisions?
- What type of personal space is customary?
- How are important events celebrated?
- Are there cultural or ethnic influences on the family's usual diet?

Examples of NANDA Nursing Diagnoses
Home Healthcare

Nursing Diagnoses	Related Factors
Risk for Infection	Presence of large draining wound and unclean living environment
Impaired Home Maintenance	Fatigue and pain during recovery from injuries in automobile crash
Caregiver Role Strain	Requirement for 24-hour attention to needs and safety of husband with Alzheimer's disease
Readiness for Enhanced Knowledge	Requests from family members for increased information about providing care and using community resources and support services
Readiness for Enhanced Parenting	Children express satisfaction with home environment

- What cultural beliefs and taboos are followed?
- What do the patient and family believe to be the cause of this illness and the treatment of this illness?
- Are traditional medical practices followed?

➤ Recall Alphonse Califano, the widowed man with several health problems. Because he is a widower, the nurse would need to identify his primary caregiver or responsible party. The nurse also would need to determine the amount of support, if any, the patient has from his family. This information would provide a basis for possible referrals to community services. ■

The nurse also assesses the physical environment of the home. Safety hazards, such as throw rugs or clutter, could easily cause falls. The home may be unsanitary, with rodent or insect infestations, or it may lack running water. Caregivers may have an alcohol or drug problem that impairs their ability to care for the patient. All of these factors must be considered because they could interfere with the patient's health and safety. Assessing the family helps the nurse to plan appropriate interventions and care for the patient.

Determining Interventions

Specific interventions are based on the patient's needs, but controlling infection and teaching the patient and caregiver are part of all home visits.

CONTROLLING INFECTION

The nurse's use of infection-control techniques is important to avoid spreading infection from one patient to the next. Of all the methods used to prevent infection, hand hygiene is the most important and is necessary before and after treating the patient. Nurses use standard precautions during home care visits, including wearing gloves when contacting blood,

body fluids, secretions, excretions, and contaminated items. Clean disposable gloves should be put on just before touching areas of broken skin or mucous membranes.

To prevent the spread of infection, nurses should also use appropriate technique when handling their equipment bags, including the following:

- Perform hand hygiene before reaching into the bag for supplies.
- Clean any equipment removed from the bag before returning it to the bag.
- Place the bag on a liner when setting it down in the patient's home.

TEACHING THE PATIENT AND CAREGIVERS

Because home healthcare is meant to be short term and intermittent, the nurse includes the family and friends in the teaching process so they can learn how to care for the patient after the nurse's home care is no longer needed. The nurse designs and implements the teaching plan based on the patient and caregiver's readiness to learn. It must be adapted to the patient's and caregiver's physical and emotional status and must be understandable and "doable."

➤ Consider Joey Marshall, the infant discharged home after 7 months. Because of the complex technology associated with his care and because his mother feels anxious and afraid, the nurse would need to provide the necessary teaching about his care, but in small sessions to avoid overwhelming the mother. ■

Teaching should identify both the positive outcomes of following instruction and the serious consequences of failing to do so. The nurse points out the major problem areas specific to care in the home, focusing on the information needed to keep the patient safe until the nurse's next home visit.

Documenting Care Given in the Home

Documenting care given in the home is mandated by regulatory and federal agencies (see Chapter 17). The nurse may document the visit on preprinted forms or checklists or may use a computer.

The documented plan of care, the visit plan, and progress notes are routinely used by regulatory agencies and payer sources (e.g., private insurance or Medicare) to determine whether various state and federal regulations are being met and if payment is warranted. Figures 10-3 and 10-4 illustrate such documentation.

During the initial home visit, the nurse documents the assessment of the patient's healthcare needs; a plan of care that includes all the information needed to meet agency policy, regulatory requirements, and payer source needs; and a schedule for subsequent visits. The plan of care accurately reflects the condition of the patient, the need for skilled care, specific physician orders, anticipated progress, the criteria for discharge, the supplies needed, a visit schedule for all healthcare providers, and a list of support systems available. The plan of care includes the patient's functional limitations and safety needs; it establishes specific measurable goals and specifies a time frame for reaching the goals.

The nurse writes progress notes to document each visit to the patient's home. These notes must accurately describe the patient's condition, the skilled care provided, the patient's response, the patient's progress toward discharge, and an ongoing plan for continued care. They also include the nurse's plan for the next visit. To meet reimbursement requirements, each progress note must indicate that the care provided requires the knowledge and skills of a professional nurse.

A further requirement of documentation in home healthcare is the **Outcome and Assessment Information Set (OASIS)**. This assessment instrument represents core items of a comprehensive assessment for adult nonmaternity home care patients and forms the basis for measuring patient outcomes for the purpose of improving the quality of care that is provided. The general categories of the items in OASIS include demographics; history; living arrangements; supportive assistance; status of senses, skin, respiratory function, elimination, neurologic, and behavioral function; activities of daily living; medications; equipment management; and information from inpatient care or agency discharge. The OASIS is completed by home health agency personnel at the start of care and every 2 months thereafter until and including discharge, and data are electronically transmitted to a state OASIS system.

THE FUTURE OF HOME HEALTHCARE

The 1990s were a time of transition, growth, and specialization for the home care industry. In this century, more complex services are being provided at home. Increasing numbers of surgical procedures are being performed on an outpatient or short-stay basis; thus, families and friends have more responsibility for providing care at home. Specialization will continue to expand in the areas of cardiac care, wound care, and high-technology services. The role of prevention will continue to grow in home healthcare through the use of health screening, immunization, and community education programs. Keeping people healthy in the home will be a goal to prevent illnesses resulting in hospitalization. Home healthcare nurses will need to expand their knowledge and skills continually to meet the challenges of providing preventive, acute, chronic, and end-of-life care to patients in their homes.

● Developing Critical Thinking Skills

1. Interview a nurse employed in a hospital setting and a nurse employed by a home healthcare agency. How are their roles and responsibilities alike? How do they differ?

2. Consider what you would do in the following home healthcare situations:
   • An 85-year-old patient cannot move by himself and refuses to eat. His 83-year-old wife tries to care for him, but she is under a great deal of stress and begins to cry when you enter their apartment.
   • A 43-year-old woman is receiving home care after surgery to repair a herniated vertebral disc ("slipped disc"). When you arrive for the scheduled visit, you find that her speech is slurred and she does not remember how much pain medication she has taken.
   • A 2-year-old has a malignant brain tumor. He is not expected to live more than 1 week and is receiving hospice care.

● Practicing for NCLEX

1. Which one of the following statements is a requirement for Medicare home healthcare reimbursement?
   a. The patient must be essentially homebound.
   b. The patient must require intravenous therapy.
   c. The caregiver must be able to provide all physical care.
   d. The caregiver must live with the patient.

2. In general, how does home care nursing compare with hospital-based nursing?
   a. Nursing care provided in the home is no different from hospital-based nursing care.
   b. Home care patients do not have the same basic needs as those in the hospital.
   c. In the home, care must be adapted to the patient's schedules and customs.
   d. The family or caregiver's role is less important in home care nursing.

3. Although the home care nurse follows an established plan of care, he or she is more independent in what role?
   a. Deciding which physician orders can be followed
   b. Assuming responsibility for decision making
   c. Shifting accountability for care to family caregivers
   d. Delegating advanced clinical skills to unlicensed personnel

4. Although all of the following skills are important, what would be the *most* important to effective coordination of care and services?
   a. Physical assessment
   b. Knowledge of the law
   c. How to use equipment
   d. Effective communication

5. Which of the following activities would the nurse do in the pre-entry phase of the home visit?
   a. Call the physician for a referral order
   b. Conduct a health history and physical assessment
   c. Collect information and schedule a visit
   d. Establish mutually acceptable goals for care

6. Before washing her hands, what might a home health nurse ask or say to the patient?
   a. "I need to wash my hands. May I use your bathroom?"
   b. "I'm going to wash my hands in your bathroom."
   c. "I will wash my hands after I leave so I don't bother you."
   d. "How often do you wash your hands?"

7. What one activity is most important in preventing infection when providing home care?
   a. Wearing gloves whenever touching the patient
   b. Following proper procedures for sterile dressing changes
   c. Asking the caregiver to step out of the room during visits
   d. Performing hand hygiene before and after care

8. How often must a home care nurse document progress notes?
   a. Once a week
   b. At the initial visit
   c. At each visit
   d. At the final visit

● Answers With Rationale

1. *a.* To be eligible for Medicare reimbursement, the patient must be essentially homebound, or normally unable to leave the home unassisted.

2. *c.* In the hospital, patients must conform to established schedules for treatments, medications, meals, and visitors. In contrast, in the home it is the patient or caregiver who establishes the schedule and controls the environment.

3. *b.* The home healthcare nurse is more independent and assumes responsibility for decision making.

4. *d.* The home healthcare nurse must use effective communication skills with other healthcare providers while coordinating services for the patient.

5. *c.* During the pre-entry phase of the home visit, the nurse collects information and schedules the first visit.

6. *a.* The nurse must ask permission before rearranging furniture or using facilities for handwashing.

7. *d.* Performing hand hygiene before and after caring for the patient is critical in preventing infection.

8. *c.* The home health nurse must document progress notes at each visit.

Taylor Suite Resources

The Taylor Suite offers these additional resources to enhance learning and facilitate understanding of this chapter:

- thePoint online resource, http://thepoint.lww.com/Taylor7E
- Student DVD included with the book
- Study Guide for Taylor's Fundamentals of Nursing

BIBLIOGRAPHY

Ahrens, J. (2005). Home care today. The need for evidence-based guidelines in home care. *Home Healthcare Nurse, 23*(3), 147–149.

American Association of Retired Persons. (2008). *Caregiving.* Available at http://www.aarpmagazine.org/family/Articles/a2003-02-25-meformeresources.html

American Nurses Association [ANA]. (2007). *Home health nursing scope and standards of practice.* Available at http://nursingworld.org

Boucher, M. (2005). "Making it": Qualities needed for rural home care nursing. *Home Healthcare Nurse, 23*(2), 103–108.

Buhler-Wilkerson, K. (2007). No place like home: A history of nursing and home care in the U.S. *Home Healthcare Nurse, 25*(4), 253–259.

Centers for Medicare & Medicaid Services. (2009). *Medicare & you.* Baltimore, MD: U.S. Department of Health and Human Services.

Centers for Medicare & Medicaid Services. (2008a). *Home health overview.* Available at http://www.cms.hhs.gov/HomeHealthPPS/

Centers for Medicare & Medicaid Services. (2008b). *OASIS background.* Available at http://www.cms.hhs.gov/OASIS/02_Background.asp

Chu, J. (2009). Undereating in the homebound elderly. *American Journal of Nursing, 109*(1), 67.

Health Care Financing Administration. (1999). *CMS manuals, Home health agency center; Participation, enrollment & certification.* Section 484.30. Available at http://www.cms.hhs.gov/center/hha.asp

Health Care Financing Administration. (2008). *Who pays for home care services.* Available at http://www.nahc.org/consumer/FAQs/whopays.html

Hospice Association of America. (2008). *Hospice facts & statistics.* Washington, DC: Author.

Leongard, A., & Boal, J. (2004). Home care of the frail elderly. *Clinics in Geriatric Medicine, 20*(4), 795–807.

MedPac. (2008). *Evaluating Medicare's hospice benefit* (Chapter 8). Available at http://www.medpac.gov/chapters/Jun08_Ch08.pdf

NANDA International. (2009). *Nursing diagnoses: Definitions and classification 2009–2011.* West Sussex, UK: Wiley-Blackwell.

National Cancer Institute. (2007). *Home care for cancer patients.* Available at http://www.cancer.gov/cancertopics/factsheet/support/home-care

National Association for Home Care & Hospice. (2009). *Consumer information: What are my rights as a patient?* Available at http://www.nahch.org/consumer/rights.htm

National Association for Home Care & Hospice. (2008). *Hospice facts & statistics; What are my rights as a patient?* Washington, DC: Author.

Onega, L. (2008). Helping those who help others: The modified care-giver strain index. *American Journal of Nursing, 108*(9), 62–69.

Schneider, J., Barkauskas, V., & Keenan, G. (2008). Evaluating home health care nursing outcomes with OASIS and NOC. *Journal of Nursing Scholarship, 40*(1), 76–82.

Smith-Temple, J., & Johnson, J. (2006). *Nurses' guide to clinical procedures.* Philadelphia: Lippincott Williams & Wilkins.

Spotlight on home health nursing. (2007). *Nursing, 37*(12), 56-R2.

Stanhope, M., & Lancaster, J. (2008). *Community & public health nursing* (7th ed.). St. Louis: Mosby Elsevier.

Taylor, E. (2008). Promoting spiritual health in home healthcare. *Home Healthcare Nurse, 26*(6), 367–374.

U. S. Department of Health and Human Services, Centers for Medicare and Medicaid Services. (2007). *Medicare and home health. Section 1 Medicare coverage of home health care.* Available at http://www.medicare.gov/Publications/Pubs/pdf/10969.pdf

U. S. Department of Health & Human Services. Centers for Medicare & Medicaid Services. (2009). *Medicare & you.* Baltimore, MD: Author.

Vasquez, S. (2009). Preventing rehospitalization through effective home health nursing care. *Professional Case Management, 14*(1), 32–38.

Wolff, J., Meadow, A., Weiss, C., Boyd, C. M., & Leff, B. (2008). Medicare home health patients' transitions through acute and post-acute care settings. (Report). *Medical Care, 46*(11), 1188–1193.

World Health Organization. (2009). *WHO definition of palliative care.* Available at http://www.who.int/cancer/palliative/definition/en/print.html

THE NURSING PROCESS

The nursing process is a systematic, patient-centered, goal-oriented method of caring that provides a framework for nursing practice. Unit III discusses each of the five steps of the nursing process—assessing, diagnosing, outcome identification and planning, implementing, and evaluating. It also describes the blended skills nurses need to use the process for promoting patient well-being, and concludes with a chapter on documentation, reporting, and conferring.

The steps of the nursing process are not actually separate items but, rather, are parts of a whole, used to identify needs, to establish priorities of care, to maximize strengths, and to resolve actual or potential alterations in human responses to health and illness, thereby promoting health to the highest level possible for each patient.

Assessment, the systematic and continuous collection and communication of data, allows analysis of data to identify problems and strengths of patients. During outcome identification and planning, the nurse and patient mutually identify expected outcomes and agree on nursing interventions necessary to meet these outcomes. The nurse implements the plan of care, adapting it to each individual, and documents nursing actions and patient responses. After implementation, the nurse and patient evaluate the effectiveness of the plan, based on achievement of outcomes, and determine if the plan should be continued, modified, or terminated.

The nursing process is nursing practice in action. Unit III provides the information necessary to begin to apply the nursing process. As blended skills are learned and practiced (both by students and by nurses), the process becomes an integral component of each nurse–patient interaction. The outcome is compassionate, comprehensive, and individualized nursing care.

" *. . . the nursing process is educative and therapeutic when nurse and patient can come to know and to respect each other, as persons who are alike, and yet different, as persons who share in the solution of problems.* "

HILDEGARD PEPLAU (1909–1999) • *had been an active participant in ANA and NLN, and a leader in recognizing the significance of interpersonal relationships in psychiatric nursing. Her landmark book integrated theory into her model at a time when nursing theory was in its infancy.*

11 Blended Skills and Critical Thinking throughout the Nursing Process

CHARLOTTE HORVATH

Charlotte is a single mother whose 5-year-old daughter will be discharged soon. Ms. Horvath is to learn how to perform wound care for her daughter at home. However, she has missed every planned teaching session thus far.

ADDIE WARNER

Addie is an elderly African American woman who had suffered a cerebrovascular accident (CVA). She is currently being cared for in a neurologic step-down unit. The patient frequently uses her call light and is called "demanding" by the staff.

JERMAINE BYRD

Jermaine is a 58-year-old man who has just returned to the medical–surgical unit after undergoing vascular surgery on the femoral artery. Orders include assessing the distal pulses to ensure adequate blood flow. However, when assessing the patient, the posterior tibial pulse is not palpable.

LEARNING OBJECTIVES

After completing the chapter, you will be able to accomplish the following:

1. Describe the historic evolution of the nursing process.

2. Describe the nursing process and each of its five steps.

3. List five characteristics of the nursing process.

4. Contrast three approaches to problem solving.

5. List three patient benefits and three nursing benefits of using the nursing process correctly.

6. Describe how to develop the four blended skills essential to nursing practice.

7. Use a model of critical thinking when making clinical judgments and decisions.

8. Identify four habits that assist in the development of technical skills.

9. Develop a personal plan to develop the interpersonal skills essential to quality care.

10. Explain the relationship between a nurse's sense of accountability and the patient's well-being.

11. Describe the steps in concept mapping care planning.

12. Identify personal strengths and weaknesses in light of nursing's essential knowledge and skills.

KEY TERMS

assess

concept mapping

critical thinking

critical thinking indicators

decision making

evaluate

expected outcomes

implement

intuitive problem solving

nursing diagnoses

nursing process

plan

scientific problem solving

standards for critical thinking

trial-and-error problem solving

Traditionally, nurses prided themselves on comforting those who were ill and on executing with precision such tasks as dressing wounds, administering medications, and bathing, feeding, and ambulating patients. Physicians ordered many of these tasks, and few nurses in the past would have charac-terized their "work" as being independent, evidence-based, or creative.

But as society and the healthcare delivery system change, so does nursing. Nurses now work with healthy and ill patients in both private and institutional settings. In addition to their role as caregivers, nurses fill specialized roles as care managers/coordinators, teachers, counselors, advocates, and researchers. Nurses are responsible for a unique dimension of healthcare—"the diagnosis and treatment of human responses to actual or potential health problems" (American Nurses Association [ANA], 2003) and, as such, are knowl-edgeable, competent, and independent professionals who work collaboratively with other healthcare professionals to design and to deliver holistic care. As the role has changed, definitions of nursing have evolved to acknowledge essential features of professional nursing:

- Provision of a caring relationship that facilitates health and healing
- Attention to the range of human experiences and responses to health and illness within the physical and social environments
- Integration of objective data with knowledge gained from an appreciation of the patient or group's subjective expe-rience
- Application of scientific knowledge to the processes of diagnosis and treatment through the use of judgment and critical thinking
- Advancement of professional nursing knowledge through scholarly inquiry
- Influence on social and public policy to promote social justice

As the practice of nursing became more complex, nurses began to study the process of nursing to both understand and improve the means nurses use to accomplish their aims. (See the accompanying Reflective Practice display for an exam-ple of this process.) This chapter provides an overview of the nursing process and then describes the blended skills needed to successfully use the nursing process.

THE NURSING PROCESS
Historical Perspective

Since Hall first used the term "nursing process" in 1955, many nurses have struggled to define exactly what constitutes the "work of nursing" and what makes nurses successful. In the 1960s, nursing theorists began to describe nursing as a distinct entity among the healthcare professions and also delineated specific steps in a process approach to nursing practice. In 1967, Yura and Walsh published the first compre-hensive book on nursing process, in which they described four steps in the nursing process: assessment, planning, inter-vention, and evaluation. They viewed the element of nursing diagnosis as the logical conclusion of the assessment phase, whereas Gebbie and Lavin (1974) made nursing diagnosis a separate step in the process. These and other studies led to the development of the five-step nursing process commonly used

REFLECTIVE PRACTICE
Challenge to Ethical and Legal Skills

Recently, I spent time working as a pediatric nurse technician. My job was to provide basic care to patients, such as giving bed baths, assisting with meals, and changing linens. One of the nicest parts of my job was that I was able to spend more time than most nurses are able to, talking with my patients and getting to know them, and hopefully making a positive difference in their days. One day I was assigned to float to the neurologic step-down unit. Here, I met Addie Warner, an elderly African American woman who had suffered a cerebrovascular accident (CVA). Because of what happened that day, I became responsible for her care for the rest of the day.

When I arrived on the unit that morning, the nurses told me what a "pain" Mrs. Warner was, describing how she kept demanding that the nurse come into her room and help her with this or that. They told me I should "ignore her," and they told me I didn't need to listen to her. I was immediately appalled. I witnessed yet another nurse stand outside her door and condescendingly tell her in an annoyed voice, "I'll be with you when I have time." As I passed her room, Ms. Warner yelled out for attention.

Thinking Outside the Box: Possible Courses of Action

- Listen to all the nurses out of personal ignorance, out of fear for being reprimanded by them, or out of selfishness, and continue to ignore this patient and her needs just like everyone else was doing.
- Ask one of the nurses to go into the room with me to determine what the patient's needs were and to help me meet them, despite the nurses' obvious dislike of the patient and obvious lack of desire to help her.
- Go into the patient's room by myself, assess her needs for the simple purpose of relaying them to the nurse, and then not do anything to meet any of her needs myself.
- Enter the patient's room by myself, assess her needs, assure her I would try to help her meet her needs once the nurse became available, and then drop the ball in the end, not helping her much myself or with the nurse.
- Go into her room by myself, assess her needs, assure her I would help her meet her needs, and take the steps to meet them later in the shift when I had more time.
- Proceed into her room by myself, assess her needs, assure her I would help her meet them, and take the steps to meet them immediately and throughout the whole shift.
- Ignore the patient, stating that meeting her needs was not my job, but encourage the nurses to go into the room to assess and meet her needs.

Evaluating a Good Outcome: How Do I Define Success?

- The patient's needs are assessed and met by the most compassionate and most qualified professional possible.
- The patient feels heard and respected.
- I feel respected, feeling that I used my professional patient-care skills to the best of my ability to facilitate resolution of the patient's situation.
- The patient's inherent dignity, worth, and uniqueness is respected by everyone who comes into contact with her.
- The patient remains the primary commitment for me and the nurses.
- The patient feels that she is the primary commitment for the nurse and me.
- The health, safety, and rights of the patient are promoted, advocated for, and protected.
- The integrity of my patient, myself, and my fellow nurses is preserved.

Personal Learning: Here's to the Future!

Immediately upon starting my shift, I went into Ms. Warner's room to see what the problem was. She told me, in tears, that she's had to go to the bathroom for the past 2 hours, and that no one would help her. As a result, she ended up urinating on herself in bed. I immediately helped her out of bed into a chair, gave her soap and towels to start washing herself, and set about changing her linens. All the while, I listened to her talk about how humiliated and upset she was about having been forced to "wet the bed." She also was upset that she'd ruined the only pair of underwear she had with her in the hospital. So, I washed the underwear in the sink for her. I asked her questions about what had happened that morning and validated her feelings. I helped her finish bathing, set her up to be sitting comfortably in the chair, and got her lunch tray, which I then set up for her. Although, for the most part, she could feed herself, her CVA had left her with some residual weakness, necessitating some help with opening containers, cutting foods, and placing items within her reach on the tray. She also wanted me to bring her the phone and help her dial, which I did. I let her eat and talk on the phone alone, promising I would come back to check on her soon.

Throughout the rest of the shift, I peeked my head into her room every half hour or so, eventually helping her back into her bed after she was comfortable, fed, and less upset. Probably the most important thing I did for her, besides resolving the wet bed situation, was to listen to her as she purged her feelings. I validated her feelings and did everything in my power to make sure that she experienced no further episodes of disrespect. Unfortunately, while the patient's needs were met by the most compassionate professional possible (me), they were not met by the most qualified professional possible (the nurse). I believe the patient did feel heard and respected after our interactions. However, she stated that she felt ignored after her interactions with the nurses and physicians.

I felt that my actions were respected because none of the nurses gave me a difficult time or made fun of me

(continued)

REFLECTIVE PRACTICE

Challenge to Ethical and Legal Skills (continued)

for taking the extra time to soothe this patient. I did feel that I provided professional patient care to this patient in the best manner I knew. I respected her inherent dignity, worth, and uniqueness, and I believe the patient felt my primary commitment was to her. Unfortunately, this only highlighted the fact that no one else's

primary commitment had been to her. I certainly promoted, advocated for, and strove to protect this patient's health, safety, and rights. However, it seemed the nurses went out of their way not to do that for this patient.

Tracey Sara Miller, Georgetown University

Reflection

How do you think you would respond in a similar situation? Why? What does this tell you about yourself and about the adequacy of your skills for professional practice? What reasons can you postulate to account for the nursing staff's actions? Would these reasons be justified? Can you think of other ways to respond? What other skills (cognitive, interpersonal, technical, ethical/legal) would you need to respond well in this situation? Do you think the nursing student should have approached the nursing staff about what she had found? Did the nursing student violate any ethical or legal principles based on her position as a nursing technician? Please explain. Do you agree with the criteria to evaluate a successful outcome? Did the nursing student meet the criteria? Please support your response.

today: assessment, diagnosis, outcome identification and planning, implementation, and evaluation.

The steps of the nursing process were legitimized in 1973, when the ANA Congress for Nursing Practice developed Standards of Practice to guide nursing performance. The following definition serves as the foundation for the scope and standards of nursing practice: *Nursing is the protection, promotion, and optimization of health and abilities, prevention of illness and injury, alleviation of suffering through the diagnosis and treatment of human response, and advocacy in the care of individuals, families, communities, and populations* (ANA, 2003, p. 6). The scope defines the range and boundaries of nursing practice (see Chapter 1 for more information). The standards are authoritative statements by which the nursing profession describes responsibilities for which its practitioners are accountable. These standards were revised in 1991, 1998, and 2004. The six *Standards of Practice* (assessment, diagnosis, outcome identification, planning, implementation, and evaluation) describe a competent level of nursing care as demonstrated by the critical thinking model of the nursing process. The nursing process encompasses all significant actions taken by registered nurses and forms the foundation of the nurse's decision making (ANA, 2004, p. 4).

Although the ANA refers to a six-step nursing process, many practitioners still commonly refer to a five-step nursing process in which outcome identification and planning are combined into one step. The five-step nursing process is presented throughout this textbook.

The Joint Commission requires that care be documented according to the nursing process, and the National League for Nursing has recommended that educational programs incorporate the nursing process as their intellectual process. In 1982, the state board examinations for professional nursing practice underwent major revisions and began to use the nursing process as an organizing concept. The revised examinations

are structured to test the practitioner's ability to assess patients, to diagnose health problems amenable to nursing therapy, and to plan, implement, and evaluate nursing care. The examinations had previously organized content on a medical model, structured according to medical specialties—medicine, surgery, maternity, pediatrics, and psychiatry.

Description of the Nursing Process

The **nursing process** is a systematic method that directs the nurse and patient, as together they accomplish the following: (1) **assess** the patient to determine the need for nursing care, (2) determine **nursing diagnoses** for actual and potential health problems, (3) identify **expected outcomes** and **plan** care, (4) **implement** the care, and (5) **evaluate** the results. The steps in this patient-centered, outcome-oriented process are interrelated; each step depends on the accuracy of the steps preceding it. The process provides a framework that enables the nurse and patient to accomplish the following:

- Systematically collect patient data (assessing)
- Clearly identify patient strengths and actual and potential problems (diagnosing)
- Develop a holistic plan of individualized care that specifies the desired patient goals and related outcomes and the nursing interventions most likely to assist the patient to meet those expected outcomes (planning)
- Execute the plan of care (implementing)
- Evaluate the effectiveness of the plan of care in terms of patient goal achievement (evaluating)

> *Consider Addie Warner, the elderly patient who had suffered a CVA and is considered "demanding" by the staff. The nurse integrates the use of this framework to determine the patient's presenting problem, that is, the reason for using the call light. By systematically collecting information,*

determining the patient's strengths and needs, quickly developing a plan for these needs, executing it, and then determining the effectiveness of the plan, the nurse provides the patient with safe, quality, effective care. ■

The five steps of the nursing process are shown in Figure 11-1 and described in Table 11-1. In each step of the process, the nurse and patient work together as partners (Fig. 11-2); the patient's health state and resources influence the patient's level of participation. When the patient is an infant or is unconscious or uncooperative, the nurse works through the steps of the process with the help of a family member or support person whenever possible.

Nursing Process Trends

Although experienced nurses might tell stories about lengthy handwritten plans of individualized care, the trend today is toward standardization and computerization. Nurses at centralized or bedside computer terminals have access to databases that allow them to plan and document care easily. Critical pathways (see Chapter 14), which target desired outcomes for particular illnesses, procedures, or conditions and accompanying multidisciplinary staff actions along a timeline, provide the standard guidelines for care in many institutions. Facilitating this work are national efforts to develop the state of nursing knowledge and science and a standard nursing language (Table 11-2). This work is described in subsequent chapters on diagnosis, planning, and implementation. Two recent milestone monographs in nursing science are *Unifying Nursing Languages: The Harmonization of NANDA, NIC, and NOC* (Dochterman & Jones, 2003) and *Clinical Information Systems: A Framework for Reaching the Vision* (Androwich, 2002).

Characteristics of the Nursing Process

Various words and phrases have been used to describe the nursing process. Key descriptors include systematic, dynamic, interpersonal, outcome oriented, and universally applicable.

Systematic

Each nursing activity is part of an ordered sequence of activities. Moreover, each activity depends on the accuracy of the activity that precedes it and influences the actions that follow it. Without a complete and accurate database, the nurse cannot identify patient strengths and problems. Lacking knowledge of these, it is impossible for the nurse and patient to develop a plan of care based on realistic and valued patient goals. Unless the goals and outcomes are well written, nursing actions and evaluation lack focus and might be ineffective. The nursing process directs each step of nursing care in a sequential, ordered manner.

Dynamic

Although the nursing process is presented as an orderly progression of steps, in reality, there is great interaction and

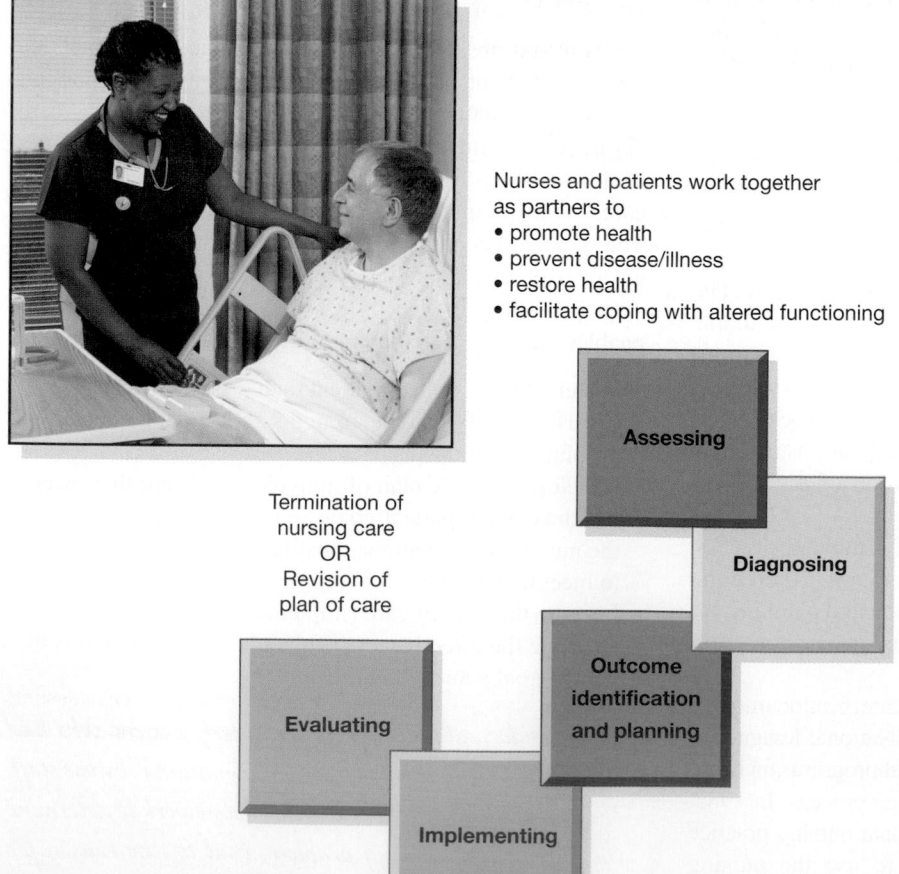

Nurses and patients work together as partners to
• promote health
• prevent disease/illness
• restore health
• facilitate coping with altered functioning

Termination of nursing care OR Revision of plan of care

Assessing

Diagnosing

Outcome identification and planning

Evaluating

Implementing

FIGURE 11-1. The steps in the patient-centered, outcome-oriented nursing process are dynamic and interrelated. Each of the five steps depends on the accuracy of the preceding step.

TABLE • 11-1	**OVERVIEW OF THE NURSING PROCESS**		
Component	**Description**	**Purpose**	**Activities**
Assessing	Collection, validation, and communication of patient data	Make a judgment about the patient's health status, ability to manage his or her own healthcare, and need for nursing. Plan individualized holistic care that draws on patient strengths and is responsive to changes in the patient's conditions.	1. Establish the database: • Nursing history • Physical assessment • Review of patient record and nursing literature • Consultation with patient's support people and healthcare professionals 2. Continuously update the database. 3. Validate data. 4. Communicate data.
Diagnosing	Analysis of patient data to identify patient strengths and health problems that independent nursing intervention can prevent or resolve	Develop a prioritized list of nursing diagnoses.	1. Interpret and analyze patient data. 2. Identify patient strengths and health problems. 3. Formulate and validate nursing diagnoses. 4. Develop prioritized list of nursing diagnoses.
Outcome identification and planning	Specification of (1) patient outcomes to prevent, reduce, or resolve the problems identified in the nursing diagnoses; and (2) related nursing interventions	Develop an individualized plan of nursing care. Identify patient strengths that can be tapped to facilitate achievement of desired outcomes.	1. Establish priorities. 2. Write outcomes, and develop an evaluative strategy. 3. Select nursing interventions. 4. Communicate plan of nursing care.
Implementing	Carrying out the plan of care	Assist patients to achieve desired outcomes—promote wellness, prevent disease and illness, restore health, and facilitate coping with altered functioning.	1. Carry out the plan of care. 2. Continue data collection, and modify the plan of care as needed. 3. Document care.
Evaluating	Measuring the extent to which the patient has achieved the outcomes specified in the plan of care; identifying factors that positively or negatively influenced outcome achievement; revising the plan of care if necessary	Continue, modify, or terminate nursing care.	1. Measure how well the patient has achieved desired outcomes. 2. Identify factors that contribute to the patient's success or failure. 3. Modify the plan of care (if indicated.)

overlapping among the five steps. No one step in the nursing process is a one-time phenomenon; each step flows into the next step. In some nursing situations, all five stages occur almost simultaneously.

Interpersonal

Always at the heart of nursing is the human being. Read one student's account of this truth in the accompanying box,

Through the Eyes of a Student. The nursing process ensures that nurses are patient centered rather than task centered (Fig. 11-3). Rather than simply approaching a patient to take vital signs, the nurse might ask, "How are you today, Mr. Byrd? Are our nursing actions helping you to achieve your goals? What are the most important things you'd like me to do?" The nurse might also consider any new data that indicate a need to modify the patient's plan of care.

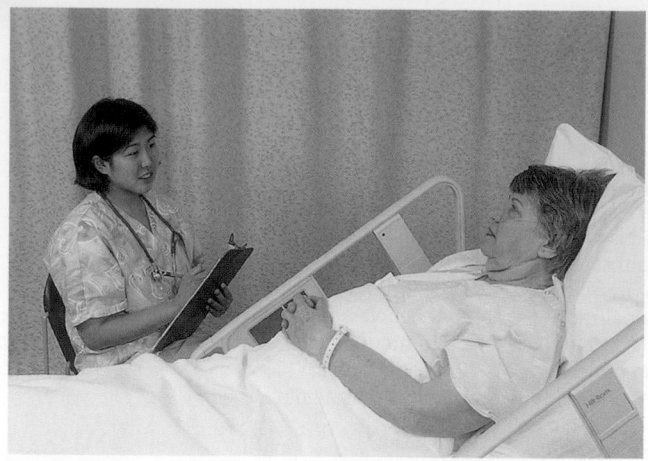

FIGURE 11-2. Nurses work collaboratively with patients when using the nursing process to plan and deliver care. *(Photo by B. Proud.)*

> *Consider Charlotte Horvath, the single mother who requires wound care teaching but has failed to attend any scheduled teaching sessions. A nurse who values the interpersonal dimensions of nursing would investigate with Ms. Horvath the reasons underlying her inability to make the teaching sessions. This investigation may reveal many reasons, possibly inability to get away from work, fear, feelings of being overwhelmed, or lack of awareness about the importance of the wound care.* ■

The nursing process encourages nurses to work together to help patients use their strengths to meet all their human health needs. This is different from viewing the patient as a "problem to be solved" and interacting mechanically to provide the solution. Working intimately with patients helps

TABLE • 11-2	**EXAMPLES OF GROUPS DEVELOPING STANDARD LANGUAGES (VOCABULARIES)**	
Group Name	**Focus**	**Purpose**
North American Nursing Diagnosis Association (NANDA) International	Diagnoses	Increase the visibility of nursing's contribution to patient care by continuing to develop, refine, and classify phenomena of concern to nurses (see Nursing Diagnosis Quick Reference section) **Web site:** http://www.nanda.org
Nursing Interventions Classification (NIC)	Interventions	Identify, label, validate, and classify actions nurses perform, including direct and indirect care interventions (interventions done directly with patients, for example, teaching, and those done indirectly, for example, obtaining laboratory studies). **Web site:** http://www.nursing.uiowa.edu/excellence/nursing_knowledge/clinical_effectiveness/index.htm
Nursing-Sensitive Outcomes Classification (NOC)	Outcomes	Identify, label, validate, and classify nursing-sensitive patient outcomes and indicators to evaluate the validity and usefulness of the classification, and define and test measurement procedures for the outcomes and indicators. **Web site:** http://www.nursing.uiowa.edu/excellence/nursing_knowledge/clinical_effectiveness/index.htm
Home Health Care Classification (HHCC)	Diagnoses, Interventions, and Outcomes	Provide a structure for documenting and classifying home health and ambulatory care. Consists of two interrelated taxonomies: HHCC of Nursing Diagnoses and HHCC of Nursing Interventions. **Web site:** http://www.sabacare.com
International Classification for Nursing Practice (ICNP®)	Diagnoses, Interventions, and Outcomes	Capture nursing's contributions to health and provide a framework into which existing vocabularies and classifications can be cross-mapped, enabling comparison of nursing data from various countries throughout the world. **Web site:** http://www.icn.ch/icnp.htm
SNOMED CT (Systematized Nomenclature Of Medicine—Clinical Terms)	Comprehensive clinical terminology	Integrate, link, and map terms from various disciplines such as medicine, nursing, and occupational therapy. **Web site:** http://www.nlm.nih.gov/research/umls/Snomed/snomed_main.html

From Alfaro-LeFevre, R. (2010). *Applying nursing process: A tool for critical thinking* (7th ed., p. 100). Philadelphia: Lippincott Williams & Wilkins. Used with permission.

Through the Eyes of a Student

My first experience with an open wound was with a woman who had a stage IV sacral decubitus. I needed to do a dressing change with packing. I was fearful of what the wound would look like. I thought for sure I was going to be "grossed out," and I was—not by the appearance of the wound, but by the odor. The stench was awful! I started to feel queasy and began to sweat, and I thought I was going to pass out and fall right over on the patient. While I was packing the wound, I kept thinking that I was never going to get out of that room. I looked over at my clinical instructor and searched her face for approval of my technique, and I wondered if she also smelled anything and if it was making her feel sick too!

After the procedure was over and I left the room, I asked my instructor if all wounds smell that awful and would the

smell always make me feel sick. Her response was that sometimes an odor will be really bad, and it might make me feel sick. With this kind of reassurance, I thought this is it—I never want to smell that again, and no way do I want to be a nurse.

Later, I realized that I had forgotten there was someone else in that room: the patient. She had to stay in there with that wound and its odor. It was for this reason I changed my mind about leaving nursing. I remembered that it was wanting to help patients to deal with their wounds that made me decide to be a nurse in the first place.

—*Barbara L. Dlugosz*
Holy Family College, Philadelphia, PA

nurses to explore their own strengths and limitations and to develop themselves personally and professionally.

Outcome Oriented

The nursing process offers a means for nurses and patients to work together to identify specific outcomes related to health promotion, disease and illness prevention, health restoration, and coping with altered functioning; to determine which outcomes are most important to the patient; and to match them with the appropriate nursing actions. When these outcomes are recorded in the plan of care and prioritized, each nurse can quickly determine the patient's priorities and begin nursing with a clear sense of how to proceed. The patient benefits from continuity of care, and each nurse's care moves the patient closer to outcome achievement.

Universally Applicable in Nursing Situations

The one constant in healthcare is change. When nurses have a working knowledge of the nursing process, they find that

FIGURE 11-3. Nurses focus on people, not problems or tasks. The nursing process is patient-centered, not task-centered.

they can practice nursing with well or ill people, young or old, in any type of practice setting. The student's efforts to master the nursing process result in possession of a valuable tool that can be used with ease in any nursing situation.

It should be clear from the preceding discussion that the nursing process provides a framework for all the nurse's activities. In each nurse–patient interaction, it is important to assess the patient, note any significant alterations in health status, determine whether the nursing action is helping the patient achieve his or her goals, and modify the plan of care as necessary. Thus, the nurse who feeds a child through a special tube as ordered by a physician continually assesses how the child is responding to the feeding and whether the child or family will be able to manage the feedings independently when the child is discharged. Depending on the results of the nursing assessment, new nursing diagnoses might be needed, along with related additions to the plan of care. The nursing process offers direction for all the activities carried out by the nurse when caring for patients.

Problem Solving and the Nursing Process

One of the strengths of the nursing process is that it is based on a methodology that is familiar to most nursing students—problem solving. Problem solving is a basic life skill; identifying a problem and then taking steps to resolve it are a matter of common sense. However, different approaches to problem solving yield different results, some of which are more successful than others.

Trial-and-Error Problem Solving

Trial-and-error problem solving involves testing any number of solutions until one is found that works for that particular problem. This method is not efficient for the nurse and can be dangerous to the patient; it is, therefore, not recommended as a guide for nursing practice. For example, although you might enjoy experimenting with different types of ethnic food as you discover and develop personal food preferences, you would not want to use the trial-and-error method of determining food preferences for a dehydrated and malnourished patient. You want to know, based on clinical research, exactly what food and fluid supplements are most likely to reverse his or her deficiencies.

> ➤ *Consider Jermaine Byrd, the patient who has returned from vascular surgery and whose posterior tibial pulse cannot be palpated. The nurse might use trial-and-error to determine if the pulse is indeed absent or just difficult to palpate or locate. For example, the nurse might try to reposition the fingers for palpation or apply less pressure during palpation to determine if the pulse can be palpated.* ■

Scientific Problem Solving

Scientific problem solving is a systematic, seven-step, problem-solving process that involves (1) problem identification, (2) data collection, (3) hypothesis formulation, (4) plan of action, (5) hypothesis testing, (6) interpretation of results, and (7) evaluation, resulting in conclusion or revision of the study. This method is used most correctly in a controlled laboratory setting but is closely related to the more general problem-solving processes commonly used by healthcare professionals as they work with patients, such as the nursing process.

> ➤ *Again, think back to Jermaine Byrd, the postoperative patient with a nonpalpable pulse. The nurse would use scientific problem solving to investigate the situation. For example, after attempts at repositioning yield no change, the nurse would collect more data, such as the temperature and the color of the patient's extremity when compared with the opposite leg, existence of pulses above and below the posterior tibial pulse, complaints of pain, numbness or tingling in the extremity, and the patient's overall condition. These findings would lead the nurse to identify if the patient was experiencing vascular compromise, the pulse was difficult to palpate, or the nurse needed more skill in palpation. In addition, the nurse could summon the assistance of another nurse to negate or validate the findings. Once the problem is identified, the nurse would then be able to plan care appropriately to meet the patient's need.* ■

Intuitive Problem Solving

For years, nurse theorists and educators argued that clinical judgments should be based on data alone (the logical, scientific, evidence-based method), in an attempt to establish nursing as a science, worthy of the respect of other professions. Today, nurses acknowledge the role of intuitive thinking in making clinical decisions. Many veteran nurses can describe situations in which an "inner prompting" led to a quick nursing intervention that saved a patient's life. When they directly apprehend a situation based on its similarity or dissimilarity to other situations, they use intuitive problem solving. **Intuitive problem solving** is thus a direct understanding of a situation based on a background of experience, knowledge, and skill that makes expert decision making possible. A recovery room nurse who realizes that a postoperative patient is "going bad" before there are measurable signs to suggest trouble is using intuitive problem solving, as is an oncology nurse who somehow senses the right moment to teach, offer encouragement, affirm, or simply listen.

Advocates of intuition recommend the following:

- Welcoming flashes of intuition as additions to logical reasoning, rather than as disruptions
- Validating intuitions: When an intuition cannot be validated (e.g., when the nurse senses that something is wrong with the patient, although there are no clinical signs), careful monitoring of the patient should be initiated
- Furthering nursing research to help find ways to (1) cultivate intuition and its typical results (accurate and early diagnosis, vigilant monitoring, better patient care) and (2) document the information intuition supplies (Rew, 1987)

Beginning nurses must use nursing knowledge and scientific problem solving as the basis of care they give; intuitive problem solving comes with years of practice and observation. If the beginning nurse has an intuition about a patient, that information should be discussed with the supervisor.

Critical Thinking: Intuitive, Logical, or Both

While this text makes a strong case for clinical reasoning that is logical, scientific, and evidence-based, it also promotes clinical reasoning that is creative and intuitive. Alfaro-LeFevre, an expert in critical thinking, is quick to note that critical thinking is contextual and changes depending on the circumstances. As examples, she cites brainstorming sessions as a good method for nurturing intuition because logical thinking might constrain and block ideas. On the other hand, developing policies, procedures, and plans of care requires more logical, evidence-based thought. In summary, when intuition is used alone, there are increased risks and fewer benefits. Intuition often moves problem solving forward quickly, but it might result in a lot of trial-and-error approaches. Logic is the safest approach, but it doesn't foster out-of-the-box ideas and might inhibit right-brain thinkers from getting started. Pairing intuitive and logical thinkers who have learned specific strategies to promote reasoning (e.g., mind mapping) can bring great results (Alfaro-LeFevre, 2009).

Decision Making and the Nursing Process

Nurses make decisions every day. We decide what to eat, where to work, whether or not to exercise. While some use the problem-solving process and decision-making process synonymously, not all decisions result from problems. Decision making is about choosing from options. Lipe and Beasley (2004) define **decision making** as "purposeful, goal directed effort applied in a systematic way to make a choice among alternatives," and they explain that even choosing not to act in a certain situation is a decision (p. 37). They also emphasize that all decisions have consequences. Since the nurse's decisions about patient care have the power to literally determine how people are born, live, suffer, and die, it is critical for nurses to be skilled in making decisions.

Potential errors in decision making include (Lipe & Beasley, 2004, p. 46):

- *Bias:*
  - Placing excess emphasis on first data received
  - Avoiding information contrary to one's opinion
  - Selecting alternatives to maintain status quo
  - Being predisposed to a single solution
  - Stating the problem in a way to support one's choices
  - Making decisions to support past choices
- *Failure to consider the total situation:*
  - Using inaccurate data
  - Not clearly identifying the problem
  - Failing to prioritize or rank the problems in order of importance
  - Using unrealistic goals
- *Impatience:*
  - Failing to identify multiple solutions
  - Incorrectly implementing the decision
  - Failing to use appropriate resources

Documenting the Nursing Process

The ability to communicate clearly is a critical nursing skill. Accurate, concise, timely, and relevant documentation provides all the members of the caregiving team with a picture of the patient. The patient record is the chief means of communication among members of the interdisciplinary team. Legally speaking, a nursing action not documented is a nursing action not performed. If accused of negligent care, a nurse might tell the court that she faithfully assessed the patient's needs, diagnosed problems, and implemented and evaluated an effective plan of care. However, unless the patient's health records contain documentation supporting her claims, the court has no reason to accept her word rather than that of the patient or family who are claiming that such care was not given.

Each chapter in this unit offers specific documentation guidelines for nursing process activities; Chapter 17 discusses documentation in general. It is helpful to practice documentation while learning any given nursing activity; like any other nursing skill, documentation improves with practice. Examples of nursing documentation, nursing assessments, plans of care, and notes are provided throughout this text.

Benefits of the Nursing Process

When used well, the nursing process achieves for the patient scientifically based, holistic, individualized care;

the opportunity to work collaboratively with nurses; and continuity of care. Nurses who use the nursing process in a thoughtful and systematic way achieve a clear, efficient, and cost-effective plan of action by which the entire nursing team can achieve the best results for patients; the satisfaction that they are making an important "difference" in the lives of their patients; and the opportunity to grow professionally as they evaluate the effectiveness of interventions and variables that contribute positively or negatively to the patient's achievement of valued outcomes. See Box 11-1 for an example of the nursing process in action. The accompanying Promoting Health Literacy box is another example of how nurses can make a difference.

Box 11-1 EXAMPLE OF THE NURSING PROCESS IN ACTION

Assessing
You are checking on a patient who had abdominal surgery yesterday and hear that the patient has considerable pain. "It kept me up all night." The patient has been reluctant to ask for any pain medication, fearing effect of the drug. "I don't want to become a junkie." The patient's blood pressure and pulse rate are slightly elevated.

Diagnosing
You analyze the data above and write the nursing diagnosis: *Unrelieved pain related to a fear of taking pain-relieving medications.* The patient agrees that this is becoming a problem.

Outcome Identification and Planning
You decide to work with the patient to achieve the outcome: *By 3:00 p.m., patient reports sufficient relief of pain to enable him to rest and to get out of bed to go to the bathroom.* The patient wants to accomplish the outcome. You identify teaching as the primary nursing intervention.

Implementing
After asking the patient about his experiences with pain-relieving medications, you explain that although many of these drugs are addictive when abused, there is no harm if they are taken as prescribed postoperatively. You also explain that it is important for him to experience enough pain relief to be able to cough and deep breathe, ambulate, and do other things important to his recovery. You suggest that the medication will be most effective if taken before his pain peaks and becomes intense. You administer the prescribed medication for pain when the patient indicates that he is willing to give it a try.

Evaluating
After enough time has elapsed for the medication to take effect, you check back with the patient to evaluate whether he has obtained relief and met his outcome. If the patient is satisfied and you both feel comfort is no longer a problem, you terminate the plan of care for this diagnosis. If the patient still feels pain or is dissatisfied with the medication, each of the preceding steps of the nursing process is re-evaluated, and necessary changes are made in the plan of care.

Promoting Health Literacy

IN PATIENTS AND FAMILIES WITH ASTHMA

Patient Scenario

Your mom calls to tell you that your neighbor back home spent the night in the emergency room with her 3-year-old son Bobby, whom you used to baby sit. When Bobby experienced chest tightness and shortness of breath, his pediatrician recommended a quick trip to the local emergency room. For the present, Bobby's parents are comforted that he was able to be discharged and is now breathing easier. They were terrified, however, to learn that he may have asthma and wanted your opinion on what they should do. They have an appointment scheduled with their pediatrician.

Nursing Considerations: *Tips for Improving Health Literacy*

Call Bobby's mom and give her an information sheet about childhood asthma and tips on finding out more

information about the disease online from a credible source. Explain that it is a potentially serious disorder if not treated properly but with good management children are able to sleep, learn, and play. Encourage her to follow the pediatrician's recommendations and to be prepared to ask her pediatrician three questions:

- What is Bobby's main problem?
- What do they need to do?
- Why is it important for them to do this?

What additional measures can you take to help increase health literacy in this patient/family? What other measures would be helpful if Bobby's parents do not speak English, cannot read, or have other learning deficits?

Evaluating the Use of the Nursing Process

The chapters that follow in this unit describe each step of the nursing process in detail. Student nurses beginning to use the nursing process should evaluate their growing skill in using the nursing process correctly. Box 11-2 presents a checklist to help evaluate this personal skill in using the nursing process.

BLENDED SKILLS AND CRITICAL THINKING

The primary purpose of the nursing process is to help nurses manage each patient's care scientifically, holistically, and creatively. To do this successfully, the nurse needs many cognitive, technical, interpersonal, and ethical/legal skills, along with the willingness to use them creatively and critically when working with patients to promote or restore health, to prevent disease or illness, and to facilitate coping with altered functioning.

Before studying each step of the nursing process in more depth, it is useful to look at the skills essential to nursing practice. Understanding their importance helps the student work consciously to develop them while beginning to master the nursing process. Cognitive and technical skills equip nurses to manage the clinical problems stemming from the patient's changing health or illness state. Interpersonal and ethical skills are essential, however, for nurses concerned about the patient's broader well-being.

Few nurses excel naturally in all four of these skills, and even experienced nurses continue working on becoming more proficient in the skills that lead to excellence. These skills are first introduced and defined in Chapter 1. The remainder of this chapter focuses on development of these skills and how they are used successfully within the nursing

process. To highlight the importance of these skills, each chapter in this text contains a feature entitled *Reflective Practice: Developing Blended Skills*. These displays are written by nursing students.

Developing Cognitive Skills

Cognitively skilled nurses are critical thinkers. **Critical thinking** is defined as "a systematic way to form and shape one's thinking. It functions purposefully and exactly. It is thought that is disciplined, comprehensive, based on intellectual standards, and, as a result, well-reasoned" (Paul, 1993, p. 20). Paul's four domains of critical thinking (Box 11-3) include elements of thought (the basic building blocks of thinking), abilities (the skills essential to higher-order thinking), affective dimensions, and intellectual standards. Central to Paul's work are carefully delineated standards, potential problems, and principles. The exercises below should help you to develop the ability to think critically in professional practice.

Developing the Method of Critical Thinking

Nurses who wish to develop the critical thinking skills essential to quality nursing practice will find it helpful when posed with a thinking challenge to work methodically through a set of five types of considerations. These are the purpose of thinking, adequacy of knowledge, potential problems, helpful resources, and critique of judgment/decision.

PURPOSE OF THINKING

The first step when thinking critically about a situation is to identify the purpose or goal of your thinking. This helps to

Box 11-2   CHECKLIST FOR EVALUATING YOUR USE OF THE NURSING PROCESS

Assessing

- [ ] The initial database is obtained by means of a nursing history and nursing examination.
- [ ] Assessment data are documented:
  - [ ] Accurately—Questionable data are validated.
  - [ ] Completely—Use of a systematic guide ensures that recorded data describe (1) the patient's functional ability to meet each basic human need, and (2) responses to health and illness.
  - [ ] Concisely—Irrelevant data and meaningless generalizations are avoided.
  - [ ] Factually—Patient behaviors are recorded rather than the nurse's interpretation of these behaviors.
  - [ ] Timely—Current data are recorded for the team.
- [ ] The initial database communicates a "real sense" of the patient that makes possible individualized care.
- [ ] Focused assessment data are recorded for each patient problem.
- [ ] Data collection and documentation are ongoing and responsive to changes in the patient's condition.

Diagnosing

- [ ] A prioritized list of nursing diagnoses is on the plan of care.
- [ ] Each nursing diagnosis describes an actual or potential patient health problem that independent nursing intervention can prevent or resolve. Each nursing diagnosis:
  - [ ] Is derived from an accurate and validated interpretation of a cluster of significant patient data or "cues"
  - [ ] Contains a precise problem statement describing what is unhealthy about the patient and what needs to change—suggests patient goals
  - [ ] Identifies factors that contribute to the problem (etiology)—these suggest nursing interventions
  - [ ] Uses nonjudgmental language and is written using legally advisable terms
- [ ] Old nursing diagnoses are deleted from the plan of care once resolved, and new diagnoses are added as soon as identified.

Outcome Identification and Planning

- [ ] A comprehensive, individualized, and up-to-date plan of care that specifies patient outcomes and nursing orders for each nursing diagnosis is developed with the assistance of the patient and family.
- [ ] Planning is comprehensive:
  - [ ] Initial

- [ ] Ongoing
- [ ] Discharge
- [ ] Long-term goals alert the entire nursing team to realistic patient expectations after discharge.
- [ ] Short-term outcomes:
  - [ ] When achieved, demonstrate a resolution of the problem specified in the nursing diagnosis
  - [ ] Describe a single, observable, and measurable patient behavior
  - [ ] Are valued by the patient and family
  - [ ] Are realistic in terms of the resources of the patient and the nurse
- [ ] Nursing orders:
  - [ ] Clearly and concisely describe the nursing intervention to be performed (ongoing assessment; nursing treatments and procedures; teaching, counseling, advocacy)
  - [ ] Are individualized to the patient
  - [ ] Are consistent with standards of care and supportive of other therapies
  - [ ] Are effective in accomplishing the desired patient outcomes
- [ ] The plan of care encourages patient and family participation.

Implementing

- [ ] The patient record contains daily documentation of the nursing measures used to (1) assist the patient to meet basic human needs, (2) resolve health problems, and (3) implement select aspects of the medical plan of care.
- [ ] The plan of care is implemented:
  - [ ] Competently
  - [ ] Confidently
  - [ ] Caringly
  - [ ] Creatively

Evaluating

- [ ] Evaluative statements are recorded on the plan of care to document the patient's level of outcome achievement at targeted times.
- [ ] Ongoing evaluation of the patient's responses to the plan of care are used to make decisions about terminating, continuing, or modifying nursing care.

---

discipline your thinking by directing all thoughts toward the goal. The purpose of critical thinking might be to make a judgment about a particular patient or situation or to make a decision about how best to intervene.

ADEQUACY OF KNOWLEDGE

At the outset of critical thinking, it is important for you to judge whether the knowledge you have is accurate, complete, factual, timely, and relevant. If you reason with false information or a lack of important data, it is impossible to draw a sound conclusion. You also want to be sure that you understand all the details relevant to the issue. What is at stake? How much time do you have to make a decision? How much room is there for error?

> *Consider Addie Warner, the patient described as "demanding" by the nursing staff. Rather than accept the staff's description, the nurse answers the patient's call light, thereby obtaining information from which to make an informed decision.* ∎

POTENTIAL PROBLEMS

As you become skilled in critical thinking, you will learn to "flag" and remedy the pitfalls to sound reasoning. Common problems include working with untested or faulty assumptions, accepting an unproven claim or line of argument, allowing bias to color your thinking, and reasoning

Box 11-3   THE FOUR DOMAINS OF CRITICAL THINKING

I. Elements of Thought: The Basic Building Blocks of Thinking

Element	Fundamental Standard	Potential Problems	Principle
Purpose	1. Clarity of purpose 2. Significance of purpose 3. Achievability of purpose 4. Consistency of purpose	1. Unclear purpose 2. Trivial purpose 3. Unrealistic purpose 4. Contradictory purposes	All reasoning has a purpose.
Question at issue or central problem	1. Clarity of question 2. Significance of question 3. Answerability 4. Relevance	1. Unclear 2. Insignificant 3. Not answerable 4. Irrelevant	To settle a question, you must understand what it requires.
Point of view	1. Flexibility in point of view 2. Fairness of point of view 3. Clarity of point of view 4. Breadth of point of view	1. Restricted 2. Biased 3. Unclear 4. Narrow	Reasoning is better when multiple, relevant points of view are sought out, articulated clearly, empathized with fairly and logically, applied consistently and dispassionately.
Empirical dimension	1. Clear evidence 2. Relevant information 3. Fairly gathered and reported evidence 4. Accurate data 5. Adequate evidence 6. Consistently applied data	1. Unclear 2. Unfairly or self-servingly gathered 3. Inaccurate 4. Insufficient	Reasoning can only be as sound as the evidence it is based on.
Concepts and ideas	1. Clarity of concepts 2. Relevance of concepts 3. Depth of concepts 4. Neutrality of concepts	1. Unclear 2. Irrelevant 3. Superficial 4. Biased	Reasoning can only be as clear, relevant, and deep as the concepts that shape it.
Assumptions	1. Clarity of assumptions 2. Justifiability of assumptions 3. Consistency of assumptions	1. Unclear 2. Unjustified 3. Contradictory	Reasoning can only be as sound as the assumptions it makes.
Implications and consequences	1. Significance of implications 2. Realistic nature of implications 3. Clarity of articulated implications 4. Precision of articulated implications 5. Completeness of articulated implications	1. Unimportant 2. Unrealistic 3. Unclear 4. Imprecise 5. Incomplete	To reason through an issue or decision, you must understand the implications and consequences that follow from it.

II. Abilities: The Skills Essential to Higher-Order Thinking

- Ability to evaluate the credibility of sources of information
- Ability to analyze arguments, interpretations, beliefs, or theories
- Ability to clarify the meaning of words and phrases
- Ability to transfer insights into new contexts
- Ability to generate and assess possible solutions
- Ability to develop criteria for evaluation: clarify values and standards
- Ability to read, listen, write, and speak critically

III. Affective Dimensions: The Attitudes, Dispositions, Passions, and Traits of Mind Essential to Higher-Order Thinking in Real Settings

- Thinking independently
- Exercising fair-mindedness
- Developing insight into egocentricity and sociocentricity
- Developing intellectual humility and suspending judgment
- Developing intellectual courage
- Developing intellectual good faith and integrity
- Developing intellectual perseverance
- Developing confidence in reason
- Developing intellectual curiosity

IV. Intellectual Standards: The Standards Used to Critique Higher-Order Thinking

Clear	Precise
Specific	Accurate
Relevant	Plausible
Consistent	Logical
Deep	Broad
Complete	Significant
Adequate (for purpose)	Fair

Content from Paul, R. W. (1993). *Critical thinking: How to prepare students for a rapidly changing world* (pp.123–132). Santa Rosa, CA: Foundation for Critical Thinking. Used with permission.

illogically, such as making a generalization on the basis of a single experience or case, or allowing emotion to rule reason. The more familiar you are with these common impediments to critical thinking, the easier it is to detect them in your own thinking.

HELPFUL RESOURCES

Wise professionals are quick to recognize their limits and to seek help in remedying their deficiencies. Experienced clinicians know that learning is continuous and expect their practice to present challenges that demand new knowledge. Critical thinkers know what help they need to assist their reasoning and what resources to tap. Key resources include experienced clinicians, texts and journals, institutional policies and procedures, and professional groups and writings.

CRITIQUE OF JUDGMENT/DECISION

Ultimately, you must identify alternative judgments or decisions, weigh the merits of each, and reach a conclusion. It is helpful to try to predict the consequences of your major options before concluding your reasoning. You will also want to evaluate the alternative you selected as your decision begins to influence your actions.

After using this method to work through an intellectually challenging situation, critique your use of the method in light of the **standards for critical thinking:** clear, precise, specific, accurate, relevant, plausible, consistent, logical, deep, broad, complete, significant, adequate (for the purpose), and fair.

FOCUSED CRITICAL THINKING GUIDES

Focused Critical Thinking Guide 11-1 illustrates the use of these five considerations to facilitate critical thinking about a care dilemma experienced by a nursing student. The merits of thinking critically about which of the options is most likely to meet that patient's needs are readily apparent. Because nurses are accountable for the well-being of their patients, sloppy reasoning is both dangerous and inexcusable—even for someone new to nursing and clinical practice. Other examples of this method are found throughout the book.

Developing the Attitudes and Dispositions to Think Critically

Certain habitual dispositions are needed by anyone who wants to be a critical thinker. Some of the most important of these are described below. Review this list, and assess the degree to which the dispositions characterize your thinking.

THINKING INDEPENDENTLY

Nurses who are independent thinkers are careful not to allow the status quo or a persuasive individual to control their thinking.

> *Remember Addie Warner, the elderly woman who was considered to be demanding by the staff? The nurse demonstrated independent thinking by not accepting the staff's description of the patient. Rather, the nurse confronted the situation, obtained information, and then acted based on this information.* ∎

When confronted with an intellectual challenge, such as "Why is this patient so resistant to change?," they proceed cautiously, consulting with the patient and respected colleagues and reviewing the literature. Only then do they reach a clinical judgment. Compare this with a nurse who makes a snap judgment that a patient is "unreasonable" based on the comments of one nurse—even if this nurse is the nurse manager.

> *Recall Charlotte Horvath, the single mother needing wound care teaching? A nurse who is not an independent thinker might quickly assume that Ms. Horvath just wasn't interested in caring for her child at home. Conversely, the nurse who is an independent thinker would investigate the situation further before making a decision.* ∎

BEING FAIR-MINDED

Nurses who are fair-minded are open to different points of view and hear all sides of an argument before making a judgment. When a patient complains about another nurse or a physician, a fair-minded nurse seeks to validate the complaint and talks with the person being complained about before reaching a decision. A fair-minded thinker recognizes the limits of being egocentric ("It's right because this is what I think!") and sociocentric ("It's right because this is the way Americans—or Philadelphians—think!").

BEING INTELLECTUALLY HUMBLE

One can easily differentiate between nurses who are convinced that "they know it all" and those who are open and willing to learn. Intellectually humble nurses are learning all the time, often from patients and their nonprofessional caregivers, other colleagues, and the media. Never be afraid to say, "I don't know the answer to that question, but I'll be happy to talk with you after I've had time to research the topic."

BEING INTELLECTUALLY COURAGEOUS

Nurses who are intellectually courageous are not afraid to challenge the status quo and "go against the flow." They resist the comment "But we've always done it that way here . . ." when their experience or intuition suggests that another way might be better. They are not afraid to ask, "Is there something we might be able to do differently that would help this patient or situation?"

DEMONSTRATING GOOD FAITH AND INTEGRITY

Commitment to integrity helps nurses who are critical thinkers remain sensitive to discrepancies in the way one

FOCUSED CRITICAL THINKING GUIDE • 11-1

Western vs. Alternative Medicine

You are a nursing student. Your friend, Amy Chang, confides to you that she is very worried about her grandmother. When you meet Mrs. Chang, she demonstrates many of the assessment findings related to heart failure. Although her family has entreated her to seek medical attention, Mrs. Chang insists on relying on herbal teas and traditional Chinese remedies. Now 88 years old, Mrs. Chang came to America from mainland China when she was 14. Although she raised a family that is now thoroughly "Americanized," Mrs. Chang has resisted embracing her new culture and now wants nothing to do with "American medicine." Amy, who is also a nursing student, loves her grandmother dearly and is frustrated by her stubborn refusal to see an internist. Both of you have reason to believe that she could be helped by medical attention. What do you do?

1. Identify Goal of Thinking

Clarify your thinking about alternative medicine so that you can decide how you ought to respond to Mrs. Chang's worsening physical condition.

2. Assess Adequacy of Knowledge

Pertinent circumstances: Although you have strong reason to believe that Mrs. Chang is suffering from congestive heart failure, she has not been medically diagnosed, and you lack definitive knowledge about her medical condition and the likelihood that she would respond to treatment. You know that she places a high value on traditional Chinese culture and strongly believes that if she is to be healed, the healing will result from herbal teas and traditional Chinese remedies. She has no confidence in American medicine. Her family describes her as being extremely strong-willed and very lovable. You do not know if she has the benefit of seeing a competent practitioner of Chinese medicine.

Prerequisite knowledge: To decide how you should respond in this situation, you need to know that traditional Western medicine is not the only beneficial system of medicine. It would be helpful for you and Mrs. Chang's family to learn more about Chinese medicine and the probability of its benefiting her (as well as the possibility of its harming her) in her present condition. You will also need to learn more about what is essential to Mrs. Chang's well-being. How much value does she place on physical health? How important is it for her to live (and possibly die) within the familiar and comforting boundaries of her culture? You will want to assess what teaching, counseling, and support Mrs. Chang needs to reach an informed and voluntary decision that is right for her.

Room for error: Because Mrs. Chang's life may literally be at stake, there is not much room for error in the manner you and her family choose to respond. Even if her condition is not life-threatening, her sense of well-being may be severely threatened if she feels forced to pursue treatment that is alien and frightening.

Time constraints: Although you are uncertain about the seriousness of her condition, you understand that the sooner Mrs. Chang receives effective therapy, the better. Unless her condition suddenly deteriorates, this is not a decision that needs to be made within the next 24 hours.

3. Address Potential Problems

The most serious obstacle to critical thinking in this situation would be an inability to weigh the respective merits of alternative healing systems. Cultural bias may result in the untested assumption that American medicine is necessarily superior to all other systems of healing and that it would be morally wrong to support a choice of anything else. The love of Mrs. Chang's family and their desire to do everything possible to keep her well may interfere with their ability to allow her the freedom to make the choice that is right for her.

4. Consult Helpful Resources

Your first challenge will be to learn more about traditional Chinese medicine by consulting with local authorities and available literature. The National Institutes of Health have now established an Office of Alternative Medicine, which may provide helpful information and which is easily accessed through their website. Your most important resource may be Mrs. Chang herself, and it will be important to try to learn from her as much as you can about what she values and what her goals are at this point in her life. You will also want to be sure that Mrs. Chang has the benefits of a competent practitioner of Chinese medicine.

5. Critique Judgment/Decision

After getting to know Mrs. Chang better, you realize that she is firmly committed to her ways and adamant about not going to an American doctor or into a hospital at this point of her life. Thus, you (with her family) have only two options: to force her to see an internist against her will, possibly deceiving her to get her to the internist's office, or to support her choice to rely on familiar remedies, which may or may not successfully resolve her problems. The first alternative may save her life, and her family can see no other choice. You realize that by making this choice, the family is imposing its values on Mrs. Chang and violating her autonomy, her right to determine the course of her life. You decide to support her and to try to explain to her family the importance of doing this. You understand that if her condition is serious and her traditional remedies prove ineffective, her death may be hastened, but she accepts this consequence and prefers it to embracing an alien and frightening culture.

reasons in different situations and with different people. This sensitivity, for example, might result in our mind "throwing out a red flag" when it catches us reasoning unfairly.

BEING CURIOUS AND PERSEVERING

Nurses who persevere intellectually resist "easy answers." When the answer to "Why is this patient so resistant to change?" comes back "Oh, that's just the way he is," the persevering nurse keeps questioning: "But why is he that way? What experiences, values, or beliefs have made him so resistant? Until we understand these things, we won't be able to help him!"

BEING DISCIPLINED

Nurses who are disciplined are thorough and take the time necessary to reach well-reasoned conclusions. When an initial conclusion or judgment does not "feel right," they are willing to go back to try to reason out a better judgment. They consult wise colleagues and are not afraid of doing the hard work of critical thinking.

BEING CREATIVE

Thinking critically might mean "thinking outside the box." The solution to a challenge might involve resources as yet untapped, effective, and cost-saving interventions as yet undiscovered and untried. The process of brainstorming might bring out, along with unworkable options, one or two realistic suggestions that would not have surfaced otherwise.

DEMONSTRATING CONFIDENCE

Nurses who routinely think critically develop confidence in their judgments and are not afraid to take and defend a position. When challenged by a patient or colleague to defend a course of action, they can reply with confidence, "I am doing it this way because research (or reason) convinced me that this is the best course of action."

Developing Technical Skills

Some people are naturally "good with their hands" and quickly master intricate procedures that involve working with technical equipment. Others have to practice procedures many times before they feel competent handling the equipment and performing clinical activities independently. Whatever your natural technical skill, you can help master the manual skills essential in the nursing process by developing the following habits:

- When a procedure demands manual dexterity, practice the necessary skill until you feel confident in its execution before attempting to perform it with a patient.
- Take time to familiarize yourself with new equipment before using it in a clinical procedure. Understand how it works and what supplies are needed to ensure optimal functioning. If possible, anticipate problems and know how to remedy them.
- Identify nurses who are technical experts, and ask them to share their secrets. Many experienced clinicians have

developed quality, time-saving techniques they are willing to share.
- Never be ashamed to ask for help when feeling unsure of how to perform a procedure or manage equipment. Don't overlook the patient or family caregiver as a source of helpful hints for care they routinely provide. Never forget that the patient's well-being and sometimes the patient's life depend on your technical competence.

Many nursing procedures are described in the clinical chapters in this text. Performance checklists break each procedure down into its component parts, allowing you to evaluate your performance of each step of the procedure. This type of self-knowledge enables you to identify quickly and remedy recurrent deficiencies in technical skills.

Developing Interpersonal Skills

Interpersonal skills are essential to the practice of nursing. Interpersonal caring involves promoting the dignity and respect of patients as people and establishing a caring relationship. As a result, both the nurse and patient experience mutual enrichment.

Promoting Human Dignity and Respect

Nurses committed to respecting the human dignity of patients find it helpful to reflect on the following questions:

- What obligates me to respect patients' human dignity? Must all patients be respected equally? Are some patients more deserving of respect? Can a patient ever forfeit the right to be respected?
- What does it mean to respect the dignity of patients? What are five concrete ways I can demonstrate respect?
- What are my strengths and deficiencies when it comes to respecting patients?
- In what ways (if any) must I change to be faithful to the duty of respecting the dignity of patients?
- What patients most challenge my ability to give care respectfully? How do I respond to this challenge? What does this teach me for the future?

Nurses often underestimate their power to help a patient heal simply through their respectful and caring presence. Each time a nurse walks into a room, he or she communicates one of two messages: (1) "You are a job to be done. You mean nothing to me." or (2) "You are a person of worth, and I care about you." Even a 60-second nurse–patient interaction can enhance or jeopardize human well-being. It is important for nurses to be sensitive to what their looks, speech, and touch communicate to patients and colleagues. The more vulnerable the patient and the more threatened the patient's sense of self, the more powerful effect the nurse's message has on the recipient's sense of worth and well-being.

> *Consider Addie Warner, the patient described in the Reflective Practice display. Imagine the message that she received from the staff when she used her call light to ask*

for help. Most likely, the message conveyed was negative. Compare this to the message communicated by the nursing student who helped get her out of bed and get washed, a more positive message supporting the patient's self-worth. ∎

The learning activity in Box 11-4 was developed for nurses caring for older patients in a nursing home. To help develop interpersonal skills, try these activities with a friend. Take turns being both the nurse and the older adult, and talk about how different types of nursing presence makes you feel.

Establishing Caring Relationships

Increasingly, nurses report that new systems of care and the demand to work "harder, faster, and smarter" to keep up in today's competitive healthcare arena are making traditional nurse–patient relationships difficult to attain. As you begin your nursing practice, ask yourself what priority you assign

to caring. Nurses who accept that there can be no excellence in nursing in the absence of this relationship commit themselves to finding creative means to establish caring relationships. Obviously, many variables influence the quality of relationships that are possible, not the least of which is the acuity level of the patient and the patient's length of stay. Helpful reflection questions include the following:

- Do I know my patients well enough to promote anything more than their physical well-being?
- If asked to describe a patient, would I be able to report on anything other than the patient's physical condition?
- Is the care I routinely provide really holistic, individualized, prioritized according to medical need and the patient's interests, and continuous? Do my care plans reflect this?
- What does the content of the patient report and nursing documentation communicate about nursing priorities in my practice setting?

Box 11-4 DEVELOPING INTERPERSONAL SKILLS

Human Dignity: How Who I Am as a Caregiver Affects Others

Description
The purpose of this exercise is to explore the notion of "therapeutic use of self." You will be challenged to reflect on the effect your looks, speech, and touch have on other people. Role play and guided discovery will be used to enable you to experience the affirming and negating influences of different means of human relating.

Objectives
Upon conclusion of this exercise, you will be able to:
1. Demonstrate how looks, words, and touch can be used to harm or benefit others
2. Describe how the way you approach others enhances or diminishes their well-being
3. Identify one care behavior you plan to modify to improve your nursing practice

Learning Activities
Invite an experienced nurse to demonstrate how looks, words, and touch can be used to communicate two different messages to others: "You are a job to be done; you mean nothing to me"; and "You are precious, and I care about you." After the demonstration, team up with another student, and experience giving and receiving these messages. Share the feelings you both experienced. After these preliminary exercises, role play the suggested nursing situations (or others of your choosing), and once again process the experience. Talk about the relevance of this experience to human interaction in general, and conclude the exercise by writing a goal for your practice.

Worksheet
A. Practice looking at a colleague two different ways:
   1. "You are a job to be done; you mean nothing to me" look
   2. "You are precious, and I care about you" look
B. Practice speaking to a colleague in two different ways:
   1. Indifferent: "Your resident, your light."
   2. Helpful: "I think Mrs. Jones' light is on again. Do you need help?"
C. Practice touching a colleague in two different ways:
   1. Indifferent: Pick up your colleague's wrist and feel for a pulse.
   2. Using warm lotion, massage your colleague's hands.
D. Talk about how each of the above looks, words, and touches made you feel. Talk about how you think they make patients or residents feel.
E. Role play each of the situations below in two different ways, trying to incorporate looks, words, and touches that communicate:
   First time: You are a job to be done; you mean nothing to me.
   Second time: You are precious, and I care about you.
   1. Student feels overwhelmed by patient care assignment and approaches clinical instructor to discuss her options.
   2. Student walks into patient's room to begin morning care.
   3. Student assists elderly patient to stand and ambulate around room.
   4. Student brings medication to patient.
   5. Student approaches another student and asks for help changing the bed linens of an obese patient who is on complete bed rest.
F. Name one thing you have decided to try to do differently when you take care of your patients as a result of this session.
G. Does what you experienced today have any implications for who you are when you are not nursing?

Through the Eyes of a Patient

I recently spent 2 months in a university teaching hospital while doctors tried to find a way to regulate my heart beats. Many of the days were filled with tests, some of which were frightening. I was given many drugs—most of which turned out not to be helpful. I was a 2-hour car ride away from my home, family, and friends—which meant there wasn't always a familiar face at my bedside.

I quickly learned I could judge what kind of day I was going to have as soon as I saw my nurse each morning. All of them brought my medicines and helped with the treatment plan. With some nurses, however, I also experienced the comfort and security of knowing that my expressed needs would be promptly and respectfully tended to. If I needed help getting up to the bathroom or asked for something for pain, I could count on help coming quickly. And finally there were those few with whom I knew I was going to have a great day because they would "make it happen" no matter how sick I was feeling. These were the nurses who offered a hug with their medicines, who had a moment to sit and listen, who teased about the "fashion statements" I was making with my nightgowns, and who "walked me through" new tests so that at least I felt better prepared to face the unknown. Most often, it wasn't what they did but how they did it.

I wish all nurses understood the power they have to influence a patient's basic sense of well-being. A hospital can be a pretty scary, lonely place. Nurses can make all the difference!

—Mildred Taylor, Pine Grove, PA

- What are my strengths and deficiencies in creating caring relationships?
- In what ways (if any) must I change to establish better caring relationships?

Nurses committed to caring relationships routinely use opportunities for conversation to communicate genuine interest in who the patient is and what the patient is experiencing to provide meaningful nursing assistance. For example, rather than just "chattering" aimlessly with a talkative patient, a nurse skilled in developing caring relationships will direct the conversation. Leading statements or questions that are often successful in eliciting useful information from older patients include the following:

- "Tell me something about your life at home. What do you miss most now that you are here?"
- "What family members and friends do you see most often? Who do you think knows you best and you would trust to speak for you if you were ever unable to speak for yourself?"
- "Most of us have some goal or dream that keeps us going. It might be owning our own home, seeing some relationship patched up, or being able to celebrate the birth of a grandchild. What is your dream?"
- "When you've had troubles in the past, what did you draw on for strength? What keeps you going?"
- "Looks like you've got a lot of time for thinking these days . . . would you like to share what's been on your mind?"
- "Looks like we'll be spending some time together . . . what would you like to do with this time? How may I help you?"
- "What would you like us to know that will help us to better meet your needs?"
- "Hospitals can be scary places . . . how can I help you?"

Nurses who are sensitive to the well-being of their patients can find many ways to communicate caring. Happily, most caring is mutually enriching, and nurses who care find themselves re-energized for the more demanding aspects of their practice. Read one patient's account of the importance to her of nurse caring in the accompanying box, Through the Eyes of a Patient.

Enjoying the Rewards of Mutual Interchange

In any helping profession, but especially in nursing, countless opportunities exist to interact with others. Those committed to interpersonal caring enrich everyday interactions by investing them with something of themselves and, in return, receiving something of the other, as shown in Figure 11-4. Think of your last encounter with a patient. Whether you were administering a medication, checking vital signs, or preparing the patient for discharge, you had the choice of merely accomplishing the given task or accomplishing the task while simultaneously communicating a personal gift of support, caring, strength, and peacefulness. Frequently overlooked, these interpersonal gifts might contribute to a patient's healing as significantly as medical interventions.

FIGURE 11-4. Interpersonal caring enriches the lives of everyone participating, providing a mutual exchange of giving and receiving.

Rather than deplete their giver, these interpersonal gifts invite similar gifts from the recipient, which in return enrich the caregiver. Nothing causes burnout faster than a practice that is reduced to the performance of multiple tasks stripped of their human significance. When a patient is given care in a way that "makes a difference" in terms of his or her well-being, the patient's gratitude, even when unspoken, helps renew the nurse's energy. Too seldom do we stop our busy practices long enough to reflect on how who we are that day is influencing the well-being of those receiving our care. It is helpful to question:

- How conscious am I of how my mood influences the well-being of others?
- Have I ever consciously tried to transmit strength, peace, support, or joy to another? What were the results?
- Am I aware of any situation in which my fatigue, anxiety, frustration, or negativity was communicated to a patient in a manner that negatively influenced his or her well-being?
- Am I conscious of ways in which patients enrich me personally or enrich my practice?
- In what ways is my practice different when I am attuned to the interpersonal dimensions of nurse–patient interactions?
- In what ways must my practice change if I am to facilitate healing by willing something of my essence to patients?

Developing Ethical/Legal Skills

Nurses who prize their role in securing patient well-being are sensitive to the ethical and legal implications of nursing practice. Chapters 6 and 7 describe essential components of ethical and legal competence for nurses. Although it can take years to master effective patient advocacy skills and to become proficient in mediating ethical conflict, even beginning nurses are responsible for certain basic ethical skills. For example, one of the greatest challenges nursing students face is balancing the competing demands of home life, school, and the hospital or practice setting. Learning to be true to oneself, to the patients for whom one is responsible, to the caregiving team, and to the profession and society is an ongoing struggle. Examining one's sense of accountability is crucial as one assumes professional responsibilities.

Developing Accountability

Nurses committed to interpersonal caring hold themselves accountable for the human well-being of patients entrusted to their care. Being accountable means being attentive and responsive to the healthcare needs of individual patients. It means that my concern for the patient transcends whatever happens during my shift, and that I ensure continuity of care when I leave a patient. In today's system of increasingly fragmented care, patients often find themselves unable to point to any one caregiver who knows their overall situation and is capable and willing to coordinate the efforts of the healthcare team. Being responsive and responsible earns a patient's trust that "all will be well" as healthcare needs are

addressed. Nurses committed to responsible caring reflect on the following:

- To what extent does my commitment to securing the human well-being of those in my care dictate my work priorities?
- How comfortable am I voicing unmet patient needs to other members of the healthcare team? Is meeting the patient's needs more important to me than remaining in my comfort zone?
- Do other caregivers listen when I present patient concerns because of my successful record of patient advocacy?
- What system variables (e.g., nurse–patient ratios, skill mix, availability of resources) need to change for us to meet the human needs of our patients adequately?
- In what ways must I change for my patients to be able to count on me to respond in a responsible way to their needs?

Nurses who are sensitive to the legal dimensions of practice are careful to develop a strong sense of both ethical and legal accountability. Competent practice is a nurse's best legal safeguard. Nurses seeking to develop legal competence might find it helpful to ask the following questions:

- Do I know the legal boundaries of my practice?
- Am I familiar with pertinent institutional procedures and policies?
- Do I "own" my personal strengths and weaknesses and seek assistance as needed?
- Am I careful never to accept responsibility for an assignment for which I am unprepared?
- Am I knowledgeable about, and respectful of, patient rights?
- Does my documentation provide a legally defensible account of my practice?

When working to develop ethical and legal accountability, nurses must recognize that both deficiencies and excesses of responsible caring are problematic. Although it is reasonable to hold oneself accountable for promoting the human well-being of patients, nurses can err by setting unrealistic standards of responsiveness and responsibility for themselves. Prudence is always necessary to balance responsible self-care with care of others. Inexperienced nurses might feel totally responsible for effecting patient outcomes beyond their control and become frustrated and sad when unable to produce the desired outcome. Conversations about what is reasonable to hold ourselves and others accountable for are always helpful. The sample learning activity in Box 11-5 was designed to explore such accountability issues.

Reporting Incompetent, Unethical, or Illegal Practices

Each employing institution or agency providing nursing services has an obligation to establish a process for reporting and handling practices by individuals or by healthcare systems that jeopardize a patient's health or safety. The ANA Code for Ethics obligates nurses to report professional conduct

Box 11-5   DEVELOPING ETHICAL/LEGAL SKILLS

Accountability

Description

The purpose of this exercise is to explore the issue of account-ability. You will be challenged to reflect on whether your every-day nursing practice demonstrates a commitment to ensuring the human well-being of those in your care. Individual patterns of responding to human need and responsible caring will be critiqued. Role playing and guided discovery will be used to invite you to experience the effects of both responsible caring and the indifferent provision of services.

Objectives

Upon conclusion of this exercise, you will be able to:
1. Describe how the way you respond (or fail to respond) to the needs of patients influences their general sense of well-being.
2. Critique the amount of responsibility you and other nurses accept for the well-being of individual patients.
3. Describe one way your practice will change in order for you to be more accountable to yourself, your patients, the nursing profession, and society.

Learning Activities

Choose another student, and work through exercises 1 to 4. Begin by describing your own positive and negative experiences of being cared for, and draw parallels to how patients feel when they believe they can count on their caregivers to recognize and respond to their needs. Then develop and discuss a list of personal, patient, and system variables that either facilitate or impede responsible caring. Finally, role play the given scenarios, and focus discussion on how different nursing responses influence patient well-being. End the discussion by developing a goal for your practice that will help you to be accountable to yourself, patients, the nursing profession, and society.

Worksheet

Objective

To critique our responsiveness to patient need and the amount of responsibility we each assume to secure patient well-being

Exercise One

Take a moment to reflect on a recent experience when you felt vulnerable (e.g., new role responsibilities: first clinical rotation, new job, new spouse, new parent; car breaks down; major purchase). Share with a colleague how the conduct of the one(s) you expected to be sensitive and responsive to your need influenced your overall sense of well-being. Draw parallels to nursing.

Exercise Two

List all the *personal* variables that enable you to care for your patients responsibly (e.g., coming to work rested, honestly caring about patients) and that impede your ability to do this (e.g., you come to work but are mentally and emotionally back home with some other problem, such as difficulties with spouse, sick child).

Positive Personal Variables	Negative Personal Variables

Next, list all the *system* variables that enable you to care for your patients responsibly (e.g., patient assignments are matched to your developing level of expertise, good team spirit among caregivers and their willingness to work together to meet complex patient needs) and that impede your doing this (e.g., student assignments are unrealistic, chronic understaffing results in staff being unavailable to direct students, sense in the healthcare institution that management has "given up" and is no longer concerned about the quality; that the bottom line is always money).

Positive System Variables	Negative System Variables

Finally, list *patient* variables that positively and negatively influence your ability/willingness to care for your patients responsibly (e.g., patient looks like me, patient is pleasant and makes few demands, patient has strong potential for complete recovery, or patient is homeless, has a history of self-abuse).

Positive Patient Variables	Negative Patient Variables

Talk about how you plan to address the negative variables that interfere with your ability to care for patients responsibly. What does it mean to be accountable to yourself, your patients, the nursing profession, and society?

(continued)

Box 11-5 DEVELOPING ETHICAL/LEGAL SKILLS *(continued)*

Exercise Three

Role play each of the scenarios below, and discuss how the nurse responds (or fails to respond) is likely to influence the patient. It would be helpful to discuss how you think nurses on your unit would respond to this type of situation and how you think they should respond. If these differ, discuss why.

1. You suspect from the blood pressure reading you just obtained that the elderly clinic patient you are examining is not taking his medication or complying with other aspects of the treatment plan. "I try to take 'em but sometimes I forgets." The clinic is understaffed, and you have many more patients to see, some of whom have waited for more than an hour.
2. You tell the resident that you don't think the pain medication one woman with metastatic cancer is receiving is adequate, and the resident tells you that it's a more than adequate dose.
3. Another nurse tells you that he's utterly frustrated because Dr. Braxton refuses to talk with a patient about advance

directives because "it might depress her." You share this nurse's belief that the patient wants to participate in decision making and that it is very possible that she will lose the ability to do this soon.
4. You are making a home visit to a 32-year-old man with end-stage AIDS. He tells you that he is tired of fighting, has no money, and no longer wants to be a bother to his friends. He asks you what he can do to end his life.

Exercise Four

Review each of the above four situations, and discuss with your colleague the legal implications of being accountable. What legal safeguards would you recommend?

Exercise Five

Name one thing about your practice that you have decided to change as a result of this session.

---

that is incompetent, unethical, or illegal (ANA, 2001). For nurses, incompetent practice is measured by nursing standards as defined in State Nurse Practice Acts and Regulations, the Scope of Practice, Professional Standards of Nursing Practice, and other practice guidelines and protocols. Unethical practice is evaluated in light of professional codes of ethics. Illegal practice is identified in terms of violations of law, including Federal and State health regulations, pharmacy laws, Occupational Safety and Health Administration standards and regulations, medical records and communicable disease laws, environmental laws, Centers for Disease Control and Prevention guidelines, antidiscrimination laws, service facility regulations, Clinical Improvement Act, and Joint Commission regulations (ANA, 1994).

As discussed in Chapter 7, *whistle-blowing* refers to efforts by employees to report their employer's violation of the law to appropriate law enforcement agencies outside the employer's facilities. Citing the inadequacies of current laws to protect whistle-blowers, the ANA offers the following caution: "because of the limits of current law, nurses should be advised that they might not be protected against retaliation for reporting the incompetent, unethical or illegal practices of their employers" (ANA, 1994, p. 12). Many individual nurses and nursing organizations are working to secure state and federal legislation to protect whistle-blowers.

CRITICAL THINKING AND CLINICAL REASONING

People use critical thinking skills whenever they want to use clear, focused thinking to achieve a result. I can think critically about how to survive the day's challenges, find a partner for life, pass a licensing exam, or become president! Critical thinking applied to clinical reasoning and judgment in nursing practice:

- Is guided by standards, policies and procedures, ethics codes, and laws (individual state practice acts).
- Is based on principles of nursing process, problem solving, and the scientific method (requires forming opinions and making decisions based on evidence).
- Carefully identifies the key problems, issues, and risks involved, including patients, families, and major care providers in decision making early.
- Is driven by patient, family, and community needs, as well as nurses' needs to give competent, efficient care (e.g., streamlining paperwork to free nurses for patient care).
- Calls for strategies that make the most of human potential and compensate for problems created by human nature (e.g., finding ways to prevent errors, using information technology, and overcoming the powerful influence of personal views).
- Is constantly re-evaluating, self-correcting, and striving to improve (Alfaro-LeFevre, 2010, p. 32).

Each of the nursing process chapters that follow has a section highlighting the type of critical thinking necessary to successfully implement that step of the nursing process.

Critical Thinking Indicators™

Alfaro-LeFevre (2009) has carefully developed a list of **critical thinking indicators** (CTIs™), that is, evidence-based descriptions of behaviors that demonstrate the knowledge, characteristics, and skills that promote critical thinking in clinical practice. See Boxes 11-6 and 11-7. If you are serious about developing the critical thinking skills needed for professional practice, now would be a good time to sit down with someone who knows you well to see which critical thinking characteristics you possess and which need work. One way to do this is to ask with each characteristic:

Box 11-6 CRITICAL THINKING INDICATORS™: BEHAVIORS DEMONSTRATING KNOWLEDGE AND INTELLECTUAL SKILLS

Knowledge
Requirements vary, depending on context (e.g., specialty practice).

Clarifies
- [ ] Nursing and medical terminology
- [ ] Nursing vs. medical and other models, roles, and responsibilities.
- [ ] Signs and symptoms of common problems and complications.
- [ ] Related anatomy, physiology, pathophysiology
- [ ] Normal and abnormal function (bio-psycho-social-cultural-spiritual)
- [ ] Factors that promote or inhibit normal function (bio-psycho-social-cultural-spiritual)
- [ ] Related pharmacology (actions, indications, side effects, nursing implications)
- [ ] Reasons behind interventions and diagnostic studies
- [ ] Normal and abnormal growth and development
- [ ] Nursing process, nursing theories, and research principles
- [ ] Applicable standards, laws, practice acts
- [ ] Policies and procedures and the reasons behind them
- [ ] Ethical and legal principles
- [ ] Spiritual, social, and cultural concepts
- [ ] Where information resources can be found

Demonstrates
- [ ] Focused nursing assessment skills (e.g., breath sounds or IV site assessment)
- [ ] Mathematical problem solving for drug calculations
- [ ] Related technical skills (e.g., n/g tube or other equipment management)

Clarifies
- [ ] Personal values, beliefs, needs
- [ ] How own thinking, personality, and learning style preferences may differ from others' preferences.
- [ ] Organizational mission and values

Intellectual Skills/Competencies
Nursing Process and Decision-Making Skills
- [ ] Applies standards, principles, laws, and ethics codes when planning, giving, and adapting care
- [ ] Identifies purpose and focus of assessment in each situation.
- [ ] Assesses systematically and comprehensively, as indicated by patient circumstances
- [ ] Detects bias; determines credibility of information sources
- [ ] Distinguishes normal from abnormal; identifies risks for abnormal
- [ ] Distinguishes relevant from irrelevant; clusters relevant data together.
- [ ] Recognizes changes in patient status—takes appropriate action.
- [ ] Identifies assumptions and inconsistencies; checks accuracy and reliability; recognizes missing information; focuses assessment as indicated
- [ ] Concludes what's known and unknown; draws reasonable conclusions—gives evidence to support them.
- [ ] Identifies both problems and their underlying cause(s) and related factors; includes patient and family perspectives
- [ ] Considers multiple explanations and solutions
- [ ] Determines individualized outcomes; focuses on results
- [ ] Manages risks, predicts complications, promotes health, function, and well-being; anticipates consequences and implications—plans ahead accordingly
- [ ] Sets priorities and makes decisions in a timely way; includes key stakeholders in making decisions
- [ ] Weighs risks and benefits; individualizes interventions
- [ ] Reassesses to check responses and monitor results (outcomes)
- [ ] Communicates effectively orally and in writing
- [ ] Identifies ethical issues and takes appropriate action
- [ ] Identifies and uses technologic, information, and human resources

Additional Related Skills
- [ ] Establishes empowered partnerships with patients, families, peers, and coworkers
- [ ] Teaches patients, self, and others
- [ ] Addresses conflicts fairly; fosters positive interpersonal relationships
- [ ] Facilitates and navigates change
- [ ] Organizes and manages time and environment
- [ ] Facilitates teamwork (focuses on common goals; helps and encourages others to contribute in their own way)
- [ ] Gives and takes constructive criticism
- [ ] Delegates appropriately; leads, inspires, and motivates others
- [ ] Demonstrates systems thinking (shows awareness of the interrelationships existing within and across healthcare systems)

Box 11-7 **PERSONAL CRITICAL THINKING INDICATORS (CTIs): BEHAVIORS DEMONSTRATING CT CHARACTERISTICS/ATTITUDES**

Personal CTIs are brief descriptions of behaviors, attitudes and qualities often seen in individuals who are critical thinkers

- ☐ **Self-aware:** Identifies own learning, personality, and communication style preferences; clarifies biases, strengths, and limitations; acknowledges when thinking may be influenced by emotions or self-interest.
- ☐ **Genuine/authentic:** Shows true self; demonstrates behaviors that indicate stated values.
- ☐ **Effective communicator:** Listens well (shows deep understanding of others' thoughts, feelings and circumstances); speaks and writes clearly (gets key points across to others).
- ☐ **Curious and inquisitive:** Asks questions; looks for reasons, explanations, and meaning; seeks new information to broaden understanding.
- ☐ **Alert to context:** Looks for changes in circumstances that warrant a need to modify thinking or approaches.
- ☐ **Analytical and insightful:** Identifies relationships; expresses deep understanding.
- ☐ **Logical and intuitive:** Draws reasonable conclusions (if this is so, then it follows that . . . because . . .); uses intuition as a guide; acts on intuition only with knowledge of risks involved.
- ☐ **Confident and resilient:** Expresses faith in ability to reason and learn; overcomes problems and disappointments.
- ☐ **Honest and upright:** Looks for the truth, even if it sheds unwanted light; demonstrates integrity (adheres to moral and ethical standards; admits flaws in thinking).
- ☐ **Autonomous/responsible:** Self-directed, self-disciplined, and accepts accountability.
- ☐ **Careful and prudent:** Seeks help as needed; suspends or revises judgment as indicated by new or incomplete data

- ☐ **Open and fair-minded:** Shows tolerance for different viewpoints; questions how own viewpoints are influencing thinking.
- ☐ **Sensitive to diversity:** Expresses appreciation of human differences related to values, culture, personality, or learning style preferences; adapts to preferences when feasible.
- ☐ **Creative:** Offers alternative solutions and approaches; comes up with useful ideas.
- ☐ **Realistic and practical:** Admits when things aren't feasible; looks for useful solutions.
- ☐ **Reflective and self-corrective:** Carefully considers meaning of data and interpersonal interactions, asks for feedback; corrects own thinking, alert to potential errors by self and others, finds ways to avoid future mistakes.
- ☐ **Proactive:** Anticipates consequences, plans ahead, acts on opportunities.
- ☐ **Courageous:** Stands up for beliefs, advocates for others, doesn't hide from challenges
- ☐ **Patient and persistent:** Waits for right moment; perseveres to achieve best results.
- ☐ **Flexible:** Changes approaches as needed to get the best results.
- ☐ **Healthy:** Promotes a healthy lifestyle; uses healthy behaviors to manage stress.
- ☐ **Improvement-oriented (self, patients, systems): Self**—Identifies learning needs; finds ways to overcome limitations, seeks out new knowledge. **Patients**—Promotes health; maximizes function, comfort, and convenience. **Systems**—Identifies risks and problems with health care systems; promotes safety, quality, satisfaction, and cost containment.

Note: The above is the ideal—no one is perfect. Even the best thinkers' characteristics vary depending on circumstances such as comfort and familiarity with the people and situations at hand. What matters is *patterns* of behavior over time (is the behavior usually evident?). If you're a critical thinker, you probably easily pick three or more of the above characteristics that to improve (critical thinkers are naturally focused on self-improvement).

---

1. On a scale of 1 to 7 (with 1 almost never and 7 always), to what degree do I demonstrate this characteristic that promotes critical thinking?
2. Think of examples of times when you both demonstrated and failed to demonstrate these characteristics. What were the consequences in these situations?

It can be helpful to see if you and others you invite to evaluate your characteristics reach the same conclusions about your strengths and areas for improvement.

Another way to use this list is to try to determine as a class which characteristics accurately describe your class! Alternatively, you can compare groups. For example, as a rule, which characteristics do nurses as a group and physicians as a group demonstrate.

As you begin clinical practice, you can also use the Critical Thinking Indicators™ Behaviors Demonstrating Knowledge and Intellectual Skills list to critique your competence for professional practice.

Concept Mapping

Concept mapping is an instructional strategy that requires learners to identify, graphically display, and link key concepts. Concept maps, also called cognitive maps, mind maps, and meta cognitive tools for learning, are a proven means to promote critical thinking and self-directed learning. McHugh Schuster (2002), who recommends concept mapping as a "critical-thinking approach to care planning," writes:

The important ideas that must be linked together during clinical care planning are the medical and nursing diagnoses, along with all pertinent clinical data. Concept map care planning can be used to promote critical thinking about patient problems and treatment of problems. Through concept mapping of diagnoses and clinical data, you can evaluate what you know about the care of a patient and what further information you need to provide safe and effective nursing care. The visual map of relationships among diagnoses allows you and your clinical faculty to exchange

(text continues on page 216)

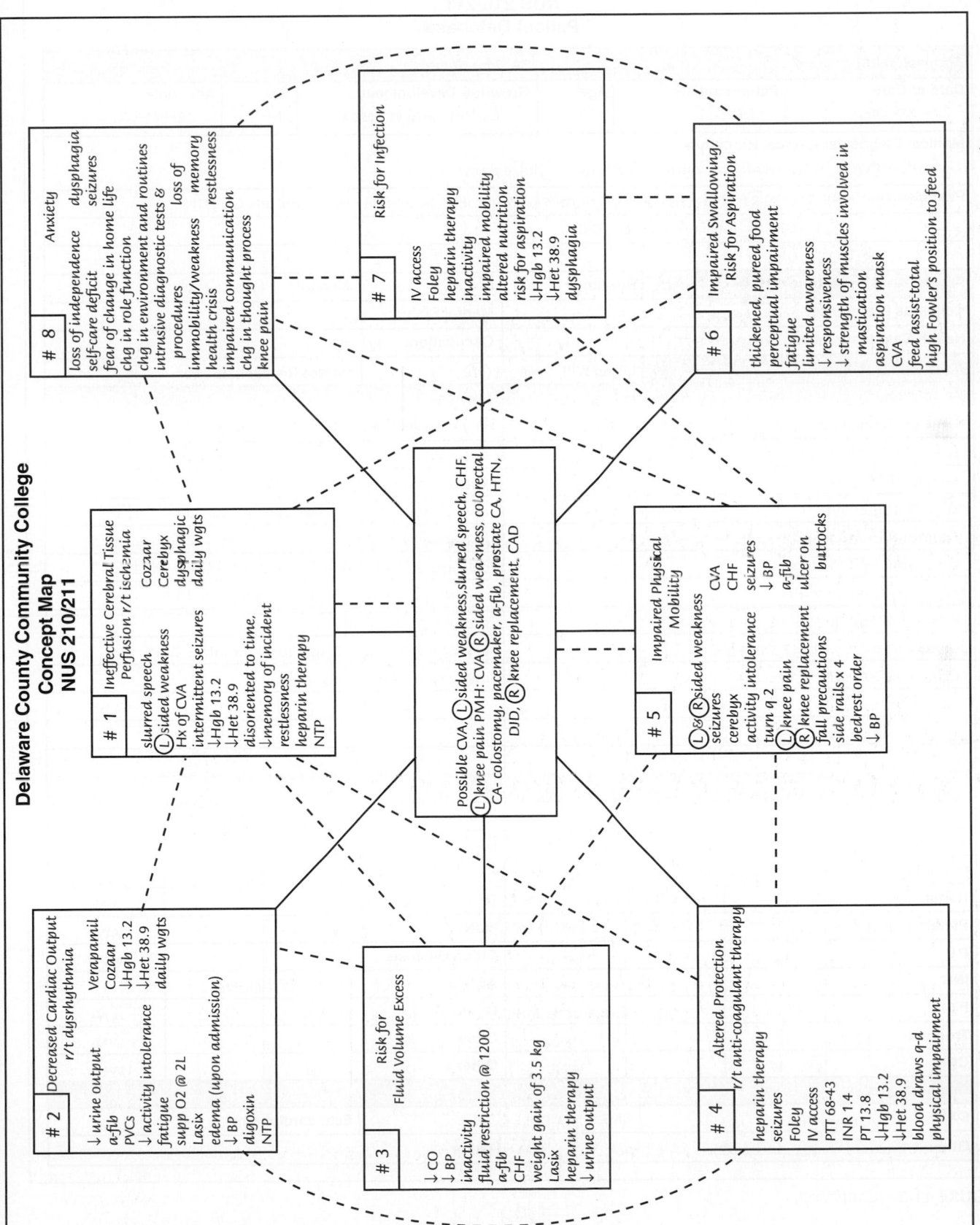

FIGURE 11-5. Sample concept map and supporting data. (Adapted from Schuster, P. M. [2002]. *Concept mapping: A critical-thinking approach to care planning*. Philadelphia: F. A. Davis. Completed forms used with permission from Janet Heck, Delaware County Community College.) *(continued)*

Delaware County Community College
NUS 210/211
Patient Database

Admission Information			Student Name: JANET HECK			
Date of Care 2—27—06	**Patient Initials** DR	**Age** 79	**Growth & Development** Ego Integrity vs Despair	**Sex** M	**Adm date** 2—24—06	

Medical Diagnosis/Surgical Procedure:
Possible CVA, (L) sided weakness, slurred speech, CHF, (L) knee pain

Past Medical History: CVA (R) sided weakness, colorectal CA—colostomy, pacemaker, A-fib, prostate CA, HTN,
DJD, (R) knee replacement, CAD

Psychosocial History	Smoking yes (no)		Alcohol yes (no)
Religious Preference: Protestant		**Marital Status:** Widower	
Health Care Insurance: Keystone 65		**Occupation:** Retired	

Advanced Directives	Living Will yes (no)	Do Not Rescucitate yes (no)

Medications:	Allergies: NKA
Name of Medication	**Why is patient taking this medication?**
IV Heparin 24 cc/hr /raised to 28 cc/hr per PTT protocol	anti-coagulant -prevention of thrombi (a-fib)
K-DUR 20 meQ qd	potassium supplement (K 3.5)
Lasix 40 mg po qd	diuretic - treat CHF/edema upon admission
Digoxin 0.25 mg po qd	to treat a-fib, ↑ CO
Verapamil SR 120 mg qd	calcium channel blocker, treat dysrhythmia (a-fib)
NTP 1" q 6 to chest wall	coronary dilator, ↑ blood flow, treat CHF ↓ BP
Protonix 40 mg qd	suppress gastric acid
Cozaar 50 mg & Het 212.5 mg qd	blocks angiotension II, acts to vasodilate & ↓ BP
Cerebyx 1000 mg IV @ 10 cc/hr	anti-convulsant; treat seizures

Laboratory Data

Lab Value	On adm	Current	Why abnormal	Lab Value	On adm	Current	Why abnormal
WBS	8.6	9.2	WNL	Na	128	NOT DONE	WNL
Hemoglobin	14.1	13.2↓	heparin; ↓nutrition	K	3.5	"	WNL (but K supp administered)
Hematocrit	42.2	38.9↓	heparin; ↓nutrition	Cr	1.2	"	WNL
Platelets	233	232	WNL	BUN	11	"	WNL
PT	13.8	—	WNL	Blood Glucose	114	"	WNL
INR	1.4	—		ABG		NOT DONE	
PTT	68	43↓	heparin therapy	Other Mg	1.9	"	WNL
Troponin	<0.5	—	WNL	Other CA	8.5	"	WNL
CPK	47	—	WNL	Other Dig	1.4	"	WNL

Diagnostic Tests

CXR ✓ shows CHF	EKG ✓ A-fib	Echocardiogram —
Other CT-scan ⊖ No △ ; bleed (x2)		Other

FIGURE 11-5. (Continued)

Treatments:	Daily wgts
	Pulse Ox q shift – > 90% (on 2L NC)
	No neuro checks ordered
	Turn q 2●

Diet

Type: Pureed, ↓NA 2 gm	Restrictions: thickened only 1200 cc po fluid	Appetite: Good
Difficulty Swallowing: (yes) no		Assist with Feeds: (yes) no

Fluid Status

IV solution & rate: Heparin 28 cc/hr	Type of IV access: Peri	Site condition: Ø swelling, Ø redness
24 hr intake: 1460	24 hr output: 1000	Balance: +460
5 hr intake: 480	5 hr output: 250	Balance: +230
Weight: 86.2 kg admin; 89.7 kg		Amount of gain or loss: +3.5 kg

Elimination

Continent:	Bladder: (yes) no	Bowel: (yes) no
Foley: (yes) no	Urine color: dark amber	Last BM: 2/27/06

Activity

Activity Order: Bedrest	Gait: N/A	Use of Assistive Devices: N/A
Risk for Falls: (yes) no	Weakness: (yes) no	Restraints: yes (no)

Vital Signs 8 am	BP 112/60	P 66	R 16	T 97 SAO₂ 99%
Any additional vs 1200	94/60	70	18	97 (AX) SAO2 99%

Narrative Assessment Notes for Clinical Day:

2/27/06 0800. Rec'd pt sleeping– responsive to verbal stimuli. Pt is oriented to person, place only. Responds slowly c̄ one word answers or head motion. Heparin infusion running at 24 cc/hr s̄ incident IV site #11 shows ↓ swelling and ↓ redness. Pt denies pain. VS BP 112/60, T 97+(0); P66, R16, Pt on 2L O₂ via nc, SAO₂ @ 99%. Pt has colostomy bag - no BM present. Foley draining c̄ dark amber urine. Pt's lungs are clear but decreased in bases. BS ⊕, Radial and DI pulses palpable +2. Skin warm and dry. Rash evident on face– pt picks and scratches at face especially nose and mouth frequently. Inspected nose and mouth, both clear c̄ no evidence of inflammation or sores. Pt weak in both LE and upper extremities, limited mvmt. Pt grimaces upon manipulation or mvmt of (L) knee. (R) arm spasms frequently– subsides c̄ touch. Pt dozes on & off but responsive to verbal stimuli. Pt has duoderm on (L) buttock - unable to inspect wound. Complete bed bath given c̄ mouthcare, pt tolerated well. Capillary refill brisk. ↓ edema present. PEARL; heart sounds S, S₂ c̄ murmur ———————————— JM DCCCSN

FIGURE 11-5. (Continued)

Delaware County Community College Concept Map Care Plan

Problem #1 Ineffective Cerebral Tissue Perfusion r/t ischemia (thrombosis)
Short-term Goal: Cerebral perfusion pressure will be maintained during hospital stay.
Long-term Goal: Pt will participate in rehabilitation exercises to regain optimal strength in (L) extremities.

Nursing Interventions:	Patient's Response:
1. Monitor VS q 4, check pupils	1. BP 112/60, T97, P66, RR16, PEARL @ 0800
2. Monitor I & O strict q shift.	2. BP 94/60, T97, P70, RR18, PEARL @ 1200
3. Monitor pulse Ox q shift	3. Pt on restricted 1200 cc fluids po, 5 hr intake=480, SAO$_2$ 99% on 2L NC.
4. Keep head of bed 30 or lower (except when feeding)	4. Pt responsive to verbal stimuli, oriented to person & place.
5. Cluster activities to ↓ ICP.	5. Pt tolerated assessment, bath and feeding before tiring.
6. Administer heparin infusion.	6. Pts PTT 68 to 43.

Summarize your impressions of patient progress towards goals Pt displays Ø worsening of symptoms of reduced of cerebral perfusion. Continue interventions.

Problem #2 Decreased Cardiac Output r/t dysrhythmia
Short-term Goal: Pt will maintain optimally compensated cardiac output evidenced by clear lung sounds, Ø SOB, increased urine output on ↑activity tolerance while hospitalized.
Long-term Goal: Pt will comply c̄ medication regimen to maintain optimal cardiac output after discharge.

Nursing Interventions:	Patient's Response:
1. Assess rate & quality of apical & peripheral pulses.	1. Pulses palpable +2, apical rate S$_1$S$_2$ c murmur; Ø pulse deficit.
2. Assess BP q 4	2. BP 112/60 @ 0800, 94/80 @ 1200.
3. Assess lung sounds q 2	3. Lungs clear but decreased in bases bilaterally.
4. Assess urine output.	4. Urine output 50 cc/hr (250 in 5 hrs)
5. Assess SAO2.	5. Pt SAO2 99% c 2L O$_2$ via nc.
6. Weigh pt daily.	6. Pt has gained 3.5 kg from 2/24 to 2/27.

Summarize your impressions of patient progress towards goals Pt is maintaining good cardiac output as evidenced by ↑ urine output, clear lung sounds and ↓ edema. Continue interventions.

Problem #3 Risk for Fluid Volume Excess
Short-term Goal: Pt will maintain optimal fluid balance as evidenced by stable wgt, clear lung sounds, Ø edema and adequate urine output.
Long-term Goal: Pt will maintain fluid balance upon discharge by compliance c̄ medication regimen and fluid intake.

Nursing Interventions:	Patient's Response:
1. Weigh pt daily.	1. Pt gained 3.5 kg since admission.
2. Monitor strict I & O (1200 cc/24 hr)	2. Pt's intake was 480, output 250 in 5 hrs.
3. Evaluate urine output.	3. Urine output is 50 cc/hr for 5 hrs (0800—1300)
4. Administer Lasix as ordered.	4. Lasix given @ 1000 40 mg po.
5. Monitor electrolytes (side effect of diuretic)	5. All electrolytes WNL.
6. Assess for edema.	6. Ø edema present.

Summarize your impressions of patient progress towards goals Pt is maintaining optimum fluid balance presently c̄ exception of wgt gain. Continue interventions.

Problem #4 Altered Protection r/t anticoagulant therapy
Short-term Goal: Pt will maintain therapeutic blood level of anticoagulant as evidenced by PTT, PT and INR WNL.
Long-term Goal: Pt will set up schedule for bloodwork to be drawn after discharge to maintain therapeutic levels.

Nursing Interventions:	Patient's Response:
1. Monitor pt for adverse effects to anti-coagulant.	1. Pt shows Ø signs of unexplained bleeding– Ø bruising, Ø petechic.
2. Monitor vs q 4.	2. Pts BP 112/60, T978, P66, RR16 @ 0800, 94/60, T974, P20, RR18@1200.
3. Ensure IV infusion & site is uninterrupted.	3. Heparin infusing s̄ incident, IV site shows Ø signs of inflammation or bleeding.
4. Monitor lab results of PTT, PT, INR and intact.	4. Pts PTT 68 to 43, PT 13.8, INR 1.4.
5. Monitor Hgb & Hct for internal bleeding.	5. Hgb ↓ 13.2, Hct 38.9 ↓

Summarize your impressions of patient progress towards goals Pt currently shows Ø signs of bleeding caused by anti-coagulant therapy. Continue to monitor –check H&H to see if continues downward trend. Continue interventions.

FIGURE 11-5. (Continued)

Delaware County Community College Concept Map Care Plan

Problem #5 Impaired Physical Mobility
Short-term Goal: Pt will maintain maximum level of function and risk of complications will be reduced while hospitalized.
Long-term Goal: Pt will regain optimal level of functioning as dictated by severity of CVA.

Nursing Interventions:	Patient's Response:
1. Assess pt's degree of weakness in both upper & lower extremities.	1. Pt's (L) side shows ↑ weakness to (R) side.
2. Determine active & passive ROM capabilities.	2. Pt can move (R) arm independently, other extremities require passive ROM.
3. Monitor skin integrity for potential breakdown.	3. Pt's skin intact c̄ exception of (L) buttock -opaque dsg- cannot assess.
4. Change pt's position q 2.	4. Pt appears comfortable, Ø breakdown present.
5. Use pressure relieving devices to ↓ stress.	5. Placed pillows under legs to elevate heels, pillow under (R) or (L) side to ↓ pressure on sacrum.
6. Implement fall precautions for pt safety.	6. Side rails x 4, bed in low, locked position.

Summarize your impressions of patient progress towards goals Pt has Ø falls. Pt shows Ø skin breakdown and passive ROM performed on lower extremities & (L) arm. Continue interventions.

Problem #6 Impaired Swallowing/Risk for Aspiration
Short-term Goal: Pt will not experience aspiration while hospitalized.
Long-term Goal: Pt will maintain adequate nutrition, as evidenced by stable wgt and albumin WNL.

Nursing Interventions:	Patient's Response:
1. Before mealtime, provide adequate rest periods.	1. Pt was able to stay alert through meal.
2. Provide oral care before feeding.	2. Pt's mouth moistened, displayed good appetite.
3. Place pt in high Fowler's position for feeding.	3. Pt swallowed and chewed well.
4. Prompt pt to chew/swallow.	4. Pt responsive to prompts.
5. Identity food given to pt before each mouthful.	5. Pt nodded recognition- frowned to display distaste.
6. Crush pills and place in pureed food.	6. Pt took all medications s̄ incident

Summarize your impressions of patient progress towards goals Pt did not aspirate and completed 75% of meals. Continue interventions.

Problem #7 Risk for Infection
Short-term Goal: Pt will remain free of infection as evidenced by VS WNL, Ø purulent drainage from tubes.
Long-term Goal: Pt will remain free of infection post discharge.

Nursing Interventions:	Patient's Response:
1. Monitor VS q 4.	1. VS WNL: Temp 97, HR66
2. Monitor WBC.	2. WBC WNL - 9.2.
3. Monitor pt for S & S of infection.	3. Pt shows Ø S & S of inflammation, swelling, drainage at any IV site.
4. Practice aseptic technique at all times.	4. Pt remains free of infection.
5. Monitor appearance of urine.	5. Pt's urine is dark, amber color. MD notified. Culture ordered.
6. Encourage intake of protein & calorie rich foods.	6. Pt completes app. 75% of food offered.

Summarize your impressions of patient progress towards goals Pt has remained free of S/S of infection—awaiting results of urine culture. Continue interventions.

Problem #8 Anxiety
Short-term Goal: Pt will demonstrate a reduced level of anxiety evidenced by ↓ seizures, ↓ restlessness.
Long-term Goal: Pt will demonstrate positive coping mechanisms.

Nursing Interventions:	Patient's Response:
1. Acknowledge awareness of pt's anxiety.	1. Pt appeared grateful, nodded affirmatively.
2. Maintain a calm manner c̄ pt.	2. Pt appears calm and responsive.
3. Maintain frequent contact c̄ pt.	3. Pt demonstrates recognition when I appear.
4. Use simple language & brief statements to explain procedures & tasks.	4. Pt followed commands appropriately.
5. Reduce sensory stimuli.	5. Pt appears calm and resting comfortably.

Summarize your impressions of patient progress towards goals Pt is experiencing less restlessness and appears more comfortable c̄ environment. Continue interventions.

FIGURE 11-5. (Continued)

views on why relationships exist among diagnoses. It also allows you to recognize missing diagnoses and linkages, thus suggesting further learning (p. 3).

Steps in concept map care planning are:

1. Develop a basic skeleton diagram.
2. Analyze and categorize data.
3. Analyze nursing diagnoses relationships.
4. Identify goals, outcomes, and interventions.
5. Evaluate patient's responses.

Examples of concept maps prepared by a student at Delaware County Community College with the related patient database problem list forms are illustrated in Figure 11-5. Simple concept maps demonstrating the nursing process for featured patients can be found in selected chapters in Units VI, VII, and VIII.

REFLECTIVE PRACTICE

Nurses who are sincerely committed to quality care learn early to make self-evaluation an integral part of their nursing practice. Self-evaluation skills promote professional devel-opment, enhance self-esteem, and help one develop self-awareness. The Reflective Practice exercises in each chapter illustrate this practice. Each exercise describes a particular challenge to the student's competence, a range of possible responses, the criteria the student used to evaluate a good response, and a brief statement about what the student learned from this experience.

The nurse who is just beginning to develop in the care-giver role might find it helpful to conclude each caregiving experience with a brief moment of reflection that identifies and celebrates the nursing skills used and targets skills that need to be developed. This practice can keep one from feel-ing overwhelmed by everything that remains to be mastered and yet strongly motivated to learn new skills.

The assessment tool in Box 11-8 helps you assess your proficiency in the skills essential for competent use of the nursing process. After completing the exercise, share your self-evaluation with a trusted colleague or clinical instructor and see whether your assessments of your abilities agree. Celebrate your natural and developed strengths. Begin now to plan a strategy to boost those skills in which you are defi-cient. This might sound trite, but it is true: Your patients will be grateful you cared enough to be your best.

Box 11-8 TAKE THE CHALLENGE

Read the professional behaviors below, and circle the number that best reflects the proficiency you now have in each of these essen-tial nursing competencies.

1 = no skills
2 = somewhat skilled
3 = moderately skilled
4 = well skilled
5 = excellent skills

Cognitive Competencies

1	2	3	4	5	• Offer a scientific rationale for the plan of care.
1	2	3	4	5	• Select those nursing interventions that are most likely to yield desired outcomes.
1	2	3	4	5	• Use critical thinking to problem solve creatively.

Technical Competencies

| 1 | 2 | 3 | 4 | 5 | • Use technical equipment with sufficient competence and ease to achieve goal with a minimum of distress to involved participants. |
| 1 | 2 | 3 | 4 | 5 | • Creatively adapt equipment and technical procedures to the needs of particular patients in diverse circumstances. |

Interpersonal Competencies

1	2	3	4	5	• Creative use of look, speech, and touch to communicate respect and to enhance sense of worth
1	2	3	4	5	• Skilled use of presence and conversation to demonstrate empathy and to obtain sufficient knowledge about the patient to personalize care and serve as an effective advocate
1	2	3	4	5	• Responsible, competent attentiveness to the holistic needs of patients such that trust is built and patients experience comfort of security
1	2	3	4	5	• Value mutual enrichment of both participants in the nurse–patient relationship

Ethical/Legal Competencies

1	2	3	4	5	• Self-motivated to act in ways that advance the interests of patients (consistently trustworthy)
1	2	3	4	5	• Accountable for practice to self, patients served, the caregiving team, and society
1	2	3	4	5	• Consistently serve as effective patient advocate
1	2	3	4	5	• Skilled in mediating ethical conflict among the patient, significant others, healthcare team, and other interested parties
1	2	3	4	5	• Practice nursing faithful to the tenets of professional codes of ethics
1	2	3	4	5	• Use legal safeguards that reduce the risk of litigation

It is helpful when planning care to identify what nursing resources are needed to ensure that you meet each challenge. Nurses sensitive to mastering both the art and the science of nursing care evaluate whether they have the prerequisite skills for each nurse–patient encounter, as well as the skills needed to perceive, respond to, and appreciate the uniqueness of each patient. Quality care is each nurse's responsibility.

● Developing Critical Thinking Skills

1. A nursing student realizes that her college roommate's behavior has changed dramatically during the past month. Once outgoing and funny, she is now withdrawn and moody, rebuffing efforts to discuss the change. Compare and contrast the processes and likely outcomes of using different methods of problem solving (trial-and-error, scientific, intuitive) and the nursing process to address the roommate's needs.

2. The nursing process is an interpersonal process that is always patient centered rather than task centered. Discuss with other students the meaning of this claim. Think through (and discuss) the implications of approaching patients as "problems to be solved."

3. Describe how you would structure an assessment of the situation described below, using critical thinking considerations: purpose of thinking, adequacy of knowledge, potential problems, helpful resources, and critique of judgment/decision.
   - A 28-year-old woman is admitted to a hospital for multiple contusions and a hairline fracture of the skull. She claims that she "fell down the steps," but on examination, it appears that several of the injuries are inconsistent with a fall. The woman sticks to her story that her fall was an accident. You are her nurse.
   - Assess whether your attitudes and dispositions would help or hinder the task of critical thinking if you were the nurse in this situation. Share your self-evaluation with another student and compare your responses.

4. Using the above scenario, identify the cognitive, technical, interpersonal, and ethical/legal skills you would need to meet the nursing needs of this woman. If possible, compare your list with that of an experienced nurse and discuss the differences.

● Practicing for NCLEX

Read the patient scenario below and then match each numbered and boldfaced nursing activity with the correct step of the nursing process.

Annie seeks your help in the student health clinic because she suspects that her roommate Angela suffered date rape. She is concerned because Angela chose not to report the rape and does not seem to be coping well. (1) ***After talking with Annie, you learn that although Angela blurted out that she had been raped when she first came home, since then she has refused verbalization about the rape ("I don't want to think or talk about it"), has stopped attending all college social activities (a marked change in behavior), and seems to be having nightmares.*** *After analyzing the data, you believe that Angela might be experiencing* (2) ***rape-trauma syndrome: silent reaction.*** *Fortunately, Angela trusts Annie and is willing to come to the student health center for help. After a conversation with Angela confirms your suspicions and problem identification, you talk with Angela* (3) ***to develop some treatment goals that you formulate as outcomes and begin to think about the types of nursing interventions most likely to yield the outcomes you both seek.*** *In your initial meeting with Angela,* (4) ***you encourage her expression of feelings and help her to identify personal coping strategies and strengths.*** *You and Angela decide to meet in 1 week* (5) ***to assess her progress toward achieving targeted outcomes.*** *If she is not making progress, you might need to modify the plan of care.*

1. The nursing activity represented as (1) is an example of which step of the nursing process?
   a. Assessing
   b. Diagnosing
   c. Evaluating
   d. Implementing
   e. Planning

2. The nursing activity represented as (2) is an example of which step of the nursing process?
   a. Assessing
   b. Diagnosing
   c. Evaluating
   d. Implementing
   e. Planning

3. The nursing activity represented as (3) is an example of which step of the nursing process?
   a. Assessing
   b. Diagnosing
   c. Evaluating
   d. Implementing
   e. Planning

4. The nursing activity represented as (4) is an example of which step of the nursing process?
   a. Assessing
   b. Diagnosing
   c. Evaluating
   d. Implementing
   e. Planning

5. The nursing activity represented as (5) is an example of which step of the nursing process?
   a. Assessing
   b. Diagnosing
   c. Evaluating
   d. Implementing
   e. Planning

6. Which of the following statements about the nursing process is most accurate?
   a. The nursing process is a four-step procedure for identifying and resolving patient problems.
   b. Beginning in Florence Nightingale's days, nursing students learned and practiced the nursing process.
   c. Use of the nursing process is optional for nurses, since there are many ways to accomplish the work of nursing.
   d. The state board examinations for professional nursing practice now use the nursing process rather than medical specialties as an organizing concept.

7. The nursing process ensures that nurses are patient centered rather than task centered. Rather than simply approaching a patient to take vital signs, the nurse thinks "How is Mrs. Barclay today? Are our nursing actions helping her to achieve her goals? How can we better help her?" This demonstrates which characteristic of the nursing process?
   a. Systematic
   b. Interpersonal
   c. Dynamic
   d. Universally applicable in nursing situations

8. An experienced nurse tells you not to bother studying too hard, since most clinical reasoning becomes "second nature" and "intuitive" once you start practicing. What thinking below should underlie your response?
   a. When intuition is used alone, there are increased risks and fewer benefits. Intuition often moves problem solving forward quickly, but it might result in a lot of trial-and-error approaches.
   b. For nursing to remain a science, nurses must continue to be vigilant about stamping out intuitive reasoning.
   c. The emphasis on logical, scientific, evidence-based reasoning has held nursing back for years. It's time to champion intuitive, creative thinking!
   d. It's simply a matter of preference. Some of us are logical, scientific thinkers, and some are intuitive, creative thinkers.

9. This text is based upon a notion of blended skills. Simply described, what does this mean?
   a. Nursing works best when nurses competently use the intellectual and technical skills that achieve patient outcomes. Nursing has been held back by outdated notions of care and compassion (interpersonal skills), which can be done by anyone.
   b. Nursing works best when each nurse competently uses the intellectual, interpersonal, technical, and ethical/legal skills demanded by each situation.
   c. All of the blended skills are important, but not every nurse has to be skilled in each area. We benefit patients by knowing what we do best. I might be utterly deficient in interpersonal skills but excellent in intellectual skills.
   d. Every nursing situation demands the same blend of basic nursing skills, intellectual, technical, interpersonal, and ethical/legal.

10. The best description of critical thinking indicators (CTIs) is which of the following?
    a. Evidence-based descriptions of behaviors that demonstrate the knowledge that promotes critical thinking in clinical practice
    b. Evidence-based descriptions of behaviors that demonstrate the knowledge and skills that promote critical thinking in clinical practice
    c. Evidence-based descriptions of behaviors that demonstrate the knowledge, characteristics, and skills that promote critical thinking in clinical practice
    d. Evidence-based descriptions of behaviors that demonstrate the knowledge, characteristics, standards, and skills that promote critical thinking in clinical practice

● Answers With Rationale

1. *a.* (1) is an illustration of the collection of patient data.

2. *b.* (2) is an illustration of the identification of a nursing diagnosis, a health problem that independent nursing intervention can resolve.

3. *e.* (3) is an illustration of outcome identification and related nursing interventions.

4. *d.* (4) is an illustration of carrying out the plan of care.

5. *c.* (5) is an illustration of measuring the extent to which Angela has achieved targeted outcomes.

6. *d.* The nursing process is a five-step process (*a*); the term nursing process was first used by Hall in 1955 (*b*); and standards demand the use of the nursing process (*c*), so it is not optional.

7. *b,* interpersonal. Each of the other options are characteristics of the nursing process, but the conversation and thinking quoted best illustrates the interpersonal dimension of the nursing process.

8. *a.* When intuition is used alone, there are increased risks and fewer benefits. Intuition often moves problem solving forward quickly, but it might result in a lot of trial-and-error approaches. Answer *b* is incorrect because there is a place for intuitive reasoning in nursing, but it will never replace logical, scientific reasoning (*c*). Critical thinking is contextual and changes depending on the circumstances, not on personal preference (*d*).

9. *b.* Every nurse must be competent in all four basic skill areas and judge what skills each situation needs. Each situation is unique and might call for a different "blend" of basic skills.

10. *c,* evidence-based descriptions of behaviors that demonstrate the knowledge, characteristics, and skills that promote critical thinking in clinical practice.

Taylor Suite Resources

The Taylor Suite offers these additional resources to enhance learning and facilitate understanding of this chapter:

- thePoint online resource, http://thepoint.lww.com/Taylor7E
- Student DVD included with the book
- Study Guide for Taylor's Fundamentals of Nursing

BIBLIOGRAPHY

Alfaro-LeFevre, R. (2009). *Critical thinking and clinical judgment: A practical approach* (4th ed.). St. Louis: Saunders Elsevier.

Alfaro-LeFevre, R. (2010). *Applying nursing process: A tool for critical thinking* (7th ed.). Philadelphia: Lippincott Williams & Wilkins.

American Association of Colleges of Nursing. (1998). *Essentials of baccalaureate education for professional nursing.* Washington, DC: Author.

American Nurses Association (ANA). (1994). *Guidelines on reporting incompetent, unethical or illegal practices.* Washington, DC: Author.

American Nurses Association (ANA). (2001). *Code for nurses with interpretive statements.* Washington, DC: Author.

American Nurses Association (ANA). (2003). *Nursing: A social policy statement* (2nd ed.). Washington, DC: Author

American Nurses Association Congress for Nursing Practice. (2004). *Standards of practice* (Rev. ed.). Washington, DC: Author.

Androwich, I. (Ed.), American Medical Informatics Association, American Nurses Association, American Nurses Pub. (2002). *Clinical information systems: A framework for reaching the vision.* Washington, DC: American Nurses Association.

Aroskar, M. A. (1993). Incompetent, unethical or illegal practice—teaching students to cope. *Journal of Professional Nursing, 9*(3), 130.

Baxter, P. E., & Boblin, S. (2008). Decision making by baccalaureate nursing students in the clinical setting. *The Journal of Nursing Education, 47*(8), 345–350.

Benner, P. (2001). *From novice to expert.* Menlo Park, CA: Addison-Wesley.

Benner, P. (2005). Extending the dialogue about classification systems and the work of professional nurses. *American Journal of Critical Care, 14*(3), 242–243, 272.

Benner, P., & Wrubel, J. (1989). *The primacy of caring in health and illness.* Menlo Park, CA: Addison-Wesley.

Bulechek, G. M., Butcher, H. K., & Dochterman, J. (Eds.). (2008). *Nursing interventions classification [NIC]* (5th ed.). St. Louis, MO: Mosby.

Craft-Rosenberg, M., & Delaney M. (1997). Nursing diagnosis extension and classification (NDEC). In M. J. Rantz & D. LeMone (Eds.), *Classification of nursing diagnoses: Proceedings of the Twelfth Conference North American Nursing Diagnosis* (pp. 26–31). Glendale, CA: CINAHL Information Services.

Daley, B. J. (1996). Concept maps: Linking nursing theory to clinical nursing practice. *Journal of Continuing Education in Nursing, 27*(1), 17–27.

Davies, E. (1995). Reflective practice: A focus for caring. *Journal of Nursing Education, 34*(4), 167–174.

Diers, D. (2004). *Speaking of nursing . . . Narratives of practice, research, policy and the profession.* Sudbury, MA: Jones and Bartlett Publishers.

DiVito-Thomas, P. (2000). Identifying critical thinking behaviors in clinical judgments. *Journal of Nursing Staff Development, 16*(3), 174–180.

DiVito-Thomas, P. (2005). Nursing student stories on learning how to think like a nurse. *Nurse Educator, 30*(3), 133.

Dochterman, J. M., & Jones, D. A. (2003). *Unifying nursing languages: The harmonization of NANDA, NIC, NOC.* Washington, DC: The American Nurses Association.

Facione, P., & Facione, N. The California Critical Thinking Skills Test. Available at http://www.insightassessment.com/test-cctst.html. Accessed August 10, 2009.

Facione, P., & Facione, N. California Critical Thinking Disposition Inventory. Available at http://www.insightassessment.com/test-cctst.html. Accessed August 10, 2009.

Facione, P. Critical Thinking: What It Is and Why It Counts (2007 Update). Available at http://www.insightassessment.com/pdf_files/what&why2007.pdf. Accessed August 10, 2009.

Ferrario, C. G. (2003). Experienced and less-experienced nurses' diagnostic reasoning: Implications for fostering students' critical thinking. *International Journal of Nursing Terminologies and Classifications, 14*(2), 41–52.

Ferrario, C. G. (2004). Developing nurses' critical thinking skills with concept mapping. *Journal for Nurses in Staff Development, 20*(6), 261–267.

Fonteyn, M. E., & Cooper, L. F. (1994). The written nursing process: Is it still useful to nursing education? *Journal of Advanced Nursing, 19*(2), 315–319.

Gebbie, K., & Lavin, M. A. (1974). Classification of nursing diagnosis. *American Journal of Nursing, 74,* 250–253.

Glaze, J. E. (2002). Stages in coming to terms with reflection: Student advanced nurse practitioners' perceptions of their reflective journeys. *Journal of Advanced Nursing, 37*(3), 265–272.

Hall, L. E. (1955). Quality of nursing care. Address given at the Department of Baccalaureate and Higher Degree Programs of the New Jersey League for Nursing. *Public Health News (June).* Trenton, NJ: New Jersey State Department of Health.

Hansten, R., & Washburn, M. (2001). Intuition in professional practice: Executive and staff perceptions. *Journal of Nursing Administration, 30*(4), 185–188.

Hill, C. (2006). Integrating clinical experiences into the concept mapping process. *Nurse Educator, 31*(1), 36.

Hinck, S. M., Webb, P., Simms-Giddens, S., Helton, C., Hope, K. L., Utley, R., et al. (2006). Student learning with concept mapping of care plans in community-based education. *Journal of Professional Nursing, 22*(1), 23.

Iowa Intervention Project. (1997). Nursing interventions classification (NIC): An overview. In M. J. Rantz & P. LeMone (Eds.), *Classification of nursing diagnoses: Proceedings of the Twelfth Conference, North American Nursing Diagnosis* (pp. 32–39). Glendale, CA: CINAHL Information Systems.

Irvine, L. (1995). Can concept mapping be used to promote meaningful learning in nurse education. *Journal of Advanced Nursing, 21,* 1175–1179.

Jackson, M., Ignatavicius, D., & Case, B. (Eds.). (2004). *Conversations in critical thinking and clinical judgment.* Pensacola, FL: Pohl Publishing.

Joint Commission on Accreditation of Healthcare Organizations (JCAHO). (2005). *Accreditation manual for hospitals.* Oakbrook Terrace, IL: Author.

King, M., & Shell, R. (2002). Teaching and evaluating critical thinking with concept maps. *Nurse Educator, 27*(5), 214.

Lamond, D., & Thompson, C. (2000). Intuition and analysis in decision making and choice. *Journal of Nursing Scholarship, 32*(3), 411–414.

Lewenson, S. B., & Truglio-Londrigan, M. (2008). *Decision-making in nursing: Thoughtful approaches for practice.* Boston: Jones and Bartlett.

Lipe, S. K., & Beasley, S. (2004). *Critical thinking in nursing: A cognitive skills workbook.* Philadelphia: Lippincott Williams & Wilkins.

Locsin, R. C. (1995). Machine technologies and caring in nursing. *Image—The Journal of Nursing Scholarship, 27*(3), 201–203.

NANDA International. (2009). *Nursing diagnoses: Definitions & classification, 2009–2011*. West Sussex, UK: Wiley-Blackwell.

Miller, M. A., & Babcock, D. E. (1996). *Critical thinking applied to nursing*. St. Louis: C. V. Mosby.

Mueller, A., Johnston, M., & Bligh, D. (2002). Joining mind and mapping care planning to enhance student critical thinking and achieve holistic nursing care. *Nursing Diagnosis, 13*(1), 24–27.

Myrick, R., & Yonge, O. (2004). Enhancing critical thinking in the preceptorship experience in nursing education. *Journal of Advanced Nursing, 45*(4), 371–380.

Paul, R. W. (1993). *Critical thinking: How to prepare students for a rapidly changing world*. Santa Rosa, CA: Foundation for Critical Thinking.

Profetto-McGrath, J. (2003). The relationship of critical thinking skills and critical thinking dispositions of baccalaureate nursing students. *Journal of Advanced Nursing, 43*(6), 569–577.

Rew, L. (1987). Nursing intuition: Too powerful—and too valuable—to ignore. *Nursing, 17*(7), 43–45.

Scheffer, B., & Rubenfeld, M. (2000). A consensus statement on critical thinking in nursing. *Journal of Nursing Education, 39*(8), 352–359.

Schraeder, B. D., & Fischer, D. K. (1986). Using knowledge to make clinical decisions. *MCN, 11,* 161–163.

Schuster, P. M. (2002). *Concept mapping: A critical-thinking approach to care planning*. Philadelphia: F. A. Davis.

Swanson, E. (2008). *Nursing Outcomes Classification (NOC)* (4th ed.). St. Louis: Mosby Elsevier.

Taylor, C. (1995). Rethinking nursing's basic competencies. *Journal of Nursing Care Quality, 9*(4), 1–13.

Welk, D. D. (2002). Designing clinical examples to promote pattern recognition: Nursing education-based research and practical applications. *Journal of Nursing Education, 41*(2), 53–60.

Wilkinson, J. (2001). *Nursing process and critical thinking* (3rd ed.). Redwood City, CA: Addison-Wesley Nursing.

Yura, H., & Walsh, M. B. (1988). *The nursing process: Assessing, planning, implementing, evaluating* (5th ed.). Norwalk, CT: Appleton-Century-Crofts.

Assessing 12

SUSAN MORGAN

Susan is a 34-year-old woman newly diagnosed with multiple sclerosis (MS). She says, "How am I going to tell my husband? We were just married last year and planned to do lots of hiking and outdoor sports. It's not fair for him to be tied down to me if I can't be the wife and partner that he thought he had married."

SYLVIA WU

Sylvia, a 17-year-old woman, has just arrived back in the United States after a visit to her family in mainland China. She comes to the emergency department because she woke up that morning with flu-like symptoms (cough, sore throat, fever, muscle aches, fatigue). "I'm scared because of everything I've seen on television and read in the newspapers about that new virus."

JAMES FARREN

James is a college junior who comes to the student health center complaining of difficulty sleeping, eating, and studying. He reveals that his mother died when he was 8 years old, and last semester his father died suddenly, a victim of a fatal car crash. "Ever since my dad died, nothing seems to mean anything anymore. All I see is gray."

LEARNING OBJECTIVES

After completing the chapter, you will be able to accomplish the following:

1. Define and describe the purpose of four types of nursing assessments.

2. Explain the relationship between nursing assessment and medical assessment.

3. Differentiate objective and subjective data.

4. Identify five sources of patient data useful to the nurse.

5. Describe the purpose of nursing observation, interview, and physical assessment.

6. Obtain a nursing history using effective interviewing techniques.

7. Plan patient assessments by identifying assessment priorities and structuring the data to be collected systematically.

8. Identify common problems encountered in data collection, noting their possible cause.

9. Explain when data need to be validated and several ways to accomplish this.

10. Describe the importance of knowing when to report significant patient data and of proper documentation.

11. Obtain and document purposeful, complete, accurate, factual, and relevant patient data.

KEY TERMS

assessing	minimum data set
cue	nursing history
data	objective data
database	observation
emergency assessment	physical assessment
focused assessment	review of systems (ROS)
inference	subjective data
initial assessment	time-lapsed assessment
interview	validation

Assessing is the systematic and continuous collection, validation, analysis, and communication of patient **data,** or information. These data reflect how health functioning is enhanced by health promotion or compromised by illness and injury. A **database** includes all the pertinent patient information collected by the nurse and other healthcare professionals.

The database enables a comprehensive and effective plan of care to be designed and implemented for the patient. Assessment is the first of six nursing standards (Box 12-1); collecting patient data is a vital step in the nursing process because the remaining steps depend on complete, accurate, factual, and relevant data.

▶ *Refer to the Reflective Practice box regarding Sylvia Wu, a patient who fears that she has a virus. The nurse's assessment would reveal possible risk factors. Additionally, the patient's statements about her fears provide further data on which to develop a plan of care.* ■

The initial comprehensive nursing assessment results in baseline data that enable the nurse to:

- Make a judgment about a patient's health status, the ability to manage his or her own healthcare, and the need for nursing
- Refer the patient to a physician or other healthcare professional, if indicated
- Plan and deliver individualized, holistic nursing care that draws on the patient's strengths

In addition to an initial assessment of the patient, the nurse makes ongoing assessments. These assessments alert the nurse to changes in the patient's responses to health and illness, and suggest necessary changes in the plan of nursing care or care offered by other healthcare professionals.

During the assessment step of the nursing process, the nurse establishes the database by interviewing the patient to obtain a nursing history. The **nursing history** identifies the patient's health status, strengths, health problems, health risks, and need for nursing care. The nurse may also perform a nursing physical examination to collect data. Other sources of patient

Box 12-1   ANA STANDARDS OF PRACTICE: STANDARD 1, ASSESSMENT

The registered nurse collects comprehensive data pertinent to the patient's health or the situation.

Measurement Criteria
The registered nurse:

Collects data in a systematic and ongoing process.

Involves the patient, family, other healthcare providers, and environment, as appropriate, in holistic data collection.

Prioritizes data collection activities based on the patient's immediate condition, or anticipated needs of the patient or situation.

Uses appropriate evidence-based assessment techniques and instruments in collecting pertinent data.

Uses analytical models and problem-solving tools.

Synthesizes available data, information, and knowledge relevant to the situation to identify patterns and variances.

Documents relevant data in a retrievable format.

REFLECTIVE PRACTICE

Challenge to Intellectual Skills

While on a clinical rotation in the emergency department, I met Sylvia Wu, a 17-year-old young woman who had just arrived back in the United States after a visit to her family in mainland China. She came to the emergency department because she woke up that morning with flu-like symptoms (cough, sore throat, fever, muscle aches, fatigue) and was terrified because of everything she had seen on television and read in the newspapers about the latest new virus. Although 64 people have died already, she knows that most of the cases are in Asia. She came to the emergency room, begging to be told that she doesn't have the virus, but, rather, that most likely her symptoms are due to fatigue or a cold. I want to calm her, but I honestly don't know what she has. Besides, I am starting to feel a bit anxious myself because the one thing everyone knows about this virus is the fact that it is extremely "contagious." I could feel myself recoil when Sylvia sneezed.

Thinking Outside the Box: Possible Courses of Action

- Reassure Sylvia and tell her not to worry because the overwhelming probability is that her symptoms aren't anything serious.
- Quickly get someone with more experience to care for Sylvia because I don't want to be anywhere near her if she does have this virus.

- Document and report her concerns, trying to keep her isolated and away from other patients, while trying to find more information about this new virus quickly, since I'm not sure about its signs and symptoms.

Evaluating a Good Outcome: How Do I Define Success?

- Sylvia gets the medical treatment she needs, and her fears are appropriately addressed.
- In the event that Sylvia does have a highly communicable disease, the risk for disease transmission to others is reduced.

- I manage to control my fears, being able to respond to Sylvia's concerns appropriately.
- I learn something about my immediate response to feeling at risk and my commitment to professionalism.

Personal Learning: Here's to the Future!

Although I am not proud of my response, I falsely reassured Sylvia that this was probably nothing. As a result, I did not report or document her fears. Unfortunately, Sylvia was diagnosed with the virus and several others in our emergency department at that time became infected. For some reason, I escaped. In the future, I hope I'll never be so insensitive to a patient's concerns or insights again.

Reflection

How do you think you would respond in a similar situation? Why? What does this tell you about yourself and about the adequacy of your skills for professional practice? What factors might have influenced this nursing student's actions? What types of data could have led the nursing student to a different course of action? How might the nursing student have assessed the patient differently? Can you think of other ways to respond? What other skills (cognitive, interpersonal, technical, ethical/legal) would you need to respond well in this situation? Do you agree with the criteria to evaluate a successful outcome? Did the nursing student meet the criteria? If not, what else might the nursing student have done to ensure a successful outcome?

information used by the nurse include the patient's family and significant others, the patient record, the patient's healthcare professionals, and nursing and other healthcare literature.

After the nurse has established the database, data about the patient are collected continuously because the patient's health status can change quickly. Questionable data are verified (validated) as part of the assessment step of the nursing process. All pertinent data are recorded and, when appropriate, communicated to other healthcare professionals so that the data can best benefit the patient (Fig. 12-1). In addition to collecting data, nurses might use intuition to assess patients (see Chapter 11).

UNIQUE FOCUS OF NURSING ASSESSMENT

When nurses make nursing assessments, they do not duplicate medical assessments. Medical assessments target data

pointing to pathologic conditions, whereas nursing assessments focus on the patient's responses to health problems. For example, is there interference with the patient's ability to meet basic human needs? Can the patient perform the activities of daily living? Although the findings from a nursing assessment may contribute to the identification of a medical diagnosis, the unique focus of nursing assessments is on the patient's responses to actual or potential health problems.

> *Remember Susan Morgan, a patient recently diagnosed with MS? By looking at the data supplied by the patient, the nurse would be able to determine that the patient's new diagnosis of MS is affecting her body image and self-esteem. The nurse then would use this information to focus assessment questions to obtain additional*

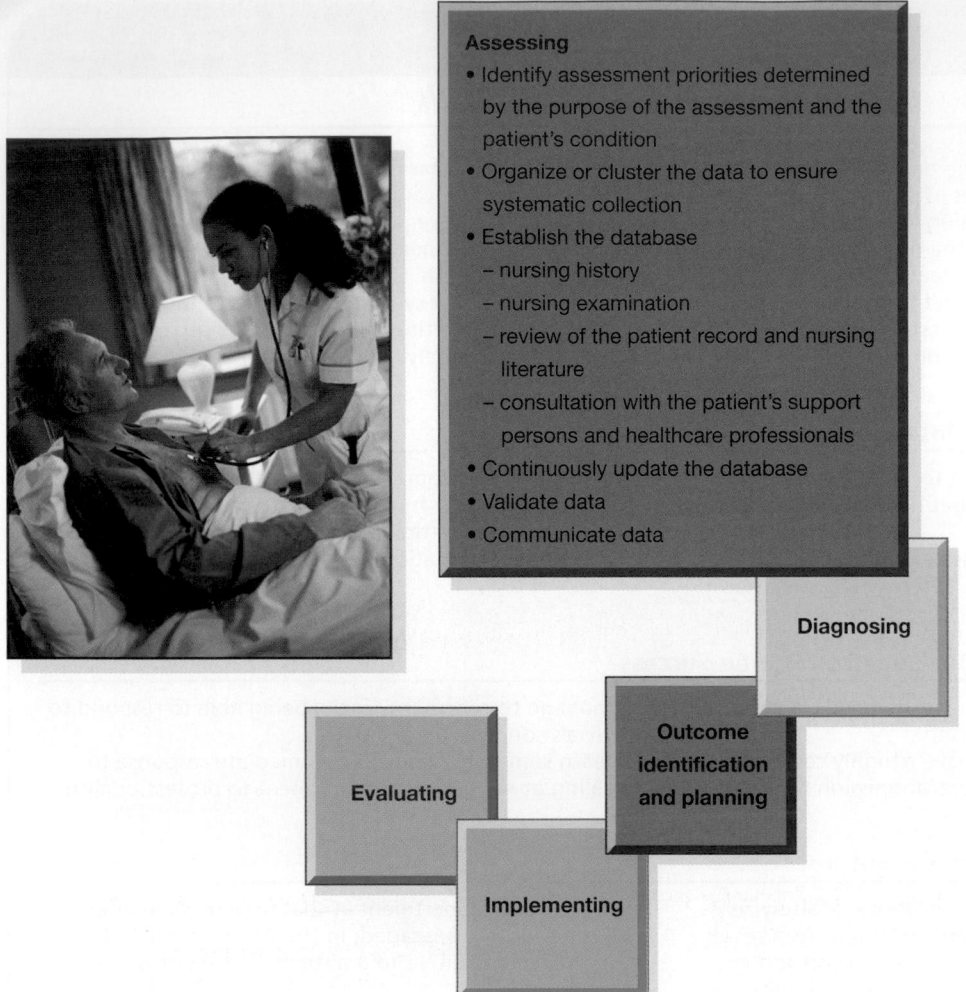

Assessing

• Identify assessment priorities determined by the purpose of the assessment and the patient's condition
• Organize or cluster the data to ensure systematic collection
• Establish the database
  – nursing history
  – nursing examination
  – review of the patient record and nursing literature
  – consultation with the patient's support persons and healthcare professionals
• Continuously update the database
• Validate data
• Communicate data

Diagnosing

Outcome identification and planning

Evaluating

Implementing

FIGURE 12-1. Assessing. The primary source of patient information is the patient. Resources include the patient's support people, the patient record, information from other healthcare professionals, and information from nursing and healthcare literature.

information to be included in the database, from which a plan of care specific to Susan's needs can be developed. ■

ASSESSMENT AND CRITICAL THINKING

Since the entire nursing process rests on the initial and ongoing assessment of the patient, it is imperative to use excellent critical thinking skills when gathering, validating, analyzing, and communicating data. Among the critical thinking activities linked to assessment are (Alfaro, 2010, p. 49):

• Assessing systematically and comprehensively, using a nursing framework to identify nursing concerns and a body systems framework to identify medical concerns
• Detecting bias and determining the credibility of information sources
• Distinguishing normal from abnormal and identifying the risks for abnormal findings
• Making judgments about the significance of data, distinguishing relevant from irrelevant
• Identifying assumptions and inconsistencies, checking accuracy and reliability, and recognizing missing information.

Many of these activities are challenging for those new to nursing who most likely lack the sorts of clinical experience

that facilitate expert clinical reasoning. Thus, students are urged to ask questions frequently about data and to test their inferences and judgments.

TYPES OF NURSING ASSESSMENTS

Nursing assessments include the comprehensive initial assessment, the focused assessment, the emergency assessment, and the time-lapsed assessment. In this chapter, we will focus on assessing the health status of an individual. As you develop expertise in nursing assessments, you will be able to assess communities and special populations, such as schoolchildren or people with AIDS or other infectious diseases.

Initial Assessment

The **initial assessment** is performed shortly after the patient is admitted to a healthcare agency or service. Most institutions have policies specifying the time interval within which the assessment must be completed. The purpose of this assessment is to establish a complete database for problem identification and care planning. The nurse collects data concerning all aspects of the patient's health, establishing priorities for ongoing focused assessments and creating a reference for future comparison. See Figure 12-2

(text continues on page 227)

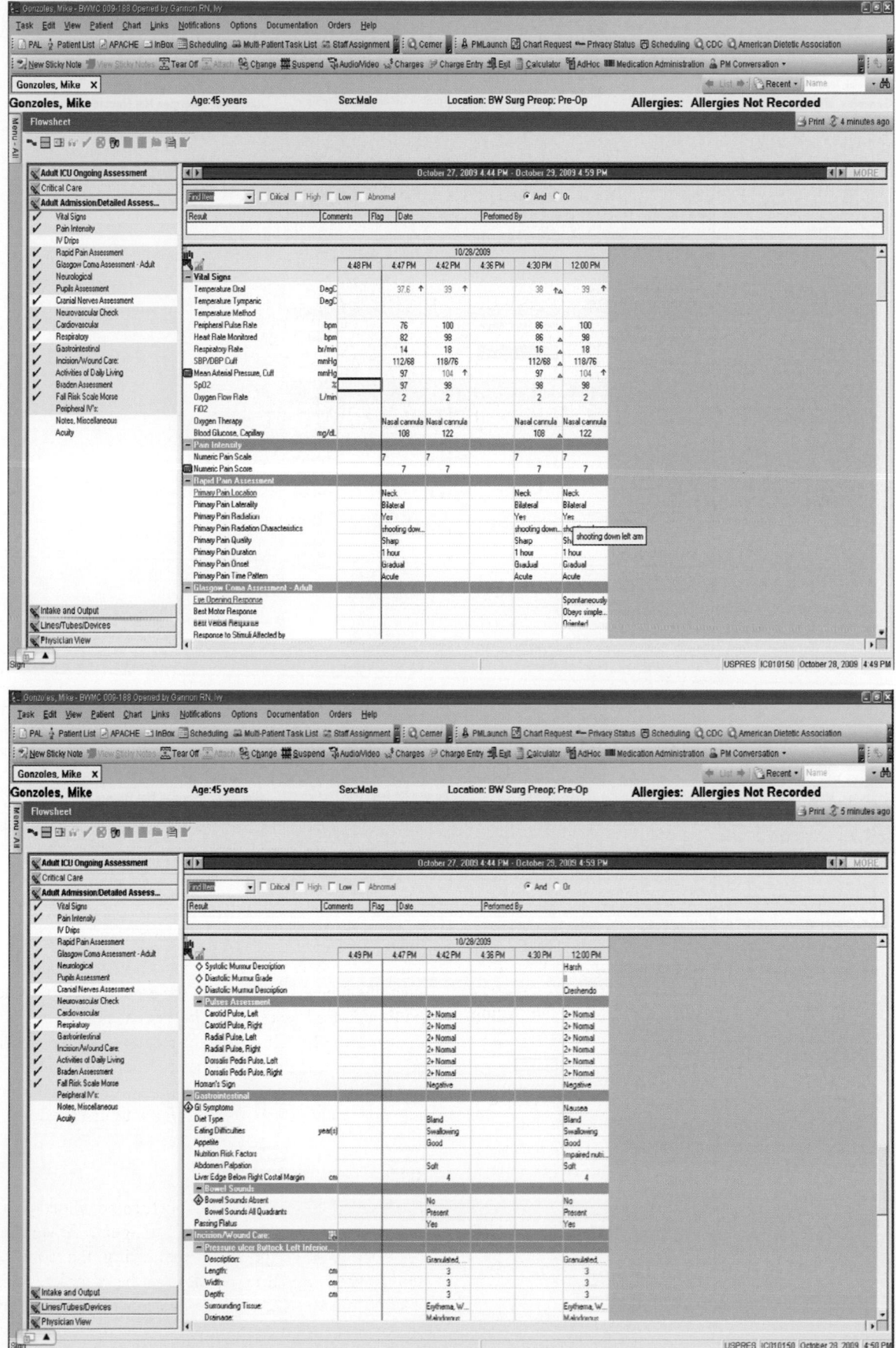

FIGURE 12-2. Sample electronic nursing admission assessment form. *(© Cerner Corporation. All rights reserved. Used with permission.)   (continued)*

FIGURE 12-2. (*Continued*)

for a sample of an initial assessment in an electronic medical record. For an example of a handwritten admission database, see Chapter 9.

Focused Assessment

In a **focused assessment,** the nurse gathers data about a specific problem that has already been identified. Helpful questions include:

- What are your symptoms?
- When did they start?
- Were you doing anything different than usual when they started?
- What makes your symptoms better? Worse?
- Are you taking any remedies (medical or natural) for your symptoms?

A focused assessment may be done during the initial assessment if patient health problems surface, but it is routinely part of ongoing data collection. Another purpose of the focused assessment is to identify new or overlooked problems.

> *Remember Sylvia Wu, the 17-year-old who comes to the emergency department because she thinks that she might have a virus? The nurse would use a focused assessment to evaluate her complaints that are specifically related to her respiratory status. This information would be supplemented by additional data about the patient's recent travel to mainland China.* ∎

Emergency Assessment

When a physiologic or psychological crisis presents, the nurse performs an **emergency assessment** to identify life-threatening problems. A nursing home resident who begins choking in the dining room, a bleeding patient brought to the emergency room with a stab wound, an unresponsive patient in the rehabilitation unit, and a factory worker threatening violence are all candidates for an emergency assessment.

Time-Lapsed Assessment

The **time-lapsed assessment** is scheduled to compare a patient's current status to baseline data obtained earlier. Most patients in residential settings and those receiving nursing care over longer periods of time, such as homebound patients with visiting nurses, are scheduled for periodic time-lapsed assessments to reassess health status and to make necessary revisions in the plan of care.

PREPARING FOR DATA COLLECTION

When preparing for data collection, establishing assessment priorities and systematically structuring data collection are two important considerations.

Establishing Assessment Priorities

Before beginning to collect data on any patient, it is helpful to think carefully about the type of data needed to develop a satisfactory plan of care. This includes identifying data that is not a priority to collect. For example, data already collected from the patient and in the patient record should not be repeatedly sought from the patient unless there is a need to validate them. Repetitious questioning can also be annoying to a patient and may cause the patient to wonder about the lack of communication among healthcare professionals. A careful review of the patient record before interviewing the patient helps prevent this problem.

Nurses spend more or less time on different components of the nursing history depending on the patient's reason for needing nursing assistance. For example, pediatric nurses are careful to establish the developmental age and milestones obtained by children admitted to a pediatric unit so that they can respect and promote these achievements. A school nurse who suspects child abuse pays careful attention to the child's statements about living conditions at home and relationships with family members and caregivers. A nurse preparing to discharge a patient from same-day surgery makes sure that the patient has the human and physical resources needed to supply appropriate postoperative care.

The purpose for which the assessment is being performed offers the best guideline about what type and how much data to collect. Assessment priorities are influenced by the patient's health orientation, developmental stage, culture, and need for nursing. After the comprehensive nursing assessment has been completed, patient health problems dictate assessment priorities for future nurse–patient interactions.

Health Orientation

Nurses may use health assessments, such as the *Health-Style Self-Test* in Chapter 3 and the Promoting Health displays in each clinical chapter, to help patients identify potential and actual health risks, and to explore their habits, behaviors, beliefs, attitudes, and values that influence levels of wellness. The literature abounds in specialized assessment tools that focus on relationships; psychological, environmental, and physical self-care; relaxation; spirituality; humor and play; movement and exercise; sleep and dreams; nutrition; and sexuality. In terms of the type of patient data gathered, these assessments are different from the assessments of patients being hospitalized for disease-related treatment.

Developmental Stage

Nursing assessments are modified according to the developmental needs of patients. For example, when assessing an infant, special attention is given to weight gain and physical growth, feeding and elimination problems, sleep–activity cycles, and the parenting skills of caregivers. When children are hospitalized, it is important to note how independent the child is with basic care measures (toileting, hygiene, dressing, eating), what words the child uses to indicate the need to void and defecate, play preferences, and so forth.

Culture

When assessing patients from different cultural backgrounds (e.g., racial, ethnic, religious, socioeconomic), it is important to remember all the ways that cultural factors can influence the process of assessment. Consideration of the patient's culture begins with how the nurse approaches the patient and whether or not one makes direct eye contact or shakes a hand. Chapter 2 offers practical guidelines for incorporating cultural considerations into nursing assessments. It is also important to assess the need for an interpreter. In what language does the patient wish to communicate? If an interpreter is necessary, it is important to be familiar with your agency's policies about the availability of professional interpreters, since it is inappropriate to rely on the patient's family members to provide this service.

Need for Nursing

Whether nurses will be interacting with the patient for a short or a long period (e.g., same-day surgery versus surgery that necessitates a long recovery in an intensive care unit) and the nature of nursing care needed by the patient (e.g., assistance with the birth of a baby versus support and home care throughout a terminal illness), both powerfully influence the type of data the nurse collects. A general guideline when assessing patients is to gather only data that are helpful when planning and delivering care. It would be inappropriate, for example, to collect a detailed sexual history on a patient admitted to the hospital overnight after a slight concussion. Conversely, a nurse should not fail to ask a pregnant woman admitted to the hospital for observation because of bleeding during her first trimester whether she has any questions about resuming sexual activity after she gets home.

> *Think back to James Farren, the college junior who was described at the beginning of the chapter. The nurse would assess his sleeping, eating, and activity habits as well as his emotional status to gain further insight into his possible problems. However, a detailed assessment of his elimination habits would probably be inappropriate at the present time.* ∎

Structuring the Assessment

Because many different types of data are collected about patients, there is a need to structure data collection systematically. Using systematic guidelines specifically developed for a nursing assessment ensures that comprehensive, holistic data are collected for each patient and lead easily to formulating nursing diagnoses. When the nurse internalizes such assessment guidelines, it is easier to focus on the patient during the assessment rather than to worry about what to assess next.

Most schools of nursing and healthcare institutions establish a **minimum data set** that specifies the information that must be collected from every patient and use a structured assessment form to organize or cluster this data. Many nursing assessment guides are based on holistic models rather than medical models. Gordon's (1994) framework identifies 11 functional health patterns and organizes patient data into these patterns. Maslow uses a hierarchy of five sets of human needs. A medical model used to organize data collection with which all nurses are familiar is the body systems model. This method organizes data collection according to organ and tissue function in various body systems. Although it is helpful in formulating diagnoses related to physiologic problems, it neglects patient problems and strengths in psychosocial and spiritual dimensions of health and well-being. Box 12-2 describes models for organizing assessment data.

DATA COLLECTION
Types of Data: Subjective and Objective

There are two types of data: subjective and objective. **Subjective data** are information perceived only by the affected person; these data cannot be perceived or verified by another person. Examples of subjective data are feeling nervous, nauseated, or chilly and experiencing pain. Subjective data also are called symptoms or covert data.

Objective data are observable and measurable data that can be seen, heard, or felt by someone other than the person experiencing them. Objective data observed by one person can be verified by another person observing the same patient. Examples of objective data are an elevated temperature reading (e.g., 101°F), skin that is moist, and refusal to look at or eat food. Objective data also are called signs or overt data. Table 12-1 compares subjective and objective data.

Paying attention to both subjective and objective data promotes critical thinking because the two types of data complement and clarify one another.

> *Review the data provided in the scenario for Sylvia Wu in the Reflective Practice display. Her complaints of flu-like symptoms provide the nurse with subjective data. Hearing her cough, noting any sputum produced, inspecting her throat for redness and irritation, and checking her temperature would provide the nurse with objective data that help to clarify and substantiate the patient's complaints.* ∎

Characteristics of Data

When collecting and recording patient data, nurses should be purposeful, complete, accurate, factual, and relevant.

Purposeful

When preparing for data collection, the nurse identifies the purpose of the nursing assessment (comprehensive, focused, emergency, time-lapsed) and then gathers the appropriate data. The circumstances of the patient situation may also dictate the nature and amount of data collected.

| Box 12-2 | MODELS FOR ORGANIZING OR CLUSTERING DATA |

Holistic			Medical
Human Needs (Maslow)	**Functional Health Patterns (Gordon)**	**Human Response Patterns (Unitary Person)**	**Body System Model**
Physiologic (Survival) Needs: Food, fluids, oxygen, elimination, warmth, physical comfort *Safety and Security Needs:* Things necessary for physical safety (e.g., a cane) and psychological security (e.g., a child's favorite toy) *Love and Belonging Needs:* Family and significant others *Self-esteem Needs:* Things that make people feel good about themselves and confident in their abilities (e.g., being well groomed, having accomplishments recognized) *Self-actualization Needs:* Need to grow, change, and accomplish goals	*Health Perception/Health Management:* Perception of general health status and well-being. Adherence to preventive health practices *Nutritional–Metabolic:* Patterns of food and fluid intake, fluid and electrolyte balance, general ability to heal *Elimination:* Patterns of excretory function (bowel, bladder, skin) and client's perception *Activity/Exercise:* Pattern of exercise, activity, leisure, recreation, and ADL; factors that interfere with desired to expected individual pattern *Cognitive–Perceptual:* Adequacy of sensory modes such as vision, hearing, taste, touch, smell, pain perception, cognitive functional abilities *Sleep/Rest:* Patterns of sleep and rest–relaxation periods during a 24-hour day, as well as quality and quantity *Self-perception/Self-concept:* Attitudes about self, perception of abilities, body image, identity, general sense of worth and emotional patterns *Role/Relationship:* Perception of major roles and responsibilities in current life situation *Sexuality and Reproductive:* Perceived satisfaction or dissatisfaction with sexuality. Reproductive state and pattern *Coping/Stress Tolerance:* General coping pattern, stress tolerance, support systems, perceived ability to control and manage situations *Value-Belief:* Values, goals, or beliefs that guide choices or decisions	*Exchanging:* Nutritional status, temperature, elimination, oxygenation, circulation, fluid balance, skin, and mucous membranes, risk for injury *Communicating:* Ability to express thoughts verbally; orientation, speech impairments, language barriers *Relating:* Establishing bonds, social interaction, support systems, role performance (including parenting, occupation, and sexual role) *Valuing:* Religious and cultural preference and practices, relationship with deity, perception of suffering; acceptance of illness *Choosing:* Ability to accept help and make decisions, adjustment to health status, desire for independence/dependence, denial of problem, adherence to therapies *Moving:* Activity tolerance, ability for self-care, sleep patterns, diversional activities, disability history, safety needs, breastfeeding *Perceiving:* Body image, self-esteem, ability to use all five senses, amount of hopefulness, perception of ability to control current situation *Knowing:* Knowledge about current illness or therapies; previous illnesses; risk factors, expectations of therapy, cognitive abilities; readiness to learn, orientation, memory *Feeling:* Pain, grieving, risk for violence, anxiety level, emotional integrity	Neurologic Cardiovascular Respiratory Gastrointestinal Musculoskeletal Genitourinary Psychosocial

Adapted from Alfaro-LeFevre, R. (2010). *Applying nursing process: A tool for critical thinking* (7th ed.). Philadelphia: Lippincott Williams & Wilkins.

TABLE • 12-1	COMPARISON OF OBJECTIVE AND SUBJECTIVE DATA

Objective Data	Subjective Data
32-year-old man Height: 5'8" Weight: 9/18/10—224 lb 2/4/11—202 lb	"I'm beginning to feel better about myself now that I'm losing weight and I seem to have more energy."
Posterior, left midcalf is warm and red.	"My leg hurts when I walk."
Patient observed fidgeting with bed covers; facial features are tightly drawn.	"I'm so afraid of what they might find when they cut me open tomorrow."

Complete

As much as possible, all the patient data needed to understand a patient health problem and develop a plan of care to maximize health and well-being should be identified. For example, knowing that a patient has lost weight is not fully meaningful until the nurse discovers (1) if the weight loss was intentional or unintentional, (2) if it was related to a change in eating or exercise patterns or to some underlying pathologic condition, and (3) how the patient views and is responding to the weight loss.

Factual and Accurate

Both the patient and the nurse may intentionally or unintentionally misrepresent or distort patient information. For example, a patient who values being thin may describe a weight gain of several pounds as the onset of obesity. Nurses concerned with accuracy and fact continually verify what they hear with what they observe, using other senses and validating all questionable data. At the outset of data collection, it is crucial to determine whether the patient or caregiver who is supplying the data is reliable. When nurses suspect that their own personal bias or stereotyping is influencing their data collection, they should consult with another nurse. It is also best to describe observed behavior rather than to interpret the behavior. Such a description may read: "Patient frequently is observed lying with his face to the wall. Attempts to engage him in conversation fail. He refused lunch today and ate only soup for dinner." On the other hand, the statement "Patient is depressed" is the nurse's interpretation of the patient's behavior; it is not a factual statement. Recording the patient's behaviors factually allows other healthcare professionals to explore causes of the behavior with the patient.

Relevant

Because recording comprehensive data can become an endless task, one challenge facing nurses is to determine what type of data and how much data to collect for each patient. This chapter describes ways to do this. The aim is to record concisely all pertinent data. Often, only experience teaches nurses what data are needed in specific cases.

Learning how to collect, validate, and communicate data that are complete, accurate, factual, and relevant is the focus of the remainder of this chapter.

Sources of Data
Patient

The patient is the primary and usually the best source of information. Unless specified otherwise, it is assumed that the data recorded in the nursing history were collected from the patient. Most patients are willing to share information when they know it is helpful for planning their care. See Through the Eyes of a Student. Although data collected from the patient are usually accurate, the nurse should be alert for certain difficulties. For example, a patient who is acutely ill may not be able to communicate adequately if the pain is severe or consciousness is altered in any way. An emotionally upset patient may distort information; for example, patients who are fearful because they think their illness may threaten their work or life may deny certain symptoms or deliberately give misleading facts. If the nurse becomes aware that a patient's report of symptoms differs from physical findings or data obtained from other sources, it is important to note this and to explore the cause of the discrepancy.

Patients with limited mental or communication capacity, such as young children and older adults with dementia, cannot be relied on to report accurately. Children and people with decreased mental capacity or impaired verbal ability should, however, be encouraged to respond to interview questions as best as they can. Bypassing these patients and automatically turning to a family member, friend, or caregiver for information communicates powerfully that the nurse either has no time for the patient to express his or her needs or mistakenly doubts the patient's ability to communicate these needs.

Through the Eyes of a Student

During my chronic medical–surgical rotation, my clinical group was placed on an oncology floor. My first thought was "Oh no, not the cancer floor!" The word *fear* didn't even begin to describe how I felt. These patients had enough problems without some "green" nursing student aggravating them all day. I kept thinking these people are extremely ill and won't want to be bothered by my intruding questions.

Nonetheless, I knew I had to do it. Not only did I have to take care of this patient all day, but I also had to develop a database and plan of care. I knew I would have to do a lot more than give him his morning care and leave him alone. I would have to carry on an extended conversation with this patient to get all the information I needed.

As if all of this wasn't enough to make me throw in the white flag, when my patient assignment was given, I discovered my patient was a man only 1 year older than me. A 28-year-old man with terminal cancer—this was too scary!

Clinical day came, as I knew it would, and I was choking. I walked in that room and together the patient and I planned his care. I explained to him the things I needed to talk about with him and I couldn't believe it—he didn't tell me to go away!

We talked at length about his disease process and how it had affected his plans and goals. He opened up to me about his spirituality, his relationships with friends and family, and other personal subjects. Periodically, he would cringe, and I could tell it was time for a break. He was hurting too badly to go on at that time.

At the end of that day, my viewpoint was totally different than it had been that morning. I walked away from that room and off that floor feeling like I had made a difference for this person. We had shared a lot and he seemed so appreciative for the time I took to talk with him. The information he shared helped me to develop a better plan of care that was more responsive to his particular needs. The amazing part was that all I had to do was just be myself and allow him to do the same and our day flowed smoothly. The lesson I learned here was important for me: Keep calm and hold on to compassion, and nursing offers many rewards!

—Nancy E. Driskill,
Southeast Missouri State University,
Cape Girardeau, Missouri

Family and Significant Others

Family members, friends, and caregivers are especially helpful sources of data when the patient is a child or has limited capacity to share information with the nurse. Husbands and wives can supply information concerning their spouses. Friends often accompany a patient to a health agency and can supply useful information. Care must be taken to determine that the patient does not object to data being gathered from friends and that the friends want to participate. Also, there should be a clear understanding by the patient, family, and friends of the confidentiality of the data collected. Whenever data are gathered from support people, this should be indicated in the nursing history.

Patient Record

Records prepared by different members of the healthcare team provide information essential to comprehensive nursing care. The nurse should review records early when gathering data—in some instances, before the first contact with the patient. Such a review helps to focus the nursing assessment and to confirm and amplify information obtained from other sources.

The patient's health record or chart, which lists such information as age, sex, occupation, religious preference, next of kin, and financial status, is one type of record. The health record includes information entered by various healthcare professionals such as physicians, social workers, dietitians, physiotherapists, and laboratory technicians.

> ▶ *For Susan Morgan, the 34-year-old patient recently diagnosed with MS, the nurse would review her medical record for information related to her diagnosis, treatment plans, including specialized consultations and therapy, as well as her current home situation. This information would be important in determining the nurse's approach to the nursing history and physical examination and in planning the patient's care.* ■

Nurses who want their care to be supportive of the patient as he or she responds to changes in health status must be familiar with the many sections of the patient record, in addition to the documentation of the nursing plan of care and nursing notes. The following parts of the patient record are important sources of data for the nurse.

MEDICAL HISTORY, PHYSICAL EXAMINATION, AND PROGRESS NOTES

These sources record the findings of physicians as they assess and treat the patient; they focus on identifying pathologic conditions and their causes and on determining the medical regimen for treatment.

CONSULTATIONS

The patient's physicians may invite specialists to assess and to work with the patient. Their focus is on identifying findings that help to establish a medical diagnosis or on planning and executing the treatment regimen.

REPORTS OF LABORATORY AND OTHER DIAGNOSTIC STUDIES

Reports of laboratory studies and other diagnostic tests, such as radiographs, offer the nurse objective data that can either confirm or conflict with data collected during the nursing history or examination. Results of diagnostic studies are helpful to physicians for establishing a diagnosis and monitoring the patient's response to treatment. The results of these same studies may also be helpful to nurses in evaluating the success of nursing interventions.

REPORTS OF THERAPIES BY OTHER HEALTHCARE PROFESSIONALS

Other healthcare professionals who interact with the patient also record their findings and note any progress the patient is making in their specific areas—for example, nutrition, physical therapy, or speech therapy. These reports help the nurse to assess the patient's progress and are useful when determining the patient's ability to return home and manage care independently.

Records of previous admissions for healthcare and records from other health agencies, such as a social service agency or a home healthcare agency, are also valuable sources of data. They contain information about the patient's previous medical or surgical problems and response patterns, which may be important determinants of the current plan of care. See Chapters 17 and 21 for a description of the critical information that should be shared when patients are "handed off" from one caregiver or team to another (SBAR Communication).

Other Healthcare Professionals

Nurses can learn a great deal about a patient's normal health habits and patterns and response to illness by talking with other nurses, physicians, social workers, and others on the healthcare team (Fig. 12-3). Although such communication is always important, it can be crucial when patients are transferred from home to an institution or from one hospital or institution to another. The only way to ensure continuity of care is to make special efforts to share pertinent information.

Nursing and Other Healthcare Literature

To obtain a comprehensive patient database, it may be necessary to consult the nursing and related literature on specific health problems. For example, if a nurse has not cared for a patient with Paget's disease before, it is important for him or her to read about the clinical manifestations of the disease and its usual progression to know what to look for when assessing the patient. In addition to information concerning the medical diagnoses, treatment, and prognosis, a literature review offers nurses important information about nursing diagnoses, developmental norms, and psychosocial and spiritual practices that is helpful when assessing and caring for patients.

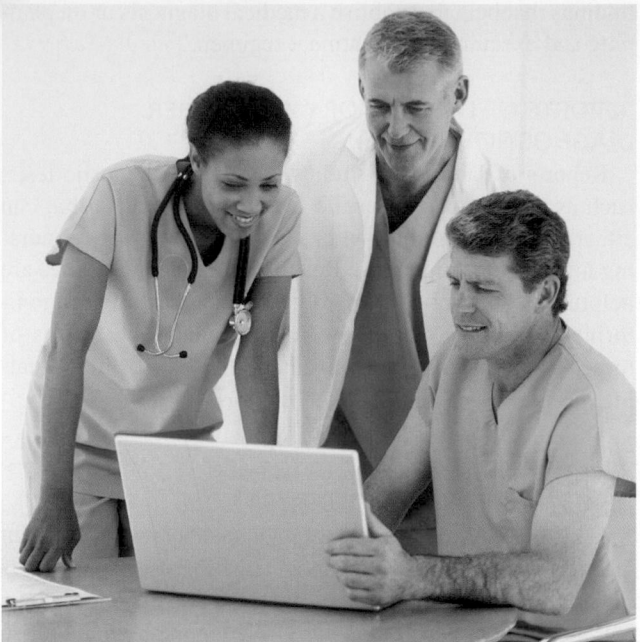

FIGURE 12-3. Nurses can learn a great deal about a patient's health habits, patterns, and responses to illness by talking with other nurses, physicians, social workers, and other members of the healthcare team. This exchange of information is particularly important when patients transfer from one healthcare setting to another, or to home.

➤ *For Sylvia Wu, the possible diagnosis of a virus that is potentially lethal can be extremely frightening. To provide the most appropriate care, the nurse would need to know as much as possible about the disease. In doing so, the nurse would be better able to act as an advocate for the patient.* ■

Methods of Data Collection

Components of data collection include the nursing history and the nursing physical assessment (see Chapter 25). These data may be documented on separate assessment tools or incorporated into a combined database assessment form, as shown in Figure 12-2.

Observation is a key nursing skill, whether gathering the nursing history or performing the physical examination. **Observation** is the conscious and deliberate use of the five senses to gather data. Skilled nurses use each nurse–patient interaction to observe and to interpret meaningful stimuli (data). You can develop such observation skills by training yourself to observe carefully for the following each time you encounter a patient:

- What are the patient's current responses (physical and emotional) to his or her situation? Be alert to signs of distress—difficulty breathing, bleeding, pain, heightened anxiety—as well as anything out of the ordinary, such as sudden eruption of rash or changes in level of consciousness.
- What is the patient's current ability to manage his or her care (need for additional information or nursing assistance)?

- What is the immediate environment? Consider the safety of the environment as well as the functioning of equipment (intravenous therapy, oxygen, drains). Who are the people in the room and at home? What are the temperature and odor of the room?
- What is the larger environment (hospital or community)?

Nursing History

Ideally, the nursing history captures and records the uniqueness of the patient so that care may be planned to meet the patient's individual needs. The nursing history should, therefore, be obtained as soon as possible after a patient presents for care and should be followed by the nursing physical assessment. The nursing history should clearly identify the patient's strengths and weaknesses; health risks, such as hereditary and environmental factors; and potential and existing health problems. The nursing history focuses on getting to know the person.

➤ *When obtaining the nursing history from Sylvia Wu, it would be important for the nurse to ascertain when the patient had traveled in China, how long she had been there, how long she had been home, with whom she may have been in contact, and if these individuals exhibited any signs and symptoms. This information would be important in determining the patient's actual risk for developing a particular virus.* ■

COMPONENTS OF A NURSING HISTORY
Components of a nursing history include:

- Profile: name, age, sex, race/ethnicity, marital status, religion, occupation, education
- Reason for seeking healthcare
- Normal health habits and patterns and related needs for nursing assistance
- Cultural considerations in relation to diet, decision making, and activities
- Current state of health, functioning of body systems, degree of pain, and past medical and surgical history
- Current medications, allergies, and record of immunizations and exposure to communicable diseases
- Perception of health status and the meaning the patient attributes to health and illness, as well as characteristic response or coping patterns
- Developmental history, family history, environmental history, and psychosocial history
- Patient's and family's expectations of nursing and of the healthcare team
- Patient's and family's educational needs and ability and willingness to learn
- Patient's and family's ability and willingness to participate in the plan of care
- Whether or not an advance directive exists, or if the patient wants help to prepare an advance directive

- Patient's personal resources (strengths) and deficits
- Patient's potential for injury

PATIENT INTERVIEW

The nurse obtains a nursing history by interviewing the patient. An **interview** is a planned communication. Strong interviewing skills are needed to establish a successful working partnership with the patient, to communicate care and concern for the patient, and to obtain the necessary patient data. The interview can be understood in terms of its four phases, which include the preparatory phase, introduction, working phase, and termination. More detailed information on interviewing techniques is provided in Chapter 21.

Preparatory Phase

Before initiating the interview, the nurse prepares to meet the patient by reading current and past records and reports, when available. During this phase, it is important not to let one's stereotypes and prejudices affect the nurse–patient relationship. Nurses who are aware of their own prejudices can deal with them constructively. Professional nurses learn to approach patients with open minds and to be sensitive to the human needs that underlie diverse behaviors.

During the preparatory phase, the nurse should ensure that the environment in which the interview is to be conducted is private and relaxed. Unless the patient wants family members or friends present during the interview, the nurse should interview the patient alone, either in the patient's room or in a quiet office.

Both the seating arrangement and the distance between nurse and patient are important (Fig. 12-4). Chairs placed at right angles to each other and about 3 to 4 feet (0.9–1.2 m) apart facilitate an easy exchange of information. If the patient is in bed, placing a chair at a 45-degree angle to the bed is helpful. If the nurse stands at the foot or side of the patient's bed and physically talks or looks down at the patient, a superior–inferior relationship is communicated and can negatively affect the interview. Whenever possible, it is best to communicate with patients at eye level.

The interview should be scheduled when both the nurse and the patient are free of concerns and distractions so that they can concentrate on the task. Ten to 15 minutes may be all that is necessary in some circumstances, whereas an hour or more may be required in others. Information can be gathered in several meetings, especially if the nurse notices that the patient is tiring or is in pain.

Introductory Phase

The interview's introduction is crucial because it sets the tone not only for the remainder of the interview but also for every following nurse–patient interaction. At the end of this phase of the interview, the patient should know the name of the primary nurse and what he or she can expect of nursing care, should sense that the nurse is competent and cares about him or her, and should know what is expected of him or her in terms of developing the plan of care and participating in its execution.

The nurse initiates the interview by stating his or her name and status, identifying the purpose of the interview, and clarifying the roles of nurse and patient. A typical introduction might run like this: "Good afternoon, Miss LeBon. My name is Lisa Gray and I'll be your student nurse. Right now I'd like to ask you a few questions about yourself so that we can plan your nursing care together. Feel free to respond only to those questions you feel comfortable answering, and know that your responses will be treated confidentially by the staff. This will take about 20 minutes. Is this time convenient for you? Do you need anything before we start?"

The initial impression the nurse creates is crucial, especially with patients who are new to the healthcare environment. *All nurses whom the patient encounters in the future may be judged in light of this first impression.* When the nurse communicates respect and genuine concern for the patient, the patient is then encouraged to discuss health concerns and problems freely. The competence and professionalism of the nurse as well as the interpersonal qualities of a respectful presence, professionalism, and caring invite the patient's confidence and ensure the patient that help is available.

During the introduction, the nurse should assess the patient's comfort and ability to participate in the interview. It is also appropriate to assure the patient of confidentiality. The patient should know where the data being recorded are stored, how they will be used, and who has access to them. Some nurses record data on the appropriate form while with the patient, whereas other nurses take notes and complete the form later. Bedside computers are facilitating quick documentation. However, documenting data should not interfere with the sharing of information during the interview. In unusual situations in which a contractual agreement that clearly identifies the responsibilities of both patient and nurse is indicated (e.g., a gerontologic nurse entrepreneur), terms are discussed at this time.

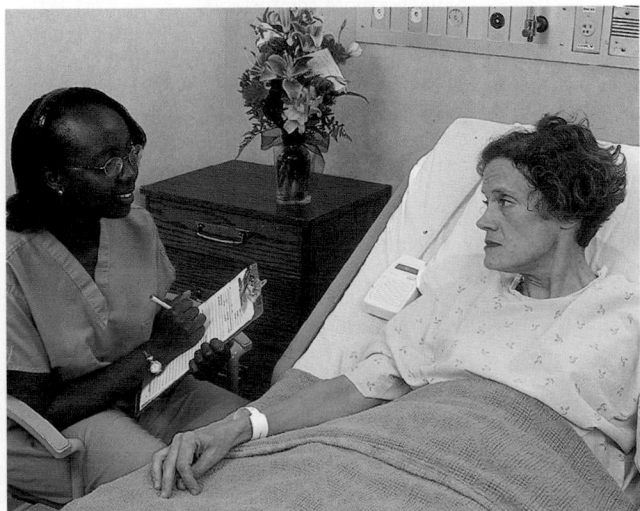

FIGURE 12-4. In the interview, both the seating arrangement and the distance from the patient are important in establishing a relaxed and comfortable environment for data collection. *(Photo © B. Proud)*

Box 12-3   COMMUNICATION TECHNIQUES FOR A SUCCESSFUL INTERVIEW

- Focus on the patient during the interview, demonstrating interest and concern: use the patient's name of choice, use eye contact appropriately, be sensitive to cultural variations, and avoid rushing the patient.
- Listen to the patient attentively; use reflection and paraphrase to communicate to the patient that you understand him or her.
- Ask about the patient's main problem first, using terminology the patient understands; save personal or delicate questions for later, when a rapport has been established. Defer less important questions until a later interview if the patient is too ill or upset to communicate easily.
- Pose questions and comments to the patient in the manner best suited to produce the desired communication (see Chapter 21):

Closed questions elicit specific information.
Open-ended questions allow the patient to verbalize freely.
Reflective questions encourage the patient to elaborate on thoughts and feelings.
Direct questions can validate information, clarify information,
    or place events into a meaningful sequence.

- Avoid comments and questions that impede communication (see Chapter 21)—clichés, questions that require a "yes" or "no" answer only, intimidating "why" or "how" questions, probing questions, giving advice, using judgmental comments, changing the subject, and giving false assurance.
- Use silence and touch appropriately.

Working Phase

During the working phase of the interview, the nurse gathers all the information needed to form the subjective database. The accuracy, completeness, and relevance of the database depend on the nurse's use of the interviewing and basic communication techniques discussed in Chapter 21. The communication techniques highlighted in Box 12-3 are important guidelines for a successful interview.

Many patient variables can positively or negatively affect the outcome of an interview. Table 12-2 identifies patient

TABLE • 12-2   PATIENT VARIABLES THAT CAN NEGATIVELY INFLUENCE AN INTERVIEW AND SUGGESTED NURSING RESPONSES

Patient Variables	Effect on Interview	Nursing Response
High anxiety	Patient may speak rapidly or incoherently and may jump from one topic to another; patient may deny or misrepresent what he or she is experiencing.	Normalize anxiety: "Many people find it difficult to talk about their health and become anxious"; approach patient gently, speak slowly and softly; underscore importance of the patient sharing what he or she is experiencing so nurses can help.
Pain	Patient offers clipped responses and "yes" or "no" answers whenever possible; overriding concern is pain relief.	Do everything possible to make patient comfortable before the interview, including obtaining an order for and administering pain medication; if pain persists, obtain only vital data and defer remainder of interview until patient is more comfortable.
Language difficulty (patient not fluent in nurse's language because patient speaks a different language, has a limited education, or fears saying the "wrong thing")	Vital patient data will not be communicated; patient may mistakenly be labeled "indifferent" or "noncommunicative."	Speak clearly (do not raise voice) using simple language; whenever possible, obtain the assistance of an interpreter (family member may help, but if patient data are confidential, a stranger may be preferable).
Previous negative experience with nurses or healthcare delivery system	Patient is aloof, unwilling to participate in interview; general attitude: "Why should I waste my time telling you anything . . . it won't do me any good."	"I know other people who have had a tough time with nurses or the system . . . life isn't perfect . . . but how about giving us a chance this time to show you what nurses can do?" Communicate respect for the patient and competence.
Unrealistic expectations of healthcare professionals	Patient expects nurses and other healthcare professionals magically to know everything about him or her and to "take care" of him or her; "surrenders" himself or herself to the system—"you know best" attitude.	Communicate clearly that no one knows or understands the patient like the patient does, and invite him or her to become involved in his or her care; "No two persons are alike, and unless you tell me a little more about yourself and how you are feeling, there is no way we'll be able to plan good care."

variables that can negatively influence an interview unless the nurse responds appropriately.

Termination

The successful interview is concluded carefully. The nurse should advise the patient that the interview is coming to an end. It is helpful to recapitulate the interview, highlighting key points. Both the patient and the nurse should be satisfied that the important data are recorded. A helpful strategy is to ask the patient after the summary: *"Is there anything else you would like us to know that will help us plan your care?"* This gives the patient an opportunity to add data the nurse did not think to include.

Before leaving the patient, it is helpful to alert the patient as to what he or she can expect. The patient should also know when the nurse will reestablish contact; for example, "Thank you for answering these questions, Miss LeBon. Please feel free to keep us informed of anything you think we should know. I'll be leaving soon, but when I return tomorrow morning, I'll discuss your plan of care. This afternoon will be busy for you—some blood tests and a chest x-ray have been ordered. Your evening will probably be quiet. Do you have any questions? Is there anything else I can do for you before I leave?"

Nursing Physical Assessment

Physical assessment is the examination of the patient for objective data that may better define the patient's condition and help the nurse in planning care. The physical assessment normally follows the nursing history and interview, and may verify data gathered during the history or yield new data. Physicians traditionally have performed the intake physical assessment, which commonly is the mechanism of entry into the healthcare delivery system, as well as the basis for medical treatment. Some nurses in advanced practice roles perform comprehensive intake physical assessments similar to those of their physician colleagues, which identify health and illness states, and then recommend or prescribe appropriate

follow-up care. In any case, all nurses conduct selected aspects of physical assessment for nursing purposes.

Unlike the physical assessment performed by the physician to identify pathologic conditions and their causes, the nursing physical assessment focuses primarily on the patient's functional abilities. If a neurologic deficit is present, the nurse is concerned with identifying how this deficit affects the patient's reasoning and sensorimotor abilities. For example, a patient who has had a cerebrovascular accident (brain attack or stroke) is examined to determine ability to comprehend and communicate information and execute the tasks of everyday life.

> ➤ *The physical assessment for Susan Morgan, the young woman newly diagnosed with MS described at the beginning of the chapter, would include investigation of the patient's muscle strength, endurance level, and the effects of MS on the patient's ability to perform daily activities. Also as part of the physical examination, the nurse would be alert to indications of fatigue or inability to complete specific activities. This information would help the nurse to respond appropriately to the patient's concerns about her marriage.* ∎

Purposes of the nursing physical assessment include the appraisal of health status, the identification of health problems, and the establishment of a database for nursing intervention. See Through the Eyes of a Student and Figure 12-5. See Chapter 25 for a detailed description of physical assessment skills.

Nurses practicing in different settings may use different physical assessment techniques for different purposes. Nurses in the coronary care unit use sophisticated, high-technology assessment techniques, whereas nurses in a rehabilitation center use a wide range of physical assessment skills that focus on identifying functional and nonfunctional response patterns to disabilities.

Through the Eyes of a Student

As a first-year nursing student, I often questioned myself on my technique in assessing a patient. Sure, I understood what my instructors taught me, but was I doing it right? So, I find my patient has an elevated temperature, or perhaps urinary output is scanty—but what does it all mean? I often wondered if I would be able to make sense of all this information, and would I *really* be able to detect a problem should one develop. Well, it works! Keep assessing, recording, and reporting.

During my second year (first semester), I realized how an assessment can aid in saving your patient's life. A continuous assessment for 2 days saved my 91-year-old patient. I detected early signs of pulmonary edema and congestive heart failure

and was able to notify appropriate medical personnel and immediately implement life-saving procedures. Sure it was scary, but how proud I felt when the nursing staff congratulated me on a job well done! I realized how significant my assessment was for my patient, when, as I stood with her in the radiology department, she looked up at me from her stretcher and thanked me for taking good care of her. Knowing my patient was aware of what I had done for her meant the world to me, and at this point, I realized why I had chosen the nursing profession.

*—Delores (Dee) C. Pascale,
Delaware County Community College,
Media, Pennsylvania*

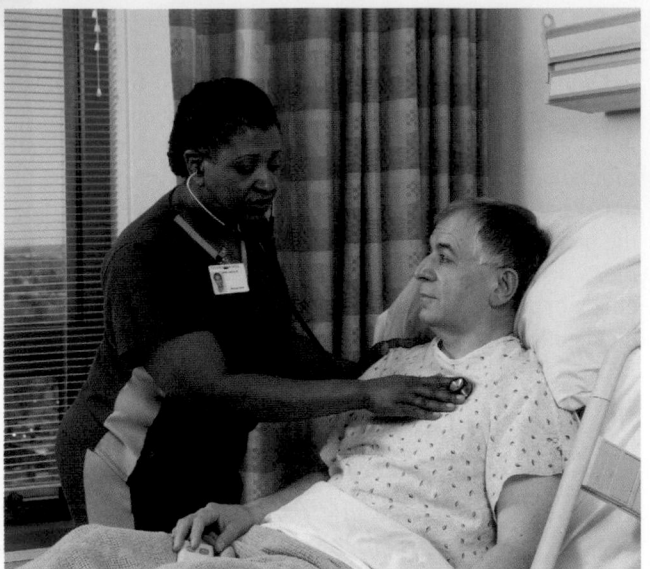

FIGURE 12-5. The nurse provides a physical examination. No matter what the setting or the age of the patient, the physical examination should include appraisal of health status, identification of health problems, and establishment of a database for nursing intervention. *(Photo by B. Proud)*

The nursing physical assessment involves the examination of all body systems, **review of systems (ROS),** in a systematic manner, commonly using a head-to-toe format. Four methods are used to collect data during a physical assessment: inspection, palpation, percussion, and auscultation. Nurses may also use physical assessment skills to evaluate selected body systems. These techniques and the basic skills for physical assessment are described in Chapter 25.

Problems Related to Data Collection

Common problems encountered during data collection include inappropriate organization of the database, omission of pertinent data, inclusion of irrelevant or duplicate data, erroneous or misinterpreted data, failure to establish rapport and partnership, recording an interpretation of data rather than observed behavior, and failure to update the database. Table 12-3 describes possible causes and remedies for such problems.

DATA VALIDATION

Validation is the act of confirming or verifying. The purpose of validating is to keep data as free from error, bias,

TABLE • 12-3	COMMON PROBLEMS OF DATA COLLECTION, POSSIBLE CAUSES, AND SUGGESTED REMEDIES	
Problem	**Possible Causes**	**Suggested Remedies**
Database inappropriately organized	Failure to plan for the assessment by identifying needed data; use of inappropriate tools for data collection	Review the guidelines for specifying pertinent data. Consider modifying tool for data collection or select an alternative tool.
Pertinent data omitted	Not following up on cues during data collection; inappropriate guidelines	Identify potentially relevant factors in advance of collection. Practice interview strategies.
Irrelevant or duplicate data collected	Failure to identify specific purpose of data collection; failure to review available patient records; use of inappropriate tools for data collection	Determine specific purpose of data collection for each patient. Consider existing data before initiating collection. Consider modifying data collection tool or selecting alternative.
Erroneous or misinterpreted data collection	Failure to observe carefully or validate during data collection; interviewer prejudices or stereotypes	Sharpen observation skills by independently observing the same situation with a peer and comparing notes afterward. Role play several validation techniques.
Failure to establish rapport	Failure to establish sufficient rapport or use appropriate communication techniques with patient; failure to know what information is wanted	Review and practice communication techniques discussed in Chapter 21. Role play several explanations of purpose of data collection. Identify general data desired before collection.
Interpretation of data is recorded rather than the observed behavior	Nurse jumps to hasty conclusion about patient's behavior and deprives others of exploring with the patient possible causes of the behavior; deficient validation	Review the distinction between data and interpretation of data. Practice documenting observed patient behavior concisely.
Failure to update the database	Erroneous belief that assessment is concluded after the initial database is recorded; low priority attached to ongoing data collection	Recollect that it is impossible to give quality, individualized care without knowledge of changes in the patient's status. Ongoing data collection is critical to the deletion or modification of old problems and the identification of new problems.

and misinterpretation as possible. Validation is an important part of assessment because invalid information can lead to inappropriate nursing care.

Identifying Data to Be Validated

Because validation of all data is neither possible nor necessary, nurses need to decide which items need verification. For example, data need to be verified when there are discrepancies: a patient tells the nurse he is fine and has no concerns, but the nurse notes that he demonstrates tense body musculature and seems curt in his responses. When there is a discrepancy between what the person is saying and what the nurse is observing, validation is necessary to determine accuracy. Validation in this instance may take the form of the nurse saying, "You tell me you feel fine, but right now your body and behaviors are telling me something else. Tell me more about this."

Data also need verification when they lack objectivity. For example, a nurse suspects that the patient hears in one ear but does not seem to hear well in the other. The nurse should validate the data before proceeding and should determine whether the patient does indeed have a hearing problem. Suspicions are not objective. In this instance, the nurse needs to test the patient's hearing in both ears. Speaking toward the suspected better ear, the nurse explains, "It seems to me that you hear better out of one ear than the other. I would like to test this. I'll bring a watch slowly toward your right ear first and then toward your left. Please look straight ahead and tell me when you first hear the watch ticking." The nurse then records how far the watch was from each ear when the patient first heard it ticking.

Identifying Cues and Making Inferences

Nurses now use the language of cues and inferences to describe the process of validation. The subjective and objective data you identify (patient does not respond when I speak to him on his left side) is a **cue** that something may be wrong. The judgment you reach about the cue (the patient's hearing may be impaired on his left side) is an **inference.** Until you check the patient's hearing, you cannot be sure that your inference is correct. Inferences may be validated in multiple ways:

- Physical examination, using the proper equipment and procedure (you may need to have an expert confirm your findings)
- Clarifying statements ("You said this is not a problem, but I sense you may still be worried.")
- Sharing your inferences with other respected members of the team and seeking consensus
- Checking your findings with research reports, textbooks, or journals
- Comparing cues to knowledge base of normal function
- Checking consistency of cues

Figure 12-6 illustrates the process for validating inferences.

The nurse may validate data as they are collected or at the end of the data-gathering process. When it is clear that the data are correct, the nurse is ready to analyze the data and formulate nursing diagnoses—the next step of the nursing process.

DATA REPORTING AND RECORDING

The patient data collected by the nurse, both initially and as patient contact continues, are of no benefit to the patient and the healthcare team unless they are appropriately communicated. See Box 12-4: Legal Alert. Appropriate communication involves correct timing and proper documentation.

Timing

Immediate verbal reporting of data is indicated whenever assessment findings reveal a critical change in the patient's health status that necessitates the involvement of other nurses or healthcare professionals. The nurse who observes an elevated temperature of 103.2°F (39.5°C) in a patient scheduled for surgery that morning must report this to the charge nurse and to the surgeon, who might then cancel surgery. Failure to communicate this finding could result in the patient's receiving preoperative sedation, being taken to the operating room, and even having the surgery performed under less than optimal conditions. Similarly, a nurse who hears a patient making suicidal remarks must communicate this information to the healthcare team so that all are alerted to the patient's danger and that suicide precautions may be taken immediately.

A nurse who is unsure of the significance of a particular finding is well advised to consult with another nurse. In some situations, years of experience are needed to distinguish significant from nonsignificant findings. Neither ignorance nor the fear of appearing less than competent justifies failure to report critical data.

> ▶ *The nurse would need to report Sylvia Wu's complaints along with the underlying history of travel to China immediately to the appropriate healthcare personnel. Doing so ensures that the necessary precautions are taken to reduce the risk of infection transmission with highly communicable viruses.* ■

Documentation

The initial database should be entered into the computer or recorded in ink, using the designated agency forms, the same

---

Box 12-4   LEGAL ALERT

Nurses are responsible for alerting the appropriate healthcare professional whenever assessment data differ significantly from the patient's baseline, indicating a potentially serious problem. Interventions for which the nurse may be legally responsible include increasing the frequency of assessments and initiating necessary changes in the treatment regimen.

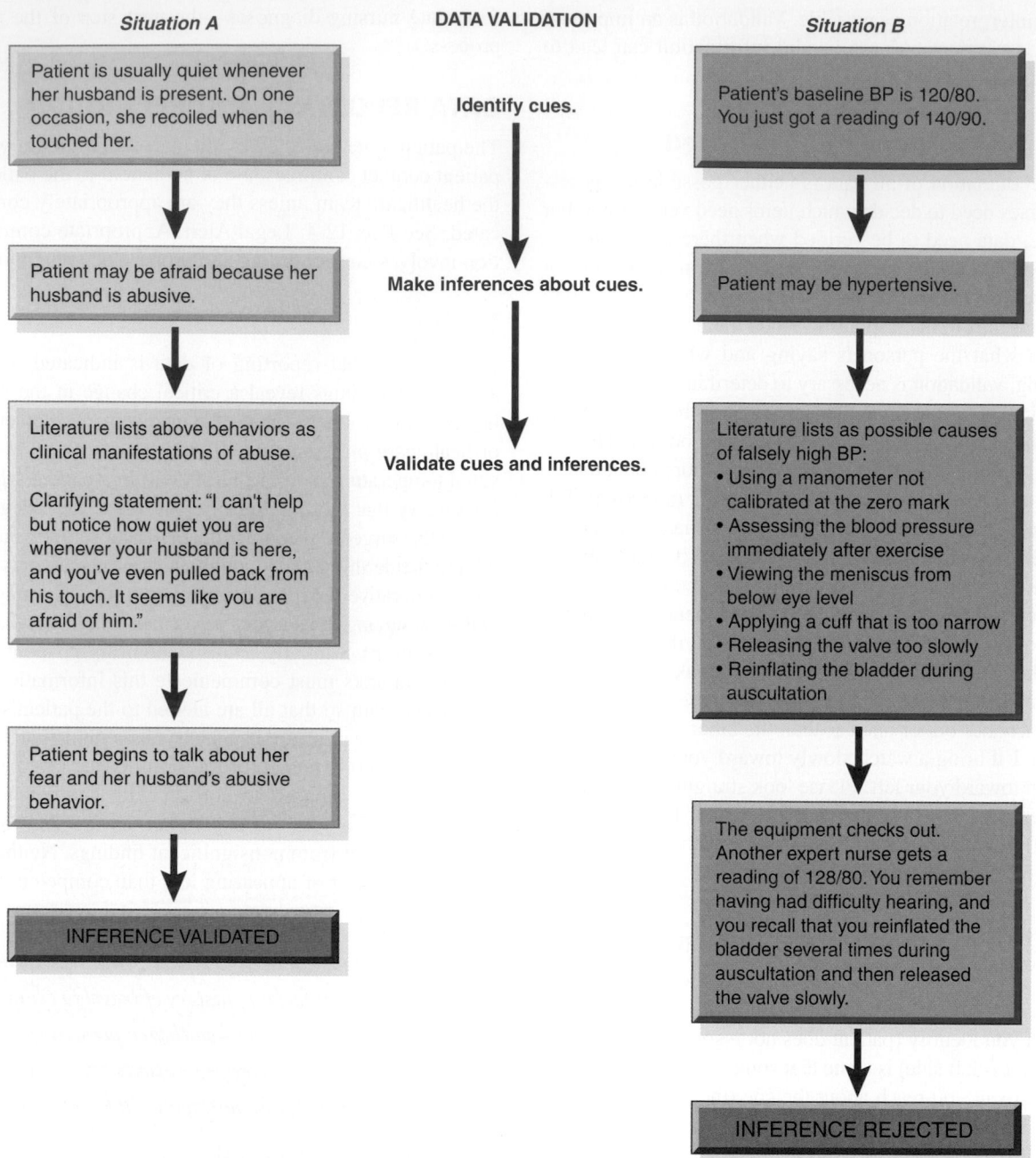

DATA VALIDATION

Situation A

Patient is usually quiet whenever her husband is present. On one occasion, she recoiled when he touched her.

↓

Identify cues.

↓

Patient may be afraid because her husband is abusive.

↓

Make inferences about cues.

↓

Literature lists above behaviors as clinical manifestations of abuse.

Clarifying statement: "I can't help but notice how quiet you are whenever your husband is here, and you've even pulled back from his touch. It seems like you are afraid of him."

↓

Validate cues and inferences.

↓

Patient begins to talk about her fear and her husband's abusive behavior.

↓

INFERENCE VALIDATED

Situation B

Patient's baseline BP is 120/80. You just got a reading of 140/90.

↓

Patient may be hypertensive.

↓

Literature lists as possible causes of falsely high BP:
• Using a manometer not calibrated at the zero mark
• Assessing the blood pressure immediately after exercise
• Viewing the meniscus from below eye level
• Applying a cuff that is too narrow
• Releasing the valve too slowly
• Reinflating the bladder during auscultation

↓

The equipment checks out. Another expert nurse gets a reading of 128/80. You remember having had difficulty hearing, and you recall that you reinflated the bladder several times during auscultation and then released the valve slowly.

↓

INFERENCE REJECTED

FIGURE 12-6. An illustration of the process used to validate cues and inferences.

day the patient is admitted to the agency. If, for any reason, important data cannot be obtained during the initial assessment, this needs to be documented so that they are obtained as soon as possible. Objective and subjective patient data should be summarized and written so that data communicate a unique sense of the patient and are comprehensive, concise, and easily retrievable. The data should be written legibly, and good grammar and only standard medical abbreviations should be used. To facilitate quick data retrieval, data should be presented under clearly marked headings.

Whenever possible, subjective data should be recorded using the patient's own words. Quotation marks should be used: "I feel tired from the moment I first get up in the morning. Any more it seems I have no energy at all." Patient reports may also be paraphrased: Patient reports feeling dyspneic, has difficulty catching breath when walking one flight of stairs.

The tendency to record data using nonspecific terms that are subject to individual definition or interpretation—words like adequate, good, average, normal, poor, small, large—should be avoided. One nurse's sense of what constitutes an average fluid intake may be very different from that of another nurse. It is important to be specific. Chapter 17 offers general documentation guidelines.

Developing Critical Thinking Skills

1. Working with another student, interview patients in both home and institutional settings, and record your findings separately. Make a list of the objective and subjective data you gather on each patient interviewed and the inferences you make from these cues. Compare your data lists and inferences. Describe to one another how you plan to validate your inferences. Explore possible reasons for the differences you discover.

2. Allow another student to perform a comprehensive nursing assessment (interview and physical assessment) on you. Reflect on what you experienced. Offer the student feedback about which of her or his behaviors were helpful, comforting, or distressing. Change roles and talk about what you learned from this experience.

3. Collect several different forms for recording the initial comprehensive nursing assessment (hospital, nursing home, home care, school of nursing forms). Identify and explain the differences you see. Experiment with using the different forms, and make a list of features that help you get all the data you need in the easiest way possible. Review Table 12-2. What other patient variables might negatively influence an interview? Nursing variables? How should you address these?

Practicing for NCLEX

1. Although the nursing process is presented as an orderly progression of steps, in reality there is great interaction and overlapping among the five steps. Which of the following describes this characteristic of the nursing process?
   a. Systematic
   b. Dynamic
   c. Interpersonal
   d. Outcome oriented

2. While administering a medication to relieve a patient's pain, you wonder if there are some nonpharmacologic interventions that would enhance relief by complementing the pain medication. When you discuss this question with your instructor, which of the following responses are you most likely to hear?
   a. "You should wait until after you evaluate the effect of the medication you just administered before planning a different intervention."
   b. "One step at a time. Don't start planning a new intervention until you evaluate the old."
   c. "Let's talk about this . . . we often get new information that we can incorporate successfully into the plan of care. Sometimes the steps of the process interact or overlap."
   d. "Think about this patient. Nonpharmacologic interventions wouldn't be effective with her."

3. When a patient you are admitting to the unit asks you why you are doing a history and exam since the doctor just did one, which of the following statements is your best reply?
   a. "In addition to providing us with valuable information about your health status, the nursing assessment will allow us to plan and deliver individualized, holistic nursing care that draws on your strengths."
   b. "It's hospital policy. I know it must be tiresome, but I will try to make this quick!"
   c. "I'm a student nurse and need to develop the skill of assessing your health status and need for nursing care. This information will help me develop a plan of care individualized to your unique needs."
   d. "We want to make sure that your responses are consistent and that all our data are accurate."

4. When you receive the shift report, you learn that your patient has no special skin care needs. You are surprised during the bath to observe reddened areas over bony prominences. What action is appropriate?
   a. Correct the initial assessment form.
   b. Redo the initial assessment and document current findings.
   c. Conduct and document an emergency assessment.
   d. Perform and document a focused assessment on skin integrity.

5. Fearful of attempting your first nursing history, you ask your instructor how anyone ever learns everything you have to ask to get good baseline data. You are most likely to hear which reply from the instructor?
   a. "There's a lot to learn at first, but once it becomes part of you, you just keep asking the same questions over and over in each situation until you can do it in your sleep!"
   b. "You make the basic questions a part of you and then learn to modify them for each unique situation, asking yourself how much you need to know to plan good care."
   c. "No one ever really learns how to do this well because each history is different! I often feel like I'm starting afresh with each new patient."
   d. "Don't worry about learning all of the questions to ask. Every agency has its own assessment form you must use."

6. A patient complains about feeling nauseated after lunch. This is an example of what type of data?
   a. Subjective
   b. Objective
   c. Signs and symptoms
   d. Overt

7. When you enter the patient's room to begin your nursing history, the patient's wife is there. What should you do?
   a. Introduce yourself to both and thank the wife for being present.
   b. Introduce yourself to both and ask the wife if she wants to remain.

c. Introduce yourself to both and ask the wife to leave.
d. Introduce yourself and ask the patient if he would like the wife to stay.

8. The patient is Vietnamese and does not speak English. Her son is with her and does speak English. How should you respond?
   a. Ask the son if he is willing to translate and be sure to thank him if he says yes.
   b. Determine if the son can translate medical information and if so, begin.
   c. After determining that the son can translate, evaluate if he can do so objectively and if the patient wants him to serve in this capacity.
   d. Explain to the son that hospital policy forbids using family members as translators and find a hospital-approved translator.

9. You are surprised to detect an elevated temperature (102°F) in a patient scheduled for surgery. The patient has been afebrile and shows no other signs of being febrile. What is the first thing you do?
   a. Inform the charge nurse
   b. Inform the surgeon
   c. Validate your finding
   d. Document your finding

10. You tell your instructor that your patient is fine and has "no complaints." You are likely to hear:
    a. "You made an inference that she is fine because she has no complaints. How did you validate this?"
    b. "She probably just doesn't trust you enough to share what she is feeling. I'd work on developing a trusting relationship."
    c. "Sometimes everyone gets lucky. Why don't you try to help another patient?"
    d. "Maybe you should reassess the patient. He has to have a problem—why else would he be here?"

● Answers With Rationale

1. **b.** The term dynamic is used to describe the fact that there is much interaction and overlap among the steps of the nursing process. In some situations, all five steps may occur almost simultaneously.

2. **c.** There may be much interaction and overlap among the steps of the nursing process. In this case, though you want to evaluate the effect of the medication you administered (options *a* and *b*), there is no reason to wait for this to happen before exploring other valid options. Answer *d* is incorrect because it is not possible to judge the effectiveness of nonpharmacologic methods before their use, and the instructor's response possibly indicates a prejudice toward complementary and alternative modalities.

3. **a.** Though it may be true that you need to develop assessment skills (*c*), the chief reason you are doing a nursing history and exam is because there needs to be a documented nursing admission assessment to serve as a basis for nursing care. The fact that this is also hospital policy (*b*) is a secondary reason.

4. **d.** Perform and document a focused assessment on skin integrity since this is a newly identified problem. The initial assessment stands as is and cannot be redone (*b*) or corrected (*a*). This is not a life-threatening event; thus, there is no need for an emergency assessment (*c*).

5. **b.** Once you learn what constitutes the minimum data set, you can adapt this to any patient situation. It is not true that each assessment is the same even when you are using the same minimum data set (*a*), nor is it true that each assessment is uniquely different (*c*). Answer *d* is incorrect because relying solely on standard agency assessment tools does not allow for individualized patient care or critical thinking.

6. **a.** A patient report of "feeling nauseated" cannot be perceived or validated by the nurse, and this is subjective data, not objective (*b*) or overt (*d*), which are observable and measurable. Answer *c* is wrong because signs are examples of objective data.

7. **d.** The patient has the right to indicate who he would like to be present for the nursing history and exam. You should neither presume that he wants his wife there (*a*), nor that he does not want her there (*c*). Similarly, the choice belongs to the patient, not the wife (*b*).

8. **c.** This is difficult, but it is important to evaluate whether or not the son can adequately translate medical information, can be trusted to translate what is said without introducing his bias, and if the patient wants him to serve in this capacity. The choice belongs to the patient, not the son (*a*) and there is no policy that prohibits family members from translating (*d*). Answer *b* is incomplete.

9. **c.** You should first validate your finding if it is unusual, deviates from normal, and is unsupported by other data. Should your initial recording prove to be in error, it would have been premature to notify the charge nurse (*a*) or the surgeon (*b*). You want to be sure that all data you record is accurate, so it should be validated before documentation if you have doubts (*d*).

10. **a.** Your instructor is most likely to challenge your inference that the patient is "fine" simply because he is telling you that he has no problems. It is appropriate for her to ask how you validated this inference. Jumping to the conclusion that the patient does not trust you (*b*) is premature and is an invalidated inference. Answer *c* is wrong because it accepts your invalidated inference. Answer *d* is wrong because it is possible that the condition is resolving.

Taylor Suite Resources

The Taylor Suite offers these additional resources to enhance learning and facilitate understanding of this chapter:

- thePoint online resource, http://thepoint.lww.com/Taylor7E
- Student DVD included with the book
- Study Guide for Taylor's Fundamentals of Nursing

BIBLIOGRAPHY

Alfaro-LeFevre, R. (2010). *Applying nursing process: A tool for critical thinking* (7th ed.). Philadelphia: Lippincott Williams & Wilkins.

American Nurses Association (ANA). (1998). *Standards of clinical nursing practice.* Washington, DC: Author.

American Nurses Association (ANA). (2003). *Nursing: A social policy statement* (2nd ed.). Washington, DC: Author.

Armstrong, J., & Mitchell, E. (2008). Comprehensive nursing assessment in the care of older people. *Nursing Older People, 20*(10), 36–40.

Bickley, L. (2008). *Bate's guide to physical examination and history taking* (10th ed.). Philadelphia: Lippincott Williams & Wilkins.

Dellefield, M. E. (2007). Implementation of the Resident Assessment Instrument/Minimum Data Set in the nursing home as organization: Implications for quality improvement in RN clinical assessment. *Geriatric Nursing, 28*(6), 377–386.

Dykes, P. C., Kim, H. E., Goldsmith, D. M., Choic, J., Esumi, K., & Goldberg, H. S. (2009). The adequacy of ICNP Version 1.0 as a representational model for electronic nursing assessment documentation. *Journal of the American Medical Informatics Association, 16*(2), 238–246.

Flores, J., & Dodier, A. (2005, May 31). HIPAA: Past, present and future implications for nurses. *Online Journal of Issues in Nursing, 10*(2), manuscript 4. Available at http://www.nursingworld.org/MainMenuCategories/ANAMarketplace/ANAPeriodicals/OJIN/TableofContents/Volume102005/No2May05/tpc27_416020.aspx

Gordon, M. (1994). *Nursing diagnosis: Process and application* (3rd ed.). St. Louis, MO: Mosby–Year Book.

Kumekawa, J. K. (2001, September 30). Health information privacy protection: Crisis or common sense? *Online Journal of Issues in Nursing, 6*(3), manuscript 2. Available at http://www.nursingworld.org/MainMenuCategories/ANAMarketplace/ANAPeriodicals/OJIN/TableofContents/Volume62001/No3Sept01/PrivacyProtectionCrisis.asp

U.S. Department of Health and Human Services, Office for Civil Rights. (2003). HIPAA: Summary of HIPAA privacy rule. Available at http://www.hhs.gov/ocr/privacy/index.html.

Weber, J., & Kelley, J. (2007). *Health assessment in nursing* (3rd ed.). Philadelphia: Lippincott Williams & Wilkins.

West, S. (2006). Physical assessment: Whose role is it anyway? *Nurse Critical Care, 11*(4), 161–167.

13 Diagnosing

MARTIN PRESCOTT

Martin, a 46-year-old man, comes to the health clinic for a routine physical examination. During the assessment, he states, "I've had problems with constipation and have seen some blood when I wipe myself after a bowel movement. It's just hemorrhoids, right? Nothing to worry about?"

ANTONIA ZUCCARELLI

Antonia is a middle-aged woman newly diagnosed with cancer that is treatable. However, she continually fails to show up for follow-up appointments for both diagnosis and treatment.

ANGIE CLARKSON

Angie, a college sophomore, tearfully reports that she believes she was a victim of date-rape. She had too much to drink at a party and can only remember waking up in a strange room with a guy she just met, unsure if she passed out because of the alcohol or date-rape drugs. A virgin, Angie was sure there was penetration because of blood and semen stains she discovered upon waking. It is now a month later and she has not been able to "get her life together" and move on.

After completing the chapter, you will be able to accomplish the following:

1. Describe the term *nursing diagnosis,* distinguishing it from a collaborative problem and a medical diagnosis.

2. Describe the four steps involved in data interpretation and analysis.

3. Use the guidelines for writing nursing diagnoses when developing diagnostic statements.

4. Identify five types of nursing diagnoses.

5. Describe means to validate nursing diagnoses.

6. Describe the benefits and limitations of nursing diagnoses.

KEY TERMS

actual nursing diagnoses
collaborative problems
cue
data cluster
diagnosing
diagnostic error
health problem
medical diagnoses
nursing diagnoses
possible nursing diagnoses
risk nursing diagnoses
standard
syndrome nursing diagnoses
wellness diagnoses

- Recognizing signs and symptoms of common health problems and those that may indicate the need for more expert diagnosis.
- Predicting problems in those at risk and taking steps to manage risks and prevent complications.
- Identifying human responses and promoting optimum function, independence, and quality of life.
- Initiating actions and referrals in a timely way to ensure appropriate, qualified treatment.

When a health problem is identified, the nurse must decide which healthcare professional can best address the problem. Actual or potential health problems that can be prevented or resolved by independent nursing intervention are termed **nursing diagnoses.** The nurse formulates, validates, and lists

FIGURE 13-1. This diagram shows how the activities of *Assessment* lead to a *pivotal* point in the nursing process: *Diagnosis.* Diagnosis is a pivotal point for the following reasons:
1. The purpose of diagnosis is to clarify the exact nature of the problems and risk factors you need to achieve the overall expected outcomes of care. If you do not completely understand the problems contributing to them, how are you going to know what to do about them?
2. The conclusions you make during this phase affect the entire plan of care. If your conclusions are correct, your plan is likely to be on target. If they are not—for example, if you are operating on *assumptions,* rather than sound reasoning that is based on evidence—your plan is likely to be flawed, maybe even dangerous.
(Used with permission from Alfaro-LeFevre, R. [2010]. *Applying the nursing process: A tool for critical thinking* [7th ed., p. 93]. Philadelphia: Lippincott Williams & Wilkins.)

Diagnosing—the second step in the nursing process—begins after the nurse has collected and recorded the patient data. The purpose of **diagnosing** is to (1) identify how an individual, group, or community responds to actual or potential health and life processes; (2) identify factors that contribute to or cause health problems (etiologies); and (3) identify resources or strengths the individual, group, or community can draw on to prevent or resolve problems. See the accompanying Reflective Practice display for an example.

In the diagnosing step of the nursing process, the nurse interprets and analyzes data gathered from the nursing assessment (Fig. 13-1). The data help the nurse identify patient strengths and health problems. A **health problem** is a condition that necessitates intervention to prevent or resolve disease or illness or to promote coping and wellness.

Alfaro-LeFevre (2010) counsels nurses to understand the types of problems they should focus on to better understand their responsibilities relating to diagnosis and management of health problems. She lists the following as the types of concerns that are clearly nursing responsibilities (2010, p. 95):

REFLECTIVE PRACTICE

Challenge to Cognitive and Interpersonal Skills

Angie Clarkson, a college sophomore, told me tearfully that she believes she was a victim of date-rape her first week in school. She knows she had too much to drink at a party and can only remember waking up in a strange room with a guy she met at the party. She is not sure if she passed out because of the alcohol or if one of the date-rape drugs was involved. A virgin, Angie was sure there had been penetration because of the blood and semen stains she discovered upon waking. It is now a month later and she has not been able to "get her life together" and move on. Angie told me that I am the first person she has told because she feels "so ashamed" and can't believe she let this happen to her. This is my first encounter with an experience like this. I don't do drugs or alcohol and am not sexually active.

Thinking Outside the Box: Possible Courses of Action

- Try to be a good friend and simply suggest she get professional help.
- Advocate for Angie by finding out what resources exist on campus.

- Inform Angie that everything she is describing sounds like the defining characteristics of rape-trauma syndrome and explain how to get professional help and why getting help is so important.

Evaluating a Good Outcome: How Do I Define Success?

- Angie gets the professional help she needs to survive this well.
- I prove worthy of her trust in me.
- I use this experience to learn more about a common problem on campus and the adequacy of existing resources.

- I learn something about my ability to diagnose a health problem and plan accordingly.

Personal Learning: Here's to the Future!

Responding to Angie's clear cry for help certainly moved me out of my comfort zone and made me aware of how my newly developing clinical skills will at times complicate something as simple as being a friend. I felt somewhat responsible for Angie's ability to cope with being raped and believed that I had to do more than simply provide a listening ear. I was pleasantly surprised to discover all the resources that exist on campus. I guess I wasn't surprised that it took quite a bit of coaxing to get Angie to seek professional help. When I showed her some of what is written about the diagnosis of rape-trauma syndrome, she seemed to find her experience validated and finally agreed to try the student health service counseling center. I felt positive about my role in helping to make this happen.

Reflection

How do you think you would respond in a similar situation? Why? What does this tell you about yourself and about the adequacy of your skills for professional practice? Can you think of other ways to respond? What if the person was a patient for whom you were providing care? Would your response be any different? Should it be? Explain your answer. What other skills (cognitive, interpersonal, technical, ethical/legal) would you need to respond well in this situation? What resources would be appropriate? Do you agree with the criteria to evaluate a successful outcome? Did the nursing student meet the criteria? Please support your response.

---

nursing diagnoses for each patient (Fig. 13-2). Nursing diagnoses provide the basis for selecting nursing interventions that will achieve valued patient outcomes for which the nurse is responsible (Fig. 13-3). See Box 13-1 for Alfaro's rule about the legal implications of diagnoses.

Alfaro recommends using both a nursing model and a body systems approach (see Chapter 12) to organize assessment data to detect both nursing and medical problems.

EVOLUTION OF NURSING DIAGNOSES

The term *nursing diagnosis* first appeared in the literature in the 1950s. As early as 1966, Hammond wrote that nurses

Box 13-1   LEGAL ALERT: ALFARO'S RULE

Legal Implications of Using the Word Diagnosis
The term *diagnosis* implies that there's a situation or problem requiring appropriate, qualified treatment. This means if you identify a problem, you must decide if you are *qualified* to treat it and willing to *accept responsibility* for treating it. If you are not, you are responsible for getting help.

Source: Alfaro-LeFevre, R. (2010). *Applying nursing process: A tool for critical thinking* (7th ed., p. 106). Philadelphia: Lippincott Williams & Wilkins.

FIGURE 13-2. Diagnosing is the interpretation and analysis of patient data to identify patient strengths and health problems that nursing intervention can prevent or resolve. Nursing diagnoses may change from day to day as the patient's responses to health and illness change. *(Photo © B. Proud.)*

need to be competent in information-seeking strategies and should have a good background of theoretical knowledge to search for cues and evaluate evidence. These skills and knowledge result in accurate diagnosing. Key elements in the evolution of nursing diagnosis as an integral component of the nursing process include the following:

- In 1953, the term "nursing diagnosis" was introduced by V. Fry (1953) to describe a step necessary in developing a care plan.
- In 1972, the New York State Nurse Practice Act identified diagnosing as part of the legal domain of professional nursing; practice acts in many other states have been revised similarly since then.

- In 1973, the American Nurses Association's Standards of Practice included diagnosing as a function of professional nursing.
- Also in 1973, Gebbie and Lavin, of St. Louis University, called the First National Conference on Classification of Nursing Diagnoses, beginning a national effort to identify, standardize, and classify health problems treated by nurses. At this first meeting, the National Group, since renamed the North American Nursing Diagnosis Association (NANDA), appointed a task force to accomplish the following goals:
  - Gather information and disseminate it through the Clearinghouse for Nursing Diagnosis.
  - Encourage educational activities at regional and state levels to promote the implementation of nursing

FIGURE 13-3. The relationship of nursing diagnosis to accountability and autonomy. (Used with permission from Carpenito-Moyet, L. J. [2008]. *Nursing diagnosis: Application to clinical practice* [12th ed.]. Philadelphia: Lippincott Williams & Wilkins.)

diagnoses. These activities include conferences to organize nurses to identify additional diagnostic labels and workshops to teach nurses about nursing diagnoses.

- Promote and organize activities to continue the development, classification, and scientific testing of nursing diagnoses. These activities include planning national conferences, identifying criteria for accepting diagnoses, surveying current research activities, and exploring varied methods for classification.
- In 1980, the American Nursing Association (ANA) Social Policy Statement defined nursing as "the diagnosis and treatment of human response to actual or potential health problems" (ANA, 1980).
- In March 1990, at the Ninth Conference of NANDA, the General Assembly approved an official definition of nursing diagnosis:

  Nursing diagnosis is a clinical judgment about individual, family, or community responses to actual or potential health problems/life processes. Nursing diagnosis provides the basis for selection of nursing interventions to achieve outcomes for which the nurse is accountable. (NANDA, 1990)

- In March 1990, the first issue of *Nursing Diagnosis*, NANDA's official journal, was published.
- In 2004, the ANA Standards of Nursing Practice revised the Standard 2 Diagnosis, to include the word *issues:* The registered nurse analyzes the assessment data to determine the diagnoses or issues (ANA, 2004) (Box 13-2). Alfaro-LeFevre (2010) believes that adding "issues" to the standard reflects the realities of today's healthcare setting. Today's nurses deal with specific problems (diagnoses) and ill-defined problems (issues).
- NANDA conferences are held every 2 years, and much progress continues to be made in defining, classifying, and describing nursing diagnoses—internationally.

Now an accepted and essential step in the nursing process, nursing diagnosis was initially confused with medical diagnosis, sparking controversy. Although this confusion has been resolved, many nurses have been slow to understand and to accept the "work" of diagnosing.

Box 13-2 **ANA STANDARDS OF PRACTICE: STANDARD 2, DIAGNOSIS**

The registered nurse analyzes the assessment data to determine the diagnoses or issues.

Measurement Criteria
The registered nurse:

Derives the diagnoses or issues based on assessment data.

Validates the diagnoses or issues with the patient, family, and other healthcare providers when possible and appropriate.

Documents diagnoses or issues in a manner that facilitates the determination of the expected outcomes and plan.

Used with permission. American Nurses Association (ANA). (2004). *Scope and standards of practice* (p. 22). Washington, DC: Author.

The most recent change in the way nurses understand the diagnosing step in the nursing process is the change in focus from nurses only diagnosing and treating nursing diagnoses, to nurses diagnosing and managing the varieties of health problems described earlier in the text.

UNIQUE FOCUS OF NURSING DIAGNOSIS

In the diagnosing step of the nursing process, the nurse identifies nursing's unique concern for a patient (i.e., what it is about the patient that gives rise to the need for nursing, as opposed to the need for medicine or for physical therapy). Nursing diagnoses are written to describe patient problems that nurses can treat independently.

> *Consider Antonia Zuccarelli, the middle-aged woman recently diagnosed with cancer but failing to maintain follow-up. Although the patient's diagnosis of cancer is important, the nurse would focus on the patient's lack of follow-up and the possible underlying reasons. For example, the patient may not realize the importance of the follow-up, thereby indicating a lack of knowledge. Or the patient may be too overwhelmed with the diagnosis, possibly denying its existence, and being unable to cope.* ∎

In her latest book on the nursing process, Alfaro-LeFevre (2010) describes the shift from diagnose and treat (DT) to predict, prevent, manage, and promote (PPMP). The latter approach focuses on early evidence-based intervention to prevent and manage problems and their potential complications. It requires three activities for nurses:

1. In the presence of known problems, predict the most common and most dangerous complications and take immediate action to (a) prevent them, and (b) manage them in case they cannot be prevented.
2. Whether problems are present or not, look for evidence of risk factors (things that we know may cause problems, such as risky sexual behaviors). If you identify risk factors, aim to reduce or control them, thereby preventing the problems themselves.
3. In all situations, encourage behaviors that promote optimum function, independence, and a sense of well-being (p. 94).

As nurses interpret and analyze patient data, they may identify health problems that are better treated by physicians (medical diagnoses) or by nurses working with other healthcare professionals (collaborative problems). In such a case, the nurse reports the findings to the physician or other appropriate healthcare professionals and works collaboratively with them to resolve the problem.

Nursing Diagnosis Versus Medical Diagnosis

Medical diagnoses identify diseases, whereas nursing diagnoses focus on unhealthy responses to health and illness.

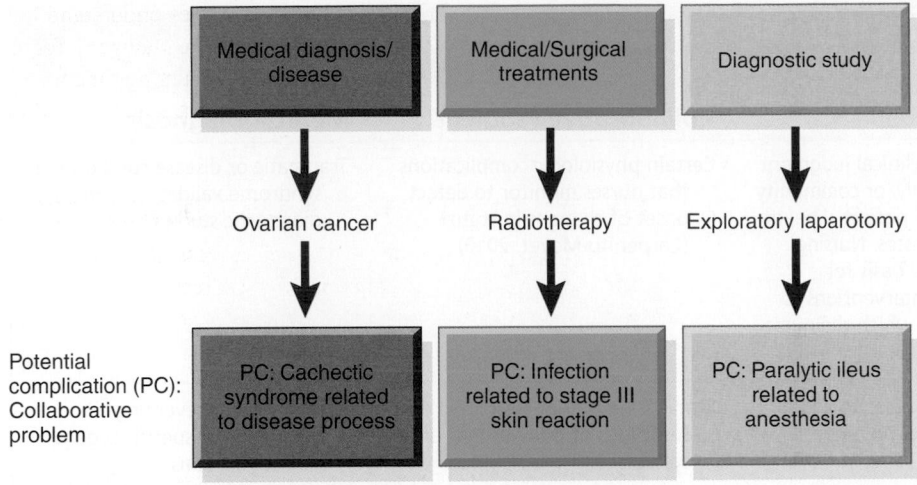

FIGURE 13-4. Collaborative problems.

Medical diagnoses describe problems for which the physician directs the primary treatment, whereas nursing diagnoses describe problems treated by nurses within the scope of independent nursing practice. A medical diagnosis remains the same for as long as the disease is present, whereas a nursing diagnosis may change from day to day as the patient's responses change. These distinctions reflect key differences in medical and nursing practices.

Myocardial infarction (heart attack) is a medical diagnosis. Examples of nursing diagnoses for a person with myocardial infarction include Fear, Altered Health Maintenance, Deficient Knowledge, Pain, and Altered Tissue Perfusion.

> ➤ *Think back to Angie Clarkson, the college sophomore who was a victim of date-rape. Possible nursing diagnoses might include Ineffective Coping, Rape-Trauma Syndrome, Post-Trauma Syndrome, Risk for Situational Low Self-Esteem, and Risk for Infection.* ∎

Nursing Diagnosis Versus Collaborative Problem

Nursing diagnoses are also different from collaborative problems. Together, nursing diagnoses and collaborative problems constitute the range of responses that nurses treat, and as such, they define the unique nature of nursing. Carpenito-Moyet defines **collaborative problems** as "certain physiologic complications that nurses monitor to detect onset or changes in status. Nurses manage collaborative problems using physician-prescribed and nurse interventions to minimize the complications of the event" (2010, p. 24).

Unlike medical diagnoses, collaborative problems are the primary responsibility of nurses. Unlike nursing diagnoses, with collaborative problems, the prescription for treatment comes from nursing, medicine, and other disciplines. When the nurse writes patient outcomes that require delegated medical orders for goal achievement, the situation is not a nursing diagnosis, but a collaborative problem. Because collaborative problems involve potential complications, they

must be identified early so that preventive nursing care can be instituted early. Figure 13-4 shows collaborative problems identified by a nurse caring for a patient with ovarian cancer. These problems are related to a medical disease, a medical treatment, and a diagnostic study.

To write a diagnostic statement for a collaborative problem, focus on the potential complications of the problem. Use "PC" (for potential complication), followed by a colon, and list the complications that might occur. For clarity, link the potential complications and the collaborative problem by using "related to." Example: PC: Paralytic ileus related to anesthesia.

Table 13-1 shows how nurses successfully interpret different clusters of data to identify a nursing diagnosis, collaborative problem, and medical diagnosis. In the first example, a nursing diagnosis is identified and successfully treated. In the next example, the nurse identifies a collaborative problem and initiates intervention within the scope of nursing practice. When this fails to resolve the problem, a physician is contacted to order medication or a catheterization. In this example, the nurse's early detection and reporting of the problem to the physician lead to the physician's prompt medical diagnosis of cystitis and successful antibiotic therapy.

DIAGNOSTIC REASONING AND CRITICAL THINKING

Successful implementation of each step of the nursing process requires high-level skills in critical thinking. To correctly diagnose health problems:

- Be familiar with nursing diagnoses and other health problems; read professional literature and keep reference guides handy.
- Trust clinical experience and judgment, but be willing to ask for help when the situation demands more than your qualifications and experience can provide.
- Respect your clinical intuitions, but before writing a diagnosis without evidence, increase the frequency of your observations and continue to search for cues to verify your intuition.
- Recognize personal biases and keep an open mind.

TABLE • 13-1 A COMPARISON: NURSING DIAGNOSIS, COLLABORATIVE PROBLEM, MEDICAL DIAGNOSIS

	Nursing Diagnosis	Collaborative Problem	Medical Diagnosis
Definition	A nursing diagnosis is a clinical judgment about individual, family, or community responses to actual or potential health problems or life processes. Nursing diagnosis provides the basis for selection of nursing interventions to achieve outcomes for which the nurse is accountable (NANDA).	Certain physiologic complications that nurses monitor to detect onset of changes in status (Carpenito-Moyet, 2010)	Traumatic or disease condition or syndrome validated by medical diagnostic studies
Focus	Monitoring human responses to actual and potential health problems	Monitoring pathophysiologic responses of body organs or systems	Correcting or preventing pathology of specific organs or body systems
Sample data cluster	56-year-old mother of seven; 5'4", 167 lb; "Whenever I sneeze lately, I dribble urine. This is embarrassing."	42-year-old woman; 1 hour after delivery; spinal anesthesia; 1,500 mL fluid infused in past 4 hours without patient voiding; unable to void	"Whenever I have to urinate it burns terribly. I also feel like I have to go all the time—real bad." Small, frequent voidings, cloudy urine; T—100.8°F
Diagnostic statement	Stress Urinary Incontinence related to degenerative changes in pelvic muscles and structural supports associated with advanced age, obesity, gravid uterus	Potential complication: Urinary Retention related to fluid overload and effects of anesthesia	Cystitis
Select nursing responses	Teach Kegel exercises to increase muscle tone; explore patient's willingness and motivation to pursue weight reduction and exercise program; evaluate need for bladder-training program.	Monitor for signs of increasing urine retention; offer bedpan, and encourage voiding with running water, warm water dripped over perineum, and so forth; if no result, administer physician-prescribed medication; if no result, perform physician-prescribed catheterization.	Report signs and symptoms to physician; obtain urine culture; report results to physician; administer appropriate physician-prescribed antibiotic.

Questions to facilitate critical thinking during diagnostic reasoning include:

- Are my data accurate and complete?
- Has the patient or the patient's surrogates validated (if able to do so) that these are important problems?
- Have I given the patient or the patient's surrogate an opportunity to identify problems that I may have missed?
- Is each diagnosis supported by evidence? Might these cues signify a different problem or diagnosis?
- Have I tried to identify what is causing the actual or potential problem, and what strengths/resources the patient might use to avoid or resolve the problem?
- Have I used agency guidelines to correctly document diagnostic statements in a way that clearly communicates patient problems to other healthcare professionals?
- Is this a problem that falls within nursing's independent domain or does it signify a medical diagnosis or collaborative problem?

DATA INTERPRETATION AND ANALYSIS

Most experienced nurses begin the work of interpreting and analyzing data while they are still collecting (assessing) it. The term **cue** is often used to denote significant data or data that influence this analysis. Significant data should "raise a red flag" for the nurse, who then looks for patterns or clusters of data that signal an actual, potential, or possible nursing diagnosis.

> Remember Martin Prescott, the 46-year-old man with bleeding associated with bowel movements? The report of bleeding accompanied by the patient's complaint of constipation should alert the nurse to a potential problem involving the patient's bowel elimination. ■

Recognizing Significant Data

Sorting out healthy patient responses from those that are not healthy is not as clear-cut as it may seem. To avoid erroneously labeling selected patient health patterns as unhealthy (**diagnostic error**) while failing to detect an actual unhealthy behavior, nurses must be familiar with comparative standards to be used in data interpretation and analysis.

A **standard,** or a norm, is a generally accepted rule, measure, pattern, or model to which data can be compared in the same class or category. For example, when determining the significance of a patient's blood pressure reading, appropriate standards include normative values for the patient's age group, race, and illness category. The patient's own normal range, if known, is an important standard. A pressure of 150/90 mm Hg may be high for someone whose pressure normally is 120/70 mm Hg, but it may be normal for a person with hypertension. Examples of how standards can be used to identify significant cues include the following (Gordon, 1994):

1. Changes in a patient's usual health patterns that are unexplained by expected norms for growth and development: *Example*—An infant who took to breastfeeding easily as a newborn suddenly stops sucking when put to the breast and begins to lose weight.
2. Deviation from an appropriate population norm: *Example*—A first-year college student begins to accelerate her exercise habits dramatically and starts inducing vomiting after binge eating. She rapidly loses weight.
3. Behavior that is nonproductive in the whole-person context: *Example*—A college student breaks up with her boyfriend and begins to believe that she is "unfit" for any other relationship, withdrawing from her friends and social activities.
4. Behavior that indicates a developmental lag or evolving dysfunctional pattern: *Example*—A 16-year-old single mother with a 6-month-old infant continues to "party hard" with her friends, hangs out at the mall, and shows no interest in caring for her son, who is repeatedly left with concerned family members.

Recognizing Patterns or Clusters

A **data cluster** is a grouping of patient data or cues that points to the existence of a patient health problem. Nursing diagnoses should always be derived from clusters of significant data rather than from a single cue. The danger of deriving a nursing diagnosis from a single cue is illustrated in the following example. Diagnosing a woman recovering from gallbladder surgery with Ineffective Coping solely on the basis of tears may misinterpret the patient's crying, which may be a healthy release of emotion. If the same patient begins to exhibit a cluster of significant cues, such as refusing to eat, preferring bed rest to scheduled ambulation, and reporting increasing discomfort, an unhealthy pattern is emerging.

➤ *Think back to Angie Clarkson, the college sophomore. Verbalization of the rape trauma is significant. However, even more significant is Angie's report that the event happened more than 1 month ago and she is having difficulty "getting her life together" and moving on.* ■

Table 13-2 offers examples of how clusters of significant data lead to formulation of accurate nursing diagnoses.

Identifying Strengths and Problems

The next step in analyzing data is to determine the patient's strengths and problems. When determining a patient's strengths and problems, it is helpful to determine whether the patient agrees with the nurse's identification of strengths and problems and is motivated to work toward problem resolution.

Determining the Patient's Strengths

If a patient appears to meet a standard, the nurse concludes that the patient has a strength in that particular area, and that this strength contributes to the patient's level of wellness. For example, a person with a history of maintaining a well-balanced diet is usually better able to cope with illness than a person who has a history of eating poorly.

Patient strengths might include healthy physiologic functioning, emotional health, cognitive abilities, coping skills, interpersonal strengths, and spiritual strengths. Resources such as the presence of support people, adequate finances, and a healthy environment may all contribute to patient strengths. Many people take their strengths for granted and might not know how to use them effectively when responding to illness. Discussing observed strengths with patients and counseling patients about ways to develop and use their strengths are important nursing measures.

Determining the Patient's Problem Areas

A person who does not meet a certain health standard probably has a limitation in this aspect of health status and may benefit from professional care. For example, a person with a long history of constipation probably needs care to help overcome this problem. As stated previously, the nurse decides whether the data represent a nursing diagnosis or a collaborative problem, or whether the data should be reported to the physician because they might lead to a medical diagnosis.

Determining Problems the Patient Is Likely to Experience

It is important for nurses to identify potential health problems. For example, a nurse notes that a patient has signs of a wound infection, but laboratory test results show that the patient's white blood cell count has not increased, as is usual when such an infection is present. The nurse concludes that the body apparently is not building up normal defenses to combat the infection. The nurse then predicts the problems this patient is likely to encounter, such as a longer-than-normal healing period. Possible nursing diagnoses alert other caregivers to problems the patient may experience if the certain trends in the patient's condition continue unreversed.

TABLE • 13-2	FORMULATING ACCURATE NURSING DIAGNOSIS BASED ON DATA CLUSTERS		
Data Interpretation and Analysis		**Formulation of Tentative Nursing Diagnosis**	**Validation of Nursing Diagnosis**
Significant Cues	*Sample Data Clusters*		
Change in a patient's usual health patterns that is unexplained by expected norms for growth and development	• "I guess I lost about 20 to 30 pounds over the last 6 months—I think I've just been too busy to eat." • Height: 5'8" • Weight: 102 lb • 35-year-old mother of 4-year-old twin boys; returned to work (executive secretary) for first time since delivery of twins 7 months ago	Imbalanced Nutrition: Less Than Body Requirements, related to stress of new job; role conflict and demands	Accurate diagnosis: Patient validates this diagnosis, agreeing with contributing factors
Deviation from an appropriate population norm	• Teacher notices and reports frequency of bruises on third-grade boy who is repeatedly observed alone during recess periods and who is withdrawn in classroom. • In conversation with the school nurse, one parent remarks: "That boy brings out the worst in me! I don't know why, but I often have to smack him hard to make him listen."	Risk for Other-Directed Violence (Child Abuse) related to? Etiology (deficient parenting skills?)	Incomplete diagnosis: Additional data collection yields new information: • Father out of work for past 18 months • Father was abused as a child Diagnosis restated: Risk For Other-Directed Violence (Child Abuse) related to increased family stress and father's history of being abused
Behavior that is nonproductive in the whole-person context	• Fiancé abruptly terminated relationship 3 months before established wedding date • Noticeable change in physical appearance; frequently wears same clothes; makeup, jewelry, hair-styling are absent; strong body odors present • No desire to be with others; goes home (lives alone) immediately after work • Stopped attending aerobics classes	Risk for Situational Low Self-esteem related to feeling rejected by fiancé	Premature diagnosis resulting from incomplete data collection. Patient has a long history of major depressive states, one of which may have resulted in the breakup of this relationship. Medical diagnosis and treatment indicated. Changes in appearance are indicative of depressive state. Need to explore related nursing diagnoses.
Behavior indicating developmental lags or evolving dysfunctional patterns	• Admitted to nursing home 2 months ago • "I have nothing to live for anymore . . . why don't I die?" • Wishes to remain in room seated in chair—will only ambulate with great urging • Anything requiring movement has become "too much bother." • Decreased muscle mass, tone, and strength, reduced joint mobility	Impaired Physical Mobility related to difficult transition to nursing home	Accurate but routinized diagnosis that may result in staff's acceptance of status quo unless a more specific cause is identified

This prediction has implications for nursing care such as measures related to the patient's diet, fluid intake, urine output, and mobility.

Identifying Potential Complications

Patients may experience many complications related to their diagnoses, medications or treatment regimens, or invasive diagnostic studies. While new to nursing, you are most likely to prevent potential complications or at least make sure that they are detected early and managed well if you research the potential complications associated with your patient's diagnoses, diagnostics and treatment, and if you report all abnormal data. For example, slurred speech, changes in skin color or moistness, inability to move an extremity or abnormal movement, and changes in levels of consciousness may all be indications of serious and life-threatening complications (Alfaro-LeFevre, 2010).

Reaching Conclusions

The nurse reaches one of four basic conclusions after interpreting and analyzing the patient data. Different nursing responses are possible for each conclusion:

No Problem
- No nursing response is indicated.
- Reinforce patient's health habits and patterns.
- Initiate health-promotion activities to prevent disease or illness or to promote a higher level of wellness.
- Wellness diagnosis might be indicated.

Possible Problem
- Collect more data to confirm or disprove suspected problem.

Actual or Potential Nursing Diagnosis
- Begin planning, implementing, and evaluating care designed to prevent, reduce, or resolve the problem.
- If unable to treat problem because patient denies problem and refuses treatment, make sure patient understands possible outcomes of this stance.

Clinical Problem Other Than Nursing Diagnosis
- Consult with appropriate healthcare professional and work collaboratively on problem.
- Refer to medicine or other services, as indicated.

Partnering with the Patient

You always want to remember that your best source of information is likely to be an aware patient. While some patients still enter the healthcare system expecting physicians and nurses to tell them what is "wrong" and to "fix it," increasingly patients want to play a leading role in identifying and treating their health problems. Be sure to ask patients what they believe their most important problems or issues are and have them confirm what your assessment is revealing and help you prioritize the resulting list of diagnoses.

FORMULATING AND VALIDATING NURSING DIAGNOSES
Terminology for Writing Nursing Diagnoses

When the nurse recognizes a cluster of significant patient data indicating a health problem that can be treated by independent nursing intervention, a nursing diagnosis should be written. If you are just beginning to understand and write nursing diagnoses, it may be helpful to consult the list of health problems accepted by NANDA for testing and study (Box 13-3). The NANDA list is a beginning list of suggested terms for health problems that might be identified and treated by nurses. Each of the diagnoses in *NANDA International Nursing Diagnoses: Definitions and Classification, 2009–2011* is presented in taxonomic order and includes the basic components of a nursing diagnosis: definition, defining characteristics, and related factors or risk factors (Box 13-4).

There are distinct advantages to nurses' use of common terminology when formulating nursing diagnoses. These range from communication advantages (everyone uses the same words to describe common problems) to promoting the development of nursing science by facilitating research and the dissemination of research findings to establishing the foundation for any cost/benefit analysis for nursing practice.

The NANDA structure has recently been simplified to facilitate the parallel development of an electronic database for nursing diagnoses. The five-digit code structure provides for the growth and development of the classification structure without having to change codes when new diagnoses, refinements, and revisions are added. The code structure is compliant with recommendations from the National Library of Medicine concerning healthcare terminology codes.

Pocket-sized handbooks of NANDA-approved nursing diagnoses are available and help students unfamiliar with this grouping of health problems. Nurses who encounter different health problems within the scope of their practice that they believe to be nursing diagnoses may submit these to the NANDA Diagnosis Review Committee.

Types of Nursing Diagnoses

NANDA describes five types of nursing diagnoses: Actual, risk, possible, wellness, and syndrome.

Actual Nursing Diagnoses

Actual nursing diagnoses represent a problem that has been validated by the presence of major defining characteristics. This type of nursing diagnosis has four components: label, definition, defining characteristics, and related factor (see Box 13-4).

Risk Nursing Diagnoses

Risk nursing diagnoses are clinical judgments that an individual, family, or community is more vulnerable to develop the problem than others in the same or similar situation.

Possible Nursing Diagnoses

Possible nursing diagnoses are statements describing a suspected problem for which additional data are needed. Additional data are used to confirm or rule out the suspected problem.

An actual nursing diagnosis for a patient who has experienced vomiting, diarrhea, and excessive diaphoresis for 3 days is Deficient Fluid Volume related to abnormal fluid loss. If the diarrhea persists and weakness interferes with the patient's normal perineal hygiene, he might be at risk for skin breakdown. This is written as the risk diagnosis, Risk for Impaired Skin Integrity. If the nurse suspects that a disturbance of self-concept is also present but lacks the necessary data (defining characteristics) to confirm this, it can be written as a possible diagnosis: Possible Chronic Low Self-Esteem. This alerts other nurses to the need to collect more data about the patient's self-esteem.

(text continues on page 254)

Box 13-3   NANDA-APPROVED NURSING DIAGNOSES

This list represents the NANDA-approved nursing diagnoses for clinical use and testing.

Domain 1: Health Promotion
Description
The awareness of well-being or normality of function and the strategies used to maintain control of and enhance that well-being or normality of function

Approved Diagnoses
Ineffective Self-Health Management
Ineffective Family Therapeutic Regimen Management
Ineffective Health Maintenance
Impaired Home Maintenance
Readiness for Enhanced Self-Health Management
Readiness for Enhanced Nutrition
Readiness for Enhanced Immunization Status
Self-Neglect

Domain 2: Nutrition
Description
The activities of taking in, assimilating, and using nutrients for the purpose of tissue maintenance, tissue repair, and the production of energy

Approved Diagnoses
Ineffective Infant Feeding Pattern
Impaired Swallowing
Imbalanced Nutrition: Less Than Body Requirements
Imbalanced Nutrition: More Than Body Requirements
Risk for Imbalanced Nutrition: More Than Body Requirements
Risk for Impaired Liver Function
Risk for Unstable Blood Glucose Level
Neonatal Jaundice
Deficient Fluid Volume
Risk for Deficient Fluid Volume
Excess Fluid Volume
Readiness for Enhanced Fluid Balance
Risk for Electrolyte Imbalance
Risk for Imbalanced Fluid Volume

Domain 3: Elimination and Exchange
Description
Secretion and excretion of waste products from the body

Approved Diagnoses
Impaired Urinary Elimination
Urinary Retention
Functional Urinary Incontinence
Stress Urinary Incontinence
Urge Urinary Incontinence
Reflex Urinary Incontinence
Risk for Urge Urinary Incontinence
Readiness for Enhanced Urinary Elimination
Overflow Urinary Incontinence
Bowel Incontinence
Diarrhea
Constipation
Risk for Constipation
Perceived Constipation
Dysfunctional Gastrointestinal Motility
Risk for Dysfunctional Gastrointestinal Motility
Impaired Gas Exchange
Ineffective Airway Clearance
Impaired Spontaneous Ventilation

Domain 4: Activity/Rest
Description
The production, conservation, expenditure, or balance of energy resources

Approved Diagnoses
Sleep Deprivation
Readiness for Enhanced Sleep
Insomnia
Disturbed Sleep Pattern
Risk for Disuse Syndrome
Impaired Physical Mobility
Impaired Bed Mobility
Impaired Wheelchair Mobility
Impaired Transfer Ability
Impaired Walking
Deficient Diversional Activity
Delayed Surgical Recovery
Sedentary Lifestyle
Disturbed Energy Field
Fatigue
Decreased Cardiac Output
Impaired Spontaneous Ventilation
Ineffective Breathing Pattern
Activity Intolerance
Risk for Activity Intolerance
Dysfunctional Ventilatory Weaning Response
Risk for Decreased Cardiac Tissue Perfusion
Risk for Ineffective Cerebral Tissue Perfusion
Risk for Ineffective Gastrointestinal Perfusion
Risk for Tissue Perfusion
Ineffective Peripheral Tissue Perfusion
Risk for Shock
Risk for Bleeding
Dressing Self-Care Deficit
Bathing Self-Care Deficit
Feeding Self-Care Deficit
Toileting Self-Care Deficit
Readiness for Enhanced Self-Care

Domain 5: Perception/Cognition
Description
The human information-processing system, including attention, orientation, sensation, perception, cognition, and communication

Approved Diagnoses
Unilateral Neglect
Impaired Environmental Interpretation Syndrome
Wandering
Disturbed Sensory Perception (specify: Visual, Auditory, Kinesthetic, Gustatory, Tactile)
Deficient Knowledge
Readiness for Enhanced Knowledge
Acute Confusion
Chronic Confusion
Impaired Memory
Disturbed Thought Processes
Readiness for Enhanced Decision Making
Risk for Acute Confusion
Ineffective Activity Planning
Impaired Verbal Communication
Readiness for Enhanced Communication

(continued)

Box 13-3   **NANDA-APPROVED NURSING DIAGNOSES**   *(continued)*

Domain 6: Self-Perception

Description
Awareness about the self

Approved Diagnoses
Disturbed Personal Identity
Powerlessness
Risk for Powerlessness
Hopelessness
Risk for Loneliness
Readiness for Enhanced Self-Concept
Readiness for Enhanced Power
Risk for Compromised Human Dignity
Readiness for Enhanced Hope
Chronic Low Self-Esteem
Situational Low Self-Esteem
Risk for Situational Low Self-Esteem
Disturbed Body Image

Domain 7: Role Relationships

Description
The positive and negative connections or associations between persons or groups of persons and the means by which those connections are demonstrated

Approved Diagnoses
Caregiver Role Strain
Risk for Caregiver Role Strain
Impaired Parenting
Risk for Impaired Parenting
Readiness for Enhanced Parenting
Interrupted Family Processes
Readiness for Enhanced Family Processes
Dysfunctional Family Processes
Risk for Impaired Attachment
Effective Breastfeeding
Ineffective Breastfeeding
Interrupted Breastfeeding
Ineffective Role Performance
Parental Role Conflict
Impaired Social Interaction
Readiness for Enhanced Relationship

Domain 8: Sexuality

Description
Sexual identity, sexual function, and reproduction

Approved Diagnoses
Sexual Dysfunction
Ineffective Sexuality Pattern
Readiness for Enhanced Childbearing Process
Risk for Disturbed Maternal/Fetal Dyad

Domain 9: Coping/Stress Tolerance

Description
Contending with life events/life processes

Approved Diagnoses
Relocation Stress Syndrome
Risk for Relocation Stress Syndrome
Rape-Trauma Syndrome
Post-Trauma Syndrome
Risk for Post-Trauma Syndrome
Fear

Anxiety
Death Anxiety
Chronic Sorrow
Ineffective Denial
Ineffective Coping
Disabled Family Coping
Compromised Family Coping
Defensive Coping
Ineffective Community Coping
Readiness for Enhanced Coping (individual)
Readiness for Enhanced Family Coping
Readiness for Enhanced Community Coping
Risk for Complicated Grieving
Stress Overload
Risk-Prone Health Behavior
Grieving
Complicated Grieving
Impaired Individual Resilience
Risk for Compromised Resilience
Readiness for Enhanced Resilience
Autonomic Dysreflexia
Risk for Autonomic Dysreflexia
Disorganized Infant Behavior
Risk for Disorganized Infant Behavior
Readiness for Enhanced Organized Infant Behavior
Decreased Intracranial Adaptive Capacity

Domain 10: Life Principles

Description
Principles underlying conduct, thought, and behavior about acts, customs, or institutions as being true or having intrinsic worth

Approved Diagnoses
Readiness for Enhanced Hope
Readiness for Enhanced Spiritual Well-Being
Spiritual Distress
Risk for Spiritual Distress
Decisional Conflict (specify)
Noncompliance (specify)
Risk for Impaired Religiosity
Impaired Religiosity
Readiness for Enhanced Religiosity
Moral Distress
Readiness for Enhanced Decision Making

Domain 11: Safety/Protection

Description
Freedom from danger, physical injury, or immune-system damage, preservation from loss, and protection of safety and security

Approved Diagnoses
Risk for Infection
Readiness for Enhanced Immunization Status
Impaired Oral Mucous Membrane
Risk for Injury
Risk for Perioperative Positioning Injury
Risk for Falls
Risk for Trauma
Impaired Skin Integrity
Risk for Impaired Skin Integrity
Impaired Tissue Integrity
Impaired Dentition

(continued)

Box 13-3   **NANDA-APPROVED NURSING DIAGNOSES**   *(continued)*

Risk for Suffocation Risk for Aspiration Ineffective Airway Clearance Risk for Peripheral Neurovascular Dysfunction Ineffective Protection Risk for Sudden Infant Death Syndrome Risk for Vascular Trauma Risk for Self-Mutilation Self-Mutilation Risk for Other-Directed Violence Risk for Self-Directed Violence Risk for Suicide Risk for Poisoning Risk for Contamination Contamination Latex Allergy Response Risk for Latex Allergy Response Readiness for Enhanced Immunization Status Risk for Imbalanced Body Temperature Ineffective Thermoregulation Hypothermia Hyperthermia	**Domain 12: Comfort** ***Description*** Sense of mental, physical, or social well-being or ease ***Approved Diagnoses*** Acute Pain Chronic Pain Nausea Readiness for Enhanced Comfort Impaired Comfort Social Isolation **Domain 13: Growth/Development** ***Description*** Age-appropriate increase in physical dimension, organ systems, and/or attainment of developmental milestones ***Approved Diagnoses*** Delayed Growth and Development Risk for Disproportionate Growth Adult Failure to Thrive Risk for Delayed Development

From NANDA International. (2009). *Nursing diagnoses: Definitions and classification, 2009–2011.* West Sussex: Wiley-Blackwell.

Wellness Diagnoses

Wellness diagnoses are clinical judgments about an individual, group, or community in transition from a specific level of wellness to a higher level of wellness. Two cues must be present for a valid wellness diagnosis:

Box 13-4   **COMPONENTS OF A NANDA NURSING DIAGNOSIS**

Label
Imbalanced Nutrition: More Than Body Requirements (1975, 2000).

Definition
Intake of nutrients that exceeds metabolic needs.

Defining Characteristics
- Concentrating food intake at the end of the day
- Dysfunctional eating pattern (e.g., pairing food with other activities)
- Eating in response to external cues (e.g., time of day, social situation)
- Eating in response to internal cues other than hunger (e.g., anxiety)
- Sedentary activity level
- Triceps skin fold greater than 25 mm in women, greater than 15 mm in men
- Weight 20% over ideal for height and frame

Related Factors
- Excessive intake in relation to metabolic need.

From North American Nursing Diagnosis Association (NANDA) International. (2009). *NANDA International nursing diagnoses: Definitions and classification, 2009–2011.* (p. 75.) Oxford, UK: Wiley-Blackwell.

- A desire for a higher level of wellness
- An effective present status or function

A persistent critique of nursing diagnoses that focuses exclusively on patient health problems is their limited applicability in nursing settings that deal primarily with healthy patients. To remedy this concern, wellness diagnoses were proposed and are now readily accepted. For an individual or group to have a wellness diagnosis, two cues should be present: (1) a desire for increased wellness and (2) effective present state or function (Carpenito-Moyet, 2010, p. 17). The diagnostic statement for wellness diagnoses is a one-part statement that contains the label Readiness for Enhanced, followed by the desired higher-level wellness. Related factors are not included. Examples include Readiness for Enhanced Family Coping, Readiness for Enhanced Health Maintenance, Readiness for Enhanced Parenting, and Readiness for Enhanced Self-Esteem.

Syndrome Nursing Diagnoses

Syndrome nursing diagnoses comprise a cluster of actual or risk nursing diagnoses that are predicted to be present because of a certain event or situation; for example, Rape-Trauma Syndrome or Post-Trauma Syndrome.

Parts of Nursing Diagnosis Statements

Most nursing diagnoses are written either as two-part statements listing the patient's problem and its cause or as three-part statements that also include the problem's defining characteristics (Table 13-3).

TABLE • 13-3   FORMULATION OF NURSING DIAGNOSIS STATEMENTS

	Definition	Purpose	Example
Problem	Identifies what is unhealthy about the patient, indicating the need for change (clear, concise statement of the patient's health problem)	Suggests the patient outcomes (expectations for change)	Bathing/Hygiene Self-Care Deficit ↓ related to ↓
Etiology	Identifies the factors that are maintaining the unhealthy state or response (contributing or causative factors)	Suggests the appropriate nursing measures	Fear of falling in the tub and obesity ↓ as manifested by ↓
Defining characteristics	Identify the subjective and objective data that signal the existence of the problem (cues that reflect the existence of a problem)	Suggest evaluative criteria	Strong body and urine odor, unclean hair: "I'm afraid I'll fall in the tub and break something." (5'4", 170 lb)

Examples:
Two-part diagnostic statement: Bathing/Hygiene Self-Care Deficit related to fear of falling in tub and obesity
Three-part diagnostic statement: Bathing/Hygiene Self-Care Deficit related to fear of falling in tub and obesity, as manifested by strong body and urine odor, unclean hair, statement of fearing fall in tub, and height and weight: 5'4", 170 lb

Problem

The purpose of the problem statement is to describe the health state or health problem of the patient as clearly and concisely as possible. Because this section of the nursing diagnosis identifies what is unhealthy about the patient and what the patient would like to change in his or her health status, it suggests patient outcomes. NANDA recommends the use of quantifiers or descriptors to limit or specify the meaning of a problem statement. For example, the descriptor "anticipatory" placed before the concept "grieving" clarifies that the nursing diagnosis for a pregnant couple who has received news prenatally that their child will most likely be stillborn and who is already grieving the death of their child. Some common descriptors are listed in Table 13-4.

Etiology

The etiology identifies the physiologic, psychological, sociologic, spiritual, and environmental factors believed to be related to the problem as either a cause or a contributing factor. Because the etiology identifies the factors that maintain the unhealthy patient state and prevent the desired change, the etiology directs nursing intervention. Unless the etiology is correctly identified, nursing actions might be inefficient and ineffective. For example, a diabetic patient who is frequently admitted to the hospital with hyperglycemia and who has a poor history of dietary and pharmacologic management is diagnosed to be noncompliant. Assuming that the noncompliance is related to a knowledge deficit, channeling all nursing activities and energies into teaching the patient how to manage the diabetes is useless if the noncompliance is actually a result of the patient's decreased will to live, which would necessitate a different group of nursing interventions.

> Recall Antonia Zuccarelli, the middle-aged woman recently diagnosed with cancer who fails to maintain follow-up? A nursing diagnosis that might be appropriate would be "Noncompliance related to repeated failure to maintain appointments for follow-up treatment and diagnostic testing." ■

Defining Characteristics

The subjective and objective data that signal the existence of the actual or potential health problem are the third component of the nursing diagnosis. NANDA has identified defining characteristics for each accepted nursing diagnosis, and familiarity with these characteristics helps nurses recognize clusters of significant data. Table 13-3 defines the three components of a nursing diagnosis statement and shows how they affect patient outcomes, nursing measures, and evaluation. Other examples of nursing diagnosis statements are found throughout the book.

Guidelines for Writing Nursing Diagnoses

Remember the following to ensure that your diagnostic statements are correctly written.

1. Phrase the nursing diagnosis as a patient problem or alteration in health state rather than as a patient need.
2. Check to make sure that the patient problem precedes the etiology and that the two are linked by the phrase "related to."
3. Defining characteristics, when included in the nursing diagnosis, should follow the etiology and be linked by the phrase "as manifested by" or "as evidenced by."

TABLE • 13-4	COMMON DESCRIPTORS USED TO CLARIFY A DIAGNOSTIC CONCEPT
Descriptor	**Meaning**
Anticipatory	Realize beforehand, foresee
Compromised	Damaged, made vulnerable
Decreased	Lessened (in size, amount, or degree)
Deficient	Insufficient, inadequate
Delayed	Late, slow or postponed
Disabled	Limited, handicapped
Disorganized	Not properly arranged or controlled
Disproportionate	Too large or too small in comparison with a norm
Disturbed	Agitated, interrupted, interfered with
Dysfunctional	Not operating normally
Effective	Producing the intended or desired result
Excessive	Greater than necessary or desirable
Imbalanced	Out of proportion or balance
Impaired	Damaged, weakened
Ineffective	Not producing the intended or desired effect
Interrupted	Having its continuity broken
Low	Below the norm
Organized	Properly arranged or controlled
Perceived	Observed through the senses
Readiness for	In a suitable state for an activity or situation
Situational	Related to a particular circumstance

From NANDA International. (2009). *Nursing diagnoses: Definitions and classification, 2009–2011.* West Sussex: Wiley-Blackwell.

4. Write in legally advisable terms.
5. Use nonjudgmental language.
6. Be sure the problem statement indicates what is unhealthy about the patient or what the patient wants to change (enhance).
7. Avoid using defining characteristics, medical diagnoses, or something that cannot be changed in the problem statement.

8. Reread the diagnosis to make sure the problem statement suggests patient outcomes and that the etiology will direct the selection of nursing measures.

▶ *Remember Angie Clarkson, the college sophomore who was a victim of date-rape? An appropriate nursing diagnosis could be "Rape-Trauma Syndrome related to feelings of embarrassment and shame as manifested by the patient's reporting of event 1 month after it happened, and by patient's statements of inability to get life together and move on."* ■

Common errors in writing nursing diagnoses are shown in Table 13-5, along with suggestions for correcting them.

What Is Not a Nursing Diagnosis

The nursing diagnosis statement is written in terms of a patient problem, alteration in health state, or patient strength for which nursing provides the primary therapy. Table 13-6 uses a patient with diabetes mellitus to illustrate what nursing diagnoses are not. For example, nursing diagnoses are not medical diagnoses or statements of patient need.

Validating Nursing Diagnoses

After a tentative nursing diagnosis is formulated, it should be validated. An affirmative response to each of the following questions validates a tentative diagnosis:

• Is my database sufficient, accurate, and supported by nursing research?
• Does my synthesis of data (significant cues) demonstrate the existence of a pattern?
• Are the subjective and objective data I used to determine the existence of a pattern characteristic of the health problem I defined?
• Is my tentative nursing diagnosis based on scientific nursing knowledge and clinical expertise?
• Is my tentative nursing diagnosis able to be prevented, reduced, or resolved by independent nursing action?
• Is my degree of confidence above 50% that other qualified practitioners would formulate the same nursing diagnosis based on my data?

Remember that you are responsible for validating the diagnoses you write, even when using computer-assisted diagnosis. The use of standardized language and electronic health records may make diagnosis writing easier by suggesting possible diagnoses to match your recorded assessment findings. However, computers cannot replace humans and critical thinking, especially when it comes to complex diagnostic reasoning. While the computer can process data faster than you can, it may not be aware of what is happening to your patient at this moment in time. You need to validate diagnoses and recognize when your computer is making an obvious error.

In addition, patients who are able to participate in decision making should be encouraged to validate the diagnosis. "It

TABLE • 13-5 **COMMON ERRORS IN WRITING NURSING DIAGNOSES AND RECOMMENDED CORRECTIONS**

Error	Example	Correction	Example
Writing the diagnosis in terms of needs and not response	Needs assistance with bathing related to bed rest	Write the diagnosis in terms of response rather than need	Bathing/Hygiene Self-Care Deficit related to immobility
Making legally inadvisable statements	Noncompliance due to hostility toward nursing staff (the words *due to* imply a direct cause-and-effect relationship)	Use "related to" rather than "due to" or "caused by" to link the etiology to the problem statement	Noncompliance related to hostility toward nursing staff (denotes a relation between the problem and etiology but not necessarily a causal relation)
	Spouse Abuse related to husband's immaturity and violent temper	Write diagnosis in legally advisable terms: statements that may be interpreted as libel or that imply nursing negligence are legally hazardous to all the nurses caring for the patient	High Risk for Violence: Spouse Abuse related to husband's reported inability to control behavior
	Impaired Skin Integrity related to patient's lying on back all night		Impaired Skin Integrity related to mobility deficit
Identifying as a problem a patient response that is not necessarily unhealthy	Mild Anxiety related to impending surgery	Include in the problem statement of the nursing diagnosis only patient responses that are unhealthy or that the patient wants to change	No need for nursing diagnosis: mild anxiety before surgery is a healthy response that motivates preoperative self-care behavior
Identifying as a problem signs and symptoms of illness	Cough related to long history of smoking	Avoid including signs and symptoms of illness in the problem statement of the nursing diagnosis	Ineffective Airway Clearance related to 20-year history of smoking
Identifying as a patient problem or etiology what cannot be changed	Alterations in Bowel Elimination: Permanent Colostomy related to cancer of bowel	Express the problem statement and etiologic factors in terms that can be changed; otherwise, nursing energies are being directed to a hopeless task	Self-Care Deficit: Care of Colostomy, related to severe anxiety about cancer and feelings of powerlessness
	Grieving related to death of spouse		Dysfunctional Grieving related to inability to accept death of spouse
Identifying environmental factors rather than patient factors as a problem	Cluttered Home related to inability to discard anything	Express the problem statement in terms of unhealthy patient responses rather than environmental conditions	Risk for Injury related to cluttered home (inability to discard anything)
Reversing clauses	Deficient Knowledge related to alteration in parenting	Avoid reversing the problem statement and etiologic statement	Impaired Parenting related to knowledge deficit: child growth and development, discipline
Having both clauses say the same thing	Impaired Comfort related to pain (pain is the comfort alteration—what is contributing to the pain?)	Be sure that the two parts of the diagnosis do not mean the same thing	Unrelieved Incisional Pain related to fear of addiction
Including value judgments in the nursing diagnosis	Poor Home Maintenance related to laziness	Write the diagnosis without value judgments; avoid words such as *poor, inadequate, abnormal, unhealthy*	Impaired Home Maintenance related to low value ascribed to home safety and cleanliness
Including the medical diagnosis in the diagnostic statement	Impaired Home Maintenance related to arthritis	Do not include the medical diagnosis in the nursing diagnosis statement	Impaired Home Maintenance related to mobility, endurance, and comfort alterations

Common errors adapted from Mundinger, M. O., & Jauron, G. D. (1975). Developing a nursing diagnosis. *Nursing Outlook, 23*(2), 94–98. Guidelines for writing nursing diagnoses adapted from Iyer, P., Taptich, B., & Bernocchi-Losey, D. (1991). *Nursing process and nursing diagnoses* (2nd ed.). Philadelphia: W. B. Saunders.

TABLE • 13-6   WHAT A NURSING DIAGNOSIS *IS NOT,* AND WHY

What a Nursing Diagnosis Is Not	Example	Rationale
Medical diagnosis	Diabetes mellitus	Although there is nursing care associated with medical illnesses, the illness is not primarily amenable to nursing intervention. Nursing's concern is the *person* who has the illness and the effect of the illness on human functioning.
Medical pathology	Hypoglycemia	Nurses need to understand the pathology underlying disease states to plan appropriate nursing care, but once again, nursing's focus is the person, not the pathology. The person's response to hypoglycemia, how hypoglycemia affects human functioning—these are the domain of *nursing* diagnoses.
Diagnostic tests, treatments, equipment	Fasting blood glucose Insulin therapy Insulin syringe Infusion pump	Nursing's concern is the person's response to the diagnostic study, treatment, or equipment. If the need for insulin therapy reveals a deficient knowledge or self-care deficit, this becomes the nursing diagnosis, not insulin therapy in and of itself.
Therapeutic patient needs	Needs to learn the relation among diet, exercise, and insulin	The diagnosis should be written as a patient health problem rather than a patient need. *Example:* Impaired Health Maintenance (Diabetic Care) related to lack of knowledge of relation among diet, exercise, and insulin.
Therapeutic nursing goals	To develop therapeutic diabetic self-care behaviors	The diagnosis should be written from the patient perspective rather than the nursing perspective and phrased as a patient health problem. *Example:* Self-Care Deficit: Diabetic Self-Care Behaviors, related to decreased value on life and decreased motivation to learn.
A single sign or symptom	After successfully administering own insulin for 3 days, patient tells nurse, "You give me my shot today."	A nursing diagnosis is not developed until a pattern or cluster of significant cues is detected. The signs and symptoms lead to the identification of the problem statement but are not the problem statement. In this situation, no nursing diagnosis is indicated until further data collection, interpretation, and analysis take place.
An *unvalidated* nursing inference	Above incident leads to the nursing inference: Noncompliance related to depression	This is a premature nursing diagnosis that may not accurately reflect a patient problem. More data and the validation of the tentative nursing diagnosis (nursing inference) are needed before the diagnoses can be recorded.

seems to me that bathing has become a problem now that you are afraid of falling in the tub. What's your sense of this?" Table 13-2 lists possible outcomes of validating tentative nursing diagnoses.

DOCUMENTING NURSING DIAGNOSES

The nurse documents validated nursing diagnoses in the patient record. Depending on the documentation system in use, nursing diagnoses might be recorded in the nursing plan of care and on the multidisciplinary problem list at the front of the patient record. Tables 13-3 and 13-4 illustrate how to document nursing diagnoses using both two- and three-part diagnostic statements.

At one time, nurses were urged to only use NANDA accepted terms to state nursing diagnoses. Today, accepted terms vary. Nurses should use the terms recommended by their school, employer, or specialty organization (e.g., Association of Perioperative Nurses [AORN] or Association of Rehabilitation Nurses [ARN]). The terms most commonly

used will be the terms chosen for standard plans and computerized systems.

NURSING DIAGNOSIS: A CRITIQUE

Current nursing diagnosis literature contains many examples of nurses writing about how using nursing diagnoses has improved their clinical practice; articles also detail the many benefits nursing diagnosis brings to the profession. Conversely, other articles point out the limitations of nursing diagnosis and urge nurses to be cautious so that an uncritical use of nursing diagnosis does not restrict their practices.

The primary benefit that nursing diagnosis offers the patient is the individualization of patient care. For example, nurses might be caring simultaneously for three women who have had a modified radical mastectomy because of breast cancer. Although the postoperative nursing management of these women is similar, priorities of care may differ. A prioritized list of nursing diagnoses enables nurses to direct their energies toward these differing patient priorities.

Patient A
- Disturbed Body Image
- Ineffective Coping

Patient B
- Pain
- Bathing/Hygiene Self-Care Deficit

Patient C
- Sexual Dysfunction
- Powerlessness

The use of nursing diagnoses also allows patients to be informed and willing participants in their care, as they validate their diagnoses and assist in prioritizing them. The process of prioritizing nursing diagnoses is the first step in planning care and is addressed in Chapter 14.

Improved communication among nurses and other healthcare professionals is probably the most important benefit that accurate, up-to-date diagnoses—expressed in well-defined and standardized terminology—offer nurses. This communication aids in planning, charting, patient data retrieval, health team conferences, change-of-shift reports, and healthcare follow-up. It also promotes nursing accountability for the problems that nurses diagnose.

Among the other benefits of nursing diagnoses for the profession is help in defining the domain of nursing for healthcare administrators, legislators, and other healthcare providers; this is important when seeking funding for nursing and reimbursement for nursing services. Nursing diagnoses are also used to define curriculum content and to direct specialization and advancement in nursing and nursing research.

When the diagnostic process is used incorrectly, a patient might be "misdiagnosed." Common sources of error include:

- *Premature diagnoses based on an incomplete database:* For example—A diagnosis of Defensive Coping is made after the patient verbally attacks one nurse who was attempting to teach him self-care for his wound.
- *Erroneous diagnoses resulting from an inaccurate database or a faulty data analysis:* For example—A diagnosis of Dysfunctional Grieving is made in a patient observed crying after learning that her cancer had returned, before anyone had time to evaluate whether this was simply an appropriate response to bad news.
- *Routine diagnoses resulting from the nurse's failure to tailor data collection and analysis to the unique needs of the patient:* For example—A diagnosis of Deficient Knowledge is made in a diabetic patient who is frequently hospitalized with diabetes-related complications, when she actually has excellent knowledge of diabetes and related self-care demands, but has lacked the motivation to care for herself appropriately.
- *Errors of omission:* Failure to modify diagnoses and to identify new diagnoses as the patient's status changes may also be problems. Failures in diagnosis lead to failures in nursing care.

> *Recall Martin Prescott, the 46-year-old man with rectal bleeding and constipation? Although an initial nursing diagnosis may involve Deficient Knowledge related to possible causes of rectal bleeding, further assessment may reveal that the patient's constipation resulting from a diet inadequate in fiber and fluids is the underlying cause of the bleeding. Thus, the nurse would need to revise the nursing diagnosis to focus on Constipation related to inadequate intake of high-fiber foods and fluids as manifested by hard stool and rectal bleeding, and Deficient Knowledge related to foods high in fiber.* ∎

These are not so much limitations of nursing diagnosis, as they are problems of nurses diagnosing incorrectly. More serious criticisms of nursing diagnoses are raised by nurses who claim that a classification of standardized nursing diagnoses limits nursing, curbing nurses' originality and ability to think things through.

Although some nurses believe that diagnosis offers a valued shortcut to practice, critics find this attitude offensive and respond that rather than invest nursing's energies in perfecting a shortcut, nurses need to change the working conditions that interfere with in-depth problem solving and thoughtful nursing care.

Critics of diagnostic labeling point out that instead of identifying what is unique and positive about nursing, nursing diagnoses make a clear statement that nurses are concerned about what is deviant, wrong, or pathologic (Hagey & McDonough, 1984). The ever-changing and dynamic human person with a need for nursing care becomes objectified (Gebbie, 1984). The practice of many experienced nurses who find nursing diagnoses helpful in targeting care for patients with diverse needs counters these concerns.

Nurses who are sensitive to transcultural issues raise important concerns about the cultural limitations of the NANDA diagnoses. Foremost among these concerns is that NANDA diagnoses and behaviors assume that the patient is "wrong" and the provider is "right" and deny the validity of cultural and healthcare beliefs and practices that are different from those of the nurse (Geissler, 1991). Examples of nursing diagnoses that often are misused in labeling such cultural deviations as abnormal include Impaired Verbal Communication, Impaired Social Interaction, and Noncompliance. Nurses who provide culturally sensitive care (see Chapter 2) and who work collaboratively with the patient as a partner avoid these problems.

In conclusion, nursing diagnosis has become a valued and essential step in the nursing process. Used correctly, it is a powerful tool for individualizing patient care and ensures that nurses' energies are being used in the most efficient way to meet patients' needs. Nurses who are as concerned about the art and spirit of nursing as they are about its science are careful to avoid labeling patients in a way that objectifies them or limits the potential range of nurse–patient interactions.

● Developing Critical Thinking Skills

1. Find a patient with a well-established medical condition. List potential medical and nursing diagnoses and collaborative problems. Explain the differing purposes of medical and nursing diagnoses and collaborative problems. What is nursing's diagnostic contribution to the interdisciplinary team's effort to care for this patient?

2. Interview several experienced nurses, and find at least one nurse who is strongly committed to using nursing diagnoses and another who believes they are a waste of time. Interview both until you can explain their different experiences with nursing diagnoses. Try to identify different patient outcomes related to their use or nonuse of nursing diagnoses. List the benefits and limitations of using nursing diagnoses.

3. Interview two patients with the same medical diagnosis. Develop a prioritized list of nursing diagnoses for both, and reflect on the differences. Compare and contrast the strengths of both patients. If you can do this exercise with another student, it would be helpful to explore why there are differences in your lists of nursing diagnoses and patient strengths.

● Practicing for NCLEX

1. Identify all of the following that are purposes of diagnosing. The purpose of diagnosing is to identify:
   (1) how an individual, group, or community responds to actual or potential health and life processes
   (2) factors that contribute to or cause health problems (etiologies)
   (3) strengths the patient can draw on to prevent or resolve problems
   (4) nursing interventions to resolve health problems
      a. (1) and (2)
      b. (3) and (4)
      c. (1), (2), and (3)
      d. All of the above

2. The terms *diagnose* and *diagnosis* have legal implications. They imply that there is a specific problem that requires management by a qualified expert. Which of the following statements is false?
   a. If you make a diagnosis, it means that you accept accountability for accurately naming and managing the problem.
   b. If you treat a problem or allow a problem to persist without ensuring that the correct diagnosis has been made, you may cause harm and be accused of negligence.
   c. You are accountable for detecting, identifying, or recognizing signs and symptoms that may indicate problems beyond your expertise.

   d. When nurses diagnose a medical problem, they are just as accountable as physicians for detecting, identifying, and managing the signs and symptoms of disease.

3. Which was the first state to identify diagnosing as part of the legal domain of professional nursing?
   a. New Jersey
   b. New York
   c. North Carolina
   d. North Dakota

4. Which group is responsible for the promotion and organization of activities to continue the development, classification, and scientific testing of nursing diagnoses?
   a. American Nurses Association
   b. National Nursing Diagnosis Association
   c. North American Nursing Diagnosis Association
   d. Clearinghouse for Nursing Diagnoses

5. Altered Health Maintenance is an example of which of the following types of problems?
   a. Collaborative problem
   b. Interdisciplinary problem
   c. Medical problem
   d. Nursing problem

6. To determine the significance of a blood pressure reading of 148/100, it is first necessary for the nurse to do which of the following?
   a. Compare this reading to standards.
   b. Check the taxonomy of nursing diagnoses for a pertinent label.
   c. Check a medical text for the signs and symptoms of high blood pressure.
   d. Consult with colleagues.

7. When the initial nursing assessment revealed that the patient had not had a bowel movement for 2 days, the student wrote the diagnostic label "constipation." Which of the following comments is she most likely to hear from her instructor?
   a. "Hold on a minute . . . Nursing diagnoses should always be derived from clusters of significant data rather than from a single cue."
   b. "Job well done . . . You've identified this problem early and we can manage it before it becomes more acute."
   c. "Is this an actual or a possible diagnosis?"
   d. "This is a medical, not a nursing problem."

8. A clinical judgment that an individual, family, or community is more vulnerable to develop the problem than others in the same or similar situation is what type of nursing diagnosis?
   a. Actual
   b. Risk
   c. Possible
   d. Wellness
   e. Syndrome

9. Which of the following nursing diagnoses are correctly written as two-part nursing diagnoses?
   (1) Ineffective Coping related to inability to maintain marriage
   (2) Defensive Coping related to loss of job and economic security
   (3) Altered Thought Processes related to panic state
   (4) Decisional Conflict related to placement of parent in nursing home
       a. (1) and (2)
       b. (3) and (4)
       c. (1), (2), and (3)
       d. All of the above

10. Which of the following nursing diagnoses are correctly written as three-part nursing diagnoses?
    (1) Disabled Family Coping related to lack of knowledge about home care of child on ventilator
    (2) Imbalanced Nutrition: Less Than Body Requirements related to inadequate caloric intake while striving to excel in gymnastics as evidenced by 20-pound weight loss since beginning the gymnastic program, and greatly less than ideal body weight when compared to standard height weight charts
    (3) Need to learn how to care for child on ventilator at home related to unexpected discharge of daughter after 3 month hospital stay as evidenced by repeated comments "I cannot do this," "I know I'll harm her because I'm not a nurse," and "I can't do medical things."
    (4) Spiritual Distress related to inability to accept diagnosis of terminal illness as evidenced by multiple comments such as "How could God do this to me?," "I don't deserve this," "I don't understand. I've tried to live my life well," "How could God make me suffer this way?"
    (5) Caregiver Role Strain related to failure of home health aides to appropriately diagnose needs of family caregivers and initiate a plan to facilitate coping as evidenced by caregiver's loss of weight and clinical depression.
        a. (1) and (3)
        b. (2) and (4)
        c. (1), (2), and (3)
        d. All of the above

● Answers With Rationale

1. *c.* Identifying nursing interventions to resolve health problems is done during the planning step of the nursing process.

2. *d.* While nurses are accountable to identify and document nursing diagnoses and the signs and symptoms suggestive of medical and collaborative problems, their responsibility for medical problems is related only to the scope of their practice and they do not share the same responsibility as their physician colleagues.

3. *b.* New York was the first state to identify diagnosing as part of the legal domain of professional nursing.

4. *c,* North American Nursing Diagnosis Association.

5. *d,* Nursing Problem, because it describes a problem that can be treated by nurses within the scope of independent nursing practice.

6. *a.* A standard, or a norm, is a generally accepted rule, measure, pattern, or model to which can be compared data in the same class or category. For example, when determining the significance of a patient's blood pressure reading, appropriate standards include normative values for the patient's age group, race, and illness category. Deviation from an appropriate norm may be the basis for writing a diagnosis.

7. *a.* A data cluster is a grouping of patient data or cues that points to the existence of a patient health problem. Nursing diagnoses should always be derived from clusters of significant data rather than from a single cue. There may be a reason for the lack of a bowel movement for 2 days, or it might be this individual's normal pattern.

8. *b.* A clinical judgment that an individual, family, or community is more vulnerable to develop the problem than others in the same or similar situation is a Risk nursing diagnosis.

9. *d.* Each of the four diagnoses is a correctly written two-part diagnostic statement that includes the problem or diagnostic label and the etiology or cause.

10. *a.* (2) is written in terms of needs and not unhealthy response and (4) is a legally inadvisable statement.

Taylor Suite Resources

The Taylor Suite offers these additional resources to enhance learning and facilitate understanding of this chapter:

- thePoint online resource, http://thepoint.lww.com/Taylor7E
- Student DVD included with the book
- Study Guide for Taylor's Fundamentals of Nursing

BIBLIOGRAPHY
Alfaro-LeFevre, R. (2009). *Critical thinking and clinical judgment: A practical approach to outcome focused thinking* (4th ed.). St. Louis: Saunders Elsevier.
Alfaro-LeFevre, R. (2010). *Applying nursing process: A tool for critical thinking* (7th ed.). Philadelphia: Lippincott Williams & Wilkins.
American Nurses Association (ANA). (1995). *Nursing: A social policy statement.* Washington, DC: Author.
American Nurses Association (ANA). (2001). *Code for nurses with interpretive statements.* Washington, DC: Author.
American Nurses Association (ANA). (2003). *Nursing: A social policy statement* (2nd ed.). Washington, DC: Author.

American Nurses Association (ANA). (2004). *Scope and standards of practice.* Washington, DC: Author.

Aspinall, M. J. (1976). Nursing diagnosis: The weak link. *Nursing Outlook, 24*(7), 433–436.

Benner, P. (2005). Extending the dialogue about classification systems and the work of professional nurses. *American Journal of Critical Care, 14*(3), 242–243, 272.

Carpenito-Moyet, L. J. (2010). *Nursing diagnosis: Application to clinical practice* (13th ed.). Philadelphia: Lippincott Williams & Wilkins.

Carroll-Johnson, R. M. (Ed.). (1991). *Classification in nursing diagnosis: Proceedings of the ninth national conference.* Philadelphia: J. B. Lippincott.

Dochterman, J. M., & Jones, D. A. (2003). *Unifying nursing languages: The harmonization of NANDA, NIC, NOC.* Washington, DC: The American Nurses Association.

Dossey, B., & Guzzetta, C. E. (1981). Nursing diagnosis. *Nursing, 11*(6), 34–38.

Dougherty, C. M., Jankin, J. J., Lunney, M. R., & Whitley, G. G. (1993). Conceptual and research-based validation of nursing diagnoses: 1950–1993. *Nursing Diagnosis, 4*(4), 156–165.

Fry, V. S. (1953). The creative approach to nursing. *American Journal of Nursing, 53,* 301–302.

Gebbie, K. M. (Ed.). (1975). *Summary of the second national conference.* St. Louis: Clearinghouse for Nursing Diagnoses.

Gebbie, K. M. (1984). Nursing diagnosis: What is it and why does it exist? *Topics in Clinical Nursing, 5*(4), 1–9.

Gebbie, K. M., & Lavin, M. A. (1973). *Summary of the first national conference.* St. Louis: C. V. Mosby.

Geissler, E. M. (1991). Transcultural nursing and diagnosis. *Nursing and Health Care, 12*(4), 190–192, 203.

Gordon, M. (1976). Nursing diagnosis and the diagnostic process. *American Journal of Nursing, 76*(8), 1298–1300.

Gordon, M. (1994). *Nursing diagnosis: Process and application* (3rd ed.). St. Louis: C. V. Mosby.

Gordon, M. (1995). *Manual of nursing diagnosis: 1995–1996 edition.* St. Louis: Mosby–Year Book.

Hagey, R. S., & McDonough, P. (1984). The problem of professional labeling. *Nursing Outlook, 32*(3), 151–157.

Hammond, K. R. (1966). Clinical inference in nursing: A psychologist's viewpoint. *Nursing Research, 15*(1), 27–38.

Herdman, T. H. (2008). Nursing diagnosis: Is it time for a new definition? *International Journal of Nursing Terminologies & Classifications, 19*(1), 2–13.

Hurley, M. (Ed.). (1986). *Classification of nursing diagnoses: Proceedings of the sixth conference.* St. Louis: C. V. Mosby.

Iyer, P., Taptich, B., & Bernocchi-Losey, D. (1991). *Nursing process and nursing diagnoses* (2nd ed.). Philadelphia: W. B. Saunders.

Kerr, M., Hoskins, L. M., Fitzpatrick, J. J., Warren, J. J., Avant, K. C., & Hurley, M., et al. (1993). Taxonomic validation: An overview. *Nursing Diagnosis, 4*(1), 6–14.

Kim, M. J., McFarland, G. K., & McLane, A. M. (Eds.). (1984). *Classification of nursing diagnosis: Proceedings of the fifth national conference.* St. Louis: C. V. Mosby.

Kim, M. J., & Moritz, D. A. (1982). *Classification of the third and fourth national conferences.* Hightstown, NJ: McGraw-Hill.

Kritek, P. B. (1985). Nursing diagnosis in perspective: Response to a critique. *Image—The Journal of Nursing Scholarship, 16*(1), 3–8.

Kurashima, S., Kobayaski, K., Toyabe, S., & Akazawa, K. (2008). Accuracy and efficiency of computer-aided nursing diagnosis. *International Journal of Nursing Terminologies & Classifications, 19*(3), 95–101.

Lindsey, A. M. (1990). Identification and labeling of human responses. *Journal of Professional Nursing, 6*(3), 143–150.

Lipe, S. L., & Beasley, S. (2004). *Critical thinking in nursing.* Philadelphia: Lippincott Williams & Wilkins.

Lunney, M. (1982). Nursing diagnosis: Refining the system. *American Journal of Nursing, 82*(3), 456–459.

Lunney, M. (2008). The need for international nursing diagnosis research and a theoretical framework. *International Journal of Nursing Terminologies & Classifications, 19*(1), 28–34.

McLane, A. M. (Ed.). (1987). *Classification of nursing diagnoses: Proceedings of the seventh conference.* St. Louis: C. V. Mosby.

Mitchell, G. J. (1991). Nursing diagnosis: An ethical analysis. *Image—The Journal of Nursing Scholarship, 23*(2), 99–103.

Mueller, A., Johnston, M., & Bligh, D. (2002). Joining mind mapping and care planning to enhance student critical thinking and achieve holistic nursing care. *Nursing Diagnosis, 13*(1), 24.

Muller-Staub, M., Lavin, M. A., Needham, I., & van Achterberg, T. (2007). Meeting the criteria of a nursing diagnosis classification: Evaluation of ICNP, ICF, NANDA and ZEFP. *International Journal of Nursing Studies, 44*(5), 702–713.

Mundinger, M. O., & Jauron, G. D. (1975). Developing a nursing diagnosis. *Nursing Outlook, 23,* 94–98.

North American Nursing Diagnosis Association (NANDA). (1990). *Taxonomy I revised with official diagnostic categories.* St. Louis: Author.

North American Nursing Diagnosis Association (NANDA) International. (2009). *NANDA international nursing diagnoses: Definitions and classification, 2009–2011.* Oxford, UK: Wiley-Blackwell.

Popkess, S. (1981). Diagnosing your patient's strengths. *Nursing, 11*(7), 34–37.

Popkess, S., & Vawter, S. (1991). Wellness nursing diagnosis: To be or not to be? *Nursing Diagnosis, 2*(1), 19–25.

Porter, E. J. (1986). Critical analysis of NANDA nursing diagnosis taxonomy I. *Image—The Journal of Nursing Scholarship, 18*(4), 136–139.

Rasch, R. F. R. (1987). The nature of taxonomy. *Image—The Journal of Nursing Scholarship, 19*(3), 147–149.

Shamansky, S. L., & Yanni, C. R. (1983). In opposition to nursing diagnosis: A minority opinion. *Image—The Journal of Nursing Scholarship, 15*(2), 47–50.

Vincent, K. G., & Coler, M. S. (1990). A unified nursing diagnostic model. *Image—The Journal of Nursing Scholarship, 22*(2), 93–95.

Warren, J., & Hoskins, L. (1990). The development of NANDA's nursing diagnosis taxonomy. *Nursing Diagnosis, 1*(4), 162–168.

Wilkinson, J. M. (2000). *Nursing diagnosis handbook with NIC interventions and NOC outcomes* (7th ed.). Upper Saddle River, NJ: Prentice Hall Health.

Wong, E. (2008). Coining and defining novel nursing technology. Part 1: Critical incident nursing diagnosis. *International Journal of Nursing Technologies and Classifications, 19*(3), 89–94.

Outcome Identification and Planning

14

GLENDA KRONK

Glenda, a 35-year-old woman, comes to the health center for a routine checkup. During the visit, she expresses a strong motivation and desire to become physically fit, lose weight, increase her muscle tone, and improve her cardiorespiratory capacity. "I know it will involve some major lifestyle changes, including diet. What's with all these diets and diet supplements now?" she asks.

DARLA JEFFERSON

Darla, a 29-year-old single woman, is about 14 weeks pregnant. She describes herself as a "hopeless addict" who has tried to stop "more times than I can remember." Although currently drug-free, she is not hopeful of preventing relapse. She does not know the baby's father and has mixed feelings about keeping the baby, saying, "On the one hand I want someone to love me, but I'm not sure I'd want me for a mother."

ELIJAH WOLINSKI

Elijah is a thin, frail, 85-year-old man who is bed-bound due to severe degenerative joint disease. He is being cared for by his 56-year-old nephew at his home. Assessment on a home visit reveals Elijah lying on soiled linens with a large pressure ulcer on his sacrum, approximately 3" in diameter and about 1" deep with purulent drainage.

After completing the chapter, you will be able to accomplish the following:

1. Describe the purpose and benefits of outcome identification and planning.

2. Identify three elements of comprehensive planning.

3. Prioritize patient health problems and nursing responses.

4. Describe how patient goals/expected outcomes and nursing orders are derived from nursing diagnoses.

5. Develop a plan of nursing care with properly constructed outcomes and related nursing interventions.

6. Differentiate nurse-initiated interventions, physician-initiated interventions, and collaborative interventions.

7. Use criteria to evaluate planning skills.

8. Describe five common problems related to planning, their possible causes, and remedies.

9. Describe the rationale for standardized outcomes (NOC) and interventions (NIC) for nursing.

clinical pathways (critical pathways, CareMaps)

computerized plans of nursing care

consultation

criteria

discharge planning

expected outcome

goal

initial planning

Kardex care plan

nursing intervention

nursing interventions classification (NIC)

nursing outcomes classification (NOC)

ongoing planning

outcome identification

patient outcome

plan of nursing care

planning

standardized care plans

After the nurse collects and interprets patient data, identifying patient strengths and health problems, it is time to plan for nursing action (see the accompanying Reflective Practice box for an example.) During the **outcome identification** and **planning** steps of the nursing process, the nurse works in partnership with the patient and family to:

• Establish priorities
• Identify and write expected patient outcomes

• Select evidence-based nursing interventions
• Communicate the plan of nursing care (Fig. 14-1)

A **goal** is an aim or an end. A **patient outcome** is an expected conclusion to a patient health problem, or in the event of a wellness diagnosis, an expected conclusion to a patient's health expectation. The words "goal," "objective," and "outcome" are often used interchangeably. In some practice settings, the term "goal" or "objective" is used to describe what is wanted, and the term "outcome" is used to describe the results achieved. In nursing, the phrase **expected outcomes** is used to refer to the more specific, measurable **criteria** used to evaluate the extent to which a goal has been met. This chapter uses "outcome" to refer to expected patient outcomes.

The nurse, patient, and family should work together as much as possible in the outcome identification and planning stage. If the outcomes specified in the plan of care are not valued by the patient or do not contribute to the prevention, resolution, or reduction of the patient's problems or the achievement of the patient's health expectations, the plan of care may be meaningless. Outcome determination is, therefore, a critical skill for successfully intervening with patients.

This chapter describes outcome identification and planning as a formal process, a deliberate step in the nursing process. A formal plan of care allows nurses to:

• Individualize care that maximizes outcome achievement
• Set priorities
• Facilitate communication among nursing personnel and their colleagues
• Promote continuity of high-quality, cost-effective care
• Coordinate care
• Evaluate the patient's responses to nursing care
• Create a record that can be used for evaluation, research, reimbursement, and legal purposes
• Promote the nurse's professional development

Nurses also engage in informal planning in practice. This is the link between identifying a patient's strength or problem and providing an appropriate nursing response. When a nurse on a busy surgical unit learns that a postoperative patient is complaining of incisional pain and quickly reshuffles priorities to allow time to assess the course and qualities of the pain and determine nursing measures to reduce discomfort, planning has occurred. When a postpartum nurse on the 3-to-11 shift realizes the evening before discharge that he or she has not seen a particular father hold his new daughter and makes a mental note to observe the father–daughter interactions that evening and facilitate their bonding, planning has occurred. When a nurse in a geriatric daycare center hears a patient choking and rushes to his side to perform the Heimlich maneuver if necessary, planning has occurred. Informal planning on a more conscious level is illustrated by a hospice nurse who drives home pondering how best to support a patient with terminal cancer who is gradually relinquishing her hold on life. She may elect to initiate a more formal process of planning the next day when she consults with colleagues who have cared for patients with similar health needs. In each of the above examples, the process of informal planning allowed an individual nurse to

REFLECTIVE PRACTICE

Challenge to Ethical and Legal Skills

While working in a women's shelter, I met Darla Jefferson, a 29-year-old single woman who was about 14 weeks pregnant. Darla described herself as a "hopeless addict" who had tried to stop "more times than I can remember." She was drug-free at the moment but not hopeful of preventing relapse. She did not know the baby's father and had mixed feelings about keeping the baby. She said, "On the one hand I want someone to love me, but I'm not sure I'd want me for a mother." I knew I needed to explore her commitment to this pregnancy, but I am strongly opposed to abortion and did not think I could talk with her objectively about her decision. I needed to develop a plan for dealing with this topic.

Thinking Outside the Box: Possible Courses of Action

- Tell Darla that I believe it is her responsibility to have this baby and to then make a decision about whether to offer the baby for adoption based upon her assessment of her parenting readiness.
- Help Darla assess her readiness to become a parent, and in light of this, explore all her options regarding continuing or terminating the pregnancy.

- Get someone else to talk with Darla so that she gets the counseling she needs and I am not morally compromised.

Evaluating a Good Outcome: How Do I Define Success?

- Darla gets the help she needs to make the decision that is right for her and her unborn baby.

- I am faithful to both my nursing responsibilities to counsel this patient and my duty to maintain my moral integrity.

Personal Learning: Here's to the Future!

Unfortunately, I overestimated my ability to counsel Darla without compromising myself, and as a result, I don't think I was as helpful to her as I should have been. Ideally, I planned to objectively explore her readiness to be a mother and then have an open and unbiased discussion about her options. When she began to talk about getting an abortion, I found myself urging her to have

the baby and then place the baby up for adoption if she still felt she couldn't care for him or her after delivery. Regrettably, I let my personal opinions come through in the discussion. Through my actions, I think she lost trust in me. I'm going to talk with other nurses to see how they handle this challenge.

Reflection

How would you respond in a similar situation? Why? What does this tell you about yourself and about the adequacy of your skills for professional practice? Can you think of other ways to respond? What actions might have proved more effective? What actions might be helpful for the nursing student so that when faced with similar situations in the future, the outcome would be more positive? What other skills (cognitive, interpersonal, technical, ethical/legal) would you need to respond well in this situation? Suggest an alternative course of action that might have been effective, and explain why. Do you agree with the criteria to evaluate a successful outcome? Did the nursing student meet the criteria? Support your response.

---

think about how best to help a particular patient—ideally, with good results. What is lacking is a coordinated plan known by everyone caring for the patient.

UNIQUE FOCUS OF NURSING OUTCOME IDENTIFICATION AND PLANNING

The primary purpose of the outcome identification and planning step of the nursing process is to design a plan of care for and with the patient that, once implemented, results in the prevention, reduction, or resolution of patient health problems and the attainment of the patient's health expectations, as identified in the patient outcomes (Box 14-1).

> *Think back to Glenda Kronk, the woman verbalizing a need to improve her fitness level. Based on a comprehensive*

patient assessment, together the nurse and patient would develop an appropriate plan to achieve this improved level of health such as planning for 20-minute walks three times a week, eating a nutritious diet, and making routine follow-ups to determine the patient's progress toward the ultimate outcome. ∎

A comprehensive plan of care additionally specifies any routine nursing assistance the patient needs to meet basic human needs (e.g., assistance with hygiene or nutrition) and describes appropriate nursing responsibilities for fulfilling the collaborative and medical plan of care. For example, physicians may delegate to nurses caring for a surgical patient the redressing of the surgical incision, the administration of

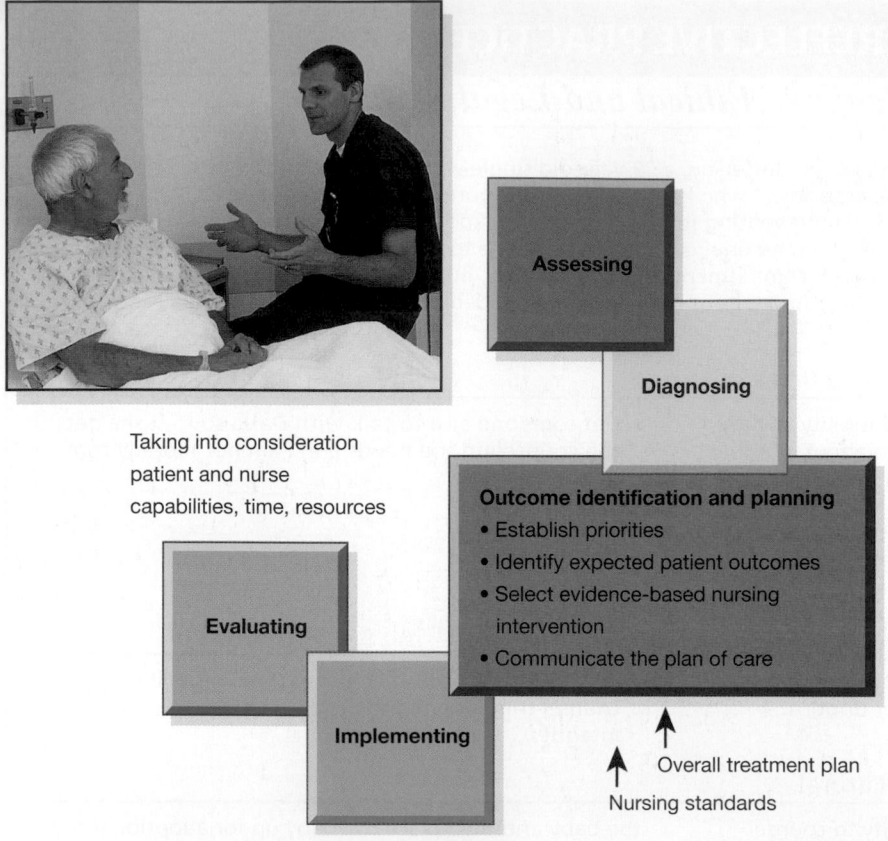

Taking into consideration
patient and nurse
capabilities, time, resources

Assessing

Diagnosing

Outcome identification and planning
- Establish priorities
- Identify expected patient outcomes
- Select evidence-based nursing
  intervention
- Communicate the plan of care

Evaluating

Implementing

↑ Overall treatment plan
↑ Nursing standards

FIGURE 14-1. Outcome Identification and Planning. The nurse and patient work together to establish priorities, identify expected patient outcomes, and select the evidence-based nursing interventions. It is important for the plan of care to be consistent with nursing standards, congruent with other planned therapies, and realistic in terms of the patient's and nurse's abilities or resources. Ensuring that the plan of care is recorded is also an important nursing responsibility. *(Photo © B. Proud.)*

Box 14-1   ANA STANDARDS OF PRACTICE: STANDARDS THREE AND FOUR, OUTCOME IDENTIFICATION AND PLANNING

Outcome Identification
The registered nurse identifies expected outcomes for a plan individualized to the patient or the situation.

Measurement Criteria
The registered nurse:

Involves the patient, family, and other healthcare providers in formulating expected outcomes when possible and appropriate.

Derives culturally appropriate expected outcomes from the diagnoses.

Considers associated risks, benefits, costs, current scientific evidence, and clinical expertise when formulating expected outcomes.

Defines expected outcomes in terms of the patient, patient values, ethical considerations, environment, or situation with such consideration as associated risks, benefits and costs, and current scientific evidence.

Includes a time estimate for attainment of expected outcomes.

Develops expected outcomes that provide direction for continuity of care.

Modifies expected outcomes based on changes in the status of the patient or evaluation of the situation.

Documents expected outcomes as measurable.

Planning
The registered nurse develops a plan that prescribes strategies and alternatives to attain expected outcomes.

Measurement Criteria
The registered nurse:

Develops an individualized plan considering patient characteristics or the situation (e.g., age and culturally appropriate, environmentally sensitive).

Develops the plan in conjunction with the patient, family, and others, as appropriate.

Includes strategies within the plan that address each of the identified diagnoses or issues, which may include strategies for promotion and restoration of health and prevention of illness, injury, and disease.

Provides for continuity within the plan.

Incorporates an implementation pathway or timeline within the plan.

Establishes the plan priorities with the patient, family, and others, as appropriate.

Utilizes the plan to provide direction to other members of the healthcare team.

Defines the plan to reflect current statutes, rules and regulations, and standards.

Integrates current trends and research affecting care in the planning process.

Considers the economic impact of the plan.

Uses standardized language or recognized terminology to document the plan.

Used with permission. American Nurses Association. (2004). *Scope and standards of practice.* Washington, DC: Author.

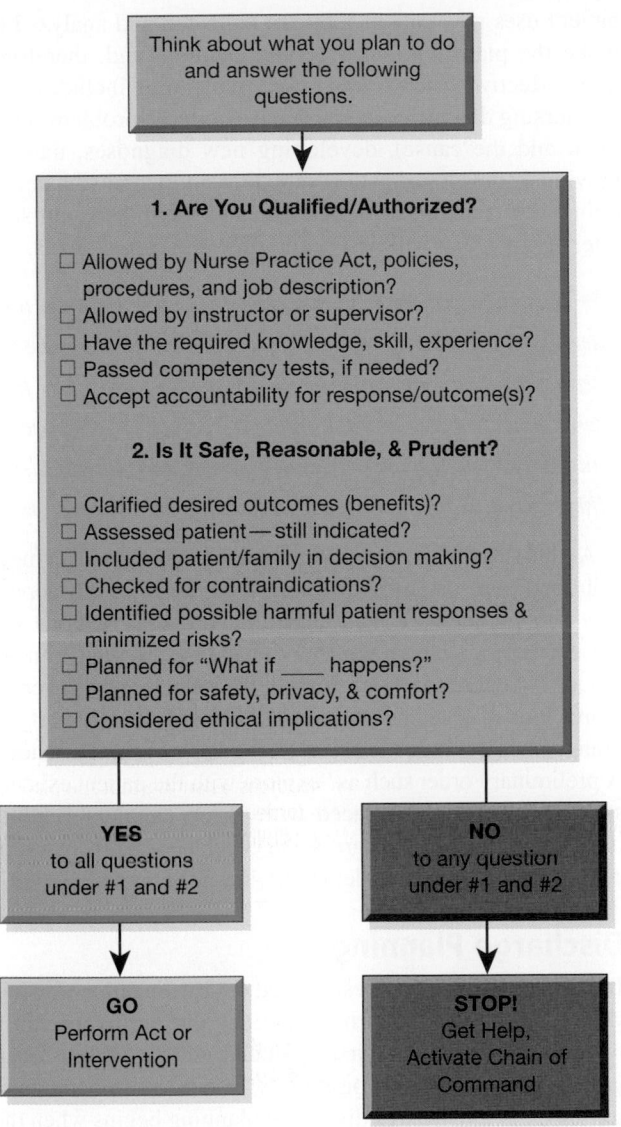

FIGURE 14-2. Clinical decision-making process for determining your ability to act independently. (© 2009 R. Alfaro-LeFevre. www.AlfaroTeachSmart.com, used with permission.)

Box 14-2 APPLYING STANDARDS TO PLAN NURSING CARE

The standards you must apply when identifying outcomes and related nursing interventions are determined by:

- *The law.* Your state's nurse practice act outlines the scope of nursing practice. Your state board of nursing also outlines what you are and are not allowed to do.
- *National practice standards*, such as those of the American Nurses Association.
- *Specialty professional organizations*, such as the American Association of Critical Care Nurses or Emergency Nurses Association, which develop standards for specialty practice.
- *The Joint Commission.* This powerful accrediting body has developed detailed standards that must be followed to keep accreditation.
- *The Agency for Health Care Research and Quality (AHRQ).* This organization develops, reviews, and updates clinical guidelines to aid healthcare providers to prevent, diagnose, and manage clinical conditions.
- *Your employer.* Each facility usually develops its own unique set of standards (standards of care, guidelines, policies, procedures, critical pathways, standard care plans, and so forth) that reflect how nursing care should be given in specific situations.

prescribed medications and intravenous therapy, and responsibility for scheduling laboratory studies. Nurses design plans of care that incorporate their independent, dependent, and collaborative responsibilities. See the clinical decision-making process illustrated in Figure 14-2 for help in determining when you can act independently. Because nursing is concerned with the patient's responses to health and illness, the plan of care is supportive of nursing's broad aims—to promote wellness, prevent disease and illness, promote recovery, and facilitate coping with altered functioning.

OUTCOME IDENTIFICATION, PLANNING, AND CRITICAL THINKING

Successful implementation of each step of the nursing process requires high-level skills in critical thinking. To plan healthcare correctly, the nurse must:

- Be familiar with standards and agency policies for setting priorities, identifying and recording expected patient

outcomes, selecting evidence-based nursing interventions, and recording the plan of care (Box 14-2)
- Remember that the goal of patient-centered care is to keep the patient and the patient's interests and preferences central in every aspect of planning and outcome identification
- Keep the "big picture" in focus: What are the discharge goals for this patient, and how should this direct each shift's interventions?
- Trust clinical experience and judgment but be willing to ask for help when the situation demands more than your qualifications and experience can provide; value collaborative practice
- Respect your clinical intuitions but before establishing priorities, identifying outcomes, and selecting nursing interventions be sure that research supports your plan
- Recognize personal biases and keep an open mind

▶ *Remember Darla Jefferson, the pregnant woman with a history of drug abuse described in the Reflective Practice box. Although the nursing student planned to engage the patient in an unbiased discussion of her alternatives, unfortunately the student was unable to adhere to the plan, inserting personal opinions in the discussion. As a result, the plan of care was thwarted and the patient lost trust in the student.* ■

Questions to facilitate critical thinking during planning and outcome identification include:

- Setting priorities: Which problems require my immediate attention or that of the team? Which problems are my responsibility, and which should I refer to someone else? Which problems are most important to the patient?

- Identifying outcomes: What must I observe in the patient to demonstrate the resolution of the problems identified by the nursing diagnoses and general problem list? What is the time frame for accomplishing these outcomes? Do the outcomes need to be modified in light of the patient's response (or lack of response) to the planned interventions?
- Selecting evidence-based nursing interventions: What do nursing science and my clinical experience suggest is the likelihood that this particular nursing intervention will help the patient realize his or her expected outcomes? How can I tailor my interventions to increase the likelihood of patient benefit? What is the worst thing that might happen with this intervention, how likely is it to happen, and what can I do to minimize the possibility of this harm?
- Communicating the plan of care: Does the plan of care adequately address the patient's priorities today? If the plan of care is computerized or standardized, does it adequately address the specific needs of this particular patient? Can anyone reading the plan of care know how to intervene effectively with this patient?

COMPREHENSIVE PLANNING

In acute care settings, three basic stages of planning are critical to comprehensive nursing care: initial, ongoing, and discharge. In other settings such as long-term care, hospice care, or a community clinic, initial and ongoing planning may be the primary stages used. If a nurse develops a comprehensive plan of care on the patient's first day but fails to update the plan, the plan will not be effective or efficient. Failure to update the plan of care as needed is a common problem in all healthcare settings.

Initial Planning

Initial planning is developed by the nurse who performs the admission nursing history and the physical assessment. This comprehensive plan addresses each problem listed in the prioritized nursing diagnoses and identifies appropriate patient goals and the related nursing care. **Standardized care plans** are prepared plans of care that identify the nursing diagnoses, outcomes, and related nursing interventions common to a specific population or health problem. (An example of a standardized care plan is shown later in the chapter.) They can provide an excellent basis for the initial plan if the nurse individualizes them. Resources for standardized plans include computerized plans, textbooks with prepared care plans, and agency-developed plans/maps/critical pathways. By using such standardized plans, the nurse is free to direct time and expertise to individualizing the plan.

Ongoing Planning

Ongoing planning is carried out by any nurse who interacts with the patient. Its chief purpose is to keep the plan up to date to facilitate the resolution of health problems, manage risk factors, and promote function. The nurse caring for the patient uses new data as they are collected and analyzed to make the plan more specific and accurate and, therefore, more effective. The work of ongoing planning includes stating nursing diagnoses more clearly (both the problem statement and the cause), developing new diagnoses, making previously developed patient outcomes more realistic, developing new outcomes as needed, and identifying nursing interventions that will best accomplish the patient goals.

> Consider Elijah Wolinski, the frail, elderly man who developed a pressure ulcer. Ongoing planning is necessary because the patient's pressure ulcer would most likely take some time to heal or at least improve. In addition, other needs might become apparent during subsequent home visits, thereby requiring the nurse to update the plan of care. ■

At this stage of planning, standardized plans based on medical conditions or procedures might be useful in developing new nursing diagnoses and related nursing interventions, but the emphasis is clearly on individualizing the plan to meet unique patient needs. For example, the standard nursing order "force fluids" would be rewritten as "offer 60 mL cranberry or orange juice between meals, and keep fresh water at bedside." A preliminary order such as "explore with the patient existing supports" might be replaced with "keep daughter Barbara informed of mother's progress and coach her in effective support strategies: Barbara Clems, (h) 448-3211, (w) 654-8999."

Discharge Planning

Discharge planning is best carried out by the nurse who has worked most closely with the patient and family, possibly in conjunction with a nurse or social worker with a broad knowledge of existing community resources. In acute care settings, comprehensive discharge planning begins when the patient is admitted for treatment. Careful planning ensures that the nurse uses teaching and counseling skills effectively to help the patient and family develop sufficient knowledge of the health problem and the therapeutic regimen to carry out necessary self-care behaviors at home competently. Discharge planning is further discussed in Chapter 9.

ESTABLISHING PRIORITIES

To develop a prioritized list of nursing diagnoses, the nurse needs guidelines for ranking diagnoses as high, medium, or low priority. High-priority diagnoses pose the greatest threat to the patient's well-being. Non–life-threatening diagnoses are ranked as medium priorities, and diagnoses that are not specifically related to the current health problem are of low priority. In all levels, psychosocial needs must be considered as well as physiologic needs.

In addition to developing a prioritized list of nursing diagnoses, nurses working within an interdisciplinary team need to set priorities for nursing care that take account of all the patient's health needs, as recorded on the general problem list. This involves looking at all problems to determine the relationships among the problems (what's causing or contributing to what). Thus, it generally makes sense to deal with medical (or suspected medical) problems first. If these can be resolved, many human response problems are gone. If a nurse sees the classic signs and symptoms of appendicitis and tries to identify and manage a nursing diagnosis of pain without consulting a physician or nurse practitioner, the patient's appendix might rupture before a nursing plan to relieve pain is even developed!

Three helpful guides to facilitate critical thinking when prioritizing patient problems include Maslow's hierarchy of human needs, patient preference, and anticipation of future problems.

Maslow's Hierarchy of Human Needs

Because basic needs must be met before a person can focus on higher ones, patient needs may be prioritized according to the following hierarchy:

1. Physiologic needs
2. Safety needs
3. Love and belonging needs
4. Self-esteem needs
5. Self-actualization needs

For example, a geriatric patient who is incontinent of urine and sitting in a wet disposable brief (physiologic need) will be unable to participate fully in a music therapy diversional activity (self-esteem need) until the more basic need is met.

Patient Preference

It is best to first meet the needs the patient thinks are most important, if this order does not interfere with other vital therapies. For example, a woman is admitted to an orthopedic unit with a fractured pelvis and multiple lacerations after an automobile accident. The morning after the accident, she complains of pain and needs assistance with bathing and attention to her lacerations, but she refuses to do anything until she calls home to find out who is caring for her 15-month-old twins. The nurse should help her to call home before beginning other care as long as it does not interfere with life-saving emergency care.

Anticipation of Future Problems

Nurses must tap their knowledge base to consider the potential effects of different nursing actions. Assigning low priority to a diagnosis that the patient wants to ignore but that can result in harmful future consequences for the patient might be nursing negligence. For example, an obese patient with multiple sclerosis and greatly decreased limb strength who spends most of her day in bed may see no value in diet modification and position changes. A nurse who is alert to the potentially serious problem of pressure ulcers would assign high priority to this diagnosis, nonetheless, and incorporate weight management and position changes into the plan of care despite the patient's reluctance.

Critical Thinking and Establishing Priorities

The work of setting priorities demands careful critical thinking. Alfaro-LeFevre (2010, p. 148) suggests that nurses ask:

1. What problems need immediate attention and which ones can wait?
2. Which problems are your responsibility, and which do you need to refer to someone else?
3. Which problems can be dealt with by using standard plans (e.g., critical paths, standards of care)?
4. Which problems aren't covered by protocols or standard plans but must be addressed to ensure a safe hospital stay and timely discharge (or simply safe care of high quality)?

> Think back to Darla Jefferson, the pregnant woman with a history of drug abuse. The nurse would incorporate critical thinking by asking these four questions, thereby ultimately arriving at the patient problems requiring the most immediate attention. ∎

When planning nursing care for each day, it is helpful to consider the following:

- Have changes in the patient's health status influenced the priority of nursing diagnoses? For example, when a routine home visit to an older adult reveals evidence of possible elder abuse, a new set of priorities for care is needed, which may even result in a new diagnosis.
- Have changes in the way the patient is responding to health and illness or the plan of care affected those nursing diagnoses that can be realistically addressed? For example, a nurse might have identified Ineffective Coping as a high-priority diagnosis for the patient after the patient learned the medical diagnosis, and planned to initiate counseling. If the patient adamantly requests to be left alone for a day to think things through, however, the nurse has to modify priorities of care for that day.
- Are there relationships among diagnoses that require that one be worked on before another can be resolved?
- Can several patient problems be dealt with together?

After answering these questions, the nurse ranks the diagnoses in the order in which they should be addressed. Setting priorities enables the nurse to make sure that time and energy are being directed first to the patient's most important problems.

IDENTIFYING AND WRITING OUTCOMES

Learning to identify and write appropriate outcomes takes practice. The text that follows and the guidelines in Box 14-1 will help you to identify outcomes that will maximize your effectiveness when working with patients.

Deriving Outcomes from Nursing Diagnoses

Outcomes are derived from the problem statement of the nursing diagnosis. For each nursing diagnosis in the plan of care, at least one outcome should be written that, if achieved, demonstrates a direct resolution of the problem statement (Table 14-1).

Other outcomes that contribute to the resolution of the problem may be written. For example, for the nursing diagnosis

TABLE • 14-1	EXAMPLES OF GOALS/OUTCOMES TO RELIEVE PROBLEMS
Problem Statement of the Nursing Diagnosis	**Related Patient Goal/Outcome**
Pain	Within 8 hours, patient will report pain is absent or diminished
Imbalanced Nutrition: More Than Body Requirements	By 12/6/12, patient will reach target weight of 122 lb
Impaired Physical Mobility	Before discharge, patient will ambulate length of hallway independently

Imbalanced Nutrition: More Than Body Requirements related to excessive snacking and inactivity, in addition to the outcome "within 12 weeks (12/6/12), the patient will lose 20 pounds and reach target weight (122 lb)," the following goals are appropriate: "within 3 days of teaching: the patient will identify 10 low-calorie snack foods he is willing to try; the patient will have 3-day diet recall consistent with nutritionally balanced 1,500-calorie diet; the patient will report incorporating three half-hour periods of walking at 5 miles per hour into each week." If the patient can identify low-calorie snack foods and adopt a more active lifestyle, there is a greater likelihood that he will reach his target weight, but it is entirely possible for a patient to achieve these secondary outcomes without resolving the chief problem. Remember, at least one outcome per nursing diagnosis must directly resolve the problem statement in the nursing diagnosis.

The **Nursing Outcomes Classification (NOC)** developed by the Iowa Outcomes Project presents the first comprehensive standardized language used to describe the patient outcomes that are responsive to nursing intervention (Moorhead, Johnson, Maas, & Swanson, 2008). The current classification lists 385 outcomes with definitions, indicators, measurement scales, and supporting references. The outcomes may be used for individuals, families, or communities. Examples of NOC outcomes are found in each clinical chapter. Explicit linkages between the North American Nursing Diagnosis Association (NANDA) diagnoses and the NOC facilitate a comprehensive approach to care planning.

Establishing Long-Term Versus Short-Term Outcomes

Outcomes might be either long term or short term. Long-term outcomes require a longer period (usually more than a week) to be achieved than do short-term outcomes. They also may be used as discharge goals, in which case they are more broadly written and communicate to the entire nursing team the desired end results of nursing care for a particular patient. For example, two women, both 77 years of age, are

Box 14-3 EXAMPLES OF LONG-TERM AND SHORT-TERM OUTCOMES

Patient on Bed Rest From Nursing Home
Long-Term Outcome
Mrs. Goldstein returns to the nursing home pain free with her incision healed and her left leg in good alignment.

Short-Term Outcomes
• Whenever observed, patient will be lying in bed with legs in correct alignment (abductor pillow in place, if ordered).
• Before discharge, Mrs. Goldstein's hip incision will show signs of healing (skin surfaces approximate, free from signs of infection—redness, swelling, heat, purulent drainage).
• Whenever observed, patient will report that comfort measures and medication are satisfactorily managing pain.

Active Patient from Private Home
Long-Term Outcome
Mrs. Silverstein returns home to her husband pain free with incision healed, fully mobile (full weight bearing on left leg), and capable of independent activities of daily living.

Short-Term Outcomes
• By 1/28/12, the patient will verbalize willingness to participate in physical therapy program.
• By 2/4/12, the patient will ambulate (with nursing assistance and walker) to bathroom (full weight bearing).
• By 2/11/12, the patient will ambulate with nursing assistance only (no walker) in her room.
• Goals for incision and pain relief same as for Mrs. Goldstein.

on a nursing unit after undergoing similar operations for fractured left hips. One woman has spent the past 2 years in bed in a nursing home; the other woman fractured her hip at the YMCA, where she swims daily. Their nursing care should not be the same because it is directed toward different long-term goals, even though their short-term goals might be similar (see Box 14-3: Examples of Long-Term and Short-Term Outcomes).

> Consider Elijah Wolinski, the frail, elderly man with a pressure ulcer. The nurse might establish a long-term outcome such as, "The patient's sacral area will exhibit no evidence of a pressure ulcer." Short-term outcomes might include, "The patient's sacral pressure ulcer demonstrates an absence of purulent drainage within 1 week of initiating wound care. By week 2, the patient's pressure ulcer has decreased in size by a quarter-inch. By week 2, the patient's caregiver demonstrates measures to relieve pressure on the skin while the patient is in bed." ■

Determining Patient-Centered Outcomes

Alfaro-LeFevre (2010) recommends that nurses be realistic and consider:

- Patient's health state, overall prognosis
- Expected length of stay
- Growth and development
- Patient values and cultural considerations
- Other planned therapies for the patient
- Available human, material, and financial resources
- Risks, benefits, and current scientific evidence
- Changes in status that indicate you need to modify usual expected outcomes (p. 153)

Moorhead et al. (2008) recommend that the following factors be considered when selecting outcomes: (1) the type of health concern, (2) the nursing or medical diagnoses and health problems, (3) patient characteristics, (4) patient resources, (5) patient preferences, (6) patient capacities, and (7) treatment potential (p. 59).

Ensuring Quality Outcomes

The Institute of Medicine (2001), in its report *Crossing the Quality Chasm*, highlights six aims to be met by healthcare systems with regard to the quality of care.

- Safe: avoiding injury
- Effective: avoiding overuse and underuse
- Patient-centered: responding to patient preferences, needs, and values
- Timely: reducing waits and delays
- Efficient: avoiding waste
- Equitable: providing care that does not vary in quality to all recipients.

Institutions measuring their achievement of these aims will welcome nursing's efforts to determine its effectiveness (Moorhead, Johnson, Maas, & Swanson, 2008, p. 69).

Using Cognitive, Psychomotor, and Affective Outcomes

Outcomes might be categorized according to the type of change they describe for the patient. Cognitive outcomes describe increases in patient knowledge or intellectual behaviors—for example: "Within 1 day after teaching, the patient will list three benefits of continuing to apply moist compresses to leg ulcer after discharge." Psychomotor outcomes describe the patient's achievement of new skills—for example, "By 6/12/12, the patient will correctly demonstrate application of wet-to-dry dressing on leg ulcer." Affective outcomes describe changes in patient values, beliefs, and attitudes. Difficult both to write and to evaluate, affective outcomes might be critical to the resolution of a complex patient problem—for example, "By 6/12/12, the patient will verbalize valuing health sufficiently to practice new health behaviors to prevent recurrence of leg ulcer." In this example, even if the patient intellectually grasps the reasons for taking care of her leg and can competently redress her ulcer, unless she is motivated to take care of herself, her knowledge and skills will not result in healthy outcomes. See Chapter 16 for other examples of these outcomes.

Involving Patient and Family in Outcome Development

One of the most important considerations in writing outcomes is to encourage the patient and family to be as involved in goal development as their abilities and interest permit. The more involved they are, the greater the probability that the goals will be achieved. When developing patient outcomes, the nurse and patient look at the problem statement of the nursing diagnosis and ask, "What patient changes or outcomes will result in the prevention or resolution of this problem?" The answer, when carefully worded, becomes the patient outcome.

Identifying Culturally Appropriate Outcomes

The ANA Standards of Practice (see Box 14-1) direct the nurse to derive *culturally appropriate expected outcomes* from the diagnoses. See Chapter 2 for a discussion of culturally appropriate care.

Identifying Outcomes Supportive of the Total Treatment Plan

When identifying outcomes, it is always important to remember that nurses nurse people, not problems. This means that every outcome you write should support the overall treatment plan and "make sense" in terms of the overall goals for the patient. For example, identifying nutritional outcomes may be appropriate for a patient who is losing weight, but if this patient is in a hospice and dying, this may not be an appropriate outcome if it is incompatible with the overall goal of a peaceful death with dignity.

Writing Patient-Centered Measurable Outcomes

To be measurable, outcomes should have the following:

- Subject: the patient or some part of the patient
- Verb: indicates the action the patient will perform
- Conditions: specifies the particular circumstances in or by which the outcome is to be achieved. Not every outcome specifies conditions.
- Performance criteria: describe in observable, measurable terms the expected patient behavior or other manifestation
- Target time: specifies when the patient is expected to be able to achieve the outcome

Verbs helpful in writing measurable outcomes include:

Define	List	Explain
Prepare	Verbalize	Select
Identify	Describe	Apply
Design	Choose	Demonstrate

The target time or time criterion may be a realistic, actual date or other statement indicating time, such as before discharge, after viewing film, whenever observed.

Following are examples of properly constructed measurable outcomes:

- During the next 24-hour period, the patient's fluid intake will total at least 2,000 mL.
- At the next visit, 12/23/12, the patient will correctly demonstrate relaxation exercises.

It might be helpful to include special conditions when writing an outcome if this information is important for other nurses (e.g., "Before discharge, the patient will ambulate independently the length of hallway and back, using a Philadelphia collar to support cervical vertebrae").

Avoiding Common Errors

Common errors when writing patient outcomes include the following:

- *Expressing the patient outcome as a nursing intervention.* Incorrect: "Offer Mr. Myer 60 mL fluid every 2 hours while awake." Correct: "Mr. Myer will drink 60 mL fluid every 2 hours while awake, beginning 2/24/12."
- *Using verbs that are not observable and measurable.* Incorrect: "Mrs. Gaston will know how to bathe her newborn." Correct: "After attending the infant care class, Mrs. Gaston will correctly demonstrate the procedure for bathing her newborn." Verbs to be avoided when writing goals include "know," "understand," "learn," and "become aware." These verbs are too general and cannot be measured. Verbs that are helpful when writing outcomes that are observable and measurable were listed previously.
- *Including more than one patient behavior/manifestation in short-term outcomes.* Incorrect: "Patient will list dangers of smoking and stop smoking." Correct: "By next meeting, 3/11/12, the patient will (1) identify three dangers of smoking and (2) describe a plan he is willing to try to stop smoking. By 6/20/12, the patient will report that he no longer smokes."
- *Writing outcomes that are so vague that other nurses are unsure of the goal of nursing care.* Incorrect: "Patient will cope better." Correct: "After teaching, 10/20/12, the patient will (1) describe two new coping strategies he is willing to try and (2) demonstrate decreased incidence of previously observed ineffective coping behaviors (chain smoking, withdrawal behavior, heavy alcohol consumption)."

IDENTIFYING NURSING INTERVENTIONS

A **nursing intervention** is any treatment, based on clinical judgment and knowledge, that a nurse performs to enhance patient outcomes (Bulechek, Butcher, & Dochterman, 2008). There are nurse-initiated, physician-initiated, and collaborative interventions.

Nurse-Initiated Interventions

A nurse-initiated intervention is an autonomous action based on scientific rationale that a nurse executes to benefit the patient in a predictable way related to the nursing diagnosis

and projected outcomes. Nursing interventions are actions performed by the nurse to:

1. Monitor health status
2. Reduce risks
3. Resolve, prevent, or manage a problem
4. Facilitate independence or assist with activities of daily living
5. Promote optimal sense of physical, psychological, and spiritual well-being (Alfaro-LeFevre, 2010, p. 160)

Nurse-initiated interventions do not require a physician's (or other team member's) order. Nurse-initiated interventions, like patient goals, are derived from the nursing diagnosis. But whereas the problem statement of the diagnosis suggests the patient goals, it is the cause of the problem (etiology) that suggests the nursing interventions (Fig. 14-3). Effective nurses select nursing interventions that specifically address factors that cause or contribute to the patient's problems. For example, many factors may contribute to obesity, such as deficient nutritional knowledge, convenience of high-calorie fast foods, lifetime snacking habits, limited food budget, little exercise, and low self-esteem. The nurse working with a patient who wants to lose weight could attempt to deal with all these factors, but this approach would be inefficient. When a carefully developed nursing

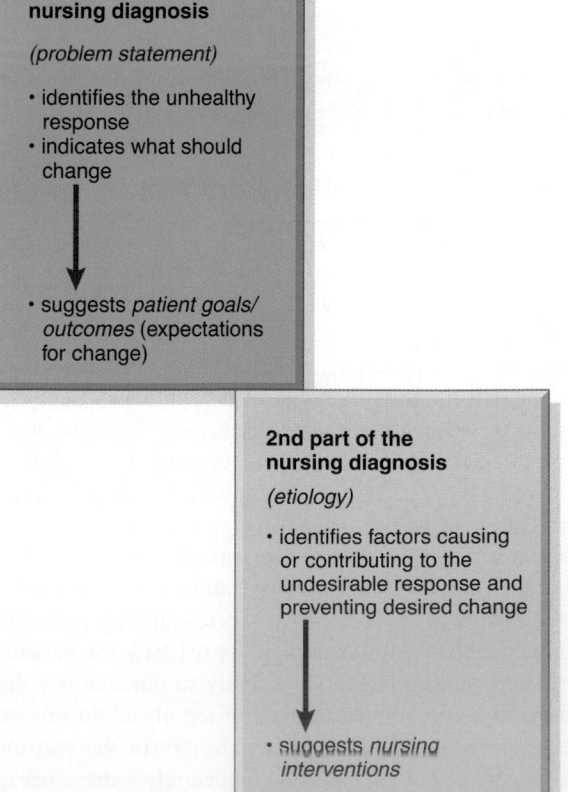

FIGURE 14-3. Deriving patient goals/outcomes and nursing orders from nursing diagnoses.

diagnosis identifies the specific factors that contribute to a particular patient's weight problem, nursing interventions can be selected to deal directly with these factors.

> *Remember Glenda Kronk, the woman desiring to improve her fitness. Based on assessment, the nurse would determine the factors that have played a role in the patient's current status, developing appropriate nursing diagnoses and outcomes from which to establish appropriate interventions. For example, if the patient has been sedentary over the past several years, interventions should focus on measures to increase the patient's activity level, thereby promoting improvement in her overall health and fitness.* ■

Similarly, nursing interventions for the patient with the diagnosis Imbalanced Nutrition: More Than Body Requirements related to lifetime snacking habits and heavy reliance on high-calorie fast foods might include education about the fat content and calories in fast foods and an exploration of ways the patient could change her eating habits to eat more nutritionally balanced meals with fewer calories. Thus, the nursing approach is not the same for every patient with a weight problem. The art of nursing involves the careful identification of the specific nursing interventions needed by particular patients to meet their individual needs.

Identifying and Selecting Appropriate Nurse-Initiated Interventions

After writing the patient outcomes, the nurse identifies various nursing interventions to help the patient achieve the outcomes. The **Nursing Intervention Classification (NIC),** the first comprehensive, validated list of nursing interventions applicable to all settings that can be used by nurses in multiple specialties, greatly facilitates the work of identifying appropriate interventions (Bulechek, Butcher, & Dochterman, 2008). Examples of using NIC to facilitate care planning for specific patient health problems may be found in each clinical chapter of this text; in addition, NIC taxonomy is included in Table 15-2 in the next chapter.

The effectiveness of the nurse is directly proportional to his or her knowledge of varied nursing strategies. Consider these different nursing care options identified by three nurses when they are asked to describe nursing care for a woman 2 days after cesarean delivery who is complaining of pain in the incisional area.

Nurse A
- Check to see what type of pain medication is ordered, and give it if the time interval is sufficient.

Nurse B
- Assess the quality of the pain, and use this time to communicate support by means of expression and squeeze of hand.
- Administer analgesic if indicated.
- Assess effectiveness of the analgesic ordered.

Nurse C
- Assess quality of the pain, and explore the possibility of contributing factors such as the effects of increased gas in the abdominal area or concern about the newborn, herself, or other family members.
- Use empathic listening (possibly touch) to communicate support and to encourage the mother to share her concerns.
- Change the patient's position in bed.
- Offer a backrub.
- If appropriate, suggest activity that will distract attention from the pain (e.g., watching a film about newborn care or listening to music).
- Give the prescribed medication for pain and observe its effect.
- When administering the medication, use the power of positive suggestion to enhance its effectiveness: "This will start taking the pain away in about 10 minutes and will help you relax."

It is possible that the patient simply needs her prescribed analgesic to achieve the outcome: "Patient will report minimal to no pain at assessment every 2 hours." In that case, all three nurses would be effective in meeting the patient's need for nursing care. It is highly possible, however, that the prescribed medication is not working or the pain is compounded by the mother's fears about caring for her new baby or by her worries that the baby will ruin her relationship with her husband. Therefore, nurse C, whose knowledge level is more comprehensive, is most likely to be effective in resolving the patient's problem.

The more varied the options available to the nurse, the more effective the nursing response. In different situations, a skilled nursing procedure, the appropriate use of silence, respectful listening, humor, teaching, counseling, and touch can all be effective nursing strategies. Nurses who are merely task-oriented and satisfied to meet every patient problem with a mechanical procedure are limiting their effectiveness.

When selecting nursing interventions for individual patients, use the guidelines in Box 14-4. Use of these guidelines increases the chances that the patient will achieve the outcome. Ongoing evaluation enables the nurse to determine the effectiveness of the selected interventions.

Box 14-4 GUIDELINES FOR SELECTING NURSING INTERVENTIONS

Nursing interventions should be:
- Appropriate in terms of the nursing diagnosis and related patient outcomes, safe and efficient
- Consistent with research findings and standards of care
- Realistic in terms of the abilities, time, and resources available to the nurse and patient
- Compatible with the patient's values, beliefs, and cultural and psychosocial background
- Valued, whenever possible, by the patient and family
- Compatible with other planned therapies

Individualizing Evidence-Based Interventions

Nurse researchers are attempting to establish a statistical pattern for predicting the probability of success of select nursing interventions. Find the student plan of care at the end of this chapter and review the scientific rationale for the selected nursing orders. You should always be prepared to explain why you are doing intervention "a" as opposed to intervention "b" or "c." You should know how likely it is that the proposed intervention will achieve the desired outcomes and what the associated risks are. Alfaro-LeFevre (2010) recommends that nurses answer four key questions if they want to determine individualized evidence-based interventions:

1. What can be done to prevent or minimize the risks or causes of this problem?
2. What can be done to manage the problem?
3. How can I tailor interventions to meet expected outcomes?
4. How likely are we to get desired versus adverse responses to the interventions, and what can we do to reduce the risks and increase the likelihood of beneficial responses? (p. 163)

You can learn more about evidence-based practice in Chapter 5 and in the Research in Nursing and PICO in Practice recurring displays in the clinical chapters. Competent nurses use research findings (science of nursing), experience, and knowledge of the patient (art of nursing) to aid in the selection of effective nursing interventions. Consultation with nurse colleagues and continuing education enable the nurse to develop effective nursing approaches to patients' problems.

Writing Nurse-Initiated Interventions in the Plan of Care

Nursing interventions describe in writing, and thus communicate to the entire nursing staff and healthcare team, the specific nursing care to be implemented for the patient. Each nursing intervention should include:

- Date
- Verb: Action to be performed
- Subject: Who is to do it
- Descriptive phrase: How, when, where, how often, how long, or how much

Well-written nursing interventions accomplish the following:

- Assist the patient to meet specific outcomes that are related directly to one outcome
- Clearly and concisely describe the nursing action to be performed (answer the questions who, what, where, when, and how)
- Are dated when written and when the plan of care is reviewed
- Are signed by the nurse prescribing the order or intervention
- Use only those abbreviations accepted in the institution (these are usually found in the agency's policy manual; a

list of commonly accepted abbreviations appears in Chapter 17)
- Refer the nurse to the agency's procedure manual or other literature for the steps of routine, lengthy procedures

Following are examples of well-stated nursing interventions:

- Offer patient 60 mL water or juice (prefers orange or cranberry juice) every 2 hours while awake for a total minimum PO intake of 500 mL.
- Teach patient the necessity of carefully monitoring fluid intake and output; remind patient each shift to mark off fluid intake on record at bedside.
- Walk with patient to bathroom for toileting every 2 hours (on even hours) while patient is awake.

The set of nursing interventions written to assist a patient to meet an outcome must be comprehensive. Comprehensive nursing interventions specify what *observations* (assessments) need to be made and how often, what nursing *interventions* need to be done and when they must be done, and what *teaching, counseling,* and *advocacy* needs patients and families have.

Many sets of nursing interventions are inadequate because they fail to indicate the ongoing assessment priority needs for a specific problem or goal. Clearly stating assessment priorities helps all nurses to be more sensitive to important patient data.

> Review the scenario at the beginning of the chapter for Glenda Kronk. The nurse would need to establish assessment priorities. For example, when assisting Glenda, who wants to lose weight to reach her target weight, appropriate nursing interventions might include the following: "6/17/12: Continue to assess (1) patient's motivation to participate in weight-loss program and (2) factors that positively or negatively influence weight loss." ■

Similarly, it is often assumed that all patients have the same teaching needs. Nothing is farther from the truth. In fact, many patients have an excellent knowledge base (which might be greater than that of the nurse for a particular disease). Their need for nursing might be a need for counseling, instead of teaching, as they learn to live with a chronic illness. However, it is important to obtain proof of the patient's knowledge or competency before proceeding with the plan of care. For example, a diabetic patient would need to state the signs and symptoms of hypo- and hyperglycemia or to give a return demonstration of doing a fingerstick blood glucose test.

Comprehensive nursing interventions relate to individual patient needs.

Physician-Initiated Interventions

A physician-initiated intervention is an intervention initiated by a physician in response to a medical diagnosis but carried out by a nurse in response to a doctor's order. For example, a physician examining a patient brought into the emergency room after a motor vehicle accident might ask the nurse to administer a medication to relieve pain and schedule the patient for radiographs and other diagnostic tests. The nurse who performs these interventions is implementing physician-initiated interventions. Both the physician and nurse are legally responsible for these interventions, and nurses are expected to be knowledgeable about how to execute these interventions safely and effectively. Nurses who question the appropriateness of physician-initiated interventions are legally responsible to seek clarification of the order with responsible parties. Under no circumstances should a nurse implement a questionable intervention, even at the urging of a physician or other professional. Chapter 7 addresses nurses' legal responsibility for their actions.

Collaborative Interventions

Nurses also carry out treatments initiated by other providers such as pharmacists, respiratory therapists, or physician assistants. For example, nurses caring for a patient who was in a motor vehicle accident might eventually be implementing interventions written by a physical therapist, occupational therapist, or other member of the healthcare team.

Structured Care Methodologies

Efforts to standardize nursing care have taken different forms. Approaches popular during different decades include procedures (1960s), standards of care (1970s), algorithms (1980s), and clinical practice guidelines (1990s). Each of

these aims to help the nurse identify and select interventions that produce optimal care, reduce legal risks, and lower healthcare costs. A description of each approach follows:

- Procedure: A set of how-to action steps for performing a clinical activity or task
- Standard of care: A description of an acceptable level of patient care or professional practice
- Algorithm: A set of steps that approximates the decision process of an expert clinician and is used to make a decision; these clinical rules are typically embedded in a branching flow chart
- Clinical practice guideline: A statement or series of statements outlining appropriate practice for a clinical condition or procedure

National guidelines such as those published by the U.S. Agency for Health Care Research and Quality (AHRQ; http://www.ahrq.gov) and the Cochrane Library (http://www.cochrane.org/cochrane/cc-broch.htm#CC and http://www.cochrane.org/reviews/clibintro.htm) are generally based on the latest, most comprehensive scientific evidence and expert analysis. They provide standards for delivering and evaluating care for patients with the same diagnosis. Box 14-5 compares structured care methodologies. Additional examples may be found in Chapter 16.

Consulting

A nurse designing the plan of care might discover that more information is needed about the nature of the problems

---

Box 14-5   STRUCTURED CARE METHODOLOGIES

Algorithm
- Useful in management of high-risk subgroups within the cohort; may be "layered" on top of a pathway to control care practices that are used to manage a specific problem
- Binary decision trees that guide stepwise assessment and intervention
- Intense specificity; no provider flexibility
- May use analytical research methods to ensure cause and effect

Critical Pathway
- Represents a sequential, interdisciplinary, minimal practice standard for a specific patient population
- Provides flexibility to alter care to meet individualized patient needs
- Abbreviated format, broad perspective
- Phase or episode driven
- Ability to measure cause-and-effect relationship between pathway and patient outcomes prohibited by lack of control; changes in patient outcomes directly attributable to the efforts of the collaborative practice team

Guideline
- Broad, research-based practice recommendations
- May or may not have been tested in clinical practice

- Practice resources helpful in construction of structured care methodologies
- No mechanism for ensuring practice implementation

Order Set
- Preprinted provider orders used to expedite the order process after a practice standard has been validated through analytical research
- Complements and increases compliance with existing practice standards
- Can be used to represent the algorithm or protocol in order format

Protocol
- Prescribes specific therapeutic interventions for a clinical problem unique to a subgroup of patients within the cohort
- Multifaceted; may be used to drive practice for more than one discipline
- Broader specificity than an algorithm; allows for minimal provider flexibility by way of treatment options
- May be "layered" on top of a pathway

Agency for Health Care Policy and Research's (now Agency for Healthcare Research and Quality) Clinical Practice Guideline Development, AHCPR program note in Publication 93-0023, 1993.

FIGURE 14-4. Consulting with a nursing colleague or other member of the healthcare team can assist the nurse in developing an effective nursing plan of care. *(Photo © B. Proud.)*

Box 14-6   **EVALUATIVE STATEMENT**

Documents that patient has met, partially met, or not met the goal/outcome

Goal/Outcome Statement
Beginning 6/8/12, the patient will ambulate half the length of hallway with assistance three times daily.

Evaluative Statement
6/8/12—Goal partially met; patient refused to ambulate in the morning but did walk to the bathroom once in the afternoon with the assistance of one nurse.
Recommendation: Review reason for progressive ambulation with patient; assess motivation to increase independence.

—*M. Stenulis, RN*

underlying the need for nursing or about specific interventions. **Consultation,** a process in which two or more individuals with varying degrees of experience and expertise discuss a problem and its solution, often proves helpful. Nurses might consult with nurse specialists and other members of the healthcare team, including physicians, nutritionists, social workers, therapists, pastoral caregivers, and ethicists (Fig. 14-4). Consultations are a valuable means for nurses to expand their nursing knowledge and repertoire of effective strategies.

➤ *Review the Reflective Practice box describing Darla Jefferson. The nurse would consult other healthcare team members for assistance. For example, the nurse might consult social services for assistance with drug treatment and rehabilitation. Should the patient decide to keep her baby, social services also would be helpful, such as with obtaining food stamps and infant formula through government programs, appropriate housing, and follow-up in the community. A consultation with a nutritionist would be helpful prenatally to ensure that Darla meets the requirements for herself and her fetus, and also postpartum to ensure that the infant is receiving adequate nutrition to grow and develop.* ▪

DEVELOPING EVALUATIVE STRATEGIES

Well-written outcomes define the evaluative strategy to be used by the nurse. Patient outcomes are meaningless unless nurses evaluate the patient's progress toward their achievement. The nurse records the date the outcome was written and the date it is achieved. Evaluative statements (Box 14-6) include a statement about achievement of the desired outcome (met, partially met, not met) and list actual patient behavior as evidence supporting the statement. If the plan is not achieved, recommendations for revising the plan of care are included in the evaluative statement. Chapter 16 deals specifically with the evaluative component of the nursing process.

COMMUNICATING AND RECORDING THE PLAN OF NURSING CARE

The **plan of nursing care** (patient care plan) is the written guide that directs the efforts of the nursing team as nurses work with patients to meet their health goals. It specifies nursing diagnoses, outcomes, and associated nursing interventions. Well-written plans of care offer many benefits to the patient, nurse, nursing unit, nursing administration, and nursing profession. Primarily, plans of nursing care ensure that the nursing team works efficiently to deliver holistic, goal-oriented, individualized care to patients. A well-written plan of nursing care accomplishes the following:

- Represents an effective philosophy of nursing and advances nursing's four aims: promotes health, prevents disease and illness, promotes recovery, facilitates coping with altered functioning
- Is prepared by the nurse who best knows the patient and is recorded on the day the patient presents for treatment and care according to agency policy; modifications to the initial plan are signed and dated
- Is responsive to the individual characteristics and needs of the patient; is culturally appropriate
- Clearly identifies the nursing assistance the patient needs and nursing's collaborative responsibilities for fulfilling the medical and interdisciplinary plan of care (clearly specifies nursing diagnoses, patient outcomes, nursing interventions, and evaluative strategies)
- Directs the nurse's assessment priorities, caregiving behaviors, and teaching, counseling, and advocacy behaviors
- Is based on scientific principles and incorporates findings of nursing research
- Meets the developmental, psychosocial, and spiritual needs of the patient, as well as his or her physiologic needs
- Is updated to reflect changes in the patient's status and related needs for nursing care
- Addresses the discharge needs of the patient and family

- Provides for as much patient and family participation as possible
- When appropriate, is compatible with the medical plan of care and that of the interdisciplinary team
- Creates a record that can be used for evaluation, research, reimbursement, and legal purposes

Many suggestions for plans of care appear in the nursing literature. Each school of nursing and each healthcare institution and agency has its own format, which may reflect a particular nursing theory. Common to all formats is a minimum of three columns for documenting nursing diagnoses, patient outcomes, and nursing interventions. Formats differ in the way assessment data and the nursing evaluation are addressed.

Institutional and Agency Plans of Care

The Joint Commission requires healthcare institutions and agencies to formulate, maintain, and support a patient-specific plan for care, treatment, and rehabilitation.

Types of Nursing Care

In most institutions and agencies, the plans of care, regardless of their format, communicate directions for three different types of nursing care: nursing care related to basic human needs, nursing care related to nursing diagnoses, and nursing care related to the medical and interdisciplinary plan of care.

NURSING CARE RELATED TO BASIC HUMAN NEEDS

The plan should concisely communicate to caregivers the data about the patient's usual health habits and patterns, obtained during the nursing history, that are needed to direct daily care. For example, it is important to know whether a toddler is toilet-trained and what words he or she uses to indicate the need to void or defecate. Directives about the patient's usual health habits and patterns might be modified by current treatment orders, such as an order to fast for a diagnostic procedure or to limit or increase activity. This information is useful to caregivers only if it is kept current as the patient's condition changes. Any nurse should be able to find in the plan of care the instructions needed to provide competent care.

NURSING CARE RELATED TO NURSING DIAGNOSES

The plan contains outcomes and nursing interventions for every nursing diagnosis, as well as a place to note the patient's responses to care. This section is the heart of the nursing care plan because it represents the independent component of nursing practice. If well developed, it demonstrates the nurse's clinical competence (knowledge of the science of nursing), sensitivity to the individual needs of the patient, and creativity in mobilizing the resources of the patient and the caregiving team to meet the patient's health needs.

NURSING CARE RELATED TO THE MEDICAL AND INTERDISCIPLINARY PLAN OF CARE

The plan of care also records current medical orders for diagnostic studies and treatment and specified related nursing care.

Formats for Plans of Care

A great variety of formats are used to communicate the plan of care.

KARDEX PLANS OF CARE

Many healthcare institutions and agencies use a **Kardex care plan,** in which the plan of nursing care for each patient is concisely recorded on a folded card and placed in a central Kardex file, where it is easily accessible. The plan is eventually placed in the patient's health record. The outside of the card contains basic information such as the patient's profile, admitting diagnosis, activity levels, diet, and routine treatments, medications, and procedures. The inside of the Kardex contains the nursing care plan specifying at the very minimum nursing diagnoses or health problems and related outcomes and nursing interventions.

COMPUTERIZED PLANS OF CARE

In an increasing number of settings, nurses use **computerized plans of nursing care** as part of the electronic medical record. The benefits of using computerized plans include ready access to a large knowledge base; improved record keeping, with resultant improvement in audits and quality assurance; documentation by all members of the healthcare team with printouts for the patient's record and for change-of-shift reports; and reduced time spent on paperwork. One nurse researcher, however, has studied the negative impact of computerized plans on the professionalization of staff nurses. Harris (1990) cautions that computerized systems for patient care planning and the larger systems in which they are embedded contribute to the loss of autonomy, loss of individualization of care, and loss of nursing expertise. Individual nurses, as well as researchers, need to respond to this challenge from Harris: "Does a lot of nursing time spent in procedural, rule-governed, step-by-step thinking processes destroy part of the nurse's ability to care, to empathize, to intuit, to gain insight, to function in the expert mode?" (1990, p. 73).

CASE MANAGEMENT PLANS OF CARE

Clinical pathways (critical pathways, CareMaps) are tools used in case management to communicate the standardized, interdisciplinary plan of care for patients. Case management is a healthcare delivery system intended to provide high-quality, cost-effective care for individuals, families, and groups. The emphasis is on clearly stating expected patient outcomes and the specific times within which it is reasonable to achieve these outcomes. Chapter 17 provides examples of how critical pathways are used with select documentation tools in a computerized system. Figure 14-5 illustrates a standardized plan of care for patients with congestive heart failure. Care guidelines and outcomes are specified for each day of the patient's stay. In this case, the patients receive a version of their own plan of care on admission, based on the rationale that knowing what to expect will result in less stress, quicker recovery, and earlier discharge.

(text continues on page 280)

Standardized Plan of Care

Chart 1
Sacred Heart—St. Mary's Hospitals, Inc.
PLAN OF CARE: CONGESTIVE HEART FAILURE
ESTIMATED LENGTH OF STAY: 4 Days
Supplies Given: Adm. Kit _PN 2-1-11_   **Urinal** _PN 2-1-11_   **Bedpan** _PN 2-1-11_   **Air Mattress** _PN 2-1-11_

FOCUS Date:	Day of Admission	Day 2	Day 3	Day 4
ACTIVITY	Activity Intolerance related to dyspnea • Restrict activity 30 min before and 60 min after meals *Expected outcome* • Activity as tolerated _PN 2-1_	• Restrict activity 30 min before and 60 min after meals • Chair 30 min t.i.d. for meals • Ambulate 60 ft in hall w/ assist • Bathroom privileges *Expected outcome* • Able to tolerate activity without distress _PN 2-2_	• Ambulate 100 ft t.i.d. *Expected outcome* • Able to perform ADLs and ambulation without the use of O_2 ____	• Prepare pt for discharge home *Expected outcome* • Able to tolerate activity without distress ____
NUTRITION Needs assist _no_ Consult needed? _no_	NAS diet or ____ _PN 2-1_	NAS diet or ____	NAS diet or ____	NAS diet or ____
TREATMENTS Skin protocol _PN 2-1_ Fall protocol _PN 2-1_	Excess Fluid Volume related to compromised cardiac output • Vital signs q4h • I&O • Daily weight • Telemetry if ordered • Heparin lock • O_2 at _3 l/min_ • Assess lung and heart sounds q shift and p.r.n. • Assess pedal edema and pulses q shift	• Vital signs q4h • I&O • Daily weight • Telemetry if ordered • Heparin lock • O_2 at _3 l/min_ • Assess lung and heart sounds q shift and p.r.n. • Assess pedal edema and pulses q shift *Expected outcomes* • Pt's foot edema is decreased or pt has lost weight (min 1 lb) _PN 2-2_ • Pt has improved breath sounds _PN 2-2_	• Vital signs q shift • I&O • Daily weight • Discontinue telemetry if previously ordered ____ • Heparin lock • O_2 p.r.n. (If still needed, consult cardio-pulmonary services for need for home O_2.) • Assess lung and heart sounds q shift • Assess pedal edema and pulses q shift	• Vital signs q shift • I&O • Daily weight • Discontinue heparin lock ____ • Discontinue O_2 ____ • Assess lung and heart sounds q shift • Assess pedal edema and pulses q shifts *Expected outcomes* • Feet/ankle edema resolved • Unlabored respirations ____
TEACHING	• Review Plan of Care with pt • Explain medications to pt • Give copy of Plan of Care to pt • Give info sheet on congestive heart failure to pt • Home health referral needed _yes_ PN 2-1-11 • Home O_2 needed _possibly_ PN 2-1-11	*Expected outcomes* • Pt can verbalize understanding of present medications _PN 2-2_	• Discharge medication sheets given ____ • Home health referral arranged if needed ____ • Home O_2 arranged if needed ____	*Expected outcomes* • Pt can verbalize understanding of present medications ____ • Discharge medication sheet reviewed and pt can verbalize understanding ____ • Discharge instructions reviewed and pt can verbalize understanding ____ • Pt can verbalize understanding for need of follow-up visit and when to call doctor ____

OTHER FOCAL AREAS
• Durable power of attorney _yes PN 2-1_
• Living will _yes PN 2-1_
• Code status _full PN 2-1_

FIGURE 14-5. Standardized plan of care for a patient with congestive heart failure. (Adapted from Rasmussen, N., & Gengler, T. [1994]. Clinical pathways of care: The route to better communication. *Nursing 94, 24*[2], 48–49. Used with permission.) *(continued)*

Chart 2
Sacred Heart—St. Mary's Hospitals, Inc.
PLAN OF CARE: CONGESTIVE HEART FAILURE   **PATIENT COPY**
ESTIMATED LENGTH OF STAY: 4 Days

FOCUS Date:	Day of Admission	Day 2	Day 3	Day 4
ACTIVITY	You can move around as you are able. Avoid becoming overtired or short of breath. You should remain in bed 30 minutes before and after your meals.	You should increase your activity slowly. Start by sitting up in the chair for meals and walking short distances with the help of the nurses twice a day.	You should be starting to feel better and should be able to do mild activities without your oxygen.	You should be able to walk in the halls and take your own bath without trouble breathing. You'll go home today if your doctor feels you're ready.
NUTRITION	You'll be on a no-added-salt diet. The dietitian will come to talk to you about this if you don't understand. A salt substitute is available if you need it. (Salt causes your body to hold in extra fluids, making your swelling worse and causing your heart to work even harder.)	Low-salt diet.	Low-salt diet.	Low-salt diet. Ask your doctor or nurse if you should continue this diet at home.
TREATMENTS	The nurse will measure the amount of fluid you take in and put out. The nurse will listen to your heart and lungs to see if they are getting better. You may have to use oxygen for the first day or two to help you breathe easier. You'll be weighed daily. You'll have an intravenous needle placed in your hand or arm. This will be used to give you medication. You may have a telemetry heart monitor on. Nurses in the intensive care unit will monitor your heart's rhythm.	Treatments will remain the same.	Some treatments will remain the same. You'll use oxygen only when you feel you need it. The heart monitor will be discontinued if previously ordered.	Some treatments will remain the same. Your oxygen may be discontinued. Your needle will be removed if you're going home.
TEACHING	You'll need to understand what is going on with your body. Please ask questions if you don't understand something. You'll be given a sheet to explain what congestive heart failure is. Ask about your medications if you're unfamiliar with them.		You'll be given information sheets that explain the medication you'll take at home. You should know about the right foods to eat and what types of food you should avoid. Your doctor may order a follow-up by a home health nurse.	You'll need to follow up with your doctor. Make sure you know when your appointment is. Know what problems may require medical attention.

FIGURE 14-5. (Continued)

CONCEPT MAP PLANS OF CARE

A concept map care plan is a diagram of patient problems and interventions. Your ideas about patient problems and treatments are the "concepts" that are diagrammed. These maps are used to organize patient data, analyze relationships in the data, and enable you to take a holistic view of the patient's situation (Schuster, 2002). Examples of concept map care plans can be found in Chapter 11 and throughout the text.

Student Plans of Care

The care plans that students are required to develop are often more detailed than those found in practice settings. The aim

---

Box 14-7 **SAMPLE STUDENT PLAN OF CARE**

Assessment/Diagnosis	Goal/Outcome	Nursing Orders

Subjective data: "Will I get a stroke now? I don't think I could handle that." "How can I help myself prevent it?"
Objective data: Admitting diagnosis: TIA
BP: 184/120
Strengths: Past pattern of adhering to prescribed health behaviors.
Nursing diagnosis: Ineffective Health Maintenance Response to TIA and Stroke Prevention related to knowledge deficit
	Before discharge, the patient will:
	• Describe the terms *TIA* and *stroke*, identifying the underlying disease process, causes, symptoms, and treatment
	
	After discussion with the physician and nurse, the patient will:
	• Correctly describe the treatment plan:
	  • Medications (drugs, intended effect, dose, time, route)
	  • Dietary modifications
	  • Exercise prescription
	  • Signs and symptoms to report
	• Follow-up appointment date
		Assess what the patient knows about TIA and stroke (correct any misinformation). Assess learning needs, readiness to learn, and factors that will influence learning.
		Plan teaching and learning sessions to involve family members designated by patient.
		Include in the teaching plan a description of TIA and stroke and the underlying disease process, causes, symptoms, and treatment plan.
		After the treatment plan has been developed, make sure the patient and family can restate it (teaching) and value the prescribed lifestyle modification (counseling).

Subjective data: Husband died 8 months ago; moved in with daughter 6 months ago after selling family home Daughter reports mother had been a very independent, strong woman in the past—seemed to "crumple" after husband's death. History of headaches *Objective data:* Clutches daughter's hand *Strengths:* History of handling life stressors well *Limitations:* In the past, her husband was her primary support *Nursing diagnosis:* Ineffective Coping related to illness, recent death of husband, and relocation with daughter	Beginning 9/7/12, the patient will: • Verbalize her feelings related to the loss of her husband, loss of family home, loss of health • Identify coping patterns that have helped her in the past • Identify three personal strengths and three outside supports that will help her now Before discharge, the patient will: • Verbalize that she feels "okay" (sufficiently in charge of her life) about returning home	Once during each shift, primary nurse should sit at patient's bedside for at least several minutes to communicate caring and to explore with the patient her current stressors and the adequacy of her coping response. • Assess factors compounding her losses. • Reinforce her personal strengths and support systems; counsel her to tap into these now. • Suggest local support groups, if indicated. Primary nurse to explore with daughter, Lisa, how her mother's moving in with her has affected the family. Recommend support systems.

Subjective data: "I move my bowels every 2 or 3 days; get constipated at least once a week. Often Metamucil helps."
"I drink plenty of fluids and eat fruits and vegetables."
History of hemorrhoids secondary to straining
Objective data: No bowel movement in past 4 days
On bed rest since hospitalized
Nursing diagnosis: Constipation related to decreased physical activity and long-term laxative use (Metamucil)
	Beginning 9/7/12, the patient will:
	• Pass soft, formed stool every 1 to 3 days without use of laxatives
	By 9/10/12, the patient will:
	• Verbalize the importance of the following natural aids to bowel elimination:
	  • Daily intake of foods high in bulk
	  • Daily fluid intake of 8 to 10 glasses
	  • Regular time for elimination
	  • Daily physical exercise: walking
		Monitor bowel elimination patterns; identify causative factors of constipation and successful corrective measures.
		Explain the importance of adhering to a regular time for defecation (patient suggests after breakfast)—adhere to this in the hospital.
		When given medical clearance, assist patient with progressive ambulation.
		Recommend that she include brisk walking into daily health habits (build strength to 20- to 30-minute brisk walk daily).
		Explain the long-term effects of laxative abuse on the bowel, and discourage use of laxatives.
		Reinforce the patient's fluid intake and ingestion of high-bulk foods, such as fresh fruits and salad.

is to assist students to assimilate each of the five steps of the nursing process. Although care plan formats vary among different nursing programs, most are designed so that the student systematically proceeds through the interrelated steps of the nursing process, and many use a five-column format.

The sample student plan of care shown in Box 14-7 demonstrates a plan developed for a 72-year-old woman who was admitted to the hospital after experiencing a mini-stroke/brain attack (transient ischemic attack) at home. Her condition is stable, and the three prioritized diagnoses written in the plan address her inability to deal with this new medical diagnosis and to prevent a major stroke (high priority), ineffective coping (medium priority), and constipation (low priority).

Scientific Rationale	Evaluation
Each person's learning needs are different; each person learns in own unique way; learning is dependent on readiness.	9/10/12—Outcome not met. Patient says her head is "too old" to learn all this stuff. Equates stroke with death. *Revision:* Reteach content in simpler terms. Reassess learning readiness. —*M. Foley, SN*
The more support people knowledgeably committed to the plan of care, the greater the probability the patient will achieve goals. New self-care behaviors are dependent on knowledge.	
New self-care behaviors are dependent on motivation. Unless the patient is committed to stroke prevention and values this outcome, she will not follow the treatment plan.	9/10/12 Too early to evaluate. —*M. Foley, SN*
The nurse's unhurried, attentive, and caring presence communicates to the patient that she is important to the nurse and that the nurse values her well-being. It is an invitation to the patient to become actively involved in recovery. Also, it is logical to explore adequacy of past and current coping mechanisms before suggesting new approaches.	9/10/12 Outcome partially met. Patient speaks freely about how much she misses her husband and how fearful this hospitalization makes her. When asked about living with her daughter, she becomes uncharacteristically quiet. —*M. Foley, SN* 9/10/12 Outcome met. Patient talks about how everything seemed better in the past after she talked it over with her husband and God. —*M. Foley, SN* 9/10/12 Outcome not met. Patient couldn't think of anything about herself that is healthy or strong. Says "maybe" her family can help her now.
Adult children of aging parents frequently experience overwhelming stress as they try to deal with their own and their parents' problems. Supporting this family is supporting the patient indirectly.	*Revision:* Counsel regarding personal strengths. Help her to experience them. —*M. Foley, SN* 9/11/12 Too early to evaluate. —*M. Foley, SN*
This patient's elimination problems will not be resolved until all the specific causes of her constipation and successful corrective measures are identified. Needs to be an ongoing assessment priority.	9/10/12 Outcome partially met. Soft, formed stool passed every 2 to 3 days with aid of Colace. —*M. Foley, SN*
This encourages positive use of circadian rhythms.	9/10/12 Outcome met. Patient correctly related value of four natural aids to elimination. Questions whether she will be strong enough to walk. *Revision:* Encourage assisted ambulation. —*M. Foley, SN*
Peristalsis is stimulated by physical exercise.	
Laxative abuse leads to decreased peristaltic response to food and loss of intestinal tone. Commenting on these positive self-care behaviors reinforces them.	

Assessing

The student records the assessment data that led to the determination of each diagnosis in the assessment/diagnosis column. Recording these data helps to link specific defining characteristics with diagnostic problem statements.

Diagnosing

Nursing diagnoses are recorded in the assessment/diagnosis column in a prioritized list beginning with the top-priority diagnosis. For each diagnosis, a clear and concise problem statement is followed by an etiology statement that identifies specific contributing factors.

Outcome Identification and Planning

The outcome identification and planning column contains the expected changes in patient health status or in patient behaviors (i.e., patient outcomes). If achieved, these resolve the problem statement in the nursing diagnosis.

Implementing

Sets of nursing orders that describe specific nursing interventions are written for each patient outcome. These specify what nursing interventions are to be performed, how they are to be performed, when they are to be performed, and who is to perform them. In many nursing programs, students are asked to document the source of the nursing interventions they propose. Although students might be able to "pull from their head" some nursing strategies, developing the practice of consulting the nursing literature is a sure means to increase nursing knowledge. Some programs also require students to provide a scientific rationale for the interventions they propose. A succinct rationale statement demonstrates that the student is deliberately choosing the nursing intervention because of its high probability to effect the desired change.

Evaluating

Incorporating evaluative statements in the plan of care clearly communicates the message that nursing care is never complete until achievement of patient outcomes is evaluated. Just as some say that teaching does not occur if learning does not take place, so nursing care is incomplete if the desired patient goals are not achieved.

PROBLEMS RELATED TO OUTCOME IDENTIFICATION AND PLANNING

Problems commonly encountered while developing plans of nursing care include failure to involve the patient in the planning process, insufficient data collection, use of inaccurate or insufficient data to develop nursing diagnoses, outcomes that are stated too broadly, outcomes that are derived from poorly developed nursing diagnoses, failure to write nursing orders clearly, written nursing orders that

do not resolve the problem, and failure to update the plan of care.

> ▶ *Recall Elijah Wolinski, the frail, elderly man with a pressure ulcer. Since the nurse is providing care in the patient's home, a written plan of care is extremely important because more than one caregiver may be involved in the patient's care. In addition, the nurse must update the plan regularly to ensure that regardless of who is providing the care, the correct care is given consistently.* ■

A FINAL WORD ABOUT NIC/NOC AND STANDARDIZED LANGUAGES

Moorhead, Johnson, Maas, and Swanson (2008) lament that while nurses' clinical-reasoning and decision-making skills are integral to quality healthcare and account for much of the healthcare system "safety net," little attention has been focused on the outcomes of nursing interventions. They write that, as part of improving healthcare quality and safety, "it is imperative that nursing define its interventions and outcomes and that these standardized nomenclatures be included in clinical nursing information systems and in large data sets used for systematic analysis" (p. 3).

The use of Nursing Interventions Classification (NIC)

- Helps demonstrate the impact that nurses have on the system of healthcare delivery
- Standardizes and defines the knowledge base for nursing curricula and practice
- Facilitates the selection of appropriate nursing intervention
- Enables researchers to examine the effectiveness and cost of nursing care
- Assists educators to develop curricula that better articulate with clinical practice
- Facilitates the teaching of clinical decision making to novice nurses
- Assists administrators in planning more effectively for staff and equipment needs
- Promotes the development and use of nursing information systems
- Communicates the nature of nursing to the public (Bulechek, Butcher, & Dochterman, 2008, p. vi).

● Developing Critical Thinking Skills

1. Write nursing diagnoses for three obese patients, and make sure that the etiologies for the problem statement (Imbalanced Nutrition: More Than Body Requirements) differ. Describe how these different etiologies result in different plans of care.

2. Use one of the nursing diagnoses from Exercise 1 and write related cognitive, psychomotor, and affective

goals. Explain the different purposes of each type of goal and why it may be necessary to include all three to resolve a patient problem successfully.

3. An alert 82-year-old widow, who has a history of unsafe behaviors, has recently been discharged from the hospital to her home. Caregivers attempted to secure her consent to be transferred to a nursing home, but she flatly refused. Responsible for her home care, you list Risk for Injury as a priority nursing diagnosis. Join several students and independently list the nursing measures that are most likely to achieve the outcome of preventing injury. Compare your lists of interventions and discuss how practicing nurses can be sure they select the best nursing interventions for each expected patient outcome.

● Practicing for NCLEX

1. During the outcome identification and planning step of the nursing process, the nurse works in partnership with the patient and family to do which of the following? *Select all that apply.*
   a. Formulate and validate prioritized nursing diagnoses
   b. Identify expected patient outcomes
   c. Select evidence-based nursing interventions
   d. Communicate the plan of nursing care

2. Mr. Price tells the nurse he fears becoming "hooked on drugs" and consequently waits until his pain becomes unbearable before requesting his PRN analgesic. The nurse plans to be more attentive to Mr. Price and to assess his needs for pain management more closely. Which of the following consequences of informal planning ought to be the major concern for this nurse?
   a. The lack of a coordinated plan known by everyone will result in uneven pain management.
   b. Faulty prioritization of patient needs
   c. Inability to evaluate the patient's responses to nursing care
   d. Lack of a record for reimbursement purposes

3. When helping Mr. Price turn in bed, the nurse notices that his heels are reddened and plans to place him on precautions for skin breakdown. This is an example of what type of planning?
   a. Initial planning
   b. Standardized planning
   c. Ongoing planning
   d. Discharge planning

4. For the following patient problems:
   (1) Disturbed Body Image
   (2) Ineffective Airway Clearance
   (3) Spiritual Distress
   (4) Impaired Social Interaction

Which answer choice below lists the problems in order of highest priority to lowest priority based on Maslow's hierarchy of human needs?
   a. 2, 4, 1, 3
   b. 3, 1, 4, 2
   c. 1, 4, 3, 2
   d. 3, 2, 4, 1

5. From which of the following are nursing outcomes derived?
   a. The problem statement of the nursing diagnosis
   b. The etiology of the problem of the nursing diagnosis
   c. The defining characteristics of the problem
   d. The evaluative statement

6. Which of the following is an example of an affective outcome?
   a. Within 1 day after teaching, the patient will list three benefits of continuing to apply moist compresses to leg ulcer after discharge.
   b. By 6/12/12, the patient will correctly demonstrate application of wet-to-dry dressing on leg ulcer.
   c. By 6/19/12, the patient's ulcer will begin to show signs of healing (e.g., size shrinks from 3″ to 2.5″).
   d. By 6/12/12, the patient will verbalize valuing health sufficiently to practice new health behaviors to prevent recurrence of leg ulcer.

7. Which of the following is an optional element in a measurable outcome?
   a. Subject
   b. Verb
   c. Performance criteria
   d. Conditions
   e. Target time

8. Which of the following outcomes are correctly written? *Select all that apply.*
   a. Offer Mr. Myer 60 mL fluid every 2 hours while awake.
   b. During the next 24-hour period, the patient's fluid intake will total at least 2,000 mL.
   c. Teach Mrs. Gaston proper newborn care by 1/15/11.
   d. By discharge, Mrs. Gaston will know how to bathe her newborn.
   e. At the next visit, 12/23/11, the patient will correctly demonstrate relaxation exercises.

9. Which of the following guidelines for outcome writing are correct? *Select all that apply.*
   a. At least one of the outcomes shows a direct resolution of the problem statement in the nursing diagnosis.
   b. The patient (and family) values the outcomes.
   c. The outcomes are supportive of the total treatment plan.
   d. Each outcome is brief and specific (clearly describes one observable, measurable patient behavior/manifestation), is phrased positively, and specifies a time line.

10. Which of the following are examples of well-stated nursing interventions? *Select all that apply.*
    a. Offer patient 60 mL water or juice (prefers orange or cranberry juice) every 2 hours while awake for a total minimum PO intake of 500 mL.
    b. Teach patient the necessity of carefully monitoring fluid intake and output; remind patient each shift to mark off fluid intake on record at bedside.
    c. Walk with patient to bathroom for toileting every 2 hours (on even hours) while patient is awake.
    d. Manage patient's pain.

● Answers with Rationale

1. *b, c,* and *d.* Formulating and validating nursing diagnoses (*a*) occur during the diagnosing step of the nursing process.

2. *a.* If this nurse fails to incorporate this learning into the formal plan of care, other professional caregivers will not be aware of the need to monitor the patient's pain needs more closely. *b, c,* and *d* may all be correct responses, but they should not be the major concern of the nurse.

3. *c.* Ongoing planning is problem oriented and has as its purpose keeping the plan up to date as new actual or potential problems are identified.

4. *a.* Maslow's hierarchy is (1) physiologic needs, (2) safety needs, (3) love and belonging needs, (4) self-esteem needs, and (5) self-actualization needs. (2) is an example of a physiologic need, (4) is an example of a love and belonging need, (1) is an example of a self-esteem need, and (3) is an example of a self-actualization need.

5. *a.* Outcomes are derived from the problem statement of the nursing diagnosis. For each nursing diagnosis in the plan of care, at least one outcome should be written that, if achieved, demonstrates a direct resolution of the problem statement.

6. *d.* Affective outcomes describe changes in patient values, beliefs, and attitudes. Cognitive outcomes (*a*) describe increases in patient knowledge or intellectual behaviors; psychomotor outcomes (*b*) describe the patient's achievement of new skills. *c* is an outcome describing a physical change in the patient.

7. *d.* Conditions specify the particular circumstances in or by which the outcome is to be achieved. Not every outcome specifies conditions.

8. *b* and *e.* The outcomes in *a* and *c* make the error of expressing the patient goal as a nursing intervention. Incorrect: "Offer Mr. Myer 60 mL fluid every 2 hours while awake." Correct: "Mr. Myer will drink 60 mL fluid every 2 hours while awake, beginning 1/3/11." The outcome in *d* makes the error of using verbs that are not observable and measurable. Incorrect: "Mrs. Gaston will know how to bathe her newborn." Correct: "After attending the infant care class, Mrs. Gaston will correctly demonstrate the procedure for bathing her newborn." Verbs to be avoided when writing goals include "know," "understand," "learn," and "become aware."

9. *a, b, c,* and *d.*

10. *a, b,* and *c.* The last item, *d*, lacks sufficient detail to effectively guide nursing intervention. The set of nursing interventions written to assist a patient to meet an outcome must be comprehensive. Comprehensive nursing interventions specify what observations (assessments) need to be made and how often, what nursing interventions need to be done and when they must be done, and what teaching, counseling, and advocacy needs patients and families have.

Taylor Suite Resources

The Taylor Suite offers these additional resources to enhance learning and facilitate understanding of this chapter:

- thePoint online resource, http://thepoint.lww.com/Taylor7E
- Student DVD included with the book
- Study Guide for Taylor's Fundamentals of Nursing

BIBLIOGRAPHY

Alfaro-LeFevre, R. (2009). *Critical thinking and clinical judgment: A practical approach to outcome-focused thinking* (4th ed.). St. Louis: Saunders Elsevier.

Alfaro-LeFevre, R. (2010). *Applying nursing process: A tool for critical thinking* (7th ed.). Philadelphia: Lippincott Williams & Wilkins.

American Nurses Association (ANA). (2004). *Scope and standards of practice*. Washington, DC: Author.

Bulechek, G. M., Butcher, H. K., & Dochterman, J. (Eds.). (2008). *Nursing interventions classification (NIC)* (5th ed.). St. Louis: Mosby.

Carpenito-Moyet, L. J. (2009). *Nursing care plans and documentation: Nursing diagnoses and collaborative problems* (5th ed.). Philadelphia: Lippincott Williams & Wilkins.

Carpenito-Moyet, L. J. (2010). *Nursing diagnosis: Application to clinical practice* (13th ed.). Philadelphia: Lippincott Williams & Wilkins.

Committee on Quality Health Care in America, Institute of Medicine. (2001). *Crossing the quality chasm: A new health system for the 21st century*. Washington, DC: National Academy Press.

Daley, B. J. (1999). Concept maps: A strategy to teach and evaluate critical thinking. *Journal of Nursing Education, 38*(1), 42.

Ferrario, C. G. (2003). Experienced and less-experienced nurses' diagnostic reasoning: Implications for fostering students' critical thinking. *International Journal of Nursing Terminologies and Classifications, 14*(2), 41–52.

Ferrario, C. G. (2004). Developing nurses' critical thinking skills with concept mapping. *Journal for Nurses in Staff Development, 20*(6), 261–267.

Glaze, J. E. (2002). Stages in coming to terms with reflection: Student advanced nurse practitioners' perceptions of their reflective journeys. *Journal of Advanced Nursing, 37*(3), 265–272.

Harris, B. L. (1990). Becoming deprofessionalized: One aspect of the staff nurse's perspective on computer-mediated nursing care plans. *Advances in Nursing Science, 13*(2), 63–74.

Hendry, C., & Walker, A. (2004). Priority setting in clinical nursing practice: Literature review. *Journal of Advanced Nursing, 47*(4), 427.

Iowa Intervention Project. (1997). Nursing interventions classification (NIC): An overview. In M. J. Rantz & P. LeMone (Eds.), *Classification of Nursing Diagnoses: Proceedings of the Twelfth Conference, North American Nursing Diagnosis* (pp. 32–39). Glendale, CA: CINAHL Information Systems.

Johnson, M., Bulechek, G., McCloskey Dochterman, J., Maas, M., & Moorhead, S. (Eds.). (2001). *Nursing diagnoses, outcomes and interventions: NANDA, NIC, NOC, linkages.* St. Louis: Mosby.

Joint Commission. (2009). Comprehensive accreditation manual for hospitals. Available at http://www.jointcommission.org/Standards/Manuals/

King, M., & Shell, R. (2002). Teaching and evaluating critical thinking with concept maps. *Nurse Educator, 27*(5), 214.

LaDuke, S. (2008). Viewpoint: Death to nursing care plans! *American Journal of Nursing, 108*(6), 13.

Lunney, M. (2006). Helping nurses use NANDA, NOC and MC: Novice to expert. *Nurse Educator, 31*(1), 40–46.

Moody, L. E., Slocumb, E., Berg, B., & Jackson, D. (2004). Electronic health records documentation in nursing: Nurses' perception, attitudes, and preferences. *Computers, Informatics, Nursing, 22*(6), 337.

Moorhead, S., Johnson, M., Maas, M. L., & Swanson, E. (Eds). (2008). *Nursing outcomes classification (NOC)* (4th ed.). St. Louis, MO: Mosby Elsevier.

Mueller, A., Johnston, M., & Bigh, D. (2002). Joining mind mapping and care mapping to enhance student critical thinking and achieve holistic nursing care. *Nursing Diagnosis, 13*(1), 24–27.

Schuster, D. M. (2002). Concept mapping: A critical thinking approach to care planning. Philadelphia: F. A. Davis.

Swanson, E. (2008). *Nursing Outcomes Classification (NOC)* (4th ed.). St Louis: Mosby Elsevier.

15 Implementing

ANTOINETTE BROWNE

Antoinette, a toddler, is brought to the well-child community clinic by her grandmother. The health history reveals recurrent nausea, vomiting, and diarrhea. Her physical examination reveals a negligible gain in height and weight, lethargy, and a delay in achieving developmental milestones.

ESTELLE MORRISSEY

Estelle is an 86-year-old woman who is in a nursing home because of multiple chronic health problems. She is alert and oriented to person, place, and time. She states, "I'm all alone. There's no one left and I want to die. Can you help me?"

JAMES McMAHON

James, a 62-year-old man, is admitted to the intensive care unit in hepatic failure. He is critically ill, being monitored continuously, and is receiving intravenous fluids and medications via central and peripheral IV catheters.

After completing this chapter, you will be able to accomplish the following:

1. List advantages of having a standard classification of nursing interventions and outcomes.

2. Distinguish nurse-initiated, physician-initiated, and collaborative nursing interventions.

3. Use cognitive, interpersonal, technical, and ethical/legal skills to implement a plan of nursing care.

4. Use eight guidelines for implementation.

5. Describe six variables that influence the way a plan of care is implemented.

6. Use ongoing data collection to determine how to safely and effectively implement a plan of care.

7. Explain why reassessment after nursing intervention is important.

8. Describe the risks and responsibilities of delegating nursing interventions.

KEY TERMS

collaborative
  interventions

delegation

evidence-based practice

implementing

nurse-initiated
  intervention

nursing interventions

physician-initiated
  intervention

protocols

standing orders

unlicensed assistive
  personnel (UAP)

During the **implementing** step of the nursing process, nursing actions planned in the previous step are carried out. The purpose of implementation is to assist the patient in achieving valued health outcomes: promote health, prevent disease and illness, restore health, and facilitate coping with altered functioning. For an example, see the accompanying Reflective Practice box. The plan of care is best implemented when patients who are able and willing to participate have maximum opportunities to provide self-care. Family members and other support people, as well as other healthcare professionals, may also be involved in successfully implementing the plan of care (Table 15-1). During the implementation step, the nurse continues to collect data and to modify the plan of care as needed (Fig. 15-1). All activities are documented in the format used by the nurse's institution or agency.

UNIQUE FOCUS OF NURSING IMPLEMENTATION

In all nurse–patient interactions, the nurse is concerned with the patient's response to health and illness and the nurse's ability to meet basic human needs. Whereas other healthcare professionals focus on selected aspects of the patient's treatment regimen, nurses are concerned with how the patient is responding to the plan of care in general. Standards of practice for implementation are described in Box 15-1.

The Nursing Interventions Taxonomy Structure

In 1992, McCloskey Dochterman and Bulechek published *Nursing Interventions Classification* (NIC), a report of research to construct a taxonomy of nursing interventions. New editions appeared in 1996, 2000, 2004, and 2008. Each of the interventions listed has a label, a definition, a set of activities that a nurse performs to carry out the intervention, and a short list of background readings. Advantages of having

---

Box 15-1 ANA STANDARDS OF PRACTICE: STANDARD 5, IMPLEMENTATION

The registered nurse implements the identified plan.
Measurement Criteria
The registered nurse:

Implements the plan in a safe and timely manner.

Documents implementation and any modifications, including changes or omissions of the identified plan.

Utilizes evidence-based interventions and treatments specific to the diagnosis or problem.

Utilizes community resources and systems to implement the plan.

Collaborates with nursing colleagues and others to implement the plan.

The registered nurse coordinates care delivery.
Measurement Criteria
The registered nurse:

Coordinates implementation of care.

Documents the coordination of care.

The registered nurse employs strategies to promote health and a safe environment.
Measurement Criteria
The registered nurse:

Provides health teaching that addresses such topics as healthy lifestyles, risk-reducing behaviors, developmental needs, activities of daily living, and preventative care.

Uses health promotion and health teaching methods appropriate to the situation and the patient's developmental level, learning needs, readiness, ability to learn, language preference, and culture.

Seeks opportunities for feedback and evaluation of the effectiveness of strategies used.

Used with permission. American Nurses Association. (2004). *Scope and standards of practice.* Washington DC: Author.

REFLECTIVE PRACTICE

Challenge to Technical Skills

James McMahon, a 62-year-old man, is admitted to the intensive care unit (ICU) in hepatic failure. He is critically ill, being monitored continuously, and receiving intravenous (IV) fluids and medications via central and peripheral IV catheters. During a recent clinical rotation in an ICU, I followed an extremely busy nurse who was caring for Mr. McMahon. He had several IV infusion lines and required numerous technologic devices for monitoring and care. The nurse asked me to hang a new bag of IV medication. I found myself completely overwhelmed and confused by the myriad tangle of IV lines and knew that I wouldn't be able to determine how to run the medication without the guidance of the nurse. I became frustrated because I should have been able to perform this task quickly and correctly if I had been working independently. I didn't want to risk hanging the IV medication and infusing it into a line with another fluid that was possibly incompatible. Nor did I want to risk running the medication through the incorrect port. The nurse was extremely busy, and I felt pressured to perform this task immediately.

Thinking Outside the Box: Possible Courses of Action

- Request that the nurse hang the medication once she was through with her other tasks.
- Hang the medication, hoping that it was compatible with the other fluids that were already infusing.
- Ask another nurse on the unit to hang the medication.

- Wait until the nurse was through with what she had to do, admit to her that I felt uncomfortable hanging the medication on my own, and then ask that she walk me through the process.

Evaluating a Successful Outcome: How Do I Define Success?

- The patient remains free from harm while receiving the necessary medication.
- The nurse recognizes the need to provide me with more guidance.

- I feel comfortable and competent in my skills.
- The patient receives efficient, safe care.

Personal Learning: Here's to the Future!

Luckily, there was a positive ending to this situation. I explained to the nurse that I was confused by the maze of IV lines and that I was uncomfortable administering the IV medication on my own. The nurse immediately recognized that the patient's lines were tangled and disorganized and some were unlabeled. With me at her side, she took the time to reorganize and label all of the lines, making it easier to visualize all of the medications and fluids the patient was receiving. We referenced a drug book to ensure that the medication was compatible with the other fluids that were running. She also walked me through the process of hanging the medication and connecting it to the appropriate port. The nurse appreciated the fact that I waited to ask her for help. As a result, the patient remained safe from injury. In addition, she realized that she shouldn't have asked me to perform this task independently. I benefited from the experience because I became more familiar with this particular skill. As of now, I still find myself feeling somewhat anxious and uncomfortable with certain technical skills. However, I am finding that with each new clinical experience, I become more comfortable and more independent in my practice.

Colleen Kilcullen, Georgetown University

Reflection

How do you think you would respond in a similar situation? Why? What does this tell you about yourself and about the adequacy of your skills for professional practice? Can you think of other ways to respond? What other skills (cognitive, interpersonal, technical, ethical/legal) would you need to respond well in this situation? What factors might have influenced the nurse in assigning this task to the student? Did the nurse effectively delegate this intervention? Why or why not? Did the student adhere to ethical and legal guidelines with the response? If so, please explain how. If not, what issues were present? Do you agree with the criteria to evaluate a successful outcome? Were the criteria appropriate for the situation and skill?

a standard classification of nursing interventions include the following:

- Helps demonstrate the impact that nurses have on the system of healthcare delivery
- Standardizes and defines the knowledge base for nursing curricula and practice
- Facilitates the appropriate selection of a nursing intervention
- Facilitates communication of nursing treatments to other nurses and other providers

- Enables researchers to examine the effectiveness and cost of nursing care
- Assists educators to develop curricula that better articulate with clinical practice
- Facilitates the teaching of clinical decision making to novice nurses
- Assists administrators in planning more effectively for staff and equipment needs
- Promotes the development of a reimbursement system for nursing services

| | TABLE • 15-1 | PROFESSIONAL NURSING RELATIONSHIPS: ROLE RESPONSIBILITIES AND RELATED COMPETENCIES | |

Relationship	Role Responsibilities	Related Competencies
Nurse–patient	• Communicate to the patient that someone is concerned about him or her (as well as the disease) and is interested in how this change in health state will affect his or her overall well-being. • Create an environment in which the patient can commit his or her energies to health promotion or restoration or peaceful dying, confident that basic human needs are being addressed. • Challenge the patient to develop self-care abilities that promote holistic health.	• Repertoire of therapeutic interpersonal behaviors—attending, listening, interviewing, nonverbal communication, touching, facilitating, coaching • Ability to establish trusting nurse–patient–family relationships • Demonstrated competence in the nursing roles of caregiver, teacher, counselor, advocate
Nurse–patient–family	• Develop in the patient and family the knowledge, attitude, and skills that will enable them to respond to the self-care challenge of their health or illness state. • Intervene as appropriate to promote healthy family functioning. • Educate the family to be wise and assertive healthcare consumers.	
Nurse–nurse	• Support one another's efforts to deliver quality nursing care; work collaboratively with nursing administration to improve quality care. • Provide creative leadership—formally or informally—to make the nursing unit a satisfying and challenging place to work. • Supervise the nursing care given by other nursing personnel; affirm the nursing strengths of others, and constructively address the nursing deficiencies encountered. • Enhance the professional development of self and other nurses through active participation in professional organizations.	Communication Teaching/counseling/advocacy Assertiveness Collaboration Coordination Group process Organization Leadership Delegation Change strategies Problem solving Decision making Conflict resolution
Nurse–healthcare team	• Communicate clearly nursing's perspective regarding the patient and family to the healthcare team. • Coordinate the inputs of the multidisciplinary team into a comprehensive plan of care. • Serve as a liaison between the patient and family and the healthcare team, as necessary.	

• Facilitates the development and use of nursing information systems
• Communicates the nature of nursing to the public (Bulechek, Butcher, & Dochterman, 2008, p. vi)

Table 15-2 illustrates the NIC taxonomy structure designed to help clinicians locate and select interventions most helpful for patients.

The researchers involved in the development of NICs are also committed to developing a classification of patient outcomes for nursing interventions, called Nursing Outcomes Classifications (NOCs). This research aims to:

1. Identify, label, validate, and classify nursing-sensitive patient outcomes and indicators
2. Evaluate the validity and usefulness of the classification in clinical field-testing
3. Define and test measurement procedures for the outcomes and indicators

This research continues in an effort to develop a common nursing language to optimize the design and delivery of safe, high-quality, and cost-effective care.

For examples of how NIC and NOC can be used to plan and implement care, see the box "Examples of Nursing Interventions and Nursing Outcomes Classifications (NIC/NOC)" in this chapter and in each clinical chapter. The examples in this chapter illustrate how NIC and NOC can be used to implement care for a patient and family who require assistance to maintain the home as a clean, safe, and pleasant place. The box lists representative nursing activities for the intervention Home Maintenance Assistance and suggested outcomes for Impaired Home Maintenance.

The Nurse as Coordinator

One of nursing's major contributions to the healthcare team is the role of coordinator. Care can easily become fragmented

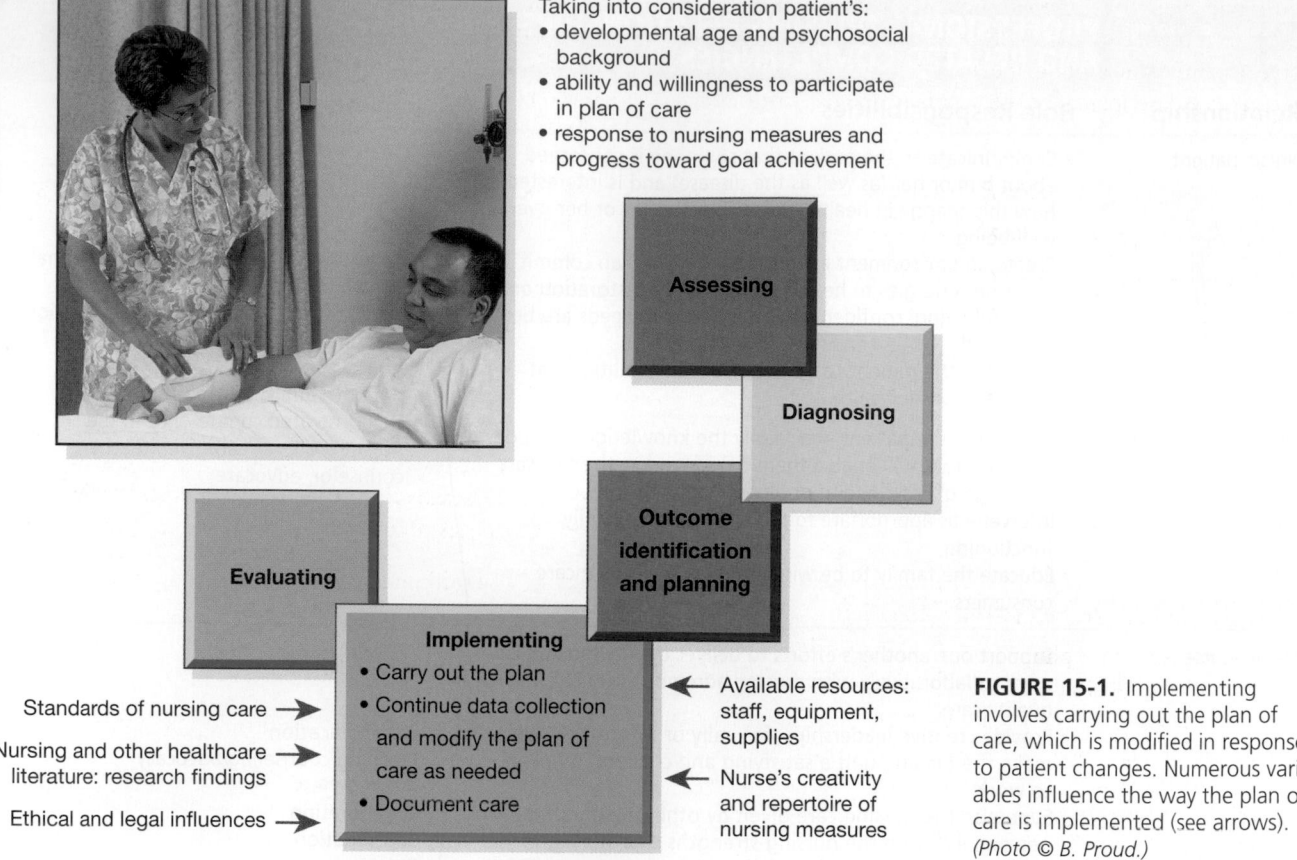

Taking into consideration patient's:
- developmental age and psychosocial background
- ability and willingness to participate in plan of care
- response to nursing measures and progress toward goal achievement

Assessing

Diagnosing

Outcome identification and planning

Evaluating

Implementing
- Carry out the plan
- Continue data collection and modify the plan of care as needed
- Document care

Standards of nursing care →

Nursing and other healthcare literature: research findings →

Ethical and legal influences →

← Available resources: staff, equipment, supplies

← Nurse's creativity and repertoire of nursing measures

FIGURE 15-1. Implementing involves carrying out the plan of care, which is modified in response to patient changes. Numerous variables influence the way the plan of care is implemented (see arrows). *(Photo © B. Proud.)*

when patients are seen by numerous specialists—each interested in a different aspect of the patient. At best, patients complain that no one person really knows them and can talk with them about what is going on and how it all may affect them in the future. At worst, the orders of different specialists may conflict with one another and be counterproductive. Therefore, it is important for you as the nurse to make rounds with other healthcare professionals and to read the results of consultations patients have had with specialists. You can then interpret the specialists' findings for patients

Examples of Nursing Interventions and Nursing Outcomes Classifications (NIC/NOC)

Home Maintenance Assistance

Nursing Interventions	**Nursing Outcomes**
• Determine patient's home maintenance requirements.	• Family Functioning
• Involve patient and family in deciding home maintenance requirements.	• Parenting Performance
• Suggest necessary structural alterations to make the home accessible.	• Parenting: Psychosocial Safety
• Provide information on how to make the home environment safe and clean.	• Role Performance
• Advise for the alleviation of all offensive odors.	• Safe Home Environment
• Suggest services for pest control, as needed.	• Self-Care: Instrumental Activities of Daily Living (IADL)
• Offer solutions to financial difficulties.	
• Order homemaker services, as appropriate.	
• Provide information on respite care, as needed.	

Bulechek, G. M., Butcher, H. K., & Dochterman, J. (Eds.). (2008). *Nursing interventions classification (NIC)* (5th ed.). St. Louis: Mosby, p. 406.
Moorhead, S., Johnson, M., Maas, M. L., & Swanson, E. (Eds.). (2008). *Nursing outcomes classification (NOC)* (4th ed.). St. Louis: Mosby Elsevier, p. 778.
   (A full listing of nursing activities for each nursing intervention and indicators for each nursing outcome can be found in these books.)

and family members, prepare patients to participate maximally in the plan of care before and after discharge, and serve as a liaison among the members of the healthcare team. Nurse case managers are specialists in the role of care coordinator.

> *Think back to Antoinette Browne, the toddler described at the beginning of the chapter. As a result of the child's delays, multiple disciplines would likely be involved in caring for the child. The nurse would play a major role as coordinator for the child's care, ensuring communication among all team members. Additionally, the nurse would act as the liaison between the other members of the team to ensure that the child's grandmother understands the plan of care.* ∎

CRITICAL THINKING AND IMPLEMENTING

As you implement the plan of care, you are constantly thinking critically about what you are doing. Since patient conditions can change dramatically in minutes, you must reassess the patient for changes in status that might dictate a different set of interventions. You also want to be sure that research supports the interventions you have selected and be open to better ways of addressing patient problems and issues. In every clinical setting, we should hear nurses and other members of the team actively questioning whether there are better ways to achieve desired patient outcomes. Finally, you are always monitoring the patient's responses to your interventions so that you can modify the plan of care if needed.

As a student, you will always need to ask if you are competent to implement the plan of care. If you doubt that your cognitive, interpersonal, or technical skills are adequate to successfully implement the plan of care, it is your responsibility to ask for help. Getting help when you need it demonstrates your primary commitment to the patient. Expert nurses understand that learning is a lifelong practice and that we need one another to continue to master clinical skills.

TYPES OF NURSING INTERVENTIONS

The Nursing Interventions Classification (NIC) project defines a **nursing intervention** as "any treatment based upon clinical judgment and knowledge that a nurse performs to enhance patient/client outcomes" (Bulechek, Butcher, & Dochterman, 2008, p. xxi). The NIC project further goes on to describe the types of interventions:

Nursing interventions include both direct and indirect care; those aimed at individuals, families and community; and those for nurse-initiated and other provider-initiated treatments.

A direct care intervention is a treatment performed through interaction with the patient(s). Direct care interventions include both physiological and psychosocial nursing actions and include both the 'laying of hands' actions and those that are more supportive and counseling in nature.

An indirect care intervention is a treatment performed away from the patient but on behalf of a patient or group of patients. Indirect care interventions include nursing actions aimed at management of the patient care environment and interdisciplinary collaboration. These actions support the effectiveness of direct care interventions.

A community (or public health) intervention is targeted to promote and preserve the health of populations. Community interventions emphasize the health promotion, health maintenance, and disease prevention of populations and include strategies to address the social and political climate in which the population resides. (Bulechek, Butcher, & Dochterman, 2008, p. xxi)

Carpenito-Moyet (2010) describes how the major focus of intervention differs according to the type of nursing diagnoses or collaborative problem being addressed. For actual nursing diagnoses, interventions seek to:

- Reduce or eliminate contributing factors of the diagnosis
- Promote higher-level wellness
- Monitor and evaluate status

For risk nursing diagnoses, interventions seek to:

- Reduce or eliminate risk factors
- Prevent the problem
- Monitor and evaluate status

For possible nursing diagnoses, interventions seek to:

- Collect additional data to rule out or confirm the diagnosis

For collaborative problems, interventions seek to:

- Monitor for changes in status
- Manage changes in status with nurse-prescribed and physician-prescribed interventions
- Evaluate response (p. 42)

When you carry out the interventions identified in the plan of care, you are implementing the plan of care. When implementing the plan of care, you function independently and collaboratively. These are the types of nursing interventions described in the preceding chapter.

Independent Nursing Action

Nurse-initiated interventions, or independent nursing actions, involve carrying out nurse-prescribed interventions resulting from their assessment of patient needs written on the nursing plan of care, as well as any other actions that nurses initiate without the direction or supervision of another healthcare professional. Nurses are legally accountable for their assessments and their nursing responses.

Protocols and standing orders expand the scope of nursing practice in certain clearly defined situations. **Protocols** are written plans that detail the nursing activities to be executed in specific situations. Although some protocols specify routine aspects of nursing care (e.g., protocols that describe

TABLE • 15-2 NURSING INTERVENTIONS CLASSIFICATION (NIC) TAXONOMY

	Domain I	Domain II	Domain III
Level 1 Domains	1. **Physiologic: Basic** Care that supports physical functioning	2. **Physiologic: Complex** Care that supports homeostatic regulation	3. **Behavioral** Care that supports psychosocial functioning and facilitates lifestyle changes
Level 2 Classes	A *Activity and Exercise Management:* Interventions to organize or assist with physical activity and energy expenditure B *Elimination Management:* Interventions to establish and maintain regular bowel and urinary elimination patterns and manage complications due to altered patterns C *Immobility Management:* Interventions to manage restricted body movement and the sequelae D *Nutrition Support:* Interventions to modify or maintain nutritional status E *Physical Comfort Promotion:* Interventions to promote comfort using physical techniques F *Self-Care Facilitation:* Interventions to provide or assist with routine activities of daily living	G *Electrolyte and Acid–Base Management:* Interventions to regulate electrolyte/ acid–base balance and prevent complications H *Drug Management:* Interventions to facilitate desired effects of pharmacologic agents I *Neurologic Management:* Interventions to optimize neurologic function J *Perioperative Care:* Interventions to provide care before, during, and immediately after surgery K *Respiratory Management:* Interventions to promote airway patency and gas exchange L *Skin/Wound Management:* Interventions to maintain or restore tissue integrity M *Thermoregulation:* Interventions to maintain body temperature within a normal range N *Tissue Perfusion Management:* Interventions to optimize circulation of blood and fluids to the tissue	O *Behavior Therapy:* Interventions to reinforce or promote desirable behaviors or alter undesirable behaviors P *Cognitive Therapy:* Interventions to reinforce or promote desirable cognitive functioning or alter undesirable cognitive functioning Q *Communication Enhancement:* Interventions to facilitate delivering and receiving verbal or nonverbal messages R *Coping Assistance:* Interventions to assist another to build on own strengths, to adapt to a change in function, or to achieve a higher level of function S *Patient Education:* Interventions to facilitate learning T *Psychological Comfort Promotion:* Interventions to promote comfort using psychological techniques

Used with permission from Bulechek, G. M., Butcher, H. K., & Dochterman, J. (Eds.). (2008). *Nursing interventions classification (NIC)* (5th ed., pp. 74–75). St. Louis: Mosby.

nursing responsibilities when a patient is admitted to or discharged from the institution), other protocols include **standing orders** that empower the nurse to initiate actions that ordinarily require the order or supervision of a physician. Examples include admission protocols for obstetric and gynecology patients, protocols for bowel programs that allow the nurse to select and administer necessary bowel interventions, standard orders for narcotic overdoses that specify the agents the nurse is to administer to reverse respiratory depression in an emergency, and standard orders for pain management that enable the nurse to select the strength of the medication to be given within preset ranges.

Dependent Nursing Action

Physician-initiated interventions, or dependent nursing actions, involve carrying out physician-prescribed orders. State Nurse Practice Acts specify from whom nurses can receive orders. Nurses are still accountable for dependent orders they implement and are thus responsible for the clarification of any questionable order.

> ▶ *Recall James McMahon, the critically ill patient in ICU? The nurse administers IV fluids and medications based on orders written by the physicians.* ∎

Domain IV	Domain V	Domain VI	Domain VII
4. Safety Care that supports protection against harm	**5. Family** Care that supports the family unit	**6. Health System** Care that supports effective use of the healthcare delivery system	**7. Community** Care that supports the health of the community
U *Crisis Management:* Interventions to provide immediate short-term help in both psychological and physiological crises V *Risk Management:* Interventions to initiate risk reduction activities and continue monitoring risk over time	W *Childbearing Care:* Interventions to assist in understanding and coping with the psychological and physiological changes during the childbearing period X *Life Span Care:* Interventions to facilitate family unit functioning and promote the health and welfare of family members throughout the life span	Y *Health System Mediation:* Interventions to facilitate the interface between patient/family and the healthcare system Z *Childrearing Care:* Interventions to assist in raising children a. *Health System Management:* Interventions to provide and enhance support services for the delivery of care b. *Information Management:* Interventions to facilitate communication among healthcare workers	c. *Community Health Promotion:* Interventions that promote the health of the whole community d. *Community Risk Management:* Interventions that assist in detecting or preventing health risks to the whole community

Interdependent Nursing Action

Collaborative interventions, or interdependent nursing actions, are those performed jointly by nurses and other members of the healthcare team. Because nurses are increasingly respected as professional colleagues with unique patient knowledge, they are increasingly involved in collaborative ventures with the healthcare team.

➤ *The three types of nursing actions can be illustrated by the example of Antoinette Browne, the toddler with gastrointestinal symptoms and delays in growth and development. If the physician orders a series of gastrointestinal studies, it is the nurse's responsibility to prepare the patient by executing the physician's order for cleansing the bowel. This nursing action is a physician-initiated intervention. When the nurse senses that the grandmother seems unusually fearful of the outcome of the studies, and explores her fears and then follows up with appropriate teaching and counseling, the nurse is using nurse-initiated interventions. When a multidisciplinary team conference is held to discuss the patient's failure to progress, the nurse works collaboratively with the psychiatrist, gastroenterologist, social worker, and child development specialist to develop a comprehensive plan of care; this involves collaborative nursing interventions.* ■

IMPLEMENTING THE PLAN OF CARE

When carrying out the plan of care, nurses use specialized abilities to (1) determine the patient's new or continuing need for nursing assistance, (2) promote self-care, and (3) assist the patient to achieve valued health outcomes.

Reassessing the Patient and Reviewing the Plan of Care

A patient's condition can change dramatically in a matter of minutes. Therefore, it is critical to assess the patient carefully before initiating any nursing intervention to make sure that the plan of care is still responsive to the patient's needs and prioritized to the most pressing of those needs. It is also important for each nurse implementing the plan:

- To be sure that each nursing intervention is supported by a sound scientific rationale, as demanded by an **evidence-based practice** (see Chapter 5)
- To be sure that each nursing intervention is consistent with professional standards of care and consistent with the protocols, policies, and procedures of the institution or agency
- To be sure that the nursing actions are safe for this particular patient and individualized to his or her preferences
- To clarify any questionable orders

Clarifying Prerequisite Nursing Skills

To implement the plan of nursing care, nurses need blended intellectual, interpersonal, technical, and ethical/legal skills. Each nurse has a unique blend of these skills and can act effectively to the extent that her or his abilities match the patient's need for nursing care.

> ➤ *Remember James McMahon, the critically ill patient in the intensive unit? Although technological skills are key in this area, the nurse also needs to implement care that integrates intellectual, interpersonal, and ethical and legal skills because of the patient's complex needs.* ■

These blended skills are described in Chapter 11. Be sure to notify your nursing instructor or nurse mentor if you believe that you lack any skills needed to safely implement the plan of care.

Organizing Resources

Successful implementation of the plan of care requires a high degree of organization and efficiency in today's hectic healthcare environments.

Patient and Patient Visitors

Make sure the patient is physically and psychologically prepared for what you are going to do. Give nursing interventions the best chance for success by making sure a patient is not in too much pain to cooperate, understands what is being attempted and why he or she should cooperate, and is not distracted (e.g., by wanting to talk with visitors or watch TV). If visitors are in the room, check with the patient to see if she or he wants the visitor(s) to stay during the procedure. If a family caregiver needs to learn new caregiving skills, try to schedule your interventions at a time both appropriate for the patient and convenient for the family caregiver.

Equipment

Anticipate all the equipment you will need to successfully carry out the intervention and arrange it so that it is easily accessible. Be sure to order sufficient supplies at the beginning of the shift for the care you expect to provide, and be thoughtful of the nurse who will follow you by leaving adequate supplies. Follow agency policy when ordering supplies to ensure proper charges. To avoid injury on the job, it is essential to take the time to use proper assistive devices, such as lifts for heavy patients or transfer boards for patients with limited mobility.

Environment

Think through the proper environment for each intervention. Pay special attention to respecting the patient's dignity, privacy, and safety needs. Remember routine measures as simple as closing a door or pulling drapes. These considerations are of special importance when patients or residents share rooms. For example, if an enema is being administered, it can be embarrassing for the patient and unpleasant for the patient's roommate. With some planning, the intervention can be scheduled in a private bathroom or at a time when the roommate is absent.

Personnel

Identify if you are able to carry out the planned intervention independently or if you are likely to need assistance. To avoid injury to both patients and professional caregivers, be sure interventions are attempted by the right person or by a sufficient number of people. Because it is easy to underestimate the strength it takes to lift or support a large patient, it is always safer to err on the side of having too much help rather than not enough. One helpful tip for teams of student nurses is to begin each rotation by asking, "Who thinks they might need help today?" The team can then plan to coordinate care so that help is available when needed.

Anticipating Unexpected Outcomes/Situations

When you learn about new nursing procedures and interventions, you often see a description of possible adverse effects listed. While everyone hopes never to encounter these complications, they do occur with some frequency. The skilled nurse knows what might happen if an intervention "goes wrong" and is prepared to deal with the new challenge. This may be as simple as accurately assessing how much support a patient will need to avoid a fall when ambulating for the first time after surgery, or being prepared to respond to complaints of burning at a new IV site. For further consideration of unexpected outcomes and situations, refer to *Taylor's Clinical Nursing Skills* by Pamela Lynn and *Taylor's Video Guide to Clinical Nursing Skills* by Lippincott Williams & Wilkins.

Promoting Self-Care: Teaching, Counseling, and Advocacy

Although most people can independently meet their basic human needs, illness and the stress of diagnostic and therapeutic measures may interfere with a person's usual practice of self-care. The nurse assesses the patient's abilities to meet his or her human needs independently. Nurses can fail patients by doing too much for them and by encouraging negative, sick-role behaviors, such as inappropriate dependence. Conversely, there is a time and a place for the "tender loving care" that says to a patient "I know you may be able to do this for yourself, but just this once, how about if I do it and we'll talk!" Balancing the need to encourage a patient's best self-care effort with the effort to make each patient feel cared for and loved is an important component of the art of nursing.

> *Recall Estelle Morrissey, the 86-year-old woman living in a nursing home, asking to die. The nurse's ability to apply knowledge of counseling and advocacy would be important in developing a plan of care that addresses the patient's needs.* ■

The plan of nursing care should include specific instructions for any nursing assistance the patient needs to meet basic human needs, including the need for significant nursing encouragement to promote greater independence in functioning. When routines of self-care (or assisted self-care) are included (e.g., colostomy management), instructions should include the time of the procedure, the equipment used, the process, and the level of patient involvement. Continuity of nursing care is essential to the patient's development of a comfortable routine.

If patients and their families want to participate actively in seeking wellness, preventing disease and illness, recovering health, and learning to cope with altered functioning, they need to possess effective self-care behaviors. Nurses sensitive to the importance of patients learning to direct and manage their own care use nurse–patient interactions for both planned and spontaneous teaching, counseling, and advocacy. These nursing roles are described in Chapter 6 and Chapter 22. (See also the accompanying Nursing Advocacy in Action box.) For example, while caring for a child recently diagnosed as having cystic fibrosis, the nurses work continuously with the parents and siblings, helping them to develop the knowledge and skills that will enable them to care for the child after discharge. Referring families such as this to a community support group or other resources further enhances the self-care behaviors being developed. See Through the Eyes of the Family Caregiver for a description of one wife's experiences when her husband was discharged home.

NURSING ADVOCACY IN ACTION

Patient Scenario

The emergency room is very rushed and overcrowded. Mrs. Penuela, who speaks little English, grabs you when you walk into the waiting area and begs someone to look at her husband, who is holding his head and moaning. When you finally get him in the unit to be assessed, he has a blood pressure of 240/150 mm Hg. He speaks a little more English than his wife, but is not fluent. However, you are able to learn that he stopped taking his blood pressure medication because he couldn't afford the prescription. He also lost his job and the family lost their house because of an inability to make mortgage payments. They are now living with her brother. Mr. Penuela is in the emergency room for several hours while intravenous medications are administered. You are shocked to discover that the only discharge orders for Mr. Penuela are a prescription for the same medication he was on previously, which he couldn't afford. His doctor tells you that the ER isn't a charity or social service—"our job is to fix medical problems."

Implications for Nursing Advocacy

How will you respond if you are Mr. Penuela's nurse? Talk with your classmates and experienced nurses about the questions that follow.

- If you elect to advocate for the Penuelas, what practical steps can you take to ensure better health outcomes?
- What is it reasonable to expect of a student nurse, a graduate nurse, and an experienced nurse in this situation?
- What advocacy skills are needed to effectively respond to this challenge?

Assisting Patients to Meet Health Outcomes

In this phase of the implementation process, the nursing team carries out the nursing orders detailed in the nursing plan of care. If the plan of care is well constructed, carrying out its orders is the nurse's most important task and should receive top priority. The nursing actions planned to promote patient goal/outcome achievement and the resolution of health problems should be carefully executed. Implementation guidelines are listed in Box 15-2.

Because understaffing is a problem in many practice settings, nurses must learn to use their time wisely and to maximize each patient encounter. A patient bath can be simply that, or it can be an opportunity to gather additional focused data, to communicate concern for what the patient is experiencing and

Through the Eyes of a Family Caregiver

"The nurses never told me there'd be days like this."

I wasn't prepared for a roller coaster ride when my husband became ill. My husband was admitted to the hospital in an emergency condition, became confused when his electrolytes were off balance, went into cardiac arrest and had CPR, was placed on a ventilator, and was sedated because he was too apprehensive about the ventilator. I had reached the lowest point as I sat by his bedside for days, talking to him and wondering if he heard me.

My spirits soared the day they brought him out of his sleep state and he recognized me and was hungry for real food. The next day when I went to the hospital, I plummeted to the low point again when he was crumpled in bed like a confused rag doll with his hospital gown up to his chest and the sheet to his ankles. I started to cry, and the nurse came and put her arm around me. She said, "Don't think he's taken a turn for the worse. There will be good days and bad days as he recovers." No one had prepared me for that—and her arm around me and her words were so consoling.

When I brought him home after 6 weeks in the hospital, I was not prepared for his anger at being confined to the house (in a heat wave) and not being allowed to drive. His reasoning that he had to get a haircut because he hadn't had one in 2 months made sense to him. My saying that no one would care about the length of his hair did not soothe his anger.

He couldn't accept the fact that he was too weak to go up and down the steps more than once a day, so he insisted on going to the basement. Going down was simple; coming up wasn't. We forgot there was no railing (which he needed to haul himself up) on the last four steps. He solved the problem by sitting on the steps and lifting himself up a step at a time. Then he got to the floor at the top and couldn't stand up. I couldn't lift him. We were stuck. Again, I took a nose dive.

I thought I understood how difficult it would be for him to readjust. I knew he would be depressed and expected him to lean on me. But I was not prepared for his frustration to come out as anger at me. It would have been helpful to have someone prepare me. Or, it would be nice to have a nurse put her arm around me now when my roller coaster plummets.

—Eleanor Faven
Philadelphia, Pennsylvania

offer support, and to teach and counsel as appropriate. How the nurse uses the 30 minutes that he or she is in the patient's room for the bath determines how effective the nurse is in helping the patient to achieve his or her goals/outcomes. See

the accompanying Through the Eyes of a Student display for one student's account of an important bath.

Variables That Influence Outcome Achievement

When working with patients to achieve the outcomes specified in the plan of care, remember that nothing about the plan of care is fixed. Some of the most important variables that influence how the plan of care is implemented follow.

PATIENT VARIABLES

Ideally, the patient is primary in determining how nursing interventions are implemented. Successful nurses modify their nursing actions according to the patient's (1) changing ability and willingness to participate in the plan of care and (2) previous responses to nursing interventions and progress toward goal/outcome achievement. Other important patient variables are developmental stage and psychosocial background.

Developmental Stage

Addressing the developmental needs of a patient involves identifying the patient's developmental stage, as well as the developmental tasks related to this stage and their relationship to nursing care. For example, a nurse may recommend that the parents of a premature infant make a tape of their voices to stimulate their infant in the neonatal intensive care unit. Be careful not to let stereotypes about developmental stages and tasks influence patient care. In nursing homes, for example, the developmental needs of older patients are ignored if a staff member makes humorous comments about "romances" among the residents; embarrasses some residents by calling them cute names or putting big, bright bows in their hair; or demeans some patients by

---

Box 15-2   IMPLEMENTING GUIDELINES

- When implementing nursing care, remember to act in partnership with the patient/family.
- Before implementing any nursing action, reassess the patient to determine whether the action is still needed.
- Approach the patient competently. Know how to perform the nursing action, why the action is being performed, and potential adverse responses. Have all equipment and supplies ready.
- Approach the patient caringly. Explain the nursing action using language the patient understands. Communicate genuine concern for what the patient is experiencing.
- Modify nursing interventions according to the patient's (1) developmental and psychosocial background, (2) ability and willingness to participate in the plan of care, and (3) responses to previous nursing measures and progress toward goal/outcome achievement.
- Check to make sure that the nursing interventions selected are consistent with standards of care and within legal and ethical guides to practice.
- Always question that the nursing intervention selected is the best of all possible alternatives. Consult colleagues and the nursing and related literature to see if other approaches might be more successful. Evaluate the effectiveness of the intervention selected, noting any factors that positively or negatively influenced the outcome.
- Develop a repertoire of skilled nursing interventions. The more options one can choose from, the greater the likelihood of success.

Through the Eyes of a Student

One of my first patients was a woman with a history of Alzheimer's disease. When I was assigned this patient, I knew that I was not going to have a good day. I had been introduced to her the week before, when I had orientation. She was sitting in a geriatric chair in the hallway, where she sang at the top of her lungs and threw tissues on the floor. Occasionally, she would curse at a person passing by.

I took a deep breath and entered her room. At her bedside, I introduced myself. With a few choice words, she told me to get out of her room. I tried to ignore her response and prepared her breakfast tray. She proceeded to throw her scrambled eggs around the room. After I took the tray away from her and finished cleaning up the mess, it was time for preconference. At preconference, my instructor told me that we were going to "tub" my patient. I had visions of a grand fiasco in the tub room, and I dreaded giving her the bath.

My instructor and I took her to the tub room by wheelchair. Once we convinced her to get in the tub, she did nothing but yell that it was cold. We started the water and she yelled even louder. I knew everyone could hear her in the hallway as she cursed and

yelled, but as the bath proceeded, she quieted down and stopped fighting me. We completed the bath and wheeled her back down the hall to her room. I bundled her up in blankets and put her in the gerry chair in the hallway. She was so relaxed from the bath that she let me brush her hair and put it in a ponytail. While I was brushing her hair, she fell asleep. I did my chart until her lunch arrived. When I set her up for her lunch and told her I would be leaving, she thanked me, and it made my day. All the struggling I went through all day with her and she thanked me. When I went home, I felt really good about helping her. During all my worrying about the day being a fiasco and the embarrassment of having a patient yell at me, I had lost sight of the patient herself and what she needed me to do for her. By her thanking me at the end of the day, I realized that when my clinical instructor forced me to do something for my patient that the regular staff of the hospital wouldn't do, I was meeting her basic needs, and my patient recognized that.

—Jeanene C. Smith
Delaware County Community College, Media, Pennsylvania

---

planning childish group activities. Perhaps the worst stereotype is the belief that all older people have to do is wait to die and that there are no developmental challenges for this age group.

> ➤ *Remember Estelle Morrissey, the nursing home resident who wants to die? Knowledge about this stereotype would be important for the nurse when implementing the patient's care.* ∎

To implement a comprehensive and holistic plan of care, nurses must find creative ways to meet developmental needs. This is of greatest importance when patients are separated from their families and home environments for long periods.

> ➤ *Think back to Antoinette Browne, the toddler with physical and developmental delays. The nurse would creatively adapt interventions to meet the needs of this toddler.* ∎

Psychosocial Background

The same is true of the psychosocial needs of patients. When choosing nursing interventions, the nurse should consider and respect the patient's socioeconomic background and culture. Confronted with a malnourished patient on a limited income who rents a single room in a boarding home, a nurse cannot simply teach the importance of including more protein in the diet. To be effective, the nurse must explore the realistic issue of whether the patient can afford and obtain foods rich in protein. Moreover, the nurse needs

to assess whether the patient values this intervention and is willing to make the necessary changes.

NURSE VARIABLES

Nurse variables that influence the implementation of the plan of care include levels of expertise, creativity (ability to match patient needs with specific nursing strategies), willingness to provide care, and available time. Focused Critical Thinking Guide 15-1 illustrates the importance of a nurse's ability to think critically about intervention strategies.

RESOURCES

The most elaborately designed plan of care cannot be fully effective without adequate staff, equipment, and supplies. These resources are all important determinants of patient care. The financial resources of the patient and adequacy of community-based resources also influence the plan of care.

CURRENT STANDARDS OF CARE

All nursing actions for implementing the plan of care must be consistent with standards of practice. See Chapter 16 for a discussion of these standards. All nurses are responsible for learning the standards that dictate practice in their specialty. Failure to practice according to these standards may result in a charge of negligence.

RESEARCH FINDINGS

Nurses concerned about improving the quality of nursing care use research findings to enhance their nursing practice. Reading professional nursing journals and attending continuing education workshops and conferences are

FOCUSED CRITICAL THINKING GUIDE • 15-1

Intervention Strategies

One of the nurses on the oncology unit where you have been working for 6 months since graduation wants to develop a "humor room" where patients, their families, and staff can "take a break" from the serious business of illness. Designed to lift the spirits, amuse, distract, and thus speed the healing process, humor rooms are gaining popularity as new therapeutic tools. Funny books, comic movies on a large-screen TV, games and puzzles—and ideally, even clowns, magicians, musicians, and stand-up comedians—are being envisaged. Several nurses have vocally expressed their lack of support for the project and think the idea is "stupid" at best, and potentially a great waste of money, time, and energy that could be devoted to "tried and true" methods of healing. You have been asked to support the project and must decide how to respond.

1. Identify Goal of Thinking

Clarify your thinking about humor as a therapeutic measure so that you can decide whether to support this project.

2. Assess Adequacy of Knowledge

Pertinent circumstances: The nurse who wants to develop the humor room is more popular with patients than she is with her colleagues. Her nurse friends are quick to point out that while it's true that she is "a bit flaky" and unorthodox, she is an efficient nurse who is well-loved by her patients and their families. The hospital is in the midst of cutting expenses and has laid off both professional and nonprofessional employees.

Prerequisite knowledge: To decide how you should respond in this situation, you need to research the healing benefits of humor. Are there clinical studies demonstrating its effectiveness as a therapeutic measure? If studies point to humor's effectiveness, you will need to determine (1) what priority it should have among other treatment modalities and (2) the feasibility of creating a humor room in the current climate of cutting expenses. Is there a creative way to finance this venture?

Room for error: Since life and death do not hinge on how you elect to respond to this plea for support, there is a relatively wide margin for error. Because personal energy and finances are limited, however, you do not want to involve your unit in a futile project.

Time constraints: There is no rush for an immediate decision on your part, which gives you adequate time to develop the knowledge base you need to make an informed decision.

3. Address Potential Problems

The most serious obstacle to critical thinking in this situation would be the lack of an open mind and refusal to weigh the merits of a new treatment modality. Complicating factors include divided loyalties among the nurses and the tendency to support or refuse support for the project on the basis of whether one likes the nurse advocating the project, rather than on the merits of the project. Finally, the lowered morale caused by lay-offs may squash all creativity and willingness to "dream new dreams."

4. Consult Helpful Resources

Your first challenge will be to learn more about humor as a healing measure. Ideally, you may be able to consult a local expert and invite her or him to meet with the staff. Alternately, you can research the literature, looking for clinical studies and reports of the first-person experiences of others.

5. Critical Judgment/Decision

After a search of the literature convinced you and some of the other nurses of the clinical benefits of humor, you decide to explore the feasibility of developing a humor room. Your options are to "play it safe" and not rock the boat during a difficult period in the hospital by trying something new, or to become an advocate for the project and commit your energies to making it happen. You decide that a creative project may be exactly what the staff needs to rediscover the "joy of nursing" and begin to explore means to fund the project. You plan to "start small" and to reassess the project every 6 months. Since your research educated you about the potential benefits *and harms* humor can create, you decide that your first objective must be to educate the staff.

excellent ways to learn about new nursing strategies that have proved effective. Evidence-based practice resources include:

- Agency for Healthcare Research and Quality (AHRQ) (http://ahrq.gov)
- Reviews on effective quality improvement and implementation (http://epoc.cochrane.org)

- Toolkit: Implementation of clinical practice guidelines (http://www.rnao.org)
- Intervention mapping step 5: Adoption and implementation. (http://interventionmapping.com)

Research in Nursing boxes throughout this text demonstrate the difference nursing research can make in improving patient outcomes. Proponents of nursing implementation science are beginning to address the challenges of implementing research findings into practice (van Achterber, Schoonhoven, & Grol, 2008).

ETHICAL AND LEGAL GUIDES TO PRACTICE

To practice good nursing, it is important to be knowledgeable about the laws and regulations that affect healthcare and the ethical dimensions of clinical practice. Without this understanding, a sincere motivation to benefit the patient and a conscientious attempt to implement nursing orders will not be sufficient. Each nurse is responsible for becoming sensitive to the ethical and legal dimensions of practice, and moral and legal accountability are inherent in the practice of professional nursing.

> ➤ *Look back on the scenario presented at the beginning of the chapter for Estelle Morrissey. Ethical and legal guidelines are crucial in determining how the nurse intervenes. Additionally, the nurse needs to evaluate the ethical and legal ramifications of his or her action in light of the patient's request to die.* ■

Chapters 6 and 7 discuss the ethical and legal dimensions of practice. Hospital risk managers and ethics committees are increasingly available as institutional resources for nurses.

CONTINUING DATA COLLECTION AND RISK MANAGEMENT

An important nursing intervention is ongoing data collection. In every patient encounter, it is important to be sensitive to both subtle and dramatic changes in the patient's condition. Skilled nurses monitor the patient's responses to planned interventions to determine if the plan of care is working. These assessment findings are used to update and revise the plan of care. Sensitivity to how the patient is responding to nursing interventions and to the patient's progress toward outcome achievement allows the nurse to modify nursing interventions appropriately.

Another vital nursing intervention is ongoing risk management. While monitoring the patient's responses to the plan of care, nurses are also alert to the development of new problems that may result in the identification of new diagnoses or collaborative problems. As nurses get to know patients and recognize clusters of significant data, they can identify problems for which the patient is at risk and intervene appropriately to promote health and to prevent disease.

DOCUMENTING NURSING CARE

Remembering the legal truth, "It wasn't done if it wasn't documented," each nurse carefully documents all nursing interventions. See Chapter 17 for a description of guidelines for written documentation and see the plans of nursing care at the end of each clinical chapter for samples of documented nursing interventions.

WHEN A PATIENT DOES NOT COOPERATE WITH THE PLAN OF CARE

When a patient does not follow the plan of care despite the nurse's best efforts, it is time to reassess strategy. The first objective is to identify why the patient is not following the therapy. One possibility is that the plan of care may not be right for this patient. In this event, what is needed is not a change in the patient but, rather, a change in the plan of care. If the nurse determines, however, that the plan of care is adequate, he or she must identify and remedy the factors contributing to the patient's noncompliance. Common reasons for noncompliance include:

- Lack of family support
- Lack of understanding about the benefits of compliance
- Low value attached to outcomes or related interventions
- Adverse physical or emotional effects of treatment (such as pain and fatigue)
- Inability to afford treatment
- Limited access to treatment

DELEGATING NURSING CARE

Because of the pressure to reduce healthcare costs and the increasing demand for nursing services in the midst of a critical shortage of professional nurses, many employers of nurses have increased their use of unlicensed assistive personnel (UAP) or "nurse extenders." **Unlicensed assistive personnel** are individuals who are trained to function in an assistive role to the licensed registered nurse (RN) in the provision of patient activities as delegated by and under the supervision of the registered professional nurse. **Delegation** is the transfer of responsibility for the performance of an activity to another individual while retaining accountability for the outcome. In some cases, the new mix of professional and nonprofessional staff is threatening patient safety. Never has it been more important for nurses to critically identify which nursing interventions require professional nurses and which can be safely delegated. This can be especially challenging for new nurses.

> ➤ *Review the patient scenario for James McMahon, the critically ill patient described at the beginning of the chapter and in "Reflective Practice: Challenge to Technical Skills." The nurse's ability to delegate effectively would be important in providing safe, efficient care.* ■

Risks and Responsibilities of Delegating

Boucher (1998) aptly describes the dangers of fewer nurses caring for sicker patients while simultaneously supervising UAPs who are performing patient care that, until recently, was reserved for professional nurses:

> Even when the delegation is appropriate (that is, the right task assigned to the right person using clear, concise communication) and the task is performed correctly, the

Box 15-3 **ESSENTIALS OF EFFECTIVE DELEGATION**

The following will help you with the essential responsibilities and techniques of delegating care tasks:
- Know your state and institutional policies on delegation (the policy and procedure manual is available on each unit; for state policies, contact the state nurse association).
- Be clear on the difference between nursing process and nursing tasks.
- Know the training and background of the unlicensed assistive personnel (UAP). (Administration must have a standard and process to validate the UAP's preparation.)
- Know the patient's needs and what he or she is at risk for.
- Know what clinical cues the UAP should be alert for and why.
- Assess which tasks can be safely delegated.
- Have the UAP repeat your instructions to be sure you have communicated them clearly.
- Make frequent walking rounds to assess patients.
- When talking with the patient, members of the patient's family, or UAPs, listen for cues that indicate changes in the patient's condition.
- Take frequent mini-reports for the UAP.
- Evaluate the UAP's performance and the patient's response.

Boucher, M. A. (1998). Delegation alert! *American Journal of Nursing, 98*(2), 26–32.

nurse–patient dynamic is absent. It's this dynamic, or contextual presence—seeing the patient within the contexts of time, location, and physical and emotional conditions—that is the core of nursing. UAPs aren't trained to see a patient within a specific context, do a focused assessment, and know the significance of what the assessment reveals . . . UAPs are prepared to do many things, but they are not prepared to know (this is the absence of the critical thinking component). (p. 28)

See Box 15-3 for Boucher's list of "Essentials of Effective Delegation." Additional content on delegation is in Chapter 23.

Delegation and the Student Nurse

Student nurses may find themselves the recipient of delegated care that they cannot safely perform. Whenever you are asked by a staff nurse to perform an intervention for which you lack training, you should consult with your instructor to see if you can safely perform it with supervision. Never attempt to perform interventions beyond your capacity without supervision, even if instructed to do so by a staff nurse. Students who work as nursing assistants while enrolled in professional programs are especially likely to be asked to perform interventions beyond their mastery. You may be able to turn these requests into learning opportunities. For example, you might say, "I've never practiced that procedure but I'd love the opportunity to observe one of the experienced nurses do this."

GUIDE FOR STUDENTS
Organizing Care

Student nurses trying in advance to organize their nursing care for a particular clinical day can use the guidelines for student clinical responsibilities in Box 15-4 to help identify nursing measures for which they will be responsible. After these have been identified, working out a time schedule may provide clear direction for the clinical day and ensure that the patient's needs are met. The accompanying Reflective Practice box presents a scenario in which a nursing student learns to better manage her time and appropriately organize care.

Nursing Oneself

It is difficult for nurses to be sincerely attentive to patient needs if their own human needs are not met. Because no one is perfectly healthy or "whole" all the time, it is important that nurses preparing for professional practice spend time getting to know themselves. Activities that promote psychological health when practiced on a regular basis include self-awareness, communication, time management, preparation for crisis and loss, developing and maintaining support systems, and concurrent practice of self-care in all areas. The characteristics of emotional health include self-esteem, self-knowledge, satisfying interpersonal relationships, environmental mastery, stress management, a positive body image, a sense of humor, and the ability to experience pleasure.

Nurses who want to be competent practitioners learn early to nurse themselves and other nurses before attempting to

Box 15-4 **ORGANIZING STUDENT CLINICAL RESPONSIBILITIES**

To organize clinical responsibilities, check:
1. Patient profile
2. Name by which patient wishes to be addressed
3. Patient's chief complaint and reason for admission
4. Patient's current health status: Note any physical or emotional changes indicating the need to modify the plan of care.
5. Routine assistance patient needs to meet basic human needs
6. Priorities for nursing care:
   - Priorities identified by the patient as "most important." The nurse might state, "I'll be your nurse until 3 PM, and I'm interested in learning what you would most like to accomplish today."
   - Prioritized nursing diagnoses, patient outcomes, and related nursing interventions
   - Medical orders that need to be implemented
   - Interdependent or collaborative nursing responsibilities
7. Special "events" of the day that may require special observation of the patient, teaching, preparation, or aftercare:
   - Diagnostic tests
   - Consultations with specialists
   - New therapies (physical therapy, medications, surgery, radiotherapy, etc.)
8. Special teaching, counseling, or advocacy needs
9. Special needs of the family

REFLECTIVE PRACTICE
Challenge to Interpersonal Competence

For our complex care clinical, we were assigned to the hospital's cardiac care unit. I missed orientation because I was instructed to attend my public health orientation and was told that it would be easy to make up. The first day of clinical, we received report and were informed that the nurse assigned to our patient was not responsible for helping us with patient care, and that it was our clinical instructor's responsibility to assist all seven of us with patient care. My patient was a 53-year-old obese, diabetic African American man who came into the ER the previous day with shortness of breath and generally not feeling well. He was scheduled for a PICC line placement the day I was assigned to care for him, so I was instructed to complete his vital signs, give his 8 AM medications, take his blood glucose, and complete my head-to-toe assessment of him, all before he was scheduled to go down. Since this was my first time on the unit, I did not know where anything was and it took me a long time to find the necessary supplies. My nurse was of little help to me. By the time I got organized and was ready to start my care at 7:30 AM, a transporter was there to take my patient down for his procedures, and none of the tasks that I needed to complete were done. My nurse told me it was fine for him to go down without having his vitals or blood glucose taken. My patient had his PICC line put in, and then was sent for a foot x-ray, an echo, and a pressure test on his extremities. By the time I got back up to the unit with my patient 3 hours later, I was overwhelmed by the amount of care I needed to catch up on, and meanwhile my nurse was yelling at me about how I should have completed my care before leaving the unit.

Thinking Outside the Box: Possible Courses of Action

- I could have asked my clinical instructor or the nurse assigned to my patient to help me with the tasks I needed to carry out before my patient went down for his procedures.
- I could have asked a fellow classmate to help me collect the necessary supplies and to assist me in carrying out my care before leaving the floor.
- I could have organized and prioritized the care that needed to be delivered to my patient before his procedures. I could have carried out the most important tasks, such as taking his blood glucose and vital signs, in the short amount of time I had before he went down, and then completed the rest of my care when we returned to the unit.
- I could have been more organized when I returned to the unit, asking for the necessary help to provide adequate care for my patient and catching up on the tasks that I missed while we were off the unit.
- I could have become flustered upon returning to the unit, since I was behind on my care and since the nurse was yelling at me about completing his care, when she initially said it was "ok" for it not to be done before leaving the unit.
- I gained skill in prioritizing care.

Evaluating a Good Outcome: How Do I Define Success?

- The patient's needs were addressed in a timely and compassionate manner.
- The patient was comfortable and content with the care provided.
- The patient was respected by all individuals who were responsible for his care.
- The patient recognized our commitment as healthcare professionals to provide the best quality of care possible to him.
- I advocated on behalf of my patient to protect his health and rights as an individual.
- The needs of the nurses to provide the best patient care possible for the patient were met.

Personal Learning: Here's to the Future!

When I got back to the floor with my patient, I was overwhelmed by the amount of patient care that I needed to catch up on. I was having difficulty finding the blood glucose machine and the vitals machine. It was as if I were running around like a chicken with my head cut off and I was accomplishing nothing productive. Finally, my instructor pulled me aside because she could see that things were spiraling out of control. We sat down and prioritized from "most important" to "least important" the tasks I needed to do for my patient. First, I took his blood glucose, which was very low since he had not eaten all morning, and I ordered him a lunch tray. Next, I gave his morning medications that he missed. I then took his vital signs and completed my head-to-toe assessment and recorded my findings in his chart. I spent the rest of my day in clinical trying to make my patient comfortable and caring for his needs.

I think I became flustered when I returned to the floor because of the way the nurse treated me. She made me feel incompetent and stupid because I had not carried out all my care in the short time I was allotted. However, she did nothing to help me or assist me in caring for our patient. Looking back, I learned a great deal from this clinical experience. I should have told my nurse that I needed help in caring for the patient because I was trying to catch up on what was missed during the morning. If she was unwilling to help me, I should have consulted my clinical instructor or classmates for their assistance. I also should have pulled my nurse aside and confronted her about how she contradicted herself, in that she initially told me that it was okay for my patient to go down to his procedures without his care being complete, and then later reprimanded me for not carrying out his care before we left. I do not think my reactions to this

(continued)

REFLECTIVE PRACTICE

Challenge to Ethical and Legal Skills (continued)

clinical situation were unusual, and I think most nursing students would have become frustrated and overwhelmed under similar circumstances. Although this situation tested my interpersonal skills in working with

this nurse, I feel as though I was able put my frustrations aside and provide quality care in a professional manner to meet the needs of my patient.

Kate Sullivan, Georgetown University

Reflection

How do you think you would respond in a similar situation? Why? What does this tell you about yourself and about the adequacy of your skills for professional practice? Can you think of other ways to respond? How might the nursing student have approached the nurse assigned to the patient's care for assistance? What could the nursing student have done to prepare for this assignment? What other skills (cognitive, interpersonal, technical, ethical/legal) would you need to respond well in this situation? What role do you think the clinical environment (a cardiac care unit) played in the nursing student's feelings of being overwhelmed? Do you agree with the criteria to evaluate a successful outcome? Were the criteria met? Please explain why or why not.

nurse patients. Good personal health enables nurses not only to practice more efficiently, but also to be a health model for patients and their families. Nurses can help patients to imitate good health behaviors and eventually integrate them into their daily life through the process of identification.

Developing Critical Thinking Skills

1. Team up with another student and take turns role-playing a nurse visiting a homebound older man who needs his vital signs and nutritional status assessed. Discuss with each other the truth or falsity of the claim "Who the nurse is, is as important as, and sometimes more important than, what the nurse does."

2. Receive the same clinical assignment as another student, and independently outline your care priorities, specifying what you plan to accomplish during each of your clinical hours. Talk with the other student about the differences in what you both hope to accomplish and how you would do this. Try to imagine what these differences would mean to the patient.

3. You are the only RN on a 50-bed wing in a long-term care facility. You have one LPN working with you and two personal care assistants. Each of the 50 residents requires assistance with activities of daily living, all take at least some medications, and most require monitoring for multiple chronic (and sometimes acute) illnesses. How will you decide which interventions to delegate? When the home is short-staffed, you are sometimes the only RN covering two 50-bed units.

4. Describe how you would probably respond, and how you would like to respond (if these are different), to hearing another nurse in the shift report say that one of the patients you are assigned to was a real "PIB" ("pain in the butt") all day and "just impossible" to care for. Reflect on the importance of the language we use to report on a patient to one another.

Practicing for NCLEX

1. A school nurse notices that Jill is losing weight and wants to perform a focused assessment on Jill's nutritional status, fearing that she might have an eating disorder. How should the nurse proceed?
   a. Perform the focused assessment. This is an independent nurse-initiated intervention.
   b. Request an order from Jill's physician since this is a physician-initiated intervention.
   c. Request an order from Jill's physician since this is a collaborative intervention.
   d. Request an order from the nutritionist since this is a collaborative intervention.

2. Which of the following would you expect to find in the Nursing Interventions Classification Taxonomy?
   a. Case studies illustrating a complete set of activities that a nurse performs to carry out nursing interventions
   b. Nursing interventions, each with a label, a definition, and a set of activities that a nurse performs to carry it out, with a short list of background readings
   c. A complete list of nursing diagnoses, outcomes, and related nursing activities for each nursing intervention
   d. A complete list of reimbursable charges for each nursing intervention

3. You are a brand new RN. When you orient to a new nursing unit that is currently understaffed, you are told that the UAPs have been trained to obtain the initial nursing assessment. What is the best response?
   a. Allow the UAPs to do the admission assessment and report the findings to you.
   b. Do your own admission assessments but don't interfere with the practice if other professional RNs seem comfortable with the practice.
   c. Tell the charge nurse that you are choosing not to delegate the admission assessment at this time until you can get further clarification from admission.
   d. Contact your labor representative and complain.

● Answers With Rationale

1. **a.** Performing a focused assessment is an independent nurse-initiated intervention. The nurse, therefore, does not need an order from the physician (*b*, *c*) or the nutritionist (*d*).

2. **b.** The Nursing Interventions Classification Taxonomy lists 336 interventions, each with a label, a definition, a set of activities that a nurse performs to carry it out, and a short list of background readings. It does not contain case studies (*a*), diagnoses (*c*), or charges (*d*).

3. **c.** You do not delegate this nursing admission assessment because you learned that only nurses can perform this intervention. You should seek clarification for this policy from nursing administration.

Taylor Suite Resources

The Taylor Suite offers these additional resources to enhance learning and facilitate understanding of this chapter:

- thePoint online resource, http://thepoint.lww.com/Taylor7E
- Student DVD included with the book
- Study Guide for Taylor's Fundamentals of Nursing

BIBLIOGRAPHY

Alfaro-LeFevre, R. (2009). *Critical thinking and clinical judgment: A practical approach* (4th ed.). St. Louis: Saunders Elsevier.

Alfaro-LeFevre, R. (2010). *Applying nursing process: A tool for critical thinking* (7th ed.). Philadelphia: Lippincott Williams & Wilkins.

American Association of Critical Care Nurses. (2005). *Standards for establishing and sustaining healthy practice environments.* Aliso Viejo, CA: Author.

American Nurses Association. (2007). *ANA's principles of environmental health for nursing practice with implementation strategies.* Washington, DC: Author.

Benner, P. (1984). *From novice to expert: Excellence and power in clinical nursing practice.* Menlo Park, CA: Addison-Wesley.

Benner, P., & Wrubel, J. (1989). *The primacy of caring: Stress and coping in health and illness.* Menlo Park, CA: Addison-Wesley.

Blegen, M. A., Gardner, D. I., & McCloskey, J. C. (1992). Who helps you with your work? *American Journal of Nursing, 92*(1), 26–31.

Boucher, M. A. (1998). Delegation alert! *American Journal of Nursing, 98*(2), 26–32.

Bulechek, G. M., Butcher, H. K., & Dochterman, J. (Eds.). (2008). *Nursing interventions classification (NIC)* (5th ed.). St. Louis: Mosby.

Carpenito-Moyet, L. J. (2010). *Nursing diagnosis: Application to clinical practice* (13th ed.). Philadelphia: Lippincott Williams & Wilkins.

Dall, T. M., Chen, Y. J., Seifert, R. F., Maddox, T. J., & Hogan, T. F. (2009). The economic value of professional nursing. *Medical Care, 47*(1), 1–8.

Davies, B., Edwards, N., Ploeg, J., & Virani, T. (2008). Insights about the process and impact of implementing nursing guidelines on delivery of care in hospitals and community settings. *BMC Health Services Research, 8,* 29.

Eisenhauer, L. A. (1994). A typology of nursing therapeutics. *Image—The Journal of Nursing Scholarship, 26*(4), 261–264.

Holleman, G., Eliens, A., Van Vliet, M., & Van Achterberg, T. (2006). Promotion of evidence-based practice by professional nursing associations: Literature review. *Journal of Advanced Nursing, 53,* 702–709.

Iowa Intervention Project. (1993). The NIC taxonomy structure. *Image—The Journal of Nursing Scholarship, 25*(3), 187–192.

Iowa Intervention Project. (1997). Nursing interventions classification (NIC): An overview. In M. J. Rantz & P. LeMone (Eds.), *Classification of nursing diagnoses: Proceedings of the Twelfth Conference, North American Nursing Diagnosis* (pp. 32–39). Glendale, CA: CINAHL Information Systems.

Joint Commission on Accreditation of Healthcare Organizations. (2006). *2006 Accreditation manual for hospitals.* Oakbrook Terrace, IL: Author.

Lavoie-Tremblay, M., Wright, D., Desforges, N., Gelinas, C., Marchionni, C., & Drevniok, U. (2008). Creating a health workplace for new-generation nurses. *The Journal of Nursing Scholarship, 40*(3), 290–297.

Maxfield, D., Grenny, J., Patterson, K., McMillan, R., & Switzler, A. (2005). *Silence kills: The seven crucial conversations in healthcare.* Available at http://www.aacn.org/WD/Practice/Docs/PublicPolicy/SilenceKillsExecSum.pdf

McCauley, K. M. (2005). A message from the American Association of Critical Care Nurses. *American Journal of Critical Care, 14*(3), 186–197.

McCloskey Dochterman, J. C., & Bulechek, G. M. (Eds.). (1992). *Nursing interventions classification (NIC).* St. Louis: Mosby–Year Book.

McCloskey Dochterman, J. C., & Bulechek, G. M. (Eds.). (1995). Validating and coding of the NIC taxonomy structure. *Image— The Journal of Nursing Scholarship, 27*(1), 43–49.

McCloskey Dochterman, J. C., & Bulechek, G. M. (Eds.). (1996). *Nursing interventions classification (NIC)* (2nd ed.). St. Louis: Mosby–Year Book.

McCloskey Dochterman, J. C., & Bulechek, G. M. (Eds.). (2000). *Nursing interventions classification (NIC)* (3rd ed.). St. Louis: Mosby–Year Book.

McCloskey Dochterman, J., & Bulechek, G. M. (Eds.). (2004). *Nursing interventions classification (NIC)* (4th ed.). St. Louis: Mosby.

Moorhead, S., Johnson, M., Maas, M. L., & Swanson, E. (Eds.). (2008). *Nursing outcomes classification (NOC)* (4th ed.). St. Louis: Mosby Elsevier.

Muller-Staub, M., Needham, I., Odenbreit, M., Lavin, M. A., & Van Achterberg, T. (2008). Implementing nursing diagnostics effectively: Cluster randomized trial. *Journal of Advanced Nursing, 63*(3), 291–301.

NANDA International. (2009). *Nursing Diagnoses: Definitions & classification, 2009–2011.* Oxford, UK: Wiley-Blackwell.

Swanson, E. (2008). *Nursing Outcomes Classification (NOC)* (4th ed.). St. Louis: Mosby Elsevier.

Titler, M. G., Kleiber, C., Steelman, V., Rakel, B., Budreau, G., Everett, L. Q., et al. (2001). The Iowa Model of evidence-based practice to promote quality care. *Critical Care Nursing Clinics of North America, 13,* 497–509.

Van Achterberg, T., Schoonhoven, L., & Grol, R. (2008). Nursing implementation science: How evidence-based nursing required evidence-based implementation. *Journal of Nursing Scholarship, 40*(4), 302–310.

16 Evaluating

TYLER JAMESON

Tyler, a term neonate born 30 hours ago, has yet to pass stool. Follow-up assessment reveals that he does not have a patent anus, a finding that was not detected in the neonate's initial assessment.

MIOSHI OTSUKI

Mioshi, an elderly woman with a history of heart failure being treated with diuretics, is receiving home care. Questioned about her prescribed drug-therapy regimen, the patient states, "I take this one labeled 'furosemide' every day in the morning along with this other one labeled 'Lasix.'"

NICHOLAS SOROS

Nicholas is a 68-year-old patient newly diagnosed with diabetes. His initial assessment revealed that he was about 50 pounds overweight due to poor diet and lack of exercise. A plan was developed to help Mr. Soros better manage his diabetes through planned weight reduction and regular exercise. At a follow-up visit, assessment reveals a weight gain of 5 pounds. He stated, "I'm too old to worry about diet and exercise. You can control my diabetes with medication, right?"

• Continue the plan of care if more time is needed to achieve the outcomes

LEARNING OBJECTIVES

After completing the chapter, you will be able to accomplish the following:

1. Describe evaluation, its purpose, and its relation to the other steps in the nursing process.

2. Evaluate the patient's achievement of four types of outcomes specified in the plan of care.

3. Manipulate factors that contribute to success or failure in outcome achievement.

4. Use the patient's response to the plan of care to modify the plan as needed.

5. Explain the relation between quality-assurance/quality-improvement programs and excellence in healthcare.

6. Describe the AACN standards for establishing and sustaining healthy work environments and describe the seven crucial conversations in healthcare.

7. Value self-evaluation as a critical element in developing the ability to deliver quality nursing care.

KEY TERMS

concurrent evaluation

criteria

evaluating

evidence-based practice

nursing audit

outcome evaluation

peer review

performance
   improvement

process evaluation

quality-assurance
   program

quality improvement

retrospective
   evaluation

standards

structure evaluation

In the fifth step of the nursing process, **evaluating,** the nurse and patient together measure how well the patient has achieved the outcomes specified in the plan of care. When evaluating patient outcome achievement, the nurse identifies factors that contribute to the patient's ability to achieve expected outcomes and, when necessary, modifies the plan of care (Fig. 16-1). The purpose of evaluation is to allow the patient's achievement of expected outcomes to direct future nurse–patient interactions. Based on the patient's responses to the plan of care, the nurse decides to:

• Terminate the plan of care when each expected outcome is achieved

• Modify the plan of care if there are difficulties achieving the outcomes

• Continue the plan of care if more time is needed to achieve the outcomes

When evaluation points to the need to modify nursing care, the nurse reviews each preceding step of the nursing process (assessing, diagnosing, planning, and implementing). Successful evaluation ensures that valued patient outcomes are attained. It also enhances the public's image of nursing and helps ensure nursing's survival by promoting continued selection and funding of nursing services in the competitive healthcare market.

UNIQUE FOCUS OF NURSING EVALUATION

As members of the healthcare team, nurses are involved in many types of evaluation. Nurses measure patient outcome achievement, how effectively nurses help targeted groups of patients to achieve their specific outcomes, the competence of individual nurses, and the degree to which external factors, such as different types of healthcare services, specialized equipment or procedures, or socioeconomic factors, influence health and wellness. *The patient, however, is always the nurse's primary concern.* A nurse may perform a nursing procedure competently, creatively, and with care, but if this nursing intervention does not help the patient reach desired outcomes, it is not fully meaningful. Either directly or indirectly, the aim of all nursing evaluation is quality nursing care that aids patient outcome achievement. Therefore, the most important act of evaluation performed by nurses is evaluating outcome achievement with the patient (see the accompanying Reflective Practice box for an example).

The Institute of Medicine's Committee on Quality of Health Care in America is educating the public on what it is reasonable for patients to expect from their healthcare (Box 16-1). Even beginning nurses can use these guidelines to evaluate the care they are providing.

CRITICAL THINKING AND MEASURING PATIENT OUTCOME ACHIEVEMENT

The five classic elements of evaluation are (1) identifying evaluative criteria and standards (what you are looking for when you evaluate, e.g., expected patient outcomes), (2) collecting data to determine whether these criteria and standards are met, (3) interpreting and summarizing findings, (4) documenting your judgment, and (5) terminating, continuing, or modifying the plan. Each element requires the nurse to *think critically* about how best to evaluate the patient's progress toward valued health outcomes. In the nursing process, evaluative criteria are the patient outcomes developed during the planning step. Because these reflect desired changes or outcomes in patient behavior and because nursing actions are directed toward these outcomes, they are the core of evaluation. Determining whether these outcomes have been or are being met and then identifying the appropriate nursing response are the functions of evaluation.

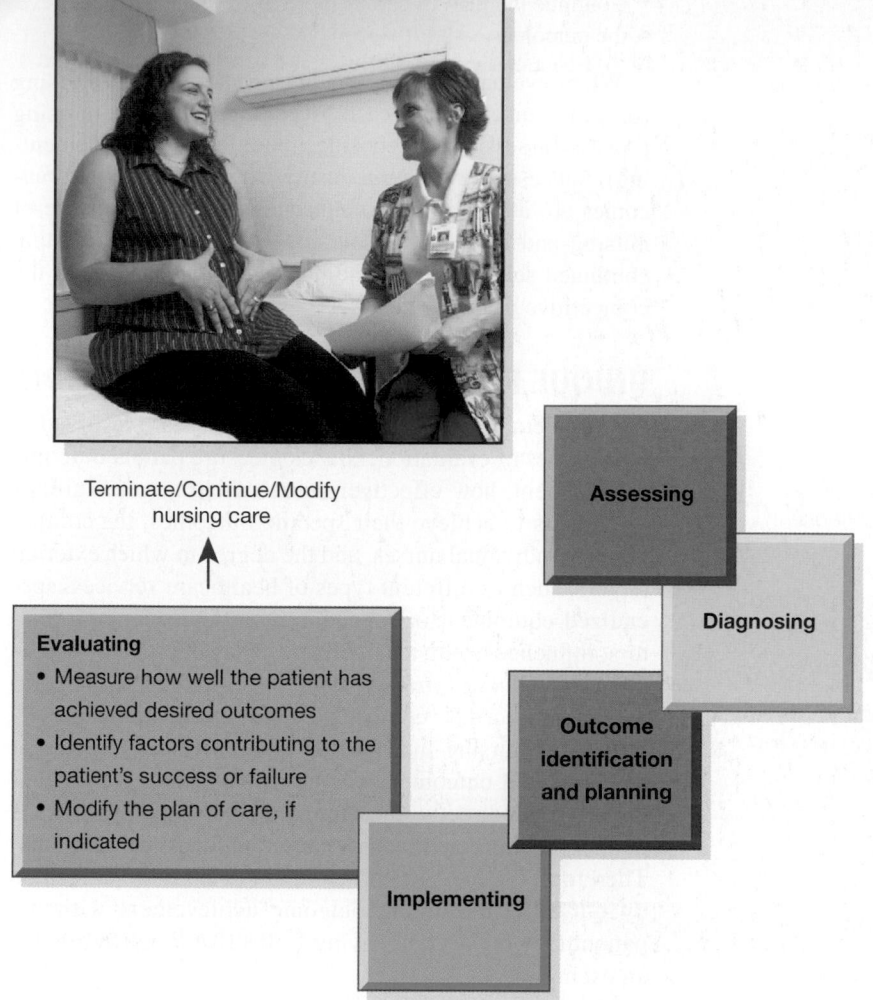

Terminate/Continue/Modify nursing care

Evaluating
- Measure how well the patient has achieved desired outcomes
- Identify factors contributing to the patient's success or failure
- Modify the plan of care, if indicated

Assessing

Diagnosing

Outcome identification and planning

Implementing

FIGURE 16-1. Evaluating. The nurse and patient together measure how well the patient has achieved the outcomes specified in the plan of care. Factors that contribute to the patient's success or failure are identified, and the plan of care is modified if necessary. Patient responses to the plan of care determine whether nursing care is to be continued as is, modified, or terminated. *(Photo by Joe Mitchell.)*

Box 16-1 WHAT PATIENTS SHOULD EXPECT FROM THEIR HEALTHCARE

1. **Beyond patient visits:** You will have the care you need when you need it . . . *whenever* you need it. You will find help in many forms, not just in face-to-face visits. You will find help on the Internet, on the telephone, from many sources, by many routes, in the form you want it.

2. **Individualization:** You will be known and respected as an individual. Your choices and preferences will be sought and honored. The usual system of care will meet most of your needs. When your needs are special, the care will adapt to meet you on your own terms.

3. **Control:** The care system will take control only if and when you freely give permission.

4. **Information:** You can know what you wish to know, when you wish to know it. Your medical record is yours to keep, to read, and to understand. The rule is: "Nothing about you without you."

5. **Science:** You will have care based on the best available scientific knowledge. The system promises you excellence as its standard. Your care will not vary illogically from doctor to doctor or from place to place. The system will promise you all

the care that can help you, and will help you avoid care that cannot help you.

6. **Safety:** Errors in care will not harm you. You will be safe in the care system.

7. **Transparency:** Your care will be confidential, but the care system will not keep secrets from you. You can know whatever you wish to know about the care that affects you and your loved ones.

8. **Anticipation:** Your care will anticipate your needs and will help you find the help you need. You will experience proactive help, not just reactions, to help you restore and maintain your health.

9. **Value:** Your care will not waste your time or money. You will benefit from constant innovations, which will increase the value of care to you.

10. **Cooperation:** Those who provide care will cooperate and coordinate their work fully with each other and with you. The walls between professions and institutions will crumble, so that your experiences will become seamless. You will never feel lost.

REFLECTIVE PRACTICE

Challenge to Interpersonal Skills

I first met Mr. Nicholas Soros, a 68-year-old client newly diagnosed with diabetes, in the clinic. He was about 50 pounds overweight, and his health history revealed the need for major dietary changes and an exercise program. The interdisciplinary team devised a plan to help Mr. Soros better manage his diabetes through planned weight reduction and regular exercise, for which I did much of the initial teaching. Unfortunately, when Mr. Soros returned for his next check-up, he had gained 5 additional pounds and reported being "too old" to worry about diet and exercise. "You can control my diabetes with medication, right?" When I reported this to the nurse practitioner, he told me that Mr. Soros knows what to do and now it is his responsibility. I wasn't perfectly comfortable with this response and thought that Mr. Soros needed more than someone wagging a finger in his face.

Thinking Outside the Box: Alternate Courses of Action

- Remind Mr. Soros of what he needs to do and tell him that responsibility for this is his!
- After I make sure that he does indeed know what to do, spend time making sure that he values his health sufficiently to try these new behaviors.

- Make sure that Mr. Soros trusts us sufficiently to value working with us to achieve his health goals.

Evaluating a Good Outcome: How Do I Define Success?

- Mr. Soros achieves his target weight and is faithful to a program of regular exercise.
- Mr. Soros feels that his independence and ability to determine his own life plan are respected, at the same time feeling that we care about his health status.

- I learn more about developing a trusting nurse–patient relationship, exploring the relationship's role in helping patients to achieve valued health outcomes.

Personal Learning: Here's to the Future!

I learned something about myself and an important distinction between teaching and counseling. Clearly, just teaching Mr. Soros about diet and exercise wasn't sufficient. Mr. Soros was in no way going to change his lifestyle until he valued his health enough to make needed changes, including understanding why these changes were important. I also learned how important

nurse–patient relationships are. When Mr. Soros came for his third visit, he asked the nurse who greeted him where I was, telling her "I want to see that nurse who cared about me!"—positive reinforcement for the relationship's importance.

Megan Kyle, Georgetown University

Reflection

How do you think you would respond in a similar situation? Why? What does this tell you about yourself and about the adequacy of your skills for professional practice? Can you think of other ways to respond? Describe the type of teaching plan that the nursing student may have used at the initial teaching session. How might that teaching plan have changed based on the patient's response at the next visit? Would the outcomes identified initially need to be revised based on any changes in the teaching plan? Please explain why or why not. What other skills (cognitive, interpersonal, technical, ethical/legal) would you need to respond well in this situation? Classify these other skills as belonging to the cognitive, affective, or psychomotor domains. Do you agree with the criteria to evaluate a successful outcome?

➤ *Think back to Nicholas Soros, the 68-year-old man diagnosed with diabetes who needed to lose weight and to exercise. The outcomes identified initially most likely focused on weight loss and adherence to an exercise program. Teaching at this initial visit also focused on ways to achieve these outcomes. However, the patient's statements and weight gain on his next clinic visit would lead the nurse to suspect that the outcomes identified were not being achieved. Therefore, some changes in the patient's plan of care are necessary. ∎*

Identifying Evaluative Criteria and Standards

Although the terms "criteria" and "standard" are often used interchangeably in reference to the evaluation step, they have distinct definitions. **Criteria** are measurable qualities, attributes, or characteristics that specify skills, knowledge, or health states. They describe acceptable levels of performance by stating the expected behaviors of the nurse or the patient. Chapter 14 describes how patient criteria are identified and formulated as patient outcomes.

Standards are the levels of performance accepted and expected by the nursing staff or other health team members. They

Box 16-2   ANA STANDARDS OF PRACTICE: STANDARD 6, EVALUATION

The registered nurse evaluates progress toward attainment of outcomes.

Measurement Criteria
The registered nurse:

Conducts a systematic ongoing, criterion-based evaluation of the outcomes in relation to the structures and processes prescribed by the plan and the indicated timeline.

Includes the patient and others involved in the care or situation in the evaluative process.

Evaluates the effectiveness of the planned strategies in relation to patient responses and the attainment of the expected outcomes.

Documents the results of the evaluation.

Uses ongoing assessment data to revise the diagnoses, outcomes, plan, and implementation, as needed.

Disseminates the results to the patient and others involved in the care or situation, as appropriate, in accordance with the state and federal laws and regulations.

Used with permission. American Nurses Association (ANA). (2004). *Scope and standards of practice.* Washington DC: Author.

are established by authority, custom, or consent. A good example of standards is the American Nurses Association's *Standards of Nursing Practice,* which are displayed in Chapter 1, this chapter, and each of the chapters in The Nursing Process unit. See Box 16-2 for ANA Standards of Practice related to evaluation. Chapters 14 and 15 describe clinical practice guidelines, a term used interchangeably with standards and protocols, all of which describe how care should be managed in certain situations. The goal is to design and deliver nursing care that evidence supports as likely to produce the expected patient outcomes (i.e., **evidence-based practice**).

Collecting Evaluative Data

The nurse collects evaluative data to determine whether or not the patient has met the desired outcomes. Whereas the nurse collects data in the nursing assessment to identify patient health problems, the data collected in the evaluation step are used to determine whether the identified health problems have been or are being resolved through outcome achievement.

➤ *Consider Mrs. Otsuki, the older adult woman who is inadvertently taking double the dose of prescribed diuretic (lasix is the generic name for furosemide). This initial assessment indicates a need for teaching. Thus, when evaluating outcome achievement for this patient, the nurse would determine whether the patient demonstrates understanding of her drug therapy regimen and is no longer taking two doses of the same drug.* ■

This section discusses (1) the different types of data collected to evaluate the achievement of different types of patient outcomes and (2) time criteria for data collection.

Types of Outcomes

The type of patient data collected to support the evaluation of outcome achievement is determined by the nature of the outcome. Four types of outcomes are discussed below. The data collected to determine the degree of outcome achievement are recorded in the corresponding evaluative statements.

COGNITIVE OUTCOMES

Cognitive outcomes involve increases in patient knowledge. These outcomes may be evaluated simply by asking patients to repeat information or, at a higher level of performance, by asking patients to apply the new knowledge to their everyday situations. For example, asking patients to describe new dietary restrictions is different from asking them to plan a weekly menu compatible with these restrictions.

PSYCHOMOTOR OUTCOMES

Psychomotor outcomes describe the patient's achievement of new skills; they are evaluated by asking the patient to demonstrate the new skill.

AFFECTIVE OUTCOMES

Affective outcomes pertain to changes in patient values, beliefs, and attitudes and are more complex to evaluate. Observation of patient behavior and conversation can determine whether affective outcomes have been achieved.

PHYSIOLOGIC OUTCOMES

In the final type of outcome statement, physiologic outcomes, physical changes in the patient are the targeted outcome. To evaluate achievement of this type of outcome, the nurse uses physical assessment skills to collect relevant data and compares these with previous patient data.

➤ *Remember Tyler Jameson, the neonate who has not passed any stool due to the lack of a patent anus? The nurse would develop a physiologic outcome focusing on bowel elimination and the passage of stool.* ■

Samples of the outcomes are shown in Box 16-3.

Time Criteria

In addition to knowing what type of data to collect to determine outcome achievement, it is important to know when to collect the data. When the patient outcomes were developed, a time frame was established for determining whether the specified changes have been achieved. At the designated time, the nurse, in collaboration with the patient, the family, and other members of the nursing team, evaluates the patient's attainment of the outcome. If outcomes are developed in observable and measurable terms, the task of collecting data for evaluation is clear-cut. Examples of three types of time criteria follow:

- By 7/8/12, the patient will walk the length of the hallway with support of a walker
- Beginning 7/8/12, the patient will demonstrate a weight loss of 3 lb per month until target weight (135 lb) is achieved (6/8/12, weight: 151 lb).

Box 16-3   EVALUATING FOUR TYPES OF OUTCOMES IN THE PLAN OF NURSING CARE

Nursing Diagnosis
High Risk for Altered Parenting related to no previous experience in childrearing (fear)

Assessment Data
Subjective: "My husband and I are both afraid we won't know what to do when we get the baby home."

Objective: Both parents are single children, report no childrearing experience; healthy newborn son delivered 2/4/12; first born

Strengths
VIB (very important baby): parents are both 38; history of infertility with one miscarriage; strong motivation to learn and use good parenting skills; strong support network

Expected Outcomes	Nursing Interventions	Evaluative Statement (Actual Outcomes)
Psychomotor Outcomes Before discharge, parents will demonstrate confidence in: • Holding baby • Diapering, dressing baby • Bathing baby • Feeding baby	Assess both parents' knowledge of childrearing practices; identify and reinforce motivation to learn; correct any misinformation. Develop and implement at a time convenient for both parents a teaching plan to include: • The primary nurse role-modeling techniques for comfortably and safely holding, talking to, and dressing baby • Parents independently viewing videocassettes on: Baby care, Baby bath, and Breastfeeding, followed by one-on-one discussion • Class for new parents: nurse to demonstrate baby bath and discuss general principles of care • Primary nurse observing mother and infant during initial feeding sessions and offering teaching and support as necessary	2/6/12 Outcome partially met. Both parents have correctly demonstrated safe techniques for holding, dressing, and bathing the baby. Mother is still concerned baby is not getting enough milk. *Revision:* Continue to spend time with mother and infant during feeding—provide positive reinforcement. *F. Morales, RN*
Cognitive Outcomes By 2/6/12, parents will report appropriate action to be taken if questions or problems arise after discharge: • Name and number of primary nurse • Name and number of pediatrician • La Leche League contact and number	Answer parents' questions and address related concerns. Assess parents' knowledge of infant problems frequently encountered by new parents. Inform parents of available community resources and describe appropriate action to take if questions or problems arise.	2/6/12 Outcome met. Parents discussed some infant problems related to feeding, elimination, and illness and reported appropriate community resource to contact. *F. Morales, RN*
Affective Outcome Before discharge, parents will verbalize decreased anxiety in regard to caring for son.	Assess parents' level of anxiety and potential negative effects on childrearing. Discuss this with parents. Explore adequacy of parents' coping strategies—increased knowledge, practice in supportive environment, community resources. Counsel as necessary. Compliment parents on new parenting skills. Allow for ventilation of anxiety or specific fears. Respond with teaching or emotional support, as necessary.	2/6/12 Outcome partially met. Except for concern about breastfeeding, *both* parents expressed feeling comfortable and eager to care for their son at home. *F. Morales, RN*
Physiologic Outcomes At 1-month postpartal telephone interview, 3/4/12 (by parents' report), the baby will demonstrate adequate: • Weight gain (birth weight, 7 lb 6 oz) • Sleep–wakefulness patterns • Comfort level indicating adequate parenting.	Use a 1-month postdelivery telephone interview to assess the adequacy of parenting skills. With positive report of growth and development, compliment (reinforce) the parents. With negative report, teach or counsel and refer as appropriate.	3/4/12 Outcome met. Parents' report of baby's weight gain and behavior indicates good parenting skills. *F. Morales, RN*

- Before discharge, parents will correctly demonstrate chest physiotherapy procedures for patient.

It is important for nurses to evaluate patient outcome achievement as early as possible. Celebrating outcome attainment with the patient usually helps encourage the patient and leads to further outcome achievement. When failure to meet designated outcomes is detected early, the plan of care can be modified to remedy the failure.

> *Think back to Nicholas Soros, the 68-year-old patient with diabetes. By recognizing the lack of outcome achievement on the next visit, the nurse can gather additional data to revise the plan of care. For example, perhaps Mr. Soros did not completely understand the teaching that was presented. Or, he may have had difficulty accepting his diagnosis, thereby interfering with his ability to comply with the plan, ultimately leading to weight gain instead of a weight loss.* ■

The most common mistake nurses make when evaluating in acute care settings is waiting until the day the patient is to be discharged before evaluating outcome achievement. At that point, it is too late to revise the plan of care.

Interpreting and Summarizing Findings

Before the nurse can make a judgment about the patient's achievement of outcomes, it is necessary to study and interpret the data collected. Just as clusters of data are interpreted before the nurse identifies and validates a nursing diagnosis, so too does evaluative data need to be interpreted. For example, a patient who is expected to walk the length of the hallway with support of a walker asks to be taken back to her room because she feels weak. The nurse must gather more data and then determine if this is a one-time incident linked to medications or a temporary metabolic imbalance, or if it signals a consistent inability to achieve this behavior. Interpreting evaluative data requires critical thinking and is a skill that must be practiced.

When interpreting and summarizing findings, it is important to consider factors that influence outcome achievement. Numerous patient, nurse, and healthcare system variables contribute positively or negatively to patient outcome achievement. Identifying these variables allows the nurse to reinforce positive factors by drawing on them in the future, as well as to deal with other variables that are creating problems. The more sensitive and responsive nurses are to these variables, the more rewarding their practices will be.

Examples of positive factors include a patient's strong motivation to learn new health behaviors, a nurse who comes to work well rested and with a new care idea learned from a nursing journal, and a healthcare institution or agency that offers incentives for quality nursing and has an optimal nurse-to-patient ratio.

When the nurse understands what factors are helpful to the patient who is trying to reach desired outcomes, she or he can often manipulate these factors. For example, if a patient is learning to ambulate independently after hip surgery and you

notice that he seems to make his best effort when his wife is present, mention this to her and plan to ambulate the patient at least once a day when she is present. Conversely, if a patient seems more fearful when his wife is present, note in the plan of care that ambulation is best attempted when the patient's wife is not on the unit. Ideally, this fear would be explored with the patient before discharge so that he can continue to make progress when he is discharged home with his wife.

Table 16-1 presents common variables that can negatively influence patient outcome achievement. Tentative nursing approaches are suggested. Nurses need to think critically about the effects of these variables and respond creatively to them.

Documenting Your Judgment

After the data have been collected and interpreted to determine patient outcome achievement, the nurse makes and documents a judgment summarizing the findings. This is termed the evaluative statement. The two-part evaluative statement includes a decision about how well the outcome was met, along with patient data or behaviors that support this decision. The nurse has three decision options for how outcomes have been met: met, partially met, or not met.

- 1/21/12—Outcome met. Patient reports 1 week of no tobacco use. C. Taylor, RN
- 1/21/12—Outcome partially met. Patient reports decreasing tobacco use from one pack per day to 4 to 6 cigarettes per day. C. Taylor, RN
- 1/21/12—Outcome not met. Patient reports no change in tobacco use. Revision: Reexplore patient's commitment to try tobacco-use control strategies and adequacy of personal support systems to eliminate tobacco use. C. Taylor, RN

The nurse signs and dates the evaluative statement (see Box 16-3). Alternatively, the nurse follows the documentation guidelines for evaluating outcome achievement specified in the institution's computerized documentation systems.

Modifying the Plan of Care

When evaluation reveals that the patient has made little or no progress toward outcome achievement, the nurse needs to reevaluate each preceding step of the nursing process to try to identify the contributing factors pointing to problems with the plan of care. New assessment data might need to be collected, diagnoses may be added or altered, outcomes might need to be modified or rewritten, nursing orders may be changed, or evaluation may be targeted more frequently.

> *Remember Tyler Jameson, the neonate who has not passed any stool after 30 hours? The initial outcome may have stated that the neonate would pass stool within 18 to 24 hours after birth. However, this outcome was developed based on data that was inaccurate. Therefore, the nurse, learning of the new data, would revise the outcome to correlate with the neonate's condition, dependent on the treatment to correct the anomaly.* ■

TABLE • 16-1	PATIENT, NURSE, AND HEALTHCARE SYSTEM VARIABLES THAT MAY DETRACT FROM QUALITY NURSING CARE	

Variables	Possible Solution
Patient Variables	
Patient who is physically and cognitively capable of self-care gives up—refuses to cooperate with therapeutic regimen or thwarts the regimen	Identify one nurse who is able to develop a trusting relationship with the patient and determine the reason underlying the observed behavior: • No longer finds meaning and purpose in life • Overwhelming sense of powerlessness • Previous history of being "hurt," "exploited," "cheated" by the healthcare system • Inability to accept illness and related lifestyle changes Counsel appropriately Use a team conference to develop a consistent plan of nursing care.
Patient who quietly accepts whatever is done or not done for him or her; seldom communicates needs or dissatisfaction	Note on the plan of care the need to assess this patient thoroughly because the patient will probably not advocate for himself or herself. Educate the patient to become a more assertive healthcare consumer.
Nurse Variables	
Nurse who sincerely desires to give 150% all the time and who becomes quickly frustrated when observing substandard care; may feel alienated from other staff; excellent candidate for burnout	Learn to give quality care during designated work period; leave on time; avoid the temptation to do the work of others; leave work concerns at work. After establishing a reputation for delivering quality nursing care, seek creative solutions for nursing problems (strategies to increase nursing resources, motivation, morale) and try them—hopefully with a support network. View concerns as challenges rather than overwhelming obstacles. Develop a realistic sense of how much nursing care and of what quality can be delivered with existing resources. If resources do not permit quality care, explore change strategies within the institution. If administration is not supportive, explore other practice settings.
Nurse with overwhelming outside concerns: • Preparation for marriage, childbirth, divorce • Illness (self or family members) • Role conflict (familial roles, school, work, etc.) • New apartment, house	During periods of peak demand, may need to accept less than optimal performance at work. If this becomes the norm rather than the exception, carefully evaluate priorities. May need to cut work hours rather than "cheat" patients.
Nurse who is bored	After reflection, write down *personal* objectives related to work. Explore avenues within work setting for professional growth and development: initiate changes in nursing unit to improve patient care and to stimulate peer development; join institutional committees; participate actively in staff development programs; develop patient and family support groups. Look for new position that offers new challenges within or outside the institution. Join professional organizations and participate actively. Evaluate educational goals and explore possibilities—continuing education programs and degree work.
Healthcare System Variables	
Inadequate staffing	Develop and use a patient classification system that incorporates an identification of the kind and amount of nursing services required. Record staffing patterns and relate to needs for nursing care and patient outcomes. Clearly demonstrate and document that adequate staffing makes a difference. Present these data to nursing administration with the request for additional staff. If necessary, use professional bargaining unit.
Nursing administration has sold out nursing; insensitivity to nursing demands within the institution	It may be impossible to practice quality, progressive nursing in this environment. If there seems to be no hope for change after appropriate channels have been explored, look for a new practice setting. Evaluate the new setting on the basis of what experience has taught you.

Review the checklist for help in evaluating your use of the nursing process in Chapter 11. Table 16-2 suggests appropriate nursing responses to common problems encountered during evaluation.

When the nurse has identified the factors contributing to the outcomes not being achieved, the evaluative statement can be used to suggest the necessary revision in the plan of care: (1) delete or modify the nursing diagnosis, (2) make the outcome statement more realistic, (3) increase the complexity of the outcome statement, (4) adjust time criteria in outcome statement, or (5) change the nursing intervention. Increasing the complexity of an outcome after it has been

TABLE • 16-2   COMMON PROBLEMS NOTED DURING EVALUATION OF THE NURSING PROCESS

Problem	Nursing Response
Assessing	
1. Inaccurate database → inaccurate nursing diagnoses and a distorted plan of care	1. a. Identify the patient or nurse variables responsible for inaccuracy. b. Revise the recorded database.
2. Database does not reflect changes in patient condition.	2. Review with the *entire* nursing staff the importance of making assessment a priority in every patient interaction as well as the recording of the new data obtained.
3. Database is superficial: • Fails to communicate uniqueness of patient • Lacks sufficient detail on major problems or developments	3. a. Rethink the critical relation between an adequate database and quality care. b. Develop interviewing and physical assessment skills. c. Begin to identify the key data that need to be collected for specific nursing diagnosis and medical diagnosis and to assess patient response to therapeutic regimen (use of a nursing diagnosis handbook may be helpful).
Diagnosing	
1. General sense that nursing diagnoses are "common sense" and, therefore, do not need to be put in writing → failure to address patient's real problems	1. Carefully develop and record priority nursing diagnoses for several patients and fairly evaluate whether this makes a difference in terms of the continuity of quality care.
2. General sense that nurses are too busy doing treatments, "passing meds," and doing paperwork to develop nursing diagnoses carefully → independent dimension of nursing remains underdeveloped	2. Examine practice and see whether *independent* nursing has a place; what percentage of every day is devoted to independent nursing functions? If this percentage is nonexistent or small, there understandably may be *no felt need* for nursing diagnoses—but a desperate need to revise practice priorities.
3. Nursing diagnoses are too vague to be helpful → routinized patient care	3. a. Revise the problem statement to describe more accurately what is *unhealthy* about the patient (the behavior that needs to be changed). b. Revise the etiology to more accurately identify what is making the problem a problem—this should be a guide to nursing intervention. c. Check NANDA lists.
4. Nursing diagnoses are not up to date → no one uses the plan of care	4. Have a process for periodically reviewing the plan of care to delete nursing diagnoses when problems have been resolved and to add a new diagnosis as needed.
Planning	
1. The plan of care contains only the standard knowledge most nurses would know without a written plan.	1. Make use of standardized (computerized) plans as a basis for care planning. Devote nursing energies to *individualizing* this plan.
2. The long-term goal is vague, standard; fails to make clear the discharge goal for this patient.	2. Practice writing specific long-term goals that clarify for all nurses the aim toward which all nursing care is directed (e.g., patient returns home ambulatory with walker, right hip incision healing, able to manage activities of daily living with minimal assistance from spouse).
3. The nursing outcomes, even if met, do not necessarily guarantee a resolution of the patient problem.	3. When writing goals, it often is helpful to develop outcomes related to etiologic factors. Because the stated etiology may be incomplete or inaccurate, it is essential that at least *one outcome* be written so that if it is achieved, the problem in the nursing diagnosis is resolved.
4. The outcomes are incorrectly developed; progress toward goal achievement is difficult to evaluate	4. After writing outcomes, check them against the following criteria: • Subject is the patient or some part of the patient. • The patient behavior is stated in observable, measurable terms. • Criteria of acceptable performance are specified. • Time criteria are included in notes.
5. Nursing orders are superficial → patient receives routinized care	5. Review nursing orders to ensure that they indicate the *specific* nursing strategies or interventions most likely to result in successful outcome achievement *for this patient* (e.g., particular comfort measures that are successful adjuncts to analgesic administration for a particular patient). In specifying the "who, what, when, where, how, and how much" of nursing interventions, be sure to list the type of equipment and supplies needed in various treatments. As new patient data are obtained, update nursing orders. Delete inappropriate or unnecessary orders.

(continued)

Problem	Nursing Response

TABLE • 16-2 COMMON PROBLEMS NOTED DURING EVALUATION OF THE NURSING PROCESS *(continued)*

Planning *(continued)*

6. The initial plan of care fails to be updated → plan of care will not be consulted by nurses—if used, it will be to patient's detriment

6. If personal accountability for updating plan fails, develop a process on the nursing unit to ensure care plan review and revision.

7. The plan of care addresses the immediate needs of the patient but fails to anticipate discharge needs → patient returns home unable to manage self-care activities

7. Work hard at developing the ability to project yourself into the patient's home after discharge. Learn to anticipate problems and concerns and prepare the patient and family for these. Use all discharge resources in the institution. Learn from patients what their needs were after previous discharge.

Implementing

1. Nurses are not aware of patient priorities and the plan of care; lack of continuity; inefficient use of nursing resources → patient fails to achieve goals/outcomes

1. a. Use shift report to update staff on status of priority nursing diagnosis and concomitant nursing care.
b. Review plan of care and nursing notes before beginning care.

2. Nursing care becomes routine and mechanized → patient never has the sense that he or she is personally known by nurses

2. Explore creative strategies to make quality nursing care on this particular unit a *challenge* rather than a *burden;* use ongoing education, problem-solving strategies by the nursing team, gaming, and other incentives.

3. Documentation is inadequate → because there is no complete written record of nursing care, *legally* this care was never provided.

3. a. Develop the philosophy that quality nursing care *deserves* to be documented. Review legal reasons for careful documentation.
b. Become familiar with the flow sheets and note format used within the work setting so that charting can be done quickly and comprehensively.

Evaluating

1. It is not done → mastery of nursing process is stunted; severely limits accomplishment of nursing aims.

1. Develop the belief that quality nursing care does not happen automatically and that only ongoing evaluation will identify needed areas of revision. Devise an evaluative strategy and carry it out. Study its effect on quality of care after 6 months' implementation.

---

achieved facilitates optimal function. For example, the initial outcome for a patient with the diagnosis "Impaired Physical Mobility" might be "patient transfers from the bed to the chair." After this is achieved, however, the outcome needs to be stepped up in complexity to "patient walks around room with support of walker."

The following evaluative statement might be noted, for example, if a patient did not meet the specified outcome: "Patient will participate in a minimum of two planned social activities per week beginning 9/16/12." "9/27/12—Outcome not met. Resident chose not to participate in any group activities this week." Many courses of action are then available to the nurse. Possible revisions to any plan of care include the following:

- *Delete or modify the nursing diagnosis.* This might not be a problem or concern for the resident. Evaluate and validate data pointing to the nursing diagnosis.
- *Make the outcome statement more realistic.* Carefully determine the resident's need for activities and ability or desire to participate in activities.
- *Adjust time criteria in outcome statement.* Reevaluate after 3 weeks; resident may need more time to adjust to being institutionalized and more encouragement.

- *Change nursing interventions.* Make a special effort to familiarize yourself with the resident's interests, and match these with available programs and activities.

Once the nurse, in partnership with the patient if possible, makes a decision about how to respond, this must be communicated to the patient or the patient's surrogate and to other members of the professional caregiving team, via the patient's record.

> *Think back to Mioshi Otsuki, the elderly woman taking too much diuretic. The home care nurse would work with the patient to develop a teaching plan about her heart failure, specifically related to her drug-therapy regimen. This plan then would be documented on the patient's record and communicated to all individuals involved in the patient's care, such as other home care agency nurses who may be on-call or filling in to visit the patient or home health aides involved in providing personal care and hygiene for the patient.* ■

EVALUATING QUALITY CARE

In addition to each nurse's evaluation of patient outcome achievement and subsequent modifications to the plan of care, many informal and formal mechanisms are used to ensure quality nursing care. See the ANA Standards for Quality of Practice and Professional Practice (Box 16-4).

Performance Improvement in Everyday Clinical Practice

It is not unusual for nurses to discover problems with the delivery of nursing care in their practice setting. The Institute of Medicine's Committee on Quality of Health Care in America (Kohn, Corrigan, & Donaldson, 2000) suggests 10 new rules to redesign and improve care:

1. Care based on continuous healing relationships
2. Customization based on patient needs and values
3. The patient as the source of control
4. Shared knowledge and the free flow of information
5. Evidence-based decision making
6. Safety as a system property
7. The need for transparency
8. Anticipation of needs
9. Continuous decrease in waste
10. Cooperation among clinicians

Each nurse must decide how to respond when it is perceived that patient care is being compromised. Nurses committed to healthier patients, quality care, reduced costs, and the personal satisfaction of knowing that they *are actually making a difference* versus merely *wishing things were different* value **performance improvement.** The following four steps are crucial in improving performance (Haase & Miller, 1999):

- Discover a problem.
- Plan a strategy using indicators.
- Implement a change.
- Assess the change; if the outcome is not met, plan a new strategy.

See Box 16-5 for an example of a performance-improvement strategy.

An important resource for nurses committed to performance improvement is *Quality and Safety Education for Nurses* (QSEN). The overall goal of QSEN initiatives is to prepare nurses who have the knowledge, skills, and attitudes

---

Box 16-4 **ANA STANDARDS OF PRACTICE: STANDARDS 7 AND 8, QUALITY OF PRACTICE AND PROFESSIONAL PRACTICE EVALUATION**

Quality of Practice
The registered nurse systematically enhances the quality and effectiveness of nursing practice.

Measurement Criteria
The registered nurse:

Demonstrates quality by documenting the application of the nursing process in a responsible, accountable, and ethical manner.

Uses the results of quality improvement activities to initiate changes in nursing practice and in the healthcare delivery system.

Incorporates new knowledge to initiate changes in nursing practice if desired outcomes are not achieved.

Participates in quality-improvement activities. Such activities may include:

Identifying aspects of practice important for quality monitoring.

Using indicators developed to monitor quality and effectiveness of nursing practice.

Collecting data to monitor quality and effectiveness of nursing practice.

Analyzing quality data to identify opportunities for improving nursing practice.

Formulating recommendations to improve nursing practice or outcomes.

Implementing activities to enhance the quality of nursing practice.

Developing, implementing, and evaluating policies, procedures, and/or guidelines to improve the quality of practice.

Participating on interdisciplinary teams to evaluate clinical care or health services.

Analyzing factors related to safety, satisfaction, effectiveness, and cost/benefit options.

Implementing processes to remove or decrease barriers within organizational systems.

Professional Practice Evaluation
The registered nurse evaluates one's own nursing practice in relation to professional practice standards and guidelines, relevant statutes, rules, and regulations.

Measurement Criteria
The registered nurse's practice reflects the application of knowledge of current practice standards, guidelines, rules, and regulations.
The registered nurse:

Provides age-appropriate care in a culturally and ethnically sensitive manner.

Engages in self-evaluation of practice on a regular basis, identifying areas of strength, as well as areas in which professional development would be beneficial.

Obtains informal feedback regarding one's own practice from patients, peers, professional colleagues, and others.

Participates in systematic peer review as appropriate.

Takes action to achieve goals identified during the evaluation process.

Provides rationales for practice beliefs, decisions, and actions as part of the informal and formal evaluation process.

Box 16-5   STEPS IN PERFORMANCE IMPROVEMENT

The following four steps are crucial in improving performance:

- **Discover a problem**
  Advance directives are a powerful legal tool for people to indicate their end-of-life care preferences. Nurses on an oncology unit are becoming frustrated because many of the patients on their unit lack advance directives. By the time decisions need to be made about ventilators, coding, dialysis, and so forth, patients are often no longer able to communicate their preferences. The hospital has a policy about advance directives, but no one seems to be taking responsibility for initiating discussions with patients when they are first admitted.
- **Plan a strategy using indicators**
  The nurses call an interdisciplinary meeting with the oncologists, social workers, and pastors, who decide that the nurse case manager will be responsible for working with patients on admission to see if they want help in preparing an advance directive. Each case manager will be responsible for

documenting within 48 hours of admission the patient's decision regarding an advance directive. Staff nurses will be able to direct patient and family requests to do advance planning to the case manager and appropriate team members. The ethics committee was asked to do an in-service on advance directives for the team.

- **Implement a change**
  Case managers begin assuming this responsibility, and one nurse volunteers to monitor progress at 3-month intervals by checking charts for advance directive content and by speaking with the staff nurses who voiced the initial frustration about decision making.
- **Assess the change**
  If the goal is not met, plan a new strategy. At the end of 6 months, everyone seems satisfied that the new plan is working, but a decision is made to schedule a 6-month follow-up evaluation to prevent backsliding.

Four-step process from Haase, R., & Miller, K. (1999). Performance improvement in everyday clinical practice. *American Journal of Nursing, 99*(5), 52, 54.

(KSAs) necessary to continuously improve the quality and safety of the healthcare systems within which they work. Visit their Web site (www.qsen.org) to view a variety of educational materials.

Peer review, the evaluation of one staff member by another staff member on the same level in the hierarchy of the organization, is an important mechanism nurses can use to improve their professional performance. This can be done formally or informally by inviting a peer you respect to give you feedback on nursing skills you are trying to develop. "How do you think that session went with the patient's daughter? She's been so critical of us and I'm trying to understand the situation from her point of view and respond appropriately."

Establishing and Sustaining Healthy Work Environments

According to the study *Silence Kills: The Seven Crucial Conversations for Healthcare* (Maxfield, Grenny, Patterson, McMillan, & Switzler, 2005), the prevalent culture of poor communication and collaboration among health professionals relates significantly to continued medical errors and staff turnover. Additionally, a lack of adequate support systems, skills, and personal accountability results in communication gaps that can cause harm to patients. Results of the national study conducted by the American Association of Critical-Care Nurses and VitalSmarts of more than 1,700 health professionals include:

- 84% of physicians and 62% of nurses and other clinical-care providers have seen coworkers taking shortcuts that could be dangerous to patients.
- 88% of physicians and 48% of nurses and other providers work with people who show poor clinical judgment.
- Fewer than 10% of physicians, nurses, and other clinical staff directly confront their colleagues about their concerns,

and one in five physicians said they have seen harm come to patients as a result.

- The 10% of healthcare workers who raise these crucial concerns observe better patient outcomes, work harder, and are more satisfied and are more committed to staying in their jobs (Executive Summary).

The study pinpoints seven categories of communication problems that are frequently encountered, yet rarely addressed. See Table 16-3 for examples of the seven crucial conversations in healthcare that nurses and other professionals must learn to master. If you find yourself in one of these situations, be sure to ask an experienced and trusted colleague how best to respond and don't accept as a response, "Spare yourself some grief and do nothing."

The American Association of Critical-Care Nurses' (AACN) commitment *to actively promote the creation of healthy work environments that support and foster excellence in patient care* is a superb example of nursing leadership. Citing the mounting evidence that unhealthy work environments contribute to medical errors, ineffective delivery of care, and conflict and stress among health professionals, AACN President Kathleen M. McCauley wrote:

> Negative, demoralizing and unsafe conditions in workplaces cannot be allowed to continue. The creation of healthy work environments is imperative to ensure patient safety, enhance staff recruitment and retention, and maintain an organization's financial viability. . . . The public has repeatedly identified nurses as the profession most trusted to act honestly and ethically. Five times since 1999 nurses have topped Gallup's annual survey of honest and ethics among professions (Moore, 2004). The public relies on nurses to bring about bold change that assures safe patient care and sets a path toward excellence. (AACN, 2005, p. 4)

See Box 16-6 for AACN's six essential standards for establishing and sustaining healthy work environments. The

TABLE • 16-3	THE SEVEN CRUCIAL CONVERSATIONS IN HEALTHCARE	
Category of Conversation	**Examples**	**Recommendations**
1. Broken rules	Colleague fails to wash hands.	Confront your colleague and tell her that you noticed that she failed to wash her hands and that this could be harmful to herself, the patient, or other patients. If the behavior continues, report your concerns to the nurse manager and work up the chain of command.
2. Mistakes	Nurse administers medication to the wrong patient and asks you to keep an eye on him or her for adverse reactions. She does not plan to report the error.	Tell your colleague that you'll be happy to help watch the patient but that a full report needs to be made. If appropriate, help your colleague identify what contributed to her giving the medication to the wrong patient.
3. Lack of support	Nurse refuses to help a colleague move an obese patient although she has time to do so.	Explain to this nurse that teamwork is essential to good outcomes and that her behavior is simply unacceptable. "When we have patients with special needs and need all hands on deck, everyone who's free is obligated to help out!" Develop and enforce zero tolerance for selfish behavior.
4. Incompetence	Nurse fails to correctly administer dialysis. She wasn't finished with her orientation to the unit and attempted a procedure before she was prepared to do it solo.	In addition to reporting the error, help the nurse identify that overconfidence in one's abilities can have deadly results for patients. The nurse manager will need to address the incompetence.
5. Poor teamwork	A particularly difficult family is splitting the team by choosing (and rewarding) favorites among the staff and complaining to them about other workers. The staff is encouraging this behavior.	Someone needs to call the team together and name the divisive behavior and get everyone working together again. If there is staff who are problematic, appropriate channels need to be used to address these behaviors.
6. Disrespect	When a student nurse asks a physician if she has time to answer a few questions for her patient, the physician screams at her and tells her that she has more important things to do than babysit her patient and tells the student to find someone else to answer the questions.	The student should calmly tell the physician that her response is inappropriate and that she is entitled to respectful conversation, then seek the counsel of an experienced nurse. The physician's behavior should be reported.
7. Micromanagement	A student asks her clinical preceptor, "will you walk me through this procedure before I do it, since it's my first time." The preceptor then takes over, and does the procedure for the student and starts watching her every move.	The student should inform her preceptor that she merely wanted to review the steps of the procedure to make sure that she would perform it correctly and that it is essential for the student to gain experience by trying new procedures. If the preceptor's behavior does not change, the student should seek the counsel of her instructor.

Adapted from Maxfield, D., Grenny, J., Patterson, K., McMillan, R., & Switzler, A. (2005). Silence Kills. Available at: http://www.aacn.org/WD/Practice/Docs/PublicPolicy/SilenceKillsExecSum.pdf

standards represent *evidence-based* and *relationship-centered* principles of professional performance. Each standard is considered essential because studies show that effective and sustainable outcomes do not emerge when any standard is considered optional. For copies of the *Silence Kills* report and the AACN Standards for Establishing and Sustaining Healthy Work Environments, visit http://www.aacn.org.

Evaluative Programs

In the United States, regulatory agencies, such as state boards of nursing, the Joint Commission, the Professional Standards Review Organization, and the National Health Planning and Resources Development Act of 1975, require nurses to document that nursing standards are being implemented and maintained. Each of these agencies is concerned with quality care and quality control. The decreased availability of resources to treat patients in hospitals and the unavailability of sufficient alternative treatment settings pose a strong challenge to the nursing profession to find ways to avoid compromising quality of care. Numerous professional organizations are working to meet this challenge (see Table 16-4: National Quality Initiatives and Table 16-5: Selected Web Resources for Patients and Families).

Box 16-6 | THE AMERICAN ASSOCIATION OF CRITICAL-CARE NURSES STANDARDS FOR ESTABLISHING AND SUSTAINING HEALTHY WORK ENVIRONMENTS

- **Skilled Communication.** Nurses must be as proficient in communication skills as they are in clinical skills.
- **True Collaboration.** Nurses must be relentless in pursuing and fostering true collaboration.
- **Effective Decision Making.** Nurses must be valued and committed partners in making policy, directing and evaluating clinical care, and leading organizational operations.

- **Appropriate Staffing.** Staffing must ensure the effective match between patient needs and nurse competencies.
- **Meaningful Recognition.** Nurses must be recognized and must recognize others for the value each brings to the work of the organization.
- **Authentic Leadership.** Nurse leaders must fully embrace the imperativeness of a healthy work environment, authentically live it, and engage others in its achievement.

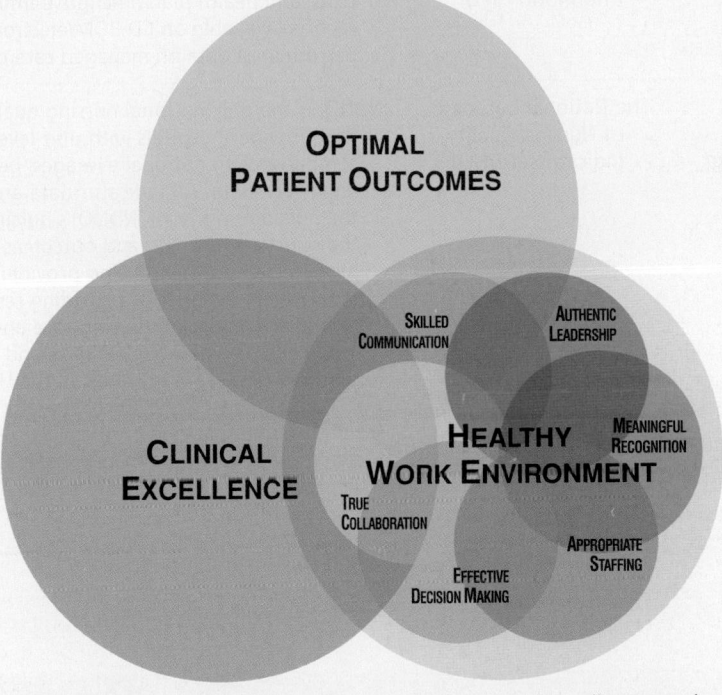

Interdependence of a healthy work environment, clinical excellence, and optimal patient outcomes.

Used with permission from American Association of Critical-Care Nurses (AACN). (2005). *AACN standards for establishing and sustaining healthy work environments: A journey to excellence* (pp. 13–14). Aliso Viejo, CA: Author.

Quality Assurance

Specially designed programs that promote excellence in nursing are called **quality-assurance programs.** These range from small programs conducted by nurses on a small nursing unit to those developed for an entire institution, state, province, or country.

Quality-assurance programs enable nursing to be accountable to society for the quality of nursing care. Such programs are also a response to the public mandate for professional accountability. They ensure survival of the profession, encourage nursing's fidelity to its moral and ethical responsibilities, and assist nursing to comply with other external pressures.

There are two different approaches to ensuring quality. *Quality by inspection* focuses on finding deficient workers and removing them. Nurses and others working in this type of setting may be afraid to admit a mistake or error and wrongly attempt to hide a problem. Such behavior is never acceptable and may result in serious harm to patients. *Quality*

as opportunity, on the other hand, focuses on finding opportunities for improvement and fosters an environment that thrives on teamwork, with people sharing the skills and lessons they have learned. Mistakes are viewed not as being caused by a lack of motivation or lack of effort by a worker but rather as a result of a problem in the system. In this work environment, nurses respond with openness and a desire to learn because their integrity and self-worth are not threatened. Our outcome should be to work in an environment in which quality measurements encourage our best efforts.

The American Nurses Association (ANA) in 1975 developed a model quality-assurance program consisting of seven steps: (1) identify values; (2) identify structure, process, and outcome standards and criteria; (3) measure the degree of attainment of criteria and standards; (4) make interpretations about strengths and weaknesses based on such measurements; (5) identify possible courses of action; (6) choose a course of action; and (7) take action. The ANA hoped the

TABLE • 16-4   NATIONAL QUALITY INITIATIVES

Organization	Initiative	Description
The Joint Commission http://www.jointcommission.org/ AccreditationPrograms/ Hospitals/ORYX/	ORYX	Integrates use of outcomes and performance measures into accreditation process; requires accredited hospitals and long-term care agencies to identify two clinical measures related to at least 20% of patient population; number of measures and percentage of patient population will increase each year.
NCQA (National Committee for Quality Assurance) Accrediting body for managed care http://www.ncqa.org	HEDIS (Health Plan Employer Data and Information Set)	HEDIS targets these areas: effectiveness of care, access and availability of care, patient satisfaction, health plan stability, use of services, costs, and health plan descriptive information. Quality Compass reports (available on CD-ROM/electronic data file) include performance data on managed care plans.
ANA (American Nurses Association) https://www.nursingquality.org/	The National Database of Nursing Quality Indicators (NDNQI®)	NDNQI is the only national nursing quality measurement program that provides hospitals with unit-level performance reports with comparisons to national averages, percentile rankings, and other important data. All indicator data are collected and reported at the nursing-unit level. NDNQI's nursing-sensitive indicators reflect the structure, process, and outcomes of nursing care. NDNQI's mission is to aid the nursing provider in patient safety and quality improvement efforts by providing research-based national comparative data on nursing care and the relationship to patient outcomes. The database collects and evaluates unit-specific nurse-sensitive data from hospitals in the United States.
Centers for Medicine and Medicaid Services http://www.cms.hhs.gov/ oasis/default.asp	OASIS (Outcome and Assessment Information Set)	Set of assessment questions to collect clinical, financial, and administrative data in home health agencies. Goals of OASIS: to improve quality of care delivered to home healthcare patients and to provide data to HCFA.

TABLE • 16-5   SELECTED WEB RESOURCES FOR PATIENTS AND FAMILIES

Organization	Internet Address	Available Information
Agency for Health Care Research and Quality (AHRQ)	http://www.ahrq.gov http://www.ahrq.gov/consumer http://www.ahrq.gov/consumer/ insuranceqa/ http://www.ahrq.gov/consumer/ qualguid.pdf *or* http://www.ahrq.gov/consumer/ qnt/ http://www.ahrq.gov/consumer/ quick.htm	Website includes links to health information for consumers. Healthfinder is a gateway for health information with many links. Consumer versions of clinical practice guidelines by condition available at site. Consumer guide for choosing and using a health plan "Your Guide to Choosing Quality Health Care" is a comprehensive consumer reference for choosing health plans, physicians, treatments, hospitals, and long-term care (PDF file). "Quick Checks for Quality" is a short guide for determining quality in healthcare.
Joint Commission	http://www.jointcommission.org http://www.qualitycheck.org	General public menu includes information about reporting a complaint about a healthcare organization, making healthcare choices, and performance measurement. With Quality Check, consumers can retrieve information about how Joint Commission-accredited organizations have been rated in areas such as patient rights, infection control, and others.
National Committee for Quality Assurance (NCQA)	http://www.ncqa.org/tabid/60/ Default.aspx	NCQA Consumer Page includes links to information on healthcare organizations. Consumers can search NCQA's accreditation status list and see if their health plan has an accreditation summary report.

model would be used to develop and implement quality-assurance programs within institutions.

The ANA model directs attention to three essential components of quality care: structure, process, and outcome. Other types of quality-assurance programs may focus only on one of these components or on a mixture of components.

STRUCTURE

A **structure evaluation** or audit focuses on the environment in which care is provided. Standards describe physical facilities and equipment; organizational characteristics, policies, and procedures; fiscal resources; and personnel resources.

PROCESS

The focus of the **process evaluation** is the nature and sequence of activities carried out by nurses implementing the nursing process. Criteria make explicit acceptable levels of performance for nursing actions related to patient assessment, diagnosis, planning, implementation, and evaluation.

OUTCOME

Outcome evaluation focuses on measurable changes in the health status of the patient or the end results of nursing care. Whereas the proper environment for care and the right nursing actions are important aspects of quality care, the critical element in evaluating care is demonstrable changes in patient health status.

From Quality Assurance to Quality Improvement

Concern about the spiraling costs of healthcare, coupled with the success of industrial models for quality improvement, led to a strong commitment to quality improvement in the 1990s. **Quality improvement** (also known as continuous quality improvement [CQI] or total quality management [TQM]) is "the commitment and approach used to continuously improve every process in every part of an organization, with the intent of meeting and exceeding customer expectations and outcomes" (Schroeder, 1994, p. 3). Unlike quality assurance, quality improvement is internally driven, focuses on patient care rather than organizational structure, focuses on processes rather than individuals, and has no end points. Its outcome is *improving* quality rather than *assuring* quality. The major premises of quality improvement are as follows (Schroeder, 1994, pp. 5–8):

- Focus on organizational mission
- Continuous improvement
- Customer orientation
- Leadership commitment
- Empowerment
- Collaboration/crossing boundaries
- Focus on process
- Focus on data and statistical thinking

From the patient's point of view, one of the most important outcomes of quality improvement is the recognition that patient satisfaction is as important as customer satisfaction in retail business. With increased competition for the healthcare dollar, providers are learning that it is important to offer services that patients value and to offer them in a way that is valued by patients. By reemphasizing the critical nature of nursing's *person* versus *task* orientation, quality improvement underscores the need for nurses to blend cognitive, technical, interpersonal, and ethical/legal skills successfully.

Patient Satisfaction

An evaluative program that focuses on patient satisfaction is a powerful tool for patients and families who want to know what care will be like before choosing a healthcare facility. Hospital Consumer Assessment of Healthcare Providers and Systems (HCAHPS), the Centers for Medicare and Medicaid Services patient satisfaction program, is the first national, standardized, publicly reported survey of patients' perspectives of hospital care. The program provides consumers with information about a hospital's performance in key areas of communication, pain control, timeliness of care, discharge instructions, hospital cleanliness, and treatment with courtesy and respect. First, the survey is designed to produce data about patients' perspectives of care that allow objective and meaningful comparisons of hospitals on topics that are important to consumers. Second, public reporting of the survey results creates new incentives for hospitals to improve quality of care. Third, public reporting serves to enhance public accountability in healthcare by increasing the transparency of the quality of hospital care provided in return for the public investment.

Are you helping or hurting your hospital? With your first clinical rotation, you can ask yourself how you think your patients would respond if asked the following questions: During this hospital stay, how often did nurses (1) treat you with courtesy and respect? (2) listen carefully to you? (3) explain things in a way you could understand? (Never, Sometimes, Usually, or Always?) And (4) During this hospital stay, after you pressed the call button, how often did you get help as soon as you wanted it? (Never, Sometimes, Usually, Always, or I never pressed the call button?) You can see how your local hospitals compare by searching the website www.hospitalcompare.hhs.gov. To learn more about HCAHPS visit www.cms.hhs.gov/HospitalQualityInits/.

Nursing Audit

A **nursing audit** is a method of evaluating nursing care that involves reviewing patient records to assess the outcomes of nursing care or the process by which these outcomes were achieved. Successful nursing audits depend on careful nursing documentation.

Concurrent Versus Retrospective Evaluation

Nursing care and patient outcomes may be evaluated while the patient is receiving care (i.e., a concurrent evaluation) or after the patient has been discharged (i.e., a retrospective evaluation). **Concurrent evaluation** is conducted by using direct observation of nursing care, patient interviews, and chart review to determine whether the specified evaluative criteria are met.

Retrospective evaluation may use postdischarge questionnaires, patient interviews (by telephone or face to face), or chart review (nursing audit) to collect data. The type of retrospective audit most familiar to nurses working in hospitals is the Joint Commission retrospective chart review. This accrediting body initially required hospitals to conduct a certain number of audits per year.

SUMMARY

The cultivation of evaluation as a critical component of the nursing process ensures nursing's continued success in achieving desired changes in patient health status.

> ➤ *Recall Nicholas Soros, the patient described in the Reflective Practice display. The nurse's commitment to teaching and follow-up demonstrates concern for the patient and his needs. Success would be possible only if the nurse modifies the plan, works with the patient, and realizes the need for the patient to value his own health while respecting his independence and individuality.* ∎

Only a firm commitment to evaluation enables nurses to answer the following questions:

- What are the patient's outcomes?
- What are nursing's values?
- How can these values be formalized in standards and evaluative criteria?
- What data exist to determine whether the specified evaluative criteria are being met?
- How can these data best be collected, analyzed, and interpreted?
- To what courses of action do the findings lead?

Nursing actions are far too valuable and costly resources to be haphazardly implemented. Evaluation that is carefully planned and executed can direct and redirect these actions to maximize the patient's benefit. This is the outcome and challenge of nursing evaluation. Criteria that might be helpful in determining the adequacy of the evaluation step of the nursing process include the following:

- Evaluation of the patient's achievement of desired outcomes
- Review of how the process is used and revision of the plan of care, if necessary
- Participation in quality-assurance programs

● Developing Critical Thinking Skills

1. Interview five students who have personal fitness outcomes. Ask them to describe what personal factors have helped or hindered their achieving their outcomes. Note commonalities and differences. Reflect on how you can help patients tap their own personal strengths to achieve their outcomes more successfully.

2. Interview several patients and ask them what qualities in a nurse are most helpful as they try to achieve their health outcomes. Similarly, ask what nurse qualities are most problematic. Reflect on how you measure up in terms of both positive and negative nurse qualities.

3. Interview three or more experienced nurses in the same practice setting. Ask them what system variables (such as philosophy of care, nurse-to-patient ratio, professional and nonprofessional staff mix, nursing management, adequacy of resources) most influence their ability to deliver quality care. Identify variables you want to look for when you interview for a job.

4. How might nurses use the AACN standards and crucial conversation recommendations to change the outcomes in the following situations:
   - A nurse knows that a patient's pain medication isn't working but decides not to call his attending physician because the physician was verbally abusive to her in the past and believes his patients "don't need analgesics."
   - A new policy was developed to make sure that obese patients are transferred safely without harm to themselves or staff. The nurse manager places the new policy in the policy manual but fails to educate staff in the new bariatric unit. Moreover, some nurses have been quite vocal about not putting themselves at risk with these patients and have refused to participate in collaborative efforts to move these patients safely.
   - Two nurses call in sick and staffing is at an all-time low. Additional patients are added to each nurse's assignment, increasing the probability that errors will be made. The nurses are frustrated and angry.

● Practicing for NCLEX

1. Jeanne is a college student who wants to lose 20 pounds. She meets with the student health nurse and develops a plan to increase her activity level and decrease the consumption of the wrong types of foods and excess calories. The nurse plans to evaluate her weight loss monthly. When Jeanne arrives for her first "weigh-in," the nurse discovers that instead of the projected weight loss of 5 pounds, Jeanne has only lost 1 pound. Which is the best nursing response?
   a. Congratulate Jeanne and continue the plan of care.
   b. Terminate the plan of care since it is not working.
   c. Try giving Jeanne more time to reach the targeted outcome.
   d. Modify the plan of care after discussing possible reasons for Jeanne's partial success.

2. The following are all classic elements of evaluation. Which item below places them in their correct sequence?
   (1) Interpreting and summarizing findings
   (2) Collecting data to determine whether evaluative criteria and standards are met
   (3) Documenting your judgment
   (4) Terminating, continuing, or modifying the plan

(5) Identifying evaluative criteria and standards (what you are looking for when you evaluate, e.g., expected patient outcomes)
  a. (1), (2), (3), (4), (5)
  b. (3), (2), (1), (4), (5)
  c. (5), (2), (1), (3), (4)
  d. (2), (3), (1), (4), (5)

3. When a new nurse is oriented to the subacute unit, she is told that each nurse is expected to observe her patients at least every hour, and more if their condition warrants extra monitoring. This expectation is best termed:
  a. Standard
  b. Criteria
  c. Custom
  d. Order

4. Remember Jeanne, the college student who wants to lose 20 pounds? When the nurse weighs her during the fifth step of the nursing process, what is she doing?
  a. Collecting assessment data to identify health problems
  b. Collecting assessment data to identify patient strengths
  c. Collecting evaluative data to justify terminating the plan of care
  d. Collecting evaluative data to measure outcome achievement

5. One of the outcomes Jeanne and the nurse planned is that Jeanne "appreciates or values a healthy body sufficiently to try to new behaviors." Which of the following best describes this type of outcome?
  a. Cognitive
  b. Psychomotor
  c. Affective
  d. Physical changes

6. Another of the outcomes Jeanne and the nurse planned is that Jeanne "can explain the relationship between weight loss, increased exercise, and decreased calorie intake." Which of the following best describes this type of outcome?
  a. Cognitive
  b. Psychomotor
  c. Affective
  d. Physical changes

7. Which of the following is the correct example of an evaluative statement?
  a. "Outcome not met."
  b. "1/21/09—Patient reports no change in tobacco use."
  c. "Outcome not met. Patient reports no change in tobacco use."
  d. "1/21/09—Outcome not met. Patient reports no change in tobacco use."

8. A quality-assurance program reveals a higher incidence of falls and other safety violations on a particular unit. A nurse manager states, "We'd better find the folks responsible for these errors and see if we can't replace them." This is an example of which of the following?
  a. Quality by inspection
  b. Quality by punishment
  c. Quality by surveillance
  d. Quality by opportunity

9. One nursing unit with an excellent safety record meets to review the findings of the audit and the nurse manager states, "We're doing well, but we can do better! Who's got an idea to foster increased patient well-being and satisfaction?" This is an example of leadership that values which of the following?
  a. Quality assurance
  b. Quality improvement
  c. Process evaluation
  d. Outcome evaluation

● Answers With Rationale

1. *d.* Since Jeanne has only partially met her outcome, the nurse should first explore the factors making it difficult for Jeanne to reach her outcome and then modify the plan of care. It would not be appropriate to continue the plan as it is since it is not working (*a*), and it is premature to terminate the plan of care (*b*) since Jeanne has not met her targeted outcome. Jeanne may need more than time to reach her outcome, which makes (*c*) the wrong response.

2. *c.* This is a sequenced list.

3. *a,* standard, the levels of performance accepted and expected by the nursing staff or other health team members. Criteria (*b*) are measurable qualities, attributes, or characteristics that specify skills, knowledge, or health states. Custom (*c*) sometimes establishes standards. Orders (*d*) are written to address the special needs of the patient.

4. *d,* collecting evaluative data to measure outcome achievement. While this may justify terminating the plan of care (*c*), that is not necessarily so. Assessment data (*a, b*) are collected during the first step of the nursing process.

5. *c.* Affective outcomes pertain to changes in patient values, beliefs, and attitudes. Cognitive outcomes (*a*) involve increases in patient knowledge; psychomotor outcomes (*b*) describe the patient's achievement of new skills; physical changes (*d*) are actually bodily changes in the patient (e.g., weight loss, increased muscle tone).

6. *a.* Cognitive outcomes involve increases in patient knowledge; psychomotor outcomes (*b*) describe the patient's achievement of new skills; affective outcomes (*c*) pertain to changes in patient values, beliefs, and attitudes; and physical changes (*d*) are actually bodily changes in the patient (e.g., weight loss, increased muscle tone).

7. *d.* The evaluative statement contains a date; the words "outcome met," "outcome partially met," or "outcome

not met," and the patient data or behaviors that support this decision. Answers *a*, *b*, and *c* are incomplete statements.

8. *a.* Quality by inspection focuses on finding deficient workers and removing them. Quality as opportunity (*d*) focuses on finding opportunities for improvement and fosters an environment that thrives on teamwork, with people sharing the skills and lessons they have learned. Answers *b* and *c* are distractors.

9. *b.* Unlike quality assurance (*a*), quality improvement is internally driven, focuses on patient care rather than organizational structure, focuses on processes rather than individuals, and has no end points. Its outcome is improving quality rather than assuring quality. Answers *c* and *d* are types of quality-assurance programs.

Taylor Suite Resources

The Taylor Suite offers these additional resources to enhance learning and facilitate understanding of this chapter:

- thePoint online resource, http://thepoint.lww.com/Taylor7E
- Student DVD-ROM included with the book
- Study Guide for Taylor's Fundamentals of Nursing

BIBLIOGRAPHY

Alfaro-LeFevre, R. (2009). *Critical thinking and clinical judgment: A practical approach* (4th ed.). St. Louis: Saunders Elsevier.

Alfaro-LeFevre, R. (2010). *Applying nursing process: A tool for critical thinking* (7th ed.). Philadelphia: Lippincott Williams & Wilkins.

American Association of Critical-Care Nurses (AACN). (2005). *AACN standards for establishing and sustaining healthy work environments: A journey to excellence.* Aliso Viejo, CA: Author.

American Nurses Association (ANA). (1975). *A plan for implementation of the standards of nursing practice.* Kansas City, MO: Author.

American Nurses Association (ANA). (1976). *ANA quality assurance workbook.* Kansas City, MO: Author.

American Nurses Association (ANA). (1994). *Guidelines on reporting incompetent, unethical or illegal practices.* Washington, DC: ANA.

American Nurses Association (ANA). (1999). *Nursing quality indicators: Guide for implementation* (2nd ed.). Washington, DC: Author.

American Nurses Association (ANA). (2001). *Code for nurses with interpretive statements.* Washington, DC: Author.

American Nurses Association (ANA). (2003). *Nursing: A social policy statement* (2nd ed.). Washington, DC: Author.

American Nurses Association (ANA). (2004). *Scope and standards of practice* (5th ed.). Washington, DC: Author.

Bloch, D. (1975). Evaluation of nursing care in terms of process and outcome: Issues in research and quality assurance. *Nursing Research, 24,* 256–263.

Donabedian, A. (1980). *The definition of quality and its approaches.* Ann Arbor, MI: Health Administration Press.

Donabedian, A. (1982). *The criteria and standards of quality: Explorations in quality assessment and monitoring.* Ann Arbor, MI: Health Administration Press.

Haase, R., & Miller, K. (1999). Performance improvement in everyday clinical practice. *American Journal of Nursing, 99*(5), 52, 54.

HealthGrades, Inc. (2004). *HealthGrades Quality Study: Patient safety in American hospitals.* Golden, CO: Author.

Institute of Medicine. (1999). *Measuring the quality of health care.* Washington, DC: National Academy Press.

Institute of Medicine. (2001). *Crossing the quality chasm: A new health system for the 21st century.* Washington, DC: National Academy Press.

Institute of Medicine. (2007). *Advancing QI research: Challenges and opportunities.* Washington, DC: National Academies Press.

Institute of Medicine. (2008). Knowing what works in healthcare: A roadmap for the nation. Washington, DC: National Academies Press.

Joint Commission. (2009). Comprehensive accreditation manual for hospitals. Available at: http://www.jointcommission.org/Standards/Manuals/

Kohn, L. T., Corrigan, J. M., & Donaldson, M. S. (Eds.), Committee on Quality of Health Care in America, Institute of Medicine. (2000). *To err is human: Building a safer health system.* Washington, DC: National Academy Press.

Manojlovich, M., & DeCicco, B. (2007). Healthy work environments, nurse-physician communication, and patients' outcomes. *American Journal of Critical Care, 16*(6), 536–543.

Maxfield, D., Grenny, J., Patterson, K., McMillan, R., & Switzler, A. (2005). *Silence kills: The seven crucial conversations for healthcare.* Available at: http://www.aacn.org/WD/Practice/Docs/PublicPolicy/SilenceKillsExecSum.pdf

Moore, D. W. (2008). Nurses top list in honesty and ethics poll. Gallup News Service. Available at: http://www.gallup.com/poll/1654/honesty-ethics-professions.aspx

Oermann, M. H., & Huber, D. (1999). Patient outcomes: A measure of nursing's value. *American Journal of Nursing, 99*(9), 40–48.

Peters, D. (1991). Measuring quality: Inspection or opportunity? *Holistic Nursing Practice, 5*(3), 1–7.

Phaneuf, M. (1976a). *The nursing audit: Self-regulation in nursing practice.* New York: Appleton-Century-Crofts.

Phaneuf, M. (1976b). Quality assurance: A nursing view. *New Zealand Nursing Journal, 69*(2), 9–11.

Ratz, M., Bostick, J., & Riggs, C. J. (2002). *Nursing quality measurement: A review of nursing studies 1995–2000.* Washington, DC: American Nurses Association.

Salmon, M. (2007). Care, quality and safety: Same old? *Nursing Outlook, 55*(3), 117–119.

Schroeder, P. (1994). *Improving quality and performance: Concepts, programs, and techniques.* St. Louis, MO: C. V. Mosby.

Wright, D. (1984). An introduction to the evaluation of nursing care: A review of literature. *Journal of Advanced Nursing, 9*(5), 457–467.

Documenting, Reporting, Conferring, and Using Informatics

17

PHILLIPPE BARON

Phillippe is a 52-year-old man being discharged from the outpatient surgery department after undergoing a colonoscopy for removal of three polyps. He will be going home with his wife, who is a nurse, and they both require discharge teaching.

MILLIE DELONG

Millie, a 44-year-old woman, develops a wound infection following abdominal surgery. Wound care with normal saline irrigations is ordered 4 times a day.

JASON CHANDLER

Jason, 15 years old and in police custody, is brought to the emergency department for treatment because he allegedly consumed a handful of individually wrapped crack rocks (estimated to be about 30 rocks) to avoid arrest. Treatment with insertion of nasogastric tube and bowel preparation solution is ordered. Jason is refusing treatment because he denies possession of drugs entirely.

After completing the chapter, you will be able to accomplish the following:

1. List guidelines for effective documentation.

2. Identify measures to protect confidential patient information.

3. Identify abbreviations and symbols commonly used for charting.

4. Describe the purposes of patient records.

5. Compare and contrast different methods of documentation: source-oriented record; problem-oriented record; PIE—problem, intervention, evaluation; focus charting; charting by exception; case management model; and computerized records.

6. Describe the purpose and correct use of each of the following formats for nursing documentation: nursing assessment, nursing care plan, critical/collaborative pathways, progress notes, flow sheets, discharge summary, and home care documentation.

7. Document nursing interventions completely, accurately, currently, concisely, and factually—avoiding legal problems.

8. Describe the nurse's role in communicating with other healthcare professionals by reporting and conferring.

9. Describe nursing informatics and its contributions to nursing and healthcare.

KEY TERMS

change-of-shift report

charting by exception (CBE)

collaborative pathway

confer

consultation

critical pathway

discharge summary

documentation

electronic medical record (EMR)

flow sheet

focus charting

graphic sheet

incident report

minimum data set

narrative notes

nursing informatics

OASIS

patient record

personal health record (PHR)

PIE charting

problem-oriented medical record (POMR)

progress notes

referral

SBAR communication

SOAP format

source-oriented record

variance charting

Effective communication among healthcare professionals is essential to the coordination and continuity of care. Communicating effectively enables personnel to support and to complement one another's services and to avoid duplications and omissions in care. This chapter describes three methods of communication central to nurses' professional role: documenting, reporting, and conferring, as well as some of the newer informatics technologies that are assisting communication. The first day you care for patients, you will find yourself conferring with colleagues, recording your interventions, and reporting on your patient's progress toward valued goals and outcomes. As you develop these skills, you will quickly see a link between communicating information and thinking critically. As you document data, you are looking for relationships and patterns—things that might otherwise be overlooked. As you confer with the patient and the patient's family and professional caregivers, you might learn something about the patient or situation that enhances your data set and clarifies the patient's health problem and related need for care (see the accompanying Reflective Practice box for an example). This chapter will help you assume these responsibilities with greater confidence and skill. The communication process itself and specific communication techniques are discussed in Chapter 21.

DOCUMENTING CARE

Documentation is the written or typed legal record of all pertinent interactions with the patient—assessing, diagnosing, planning, implementing, and evaluating. Increasingly sophisticated management information systems are being designed to manage patient-specific data and information. These records contain data used to facilitate patient care, serve as financial and legal records, help in clinical research, and support decision analysis. Information specialists aim to create an environment that supports timely, accurate, secure, and confidential recording and use of patient-specific information.

The **patient record** is a compilation of a patient's health information. Each healthcare institution or agency has policies that specify the nurse's documentation responsibilities. The Joint Commission (2010) specifies that nursing care data related to patient assessments, nursing diagnoses or patient needs, nursing interventions, and patient outcomes are permanently integrated into the patient record. Each nurse is expected to practice according to local policies and professional standards.

Guidelines for Effective Documentation

The patient record is the only permanent legal document that details the nurse's interactions with the patient and is the nurse's best defense if a patient or patient surrogate alleges nursing negligence. Unfortunately, there are often crucial omissions in the nursing documentation, along with meaningless repetitious or inaccurate entries. Although these errors might go undetected and have no effect on the patient, they might also seriously affect the care the patient receives,

(text continues on page 327)

REFLECTIVE PRACTICE
Challenge to Ethical and Legal Skills

Working in the emergency department (ED) this summer never ceased to amaze me. Police brought Jason Chandler to the ED, a 15-year-old male who was in custody for drug charges. Apparently, as police approached Jason, he consumed a handful of individually wrapped crack rocks (estimated to be about 30 rocks) to avoid arrest. He was brought to the ED as a precaution. If this bag broke inside his gastrointestinal tract, it would obviously have serious consequences. Jason was refusing treatment because he denied the possession of drugs entirely. The ED attending physician was unsure of his legal rights for treating the boy and called the hospital attorney. The attorney said the doctor could force treatment if there were probable signs that ingestion had occurred. However, the boy was not showing any clinical manifestations of chemical ingestion. This was a dilemma because if the bag of drugs burst open inside the boy, the physician stated that he most likely would not survive. The legal issue was whether or not the officer's statement of witnessing the ingestion was enough to constitute the need for treatment. The doctor was about to begin treating the patient when his mother arrived, threatening to sue anyone and everyone who "touched her little boy."

My preceptor and I were assigned to this patient and were given orders to insert a nasogastric (NG) tube so that a bowel preparation solution (GoLYTELY) could be used to flush out the drugs. The hospital attorney concluded that there was probable cause to justify forced treatment. However, the mother was furious and said she would sue under these circumstances, despite what the doctor or attorney said. As we entered the room to insert the NG tube and begin treatment, the boy, who was handcuffed to the bed, was screaming at us not to touch him.

Thinking Outside the Box: Possible Courses of Action

- Go with my preceptor and assist with the NG tube insertion.
- Refuse to treat the patient for fear of becoming part of a lawsuit.
- Allow my preceptor to sedate the patient against his will, to make the NG tube insertion easier.

- Inform the physician that I do not feel comfortable proceeding with treatment on a patient who refuses it and shows no clinical manifestations of drug toxicity.

Evaluating a Good Outcome: How Do I Define Success?

- The patient is benefited or, at the very least, not harmed by our actions.
- The hospital and its employees act in a legally defensible manner and (hopefully!) are not sued by the patient's family.

- The patient accepts treatment.
- The mother is able to realize the need for medical intervention.
- Hospital policy is maintained.
- I learn more about my legal and ethical responsibilities.

Personal Learning: Here's to the Future!

My preceptor and I went into the room and explained to the patient and his mother the procedure of NG tube insertion and what the bowel preparation solution was expected to do. I think the mother appreciated that we were not talking to them in a condescending fashion and, therefore, began to see us as trying to help her son, not harm him. She asked a couple of questions about side effects of the medication and how the NG tube worked. She began to show signs of calming down until the physician walked into the room. Then she started to show her frustration again. Therefore, my preceptor politely asked the doctor to leave. Subsequently, we were able to insert the NG tube, despite some resistance from the patient. Several hours later, the patient passed a bag of crack rocks intact.

Obviously, this situation was very new to me. I had never dealt with a patient who was threatening to sue and who was clearly upset by what was happening. I was able to see the collaboration between the attending physician, the toxicologist, the hospital attorney, and the nurses and myself. This was an interesting case because the treatments were clearly necessary for the patient's well-being, but everyone wanted to make sure they were legally able to impose treatment. I learned that a hospital attorney is a good resource when legal questions or ambiguous situations arise.

I think that my professional legal skills need a fair amount of work. Unfortunately, I also believe that nurses violate the law more often than is recognized— for example, subtle breaches of the law such as failure to ensure patient safety and failure to follow agency policy. Although I feel that I understand many of the obvious legal violations, I think I have a lot to learn regarding legal issues in the nursing practice.

Julia Strobel, Georgetown University

Reflection

How do you think you would respond in a similar situation? Why? What does this tell you about yourself and about the adequacy of your skills for professional practice? Can you think of other ways to respond? What legal and ethical principles were involved in this situation? Which ones had the potential to be violated? Did the preceptor and nursing student ensure the patient's rights? How might this situation have been different if the patient were over 18 years of age? What other skills (cognitive, interpersonal, technical, ethical/legal) would you need to respond well in this situation? Do you agree with the criteria to evaluate a successful outcome? Did the nursing student meet the criteria? Please explain your answer.

Box 17-1 DOCUMENTATION GUIDELINES

Aim: Complete, accurate, concise, current, factual, and organized data communicated in a timely and confidential manner to facilitate care coordination and serve as a legal document.

Content

- Enter information in a *complete, accurate, concise, current,* and *factual* manner.
- Make sure your documentation reflects the nursing process and your professional responsibilities.
- Record patient findings (observations of behavior) rather than your interpretation of these findings.
- Avoid words such as "good," "average," "normal," or "sufficient," which may mean different things to different readers.
- Avoid generalizations such as "seems comfortable today." A better entry would be "on a scale of 1 to 10, patient rates back pain 2 to 3 today as compared with 7 to 9 yesterday; vital signs returned to baseline."
- Note problems as they occur in an *orderly, sequential manner;* record the nursing intervention and the patient's response; update problems or delete as appropriate.
- Chart precautions or preventive measures used.
- Document all medical visits and consultations of which other nurses should be aware, either because of their impact on the patient or because of the nursing care the patient now requires.
- Document in a *legally prudent manner.* Know and adhere to professional standards and agency/institutional policy for documentation.
- Document the nursing response to questionable medical orders or treatment (or failure to treat). Factually record the date and time the physician was notified of the concern and the exact physician response. If this occurs by phone, have a second nurse listen to the conversation and cosign the note. If a nurse administrator was contacted, document this. Documentation should give legal protection to the nurse, other caregivers, the healthcare agency or institution, and the patient.
- Avoid the use of stereotypes or derogatory terms when charting.

Timing

- Chart in a *timely* manner. Follow agency policy regarding the frequency of documentation and *modify this if changes in the patient's status warrant more frequent documentation.*
- Indicate in each entry the date and both the time the entry was written and the time of pertinent observations and interventions. This is crucial when a case is being reconstructed for legal purposes.
- Most agencies use military time, one 24-hour time cycle, to avoid confusion between a.m. and p.m. times (see accompanying figure).
- Document nursing interventions as closely as possible to the time of their execution. The more seriously ill the patient, the greater the need to keep documentation current. Never leave the unit for a break when caring for a seriously ill patient until all significant data are recorded.
- Never document interventions before carrying them out.
- Write a progress note for each of these instances:
  - Upon admission, transfer to another unit, and discharge.
  - When a procedure is performed.
  - Upon receiving a patient postoperatively or postprocedure.
  - Upon communicating with physicians regarding critical patient information (e.g., abnormal lab value result).
  - For any change in patient status.

Format

- Check to make sure you have the correct chart before writing.
- Chart on the proper form as designated by agency policy.
- Print or write legibly in *dark* ink to ensure permanence. Use correct grammar and spelling. Use *standard terminology*, only commonly accepted terms and abbreviations and symbols (see Box 17-3). Alternately, follow computer documentation guidelines.
- Date and time each entry.
- Chart nursing interventions chronologically on consecutive lines. Never skip lines. Draw a single line through blank spaces.

Accountability

- Sign your first initial, last name, and title to each entry. Do not sign notes describing interventions not performed by you that you have no way of verifying.
- Do not use dittos, erasures, or correcting fluids. A single line should be drawn through an incorrect entry and words "mistaken entry" or "error in charting" should be printed above or beside the entry and signed. The entry should then be rewritten correctly.
- Identify each page of the record with the patient's name and identification number.
- Recognize that the patient record is *permanent*. Follow agency policy pertaining to the color of ink and the type of pen or ink to be used. Ensure that the patient record is complete before sending it to medical records.

Confidentiality

- Patients have a moral and legal right to expect that the information contained in their patient health record will be kept private. Students should be familiar with agency policy and pertinent legislation about who has access to patient records, other than the immediate caregiving team, and the process used to obtain access (see HIPAA guidelines).
- Most agencies allow students access to patient records for educational reasons. Students using patient records are bound professionally and ethically to keep in strict confidence all the information they learn by reading patient records. Actual patient names and other identifiers should not be used in written or oral student reports.

The military clock uses one 24-hour time cycle instead of two 12-hour cycles (e.g., 9:00 a.m. is 0900 and 9:00 p.m. is 2100).

undermine nursing's credibility as a professional discipline, and cause legal problems for the nurses responsible. Adherence to the documentation guidelines shown in Box 17-1 helps to prevent errors. In brief, documentation should be consistent with professional and agency standards; complete, accurate, concise, factual, organized, and timely; legally prudent; and confidential.

Responding to the widespread nursing concern that the time spent documenting nursing care comes at the expense of providing safe, quality patient care, the American Nurses Association (ANA) introduced a new tool to streamline the nursing documentation process in 2003. Available as a brochure titled *Principles for Documentation,* this guide includes policy statements, principles, and recommendations to assist nurses with documentation and to comply with institutional and regulatory requirements.

The policy statements and principles outlined in the guide are based on the *ANA Code of Ethics for Nurses With Interpretive Statements* (American Nurses Association [ANA], 2001) and *Standards of Clinical Nursing Practice,* 2nd edition (ANA, 1998). In addition, the formulated principles in many instances are based on standards set forth by state and federal regulatory agencies, the Centers for Medicare and Medicaid Services (CMS), and through accrediting organizations, such as the Joint Commission and the National Committee for Quality Assurance (NCQA).

In addition, in February 2006, the ANA CNPII (Committee for the Nursing Practice Information Infrastructure Committee) launched a new website dedicated to promoting awareness, use, and further development of standardized data elements and terminologies (www.nursingworld.org/npii). The website lists recognized terminologies and data element sets.

Privacy and Confidentiality

Nurses and other professional caregivers learn and communicate private information about patients and their families every day.

WHAT INFORMATION IS CONFIDENTIAL?

All information about patients is considered private or confidential, whether written on paper, saved on a computer, or spoken aloud. This includes their names and all identifiers such as address, telephone and fax number, Social Security number, and any other personal information. It also includes the reason the patient is sick or in the hospital, office, or clinic, the treatments he or she receives, and information about past health conditions. Protected health information might be found in the patient medical record, computer systems, telephone calls, voice mails, fax transmissions, e-mails that contain patient information, and conversations about patients between clinical staff.

While most nurses are staunch advocates of a patient's right to privacy and confidentiality, it is possible to violate these rights thoughtlessly. For example, one nurse gives patient information over the phone to a patient's alleged spouse without knowing whether or not the patient wants his wife to know, another talks about a difficult patient in the elevator on the way to dinner, and another gives patient information to a professional caregiver who "knows" the patient but is not involved in the patient's care. Additional examples of breaches of confidentiality and security include the following:

- Discussing patient information in any public area where those who have no need to know the information can overhear.
- Leaving patient medical information in a public area.
- Leaving a computer unattended in an accessible area with medical record information unsecured.
- Failing to log off a computer terminal.
- Sharing or exposing passwords.
- Copying or providing data, either in hard copy or machine-readable form, for one's self, coworkers, or any other party, except as required to fulfill job responsibilities.
- Improperly accessing, reviewing, and/or releasing birth dates and addresses of friends or relatives, or requesting another individual to do so.
- Improperly accessing, reviewing, and/or releasing the record of a patient out of concern or curiosity, or requesting another individual to do so.
- Improperly accessing, reviewing, and/or releasing a patient record to use information in a personal relationship.
- Improperly accessing, reviewing, and/or releasing the patient record of a public personality for the intent of giving or selling information to the media.
- Improperly accessing, reviewing, and/or releasing confidential information of another member of the workforce who is also a patient.
- Improperly accessing, reviewing, and/or releasing confidential information that may bring harm to the organization or individuals associated with it.

Table 17-1 provides specific measures to use to ensure information about your patients remains confidential.

Professional codes of ethics, agency policies, and state and federal privacy legislation dictate how patient information can be communicated (verbally and in writing), where and how it can be stored, the appropriate persons and entities to whom it may be divulged, and the purposes for which it may be divulged. It is essential for nurses to be familiar with these guidelines.

Take note! There have been reports of school suspensions for nursing and medical students who are using Facebook, MySpace, Blogs, and YouTube to unprofessionally share patient experiences. What may start as a prank may lead to your suspension or dismissal.

HEALTH INSURANCE PORTABILITY AND ACCOUNTABILITY ACT (HIPAA)

Congress passed the Health Insurance Portability and Accountability Act (HIPAA) in 1996. The final regulations were published in December 2000, modified by the Bush administration, and released in August 2002. Most agencies now require workers to undergo HIPAA training and to

TABLE • 17-1 TIPS FOR PREVENTING BREACHES IN PATIENT CONFIDENTIALITY	
Type of Breach	**How to Prevent It**
Computers Displaying information on a screen (especially handheld computers) that is viewed by unauthorized users	Make sure display screens do not face public areas. For portable devices, install encryption software that makes information unreadable or inaccessible.
Sending confidential e-mail messages via public networks such as the Internet, where they can be read by unauthorized users	Use encryption software when sending e-mail over public networks.
Sharing printers among units with differing functions and information (unauthorized users can read printouts)	Request that your unit have a separate printer not shared with another unit.
Copiers Discarded copies of patient health information in trash cans adjacent to copiers	Use secure disposal containers (similar to mailboxes) adjacent to copiers.
Cordless and Cellular Phones Holding conversations vulnerable to eavesdropping outsiders with scanning equipment	Use phones with built-in encryption technology.
Fax Machines Faxing confidential information to unauthorized persons	Before transmission, verify the fax number and that the recipient is authorized to receive confidential information.
Voice Pagers Sending confidential messages that can be overheard on the pager	Restrict use of voice pagers to nonconfidential messages.

Used with permission. Holmes, H. N. (Ed.). (2006). *Documentation in action.* Philadelphia: Lippincott Williams & Wilkins.

review and sign a confidentiality agreement both when hired and at each performance review. As a student in a healthcare setting, it is important for you to discuss privacy guidelines with your instructor and nurse mentors. According to HIPAA, patients have a right to:

• See and copy their health record
• Update their health record
• Get a list of the disclosures a healthcare institution has made independent of disclosures made for the purposes of treatment, payment, and healthcare operations
• Request a restriction on certain uses or disclosures
• Choose how to receive health information

➤ *Consider Jason Chandler, the adolescent brought to the emergency department by the police. The nurse would need to be knowledgeable about HIPAA regulations to ensure Jason's confidentiality is maintained. In addition, the nurse would need to keep in mind that Jason is a minor, and any authorizations would probably require a parent's consent.* ■

If a health institution wants to release a patient's health information for purposes other than treatment, payment, or routine healthcare operations, the patient must be asked to sign an authorization (see Box 17-2 for a list of permitted disclosures of patient health information and incidental disclosures).

Take note! HIPAA legislation includes punishments for anyone caught violating patient privacy. Those who do so for

financial gain can be fined as much as $250,000 or go to jail for as many as 10 years! Even accidentally breaking the rules can result in penalties—and embarrassment—for you and your organization.

Agency Policies

Most agencies have specific policies for patient records. Everyone who has access to the record (direct caregivers) is expected to maintain its confidentiality (see the discussion about privacy above). Most agencies grant student nurses access to patient records for education purposes. In this instance, *the student assumes responsibility to hold patient information in confidence.* Never use a patient's name when preparing written or oral reports for school.

Agency policies also indicate which personnel are responsible for recording on each form in the record, and such policies might also describe the order in which the forms are to appear in the record. Additional policies might concern the frequency with which entries are to be made, whether routine care is recorded, the manner in which health personnel identify themselves after making an entry, which types of abbreviations are acceptable, and the manner in which recording errors are handled. Box 17-3 provides a list of commonly used abbreviations. One of the strategies the Joint Commission (2009) is using to achieve National Patient Safety Goals is a list of "do not use" abbreviations, acronyms, and symbols (Table 17-2). Be sure to know the latest Joint Commission and agency policies regarding the

Box 17-2 THE HEALTH INSURANCE PORTABILITY AND ACCOUNTABILITY ACT OF 1996 AUTHORIZATION RULE

If a health institution wants to release a patient's health information (PHI) for purposes other than treatment, payment, and routine health care operations, the patient must be asked to sign an authorization.

Permitted Disclosure of PHI

While the authorization rule covers most situations where we need to release patient information for purposes other than treatment, payment, and routine healthcare operations, there are some exceptions to the authorization rule for the good of the general population.

These three exceptions show situations where authorization is *not* required prior to releasing the patient's information:

Public health activities	• Tracking and notification of disease outbreaks • Infection control • Statistics related to dangerous problems with drugs or medical equipment
Law enforcement and judicial proceedings	• Medical records crucial to the investigation and prosecution of a crime • Medical records to identify victims of crime or disasters • Medical personnel reporting incidents of child abuse, neglect, or domestic violence • Medical records released according to a valid subpoena
Deceased individuals	• PHI needed by coroners, medical examiners, and funeral directors • PHI needed to facilitate organ donations • PHI provided to law enforcement in the case of a death from a potential crime

Incidental Disclosure of PHI

Incidental Disclosure of PHI is defined as a secondary disclosure that cannot reasonably be prevented, is limited in nature, and occurs as a byproduct of an otherwise permitted use or disclosure of PHI.

Examples of incidental disclosures that are permitted:

Permitted Disclosure	Necessary Conditions
• Use of sign-in sheets	• Provided that the sign-in sheet does not contain information on the reason for the patient's visit
• The possibility of a confidential conversation being overheard	• Provided that the surroundings are appropriate for a confidential conversation and voices are kept down
• Placing patient charts outside exam rooms	• Provided that unauthorized public traffic is not permitted in the area of the exam rooms and face sheets are turned toward the wall
• Use of white boards	• Provided that only the minimum information needed for the purpose of the white board is used
• X-ray light boards that can be seen by passers-by	• Provided that patient x-rays are not left unattended on the light board
• Calling out names in the waiting room	• Provided that the reason for the patient's visit is not mentioned
• Leaving appointment reminder voicemail messages	• Provided that the minimum amount of information is disclosed

use of abbreviations, acronyms, and symbols in your practice setting. An issue of growing importance concerns documentation made by unlicensed personnel. Because professional nurses frequently supervise the care that unlicensed personnel give, it is essential to clarify which assessments and interventions may be charted by unlicensed personnel and which require documentation by a professional nurse.

The storage of patient records when a patient is no longer receiving treatment is a function of the health agency's record department. Many patient records are microfilmed for compact storage or are entered into a computer to expedite accessibility of information.

You will also want to be aware of agency policies regarding the patient's right to access records. Be sure to check the policy where you work to find out answers to the following frequently asked questions:

• Can I take my chart home?
• How long do you retain records?
• How long will it take to get a copy of my record?
• How much does it cost?

• I do not want some parts of my record (e.g., psychiatric information) released to anyone. What do I do?
• May I look at my family's medical record?
• Who can look at my record?
• Who do I tell if my name has changed?

To see one hospital's policies regarding these questions, visit www.dukehealth.org/AboutDuke/AboutWebsite/Privacy/PatientConfidentiality.

Purposes of Patient Records

Patient records serve many purposes such as communication with other healthcare professionals, recording of diagnostic and therapeutic orders, care planning, quality-of-care reviewing, research, decision analysis, education, legal documentation, reimbursement, and historical documentation.

Communication

The primary purpose of the patient record is to help healthcare professionals from different disciplines (who interact

Box 17-3   ABBREVIATIONS AND SYMBOLS COMMONLY USED BY HEALTH PRACTITIONERS*

Activities
AMB	ambulatory
BRP	bathroom privileges
CBR	complete bed rest
OOB	out of bed
up ad lib	up as desired

Assessment Data
abd	abdomen
BP	blood pressure
bx	biopsy
C	Celsius (centigrade)
c/o	complains of
CTA	clear to auscultation
dx	diagnosis
F	Fahrenheit
FUO	fever of unknown origin
GI	gastrointestinal
GU	genitourinary
H/A	headache
h/o	history of
HPI	history of present illness
Imp	impressions
lt or Ⓛ	left
MAE	moves all extremities
NAD	no apparent distress
NKA	no known allergies
N/V	nausea and vomiting
neg	negative
P	pulse
PE	physical examination
PMH	past medical history
R	respirations
R/O	rule out
ROS	review of systems
rt or ®	right
SOB	short of breath
Sx	symptoms
T	temperature
⊕	positive
⊖	negative

Diseases
ASCVD	arteriosclerotic cardio-vascular disease
ASHD	arteriosclerotic heart disease
BPH	benign prostatic hypertrophy
CA	cancer
CAD	coronary artery disease

CHF	congestive heart failure
COPD	chronic obstructive pulmonary disease
CVA	cerebrovascular accident
DM	diabetes mellitus
HTN (↑ BP)	hypertension
MI	myocardial infarction
PE	pulmonary emboli
PVD	peripheral vascular disease
STD	sexually transmitted disease
URI	upper respiratory infection

Diagnostic Studies
ABG	arterial blood gases
BE	barium enema
CBC	complete blood count
CO₂	carbon dioxide
C&S	culture and sensitivity
CXR	chest x-ray
ECG (EKG)	cardiogram
lytes	electrolytes
RBC	red blood cells
UA	urinalysis
UGI	upper GI
WBC	white blood cells

Symbols
>	greater than
<	less than
↑	increase
↗	increasing
↓	decrease
↙	decreasing
2°	secondary to
=	equal to
≠	unequal
♀	female
♂	male
°	degree
▲	change
x̄	except

Miscellaneous
ā	before
ad lib	as desired
AMA	against medical advice
ASAP	as soon as possible
BM	bowel movement
BSD	bedside drainage

c̄ (C)	with
CABG	coronary artery bypass graft
CPR	cardiopulmonary resuscitation
dc (disc)	discontinue
DNR (no code)	do not resuscitate
Dsg	dressing
dx	diagnosis
FOB	foot of bed
Fx	fracture
GHWT	good handwashing technique
HOB	head of bed
hs	hour of sleep
Hx	history
I&O	intake and output
IV	intravenous
KVO	keep vein open
NG	nasogastric
noc	night
NPO (npo)	nothing by mouth
NS (NIS) (N/S)	normal saline
O₂	oxygen
OT	occupational therapy
p̄	after
postop	postoperative
preop	preoperative
prep	preparation
PRN (p.r.n.)	as needed
PT	physical therapy
pt	patient
q	every
ROM	range of motion
RX	treatment
s̄ (S)	without
SOB	side of bed
S/P	status post
STAT	immediately
TF	tube feeding
TPR	temperature, pulse, respirations
TURP	transurethral resection of prostate
TX	treatment
VS	vital signs
WA	while awake
×	times

*Use only those abbreviations and symbols accepted by your institution.

with the patient at different times) communicate with one another. Communication fosters continuity of care. For example, it is not unusual for a critically ill patient in an academic health center to be seen by an attending physician, seven consulting physicians, different teams of residents, an assigned social worker or case manager, assorted therapists, a hospital chaplain, and many nurses. Because these individuals are never all in the same room at the same time, it is crit-

ical to use the patient record as a means of communication. A nurse may check the patient record to see if the physician has spoken with the patient or the patient's surrogate about a do-not-resuscitate order. The physician may read the nurse's note to see how the family is responding to the recommendation to withhold or withdraw life-sustaining treatment.

It is helpful to keep in mind that other healthcare professionals make judgments about nurses and nursing's contributions

TABLE • 17-2	JOINT COMMISSION "DO NOT USE" ABBREVIATIONS, ACRONYMS, AND SYMBOLS	
Abbreviation	**Potential Problem**	**Use Instead**
Official "Do Not Use" List[1]		
U (for unit)	Mistaken as 0 (zero), 4 (four), or cc	Write "unit."
IU (for international unit)	Mistaken as IV (intravenous) or 10 (ten)	Write "international unit."
Q.D., QD, q.d., qd (daily) Q.O.D., QOD, q.o.d, qod (every other day)	Mistaken for each other. The period after the Q can be mistaken for an "I" and the "O" can be mistaken for "I."	Write "daily" and "every other day."
Trailing zero (X.0 mg)*	Decimal point is missed.	Write X mg
Lack of leading zero (.X mg)		Write 0.X mg
MS	Can mean morphine sulfate or magnesium sulfate.	Write "morphine sulfate" or "magnesium sulfate."
MSO_4 and $MgSO_4$	Confused for one another.	
Additional Items (For *Possible* Future Inclusion in the Official "Do Not Use" List)		
> (greater than) < (less than)	Misinterpreted as the number "7" or the letter "L"; confused with one another	Write "greater than" or "less than."
Abbreviations for drug names	Misinterpreted due to similar abbreviations for multiple drug	Write drug names in full.
Apothecary units	Unfamiliar to many practitioners; confused with metric units	Use metric units.
@	Mistaken for the number "2"	Write "at."
cc (for cubic centimeter)	Mistaken for U (units) when poorly written	Write "mL" or "ml" or "milliliters" ("mL" is preferred).
μg (for microgram)	Mistaken for mg (milligrams), resulting in one thousand-fold dosing overdose.	Write "mcg" or "micrograms."

[1]Applies to all orders and all medication-related documentation that is handwritten (including free-text computer entry) or on preprinted forms.
   *Exception: A "trailing zero" may be used only where required to demonstrate the level of precision of the value being reported such as for laboratory results, imaging studies that report the size of lesions, or catheter/tube sizes. It may not be used in medication orders or other medication-related documentation.
   ©The Joint Commission, 2010. Reprinted with permission. Available at http://www.jointcommission.org/PatientSafety/DoNotUseList/.

to the healthcare team partially on the basis of what is documented in the patient record.

Diagnostic and Therapeutic Orders

Patient records also include diagnostic and therapeutic orders. Anyone reviewing the chart can find all the diagnostic studies ordered for the patient since admission, the results of these studies, and related orders for care. Nurses are responsible for ensuring that these orders are entered in the patient record and implemented. It is the policy of most agencies that diagnostic and therapeutic orders should be accepted and executed only when written and signed by the member of the house or professional staff who issued the orders, except in medical emergencies (verbal orders) or when the practitioner is unable to be present on the unit (telephone or faxed orders). Nurses may take orders only from physicians, dentists, psychologists, podiatrists, and advanced practice nurses who are licensed and have credentials. Medical students' orders may be executed only when countersigned by the attending physician, nurse practitioner, or a house officer assigned to the clinical department.

Illegible notes are the source of many errors. Whenever you are unsure of what has been written, check the order. Never guess about what is written. A patient's life and your license are literally at risk if you incorrectly transcribe an order.

VERBAL ORDERS

In most agencies, the only circumstance in which an attending physician, nurse practitioner, or house officer may issue orders verbally is in a medical emergency when the physician/nurse practitioner is present but finds it impossible, due to the emergency situation, to write the order. The order must be given directly by the physician or nurse practitioner to a registered professional nurse or registered professional pharmacist, who receives, documents, and executes the order. Verbal orders may not be given, received, or executed under any other circumstances. A sample policy for verbal orders follows:

A. The registered professional nurse or registered professional pharmacist who receives the verbal order will:
   1. Record the orders in the patient's medical record.
   2. Read back the order to verify accuracy of the order.

3. Date and note the time the orders were issued during the emergency.

4. Record V.O. (verbal orders), the name of the physician or nurse practitioner who issued the orders, followed by the nurse's own name and title.

B. Immediately after the conclusion of the emergency, it is the responsibility of the physician or nurse practitioner who has issued the verbal orders to:

1. Review the orders to ascertain whether they are correct.

2. Sign the orders with his or her name, title, and pager number.

3. Date and note the time he or she signs the orders.

C. It is the responsibility of the unit secretary and/or the registered professional nurse to see that the orders are transcribed according to procedure.

TELEPHONE AND FAX ORDERS

Agency policy must be followed regarding telephone orders. Every telephone order should be repeated back to the physician to ensure that the order is correctly understood. If you are unsure of an order given by phone, ask the physician to repeat it. Telephone orders must be transcribed on an order sheet; policy usually dictates that they be cosigned by the physician within a set time. If a telephone order is judged to be inappropriate, another nurse should also listen to the order. Then, agency guidelines for questioning inappropriate orders are followed. Fax orders are acceptable as long as they are legible and issued from a credentialed and privileged individual. As always, if there are any concerns, the ordering physician should be contacted. Sample policy follows:

A. An attending physician or nurse practitioner who finds it necessary to issue orders via telephone should be referred to a house officer or, in the absence of a

PATIENT CARE FLOW SHEET

Date 1/22/11	2300–0700	0700–1500	1500–2300
Respiratory			
Breath sounds	Clear 2330 PW	Crackles ©LL 0800 SR	Clear 1600 MLF
Treatments/results	———	Nebulizer 0830 SR	———
Cough/results	———	Mod. amt. tenacious yellow mucus, 0900 SR	———
O₂ therapy	Nasal cannula @ 2 L/min PW	Nasal cannula @ 2 L/min SR	Nasal cannula @ 2 L/min MLF
Cardiac			
Chest pain	÷ PW	÷ SR	÷ MLF
Heart sounds	Normal S₁ and S₂ PW	Normal S₁ and S₂ SR	Normal S₁ and S₂ MLF
Telemetry	N/A	N/A	N/A
Pain			
Type and location	© flank 0400 PW	© flank 1000 SR	© flank 0400 MLF
Intervention	Meperidine 0415 PW	Repositioned and meperidine 1010 SR	Meperidine 1615 MLF
Pt. response	Improved from #9 to #3 in 1/2 hr PW	Improved from #8 to #2 in 45 min. SR	Complete relief in 1 hr MLF
Nutrition			
Type	———	Regular SR	Regular MLF
Toleration %	———	90% SR	80% MLF
Supplement	———	1 can Ensure SR	———
Elimination			
Stool appearance	÷ PW	÷ SR	+ soft dark brown MLF
Enema	N/A	N/A	N/A
Results	———	———	———
Bowel sounds	Present all quadrants 2330 PW	Present all quadrants 0800 SR	Hyperactive all quadrants 1600 MLF
Urine appearance	Clear, amber 0400 PW	Clear, amber 1000 SR	Dark yellow 1500 MLF
Indwelling urinary catheter	N/A	N/A	N/A
Catheter irrigations	———	———	———

FIGURE 17-1. Using a flow sheet to record routine care. (Used with permission. *Documentation in Action.* [2006] Philadelphia: Lippincott Williams & Wilkins, p. 236–241.) *(continued)*

house officer, to a registered professional nurse or a registered professional pharmacist.

B. If a registered professional nurse accepts the orders, he or she must:

1. Record the orders in the patient's medical record.
2. Read the order back to the ordering practitioner to verify accuracy.
3. Date and note the time the orders were issued.
4. Record T.O. (telephone orders) and the full name and title of the physician or nurse practitioner who issued the orders.
5. Sign the orders with name and title (*Example:* "Demerol 100 mg IM now and q 4 hr p.r.n. for pain. T.O. James E. Walker, MD/Mary Pint, RN").

It is the responsibility of the physician or nurse practitioner dictating the orders to sign them as soon as practical, with the exception of orders for restraints, narcotics, anticoagulants, and antibiotics, which many policies dictate must be signed within 24 hours. He or she must also note the date and time the order is signed.

Care Planning

Each professional working with the patient has access to the patient's baseline and ongoing data and can see how the patient is responding to the treatment plan from day to day (see Fig. 17-1). For example, if recorded data indicate that a patient is gradually becoming weaker and is now unable to tolerate ambulation, orders for physical therapy and other

PATIENT CARE FLOW SHEET

Date 1/22/11	2300–0700	0700–1500	1500–2300
I.V. therapy			
Tubing change	—	1100 SR	—
Dressing change	—	1100 SR	—
Site appearance	No edema, no redness 2330 PW	No redness, no edema, no drainage 0800 SR	No redness, no edema, 1600 MLF
Wound			
Type	@ flank incision 2330 PW	@ flank incision 1200 SR	@ flank incision 2000 PW
Dressing change	Dressing dry and intact 2330 PW	1200 SR	2000 MLF
Appearance	Wound not observed PW	See progress note. SR	See progress note. MLF
Tubes			
Type	N/A	N/A	N/A
Irrigation	—	—	—
Drainage appearance	—	—	—
Hygiene			
Self/partial/complete	—	Partial 1000 SR	Partial 2100 MLF
Oral care	—	1000 SR	2100 MLF
Back care	0400 PW	1000 SR	2100 MLF
Foot care	—	1000 SR	—
Remove / reapply elastic stockings	0400 PW	1000 SR	2100 MLF
Activity			
Type	Bed rest PW	OOB to chair X 20 min. 1000 SR	OOB to chair X 20 min. 1800 MLF
Toleration	Turns self PW	Tol. well SR	Tol. well MLF
Repositioned	2330 supine PW 0400 @ side PW	@ side 0800 SR @ side 1400 SR	self MLF
ROM	—	1000 (active) SR 0800 (active) SR	1800 (active) MLF 2200 (active) MLF

FIGURE 17-1. (*Continued*)

PATIENT CARE FLOW SHEET

Date 1/22/11	2300–0700	0700–1500	1500–2300
Sleep			
Sleeps well	0400 PW / 0600 PW	N/A	N/A
Awake at intervals	2330 PW / 0400 PW	———	———
Awake most of the time	———	———	———
Safety			
ID bracelet on	2330 PW 0200 PW / 0400 PW	0800 SR 1500 SR / 1200 SR	1600 MLF 2200 MLF
Side rails up	2330 PW 0200 PW / 0400 PW	0800 SR 1500 SR / 1200 SR	1600 MLF 2200 MLF
Call button in reach	2330 PW 0200 PW / 0400 PW	0800 SR 1500 SR / 1200 SR	1600 MLF 2200 MLF
Equipment			
Type IVAC pump	Continuous 2300 PW	Continuous 0800 SR	Continuous 1600 MLF
Teaching			
Wound splinting	0400 PW	1000 SR	———
Deep breathing	0400 PW	1000 SR	1600 MLF
Initials/Signatures/Titles	PW / Pam Watts, RN	SR / Susan Reynolds, RN	MLF / Mary La Forge, RN

PROGRESS SHEET

Date	Time	Comments
1/22/11	1200	ⓇRight flank dressing saturated with serosang. drng. Dressing removed. Wound edges well-approximated except for 2-cm opening noted at lower edge of incision. Small amount sersang. drng noted oozing from this area. No redness noted along incision line. Sutures intact. Incision line painted with povidone-iodine. Five 4" X 4" gauze pads applied and taped in place. Dr. Wong notified of increased amt. of drng. ——— Susan Reynolds, RN
1/22/11	2000	Dr. Wong to see pt. Ⓡ flank drsg. removed. 2-cm opening noted at lower edges of incision. Otherwise, wound edges well-approximated. Dr. Wong sutured opening with one 3-0 silk suture. No redness or drng. noted along incision line. Painted incision line with povidone-iodine and applied two 4" X 4" gauze pads. Taped drsg. in place. ——— Mary La Forge, RN

FIGURE 17-1. (Continued)

nurse-initiated ambulation will need to be modified. Modifications of the plan of care are based on these data.

▶ Think back to Phillippe Baron, the patient who had undergone a colonoscopy. The nurse would use the patient's chart to obtain information about the patient, including events of the colonoscopy and how the patient responded, so that an individualized discharge teaching plan could be developed. ■

Quality Review

Charts might be reviewed to evaluate the quality of care patients have received and the competence of the nurses providing that care. For example, in a nursing audit, a committee decides in advance certain standards of care it wants to evaluate (e.g., pertaining to nursing assessment, nursing documentation, or safety measures). A number of charts are then randomly selected and reviewed for evidence that the nurses met the selected standards of care. If deficiencies are found, in-service training can be used to remedy the problem and to improve the quality of care. Accrediting agencies, such as the Joint Commission, might also use chart review to determine whether a particular agency or healthcare institution is meeting its standards.

Research

Researchers might study patient records, hoping to learn how best to recognize or treat identified health problems from the study of similar cases.

Decision Analysis

Information from record review often provides the data needed by administrative strategic planners to identify needs and the means and strategies most likely to address these needs. Record review might reveal both underused and overused services, patients with prolonged stays who require special assistance, and financial information about which services generate revenue compared with those that cost the institution or agency money.

Education

Healthcare professionals and students reading a patient's chart can learn a great deal about the clinical manifestations of particular health problems, effective treatment modalities, and factors that affect patient goal achievement.

Legal Documentation

Patient records are legal documents that might be used as evidence in court proceedings; therefore, they play an important role in implicating or absolving health practitioners charged with improper care. The record can also be used in accident or injury claims made by the patient.

Reimbursement

Patient records are used to demonstrate to payers (insurance companies) that patients received the care for which reimbursement is being sought.

Historical Documentation

Because the dates of entries on records are specified, the record has value as a historical document. Years later, information concerning a patient's past healthcare might be pertinent.

Methods of Documentation

While the different methods of documentation systems might initially seem confusing, each is designed to achieve certain aims. Familiarity with a variety of systems allows nurses to adapt quickly when in different practice settings.

Source-Oriented Records

A **source-oriented record** is one in which each healthcare group keeps data on its own separate form. Sections of the record are designated for nurses, physicians, laboratory, x-ray personnel, and so on. Notations are entered chronologically, with the most recent entry being nearest the front of the record. An advantage of the source-oriented record is that each discipline can easily find and chart pertinent data. The main disadvantage is that data are fragmented, making it difficult to track problems chronologically with input from different groups of professionals.

Although the specifics vary among health agencies, the general characteristics of the source-oriented record have essentially remained the same. Types of forms typically used in a source-oriented patient record are shown in Table 17-3. Notes written to inform caregivers of the progress a patient is making toward achieving expected outcomes are called **progress notes.** Progress notes written by nurses in a source-oriented record are **narrative notes** and address routine care, normal findings (findings that do not call for changes in the plan of care), and patient problems identified in the plan of care. They include a description of the status of the problem, related nursing interventions, patient responses, and needed revisions to the plan of care.

Problem-Oriented Medical Records

Another type of record used in some health agencies is the **problem-oriented medical record (POMR),** or problem-oriented record, originated by Dr. Lawrence Weed in the 1960s. The POMR is organized around a patient's problems rather than around sources of information. With POMRs, all healthcare professionals record information on the same forms. The advantages of this type of record are that the entire healthcare team works together in identifying a master list of patient problems and contributes collaboratively to the plan of care. Progress notes clearly focus on patient problems. Box 17-4 describes and illustrates the major parts of the POMR: the defined database, problem list, care plans, and progress notes.

The **SOAP format** (**S**ubjective data, **O**bjective data, **A**ssessment [the caregiver's judgment about the situation], **P**lan) is used to organize data entries in the progress notes of the POMR. Caregivers select numbered problems from the master list on the front of the patient record and then work up the problem or "SOAP it" on the progress sheet. Some nurses believe that the SOAP method of charting focuses too narrowly on problems and advocate a return to the traditional narrative format. Variants of the SOAP format include SOAPE, SOAPIE, and SOAPIER (**I**ntervention, **E**valuation, and **R**esponse).

PIE—Problem, Intervention, Evaluation

The **PIE charting** system is unique in that it does not develop a separate plan of care. The plan of care is incorporated into the progress notes in which problems are identified by number (in the order they are identified). In this documentation system, a complete patient assessment is performed and documented at the beginning of each shift using preprinted fill-in-the-blank assessment forms (flow sheets). Patient problems identified in these assessments are numbered, documented in the progress notes, worked up using the **P**roblem, **I**ntervention, **E**valuation (PIE) format, and evaluated each shift. Resolved problems are dropped from daily documentation following the nurse's review. Figure 17-2 is an example. Continuing problems are documented and numbered each day. One advantage of this system is that it promotes continuity of care. It also saves time because there is no separate plan of care. The disadvantage of not having a formal care plan is that nurses need to read all the nursing

(text continues on page 338)

TABLE • 17-3   EXAMPLES OF FORMS AND INFORMATION IN SOURCE-ORIENTED PATIENT RECORDS

Form	Typical Client Information
Admission sheet	Legal name, identification number Age, birth date, sex Marital status Occupation and employer Religious preference Next of kin and person to notify in case of emergency Date, time, reason for admission Name of the attending physician Insurance information Discharge data
Admission nursing assessment	Results of nursing history and physical assessment
Graphic sheet (see Fig. 17-7)	Daily temperatures, pulse and respiratory rates, blood pressure (vital signs), pain level Daily weight Special measurements, such as the patient's fluid intake and output
Flow sheet to record routine care (see Fig. 17-1)	Respiratory Hygiene Cardiac Activity Pain Sleep Nutrition Safety Elimination Equipment I.V. therapy Teaching Wound Progress sheet Tubes
Narrative nurse's notes (see Fig. 17-1)	Descriptions of pertinent observations of patient Statements that specify the nursing care, including teaching, received by patient and his or her responses to nursing care Statements that describe patient's condition and progress, or lack of progress, toward recovery and goal achievement Descriptions of patient's complaints and how patient is coping, or failing to cope, with them and nursing's response
Medication sheet (see Chapter 29)	Name of prescribed medications administered on a regular or p.r.n. basis Dosage of medication administered Route by which medication was administered, unless given orally Time medication was administered Name or initials of person administering the medication
Medical history and examination sheet	Results of physical examination performed by physician Current medical condition Health history, including previous illnesses Family medical history Confirmed or tentative diagnosis Plan of medical therapy
Physician's order sheet	Orders for medications Orders for treatments Other directives pertinent to a particular patient's care
Physician's progress notes	Interpretations of patient's pathology Responses of patient to medical therapy
Miscellaneous forms	Laboratory reports X-ray film reports Consultation reports Dietary requirements Results of social service consultations Types and results of physical, respiratory, and x-ray therapy

Box 17-4   ORGANIZATION OF THE PROBLEM-ORIENTED MEDICAL RECORD (POMR)

The POMR includes a database, problem list, plan of care, progress notes, flow sheets, and discharge notes.

Database

The database (Figure A) is a compilation of all initial information about the patient and includes the following:

- Health state profile prepared by the nurse
- Medical history and the physical examination, prepared by the physician
- Social history
- Initial diagnostic test results

> 72 year old, white, recently widowed female
>
> brought to hospital after sudden fall caused by temporary paralysis of left leg; admitting diagnosis: transient ischemic attack (TIA), R/O cerebrovascular accident
>
> treated for hypertension since 1990, otherwise in good health; history of headaches—once or twice a week (increasing in severity)—for last six months
>
> ht 5'2"   wt 63.6 kg   98.2 F-88-18   BP L—184/120 R—180/120
>
> ↓ strength ↓ movement left lower extremity (LLE)

FIGURE A.   Summary of database for patient.

Problem List

The multidisciplinary problem list (Figure B) itemizes major aspects of the patient's life that require health attention and includes the following: socioeconomic, demographic, psychological, and physiologic problems. Each problem is labeled, numbered, and categorized as active or inactive.

Date	No. Problem	Identified	Resolved
9/2/11	#1 transient ischemic attack (TIA) R/O cerebro-vascular accident	J. Gleer MD	
	#1A impaired physical mobility related to weakness in left lower extremity	D. Kande RN	
9/4/11	#2 impaired adjustment related to major life stressors and decreased supports	D. Kande RN	

FIGURE B.   Problem list.

Plan of Care

An initial plan is formulated for each specifically numbered problem on the problem list. The nursing plan (Figure C), whether therapeutic, diagnostic, or educational, is expressed through nursing orders.

Date	Problem
9/4/11 1500	#2 impaired adjustment related to major life stressors (including illness) and decreased supporters Goal: Prior to discharge, patient reports feeling able to go home and take one day at a time Plan: *Diagnostic:* explore adequacy of patient's usual patterns of coping and motivation to learn new strategies *Therapeutic:* 1) explain all tests/procedures to patient who wants to know and understand what is happening to her 2) create a restful environment 3) talk with patient's home minister (daughter will contact) *Educative:* Teach patient new coping skills (e.g., relaxation exercises). Refer to community support group for widows. ————————— D. Kande RN

FIGURE C.   Plan of care.

Progress Notes

Progress notes (Figure D) consist of narrative progress notes, flow sheets, and discharge notes.

Date	Problem-Oriented Progress Notes
9/6/11 1000	Impaired mobility related to weakness left lower extremity (LLE) **S** "My left leg still feels queer, pins and needles—but I can move it alright." **O** Able to lift left leg off bed, positive flexion, positive extension; muscle strength in LLE 3/5 (normal movement against gravity) **A** recovering mobility as strength returns **P** *therapeutic:* consult with physician about complete bed rest order; *diagnostic:* continue to monitor muscle strength and movement at least once/shift; be alert for any signs of recurrent TIA; *educative;* instruct not to try to get out of bed without assistance until diagnostic work-up is complete; reinforce need for safety precautions. ————— D. Kande RN

FIGURE D.   Progress notes.

(continued)

Box 17-4   ORGANIZATION OF THE PROBLEM-ORIENTED MEDICAL RECORD (POMR) *(continued)*

The *narrative progress notes* on the patient follow the SOAP format, as follows:
- S—Subjective information reported by the patient
- O—Objective observations made by health practitioners
- A—Assessments drawn from new data
- P—Plans or goals for action related to the patient's problems

Flow sheets are used for recording information that is monitored over time. This information provides data for making comparisons of a patient's status at one time with that patient's status later.

Discharge notes are the entries made at the time an episode of the patient's care is terminated and include the following information:
- The date of the resolution of each problem, as had been described while using the SOAP format
- Referrals made for the patient
- Recommendations for unresolved or partially resolved problems

notes to determine problems and planned interventions before initiating care. Unlike the SOAP method, which originated from the medical record, the PIE format has a nursing origin.

Focus Charting

The purpose of **focus charting** is to bring the focus of care back to the patient and the patient's concerns. Instead of a problem list or list of nursing or medical diagnoses, a focus column is used that incorporates many aspects of a patient and patient care. The focus might be a patient strength, problem, or need. Topics that may appear in the focus column include patient concerns and behaviors, therapies and responses, changes of condition, and significant events such as teaching, consultations, monitoring, management of activities of daily living, or assessment of functional health patterns. The narrative portion of focus charting uses the **D**ata, **A**ction, **R**esponse (DAR) format (Fig. 17-3). The principal advantage of focus charting is the holistic emphasis on the patient and the patient's priorities. Ease of charting is also cited as an advantage of focus charting because it is not required that each note incorporate data, action, and response. Some nurses report, however, that the DAR categories are artificial and not helpful when documenting care.

> For Mr. Baron, the nurse would use focus charting to document specific aspects of teaching related to the colonoscopy and postprocedural care. In addition, due to the effects of anesthesia from the colonoscopy procedure, Mr. Baron might not completely remember all that is taught. Therefore, the nurse would document to include the patient's wife in the discharge teaching to ensure that the information presented was indeed understood. Remember that Mrs. Baron is a nurse. Her clinical knowledge and any necessary reinforcement of information would also be documented. ■

Charting by Exception

Charting by exception (CBE) is a shorthand documentation method that makes use of well-defined standards of practice; only significant findings or "exceptions" to these standards are documented in narrative notes. Benefits of this approach include decreased charting time (freeing more time for direct patient care), a greater emphasis on significant data, easy retrieval of significant data, timely bedside charting, standardized assessment, greater interdisciplinary communication, better tracking of important patient responses, and lower costs.

A significant drawback to charting by exception is its limited usefulness when trying to prove high-quality safe care in response to a negligence claim made against nursing. As an increasing number of facilities move to a totally electronic medical record, even facilities that had not previously adopted a system of charting by exception (CBE) are considering doing so. Although most nurses' initial discomforts with CBE may have been settled, Murphy (2003) reports that enough questions remain to make a comprehensive look at the legality of CBE useful. Figure 17-4 shows one example of this type of charting.

Case Management Model

Managed care's emphasis on quality, cost-effective care delivered within a limited time frame has led to the development of interdisciplinary documentation tools that clearly identify those outcomes that select groups of patients are

P#1: 4/02/11 1300
Caregiver role strain related to patient's new safety needs and increased need for assistance with activities of daily living upon discharge.

I: Sat with patient's daughter and made a list of patient's safety and basic needs upon discharge. Identified what patient already knows and feels comfortable providing and developed a teaching plan to address deficiencies. Patient is highly motivated. Explored community-based resources available to daughter and made referrals to support group for family members of persons with Alzheimer's disease. Social work will talk with daughter 4/03/11 to explore care options should it become impossible to continue providing care at home.

E: Daughter verbalized feeling more in control and less anxious about her father's return home.—C. Taylor, RN

FIGURE 17-2. Sample PIE patient care note

Date/Time	Focus	Patient Care Notes
7/11/11 9:15 am	High risk for trauma	**DATA:** *Patient crying when I entered room; confided that she is afraid to go home because her injuries are the result of husband's battery* **ACTION:** *Attending notified and discharge cancelled; Abuse network called with patient's permission and they are sending a counselor this afternoon to talk with her.* ——— *C. Taylor, RN*
10:00 am	Pain	**DATA:** *Patient complaining of pain in right rib area* **ACTION:** *Tylenol 3 administered as ordered.* ——— *C. Taylor, RN*
10:30 am	Pain	**RESPONSE:** *Patient reports relief from rib pain, still anxious about aftermath of discharge.* ——— *C. Taylor, RN*

FIGURE 17-3. Sample focus patient care notes.

expected to achieve on each day of care. The case management model promotes collaboration, communication, and teamwork among caregivers; makes efficient use of time; and increases quality by focusing care on carefully developed outcomes. One limitation of this model, however, is that it works best for "typical" patients with few individualized needs. At present, there is little consensus about which documentation tools are best for recording routine aspects of care and avoiding repetition.

COLLABORATIVE PATHWAYS

Collaborative pathways (may also be called **critical pathways** or care maps) are used in the case management model. The collaborative pathway specifies the plan of care linked to expected outcomes along a timeline. In some documentation systems, the collaborative pathway is part of a computerized documentation system that integrates the collaborative pathway and documentation flow sheets designed to match each day's expected outcomes. Charting by exception is frequently used with collaborative pathway documentation systems.

VARIANCE CHARTING

When a patient fails to meet an expected outcome or a planned intervention is not implemented in the case management model, this variance from the plan is documented. The usual format for **variance charting** is the unexpected event, the cause of the event, actions taken in response to the event, and discharge planning, when appropriate. The variances most likely to be documented are those that affect quality, cost, or length of stay.

> *Consider Millie Delong, the woman who developed a wound infection. Typically, after abdominal surgery, infection is a complication, not a normal or expected occurrence. Therefore, using the case management model, the nurse would need to document this unexpected outcome with variance charting.* ∎

Computerized Documentation and Electronic Medical Records (EMR)

In an increasing number of healthcare institutions, comprehensive computer systems have revolutionized nursing documentation in the patient record (Fig. 17-5). In these settings, computer capacities exist in which the nurse:

1. Calls up the admission assessment tool on the computer screen and keys in patient data (see Chapter 12)
2. Develops the plan of care using computerized care plans available for each North American Nursing Diagnosis Association (NANDA)-approved diagnosis
3. Adds to the patient database as new data are identified and modifies the plan of care accordingly
4. Receives a work list showing the treatments, procedures, and medications necessary for the patient throughout the shift
5. Documents care immediately using the computer terminal at the patient's bedside

The ANA has been instrumental in developing the Computer-Based Patient Record Institute (CPRI) in response to a recommendation by the Institute of Medicine that a computer-based patient record be adopted nationwide by all healthcare providers and systems.

As healthcare reform initiatives evolve, patient outcomes will become the primary focus when evaluating the effectiveness of care. This focus will intensify as the Health Care Financing Administration and other reimbursement-management sources develop standard outcome measurements for all healthcare organizations. Outcome evaluations will be an important part of the healthcare agency's report card for consumers buying healthcare in this managed-care environment. A key component to facilitate data and outcome comparisons will be the **minimum data sets.** These specific categories of information will use uniform definitions to create a common language among multiple healthcare data users.

FIGURE 17-4. Sample documentation of nursing care using charting by exception. (Courtesy of the Department of Nursing, Williamsport Hospital and Medical Center, Williamsport, PA.)

FIGURE 17-5. Computerized bedside charting allows the nurse to remain in contact with the data source while electronically documenting patient information. *(Photo by B. Proud)*

The nursing minimum data set is organized into three categories:

- Nursing care elements (such as nursing diagnoses and interventions)
- Patient demographic elements (such as sex, date of birth, and ethnicity)
- Service elements (such as admission and discharge dates and expected payer for services)

With computer-based records, or **electronic medical records (EMR),** these data can be distributed among many caregivers in a standardized format, allowing them to compare and uniformly evaluate patient progress easily. Besides tracking the progress of individual patients, computerized outcome information can compare the progress of groups of patients with similar diagnoses. These results will contribute to research, education, and, ultimately, better and more efficient nursing practice. Table 17-4 describes terms used to discuss electronic records in healthcare.

The increasing use of computerized patient information systems to store and analyze patient data has necessitated the development of policies and procedures to ensure the privacy and confidentiality of patient information. Policies should specify what types of patient information can be retrieved, by whom, and for what purpose. Patient consent is necessary for the use and release of any stored information that can be linked to the patient. According to McGraw, Dempsey, Harris, and Goldman (2009), the privacy issue, which for too long was seen as a barrier to electronic health information exchange, "can be resolved through a comprehensive framework that implements core privacy principles, adopts trusted network design characteristics, and establishes oversight and accountability mechanisms" (p. 416).

The American Nurses Association, the American Medical Record Association, and the Canadian Nurses Association offer the following guidelines and strategies for safe computer charting:

- Never give your personal password or computer signature to anyone, including another nurse in the unit, a float nurse, or a doctor.
- Don't leave a computer terminal unattended after you have logged on.
- Follow the correct protocol for correcting errors. To correct an error after storage, mark the entry "mistaken entry" add the correct information and date and initial the entry. If you record information in the wrong chart, write "mistaken entry—wrong chart" and sign off.

TABLE · 17-4	DESCRIPTIONS OF TERMS USED TO DISCUSS ELECTRONIC RECORDS IN HEALTHCARE
Entity	**Description**
Healthcare Smartcard	The healthcare smartcard is a card, similar to a credit card, with a magnetic strip that either contains vital emergency healthcare information or creates a link to information in another location. Using the cardholder's PIN number and entering the card into a reader enables emergency providers to retrieve designated, health-related information about a given patient. Individuals should always carry their PIN number with them to permit access in an emergency.
Electronic Health Record (EHR)	The EHR is the patient care record created when agencies under different ownership share their data. The goal is for this sharing to be nationwide, creating a situation in which a person's healthcare record is accessible by designated healthcare providers anywhere in the nation. The patient will decide which portions of a record will be available to whom.
Electronic Medical Record (EMR)	An EMR is an electronic patient care record created by an agency or agencies having common ownership. Although these EMRs today are often called EHRs, they are not true EHRs because the data is not shared between providers in agencies under different ownership.
Electronic database	An electronic database is an electronic collection of data that allows easy searching and easy retrieval of similar pieces of data from many records.

- Never create, change, or delete records unless you have specific authority to do so.
- Make sure that stored records have back-up files—an important safety check. If you inadvertently delete part of the permanent record, type an explanation into the computer file with the date, time, and your initials and submit an explanation in writing to your manager.
- Don't leave information about a patient displayed on a monitor where others may see it. Keep a log that accounts for every copy of a computerized file that you've generated from the system.
- Never use e-mail to send protected health information unless it has been encrypted to protect it from unauthorized access.
- Follow the agency's confidentiality procedures for documenting sensitive material, such as a diagnosis of acquired immunodeficiency syndrome or human immunodeficiency virus infection.

Personal Health Records (PHRs)

Many individuals today are preparing **personal health records (PHRs)** on the Web to manage their healthcare via computer. These records contain the individual's medical history, including diagnoses, symptoms, and medications. Some patients are scanning in doctors' notes, test results, CT images, and insurance information. They may give healthcare professionals passwords so they can log on, and the permission to share the record with other family members. The chief reason for creating a personal health record is to provide easy access to up-to-date, complete health information to assist in self-care and communication with providers. Patients with chronic illnesses and caregivers who care for children or aging adults with complex medical histories and needs are most likely to benefit from digital, comprehensive medical records.

Kahn, Aulak, and Bosworth (2009) list as current barriers to personal health record adoption among patients: cost, concerns that information is not protected or private, inconvenience, design shortcomings, and the inability to share information across organizations. They do believe, however, that once these concerns are addressed and health data are portable and understandable (both in content and format), PHRs are likely to prove invaluable.

When talking with patients considering using a personal health record, be sure to advise them to do the following: Check the service's privacy policy carefully to see how much control they will have over their information and whether the service can share or exchange their data, and ask their healthcare providers if they are willing to read their PHR (Gearon, 2005).

An informational website, www.myPHR.com, offers a guide to creating a personal healthcare record, how-to information on obtaining medical records, privacy rights, and downloadable health record forms. Other suggestions for Web-based and password-protected PHR products that let users upload and input a wide variety of personal health information include:

- www.medicare.gov/PHR/Overview.asp
- www.thesmartphr.com
- www.webmd.com

Formats for Nursing Documentation

When the nursing process is fully implemented, nursing documentation in the patient's permanent record includes the following formats.

Initial Nursing Assessment

A typical form used to record the initial database obtained from the nursing history and physical assessment is illustrated in Chapter 12. Accurate documentation of these data is important because it provides a baseline for later comparisons as a patient's condition changes.

> Think back to Jason Chandler, the adolescent brought to the emergency department in police custody. Due to the nature of the admission, a complete nursing assessment would be inappropriate. However, the nurse would need to thoroughly assess the patient for signs and symptoms indicating problems associated with swallowing the bag of drugs. Later on, once the initial situation is resolved, an initial history and physical examination would be performed.

Kardex and Patient Care Summary

Many healthcare institutions and agencies use a Kardex care plan to communicate conveniently and concisely the plan of nursing care for each patient. The Kardex is recorded on a folded card and placed in a central Kardex file where it is easily accessible. The plan is eventually placed in the patient's health record. The outside of the card (activity and treatment section) contains basic information such as the patient's profile, admitting diagnosis, and orders concerning activity levels, diet, vital signs, diagnostic tests, medications, and other treatments and procedures. The inside of the Kardex contains the nursing care plan specifying nursing diagnoses and health problems, related outcomes and nursing interventions, and special safety precautions. Some agencies now have computerized systems that are able to generate this same information in the form of a patient care summary for each shift (see Fig. 17-6).

Plan of Nursing Care

Patient records must communicate the patient's problems or diagnoses; related goals, outcomes, and interventions; and progress or resolution of the problems. The plan of nursing care may be written separately or incorporated into a multidisciplinary plan. In a traditional plan of nursing care, nursing diagnoses, goals and expected outcomes, and nursing interventions are written for each patient (see the sample student plan in Chapter 14 and the plans of care at the end of each clinical chapter). Standardized plans of care may also

```
3/10/11      539                          Page 001

Stevens, James                             M 65
MR #: 00310593                  Acct #: 9400037290
DR: J. Carrio                              2/W 204-01
DX: Unstable angina             Date: 3/10/11

SUMMARY : 3/10              0701 to 1501

PATIENT INFORMATION
     3/10      ADVANCE DIRECTIVE:  No.
               Advance directive does not exist
     3/10      ORGAN DONOR: Yes
     3/10      ADMIT DX:  Unstable angina
     3/10      MED ALLERGY:  None known
     3/10      ISOLATION:  Standard precautions

MISC. PATIENT DATA

NURSING CARE PLAN PROBLEMS
3/10      Acute pain  R/T:  anginal pain

ALL CURRENT MEDICAL ORDERS

NURSING ORDERS:
3/10      Activity, OOB, up as tol.
3/10      Routine V/S q & h
3/10      Telemetry
3/10      If 1800 PTT < 50, increase heparin drip to 1200 units/hr. If
          50 to 100, maintain 1000 units/hr. If > 100, reduce to 900
          units/hr.
DIET:
     3/10      Diabetic:  1600 cal., start with lunch today
I.V.s.:
     3/10      Peripheral line #1.... Start D2W 250 ml with heprin 25,000
               units: rate, 1000 units/hr.

                                            (continued)
```

```
3/10/11      539                          Page 002

Stevens, James                             M 65
MR #: 00310593                  Acct #: 9400037290
DR: J. Carrio                              2/W 204-01
DX: Unstable angina             Date: 3/10/11

SUMMARY : 3/10              0701 to 1501

SCHEDULED MEDICATIONS:
     3/10      Nitroglycerin oint 2%, 1-1/2 inches, apply to chest wall
               q 8 h, starting on 3/10, 1800 hrs.
     3/10      Diltiazem tab 90 mg, #1, P.O., q 6 h 0800, 1400, 2000, 0200
     3/10      Furosemide tab 40 mg, #1, P.O., daily 0900
     3/10      Potassium chloride tab 10 mEq, #1, P.O. daily 0900
     3/10      Labetalol tab 100mg, #1/2, P.O. bid 0900, 1800

STAT/NOW MEDICATIONS:
3/10      Furosemide tab 40 mg, #1, P.O. now
3/10      Potassium chloride tab 10 mEq, #1, P.O., now

PRN MEDICATIONS:
     3/10      Procardia nifedipine cap 10 mg, #1, subling. q 6 n, prn
               SBP > 170 or DSBP > 105
     3/10      Acetaminophen tab 325 mg, #2, P.O., q 4 h, prn for pain
     3/10      Temazepan cap 15 mg, #1, P.O. q  HS, prn
     3/10      Alprazolam tab 0.25 mg, #1/2, P.O., q 8 h, prn

LABORATORY:
3/10      CK & MB 1800 today
3/10      CK & MB 0200 tomorrow
3/10      Urinalysis floor to collect
3/10      PTT 1800 today

LABORATORY:
3/10      Stress test persantine, perp H1, Patient handling:
          Wheelchair, Schedule:  tomorrow

                      Last page
```

FIGURE 17-6. Computer generated Kardex. (Used with permission. Holmes, H. N. [Ed.]. [2006]. *Documentation in action* [pp. 231–232]. Philadelphia: Lippincott Williams & Wilkins.)

be used that identify common problems and related care for select patient groups. These generally incorporate standards of high-quality care, but unless such care plans are individualized, they might not sufficiently address individual patient needs. Formats for plans of care vary greatly.

Critical/Collaborative Pathways

The case management plan is a detailed, standardized plan of care that is developed for a patient population with a designated diagnosis or procedure. It includes expected outcomes, a list of interventions to be performed, and the sequence and timing of those interventions. The critical/collaborative pathway, illustrated in Chapter 14, is an abbreviated summary of key information taken from the more detailed case management plan.

Progress Notes

The purpose of progress notes is to inform caregivers of the progress a patient is making toward achieving expected outcomes. The method used to record the patient's progress depends on the documentation system being used. Common examples include narrative nursing notes, SOAP notes, PIE notes, focus charting, charting by exception, and the case management model. The advantages and disadvantages of each are listed in Table 17-5.

Flow Sheets

Flow sheets are documentation tools used to record routine aspects of nursing care. Refer back to Figure 17-1 for an example.

GRAPHIC (CLINICAL) RECORD

The **graphic sheet** is a form used to record specific patient variables such as pulse, respiratory rate, blood pressure readings, body temperature, weight, fluid intake and output, bowel movements, and other patient characteristics (see Fig. 17-7).

> ➤ *A graphic record would be used for both Millie Delong and Phillippe Baron, described at the beginning of the chapter. Specifically for Ms. Delong, documentation of vital signs would be significant because she has wound infection. Because Mr. Baron is postcolonoscopy, his vital signs also need to be assessed frequently. In addition, fluid intake and output are key postoperative assessment findings to document.* ■

24-HOUR FLUID BALANCE RECORD

Forms are available to document the 24-hour intake and output of fluids for patients with special needs. The forms

(text continues on page 347)

TABLE • 17-5	ADVANTAGES AND DISADVANTAGES OF DIFFERENT DOCUMENTATION FORMATS	
Format	**Advantages**	**Disadvantages**
Narrative notes	Narrative notes allow nurses to describe a condition, situation, or response in their own terms, as they understand it.	It is time-consuming and difficult to read days and weeks of narrative notes to find a specific problem, its treatment, and patient response.
SOAP notes (subjective data, objective data, assessment–judgment, plan)	The location of the problem list at the front of the chart alerts all caregivers to patient priorities. Care and documentation of care is problem focused. Easy retrieval of information facilitates quality review and research. Healthcare professionals from different disciplines chart on same progress notes. SOAP format is consistent with nursing process.	The level of ability and consistency of caregivers in organizing data into the SOAP format may vary. Problem focus may reduce patients to "problems to be solved." Maintaining a neat, up-to-date problem list takes constant vigilance and routine review.
PIE (problem, intervention, evaluation)	Without a formal, separate care plan, the method saves time because a nurse does not have to create or update a plan. Consistent with nursing process	Because there is no formal care plan, the nurse preparing to provide care will need to read all the nursing notes to determine problems, planned interventions, and evaluations to see if those interventions are effective.
Focus charting	Ease of charting with DAR is an advantage because categories of data, action, and response are not required for each focus cited. Components of DAR can be cited alone or out of sequence.	Many nurses have difficulty documenting information by separating the data into DAR categories. The "result" portion of the note seems to be a particularly difficult area because some nurses relate this portion to the resulting problems identified from the assessment data rather than to the patient outcome of care after nursing intervention.
Charting by exception	Abnormal status can be seen immediately, with narrative easily retrieved. The flow-sheet format shows overall trends in the patient's condition. Guidelines provide specific but concise standard information regarding "normal" assessments and expected outcomes. Documentation time is decreased because standard care is not written in narrative and duplication of charting is eliminated. This results in charting being done in a timelier manner.	Preventive and wellness-promoting functions of nursing are not documented on this format because they do not address problems. The system requires predictable, defined patient outcomes, which are more difficult to predict for some patients and in some settings than in others. More difficult to computerize
Case management model	Makes efficient use of time because each day has planned interventions and patient expected outcomes written on the plan. Increases the probability that a patient will be discharged in a timely fashion. Care is goal focused, which potentially increases quality. Promotes collaboration, communication, and teamwork among caregivers	Effective for patients with one or two diagnoses and few complications; less helpful for patients with multiple variances. Space to document is limited on critical pathways, and too much writing causes illegibility. Space for individualization is limited. Separate narrative notes must be used for documentation of care. The intervention flow sheet, nursing notes, and critical path must all be reviewed to get a picture of a patient's condition.

Data for this chart were adapted in part from Eggland, E. T., & Heinemann, D. S. (1995). *Nursing documentation: Charting, recording and reporting.* Philadelphia: J. B. Lippincott.

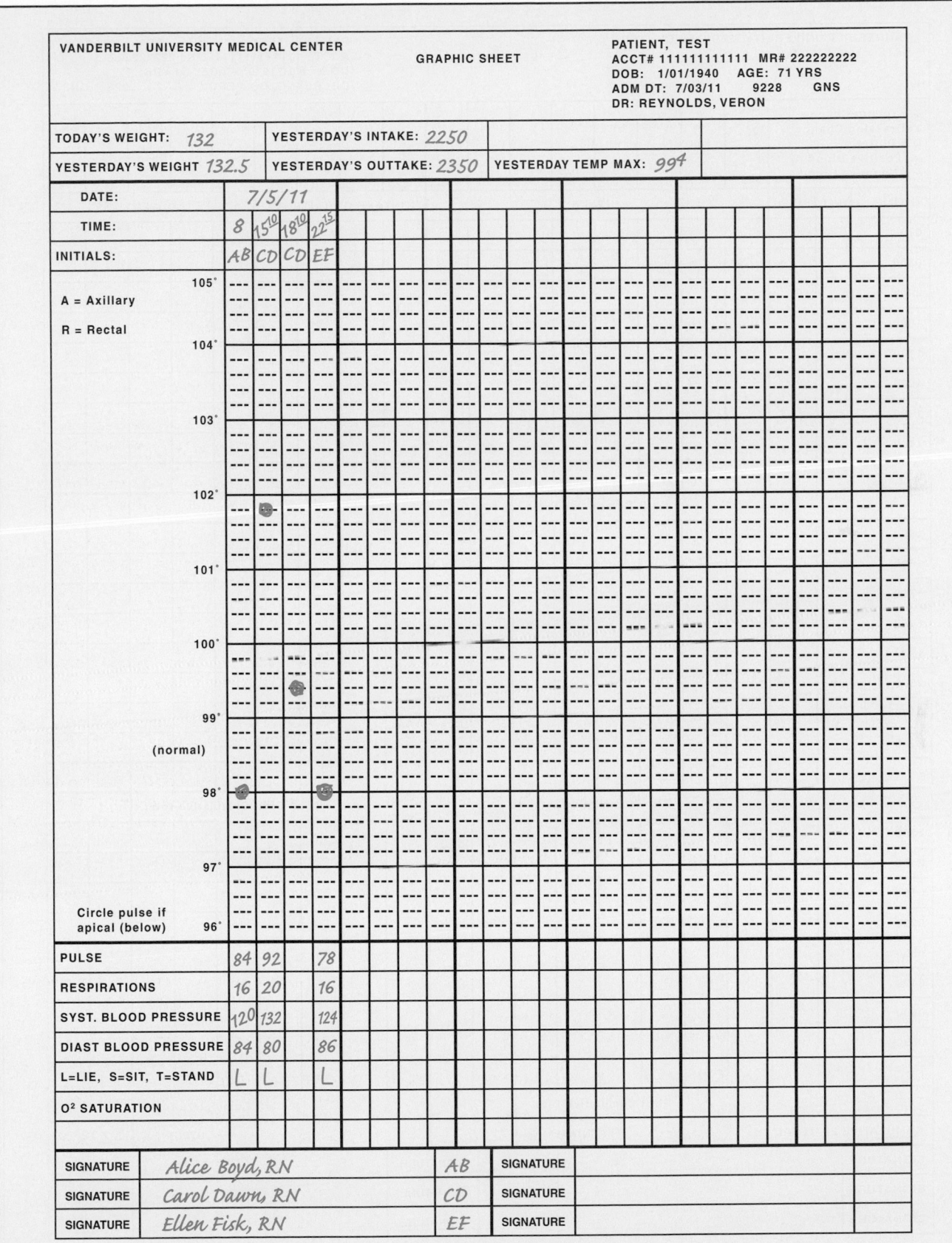

FIGURE 17-7. Example of a graphic record. (Courtesy of Vanderbilt University Medical Center, Nashville, TN.)   *(continued)*

VANDERBILT UNIVERSITY MEDICAL CENTER
DATE : _7_,_5_,_11_

I & O SHEET

PATIENT, TEST   ADM: 7/03/11
ACCT# 111111111111 MR# 222222222
DOB: 1/01/1940   AGE: 71 YRS
DR: REYNOLDS, VERON   9228   GNS

T = Tubing Change
▲=Dressing Change
D = Diuretic
+= Positive Blood
− = Negative Blood

TIME	INIT	SITE	D5 1/2 NS W 20 K	Meds	PO						urine	JP#1	JP#2		BM
			INTAKE							INTAKE OR OUTPUT	OUTPUT				
0700															
0800	AB	√	240/60		400						200				
0900															T
1000	AB	√	180/60	50	100										
1100															
1200	AB	√	120/60		400						400				
1300															
1400	AB	√	60/60	50								15	25		
			240	100	900						600	15	25		
			Shift Cumulative Total			1240					Shift Cumulative Total			640		
1500															
1600	CD	√	1000/60								400				
1700															
1800	CD	√	930/70	100	240										
1900															
2000	CD	√	880/50		100										
2100												500				
2200	CD	√	820/60	50								15	30		
			240	150	340						900	15	30		
			Shift Cumulative Total			730					Shift Cumulative Total			945		
2300												400				
2400	EE	√	770/60	50											
0100															
0200	EE	√	705/65												
0300															
0400	EE	√	650/55												
0500															
0600	EE	√	580/60									10	25		
			240	50							400	10	25		
			Shift Cumulative Total			290					Shift Cumulative Total			440		
CUMULATIVE 24° TOTAL					INTAKE		2260				OUTPUT			2030		
SIGNATURE						SIGNATURE									
SIGNATURE						SIGNATURE									
SIGNATURE						SIGNATURE									

FIGURE 17-7. (Continued)

include shift and daily fluid intake and output totals. A sample tool is shown in Chapter 40.

MEDICATION RECORD

The patient's medication record must include documentation of all the medications administered to the patient (drug, dose, route, time), the nurse administering the drug, and for some medications (e.g., analgesics), the reason the drug was administered and its effectiveness. Sample medication records are shown in Chapter 29.

24-HOUR PATIENT CARE RECORDS AND ACUITY CHARTING FORMS

Flow sheets, such as the one illustrated in Figure 17-1, are often used to document routine aspects of nursing care efficiently throughout a 24-hour period. When well designed, they enable nurses to quickly document the routine aspects of care that promote patient goal achievement, safety, and well-being.

Twenty-four-hour reports are increasingly used in conjunction with acuity reports, which allow nurses to rank patients as high-to-low acuity in relation to both the patient's condition and need for nursing assistance or intervention. A trauma patient whose condition is changing rapidly and who requires intensive nurse monitoring and intervention will merit a higher acuity rank than a patient whose condition is stable. Acuity rankings are often used to determine staffing requirements. A nursing unit with patients with higher acuity rankings requires more professional nurses than a unit with the same number of patients, but with lower acuity ranks.

Discharge and Transfer Summary

At the time a patient is discharged from care or transferred from one unit or institution or agency to another, a **discharge summary** should be written that concisely summarizes the reason for treatment, significant findings, the procedures performed and treatment rendered, the patient's condition on discharge or transfer, and any specific pertinent instructions given to the patient and family. You can imagine how frustrating it is for patients and their family caregivers to arrive in a new treatment setting and have to start informing professional caregivers about their needs from square one because the plan of care didn't accompany them.

> ► *Consider Phillippe Baron, the man who had undergone a colonoscopy. The nurse would be responsible for completing the discharge summary, making sure to include specific aspects of self-care teaching and both the patient's and wife's understanding of the teaching.* ■

Home Healthcare Documentation

Documentation of home care visits that reports the patient's progress serves multiple purposes. Sent to the attending physician with a request for signed medical orders to continue treatment, these records ensure continuity of care. Sent to third-party payers, they establish the need for continuing home care that results in continued reimbursement for necessary services. Medicare, for example, reviews progress summaries to determine whether a patient meets one of these Medicare requirements:

- The patient is homebound and still needs skilled nursing care.
- Rehabilitation potential is good (or the patient is dying).
- The patient's status is not stabilized.
- The patient is making progress in expected outcomes of care.

The Outcome and Assessment Information Set, or **OASIS,** is a group of data elements that:

- Represent core items of a comprehensive assessment for an adult home care patient
- Form the basis for measuring patient outcomes for purposes of outcome-based quality improvement (OBQI)

The OASIS is a key component of Medicare's partnership with the home care industry to foster and monitor improved home healthcare outcomes. It is proposed to be an integral part of the revised *Conditions of Participation* for Medicare-certified home health agencies (HHAs). Overall, the OASIS items are useful for outcome monitoring, clinical assessment, care planning, and other internal agency-level applications. OASIS data items encompass sociodemographic, environmental, support system, health status, and functional status attributes of adult (nonmaternity) patients. In addition, selected attributes of health service use are included (see http://cms.hhs.gov/oasis). Chapter 10 shows a sample home health certification and a skilled nursing note.

Long-Term Care Documentation

Documentation in long-term care settings is specified by the Resident Assessment Instrument (RAI), which helps staff gather definitive information on a resident's strengths and needs, and addresses these in an individualized plan of care. The RAI helps staff track changes in a resident's status by evaluating resident goal achievement and making appropriate revisions in the plan of care. The goal is to coordinate the efforts of the multidisciplinary team to ensure that residents achieve the highest level of functioning possible (Quality of Care) and maintain their sense of individuality (Quality of Life).

The RAI consists of four basic components:

- *Minimum data set*—a core set of screening, clinical, and functional status elements that forms the foundation of the comprehensive assessment of all residents in long-term care facilities certified to participate in Medicare or Medicaid. The items in the minimum data set standardize communication about resident problems and condition.
- *Triggers*—specific resident responses for one or a combination of minimum data set elements that identify residents who either have or are at risk for developing specific functional problems and who require further evaluation using resident assessment protocols.

• *Resident assessment protocols*—structured, problem-oriented frameworks for organizing minimum data set information and examining additional clinically relevant information about a resident. Resident assessment protocols help identify social, medical, nursing, and psychological problems and form the basis for individualized care planning.
• *Utilization guidelines*—specified in state operation manuals that instruct when and how to use the RAI.

Statutory law, federal regulations, and the Health Care Financing Administration specify how the RAI is implemented. An RAI must be completed for residents of Medicare skilled nursing facilities or Medicaid nursing facilities, hospice residents, and short-term stay or respite residents who are residing in a facility for longer than 14 days.

Benefits of using the RAI process according to Health Care Financing Administration (1998) include the following:

• Residents respond to individualized care.
• Staff communication becomes more effective.
• Resident and family involvement increases.
• Documentation becomes clearer.

Potential Legal Problems in Documentation

The results of one in four malpractice suits are determined on the basis of the patient's record. In Box 17-5, Potential Legal Problems in Documentation, Eggland and Heinemann (1995) outline documentation content and mechanics that increase a nurse's legal risk. No nurse can afford to be ignorant or careless with respect to agency policies and professional standards for documentation.

REPORTING CARE

To report is to give an account of something that has been seen, heard, done, or considered. Reporting is the oral, written, or computer-based communication of patient data to others. A laboratory report, for example, might communicate to the healthcare team that a patient's cardiac enzymes are normal or that a biopsy of breast tissue revealed malignant or atypical cells. A nurse's shift report or nursing note might communicate the progress a patient is making toward goal achievement. Common methods for reporting among health practitioners, in addition to the patient record, include face-to-face meetings, telephone conversations, messengers, written messages, audiotaped messages, and computer messages. Each of these methods has certain benefits and limitations, as detailed in Table 17-6.

The Joint Commission included "managing hand-off communications" among its 2009 national patient-safety goals. The Institute for Health Care Improvement (www.ihi.org) is promoting the SBAR Communication (Situation, Background, Assessment, Recommendation) technique as a framework for communication between members of the healthcare team about a patient's condition.

Box 17-5   POTENTIAL LEGAL PROBLEMS IN DOCUMENTATION

Documentation Content That Increases Risk for Legal Problems
• The content is not in accordance with professional or healthcare organization standards.
• The content does not reflect patient needs.
• The content does not include description(s) of situations that are out of the ordinary.
• The content overgeneralizes patient assessment or nursing interventions.
• The content is incomplete or inconsistent.
• The content does not include appropriate medical orders.
• The content implies a potential or actual risk situation.
• The content implies attitudinal bias.

Documentation Mechanics That Increase Risk for Legal Problems
• Lines between entries
• Countersigning documentation
• Tampering
• Different handwriting or obliterations
• Illegibility
• Sloppiness (some lawyers infer sloppy care from sloppy charting)
• Dates and times of entries omitted or inconsistently documented
• Improper nurse signature or unidentifiable initials
• Transcription errors (notes are made at bedside and later transcribed into patient record; problems include the amount of time that elapses between the event and when it is recorded and errors associated with recopying)

Eggland, E. T., & Heinemann, D. S. (1995). *Nursing documentation: Charting, recording and reporting*. Philadelphia: J. B. Lippincott. Used with permission.

• Situation—Communicate what is occurring and why the patient is being handed off to another department or unit.
• Background—Explain what led up to the current situation and put in context if necessary.
• Assessment—Give your impression of the problem.
• Recommendation—Explain what you would do to correct the problem

SBAR (described in Chapter 21) is an easy-to-remember, concrete mechanism useful for framing any conversation, especially critical ones, requiring a clinician's immediate attention and action. It allows for an easy and focused way to set expectations for what will be communicated and how between members of the team, which is essential for developing teamwork and fostering a culture of patient safety.

Be professional whenever making a report about care. Ensure that you have all the pertinent data and be concise. Most importantly, keep the report focused on the patient and avoid gossip, floor politics, and social plans. It is never professional to speak disrespectfully about a patient or family, and such comments have the power to negatively dispose a colleague to patients and the coming shift.

TABLE • 17-6	COMMON METHODS OF COMMUNICATION AMONG HEALTHCARE PROFESSIONALS		
Method	**Advantages**		**Disadvantages**
Face-to-face meeting	• Message can be delivered immediately. • Nonverbal messages are readily conveyed. • Message can be clarified; receiver's questions can be raised and answered.		• Both the communicating and the receiving people must be available at the same time, in the same place. • Ordinarily, there is no permanent record for later use.
Telephone conversation	• Message can be delivered immediately. • Message can be clarified; receiver's questions can be raised and answered. • Two parties need not be present in same place.		• Only the tone of voice and voice inflections can be communicated—no nonverbal messages. • Ordinarily, there is no permanent record.
Written message	• Message can be exchanged at times convenient for the people involved. • Record is available. • Time-efficient if message is understood		• Message usually cannot be validated with the sender.
Audiotaped message	• Message can be exchanged at times convenient for the people involved. • Record is available. • Time-efficient if information communicated is complete		• Message usually cannot be validated with the sender.
Computer message	• Message can be delivered immediately—even to those at a great distance. • Parties need not be present in same place. • Two-way communication is possible by e-mail. • Record is available • Many people can participate in exchange.		• No nonverbal messages can be communicated. • Privacy concerns remain an issue.

Change-of-Shift Reports

A **change-of-shift report** is given by a primary nurse to the nurse replacing him or her or by the charge nurse to the nurse who assumes responsibility for continuing care of the patient. The change-of-shift report might be given in written form or orally in a meeting (Fig. 17-8), or it may be audio- or video-

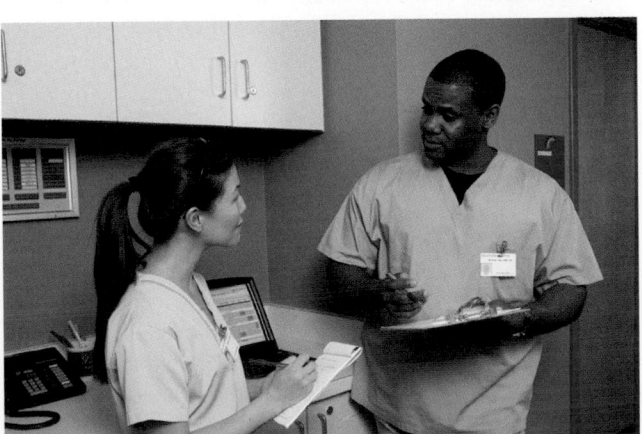

FIGURE 17-8. During a change-of-shift report, a nurse from the ending shift provides a summary of the patient's condition and current status of care to the nurse coming on duty. *(Photo by B. Proud)*

taped. Many charge nurses find that taped reports decrease the amount of time spent reporting and allow more time for last-minute details.

Typical information shared among nurses in a change-of-shift report includes the following:

• Basic identifying information about each patient—name, room number, bed designation, diagnosis, and attending and consulting physicians
• Current appraisal of each patient's health status:
  • Changes in patient's status during your shift and the patient's response to medical therapy
  • Pertinent monitoring, lab, and/or radiology data; data that is irregular or data that has been noted to be irregular in the past and has now been resolved
  • Abnormal findings in your physical/head-to-toe assessment
  • Where the patient stands in relation to identified nursing diagnoses and goal achievement
  • Pain level and pain management needs
• Current orders (especially any newly changed orders):
  • Changes in medications, intravenous fluids, diet, toileting, and activity level
  • Upcoming or ongoing tests and procedures, and specific instructions for these such as NPO after midnight
• Abnormal occurrences during your shift

- Any unfilled orders that need to be continued onto the next shift
- Reports on patients who have been transferred or discharged

Some hospitals are now implementing a standardized, streamlined shift report system at the bedside, which has patient safety as its primary driver (Trossman, 2009). Vital elements of the bedside report include the oncoming and outgoing nurse visualizing the patient together, reviewing medication records and the physician and nursing orders, establishing patient goals for the shift, and inviting patients and their families to participate.

Telephone/Telemedicine Reports

Telephones and telemedicine equipment can link healthcare professionals immediately and enable nurses to receive and give critical information about patients in a timely fashion. For example, the hematology lab might call to report a dangerously low platelet count, and the nurse might in turn notify the attending physician to obtain new medical orders. When reporting significant changes in a patient's condition to physicians and other healthcare professionals, be prepared to do the following:

- Identify yourself and the patient, and state your relationship to the patient. ("Dr. Gomez-Lobo, this is Ellen McLouglin, and I'm calling about Mr. Clouser, a patient of yours who was just discharged home following a work-up for recurrent chest pain. I'm his new nurse case manager.")
- Report concisely and accurately the change in the patient's condition that is of concern and what has already been done in response to this condition. ("When I first arrived in his home, he was complaining of feeling dizzy, and his blood pressure was 190/110. Yesterday morning in the hospital, it was 150/90. His wife appears very flustered and says she doesn't know how she is going to take care of him. I had him rest for 30 minutes, and when I checked his pressure at that time, it was still 186/110.")
- Report the patient's current vital signs and clinical manifestations.
- Have the patient's record at hand to make knowledgeable responses to any physician's inquiries. In this example, the physician will probably want to know all the vital signs and may ask questions about the treatment regimen, both in the hospital and upon discharge.
- Concisely record the time and date of the call, what was communicated to the physician, and the physician's response.

Transfer and Discharge Reports

Nurses report a summary of a patient's condition and care when transferring patients from one unit or institution or agency to another (e.g., from the postanesthesia care unit to a surgical floor) and when discharging patients. The nurse making the report should concisely summarize all the patient data that caregivers need to provide immediate care. See Chapter 9 for transfer and discharge reporting guidelines.

Reports to Family Members and Significant Others

Nurses play a crucial role in keeping the patient's family and significant others updated about the patient's condition and progress toward goal achievement. Always clarify with the patient which visitors, if any, are entitled to progress reports. "Mrs. Neale, do you object to our disclosing your health information to family or friends?" Similarly, clarify what types of information may be communicated and be familiar with agency policy about such communications. Some agencies provide family members approved by the patient a "code" to use when calling the agency to ask about the patient's condition. If the patient objects to disclosure, nurses are not permitted to discuss the patient's health condition with family or friends. If a patient is not able to communicate that he or she objects, such as in an emergency situation or when a patient is unconscious, professional caregivers must use their best professional judgment to decide whether to talk to family and friends.

For example, the nurse is generally not the caregiver who informs family members that a patient's biopsy has revealed a malignancy. The nurse does, however, often explain what this will mean for the patient after the family has this information. Information should be shared in a manner that is honest, compassionate, and respectful of the person's ability to understand medical concepts.

Incident Reports

An **incident report,** also termed a variance or occurrence report, is a tool used by healthcare agencies to document the occurrence of anything out of the ordinary that results in or has the potential to result in harm to a patient, employee, or visitor. These reports are used for quality improvement and should not be used for disciplinary action against staff members. They are a means of identifying risks. More harm than good results from ignoring mistakes. Incident reports improve the management and treatment of patients by identifying high-risk patterns and initiating in-service programs to prevent future problems. These forms also make all the facts about an incident available to the agency in case of litigation. It is important to be familiar with agency policy about your responsibilities and obligations if involved personally in an incident that results in or has the potential to result in harm to a patient, employee, or visitor, or if you witness such an incident. An example of an incident report form and a fuller discussion of this topic appear in Chapter 7.

CONFERRING ABOUT CARE

To **confer** is to consult with someone to exchange ideas or to seek information, advice, or instructions. A nurse might consult with another nurse, such as when a primary care nurse consults with a nurse clinical specialist about a particular patient's care. A school nurse might confer with a child's teacher or a psychologist about a behavior problem. A community health nurse and a physician might confer about a patient's activity regimen. Health practitioners also confer with each other to validate information. Healthcare professionals increasingly use electronic support groups to consult with clinicians who share similar interests or who have expertise in other specialty areas.

> ➤ *Think back to Jason Chandler, the adolescent who was brought into the emergency department by the police. He was refusing treatment. To determine the legal implications of administering treatment to the patient, the physician consulted the hospital's attorney for legal guidance. Doing so helped to clarify what actions were and were not acceptable.* ■

Consultations and Referrals

When nurses detect problems they cannot resolve because they lie outside the scope of independent nursing practice or their expertise, they make consultations or referrals to other professionals. The process of inviting another professional to evaluate the patient and make recommendations to you about his or her treatment is called a **consultation.** The process of sending or guiding the patient to another source for assistance is called a **referral.** A patient might be referred by a hospital to a community health nursing service for assistance with home care. A school nurse might refer a student to a hospital emergency department. A community health nurse who learns that a patient with multiple sexual contacts is HIV positive will refer to the Department of Health for tracking of these contacts.

Most health agencies have policies for referrals. An agency may have a special form that personnel are to use when making referrals. Referral policies usually indicate who may initiate a referral, how it is to be done, and so on. Referrals are especially important in providing continuity of care for people who need a variety of services. It is essential that health practitioners to whom a patient is referred receive the information that is most useful to the continuity of care. The key question is "What would I want to know about this patient if I were the person who had to continue his or her care?" The patient must know and approve of a referral to another agency or to other health personnel.

Before requesting a consultation or making a referral, determine which profession has the needed expertise and which of its practitioners are appropriate for consultation or referral. A great disservice is done to patients when referrals are poorly made. Patients and family members also appreciate a phone number and practical tips about how to easily reach the referred practitioner.

> ➤ *Recall Millie Delong, the woman with the wound infection. Obtaining a consultation from a wound, ostomy, and continence nurse might be appropriate to assist with measures for wound care. Additionally, consultation with an infection-control nurse may be necessary if the patient's wound remains infected or fails to heal.* ■

Nursing and Interdisciplinary Team Care Conferences

Nurses and other healthcare professionals frequently confer in groups to plan and coordinate patient care. Such conferences are also used for instructing students and practitioners. A nursing care conference is a meeting of nurses to discuss some aspect of a patient's care. For example, several nurses who are caring for a generally uncooperative patient might initiate a conference. This would allow each nurse an opportunity to offer his or her opinion about the patient's problem and its cause, and then together they could discuss possible solutions to the problem.

Nurses might invite other healthcare practitioners to a nursing care conference concerning a patient's care. For example, a clinical psychologist might be invited in the preceding example to address the possibility that a mental disorder is influencing this patient's behavior.

Nursing Care Rounds

Nursing care rounds are procedures in which a group of nurses visit selected patients individually, at each patient's bedside. The primary purposes of nursing care rounds are to gather information to help plan nursing care, to evaluate the nursing care the patient has received, and to provide the patient with an opportunity to discuss his or her care with those administering it. As each patient is visited, the nurse assigned provides a short summary of the patient's nursing diagnoses and goals and the care being given. Nursing care rounds have two principal advantages over discussions in a meeting room: Nursing personnel can actually see the patient as a report of care is given, and the patient can participate in discussions of his or her care.

Nurses should use language the patient can understand when holding discussions at the bedside. Otherwise, the patient is likely to feel excluded and that they cannot intelligently participate in the discussion. Nurses might also make rounds with physicians to share nursing's perspective with them.

USING NURSING INFORMATICS

According to the ANA Scope and Standards of Nursing Informatics Practice, **nursing informatics** is a specialty that integrates nursing science, computer science, and information science to manage and communicate data, information, and knowledge in nursing practice. Nursing informatics facilitates the integration of data, information, and knowledge to support patients, nurses, and other providers in their decision making in all roles and settings. This support is accomplished through the use of information structures, information processes, and information technology (American Nurses Association, 2008). As more nurses become informaticists, we are beginning to see tangible benefits of their efforts:

- Increases in the accuracy and completeness of nursing documentation

TABLE • 17-7   HEALTHCARE TECHNOLOGIES DEVELOPED AND IMPLEMENTED BY NURSES

Technology	Description
Smart phones for perioperative nurses	Plans for the iPhone include loading the most up-to-date policies and procedures and educational materials onto an iPhone application for all nurses to access. These include the facility's orientation materials, notes on surgeons' preferences, patient positioning, troubleshooting equipment, PowerPoint presentations, and videos about surgical equipment, instruments, and procedures. Applications also can be developed for quick references for lab values, drug information and calculations, medical terminology, best practices, and numerous other teaching tools.
AccuNurse, a wireless, hands-free voice recognition documentation and communication system for infusion nurses	AccuNurse consists of a wearable computer headset, a speech recognition engine, and a software application. The system prioritizes interventions on a task list and allows nurses to rapidly dictate documentation into the electronic medical record system. It can also remind nurses and staff when interventions need to be performed, such as when to assess or change an IV site.
Bedside medication system on a PDA device	Nurses use the bedside medication administration system to scan patients' bar-coded identification bracelets and medications. The PDA brings up all the necessary medication information, such as the critical five rights: the right patient, drug, dose, route, and time. The PDA allows nurses to document medication administration at the bedside and features automated alerts for such information as vital signs, pain score assessments, and lab results. In addition, nurses can communicate with the pharmacy via the PDA about orders and missing medications.
Vocera B2000 communications badge	This system includes a small wearable device ("Star Trek badge") that is controlled using hands-free instant two-way voice conversation. The system allows nurses to answer calls using their voices without breaking sterile technique or stopping what they are doing. In addition, the system can relay text messages and alerts to a display on the back of the badge. A study done at the University of California Davis found the system eliminated 2 miles of walking per nurse per shift on the nursing units.

Adapted from Spader, C. (2009, August 10). Cool tools. Cutting-edge gadgets sharpen nurses' efficiency. *Nursing Spectrum. Washington, DC/MD/VA, 19*(11), 20–21.

- Improvement in the nurse's workflow and an elimination of redundant documentation
- Automation of the collection and reuse of nursing data
- Facilitation of the analysis of clinical data (Joint Commission indicators, Core measures, federal or state mandated data and facility specific data) (Barthold, Duecker, Guinn, & MacCallum, 2009).

Table 17-7 describes ways that nurses in different areas and specialties are "involved with developing and implementing cutting-edge technologies and tools that are revolutionizing the way they work while improving safety and quality of care for patients" (Spader, 2009). If you are interested in learning about how your personal digital assistant (PDA) can make you more efficient at work and in your personal life, increase your knowledge and understanding of the rapidly changing healthcare environment, and help you keep patients safe, check out the article by Gendreau-Webb (2007) listed in the bibliography. She recommends visiting http://PDACortex.com, a website built specifically for nurses who are considering or already using PDAs and suggests using a search engine, such as Google, to discover available applications. Combine the search terms "freeware" or "shareware" with "nursing" or "medical" and "PDA."

● Developing Critical Thinking Skills

1. Interview three practicing nurses and ask them to describe the documentation methods they have used in their practice. Which methods did they prefer? Which method was more effective, time efficient, and easiest to use?

2. A nurse overhears you complaining about writing narrative nursing notes and says to you, "Don't sweat it. I never worry about documentation—it's a waste of time. I'd rather spend my time doing things for patients than writing up what I did." Think about what you would like to say to this nurse and your rationale for this. Ask other students for their response, and compare your answers.

3. Imagine that you are a nurse in a nursing home and that you and the home are being sued for negligence by the family of an elderly resident who fell and fractured her hip last year. You know the resident but do not remember much about the day she fell. What data do you hope to find recorded in her health record? Which documentation system would most likely provide the type of information you think you need to reconstruct the events surrounding her fall?

4. How would you respond to each of the following requests for patient information? Compare your responses with those of another student and talk about any differences.
   - The mayor of your town, who is up for reelection, was just admitted to your unit after an acute myocardial infarction. You receive a phone call from his office requesting information about his condition.
   - A woman you have never seen approaches you in the hallway, identifies herself as the sexual partner of a married male patient on your unit, and requests information about his condition.
   - A case manager from a managed care organization calls you to ask about the progress an elderly surgical patient is making postoperatively. You have heard that the organization is eager to discharge her quickly, and you feel uncomfortable reporting any information over the phone.
   - A family member asks your advice about developing a personal health record. She says she has heard that there are privacy concerns. How do you respond?

● Practicing for NCLEX

1. Which of the following documentation guidelines are correct? Select all that apply.
   a. Enter information in a complete, accurate, concise, factual, and organized manner.
   b. Use words such as "good," "average," "normal," or "sufficient" to communicate judgments about data.
   c. Wait until the end of the shift to document nursing interventions to ensure comprehensive charting.
   d. Date and time each entry.

2. Which of the following documentation guidelines are correct? Select all that apply.
   a. Erase or use correcting fluid to completely delete mistaken entries.
   b. Document nursing interventions as closely as possible to the time of their execution.
   c. Note problems as they occur in an orderly, sequential manner.
   d. Carefully document all the factors that compromise patient safety and contribute to patient harm.

3. According to the Health Insurance Portability and Accountability Act of 1996, patients have a right to which of the following? Select all that apply.
   a. To see and copy their health record
   b. To update their health record
   c. To get a list of the disclosures a healthcare institution has made independent of disclosures made for the purposes of treatment, payment, and healthcare operations
   d. To request a restriction on certain uses or disclosures
   e. To choose how to receive health information

4. According to the Health Insurance Portability and Accountability Act of 1996, if a health institution wants to release a patient's health information for purposes other than treatment, payment, and routine healthcare operations, the patient must be asked to sign an authorization. There are exceptions to this requirement. In which case below is an authorization needed?
   a. The patient is a public figure and the local news media are preparing a news report.
   b. Data are needed for the tracking and notification of disease outbreaks.
   c. Child abuse and neglect are suspected.
   d. Protected health information is needed to facilitate organ donations.

5. A friend of yours calls you and asks if you are still working at Memorial Hospital. You reply "yes." He tells you that his girlfriend's father was just admitted as a patient, and he wants you to find out how he is. "Sue (his girlfriend) seems unusually worried about her dad, but she won't talk to me and I want to be able to help her." What is the best response you can make to your friend?
   a. "Listen, you shouldn't be asking me to do this. I could be fined big bucks or even lose my job for disclosing this information."
   b. "Sorry, but I'm not able to give information about patients to the public—even when my best friend or a family member asks."
   c. "Because of the Health Insurance Portability and Accountability Act, you shouldn't be asking for this information unless the patient has authorized you to receive it! This could get you in trouble!"
   d. "Why do you think Sue isn't talking about her worries?"

6. Your patient has an order for an analgesic medication to be given as needed. The correct abbreviation for "as needed" is:
   a. TURP
   b. PMH
   c. PRN
   d. TPR

7. If you were looking for trends in a patient's vital signs, what form should you consult first?
   a. Admission sheet
   b. Admission nursing assessment
   c. Activity flow sheet
   d. Graphic sheet

8. This method of documentation uses the categories data, action, and response (DAR) to facilitate charting.
   a. Narrative notes
   b. Focus charting
   c. Charting by exception
   d. Case management model

9. A resident called to see a patient in the middle of the night is leaving the unit and remembers that he forgot to write a new order for a pain medication you had

requested for another patient. Tired and already being paged to another unit, he verbally tells you the order and asks you to document it on the physician's order sheet. Your best response is:

a. "Thank you!"

b. Get a second nurse to listen to the order, and after writing the order on the physician order sheet, have both nurses sign.

c. "I am sorry but verbal orders can only be given in an emergency situation that prevents us from writing them out. I'll bring the chart and we can do this quickly."

d. Try calling another resident for the order or wait until the next shift.

● Answers With Rationale

1. **a** and **d.** Both of these answers represent documentation guidelines that all nurses should follow.

2. **b** and **c.** Both of these answers represent documentation guidelines that all nurses should follow.

3. **a, b, c, d,** and **e.** Each item is correct.

4. **a.** Under no circumstance can a nurse provide information to a news reporter without the patient's express authorization. Items **b, c,** and **d,** however, are legitimate exceptions to the authorization rule.

5. **b.** You should immediately clarify what you can and cannot do. Since your primary reason for refusing to help is linked to your responsibility to protect patient privacy and confidentiality, you should not begin by mentioning the real penalties linked to abuses of privacy (**a, c**). Finally, it is appropriate to ask about Sue and her worries, but this should be done after you clarify what you are able to do (**d**).

6. **c.** PRN means "as needed". TURP (**a**) is transurethral resection of prostate; PMH (**b**) is past medical history; and TPR (**d**) is temperature, pulse, respiration.

7. **d.** While one recording of vital signs should appear on the admission nursing assessment (**b**), the best place to find sequential recordings that show a pattern or trend is the graphic sheet. The admission sheet (**a**) does not include vital sign documentation and neither does the activity flow sheet (**c**).

8. **b.** Focus charting is the only method of documentation that uses the categories data, action, and response (DAR) to facilitate charting.

9. **c.** In most agencies, the only circumstance in which an attending physician, nurse practitioner, or house officer may issue orders verbally is in a medical emergency, which the physician/nurse practitioner is present but finds it impossible, due to the emergency situation, to write the order.

Taylor Suite Resources

The Taylor Suite offers these additional resources to enhance learning and facilitate understanding of this chapter:

- thePoint online resource, http://thepoint.lww.com/Taylor7E
- Student DVD-ROM included with the book
- Study Guide for Taylor's Fundamentals of Nursing

BIBLIOGRAPHY

American Nurses Association (ANA). (1998). *Standards of clinical nursing practice* (2nd ed.). Washington, DC: Author.

American Nurses Association (ANA). (2001). *Code of ethics for nurses with interpretive statements.* Washington, DC: Author.

American Nurses Association (ANA). (2003). *Principles for documentation.* Washington, DC: Author.

American Nurses Association (ANA). (2008). *Nursing informatics: Scope and standards of practice.* Silver Spring, MD: Author.

Baker, L., Wagner, T. H., Singer, S., & Bundorf, M. K. (2003). Use of the Internet and e-mail for health care information: Results from a national survey. *JAMA, 289,* 2400–2406.

Barthold, M. F., Duecker, T., Guinn, P., & MacCallum, R. (2009). Nursing Informatics 101 [Powerpoint]. Available at http://www.himss.org/handouts/NI101.pdf.

Buckley-Womack, C., & Gidney, B. (1987). A new dimension in documentation: The PIE method. *Journal of Neuroscience Nursing, 19*(5), 256–260.

Burke, L., & Murphy, J. (1988). *Charting by exception: A cost-effective quality approach.* Albany, NY: Delmar.

Capuano, T. A. (1995). Clinical pathways: Practical approaches, positive outcomes. *Nursing Management, 26*(1), 34–37.

Clarke, E. B., Luce, J. M., Curtis, J. R., Danis, M., Levy, M., Nelson, J., & Solomon, M. Z. (2004). A content analysis of forms, guidelines, and other materials documenting end-of-life care in intensive care units. *Journal of Critical Care, 19*(2), 108–117.

Eggland, E. T. (1995). Charting smarter. *Nursing, 25*(9), 35–41.

Eggland, E. T., & Heinemann, D. S. (1995). *Nursing documentation: Charting, recording, and reporting.* Philadelphia: J. B. Lippincott.

Gearon, C. J. (2005, March 15). A personal record. *The Washington Post,* pp. F1, F5.

Gendreau-Webb, R. (2007). Put PDAs to work in your practice. *Nursing, 37*(10), 62–63.

George, L., & Davidson, L. (2005). PDA use in nursing education: Prepared for today, poised for tomorrow. *Online Journal Nursing Informatics, 9*(2). Available at http://ojni.org/9_2/george.htm

Greenfield, S. (2007) Medication error reduction and the use of PDA technology. *Journal of Nursing Education, 46*(3), 127–131.

Hamilton, A. V., Coyle, G. A., & Heinen, M. G. (2000). Applied technology rounds out e-documentation: Electronic options keep staff informed and patients updated. *Nursing Management, 35*(9), 44–47.

Health Care Financing Administration. (1995). *Long-term care facility resident assessment instrument (RAI) user's manual.* Washington, DC: Author.

The Health Insurance Portability and Accountability Act of 1996. (1996). Public Law, 104–191. http://www.hhs.gov/ocr/hipaa.

Holmes, H. N. (Ed.). (2006). *Documentation in action.* Philadelphia: Lippincott Williams & Wilkins.

Joint Commission. (2009). Patient safety. Available at http://www.jointcommission.org/PatientSafety/

The Joint Commission. (2010). 2010 Hospital Accreditation Standards. Available at: http://www.jcrinc.com/Accreditation-Manuals/2010-Hospital-Accreditation-Standards/1388/

Karch, A. M. (2004). Practice errors. What's wrong with U? JCAHO places limits on abbreviations used in practice. *American Journal of Nursing, 104*(6), 65–66.

Kahn, J., Aulak, V., & Bosworth, A. (2009). What it takes: Characteristics of the ideal personal health record. *Health Affairs, 28*(2), 369–376.

Keys to successful adoption of electronic medical record systems. (2009, August). *AACN Bold Voices, 1*(2), 11.

Laughlin, J., & Van Nuil, M. (2003). Information systems. Boost regulatory compliance with electronic nursing documentation. *Nursing Management, 34*(12), 51–52, 57–58.

Lefcourt, N. (2005). Reduce charting risks. *Nursing Network, 8*(4), 3.

McGraw, D., Dempsey, J. X., Harris, L., & Goldman, J. (2009). Privacy as an enabler, not an impediment: Building trust into health information exchange. *Health Affairs, 28*(2), 416–427.

Miller, J., & Glusko, J. (2003). Legal checkpoints. Standing up to the scrutiny of medical malpractice. *Nursing Management, 34*(10), 20, 22, 80.

Miller, J., Shaw-Kokot, J., Arnold, M., Boggin, T., Crowell, K., Aellegri, F., et al. (2005). A study of personal digital assistants to enhance undergraduate clinical nursing practice. *Journal of Nursing Education, 44*(1), 19–26.

Muller-Staub, M., Lunney, M., Odenbreit, M., Needham, I., Lavin, M. A., & van Achterberg, T. (2009). Development of an instrument to measure the quality of documented nursing diagnoses, interventions and outcomes: The Q-DIO. *Journal of Clinical Nursing, 18*(7), 1027–1037.

Murphy, E. K. (2003). Charting by exception—OR nursing law. *AORN Journal.* Available at http://www.findarticles.com/p/articles/mi_m0FSL/is_5_78/ai_111011830.

National Alliance for Health Information Technology. (2008, May 20). *Health IT terms established.* Available at www.endonurse.com/hotnews/health-it-terms-set-alliance.html.

Pugno, P. A. (2002). Ethical considerations of electronic communication in the clinical outpatient setting. *Journal of Clinical Ethics, 13*(4), 324–329.

Rashbass, J. (2001). The patient-owned, population-based electronic medical record: A revolutionary resource for clinical medicine. *JAMA: Journal of the American Medical Association, 285*(13), 1769.

Saranto, K., & Kinnunen, U. (2009). Evaluation nursing documentation—Research designs and methods: Systematic review. *Journal of Advanced Nursing, 65*(3), 464–476.

Sensmeier, J., & Lewis, D. (2007). Survey demonstrates importance of nurse informaticist role in health information technology design and implementation. *CIN: Computers, Informatics, Nursing, 25*(3), 180–182.

Siegrist, L., Stocks, B., & Dettor, R. (1985). The PIE system: Complete planning and documentation of nursing care. *QRB, 11*(6), 186–189.

Simpson, R. L. (2007, February). Easing the way for the electronic health record. *American Nurse Today, 2,* 48–50.

Spader, C. (2009, August 10). Cool tools. Cutting-edge gadgets sharpen nurses' efficiency. *Nursing Spectrum.* Washington, DC/MD/VA, *19*(11), 20–21.

Staff, E. J. (1997). Privacy, confidentiality, and security in clinical information systems. *Nursing Administration Quarterly, 21*(3), 21–28.

Thede, L. (2008, Aug 18). The electronic health record: Will nursing be on board when the ship leaves? *OJIN: The Online Journal of Issues in Nursing, 13*(3). Available: http://www.nursingworld.org/MainMenuCategories/ANAMarketplace/ANAPeriodicals/OJIN/Columns/Informatics/ElectronicHealthRecord.aspx

Thede, L. Q. (2006). *Nursing classifications.* Available at http://dlthede.net/Informatics/Chap13/Chap13.htm

Thede, L. Q. (2010). *Informatics and nursing: Competencies and applications* (3rd Ed.). Philadelphia: Lippincott Williams & Wilkins.

Thompson, P., & Bell, P. (2007) Potential student abuse of technology in the clinical setting. *Nurse Educator, 32*(4), 145–146.

Trossman, S. (2009, March/April). Shifting to the bedside for report. *The American Nurse,* 7.

United States Department of Health and Human Services. (n.d.). Nationwide Health Information Network (NHIN): Background. Available at http://healthit.hhs.gov/portal/server.pt?open=512&mode=2&cached=true&objID=1142

von Krogh, G., Dale, C., & Naden, D. (2005). A framework for integrating NANDA, NIC, and NOC terminologies in electronic patient records. *Journal of Nursing Scholarship, 37*(3), 275–281.

von Krogh, G., & Naden, D. (2008). A nursing-specific model of EPR documentation: Organizational and professional requirements. *Journal of Nursing Scholarship, 40*(1), 68–75.

Weaver, C. A., Delaney, C. W., Weber, P., & Carr, R. (Eds.). (2006). *Nursing and informatics for the 21st Century: An international look at practice, trends and the future.* Chicago: HiMSS.

Welton, J., Halloran, E. J., & Zone-Smith, L. (2006). Nursing intensity: In the footsteps of John Thompson. In H. A. Park, P. Murray, & C. Delaney (Eds.), *Consumer centered computer-supported care for healthy people* (pp. 367–371). Amsterdam, Netherlands: IOS Press.

White, A., Allen, P., Goodwin, L., Breckinridge, D., Dowell, J., & Garvey, R. (2005) Infusing PDA technology into nursing education. *Nurse Educator, 30*(4),150–154.

Windle, P. E. (1994). Critical pathways: An integrated documentation tool. *Nursing Management, 25*(9), 80F–L, 80P.

PROMOTING HEALTH ACROSS THE LIFE SPAN

The chapters in Unit IV focus on growth and development through the life cycle. By considering all aspects of the individual, nurses provide healthcare oriented toward wellness and maximize the patient's strengths to reach his or her potential. (Information specific to the influences of the family on growth and development is provided in Chapter 4.)

Chapter 18 gives an overview of developmental concepts and theories necessary to understanding growth and development across the life span. Major theorists and their contributions to the understanding of psychosocial, physical, cognitive, moral, and faith development are described.

Chapter 19 provides information about the individual from conception through young adulthood. Influences on growth and development, as well as physiologic, cognitive, psychosocial, moral, and spiritual development are discussed. Common health problems of each age group and the role of the nurse in health promotion and illness prevention for each age group are considered.

In Chapter 20, the adult years are divided into early, middle, and older-adult stages. Common health problems and the nurse's role in healthcare for the adult continue through older adulthood. The chapter ends with a look at the paradigm of aging and stereotypes common to the older adult. Gerontology and the healthcare system related to this field are discussed.

"The concern of nursing is with man in his entirety, his wholeness. Nursing's body of scientific knowledge seeks to describe, explain, and predict about human beings."

MARTHA ROGERS (1914–1994) • *a nationally renowned nurse theoretician, author, lecturer, and consultant, whose "theory of man" inspired tremendous creativity, research activity, and intellectual growth in the nursing profession*

18 Developmental Concepts

MELANIE KIMBER

Melanie, a 24-year-old single mother, voices concerns about rearing her 12-month-old son by herself. "He is just so active, putting toys in his mouth, and getting into everything. I'm afraid to look away for even a second because he might get hurt. I don't know how other parents do it."

JUAN ALVAREZ

Juan, an 8-year-old boy with encephalitis, becomes violent and combative at times, throwing himself against the bed and muttering words. He immediately calms down when an interpreter visits with him who speaks to him in Spanish and when some of the nurses use Spanish words with him.

JOSEPH LOGAN

Joseph, a 70-year-old man who fell and fractured his hip while repairing the exterior of his home, states, "Go away and leave me alone. I'm a grown man, I can take care of myself . . . and get rid of this tray. I'm not hungry." Further investigation reveals that Mr. Logan has been the traditional head of his household and is now troubled by needing others, including his wife, to care for him.

LEARNING OBJECTIVES

After completing the chapter, you will be able to accomplish the following:

1. Summarize basic principles of growth and development.

2. Discuss the theories of Freud, Erikson, Havighurst, Gould, Levinson, Piaget, Kohlberg, Gilligan, and Fowler.

3. Describe the importance of incorporating theories of growth and development in assessing and planning nursing care for individuals.

4. Explain implications for nursing practice based on an understanding of growth and development.

KEY TERMS

accommodation	faith
assimilation	genomics
cognitive development	growth
development	moral development
developmental task	

Humans grow and develop throughout life. **Growth** is an increase in body size, or changes in body cell structure, function, and complexity. **Development** is an orderly pattern of changes in structure, thoughts, feelings, or behaviors resulting from maturation, experiences, and learning. Development is a dynamic and continuous process as one proceeds through life, characterized by a series of ascents, plateaus, and declines. The human processes of growth and development result from the interrelated effects of heredity and environment. Humans simultaneously grow and develop in physical, cognitive, psychosocial, moral, and spiritual dimensions, with each dimension being an essential part of the whole person.

Nurses promote health in people from birth to death. All people, regardless of age, have unique healthcare needs that result from their physical, intellectual, emotional, sociocultural, spiritual, and environmental dimensions at their developmental level. To plan and give holistic and individualized care, the nurse must understand typical growth and development characteristics, tasks, and needs of patients of all ages. (See the accompanying Reflective Practice box.)

This chapter presents theories and principles of growth and development across the life span that help us understand both healthy and ill people at various life stages. The major theories examining cognitive, psychosocial, spiritual, and moral development are discussed.

PRINCIPLES OF GROWTH AND DEVELOPMENT

Everyone's physical development has a predetermined genetic base because of inheritance patterns carried on the chromosomes. Thus, an unborn child begins life with specific physical attributes. Environmental factors from birth through the early years of growth provide initial psychological and social contact through positive or negative experiences with caregivers. As environmental influences expand beyond the immediate caregivers or family, development is influenced by a wide variety of psychosocial experiences. Cognitive, moral, and spiritual development are fostered through interactions within the family, school, and community. The nurse can better understand these interrelated variables at specific life stages through theories of human growth and development.

Growth and development are orderly and sequential as well as continuous and complex. All humans experience the same growth patterns and developmental levels, but because these patterns and levels are individualized, a wide variation in biologic and behavioral changes is considered normal. Within each developmental level, certain milestones can be identified; for example, the first time the infant rolls over, crawls, walks, or says his or her first words. Although growth and development occur in individual ways for different people, certain generalizations can be made about the nature of human development for everyone. These generalizations, outlined in Box 18-1, form the principles that help us understand growth and development.

FACTORS INFLUENCING GROWTH AND DEVELOPMENT

Many different factors influence both growth and development. One's growth and development might be facilitated or delayed by genetic heredity; prenatal, individual, and caregiver factors; and environment and nutrition. Other factors influencing growth and development are health–illness state (discussed in Chapters 3, 4, 19, 20) and culture (discussed in Chapter 2).

> *Think back to Juan, the 8-year-old boy with encephalitis described in the case file at the beginning of the chapter. Although his behavior could be attributed to his infection, culture also may be a contributory factor for his behavior.* ■

Because of these often interrelated and interdependent factors, each person's growth and development is individualized.

Genetic Heredity

At conception, every human receives an equal number of chromosomes from each parent. The characteristics inherited from each parent are carried in gene pairs on the 23 pairs of chromosomes, which carry the genetic information that determine the person's cellular differentiation, growth, and function. As a result, physical characteristics such as height, bone size, and eye and hair color are inherited from our family of origin. Other characteristics, such as personality, are not as clearly identified with genetic heredity, but research is ongoing in this area. It is well known that genetic heredity influences the development of many diseases, such as cancer and diabetes. The Human Genome Project, completed in 2003, was a national and international research project to map the estimated 35,000 to 140,000 genes in the human chromosomes.

REFLECTIVE PRACTICE
Challenge to Ethical Skills

Two summers ago, while working in a nurse externship program, I worked with Juan, a Spanish-speaking 8-year-old boy diagnosed with encephalitis. The boy would become violent and combative at times, throwing himself against the bed and muttering words. Although his underlying disease was a likely cause of this behavior, he became calm when an interpreter was with him. The interpreter would speak to him in Spanish and he seemed to calm down. He also would appear calmer when nurses spoke Spanish words to him. Unfortunately, most nurses and physicians would ignore his screams in a language they did not understand, complaining about his behavior, and relying on medication to calm him.

On one particular day, I was in the room with a physician who was writing an assessment note for Juan while I was getting his bath water ready for morning care. As usual, Juan was muttering words and thrashing in the bed. I knew some measures to calm him; for example, speaking the few Spanish words I knew. The physician remained in her chair, looking at me and complaining about Juan's behavior, not making any effort to calm him. She said that she could not do anything to calm him down except prescribe sedative medications. I felt bad for the patient and knew he was frustrated. I knew that I could possibly help in this situation, but did not want to show disrespect to the physician.

Thinking Outside the Box: Possible Courses of Action

- I could nod in agreement with the physician. After all, I was only a nursing student and "didn't know better" than she did.
- I could tell her what measures I had used to help calm Juan.
- I could refrain from saying anything at all, wait until the physician had left, and then try to calm Juan.

Evaluating a Good Outcome: How Do I Define Success?

- Patient benefited from my actions.
- I did not disrespect the physician.
- I was able to use my intuition, authority, and common sense to the best of my ability.
- Did I have the authority to jump in and give the physician advice on how to care for the patient?
- In this situation, my intuition and common sense told me to jump up and take action to calm down poor Juan, who was frustrated and upset.

Personal Learning: Here's to the Future!

Unfortunately, in this situation, I did not respond as I would have liked to. I did not say anything, but watched Juan become upset and mutter Spanish words. During this whole time, the physician shook her head, looked down on him, and told me she just "couldn't do anything about him" except to give him medications. I waited until the physician left, and then tried to calm Juan myself. In this situation, I should have let the physician know about the methods used to calm Juan previously, not just the simple use of drugs to sedate him.

However, as a junior level nursing student, I did not feel comfortable enough to use this type of authority. I now see how important it is for nurses and all staff members to communicate their opinions, beliefs, and observations about patients for the benefit of the patient. These suggestions and opinions need to be heard so that patients receive the best possible care. In the future, as a practicing nurse, I will respect my fellow staff members, but always make sure that my voice is heard concerning a patient's needs.

Reflection

How do you think you would respond in a similar situation? Why? What do you think Juan might have been experiencing and why? What if the nursing student did approach the physician about using other methods to calm Juan? Would you consider this action to be disrespectful? How do you think the physician would have responded to the nursing student's feedback about the use of the Spanish language to calm Juan? What does this tell you about yourself and about the adequacy of your skills for professional practice? Do you think that you would act differently if the physician were male? At a different stage of development? For example, a 60-year-old physician instead of one that might be 45 years old? What would influence your actions in each of these situations? Can you think of other ways to respond or approach the situation? What other skills (cognitive, interpersonal, technical, ethical/legal) would you need to respond well in this situation? Would Juan's stage of growth and development influence your nursing care? Do you think that the nursing student's stage of growth and development may have played a role in the student's response? Why or why not? Do you agree with the criteria that the nursing student used to evaluate a successful outcome? Explain your answer.

Box 18-1 PRINCIPLES OF GROWTH AND DEVELOPMENT

Growth and development are orderly and sequential, as well as continuous and complex. All humans experience the same growth patterns and developmental levels. Because these patterns and levels are individualized, a wide variation in biologic and behavioral changes is considered normal. Within each developmental level, certain milestones can be identified; for example, the time the infant rolls over, crawls, walks, and says his or her first words.

Growth and development follow regular and predictable trends. Cephalocaudal (proceeding from head to tail) development is the first trend, with the head and brain developing first, followed by the trunk, legs, and feet. The second trend is proximodistal development, which means that growth progresses from gross motor movements (such as learning to lift one's head) to fine motor movements (such as learning to pick up a toy with the fingers). The last trend is symmetric development of the body, with both sides of the body developing equally.

Growth and development are both differentiated and integrated. As nerve pathways develop, they become more specialized, allowing the growing child to respond to different stimuli. Throughout the life span, each new learned ability builds on previously learned abilities so that increasingly complex tasks can be accomplished. For example, the toddler learning to use a spoon combines motor skills, hand–eye coordination, cog-

nitive patterning, and social imitation from watching others. As children grow and develop, the task of learning to use a spoon becomes basic, forming the foundation for learning skills requiring more manual dexterity.

Different aspects of growth and development occur at different stages and at different rates, and can be modified. For example, muscles and bones both grow most rapidly during the first year of life. During the toddler and preschool years, bone growth slows, but muscle fibers increase in size and strength. The most intense period of speech development is between 3 and 5 years of age. Sexual maturity begins during the preadolescent years and progresses into the adult years, but is based on gender and sex role identity established from birth. Many factors can modify growth and development, including nutrition, love and affection from caregivers, and illnesses.

The pace of growth and development is specific for each person. Both physical and psychological skills and maturation vary among people. For example, while learning to walk, a child may concentrate energies on the task and temporarily slow down in language development. Racial variations may also be seen; Asian children tend to be smaller than white children of the same age. In addition, one's genetic heredity places restrictions on the upper limits that can be achieved in growth and development.

Ongoing analysis of the results of this project aim to identify the chemical basis for as many as 4,000 genetic diseases, and to provide tests to screen for, diagnose, and treat genetic disorders (Williams, Skirton, & Masny, 2006; Porth, 2007).

Genomics is the study of the structure and interactions of all the genes in the human body, including their interactions with each other as well as the environment. In the very near future, all healthcare providers will be challenged to integrate genomics into their research, education, and practice (Goldberg & Jenkins, 2008). Nurses must be prepared to answer questions and discuss the impact of genetic findings on health and illness. Their patient assessments, nursing care, and health teaching will depend on this knowledge base (see the accompanying Research in Nursing box) Organizations that serve as resources for genetic technology and information are included in Table 18-1.

Prenatal, Individual, and Caregiver Factors

Prenatal, individual, and caregiver factors influence development. Fetal development can be altered by maternal age (with risk greater in those younger than 15 years of age or older than 35 years of age), substance abuse, inadequate prenatal care, inadequate maternal nutrition, and maternal substance abuse. Individual factors that might result in altered development from birth through adolescence include congenital or genetic disorders, brain damage from accidents or abuse, vision and hearing impairments, chronic illness, inadequate nutrition, chemotherapy or radiation therapy, lead poisoning, poverty, and substance abuse. Caregiver factors that negatively affect development are neglect and abuse, mental illness, mental retardation, or a severe learning disability.

Environment and Nutrition

Environment and nutrition influence all stages of development. Environmental factors that might alter development include poverty and violence. The effect of each can occur independently, but they are more likely to be interrelated, as seen in these examples:

- Infants who are malnourished in utero develop fewer brain cells than infants who have had adequate prenatal nutrition.

TABLE • 18-1 **GENETIC TECHNOLOGY AND INFORMATION RESOURCES**

Organization	Activities
Human Genome Project www.genome.gov	Helps healthcare practitioner understand concepts and issues related to genetic services
My Family Health Portrait https://familyhistory.hhs.gov	Aids in construction of a family pattern of diseases
Gene Tests www.genetests.org	Provides information on breast cancer screening and government-related labs
National Society of Genetic Counselors www.nsgc.org/resourcelink.cfm	Locates genetic nurse counseling services according to zip code location

RESEARCH IN NURSING
Bridging the Gap to Evidence-Based Practice

USING GENOMIC INFORMATION TO EDUCATE PATIENTS ABOUT PREGNANCY RISKS

Both before pregnancy occurs and during a pregnancy are critical times to incorporate health teaching that has the potential to reduce risks and lead to the birth of a healthy child. Genomic information can identify gene mutations and environmental influences that can impact a pregnancy and help families to make more informed decisions about these pregnancy risks.

Related Research

Dolan, S., Biermann, J., & Damus, K. (2007). Genomics for health in preconception and prenatal periods. *Journal of Nursing Scholarship, 39*(1), 4–9.

This research was designed to review and report the effect of genomic-based knowledge on nursing interactions and care during the prenatal and pregnancy period. Genomic research continues to identify populations at risk for certain diseases, and nurses need the knowledge base to be able to answer questions, provide appropriate health teaching, and counsel or direct patients at risk to available resources. Genetic testing and screening have enhanced risk assessment. For example, women who have a family history of cystic fibrosis (CF) or a partner with a history of CF can participate in carrier screening for this disease. The ability to predict with certainty the severity of a disease based on genotype (the inherited genetic informa-

tion carried by all living organisms) is more difficult. Nurses, in collaboration with genetics professionals, may be involved in communicating and explaining particular risks to women and their families. Extensive research has attempted to identify the exact determinants of preterm birth. Many potential causes have been studied, including the interaction of environmental factors with various genetic factors. Some studies reported that the genetic component was responsible for one-quarter to one-third of preterm births, but the value of risk assessment strategies that take into account the effect of personal and family history and environmental factors is yet to be determined. More research is needed to accurately predict particular populations that will be impacted by disease and the complex relationship between genetics and environment.

Relevance to Nursing Practice

This study is one example of how research impacts nursing practice. Nurses need to effectively interact with individuals and families to better define risks and promote health in these vulnerable populations. New genetic technologies and information require nurses to continue to expand their knowledge base by taking advantage of ever expanding resources. Nurses must be prepared to become a driving force in this genomic approach to targeting many diseases.

For additional research, visit thePoint.

- Substance abuse by a pregnant woman increases the risk for congenital anomalies, low birthweight, and prematurity in her developing fetus.
- Federally sponsored school meal programs support enhanced learning with adequate nutrition.
- Failure to thrive, a condition of early infancy, has been linked to both nutritional and emotional deprivation.
- Environmental challenges, such as substandard housing and inadequate medical care, can further compound the effects of poor nutrition.
- Child abuse is an extreme example of physical and emotional harm or deprivation, leading to deficits in physical or psychosocial development, or both.
- Substance abuse by adolescents and young adults is associated with an increased incidence of teenage pregnancy, violence, accidents, and suicide. Abuse of alcohol and drugs is more prevalent in teenagers who have poor family relationships, low self-esteem, and poor social skills.

OVERVIEW OF DEVELOPMENTAL THEORIES

Human development and behavior have been studied since the beginning of the 20th century, and theories that explain human responses expected at certain ages during life have been developed. Although a psychological approach is common to all developmental theories, each theory has a different focus. The theories discussed in the following sections

examine cognitive, social, and instinctual influences on human growth and development, and key points are summarized in Table 18-2.

Theory of Psychoanalytic Development: Sigmund Freud

Freud's theory emphasizes the effect of instinctual human drives on behavior. Freud identified the underlying stimulus for human behavior as sexuality, which he called *libido*. Libido is defined as general pleasure-seeking instincts rather than purely genital gratification.

Four major components of Freud's theory are:

- the unconscious mind
- the id
- the ego
- the superego

The unconscious mind contains memories, motives, fantasies, and fears that are not easily recalled but that directly affect behavior. The id is the part of the mind concerned with self-gratification by the easiest and quickest available means. Defense mechanisms are a means of unconscious coping to reduce stress in the conscious mind when the id's impulses cannot be satisfied. (Defense mechanisms are discussed in Chapter 42.)

The ego is the conscious part of the mind that serves as a mediator between the desires of the id and the constraints of

TABLE • 18-2	KEY POINTS OF DEVELOPMENTAL THEORIES				
	Freud	Erikson	Havighurst	Piaget	Fowler	Kohlberg
Theme	Psychosexual	Psychosocial	Developmental	Cognitive	Faith	Moral
Infancy to toddlerhood	Oral stage; anal stage	Trust versus mistrust; autonomy versus shame and doubt	Learning to walk; learning to talk; learning to control body waste elimination	Basic reflexes; coordinates more than one thought at a time; begins to reason and anticipate events	Centers on relationship with primary caregiver	Oriented to obedience and punishment
Preschool to early school years	Phallic stage	Initiative versus guilt	Learning sex differences; forming concepts; getting ready to read	Increased language; increased understanding of life events and relationships	Imitates religious behaviors of others	Defines acts satisfying to self and some satisfying to others as right
School years	Latent stage	Industry versus inferiority	Learning physical skills; learning to get along with others; developing conscience and morality	Develops logical thinking; incorporates others' perspectives; uses abstract thinking and deductive reasoning; tests beliefs to establish values	Accepts existence of deity; stories define religious and moral beliefs	Morality of maintaining good relations and approval of others; aware of need to respect authority
Adolescent to adult years	Genital stage	Intimacy versus generation	Achieving gender-specific social role; achieving independence; acquiring a set of values and an ethical system to guide behavior	Adopts life-guiding values or religious practices	Selects principles to follow; concern for the rights and needs of others	
Middle adult years		Generativity versus stagnation	Achieving social and civic responsibility; accepting and adjusting to physical changes	Integrates others' viewpoints into own understanding of truth		
Later adult years		Ego integrity versus despair	Adjusting to decreasing physical status and health; adjusting to retirement	Values absolute love and justice of all; believes in the existence of the future		

reality so that one might live effectively within one's social, physical, and psychological environment. The ego includes one's intelligence, memory, problem solving, separation of reality from fantasy, and incorporation of experiences and learning into future behavior. Development of the ego allows the infant, by 6 months of age, to view self as separate from others and to begin to alter behaviors in response to cues. Ego development continues throughout life.

The superego is the part of the mind that represents one's conscience. It develops from the ego during the first year of life, as the child learns praise versus punishment for actions. The superego represents the internalization of rules and values so that socially acceptable behavior is practiced.

In addition, Freud described a series of developmental stages through which all people must pass. The stages of development are based on sexual motivation (Freud & Strachey, 1960). A discussion of the developmental stages follows.

Oral Stage (Ages 0 to 18 Months)

During the oral stage, the infant uses his or her mouth as the major source of gratification and exploration. Pleasure is experienced from eating, biting, chewing, and sucking. The infant's primary need is for security. A major conflict occurs with weaning.

> ➤ *Recall Ms. Kimber, the young, single, frustrated mother of a 12-month-old child. The nurse might apply the concepts of Freud's theory in the nursing care of Ms. Kimber and her child by explaining the oral behaviors typical of the stage of her child's development.* ∎

Anal Stage (Ages 8 Months to 4 Years)

This stage begins with the development of neuromuscular control to allow control of the anal sphincter. Toilet training is a crucial issue, requiring delayed gratification as the child compromises between enjoyment of bowel function and limits set by social expectations.

Phallic Stage (Ages 3 to 7 Years)

The child has increased interest in gender differences and his or her own gender (Fig. 18-1). The child experiences conflict and resolution of that conflict with the parent of the same sex (named the Oedipus complex in boys and the Electra complex in girls, based on feelings of intimate sexual possessiveness for the opposite-sex parent). Curiosity about the genitals and masturbation increase during this stage.

Latency Stage (Ages 7 to 12 Years)

This stage marks the transition to the genital stage during adolescence. Increasing sex-role identification with the parent of the same sex prepares the child for adult roles and relationships.

FIGURE 18-1. This preschool girl enjoys imitating her mother as she learns about the world around her. *(Photo by Joe Mitchell.)*

Genital Stage (Ages 12 to 20 Years)

At this stage, sexual interest can be expressed in overt sexual relationships. Sexual pressures and conflicts typically cause turmoil as the adolescent makes adjustments in relationships.

Theory of Cognitive Development: Jean Piaget

Piaget and Inhelder (1969) developed a theory of **cognitive development** from infancy through adolescence. Piaget believed that learning occurs as a result of the internal organization of an event, forming a mental schema (plan) and serving as a base for further schemata as one grows and develops. Intellectual growth is a continual restructuring of knowledge to progress to higher levels of problem solving and critical thinking. Two continual processes of restructuring knowledge, assimilation and accommodation, stimulate intellectual growth in the child. **Assimilation** is the process of integrating new experiences into existing schemata. **Accommodation** is an alteration of existing thought processes to manage more complex information. Piaget described four stages of cognitive development, which are discussed here.

Sensorimotor Stage (Birth to 24 Months)

This stage is marked by progression through a series of developmental stages; for example:

- 0 to 1 month—Demonstrates basic reflexes, such as sucking
- 1 to 4 months—Discovers enjoyment of random behaviors (such as smiling or sucking thumb) and repeats them
- 4 to 8 months—Relates own behavior to a change in environment, such as shaking a rattle to hear the sound or manipulating a spoon to eat
- 8 to 12 months—Coordinates more than one thought pattern at a time to reach a goal, such as repeatedly throwing an object on the floor; only objects in sight are considered permanent

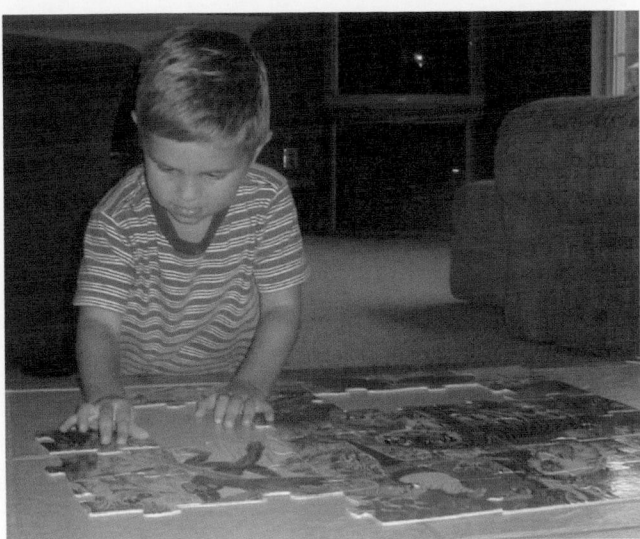

FIGURE 18-2. This child's cognitive development is characterized by the ability to learn simple sequences and relationships.

- 12 to 18 months—Recognizes the permanence of objects, even if out of sight; can understand simple commands
- 18 to 24 months—Begins to develop reasoning and can anticipate events

➤ *Recall Ms. Kimber, the single mother of a 12-month-old infant. Applying the knowledge of Piaget's theory, the nurse could develop a teaching plan for the mother that addresses appropriate anticipatory guidance to prevent injury while fostering the child's cognitive development.* ■

Preoperational Stage (Ages 2 to 7 Years)

This stage is characterized by the beginning use of symbols, through increased language skills and pictures, to represent the preschooler's world (Fig. 18-2). This stage is divided into two parts: the preconceptual stage (ages 2 to 4 years) and the intuitive stage (ages 4 to 7 years). Play activities during this time help the child to understand life events and relationships.

Concrete Operational Stage (Ages 7 to 11 Years)

During this stage, children learn by manipulating concrete or tangible objects and can classify articles according to two or more characteristics. Logical thinking is developing, with an understanding of reversibility, relations between numbers, and loss of egocentricity, in addition to the ability to incorporate another's perspective.

Formal Operational Stage (Age 11 Years or Older)

This stage is characterized by the use of abstract thinking and deductive reasoning. General concepts are related to

specific situations and alternatives are considered. The world is evaluated by testing beliefs in an attempt to establish values and meaning in life.

Theories of Psychosocial Development
Erik Erikson

Erikson's (1963) developmental theory was based on Freud's work but was expanded to include cultural and social influences in addition to biologic processes. His psychosocial theory is based on four major organizing concepts:

- Stages of development
- Developmental goals or tasks
- Psychosocial crises
- The process of coping

Erikson believed that development is a continuous process made up of distinct stages, characterized by the achievement of developmental goals that are affected by the social environment and significant others. He identified eight stages that progress from birth to old age and death. Each stage is characterized by a developmental crisis to be mastered, with possible successful or unsuccessful resolution of the crisis. Unsuccessful resolution at any one stage might delay progress through the next stage, but mastery can occur later. A discussion of the developmental stages follows.

TRUST VERSUS MISTRUST (INFANCY)

The infant learns to rely on caregivers to meet basic needs of warmth, food, and comfort, forming trust in others. Mistrust is the result of inconsistent, inadequate, or unsafe care (Fig. 18-3).

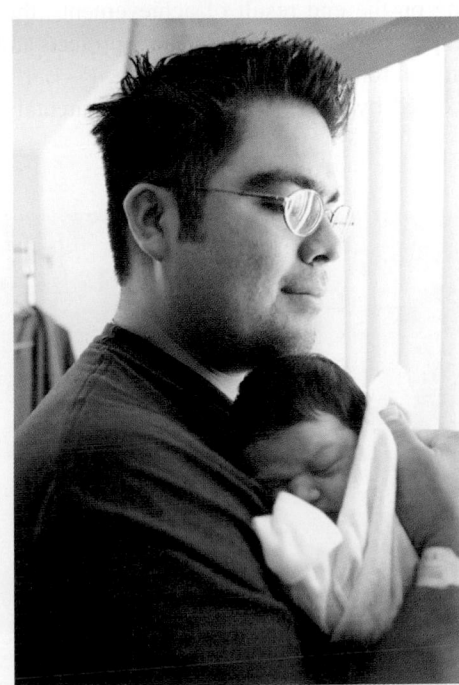

FIGURE 18-3. This caregiver provides comfort and affection to his daughter, teaching her to trust in others. *(Photo by Joe Mitchell.)*

AUTONOMY VERSUS SHAME AND DOUBT (TODDLER)

As motor and language skills develop, the toddler (ages 1 to 3 years) learns from the environment and gains independence through encouragement from caregivers to feed, dress, and toilet self. If the caregivers are overprotective or have expectations that are too high, shame and doubt, as well as feelings of inadequacy, might develop in the child.

▶ *Think back to Ms. Kimber, the single mother. The nurse could apply Erikson's theory to explain the child's "getting into everything" as his need for learning about the environment and gaining independence. Additionally, the mother's anxiety level and the child's attempts to investigate the environment through locomotion and oral exploration place the child at risk for injury from a fall or aspiration of a small object. With astute observation and knowledge of child development, the nurse plays a primary role in prevention by educating the mother.* ■

INITIATIVE VERSUS GUILT (PRESCHOOL)

Confidence gained as a toddler allows the preschooler (ages 4 to 6 years) to take the initiative in learning so that the child actively seeks out new experiences and explores the how and why of activities. If the child experiences restrictions or reprimands for seeking new experiences and learning, guilt results, and the child hesitates to attempt more challenging skills in motor or language development.

INDUSTRY VERSUS INFERIORITY (SCHOOL-AGED CHILDREN)

Focusing on the end result of achievements, the school-aged child gains pleasure from finishing projects and receiving recognition for accomplishments (Fig. 18-4). If the child is not accepted by peers or cannot meet parental expecta-

tions, a feeling of inferiority and lack of self-worth might develop.

▶ *Think back to Juan, the 8-year-old boy described in the case file at the beginning of the chapter. The nurse could help to foster Juan's industry by offering positive reinforcement for his ability to calm down when spoken to in Spanish. The nurse also could incorporate activities into Juan's plan of care that would provide him with opportunities to succeed.* ■

IDENTITY VERSUS ROLE CONFUSION (ADOLESCENCE)

With many physical changes occurring, the adolescent is in transition from childhood to adulthood. Hormonal changes produce secondary sex characteristics and mood swings. Trying on roles and even rebellion are considered normal behaviors as the adolescent acquires a sense of self and deciding what direction will be taken in life. Role confusion occurs when the adolescent is unable to establish identity and a sense of direction.

INTIMACY VERSUS ISOLATION (YOUNG ADULTHOOD)

The tasks for the young adult are to unite self-identity with identities of friends and to make commitments to others. Fear of such commitments results in isolation and loneliness.

▶ *Remember Ms. Kimber, the single mother described at the beginning of the chapter. She appears to have a limited support system. Recognizing this, the nurse can assess further to identify the mother's potential problems with intimacy and subsequently, her progression toward generativity.* ■

GENERATIVITY VERSUS STAGNATION (MIDDLE ADULTHOOD)

The middle adult years are marked by involvement with family, friends, and community. This is also a time of having concern for the next generation and a desire to make a contribution to the world. If this task is not met, stagnation results, and the person becomes self-absorbed and obsessed with her or his own needs or regresses to an earlier level of coping.

EGO INTEGRITY VERSUS DESPAIR (LATER ADULTHOOD)

As one enters the older years, reminiscence about life events provides a sense of fulfillment and purpose. If one believes that one's life has been a series of failures or missed directions, a sense of despair might prevail.

▶ *Think back to Mr. Logan, the 70-year-old man who broke his hip. Applying Erikson's theory, the nurse could*

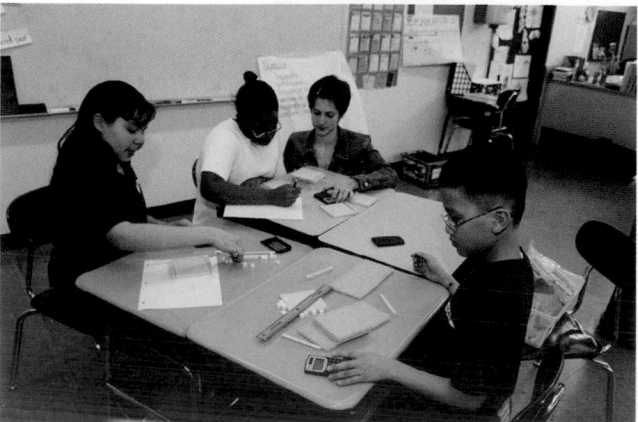

FIGURE 18-4. School-aged children focus on the end results of accomplishments—recognition and praise from family, teachers, and peers—in their development of a sense of competition and industry.

assess Mr. Logan for indications of despair due to his feelings of dependency on others, and plan appropriate interventions to foster a sense of fulfillment and purpose. ■

Robert J. Havighurst

Havighurst (1972) believed that living and growing are based on learning, and that a person must continuously learn to adjust to changing societal conditions. He described learned behaviors as **developmental tasks** that occur at certain periods in life. Successful achievement leads to happiness and success in later tasks, whereas unsuccessful achievement leads to unhappiness, societal disapproval, and difficulty in later tasks. The developmental tasks arise from maturation, personal motives, and values that determine occupational and family choices and civic responsibility. The developmental tasks, by age, follow.

INFANCY AND EARLY CHILDHOOD

Developmental tasks for infancy and early childhood include:

- Achieving physiologic stability
- Learning to eat solid foods
- Learning to walk and talk
- Forming simple concepts of social and physical reality
- Learning to relate emotionally to parents, siblings, and other people
- Learning to control the elimination of body wastes
- Learning to distinguish between right and wrong
- Learning sex differences and sexual modesty

MIDDLE CHILDHOOD

Developmental tasks for middle childhood include:

- Learning physical skills necessary for games
- Learning to get along with age-mates
- Developing fundamental skills in reading, writing, and mathematics
- Developing a conscience, morality, and a scale of values
- Achieving personal independence

ADOLESCENCE

Developmental tasks for adolescence include:

- Accepting one's body and using it effectively
- Achieving a masculine or feminine gender role
- Achieving emotional independence from parents and other adults
- Preparing for a career
- Preparing for marriage and family life
- Desiring and achieving socially responsible behavior
- Acquiring an ethical system as a guide to behavior

YOUNG ADULTHOOD

Developmental tasks for young adulthood include:

- Selecting a mate (Fig. 18-5)
- Learning to live with a marriage partner

FIGURE 18-5. Choosing a life partner is often an important developmental task for young adults.

- Starting a family and rearing children
- Managing a home
- Getting started in an occupation
- Taking on civic responsibility
- Finding a congenial social group

MIDDLE ADULTHOOD

Developmental tasks for middle adulthood include:

- Accepting and adjusting to physical changes
- Attaining and maintaining a satisfactory occupational performance
- Assisting children to become responsible adults
- Relating to one's spouse as a person
- Adjusting to aging parents
- Achieving adult social and civic responsibility

LATER MATURITY

Developmental tasks for later maturity include:

- Adjusting to decreasing physical strength and health
- Adjusting to retirement and reduced income
- Adjusting to death of a spouse
- Establishing an explicit affiliation with one's age group
- Adjusting and adapting social roles in a flexible way
- Establishing satisfactory physical living arrangements

➤ *Recall Mr. Logan, the older adult male with the fractured hip described at the beginning of the chapter. Based on his comments, the nurse could apply Havighurst's theory to conclude that Mr. Logan might be fluctuating between feelings of nonadjustment and feelings of acceptance of his declining health.* ■

Roger Gould

Gould (1978) studied men and women between the ages of 16 and 60 years, labeling the central theme for the adult years as "transformation," with specific beliefs and developmental phases.

AGES 18 TO 22

During the young adult years, individuals typically struggle with leaving their parents' world and challenging false assumptions from their child-like consciousness (e.g., "Only my parents can guarantee my safety."). However, these assumptions are replaced with new false assumptions, such as "Rewards will come automatically if we do what we are supposed to do."

AGES 22 TO 28

Individuals in their 20s feel established as adults and separate from their families, but believe they must still demonstrate their competence as independent adults to their parents. They want to enjoy the present but build for the future.

AGES 29 TO 34

Self-acceptance increases as the need to prove oneself disappears. Marriage and careers are well established, and young parents want to accept their own children for what they are becoming without imposing rules. Questions about life in general are still present.

AGES 35 TO 43

Adults in this age group tend to continually look inward and question themselves, their values, and life. They see time as having an end and believe they have little time left to shape the behavior of their adolescent children (Fig. 18-6). They may be critical of their own parents, blaming them for many of their own problems.

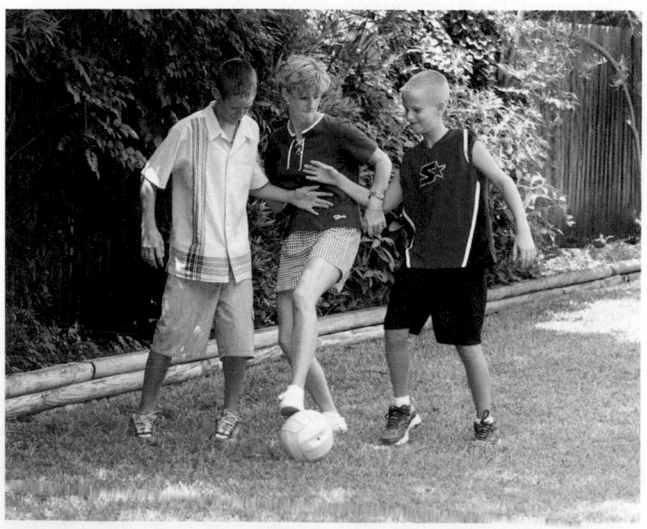

FIGURE 18-6. As her sons grow into young adults, this mom adapts to remain a positive influence in their lives. *(Photo by Joe Mitchell.)*

AGES 43 TO 50

At this phase, the adult accepts the reality of boundaries for the life span, and believes personalities are set. They are interested in an active social life, church activities, community service, friends, and spouse. Life is viewed as neither simple nor controllable, which might result in periods of passivity, rage, depression, and despair.

AGES 50 TO 60

Previous patterns of reflection and contemplation result in increased self-approval and self-acceptance. Increased marital happiness and contentment were associated with seeing spouse as a valued companion.

Daniel Levinson and Associates

Levinson and associates (1978) based their theory on the organizing concept of "individual life structure." The theory centered on the belief that the pattern of life at any point in time is formed by the interaction of three components: the self (values, motives), the social and cultural aspects of one's life (family, career, religion, ethnic background), and the particular set of roles in which one participates (husband, father, friend, student). When anything changes in one component, the whole life structure must then reorganize. According to Levinson and associates, the major phases in young and middle adult life are (1) early adult transition, (2) entering the adult world, (3) settling down, (4) midlife transition, and (5) pay-off years.

EARLY ADULT TRANSITION

The major concerns of the young adult (age 18–22) are to break away from one's parents, to make initial career choices, and to establish intimate relationships. Many separations, losses, and transformations are necessary to terminate old relationships. This is also a time to begin to select personal values and establish goals, as one's life structure begins to be more integrated.

ENTERING THE ADULT WORLD

The years of the middle to late 20s (age 22–28) are a time to build on previous decisions and choices, and to try different careers and lifestyles. By the late 20s, the young adult enters the age-30 transition period. The individual often feels uneasy that something is missing. During this transition, decisions are made either to find a new direction in life or to make a stronger commitment to previous choices.

SETTLING DOWN

In the settling-down phase (age 30–40), the adult invests energy into the areas of life that are most personally important. The areas of investment are primarily family, work, and community. The individual strives to gain respect, status, and a sense of authority.

MIDLIFE TRANSITION

Midlife transition (age 40–45) involves a reappraisal of one's goals and values. The established lifestyle may continue, or the individual may choose to reorganize and change careers. This is an unsettled time, with the individual often anxious and fearful.

THE PAY-OFF YEARS

The years from 45 to 65 are a time of maximum self-direction and self-approval. Physical and mental changes increase an awareness of one's aging and mortality.

Theories of Moral Development
Lawrence Kohlberg

Kohlberg (1969) developed a theory of **moral development** in levels that closely follow Piaget's theory of cognitive development. Kohlberg recognized that a person's moral development is influenced by cultural effects on one's perceptions of justice in interpersonal relationships. A child's beginnings of moral development result from caregiver and child communications during the early childhood years, as the young child tries to please his or her parents (Fig. 18-7). The concept of morality emerges as a subset of a person's beliefs or values and governs choices made throughout life. Rules and regulations established by society are eventually challenged and evaluated as a person either accepts societal rules into his or her own internal set of values or rejects them.

> *Remember Juan, the 8-year-old with encephalitis. Juan's language barrier and cultural heritage may be adding to the child's already heightened fears and anxieties due to hospitalization. Astute observation and knowledge of Kohlberg's theory by the nurse can help toward understanding the child's perceptions, beliefs, and, ultimately, his choices and actions.* ■

The levels of moral development include preconventional, conventional, and postconventional. Each level is further divided into separate stages.

PRECONVENTIONAL LEVEL

The preconventional level is based on external control, as the child learns to conform to rules imposed by authority figures. At stage 1, punishment and obedience orientation, the motivation for choices of action is fear of physical consequences of authority's disapproval. As a result of the consequences, a perception of goodness or badness develops. At stage 2, instrumental relativist orientation, the thought of receiving a reward overcomes fear of punishment, so actions that satisfy this desire are selected.

CONVENTIONAL LEVEL

The conventional level involves identifying with significant others and conforming to their expectations. The person respects the values and ideals of family and friends, regardless of consequences. In stage 3, "good boy–good girl" orientation, the person strives for approval in an attempt to be viewed as "good." At stage 4, "law and order" orientation, behavior follows social or religious rules from a respect for authority. In his later work, Kohlberg maintained that many adults are at this stage because they think abstractly and view themselves as members of society.

POSTCONVENTIONAL LEVEL

The postconventional level involves moral judgment that is rational and internalized into one's standards or values. At stage 5, social contract and utilitarian orientation, correct behavior is defined in terms of society's laws. Laws can be changed, however, to meet society's needs, while maintaining respect for self and others. Stage 6, universal ethical principle orientation, represents the person's concern for equality for all human beings, guided by personal values and standards, regardless of those set by society or laws. Justice might be internalized at an even higher level than society. Few adults ever reach this stage of development.

Carol Gilligan

Gilligan (1977;1982) originally worked with Kohlberg. As she listened to women discuss their own real-life moral conflicts, she recognized that there was a conception of morality from the female viewpoint that was not represented in Kohlberg's work. Gilligan's theory views females as developing a morality of response and care, and males as developing a morality of justice.

In Gilligan's theory, males and females have different ways of looking at the world. Males are more likely to associate morality with obligations, rights, and justice. Females are

FIGURE 18-7. This grandfather reads traditional stories to his young granddaughter, teaching her important cultural values and beliefs and thereby influencing her moral development. *(Photo by Joe Mitchell.)*

more likely to see moral requirements emerging from the needs of others within the context of a relationship. This moral orientation of females is called the ethic of care, which develops through three levels. Each level ends with a transitional period—a time when the female considers new approaches to moral considerations and moves to a new level.

LEVEL 1—SELFISHNESS

In level 1, the focus is on one's own needs. "Should" and "would" are the same. Morality is seen in terms of sanctions by society. Relationships are often disappointing, and as a result, a woman might isolate herself to avoid getting hurt. The transition that follows this level is characterized by the move from selfishness to responsibility—a move that integrates the responsibility to care for oneself with the desire to care for others.

LEVEL 2—GOODNESS

In level 2, moral judgment is based on shared norms and expectations, and societal values are adopted. Acceptance by others becomes critical, and the ability to protect and care for others is seen as the defining characteristic of female goodness. This characteristic is upheld through beliefs that one is responsible for the actions of others but that others are responsible for the choices they make. As a woman examines her self-sacrifice, the second transition occurs, with the woman asking if her own needs are not also important. A shift from goodness to truth (as well as a new conception of goodness) takes place.

> *Think back to Ms. Kimber, the single mother. The nurse could apply Gilligan's theory to assist Ms. Kimber in adjusting to her role as both a single parent caring for a child and as a woman with her own set of needs.* ■

LEVEL 3—NONVIOLENCE

In level 3, a changed understanding of self and a redefinition of morality allow reconciliation of selfishness and responsibility. Nonviolence (the injunction against hurting) governs all moral judgments and actions. Care becomes a universal obligation toward self and others. Moral problems are usually considered within the contexts of maintaining relationships and of promoting the welfare or preventing the harm of others.

Theory of Faith Development: James Fowler

Fowler (1981) postulated a developmental theory of the spiritual identity of humans, based on work by Piaget, Kohlberg, and Erikson. Fowler describes **faith** as follows:

Faith is not always religious in its content or context. . . . Faith is a person's or group's way of moving into the force field of life. It is our way of finding coherence in and giving meaning to the multiple forces and relations that make up our lives. Faith is a person's way of seeing him or herself in relation to others against a background of shared meaning

and purpose. Faith, therefore, is not necessarily religious, but it comprises the reasons one finds life worth living. (p. 4)

Fowler's theory is composed of a prestage and six stages of faith development. The age when a certain stage occurs varies, but the sequence does not. Fowler explained that a relationship among self, shared causes or values, and others is the unifying factor in all stages and is based on trust. Equilibrium, or a plateau in faith development, can occur at any stage from stage 2 and beyond.

Prestage—Undifferentiated Faith

During the prestage, trust, courage, hope, and love compete with threats of abandonment and inconsistencies in the infant's environment. The strength of faith in this stage is based on the infant's relationship with the primary caregiver.

Stage 1—Intuitive–Projective Faith

Intuitive–projective faith is most typical of the 3- to 7-year-old child. Children imitate religious gestures and behaviors of others, primarily their parents. They take on their parents' attitudes toward religious or moral beliefs without a thorough understanding of them. Imagination in this stage leads to long-lived images and feelings that they must question and reintegrate in later stages.

Stage 2—Mythical–Literal Faith

Mythical–literal faith predominates in the school-aged child, who is having more social interaction. Stories represent religious and moral beliefs, and the child accepts the existence of a deity. The child can appreciate the perspectives of others as well as the concept of reciprocal fairness.

Stage 3—Synthetic–Conventional Faith

Synthetic–conventional faith is the characteristic stage for many adolescents. As the person experiences increasing demands from work, school, family, and peers, the basis for identity becomes more complex. The person has an emerging ideology but has not closely examined it until now. The person begins to question life-guiding values or religious practices in an attempt to stabilize his or her own identity.

Stage 4—Individuative–Reflective Faith

Individuative–reflective faith is crucial for older adolescents and young adults because they become responsible for their own commitments, beliefs, and attitudes. Many adults do not develop to this stage, and for some people, it does not emerge until they are in their 30s or 40s. Searching for self-identity no longer defined by the faith compositions of significant others is a primary concern.

Stage 5—Conjunctive Faith

Conjunctive faith integrates other viewpoints about faith into one's understanding of truth. One is able to see the

FIGURE 18-8. To provide holistic and individualized care, the nurse applies theories of growth and development. (**A**) The nurse caring for young children uses dramatic play to teach them about their hospital experience. (**B**) The nurse caring for an older adult includes the daughter, with whom the patient now lives, in discharge teaching. *(B: Photo by B. Proud.)*

nature of the reality of one's own beliefs. Along with this realization, one observes the divisions of faith development among people.

Stage 6—Universalizing Faith

Universalizing faith involves making tangible the values of absolute love and justice for humankind. The faith relationship is characterized by total trust in the principle of actively "being-in-relation" to others in whom we invest commitment, belief, love, risk, and hope, and in the existence of the future, regardless of what religion or image of faith is involved.

APPLYING THEORIES OF GROWTH AND DEVELOPMENT TO NURSING CARE

The complex and interrelated elements that contribute to human growth and development involve not only biophysi-

cal factors, but also factors of personality development. The theories summarized in this chapter help us understand cognitive, psychosocial, moral, and spiritual development. To understand the whole person, nurses need to evaluate all the components of growth and development to understand certain life events or concerns (Fig. 18-8).

Although these theories offer a great deal of insight into the processes of human growth and development, they do have some limitations. When planning holistic nursing care for patients with diverse needs, backgrounds, and ages, nurses should assess the patient as an individual and use interventions based on rationales from multiple developmental theories to provide comprehensive health promotion. Guidelines for incorporating the principles and theories of growth and development in nursing care are listed in Box 18-2.

Healthcare needs change quickly as a person grows and passes through life. These needs are unique for each person

---

Box 18-2   INCORPORATING PRINCIPLES AND THEORIES OF GROWTH AND DEVELOPMENT

General guidelines for incorporating principles and theories of growth and development and family dynamics into daily practice of nursing care are listed below. They are provided as suggestions for working with patients of all ages.

- Be knowledgeable about the various stages of cognitive, psychosocial, moral, and spiritual development and prepared to support developmental stages typical of certain ages.
- Maintain flexibility in assessing people, and respect the uniqueness of each person. Although the literature describes development typical of a particular age, not everyone fits into an exact mold.
- Anticipate possible regression during difficult periods or times of crisis, accepting and supporting a person's return to a forward progression in development.
- Become cognizant that environmental and cultural influences have a strong effect on development, especially psychosocial development. A deprived environment can be detrimental, whereas an enriched environment enhances development.
- Assess each person with an awareness that within each stage of development, a person may retain some behaviors of a

previous stage, attain goals of the current stage, and begin to exhibit behaviors of the next stage. There is a time of transition to the next stage with no definite beginning or ending to the particular stage of development.

- Remember that patients are members of families and that the family unit can have both positive and negative influences on the development of individual members. Attempt to support good family relationships and healthy environments that assist members to reach their greatest potential for growth. Provide patient teaching to individuals and their families to aid in their understanding of periods of development.
- Be ready to provide healthcare to patients who are ill or who fail to meet developmental goals. Collaborate with other members of the healthcare team in providing care to prevent or minimize disruption of development and to promote optimal health throughout life.
- Provide environments and experiences that are developmentally challenging.

but include certain similarities at specific periods. The nurse must plan care based on the patient's general and unique health needs and must continually revise aspects of care as the growth process evolves or alterations in health status occur.

The nurse is also uniquely positioned to address the sensitive emotional, psychological, and educational issues related to genomic discoveries. This focus on health, rather than disease, has the potential to result in significantly positive outcomes for the growth and development of all individuals.

● Developing Critical Thinking Skills

1. Identify developmental challenges for five of your family members or friends at different ages across the life span. Explain why meeting developmental needs is an essential role of nursing.

2. Compare and contrast the psychosocial theories of Erikson and Gould. Are the concepts in these theories relevant today? If your answer is no, what would you delete and what would you add?

3. Using Piaget's theory of cognitive development, describe how you would explain the death of a parent to children 4, 9, and 13 years of age.

● Practicing for NCLEX

1. Sue has blue eyes and is 5 feet tall. Tom has brown eyes and is 6 feet tall. These physical characteristics are primarily determined by which of the following?
   a. Socialization with caregivers
   b. Maternal nutrition during pregnancy
   c. Genetic information on chromosomes
   d. Meeting developmental tasks

2. The developing fetus exhibits a common trend in growth and development. Which of the following growth and development trends initially occurs?
   a. Symmetric
   b. Cephalocaudal
   c. Proximodistal
   d. Lateral

3. A 2-year-old grabs a handful of cake sitting on the table and stuffs it in his mouth. According to Freud, what part of the mind is the child satisfying?
   a. Id
   b. Superego
   c. Ego
   d. Unconscious mind

4. What is the primary developmental stage of the preschool-aged child, as described by Erikson?
   a. Industry versus inferiority
   b. Autonomy versus shame and doubt
   c. Trust versus mistrust
   d. Initiative versus guilt

5. An older adult smiles as she talks about her life events. This, according to Erikson, is demonstrating what developmental stage?
   a. Ego integrity
   b. Generativity
   c. Intimacy
   d. Identity

6. What did Havighurst define as a developmental task of the adolescent?
   a. Learning sex differences and sexual modesty
   b. Taking on civic responsibility
   c. Accepting one's body and using it effectively
   d. Achieving personal independence

7. Based on Piaget's theory, children between the ages of 2 and 7 years use play for what purpose?
   a. To classify objects based on characteristics
   b. To understand life events and relationships
   c. To relate own enjoyment of random behaviors
   d. To incorporate the perspective of others

8. Which of the following factors initially influences moral development as defined in Kohlberg's theory?
   a. Parent–child communications
   b. Societal rules and regulations
   c. Social and religious rules
   d. One's beliefs and values

9. In Gilligan's theory, women develop morality differently than do men. How did she describe this morality in women?
   a. Law and justice
   b. Obligations and rights
   c. Order and selfishness
   d. Response and care

10. During the development of faith, described by Fowler, the teenager commonly does which of the following?
    a. Accepts parental attitudes and beliefs
    b. Exhibits a value of justice for others
    c. Questions previously accepted values
    d. Demonstrates responsibility for own beliefs

● Answers With Rationale

1. *c.* Physical appearance and growth have a predetermined genetic base from inheritance patterns carried on the chromosomes.

2. *b.* The head and brain (cephalocaudal) grow and develop first in the fetus.

3. *a.* Freud defined the id as the part of the mind concerned with self-gratification by the easiest and quickest available means.

4. *d.* The preschool child seeks new learning experiences (initiative); if restrictions or reprimands result, the child feels guilty and is hesitant to try new skills.

5. *a.* Reminiscence during the older years of one's life provides a sense of fulfillment and purpose (ego integrity).

6. *c.* The adolescent must learn to accept his or her body and use it effectively.

7. *b.* Children ages 2 to 7 years are in the preoperational stage, and use play to help understand life events and relationships.

8. *a.* Moral development in the young child results from communications as the child tries to please his or her parents.

9. *d.* Gilligan believed that, for women, response and care are a universal obligation toward self and others.

10. *c.* Synthetic–conventional faith is characteristic of many adolescents, as they begin to question values in an attempt to stabilize their own identity.

Taylor Suite Resources

The Taylor Suite offers these additional resources to enhance learning and facilitate understanding of this chapter:

- thePoint online resource, http://thepoint.lww.com/Taylor7E
- Student DVD-ROM included with the book
- Study Guide for Taylor's Fundamentals of Nursing

BIBLIOGRAPHY

Calzone, K., Jenkins, J., Yates, J., Cusack, G., & McBride, C. (2008). Evaluation of the integration of genetics and genomics into nursing practice. *Oncology Nursing Forum, 35*(3), 539.

DeSevo, M. (2006). A genetic disorder hits home. *RN, 69*(2), 46–50.

Dolan, S., Biermann, J., & Damus, K. (2007). Genomics for health in preconception and prenatal periods. *Journal of Nursing Scholarship, 39*(1), 4–9.

Erikson, E. H. (1963). *Childhood and society* (2nd ed.). New York: Norton.

Fowler, J. W. (1981). *Stages of faith: The psychology of human development and the quest for meaning.* New York: Harper & Row.

Fowler, J. W. (1991). *Weaving the new creation: Stages of faith and the public church.* San Francisco: Harper Collins.

Freud, S., & Strachey, J. (1960). *The ego and the id: The standard edition of the complete psychological works of Sigmund Freud.* New York: Norton.

Friedman, M. M., Bowden, V., & Jones, E. (2003). *Family nursing: Research, theory and practice* (5th ed.). Upper Saddle River, NJ: Prentice Hall.

Gilligan, C. (1977). In a different voice: Women's conceptions of the self and of morality. *Harvard Educational Review, 47,* 481–517.

Gilligan, C. (1982). *In a different voice.* Cambridge, MA: Harvard University Press.

Goldberg, P., & Jenkins, S. (2008). Genetics: Soon to be a part of nursing practice. *Nursing Spectrum, 17*(10), 28–33.

Gould, R. (1978). *Transformations.* New York: Simon & Schuster.

Havighurst, R. J. (1972). *Developmental tasks and education.* New York: David McKay.

James, E. (2008). 0.1 Percent Different. *Advance for Nurses, 10*(14), 14.

Johnson, R., Williams, S., & Spruill, I. (2006). Genomics, nutrition, obesity, and diabetes. *Journal of Nursing Scholarship, 38*(1), 11–18.

Kohlberg, L. (1969). Stage and sequence: The cognitive–developmental approach to socialization. In D. Gaslin (Ed.), *Handbook of socialization: Theory and research* (pp. 347–380). Chicago: Rand McNally.

Levinson, D., Darrow, C., Klein, E., Levinson, M., & McKee, B. (1978). *The seasons of a man's life.* New York: Knopf.

Murray, R., Zentner, J., & Yakimo, R. (2001). *Health promotion strategies through the life span.* Upper Saddle River, NJ: Prentice Hall.

NANDA International. (2009). *Nursing diagnoses: Definitions & classification 2009–2011.* West Sussex, UK: Wiley-Blackwell.

Piaget, J., & Inhelder, B. (1969). *The psychology of the child.* New York: Basic Books.

Porth, C. M. (2007). *Essentials of pathophysiology: Concepts of altered health states* (2nd ed.). Philadelphia: Lippincott Williams & Wilkins.

Thies, K., & Travers, J. (2001). *Human growth and development through the lifespan.* Thorofare, NJ: Slack Inc.

Williams, J., Skirton, H., & Masny, A. (2006). Ethics, policy, and educational issues in genetic testing. *Journal of Nursing Scholarship, 38*(2), 119–125.

19 Conception Through Young Adult

PATRICIA LEMMING

Patricia is a 26-year-old woman in the first trimester of her pregnancy. At a recent clinic visit, she states, "I've been trying to cut back on smoking and drinking alcohol, but I haven't had much success."

DARLENE JENKINS

Darlene, a pregnant 14-year-old in her third trimester, comes to the prenatal clinic for the first time. Her history reveals sexual activity with multiple partners, smoking two packs of cigarettes per day, beer "4 or 5 nights a week," and eating mostly "fast foods." She has had no prenatal care and hasn't been taking any prenatal vitamins. She is homeless but occasionally stays with an older girlfriend since her parents "threw her out of the house."

HILLARIE BROWNING

Hillarie, who is 2 years old, is brought to the emergency room by her father, James Browning. She is unresponsive. Mr. Browning says that she "took a tumble" down the stairs, but assessment reveals that her injuries are inconsistent with this type of fall.

LEARNING OBJECTIVES

After completing the chapter, you will be able to accomplish the following:

1. Summarize major physiologic, cognitive, psychosocial, moral, and spiritual developments from conception through the young adult.

2. List common health problems of each age period from conception through the young adult.

3. Describe nursing interventions to promote health in patients from conception through the young adult.

KEY TERMS

adolescence	puberty
attachment	regression
bonding	school-aged child
child maltreatment	separation anxiety
colic	sexually transmitted infection (STI)
failure to thrive (FTT)	sudden infant death syndrome (SIDS)
infant	temperament
negativism	toddler
neonate	young adult
preschooler	

Growth and development occur throughout the life span. The nurse's knowledge of growth and developmental milestones provides a base for planning and implementing holistic, individualized nursing care. This chapter continues the discussion of developmental theories introduced in Chapter 18, with specific information related to the sequential stages of growth and development from conception through young adulthood.

Although divided into different stages, childhood encompasses the entire period before young adulthood. Included within this time span are the fetus, the neonate, the infant, the toddler, the preschooler, the school-aged child, and the adolescent. The discussion of each of these stages includes, as appropriate, physiologic, cognitive, psychosocial, and moral and spiritual development; health; and the nurse's role in promoting health. For an example addressing the adolescent, see the accompanying Reflective Practice box.

CONCEPTION AND PRENATAL DEVELOPMENT

Human growth and development begin at the moment the ovum is fertilized by the sperm. The fertilized ovum (zygote) contains the full complement of genetic information provided by each parent that determines gender and influences

personality, intellect, and physical and psychological traits. The growth and development stages of the fetus are orderly and continuous, and proceed as follows.

Preembryonic Stage

The preembryonic stage lasts for about 3 weeks. The zygote, which implants in the uterine wall, has three distinct cell layers. The endoderm (inner layer) becomes the respiratory system, the digestive system, the liver, and the pancreas. The mesoderm (middle layer) becomes the skeleton, connective tissue, cartilage, muscles, and the circulatory, lymphoid, reproductive, and urinary systems. The ectoderm (outer layer) becomes the brain, spinal cord, nervous system, and outer body parts (skin, hair, and nails).

Embryonic Stage

The embryonic stage occurs from the 4th through the 8th week. Rapid growth and differentiation of the cell layers take place. By the end of this stage, all basic organs have been established, the bones have begun to ossify, and some human features are recognizable. Because this is a period of such rapid growth and change, the fetus is especially vulnerable to any factor that might cause congenital anomalies (such as maternal use of alcohol, nicotine, over-the-counter medications, or drugs).

> ➤ *Recall Patricia Lemming, the 26-year-old pregnant woman in her first trimester described at the beginning of the chapter. The nurse could incorporate knowledge about fetal growth during the embryonic stage when teaching her about the effects of alcohol and nicotine on the fetus, with the goal of fostering an even greater desire in the patient to stop using these substances.* ■

Fetal Stage

The fetal stage lasts from 9 weeks to birth. All body organs and systems continue to grow and develop. At the end of the first trimester (12 weeks' gestation), some reflexes are present, kidney secretion begins, the heartbeat can be heard by Doppler, and the sex of the infant is distinguishable by outward appearance. At the end of the second trimester (24 weeks' gestation), fetal heart tones are audible by stethoscope, the liver and pancreas are functioning, hair forms, sleep–wake patterns are established, lung surfactant is produced, and eyelids open. At the end of the third trimester (40 weeks' gestation), testes have descended, lung alveoli are formed, subcutaneous fat is deposited, and the fetus actively kicks. By birth, the average neonate weighs 7.5 lb (3.4 kg) and is 20 inches (50.8 cm) long.

During pregnancy, adequate maternal nutrition is essential for normal growth and development of the fetus. A fetus that does not have adequate nutrition might be small for gestational age, fail to have normal brain development, have learning disabilities as a child, and be at increased risk for chronic illnesses as an adult. Vitamin and mineral deficiencies can result in fetal

REFLECTIVE PRACTICE

Challenge to Interpersonal Skills

I was admitting Darlene Jenkins, a pregnant, unmarried, 14-year-old to the prenatal clinic. This was her first visit and she was already in her third trimester. A quick history revealed multiple factors putting both her and her fetus at risk for health problems: lack of family (or other) support (homeless, occasionally staying with an older girlfriend), father of the baby unknown, multiple sexual partners, diet consisting mainly of fast food, no prenatal vitamins, little to no exercise, and history of smoking (2 packs of cigarettes per day) and alcohol consumption ("beer 4 to 5 times a week"). When she was seen by the medical resident, he asked her quite curtly if she was trying to "kill her baby," telling her that it was probably too late for her to get the care she needed. "Why should we waste our time on you when other women here really want to be helped?" Although Darlene was acting "tough," I could tell from her expression that she was both angry and hurt. While I was upset by the choices that she had made so far and shared some of the resident's frustration, I knew we had to give her a reason to trust us if we wanted her to start taking better care of herself and her baby. I was also upset by the resident's lack of professionalism and wondered if I should say something to him.

Thinking Outside the Box: Possible Courses of Action

- Play the "good cop–bad cop" routine; after the resident finished his visit, I could try to be especially caring and explain why we were all concerned about her and her baby. Then I could talk to her about what she needed to do to maximize good outcomes.
- Challenge the resident in the patient's presence, thereby showing her that at least I honestly cared about her.

- Confront the resident later in a "cooler moment," hoping that this behavior doesn't repeat itself, while being prepared to report my concerns to a "higher authority" should this behavior occur again.
- Approach the resident outside the patient's presence and explain my concerns. Persuade the resident to apologize to Darlene in the interests of winning the patient's trust and compliance with prenatal care program.

Evaluating a Good Outcome: How Do I Define Success?

- The respect for each person's human dignity (Darlene, the resident, myself) is affirmed.
- Each person feels empowered to make personal decisions that advance her/his interests and goals.
- The patient makes the needed lifestyle changes, with good outcomes for herself and her baby.

- Personal integrity is maintained; no one has to sacrifice her or his beliefs and values.
- Professional integrity is maintained.

Personal Learning: Here's to the Future!

In this situation, I don't think that I chose the best alternative because I tried to comfort Darlene and make "excuses" for the resident's behavior. I tried to explain that the resident was very busy and simply "out of sorts." I have to admit that, initially, I was probably just as shocked by the resident's response as Darlene. Personally, I knew that I'd die if someone said something like that to me. After I spoke with the resident, I realized there might be some value in shocking a patient into seeing the harm of her ways. However, in this encounter, Darlene had no way of knowing whether this response was well-intended (if indeed it was!) or not. While talking further with Darlene, I became convinced that she wouldn't start listening to us until she could trust us. I wish I had the courage to ask the resident to apologize to Darlene. His apology might have been exactly what was needed to get her to trust us. I'm learning that when patient welfare is at stake, I might have to sacrifice my own comfort level to challenge other professional caregivers. Hopefully, I'll learn how to do this in a way that promotes respectful, collaborative relationships.

Reflection

How do you think you would respond in a similar situation? Why? What if the nurse confronted the resident in front of the patient? Would you consider this professional behavior? Do you feel that the resident acted in a professional manner? Could the resident's developmental stage have influenced his response to the patient? Please explain your answer. How might the nurse's developmental stage affect the actions taken toward the resident? Toward the patient? Do you agree with the nurse in the thinking that an apology from the resident would help in fostering trust? Why or why not? What does this tell you about yourself and about the adequacy of your skills for professional practice? Can you think of other ways to respond? What would the basis be for these other ways? What other skills (cognitive, interpersonal, technical, ethical/legal) would you need to respond well in this situation? Do you agree with the criteria proposed for use to evaluate a successful outcome?

megaloblastic anemia and neural tube defects (folic acid deficiency), inadequate bone calcification (vitamin D and calcium deficits), and hypothyroidism (iodine deficiency).

During the past decade, there has been a significant increase in the number of premature births (those occurring before 37 weeks' gestation). Approximately 12.8% of the births in the United States in 2006 were premature, and this rate has increased 20% since 1990 (Martin, Hamilton, Sutton, Ventura, Menacker, Kirmeyer, et al., 2009). Low birth weight is one of the leading causes of infant mortality and the leading cause of infant death during the first month of life. Infants born prematurely are at increased risk for disorders such as cerebral palsy, mental retardation, and chronic respiratory problems. Many people, including healthcare workers, are unaware of the magnitude of this problem.

Other health risks for the developing fetus are discussed later in this chapter.

NEONATE: BIRTH TO 28 DAYS

At birth, the **neonate** must adapt to extrauterine life through several significant physiologic adjustments. The most important occur in the respiratory and circulatory systems as the neonate begins breathing and becomes independent of the umbilical cord. The neonate is assessed immediately after birth. Of several existing measurement scales, the Apgar rating scale is the most commonly used. This scale is used to assess neonates 1 minute and 5 minutes after birth (Table 19-1).

Physiologic Development

The physical characteristics and behaviors of normal neonates include:

- Reflexes include the Moro reflex, the stepping reflex, grasp reflex, hand-to-mouth activity, sucking, swallowing, blinking, sneezing, and yawning (Fig. 19-1).
- Body temperature responds quickly to the environmental temperature.
- Senses are used to respond to the environment, see color and form, hear and turn toward sound, smell and taste, and feel touch and pain.

- Stool and urine are eliminated.
- Both an active crying state and a quiet alert state are exhibited (see Fig. 19-1).

The neonate inherits a transient immunity from infections as a result of immunoglobulins that cross the placenta. Breastfeeding provides further protection against bacterial and viral infections through antibodies, immunoglobulins, and leukocytes in breast milk. The high lactose content in breast milk, combined with limited protein, promotes an acid environment that is unsuitable for bacterial growth.

Health of the Neonate

Difficulties related to the birth process, the transition to extrauterine life, or congenital anomalies might require intervention by healthcare personnel.

Respiratory difficulties might occur, especially if drugs given to the mother during labor and delivery have sedated the neonate. Premature neonates are vulnerable to respiratory distress syndrome because of the relative immature lung function. Neonates delivered by cesarean birth are at risk for respiratory difficulties because of excess mucus in the lungs and might require frequent suctioning.

Incompatibility between the neonate's and mother's blood groups requires prompt care at birth. Congenital malformations, such as cleft palate and cleft lip or neural tube defects (such as spina bifida) and hydrocephalus, might result in long-term health problems. Birth traumas that cause temporary symptoms are of concern because the parents need to be reassured that the symptoms will disappear. Examples include caput succedaneum (localized edema of the scalp), molding (elongation of the skull as the baby passes through the birth canal), and subconjunctival hemorrhage. The nonthreatening nature of physiologic jaundice, which commonly occurs in the neonate's first days, should also be explained to the parents.

Neonates born to mothers who smoke cigarettes, drink alcohol, or use drugs are at risk for developmental deficits as well as complications during birth. Smoking during pregnancy might cause low birth weight. Fetal alcohol syndrome

TABLE • 19-1	**APGAR SCORING CHART**		
Category*	**0**	**1**	**2**
Heart rate	Absent	Slow (less than 100 beats/min)	More than 100 beats/min
Respiratory effort	Absent	Slow, irregular	Good, crying
Muscle tone	Flaccid	Some flexion of extremities	Active motion
Reflex irritability	No response	Weak cry or grimace	Vigorous cry
Color	Blue, pale	Body pink, extremities blue	Completely pink

*Each category is rated as 0, 1, or 2. The rating for each category is then totaled to a maximum score of 10. Normal neonates score between 7 and 10. Neonates who score between 4 and 6 require special assistance; those who score below 4 are in need of immediate life-saving support.

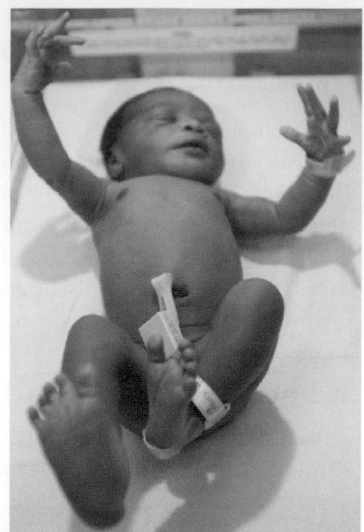

Moro reflex *(Photo by Joe Mitchell.)*

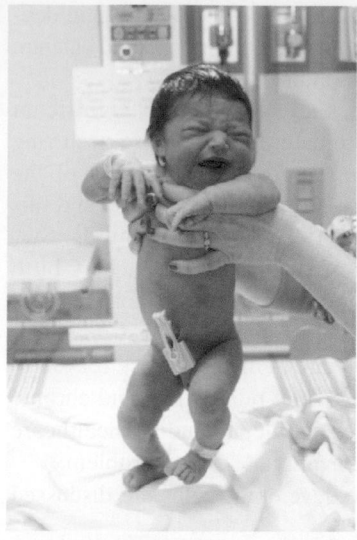

Stepping reflex *(Photo by Joe Mitchell.)*

Grasp reflex *(Photo by Joe Mitchell.)*

Hand to mouth and sucking activity

Quiet alert state

Active crying state *(Photo by Joe Mitchell.)*

FIGURE 19-1. Reflexes and behaviors of the neonate.

caused by maternal drinking is believed to be a leading cause of birth defects, including growth retardation, developmental delay, and impaired intellectual ability.

> ➤ *Think back to Patricia Lemming, the 26-year-old mother in her first trimester. The nurse could integrate information about the typical effects occurring in neonates secondary to nicotine and alcohol use as a basis for planning care for Patricia as she progresses through her pregnancy.* ■

The woman who uses drugs during pregnancy puts herself as well as her baby at risk. For example, maternal use of methamphetamine increases the probability of congenital anomalies, prematurity, low birth weight, and drug withdrawal symptoms. Methamphetamine use can result in abrupt changes in the mother's blood pressure, resulting in decreased fetal blood flow and oxygenation. Babies born to meth-addicted mothers are jittery, irritable, intolerant of cuddling, feed poorly, and experience difficulty sleeping (Clark, 2008).

INFANT: 1 MONTH TO 1 YEAR

The neonate becomes an **infant** at 1 month, a period lasting until the first birthday (Fig. 19-2).

Bonding might occur in the first few hours after birth or later in the first few months and is necessary for later attachment. *(Photo by Joe Mitchell.)*

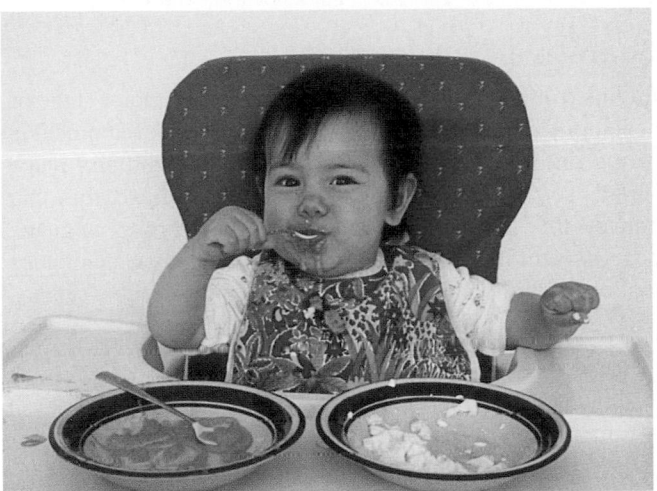

Developmental tasks of the first year include taking solid food.

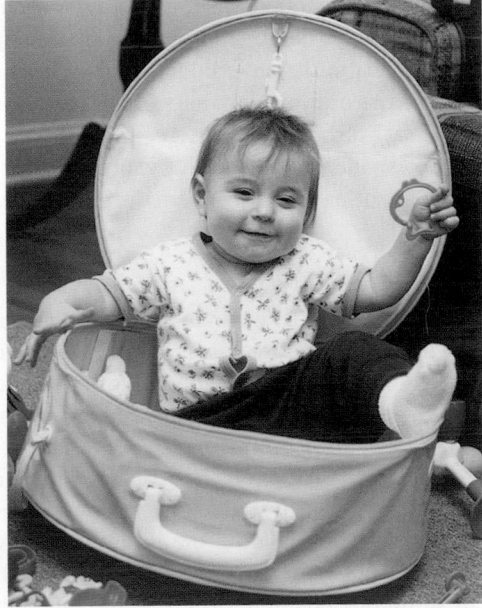

As the infant enters the second half of her first year, play will begin to involve manipulation of objects and the environment.

Later infancy is characterized by the ability to pull-to-stand, cruise, and often walk.

FIGURE 19-2. Development in the infant.

Physiologic Development

The physical characteristics of the infant include the following:

- Brain grows to about half the adult size.
- Body temperature stabilizes.
- Motor abilities develop, allowing use of building blocks, attempting to feed self, crawling, and walking.
- Eyes begin to focus and fixate.
- Heart doubles in weight, heart rate slows, and blood pressure rises.
- Deciduous teeth begin to erupt at 4 to 6 months.
- Birth weight usually triples by 1 year, when the average male infant weighs 22 lb (10 kg) and the average female infant weighs 21 lb (9.5 kg). Length increases by 50%.

Cognitive Development

Infants from birth to 1 year are in the sensorimotor stage of development described by Piaget. Language development is in the prelinguistic phase. Babies begin to coo and make sounds soon after birth, and by 12 months of age, they can convey their wishes through a few key words. Language development in infants has several consistent characteristics that occur with all languages:

- Use of syllable repetition (such as ma-ma, da-da, bye-bye)
- Universal early phonetic expressions (babbling sounds)
- Imitation of sounds and intonations spoken by caregivers

Psychosocial Development
Developmental Theories

In terms of the developmental theories discussed in Chapter 18, the infant has the following characteristics:

- Is in the oral stage (Freud), striving for immediate gratification of needs and having a strong sucking need
- Develops trust (Erikson) if the caregiver can be counted on to provide food when the infant is hungry; trust is also facilitated by diaper changing, warmth, and comforting
- Meets developmental tasks (Havighurst) by learning to take solid food, walk, and talk

Special Considerations

Other components of psychosocial development in the neonate and infant include attachment, bonding, play, and temperament.

ATTACHMENT AND BONDING

Attachment is an active, affectionate, reciprocal relationship between two people, which is somewhat different from bonding. **Bonding,** described by Klaus and Kennell (1982), occurs during a sensitive period in the first few hours after birth (although bonding also might occur later in the first few months) and is necessary for later attachment. Bonding might be considered the emotional linkage of two people,

and attachment the long-term maintenance and strengthening of the linked state.

PLAY

Infants and children discover their environment and begin to learn how to control it through play. Beginning as soon as the baby is aware of sensations and the pleasure they produce, play progresses from self-pleasure to interaction with others. The two dimensions of play are social play and cognitive play. Social play, such as rolling a ball back and forth between two children, is motivated by a desire for fun, pleasure, and relationships with others. Cognitive play, as when a child puts a puzzle together, is motivated by the desire to learn.

TEMPERAMENT

Temperament is primarily inborn, although it is influenced by environment. A baby or child might be said to be "easy," "slow to warm," or "difficult" (Thomas, Chess, & Birch, 1968). The "easy" infant sleeps, eats, and eliminates easily; smiles spontaneously; and cries in response to significant needs. The "slow-to-warm" infant is more passive and distant. The "difficult" infant has volatile and labile responses, often is a restless sleeper, is highly sensitive to noises, and eats poorly. These traits often remain fairly consistent throughout the individual's life. The behavior of caregivers as they care for the baby can positively or negatively influence the degree to which temperament dictates behavioral style.

Health of the Infant

Various health problems in infancy might require the intervention of healthcare personnel. Gastroenteritis and food allergies are common. Skin disorders, such as diaper dermatitis (diaper rash), seborrheic dermatitis (infant dandruff), prickly heat rash, acute infantile eczema, and thrush (infection of the oral mucous membrane by the fungus *Candida albicans*), also often occur. Accidents, infant colic, failure to thrive, sudden infant death syndrome, and child maltreatment are of particular concern during infancy.

Accidental Injuries

Safety issues must be addressed during infancy. The swallowing reflex matures progressively from birth, but until it is fully developed, aspiration is a risk. Because infants put small objects in their mouths, choking is a risk. Choking might also result from small pieces of food, nuts, and popcorn. If the airway is obstructed, parents and caregivers need instruction to use five quick back blows between the infant's shoulders while holding the infant prone over one arm. If this does not dislodge the object, the infant should be placed in a supine position over the rescuer's thighs with the infant's head lower than the chest. Five downward chest thrusts to the lower third of the sternum should be given quickly. If still ineffective, rescue breathing needs to be initiated (Pillitteri, 2009).

Examples of NANDA Nursing Diagnoses
Infancy Through School Age

Nursing Diagnoses	Possible Related Factor
Risk for Infection	Exposure to other children in childcare and at school
Diarrhea	Milk intolerance
Deficient Fluid Volume	Severe case of vomiting and diarrhea
Risk for Suffocation	Caregiver's lack of knowledge of safety precautions
Disorganized Infant Behavior	Environmental overstimulation
Risk for Poisoning	Caregiver's lack of knowledge of proper storage of hazardous liquids
Risk for Injury	Lack of knowledge about proper use of skates, bicycles, roller blades, and trampolines
Risk for Situational Low Self-Esteem	History of physical abuse by caregiver

Death rates for infants due to strangulation and suffocation have increased dramatically since the 1980s. These accidental deaths occur most commonly when infants share a bed with parents (cosleeping) and are inadvertently wedged beneath another person, trapped in a dangerous position, such as between the bed and the wall, or suffocated by bedding. The reason for this rise in accidental strangulation or suffocation is unknown but may be related to an increase in cosleeping. In earlier years, the cause of some of these deaths may also have been listed as unknown. In an effort to reduce infant risk for suffocation, nurses need to speak to parents about safe cosleeping strategies, possible use of a cosleeper three-sided bassinet placed next to the bed, and the selection of safe, nonpuffy bedding (Kennedy & Jacobsen, 2009).

As the infant becomes more mobile, the risk for falls or for being caught in dangling cords (such as in mini-blinds) increases. Preventive measures against such safety hazards must be taught to new parents. In addition, law mandates the use of special car safety seats and restraints for infants. See Examples of NANDA Nursing Diagnoses: Infancy Through School Age.

Infant Colic

Colic is uncontrollable, extended crying in an otherwise healthy and well-fed baby. Colic generally occurs during the first 3 months of life and has been referred to as the "100-day syndrome." This continuous crying can occur at any time but usually worsens in the evening. The infant cries loudly and draws the legs up to the abdomen. Despite the symptoms, the infant gains weight. Parents and other family members might experience stress and anxiety due to the constant crying (see Through the Eyes of a Caregiver).

The exact cause of colic is not known. One common belief is that an immature digestive system might be the cause. Swallowing excess air, feeding too rapidly or too much, improper feeding techniques, or allergies might lead to spasmodic contractions of the intestines, with acute abdominal pain. Another belief is that an immature nervous system might be the cause. Normal external stimulation might cause the baby to tense up.

Failure to Thrive

Failure to thrive (FTT) is a condition of inadequate growth in height and weight resulting from the infant's inability to obtain or use calories needed for growth. Infants with FTT have signs of malnutrition and delayed development. Causes and contributing factors might include physiologic causes, inadequate funds to buy sufficient food, the use of a fad diet, inadequate nutritional knowledge, insufficient breast milk, and disturbances in maternal–child attachment. In most cases of FTT not caused by a physiologic problem, a team of healthcare providers is needed to meet the complex needs of the infant and caregivers.

Sudden Infant Death Syndrome

Sudden infant death syndrome (SIDS) is the sudden death of an infant under the age of 1 year, unexpected in light of the infant's history, in which a postmortem examination fails to reveal a cause of death. Incidences of SIDS has declined significantly in the past decade, but it is still the leading cause of death in infants ages 1 month to 1 year, with most deaths occurring between 2 and 4 months of age (National Institute of Child Health and Human Development, 2008). The exact cause is still unknown, but it is believed to be associated with

Through the Eyes of a Caregiver

When my son Luke was first born, he was an easy-going, pleasant baby. Then, when he was about 3 weeks old, it started. He cried inconsolably every night from 5 p.m. until 12 a.m. We could do nothing to comfort him. We took him to the pediatrician. The doctor said the word we already expected to hear: "colic." He gave us a prescription for an antacid and a muscle relaxant. He gave us some advice on how to comfort him . . . wrap him snugly, hold him like a football, eliminate milk and dairy from your diet (I was breast-feeding), and put pressure on his belly. None of these things worked. Eventually, we discovered that rocking him in our arms as we ran the shower seemed to calm him. Pink Floyd and Dark Side of the Moon also comforted him. We found this out quite accidentally when we played the CD in an attempt to drown out his crying. These methods somewhat helped with the crying, but little helped my anxiety. I was concerned for my little son, who was clearly upset or in pain. At the same time, I found it very difficult to bond with him. I'd find myself dreading the evening; dreading being with my baby. When I'd come home from work, I'd take a deep breath and stand paralyzed at the front door, wondering if I had to go in. I could hear his crying from the

doorstep. I felt horrible about these feelings. I questioned my parenting skills. At one point, I spoke with a nurse whose daughter had colic. She said "My daughter's colic lasted 100 days, but it has taken me 14 years to forgive her!" This made me laugh for the first time in weeks. Then she asked how I was doing and if I wanted to talk about how I was feeling. I hadn't told anyone how I was feeling toward my son. How could I? I confided in her, though. I knew she wouldn't judge me. I knew she'd understand. After speaking with the nurse, I felt a lot better knowing that it was OK to feel the way I did. As time went on, Luke's crying spells got shorter and shorter, until the 99th day; then, miraculously, it ended. We had a party the next day, with a cake that said "Day 100. We made it." Today, he is a sweet, healthy child. He is no fussier than any other 3-year-old child. We have bonded exceptionally well. My husband and family were supportive and helped care for Luke when he had colic, but it was the nurse who helped care for me!

—Dana Jameson
Philadelphia, PA

neurologic regulation of cardiac and respiratory control. African American infants are at a greater risk for SIDS. Because sleep habits have been implicated with SIDS, it is recommended that healthy infants up to the age of 6 months sleep on their back (rather than the stomach) on a firm surface in a safety-approved crib. Placing infants in a side-lying position is not recommended because babies who sleep on their sides are more likely to roll onto their abdomen. Other risk factors include smoke exposure, overheating, and soft bedding or stuffed toys.

Child Maltreatment

Although **child maltreatment** may occur at any age, the greatest numbers of victims are from birth to age 3 years. The Centers for Disease Control and Prevention (CDC) define child maltreatment as "an act or series of acts of commission or omission by a parent or other caregiver that results in harm, potential for harm, or threat of harm to a child" (CDC, 2007a). Forms of child maltreatment include child abuse (acts of commission) and child neglect (acts of omission). In the United States in 2007, over 750,000 children were victims of maltreatment, and approximately 1,760 children died from abuse and neglect (CDC, 2009a).

Neglect, the most common form of maltreatment, is the failure of a caregiver to provide for the child's basic needs with an adequate level of care or the failure to supervise (Anbarghalami, Yang, Van Sell, & Miller-Anderson, 2007). Child abuse can be physical, sexual, or psychological in nature. Physical abuse, often referred to as the battered child syndrome, refers to deliberate physical abuse and is typically inflicted by a parent or caregiver. Sexual abuse includes incest, molestation, exhibitionism, child pornography, child

prostitution, and pedophilia. These acts, when committed by a caregiver, such as a parent or babysitter, are considered sexual abuse. When a stranger commits such an act, it is considered sexual assault (a criminal act). Psychological or emotional abuse includes belittling behavior on the part of the parent or caregiver, placing a child in a dangerous situation, unreasonable confinement, exploiting or corrupting a child, and failing to express any emotion toward a child (Child Welfare Information Gateway, 2009). Other forms of child maltreatment include violent shaking, called shaken baby syndrome, especially in infants younger than 6 months of age (resulting in brain trauma), and Munchausen syndrome by proxy, which is an illness fabricated or induced in another person. It is most often the mother who fabricates or causes an illness in a child to gain attention from healthcare providers.

Although child abuse occurs in all ethnic groups and at all levels of society, certain factors increase the risk, including the following:

- Parents experiencing stress from unemployment, depression, poor social and marital relationships, substance abuse, or health problems
- Children who cry frequently, have sleep difficulties, wet the bed, are hyperactive or aggressive, have difficult temperaments, or have physical, emotional, or cognitive disabilities
- Caregivers' lack of knowledge about parenting and the normal behaviors of children
- Lack of family and social support for caregivers

The number of reported cases of child abuse has increased dramatically and is a cause of national concern. Healthcare providers and facilities, teachers, daycare providers, and

TABLE • 19-2	CHILD ABUSE RESOURCES
Organization	**Activities**
U.S. Department of Health and Human Services Children's Bureau http://www.acf.hhs.gov/programs/cb/index.htm	Assists states in the delivery of child welfare services.
Childhelp National Child Abuse Hotline http://www.childhelp.org/ Phone: 1-800-4-A-CHILD (1-800-422-4453)	Hotline counselors are available and can provide phone numbers for reporting abuse situations.
Prevent Child Abuse America http://www.preventchildabuse.org Phone: 1-800-244-5373 or 312-663-3520	National organization that provides access to hotlines, self-help groups, publications, and volunteer opportunities.
Child Welfare Information Gateway http://www.childwelfare.gov/ Phone: 1-800-394-3366 or 703-385-7565	Provides access to information and resources to help protect children and strengthen families.

social workers are in an excellent position to recognize families at risk and offer interventions, and in all 50 states, they have a legal obligation to report suspected maltreatment (see Chapter 7). Organizations that serve as resources for child abuse concerns are listed in Table 19-2. The long-term treatment of abused children and their families is complex and multidisciplinary.

Role of the Nurse in Promoting Health and Preventing Illness

The most essential role of the nurse in promoting health of the infant is teaching family members and caregivers. Teaching ranges from providing basic information about prevention of diaper rash to facilitating grieving in parents who have lost a baby to SIDS. Examples of specific areas of preventive teaching for parents of infants are given in Teaching Tips 19-1.

Immunization against contagious diseases begins during the first year of life and should follow a regular schedule, as outlined in Figure 19-3. In recent years, controversy has arisen regarding the relationship of immunization vaccines and the development of autism disorders. Some parents have also been concerned with a vaccine preservative, thimerosal, which contains mercury. Research by both the Food and Drug Administration and the Institute of Medicine shows that thimerosal poses no threat to children, but as a precaution, vaccines in which thimerosal has been eliminated or significantly reduced are now available. Healthcare providers need to listen to parent concerns about immunization and guide them to resources with current immunization information and schedules (Fraleigh, 2009). Vaccine information is available at the following CDC website: http://www.cdc.gov/vaccines/programs/vfc/default.htm.

It is also important to assess the infant's growth and development. Growth rate is assessed in comparison with standardized growth charts developed for boys and girls, whose growth rates differ. Be careful when comparing an individual child's growth to standards on a chart for the following reasons:

- Every child has individual variations and short-term spurts and lags in growth.
- Atypical infants, such as those who are premature or have low birth weight, are not taken into account in such charts.
- Growth charts might be ethically and socioeconomically weighted in favor of white, middle-class children.

The Denver Developmental Screening Test (DDST) is commonly used to determine quickly and inexpensively atypical developmental patterns in infants and children. The crucial areas of development assessed in the DDST are gross motor behavior and skills, fine motor behavior and skills, language acquisition, and personal and social interaction. The test identifies problem areas that require more precise assessments. The DDST is described in more detail in most pediatric nursing texts.

When an infant in late infancy is hospitalized, separation anxiety behaviors are common. **Separation anxiety** occurs when a child is afraid of being sent away from loved ones who offer security. The infant might initially cry and scream in the phase of protest but then stop crying and appear depressed (despair phase) (Wong, Perry, Hockenberry, Lowdermilk, & Wilson, 2006). Nurses should encourage parents to stay with the hospitalized infant and provide care, or if that is not possible, consistent healthcare providers are important to maintain the infant's trust in others.

TODDLER: 1 TO 3 YEARS

From 1 to 3 years of age, the child is considered a **toddler** (Fig. 19-4).

Physiologic Development

Physiologic development continues steadily through the toddler years, but the pace is considerably slower than that in

Tips

TEACHING TIPS · 19-1

INFANTS

Health Topic	Teaching Tip	Why Is This Important?
Safety	• Feed the baby slowly and "burp" often. • Do not prop bottles and leave the baby unattended. • If choking occurs, follow procedure for giving 5 back blows followed by 5 chest thrusts until the object is dislodged. • Crib bumper pads are not recommended until 6 months of age. Keep the crib rails up at all times. Do not use pillows or fluffy covers in the crib. • Never leave the baby unattended in or near water. • Use approved car seat. • Keep small objects out of reach. • Never leave the baby unattended on a table, chair, or regular bed. • Place the baby on his or her back for sleeping. • Keep plastic bags and mini-blind cords out of reach. • Block stairs with gates. • Cover electrical outlets.	The leading causes of death in infants are drowning, suffocation, and falls. Infants wiggle, roll, creep, crawl, walk, and reach for objects. Propping bottles, even in later infancy, might increase the risk of aspiration and tooth decay. Placing babies on their back to sleep has significantly reduced the incidence of SIDS.
Nutrition	• How to breastfeed, if chosen. • Preparing formula, information about positioning for feeding, and the importance of holding the baby for feeding, if this method is chosen. • Introducing solid foods, as prescribed by the healthcare provider. Do not add sugar, salt, or honey to foods. • Weaning is usually completed by the end of the first year.	Feeding is a time for the caregiver and baby to strengthen attachment and bonding. There is no one best time to introduce solid foods, but they should be started one at a time. Overfeeding or adding extra calories might cause obesity in the infant or in later life.
Hygiene	• Bathing the baby and caring for the umbilical cord. • Provide circumcision care for boys. • Keep the diaper area clean and dry.	Skin care, as well as care for the umbilical cord and circumcision site, are necessary in preventing infections and excoriations.
Elimination	• By 2 months, babies usually have 2 stools a day. • Breastfed babies vary more in bowel consistency, color, and times than do babies fed formula.	Renal and intestinal physiology develop throughout the first year of life.
Growth and Development	• Provide consistent care and love. • Growth and development differ for each infant, but there are some predictable milestones. • Provide educational toys appropriate to the age of the infant. • Talk and read to the baby. • Allow the baby to explore different shapes, sizes, tastes, and experiences.	The infant must be consistently loved and cared for in order to thrive, learn to trust, and achieve developmental tasks. Stimulation with age-appropriate toys and the freedom to explore influence intellectual development.
Promoting Health and Preventing Illness	• If a danger of lead ingestion exists, take appropriate measures and have the baby screened. • Maintain schedule of immunizations. • Contact healthcare provider for care of respiratory infections. • Stress importance of supplemental fluoride if water is not fluoridated. • Continue well-baby check-ups as recommended. • Do not smoke in the house or car with the baby.	Infants who ingest lead, as from eating peeling lead-based paint, are at risk for brain damage, behavioral problems, and mental deficiency. Immunizations are an essential part of healthcare. Upper respiratory infections may spread to involve the middle ear or lungs. Fluoride is necessary for tooth structure. Cigarette smoke of any type (active or passive) is dangerous, and might increase the risk of respiratory illnesses, asthma, and ear infections. Infants in day care have increased exposure to respiratory and skin infections and infestations.

Recommended Immunization Schedule for Persons Aged 0 Through 6 Years—United States • 2010

For those who fall behind or start late, see the catch-up schedule

Vaccine ▼	Age ▶	Birth	1 month	2 months	4 months	6 months	12 months	15 months	18 months	19–23 months	2–3 years	4–6 years
Hepatitis B[1]		HepB	HepB				HepB					
Rotavirus[2]				RV	RV	RV[2]						
Diphtheria, Tetanus, Pertussis[3]				DTaP	DTaP	DTaP	see footnote[3]	DTaP				DTaP
Haemophilus influenzae type b[4]				Hib	Hib	Hib[4]	Hib					
Pneumococcal[5]				PCV	PCV	PCV	PCV				PPSV	
Inactivated Poliovirus[6]				IPV	IPV		IPV					IPV
Influenza[7]							Influenza (Yearly)					
Measles, Mumps, Rubella[8]							MMR		see footnote[8]			MMR
Varicella[9]							Varicella		see footnote[9]			Varicella
Hepatitis A[10]							HepA (2 doses)				HepA Series	
Meningococcal[11]											MCV	

Range of recommended ages for all children except certain high-risk groups

Range of recommended ages for certain high-risk groups

This schedule includes recommendations in effect as of December 15, 2009. Any dose not administered at the recommended age should be administered at a subsequent visit, when indicated and feasible. The use of a combination vaccine generally is preferred over separate injections of its equivalent component vaccines. Considerations should include provider assessment, patient preference, and the potential for adverse events. Providers should consult the relevant Advisory Committee on Immunization Practices statement for detailed recommendations: **http://www.cdc.gov/vaccines/pubs/acip-list.htm.** Clinically significant adverse events that follow immunization should be reported to the Vaccine Adverse Event Reporting System (VAERS) at **http://www.vaers.hhs.gov** or by telephone, **800-822-7967.**

Recommended Immunization Schedule for Persons Aged 7 Through 18 Years—United States • 2010

For those who fall behind or start late, see the schedule below and the catch-up schedule

Vaccine ▼ Age ▶	7–10 years	11–12 years	13–18 years
Tetanus, Diphtheria, Pertussis[1]		Tdap	Tdap
Human Papillomavirus[2]	see footnote 2	HPV (3 doses)	HPV series
Meningococcal[3]	MCV	MCV	MCV
Influenza[4]		Influenza (Yearly)	
Pneumococcal[5]		PPSV	
Hepatitis A[6]		HepA Series	
Hepatitis B[7]		Hep B Series	
Inactivated Poliovirus[8]		IPV Series	
Measles, Mumps, Rubella[9]		MMR Series	
Varicella[10]		Varicella Series	

Range of recommended ages for all children except certain high-risk groups

Range of recommended ages for catch-up immunization

Range of recommended ages for certain high-risk groups

This schedule includes recommendations in effect as of December 15, 2009. Any dose not administered at the recommended age should be administered at a subsequent visit, when indicated and feasible. The use of a combination vaccine generally is preferred over separate injections of its equivalent component vaccines. Considerations should include provider assessment, patient preference, and the potential for adverse events. Providers should consult the relevant Advisory Committee on Immunization Practices statement for detailed recommendations: **http://www.cdc.gov/vaccines/pubs/acip-list.htm.** Clinically significant adverse events that follow immunization should be reported to the Vaccine Adverse Event Reporting System (VAERS) at **http://www.vaers.hhs.gov** or by telephone, **800-822-7967.**

FIGURE 19-3. Recommended childhood and adolescent immunization schedules—United States, 2010. Footnote information available online. (From Centers for Disease Control and Prevention, available at www.cdc.gov/vaccines/recs/schedules.)

infancy. Growth and development highlights include the following:

- Has rapid brain growth; increase in length of long bones of the arms and legs; growth of muscles
- Uses fingers to pick up small objects
- Walks forward and backward, runs, kicks, climbs stairs, and rides a tricycle

- Drinks from a cup and uses a spoon
- At 2 years of age, the toddler is typically four times the birth weight, averaging 30 to 35 lb (13.6 to 15.9 kg) and 23 to 37 inches (58.4 to 94 cm) in height.
- Has bladder control during the day and sometimes during the night (2.5–3 years of age)
- Turns pages in a book, and by 3 years of age, draws stick people

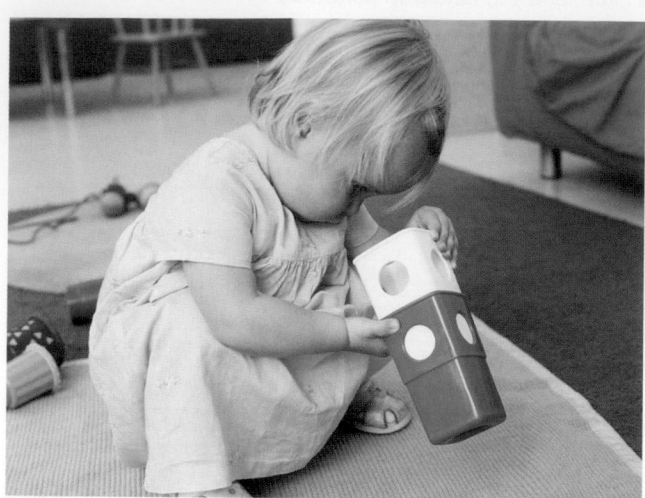

Toddlers enter a stage of autonomy, promoting exploration.

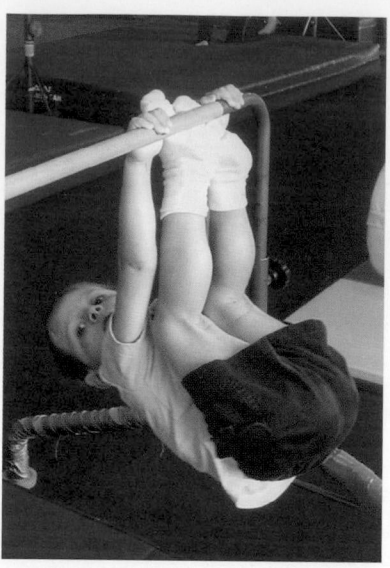

The curious and independent toddler often has a desire to do things by himself.

Discipline helps toddlers learn inner control and understand limits.

Cognitive development can be promoted by allowing the toddler the opportunity to observe and imitate. Younger siblings particularly enjoy mimicking older siblings.

Play in toddlerhood might be solitary or parallel. *(Photo by Joe Mitchell.)*

FIGURE 19-4. Development in the toddler.

Cognitive Development

Toddlers are in Piaget's last two stages of sensorimotor development: beginning to understand object permanence, following simple commands, and anticipating events. Toddlers can understand self as separate from others and have a beginning perception of body image. Toddlers can identify and name several body parts and have a sense of gender identity. Language begins at about 1 year of age, with the use of single or bisyllable sounds. At about 2 years of age, children begin to use short sentences.

Psychosocial Development

Freud's Theory

The toddler is in Freud's anal stage. Increased muscle development and sphincter control encourage the child to focus on the pleasure of sphincter contraction and relaxation. Toilet training becomes a major focus during this period.

Erikson's Theory

The toddler enters Erikson's stage of autonomy versus shame and doubt. Autonomy is developing from independence in feeding, walking, dressing, and toileting, as well as the ability to express wishes verbally. Children who do not feel autonomous might be reluctant to explore and might be fearful of activities and people.

Negativism (characteristically expressed by saying no) and outbursts of temper result from the toddler's efforts at control over the environment. **Regression,** or behavior that is more characteristic of a younger age, can occur at any time in response to stressful circumstances. The most common regressive behaviors are excessive clinging to caregivers, loss of control over elimination, and the use of more infantile speech patterns.

Separation anxiety in response to separation from the mother figure intensifies at about 18 to 24 months, and can be as intense for the toddler as it was for the infant. The child might have feelings of anger, fear, grief, and revenge during this period, but by 24 months, the toddler begins to demonstrate increased independence from the mother (Pillitteri, 2009).

Havighurst's Theory

The toddler has the developmental task of learning to control the elimination of urine and feces and begins to learn sex differences, form concepts, learn language, and distinguish right from wrong. (See the accompanying PICO in Practice display.)

Health of the Toddler

Accidents, such as motor vehicle crashes, poisonings, burns, drowning, choking and aspirations, and falls, are the major cause of death in toddlers. Dental problems can occur, espe-

PICO IN PRACTICE
Asking Clinical Questions

Scenario: Your cousin Lauren is a first-time parent of a 25-month-old toddler named Isabella. One Saturday morning, you pay a visit to your cousin in her home. Lauren has been trying to toilet-train Isabella for the past month. You note that when Lauren discovers that Isabella's pull-up diaper is soiled with urine, she expresses her frustration and displeasure with the child by loudly proclaiming "Icky, smelly, diaper, Isabella!" and turning up her nose in disgust. After Lauren changes Isabella's diaper, she asks you what method of toilet training is the quickest and most effective for toilet-training toddlers such as Isabella.

- Population: Toddlers
- Intervention: Toilet training
- Comparison: Various methods of toilet training
- Outcome: Quick achievement of sustained continence

PICO Question: Which method of toilet training toddlers results in the quickest achievement of sustained continence?

Finding: From the Agency for Healthcare Research and Quality (AHRQ): Kiddoo, D., Klassen, T. P., Lang, M. E., Friesen, C., Russell, K., Spooner, C., et al. (2006, December). The effectiveness of different methods of toilet training for bowel and bladder control. *Evidence Report/Technology Assessment No. 147.* (Prepared by the University of Alberta Evidence-based Practice Center, under contract number 290-02-0023). AHRQ Publication No. 07-E003. Rockville, MD: AHRQ.

The Azrin and Foxx method of toilet training is the superior method of toilet training toddlers. In addition, child-oriented approaches with avoidance of negative terms result in generally greater toilet training success.

Strength of Evidence: Level II

Recommendation: You download *Appendix H: Toilet Training Methods* from the AHRQ evidence-based report 147, review it, and share it with Lauren, reinforcing key concepts and recommendations that detail the Azrin and Foxx method of toilet training. You also note to your cousin that expressing disgust and use of negative terms when Isabella has relapses or episodes of incontinence are not associated with toilet-training success.

cially if the toddler is allowed to go to sleep while sucking on a bottle of milk or sweetened liquid. Respiratory tract and middle ear infections are common. Some surgeries, such as repair of a cleft lip and palate, might be done in the toddler years. Autistic disorder, with abnormal behavior, social interactions, and communication, is usually diagnosed by the time the child is 3 years old.

Recent evidence has indicated that over-the-counter (OTC) cold medications can have serious adverse effects in infants and toddlers. The initial recommendation from the CDC cautioned about use of these drugs in children younger than 2 years of age. Both the Consumer Healthcare Products Association (CHPA) and the FDA are now voluntarily supporting product labels on OTC cough and cold medicines that state "do not use" in children under the age of 4 (U.S. Food and Drug Administration, 2008). In addition to the concerns about misuse of the drugs, there is also data indicating that they have minimal therapeutic value for this age group (Mennick, 2007).

Role of the Nurse in Promoting Health and Preventing Illness

The role of the nurse in promoting health in the toddler continues to be primarily teaching, as shown by the examples in Teaching Tips 19-2. An important part of teaching is helping caregivers encourage their toddler's independence while setting firm limits.

Toddlers who require care in the hospital setting experience stress and separation anxiety when parents are not present. To decrease stress from unfamiliar surroundings and caregivers, parents should be encouraged to provide care and remain with the toddler as much as possible. Every effort should be made to have consistency of healthcare providers and to maintain familiar routines and rituals. When ill or in pain, toddlers often regress to earlier behaviors, such as wanting a bottle to drink from.

> *Recall 2-year-old Hillarie Browning, who is unresponsive. The nurse could apply knowledge about the feelings of stress and separation for a hospitalized toddler when developing the plan of care for this child, especially in light of the possible child abuse. Consistency in staff members caring for the child and maintaining rituals would be helpful in fostering trust and minimizing upset.* ■

PRESCHOOLER: 3 TO 6 YEARS

At around age 3, toddlers begin to move into the next stage: **preschooler.** Although growth and development are slower than in infancy and toddlerhood, they are still steady (Fig. 19-5).

Physiologic Development

The physical characteristics of the preschooler include the following:

- Head is close to adult size by 6 years of age.
- The body is less chubby and becomes leaner and more coordinated.
- Motor abilities include skipping, throwing and catching a ball, copying figures, and printing letters and numbers.

- Full set of 20 deciduous teeth is present; baby teeth begin to fall out and are replaced by permanent teeth.
- Average weight at 5 to 6 years of age is 45 lb (20.4 kg), with boys being slightly heavier than girls.

Cognitive Development

Preschoolers are in Piaget's preoperational stage of development. Passing through the preconceptual and the intuitive phases, preschoolers demonstrate the following transitional changes:

- Egocentrism decreases as socialization with other children increases, and the ability to express self verbally improves.
- Play is more related to real-life events (rather than fantasy).
- Basic curiosity results in constant questions and improved reasoning ability.

Language development is seen in more elaborate and grammatically correct sentences, with 6- to 18-word sentences becoming common by 6 years of age. Incessantly asking "Why?" increases the child's knowledge, encourages further conversations, and helps develop language abilities.

Preschoolers clearly identify themselves as male or female, can understand basic body functions, and have a curiosity about sex differences. This curiosity often leads to "playing doctor," which is normal behavior at this stage. Many children in this age group want to look special or dressed up and gain increased self-esteem by receiving compliments about their appearance.

Psychosocial Development
Freud's Theory

The preschooler is in Freud's phallic stage, with the biologic focus primarily genital. The child has a sexual desire for the opposite-sex parent but, as a means of defense, strongly identifies with the same-sex parent; as a result of this conflict resolution, the superego and conscience begin to develop.

Erikson's Theory

The preschooler is in Erikson's stage of initiative versus guilt. Inner turmoil occurs when natural curiosity is pitted against a constant examination of the propriety of one's actions by a rigid conscience. Realistic self-limits are learned through social interactions.

Havighurst's Theory

According to Havighurst, the preschooler has four developmental tasks to accomplish: to learn sex differences and modesty, to describe social and physical reality through concept formation and language development, to get ready to read, and to learn to distinguish right from wrong.

TEACHING TIPS • 19-2

TODDLERS

Health Topic	Teaching Tip	Why Is This Important?
Safety	• Lock medicines, cleaning supplies, and yard-care products out of reach. • Use safety plugs in electrical outlets. • Block stairs with gates. • Use approved car seat. • Never leave unattended near water. • Do not give small hard foods, small toys or toy parts, or balloons. • Keep plastic bags and mini-blind cords out of reach. • Teach danger in simple terms ("stove hot"). • Do not toss in the air or swing by the arms.	Accidents are a leading cause of injuries and death in toddlers. It is necessary to child-proof the home to prevent injury, as the toddler moves quickly, lacks judgment, and explores his or her world by seeing, touching, and tasting. Small objects or balloons might be aspirated and cause suffocation. Joints might be dislocated by swinging the child.
Nutrition	• Do not scold for messiness while eating. • Provide finger foods. • Short periods of loss of appetite are normal. • Avoid foods that are high in fat, sugar, and salt content (often found in fast foods). • Watch for signs of food allergies. Reactions to milk, egg, peanuts, tree nuts, fish, shellfish, soy, and wheat are the most common.	The toddler is growing less rapidly than the infant and does not require as many calories. Feeding self, even if messy, promotes independence. Giving too much food or food that is high in calories might result in obesity. In recent years, food allergies have increased almost 20% in children under 18 months. Children with food allergies are more likely to develop asthma or other allergies.
Hygiene	• Teach handwashing after eating and toileting. • Teach how to brush teeth. • Schedule dentist visit.	It is important to establish good hygiene and to serve as a role model. The first dentist visit might be just to become familiar with the office and provider.
Elimination	• Physical development is necessary for toilet training. • Begin training with bowel elimination. • Watch for signs of readiness (realizing wetness, staying dry for 2 or more hours). • Night dryness takes longer than day dryness.	The neuromuscular control necessary for elimination occurs between 1 and 3 years. Bowel training is a less complex task than bladder training.
Growth and Development	• Encourage independence in eating, dressing, and toileting. • Provide toys that emphasize gross motor skills and creativity. • Parallel play with other children is normal. • The concept of sharing is not yet developed. • Saying "no" to almost everything is normal.	The toddler gains a sense of security and control by being able to eat, dress, toilet self, and say "no."
Promoting Health and Preventing Illness	• If a danger of lead ingestion exists, take appropriate measures and have the toddler screened. • Complete immunizations. • See healthcare professionals for treatment of respiratory infections. • Do not smoke in the house or car with the child.	Toddlers who ingest lead, as from eating peeling lead-based paint, are at risk for brain damage, behavioral problems and mental deficiency. Immunizations are an essential part of healthcare. Respiratory infections might lead to ear infections. Avoid smoking to reduce risk of respiratory illness, asthma, and ear infections. Passive smoke is dangerous. Infants in day care have increased exposure to respiratory and skin infections and infestations.

Preschooler play is associative and cooperative in its social dimension, and cognitive development is demonstrated in constructive and pretend play.

Motor abilities include throwing and catching a ball.

Safety is a common concern for caregivers.

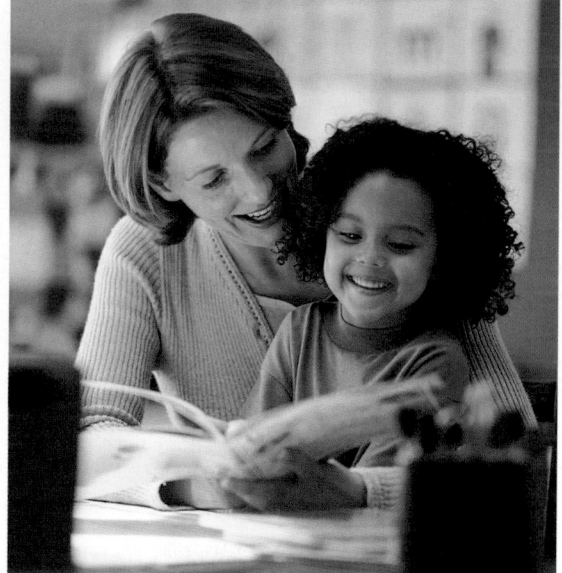

Cognitive development produces improved reasoning ability and readiness to read.

Preschoolers enjoy imitative play.

FIGURE 19-5. Development in the preschooler.

Special Considerations

Preschoolers often have fears—most commonly fear of new places, fear of the dark, and fear during nightmares. These fears are often made worse by the child's own fertile imagination and ability to fantasize. Support and validation of the preschooler's feelings by caregivers are essential.

Moral and Spiritual Development

Kohlberg's preconventional phase of moral reasoning dominates this age. The focus of this stage is obeying rules to avoid punishment or receive a reward. The cognitive, psy-

chosocial, and moral developments of the preschooler provide a base for spiritual development, as described by Fowler. The preschooler might attend activities at church or synagogue with the family, but does not understand religious concepts. The concept of a deity is literal, with God usually being viewed as a male human. Concepts such as heaven, hell, and holy spirits are incomprehensible and often frightening.

Health of the Preschooler

Preschoolers continue to have the health problems that are common in toddlerhood. Communicable diseases and respiratory tract infections are common, especially with increased interaction with other children at nursery schools and daycare. Preschoolers are prone to accidents because of their increased curiosity about the world. Some congenital disorders, such as hypospadias, inguinal hernias, and cardiac anomalies require surgery at this time. Dental caries become common if teeth are neglected. As language becomes more sophisticated, speech disorders might become apparent.

In the United States as well as worldwide, obesity is a significant threat to the health of children. The incidence of obesity has risen more significantly for African American, Hispanic, and American Indian children than for Caucasian children, where its occurrence has increased 50% (Paoletti, 2007). The alarming rise in type 2 diabetes and cardiovascular disease, in addition to other conditions seen typically during the adult years, is further evidence of the devastating toll of obesity. Body mass index (BMI) is now recommended for basic screening and identification of obesity in children. The BMI measurement is discussed in detail in Chapter 36.

Role of the Nurse in Promoting Health and Preventing Illness

Teaching Tips 19-3 provides examples of teaching to promote health in preschoolers. Nurses play a vital role in identifying children at risk for obesity, teaching families about the health consequences, providing information and health teaching, and promoting wellness in this vulnerable population. Assessments of dietary patterns and physical activity level of family members will guide nursing interventions. The CDC provides weight management guidelines and tips on the following Web site: http://www.cdc.gov/nccdphp/dnpa/obesity/childhood/tips_for_parents.htm.

When caring for a preschool-aged child who is scheduled for surgery or requires hospitalization, nurses must recognize the importance of the child's fear of pain, as well as separation anxiety. The nurse can help decrease fears by explaining procedures in language the child can understand and by being honest about how much pain a procedure will cause. Many healthcare institutions and agencies have preprocedure visits so that the child having surgery becomes familiar with the setting and with the activities that will be done. Allowing the child to practice procedures on a doll and encouraging the child to express his or her feelings openly are also beneficial (Fig. 19-6). Encouraging caregivers to take an active role in the child's care helps to reduce fear and separation anxiety.

SCHOOL-AGED CHILD: 6 TO 12 YEARS

School-aged children, from 6 to 12 years of age, are typically sturdy and strong. Physical growth during this time is relatively slow but continues steadily, with both refinement and subtle changes taking place (Fig. 19-7).

Physiologic Development

Physiologic development of school-aged children includes the following:

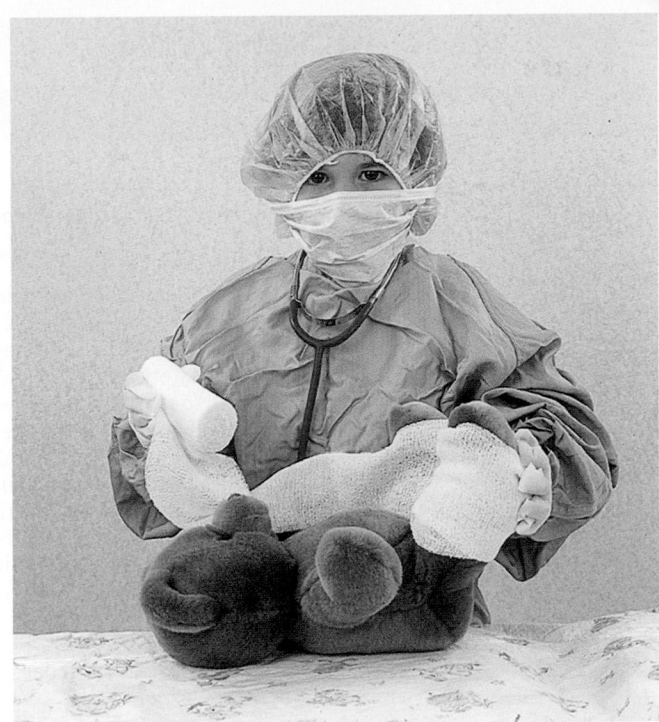

FIGURE 19-6. Abstract reasoning is necessary for children to understand that painful medical treatments given now will make them feel better later. Dramatic play may help the preschool child, who is not old enough to have developed abstract reasoning, to understand the uncomfortable experiences of the hospital stay. *(Photo by B. Proud.)*

- The brain reaches 90% to 95% of adult size; by 12 years of age, the nervous system is almost completely matured, resulting in coordinated body movements.
- Motor abilities progress from the ability to hold a pencil and print words at 6 years of age to the ability to write in script and in sentences at 12 years of age.
- Sexual organs grow but are dormant until late in this period, when hormonal changes begin.
- All permanent teeth are present, except for the second and third molars, by 12 years of age.
- Height increases 2 to 3 inches (5.1 to 7.6 cm) and weight increases 3 to 6 lb (1.4 to 2.7 kg) a year.

Cognitive Development

The school-aged child is at Piaget's concrete operational stage of development, organizing facts about the environment to use for problem solving. In this period, the child has the following characteristics:

- Thinks logically and develops concepts of mass, volume, weight, and measurement
- Deals best with actual objects and people, but can relate concepts and compare events
- Uses inductive reasoning to solve new problems
- Generalizes about people, places, and things

Tips

TEACHING TIPS • 19-3

PRESCHOOLERS

Health Topic	Teaching Tip	Why Is This Important?
Safety	• Lock medicines and cleaning and gardening supplies out of reach. • Use safety plugs in electrical outlets. • Teach child how to go up and down stairs. • Do not give small hard foods, small toys, or balloons. • Use approved car seat and bicycle helmets. • Teach simple traffic safety. • Teach to never talk to or get in the car with a stranger. Include information about inappropriate touching. • Never leave the child alone in public or unattended in a car. • Begin swimming lessons and teach water safety. • Teach danger of fire, and have a home fire safety plan.	Accidents are the leading cause of injury and death in preschoolers, most often from motor vehicles, drowning, burns, and poisoning. Even minor head trauma may cause hematoma formation. Children are at risk for harm from physical and sexual abuse and must be taught how to avoid situations that might increase that risk.
Nutrition	• A gradual increase in calories, with nutritious snacks, is necessary • Children who follow their own appetite patterns are less likely to be overweight. • Avoid foods that are high in fat, sugar, and salt (found in most fast foods). • Preschoolers like to eat one food at a time, and prefer those that are mildly flavored and lukewarm.	The preschool child needs the same food group nutrition as the adult, but in lesser amounts.
Hygiene	• Stress importance of handwashing before meals and after toileting. • Assist with brushing and flossing teeth after eating. • Teach disposal of used tissues. • Maintain regular dental checkups and care.	Preschoolers are able to carry out basic hygiene, but continue to need assistance and reminders. Dental caries often begins during this age.
Elimination	• Toilet training is completed, but night wetting may persist.	Recognizing the need to empty the bladder during sleep takes a longer time in some children. They should not be punished for wetting the bed.
Growth and Development	• Night fears and bad dreams are common. • Make-believe play and imaginary friends are normal. • Although each child grows and develops differently, there are ranges of normal. • Play occupies most of the child's time; the child can play with others for periods of time. • Provide play materials that encourage physical activity, dramatic play, quiet play, and creativity. • Provide consistent, fair, and kind limits for behavior. • Masturbation is normal, although the child should learn that it is not acceptable in public.	Sleep problems usually resolve on their own; calm reassurance by parents is appropriate when they occur. Play is the work of the child; adults should provide time, space, equipment, and safety, but should not structure the child's play.
Promoting Health and Preventing Illness	• If a danger of lead ingestion or poisoning exists, take appropriate measures and have the child screened. • Maintain immunizations. • Have vision tested. • Have hearing tested if necessary (e.g., child does not seem to listen). • Maintain regular well-child checkups. • Preschoolers often fear dental and medical treatments. Avoid hospitalization if possible, but if necessary, prepare the child before the procedure.	Lead poisoning in preschoolers causes brain dysfunction. Immunizations and health-related checkups are essential in promoting health. Preschoolers often see dental or medical procedures as a punishment and fear damage to their bodies. Parents should set a good example, be honest with the child. Preparation for procedures and hospitalization can help decrease fear and separation anxiety.

Play involves development of skill, games with rules, and competitive activities.

Making friends is important to a school-aged child.

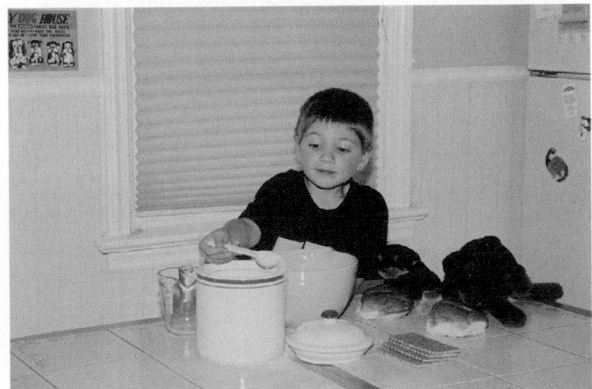

The school-aged child is aware of and understands a sequence of events.

FIGURE 19-7. Development in the school-aged child.

- Develops classification systems
- Develops an awareness and understanding of other people's feelings and points of view
- Understands reversal of events

School-aged children have well-developed language skills, using language in a more sophisticated manner. Their ability to store information in long-term memory and retrieve it in the remembering (recall) process is more efficient.

Psychosocial Development
Freud's Theory

The school-aged child is in the latency stage of Freud's theory, with psychosocial energies being channeled toward strong identification with one's own sex and creative activities. Privacy and understanding one's body are important at this age.

Erikson's Theory

The school-aged child is in the industry-versus-inferiority stage of Erikson's theory, with the child focused on learning useful skills and thereby developing positive self-esteem. A sense of identity begins to emerge, and values are integrated. The emphasis is on doing, succeeding, and accomplishing.

Havighurst's Theory

According to Havighurst, the school-aged child has the following developmental tasks:

- Learning physical game skills
- Learning appropriate masculine or feminine social role
- Developing fundamental skills in reading, writing, and calculating
- Developing concepts necessary for everyday living
- Achieving personal independence
- Developing conscience, morality, and a scale of values

Special Considerations

Peer relationships become the major gauge for determining status, skill, and personableness. Peer groups in middle childhood help prepare the child for getting along in the larger world and teach appropriate sex role behavior. They also act as transition modes for the child as he or she leaves the total caregiver influence and heads toward adult independence. Unfortunately, as children become members of social groups, they may experience some form of bullying. Data indicates that bullying behavior becomes more common during the third and fourth grades and may be related to gender, physical appearance, disability or ability, and intellect (Governo & Siewers, 2008).

Body image, self-concept, and sexuality are interrelated. Sexual development results in a strong need to understand body function and to have accurate information about sexuality.

Moral Development

Most of middle childhood is spent in the conventional phase of moral development. Behavior is based on familial and peer group beliefs, and conformity to the norm is common. Following school regulations, respecting teachers, and viewing justice as a means of fair play are all important.

Spiritual Development

In Fowler's theory, school-aged children view religious faith as a relationship that involves reciprocal fairness. They take part in rituals of their faith, with a basic understanding of the ritual's significance. The importance of spiritual beliefs and the possibility of life after death is accepted, even if not totally understood.

Health of the School-Aged Child

Accidents continue to be common in school-aged children. With increased interactions with other children in school, communicable conditions such as scabies, impetigo, and head lice are more prevalent. Other common health-related problems of the school-aged child include obesity, attention deficit hyperactivity disorder (ADHD) and learning disability (LD), and enuresis (bed wetting). In addition, chronic conditions such as sickle cell anemia, hyperactivity, seizure disorders, hypertension, diabetes mellitus, and obesity might affect the school-aged child. Scoliosis, an abnormal curvature of the spine, occurs most often in girls between the ages of 10 and 13 years.

Obesity

Over the past 20 years, obesity among children in this age group has more than doubled. The rate has grown from 6.5% in 1980 to 17% in 2006 (CDC, 2008a). Many of these obese school-aged children have diets that are high in saturated fats, do not meet fruit and vegetable daily requirements, are low in fiber, and also low in calcium. As with adults, obesity in children is the result of more calories consumed than expended. Genetics and health factors may be a contributing factor.

ADHD and Learning Disabilities

ADHD is a developmentally inappropriate degree of inattention, impulsiveness, and hyperactivity. To be diagnosed with this disorder, the child must have manifested symptoms before 7 years of age, and they must be present in at least two settings. LD is a group of disorders in which the child has significant difficulty in listening, speaking, reading, writing, reasoning, mathematic abilities, or social skills (Wong et al., 2006). Both of these conditions affect all areas of the life of the child, but they are most noticeable in the classroom. Multiple approaches are used in management, including medication, environmental strategies, and classroom education. Based on the Education for All Handicapped Children's Act, children with ADHD and LD must receive free public education in the least restrictive environment.

Enuresis

Enuresis is diagnosed when a child is at least 5 years of age and is still having involuntary urination, usually at night. Although this problem is significant to the child and his or her parents, it is defined as a benign and self-limiting disorder, usually ending between 6 and 8 years of age.

Role of the Nurse in Promoting Health and Preventing Illness

The nurse's role in promoting health for the school-aged child involves individual and family teaching, often conducted by school nurses. Multiple strategies can be implemented in schools to address the obesity epidemic. Parents, teachers, administrators, and the school nurse can collaborate to assess the current programs available in the school and take action. Some recommended approaches include increasing opportunities for students to become involved in physical activities and ensuring that students have healthy food and beverage choices while at school. Because school violence has become more common, school nurses must be prepared for a potential crisis. They need to be alert for warning signs of bullying and other dangerous behaviors and be involved in efforts to promote a safe environment in playgrounds, buses, and schools. This will most likely include collaboration between the school nurse, parents, and educators to determine creative strategies that promote healthier lifestyles and environments for school-aged children. Teaching Tips 19-4 provides examples of nursing activities specific for this age group. In addition, nurses often function as advocates for vulnerable populations (see the Nursing Advocacy in Action display).

Because school-aged children are striving for independence and control, hospitalization might mean a loss of freedom of choice (e.g., types of food, clothing, activities). Children of this age should be allowed to have some measure of control over allowable activities and should be encouraged to do what they can, such as playing competitive games and making their own bed (Fig. 19-8).

THE ADOLESCENT AND YOUNG ADULT

The adolescent and young adult years are a time of both change and stability. **Adolescence** begins with puberty and extends from 12 to 20 years of age; the **young adult** period is considered to be the 20s and 30s. However, these time periods are highly individualized. A person is defined as an adult when he or she is "physically and psychologically mature, ready to assume adult responsibilities and be self-sufficient" (Murray & Zentner, 2001, p. 525).

After experiencing rapid growth and development during adolescence, the young adult completes physical growth and develops internal and external controls and values acceptable to society. There are no specific measurements of maturity; each person is an individual and a wide range of normal values and behaviors are considered healthy (Fig. 19-9).

NURSING ADVOCACY IN ACTION

Patient Scenario

You are working as a school nurse in a district where there are many poor families who have come to the United States (many illegally) to find work. At present, there is a lively debate in the country about whether these families should be identified and "shipped home" or supported. Many of the parents are afraid of being deported and you learn that some have taken their children out of school. You know that the children benefit from being in school. In addition to the education, there is a free lunch program that for many children is the one meal of the day they can count on.

Implications for Nursing Advocacy

How will you respond if you are the school nurse approached by faculty who want to help the children? Talk with your classmates and experienced nurses about the questions that follow.

- If you elect to advocate for these children what practical steps can you take to ensure better health outcomes?
- What is it reasonable to expect of a student nurse, a graduate nurse, and an experienced nurse in this situation?
- What advocacy skills are needed to effectively respond to this challenge?

Physiologic Development

Changes in the adolescent's body transform him or her from a child to an adult in appearance. Physiologic development includes the following:

- The feet, hands, and long bones grow rapidly, accompanied by an increase in muscle mass (especially in boys).

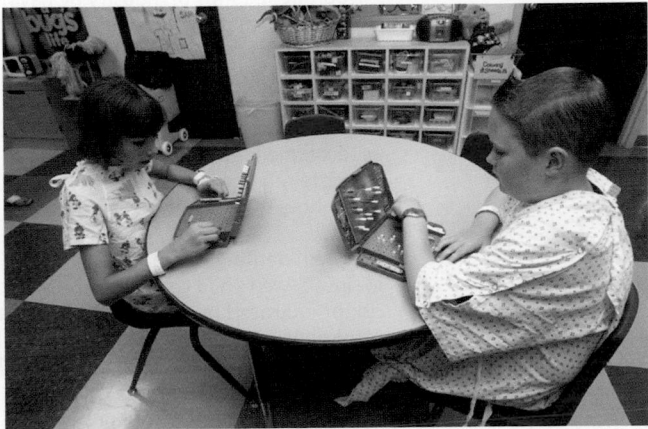

FIGURE 19-8. Allowing school-aged children to play competitive games promotes a positive hospital experience. *(Photo by Joe Mitchell.)*

Tips   **TEACHING TIPS • 19-4**

SCHOOL-AGED CHILDREN

Health Topic	Teaching Tip	Why Is This Important?
Safety	• Teach and require pedestrian traffic safety. • Wear seat belts and bicycle helmets. • Emphasize bicycle, scooter, skate, and skateboard safety. • Provide swimming lessons and water safety rules. • Rural children should be taught farm safety. • Teach how to "stop, drop, and roll" to extinguish clothing fire. • Teach the dangers of dangerous products and chemicals. • Keep guns locked up. Teach gun safety rules. • Teach use of proper equipment for contact sports.	Accidents are the leading cause of death in school-aged children, most often caused by motor vehicle crashes, fires, falls, drowning, and poisonings. Gun accidents to themselves and others occur in school-aged children. Accident prevention and safety education should be taught and reinforced both at home and at school.
Nutrition	• School-aged children need adequate calories, and might also require increased amounts of vitamin D and calcium. • Provide foods that meet nutritional needs and do not supply empty calories (as found in junk food and fast food). • Do not overemphasize table manners to keep meal times more pleasant.	Increased vitamin D and calcium are needed as bones enlarge and for girls to prevent later osteoporosis. American children eat too much salt, sugar, and fats; nearly 1/4 of all school-aged children have an elevated cholesterol level. Eating patterns for school-aged children will improve over time. Both undernutrition and overnutrition are seen in this age group.
Hygiene	• Teach girls how to wipe from front to back after urination. • Teach children not to share hats or combs.	Girls are prone to urinary infections because of their short urethra. Head lice and ringworm are common in school-aged children and are easily spread to others.
Sexual Development	• Both girls and boys have characteristics of sexual maturity, including a growth spurt, growth of body hair, changes in body proportion, and the beginning of secondary physical sex changes. • Provide accurate information and answer questions honestly about sex, including anatomy, physiology, birth control, and STIs (including AIDS). • Monitor TV watching and computer use.	Girls have breast development, grow axillary and pubic hair, and may begin to menstruate. Boys have testicular growth, grow axillary and pubic hair, and the penis enlarges. Boys may also have temporary breast enlargement. School-aged children are curious, and if unsupervised, may watch pornographic television or computer material. In addition, the violence in television shows or video games may lead to aggressive behavior.
Growth and Development	• Best friends and groups of peer friends are important to the school-aged child. • Rules are rigidly followed during games with peers. • Encourage both quiet and active play activities. • Provide guidance and set limits for behavior, focusing on only one incident at a time. • Encourage feelings of industry by having realistic expectations and recognizing unique abilities and talents. • Provide positive statements that demonstrate the child is valued, loved, and important.	From ages 7 to 9, close friends are usually the same gender and age. This is not as important from ages 10 to 12. Unrealistic expectations or excessive discipline might result in stress and feelings of inferiority.
Promoting Health and Preventing Illness	• Maintain records of immunizations, and have boosters as recommended. • Promote regular physical activity and exercise. • Teach how to "just say no" to smoking, alcohol, and drugs. • Maintain dental examinations. • Maintain well-child checkups, and have screenings (if at risk or indicated by symptoms) and treatment for chronic conditions such as asthma, diabetes mellitus, sickle cell anemia, hypertension, seizure disorder, hyperactivity, and obesity. • Have vision tested if school problems with reading, coordination, or inability to see screen or monitor in front of the room occur.	Maintaining immunizations is essential to health; records are required for enrollment in school. Children need to know how to handle peer pressure to smoke, drink, and take drugs. Many school-aged children are at risk for and exhibit symptoms of chronic illnesses.

Peer relationships are particularly influential during adolescence. *(Photo by Joe Mitchell.)*

Babysitting offers an opportunity to practice formal adult skills. *(Photo by Joe Mitchell.)*

The development of self-identity in adolescence involves discovering talents and becoming emotionally independent.

FIGURE 19-9. Development in the adolescent.

A primary developmental task of adolescence is to achieve new and more-mature relationships. *(Photo by Joe Mitchell.)*

- Primary and secondary sexual development occurs, with maturation of the genitalia; presence of body hair; breast development and menstruation in girls; facial hair growth, voice changes, and spermatogenesis in boys.
- **Puberty** (the time when the ability to reproduce begins) begins at 9 to 13 years of age in girls (with menstruation usually beginning between 10 and 14 years of age) and at 11 to 14 years of age in boys.
- Sebaceous and axillary sweat glands become active.
- Full adult size is reached, although some young men might continue to grow in their 20s.

Puberty can be divided into the following three stages (Table 19-3):

- *Prepubescence:* Secondary sex characteristics begin to develop, but the reproductive organs do not yet function.

- *Pubescence:* Secondary sex characteristics continue to develop, and ova and sperm begin to be produced by the reproductive organs.
- *Postpubescence:* Reproductive functioning and the development of secondary sex characteristics reach adult maturity.

Cognitive Development

According to Piaget, adolescence is the stage when the cognitive development of formal operations is developed. Deductive, reflective, and hypothetical reasoning are possible, and abstract concepts can be used. Long-term goals can be set as the concept of time, its passage, and the future become real. Challenging the decision making of adults is common. Egocentrism returns, and imaginary audiences and daydreaming are common.

TABLE • 19-3	ADOLESCENT SEXUAL DEVELOPMENT	
Stage	**Males**	**Females**
Prepubescence	• Progressive enlargement of testicles, seminal ducts, prostate gland • Enlargement and reddening of the scrotal sac • Increase in length and circumference of penis • Appearance of downy pubic hair	• Progressive enlargement of the ovaries • Ripening of graafian follicles • Rounding of the hips • Appearance of breast buds • Enlargement of the fallopian tubes, vagina, and uterus • Appearance of downy pubic hair
Pubescence	• Increase in amount, pigmentation, and curling of pubic hair • Growth spurt involving height and weight increase • Deepening of the voice due to growth of larynx • Enlargement of testicles • Increased pigmentation and growth of scrotum • Growth of penis in length and circumference • Beginning of spermatogenesis	• Increase in amount, pigmentation, and curling of pubic hair • Growth spurt involving height and weight increase • Menarche • Appearance of axillary hair • Enlargement of vulva and clitoris • Development of breast tissue • Ovulation
Postpubescence	• Completion of sexual growth and development • Fertility	• Completion of sexual growth and development • Fertility

Young adults, in comparison to the adolescent, are more creative in thought, are objective and realistic, and are less self-centered. Their learning is enhanced through educational and life experiences.

Psychosocial Development
Freud's Theory

The adolescent and young adult are in Freud's genital stage. The libido reemerges in a mature, adult form, and the individual is capable of full sexual function. There is a sense of self and others, extending to other adults and peers of the opposite gender. Creativity and pleasure are found in love and in work.

Erikson's Theory

Based on Erikson's theory, the adolescent tries out different roles, personal choices, and beliefs in the stage called identity versus role confusion. Self-concept is being stabilized, with the peer group acting as the greatest influence.

> *Think back to Darlene Jenkins, the 14-year-old pregnant teenager. The nurse could apply knowledge of Erikson's theory to foster a sense of identity in Darlene by explaining about important self-care measures and encouraging her participation in her pregnancy. In addition, establishing a trusting relationship with Darlene and subsequently with her and other members of the health-care staff would help to further promote her identity.* ■

The young adult, in the intimacy-versus-isolation stage, needs to complete tasks such as achieving independence from parents, establishing intimate relationships, and choos-

ing an occupation or career. If such developmental tasks are not accomplished, the young adult becomes isolated and self-absorbed.

Havighurst's Theory

According to Havighurst, more mature relationships with both boys and girls of the same age are achieved, a masculine or feminine social role is developed, one's personal appearance is accepted, and a set of values and an ethical system as a guide to behavior are internalized.

Levinson's Theory

Based on Levinson's theory of individual life structure, the years from 18 to 22 are characterized by early adult transition (Levinson, Darrow, Klein, Levinson, & McKee, 1978). This is a time of making initial career choices, establishing personal relationships, and selecting personal values and lifestyles. During the years from 22 to 28, the young adult builds on previous choices, but there might be a transient quality to occupational choices and friendships.

Gould's Theory

Gould's (1972) theory of transformation views young adults as having established their own control as adults separate from the family. They want to enjoy the present but also build for the future.

> *Remember Patricia Lemming, the 26-year-old pregnant woman described at the beginning of the chapter. Applying Gould's theory, the nurse could interpret Patricia's desire to stop smoking and drinking as an example of her attempt to establish control as an adult, thus securing*

the future for herself and her baby. The nurse could build on this desire by teaching Patricia about appropriate and effective methods for smoking and drinking cessation. ∎

Special Considerations

CHOOSING AN OCCUPATION OR CAREER

A major psychosocial developmental requirement for the young adult is choosing a vocation. The decision to enter the world of work is strongly influenced initially by the need to become independent of one's family and to be self-sufficient. The choice of an occupation or a career is also guided by factors such as the desire to get married, raise a family, and become part of the community (Fig. 19-10).

Occupational and career choices are largely tied to educational choices. Many careers require a college education. Adults learn from both informal and formal experiences and are largely goal-directed learners. If the person's identified goals are to increase career opportunities, maintain financial stability, and pursue upward mobility, the adult will be motivated to learn and change. The major factor in achieving satisfaction with one's vocational choice is the belief that one is functioning to capacity and making a contribution to society.

ESTABLISHING A FAMILY

Establishing a family involves both parents, even though the physiologic changes of pregnancy take place in the woman. Pregnancy might be considered a period of developmental crisis, during which certain tasks must be completed

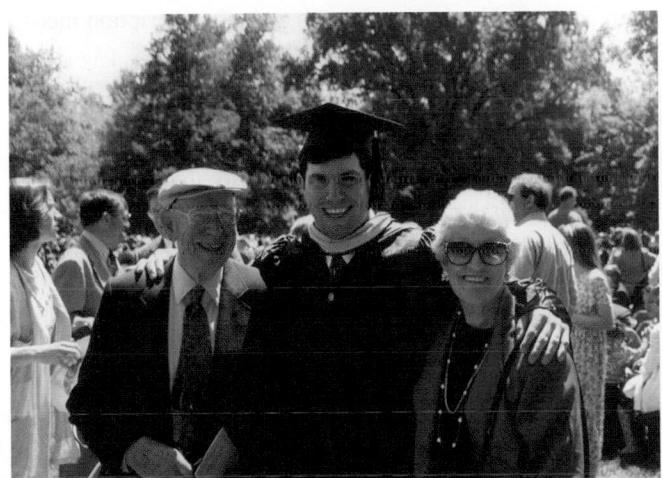

Graduating college or trade school is an important developmental milestone.

Choosing an occupation and starting a career are also important developmental milestones.

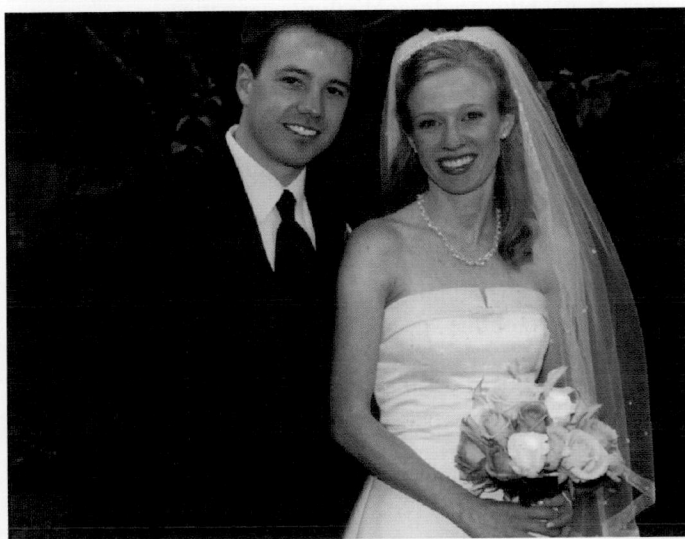

Developmental tasks of the young adult center on establishing intimate relationships, a home, and a family.

FIGURE 19-10. Development in the young adult.

for acceptance and coping by the expanding family. The cognitive, psychosocial, cultural, and educational dimensions of the prospective parents influence completion of the tasks.

The verification of pregnancy might raise conflicting emotions in the woman, influenced by such factors as whether the pregnancy was planned or unplanned and how the baby will affect career goals. As body changes occur and fetal movement is felt, the woman begins to visualize herself as a mother and normally assumes responsibility for the health of the growing baby. As the time for delivery becomes closer, the woman centers on maternal tasks (such as preparing the baby's room and having clothing ready) and prepares herself for labor and delivery. During the pregnancy, the expectant father needs to learn the normal physiologic and psychological changes of pregnancy, accept his supportive role in meeting maternal needs, and explore his feelings about the developing infant and the birth.

Moral Development

The child enters adolescence with a law-and-order orientation and might never progress beyond that point. Young adults who have mastered previous levels of moral development reach the conventional level and are concerned with maintaining expectations. They also value conformity, loyalty, and social order. Some people might enter the postconventional stage, in which they make moral judgments on the basis of universal beliefs.

Spiritual Development

Adolescents and young adults can think in the abstract and might question beliefs and practices that no longer serve to stabilize their identity or purpose. The individuating-reflective period in the young adult (defined by Fowler) brings discovery of the meaning of values as they relate to the achievement of social purposes and the acceptance of the value systems of others. Often, adolescents or young adults temporarily abandon traditional religious practices.

Health of the Adolescent and Young Adult

Although adolescence and young adulthood are times of maximum physiologic development and health, a wide variety of health problems can occur. Health promotion focuses on nutrition, relationships with self and others, and safety. The Advisory Committee on Immunization Practices now recommends routine vaccination with one dose of Meningococcal Conjugate Vaccine for all persons 11 to 18 years of age (CDC, 2007b). College freshmen living in dormitories are at risk for meningococcal disease and require the vaccine for protection from it. Young adults should have a tetanus and diphtheria booster every 10 years. Since 2000, there has been a recurrence of pertussis (whooping cough), and a tetanus, diphtheria, and acellular pertussis vaccine (Tdap) has been developed to provide immunity against pertussis. Tdap should replace one dose of Td when it is recommended

for this age group (Curry, 2009). See Examples of NANDA Nursing Diagnoses: Adolescence.

Injuries

Injuries are the leading cause of death for adolescents and young adults. Motor vehicle crashes are the most common cause of mortality, often associated with the use of alcohol or other drugs. According to the CDC (2009b), homicide is the second leading cause of death in the 10 to 24 year age group. In 2006, more than 720,000 youths in this age group were treated in emergency rooms for injuries related to violence (CDC, 2008g).

Substance Abuse

Smoking and the use of illegal drugs (such as marijuana and cocaine) might be a problem, and the use of alcohol is significantly related to risk-taking behavior. In addition, the use of crack-cocaine, as well as other relatively inexpensive and highly addictive drugs, has reached epidemic proportions in many areas of North America. Misuse of prescription medications among adolescents has increased in the past few years. Emergency departments have treated adolescents for overdose, with fatal results at times, following attendance at a "pharm party," at which everyone shares prescription drugs obtained from home or other sources with the intent of getting "high" (Graham-Knight & Karch, 2007). Other products that have potential for abuse in this age group include easily available household agents. Inhaling the vapors of these toxic substances with the intent of causing a mind-altering effect or "high" can damage the kidneys, brain, and liver and lead to cardiopulmonary arrest. Types of products abused include solvents such as glue and paint thinners, aerosols such as spray paint and hair spray, gas inhalants that can be found in whip cream containers, and nitrites also referred to as "poppers." Because they are easily available, survey results indicate that eighth graders try inhalants more than any other illicit drug (National Institute on Drug Abuse, 2008).

Suicide

The suicide rate of adolescents has increased drastically, with suicide being more prevalent in adolescents than in any other age group. Suicide is the third leading cause of death of 15- to 24-year-olds and the second leading cause of death for adults 25 to 34 years of age (CDC, 2008e). Although females attempt suicide more often than males, males are more likely to succeed. Depression is a possible contributing factor. Verbal or nonverbal indicators of suicide should not be ignored; rather, an immediate referral should be made to a professional trained in suicide intervention.

Pregnancy

The United States leads the developed countries in the number of pregnancies among adolescents 15 to 19 years old. These pregnancies are physically, psychologically, and economically

Examples of NANDA Nursing Diagnoses

Adolescence

Nursing Diagnoses	Possible Related Factor
Imbalanced Nutrition: More Than Body Requirements	Compulsive overeating
Imbalanced Nutrition: Less Than Body Requirements	Self-imposed dieting
Risk for Deficient Fluid Volume	Extended hours of football practice in heat
Risk for Injury	Risk-taking behavior while driving
Risk for Trauma	Lack of knowledge about water safety
Social Isolation	Perceived inability to be popular
Risk for Impaired Parenting	Teenage pregnancy
Disturbed Body Image	Obesity
Anxiety	Fear of failure in school
Ineffective Health Maintenance	Frequent use of alcohol and drugs
Risk-Prone Health Behavior	Smoking

costly for the adolescent mother, the infant, the family, and society. Many adolescent mothers are poor, do not complete high school, and are at high risk for complications involving the pregnancy and the infant.

Nutritional Problems

Fad dieting and habitually eating fast foods are common among adolescents and young adults. For those obsessed with body image (particularly girls and young women), severe eating disorders can result. The most common are anorexia nervosa (compulsive dieting to the point of self-starvation) and bulimia (a destructive cycle of binge eating followed by self-induced vomiting in an effort to prevent weight gain). The psychodynamics of these conditions are complex but almost always involve a negative self-concept. Although these disorders were once considered uncommon, 1% of adolescent girls report symptoms of anorexia and 4% of college-aged women have bulimia. New data suggest that males account for up to 15% of all persons with anorexia and bulimia (National Institute of Mental Health, 2009).

In the adolescent and young adult years, fast foods and busy lifestyles have the potential to lead to increased caloric intake with minimal exercise. This has resulted in an increase in the rate of obesity from 6% to almost 19% for people 12 to 19 years of age in the United States (CDC, 2008a). The CDC also reports that research indicates overweight children and adolescents are more likely to become obese adults.

Sexually Transmitted Infections

Adolescents and young adults who engage in unprotected sexual intercourse are at a higher risk for contracting **sexually transmitted infections (STIs)** and their complications than are adults. Lack of knowledge, lack of psychosocial maturity, embarrassment, and the denial of the need to plan ahead and use condoms are the most common reasons for this increased risk. Trichomonal and monilial infections, as well as human *Papillomavirus,* are common.

Chlamydia, an infection of the genital tract, is the most common STI in the United States (Toro, 2008). Chlamydial infections occur in both genders, as do syphilis and herpes simplex type II (genital herpes). These STIs pose serious health threats.

Acquired immunodeficiency syndrome (AIDS) poses the greatest single threat to individuals and society as a whole. Although AIDS can be transmitted through means other than sexual contact, transmission is primarily through genital, oral, or anal sexual activities. AIDS is a major cause of death in the world, and its incidence is predicted to increase still further.

Developmental and Situational Stressors

Adolescents and young adults have to deal with many stressors as a result of their choices about lifestyle, occupation, and relationships. Family-centered stressors might be either positive or negative factors such as marriage, divorce, parenthood, and death of a parent. Stress might precipitate mental or physical health problems, aggravated by ineffective coping mechanisms such as substance abuse, child abuse, spousal abuse, decreased nutrition and rest, and risk-taking behavior.

> *Consider Darlene Jenkins, the 14-year-old pregnant adolescent described in the case file at the beginning of the* chapter. *Analysis of this patient's assessment reveals multiple developmental and situational stressors affecting Darlene that place her and her fetus at high risk for problems. Using this information, the nurse could develop a highly individualized plan of care that focuses on these stressors (e.g., her lack of adequate supports, multiple sexual*

Tips   TEACHING TIPS • 19-5

ADOLESCENTS AND YOUNG ADULTS

Health Topic	Teaching Tip	Why Is This Important?
Safety	• Encourage drivers' education classes for adolescents, if available. • Discuss the relationship of alcohol and drug consumption to motor vehicle crashes. • Provide information about water safety, gun safety, and sports safety. • Provide information about emergency care measures.	Most deaths in people between the ages of 15 and 24 are the result of motor vehicle crashes, homicide, and suicide.
Nutrition	• Encourage a diet based on the food groups, with added calories during the adolescent growth spurt. • Refer for counseling for extremes in either underweight or overweight. • Discuss nutritional problems that may result from too much fast food and too many soft drinks. • A balance of food intake, exercise, and rest is important.	Nutritional needs increase to meet the accelerated physical growth and development during adolescence. Underweight may result from an inadequate intake of calories, or in extreme cases from anorexia nervosa or bulimia. Overweight results from an intake of calories in excess of metabolic needs.
Sexual Development	• Secondary sex characteristics are fully developed. • Both males and females are physically capable of reproduction. • Discuss sexual behavior openly and honestly with adolescents.	The development of secondary sex characteristics that began in the school-aged child is completed during adolescence. Sexual behavior in adolescents and young adults might result in disease or pregnancy, as well as decreased self-esteem.
Growth and Development	• The adolescent is primarily influenced by the peer group. • Risk-taking behavior, especially in males, is common. • Maintaining open communications with teens is important. • Encourage increasing independence in the adolescent and young adult, but continue to provide love and support. • Assist with clarifying values and goals for future occupation.	Peer groups may have positive or negative effects. The rapid physical and emotional changes of adolescence require revising self-concept and body image. These should stabilize by late adolescence. The young adult is usually living independently and has an occupation of choice.
Promoting Health and Preventing Illness	• Have immunizations and boosters as recommended. • Have regular physical, vision and dental examinations. • Always have a physical examination before participating in sports activities. • Do a breast self-exam (females) and a testicular self-exam (males) each month. • Learn to say "no" to pressures to have sexual activity. • Practice safer sex practices if sexually active. • Have an annual Pap test and pelvic examination if sexually active. • Know the dangers of STIs (from genital, oral, and anal sex) and have HIV testing if safer sex is not practiced.	Immunizations and regular health-related examinations are essential to maintaining health. Chronic illnesses such as hypertension, cardiovascular disease, and diabetes mellitus might appear during adolescence and young adulthood. Sexual desires are high, and sexual activity is common. Sexually-transmitted diseases, including HIV and AIDS, are a major health problem, with more than two thirds of those infected younger than 25. Untreated STIs may result in sterility in females and males or infection of an unborn baby.

partners, poor nutritional habits), ultimately to the benefit of Darlene and her baby. ■

An increasing number of men and women are remaining single, either by choice or situation. Singlehood status has advantages and disadvantages. Being single gives one the freedom to come and go as one chooses, to have more autonomy, and to spend money and time as one wishes. On the other hand, external pressures to marry and the desire for love, to belong, and to raise a family might make a young adult question his or her decision to remain single.

Couples might encounter difficulties conceiving, delay childbearing until their careers are established, or choose not to have children. If they want to have children, infertility (defined as the inability to conceive after 1 year of coitus without contraception) might add even more stress. Women who have postponed having children might realize in their middle to late 30s that their so-called biologic clock is winding down; an increasing number of women in this age group are having their first child.

Divorce is common in our society, with rates being highest among those marrying young, having low income, and having low educational levels. It separates children from their families, has long-term emotional costs, and increases the number of single-parent families headed by women.

Role of the Nurse in Promoting Health and Preventing Illness

A true assessment of adolescent development must include the profound changes in reproductive functioning. Teaching activities to promote health for adolescents and young adults are listed in Teaching Tips 19-5. Perhaps one of the more significant nursing activities for individuals in this stage is facilitating healthy family relationships. Mutual respect, open communications, and accurate information exchange among family members pave the road for a healthy transition from adolescence to adulthood. (See Research in Nursing box).

Acute illness is often more of an annoyance than of serious consequence. If hospitalized, an adolescent's and young adult's motivation to recover and to resume normal activities is strong. Because independence and self-sufficiency are important to adolescents and young adults, they will not easily accept the dependent sick role.

Although chronic illnesses are less common, their occurrence can lead to delayed development, loss of independence, and permanent changes in personal and career goals. Prolonged hospitalization, long-term care, or home care increases the adolescent's feelings of isolation and may disrupt normal development. Educational and recreational activities should be provided, if at all possible (Fig. 19-11).

RESEARCH IN NURSING
Bridging The Gap To Evidence-Based Practice

INVESTIGATING THE BEHAVIOR AND PERFORMANCE OF ADOLESCENTS WHO HAVE A TELEVISION IN THEIR BEDROOM

Pediatricians have advocated for parents to limit TV usage for their children, yet a majority of adolescents have a TV in their bedroom. The concern is less time spent exercising, less attention to school responsibilities, and less interaction with family members. Habits that develop during these adolescent years can set a trend for lifestyle during later years. Nurses, through various health-teaching opportunities, must demonstrate an awareness of developmental milestones for adolescents and promote strategies that foster healthy habits and enable them to reach their potential.

Related Research

Barr-Anderson, D., van den Berg, P., Neumark-Sztainer, D., & Story, M. (2008). Characteristics associated with older adolescents who have a television in their bedrooms. *Pediatrics, 121*(4), 718–724.

This study was designed to examine and compare the behavior of teenagers who have a television in their bedroom versus those who do not have one. Seven hundred and eighty-one (781) high school juniors and seniors in Minnesota completed surveys regarding their TV-viewing habits. These student participants were from a variety of ethnic and socioeconomic backgrounds. They also responded to questions about their grades, study habits, pattern of exercise, diet, and family relationships. Teenagers from lower income families, males, and black teens

had the highest proportion of bedroom TVs. Girls with bedroom TVs spent less time exercising, consumed more sweetened soft drinks, ate less vegetables, and spent less time eating meals with their family than those without a TV in their bedroom. Boys with TVs in the bedroom also participated in fewer family meals, had less fruit intake, and also had lower GPAs than teens without TVs in the bedroom. The findings of these researchers verify that excessive TV time can have a detrimental effect on an adolescent's personal and social behaviors.

Relevance to Nursing Practice

Promoting good health habits and healthy family and peer relationships are factors that facilitate optimal growth and development for adolescents. Nurses, with their focus on providing holistic healthcare and maximizing an individual's potential, have various opportunities to contribute to the growth and development of children in this age group. Interactions may involve discussion about the advantage of limiting TV usage for teenagers and an opportunity to introduce this research as evidence of the beneficial effects of limiting TV usage. Though eager to demonstrate their independence from their parents, adolescents are more likely to respond positively to health teaching when they feel their opinions are respected and valued and understand the rationale for parental decisions.

For additional research, visit the Point.

FIGURE 19-11. Allowing teens to "surf the net" and instant-message friends at home promotes a positive hospital experience. *(Photo by Joe Mitchell.)*

● Developing Critical Thinking Skills

1. Based on the information presented in Chapters 18 and 19, describe nursing interventions to meet developmental needs for the following:
   - An infant hospitalized for treatment of a serious birth defect involving the heart and lungs
   - A toddler with a fracture of the left leg, treated in the emergency room, and then sent home
   - A school-aged child, now in rehabilitation, with burns on both arms
   - A 20-year-old hospitalized for injuries resulting from an automobile accident after drinking alcohol

2. During your home visit for a 16-year-old with cancer, she says, "I don't believe in God." What would you reply? Why would you respond this way?

3. During a clinic visit, a 2-month-old appears listless and constantly cries. The mother tells you that he has colic, so she has been diluting his formula with water. What would you do now?

● Practicing for NCLEX

1. Infections in the neonate are less likely in mothers who provided nutrition through which of the following?
   a. Breast milk
   b. Water
   c. Formula
   d. Solid food

2. At what point during the first year of life would you normally expect bonding to occur?
   a. At 6 months
   b. At 3 weeks
   c. Soon after birth
   d. Not until 12 months

3. Parents of hospitalized infants should be encouraged to stay with their child to help decrease what potential problem?
   a. Problems with attachment
   b. Separation anxiety
   c. Risk for injury
   d. Failure to thrive

4. The toddler has the cognitive development necessary to do which of the following?
   a. Use fingers to pick up small objects
   b. Have bladder control during the day
   c. Develop independence in feeding self
   d. Identify and name body parts

5. Based on Freud's theory, the preschool-aged child is in which stage?
   a. Phallic stage
   b. Anal stage
   c. Oral stage
   d. Latency stage

6. Which of the following best describes the moral and spiritual development of the school-aged child?
   a. Obeying rules to avoid punishment
   b. Valuing loyalty and social order
   c. Accepting the value system of others
   d. Faith involves reciprocal fairness

7. The ability to reproduce in the adolescent is defined as which of the following?
   a. Maturation
   b. Adulthood
   c. Puberty
   d. Latency

8. Which of the following is a primary developmental task of the adolescent?
   a. To succeed in school
   b. To achieve new and more mature relationships
   c. To develop athletic activities and skills
   d. To accept the decisions of parents

9. Which of the following nursing diagnoses should be considered for the obese adolescent?
   a. Risk for Injury
   b. Risk for Delayed Development
   c. Acute Confusion
   d. Disturbed Body Image

10. What is the leading cause of death in adolescents and young adults?
    a. Accidents
    b. Sexually transmitted diseases
    c. Substance abuse
    d. Unsound dieting

● Answers With Rationale

1. *a.* Breast milk contains antibodies, immunoglobulins, and leukocytes that provide protection against

infections. It has a high lactose content, promoting an acid environment that hinders bacterial growth.

2. *c.* Although bonding might occur later, it normally occurs during a sensitive period in the first few hours after birth.

3. *b.* Separation anxiety, with crying initially and then appearing depressed, is common during late infancy in infants who are hospitalized.

4. *d.* Both *a* and *b* are examples of physiologic development; *c* is an example of the development of autonomy. Toddlers can identify and name several body parts and are beginning to have a sense of gender identity.

5. *a.* Preschoolers, according to Freud, have a biologic focus that is primarily genital, with a sexual desire for the opposite-sex parent.

6. *d.* School-aged children view religious faith as involving reciprocal fairness and accept the importance of spiritual beliefs.

7. *c.* Puberty is defined by reproductive function in the adolescent.

8. *b.* Adolescence is a time to establish more mature relationships with both boys and girls of the same age.

9. *d.* Adolescents who are obese are at high risk for an altered body image.

10. *a.* Accidents are the leading cause of death in adolescents and young adults. They most often are the result of motor vehicle crashes and are frequently associated with an intake of alcohol or other drugs.

Taylor Suite Resources

The Taylor Suite offers these additional resources to enhance learning and facilitate understanding of this chapter:

- thePoint online resource, http://thepoint.lww.com/Taylor7E
- Student DVD-ROM included with the book
- Study Guide for Taylor's Fundamentals of Nursing

BIBLIOGRAPHY

Anbarghalami, R., Yang, L. T., Van Sell, S. L., & Miller-Anderson M. (2007). When to suspect child abuse. *RN, 70*(4), 34–39.

Barr-Anderson, D. J., van den Berg, P., Neumark-Sztainer, D., & Story, M. (2008). Characteristics associated with older adolescents who have a television in their bedrooms. *Pediatrics, 121*(4), 718–724.

Centers for Disease Control and Prevention (CDC). (2007a). Child maltreatment prevention scientific information: Definitions. Available at http://www.cdc.gov/ncipc/dvp/CMP/CMP-def.htm.

Centers for Disease Control and Prevention (CDC). (2007b, August 10). Revised recommendations of the Advisory Committee on Immunization Practices to vaccinate all persons aged 11–18 years with meningococcal conjugate vaccine. *MMWR, 56*(31), 794–795.

Centers for Disease Control and Prevention (CDC). (2008a). Healthy youth! Childhood obesity. Available at http://www.cdc.gov/HealthyYouth/obesity/

Centers for Disease Control and Prevention (CDC). (2008b). Healthy youth! Make a difference at your school. Available at http://www.cdc.gov/HealthyYouth/keystrategies/index.htm.

Centers for Disease Control and Prevention (CDC). (2008c). Healthy youth! Nutrition and the health of young people. Available at http://www.cdc.gov/HealthyYouth/nutrition/facts.htm.

Centers for Disease Control and Prevention (CDC). (2008d). Overweight and obesity: Childhood overweight. Available at http://www.cdc.gov/nccdphp/dnpa/obesity/childhood/index.htm.

Centers for Disease Control and Prevention (CDC). (2008e). Suicide: Facts at a glance. Available at http://cdc.gov/violenceprevention/pdf/Suicide-DataSheet-a.pdf.

Centers for Disease Control and Prevention (CDC). (2008f). Understanding child maltreatment: Factsheet. Available at http://cdc.gov/violenceprevention/pdf/CM-FactSheet-a.pdf.

Centers for Disease Control and Prevention (CDC). (2008g). Youth violence. Available at http://cdc.gov/injury.

Centers for Disease Control and Prevention (CDC). (2009a). Child maltreatment: Facts at a glance. Available at http://www.cdc.gov/violenceprevention/pdf/CM-DataSheet-a.pdf.

Centers for Disease Control and Prevention (CDC). (2009b). Youth violence national and state statistics at a glance. Available at http://www.cdc.gov/ViolencePrevention/youthviolence/stats_at-a_glance/index.html.

Clark, J. (2008). The danger next door: Methamphetamine. *RN, 71*(5), 22–27.

Child Welfare Information Gateway. (2009). Child abuse & neglect: Emotional abuse. Available at http://www.childwelfare.gov/can/types/emotionalabuse/

Curry, K. (2009). Adult immunizations: Growing needs, growing numbers. *Nursing Spectrum, 18*(15), 18–22.

Daniels, J. (2006). Obesity: America's epidemic. *American Journal of Nursing, 106*(1), 40–49.

Erikson, E. (1963). *Childhood and society.* New York: Norton.

Fraleigh, J. (2009). Vaccination: Compliance controversy. *RN, 72*(5), 36–40.

Getting high on household products. (2007). *Nursing, 37*(11), 66.

Governo, M., & Siewers, M. (2008). Childhood bullying. *Advance for Nurses, 10*(8), 31–33.

Gould, R. (1972). The phases of adult life: A study in developmental psychology. *American Psychiatry, 129,* 33–43.

Graham-Knight, D., & Karch, A. (2007). Pharm party: Prescription drug abuse among teens. *American Journal of Nursing, 107*(12), 79.

Kennedy, M. (2006). SIDS: More guidelines, more controversy. *American Journal of Nursing, 106*(1), 19.

Kennedy, M., & Jacobsen, J. (2009). Infant bed deaths are on the rise. *American Journal of Nursing, 109*(5), 17.

Klaus, M. H., & Kennell, J. H. (1982). *Parent–infant bonding.* St. Louis: C. V. Mosby.

Levinson, D., Darrow, C., Klein, E., Levinson, M., & McKee, B. (1978). *The seasons of a man's life.* New York: Knopf.

Martin, J., Hamilton, B., Sutton, P. D., Ventura, S. J., Menacker, F., Kirmeyer, S., & Mathews, T. J. (2009). Births: Final data for 2006. *National Vital Statistics Reports, 57*(7). Hyattsville, MD: National Center for Health Statistics.

Mennick, F. (2007). New warnings about over-the-counter cold medicines. *American Journal of Nursing, 107*(3), 22.

Michael, M., Helm, E., Van Graafeiland, B., Malinoski, F., & Bauman, J. (2009). Influenza vaccination with a live attenuated vaccine. *American Journal of Nursing, 109*(10), 44–48.

Murray, R., & Zentner, J. (2001). *Health promotion strategies through the life span* (7th ed.). Upper Saddle River, NJ: Prentice Hall.

National Institute of Child Health and Human Development (NICHD). National Institutes of Health. (2008). Sudden infant death syndrome (SIDS). Available at http://www.nichd.nih.gov/health/topics/Sudden_Infant_Death_Syndrome.cfm.

National Institute on Drug Abuse (NIDA). (2008). NIDA InfoFacts: Inhalants. Available at http://www.drugabuse.gov/Infofacts/Inhalants.html.

National Institute of Mental Health (NIMH). National Institutes of Health. (2009). What are eating disorders? Available at http://www.nimh.nih.gov/health/publications/eating-disorders/complete-index.shtml.

NANDA International. (2009). *Nursing diagnoses: Definitions & classification 2009–2011.* West Sussex, UK. Wiley-Blackwell.

Paoletti, J. (2007). Tipping the scales: What nurses need to know about the obesity epidemic. *RN, 70*(11), 35–41.

Pillitteri, A. (2009). *Maternal & child health nursing: Care of the childbearing & childrearing family* (6th ed.). Philadelphia: Lippincott Williams & Wilkins.

Potera, C. (2008). Teens, TV, and bad habits. *American Journal of Nursing, 108*(8), 20.

Rose, J. (2009). Childhood allergies. *RN, 72*(4), 30–35.

Thomas, A., Chess, S., & Birch, H. G. (1968). *Temperament and behavior discussed in children.* New York: New York University Press.

Toro, M. (2008). Combating infection: Closing in on chlamydia. *Nursing, 38*(9), 61.

U.S. Food and Drug Administration (FDA). (2008). FDA statement following CHPA's announcement on nonprescription over-the-counter cough and cold medicines in children. Available at http://www.fda.gov/NewsEvents/Newsroom/PressAnnouncements/2008/ucm116964.htm

Wilson, S., & Giddens, J. (2005). *Health assessment for nursing practice* (3rd ed.). St. Louis: Mosby.

Wong, D., Perry, S., Hockenberry, M., Lowdermilk, D., & Wilson, D. (2006). *Maternal child nursing* (3rd ed.). St. Louis: Mosby.

The Aging Adult

20

ETHEL PEABODY

Ethel, an 88-year-old single woman with beginning dementia who was treated for cardiac problems, is being discharged. She has no family and lives in a small two-story house with her three cats. There is some concern about her safety at home. She depends on a neighbor for some help and refuses to consider moving to a retirement community or extended-care facility.

ROSEMARY MASON

Rosemary, a 59-year-old woman who comes to the clinic with her 64-year-old husband, confides that she wishes that Viagra had never been discovered. "I was happier when we just cuddled at night. Now he wants to try all sorts of things, and I'm just not ready for this!"

LARRY JENKINS

Larry, a 67-year-old man with diabetes, states "Everything's gone downhill since I retired 5 months ago. The patient reports being "bored out of my mind" and drinking more alcohol simply because "there's nothing else to do!"

407

After completing the chapter, you will be able to accomplish the following:

1. Summarize the theories that describe how and why aging occurs.

2. Describe major physiologic, cognitive, psychosocial, moral, and spiritual developments and tasks of middle and older adulthood.

3. Describe common health problems of middle and older adults.

4. Discuss physiologic and functional changes that occur with aging.

5. Describe common myths and stereotypes that perpetuate ageism.

6. Describe nursing interventions to promote health for middle and older adults.

7. Identify the healthcare needs of older adults in terms of chronic illnesses, accidental injuries, and acute care needs.

KEY TERMS

ageism	life review
Alzheimer's disease	middle adult
cascade iatrogenesis	older adult
delirium	polypharmacy
dementia	reality orientation
functional health	reminiscence
gerontologic nursing	social isolation
gerontology	sundowning syndrome

Aging is a gradual process, characterized by continued development and maturation. The changes of aging begin as one enters middle adulthood. The onset and the effect of those changes throughout the middle and older adult years are influenced by numerous biologic, psychosocial, and environmental factors (described in the Theories of Aging section). The physiologic changes of aging, first experienced in middle adulthood, become more obvious in older adults. Continued development throughout one's adult life depends to a great extent on a person's sense of self-concept and prior ability to adapt. This chapter continues the discussion of growth and development from previous chapters, focusing on the aging years. For an example addressing the older adult, see the accompanying Reflective Practice box.

THEORIES OF AGING

As one ages, changes in cells, tissues, organs, and organ systems occur. Scientists do not fully understand why some people, even within the same family or environment, age much more rapidly than others. Although internal processes may in part determine aging, other factors, such as nutrition and the environment, may also play a role. Numerous theories describe how and why aging occurs, but none is universally accepted. These theories focus on a variety of factors, including genetic inheritance, cell metabolism and function, and the immune system.

Genetic Theory of Aging

The genetic theory of aging holds that life span depends to a great extent on genetic factors. Genes within the organism control "genetic clocks," which determine the occurrence and rate of metabolic processes, including cell division. According to the wear-and-tear theory, organisms wear out from increased metabolic functioning, and cells become exhausted from continual energy depletion from adapting to stressors (Eliopoulos, 2010).

Immunity Theory of Aging

The immunity theory of aging focuses on the functions of the immune system. This system, composed primarily of the bone marrow, thymus, spleen, and lymph nodes, seeks out and destroys foreign agents (such as viruses, bacteria, and perhaps cells undergoing neoplastic changes). The immune response declines steadily after younger adulthood as the thymus loses size and function. These age-associated changes in the immune system, also known as *immunosenescence*, are thought to be responsible for the increase in infections such as pneumonia and septicemia, immune disorders, and cancer as adults age (Chettle, 2009). Some authorities believe that nutrition plays an important role in maintaining the immune response; therefore, there is much interest in vitamin supplements (such as vitamin E) to improve immune function.

Cross-Linkage Theory

Cross-linkage is a chemical reaction that produces damage to the DNA and cell death. As one ages, cross-links accumulate, leading to essential molecules in the cell binding together and interfering with normal cell function.

Free Radical Theory

Free radicals, formed during cellular metabolism, are molecules with separated high-energy electrons, which can have adverse effects on adjacent molecules. Lipids, found in cell membranes, as well as proteins and cell organelles, are affected. Over time, irreversible damage results from the accumulated effects of this damage.

THE MIDDLE ADULT

The **middle adult** years are generally considered to be ages 40 to 65. This is a period of gradual and individualized

REFLECTIVE PRACTICE

Challenge to Ethical and Legal Skills

Mrs. Ethel Peabody is an 88-year-old single woman with beginning dementia hospitalized for cardiac problems. She has no family and her only visitor is a neighbor. She lives alone in a small two-story home with her three cats.

When the doctor ordered her discharge, I had grave worries about her ability to live safely on her own. When I asked her if she had ever thought about moving to a nursing home or retirement community, she said, "I'd rather die than go to one of those places!" When I told her I was worried about her safety, she told me her cats would take care of her! When I repeated this conversation to the charge nurse, she said, "There is nothing we can do if the patient isn't willing to explore other options."

Thinking Outside the Box: Possible Courses of Action

- Feel satisfied that I had reported my concerns to the charge nurse and let whatever happens happen
- Explore hospital and other resources to determine realistic options for someone like Mrs. Peabody and the obligations of caregivers and the hospital

- Find my instructor and seek her counsel
- Seek out the unit's social worker, confide my worries, and see if she has other recommendations

Evaluating a Good Outcome: How Do I Define Success?

- Both Mrs. Peabody's safety and ability to make decisions (autonomy) are respected.
- I feel at peace with the decision that was made for the patient and the role I played in this decision.

- My personal and professional integrity are intact.
- My legal responsibilities and those of the institution are met.

Personal Learning: Here's to the Future!

Sadly, I must confess that I was invited to accompany another patient for a diagnostic study off the unit, so I never followed through on my concerns. Mrs. Peabody was discharged to her home, and I never learned what happened to her. However, I was troubled by my inaction and discussed this situation with my instructor. As a result, I am now aware of more options available that I can use when faced with similar situations in the future.

The number of older adults will continue to grow, presenting many similar challenges in the future. I want to make sure I'm prepared for my next "Mrs. Peabody." Meanwhile, I will be talking with our patient-relations person, the social worker, hospital risk manager, and our office on aging to increase my knowledge of support services for older adults.

Reflection

How do you think you would respond in a similar situation? Why? What does this tell you about yourself and about the adequacy of your skills for professional practice? Can you think of other ways to respond? What could the nursing student have done differently? Imagine if the nursing student was a young adult. Do you think that the developmental stage would affect the student's action? What if the nursing student were a middle adult? How might this affect what was or was not done? What other skills (cognitive, interpersonal, technical, ethical/legal) would you need to respond well in this situation? What skills would be of particular importance when dealing with the charge nurse? Do you agree with the criteria to evaluate a successful outcome? What other criteria would you include and why?

---

change in both physical and psychosocial dimensions. As the average life span increases, most people in this age group still consider themselves young compared with the older population. Visible signs of aging and a heightened awareness of the time left to live, however, lead middle adults to evaluate their achievement of goals and influence their adaptation to older age.

Physiologic Development

In the early years of this period of life, physical functions are usually still effective. As time passes, gradual internal and external physiologic changes occur. These are not pathologic changes, but normal changes that result from aging. The

person must modify his or her self-image and self-concept to adapt successfully to and to accept these normal changes. Physical changes of the middle adult are outlined in Box 20-1.

The hormonal changes that take place in midlife affect men and women differently. Women undergo menopause, a gradual decrease in ovarian function, with subsequent depletion of estrogen and progesterone. This change usually occurs between 40 and 55 years of age. With the cessation of ovulation, menstrual periods stop either gradually or abruptly, and many women experience hot flashes, mood swings, and fatigue. The loss of estrogen also increases the risk for osteoporosis and heart disease. The process can last for several years, and afterward, the woman can no longer become pregnant. Men do not experience physical symptoms

Box 20-1 PHYSICAL CHANGES IN THE MIDDLE ADULT

- Fatty tissue is redistributed; men tend to develop abdominal fat, women thicken through the middle.
- The skin is drier.
- Wrinkle lines appear on the face.
- Gray hair appears, and men may lose hair on the head.
- Cardiac output begins to decrease.
- Muscle mass, strength, and agility gradually decrease.
- There is a loss of calcium from bones, especially in perimenopausal women.
- Fatigue increases.
- Visual acuity diminishes, especially for near vision (presbyopia).
- Hearing acuity diminishes, especially for high-pitched sounds.
- Hormone production decreases, resulting in menopause or andropause.

from the decreased levels of hormones, called andropause. Androgen levels diminish slowly; the man may have some loss of sexual potency but is still capable of reproduction.

> *Remember Rosemary Mason, the 59-year-old woman described at the beginning of the chapter. The nurse could incorporate information about the differences in hormonal changes for men and women into a teaching plan to help Rosemary understand and adjust to the changes that are occurring.* ■

Cognitive Development

Cognitive and intellectual abilities of middle adults change little from young adulthood. There often is increased motivation to learn, especially if the knowledge gained can be applied immediately and has personal relevance. Problem-solving abilities remain throughout adulthood, although response time may be slightly longer. This is due not to any decreased ability but, rather, to a longer search through more memories and to a desire to think a problem through before responding.

Psychosocial Development

The middle adult years often are a time of increased personal freedom, economic stability, and social relationships (Fig. 20-1). This is also a time of increased responsibility and an awareness of one's own mortality. One realizes that one's life may be half or more past and may feel many things are still undone. This realization can lead to a developmental crisis and situational stressors. Several theorists describe developmental tasks of middle adulthood, as follows.

Erikson's Theory

According to Erikson's theory (1963), the middle adult is in a period of generativity versus stagnation. The tasks are to establish and guide the next generation, accept middle-age changes, adjust to the needs of aging parents, and reevaluate one's goals and accomplishments. Adults who do not achieve these tasks tend to focus on themselves, becoming overly concerned with their own physical and emotional health needs.

Havighurst's Theory

The developmental tasks of the middle adult described by Havighurst (1972) are learned behaviors arising from maturation, personal motives and values, and civic responsibility. To successfully master this developmental stage, the middle adult must accept and adjust to physical changes, maintain a satisfactory occupation, assist children to become responsible adults, adjust to aging parents, and relate to one's spouse or partner as a person.

Levinson's Theory

Levinson (Levinson, Darrow, Klein, Levinson, & McKee, 1978) theorized that the middle adult may choose either to continue an established lifestyle or to reorganize one's life in a period of midlife transition.

Gould's Theory

Gould (1972) viewed the middle years as a time when adults look inward (ages 35 to 43); accept their life span as having definite boundaries, and have a special interest in spouse, friends, and community (ages 43 to 50); and increase their feelings of self-satisfaction, value spouse as a companion, and become more concerned with health (ages 50 to 60).

Adjusting to the Changes of Middle Adulthood

Various changes can take place during the middle years. These changes include changes in employment, relationships with a spouse, relationships with children who are becoming adults, and relationships with aging parents. Midlife transition might occur in both men and women in their 40s. Although one does not feel that one is aging, realizing that others consider you older can be stressful.

Employment

Middle-aged adults might experience changes in employment. They may opt for a career change and return to school to obtain new knowledge and skills. These changes are often based on a need to have increased job satisfaction or to satisfy a life-long goal. Women who have been immersed in a career may decide to have children and either become "stay at home moms" or reduce their workload. Increasing numbers of middle-aged adults are self-employed, often working from home.

As the 50s approach, questions about retirement and economic security become more prevalent, with an increased interest in the benefits of financial and retirement plans.

FIGURE 20-1. The middle adult years are characterized by greater expendable wealth, renewed relationship with one's spouse, and expanded social relationships and family roles.

These concerns can be heightened by overall economic conditions. For example, the economic turmoil that occurred in 2008 led many people who had planned on an early retirement to decide to continue their active employment status. The security of retirement investments and income is critical to ensure that individuals remain financially stable and that workers receive the pensions they are working toward or have already achieved.

Spousal Relationships

Relationships with one's spouse may change. Although for many this is a time of greater security and stability, with stronger emotional commitment and sharing, for some it is a time of disenchantment. A husband or wife may develop negative or critical feelings and attitudes as a result of changes in physical appearance, energy levels, or sexual needs and abilities.

> ➤ *Recall Rosemary Mason, the 59-year-old woman, voicing displeasure with her husband's desire to "try all sorts of things" sexually. The nurse could use this information about spousal relationships as a means to gather additional assessment data about the couple's relationship before Viagra was started. This would help develop an appropriate plan of care that addresses Rosemary's current displeasure.* ■

Dissatisfaction with not achieving career or family goals contributes to the stresses placed on the marriage. Extramarital affairs and divorce may result.

Widowhood is more likely to occur in the middle adult years. The loss of a spouse is a major crisis and a threat to one's self-concept, as well as a major role change. A multitude of changes may occur, including a reduced income, changes in lifestyle and social relationships, and the need for help to work through the loss and grief (see Chapter 43).

Relationships With Children and Aging Family Members

Middle-aged adults may be caught in a "generation sandwich." Their children are often independent and married, with children of their own. Although much has been written about the "empty-nest syndrome" that occurs when the last child leaves home, most middle-aged parents welcome the increased space, time, and independence they have when active parenting ceases. As their involvement with and responsibility for children decrease, they may have an increased need to help care for aging parents and other family members. The physical aging or death of a parent makes one's own aging and inevitable death a reality.

Moral Development

According to Kohlberg (1969), a middle adult may either remain at the conventional level or move to the postconventional level of moral development, especially if he or she has had sustained responsibility for the welfare of others and has consistently applied ethical principles developed in adolescence. At this level, the adult believes that the rights of others take precedence and takes steps to support those rights.

Spiritual Development

As with moral development, not all adults progress to Fowler's (1991) paradoxical–consolidative state of spiritual development. Fowler believed that only some people reach this stage and only after 30 years of age. Most middle adults are less rigid in their beliefs and have increased faith in a supreme being as well as trust in spiritual strength.

Health of the Middle Adult

Middle adults are subject to physical and emotional health problems associated with lifestyle behaviors, developmental or situational crises, family history, and the environment. Both acute and chronic illnesses are more likely to occur, and recovery takes longer. This is a result of slower and more prolonged responses to stressors, more pronounced reactions to an illness, and the possibility of more than one illness being present at a time.

The leading causes of death in the middle adult years, according to 2006 statistics, are malignant neoplasms; cardiovascular disease; unintentional injury including poisoning, motor vehicle accidents, and falls; diabetes mellitus; and cerebrovascular causes (Centers for Disease Control and Prevention [CDC], 2009). Other major health problems include rheumatoid arthritis, obesity, alcoholism, and depression.

The risk for these common health problems often depends on a combination of lifestyle factors and aging. As one gets older, energy requirements decrease. Middle adults tend to maintain previous eating patterns and caloric intake while being less physically active. This trend can result in obesity and atherosclerosis, with an increased risk for high blood pressure, coronary artery disease, renal failure, and diabetes. Additionally, smoking and alcohol consumption put the person at greater risk for cancer, chronic respiratory diseases, and liver disease.

Chronic illness in middle adults has a major effect on self-concept and may precipitate changes in life structure. For example, after a serious heart attack, a man may face changes in his family role, his earning capacity, and his social relationships. Such changes usually cause great stress.

Middle age does not automatically result in physical or emotional health problems. Many men and women remain healthy throughout their lives, but knowing preventive health-care practices and their special needs at this age can help middle adults have improved quality and quantity of life.

Role of the Nurse in Promoting Health and Preventing Illness

The nurse has a major role in promoting health and preventing illness in middle adults by teaching, serving as a role

Examples of NANDA Nursing Diagnoses
The Middle Adult

Nursing Diagnoses	Possible Related Factor
Risk for Imbalanced Nutrition: More Than Body Requirements	High calorie diet and sedentary lifestyle
Constipation	Diet low in fiber and lack of exercise
Risk for Impaired Skin Integrity	Lifetime of sun exposure
Sexual Dysfunction	Alcohol abuse
Caregiver Role Strain	Long-term care of aging parents
Ineffective Denial	Continued smoking despite family history of lung cancer
Fear	Diagnosis of breast cancer
Sedentary Lifestyle	Lack of resources (time, money, facilities)
Stress Overload	Chronic illness
Insomnia	Intake of alcohol or stimulants
Risk Prone Health Behavior	Inadequate comprehension

model, and encouraging self-care responsibilities. See Examples of NANDA Nursing Diagnoses: The Middle Adult.

Health-related screenings, examinations, and immunizations for adults are outlined in Table 20-1. Additionally, the following health-promotion activities are recommended:

- Eat a diet low in fat and cholesterol, including fruits, vegetables, and fiber, and use sugar, salt, and sodium in moderation.
- Make regular exercise a part of life.
- Drink alcohol in moderation, if at all.
- Do not smoke.

The middle adult needs to know the dangers of substance abuse. Referrals to support groups and individual counseling may be necessary to strengthen a middle adult's coping mechanisms and promote acceptance of personal and family changes. Having successfully met developmental tasks, the middle adult is ready to enjoy the rest of life. A sense of continuity and adaptability from the early 20s through the 50s is essential to meeting the developmental tasks of aging satisfactorily and to enjoying one's remaining years.

THE OLDER ADULT

Society has arbitrarily labeled the **older adult** as one older than 65 years of age. The older adult period is often further divided into the young-old (ages 60 to 74 years), the middle-old (ages 75 to 84 years), and the old-old (ages 85 years and older).

American society is aging—dramatically, rapidly, and largely well. With birthrates down and baby boomers approaching retirement, we are on the threshold of the first-ever "mass geriatric society." In 2004, life expectancy at birth for the total population increased to 77.8 years from an expectancy of 75.4 years in 1990. Between 1990 and 2004, the life expectancy at birth has increased more for the black population than the white population, thus narrowing the gap between the two groups from 7.0 years to 5.2 years (National Center for Health Statistics, 2007). In 2002, there were more than 35 million older Americans, with the number estimated to more than double to about 71.5 million by 2030 (Federal Interagency Forum on Aging-Related Statistics, 2008). By 2030, people ages 65 and older are predicted to comprise 20% of the population (as compared to 12.4% in 2000). After 2030, as the Baby Boomer group ages, the number of people age 85 and older is expected to increase from 5.3 million in 2006 to approximately 21 million by 2050. Also in 2050, according to the U.S. Department of Health and Human Services (USDHHS), for the first time in history, the population of Americans over 60 years old will be larger than the population of children 0 to 14 years of age (USDHHS, 2008b).

TABLE • 20-1	GUIDELINES FOR HEALTH-RELATED SCREENINGS, EXAMINATIONS, AND IMMUNIZATIONS FOR THE AGING ADULT
Health-related Area	**Recommendations**
Physical examination	• Every 3 years to age 40 • Every year from age 40
Breast cancer (women)	• Breast self-examination each month • Breast clinical examination every 3 years to age 40, then every year • Mammogram every year beginning age 40
Cervical cancer (women)	• Pelvic examination with Papanicolaou (Pap) exam at least every 3 years • Women who have had a total hysterectomy (removal of the uterus and cervix) do not need cervical cancer screening, unless the surgery was for cervical precancer or cancer. • Women over age 65 to 70 with at least 3 normal Pap tests and no abnormal Pap tests in the last 10 years should consult with their healthcare provider about continuing cervical cancer screening.

Prostate (men, beginning age 50)	• Prostate-specific antigen (PSA) test every year
	• Digital rectal examination (DRE) every year
	  • Begin at age 45 if African American or a family history of prostate cancer.
	  • Screening is individualized based on healthcare provider and individual's concerns.

Testicular cancer (men) Colorectal cancer (men and women, beginning age 50)	• Testicular self-examination every month • Fecal occult blood test every year • Digital rectal examination (DRE) every year • Flexible sigmoidoscopy every 3–5 years, OR • Colonoscopy with follow-up every 3–5 years depending on size of polyps
Skin cancer (men and women)	• Self-examination every month • Clinical skin examination every year
Oral cancer (men and women)	• Every year as part of medical or dental checkups
Bone density	• Those at risk: postmenopausal women, maternal history of hip fracture, fracture after age 50, tall height at age 25
Vision	• Eye examination, with a test for glaucoma, every year
Immunizations	• Tetanus, diphtheria (Td): 1-dose booster every 10 years • Influenza: 1 dose every year • Pneumococcal polysaccharide vaccine (PPV): 1 dose every year up to age 64 for those with medical indications; 1 dose for those unvaccinated by age 65, or who received the first dose more than 5 years previously (before age 65) • Zoster vaccine, live (Zostavax): Recommended for adults 60 years and older to prevent herpes zoster (shingles)

In 2006, women comprised approximately 60% of the population over age 65 and the proportion of females to males increases to 213 females to every 100 males by age 85. The proportion of older people is higher in whites than in minority populations, although the number of minority older adults is projected to increase from 16% in 2010 to 23% of the elderly population by 2020 (USDHHS, 2010).

A Unique Population

The older adult population is the most unique group in today's society because its members have lived the longest and have participated in and adapted to complex societal changes. Within the life span of many older adults, society developed from a rural agricultural culture through industri-

alization to a service-oriented, high-technology culture. In the early 1900s, a 20-mile trip meant an all-day undertaking in a horse-drawn wagon; today, a person can fly across the continent in less time and with considerably less effort. Lighting has progressed from kerosene and gas lamps to electricity. Information that once took weeks or months to be received now is instantaneous. Most older adults have lived through the trauma of world wars. Many had parents with strong ethnic ties to another country, and many were immigrants themselves. Older adults have lived through the Great Depression of the 1930s and developed self-sufficiency.

Further adaptations become necessary with advancing age because of physical or cognitive limitations, retirement, loss of a spouse or family members, or changing income. Older adults face numerous role changes related to their age or health status. Lost roles must be replaced with new roles and activities that are acceptable and satisfying to the person.

➤ *Recall Larry Jenkins, the 67-year-old complaining of his life going downhill since he retired. The nurse could incorporate knowledge of role changes to develop an appropriate plan of care for the patient that fosters adjustment to his role changes.* ■

Older people are thus living in a world that requires them to change and to adapt. Senior years are a time to reach one's potential and to satisfy long-range goals that may have been delayed because of other responsibilities. It can also be a time for older adults to turn over to others tasks, such as career or community leadership. Research has shown that most older adults do adjust and adapt to new roles, and most are satisfied with their lives and with what they have. Depending on the older adult's adaptability and supportive resources, older adulthood may be a time of happiness, peace, and understanding or of sorrow, conflict, and confusion.

Ageism and Common Stereotypes

Sometimes, older adults are a victim of ageism. **Ageism** is a form of prejudice, like racism, in which older adults are stereotyped by characteristics found in only a few members of their group. Fundamental to ageism is the view that older people are different and will remain different; therefore, they do not experience the same desires, needs, and concerns. Our industrial technologic world places a high priority on productivity, and some may think that retired people have "outlived their usefulness."

➤ *Think back to Larry Jenkins, the 67-year-old retiree. The nurse could incorporate knowledge of ageism as a basis for obtaining additional assessment data, examining possible factors contributing to the patient's feelings of boredom and uselessness.* ■

As well, younger generations often have lost ties to the older generation because of increased mobility of the family, and thus, many young adults lack experiences with older relatives and their friends.

Older people may be incorrectly depicted as being rigid or narrow-minded, unable to learn, unreliable because of memory loss, too old to enjoy sexual pleasure, or child-like and dependent. Many people fear advancing age because of pervasive views that older people are poor, lonely, in frail health, and headed for institutionalization in a nursing home. These descriptors are not true for most older adults (Fig. 20-2). Common myths are compared with the realities in Table 20-2.

Most older adults are satisfied with their lives, finding retirement and old age more enjoyable than they had anticipated. Three fourths live in their own homes, and one third of these live alone. Most older adults maintain close ties with their families and have incomes above the poverty level (Eliopoulos, 2010).

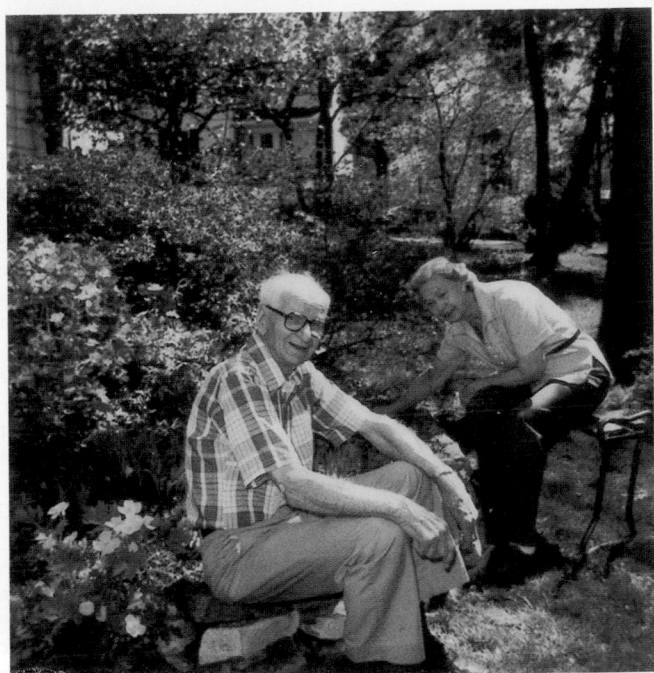

FIGURE 20-2. This couple, married 61 years, enjoys gardening together. They've found that they can continue most activities with only minor adjustments.

Physiologic Development

In older adults, all organ systems undergo some degree of decline in overall functioning, and the body becomes less efficient. Normal physiologic changes in structure and function of the body with aging are outlined in Box 20-2. Body functions that require integrated activity of several organ systems are affected the most. For example, aging of the cardiac muscles causes fluid retention in both peripheral tissues and the lungs, causing swelling of the legs and making breathing more difficult. The most commonly encountered chronic disorders are cardiovascular diseases, such as hypertension and strokes, and men have higher levels of heart disease than women (Federal Interagency Forum on Aging-Related Statistics, 2008).

➤ *Recall Ethel Peabody, the 88-year-old woman with dementia and cardiac problems. Knowledge of physiologic changes associated with aging could help with developing an appropriate plan of care for this patient after discharge.* ■

Most older adults regard themselves as healthy and deny they experience severe limitations in activities. Most are never institutionalized nor do they suffer the effects of senility. Being healthy, however, does not necessarily mean without disease. More than four of five older adults suffer from at least one chronic illness. Like younger adults, they define their health in relation to how well they function. Functional health includes a person's ability to remain self-reliant, to "make do," and to maintain a sense of control and independence over self and environment. There is a trend in health-care today toward fostering increasing independence and

TABLE • 20-2 MYTHS AND REALITIES ABOUT OLDER ADULTS	
Myth	**Reality**
Old age begins at 65 years of age.	Defining 65 years of age as "old age" happened arbitrarily when 65 years of age was set for Social Security payments in the 1930s, based on the labor market and the economy of that time.
Most older adults live in nursing homes.	Only about 7% of older adults live in nursing homes. Most older adults own their own homes; 30% live alone, 54% live with spouses, and the rest live with family or friends.
Most older adults are sick.	Fully 65% of all older adults rate their health as good or excellent.
Old age means mental deterioration.	Although response time may be prolonged from a longer processing time, neither intelligence nor personality normally decreases because of aging.
Older adults are not interested in sex.	Although sexual activity may be less frequent, the ability to perform and enjoy sexual activity lasts well into the 90s in healthy older adults.
Older adults don't care how they look.	Older adults want to be attractive to others.
Most older adults are isolated and lonely.	Loneliness results from death of loved ones or other losses, just as it does for people of all ages. Many older adults are active in social and community activities.
Bladder problems are a problem of aging.	Incontinence is not a part of aging; it requires medical attention.
Older adults do not deserve aggressive treatment for serious illnesses.	Older adults deserve aggressive treatment if they want aggressive treatment.

self-care in older adults. Those who live alone are at greatest risk for loss of independence and increased need for assisted living or long-term care.

> ➤ *Remember Ethel Peabody, the woman described in the Reflective Practice box. The nurse can apply knowledge about functional health to determine the patient's needs for safety and independence while, at the same time, fostering the patient's view of herself.* ■

There is growing evidence that aging is not synonymous with loss of function and disability. At least 80% of older adults have at least one chronic disorder, and 60% of this age group have at least two; yet their ability to adapt determines whether they are ill or healthy (CDC, 2007). Most continue their activities from middle age and adapt intuitively to the gradual limitations of aging, although it may take longer to complete an activity or the activity may need to be modified. For example, an older adult with arthritis may need to use an electric can opener rather than a manual one, or a person with heart disease may need 3 hours to garden, resting several times, rather than the former 1 hour.

The greatest threat to the health of older adults is loss of the physiologic reserve of the various organ systems. When illness occurs, increased physical and emotional stress places an older adult at risk for complex reactions. An older adult is more likely to develop complications and to recover more slowly (Fig. 20-3). For instance, an older patient with a hip fracture is at high risk for pneumonia and skin break-

down because of immobility, a decreased ability to expel pulmonary secretions, and thinner, more fragile skin.

Cognitive Development

The term *cognition* indicates cerebral functioning, including the ability to perceive and understand one's world. Cognition does not change appreciably with aging. In fact, intelligence increases into the 60s, and learning continues through life. It is normal for an older adult to take longer to respond and react, however, particularly in new or unfamiliar surroundings. Knowing this, the nurse should slow the pace of care and allow

FIGURE 20-3. The hospitalized older adult requires nursing interventions to prevent complications. (*Photo © Kathy Sloane.*)

Box 20-2   NORMAL PHYSIOLOGIC CHANGES OF OLDER ADULTS

General Status

- Progressively decreasing efficiency of physiologic processes results in a fragile balance and hinders the body's ability to maintain homeostasis.
- Physical or emotional stressors cause the older adult to be more vulnerable because of decreased physiologic reserves.
- The older adult may continue to engage in all activities of middle age but intuitively adjusts to a modified pace and more frequent rest periods.

Integument

- Wrinkling and sagging of skin occur with decreased skin elasticity; dryness and scaling are common.
- Balding becomes common in men, and women also experience thinning of hair; hair loses pigmentation.
- Skin pigmentation and moles are common, although the skin may become pale because of loss of melanocytes.
- Nails typically thicken, becoming brittle and yellowed.

Musculoskeletal

- Decreases in subcutaneous tissue and weight commonly are found in the old-old.
- Muscle mass and strength decrease.
- Bone demineralization occurs, and bones become porous and brittle. Fracture is more common.
- Joints tend to stiffen and lose flexibility, and range of motion may decrease.
- Overall mobility commonly slows, and posture tends to stoop. Height decreases slightly.

Neurologic

- The central nervous system responds more slowly to multiple stimuli. Hence, the cognitive and behavioral response of the older adult may be delayed.
- Rate of reflex response decreases.
- Temperature regulation and pain/pressure perception become less efficient.
- There may be a loss of sensation in the extremities.
- The older adult may also experience difficulty with balance, coordination, fine movements, and spatial orientation, resulting in an increased risk for falls.
- Sleep at night typically shortens, and the older adult may awaken more easily. Catnaps become common.

Special Senses

- Diminished visual acuity (presbyopia) occurs, with increased sensitivity to glare, decreased ability to adjust to darkness, decreased accommodation, decreased depth perception, and decreased color discrimination. Cataracts may further obscure vision. Difficulty reading small print might result. Daytime or night driving might be compromised.
- Diminished hearing acuity (presbyacusis) occurs, particularly diminished pitch discrimination in the presence of environmental noises. As a result of hearing problems, the older adult may withdraw from social events.
- The senses of taste and smell are decreased. Sensitivity to odors might be reduced. Problems with nutrition may result.

Cardiopulmonary

- Blood vessels become less elastic and often rigid and tortuous. Venous return becomes less efficient. Fatty plaque deposits continue to occur in the linings of the blood vessels. Lower-extremity edema and cooling may occur, particularly with decreased mobility. Peripheral pulses are not always palpable.
- The body is less able to increase heart rate and cardiac output with activity.
- Pulmonary elasticity and ciliary action decrease, so that clearing of the lungs becomes less efficient. Respiratory rate may increase, accompanied by diminished depth.

Gastrointestinal

- Digestive juices continue to diminish, and nutrient absorption decreases.
- Malnutrition and anemia become more common.
- With reduced muscle tone and decreased peristalsis, constipation and indigestion are common complaints.

Dentition

- Tooth decay and loss continue for most older adults.
- Eating habits may change, particularly if the older adult lacks teeth or has ill-fitting dentures.

Genitourinary

- Blood flow to the kidneys decreases with diminished cardiac output.
- The number of functioning nephron units decreases by 50%; waste products may be filtered and excreted more slowly.
- Fluids and electrolytes remain within normal ranges, but the balance is fragile.
- Bladder capacity decreases by 50%. Voiding becomes more frequent; two or three times a night is usual. A decrease in bladder and sphincter muscle control may result in stress incontinence or incomplete bladder emptying.
- About 75% of men over 65 years of age experience hypertrophy of the prostate gland; surgery may be required if urinary retention occurs.
- There is atrophy, decrease of secretions, and thinning of the older woman's genital tract.

older patients extra time to ask questions or complete activities. Mild short-term (recent) memory loss is common but can be remedied by an older adult using notes, schedules, and calendars. Long-term memory usually remains intact. Dementia, Alzheimer's disease, depression, and delirium might occur and cause cognitive impairment. These conditions are discussed later in relation to health of the older adult.

Psychosocial Development

Most theorists agree that a person's self-concept is relatively stable throughout adult life. An older adult who has a strong sense of self-identity and has successfully met challenges earlier in life will probably continue to do so. This person substitutes new roles for old roles and perhaps continues former roles in a new context. For example, a business manager after retirement may continue to use his or her leadership talents in community or volunteer organizations. Older adults with a strong self-concept typically describe themselves as being healthier than others or "young for my years." On the other hand, events that may accompany aging can threaten a person's self-concept. Depending on the person's outlook on life and past ability to cope, events such as retirement, loss of health or income, and isolation can be devastating. For example, a retired teacher whose sense of identity was closely tied to career may suddenly find that he or she has lost friends, income, and sense of accomplishment and may consequently feel a great loss of control and self-identity.

Disengagement Theory

An early psychosocial theory, called the disengagement theory, maintained that older adults often withdraw from usual roles and become more introspective and self-focused. This withdrawal was theorized as intrinsic and inevitable, necessary for successful aging, and beneficial for both the person and for society.

Later studies have shown that isolation is not desired or acceptable and that as societal interactions decrease, healthy older adults increase their close relationships with family and friends. According to the activity theory, successful aging involves the ability to maintain high levels of activity and functioning. An older adult may substitute activities but does not slow down or disengage from society. The identity-continuity theory assumes that healthy aging is related to the older adult's ability to continue similar patterns of behavior from young and middle adulthood.

Erikson's Theory

Erikson (1963) identified ego integrity versus despair and disgust as the last stage of human development, which begins at about 60 years of age. Older adults continue to look forward but now also look back and begin to reflect on their life. It is a time for realization of a "wholeness" perspective, with an inner search for meaning and order in the life cycle. Older adults search for emotional integration and acceptance of the past and present, as well as acceptance of physiologic decline without fear of death. Older adults often like to tell stories of past events. This phenomenon is called **life review** or **reminiscence** and has been identified worldwide. In a sense, this is a way for an older adult to relive and restructure life experiences and is part of achieving ego integrity (Fig. 20-4). Nurses can also use reminiscence as a therapy to facilitate adaptation to present circumstances.

> *Think back to Larry Jenkins, the 67-year-old male described at the beginning of the chapter. The nurse could use life review to foster the patient's ego integrity.* ∎

Ego integrity is facilitated when an older adult has successfully accomplished tasks earlier in life. Older adulthood can be a time for the person to look backward with pride and without regrets and forward with optimism and enthusiasm. A person who regrets the past and sees current problems as insurmountable, however, may despair. This person may view life as a series of unresolved problems and missed opportunities and feel worthless or hopeless. The despairing person may want to do things over but fears the lack of time before death.

The tasks of midlife continue or may resurface. Older adults still strive to guide the coming generations and to

FIGURE 20-4. Reminiscing is a culturally universal phenomenon of aging. It is a way for the older adult to reassess life experiences and further develop a sense of accomplishment, fulfillment, and reward in life.

leave something behind (generativity versus stagnation). Their need for love and closeness continues (intimacy versus isolation), as does a strong sense of who one is in relation to family and community (identity versus role diffusion). Because of physical and social changes associated with aging, older adults are repeatedly faced with the need to adapt and to again face already completed tasks.

Havighurst's Theory

According to Havighurst (1972), the major tasks of old age are primarily concerned with the maintenance of social contacts and relationships. Successful aging depends on a person's ability to be flexible and adapt to new age-related roles. The person must find new and meaningful roles in old age while being reasonably comfortable with the social customs of the times.

Adjusting to the Changes of Older Adulthood

Older adults use their years of experience as a guide to adjusting to the changes that come with increasing age. These changes, based on Havighurst's tasks for later life, involve many areas of life, as described in the following sections.

Physical Strength and Health

Most older adults gradually modify their lifestyle to accommodate for declining strength and health. They rest more frequently, although continued activity and exercise are important for maintaining all physiologic functions. The potential with this age group for sleep disorders accompanied by daytime sleepiness contributes to slower response time, impaired memory, as well as behavior that may be mistaken for some form of cognitive impairment (Gerber, 2009). An older adult is at high risk for accidents and falls and may need to curtail driving or use a cane or other aid to remain mobile. Diet modifications and prescribed medications may be necessary, and because of chronic illness, an older adult may need to adjust to living with some pain. Pain should not be assumed to be a normal consequence of aging, but it is often experienced by older adults. Attitudes toward treating pain in this population may interfere with optimum pain relief (D'Arcy, 2009). With severe illness, loss of independence can occur. The loss of health is difficult to adjust to because it affects every aspect of life.

Retirement and Reduced Income

Retirement brings a change in a person's concept of time. Older adults must learn to occupy their leisure time in ways that maintain their self-esteem while being personally satisfying. Satisfaction with retirement is closely tied to income and the relationships one has outside of work. Many older adults have adequate retirement income, but a lack of adequate income can affect an older adult's ability to meet his or her needs, such as for medical care and housing or social and creative interests.

The Health of One's Spouse

When one's spouse becomes ill, numerous and difficult adjustments must be made. An older adult may face new roles for the first time. A husband may begin to cook meals; a wife may learn to handle family finances. These role changes come at a time when stress is already high. Giving physical care can be an overwhelming task if the other spouse is also frail or in poor health. Adaptations may be needed in living conditions and lifestyle, and the spouse may need to plan social and recreational events alone.

The need for love and belonging does not diminish with age and may become acute with the loss of one's spouse through illness or institutionalization. Humans are sexual beings, and sexual behavior does not necessarily stop in old age. Sexuality is part of who we are, and older adults are no exception. Like younger adults, older adults need to express their intimacy physically by touching and sexual activity and emotionally by sharing joys, sorrows, ideas, and values (Fig. 20-5).

Relating to One's Age Group

With an aging population, social organizations for older adults are becoming more numerous. For example, most communities have senior citizens' centers that offer meals, social and informational programs, and other activities for a

FIGURE 20-5. Stereotypical images of the older adult as narrow-minded, forgetful, sexless, and dependent are untrue for most of the older adult population. This couple exhibits the vitality, sensuality, joy, and playfulness of a young couple.

nominal fee. Other organizations offer opportunities for travel, cultural events, and political involvement. Affiliation with others of the same age allows older adults to share common interests and concerns and to find status among their peers. It should not be assumed, however, that older adults want to associate only with others their age (Fig. 20-6).

Social Roles

Social roles change with the developmental tasks and adjustments of older adulthood, but the need to feel valued, useful, and productive continues. An older adult may develop new hobbies or increase his or her involvement in community, church, or family affairs. He or she may do volunteer work or even begin a new career. If an older adult cannot adjust and form new relationships, social isolation can become a problem. **Social isolation** is a sense of being alone and lonely as a result of having fewer meaningful relationships. It may occur because of declining health or income, transportation problems, or ageism. Whatever the cause, prolonged social isolation has been associated with declining health and higher mortality rates.

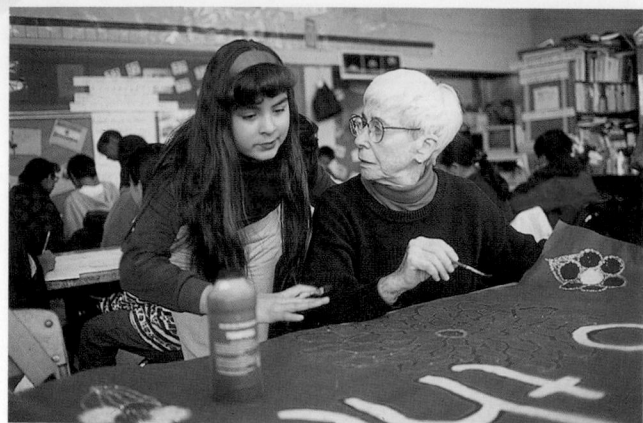

FIGURE 20-6. Social relationships and satisfying leisure activities remain important throughout life. This older adult volunteers in art class with 6th-grade Asian and Latina girls. *(Photo © Kathy Sloane.)*

Living Arrangements

Various types of housing options for older adults are outlined in Table 20-3. The ability to function safely and independently at home depends a great deal on one's functional health, transportation, income, and family. An older adult, for example, may need assistance with home repairs, house cleaning, or grocery shopping. Architectural barriers, such as steps, may need to be modified. Easy access to medical and recreational facilities and churches may become more important. Many older adults in poor health can continue living at home with some assistance from visiting nurses or with the aid of other services, such as home-delivered meals and senior transportation. Assisted-living housing is becoming more common, providing such requirements as meals, healthcare services, and housekeeping services.

Most older adults prefer to live in their own home and find it difficult to move. Moving in with adult children creates changes in roles and authority. If the older adult is chronically ill or cognitively impaired, the family caregivers face the need for daily caregiving, lack of freedom, and emotional stress. When one moves to an extended-care facility, such as a nursing home, the loss of one's home and possessions and the need to conform to the routines of institutional living can be traumatic for the person and family. Some people, however, choose to move for convenience, social relationships, or needed healthcare.

Additional options for older adults include quality patient-centered programs with a focus on providing long-term care to older adults who want to remain in the community. Several examples include:

- PACE, the Program of All-Inclusive Care for the Elderly, where adults age 55 years or older who meet specific criteria can receive comprehensive care that is interdisciplinary. They also receive support to live in the community as long as possible. In 2008, 61 PACE programs were active in 29 states (National PACE Association, 2008).

- VNS Choice, a subsidiary of the Visiting Nurse Service of New York City, is led by nurse consultant care managers and provides services to older adults primarily in home and community settings. Covered services for elderly adults include comprehensive home healthcare, adult daycare and ambulatory health services, transportation, prescription drugs, and coordination of benefits (VNS Choice, 2008).

- REACH U.S. programs (Racial and Ethnic Approaches to Community Health) represent an effort by the CDC to establish community-based, culturally appropriate programs and eliminate health disparities among racial and ethnic groups. One particular REACH project, the Latino Education Project (LEP), uses innovative approaches to promote awareness of the importance of early screening and treatment of diabetes among Hispanic older adults and their families living in a 12-county area along the south-central Gulf coast shore of Texas (CDC, 2008b).

Retirement centers and senior citizens' housing have become common. For the family members of older adults who need healthcare, alternative methods of care have become available. Examples of alternative care are respite care facilities, which allow the family a needed rest by temporarily housing and caring for an ailing older family member, and daycare centers, which provide a safe, stimulating environment during the day when family caregivers must work. Nurses should be knowledgeable about what healthcare and social services are available in the patient's community so that the patient and family can be referred.

The old-old have special significance for nursing care because they are more likely to need help with mobility and basic activities of daily living. They may need increasing assistance to maintain a safe and comfortable living environment. The older the person, the more likely that he or she needs family and community support to maintain functional health. Additional resources for community support services that help older adults live independently are located in Table 20-4.

▶ *Remember Ethel Peabody, the 88-year-old woman with beginning dementia who lives alone. The nurse could work with social services to investigate possible community support resources available for the patient so that she can safely maintain her independence as much as possible.* ■

Family and Role Reversal

An older adult's spouse and other family members are natural support systems that help the person maintain functional health and independence and meet the developmental tasks of old age. Supportive assistance may include providing transportation, food, shelter, social interactions, and even complex medical and nursing treatments. Significant others, such as close friends and neighbors, may also take on tasks formerly assumed to be the responsibilities of the traditional family.

TABLE • 20-3	HOUSING OPTIONS FOR OLDER ADULTS
Type of Living Arrangement	**Description**
Home modification	By making changes, older adults may be able to stay in their own homes. Examples of modification are replacing doorknobs with handles, replacing faucet handles with levers, and installing grab bars in bathtubs.
Homesharing	Two or more people may share an apartment or house. Each person usually has a private bedroom and shares the other living spaces. These homes may be sponsored by faith-based groups or community agencies.
Accessory apartments	A separate apartment is constructed in part of an existing house, such as a basement or attic. This allows older adults to live independently and privately, but they are not alone.
Elderly cottage housing opportunities (ECHO)	ECHO homes are small portable cottages that are placed (most often) in the yard of an adult child's home. These units typically cost $28,000 or more, but do allow living independently but close to support.
Senior retirement communities	A grouping of rental apartments or houses for residents who can take care of themselves and are mobile. Meals may be available in a central dining room, and housekeeping services may be offered (although there are additional costs for these services). Social and recreational activities are usually offered.
Continuing care retirement communities (CCRC)	This type of housing community offers several options and services, depending on the needs of the resident. Residents usually begin by living independently in apartments, and then move to an assisted-living facility on the same grounds. A skilled nursing center is also part of the community and available when needed. Sometimes called "aging-in-place" models, this type of housing tends to be expensive.
Assisted living	These facilities generally provide housing, group meals, personal care and support services, and social activities in a social setting. There may be some healthcare provided. Costs vary from around $1,000 up to $3,000 or more a month. Some states pay for personal care services for those with limited incomes.
Board and care homes Adult family home Adult group homes	Smaller in scale than assisted-living facilities, these services provide a room, meals, and help with daily activities. They may be licensed or unlicensed. Costs average $33,000 per year for a private room; Supplemental Security Income (SSI) will help pay for those with very limited incomes.
Nursing homes	Nursing homes provide skilled nursing care and/or long-term care, including meals, personal care, and medical care. Bedrooms and bathrooms may be shared. Costs average $66,000 per year, but many are more expensive. Medicare provides only short-term coverage following a hospitalization. Medicaid provides coverage for low-income, low-asset individuals.

Additional information about these housing options is provided by AARP at http://www.aarp.org/family/housing/.

Not all families can assist an aged member satisfactorily because of geographic distance, low income, poor health, strained marital relationships, or infringement on career or lifestyle. Adult children may feel "sandwiched" between responsibilities for their own children and careers and the needs of older parents. It can be a guilt-ridden and emotionally draining time for all involved when an older adult's physical or emotional illness reverses roles (with the child now assuming the role of parent, while the parent becomes dependent as the "child") and strains family resources.

The nurse must view the whole family as the recipient of care and assess the family for capabilities and limitations for assisting the aged member. The nurse can help ease the strain by listening to the patient's and family's concerns and by validating the importance of family needs. The nurse assists the patient and family to find workable solutions and may refer the family to community support services.

Moral and Spiritual Development

Older adults, according to Kohlberg (1969), have completed their moral development. Most are at the conventional level, following society's rules in response to others' expectations. Spiritually, an older adult may remain at an earlier level, often at the individuative-reflective level. Many older adults, however, demonstrate conjunctive faith, integrating faith and truth to see the reality of their own beliefs, or universalizing faith, in which they trust a greater power and believe in the future.

Self-transcendence is a characteristic of later life that helps one expand beyond personal limits to reach out to others and

TABLE • 20-4 RESOURCES FOR OLDER ADULTS	
Organization	**Activities**
U.S. Department of Health and Human Services (DHHS) http://www.hhs.gov	Government agency charged with protecting health through the delivery of human services
Administration on Aging (AoA) http://www.aoa.gov	Provides home- and community-based services to older adults through programs funded under the Older Americans Act.
Centers for Medicare and Medicaid Services (CMS) http://www.cms.hhs.gov	DHHS agency assigned to maintain healthcare security for its beneficiaries.
Eldercare Locator http://www.eldercare.gov	Connects older adults and families by zip code, city, state or county to eldercare resources in the community.
National Association for Area Agencies on Aging (n4a) http://www.n4a.org	Helps older persons and those with disabilities to live with dignity and choices in their homes and communities for as long as possible.
Meals on Wheels Association of America (MOWAA) http://www.mowaa.org	Provides lunch and dinner to older adults and people with disabilities.
NIH Senior Health http://www.nihseniorhealth.gov	Includes health and wellness information for older adults.
Senior Housing Finder http://www.alz.org/we_can_help_senior_ housing_finder.asp	The Alzheimer's Association Senior Housing Finder searches a current list of licensed assisted-living residences, nursing homes, and other types of senior housing.
Lotsa Helping Hands http://www.lotsahelpinghands.com	Provides communication resources to support family caregivers including help from volunteers and community.

the environment and a greater awareness of others' beliefs and values. Integration of the past and future in the present facilitates acceptance of where one is in life without regretting past mistakes or fearing the future (Reed, 1996). As a person ages, spirituality and transcendence are a resource and a source of strength when faced with inevitable change and loss.

Health of the Older Adult

As the number of older adults increases, nurses will spend more time providing care for this population. Older adults who require care are in all types of healthcare settings, including hospitals, long-term care facilities, emergency departments, outpatient surgeries, and homes. Nursing care for older adults should be based on two principles:

- Most older people are not impaired but are functional in the community, thereby benefiting from health-oriented interventions.
- Older people are more vulnerable to physical, emotional, and socioeconomic problems than people in other age groups and may require special attention to health promotion and maintenance.

This section provides a broad introduction to the healthcare needs of the older adult in terms of chronic illness, accidental injuries, and acute illness.

Chronic Illness

The probability and incidence of a person becoming ill increase with age. The most common chronic illnesses in older adults are hypertension, diagnosed arthritis, heart disease, any cancer, diabetes, and sinusitis (USDHHS, 2008a). Chronic health problems or disability also may result from acute illnesses or accidents such as fractures, pneumonia, motor vehicle accidents, and falls. The leading causes of death in the elderly are heart disease, cancer, and stroke.

Although illness affects all dimensions of a person regardless of age, older adults have to contend with a variety of problems as they live with chronic illness. Aging is a normal process, and chronic illness is a pathologic process, but both often occur at the same time. The changes of aging and the needs imposed by chronic illness interrelate to increase the risk for problems in all areas of life, including—but not limited to—self-care, lifestyle, economics, social factors, and living arrangements.

> *Think back to Ethel Peabody, the 88-year-old woman with beginning dementia and cardiac disease. The nurse could use the knowledge of chronic illness as a basis for a teaching plan that addresses the patient's increased needs for safety.* ■

IMPLICATIONS FOR HEALTHCARE

Consider the following:

- Ninety-five percent (95%) of healthcare expenditures for older Americans are for treatment of chronic illnesses (CDC, 2007).
- Meeting the expenses of healthcare is often difficult for older adults and their families.
- Medication costs related to chronic illness continue for the rest of a person's life, with multiple medications being the rule rather than the exception. **Polypharmacy,** the use of many medications at the same time, can pose many hazards for older adults. Complicated regimens need careful review to minimize risks and complications and maximize benefits. Alternative therapies such as herbal remedies have the potential to interact with prescribed drugs and cause dangerous effects (Lilley, Harrington, & Snyder, 2007). Refer to Chapter 29 for additional information regarding altered drug response in older adults.
- Hospitalization costs continue to rise, and the price of high-quality, long-term care may well be beyond the patient's or family members' ability to pay.
- Special diets, special equipment, and medical supplies increase economic difficulties.
- Family members must learn how to cope with the needs of the ill person. Included are personal hygiene, medication administration, special diets, elimination, activities of daily living, and recognition of symptoms that necessitate medical attention.
- Family members must also adapt to psychological stressors such as changes in communications, changes in roles (e.g., an older mother becomes dependent), and changes in their own lifestyle as they become the caregivers.

DIVERSITY AND CHRONIC ILLNESS

As the U.S. population ages dramatically and becomes more diverse, it is important to consider how cultural differences can affect future patterns of disease, disability, and healthcare use (National Center for Health Statistics, 2007). By 2030, it is predicted that 72% of the older adults in the United States will be non-Hispanic whites, 11% will be Hispanic, 10% will be black, and 5% will be Asian. This represents an 11% decrease in non-Hispanic whites, a 5% increase in the Hispanic population, and a 2% increase in blacks and Asians when compared to 2003 figures (CDC, 2007).

The prevalence of certain diseases varies among racial and ethnic groups, and research has not yet proven definitively what effect early health behaviors and practices have on the disease patterns of older adults in these various groups. Health disparities that exist between nonminority populations and racial and ethnic minorities are recognized and are particularly prevalent in the older populations. Poverty, the presence of chronic illnesses, and difficulty accessing the healthcare system make older adults much more vulnerable to a diminished quality of life caused by disease.

Profiles of various racial and ethnic groups indicate the following patterns of diseases:

- *Black American* men are 30% more likely to die from heart disease than non-Hispanic white men. Black adults are diagnosed with diabetes and die from diabetes almost twice as often as white adults. Lung, prostate, and gastric cancer are also more prevalent in this group and they account for 47% of HIV/AIDS cases (The Office of Minority Health, 2008a).
- The leading causes of illness and death for *Hispanic Americans* are heart disease, cancer, unintentional injuries (accidents), stroke, and diabetes. Hispanics have higher rates of obesity and are two times more likely to be diagnosed with diabetes than whites (The Office of Minority Health, 2008c).
- *Asian Americans* are most at risk for cancer, heart disease, stroke, accidents, and diabetes. Tuberculosis is 24 times more common in this group than the white population. Compared to the white population, Asian Americans have lower incidence of prostate and breast cancer, but they are at higher risk for stomach and liver cancer (The Office of Minority Health, 2008b).

Refer to Chapter 2 for additional discussion of cultural variations and influences on healthcare.

Accidental Injuries

The older adult is at increased risk for accidental injury because of changes in vision and hearing, loss of mass and strength of muscles, slower reflexes and reaction time, and decreased sensory ability. A significant percentage of older adults limit their activities because of fear of falling that might result in serious health consequences. Falls are the most common cause of injuries and hospital admission in older adults. Many falls result in fractures, with hip fracture being the most disabling injury (CDC, 2007). (See Examples of Nursing Interventions and Nursing Outcomes Classifications (NIC/NOC): Fall Prevention.)

In addition, the combined effects of chronic illness and medications may make an older adult more prone to accidents. Older adults with reduced income may live in inadequate housing in neighborhoods with heavy traffic and high crime rates. They may be isolated from family members, and many live alone. Combined with the normal changes of aging and the effects of any illness, older people not only are at increased risk, but also have a more difficult time regaining health after an injury. Refer to Chapter 26 for additional information related to risk for accidental injuries in older adults.

Dementia, Depression, and Delirium

When a serious mental impairment occurs, the effect on the patient and family can be devastating. **Dementia** refers to various organic disorders that progressively affect cognitive functioning. Dementia is chronic and usually develops gradually. Of the dementias that affect older adults, **Alzheimer's disease** (AD) is the most common degenerative neurologic illness and the most common cause of cognitive impairment (CDC, 2008a). It accounts for about two thirds of the cases

Examples of Nursing Interventions and Nursing Outcomes Classifications (NIC/NOC)

Fall Prevention

Nursing Interventions

- Identify behaviors and factors that affect risk of falls.
- Monitor gait, balance, and fatigue level with ambulation.
- Assist unsteady individual with ambulation.
- Post signs to alert staff that patient is at high risk for falls.
- Instruct patient to wear prescription glasses, as appropriate, when out of bed.
- Avoid clutter on floor surfaces.
- Educate family members about risk factors that contribute to falls and how they can decrease these risks.

Nursing Outcomes

- Balance
- Fall Prevention Behavior
- Knowledge: Fall Prevention
- Mobility
- Risk Control
- Safe Home Environment
- Sensory Function: Vision
- Ambulation

Bulechek, G., Butcher, H., & Dochterman, J. (2008). *Nursing interventions classification (NIC)* (pp. 342–343) (5th ed.). St. Louis: C.V. Mosby. A full listing of nursing activities for each nursing intervention can be found in this book.
Moorhead, S., Johnson, M., Maas, M., & Swanson, E. (2008). *Nursing outcomes classification (NOC)* (p. 766–767). St. Louis: C.V. Mosby. A full listing of nursing outcomes for each nursing diagnosis can be found in this book.

of dementia in the United States, affecting adults in middle to late life (Maslow & Mezey, 2008). Scientists estimate that more than 5 million people (98% of them over 65 years of age) have AD, and that the number of new cases of AD will double every 20 years (Doerflinger, 2007).

Alzheimer's disease affects brain cells and is characterized by patchy areas of the brain that degenerate. It is a progressively serious and ultimately fatal disorder. At first, forgetfulness and impaired judgment may be evident. Over a period of several years, the person becomes progressively more confused, forgetting family and becoming disoriented in familiar surroundings. A common problem in patients with dementia is **sundowning syndrome,** in which an older adult habitually becomes confused, restless, and agitated after dark. When the ability to perform simple activities of daily living is lost, the person requires constant supervision and care, often in a nursing home. There is no effective medical treatment for AD at this time.

Individuals with dementia are hospitalized more frequently than other older adults are. The precipitating factor may be a medical–surgical problem or behavioral or psychiatric symptoms that occur with dementia. Often, a medical or nursing intervention can trigger a sequence of adverse events in an older frail adult. This downward spiral and decline is referred to as **cascade iatrogenesis.** An episode of confusion and wandering at night may lead to a fall that results in a hip fracture. During the resulting hospitalization, the insertion of an indwelling catheter can precipitate a urinary tract infection that requires use of an antibiotic and possibly the development of antibiotic-resistant organisms.

Recognizing patients at risk for cascade iatrogenesis may help avoid its occurrence (Robinson &Weitzel, 2008). Communication with family members and a systematic approach

to assessment is required. The Fulmer SPICES tool is an instrument that has proved effective in identifying common problems experienced in older adults that can lead to negative outcomes. The acronym SPICES facilitates assessment and information gathering about the following:

- **S** – Sleep disorders
- **P** – Problems with eating or feeding
- **I** – Incontinence
- **C** – Confusion
- **E** – Evidence of falls
- **S** – Skin breakdown (Fulmer, 2007; Wallace & Fulmer, 2007).

This instrument can be used in all settings and acts as an alert for nurses to quickly identify interventions to individualize an older patient's care.

Comprehensive and empathetic nursing care is important. Both the patient and family caregivers need emotional support and teaching and may benefit from community resources that can ease the family's burden.

Sometimes delirium and depression in an older adult are mistaken for true dementia. **Delirium,** a temporary state of confusion, is an acute illness that can last from hours to weeks and resolves with treatment. Drug interactions, circulatory or metabolic problems, nutritional deficiencies, or a worsening illness are likely the real cause. An older adult may also become confused when too many changes or losses occur at one time or when moved to a different environment (see Research in Nursing: Bridging the Gap to Evidence-Based Practice). As many as 30% of adults 65 years of age and older experience an episode of delirium during a hospitalization. More incidences of delirium occur in hospitalized patients following cardiac or orthopedic surgery, an ICU

RESEARCH IN NURSING
Bridging The Gap to Evidence-Based Practice

MANAGING DELIRIUM IN HOSPITALIZED OLDER ADULTS

Older adults admitted to the hospital are at risk for experiencing delirium. Often, it is not diagnosed and thought by healthcare givers to be a normal progression of the aging process. In addition to advanced age, other risk factors include dementia, sensory deprivations, mobility impairments, unfamiliar environments, and multiple medications. Delirium is a leading complication of hospitalization for older adults. It is a treatable condition and the confusion associated with delirium is reversible.

Related Research

Dahlke, S., & Phinney, A. (2008). Caring for hospitalized older adults at risk for delirium. *Journal of Gerontological Nursing, 34*(6), 41–47.

The purpose of this study was to investigate how nurses respond to the challenges of caring for hospitalized older adults at risk for delirium. This qualitative study interviewed 12 nurses who worked on either medical or surgical units in a mid-sized hospital in Canada. There were a significant number of elderly patients on all units. An interviewer asked all nurses open-ended questions about their practice and specifically asked for responses to how each nurse recognized and cared for patients who became delirious. Analysis of the responses revealed three main nursing

For additional research, visit thePoint.

strategies: taking a quick look, keeping an eye on patients, and controlling the situation. The barriers to care that nurses identified include negative beliefs and attitudes about the elderly and an environment that does not recognize the unique needs of older adults. The current fast-paced hospital setting was definitely an impediment to careful assessments and individualized care for this population. Nurses also agreed that they had insufficient knowledge and resources to work effectively with delirious patients. They reinforced beliefs that caring for younger adults is less burdensome than caring for older adults.

Relevance to Nursing Practice

Given the increases that will occur in the older population, education curricula need to include information regarding the normal physiologic and cognitive changes that occur with aging, as well as knowledge about delirium and its care. Nurses in clinical settings need an awareness of best practice guidelines for assessments and interventions that target the prevention of delirium. Understanding and meeting the needs of these older patients can be challenging but appropriate responses by caregivers keep patients safe and prevent the occurrence of the cascade of adverse events that can occur in frail older adults.

stay, or during the later stages of a terminal illness (Waszynski, 2007). Treatment of delirium may include stopping unnecessary medications, as well as interventions to resolve infection and metabolic alterations. Medications that reduce agitation may be prescribed in certain circumstances. National guidelines recommend that psychotropic drugs such as haloperidol (Haldol) be used only when necessary to treat severe agitation. The benzodiazepines are usually avoided because they may increase confusion and cause oversedation (Lyons, Grimley, & Sydnor, 2008).

The nurse can help other members of the health team determine the cause of a patient's confusion and help reorient the patient. One technique the nurse can use is **reality orientation,** which involves interventions to redirect the patient's attention to what is real in the environment. See Table 20-5 for online resources that nurses can use to assess for dementia and delirium. When assessing behavioral changes, it is important to remember that an older adult with dementia may also develop delirium or depression.

Extreme or prolonged sadness in an older adult may be a warning sign of depression. Death of a spouse or friends and changes in living environment and financial resources can precipitate feelings of depression. There is usually a distinct change of behavior accompanied by other specific signs and symptoms of depression, such as altered sleep pattern, weight loss, difficulty with concentration, and suicidal thoughts or

TABLE • 20-5	ONLINE TOOLS FOR ASSESSMENT OF DELIRIUM AND DEMENTIA
Assessment Tool	**Description**
CAM (Confusion Assessment Method) http://www.consultgerirn.org/uploads/File/trythis/issue13_cam.pdf	Identifies delirium quickly. Long and short version are available.
NEECHAM Confusion Scale http://www.unc.edu/courses/2005fall/nurs/213/001/neuropsychiatric/neecham.html	Consists of nine items and is used to detect early stages of delirium. Does not differentiate between dementia and delirium
Mini-Cog http://alzheimers.about.com/od/diagnosisissues/a/Mini_Cog.htm	Two-part test to determine if dementia or cognitive impairment is present (even in early stages). Takes 3–5 minutes to administer.

preoccupation with death (Murphy, 2007). Depression usually does not resolve without treatment and is frequently underdiagnosed. The Geriatric Depression Scale (short form) is a screening tool that can be used effectively in older adults in any setting. It consists of 15 questions and, when combined with a mental health assessment by a professional, can facilitate a diagnosis of depression (Greenberg, 2007). The Geriatric Depression Scale: Short Form is available at www.chcr.brown.edu/GDS_SHORT_FORM. PDF.

Treatment of depression usually involves psychotherapy or counseling and antidepressant medication. In an older adult, hopelessness rather than sadness is more often associated with suicidal intent. The rate of suicide in older white males is six times higher than in the rest of the population (Spires, 2006).

Elder Maltreatment

The increase in the number of older adults coupled with the lengthening of the life span has resulted in greater awareness about the problem of elder maltreatment, including abuse and neglect. Some estimate that as many as 4% to 6% of older adults or 700,000 to 1.2 million individuals older than 65 years of age suffer from abuse or neglect, most often inflicted by family members (National Committee for the Prevention of Elder Abuse, 2008; Fulmer, 2008). It is difficult to determine an accurate number of elder abuse incidents because only 1 in 10 cases is reported (Fulmer, 2008). Elder abuse most commonly occurs in women who are older than 80 years of age. Physical abuse, sexual abuse, emotional or psychological abuse, neglect, abandonment, and financial or material exploitation are all types of elder maltreatment (CDC, 2008c).

Neglect accounts for more than half of all elder maltreatment reports made to adult protective service agencies. It can be active or passive and occurs when a caregiver fails to adequately meet the physical, social, or emotional needs of an older adult resulting in harm to that person. Poor hygiene, inadequate nutrition, untreated injuries, and lack of assistance with care needs are indicators of neglect. Physical abuse causes pain, impairment, or deliberate physical injury to an older adult. Hitting, assault of any kind, slapping, and restraining are all examples of forms of physical abuse. Older adults who have been physically abused present with injuries that are incompatible with the older adult or caregiver's version of how the injury occurred. Evidence of previously untreated injuries or suspicious cuts and bruises should alert healthcare providers to the possibility of physical abuse. Sexual abuse involves nonconsensual sexual contact of any kind with an elderly person (National Center on Elder Abuse, 2007). Emotional abuse occurs when threats, intimidation, or isolation result in anguish for the elder person, while financial abuse involves exploitation or misuse of another's property.

Identification of elder abuse requires an alert healthcare provider. It is not uncommon to misinterpret indications of abuse as normal signs of aging. Careful observation of the relationship between the older adult and the caregiver may be the first evidence that the older adult is a victim of abuse. Pay attention to interactions involving voice tone, caring

TABLE • 20-6	ELDER ABUSE RESOURCES
Organization	**Activities**
National Center on Elder Abuse http://www.ncea.aoa.gov Phone: 1-800-677-1116	This site is a gateway to resources on elder abuse, neglect, and exploitation.
U.S. Administration on Aging, Eldercare Locator http:www.eldercare.gov/ Eldercare.NET/Public/Home.aspx Phone: 1-800-677-1116	Connects older adults and caregivers with sources of information on senior services.
Law Enforcement Agencies Dial 911	For use when an older adult is in immediate, life-threatening danger or when reporting suspected abuse is mandatory.

behaviors, and personal touch. If you suspect abuse, attempt to speak to the older adult in a private setting away from the caregiver. A victim may deny abuse or choose not to report it because of shame, fear of abandonment, worry about retaliation, or dementia. All assessment data should be objectively documented, including direct quotes from both parties. The Elder Assessment Instrument allows practicing nurses to screen for maltreatment in suspected cases (Fulmer, 2008). It requires an interview and physical assessment for data collection and is available at: http://consultgerirn.org/uploads/File/trythis/issue15.pdf. Most states require that healthcare professionals report any suspected cases of elder abuse to officially designated agencies. Table 20-6 lists various organizations that provide additional information and support about elder abuse.

Older Adults and the Healthcare System

Our knowledge of aging has increased dramatically in the past 40 years. **Gerontology** is the scientific and behavioral study of all aspects of aging and its consequences. Normal changes that occur with aging are the result of complex interactions among genetics, biologic systems, and physical and social environments. Disease complicates a person's ability to adapt and maintain **functional health** (the ability to carry out usual and desired daily activities). Mental or physical decline in older adults often may not be directly related to the aging process but may result from the absence of supportive care and services that could prevent disease and help maintain the older adult's ability to function.

The increasing aging population has greatly strained a healthcare system that has traditionally focused on cures and acute disease processes. For an older patient with chronic disorders, the focus of care should include the patient's and family's goals and promote functional health and independent living to the greatest extent possible. **Gerontologic nursing** combines the basic knowledge and skills of nursing with a specialized knowledge of aging in both illness and health.

Role of the Nurse in Promoting Health and Preventing Illness

The nurse should teach the patient and family general health-promotion activities. This is important because older people often believe themselves "too old" to worry about nutrition, exercise, health screenings, and immunizations. In addition to the recommended screenings, examinations, and immunizations outlined in Table 20-1, the following areas should be stressed:

- Eat a diet that includes all food groups; is low in fat, saturated fat, and cholesterol; balances calories with physical activity; has recommended amounts of fruits, vegetables, and grains; and uses sugar and salt in moderation.
- Make exercise a part of daily activities.
- Drink alcohol in moderation.
- Do not smoke.

An older adult who requires surgery or medical treatment for chronic or acute illness has special, age-related needs regardless of the setting for care. Nursing care to meet age-related needs in any setting are outlined in Table 20-7.

Although nursing care adapted to the needs of older patients is described throughout this text, general principles for care are included here. Nurses must recognize physiologic and psychosocial interrelationships and view older patients holistically. See Examples of NANDA Nursing Diagnoses: The Older Adult.

Illness can severely disrupt an older adult's ability to function independently. The ill patient is under increased physical and emotional stress, which increases the risk for complications because of the lack of physiologic reserves. When a patient is hospitalized or institutionalized, family and community interactions are severely inhibited. The acute care environment itself adds new stressors such as diagnostic tests, treatments, and surgery. In the face of new and unfamiliar routines and sensory stimulation, prior coping skills may not work, and an older patient may feel less able to understand and control the new environment. An older patient is more likely than a younger patient to suffer multisystem dysfunctions, iatrogenic complications (caused by medications or treatments), accidents such as falls, and increasing dependence and confusion.

Examples of NANDA Nursing Diagnoses
The Older Adult

Nursing Diagnoses	Possible Related Factor
Risk for Infection	Dry, thin skin
Risk for Imbalanced Body Temperature	Very high environmental temperatures and lack of air conditioning or fans
Risk for Injury	Unstable gait and decreased vision from cataracts
Risk for Loneliness	Death of spouse
Ineffective Coping	Diagnosis of chronic illness
Impaired Physical Mobility	Severe arthritic changes in legs
Impaired Home Maintenance	Insufficient finances
Impaired Memory	Cognitive impairment from onset of Alzheimer's disease
Anxiety	Increase of crime and violence in neighborhood
Sedentary Lifestyle	Lack of motivation and insufficient knowledge of health benefits of exercise
Risk for Acute Confusion	Dementia
Risk for Compromised Human Dignity	Loss of control of body functions
Risk for Bleeding	History of falls

TABLE • 20-7	PROMOTING HEALTH IN OLDER ADULTS
Area of Concern	**Nursing Actions**
Physiologic function	• Maintain physiologic reserves. Maintain ongoing assessments for early detection of problems. • Review perceptions of current health status, health problems, and prescribed or over-the-counter medications. • Include nursing care that maintains physical status, such as skin care and planned rest and activity.
Cognitive function	• Slow pace of activity and wait for responses. • Be sure eyeglasses and hearing aids are used; ensure lenses are clean and batteries are strong.
Psychosocial needs	• Be aware that illness, hospitalization, or changes in living arrangements are major stressors. • Assess and support sources of strength, including cultural and spiritual values and rituals. • Encourage use of support systems: family, friends, community resources, and pets. • Set mutual goals and encourage the patient's role in making decisions about care. • Encourage life review and reminiscence. • Encourage self-care. • Consider the patient's background, interests, capabilities, values, culture, and lifestyle when planning care.
Nutrition	• Assess for lost or damaged teeth; ensure dentures fit properly. Provide foods appropriate to the patient's ability to chew. • Assess height, weight, eating patterns, and food choices. If weight is being lost, assess income, storage, and transportation. • Assess swallowing ability. • Consider using supplements.
Sleep and rest	• Discourage excessive napping. • Assess normal bedtime, time for rising, bedtime rituals, effects of pain, medications, anxiety, and depression.
Elimination	• Assess frequency of bladder elimination as well as problems with incontinence. • Assess normal times for bowel movements, changes in activity, privacy, and medications. • Ensure that the floor is not cluttered, the toilet is easily accessible, lighting is adequate, and privacy is provided. • Suggest having safety bars installed in the bathroom. • Review diet for necessary fluid and fiber content.
Activity and exercise	• Assess ability to walk; ensure that assistive devices (such as a walker or cane) are available. • Consider effects of illness, surgery, medications, and changes in diet and fluid intake on strength and motor function. • Ensure an uncluttered environment with good lighting; suggest using a night light and removing throw rugs. • Slow the pace of care, allowing extra time to carry out activities.
Sexuality	• Assist as necessary with hygiene, hair care, oral care, clean clothing and bedding, makeup, and shaving. • Maintain a clean, odor-free environment. • Demonstrate genuine caring: ask preferred name, listen carefully, and respect belongings. • Discuss safer sex if appropriate. • Discuss water-soluble lubricants with women; refer men for evaluation if erectile dysfunction is a concern.
Meeting developmental tasks	• Promote continued development and maintenance of functional health by identifying unmet tasks, feelings of isolation, and physical or sensory limitations. • Assist in finding creative solutions to developmental tasks. • Collaborate with other healthcare providers to provide information and referral to community resources for the patient and family.

The focus of nursing care is to assist older patients to function as independently as possible and to support their individual strengths. The nurse collaborates with the family and other disciplines to prevent complications of illness, to secure a safe and comfortable environment, and to promote the patient's return to health.

CARING FOR AN AGING POPULATION

Medical advances have enabled elderly and frail patients with serious and chronic illnesses and disabilities to survive much longer than they could in the past. American society is faced with the dilemma of how to care for this population. Already millions of American families are struggling nobly to provide steady and demanding long-term care for their incapacitated loved ones, often with little respite or communal support and usually for many years. It does not seem likely that an increase in paid caregiving will be able to alleviate the growing strains on family caregivers. There is an ever-shrinking pool of workers available for paid home healthcare. Factors reducing the number of home health aides and nurses include the strenuousness of the work involved, inadequate financial compensation, difficult relationships with patients, language barriers, and the lack of health insurance and other benefits.

In 2005, the President's Council on Bioethics aptly described the moral challenges confronting Americans as we struggle to care for our aging society:

How we care for the dependent elderly will test whether modern life has not only made things better for us but also made us better human beings, more willing to accept the obligations to care and more able to cope with the burdens of caregiving. Put simply, can a society that values self-reliance, personal freedom, and careerism reconcile itself to the realities of dependence, diminished autonomy, and responsibility for others? (The President's Council on Bioethics, 2005)

● Developing Critical Thinking Skills

1. Complete the following sentences, and then analyze the reasons for your answers:
   a. When my parents can no longer care for themselves, I will _____.
   b. If my parents were living in a nursing home, I would want the nurses to _____.
   c. When I am old, I want my family to _____.

2. Consider your own family. Can you identify developmental tasks for family members who are middle adults and older adults? What factors in your family facilitate or are barriers to meeting these tasks?

● Practicing for NCLEX

1. During an assessment, a 48-year-old woman tells the nurse that she is having hot flashes, fatigue, and mood swings. The nurse recognizes these symptoms as manifestations of which of the following?
   a. Andropause
   b. Puberty
   c. Menopause
   d. Senility

2. Based on Erikson's theory, middle adults who do not achieve their developmental tasks may be termed as being in stagnation. Which of the following statements would be one example of this finding?
   a. "I am helping my parents move into an assisted-living facility."

b. "I spend all of my time going to the doctor to be sure I am not sick."
   c. "I have enough money to help my son and his wife when they need it."
   d. "I earned this gray hair and I like it!"

3. Which of the following nursing diagnoses would be appropriate for the middle adult?
   a. Risk for Imbalanced Nutrition: More Than Body Requirements
   b. Delayed Growth and Development
   c. Self-Care Deficit
   d. Disturbed Thought Processes

4. Older adults may be stereotyped as different from other age groups and having outlived their usefulness. What is the term for this?
   a. Harassment
   b. World-view
   c. Racism
   d. Ageism

5. Which of the following statements is a myth about older adults?
   a. Most older adults live in their own homes.
   b. Healthy older adults enjoy sexual activity.
   c. Old age means mental deterioration.
   d. Older adults want to be attractive to others.

6. Which of the following is the leading cause of cognitive impairment in old age?
   a. Stroke
   b. Malnutrition
   c. Alzheimer's disease
   d. Loss of cardiac reserve

7. Which of the following questions would encourage reminiscence?
   a. "Tell me about how you celebrated Christmas when you were young."
   b. "Tell me how you plan to spend your time this weekend."
   c. "Did you enjoy your life when you were married?"
   d. "Why don't you want to talk about your feelings?"

8. A 90-year-old man who lives alone tells you he has no family or friends. Based on this information, what nursing diagnoses would be appropriate for him?
   a. Social Isolation
   b. Powerlessness
   c. Risk for Injury
   d. Risk for Falls

9. When teaching the older adult who is recovering from surgery, which of the following is important for the nurse to remember?
   a. Talk in a much louder voice
   b. Repeat information as often as necessary
   c. Teach caregivers rather than the patient
   d. Provide information rapidly

10. Which statement by an 85-year-old woman would demonstrate that she has met an expected outcome of the plan of care for safety?
    a. "I only wear my glasses when I go to the store."
    b. "I am going to ask my daughter to come and give me a bath."
    c. "Would you please get me a drink of water for my pills."
    d. "I am going to take up all my little scatter rugs."

● Answers With Rationale

1. *c.* During menopause, the loss of estrogen often results in women experiencing hot flashes, fatigue, and changes in mood.

2. *b.* Middle adults who do not reach generativity tend to become overly concerned about their own physical and emotional health needs.

3. *a.* Middle adults tend to continue to maintain previous eating patterns while being less active, increasing the risk of obesity.

4. *d.* Ageism is a form of prejudice in which older adults are stereotyped by characteristics found in only a few members of their age group.

5. *c.* Although response time may be longer, intelligence does not normally decrease because of aging.

6. *c.* Alzheimer's disease affects approximately 4 million older adults.

7. *a.* Asking open-ended questions about events in the past can encourage the older adult to relive and restructure life experiences.

8. *a.* Social isolation is a sense of being alone or lonely as a result of having few meaningful relationships.

9. *b.* The stress of illness and hospitalization often makes the older patient feel less able to understand teaching. It is important to repeat the information as often as necessary.

10. *d.* Removing throw rugs is one means of preventing falls and injury.

Taylor Suite Resources

The Taylor Suite offers these additional resources to enhance learning and facilitate understanding of this chapter:

- thePoint online resource, http://thepoint.lww.com/Taylor7E
- Student DVD-ROM included with the book
- Study Guide for Taylor's Fundamentals of Nursing

BIBLIOGRAPHY

Beeber, A. (2007). When your patient needs long-term care services. *Nursing, 37*(12), 62–63.

Bertera, E., & Bertera, R. (2008). Fear of falling and activity avoidance in a national sample of older adults in the United States. *Health & Social Work, 33*(1), 54–61.

Bradway, C., & Hirschman, K. (2008). Working with families of hospitalized older adults with dementia. *American Journal of Nursing, 108*(10), 52–61.

Bulechek, G., Butcher, H., & Dochterman, J. (Eds.). (2008). *Nursing Interventions Classification (NIC)* (5th ed.). St. Louis: Mosby.

Centers for Disease Control and Prevention (CDC), National Center for Health Statistics. (2005). Life expectancy hits record high: Gender gap narrows. Available at http://www.cdc.gov/nchs/pressroom/05facts/lifeexpectancy.htm.

Centers for Disease Control and Prevention (CDC) and The Merck Company Foundation. (2007). *The state of aging and health in America 2007.* Available at http://www.cdc.gov/aging/pdf/saha_2007.pdf

Centers for Disease Control and Prevention (CDC). (2008a). Alzheimer's disease. Available at http://www.cdc.gov/Features/Alzheimers/

Centers for Disease Control and Prevention (CDC). (2008b). REACH U.S.: Racial and ethnic approaches to community health. Available at http://www.cdc.gov/reach/

Centers for Disease Control and Prevention (CDC). (2008c). *Understanding elder maltreatment.* Available at http://www.cdc.gov/violenceprevention/pdf/EM-FactSheet-a.pdf

Centers for Disease Control and Prevention (CDC). (2009). National Center for Injury Prevention and Control. *Welcome to WISQARS (Web-based injury statistics query and reporting system).* Available at http://www.cdc.gov/injury/wisqars/index.html

Chettle, C. (2009). Aging immune systems more vulnerable to attack. *Nursing Spectrum, 18*(6), 20–25.

Cole, C., & Richards, K. (2007). Sleep disruption in older adults. *American Journal of Nursing, 107*(5), 40–49.

Dahlke, S., & Phinney, A. (2008). Caring for hospitalized older adults at risk for delirium. *Journal of Gerontological Nursing, 34*(6), 41–47.

D'Arcy, Y. (2009). Overturning barriers to pain relief in older adults. *Nursing, 39*(10), 32–38.

DiMaria-Ghalili, R., & Guenter, P. (2008). The mini nutritional assessment. *American Journal of Nursing, 108*(2), 50–60.

Doerflinger, D. (2007). The Mini-Cog. *American Journal of Nursing, 107*(12), 62–72.

Eliopoulos, C. (2010). *Gerontological nursing* (7th ed.). Philadelphia: Lippincott Williams & Wilkins.

Erikson, E. (1963). *Childhood and society* (2nd ed.). New York: Norton.

Federal Interagency Forum on Aging-Related Statistics. (2008). *Older Americans 2008: Key indicators of well-being.* Available at http://www.socoaaa.org/pdf/OA_2008.pdf

Fick, D., & Mion, L. (2008). Delirium superimposed on dementia. *American Journal of Nursing, 108*(1), 52–61.

Fowler, J. W. (1991). *Weaving the new creation: Stages of faith and the public church.* San Francisco: Harper Collins.

Fulmer, T. (2007). Fulmer SPICES. *American Journal of Nursing, 107*(10), 40–49.

Fulmer, T. (2008). Screening for mistreatment of older adults. *American Journal of Nursing, 108*(12), 52–60.

Gerber, L. (2008). Help your older patient blossom socially. *Nursing, 38*(2), 24–25.

Gerber, L. (2009). Putting older patients' sleep concerns to rest. *Nursing, 39*(4), 60–61.

Gould, R. (1972). The phases of adult life: A study in developmental psychology. *American Psychiatry, 129,* 33–43.

Greenberg, S. (2007). The geriatric depression scale: Short form. *American Journal of Nursing, 107*(10), 60–70.

Havighurst, R. J. (1972). *Developmental tasks and education* (3rd ed.). New York: David McKay.

Kohlberg, L. (1969). Stage and sequence: The cognitive–developmental approach to socialization. In D. Gaslin (Ed.), *Handbook of socialization: Theory and research* (pp. 347–380). Chicago: Rand McNally.

Levinson, D. J., Darrow, C. N., Klein, E. B., Levinson, M. H., & McKee, B. (1978). *The seasons of a man's life.* New York: Knopf.

Lilley, L., Harrington, S., & Snyder, J. (2007). *Pharmacology and the nursing process* (5th ed.). St. Louis: Mosby.

Lyons, D., Grimley, S., & Sydnor, L. (2008). Double trouble when delirium complicates dementia. *Nursing, 38*(9), 48–54.

Maslow, K., & Mezey, M. (2008). Recognition of dementia in hospitalized older adults. *American Journal of Nursing, 108*(1), 40–50.

McCloskey Dochterman, J., & Bulechek, G. (Eds.). (2004). *Nursing interventions classification (NIC)* (4th ed.). St. Louis: Mosby.

Messecar, D., Powers, B., & Nagel, C. (2008). The family preferences index. *American Journal of Nursing, 108*(9), 52–60.

Moorhead, S., Johnson, M., Maas, M., & Swanson, E. (Eds.). (2008). *Nursing outcomes classification (NOC)* (4th ed.). St. Louis: Mosby.

Murphy, K. (2007). Is your older patient depressed? *Nursing, 37*(6), 22–23.

Nagle, M. (2008). Screening for alcohol use and misuse in older adults. *American Journal of Nursing, 108*(11), 50–59.

National Center on Elder Abuse. US. Administration on Aging. (2007). Major types of elder abuse. Available at http://www.ncea.aoa.gov/NCEAroot/Main_Site/FAQ/Basics/Types_Of_Abuse.aspx

National Center for Health Statistics. (2007). *Health, United States, 2007.* Available at http://www.cdc.gov/nchs/data/hus/hus07.pdf

National Committee for the Prevention of Elder Abuse (NCPEA). (2008). *What is elder abuse?* Available at http://www.preventelderabuse.org/elderabuse/

National PACE Association. (2008). *What is PACE?* Available at http://www.npaonline.org/website/article.asp?id=12

NANDA International. (2009). *Nursing diagnoses: Definitions & classification 2009–2011.* West Sussex, UK: Wiley-Blackwell.

Porth, C. M. (2007). *Essentials of pathophysiology: Concepts of altered health states* (2nd ed.). Philadelphia: Lippincott Williams & Wilkins.

Reed, P. (1996). Transcendence: Formulating nursing perspectives. *Nursing Science Quarterly, 9*(1), 2–4.

Robinson, S., & Weitzel, T. (2008). Going downhill: Preventing cascade iatrogenesis. *Nursing, 38*(4), 62–63.

Rowe, M. (2008). Wandering in hospitalized older adults. *American Journal of Nursing, 108*(10), 62–71.

Spires, R. (2006). Depression in the elderly. *RN, 69*(6), 38–43.

The Office of Minority Health. (2008a). *African American profile.* Available at http://www.omhrc.gov/templates/browse.aspx?lvl=3&lvlid=23

The Office of Minority Health. (2008b). *Asian American/Pacific Islander profile.* Available at http://www.omhrc.gov/templates/browse.aspx?lvl=3&lvlid=29

The Office of Minority Health. (2008c). *Hispanic/Latino profile.* Available at http://www.omhrc.gov/templates/browse.aspx?lvl=3&lvlid=31

The President's Council on Bioethics. (2005). *Taking care: Ethical caregiving in our aging society.* Washington, DC: Author.

U.S. National Center for Health Statistics. (2008). *National vital statistics reports (NVSR), Deaths: final data for 2005.* Available at http://www.cdc.gov/nchs/data/nvsr/nvsr56/nvsr56_10.pdf

U.S. Department of Health and Human Services (USDHHS), Administration on Aging. (2008a). *A statistical profile of older Americans aged 65+.* Washington, DC: Author.

U.S. Department of Health and Human Services (USDHHS), Administration on Aging. (2008b). *Challenging of global aging.* Washington, DC: Author.

U.S. Department of Health and Human Services (USDHHS). National Vaccine Advisory Committee. (2009). Recommendations for Federal Adult Immunization Programs regarding Immunization Delivery, Assessment, Research and Safety Monitoring. Available at http://www.hhs.gov/nvpo/nvac/subgroups/nvacadultimmunizationsworkinggroupjune2009.html

U.S. Department of Health and Human Services (USDHHS), Administration on Aging. (2010). Minority aging. Available at http://www.aoa.gov/AoARoot/Aging_Statistics/Minority_Aging/index.aspx

VNS Choice. (2008). *VNS CHOICE managed long term care.* Available at http://www.vnsny.org/our-services/by-service/medical/long-term-care/vns-choice-managed-long-term-care/

Volmer, C., Rich, C., & Robinson, S. (2007). How to prevent delirium: A practical protocol. *Nursing, 37*(8), 26–28.

Wallace, M. (2008). Assessment of sexual health in older adults. *American Journal of Nursing, 108*(7), 52–61.

Wallace, M., & Fulmer, T. (2007). Fulmer SPICES: An overall assessment tool for older adults. Available at www.consultgerirn.org/uploads/File/trythis/issue01.pdf

Wallace, M. (2008). Monitoring functional status in hospitalized older adults. *American Journal of Nursing, 108*(4), 64–72.

Waszynski, C. (2007). Detecting delirium. *American Journal of Nursing, 107*(12), 50–60.

Wilson, S., & Giddens, J. (2005). *Health assessment for nursing practice* (3rd ed.). St. Louis: Elsevier Mosby.

ROLES BASIC TO NURSING CARE

Unit V discusses the nurse's professional roles of communicator, teacher, counselor, leader, and manager. These roles are interdependent, and each is an integral part of the broad nursing role of caregiver. The nurse in these roles helps patients of all ages to meet needs along the health continuum.

To be effective as a caregiver, the nurse must be proficient in both the art and the science of nursing. Communication is essential to each professional nursing role and is the heart of caring. Nursing is a person-centered service, based on relationships with patients, peers, and other members of the healthcare team. By developing effective interpersonal skills and using therapeutic communication skills, nurses can establish and maintain helping relationships.

As teacher, the nurse uses communication skills to teach individuals and families. Teaching, implemented throughout the nursing process, is used to meet learning needs. As counselor, the nurse provides information, makes appropriate referrals, and assists the patient in developing a systematic approach to problem solving and decision making. The nurse as a leader and/or manager practices assertive, self-directed nursing. Abilities to lead and to bring about change begin with the student nurse and progress as the nurse develops self-confidence and skill in interpersonal relationships and experience in healthcare settings. Unit V, therefore, enables beginning nurse caregivers to enrich their professional practice by integrating the professional nursing roles of communicator, teacher, counselor, leader, and manager. Nursing practice, as a specialized and unique service to others, is based on the application of knowledge and skills presented in this unit.

> "Clinical competence . . . has three dimensions. . . . Care is the fundamental things we do to make a patient comfortable. . . . curative nursing, . . . the broader group of restorative and rehabilitative activities . . . and counseling, . . . [providing] emotional, intellectual, and psychological support . . ."

FRANCES REITER (1904–1977) • *the first chairperson of the American Nurses Association Committee on Education, she coined the term "nurse clinician" and advocated advanced preparation of nurse clinicians.*

21 | Communicator

SUSIE MUSASHI

Susie is a 3-year-old patient with second-degree burns on both legs who currently is receiving débridement. Every time a health-care provider enters her room, she begins to cry, turning her body toward the wall and curling up with her knees to her chest. Her family lives approximately 1 $^1/_2$ hours away and can only visit her about once or twice a week.

IRWINA RUSSELLINSKI

Irwina, a 75-year-old woman transferred from the emergency department, is diagnosed with pneumonia. Her chart reveals that she is hard of hearing, "pleasantly confused" at times, and speaks "broken English." A nursing assessment is needed.

RANDOLPH GORDON

Randolph, a middle-aged man diagnosed with end-stage liver failure, is being cared for in the intensive care unit. He has been comatose for several weeks. He has numerous tubes and drainage devices in place and is receiving multiple therapies that require continuous electronic monitoring.

LEARNING OBJECTIVES

After completing the chapter, you will be able to accomplish the following:

1. Describe the communication process, identifying factors that influence communication.

2. List at least eight ways in which people communicate nonverbally.

3. Describe the interrelation between communication and the nursing process.

4. Identify patient goals for each phase of the helping relationship.

5. Use effective communication techniques when interacting with patients from different cultures.

6. Use a standardized communication technique (SBAR) to communicate with physicians and transfer patient information to other nurses.

7. Evaluate yourself in terms of the interpersonal competencies needed in nursing.

8. Describe how each type of ineffective communication hinders communication.

9. Establish therapeutic relationships with patients assigned to your care and describe effective interventions for patients with impaired verbal communication.

KEY TERMS

assertive behaviors	message
body language	noise
channel	nonverbal communication
cliché	
communication	organizational communication
empathy	
feedback	professionalism
group dynamics	rapport
helping relationship	receiver (decoder)
horizontal violence	SBAR
interpersonal communication	semantics
	small-group communication
interviewing techniques	source (encoder)
intrapersonal communication	stimulus
	therapeutic touch
language	verbal communication

Any nurse who wishes to be an effective caregiver must first learn how to be an effective communicator. Good communication skills enable nurses to get to know their patients and, ultimately, to diagnose and to meet their needs for nursing care. Nursing students who sit face to face with patients to obtain a comprehensive nursing history intuitively grasp the importance of the nurse's communicator role. To adequately document the patient's health history, the nursing student must understand and implement proper communication techniques. Communication skills are the building blocks of professional relationships between nurse and patient, nurse and nurse, and nurse and other health-team members. (See the accompanying Reflective Practice box for an example.)

Many experienced nurses identify the quality of their interpersonal relationships as the single most significant element in determining their helper effectiveness. Studies have shown that on nursing units where nurses freely exchange ideas and information, solve problems together when something goes wrong rather than assigning blame, complement one another, and use humor creatively, staff morale is high, and there is a higher level of attainment of patient outcomes.

THE PROCESS OF COMMUNICATION

Communication is the process of exchanging information and generating and transmitting meanings between two or more individuals. It is the foundation of society and the most primary aspect of a nurse–patient interaction. Without communication, it would be impossible to share family experiences, gain knowledge, establish and maintain practice protocols, and enhance caregiving. By nature, humans are social beings, and human needs are met in collaboration with other humans. Human relationships enable us to meet our physical and safety needs. Communication also assists in meeting our psychosocial needs of love, belonging, and self-esteem. The ability to communicate is basic to human functioning and well-being.

David K. Berlo (1960) is credited with the classic description of the communication process, which involves a source (encoder), message, channel, and receiver (decoder).

This communication process is initiated based on a **stimulus,** in this case a patient need that must be addressed. The need might be due to a patient's discomfort, a desire for information, or to address any uncertainty the patient might be experiencing. The sender or **source (encoder)** of the message is a person or group who initiates or begins the communication process.

The **message** is the actual physiologic product of the source. It might be a speech interview, conversation, chart, gesture, memorandum, or nursing note. The **channel** of communication is the medium the sender has selected to send the message. The channel might target any of the receiver's senses. The message can be sent to the receiver through the following channels:

- Auditory—spoken words and cues
- Visual—sight, observations, and perception
- Kinesthetic—touch

REFLECTIVE PRACTICE
Challenge to Interpersonal Skills

Recently, I was accompanying a nurse in the intensive care unit (ICU) when I encountered some behaviors that I found to be unprofessional and lacking in interpersonal skills. We were caring for Mr. Randolph Gordon, a middle-aged patient who was in end-stage liver failure and had been comatose for several weeks. The extent of drains, tubes, and technologies being used to care for Mr. Gordon was overwhelming. It was almost difficult to recognize him as a human being. I was taken aback when the nurse and some residents entered the patient's room and immediately began to assess the technological equipment, without any regard for or recognition of the patient. They proceeded to have a conversation about the patient's poor condition, unsightly appearance, and foul smell at the bedside, in the direct presence of the patient. They did not speak to the patient and they made no attempt to interact with the patient, not even the slightest touch of a hand.

Thinking Outside the Box: Possible Courses of Action

- Ignore the conversation between the nurse and residents and acknowledge the patient through words or touch.
- Calmly ask the nurse and residents to leave the room before discussing the patient's condition.
- Confront the nurse and residents, stating that they need to pay attention to the patient and his psychosocial and emotional well-being.

Evaluating a Good Outcome: How Do I Define Success?

- The patient's healthcare team will act with professionalism.
- Healthcare team will demonstrate respect for the patient's human dignity.
- We will have regard for the whole patient, with attention to spiritual, emotional, and social issues.
- We will set a good example for others in our expression of caring.

Personal Learning: Here's to the Future!

I was somewhat disappointed by my actions in this situation because I did not confront the nurse and the residents when they were acting unethically and unprofessionally. I did, however, ask the nurse if this was common behavior in ICU, that is, demonstrating little regard for the patient's holistic well-being. The nurse stated that unfortunately this was the case. The patients in the ICU are critically ill and many healthcare professionals become extremely focused on the physical and technological aspects of care. I was hesitant to interrupt the nurse and the residents because of my status as a nursing student.

I feared that my opinion would not be respected. I know that I will not be able to change the actions of everyone. However, in the future, I will demonstrate my concern for the patient, hoping that those around me will follow my example. I think that I should have immediately gone to the patient and said hello or touched his hand, even if he was comatose. Maybe my actions would have reminded the nurse and residents that there was a person in that bed. Then, possibly, they might have followed my lead.

Colleen Kilcullen, Georgetown University

Reflection

How do you think you would respond in a similar situation? Why? What does this tell you about yourself and about the adequacy of your skills for professional practice? What reasons can you propose to suggest the rationale for the nurse's and residents' behavior? How do you think that the residents would have reacted had the nursing student approached them about their behavior? Can you think of other ways to respond? What other skills (cognitive, interpersonal, technical, ethical/legal) would you need to respond well in this situation? Describe a plan that the nursing student could use to go about changing the staff's behavior. Do you agree with the criteria to evaluate a successful outcome? Did the nursing student meet the criteria? Please explain why or why not.

Nurses use all three of these channels to communicate with patients.

The **receiver (decoder)** must translate and interpret the message sent. Through the translation of the message, the receiver must then make a decision about an accurate response. To be an effective communicator, the nurse needs to be considerate of the receiver, and select a message that appeals to the client's interests and that requires minimal effort and time to decode.

> *Recall Randolph Gordon, the middle-aged man who was comatose. When planning Mr. Gordon's care, the nurse would need to incorporate knowledge about changes*

in mental status and their effect on communication. The patient's current mental status mandates that the messages sent by the nurse and other healthcare providers be simple, clear, and easy to understand. ■

Confirmation of the message provides **feedback** (i.e., evidence) that the receiver has understood the intended message. Noise—factors that distort the quality of a message—can interfere with communication at any point in the process. These distractors might be from the television, or from pain or discomfort experienced by the patient.

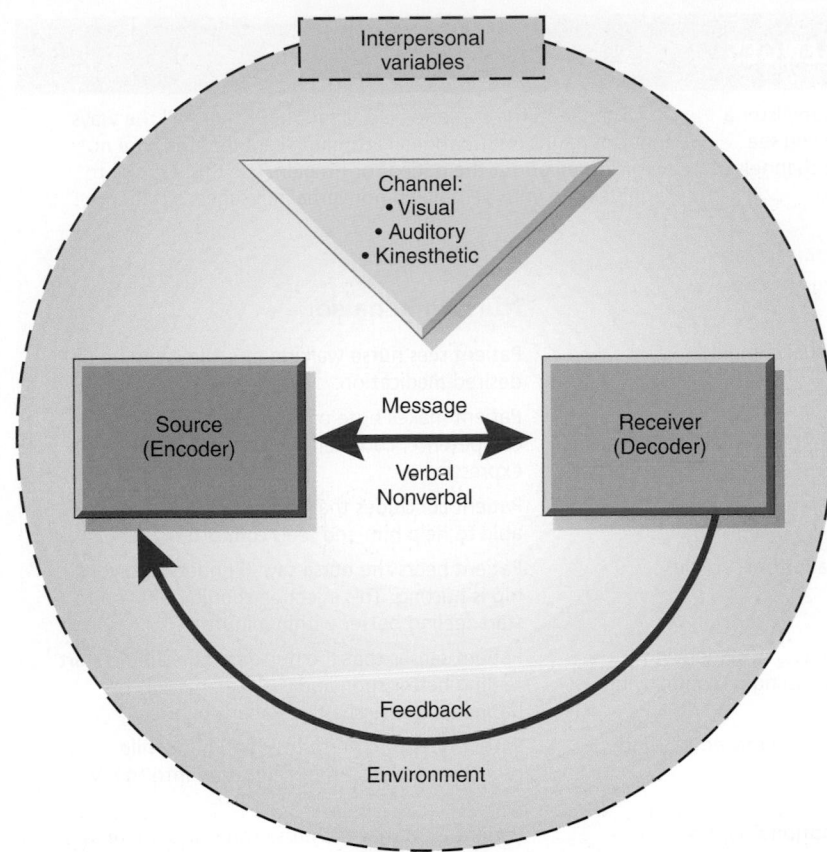

FIGURE 21-1. The various components in the process of communication.

Communication is a reciprocal process in which both the sender and the receiver of messages participate simultaneously. The communication process is illustrated in Figure 21-1. Messages might be influenced on either end by the person's previous knowledge, past experiences, feelings, or sociocultural level.

Test your knowledge of communication by reading the situation in Box 21-1.

FORMS OF COMMUNICATION

The sending and receiving of messages can be accomplished through verbal and nonverbal communication techniques. These can occur separately or simultaneously.

Verbal Communication

Verbal communication is an exchange of information using words, including both the spoken and written word. Verbal communication depends on **language,** or a prescribed way of using words so that people can share information effectively. Language includes a common definition of words and a method of arranging the words in a certain order.

A person's use of written and spoken language forms reveals aspects of the person's intellectual development, educational level, and geographic and ethnic origin. Nurses must also consider if English is a second language for the patient. Language helps nurses assess what the patient knows and feels. In turn, nurses must develop their own language skills to assist in reciprocal responses in the communication process.

> *Think back to Irwina Russellinski, the older adult woman admitted with pneumonia. According to her medical record, the patient speaks "broken English." Therefore, the nurse must incorporate knowledge of this when attempting to communicate verbally with the patient, making adaptations during the interaction to ensure that messages are clear.* ■

Nurses use verbal communication extensively when providing patient care. Aspects of nursing in which this form of communication is imperative include verbal interactions with patients and family, giving oral reports to other nurses, writing care plans, and recording progress in the patient's chart. Other examples of verbal communication include public speaking, writing for publication, and composing signs and posters. Words and language in the previous examples communicate messages to others.

Nonverbal Communication

The transmission of information without the use of words is termed **nonverbal communication,** also known as **body language.** It often helps nurses to understand subtle and hidden meanings in what is being said verbally. For example, a nurse asks the patient, "How do you feel today?" The patient responds, "I feel all right." However, the nurse notes the patient does not maintain eye contact and his facial expression is tense. This would indicate that the nurse should investigate further because of the incongruence of the patient's verbal and nonverbal communication (Fig. 21-2).

Box 21-1 COMMUNICATION CHALLENGES

Picture yourself walking into a patient's room to administer a pain medication by intravenous injection. What do you see yourself communicating through each of the three channels of communication?

Then read the scenario below and think about all the ways nurses might unintentionally communicate that they are not concerned about the patient or his pain. Use this exercise to guide both your verbal and nonverbal messages to patients.

Channel	Mode of Transmission	Outcome	Nursing Behavior
Visual	Sight	Receiving a visual stimulus	Patient sees nurse walking into the room holding desired medication.
	Observation	Interpreting a visual stimulation by making note of nonverbal enhancement	Patient makes note of the nurse's sense of competence, confidence, and sympathetic expression.
	Perception	Assigning meaning to a visual event	Patient concludes that the nurse is willing and able to help him and feels comforted.
Auditory	Hearing	Receiving an auditory stimulus	Patient hears the nurse say, "I understand your hip is hurting. This injection should help you to start feeling better within minutes."
	Listening	Gaining awareness of underlying messages and feelings accompanying auditory events	Patient senses that the nurse said he should start feeling better soon and really wants this to happen because she cares about him.
Kinesthetic	Procedural touch	Performing nursing procedures and techniques	Patient feels the nurse touching him while preparing to inject the medication into the IV access.
	Caring touch	Conveying emotional support	Patient feels that the nurse cares about him as a person when she touches his shoulder upon first entering the room while asking about his pain.

FIGURE 21-2. Eye contact, the lack of it, facial expression, posture, gesture, and silence send nonverbal messages to the receiver. What messages do you receive from each of these photographs?

> *Consider Susie Musashi, the 3-year-old described at the beginning of the chapter. Interpretation of her nonverbal behavior is essential to implementing an effective plan of care. For example, the nurse needs to interpret what her crying indicates such as fear, pain, or loneliness. In addition, the nurse needs to examine the meaning of the child's turning away from the door. Does she want to be left alone? Is she frightened? Once this information is obtained and analyzed, the nurse is better equipped to develop a plan of care to meet the child's needs.* ■

Information is exchanged through nonverbal communication in various ways. It is generally accepted that nonverbal communication expresses more of the true meaning of a message than verbal communication. Therefore, nurses must be aware of both the nonverbal messages they send and the nonverbal messages they receive from patients. Nurses working with patients from diverse cultural backgrounds should attempt to understand cultural variations to avoid misunderstanding nonverbal communication. The various forms of nonverbal communication follow.

Touch

Tactile sense has been studied seriously as a form of nonverbal communication only since the 1960s. Touch is a personal behavior and means different things to different people. Familial, regional, class, and cultural influences largely shape tactile experiences. Factors such as age and sex also play a key role in meanings associated with touch. Despite its individuality, touch is viewed as one of the most effective nonverbal ways to express feelings of comfort, love, affection, security, anger, frustration, aggression, excitement, and many others.

> *Recall Mr. Gordon, the patient with end-stage liver disease who is in a coma. Although the patient may not respond verbally or be able to comprehend, the nurse could use touch to indicate concern and respect for the patient, thus sending a message that someone is there for him.* ■

Eye Contact

Communication often begins with eye contact. A glance, for example, is often an attention-getting method to open conversation. In many cultures, eye contact suggests respect and a willingness to listen and to keep communication open. Its absence often indicates anxiety or defenselessness, or avoidance of communication. Some view eye contact as the nonverbal communication that reveals a person's true nature. However, some Asian and Native American cultures view eye contact as an invasion of an individual's privacy. In other cultures, people are taught to avoid eye contact or, out of respect, not to make eye contact with a superior.

In addition to the messages sent by eye contact, the eyes carry other nonverbal messages. For example, the eyes fix in a stare during anger, tend to narrow in disgust, and ordinarily open wide in fear. Some individuals who experience fear might be unable to speak and only their eyes will send the message of anxiety. A blank stare can indicate daydreaming or inattentiveness.

Facial Expressions

The face is the most expressive part of the body. Examples of the various messages facial expressions convey are anger, joy, suspicion, sadness, fear, and contempt. Some people have extremely expressive faces, whereas others mask their feelings, making it more difficult to determine what the person is really thinking. Nurses need to learn to control their own facial expressions.

> *Take, for example, Susie Musashi, the 3-year-old with burns. Preschoolers are naturally curious. So, she might watch the nurse's reaction when the nurse changes the burn dressings for the first time. Any sign of repulsion or disgust could greatly impact the child's self-image and recovery.* ■

Posture

The way a person holds the body carries nonverbal messages. People in good health and with a positive attitude usually hold their bodies in good alignment. Depressed or tired people are more likely to slouch. Posture also often provides nonverbal clues concerning pain and physical limitations, for instance, a rigid, stiff appearance might be a good indicator of tension and pain.

Gait

A bouncy, purposeful walk usually carries a message of well-being. A less purposeful, shuffling gait often means the person is sad or discouraged. Certain gaits are associated with illness. For example, patients recovering from recent abdominal surgery usually walk slightly bent over and slowly and might need the assistance of handrails or a helping person.

Gestures

Gestures using various parts of the body can carry numerous messages—for example, thumbs up means victory, kicking an object often expresses anger, wringing the hands or tapping a foot usually indicates anxiety or anger, and a waving hand serves to beckon someone to come on, or if waved in another way, signifies that someone should leave. Gestures are often used extensively when two people speaking in different languages attempt to communicate with each other.

> *Remember Mrs. Russellinski, the 75-year-old with pneumonia? Gestures would be very helpful in communicating with the patient, especially in light of the patient's hearing and language deficits.* ■

General Physical Appearance

Most illnesses cause at least some alterations in general physical appearance. Observing for changes in appearance is an important nursing responsibility for detecting illness or evaluating the effectiveness of care and therapy. For example, a person with an insufficient intake of fluids has dry skin that wrinkles easily, eyes that might be sunken and dull in appearance, and poor muscle tone. On the other hand, the person in good health tends to radiate his or her healthy status through general appearance.

Mode of Dress and Grooming

A person's clothing and grooming practices carry significant nonverbal messages. For example, healthy people with high self-esteem tend to pay attention to details of dress and grooming, whereas those with low self-esteem often show much less interest to them. People feeling ill often demonstrate little interest in personal appearance, and it is often a sign of returning health when interest in their physical appearance and mode of dress returns.

Sounds

Crying, moaning, gasping, and sighing are oral but nonverbal forms of communication. Such sounds can be interpreted in numerous ways. For example, a person might cry because of sadness or joy. Gasping often indicates fear, pain, or surprise. A sigh might be a sign of reluctant agreement to do something or of relief.

Silence

Periods of silence during a conversation often carry important nonverbal messages. A silence between two people might indicate complete understanding of each other, that the individuals are thinking, or it might mean that they are angry with each other. Silence and its possible uses and meanings are discussed later in this chapter.

LEVELS OF COMMUNICATION

Throughout our lives and the lives of our patients, communication occurs at varying levels. There are four levels of communication in which nurses engage during practice: intrapersonal communication, interpersonal communication, small-group communication, and organizational communication.

Intrapersonal Communication

Intrapersonal communication, or self-talk, is the communication that happens within the individual. This communication is crucial because it affects the nurse's behavior and has the ability to enhance or detract from positive interactions with the patient and family. Imagine two different nursing students preparing for the first experience with a critically ill patient. Both are frightened. One tells herself, "Calm down, you've been in challenging situations before and always survived. You can handle this." The other repeatedly

tells himself, "There's no way you can survive this experience. The instructor will be all over you, and you might as well admit defeat before you start." Obviously, the first student's positive self-talk is more helpful than that of the second student.

> *Consider Susie Musashi, the 3-year-old receiving treatment for her burns. The nurse would use self-talk when preparing to interact with the child, thereby helping her to focus on the child and her behaviors. In doing so, the nurse may be better able to interpret the child's messages. The nurse might say to herself, "I will use broad opening statements to help the patient and family express their feelings. I will talk to the patient on her level. I must maintain eye contact with the patient and family and answer their questions. I will not make light of the situation or appear unconcerned."* ∎

Understanding the importance of intrapersonal communication can also help you to work with patients and families whose negative self-talk affects their health and self-care abilities.

Interpersonal Communication

Interpersonal communication occurs between two or more people with a goal to exchange messages. Most of the nurse's day is spent communicating with patients, family members, and members of the healthcare team. The ability to communicate effectively at this level will influence your sharing, problem solving, goal attainment, team building, and effectiveness in critical nursing roles (e.g., caregiver, teacher, counselor, leader, manager, patient advocate).

Group Communication

Group communication includes small-group and organizational group communication. When making a determination about the effectiveness or ineffectiveness of a group, one studies the group dynamics.

Small-Group Communication

Small-group communication occurs when nurses interact with two or more individuals. To be functional, members of the small group must communicate to achieve their goal. Some examples of small-group communication include staff meetings, patient care conferences, teaching sessions, or support groups. The more people involved in the communication process, the more complex it becomes.

Organizational Communication

Organizational communication occurs when individuals and groups within an organization communicate to achieve established goals. Nurses on a practice council meeting to review unit policies, or nurses working with interdisciplinary groups on strategic planning or quality assurance will use organizational communication to achieve their aims.

Group Dynamics

When making a determination about the effectiveness or ineffectiveness of a group, one studies the group dynamics. **Group dynamics** can be described most simply as how individual group members relate to one another during the process of working toward group goals.

Although effective leadership facilitates a group's achievement of its goals, success or failure is largely a function of its members' behavior. Ideally, each group member uses his or her talents and interpersonal strengths to help the group to accomplish its goals. The group's ability to function at a high level depends on each member's sensitivity to the needs of the group and its individual members. Effective groups possess members who are mutually respectful. If a group member dominates or thwarts the group process, then the leader or other group members must confront the member to promote the needed collegial relationship. Effective and ineffective groups are contrasted in Table 21-1. Individual group-member roles can be categorized in one of three ways:

1. *Task-oriented roles,* focusing on the work to be done. For example, information giver, information seeker, clarifier, coordinator, delegator, energizer, or evaluator
2. *Group-building or maintenance roles,* focusing on the well-being of people doing the work. For example, active listener, harmonizer, trust builder, tension reliever, or supporter
3. *Self-serving roles,* which advance the needs of individual members at the group's expense. For example, attention seeker, dominator, blocker, special pleader, withdrawer, or aggressor

Think about groups in which you are a member, and identify the roles that you and other members play.

FACTORS INFLUENCING COMMUNICATION

Factors influencing communication include level of development; gender; sociocultural differences; roles and responsibilities; space and territoriality; physical, mental, and emotional state; and environment.

Developmental Level

The rate of language development is directly correlated with the patient's neurologic competence and cognitive development. Thus, it is helpful to understand the process of language development and the stages of intellectual and psychosocial development. This understanding assists in your ability to communicate effectively with patients and family of all age ranges.

> *Remember Susie Musashi, the 3-year-old child with burns? The nurse would incorporate knowledge of the typical preschooler fears (such as fear of new places and fear of*

TABLE • 21-1	CHARACTERISTICS OF EFFECTIVE AND INEFFECTIVE GROUPS	
Variable	**Effective Group**	**Ineffective Group**
Group identity	Members value and "own" the aims of the group; aims are clearly articulated	Group's aims are not of major importance to members
Cohesiveness	Members generally trust and like one another and are loyal to the group; high commitment; high degree of cooperation	Members often feel alienated from the group and from one another; low commitment; members tend to work better alone than with the group
Patterns of interaction	Honest, direct communication flows freely; members support, praise, and critique one another	Communication is sparing; little self-disclosure; self-serving roles (i.e., dominator, blocker, or aggressor) may be unchecked
Decision making	Problems are identified, appropriate method of decision making is used (i.e., individual, minority, majority, consensus, or unanimous); decision is implemented and followed through; group commitment to decision is high	Problems are allowed to build without resolution; little responsibility is shown for problem solving; group commitment to decision is low
Responsibility	Members feel strong sense of responsibility for group outcomes	Little responsibility for group felt by group members
Leadership	Effective style of leadership to meet desired aims	Ineffective leadership styles
Power	Sources of power are recognized and used appropriately; needs or interests of those with little power are considered	Power is used and abused to "fix" immediate problems; little attention to needs of powerless

the dark) when developing the child's plan of care. Preschoolers gain self-esteem by receiving compliments about their appearance. The presence of the burns directly affects the child's appearance, possibly threatening self-esteem. Therefore, the nurse also needs to consider the child's current fears related to her burns and burn treatment and their effect on the child's self-esteem. ■

The stages of development are presented in Chapters 18, 19, and 20. Knowing how each age group commonly perceives health, illness, and body functions should guide your interactions with your patients. For instance, a 10-year-old child has limited understanding of what an infection is; therefore, explain things in simple terms so that the child cooperates with the treatment without being frightened. Because adolescents are developing abstract thinking, more detailed and accurate explanations can be given to them. Being familiar with commonly used slang usually helps when communicating with adolescents. Communicating with adults can be affected by years of positive or negative health-related experiences and by inaccurate information. When communicating with older patients, assess for any problems with hearing or sight (discussed later in this chapter), confusion, or depression, any of which could affect nurse–patient interaction.

Gender

Men and women possess differing communication styles and might give different interpretations to the same conversation. Tannen (1990) believes that this is because girls and boys grow up communicating differently. Whereas girls generally play with "best friends" and use language to seek confirmation, minimize differences, and establish or reinforce intimacy, boys use language to establish their independence and to negotiate status activities in large groups. In contrast, Townsend (2009) states that gender roles are changing in American society because sexual roles are becoming less distinct. Factors contributing to this change are the use of the term "unisex" within our language and the fact women and men enter professions previously dominated by the other sex. It is necessary to be sensitive to the fact that men and women might communicate differently. As such, when working with patients of the opposite gender, you'll need to validate that both you and your patient are accurately receiving the message the other is trying to communicate.

Sociocultural Differences

Nurses need to develop skills in recognizing the ways in which culture, economic condition, and overall lifestyle influence a patient's preferred mode of communicating. This helps in understanding what the patient understands.

Culture refers to the common lifestyles, languages, behavior patterns, traditions, and beliefs that are learned and passed from one generation to the next. The first step toward cultural competence requires becoming aware of your own personal cultural beliefs and identifying "prejudices or attitudes that

could be a barrier to good communication" (Pullen, 2007). Likewise, understanding a patient's culture assists in understanding nonverbal communication and enables the delivery of accurate nursing care to the patient and family. For example, women in some cultures might speak of personal things only to their spouses. For this reason, a maternal care nurse might talk with the patient's husband about the woman's postdelivery care.

The healthcare system is a culture with its own customs, values, and language. Try to remain aware of these cultural variations and be careful to use lay terminology when speaking with patients, unless the patient is known to be a healthcare professional. Use of medical terminology (e.g., myocardial infarction for heart attack, cerebrovascular accident for stroke [brain attack], or cholecystectomy for gall bladder operation) usually alienates patients and can inhibit further communication. A patient's language proficiency should be evaluated upon admission to a healthcare facility and medical interpreters should be available to facilitate any communication and improve the quality of care (Oliva, 2008).

Roles and Responsibilities

A person's occupation might give the nurse a general supposition of his or her abilities, talents, interests, and economic status. Stereotyping a person according to occupation, however, can be misleading and should be avoided. This can be particularly dangerous when nurses assume that patients who are healthcare professionals know everything about their condition and need little nursing assistance, teaching, and counseling. The challenge in the provision of care is to respect the patient's roles and responsibilities, especially because these influence their preferred manner of communicating, without denying the patient needed care. For example, a successful attorney might have a "take-charge" demeanor and seem utterly self-sufficient; a skilled nurse will note this but still provide an opening for the patient to verbalize his or her needs. "You seem well prepared for this procedure and in control, but I know that patients often have questions that never get answered or fears that remain unvoiced. Is there anything I can help you with while I'm here?" Similarly, be careful not to ignore an uncomplaining patient who never asks for anything, because the power differences in the healthcare-professional–patient relationship may make communication intimidating.

Space and Territoriality

Individuals are most comfortable in areas they consider their own. We generally feel relief when we come home, take our shoes and professional's clothes off, and relax. This urge to maintain an exclusive right to certain space is termed territoriality. You might have already noticed that patients behave differently when being interviewed in their homes, at a health fair in the mall, or in an institutional setting. Similarly, healthcare professionals might behave differently when they are "on their own turf" in a healthcare setting compared to when they enter a patient's home as a guest caregiver. It is important to understand how territoriality influences the nurse–patient relationship.

The actual physical difference between the nurse and patient during interaction is also important. Each person has a sense of how much personal or private space is needed and what distance between individuals is optimum. Some of this is dictated through culture and some is idiosyncratic. Anywhere from 18 inches to 4 feet might be optimal distance to sit from a patient during an intake interview. For example, European Americans and African Americans require more personal space between two people who are speaking whereas other cultures (Mediterranean, Hispanic, Asian, Middle Eastern, East Indian) are comfortable with a closer interval when speaking (Videbeck, 2008). It is best to take cues from patients, noting whether they are moving backward from you if you are too near or leaning forward to get closer to you. Because many nursing interventions place one in proximity to a patient and entail forced intimacy, it is crucial to develop sensitivity to how offensive this might be to certain patients who are accustomed to large areas of private space. Develop the habit of seeking the patient's permission before touching areas within a patient's private zones. Although most people consider their hands, arms, shoulders, and back within a social zone, increasing levels of privacy are according to (1) mouth and feet; (2) face, neck, and front of body; and (3) genitalia.

Physical, Mental, and Emotional State

The degree to which people are physically comfortable and mentally and emotionally free to engage in interactions also influences communication. A full bladder, a dull headache, crushing chest pain, anxiety about a pending diagnosis, or concern about what is happening at home or at work, and fear can all negatively influence communication. For example, a patient who thinks that a nurse wants to hurt him or her will be difficult to interview. It is important to develop sensitivity to the physical, mental, and emotional barriers to effective communication.

Cognitively impaired patients present special communication challenges. For example, an elderly patient who has aphasia and is agitated due to pain from an abscessed tooth might be unable to communicate with the nurse.

The accompanying box, Examples of Nursing Interventions and Nursing Outcomes Classifications (NIC/NOC), suggests helpful cognitive stimulation activities and expected outcomes when communicating with these patients.

> ➤ *Remember Irwina Russellinski, the 75-year-old woman who was described as "being pleasantly confused" at times and requiring a nursing assessment? The patient's level of confusion would present challenges for the nurse when eliciting information for the nursing history. This challenge could be further complicated by the patient's difficulty speaking English. The nurse would need to speak clearly, distinctly, and in terms that the patient would understand. In addition, the nurse would need to allow ample time for the patient to respond and explore other sources for needed information.* ■

Values

Communication is influenced by the way people value themselves, one another, and the purpose of any human interaction.

Examples of Nursing Interventions and Nursing Outcomes Classifications (NIC/NOC)

Cognitive Stimulation Activities and Cognitive Orientation

Nursing Interventions	Nursing Outcomes

• Consult with family to establish patient's preinjury cognitive baseline.
• Inform patient of nonthreatening news events.
• Offer environmental stimulation through contact with varied personnel.
• Provide a calendar.
• Orient to time, place, and person.
• Provide planned sensory stimulation.
• Use TV, radio, or music as part of planned stimuli program.
• Reinforce or repeat information.
• Present information in small, concrete portions.
• Provide verbal and written instruction.
	• Cognitive Orientation
	  • Identifies significant current events.
	  • Identifies self.
	  • Identifies significant other.
	  • Identifies current place.
	  • Identifies current day.
	  • Identifies current month.
	  • Identifies current year.

Bulechek, G., Butcher, H., & Dochterman, J. (2008). *Nursing interventions classification (NIC)* (5th ed., p. 224). St. Louis: Mosby, Inc. A full listing of nursing activities for each nursing intervention can be found in this book.

Moorhead, S., Johnson, M., Maas, M., & Swanson, E. (2008). *Nursing outcomes classification (NOC)* (4th ed., p. 279). St. Louis: Mosby, Inc. A full listing of indicators for each nursing outcome can be found in this book.

Nurses who believe that teaching is an important aspect of nursing and who value empowering patients will communicate this to patients. Conversely, a nurse who believes teaching is an unimportant chore is unlikely to be an effective teacher. Similarly, the patient's motivation (or lack of motivation) to develop new self-care behaviors cannot help but influence nurse–patient communication.

Environment

Communication happens best when the environment facilitates an easy exchange of needed information. The environment most conducive to communication is one that is calm and nonthreatening. The goal is to minimize distractions and ensure privacy. The use of music, art, and interior design decorations might assist in placing the patient at ease. A patient with newly diagnosed human immunodeficiency virus (HIV) infection will find it difficult to discuss sexual history or genital warts in an area that lacks privacy. A toddler might find it easier to communicate if a parent, favorite stuffed animal, or blanket is nearby.

USING THERAPEUTIC COMMUNICATION IN THE NURSING PROCESS

The ability to communicate with patients and with other nurses is essential for effective use of the nursing process. (See the accompanying Research in Nursing box.) Knowledge of the communication process and of effective communication techniques is fundamental to all steps of the nursing process. At the same time, the nursing process provides the guidance and direction needed to communicate with patients effectively.

Assessing

The major focus of assessment is to gather information in both verbal and nonverbal communication forms. The written word is used to obtain data concerning patients and when reading a patient's records or charts before meeting them. The spoken word is used to give and to receive reports to and from other health personnel. This is commonplace when admitting a patient to a hospital unit or before visiting the patient at home. One-to-one communication is used with patients to obtain thorough nursing histories and physical

RESEARCH IN NURSING
Bridging the Gap to Evidence-Based Practice

DETERMINING BEST COMMUNICATION PRACTICES WITH FAMILIES THAT IMPROVE END-OF-LIFE CARE IN NURSING HOMES

With a growing number of older adults residing in nursing homes, facilities need to be aware of measures that improve the quality of care in end-of-life situations. In addition to the care given to the resident, family members also need support and care as they experience the loss of a loved one. In many cases, the residents are unable to provide any feedback on care, and family members interact regularly with staff and are the main determinants of satisfaction with care. Most research regarding end-of-life care and communication with family members has occurred in hospice settings. Very little information is available regarding satisfaction with care and families' communication needs in a nursing home setting. This qualitative study sought to provide caregivers with research regarding effective communication measures for this situation in a nursing home situation.

Related Research

Thompson, G., Menec, V., Chochinov, H., & McClement, S. (2008). Family satisfaction with care of a dying loved one in nursing homes: What makes the difference? *Journal of Gerontological Nursing, 34*(12), 37–44.

If accurate information is available regarding the communication preferences of family members, specific information can be provided and individualized as family members cope with a dying loved one in the nursing home setting. This research was conducted with focus groups from 12 nursing homes located in an urban area of central Canada. Candidates who agreed to participate were placed in one of two groups: those satisfied or those dissatisfied with the care their family mem-

ber received. Satisfaction was measured using the modified Toolkit of Instruments to Measure End-of-Life Care (TIME) available at: http://www.chcr.brown.edu/pcoc/toolkit.htm. One focus group (n=6) was composed of those dissatisfied with care while two focus groups (each n=8) were satisfied with care. The prevailing determinant of satisfaction with care was the fact that staff recognized and acknowledged to the family the terminal status of the resident. Once this was recognized, staff members engaged family members in discussions related to what to expect at the end of life and alterations in the plan of care. Dissatisfied family members reported that they were not adequately informed regarding the progression of the resident's illness and that all caregivers were not aware of this change of status. Inadequate communication with physicians was mentioned as a concern by both groups. This current research demonstrates that effective communication by nurses and intervention with residents' families plays a significant role in determining their satisfaction with care.

Relevance to Nursing Practice

Long-term care nurses have a responsibility to residents and their families to provide accurate, timely care that limits undue suffering and dissatisfaction with care. Communication with family that indicates the imminent death of a loved one, frequent updates on the resident's condition, and attention to pain and symptom management contribute to quality end-of-life care. This level of care better prepared families for the actual death whenever it occurred.

For additional research, visit thePoint.

examinations. Effective communication techniques, as well as observational skills, are used extensively during this phase. The data collected verbally and nonverbally are analyzed and then passed on to the appropriate people through oral and written communication.

Diagnosing

Following the formulation of the nursing diagnoses, you'll communicate findings to other nursing professionals through the use of the written and spoken word. The written diagnosis becomes a permanent part of the patient's record.

Outcome Identification and Planning

The planning step requires communication among the patient, nurse, and other team members as mutually agreed-upon outcomes are developed and interventions are determined. Because a nurse is rarely able to implement all parts of a plan alone, oral and written communication is needed to inform others of what needs to be done to meet the set objectives or goals. The formal written plan of care is a form of communication. Without communication, the nursing plan could not be implemented.

Implementing

Nurses assume many roles when they implement the plan of care. Verbal and nonverbal communication are employed to enhance basic caregiving measures and to teach, counsel, and support patients and their families during the implementation phase. Even a simple nursing order, such as "encourage patient to drink 100 mL of fluid every hour while awake," requires countless messages to be sent and received between you and the patient. You'll need to explain the importance of an adequate fluid intake, along with the amount and frequency of intake. The patient, in turn, informs you of his or her ability or inability to meet targeted objectives. The patient's verbal and nonverbal messages are assessed during each nurse–patient interaction. The implementation of the plan of care is then documented in the patient's record.

Evaluating

Nurses often rely on the verbal and nonverbal cues they receive from their patients to verify whether patient objectives or goals have been achieved. Communication, through the exchange of positive and negative messages between the nurse and the patient, also facilitates the revision of parts of the care plan.

Documenting Communication

Continual assessment of the patient's needs and conditions requires accurate documentation in the appropriate place, unless the information is confidential. This documentation helps promote the continuity of care given by nurses and other healthcare providers. Because one nurse cannot provide 24-hour coverage for patients, significant information must be passed on to others through nursing progress notes and care plans. Documentation and the use of electronic communication are discussed in detail in Chapter 17.

Hand-off Communication: SBAR Technique

Hand-off communication involves the accurate presentation of all patient-related information to another caregiver (Mascioli, Laskowski-Jones, Urban, & Moran, 2009). It may include communication with other hospital departments, nurse-to-nurse report, or nurse-to-physician discussions. In an effort to eliminate breakdowns in communication and potential adverse events, the Joint Commission (TJC) has mandated a National Patient Safety Goal that requires organizations to "implement a standardized approach to hand-off communications, including an opportunity to ask and respond to questions" (TJC, 2008). Both TJC and the Institute for Healthcare Improvement (IHI) have recommended the use of SBAR reports to improve hand-off communication. **SBAR,** which stands for **S**ituation, **B**ackground, **A**ssessment, and **R**ecommendations, provides a consistent method for hand-off communication that is clear, structured, and easy to use. This technique was originally developed by the U.S. Navy to accurately transmit critical information and then implemented by healthcare personnel at Kaiser Permanente in Colorado (Hohenhaus, Powell, & Hohenhaus, 2006). The S (Situation) and B (Background) provide objective data, whereas the A (Assessment) and R (Recommendations) allow for presentation of subjective information. The SBAR format can be modified to meet the specific situations related to shift report, conversations with physicians, and transfer of patients. Figure 21-3 provides an example of SBAR communication between a nurse and physician.

The SBAR technique has been adopted by a significant number of hospitals, but this new form of communication requires education and practice by nurses and physicians. Some methods of education include the use of posters, stickers on phones, peer observation, and inclusion of SBAR in orientation and safety training. Research on the effectiveness of SBAR communication is limited, and more studies are needed. One study reported a reduction in adverse events and improvement in medication reconciliation procedures (Pope, Rodzen, & Spross, 2007). Using SBAR is another tool that enables nurses to communicate in a collegial, collaborative manner with the focus on patient safety.

USING THERAPEUTIC COMMUNICATION IN THE HELPING RELATIONSHIP

Nurses and other healthcare personnel enter healthcare in order to help people. Relationships between healthcare providers and patients are not accomplished randomly, but through purposeful communication. A **helping relationship** exists among people who provide and receive assistance in meeting human needs. It sets the climate for the participants to move towards common goals. Therefore, need gratification occurs as the result of a successful helping relationship.

S	<u>Situation</u>
	I am calling about <u><patient name and location></u>.
	The patient's code status is <u><code status></u>
	The problem I am calling about is _____.
	           (e.g., I am afraid the patient is going to arrest.)
	
	I have just assessed the patient personally:
	
	Vital signs are: Blood pressure _____/_____, Pulse _____, Respiration_____, and Temperature _____
	
	I am concerned about the:
	        Blood pressure because it is over 200 or less than 100 or 30 mmHg below usual
	        Pulse because it is over 140 or less than 50
	        Respiration because it is less than 5 or over 40.
	        Temperature because it is less than 96 or over 104.

B	<u>Background</u>
	The patient's mental status is:
	        Alert and oriented to person place and time.
	        Confused and cooperative or noncooperative
	        Agitated or combative
	        Lethargic but conversant and able to swallow
	        Stuporous and not talking clearly and possibly not able to swallow
	        Comatose. Eyes closed. Not responding to stimulation.
	The skin is:
	        Warm and dry
	        Pale
	        Mottled
	        Diaphoretic
	        Extremities are cold
	        Extremities are warm
	The patient is not or is on oxygen.
	        The patient has been on _____ (l/min) or (%) oxygen for _____ minutes (hours)
	        The oximeter is reading _____%
	        The oximeter does not detect a good pulse and is giving erratic readings.

A	<u>Assessment</u>
	        This is what I think the problem is: <u><say what you think is the problem></u>
	        The problem seems to be cardiac infection neurologic respiratory _____
	        I am not sure what the problem is but the patient is deteriorating.
	        The patient seems to be unstable and may get worse, we need to do something.

R	<u>Recommendation</u>
	I suggest or request that you <u><say what you would like to see done></u>.
	        Transfer the patient to critical care.
	        Come to see the patient at this time.
	        Talk to the patient or family about code status.
	        Ask the on-call family practice resident to see the patient now.
	        Ask for a consultant to see the patient now.
	Are any tests needed:
	        Do you need any tests like CXR, ABG, EKG, CBC, or BMP?
	        Others?
	If a change in treatment is ordered then ask:
	        How often do you want vital signs?
	        How long to you expect this problem will last?
	        If the patient does not get better, when would you want us to call again?

This SBAR tool was developed by Kaiser Permanente. Please feel free to use and reproduce these materials in the spirit of patient safety, and please retain this footer in the spirit of appropriate recognition.

FIGURE 21-3. SBAR report to physician about a critical situation. (From Institute for Healthcare Improvement. Available at http://www.ihi.org/IHI/Topics/PatientSafety/SafetyGeneral/Tools/SBARTechniqueforCommunicationASituationalBriefingModel.htm.)

FIGURE 21-4. A helping relationship between the nurse and patient sets the climate for participants to move toward common goals.

In this book, the term is used to refer to helping relationships between nurses and patients (Fig. 21-4).

When a nurse and patient are involved in a helping relationship, sometimes called the nurse–patient relationship, the nurse is the helper, and the patient is the person being helped. The quality of the relationship between these individuals is the most significant element in determining helping effectiveness. "Of all the problems that can arise in nursing care, perhaps the most common is failure to establish rapport and a helping–trust relationship with the other person" (Watson, 1985, p. 24). Communication is the means used to establish rapport and helping–trust relationships.

A Helping Relationship Versus a Social Relationship

The difference between a helping relationship and a friendship is important. Helping relationships contain many of the qualities of a social relationship—they have in common the components of care, concern, trust, and growth. They are also very different:

- The helping relationship does not occur spontaneously, as do most social relationships. It occurs for a specific purpose with a specific person.
- The helping relationship is characterized by an unequal sharing of information. The patient shares information related to personal health problems, whereas the nurse shares information in terms of a professional role. In a friendship, information sharing is more likely to be similar in quantity and type.
- The helping relationship is built on the patient's needs, not on those of the helping person. In a friendship, needs of both participants are generally considered. A friendship might grow out of a helping relationship, but this is separate from the purposeful, time-limited interaction described as a helping relationship.

It is of great importance to remember that helping relations are professional relationships. It can be helpful to identify nurse models who, through their appearance, demeanor,

and behavior, communicate a clear sense of **professionalism** or confidence and expertise in their practice. Patients and the public are more likely to trust and value nurses who appear competent and confident and who are focused on the patients entrusted to their care. Rudeness, sloppiness, inattention to person, sexually inappropriate behavior, and other breaches of professionalism undermine nursing's professional image and the effectiveness of individual nurses.

> *Think back to Mr. Gordon, the patient described in the Reflective Practice display, and consider the behavior of the nurse and residents caring for the patient. Unfortunately, their focus was not on the patient as a whole, but, rather, on the patient's devices and technologic equipment. The nurse would need to keep in mind the highly technical nature of the intensive care unit and work to implement a plan of care that focuses on the "whole" patient.* ■

Characteristics of the Helping Relationship

The helping relationship is intangible and, therefore, difficult to describe. Most authorities agree, however, that it has at least the following three basic characteristics:

- It is dynamic. Both the person providing the assistance and the person being helped are active participants to the extent each is able.
- It is purposeful and time limited. This means there are specific goals that are intended to be met within a certain period.
- Although both parties in the helping relationship have responsibilities, the person providing the assistance is professionally accountable for the outcomes of the relationship and the means used to attain them. The helping person should present his or her helping abilities as honestly as possible and not promise to provide more assistance than he or she can offer.

Goals of the Helping Relationship

The goals of a helping relationship between a nurse and a patient are determined cooperatively and are defined in terms of the patient's needs. Broadly speaking, common goals might include increased independence for the patient, greater feelings of worth, and improved health and well-being. Selected nursing interventions will help the person move toward the goal. As the patient's needs and goals change, so do the nursing care interventions implemented to attain the patient's goals. You might also have many needs to be met, but in the helping relationship between the nurse and the patient, those are temporarily set aside, and the focus is on the patient's needs.

Phases of the Helping Relationship

The helping relationship is ordinarily described as having three phases: (1) the orientation phase, (2) the working phase,

<table>
<tr><td>

Box 21-2 **SUMMARY OF PATIENT GOALS FOR THE THREE PHASES OF THE HELPING RELATIONSHIP**

Orientation Phase
- The patient will call the nurse by name.
- The patient will accurately describe the roles of the participants in the relationship.
- The patient and nurse will establish an agreement about:
  - Goals of the relationship
  - Location, frequency, and length of the contacts
  - Duration of the relationship

Working Phase
- The patient will actively participate in the relationship.
- The patient will cooperate in activities that work toward achieving mutually acceptable goals.
- The patient will express feelings and concerns to the nurse.

Termination
- The patient will participate in identifying the goals accomplished or the progress made toward goals.
- The patient will verbalize feelings about the termination of the relationship.

</td></tr>
</table>

and (3) the termination phase. In the helping relationship, the communication process follows the sequence of the nursing process. Both processes are continuous and reciprocal. Box 21-2 summarizes goals for patients during the three phases of an effective helping relationship. In some situations, one nurse initiates the helping relationship and works with the patient and family through to termination. More often (e.g., in hospital settings), there are different nurses at different times implementing different phases of the relationship. In preparation for the orientation phase, you might use interpersonal communication to prepare for the data-gathering phase of the interaction with the patient.

Orientation Phase

The helping relationship ideally begins between the nurse and patient during the data-gathering part of the nursing process. It can also be initiated at other times during the nurse–patient relationship. In the orientation phase, the tone and guidelines for the relationship are established. You and the patient meet and learn to identify each other by name. It is especially important to introduce yourself to the patient; it might even be helpful to write your name for the patient. Failure to do so might result in the patient becoming confused and mistrustful because of the number of caregivers with whom most patients come in contact.

The following activities generally occur during the orientation phase of the helping relationship:

- The roles of both people in the relationship are clarified. A successful relationship is more likely to occur when each participant's responsibilities are known and accepted and when the nurse, by virtue of role, generally assumes leadership. Leadership does not mean control in a restrictive or manipulative sense but, rather, involves taking the initiative

to enlist the patient's point of view. When cooperative planning occurs with consideration for the patient's needs, the nurse–patient relationship is more likely to be mutually satisfactory.

- An agreement or contract about the relationship is established. The agreement is usually a simple verbal exchange or, occasionally, a written document, especially if the relationship extends over a long period of time. Elements in the agreement include the goals of the relationship; location, frequency, and length of the contacts; and duration of the relationship. The agreement might also include the way in which personal information that the patient divulges will be handled.

- The patient is provided with an orientation to the healthcare facility, its services, admission routines, and any pertinent information the patient requires to decrease anxiety. This orientation should be identified as one of the goals in the nurse–patient helping relationship.

The development of a trusting relationship is critical to the development of the nurse–patient relationship. During the orientation phase, the patient might engage in behavior to test the nursing and healthcare staff. This might occur if the patient or family previously had negative healthcare experiences. Exhibiting openness and interest in the concerns of the patient paves the way for developing trust and communicating care and respect.

Working Phase

The working phase is usually the longest phase of the helping relationship. During this phase, you will work together with the patient to meet the patient's physical and psychosocial needs. Interaction is the essence of the working phase. Nurse–patient interactions that occur at this time are purposeful in that they are designed to ensure achievement of health goals or objectives that were mutually agreed upon.

As examples of the working phase, the nurse provides whatever assistance might be needed to achieve each goal. For example, if an older patient has a poor appetite and the goal is to increase food intake, the nurse discusses the idea of small, more frequent meals with the patient. With the patient's approval, the nurse makes the necessary arrangements. In another instance, a mother explains to a school nurse that she cannot afford the dental care recommended for her child, although she would like to have the work done. The nurse asks if a referral to a social agency for financial assistance would be acceptable. With the mother's permission, the nurse contacts the agency.

When sentiments and feelings between people are unsatisfactory, these people often cannot work cooperatively toward achieving a common goal. When sentiments and feelings are satisfactory, they can usually work together. In the preceding examples, satisfactory sentiments and feelings between the nurse and patients might be the key aspects. The older person's relationship with the nurse might allow a positive response to the small, more frequent meals. The mother's feelings about the nurse might allow her to accept financial assistance for dental care without feeling embarrassed.

In addition, the nurse as caregiver provides the patient with whatever assistance might be needed to perform activities of daily living. For example, if a patient with impaired mobility is unable to get out of bed except to use a bedside commode, the nurse needs to help with daily hygiene.

The nursing roles of teacher and counselor (see Chapter 22) are performed primarily during this phase. These roles involve motivating the patient to learn and to implement health promotion activities, to facilitate the patient's ability to execute the plan of care, and to express feelings about health problems, nursing care, any progress or setbacks, and any other areas of concern. This is where your interpersonal skills are used to their fullest (see the discussions of interpersonal skills and effective communication techniques later in this chapter). A breakdown of the helping relationship on one of these levels could result in serious consequences. For instance, a patient begins to break clinic appointments, although he previously seemed to be interested in his health when he visited the clinic. "The nurse at the clinic seems too busy; she doesn't seem to care if I come or go to that clinic." The lack of satisfactory interaction between the nurse and the patient discouraged him from continuing the relationship, even at the expense of his health. Had the nurse–patient interaction been satisfactory, the problem most likely would not have occurred.

Satisfactory interaction preserves people's integrity while promoting an atmosphere characterized by minimal fear, anxiety, distrust, and tension. People feel harmonious and contented with each other as they work cooperatively to reach common goals.

Termination Phase

The termination phase occurs when the conclusion of the initial agreement is acknowledged. This might happen at change-of-shift time, when the patient is discharged, or when a nurse leaves on vacation or for employment elsewhere. At this point, you'll examine with the patient the goals of the helping relationship for indications of their attainment or for evidence of progress toward them. If the goals/outcomes have been reached, this fact should be acknowledged. Such acknowledgment generally results in a feeling of satisfaction for the patient and nurse. If the goals/outcomes have not been reached, the progress can be acknowledged and either the patient or you might make suggestions for future efforts.

Ordinarily, emotions are associated with the termination of a helping relationship. If the goals have been met, there is often regret about ending a satisfying relationship, even though a sense of accomplishment persists. If the goals have not been achieved, the patient might experience anxiety and fear about the future. Whatever the feelings, the patient should be encouraged to express his or her emotions about the termination.

You can prepare for the termination of the helping relationship in various ways. It is thoughtful to set the stage for the patient to establish a helping relationship with another nurse, if appropriate. You can also assist the patient transferring from one agency to another or from one unit in an agency to another by offering explanations concerning the transfer. In some instances, you might introduce the patient to personnel who will be giving care.

Occasionally, termination of the helping relationship causes a negative emotional reaction. The patient might feel angry, rejected by the nurse, or depressed and helpless, or might deny that a relationship ever really existed. If such a reaction occurs, try to help and to support the patient rather than make him or her feel bad or guilty for having such a view. Emotional reactions of this sort are less likely to occur, however, if the patient has been involved in establishing goals and has been helped to anticipate termination of the helping relationship.

Interpersonal relations are discussed in greater detail in the classic works of nursing theorists Orlando (1961), Paterson and Zderad (1976), Peplau (1952), Travelbee (1971), and Watson (1985).

Factors Promoting Effective Communication Within the Helping Relationship

Despite the fact that patient stays in healthcare facilities are shorter and there is an increased reliance on technology, therapeutic communication with patients and their families is essential and remains a vital part of a helping relationship. Nurses who are competent, honest, skilled communicators are viewed as effective and compassionate caregivers. This focus on helping relationships is a critical component of what nurses do and plays a vital role in promoting healing, enhancing safety, and improving clinical outcomes.

Dispositional Traits

A dispositional trait is a characteristic or customary way of behaving. Nurses who consistently demonstrate warmth and friendliness; openness and rapport; empathy, honesty, authenticity and trust; caring; and competence are well disposed to communicate effectively.

WARMTH AND FRIENDLINESS

The helping relationship depends on the nurse's ability to begin the orientation phase successfully. A pleasant greeting and friendly smile can facilitate this phase and place the patient at ease. By maintaining qualities of warmth and friendliness throughout the helping relationship, you will convey continuous acceptance of the patient and interest in discussing the patient's feelings and concern.

OPENNESS AND RESPECT

One key factor to effective communication is to be open, accepting, frank, respectful, and without prejudice. When a patient feels that a nurse is being judgmental, he or she might withhold significant information. You need to develop sensitivity to the unique challenges presented by each patient. Attention to patient variables that might influence the process of communicating (e.g., gender, developmental level, culture, life experience) can make the difference between effective and

Box 21-3   RELATING TO PATIENTS FROM DIFFERENT CULTURES

Assess your personal beliefs surrounding people from different cultures.
- Review your personal beliefs and past experiences.
- Set aside any values, biases, ideas, and attitudes that are judgmental and may negatively affect care.

Assess communication variables from a cultural perspective.
- Determine the ethnic identity of the patient, including generation in America.
- Use the patient as a source of information when possible.
- Assess cultural factors that may affect your relationship with the patient and respond appropriately.

Plan care based on the communicated needs and cultural background.
- Learn as much as possible about the patient's cultural customs and beliefs.
- Encourage the patient to reveal cultural interpretation of health, illness, and healthcare.
- Be sensitive to the uniqueness of the patient.
- Identify sources of discrepancy between the patient's and your own concepts of health and illness.
- Communicate at the patient's personal level of functioning.
- Evaluate effectiveness of nursing actions and modify nursing care plan when necessary.

Modify communication approaches to meet cultural needs.
- Be attentive to signs of fear, anxiety, and confusion in the patient.
- Respond in a reassuring manner in keeping with the patient's cultural orientation.
- Be aware that in some cultural groups, discussion concerning the patient with others may be offensive and may impede the nursing process.

Understand that respect for the patient and communicated needs is central to the therapeutic relationship.
- Communicate respect by using a kind and attentive approach.
- Learn how listening is communicated in the patient's culture.

- Use appropriate active listening techniques.
- Adopt an attitude of flexibility, respect, and interest to help bridge barriers imposed by culture.

Communicate in a nonthreatening manner.
- Conduct the interview in an unhurried manner.
- Follow acceptable social and cultural amenities.
- Ask general questions during the information-gathering stage.
- Be patient with a respondent who gives information that may seem unrelated to the patient's health problem.
- Develop a trusting relationship by listening carefully, allowing time, and giving the patient your full attention.

Use validating techniques in communication.
- Be alert for feedback that the patient is not understanding.
- Do not assume meaning is interpreted without distortion.

Be considerate of reluctance to talk when the subject involves sexual matters.
- Be aware that in some cultures, sexual matters are not discussed freely with members of the opposite sex.

Adopt special approaches when the patient speaks a different language.
- Use a caring tone of voice and facial expression to help alleviate the patient's fears.
- Speak slowly and distinctly, but not loudly.
- Use gestures, pictures, and play acting to help the patient understand.
- Repeat the message in different ways if necessary.
- Be alert to words the patient seems to understand and use them frequently.
- Keep messages simple and repeat them frequently.
- Avoid using medical terms and abbreviations that the patient may not understand.
- Use an appropriate language dictionary.

Use interpreters to improve communication.
- Ask the interpreter to translate the message, not just the individual words.
- Obtain feedback to confirm understanding.
- Use an interpreter who is culturally sensitive.

Used with permission from Gieger, J. N., & Davidhizar, R. E. (2008). *Transcultural nursing: Assessment and intervention* (5th ed.). St. Louis: Mosby.

ineffective interactions. Box 21-3 highlights guidelines for relating to patients from different cultures (see also Chapter 2).

EMPATHY

Empathy is identifying with the way another person feels. An empathic nurse is sensitive to the patient's feelings and problems, but remains objective enough to help the patient work to attain positive outcomes. By retaining this quality, you can establish successful helping relationships without appearing cold or stern. Sympathy differs from empathy because it shifts the emphasis from the patient to the nurse as he or she shares feelings and personal concerns and projects them onto the patient limiting ability to focus objectively on the patient's needs (Videbeck, 2008). For example, although it is understandable for team members to become impatient with family members who never seem satisfied with the care their loved one is receiving, it is helpful

to empathize with the family who might be feeling frightened and helpless. "This must be a hard time for you . . . how are you coping?" "Is there any way I can be of help?" When the patient and family sense that you have some idea of what they are experiencing and are committed to helping, the basis is set for a trusting therapeutic relationship.

HONESTY, AUTHENTICITY, AND TRUST

Patients should be able to trust that nurses are who they say they are (professional helpers), and that they can be trusted to do everything within their level of expertise to secure the resources and to help meet the patient needs.

CARING

Patients quickly sense whether they are merely a "task to be performed (task-centered caring) or a person of worth who is both cared about and cared for (relation-centered caring). Expert nurses know how to communicate genuine caring the minute they step into a patient's space by how they look at and touch the patient and what they say and do. Patients who feel cared for will feel accepted.

> ▶ *Think back to Susie Musashi, the 3-year-old child with burns. How the nurse approaches the child will set the stage for the interaction. Consider how the child would respond to a nurse who enters the room and scolds the child for crying as compared to the nurse who enters the room and approaches the child's bed, touching the child's shoulder or hand gently and softly. The message conveyed by the second action would be much more caring.* ■

COMPETENCE

Competent nurses are skilled in all aspects of basic nursing and can meet their patients' healthcare needs through their technical, cognitive, interpersonal, and ethical/legal skills. Take responsibility for evaluating your own strengths and weaknesses so that your patient will receive optimal care. Consequently, your patients will develop trust in and respect for you as their nurse, facilitating helping relationships and good communication.

Rapport Builders

Rapport, a feeling of mutual trust experienced by people in a satisfactory relationship (Fig. 21-5), facilitates open communication. Good rapport can be achieved by paying attention to the following variables.

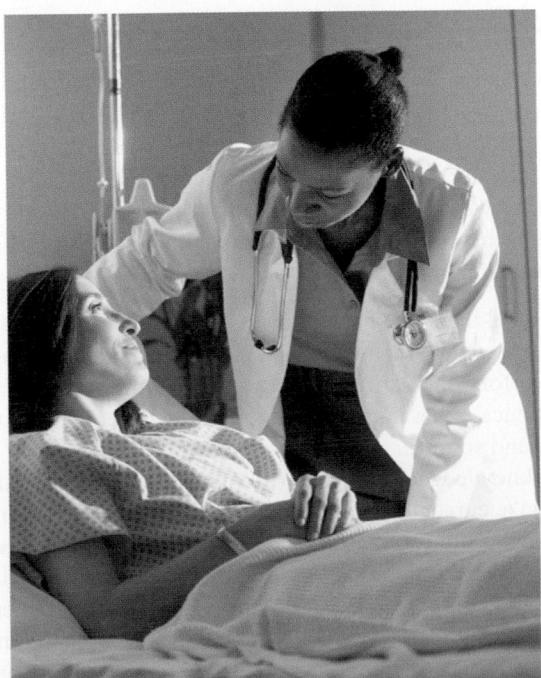

FIGURE 21-5. Rapport between the nurse and the patient/family is a necessary first step in planning care.

SPECIFIC OBJECTIVES

Having a purpose for an interaction provides guidance toward achieving a meaningful encounter with the patient. One objective might be to perform a head-to-toe physical assessment when greeting the patient and at the beginning of each shift. Another objective might be the discussion of a patient's feelings about being newly diagnosed with diabetes. The shortest encounter with a patient can have an objective, even if it is as simple as conveying a feeling of friendliness. Be flexible at all times, and follow the patient's cues to work toward meeting all needs.

COMFORTABLE ENVIRONMENT

A comfortable environment, in which both the patient and the nurse are at ease, helps to promote interactions. Suitable furniture, proper lighting, and a moderate temperature are important. Also, effective relationships are enhanced when the atmosphere is relaxed and unhurried. If you seem preoccupied and on the run, or if the patient is ill at ease for fear of missing visitors or because of another commitment, communication is impaired.

PRIVACY

It might not always be possible to carry on conversations alone with the patient in a room, but every effort should be made to provide privacy and to prevent conversations from being overheard by others. Sometimes merely drawing the curtains around the bed in a hospital or nursing home or sitting in a corner of the waiting room or lounge can provide the sense of privacy that is so important in most interactions. Home visits might need to be timed to ensure the privacy the patient desires and needs.

CONFIDENTIALITY

The confidentiality with which patient information is to be treated should be established with the patient. Indicate with whom the information that the patient gives will be shared. The patient should know about the right to specify who might have access to the information. Failure to consider this factor can be considered a breach of the patient's right to privacy. See Chapter 17 for guidelines concerning patient confidentiality.

PATIENT VERSUS TASK FOCUS

Communication in the nurse–patient relationship should focus on the patient and patient needs, not on the nurse or an activity in which the nurse is engaged (see the accompanying box: Through the Eyes of a Patient). Consider the following example, in which the nurse's comment focuses on the patient and the patient needs:

Patient: I don't know why these injections scare me, but they do.
Nurse: You are afraid of these injections?

In contrast, consider this example, in which the nurse's comment focuses instead on the nursing activity:

Patient: I don't know why these injections scare me, but they do.
Nurse: I give hundreds of injections. Don't be so immature.

Through the Eyes of a Patient

I know you come to clinical every day with your head full of all the important things you need to do for me. Probably you worry about whether or not you will remember the steps to both simple and complex procedures and fear that you will never get everything done in the time allotted. I'm sure that there are many things that your clinical instructor will use as a basis for your evaluation and perhaps other things that are important to you for your self-evaluation. But I thought you might like to know what's important to me. Most of what I've listed are simple things that you can communicate each time you walk into my home or room.*

- Really listen to me.
- Ask me what I think.
- Don't dismiss my concerns.
- Don't treat me like a disease, treat me like a person.

- Talk *to* me, not *at* me.
- Respect my privacy.
- Don't keep me waiting.
- Don't tell me what to do without telling me how to do it.
- Keep me informed.
- Remember who I used to be.
- Let me know you care.

Thanks for giving me this chance to share with you what matters to me.

The list of nursing interventions that are valued highly by patients was compiled by Roberta Messner after a review of many patient satisfaction studies. These are cited in Messner, R. L. (1993). What patients really want from their nurses. American Journal of Nursing, 93(8), 38–41.

USING NURSING OBSERVATIONS

Observations, which involve both seeing and interpreting, are especially useful for validating information. For example, a nurse suspects that a patient is afraid to hear the results of certain blood tests, but the patient insists that the results are unimportant. The nurse then observes the patient pacing in the corridor, apparently deep in thought. Observing the patient's behavior helps validate the nurse's suspicion that the patient is fearful, and the patient assertion that he or she is unconcerned appears to be a cover-up for truer feelings.

Observation serves several important purposes:

- It helps increase awareness of a patient's nonverbal messages.
- It is the primary source of information when a patient is unwilling or unable to communicate verbally.
- It demonstrates caring and interest in the patient. (Patients often recognize when a nurse is unobservant and, rightly or wrongly, usually conclude that the nurse does not care.)

OPTIMAL PACING

Consider the pace of any conversation or encounter with a patient. For instance, it would be ineffective to rush through a list of questions when obtaining a nursing history; it is more effective to let the patient set the pace. Let the patient know at the beginning of the interaction if time is limited so that the patient does not feel that you are rushing because of a lack of concern or personal interest.

RESPECTING PERSONAL SPACE

Perceptions of personal space vary. Assess a patient's personal space through careful observations of nonverbal communication. For example, when a person is speaking in close proximity, this might cause the person to back away because of feelings of discomfort in the close proximity. Other times, the person speaking might touch the person during the conversation. This interaction of close proximity might be very comfortable for both individuals. It is important to be sensitive to personal space so that patients feel comfortable during interactions (Videbeck, 2008).

DEVELOPING THERAPEUTIC COMMUNICATION SKILLS

Although humans communicate during virtually all waking moments, the therapeutic use of communication requires training and practice. Box 21-4 contrasts therapeutic and nontherapeutic communication. Nursing students might feel awkward when first trying to develop therapeutic relationships. Practice makes perfect, however, and you will soon feel at ease if you work on developing the following communication skills.

Conversation Skills

Conversation, or the exchange of verbal communication, is a social interaction. As social beings, humans learn as children how to converse with others, and nursing students, therefore, have already had years of experience communicating verbally. However, you can improve your communications with patients and achieve a more effective helping relationship in the following ways:

- Control the tone of your voice so that you are conveying exactly what you mean to say and not a hidden message. Your tone should indicate interest rather than boredom, patience rather than anger, acceptance rather than hostility, and so forth.
- Be knowledgeable about the topic of conversation and have accurate information. When possible, be familiar with the subject of conversation before discussing it with the patient. If the topic is unfamiliar (e.g., the availability of community resources for family caregivers of patients with special needs), it is best to tell the patient and family and to direct them to other resources. Convey confidence and honesty to the patient.

Box 21-4   THERAPEUTIC VERSUS NONTHERAPEUTIC COMMUNICATION

Patient Scenario

Mr. Commens is a 65-year-old divorced man who lives alone. His grown children are married and live out of town. He was recently diagnosed with cancer of the colon and underwent a colon resection. He is now home recuperating and has received a new diagnosis. The home health nurse is scheduled to visit Mr. Commens.

Nontherapeutic Communication

Nurse: Hello, Mr. Commens! I'm glad you're home. I only have 30 minutes to visit with you. It's been a very busy day.

Mr. Commens: I'm sorry you are having a bad day. I have been to the doctor and I'm very concerned about the report I received.

Nurse: Yes, I've had a busy day but not a bad day. I guess your day has been busy too. What report are you talking about?

Mr. Commens: Well, I need more tests because they think the cancer has spread.

Nurse: Now, who told you that? Maybe the test was wrong or you misunderstood the physician. Mr. Commens, I'll call your physician. Is there anything else bothering you?

Mr. Commens: No.

Nurse: I'll call your doctor and then call you tomorrow.

In this scenario, the nurse seems unconcerned about Mr. Commens' test results and gives him the idea that he/she does not believe the information he has relayed. The nurse is more concerned about his/her busy day and less concerned about the patient.

Therapeutic Communication

Nurse: Hello, Mr. Commens! I'm sorry I am running a little behind schedule. Now that I'm here, we will have as much time as we need to discuss how you're feeling and your visit to the physician. How are you feeling?

Mr. Commens: (His eyes are cast down to the floor and he is wringing his hands.) Well, I feel all right. I've had some pain in my right side.

Nurse: Mr. Commens, how would you rate your pain on a scale of 1 to 10?

Mr. Commens: About an 8.

Nurse: Mr. Commens, you seem concerned and a little preoccupied. Is there something bothering you?

Mr. Commens: Yes, I suppose there is. My doctor said my cancer has spread to my hip. I guess that's why I have pain in my right side. I have so many decisions to make and I'm very confused. The doctor said I need to start chemotherapy. I don't even know how I'll get there. My family is out of town.

Nurse: Mr. Commens, would it help if I spoke to your physician to obtain specific details about your treatment plan? This would then assist me in obtaining some help when you begin your chemotherapy.

Mr. Commens: That would be wonderful! If you call the doctor, then you can explain everything to me, and maybe it will help me to understand what I'll need to experience. Also, it might help me in making the decisions regarding my treatments.

Nurse: Mr. Commens, would you then like me to be here when you call your children about your diagnosis and treatment plan? I might be able to answer some of the questions they might have about your treatments.

Mr. Commens: That would be wonderful. I feel so much more relaxed knowing you are going to help me. Thank you so much.

Nurse: Mr. Commens, I'll call your physician and clarify the information you have received, and I'll be back at 5 p.m. Maybe at that time, we can call your family.

Mr. Commens: That sounds like a good plan, but we might need to call my children at 6 p.m.

Nurse: That's just fine. I will be back at 5 p.m. to discuss the information I have, and we will call your children at 6 p.m.

Interpretation

The first example of communication focuses on the nurse's needs, not the patient's needs. Most of the interaction in the first scenario blocks the communication process. The second example allows the patient to verbalize his concerns and his lack of decision making. The nurse provides the patient with broad opening statements and patient goals to assist in his planning and decision making.

- Be flexible. You might want to discuss a certain subject but learn that the patient wishes to discuss something else. It is better to follow the patient's lead whenever possible; in due time, you can return to the subject. For example, you arrive at the patient's bedside to administer a medication, but the patient begins to talk about his or her diet. It is better to take a little time to talk about the patient's interest than to insist on talking about only the procedure at hand, as long as there is enough time for the conversation.
- Be clear and concise, and make statements as simple as possible. Patients are often anxious and fail to understand the message unless the conversation is geared to a level the patient understands. Stay on one subject at a time. This will help decrease confusion.
- Avoid words that might have different interpretations. The study of the meaning of words is called **semantics.** Even when two people speak the same language, some words—such as love, hate, freedom, and health—might have different meanings to different people.
- Be truthful. A patient who is given false information will soon distrust the nurse. If you're not sure about something, admit you don't know and seek an answer rather than make a comment that is likely to be an error.
- Keep an open mind. An attitude of "I know better than the patient" is quickly discerned by the patient. Patients can make valuable contributions to their own healthcare.
- Take advantage of available opportunities. During most caregiving situations, you can facilitate conversation that makes even the most routine task meaningful. For instance, when giving a bed bath to a patient, ask about the patient's employment. This would allow the patient to verbalize any positive or negative feelings about the job and his or her temporary absence from it, reducing the anxiety that often occurs with the loss of work. It is often comforting to know that someone understands and cares.

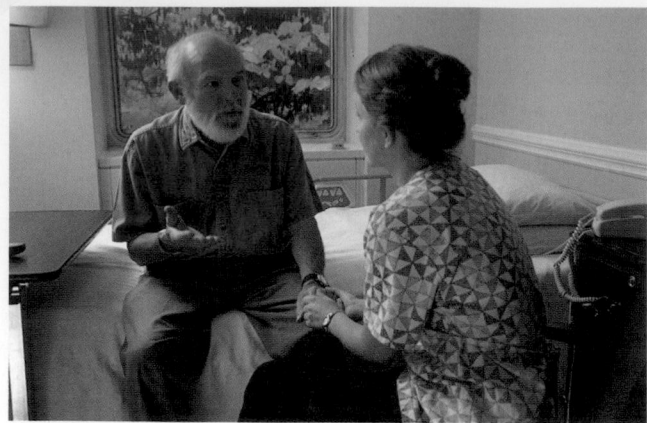

FIGURE 21-6. Listening attentively, with concentration and genuine concern, is key to productive communication.

Listening Skills

Listening is a skill that involves both hearing and interpreting what the other says. It requires attention and concentration to sort out, evaluate, and validate clues to better understand the true meaning of what is being said (Fig. 21-6). The accompanying box, Through the Eyes of a Student, relates one student's experience with attentive listening. The following recommended techniques might help to improve listening skills:

- When possible, sit when communicating with a patient. Do not cross your arms or legs because that body language conveys a message of being closed to the patient's comments.

- Be alert and relaxed and take sufficient time so that the patient feels at ease during the conversation.
- Keep the conversation as natural as possible, and avoid sounding overly eager.
- If culturally appropriate, maintain eye contact with the patient, without staring, in a face-to-face pose. This technique conveys interest in the conversation and willingness to listen.
- Indicate that you are paying attention to what the patient is saying by using appropriate facial expressions and body gestures. Be attentive to both your own and the patient's verbal and nonverbal communication.
- Think before responding to the patient. Responding impulsively tends to disrupt communication and listening.
- Do not pretend to listen. Most patients are sensitive to an attitude of feigned attention or to boredom and apathy.
- Listen for themes in the patient's comments. What are the repeated themes in the person's speech and behavior? What topics does the patient tend to avoid? What subjects tend to make the patient shift the conversation to other subjects? What inconsistencies and gaps appear in the patient's conversations?

Silence

The nurse can use silence appropriately by taking the time to wait for the patient to initiate or to continue speaking (Mullens, 2006). During periods of silence, reflect on what has already been shared and observe the patient without having to concentrate simultaneously on the spoken word. Periods

Through the Eyes of a Student

It was my first day of clinical rotation and I was assigned to Mr. Anderson, who was in his early 90s. He was in the hospital because he had a second heart attack. Mr. Anderson had lived alone for 5 years after the death of his wife. He wanted to remain independent, but his daughter, who was herself in her late 60s, and his doctor believed that he would not be able to function well on his own any longer. Mr. Anderson was distressed about this belief.

Because it was my first day and, unlike some of my classmates, I had never worked in a hospital before, I felt insecure and nervous. There really wasn't a lot of work for us to do. We weren't allowed to give medication yet, and my patient was pretty self-sufficient. Because my skills were shaky, I took my time taking vital signs, assisted Mr. Anderson with his bath and toileting, and made his bed. After checking his chart, I began my nursing interview with him. I was overjoyed to discover that he was a real talker! His memory was tremendous—either that or he was a great improvisor! He recalled stories about his childhood and his wife with great detail and emotion. He smiled and laughed when he spoke of his daughter and grandchildren. He told me about his daughter's childhood illnesses, as well as his

own. We talked about the Depression and world wars and about music, art, and education. He asked me about my family, and I felt like I had made a friend.

The next day, Mr. Anderson told me about his fears. He talked about losing his wife, about his health and body deteriorating, and about losing his independence and home. He despised having to be sent to a nursing home and having to depend on others. It hurt him a lot and made me sad. Mr. Anderson left on my second day, and as I said goodbye I wished I could do something for him.

I thought about him a lot since then, and I've come to realize that in those 2 days that I knew Mr. Anderson, I did do something for him besides washing him and changing his sheets. I listened to him. Although his family had little time for him and the doctors quickly flew in and out of the room, I let him talk and heard all he said, both in words and in his eyes. He will always be a good memory for me—and I think I'll be a good memory for him.

—*Kristina Hofmeister*
Holy Family College, Philadelphia, PA

of silence during communication can carry a variety of meanings, including the following:

- The patient might be comfortable and content in the nurse–patient relationship. Continuous talking is unnecessary.
- The patient might be trying to demonstrate stoicism and the ability to cope without help.
- The patient might be exploring his or her inner thoughts or feelings, and conversation would disrupt this. In effect, the patient is really saying, "I need some time to think."
- The patient might be fearful and use silence as an escape from a threat.
- The patient might be angry and use silence to display this emotion.

In due time, you might discuss the silence with the patient, especially if you wish to understand its meaning. Fear of silence sometimes leads to too much talking by the nurse. Also, excessive talking tends to place the focus on the nurse rather than on the patient.

Touch

Touch is a powerful means of communication with multiple meanings. It can connect people; provide affirmation, reassurance, and stimulation; decrease loneliness; increase self-esteem; and share warmth, intimacy, approval, and emotional support. It can also communicate frustration, anger, aggression, and punishment; invade personal space and privacy; and convey a negative (e.g., subservient) type of relationship with another (Gieger & Davidhizar, 2008). Because of the personal nature of touching, be sure to weigh the benefit of touch against the detrimental use of touch for each patient. Touch can be a powerful therapeutic tool when used at the right time. Anxiety or discomfort might result, however, when a patient does not understand the meaning of a tactile gesture or when the patient simply dislikes being touched.

Touch is the most highly developed sense at birth. Tactile experiences of infants and young children appear essential for the normal development of self and awareness of others. It has also been found that many elderly people long for touch, especially when isolated from loved ones because of hospitalization or nursing home care. Many older people have no living family to provide them with the caring touch so necessary for the sense of well-being. In such an instance, you can provide some special care by holding the patient's hand (Fig. 21-7).

Many situations require touching the patient while implementing nursing care. Physical closeness between the patient and the nurse is essential and inevitable. Therefore, every nurse needs to become comfortable with the judicious use of this nonverbal communication technique so that a sense of security, rather than anxiety, results. As well, dexterity and sureness in the use of the hands help to assure the patient of your expertise when measuring blood pressure or giving an injection.

Interest has continued to grow in the phenomenon known as **therapeutic touch.** Therapeutic touch involves "unruffling," or clearing, congested areas of energy in the body and redirecting this energy. After assessing a patient's "energy field," the nurse uses therapeutic touch to promote comfort,

FIGURE 21-7. A reassuring handclasp uses touch to convey a message. Sometimes touch can be a more effective way of expressing concern and interest than verbal communication. *(Photo © B. Proud.)*

relaxation, healing, and a sense of well-being. Many nurses are studying therapeutic touch in nursing educational programs and through special courses or workshops. It is becoming a widely accepted form of therapy, as well as a subject for nursing research. Many patients testify to the benefits of therapeutic touch, but research is needed to verify its effect on mood and outlook, pain control, and illness and disease (Frisch & Frisch, 2006). Refer to Chapters 28 and 35 for additional discussion of therapeutic touch.

Humor

Humor is increasingly valued as both an interpersonal skill for the nurse and a healing strategy for patients. Nurses have a valuable tool when they can use humor effectively to maintain a balanced perspective in their work and to encourage patients to do the same. Nurses with a sense of humor are able to laugh at themselves and accept their failures, confront the absurdities of everyday practice without falling apart, and challenge patients to situate their current dilemma within the context of their larger life experiences. Laughter releases excess physical and psychological energy and reduces stress, anxiety, worry, and frustration. Humor, like other interpersonal competencies, is a learned skill. When used inappropriately, however, it can be destructive. You'll need an awareness of how various cultures perceive the use of humor in the presence of an illness (Facente, 2006). You might also find it helpful to identify nurses who use humor well and to "try on" observed behaviors.

Interviewing Techniques

The purpose of the interview is to obtain accurate and thorough information. In nursing, the interview is a major tool for collecting data during the assessment step of the nursing process (see Chapter 12). Consequently, every nurse needs to become proficient in the use of the communication techniques described previously as well as interviewing techniques designed to gather and validate information.

All interviews should begin with an explanation of the purpose of the interview. During the interview, you'll use **interviewing techniques** to obtain needed information while remaining flexible in approach. The interview itself is a therapeutic interaction and might be an essential part of the orientation phase of the helping relationship. At the end of the interview, plans for further interactions can be made. The following interviewing techniques are useful in nearly all nurse–patient interactions, especially the interview.

Open-Ended Question or Comment

When obtaining a nursing history, use the open-ended question technique to allow the patient a wide range of possible responses. It allows the patient to express what he or she understands to be true, yet is specific enough to prevent digressing from the issue at hand. It encourages free verbalization. The greatest advantage of this technique is that it prevents the patient from answering with a simple yes or no. The following is an example of an open-ended question and the response:

> *Nurse:* What did your physician tell you about your need for this hospitalization?
>
> *Patient:* He told me that my blood pressure is dangerously high and that I need some special tests done while I am here.

Closed Question or Comment

The closed question provides the receiver with limited choices of possible responses and might often be answered by one or two words, "yes" or "no." Closed questions are used to gather specific information from a patient and to allow the nurse and patient to focus on a particular area. Closed questions are often a barrier to effective communication. The following is an example of an appropriate use of a closed question:

> *Nurse:* What medicines have you been taking at home?
>
> *Patient:* Let me see, my doctor gave me a water pill and a blood pressure pill to take every day.

Validating Question or Comment

This type of question or comment serves to validate what the nurse believes is heard or observed. Overusing validating questions and comments might lead the patient to think the nurse is not listening. To continue the example used in the previous technique, the nurse could validate the patient's reply as follows:

> *Nurse:* At home, you have been taking both a water pill and a blood pressure pill every day. Did you take them today?
>
> *Patient:* Yes, I took one of each with my breakfast.

Clarifying Question or Comment

The use of the clarifying question or comment allows the nurse to gain an understanding of a patient's comment. When used properly, this technique can avert possible misconceptions that could lead to an inappropriate nursing diagnosis. However, overuse of clarifying questions or comments can lead the patient to believe that the nurse is not listening or lacks appropriate knowledge. The following is an example:

> *Patient:* I have never needed to take medicine before in my life.
>
> *Nurse:* Is this the first health problem you have had?
>
> *Patient:* Yes, I've always been healthy.

Reflective Question or Comment

The reflective question technique involves repeating what the person has said or describing the person's feelings. It encourages the patient to elaborate on his or her thoughts and feelings. An example of this technique follows:

> *Patient:* I've been really upset about my blood pressure and have to take these pills.
>
> *Nurse:* You've been upset . . .
>
> *Patient:* I guess I'm worried about what could happen if my blood pressure gets too bad.

Sequencing Question or Comment

Sequencing is used to place events in a chronologic order or to investigate a possible cause-and-effect relationship between events. Nursing assessment is facilitated when events leading to a problem are placed in sequence. This technique is evident in the following example:

> *Patient:* I don't feel like myself anymore since I've been taking my blood pressure medicine. I'm tired and don't have any energy.
>
> *Nurse:* Your tiredness began after you started taking your medicine?

Directing Question or Comment

It might become necessary at times to obtain more information about a topic brought up earlier in the interview or to introduce a new aspect of the current topic. In such an instance, the nurse has gained additional valuable information to consider in assessing the patient's health status and educational or counseling needs. The following is an example of this technique:

> *Nurse:* You mentioned your dad earlier. Did he develop complications related to high blood pressure?
>
> *Patient:* Yes.
>
> *Nurse:* What sort of complications?
>
> *Patient:* Kidney failure. He was on dialysis for years before getting a transplant.
>
> *Nurse:* Are you afraid this might happen to you?

Assertiveness Skills

When interacting with patients, family members, other nurses, physicians, and other members of the healthcare team, it is important to communicate in a way that demonstrates respect

TABLE • 21-2 EXAMPLES OF ASSERTIVE AND NONASSERTIVE SPEECH

	Assertive	Nonassertive
Nurse to Nurse	"I know we all lose track of time occasionally, but I'm finding it harder and harder to cover for you when you take extra time for lunch. I don't think it's fair for your patient and I to have to wait an extra 30 minutes every day for you to come back from lunch. Can we talk about this?"	"Huh? No, I didn't really mind. Luckily I wasn't too busy today." Thought: "What a sucker I am. Now I'll have to grab a quick bite so that I can get back to the unit in time to do 2 p.m. treatments."
Nurse to Physician	"I know we talked about Mr. Esposito's pain medication before but I've collected some new data. Even with the change in dosage, he is only getting 1 to 1½ hours of relief. I believe a different analgesic agent might work better for him."	"Um . . . yes I know you already changed the dosage. It's just that I thought it still wasn't working. Maybe I didn't give it enough time. Thanks for listening to me anyway. I'm sorry to bother you with this."
Student Nurse to Preceptor	"Miss Cheng has a new order to be straight cathed. I reviewed the procedure, but I'd sure appreciate your talking me through this because I've never done it before and I'm terrified."	"Uh . . . I'm sorry to be such a pain again. I have to do this cath and don't know where to begin. I know you must be busy, but, uh, is there any way you might have time for me?"

for all parties. **Assertive behaviors,** which are one hallmark of professional nursing relationships, need to be distinguished from aggressive (i.e., harsh, injurious, or destructive) behaviors, which are very different and are discussed later in this chapter. They also differ greatly from avoidance or acquiescent behaviors. The key to assertiveness is open, honest, and direct communication. "I" statements—"I feel . . ." and "I think . . ."—play an important role in assertive statements. Table 21-2 gives examples of assertive and nonassertive speech.

Four basic components of the assertive response or approach are as follows: (1) having empathy, (2) describing one's feelings or the situation, (3) clarifying one's expectations, and (4) anticipating consequences (Angel & Petronko, 1983). For example, a student who is feeling overwhelmed by her weekly clinical assignments might communicate the following to her instructor:

Empathy: "I guess it must be hard for you to make our clinical assignments each week and to know what each one of us needs."

Description: "I have to share with you that right now I feel so overwhelmed that I go home from clinical in tears each week."

Expectation: "I am wondering if we could talk about this. I am willing to work hard, but I seem to need some help pulling everything together."

Consequences: "I expect to do well in clinical but I am afraid that if things continue the way they are right now, I might not last the semester. I would appreciate any help you can give me."

Characteristics of the assertive nurse's self-presentation include a confident, open body posture; eye contact; use of clear, concise "I" statements; and the ability to share honestly one's thoughts, feelings, and emotions. The assertive nurse's attitude toward work is characterized by working to capacity

with or without supervision, the ability to remain calm under supervision, the freedom to ask for help when necessary, the ability to give and accept compliments, and honesty in admitting mistakes and taking responsibility for them.

BLOCKS TO COMMUNICATION

Failure to Perceive the Patient as a Human Being

It is of primary importance to focus on the whole patient and not merely the patient's diagnosis. Patients report that nothing is more discomforting than to be treated as merely an object of care rather than a patient. It is also of primary importance that the patient is addressed by a formal name such as Mr., Mrs., Ms., or Dr. rather than slang terminology such "honey" or "sweetie." What distinguishes nursing from other health professions is its focus on the whole person, not simply the illness or dysfunction.

> ➤ *Think back to Mr. Gordon, the patient with end-stage liver disease. In the scenario, the nursing student voiced concerns about the staff nurse and residents focusing only on the technical aspects of the patient's care. To effectively communicate this concern to these individuals, the nurse would incorporate the four components of the assertive approach when speaking with them, stressing the need for providing care to the whole patient.* ■

Failure to Listen

Patients might or might not feel able to speak freely to the nurse. Often, the signals indicating their readiness to talk are subtle. Don't miss valuable opportunities for important communication by approaching patients with a closed mind or focusing on your own needs rather than on the patient's needs. Nurses who lack confidence in their own ability to meet the challenges a patient presents might become defensive in response to a patient's comments. Nurse defensiveness is a huge barrier to open and trusting communication.

Inappropriate Comments and Questions

Certain types of comments and questions should be avoided in most situations because they tend to impede effective communications. A description of each type follows.

Using Clichés

A **cliché** is a stereotyped, trite, or pat answer. Most healthcare clichés suggest that there is no cause for anxiety or concern, or they offer false assurance. Their use tends to be interpreted as a lack of real interest in what has been said. For example, even though the common question "How are you?" could start a conversation, it can cause a problem if the patient hearing this suspects that the nurse is not sincerely interested in how he or she feels. Following are some common clichés that are best not said because they tend to impede effective communications:

"Everything will be all right."
"Don't worry. You will be just fine in another day or two."
"Your doctor knows best."
"Cheer up. Tomorrow is another day."

Another type of cliché makes a sweeping generalization that does not necessarily apply to a specific patient. It also tends to cut off communications and makes the person feel as though he or she is just another insignificant being. Consider the following examples:

"Men tolerate pain poorly. That must be why you are complaining of severe pain."
"Everybody is afraid of surgery. Why should you be any different?"
"You teenagers are all alike. You aren't cooperative because you deny authority."

Such comments rarely promote communication with the patient to whom they are addressed.

Using Questions Requiring Only a Yes or No Answer

Questions that can be answered by simply saying yes or no tend to cut off discussion, even when the person might wish to continue. Consider the following question:

Nurse: Did you have a good day?

The question begs for a noncommittal answer, which tells the nurse little. A better comment is as follows:

Nurse: Tell me about your sessions in therapy, how did you feel they went today?

Another pitfall is to pose a question to which the patient can say no when that answer could present a problem.

Consider the following question that a nurse asks a postoperative patient:

Nurse: Are you ready to get out of bed?

By offering the patient the chance to say no, the nurse might have created difficulties if the patient is to be out of bed.

There are times when questions that can be answered with yes or no are legitimate. Following are examples:

Nurse: Did you take your insulin before breakfast this morning?
Nurse: Do you have pain when I move your arm this way?

The problem with yes or no questions arises when seeking more detailed information or when the question might create difficulty.

Using Questions Containing the Words Why and How

Questions using why and how are intimidating to many patients. Consider the following questions:

Nurse: Why were you not tired enough to sleep?
Nurse: How did you ever decide to go on a crash diet?

These two questions would be better stated as follows:

Nurse: What were you doing while you were unable to sleep?
Nurse: What things prompted you to decide to go on a crash diet?

Using Questions That Probe for Information

Questions that too obviously probe for information might cut off communication. Patients who are made to feel as though they are receiving the "third degree" become resentful and usually stop talking and try to avoid further conversation. Although more information might be needed, it is better to follow the patient's lead. Letting the patient take the initiative allows you to delve more deeply at a time when the patient is ready. A nurse who says, "Let's get to the bottom of this" is likely to destroy conversation, unless the patient is ready to face the real cause of the problem.

Using Leading Questions

A leading question suggests what response the speaker wishes to hear. Leading questions tend to produce answers that might please the nurse but are unlikely to encourage the patient to respond honestly without feeling intimidated. Consider the following examples:

Nurse: You aren't going to smoke that cigarette, are you?
Nurse: You have been well cared for by your nurses, haven't you?

These questions direct the patient to give an answer that pleases the nurse rather than to express his or her own thoughts.

Using Comments That Give Advice

Giving advice often implies that the nurse knows what is best for the patient and denies him or her the right to make decisions and have feelings. It also tends to increase the patient's dependence on caregivers. However, advice does have a rightful place when it is requested and when the person giving the advice has expert knowledge that the patient does not.

Using Judgmental Comments

Using judgmental comments tends to impose the nurse's standards on the patient. Consider the comment of a nurse who notes that a young woman is crying:

Nurse: You aren't acting very grown up. How do you think your husband would feel if he saw you crying like this?

The nurse judges the patient as being immature, and the nurse's apparent hostility could end effective communication. A better comment in this situation might be as follows:

Nurse: I would like to help. Tell me, what is making you cry?

Consider the following exchange between a nurse and a patient about to have surgery:

Patient: I think I have a right to be afraid of this operation.
Nurse: Tell me what makes you feel afraid.

This patient is likely to feel safe when allowed to express his or her feelings without being judged.

> *Remember Susie Musashi, the 3-year-old with burns who is crying? Using a response such as "You're acting like a baby. You're a big girl now" would be intimidating, especially to a young child who is striving for acceptance. Instead, a response such as "Can you tell me what is making you cry or feel so sad?" would allow the child to verbalize her concerns without feeling intimidated or scolded. This response also would help in establishing a trusting nurse–patient relationship.* ∎

Changing the Subject

A quick way to stop conversation is to change the subject. The patient might be at a point of readiness to discuss something and can be expected to feel frustrated if put off by a change in the topic of conversation. The following example illustrates this:

Patient: When can I expect to be told about my insulin?
Nurse: Let's discuss your diet now so that you will know what to eat when you get home. We can discuss your insulin some other time.

A nurse might also change the subject when feeling uncomfortable about the topic of conversation. For example, the patient's needs are being met when the nurse allows the patient to speak of impending death, thoughts of suicide, or contemplated abortion. The nurse is ignoring the patient, however, when the subject is changed because the nurse feels uncomfortable talking about it.

Giving False Assurance

It is easier and more pleasant to deal with positive outcomes than negative outcomes. As such, nurses might try to convince the patient that things are going to turn out well even when knowing the chances are not good. False assurance might give patients the impression that the nurse is not interested in their problems. The use of clichés gives a patient false assurance. Communication might be impeded when providing the patient and family with false assurance. If you inadvertently do use false assurance, then you should explain with an apology and implement effective communication techniques.

Gossip and Rumor

Gossip and rumor are common forms of communication, particularly in healthcare settings. This can also be referred to as communication via the grapevine. Gossip and rumor can produce detrimental effects on relationships and group building. Gossiping might be used to inform, influence others, entertain, or ventilate. It can be harmless but could also damage the reputation of others. Rumors serve similar functions but tend to be widespread. It is important to understand that rumors and gossip might cause blocks to team building and damage the reputations of the individuals who are the subject of the information.

Aggressive Interpersonal Behavior

Disruptive behavior has a negative effect on clinical outcomes and interpersonal relationships. Adverse events occur when communication between healthcare professionals is ineffective, abusive, or negative. The Joint Commission (TJC), in an effort to eliminate disruptive behavior in hospitals, has issued a new leadership standard for 2009 that requires hospitals to establish a code of conduct defining acceptable and unacceptable behavior. Hospitals are also required to have policies in place to address these incidents when they occur. Aggressive interpersonal behavior compromises patient safety, influences satisfaction with care, and contributes to medical errors. Additional recommendations from TJC advise hospitals to educate all staff about the code of conduct, develop reporting systems, use mediators when necessary, and document all efforts to address unacceptable behavior (Potera, 2008).

The American Association of Critical-Care Nurses (AACN), in recognition of the need for healthy work environments, has established six standards that support excellence in nursing practice. These essential standards that reaffirm a culture of safety, authority, and accountability are:

- Skilled communication
- True collaboration
- Effective decision making
- Appropriate staffing

- Meaningful recognition
- Authentic leadership

The standards are all interrelated and dependent on each other and represent an opportunity for a committed partnership between nurses and the work environment (AACN, 2005).

Nurses continue to report the occurrence of negative communication with physicians. This factor is often cited as a contributor to poor job satisfaction and it jeopardizes nurse retention. Nurses describe this disruptive behavior by physicians as rude, intimidating, and belittling and state that it occurs more frequently with older physicians than among younger ones. In settings where teamwork is essential, such as operating rooms and intensive care areas, the relationship between nurse and physician is more positive. Nurses who remain current in their field of expertise, become involved in informal collaborative work groups, participate in interdisciplinary hospital committees, and feel more empowered in their encounters with physicians. It is a mistake to permit negative behavior by a physician to discourage any future communication. Nurses who stay focused and professional and approach physicians in a collegial manner will be better prepared to avoid negative communication. If it occurs, the hospital administration policies and procedures should be implemented to deal with individual situations in a constructive manner (Sirota, 2007).

Anger and aggressive behavior between nurses, or nurse-to-nurse hostility, has been labeled **horizontal violence.** It can take the form of bullying, criticizing, blaming, or bickering. In a survey of almost 700 nurses, 72% reported having experienced some form of disruptive behavior by other nurses (Martin, 2007). Failure to address this disruptive communication can result in anger, frustration, and a feeling of vulnerability. Nurses who refuse to be a victim can help break this cycle of violence. Proactive behavior includes learning how to react professionally and protectively "in the moment," documenting and reporting the incident, and insisting that this abuse is

addressed. Nurses who have always cared for others need to also care for themselves and their peers.

Angry, hostile patients can also subject nurses to verbal and physical abuse. According to a national survey, emergency department nurses are most at risk and 83% had experienced a physical assault (Thrall, 2006). Aggressive behavior may progress according to the following stages: anxiety, verbal aggression, and physical aggression. Suggestions for techniques to diffuse the behavior of an angry patient include:

- Remain with an anxious patient unless your safety is at risk.
- Use a calm, assertive approach with a verbally abusive patient.
- Remove yourself from a dangerous situation or move to a safe distance and call for help.
- Physical restraints should be used as a last resort. They require a written order, proper documentation, and an established time frame for use.

Nurses feel more confident when they attend aggression management workshops to practice the particular skills needed to handle aggressive patients (Flores, 2008).

IMPAIRED VERBAL COMMUNICATION

The ability to communicate is our most human characteristic. Human communication is essential for learning, working, and social interaction. Impaired communication can affect every aspect of a person's life. Impaired Verbal Communication is an approved North American Nursing Diagnosis Association (NANDA) nursing diagnosis. According to NANDA, Impaired Verbal Communication is defined as decreased, delayed, or absent ability to receive, process, transmit, and/or use a system of symbols. (See Examples of NANDA Nursing Diagnoses: Communication.)

The Focus on the Older Adult box describes speech, language, and hearing disorders that most frequently affect older

Examples of NANDA Nursing Diagnoses
Communication

Nursing Diagnoses	Related Factors	Sample Defining Characteristics
Impaired Verbal Communication	Decrease in circulation to the brain; brain tumor; physical barrier (tracheostomy, intubation); anatomic defect, cleft palate; psychological barriers (psychosis, lack of stimuli); cultural differences; developmental or age related	Individual is able to speak dominant language; speaks or verbalizes with difficulty; does not or cannot speak; stutters; slurs; has difficulty forming words or sentences; has difficulty expressing thought verbally; uses inappropriate verbalization; has dyspnea; is disoriented
Disturbed Energy Field	Slowing or blocking of energy flows secondary to illness, injury, immobility, pain, anxiety, or age-related developmental crises	Perceptions of changes in patterns of energy flow such as movement, sounds, temperature, visual change, and disruption of the field

FOCUS ON THE OLDER ADULT

WHAT ARE THE DISORDERS OF COMMUNICATION THAT MOST FREQUENTLY AFFECT OLDER PEOPLE?

Our communication system, which involves speaking, hearing, and understanding the speech of others; reading, and writing, is a unique human achievement. It plays a vital role in all aspects of everyday life—in our jobs, our families, and our recreation. When communication processes are damaged by disorders of speech, language, or hearing, the effects are always serious.

Disorders of speech, language, and hearing are frequently found among older adults. These individuals often find themselves at a distinct disadvantage on social, economic, and personal levels. With the number of older adults growing rapidly, and with the increased numbers of survivors of illnesses and accidents that can result in speech, language, or hearing

disorders, more and more older adults with communication problems will be encountered. They require the understanding of family and friends as well as services from professionals in communication disorders.

Disorders of communication that affect older people may result from hearing impairment, stroke, cancer or other disease of the larynx, parkinsonism, or other neurologic disorders. The communication disorders vary widely and include difficulty with speaking and with understanding verbal messages. The effects of these disorders may be frustrating and bewildering and may lead to withdrawal and isolation. Participation on any social or economic level may become difficult or impossible either because of the disorder itself or the emotional consequences.

SPEECH, LANGUAGE, AND HEARING DISORDERS

APHASIA: Aphasia is a complex problem which may result, in varying degrees, in a reduced ability to understand what others are saying, to express oneself, or to be understood. Some individuals with this disorder may have no speech, while others may have only mild difficulties recalling names or words. Others may have problems putting words in their proper order in a sentence. The ability to understand oral directions, to read, to write, and to deal with numbers may also be disturbed. Strokes are the major cause of aphasia in the older population. It has been estimated that there are over one million adults with aphasia in the United States today. Many can be helped to communicate more effectively.

DYSARTHRIA: Dysarthria interferes with normal control of the speech mechanism. Speech may be slurred or otherwise difficult to understand due to lack of ability to produce speech sounds correctly, maintain good breath control, and coordinate the movements of the lips, tongue, palate, and larynx. Diseases such as parkinsonism, multiple sclerosis, and bulbar palsy, as well as strokes and accidents, can cause dysarthria. Many individuals with dysarthria are over 65. Their communication skills often may be improved by appropriate treatment.

HEARING PROBLEMS: It is estimated that of the approximately 27 million Americans over the age of 65, as many as 50% may be affected by hearing impairment. The hearing loss observed as a part of the aging process is called "presbycusis." Many of those with presbycusis describe the problem as being able to "hear" what others are saying, but being unable to understand what is being said. This condition can lead to withdrawal from personal interactions of all types. Family or friends may confuse the disorder with "forgetfulness" or "senility." A hearing aid can often improve communication for older people with hearing loss.

VOICE PROBLEMS: Laryngectomy, the surgical removal of the larynx (voice box) due to cancer, affects approximately 9,000 individuals each year, most of whom are older. They can usually learn to speak again by learning esophageal speech, by using an electronic device or by surgical implant of voice prosthesis. Other forms of disease may result in complete or partial loss of the voice. Most of these problems can be treated.

OTHER COMMUNICATION PROBLEMS: Brain diseases that result in progressive loss of mental faculties may affect memory, orientation to time, place and people, and organization of thought processes, all of which may result in reduced ability to communicate.

From *Communication Disorders and Aging.* American Speech-Language-Hearing Association, Rockville, Md. Reprinted with permission.

people. Nurses and other caregivers need to avoid "elderspeak" when communicating with older adults. "Elderspeak" involves using speaking patterns and words that mimic "baby talk" that imply that the older person is not competent. It is actually a form of ageism and used more commonly with the frail elderly in nursing homes. Communication adjustments may be necessary but must be respectful, positive, and individualized.

Box 21-5 offers guidelines for communicating with patients with special needs. The causes of hearing loss include chronic ear infections, heredity, birth defects, health problems at home, certain drugs, head injury, viral or bacterial infection, exposure to loud noise, aging, and tumors. Causes of speech and language disorders are related to hearing loss, cerebral palsy, and other nerve and muscle disorders; severe head injury; stroke (brain attack); viral diseases; mental retarda-

tion; certain drugs; physical impairments, such as cleft lip or palate; vocal abuse or misuse; and inadequate speech and language.

> *For Irwina Russellinski, the older adult woman admitted with pneumonia, the nurse would need to investigate the cause and degree of the patient's hearing loss and what, if any, treatments or measures have been used to manage the problem. The nurse would also need to gather additional data about the patient's confusion and her cultural background. Based on this information, the nurse would be able to develop a plan of care that addresses Mrs. Russellinski's needs.* ■

Box 21-5   COMMUNICATING WITH PATIENTS WHO HAVE SPECIAL NEEDS

Patients Who Are Visually Impaired
- Acknowledge your presence in the patient's room.
- Identify yourself by name.
- Remember that the visually impaired patient will be unable to pick up most nonverbal cues during communication. Speak in a normal tone of voice.
- Explain the reason for touching the patient before doing so.
- Indicate to the patient when the conversation has ended and when you are leaving the room.
- Keep a call light or bell within easy reach of the patient.
- Orient the patient to the sounds in the environment and to the arrangement of the room and its furnishings.
- Be sure eyeglasses are clean and intact or that contacts are in place.

Patients Who Are Hearing Impaired
- Orient the patient to your presence before initiating conversation. This may be done by gently touching the patient or moving so you can be seen.
- Talk directly to the patient while facing him or her. If the patient is able to lip read, use simple sentences and speak in a quiet, natural manner and pace. Be aware of nonverbal communication.
- Do not chew gum or cover your mouth when talking with the patient.
- Demonstrate or pantomime ideas you wish to express, as appropriate.
- Use sign language or finger spelling, as appropriate.
- Write any ideas that you cannot convey to the patient in another manner.
- Be sure that hearing aids are clean, functioning, and inserted properly.

Patients With a Physical Barrier (Laryngectomy or Endotracheal Tube)
- Select one or more simple means of communication that the patient is physically able to use. Options include eye blinks or hand squeezes to communicate yes or no; writing pads or magic slates; communication boards with words, letters, or pictures; flash cards; sign language.
- Be sure that everyone communicating with the patient—family, friends, and caregivers—understands and is able to use the communication devices selected.
- Demonstrate patience with the time needed to communicate effectively, and reinforce the efforts made by the patient.

- Ensure that the patient has an effective means of signaling need for assistance, such as call bells or alarms.

Patients Who Are Cognitively Impaired
- Establish and maintain eye contact with the patient to hold attention.
- Communicate important information in a quiet environment where there is little to distract the patient's attention.
- Keep communication simple and concrete. Break down instructions into simple tasks and avoid lengthy explanations. Do not use pronouns or abstract terms. Use pictures or drawings when appropriate.
- Whenever possible, avoid open-ended questions. Ask "Would you like to wear the brown pants or the gray pants?" instead of "What would you like to wear?"
- Be patient and give the patient time to respond. If the patient does not respond after 2 minutes, repeat what you said. If there is still no response, take a break before continuing the conversation so that neither you nor the patient becomes frustrated.

Patients Who Are Unconscious
- Be careful of what is said in the patient's presence. Hearing is believed to be the last sense lost; therefore, the unconscious patient is often likely to hear even though there is no apparent response.
- Assume the patient can hear you. Talk in a normal tone of voice about things you would ordinarily discuss.
- Speak with the patient before touching. Remember that touch can be an effective means of communication with the unconscious patient.
- Keep environment noises at as low a level as possible. This helps the patient focus on the communication.

Patients Who Do Not Speak English
- Use an interpreter whenever possible.
- Use a dictionary that translates words from one language to another so that you can speak at least some words in the patient's language.
- Speak in simple sentences and in a normal tone of voice.
- Demonstrate or pantomime ideas you wish to convey, as appropriate.
- Be aware of nonverbal communication. Remember that many nonverbal communication cues are universal.

A nurse who suspects a speech, language, or hearing problem should refer the patient to a speech-language pathologist or audiologist. A speech-language pathologist is a professional educated in the study of human communication, its development, and its disorders. An audiologist is a professional educated in the study of normal and impaired hearing.

● Developing Critical Thinking Skills

1. Think about your class as a group and evaluate how effectively it is functioning (fair, average, good, exceptional). Identify positive and negative factors influencing your effectiveness. Talk with your classmates and see if they agree or disagree with your evaluation. Talk about how your class compares with classes of other years. What roles do you see yourself playing in your class group? Do others agree with your self-assessment?

2. Working with another student, attempt to express the following without using any form of verbal communication:
   - I am in pain.
   - I am genuinely concerned about your well-being.
   - I couldn't care less that you are my patient, and I wish I were anywhere else but here caring for you.
   - I am afraid that you will hurt me.

   Try to put into words what this exercise can teach you about the importance of nonverbal communication. Explain how this understanding will influence your nursing practice.

3. Conversation is both an art and an essential nursing tool. If you had 30 minutes to spend with each of the following patients while doing a procedure that allows you to communicate, what would you talk about (communicate) and why? Compare your answers with another student's, and explore what your conversations would communicate to the patients involved.
   - An older adult recently admitted to a nursing home
   - A 6-year-old boy newly admitted to a hospital for asthma
   - An HIV-positive 33-year-old man who has just been given the news that he has acquired immunodeficiency syndrome (AIDS)
   - A 45-year-old amputee who has been in a rehabilitation hospital for 3 weeks after a motorcycle accident
   - A 19-year-old woman who has just had an elective abortion and is in the recovery unit
   - An unconscious patient in a critical care unit

4. An experienced nurse observes your distress after leaving the room of a patient who has just told her family that her cancer has recurred and is in an advanced state. She tells you that you better "toughen up" if you want to survive in nursing. She counsels not getting emotionally involved with patients and families: "Become a rock." How do you respond to this nurse and why? Of what value, if any, is empathy?

● Practicing for NCLEX

1. You are the charge nurse responsible for the evening shift. During rounds, you hear the patient care technician yelling loudly to a patient regarding his transfer from the bed to chair. When entering the room, which of the following is your best response?
   a. "You need to speak to the patient quietly. You are disturbing the patient."
   b. "Let me help you with your transfer technique."
   c. "When you are finished, be sure to apologize for your rough demeanor."
   d. "When your patient is safe and comfortable, meet me at the desk."

2. The public health nurse is leaving the home of a young mother who has a special needs baby. The neighbor states, "How is she doing, since the baby's father is no help?" What is the nurse's best response to the neighbor?
   a. "New mothers need support."
   b. "The lack of a father is difficult."
   c. "How are you today?"
   d. "It is a very sad situation."

3. A 3-year-old child is being admitted to the medical division for vomiting, diarrhea, and dehydration. During the admission interview, the nurse should implement which of the following communication techniques to elicit the most information from the parents?
   a. The use of statements that indicate the patient will be all right
   b. The use of questions that contain the word how
   c. The use of a leading question and those involving yes or no
   d. The use of questions that direct comments to clarify

4. The nurse enters the patient's room and examines the patient's IV fluids and cardiac monitor. The patient states, "Well, I haven't seen you before. Who are you?" Which of the following is the nurse's best response?
   a. "I'm just the IV therapist checking your IV."
   b. "I've been transferred to this division and will be caring for you."
   c. "I'm sorry, my name is John Smith. I'm responsible for your IV."
   d. "My name is John Smith. I'll be caring for you until 11 p.m."

5. The nurse enters the room of a patient with cancer. He is crying and states, "I feel so alone." Of the following statements, which is the most therapeutic?
   a. The nurse stands at the patient's bedside and states, "I understand how you feel. My mother said the same thing when she was ill."
   b. The nurse places a hand on the patient's arm and states, "You feel so alone."
   c. The nurse stands in the patient's room and asks, "Why do you feel so alone? Your wife has been here every day."
   d. The nurse holds the patient's hand and asks, "What makes you feel so alone?"

6. During discharge teaching, the nurse should:
   a. Determine the progress made in established goals
   b. Clarify when the patient should take medications
   c. Report the progress made in teaching to the staff
   d. Include all family members in the teaching session

7. The nursing student is nervous and concerned about the work she is about to do at the clinical facility. To allay anxiety and be successful in her provision of care, it is important for her to:
   a. Determine the established goals of the institution
   b. Be sure her verbal and nonverbal communication is congruent
   c. Engage in self-talk to plan her day and decrease her fear
   d. Speak with her fellow colleagues about how they feel

8. A nurse on the rehabilitation division states to her head nurse, "I need the day off and you didn't give it to me!" The head nurse replies, "Well, I wasn't aware you needed the day off, and it isn't possible since staffing is so inadequate." In the act of sending the message, which statement would be considered more effective?
   a. "Mr. Tyler, I placed a request to have August 8th off, but I'm working and I have a doctor's appointment."
   b. "Mr. Tyler, I would like to discuss my schedule with you. I requested the 8th of August off for a doctor's appointment. Could I make an appointment?"
   c. "Mr. Tyler, I will need to call in on the 8th of August because I have a doctor's appointment."
   d. "Mr. Tyler, since you didn't give me the 8th of August off, will I need to find someone to work for me?"

9. During a nursing staff meeting, the nurses determine that they will make sure all vital signs are reported and charted within 15 minutes following assessment. This is an example of:
   a. Group Decision Making
   b. Group Leadership
   c. Group Identity
   d. Group Patterns of Interaction

10. A patient walking to the bathroom with a stooped gait is noted with facial grimacing. It is important that the nurse assess the patient for which of the following?
    a. Pain
    b. Anxiety
    c. Depression
    d. Fluid Volume Deficit

11. A nursing student is preparing to administer morning care to the patient. What is the most important question that the nursing student should ask the patient?
    a. "Would you prefer a bath or a shower?"
    b. "May I help you with a bed bath now or later this morning?"
    c. "I will be giving you your bath. Do you use soap or shower gel?"
    d. "I prefer a shower in the evening. When would you like your bath?"

12. A nurse is providing instruction to the patient regarding the procedure to change his colostomy bag. During the teaching session, he asks, "What type of foods should I avoid to prevent gas?" The question the patient has asked allows for which of the following?
    a. A closed-ended answer
    b. Information clarification
    c. The nurse to give advice
    d. A yes or no answer

13. When interacting with a patient, the nurse answers, "I am sure everything will be fine. You have nothing to worry about." This is an example of which of the following inappropriate communication techniques?
    a. Cliché
    b. Giving advice
    c. Being judgmental
    d. Changing the subject

14. A 76-year-old patient states, "I have been experiencing complications of diabetes." The nurse needs to direct the patient to gain more information. What is the most appropriate comment or question to elicit additional information?
    a. "Do you take two injections of insulin to decrease the complications?"
    b. "Most physicians recommend diet and exercise to regulate blood sugar."
    c. "Most complications of diabetes are related to neuropathy."
    d. "What specific complications have you experienced?"

15. During an interaction with a critically ill patient's family, the nurse uses the communication technique of silence. This technique assists the family to:
    a. Communicate with the patient
    b. Plan for discharge
    c. Organize their thoughts
    d. Decrease anxiety

● Answers With Rationale

1. *d.* The charge nurse should direct the patient care technician to determine the patient's safety. Then she or he should address any concerns regarding the patient care technician's communication techniques privately. It is important that the nurse directs the patient care technician on aspects of therapeutic communication.

2. *a.* It is important that the nurse maintain confidentiality when providing care. The statement of "New mothers need support" is a general statement that all new parents need help. The statement is not judgmental of the family's roles.

3. *d.* Direct comments that clarify will assist the nurse in obtaining adequate information.

4. *d.* The nurse should identify himself, be sure the patient knows what will be happening, and the time period he will be with his patient.

5. *d.* The use of Therapeutic Touch conveys acceptance, and the implementation of an open-ended question allows the patient time to verbalize freely.

6. *a.* The discharge planning phase coordinates with the termination phase of a helping relationship. It is important that the nurse determine the progress made in achieving the goals related to the patient's care.

7. *c.* By engaging in self-talk, or intrapersonal communication, the nursing student can plan her day and enhance her clinical performance to decrease fear and anxiety.

8. *b.* Effective communication by the sender involves the implementation of nonthreatening information by showing respect to the receiver. The nurse should identify the subject of the meeting and be sure it occurs at a mutually agreed upon time.

9. *c.* Ascertaining that the staff completes a task on time and that all members agree the task is important is a characteristic of group identity.

10. *a.* A patient who presents with nonverbal communication of a stooped gait and facial grimacing is most likely experiencing pain. It is important that the nurse clarify this nonverbal behavior.

11. *b.* It is important that the nurse asks permission to assist the patient with a bath. This allows for consent to assist the patient with care that invades the patient's private zones.

12. *b.* The patient's question allows the nurse to clarify information that is new to the patient or that requires further explanation.

13. *a.* Telling a patient that everything is going to be all right is a cliché. The use of this statement is giving false assurance. The use of clichés gives the patient the impression that the nurse is not interested in the patient's condition.

14. *d.* Requesting specific information regarding complications of diabetes will elicit specific information to guide the nurse in further interview questions and specific assessment techniques.

15. *c.* Silence allows the family to organize their thoughts and develop any questions specific to understanding the patient's care.

Taylor Suite Resources

The Taylor Suite offers these additional resources to enhance learning and facilitate understanding of this chapter:

- thePoint online resource, http://thepoint.lww.com/Taylor7E
- Student DVD-ROM included with the book
- Study Guide for Taylor's Fundamentals of Nursing

BIBLIOGRAPHY

American Association of Critical-Care Nurses (AACN). (2005). AACN standards for establishing and sustaining healthy work environments. Available at http://www.aacn.org/WD/HWE/Docs/HWEStandards.pdf

Angel, G., & Petronko, D. K. (1983). *Developing the new assertive nurse: Essentials for advancement.* New York: Springer-Verlag.

Austin, S. (2008). Safe nursing practice. *Nursing, 38*(3), 35–39.

Berlo, D. (1960). *The process of communication: An introduction to theory and practice.* New York: Holt, Rinehart & Winston.

Bulechek, G., Butcher, H., & Dochterman, J. (2008). *Nursing interventions classification (NIC)* (5th ed.). St. Louis: Mosby Inc.

Eliopoulos, C. (2010). *Gerontological nursing* (7th ed.). Philadelphia: Lippincott Williams & Wilkins.

Facente, A. (2006). Humor in health care: Irreverent or invaluable? *Nursing, 36*(4), 64hn6–64hn7.

Flores, N. (2008). Dealing with an angry patient. *Nursing, 38*(5), 30–31.

Frisch, N., & Frisch, L. (2006). *Psychiatric mental health nursing.* Clifton Park, NY: Thomson Delmar Learning.

Gieger, J. N., & Davidhizar, R. E. (2008). *Transcultural nursing: Assessment and intervention* (5th ed.). St. Louis: Mosby.

Hohenhaus, S., Powell, S., & Hohenhaus, J. (2006). Enhancing patient safety during hand-offs. *American Journal of Nursing, 106*(8), 72A–72C.

Hurley, J. (2006). Nurse-to-nurse horizontal violence: Recognizing it and preventing it. *Imprint, 53*(4), 68–71.

Hutchison, C. P. (1999). Healing touch: An energetic approach. *American Journal of Nursing, 99*(4), 43–48.

Institute for Healthcare Improvement (IHI). (2008). *SBAR report to physician about a critical condition.* Available at http://www.ihi.org/IHI/Topics/PatientSafety/SafetyGeneral/Tools/SBARTechniqueforCommunicationASituationalBriefingModel.htm

Leiper, J. (2005). Nurse against nurse: How to stop horizontal violence. *Nursing, 35*(3), 44–45.

Mackey, R. B. (1995). Discover the healing power of therapeutic touch. *American Journal of Nursing, 95*(4), 26–33.

Manojlovich, M., Antonakos, C., & Ronis, D. (2009). Intensive care units, communication between nurses and physicians, and patients' outcomes. *American Journal of Critical Care, 18*(1), 21–30.

Martin, S. (2007). Stopping verbal abuse in the workplace. *American Journal of Nursing, 107*(4), 32–34.

Mascioli, S., Laskowski-Jones, L., Urban, S., & Moran, S. (2009). Improving handoff communication. *Nursing, 39*(2), 52–55.

Messner, R. L. (1993). What patients really want from their nurses. *American Journal of Nursing, 93*(8), 38–41.

Montagu, A. (1986). *Touching: The human significance of the skin* (3rd ed.). New York: Harper & Row.

Moorhead, S., Johnson, M., Maas, M., & Swanson, E. (2008). *Nursing outcomes classification (NOC)* (4th ed.). St. Louis: Mosby, Inc.

Mullens, M. (2006). Listening to the silence. *Nursing, 36*(4), 43.

Negley, K., Ness, S., Fee-Schroeder, K., Kokal, J., & Voll, J. (2009). Building a collaborative nursing practice to promote patient education: An inpatient and outpatient partnership. *Oncology Nursing Forum, 36*(1), 19–23.

North American Nursing Diagnosis Association–International (NANDA-I). (2009). *Nursing diagnoses: Definitions and classification, 2009–2011.* Oxford, UK: Wiley-Blackwell.

Oliva, N. (2008). When language intervenes. *American Journal of Nursing, 108*(3), 73–75.

Orlando, I. J. (1961). *The dynamic nurse–patient relationship.* New York: G. P. Putnam's Sons.

Paterson, J., & Zderad, L. (1976). *Humanistic nursing.* New York: Wiley.

Peplau, H. (1952). *Interpersonal relations in nursing.* New York: Putnam.

Pope, B., Rodzen, L., & Spross, G. (2007). Raising the SBAR: How better communication improves patient outcomes. *Nursing, 37*(3), 41–43.

Potera, C. (2008). Hospitals must address bad behavior. *American Journal of Nursing, 108*(10), 19.

Pullen, R. (2007). Tips for communicating with a patient from another culture. *Nursing, 37*(10), 48–49.

Ruffinen, M. (2007). 10 Steps to improve patient satisfaction. *Nursing, 37*(5), 22–24.

Schroeder, S. (2006). Picking up the PACE: A new template for shift report. *Nursing, 36*(10), 22–23.

Sirota, T. (2007). Nurse/physician relationships: Improving or not? *Nursing, 37*(1), 52–55.

Tannen, D. (1990). *You just don't understand: Women and men in conversation.* New York: Morrow.

The Joint Commission (TJC). (2008). *National patient safety goals.* Available at http://www.jointcommission.org/NR/rdonlyres/31666E86-E7F4-423E-9BE8-F05BD1CB0AA8/0/HAP_NPSG.pdf

Thompson, G., Menec, V., Chochinov, H., & McClement, S. (2008). Family satisfaction with care of a dying loved one in nursing homes: What makes the difference? *Journal of Gerontological Nursing, 34*(12), 37–44.

Thrall, T. (2006). Stopping ED violence before it happens. *Hospitals & Health Networks, 80*(9), 56–58.

Travelbee, J. (1971). *Interpersonal aspects of nursing* (2nd ed.). Philadelphia: F. A. Davis.

Townsend, M. (2009). *Psychiatric mental health nursing: Concepts of care* (6th ed.). Philadelphia: F. A. Davis.

Videbeck, S. (2008). *Psychiatric mental health nursing* (4th ed.). Philadelphia: Lippincott Williams & Wilkins.

Watson, J. (1985). *Nursing: The philosophy and science of caring.* Boulder, CO: Colorado Associated University Press.

Teacher and Counselor | 22

MARCO GARCÍA RAMÍREZ

Marco accompanies his wife, Claudia, to the antepartal clinic for a routine visit. They are expecting their first child in 5 months. He reports that they are happy and excited but also scared and very nervous. They are planning for a home birth, asking lots of questions about childbirth and their new responsibilities as parents: "We're both wondering if we'll be good parents."

RACHEL BLUMENTHAL

Rachel, age 40, is the second wife of a 57-year-old man who has suffered a serious myocardial infarction. They have been married for only 1 year. She says, "I'm a little embarrassed to talk with the cardiologist, but I have lots of questions about what my husband will be able to do after he gets home. I'm also wondering about resuming sexual activity."

ALICIA BONET

Alicia is the young mother of a baby boy; the baby's physician is recommending that he start long-term aspirin therapy. Ms. Bonet is quite concerned about agreeing to long-term aspirin therapy and asks, "I've heard so much about Reye's syndrome and aspirin. What should I do? What would you recommend?"

LEARNING OBJECTIVES

After completing the chapter, you will be able to accomplish the following:

1. Describe the teaching–learning process, including domains, developmental concerns, and specific principles.

2. Describe the factors that should be assessed in the learning process.

3. Discuss strategies that improve health literacy and promote patient safety.

4. Describe the factors that influence patient compliance with the therapeutic plan.

5. Formulate diagnoses for identified learning needs.

6. Explain how to create and implement a culturally competent, age-specific teaching plan for a patient.

7. Name three methods for evaluating learning.

8. Explain what should be included in the documentation of the teaching–learning process.

9. Discuss the nurse's role as a counselor.

10. Summarize how the nursing process is used to help patients solve problems.

11. Describe how to use the counseling role to motivate a patient toward health promotion.

KEY TERMS

affective learning
andragogy
cognitive learning
contractual agreement
counseling
developmental crisis
formal teaching
health literacy
informal teaching
learning

learning readiness
literacy
negative reinforcement
patient education
pedagogy
positive reinforcement
psychomotor learning
situational crisis
teaching–learning process

Helping patients and their families learn how to respond to their healthcare problems and how to protect their health is one of the most important nursing functions. Many patients lack the knowledge and self-care abilities they need to achieve their health goals. To work effectively with these patients, nurses must be skilled teachers and counselors. Both roles require strong communication skills. Current

trends toward shorter hospital stays and decreased time for interactions between healthcare professionals and patients, dependence on complex technologies, evidence of health promotion/consumer empowerment, cost containment, and an increase in chronic illnesses have increased the need for effective teaching and counseling. Nurses are challenged with the task of teaching copious amounts of information, with limited time and resources, to patients who might or might not be ready, willing, or able to learn. (See the accompanying Reflective Practice box for an example.)

Never has the demand for quality education and counseling been greater. Nurses who are skilled educators and counselors can improve patients' health and well-being and reduce the demand for professional services. The Joint Commission, an agency that evaluates the quality of patient care provided by hospitals, has identified goals and standards for patient and family teaching and included them throughout their accreditation manual. These standards ensure that the patient and family receive the information they need to maintain optimal health. They address an understanding of health status including disease and its treatment, informed decision making, and the promotion of healthy lifestyles. In 2002, The Joint Commission began sponsoring the "Speak Up" initiative. This is an effort to educate patients how to get involved in their care and prevent healthcare errors. The Speak Up campaign now includes 11 brochures that address topics such as things you can do to prevent infection, pain management recommendations, and how patients can avoid mistakes with their medications. The complete list of "Speak Up" informational brochures is available at http://www.jointcommission.org/GeneralPublic/Speak+Up/about_speakup.htm.

AIMS OF TEACHING AND COUNSELING

Patient education is the process of influencing the patient's behavior to effect changes in knowledge, attitudes, and skills needed to maintain and improve health. Research supports the fact that educated patients experience better health and have fewer complications. This results in fewer hospitalizations and emergency department, clinic, and physician visits. To be successful, patient education must be ongoing and interactive. It must also take into account the patient's plan of care, educational level, and need for care across the continuum from the hospital to home care to long-term care. Patient education plans should be developed in collaboration with the entire healthcare team, including members of the hospital team (e.g., dietitians, respiratory therapists, social workers, pharmacists) as well as home care agencies, wellness facilities, and long-term care agencies.

The basic purpose of teaching and counseling is to help patients and families develop the self-care abilities (knowledge, attitude, skills) they need to maximize their functioning and quality of life (or to have a dignified death). For example, a patient newly diagnosed with diabetes must: (1) acquire knowledge about diabetes as a disease process and related medical management and self-care, (2) value health sufficiently to make certain lifestyle modifications (attitude), and (3) master certain skills, such as insulin injection. When

REFLECTIVE PRACTICE
Challenge to Intellectual Skills

It was during my senior practicum in pediatrics last spring that I met Alicia Bonet, the young mother of a baby boy for whom I was caring. The baby's physician was recommending long-term aspirin therapy (unfortunately, I cannot remember what condition the child had for which long-term aspirin therapy was being recommended). Ms. Bonet was quite concerned about agreeing to aspirin therapy, asking me if I knew much about Reye's syndrome. Then she asked me what I would recommend about whether or not to agree to long-term aspirin therapy. Not really understanding the risks versus the benefits of aspirin therapy or how it actually ties into Reye's syndrome, I did not feel competent to answer Ms. Bonet's questions, let alone make an educated recommendation to her.

Thinking Outside the Box: Possible Courses of Action

- Tell the mother that I could not be of help to her in making this decision because of my lack of knowledge about either topic.
- Inform her that I would have to ask other nurses and physicians to explain both topics to me (due to my lack of knowledge) before I could give her my opinion.
- Tell her that because I didn't know very much about either aspirin therapy or Reye's syndrome, I would research the topics in books and on the Internet when I had time and would get back to her with a recommendation based on my research.
- Be honest with the mother about my lack of knowledge about either aspirin therapy or Reye's syndrome and

offer to gather information from reputable sources for both of us so that we could discuss the topics.
- Provide her with information from the hospital library or the Internet so that she could educate herself (but not for my education so that I could assist her in making her decision).
- Lie to the mother (or withhold the fact that I did not know much about aspirin therapy or Reye's syndrome) and make an uneducated recommendation simply because I had the "authority" to do so.
- Ignore the mother's request, pretending not to have time to discuss her questions, rather than admitting my own ignorance or taking the time to educate myself.

Evaluating a Good Outcome: How Do I Define Success?

- The mother's needs are met. Not only does she receive a professional, educated, and competent recommendation, but she also is given the opportunity to make her own educated decisions by being given the information she needs.
- My intellectual competence is challenged and improved. I am able to admit a deficit in my knowledge and embrace the opportunity to improve it.
- The mother and patient benefit from my actions (or at least are not harmed) by the mother's informed choice.

- The mother's autonomy is encouraged—by providing her with all the necessary information, I enable her to make a healthy, educated decision.
- Quality care is provided to the patient and his family by competent professionals.
- The mother expresses an understanding of the information presented to her, feels comfortable asking additional questions, and makes an educated decision with which she is comfortable.

Personal Learning: Here's to the Future!

After explaining to the mother that I was not very familiar with aspirin therapy or Reye's syndrome, I first attempted to gather research information off the Internet for her. However, because I did not have a password to access the Internet from the nurse's station, I could not obtain the research I needed on my own. My next step was to ask my preceptor how to gather data for the mother if I could not get it off the Internet. She suggested calling down to the hospital library and asking them to put together an information packet that could be easily understood by a patient. I did this, and several hours later, the packet arrived on the floor. After flipping through it briefly, I was satisfied with its contents and delivered it to Ms. Bonet. While I wished I had had the time to read all the information myself so that I could sit down with the mother and discuss it in detail, the day had been particularly busy. The best I could do was to pass the information on to the mother and hope she would read it herself. She was very grateful that I went to the trouble of gathering so much information for her, and she did not seem at all annoyed or disappointed that I did not have time to sit down with her to review the material. I did let her know that she could feel free to ask me any questions after she read the material, but she

never got a chance to read the packet before my shift ended (because her son had visitors). As a result, we never got around to discussing her concerns.

One of the things that I learned from this experience is that it is okay to admit to a patient that you do not have all the answers. Moreover, admitting this helps to allay any doubt that he or she may have about my intellect or abilities as a nurse. Admitting a lack of knowledge is not a weakness, but a strength, for half the battle is knowing what you do not know. If anything, my willingness to admit my lack of knowledge and eagerness to educate both myself and my patient (by doing research) helped inspire trust and faith in me by my patient. I also learned that sometimes doing the best we can is better than doing nothing at all, even if the best we can do is not very much. Although I really needed to be able to sit down with Ms. Bonet and review the research with her, simply providing her with the material was enough to enable her to make an informed decision on her own. That simple act most likely empowered her to be much more comfortable with her decision in the end.

Although this occurred only a few months ago, I feel safe saying that my professional intellectual skills are quite adequate now—actually, they were quite adequate

(continued)

REFLECTIVE PRACTICE

Challenge to Intellectual Skills (continued)

back then, too. Not knowing everything in nursing is not a reflection of inadequate professional intellectual skills, because it is impossible to know everything in this field. The fact that I knew that my knowledge was lacking, but that I knew where to go to find an answer, tells me my professional intellectual skills are more than adequate.

Tracey Sara Miller, Georgetown University

Reflection

How do you think you would respond in a similar situation? Why? What does this tell you about yourself and about the adequacy of your skills for professional practice? Imagine if the nursing student had not informed Ms. Bonet about her lack of knowledge. Would the student's actions have been ethical? Legal? Professional? Please explain. Can you think of other ways to respond? What other skills (cognitive, interpersonal, technical, ethical/legal) would you need to respond well in this situation? How did the nursing student's communication skills improve the nurse–patient relationship? What, if any, teaching and learning principles did the nursing student use? Would any referrals be appropriate in this situation? If so, please describe. Do you agree with the criteria to evaluate a successful outcome? Did the nursing student meet the criteria? Please explain your answer.

used effectively, teaching and counseling are powerful tools for helping patients achieve health goals. Teaching provides the knowledge patients need to make informed healthcare decisions and to implement a plan of care.

> Recall Alicia Bonet, the young mother worried about long-term aspirin therapy and Reye's syndrome. By providing Ms. Bonet with information, the nurse enables her to reach a decision that is based on sound knowledge and one with which she is comfortable. ■

Counseling provides the resources and support patients need to participate actively in self-care and to facilitate their coping with what cannot be changed.

Maintaining and Promoting Health

Nurses can help patients to value health and develop specific health practices that promote wellness. Health teaching is varied and ranges from teaching passive exercises to a patient with left-sided paralysis to designing a safe exercise program for a young athlete.

Preventing Illness

Illness prevention, a major theme in health teaching and counseling, takes many forms. You can counsel women of childbearing age about health practices that promote optimal fetal development, teach parents how to make their home safe for a toddler, or counsel individuals at high risk for heart disease, cancer, or communicable diseases.

Restoring Health

Once a patient is ill, teaching and counseling focus on developing self-care practices that promote recovery. Preoperative and postoperative teaching, sexual counseling for a patient recovering from a myocardial infarction, and lifestyle coun-

seling for a patient with an ostomy are all examples of teaching and counseling directed at restoring health.

> Consider Rachel Blumenthal, the wife of the patient who had suffered a myocardial infarction. She is concerned about his activity level. When developing an appropriate teaching plan, the nurse would need to assess Mrs. Blumenthal's knowledge base before determining her actual teaching needs. In addition, the nurse would need to consult with the patient's cardiologist to determine what the patient's status is and what he will be allowed to do. These actions help to ensure that the teaching plan includes accurate information and is individualized to Mrs. Blumenthal's needs. ■

Facilitating Coping

Developmental lifestyle changes and acute, chronic, and terminal illness all place demands on patients and families that may become overwhelming. As a nurse, you will work not only with patients, but also with their families and friends to help them to come to terms with illness and whatever lifestyle modifications it entails. Not all patients fully recover from their illness or injury; many patients will need to learn to cope with permanent health alterations.

Summary

Nurse caregivers who are skilled teachers and counselors can promote the following outcomes:

- High-level wellness and related self-care practices
- Disease prevention or early detection
- Quick recovery from trauma or illness with minimal or no complications

- Enhanced ability to adjust to developmental lifestyle changes and acute, chronic, and terminal illness
- Family acceptance of the lifestyle changes necessitated by illness or disability

▶ *Remember Marco García Ramírez, the father-to-be described in the beginning of the chapter. Pregnancy and childbirth are considered developmental lifestyle changes. The nurse would need to incorporate knowledge of these changes when preparing an appropriate teaching plan for Mr. García Ramírez and his wife. The goal of teaching would be a positive adaptation to their new role as parents.* ■

General topics for health teaching are highlighted in Box 22-1.

THE NURSE AS TEACHER

Teaching is a planned method or series of methods used to help someone learn. The person using these methods is the teacher. **Learning** is the process by which a person acquires or increases knowledge or changes behavior in a measurable way as a result of the experience. You assume the role of teacher and your patient assumes the role of learner when there are identifiable learning needs. This teacher–learner relationship is enhanced by the helping relationship (see Chapter 21) in which mutual respect and trust are established. You build on this trust by sharing information that you and your patient have mutually identified as important.

▶ *Think back to Alicia Bonet, the young mother with questions about long-term aspirin therapy. The nurse was able to develop trust with Ms. Bonet by honestly admitting that she lacked the necessary knowledge about the therapy. The nurse was able to promote an ongoing therapeutic relationship by seeking the information, thereby solidifying the trust.* ■

The patient may ask for this information, or you may initiate teaching after assessing and diagnosing a learning need. Much patient education focuses on three critical areas:

- Preparation for receiving care
- Preparation before discharge from a healthcare facility
- Documentation of patient education activity

As with other clinical interventions, effective patient teaching demands analytic and problem-solving skills. To maximize the effectiveness of patient teaching, remember the acronym TEACH:

T: tune into the patient

E: edit patient information

A: act on every teaching moment

C: clarify often

H: honor the patient as a partner in the education process

Learning to be an effective teacher is a critical component of professional development. A basic understanding of the **teaching–learning process** aids in developing your own teaching and learning skills. The process of patient teaching, which resembles the nursing process, consists of several steps that are necessary to provide teaching and to measure learning (Box 22-2). This process is often condensed because of limited time or resources, but the basic principles apply each time teaching–learning occurs.

Being a successful teacher requires excellent communication skills and sensitivity to all the factors that affect the patient's ability to learn (Fig. 22-1).

Factors Affecting Patient Learning

By taking into consideration the patient's age and developmental level, family support networks and financial resources, cultural influences and language deficits, and health literacy level you can individualize the teaching plan and maximize learning. This will support the nursing goal of helping the patient to manage his or her own healthcare needs.

Box 22-1 TOPICS FOR HEALTH TEACHING AND COUNSELING

Promoting Health
- Developmental and maturational issues
- Normal childbearing
- Hygiene
- Nutrition
- Exercise
- Mental health
- Spiritual health

Preventing Illness
- First aid
- Safety
- Immunizations
- Screening
- Identification and management of risk factors

Restoring Health
- Orientation to treatment center and staff
- Patients' and nurses' expectations of one another
- The illness and physical condition: anatomy and physiology, etiology of problem, significance of symptoms, prognosis
- The medical and nursing regimens and how the patient can participate in care
- Self-care practices the patient and family need to manage the patient's condition independently

Facilitating Coping
- How the patient's physical and mental condition affects other areas of functioning; lifestyle counseling
- Measures that maximize independence and enhance self-concept
- Stress management
- Environmental alterations
- Community resources
- Appropriate referrals (e.g., physical therapy, occupational therapy, self-help groups, psychiatric–mental health counselor)
- Grief and bereavement counseling

Box 22-2 STEPS OF THE TEACHING–LEARNING PROCESS

Assess Learning Needs and Learning Readiness

1. Use all appropriate sources of information.
2. Identify the knowledge, attitudes, or skills needed by the patient and family.
3. Assess the patient's emotional and experiential readiness to learn.
4. Assess factors affecting the patient's ability to learn, including age and development level, family support networks and financial resources, cultural influences, literacy, and language barriers.
5. Develop critical pathways or teaching plans that span care delivery settings from hospital to home to take advantage of optimal learning readiness.
6. Identify the patient's strengths.
7. Use anticipatory guidance.

Diagnose the Patient's Learning Needs

1. Be realistic.
2. Validate with patient or family through conversations, questionnaires, and checklists.

Develop Learning Outcomes

1. Identify specific, attainable, measurable, and short-term outcomes for patient learning.
2. Make sure that proposed behavioral changes are realistic and explored in the context of the patient's resources and lifestyle.
3. Decide which domain of learning is involved (cognitive, psychomotor, affective).
4. Prioritize.
5. Include the patient and family. Unless the patient values these outcomes, little learning is likely to occur.

Develop a Teaching Plan

1. Select content, content sequencing, and appropriate teaching strategies/activities.
2. Relate the teaching content to the patient's learning style, interests, resources, and patterns of everyday living.
3. Pay careful attention to time constraints, scheduling, and the physical environment.
4. Decide on group versus individual teaching and formal versus informal methodologies.
5. Formulate a verbal or written contract with the patient.

Implement Teaching Plan and Strategies

1. Prepare the physical environment, with attention to comfort and privacy.
2. Communicate effectively with individuals, small groups, and, in some instances, large groups.
3. Gather all audiovisual materials and equipment.
4. Deliver the content in an organized manner using the selected teaching strategies.
5. Be flexible.
6. Keep teaching sessions short.
7. Vary strategies for sensory stimulation, which promotes learning.
8. Relate the material to the patients' life experiences, which will help them assimilate new knowledge.
9. Plan how you will evaluate learning.
10. Assess verbal and nonverbal feedback.

Evaluate Learning

1. Evaluate whether the learner outcomes were met:
   - Observe a return demonstration.
   - Ask the patient to restate the instructions.
   - Ask the patient questions to determine whether teaching reinforcement is needed.
   - Use written test or questionnaires.
   - Consult with the patient's family.
   - Consider patient feedback and comments.
2. Reinforce and celebrate learning.
3. Evaluate teaching:
   - Self-evaluation
   - Patient questionnaires
4. Revise the plan if the learner outcome is not met:
   - Alter content and teaching strategies.
   - Use motivational counseling.
   - Reschedule teaching sessions.
5. Document the teaching–learning process:
   - Patient and family learning needs and identified barriers to learning
   - Mechanisms used to overcome learning barriers
   - Patient and family readiness to learn
   - Current knowledge regarding the patient's condition and health status
   - Learning outcomes agreed on by the nurse, patient, and family
   - Identification of learning outcomes
   - Information and skills taught
   - Teaching methods used
   - Patient and family response
   - Evaluation of what patient and family learned and need for follow-up

Age and Developmental Level

People learn throughout life, although what they learn and how learning occurs changes according to developmental stages. Three critical developmental areas to consider when developing a teaching plan are the patient's physical maturation and abilities, psychosocial development, and cognitive capacity. Other concerns related to the teaching–learning process include the patient's emotional maturity and moral and spiritual development.

CHILD AND ADOLESCENT LEARNERS

Piaget's theory of intellectual development is a major learning theory (see Chapter 18). By understanding how children and adolescents develop learning abilities, you can use this knowledge when teaching patients. When the patient is an infant, teaching is directed toward the parents. Toddlers and preschoolers may have some degree of understanding about medical tests or procedures, but health teaching continues to be directed toward the parents. For patients of this age, it is helpful for one nurse to establish a relationship with the patient and family and to be consistently involved in patient teaching activities. As an example of teaching considerations for young children, if a 4-year-old girl must begin to take insulin every day, it is important to recognize her limitations in understanding diabetes. Information should be simplified to include only the most basic facts, with concrete examples or demonstrations; a detailed discussion of the pathophysiology

FIGURE 22-1. Effective communication is essential in the teaching–learning process. *(Photo by Rick Brady.)*

of diabetes would not be appropriate. The girl could be told that she needs a shot every day to keep her from getting sick or feeling "funny." She could be allowed to play with the syringes and to give shots to a doll. Compared to adults, children have shorter attention spans, combined with a great need for nurturing, support, and creative participation in learning activities.

School-aged children are capable of logical reasoning and should be included in the teaching–learning process whenever possible. Teaching strategies that include clear explanations and reasons for procedures, stated in a simple and logical manner, are most successful.

The cognitive processes of adolescents are similar to those of adults, so the content and strategies of patient teaching resemble those used for teaching adults. There are some important considerations to keep in mind though. For example, if teaching a sexually active 16-year-old girl about contraceptive methods, you will need to assess whether the young patient has reached the stage Piaget refers to as formal operations (the ability to use logical reasoning to solve hypothetical problems). If the patient's intellectual development is delayed and she is still in the period of concrete operations (use of logical reasoning to solve concrete problems), she may be unable to think abstractly—that is, she may not perceive pregnancy as a real possibility and, therefore, may not understand the need for contraception. If so, you can alter the teaching plan to include online teaching aids that are easily accessible and explain the topic in concrete terms. Peer group acceptance is a critical issue for adolescents. Teaching strategies designed for an adolescent patient should recognize the adolescent's need for independence, as well as the need to establish a trusting relationship that demonstrates respect for the adolescent's opinions.

Motor development is also a concern in the teaching–learning process. The 4-year-old girl diagnosed with diabetes may not be able to give her own insulin shots if she lacks the fine motor skills needed to manipulate the equipment, but a 13-year-old patient could probably master the technique quickly.

ADULT LEARNERS

As people age, their personalities and learning abilities change. Most psychologists who have studied the teaching–learning process base their work on children and adolescents because a large amount of learning occurs early in life. The science of teaching (called **pedagogy**) generally refers to the teaching of children and adolescents. In recent years, however, the study of teaching adults (**andragogy**) has gained more attention.

Adults need to be taught differently than children. Knowles (1990) listed the following four assumptions about adult learners:

1. As a person matures, his or her self-concept is likely to move from dependence to independence.
2. The previous experience of the adult is a rich resource for learning.
3. An adult's readiness to learn is often related to a developmental task or a social role.
4. Most adults' orientation to learning is that material should be useful immediately, rather than at some time in the future.

Thus, andragogy focuses on a specific problem or need and on the immediate application of new material. In general, adult learners must believe that they need to learn before they are willing to learn. Nurses often must use their counseling skills (discussed later) to motivate patients to participate in the teaching–learning process. Adults may need to be shown the importance of learning new information, health practices, or skills.

As health promotion and injury avoidance are important activities throughout the life span, teaching methods need to be further modified when working with older patients. When developing a teaching plan for older adults, first identify any learning barriers such as sensory loss, limited physical mobility, or inability to comply with the recommended therapeutic regimen. Sensory deficits that can affect learning in older adults include the presence of cataracts that can cloud vision, a decrease in lens accommodation that necessitates adequate lighting, a decrease in peripheral vision that requires that teaching materials be kept immediately in front of learners, and hearing loss that make it imperative for teachers to speak slowly and clearly (Mauk, 2006). Successful teaching plans for older adults incorporate extra time, short teaching sessions, accommodation for sensory deficits, and reduction of environmental distractions. Older adults also benefit from instruction that relates new information to familiar activities or information.

Family Support Networks and Financial Resources

No matter what the patient's age, working with the patient's family can be a great help in patient teaching. Assess the family's function and style by talking with them and observing how the patient and family interact. This assessment will yield information about family function, stress, transitions, and expectations. Informal conversations with both the

Box 22-3   THE COPE MODEL

C: Creativity
Help the family to overcome obstacles to carrying out healthcare management and learning how to generate alternatives.

O: Optimism
Help the family caregivers learn how to view the caregiving situation with confidence.

P: Planning
Help the family learn how to plan for future problems and how to develop contingency plans that reduce uncertainty.

E: Expert Information
Help the family learn how to obtain expert information from healthcare providers about what to do in specific situations. This information empowers caregivers by encouraging them to develop plans for solving caregiving problems.

patient and family can provide data that will help in developing the teaching plan. The COPE model described in Box 22-3 is one method of helping family members to become effective problem solvers and support your teaching efforts.

When teaching long-term family caregivers, include information about the disease process and resources available in the community that can help them with disease management and education, with a focus on planning, caregiving, decision making, and problem solving. It is important to view the family caregiver as a partner in providing care and to view yourself as a health educator who teaches families how to solve problems, rather than as an expert meant to solve problems for them.

In addition, evaluate the family's financial resources, because the patient may be unable to afford to follow a new treatment regimen. If needed, refer patients and families to community-based support groups and funding sources.

Cultural Influences and Language Deficits

As our society becomes more ethnically diverse, nurses are continuously faced with the challenge of providing care and education to patients from many different cultural and ethnic backgrounds. To do so successfully, you may need to seek information from a variety of sources, such as the nursing literature and textbooks that describe the health practices and values of other cultures. Box 22-4 outlines strategies for providing patient education in a culturally competent manner.

In addition, be sure to identify language deficits or barriers and develop strategies to address them, clearly communicating this in the plan of care. One of the strategies is to develop written materials in the native language of the patient. Do not assume that a family member is adequately translating information critical to the patient's learning. As many as one in every 15 people either do not speak English or understand very little and this necessitates the need for trained interpreters who can present health teaching information in a clear, objective manner (Vesterlund, 2008).

Health Literacy

According to information contained in a report by The Joint Commission (2007b), approximately half of the adults in the United States, or 90 million people, lack the basic **literacy** skills (the ability to read and write) needed to function successfully in our society. Given the complexity of the many facets of healthcare, it follows then that many people are unable to understand basic health information and make appropriate healthcare decisions. **Health literacy** is defined as the ability to read, understand, and act on health information. Twenty percent (20%) of American adults read at the 5th-grade level or below, while the average American reads at an 8th- or 9th-grade level (Partnership for Clear Health Communication at the National Patient Safety Foundation, 2006). The scope of the problem becomes even more challenging with the knowledge that most healthcare information and directions are written at a 10th-grade level or greater. Research indicates that health literacy is a stronger predictor of health status than other factors such as socioeconomic status, age, or ethnic background (Nath, 2007). Low health literacy is believed to cost more than $58 billion annually in the United States (Partnership for Clear Health Communication at the National Patient Safety Foundation, 2006). It affects all segments of our population and threatens the quality and safety of our healthcare.

The National Patient Safety Foundation recently collaborated with the Partnership for Clear Health Communication (2007) to create awareness of the need for improved health literacy and to seek solutions that result in more positive patient outcomes. One of their first initiatives was the development of Ask Me 3. Ask Me 3 is a brief tool intended to promote understanding and improve communication between patients and their providers. It involves three simple questions that patients should ask their healthcare providers during every encounter. Providers are encouraged to answer these questions in a clear, forthright manner. The Ask Me 3 questions are:

- What is my main problem?
- What do I need to do?
- Why is it important for me to do this?

The healthcare provider's response should include plain language without the use of medical jargon, may incorporate the

Box 22-4   CULTURALLY COMPETENT PATIENT TEACHING

- Develop an understanding of the patient's culture.
- Work with a multicultural team in developing educational programs.
- Be aware of personal assumptions, biases, and prejudices.
- Understand the core cultural values of the patient or group.
- Develop written materials in the patient's native language.
- Use testimonials of persons with the same cultural background as the patient.

Promoting Health Literacy

IN PATIENTS WHO SMOKE

Patient Scenario

Jack Boyer is 37 years old and has been smoking since he was 17 years of age. During a routine physical, he admits to a one pack/day habit. In response to a question from his physician, Jack admits that several previous attempts to stop smoking failed after a day or two. He states on his history form that he is married and has two sons who are 7 and 3 years of age and also listed that his father died following a heart attack at the age of 60. Jack tells his physician that he is essentially healthy but is under a lot of stress. Because of the downturn in the economy, his job in automotive sales is at risk. His wife works full-time as an administrative assistant. The physician expresses concern to Jack about the effects of second-hand smoke on his family. Jack states "I know all about that and when I smoke in the car, I keep the window down and blow the smoke outside. At home, I try to smoke outside most of the time except when the weather is bad." The physical examination reveals that Jack has hypertension (BP 164/92), is 15 pounds overweight, and is currently having difficulty sleeping. The physician explains that he would like to monitor Jack's blood pressure for 1 month before prescribing antihypertensive medication. He recommends that Jack make a serious effort to stop smoking and reviews the harmful effects of nicotine use and the long-term benefits for Jack as well as his family if he stops smoking. He explains that the nurse will give him information about quitting smoking when he makes an appointment for his next visit. As Jack is speaking with the nurse, he comments that maybe he'll have to switch to chewing tobacco since there's no smoke involved with that.

Nursing Considerations: *Tips for Improving Health Literacy*

Provide Jack with information about ways to help him quit smoking. Mention that counseling and behavior cessation therapies have proven effective and that oftentimes it takes repeated attempts to quit. Jack needs to understand the harmful effects the second-hand smoke can have on his family, as well as the fact that people who stop smoking greatly reduce their risk of lung cancer, heart disease, and respiratory symptoms. Explain to him that smokeless tobacco is also a significant health risk and not a safe substitute for smoking cigarettes. Give him information about nicotine replacement products (gum, inhalers, patches) found effective in treating tobacco dependence. Several nonnicotine medications are also available but need to be prescribed by his physician. For extra help, tell him to call 1-800 QUIT NOW. When Jack returns for his follow-up appointment, he needs to be prepared to ask his physician the following questions to help him understand that tobacco addiction is a chronic condition and what the positive outcomes of quitting will be:

- What is my main problem?
- What do I need to do?
- Why is it important for me to do this?

What additional measures can you take to help increase health literacy in this patient? What other measures would be helpful if Jack did not speak English, could not read, or had other learning deficits?

---

use of visual models to explain a disease or procedure, and may involve patients in a "teach back" demonstration that verifies their understanding of the information presented. See the accompanying Promoting Health Literacy display in this and other chapters throughout this book for an example in action.

In 2007, The Joint Commission (2007b) issued a public policy paper entitled "What Did the Doctor Say?: Improving Health Literacy to Protect Patient Safety." This initiative addresses the gathering of information and the formulation of solutions to this silent epidemic of low health literacy. Recommendations range from enhanced training for patient interpreters to redesign of consent forms and the informed consent process (see the accompanying Research in Nursing box) to assessment of literacy levels and language needs in communities by local healthcare organizations. The multiple recommendations in this report underscore the necessity to "improve health literacy, reduce communications-related errors, and better support the interests of patients and providers of care alike" (The Joint Commission, 2007b).

Nurses, as key players in this endeavor, need an awareness of the extent of the health literacy problem. This includes efforts to assess patients' ability to understand health information, address the use of simple and effective communication, and limit the negative effects of low health literacy. Two effective tools that can be used to determine health literacy level include a Rapid Estimate of Adult Literacy in Medicine–Short Form and the Short Assessment of Health Literacy for Spanish Adults. They are available on the Agency for Healthcare Research and Quality Web site: http:www.ahrq.gov/populations/sahlsatool.htm. Specific nursing strategies that target health literacy are included in Box 22-5.

Learning Domains

Patients learn in three domains: cognitive, psychomotor, and affective (Bloom, 1956). The ability of patients to manage their daily life and resume their former roles depends on the degree to which cognitive, psychomotor, and affective

RESEARCH IN NURSING
Bridging the Gap to Evidence-Based Practice

PROMOTING HEALTH LITERACY WITH IMPROVED SURGICAL CONSENT FORMS

It is estimated that more than one-third of adults have either basic or below-basic health literacy. Healthcare related information is often complex and difficult to comprehend with basic health literacy abilities. Materials such as prescription bottle labels, procedural consents, dietary guidelines, and insurance forms are challenging and often misunderstood under normal conditions. The use of medical terminology, illness, pain, and fear often compound stress for patients and further decrease their understanding and health literacy. This research documents an effort initiated by nurses to improve the clarity of surgical consent documents thus ensuring that a patient's signature on a consent form indicates that they understand and are indeed "informed" regarding procedures.

Related Research

Lorenzen, B., Melby, C., & Earles, B. (2008). Using principles of health literacy to enhance the informed consent process. *AORN Journal, 88*(1), 23–29.

As part of its Strategic Plan for Improvement, the Iowa Health System initiated health literacy goals aimed at creating improved communication and a patient-centered environment. This three-campus regional health system selected the improvement of consent forms and processes as one of their initiatives. Each location had a health literacy team who initially participated in health literacy learning sessions, added health literacy information to learning modules for new employees and staff, and presented this information to physicians.

Review of a report from the Institute of Medicine Committee on Health Literacy and the institution's informed consent documents indicated that the forms are lengthy, crowded with

detail, use a small font size, and include unexplained medical and legal terms. Initial improvement efforts involved development of a plain language consent form that was reader friendly. Key improvements included the use of short sentences and simple words, minimal medical terms, clear headings, and a limitation to one page. A section also provided for a description of the procedure in the patient's own words as part of the teach-back process.

Baseline data was collected and results were compared between 41 patients on an ambulatory surgical unit, who used the original consent form, and 88 patients in two pilot groups who signed the revised consent form. Survey data confirmed that 25% of the patients read the original consent form while 66% just asked where to sign and did not read it. In the pilot groups, 77% and 91% of the patients read the consent while only 14% and 10% asked where to sign and did not read the "user friendly" new form. After review by all involved parties, the revised consent documents were approved for use at all sites and provision was also made to have a Spanish version available as well.

Relevance to Nursing Practice

Collaboration on this project resulted in improved patient knowledge prior to consent for procedures and contributed to the development of best practices related to health literacy. Since health literacy levels are difficult to verify, the effect of the teach-back strategy provides nurses an opportunity to confirm and document patient understanding. Each effort at improving health literacy is ultimately linked to improving patient safety.

For additional research, visit the Point.

---

learning results in behavioral changes. These domains influence the teaching and evaluation strategies that are selected. Effective teaching often involves the promotion of behaviors in all three domains.

Cognitive learning involves the storing and recalling of new knowledge in the brain (e.g., the patient describes how salt intake affects blood pressure). Cognitive learning includes intellectual behaviors such as the acquisition of knowledge, comprehension, application (using abstract ideas in concrete situations), analysis (relating ideas in an organized way), synthesis (assimilating parts of information as a whole), and evaluation (judging the worth of a body of information).

Learning a physical skill involving the integration of mental and muscular activity is called **psychomotor learning** (e.g., the patient demonstrates how to change dressings using clean technique).

Affective learning includes changes in attitudes, values, and feelings (e.g., the patient expresses renewed self-confidence after physical therapy).

Box 22-5 NURSING STRATEGIES THAT ADDRESS INADEQUATE HEALTH LITERACY

Strategies include:
- Increase health caregivers' sensitivity to health literacy issues.
- Develop literacy-assessment protocols.
- Create and evaluate health education materials that target specific ethnic and cultural populations.
- Ensure clear communication with patients.
- Include health literacy information for student nurses as they participate in various roles including direct patient care in various settings.
- Facilitate decision making with patients by encouraging them to consider alternative options and choices.
- Conduct research about literacy.

Adapted from Nath, C. (2007). Literacy and diabetes self-management. *American Journal of Nursing, 107*(6), 43–49.

> ➤ *Recall Marco Garcia Ramirez, the father-to-be with concerns about his new role. The nurse would develop a teaching plan that focuses on the three domains of learning. The nurse would address the cognitive domain by teaching Mr. Garcia Ramirez and his wife about labor and delivery, including the labor process and what events will*

occur. Teaching the couple about newborn care and breathing techniques to use during labor would address the psychomotor domain. Learning in the affective domain would be demonstrated if Mr. García Ramírez reports that the couple do not fear labor and feel comfortable handling a newborn. ∎

Effective Communication Techniques

A critical component of effective patient education is the nurse's ability to be an effective communicator. Key points of effective communication associated with patient teaching include the following:

- Be sincere and honest; show genuine interest.
- Avoid giving too much detail; stick to the basics.
- Ask if the patient has any questions.
- Be a "cheerleader" for the patient. Avoid lecturing.
- Use simple words.
- Vary your tone of voice.
- Keep the content clear.
- Listen and do not interrupt when the patient speaks.

NURSING PROCESS FOR PATIENT AND CAREGIVER TEACHING

Patient teaching is approached most effectively using the steps of the nursing process. The teaching–learning process and the nursing process are interdependent.

Assessing
Sources of Information

Usually, patients themselves are the best source of assessment information. Patients are considered primary sources of information. By using effective interviewing techniques (see Chapter 21), you can obtain the data needed to identify learning needs. In addition, relevant information can be obtained before actually meeting the patient by reviewing the patient's past and current medical records. These records are considered secondary sources of information and can provide a history of medical problems as well as documentation of the nursing assessments, nursing diagnoses, nursing physical examinations, and nursing interventions that have been performed.

The patient's family and significant others are also valuable sources of assessment data. They are sometimes needed to provide assessment data when the patient cannot communicate because of health problems, language barriers, or impaired sensory functions. At other times, family members or significant others might be the most appropriate source of certain information; for example, if seeking information about how much salt is used in the family's cooking, it is helpful to speak with the person who prepares the meals at home and to include that person in any teaching about food preparation. The patient's permission is needed before family members are involved in the teaching–learning process.

Box 22-6 ASSESSMENT PARAMETERS: FACTORS THAT AFFECT LEARNING

1. **Knowledge, attitudes, and skills needed for the patient and family to manage healthcare independently**
2. **Readiness to learn**
   - Emotional readiness
     Emotional health
     Motivation for learning
     Self-concept and body image
     Sense of responsibility for self
   - Experiential readiness
     Social and economic stability
     Past experiences with learning
     Attitude toward learning
     Culture
3. **Ability to learn**
   - Physical condition
   - Cognitive ability to learn
   - Acuity of senses
   - Developmental considerations
   - Level of education
   - Literacy
   - Communication skills
   - Primary language
4. **Learning strengths**
   - Successful learning in the past
   - Above-average comprehension, reasoning, memory, or psychomotor skills
   - High motivation
   - Strong network
   - Adequate financing

Assessment Parameters

Four elements should be considered in each assessment of patient learning needs (Box 22-6). First, identify what new knowledge, attitudes, or skills are necessary for patients and families to learn in order to manage their healthcare. Second, focus on **learning readiness,** the patient's willingness to engage in the teaching–learning process (emotional readiness) and to begin the challenge of learning. Barriers to learning readiness include a patient's denial of his or her illness, lack of physical endurance, lack of human or financial resources, perceived benefit to continue in the sick role, and disparity of values between the patient and the healthcare provider. Readiness is distinguished from the patient's actual ability to learn, which is the third element. The fourth element of assessment is the patient's strengths, which are the personal resources that you can help the patient to tap.

MOTIVATION

When assessing a patient's learning readiness, it is important to consider his or her motivation. Patients who are ready to learn are able and motivated to process new information, develop new skills, and explore new attitudes and behaviors. Motivation is an internal impulse (such as emotion or physical pain) that encourages the patient to take action or change behavior.

> *Think back to Rachel Blumenthal, the wife of the patient who had a myocardial infarction. Although further assessment is necessary, analysis of Mrs. Blumenthal's questions would lead the nurse to suspect that she is interested in finding out information, showing motivation and a beginning readiness to learn.* ∎

A patient's health beliefs can have great influence on motivation. The health belief model identifies several health beliefs as critical for patient motivation (Rosenstock, 1974). Motivation is enhanced when:

- Patients view themselves as susceptible to the disease in question
- Patients view the disease as a serious threat
- Patients believe there are actions they can take to reduce the probability of contracting the disease
- Patients believe the threat of taking these actions is not as great as the disease itself

The health belief model was designed to explain why persons are willing to take actions to support their health, but it evolved into a strategy for predicting the likelihood that patients would comply with therapies. Motivation plays a key role in the health belief model because it spurs the client to adopt health promotion and disease protection actions. Examples of motivational triggers include personal crisis and loss of social role due to disease symptoms. You can use the health belief model when developing teaching plans, evaluating the ideas or beliefs that motivate a patient and applying these to the teaching plan. For example, if you are able to modify a patient's perception of disease susceptibility, the patient might become more receptive to learning.

COMPLIANCE

Nursing assessment of the patient's learning needs is vital to developing a plan of care with which the patient can comply. Patients are considered compliant when they follow the treatment plan and use the information they have been taught. When patients understand their diagnosis, treatment rationale, medication regimen, and the benefits of compliance, they are more likely to comply. Noncompliance occurs when patients ignore instructions or do not follow them appropriately. Noncompliance can be associated with a lack of learning readiness and motivation, confusion, disappointment, misunderstanding, fear, inability to learn, or inadequate finances. Noncompliance can hurt the patient's health.

Patients control the choices they make about following the plan of care and using what they have been taught, but it is your responsibility as a nurse to help patients improve their health by sharing knowledge, solving problems, and providing support while the patient integrates the new knowledge and practices the new skills. Increased patient compliance is a direct outcome of effective patient teaching. Box 22-7 lists ways to help patients and families become compliant with the plan of care.

Box 22-7   PROMOTING PATIENT AND FAMILY COMPLIANCE

- Be certain that healthcare instructions are understandable and designed to support patient goals.
- Include the patient and family as partners in the teaching–learning process.
- Use interactive teaching strategies.
- Remember that teaching and learning are processes that rely on strong interpersonal relationships with patients and their families.

Diagnosing

If the patient lacks the required knowledge, attitudes, or skills to support health promotion, you should diagnose the deficit. Use diagnoses or problem statements approved by the North American Nursing Diagnosis Association (NANDA) as a guide when diagnosing learning needs (see Chapter 13). If you believe that a patient's knowledge deficit is the primary problem, write a diagnosis identifying a specific knowledge deficit as the problem, followed by its etiology and the related signs and symptoms. For example, Deficient Knowledge: Breastfeeding related to inexperience, as manifested by anxiety and multiple questions.

More often, a knowledge deficit results in an actual or potential problem; therefore, the knowledge deficit is written as the etiology (second part of the diagnostic statement): for example, Imbalanced Nutrition: Less Than Body Requirements related to mother's lack of knowledge about infant feeding and deficient learning readiness (as manifested by mother's quick frustration when breastfeeding, refusal to engage in learning process, infant's weight loss).

If you learn that a pregnant woman plans to breastfeed and knows nothing about breastfeeding, "Deficient Knowledge: Breastfeeding" is the problem statement. The goal is to increase the mother's knowledge. If, on the other hand, you observe a newborn failing to gain weight appropriately, and it is reasonable to suspect that the mother's lack of knowledge about how to breastfeed is interfering with the infant's nutritional intake, "Deficient Knowledge: Breastfeeding" is the etiology. The goal is to ensure the infant's proper nutrition.

Related nursing diagnoses include the following:

- Ineffective Health Maintenance
- Ineffective Therapeutic Regimen Management
- Noncompliance
- Self-Care Deficit (specify)

Wellness diagnoses, such as Readiness for Enhanced Parenting or Readiness for Enhanced Self-Concept, are written as one-part statements. Teaching and counseling are the primary nursing interventions used to achieve related outcome criteria.

In addition to identifying the patient's learning needs, it is important to assess your own knowledge base and teaching skills. Nurses cannot teach information and skills to patients if they themselves lack the information and skills to be taught. Often, knowing where to find information or an appropriate resource person is the first step in correcting one's own knowledge deficits.

Outcome Identification and Planning

Planning for learning involves the development of a teaching plan. Teaching plans are similar to nursing care plans—both follow the steps of the nursing process. One type of teaching plan is presented in Box 22-8. It is directed toward teaching appropriate nipple care to reduce the likelihood of nipple cracking and redness in breastfeeding women.

Standardized teaching plans are available for major topics of health teaching. Such plans must be tailored to the patient's learning needs and abilities. Remember that factors such as age, developmental level, family support networks, financial resources, cultural influences, language deficits, and health literacy affect the patient's ability to learn; consider them when individualizing the teaching plan. Examples of teaching plans that are incorporated into critical path documentation systems are featured in Chapters 14 and 17.

Thoughtful planning of patient teaching maximizes the patient's learning while ensuring the most efficient use of your time and talents. Learner outcomes are developed for each diagnosis of a learning need. The nursing orders become the content, teaching strategy, and learner activity columns of the written plan. This phase requires thought and creativity. Your efforts are rewarded when the patient meets the outcomes at the end of the implementation phase.

When planning for learning, decide together with the patient who should be included in the learning sessions. When the patient is a young child, one or both parents may be the primary learners. For an adult patient, a spouse or close friend who will be giving the care that is to be learned

---

Box 22-8   SAMPLE TEACHING PLAN

Diagnosis: Risk for Impaired Skin Integrity: Nipples related to knowledge and skill deficit (nipple care)
Signs and Symptoms: complaints of sore nipples, redness, cracking

Long-term Outcome: woman will be able to breastfeed as long as desired without nipple problems

Learner Outcome	Met	Content	Teaching Strategy	Learner Activity
Woman describes measures to prevent nipple cracking (cognitive)	8/10/11 L.I.	Protective measures: • Avoid soap • Avoid exposure to air and sunlight	Lecture with discussion Audiovisual: flip chart on breastfeeding	Read handout: Nipple care
Woman begins protective measures immediately (psychomotor)	8/10/11 L.I.	• Apply lanolin or vegetable oil • Avoid plastic liners in bra or bra pads		
Woman describes the correct procedure for breastfeeding (cognitive)	8/10/11 L.I.	Preparation for breastfeeding • Nipple roll before the feeding	Discussion Audiovisual: flip chart on breastfeeding	Read handout: Sore nipples
Woman explains why feedings should be shorter and more frequent (cognitive)	8/10/11 L.I.	Breastfeeding the baby • Feed baby every 2 hours during the day • Start baby on less sore side	Discovery: guide through each step; assist as necessary Return demonstration	Read handout: Positioning baby for breastfeeding Borrow books on breastfeeding from reference library
Woman demonstrates correct procedure for breastfeeding (psychomotor)	8/10/11 L.I.	• Get baby onto areola area • Position properly • Change position for each feeding • Remove baby from breast		
Display increasing confidence in breastfeeding skills and self-care (affective)	8/10/11 L.I.	After feeding • Air dry the nipples • Inspect for open or cracked areas • Apply lanolin or vegetable oil	Discovery	
Value good nutrition and rest at home (affective)	8/10/11 L.I.	Home considerations • Maintain "demand feedings" • Ensure good nutrition • Get adequate rest • Know the signs and symptoms of thrush	Lecture with discussion Audiovisual: poster	Refer to handouts at home as needed; call maternity department's information number for any questions
List the signs of thrush (cognitive)	8/10/11 L.I.			

may be included. For instance, the person who does the household's cooking is usually asked to be present for nutritional teaching. Teaching plans are developed according to the needs of the individuals being taught.

One nurse or several nurses can prepare and use a teaching plan. When two or more nurses plan and coordinate the implementation of the plan, this is called team teaching. An advantage of team teaching is that it takes advantage of the talents of more than one nurse.

Duplicating teaching that has already been completed by other members of the healthcare team wastes time and causes frustration. Accurate and thorough documentation of all patient teaching, along with review of the medical record before teaching sessions and effective communication with members of the interdisciplinary team, can eliminate this problem.

Several factors should be considered while formulating any teaching plan, as discussed in the next sections.

PATIENT LEARNING OUTCOMES

Learner outcomes are written in the same manner as the patient outcomes in the nursing process (see Chapter 14). When planning for the patient's learning, first determine which of the three learning domains (cognitive, psychomotor, or affective) will be the focus of teaching. Then write learning outcomes that reflect what learning is to occur. A well-constructed learning outcome serves as a guide for planning evaluation methods.

Choosing the verb for a learning outcome is probably the most difficult part of writing outcomes (Box 22-9). But a careful choice makes it easier to plan the content, teaching strategies, learner activities, and evaluation.

The number of outcomes needed for each diagnosis varies. It is better to have several specific outcomes than to try to cover everything with only one or two broad outcomes. Many nurses write one long-term, general outcome for each diagnosis, followed by several short-term, specific outcomes. For example, a long-term outcome for the sample teaching plan could be: "The patient will be able to breast-feed her infant as long as desired without sore nipples." This outcome could be met in 2 weeks or 2 years, depending on how long the woman decides to breastfeed. Long-term outcomes are general statements. On the other hand, the outcomes written in the learner outcome column of the sample teaching plan are short-term, specific behaviors to be accomplished within a specified time.

Patients and appropriate family members or significant others should be included in planning the outcomes. When patients value the learning outcomes, their readiness to learn is enhanced, increasing the likelihood that they will achieve the goals.

CONTENT

After writing the learner outcomes, you must decide what information the patient needs to complete them. This information is the content of the teaching plan. The most effective teaching plans address the most important topics relevant to the patient's care. New nurses usually need to research the subject to be taught to determine what information exists about the topic. Extensive information is easily accessible online, and books, journal articles, and manuals are also available in many nursing units. Current nursing literature and research materials are also available through several Web-based databases. The most complete database of nursing journals is "The Cumulative Index to Nursing and Allied Health Literature" (CINAHL). The CINAHL database index includes approximately 3,000 nursing and allied health journals as well as the publications of the American Nurses Association (ANA) and National League for Nursing (NLN). Additionally, CINAHL includes the Nursing Reference Center. This database offers the most recent best practice guidelines and is a valuable resource for staff nurses, administrators, student nurses, and faculty. Content supported by nursing research is called evidence-based and reflects the most accurate and clinically supported information.

Nurses are often concerned about just how much patients should learn about topics such as illness, procedures, medications, and surgeries. Patients have been found to benefit from explanations of the physical sensations they will experience during a procedure. They appreciate knowing in advance what they will feel, taste, hear, see, and smell.

Content explaining why certain treatments and medications are needed is included in a teaching plan. Information on the prevention of illness or its complications should also be covered. Again, patients are more likely to implement a plan that they understand and value.

TEACHING STRATEGIES

The techniques used by a teacher to promote learning are called teaching strategies. Teaching strategies are planned before the actual teaching sessions so that every content area

---

Box 22-9 VERBS THAT CAN BE USED WHEN WRITING LEARNER OUTCOMES

Cognitive Domain

compares	identifies
defines	names
describes	prepares
designs	plans
differentiates	solves
explains	states
gives examples	summarizes

Psychomotor Domain

adapts	manipulates
arranges	moves
assembles	organizes
begins	rearranges
changes	shows
constructs	starts
creates	works
demonstrates	

Affective Domain

chooses	justifies
defends	relates
displays	revises
forms	selects
gives	shares
helps	uses
initiates	values

Box 22-10　SUGGESTED TEACHING STRATEGIES FOR THE THREE LEARNING DOMAINS

Cognitive Domain
Lecture or discussion
Panel discussion
Discovery
Audiovisual materials
Printed materials
Programmed instruction
Computer-assisted instruction programs

Affective Domain
Role modeling
Discussion
Panel discussion
Audiovisual materials
Role playing
Printed materials

Psychomotor Domain
Demonstration
Discovery
Audiovisual materials
Printed materials

and learner outcome can be matched with an effective teaching technique. The strategies chosen depend on your familiarity with the method, the availability of educational resources and teaching aids, and factors affecting the patient's learning, such as educational level and cultural background. The use of age-appropriate methods is also a must; for example, a 10-year-old will be receptive to a comic book on personal safety, whereas an adult could learn similar material by discussing safety measures with you.

Education experts generally agree that using a variety of teaching strategies enhances learning. In addition, some methods are better suited for certain learning outcomes. Box 22-10 gives suggested teaching strategies for the three learning domains. The sample teaching plan shows how teaching strategies vary according to the learner outcomes and content of that particular plan. Again, be creative in choosing the methods. You should try to stimulate as many of the patient's senses as possible when teaching. Seeing, hearing, and touching are superior to reading or hearing alone. We reportedly remember 10% of what we read, 20% of what we hear, 30% of what we see, 50% of what we see and hear, and 80% of what we say and do. Descriptions of common teaching strategies follow.

Role Modeling

The old saying "actions speak louder than words" explains why role modeling is effective. Patients watch their nurses closely; use this as an opportunity to improve a patient's behavior. For example, nurses who formerly smoked can be role models for patients who are trying to quit smoking.

➤ *Consider Marco Garcia Ramirez, the father-to-be concerned about his role as a parent. The nurse would act as a role model to the couple when demonstrating newborn care.* ∎

Lecture

The term "lecture" means a presentation of information by a teacher to a learner. To be more effective, lectures usually include question-and-answer periods. This strategy can be used to deliver information to a large group of patients; it is rarely used for individual instruction, except in combination with other strategies.

Discussion

Discussion involves a two-way exchange of information, ideas, and feelings between the teacher and the learners. It is an effective method when used by a nurse who is comfortable with leading a group and knowledgeable about group processes (see Chapter 21). It can also be an effective method for one-on-one instruction.

➤ *Remember Alicia Bonet, the young mother who had to make a decision about long-term aspirin therapy for her baby. The nurse could use a discussion to present information to Ms. Bonet about aspirin therapy, its risks and benefits, and Reye's syndrome. The nurse would also provide time for Ms. Bonet to ask questions and think about the information presented.* ∎

Panel Discussion

A panel discussion involves a presentation of information by two or more people. Panel discussions can be used to impart factual material but are also effective for sharing experiences and emotions. Debates are a form of panel discussion that includes multiple sides of a controversial topic.

Demonstration

Demonstration of techniques, procedures, exercises, and the use of special equipment, combined with a lecture and discussion, is an effective strategy. The patient's learning can be evaluated by a return demonstration, often referred to as teach-back that promotes health literacy. Practice sessions are often included for the learner. Models of body parts or practice models, such as a resuscitation model, are frequently used. When teaching breast self-examinations, the use of a breast model allows the learner to feel different types of lumps commonly found in breast tissue. Childbirth educators usually demonstrate the birth of a baby by using a pelvic model, knitted uterus, and baby doll.

Discovery

In discovery learning, a problem or situation is presented to the patient or group of patients, who are then guided to discover the solution or approach. Discussion of other possible approaches and solutions can follow the patient's own solutions. This is a good method for teaching problem-solving techniques and independent thinking. For instance, you could give a group of diabetic patients a short description of a situation that includes signs and symptoms. The group would decide whether the signs and symptoms indicate hypoglycemia (low blood sugar) or hyperglycemia (high blood sugar) and would choose what measures to take. The group's decision can then be discussed as a further learning experience. Even if the patients chose a poor solution, it can be turned into an effective learning experience.

> *Recall Rachel Blumenthal, the wife of the patient who had a myocardial infarction. The nurse could present Mrs. Blumenthal with a "what-if" situation: for example, What if your husband started to have chest pain while you were cuddling and kissing? How would you handle the situation? From her answer, the nurse would be able to tell how well she understands her husband's condition. The nurse would also have an opportunity for reinstruction, reinforcement, and validation of learning.* ■

Role Playing

Role playing gives the learner a chance to experience, relive, or anticipate an event. To use this method, you would explain a scenario and then allow the patient to play out the scene with you or with one or more other learners. Role playing can be used to work through emotional traumas or to plan for possible traumas. For example, role playing could help a teenaged girl prepare to tell her parent about her pregnancy by letting the girl play herself while you play the girl's parent. This would help the patient rehearse what she wanted to say and anticipate the emotional atmosphere that she will experience. Role playing is a good strategy for adults as well as children. Puppets and dolls can be used as part of the process to help young children express negative feelings about hospitalization and traumatic procedures (Fig. 22-2).

Audiovisual Materials

AV materials such as computer programs, online courses, PowerPoint presentations, films, television programs, videotapes, overhead transparencies, flip charts, posters, and diagrams are popular and effective teaching strategies when combined with a lecture or discussion. As noted, never assume the patient is literate. AV materials should never be the sole source of learning for a patient. The patient may view the AV material alone, but it should be preceded and followed with a discussion of the material.

Printed Material

The use of printed material depends on its availability. Many brochures, fact sheets, and pamphlets are available at no cost from online sources. Many nurses have also written materials for distribution to patients. Writing instruction

FIGURE 22-2. Role playing can help children learn and express negative feelings resulting from hospitalization and traumatic procedures. *(Photo by Joe Mitchell.)*

sheets, books, and comic books for health teaching can be rewarding as well as useful. As with AV materials, printed materials are generally used in conjunction with other strategies. Specially prepared games, which are relatively easy to make, are a popular and fun way for patients to learn. For instance, cards with pictures of foods can be used to create a nutritional instruction game.

Printed materials should be selected carefully based on how well they present the needed content in a format that is attractive, understandable, and helpful. A sample of patient education material appears in Box 22-11.

> *Consider how the nurse handled the situation of Alicia Bonet, the young mother described in the Reflective Practice box. The nurse provided Ms. Bonet with written materials that were at a level she could understand, thereby helping her make her decision.* ■

Programmed Instruction

Most programmed instruction books or booklets are prepared so that learners can use them independently of a teacher. However, educators generally agree on the need to spend time with the learner before and after the program to clarify the information, answer questions, and provide the personal touch necessary for a learner's motivation. Because this is a self-paced strategy, it can be beneficial for many learners.

Web-Based Instruction

Web sites appropriate to the patient's disease process, wellness interests, or health promotion focus can be valuable teaching and learning resources. These sites provide consumer information that is formatted for easy reading and access. Be sure to evaluate the Web site chosen by the patient and advise him or her about its suitability and accuracy because some information found on the Internet is not grounded in scientific, medical, or nursing research.

Box 22-11 **WHAT TO DO IF YOU HAVE ONE OR MORE HEART ATTACK WARNING SIGNS**

Patient's Name: _____

Physicians now have treatments that can stop heart attacks and lessen damage to the heart. To make sure you can benefit from these treatments, you need to act promptly if you begin to experience symptoms that might signal a heart attack.

1. **This is what you may feel:**
   - Chest pain, discomfort, or pressure
   - Left arm pain or discomfort
   - Pain radiating to your neck or jaw
   - Shortness of breath
   - Sweating
   - Upset stomach
   - Discomfort in the area between your breastbone and navel
   - A sense of dread
   - Other:

2. **Medication instructions:**
   - Chew one 325-mg tablet of uncoated adult aspirin.
   - Place one tablet of nitroglycerin under your tongue as soon as you feel discomfort. Take a second tablet if the discomfort does not go away in 5 minutes. Take a third tablet after 5 more minutes if the discomfort does not go away.
   - Other: _____

3. **If the symptoms stop, call your physician at:** _____

4. **If symptoms continue for more than 15 minutes, call the emergency medical services phone number below immediately. (Often this is 9-1-1, but you should check to make sure.) Never wait longer than 15 minutes.**

   At home, the emergency phone number is: _____

   At work, the emergency phone number is: _____

   At _____, the emergency phone number is: _____

5. **Know the location of the nearest 24-hour emergency department.**

   At home, the closest emergency department is: _____

   At work, the closest emergency department is: _____

   At _____, the closest emergency department is: _____

Place this form next to the phone, near your other emergency numbers!

Signed: _____   MD/RN

Box 22-12 **EXAMPLE OF A CONTRACTUAL AGREEMENT BETWEEN A NURSE AND A CLIENT**

I will participate in the learning activities needed to help me learn about my low-salt diet. During my hospital stay, I will attend the class on low-salt diets, read the materials given to me, and ask questions as I need to. I will work with S. Moore, RN, to plan my meals and food preparation at home. If I need help when I get home, I will contact S. Moore.

Jim Mall

I will provide Jim Mall with the experiences needed for him to follow his low-salt diet accurately.

S. Moore, RN

CONTRACTUAL AGREEMENTS

A **contractual agreement** is a pact between two people setting out mutually agreed-on goals. Contracts between nurses and patients are becoming a common practice in many healthcare settings. The contracts are usually informal and not legally binding. When teaching a patient, such an agreement can serve to motivate both the patient and you as the teacher to do what is necessary to meet the patient's learning outcomes. The agreement notes the responsibilities of both the teacher and the learner, emphasizing the importance of the mutual commitment (Box 22-12). If the contracted outcomes are achieved, you can boost the patient's self-esteem with rewards; if the outcomes are not achieved, you can try different teaching techniques.

LEARNING ACTIVITIES

While planning teaching strategies, you will also decide what learning activities the patient will be doing independently. There are many ways that the patient can preview new material or reinforce what has already been taught. Printed materials, AV materials, and programmed instruction materials are often assigned in the learning activity column of the teaching plan. This column is used to guide the patient in learning activities that can be done before, between, and after planned learning sessions. Practical considerations for planning learning activities are discussed below.

Time Constraints

Time constraints must be considered when planning for the patient's learning as nurses often have a problem finding time to meet patients' needs. Priorities must be set so that essential content is taught thoroughly. Less important content is taught last so that the more important learner outcomes can be met within the time available. If time permits, the remaining content can be addressed.

To meet time constraints, nurses often plan together. Teamwork and cooperation allow nurses to meet deadlines. If teaching must continue beyond the hospitalization, home visit, or clinic visit, schedule additional learning opportunities through outpatient programs or referrals to community-based programs. Home healthcare nurses often receive referrals from hospital nurses to continue the teaching begun during a patient's hospitalization. Discharge planning must be started early to ensure continuity of teaching.

Scheduling

It is better to plan for shorter, more frequent teaching sessions than for one or two longer sessions. Short sessions allow patients to digest the new material and prevent them from becoming too tired or uncomfortable because of a health problem. Sessions of 15 to 30 minutes are generally well tolerated. Usually, more formal classroom programs last for more than 1 hour. In such cases, provide breaks after every 50 minutes of class time. The patient should be included in planning for the time and frequency of lessons. Scheduling teaching sessions when the patient is least stressed will enhance teaching.

Group Versus Individual Teaching

Several factors must be considered when choosing the teaching setting. Some learner outcomes are met more readily in a one-to-one encounter (Fig. 22-3), whereas others are achieved more easily in a group. For example, the outcome "The patient will change the dressing using sterile technique" would be taught and evaluated during a private session. The outcome "The patient will discuss feelings about returning home after a heart attack" might be met more easily in a group discussion with other patients.

Formal Versus Informal Teaching

Most nurse–patient interactions can include **informal teaching** by the nurse. These unplanned teaching sessions are often effective because they deal with the patient's immediate learning needs and concerns. Informal teaching might also lead to additional planned, formal sessions. **Formal teaching** is the planned teaching done to fulfill learner outcomes. Both forms are effective when used appropriately.

Implementing

Implementing the teaching plan requires use of interpersonal skills and effective communication techniques. Teaching the

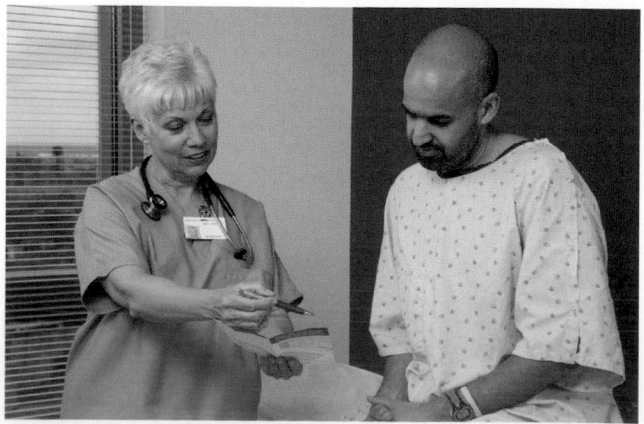

FIGURE 22-3. One-to-one teaching is used in many nurse–patient situations. The nurse must be able to assess whether individual teaching is needed or whether learning can occur in a group. *(Photo by B. Proud.)*

FIGURE 22-4. The nurse's warm approach is an important factor in interpersonal relationships. *(Photo by Rick Brady.)*

patient can be a major part of the working phase of the helping relationship (see Chapter 21). You must continually observe the patient for additional assessment data that could alter the original teaching plan. This requires skill in adapting and reorganizing the teaching plan.

Promote patient learning by using a warm and accepting approach. Your attitude has more effect on the patient than any other factor (Fig. 22-4). Avoid taking a condescending attitude and using technical and medical terms (unless the patient has a background in this area). A nonthreatening teaching–learning atmosphere allows learning to occur.

The physical environment is another important consideration when implementing the teaching plan. Some planning may be needed to ensure adequate space and lighting, comfortable chairs, and good ventilation. Privacy is also important, as is freedom from distractions and interruptions.

In the implementation phase, the patient as a learner has certain role functions. To avoid any misunderstandings, it is helpful to review the contractual agreement before implementing the teaching plan. The patient is expected to listen, observe, and attempt to understand what is being taught.

Some people are uncomfortable in the role of learner; this problem must be assessed so that the patient can be assisted to assume the role more easily. If special techniques or procedures must be learned (e.g., colostomy care, self-injections, or eye medication instillation), assure the patient that it takes time and practice before anyone can perform new skills confidently.

Be prepared and organized before implementing the teaching plan. Gather and organize all teaching aids (e.g., posters, films, or printed materials) before the teaching session. A disorganized teacher distracts the learner and hinders learning. Also, a procedure or skill must be taught in the correct sequence so that the patient does not become confused.

An important nursing responsibility is to make each learning session interesting and enjoyable for the patient. Have an enthusiastic and positive attitude and make learning fun by creative use of planned teaching strategies. When you approach teaching positively, the patient is more likely to approach learning in a similar way.

Evaluating
Evaluating Learning

Nurses cannot be sure that patients have actually learned the content without some type of proof or feedback. The key to evaluation is the learner outcomes in the teaching plan that describe what behaviors to measure. Methods for obtaining feedback about learning are discussed in the following section.

METHODS OF EVALUATION

There are several methods of evaluation. For instance, cognitive domain learning may be evaluated through oral questioning, affective domain learning through the patient's response, and psychomotor domain learning by a return demonstration. Consider the following learner outcome in the cognitive domain: "The patient will be able to describe what a blood pressure reading represents." To evaluate this, you could say to the patient, "Tell me what this blood pressure reading means to you." The patient then has a chance to talk about the reading while you evaluate the patient's understanding of it.

Asking direct questions is often an efficient method of evaluating learner outcomes. Simply ask the patient a question, and the answer reflects the patient's level of knowledge about a topic. Direct questions can also be used to evaluate the patient's affective learning.

Another way to decide whether learner outcomes have been met is to use the patient's own comments. The patient may verbalize his or her understanding of the information while avoiding further discussion of the topic. In such instances, using effective communication techniques when reintroducing the topic at a later time might provide the evaluation data needed.

Sometimes observational skills can be used to determine whether the patient is using the material learned. For example, observing what the patient has ordered for lunch shows whether dietary lessons are being put into practice. You will also depend on observation when evaluating the patient's psychomotor skills. A return demonstration is an excellent way of evaluating psychomotor domain learning (Fig. 22-5). Letting the patient change his or her own dressing, for example, provides concrete evidence of satisfactory or unsatisfactory performance of the procedure. However, you must take care to promote a nonstressful environment when the time comes for the patient's return demonstration.

TIMING OF EVALUATION

Evaluation of learning is ongoing. If learning is only evaluated as soon as teaching is completed, the results may be misleading. Home healthcare nurses may evaluate what the patient learned in the hospital, as well as what is being taught during home visits. Hospital nurses often check with family members or significant others after discharge to evaluate whether learner outcomes have been met.

Reinforcing and Celebrating Learning

Most people feel encouraged and supported when their efforts are acknowledged by another person, especially when they trust and value the other person. This is especially true in healthcare, where patients often feel overwhelmed by their illness. To make the most of this dynamic, use **positive reinforcement** to affirm the efforts of patients who have mastered new knowledge, attitudes, or skills. Reinforcement may be as simple as a few words of acknowledgment ("You've mastered this diet quickly"), as spontaneous as a warm hug, or as planned as the entire staff joining to celebrate a patient's independent ambulation. **Negative reinforcement**—criticism or punishment—is generally ineffective; undesirable behavior is usually best ignored. Behavior modification programs that reward desired behaviors and ignore undesired behaviors might be designed for some patients.

Evaluating Teaching

Evaluation of teaching must occur so you can capitalize on your strengths and work on improving weaknesses. Like all nursing roles, effective teaching requires practice and experience. Even nurse educators agree that they are always learning better ways to promote learning. It is important to avoid becoming discouraged when evaluations of one's teaching are less than perfect.

It is best to evaluate one's own teaching effectiveness immediately after a teaching session. This involves a quick review of how well you feel the plan was implemented. Mentally noting both the strengths and weaknesses of the teaching session helps you plan better for subsequent sessions.

You can also seek feedback from patients. A simple questionnaire can be used at the end of a teaching session or after discharge to gain the patient's perception of your teaching effectiveness. The questionnaire may be a standardized form used throughout the hospital or agency or one prepared by you. When using an outcome format that requires only circles or checkmarks as answers, space should be provided for comments.

FIGURE 22-5. If the patient can correctly demonstrate what you've taught, you know learning has occurred. *(Photo by B. Proud)*

> ### Box 22-13   COMMON TEACHING MISTAKES
>
> - Ignoring the restrictions of the patient's environment
> - Failing to accept that patients have the right to change their mind
> - Using medical jargon
> - Failing to negotiate goals
> - Duplicating teaching that other team members have done
> - Overloading the patient with information
> - Choosing the wrong time for teaching
> - Not evaluating what the patient has learned
> - Not reviewing educational media, or relying exclusively on media
> - Failing to document patient teaching and plan for follow-up or teaching reinforcement

Revising the Plan

During evaluation, you or your patient might decide that revisions are needed in the teaching plan. When revising the plan, it is important to identify teaching factors that might have reduced teaching effectiveness (Box 22-13). A reassessment might indicate that some patient factors were not considered in the original plan, and adjustments might be made accordingly to meet the patient's needs. Often, the use of a different teaching strategy is all that is needed for a patient to achieve the learner outcomes.

Revision is a natural part of the teaching–learning process and should not be viewed negatively. Neither you nor the patient has "failed" when an outcome is not met. Most outcomes can be met with a change in approach, although sometimes the learner outcomes are unrealistic. Further assessment might reveal that the content might be too complex or the time too short for successful achievement.

Documenting

The nurse is legally responsible for documenting teaching in the patient's record. Documentation of the teaching–learning process includes a summary of the learning need, the plan, the implementation of the plan, and the evaluation results. The evaluative statement is crucial and must show concrete evidence that demonstrates that learning has occurred. If the desired learning has not occurred, your notes should indicate how the problem was resolved. It is insufficient to document only what was taught; the charting must show evidence that the patient or significant other has actually learned the material taught. Box 22-14 gives an example of documentation.

THE NURSE AS COUNSELOR

Counseling is the interpersonal process of helping patients to make decisions that promote their overall well-being. Family members or significant others are often included in counseling sessions. Everyone participating must feel comfortable in the situation and surroundings. Like teaching, counseling may be formal or informal.

DOCUMENTATION USING A PROBLEM-ORIENTED PROGRESS NOTE TO MEET A LEARNING NEED

1/3/11   #2   New Problem—High Risk for Impaired Skin Integrity: Nipples

S   Patient stated that her nipples were sore during and after her newborn's first feeding

O   First day postpartum; patient is fair skinned with freckles; no reddened areas, no cracking yet; no nipple preparation before delivery

A   At high risk for cracked, open areas; patient lacks experience and knowledge of preventive measures

P   Reinforce teaching plan for nipple care

I   Teaching plan implemented

E   Patient able to meet all of the objectives satisfactorily as recorded on the teaching plan; she is currently doing protective and preparatory care for her nipples; when breastfeeding, she uses the correct feeding technique with good aftercare; she states that her nipples are no longer sore, and she is able to explain what she should do when she goes home

R   None needed, but reinforcement of content will be continued

—L. Sweeney, RN

The interpersonal skills of warmth, friendliness, openness, and empathy are necessary for successful counseling. An effective counselor needs to be a caring individual. Caring is based on a humanistic philosophy (Watson, 1985), which is the core of nursing practice. A humanistic approach to counseling rooted in professional caring helps the patient strive toward the greatest health potential. Caring is important in all nursing roles but is fundamental in the counseling role.

Some advanced-practice psychiatric mental health nurses specialize in counseling, and this form of counseling has an important professional role. The focus in this chapter, however, is on the everyday counseling that is a basic component of all nurses' practice. This counseling involves listening carefully to the patient's or family's questions, concerns, demands, and complaints and then responding in an effective manner.

> *Consider Rachel Blumenthal, the wife of the patient who had a myocardial infarction. By carefully listening to Mrs. Blumenthal's concerns, including her comment about being embarrassed to ask her husband's cardiologist, the nurse helps to establish a trusting relationship that forms the basis for counseling. ∎*

Knowing the appropriate responses might be difficult at first, but practice helps develop this skill. Each nurse–patient (or nurse–family) interaction is unique; a nursing response that works well with one patient might intimidate or anger another. Sensitivity to the unique needs of each patient and a willingness to get involved and make a difference are essential for effective counseling.

Table 22-1 presents typical counseling situations you might experience in your first year of nursing and analyzes both effective and ineffective nursing responses. You might want to role-play these situations with a friend. Nurses who wish to succeed as caregivers and counselors need to master the communication techniques described in Chapter 21.

In counseling situations, you do not tell the patient what to do to solve the problem but instead assist and guide them to solve problems and make decisions. If the patient lacks the knowledge and skills to approach a problem systematically, you can combine the teaching and counseling roles to help the patient solve the dilemma successfully.

The nursing process is an essential tool when guiding and teaching patients. Nurses are educated to approach all nursing situations in a logical, systematic way. In a crisis situation, whether minor or major, share your problem-solving abilities with patients. The nursing process is used to organize the nurse–patient counseling situation described in Box 22-15. See Examples of NANDA Nursing Diagnoses: Counseling Needs for diagnoses for which counseling may be indicated.

Types of Counseling

Counseling may be situational, developmental, or motivational, and short-term or long-term.

Short-Term Counseling

Short-term counseling focuses on the immediate problem or concern of the patient or family. It can be a relatively minor concern or a major crisis, but in any case, it needs immediate attention (Fig. 22-6). Short-term counseling might be used during a **situational crisis,** which occurs when a patient faces an event or situation that causes a disruption in life. For example, a male patient in the hospital finds out that his wife has been involved in a car accident; she received only a few scratches, but their only car was demolished. As a nurse, you are in an excellent position to help the patient decide what can be done to solve this situational crisis. You can guide the patient to resources to help solve the travel, financial, and

FIGURE 22-6. Counseling may involve a concern that needs immediate attention. *(Photo by Rick Brady.)*

TABLE • 22-1 ANALYSIS OF NURSING RESPONSES IN COMMON COUNSELING SITUATIONS

Ineffective Response	Analysis	Effective Response	Analysis
Situation A: You walk into the room of Ms. Goldstein, who learned earlier in the day that her tumor is malignant. She is crying.			
"Oh cheer up! Tomorrow's got to be a brighter day."	Provides false reassurance; communicates insensitivity to patient's feelings	Touch forearm and sit next to her quietly. After several minutes, say, "I can't even begin to imagine how difficult this must be for you. Please let me know if there is anything I can do to help."	Uses touch, silence, and caring appropriately
Situation B: You have been teaching 60-year-old Mr. Hyong diabetic self-care for 4 days, and he is still asking the same questions and refusing to administer his own insulin or check his blood sugar.			
"Well, I guess we are getting nowhere here. Is there anyone else who might be able to do this for you?"	Rejects patient without first evaluating the teaching plan and exploring patient variables that might be hindering learning	"We may have a bit of a problem here. . . . I hear you asking the same questions every day. Let's see if together we can figure out why this isn't making sense to you."	Enlists patient in problem solving
Situation C: One morning, you walk into the room of an older resident who had withdrawn and become totally dependent on the nurses for basic care on her transfer into the nursing home. You are surprised to discover that she has washed and dressed herself—for the first time.			
"Well, I'm happy to see that you have rejoined the ranks of the living. Did you wash off your glasses?"	Misses opportunity to celebrate the resident's achievement of an important goal	Hugs resident warmly, looks her in the eye, and exclaims, "Don't you look wonderful today? What are you celebrating?" Defers an assessment of how thorough the morning care has been until later.	Rejoices spontaneously in the resident's achievement and reinforces this behavior. Gives the resident a reason to continue to make progress. Uses touch appropriately
Situation D: You are helping Mr. Stein out of bed; he has been on bed rest for 2 weeks because of a painful and debilitating illness. A fiercely independent man, he is embarrassed to need your support and looks disgusted with himself when he steps on your foot.			
"What's the problem, Honey? Haven't been eating your Wheaties?"	Uses terms of endearment, which often denote disrespect and condescension to patients, no matter in what spirit they are uttered	"No problem, Mr. Stein, my husband steps on my toes all the time when we go dancing!" After a few minutes . . . "It must be hard when you are used to doing everything for yourself to all of a sudden find yourself needing others for simple things . . . ?"	Uses humor and empathy appropriately; invites the patient to share his feelings
Situation E: Ms. Berretta recently underwent surgery resulting in a urinary diversion. She should be able to change her own ostomy bag by this time, but she is still unwilling to look at the stoma, and participate alone in her care. The nurses are getting impatient with her "childish" refusals to learn.			
"Really Helen, I'll do it myself but you'll be the loser once you get home with this thing and there's no one around to help."	Uses a threat in an attempt to coerce learning (negative reinforcement). Displays unwillingness to explore what is blocking Ms. Berretta's readiness to learn	Before beginning Ms. Berretta's care: "I think we need to talk before your treatment today. You will be discharged soon, and I want you to feel confident about caring for your stoma. I understand that until you can accept it, you don't want to learn anything about it. Would you like to talk about this with me, or would you prefer me to make a referral to someone else?"	Communicates respect for patient and sensitivity to her needs, without ignoring what is a real problem. Offers the possibility of a referral to another healthcare professional if the patient so wishes

Box 22-15   AN EXAMPLE OF PROBLEM SOLVING THAT FOLLOWS THE NURSING PROCESS

Situation
Monday, 7:30 p.m., Amy Purcell has been admitted to the children's unit with dehydration resulting from diarrhea. Amy is responding well to intravenous (IV) fluids. Her mother is visibly distraught.

Assessing
Amy is doing well but will need 24 hours of IV therapy.

Amy and her twin sister Susan have never been separated from their parents or each other. They are 2 years old.

Ms. Purcell has no idea who will care for Susan when Mr. Purcell goes to work in the morning.

The Purcells have no regular childcare arrangements and have no family members in the area.

Ms. Purcell wants to stay with Amy during her hospitalization.

The Purcells' neighbor is home during the day. Sometimes Amy and Susan play at her house.

There is a daycare center near their home, but Susan might be upset about going there. It's also expensive.

Mr. Purcell cannot afford to take Tuesday off but will take Wednesday morning off.

Insurance does not cover a private room, which would allow Susan to come to stay in the hospital too.

Diagnosing
Anxiety related to stress of daughter's hospitalization, need for childcare for Susan, and uncertain resources.

Planning Goal
Ms. Purcell will demonstrate decreased anxiety over the care of Susan during Amy's hospitalization.

Together, Ms. Purcell and the nurse have planned the following:
- The neighbor will come to the Purcell home to care for Susan when Mr. Purcell leaves for work on Tuesday morning.
- The neighbor will bring Susan to the hospital for the afternoon visiting hours to be with Ms. Purcell and Amy.
- Mr. Purcell will come to the hospital after work to have dinner with the family.
- Mr. Purcell will take Susan home for bedtime.
- On Wednesday morning, Mr. Purcell will take off work in the morning. He and Susan will go to the hospital to pick up Ms. Purcell and Amy.

Implementing
Plan implemented by the Purcells with support of the nursing staff.

Evaluating
Ms. Purcell told the nurse that she feels that both Amy and Susan did well with the care they received from their parents. The family's stress was minimized, and she is relieved that everything went so well. The nurse decides that the goals were met.

---

emotional difficulties that arise as a result of the accident. This holistic approach is especially important because the crisis could hinder the patient's recovery.

Long-Term Counseling

Long-term counseling extends over a prolonged period. A patient might need the counsel of the nurse at daily, weekly, or monthly intervals. A patient experiencing a developmental crisis, for example, might need long-term counseling. A **developmental crisis** can occur when a person is going through a developmental stage or passage. For example, many women going through menopause need assistance when adjusting to the changes they experience. Long-term counseling may occur in nurse-led support groups.

Motivational Interviewing

Motivational interviewing is an evidence-based counseling approach that involves discussing feelings and incentives with the patient. Nurses often become frustrated because their patients do not seem to want to get better or to learn how to care for themselves. Perhaps some patients do not have the inner drive or motivation to cooperate in their own healthcare. Some patients say, "I have nothing to live for." By establishing a helping relationship with the patient early on, you can help him or her work through these feelings of despair. You might be able to get the patient to talk about what is generating his or her lack of interest in recovery. If

a problem is identified, you can use the problem-solving technique with the patient to work toward an acceptable solution.

If a patient is unwilling to participate in learning activities, assess any factors from the past or present that might be decreasing his or her motivation for learning. Sometimes, just by having you explain the need for certain knowledge and the consequences of not learning the material, the patient will become more receptive to the teaching–learning process. A trial learning session can be suggested to allow the patient to see what the sessions will be like. With use of the nursing process approach for counseling, the patient might become more motivated. Four skills have proved effective in motivational interviewing. These include:

- Reflective listening—restate the patient's response back to him or her
- Asking open questions—encourages discussion of the reason for making desired changes
- Affirming—supports the patient's efforts and encourages further exploration
- Summarizing—links and reinforces material that has been discussed (Levensky, Forcehimes, O'Donohue, & Bietz, 2007).

When assessing a motivational problem, always consider the patient's cultural values. Often the way a person feels about something is strongly influenced by his or her cultural background. For instance, if a person has grown up in a family

Examples of NANDA Nursing Diagnoses
Counseling Needs

Nursing Diagnoses	Related Factors
Anxiety	Change in health status
Disabled Family Coping	Prolonged disability progression that is exhausting the caregiving capacity of family members
Decisional Conflict	Inability to authorize withdrawal of life-sustaining treatment despite believing this to be in the patient's best interests
Disturbed Body Image	Amputation of left leg
Grieving	Inability to accept child's impending death
Fear	Strangeness of modern U.S. hospital environment and language barrier
Hopelessness	Progression of debilitating symptoms and belief that "even God has abandoned me"
Impaired Individual Resilience	Inconsistent parenting
Impaired Parenting	High number of closely spaced pregnancies and absent social supports
Impaired Social Interaction	Communication barriers
Ineffective Role Performance	History of substance abuse and mental illness
Ineffective Denial	Refusal to acknowledge substance abuse problems
Ineffective Coping	High degree of threat and poor concentration, fatigue
Powerlessness	Lifestyle of helplessness
Risk-Prone Health Behavior	Inadequate social support
Situational Low Self-Esteem	Recent lay-off and divorce
Social Isolation	Inability to engage in satisfying personal relationships
Spiritual Distress	Challenged belief and value system

in which illness is perceived as an inevitable result of aging, it will be difficult to motivate that person to practice preventive measures for health (see Chapter 2). These problems seem insurmountable, yet a caring nurse can work toward helping the patient become interested in promoting his or her own health. When discouraged, confer with a colleague to help solve patient-centered problems.

Referrals

Sometimes a patient needs specialized counseling by nurses with advanced training or by other healthcare professionals. In

these cases, offer to refer the patient to the appropriate professional (e.g., psychiatric or mental health nurse, psychologist or psychiatrist, social worker, clergy, financial counselor, sex therapist, or occupational therapist). In other cases, a simple referral to a community resource, such as a neighborhood support group, may be all the patient needs. When making a referral, be sure to address any barriers that might prevent the patient from acting on the referral. Patients might fail to follow up with a referral for financial reasons, because they do not understand the reason for or value the referral, because they lack transportation, or because the agency is not open at times when they are free.

Developing Critical Thinking Skills

1. Explain what is meant by the following statement: "It is as important for patients to understand and value the proposed treatment regimen as it is for them to understand how to implement the proposed regimen." What are the implications of this for teaching and counseling?

2. A patient your age has just learned that she has tested positive for the human immunodeficiency virus. Make a list of some of the learning (cognitive, psychomotor, affective) that you think should take place. What sorts of things might affect her readiness to learn? How would you tailor your nursing in response to these variables?

3. Mrs. Riley is being readmitted to your hospital unit with complications related to her diabetes. A coworker voices her frustrations and says, "We've taught her everything she needs to know to do a better job of managing her diabetes. I don't know what more we can do." How do you respond?

Practicing for NCLEX

1. Noncompliance with a therapeutic regimen can be a significant problem for elderly people. Which of the following is one of the common reasons for noncompliance in the elderly?
   a. Lack of time
   b. Religious practice
   c. Childlike behavior
   d. Inadequate financial resources

2. A nurse is preparing to teach a 45-year-old patient with asthma how to use his inhaler. One of the best methods to teach the patient this skill is by:
   a. Demonstration
   b. Lecture
   c. Discussion
   d. Panel session

3. A nurse has taught a diabetic patient how to administer his daily insulin. The nurse should evaluate the teaching–learning process by:
   a. Determining the patient's motivation to learn
   b. Deciding if the learning outcomes have been achieved
   c. Allowing the patient to practice the skill he has just learned
   d. Documenting the teaching session in the patient's medical record

4. A nurse is using the health belief model to assess a patient. Using this model, what should the nurse begin to understand?
   a. Which clinical and financial resources the patient requires to improve his lifestyle
   b. What motivates the patient to learn new behaviors
   c. The effects the health delivery system has on the patient's health patterns
   d. Whether the patient is willing to take actions to support health

5. Nurses play a vital role in patient teaching because of their:
   a. Need for self-actualization
   b. Expertise in healthcare
   c. Desire to help others
   d. Ability to provide illness care

6. A nurse instructs a group of parents about how to make their home safe for their toddlers. This is an example of teaching aimed toward which of the following?
   a. Restoring health
   b. Facilitating coping
   c. Preventing illness
   d. Promoting health

7. When preparing a health promotion program for patients in an adult daycare center, what is the first step the nurse must take?
   a. Develop learning outcomes
   b. Develop a teaching plan
   c. Assess the patients' learning needs and learning readiness
   d. Diagnose the patients' learning needs

8. When using facts from the patient's medical record as part of the necessary information to assess learning needs, the nurse is using which type of data source?
   a. Primary
   b. Historic
   c. Secondary
   d. Hospital-owned

9. The primary purpose of a contractual agreement between nurses and patients when beginning a teaching plan is to:
   a. Create a formal and legal bond between the nurse and patient
   b. Motivate both the patient and nurse to do what is necessary to meet the patient's learning outcomes
   c. Outline the patient's learning outcomes
   d. Limit the scope of the teaching session

10. One of the best ways to affirm the efforts of patients who master new knowledge, attitudes, or skills is through:
   a. Dialog and discussion
   b. A grading scale
   c. Positive reinforcement
   d. Encouraging the family to learn with the patient

Answers With Rationale

1. *d.* Noncompliance is often associated with inadequate finances, along with factors such as patient confusion, disappointment, misunderstanding, or fear.

2. *a.* Demonstration of techniques, procedures, exercises, and the use of special equipment is an effective patient teaching strategy.

3. *b.* The nurse cannot assume that the patient has actually learned the content unless there is some type of proof of learning. The key to evaluation is meeting the learner outcomes stated in the teaching plan.

4. *d.* The health belief model is designed to explain why persons are willing to take action to support their health.

5. *b.* Nurses who are skilled educators and counselors can improve patients' health and well-being. This is a function of their education and experience and their use of cognitive, technical, interpersonal, and ethical/legal skills.

6. *c.* Thorough assessment of the patients' learning needs may reveal the need for vehicular safety, home safety, domestic-violence recognition, recreational safety, and occupational safety and health education. This type of patient education is aimed at enhancing health-protecting behaviors.

7. *c.* The first step of the teaching–learning process is to assess the patient's learning needs and learning readiness.

8. *c.* Past and current patient medical records are considered secondary sources of information and can provide a history of medical problems, as well as documentation of nursing assessments, diagnoses, and interventions.

9. *b.* A contractual agreement is a pact two people make setting out mutually agreed-on goals.

10. *c.* People feel encouraged and supported when their efforts are acknowledged by another person, especially when they trust and value that other person.

Taylor Suite Resources

The Taylor Suite offers these additional resources to enhance learning and facilitate understanding of this chapter:

- thePoint online resource, http://thepoint.lww.com/Taylor7E
- Student DVD-ROM included with the book
- Study Guide for Taylor's Fundamentals of Nursing

BIBLIOGRAPHY

Benner, J. (2007). Finding Spanish patient-education materials online. *Nursing, 37*(9), 20–21.

Blakely, G., Skirton, H., Cooper, S., Allum, P., & Nelmes, P. (2009). Educational gaming in the health sciences: Systematic review. *Journal of Advanced Nursing, 65*(2), 259–269.

Bloom, B. S. (1956). *Taxonomy of educational objectives: The classification of educational goals.* New York: David McKay.

Burkhart, J. (2008). Training nurses to be teachers. *The Journal of Continuing Education in Nursing, 39*(11), 503–510.

Canobbio, M. (2006). *Mosby's handbook of patient teaching* (3rd ed.). St. Louis: Elsevier.

Chang, M. (2007). Patient education: Addressing cultural diversity and health literacy. *Urology Nursing, 27*(5), 411–417.

Chapman, L. (2007). Discharge planning: A family affair. *Nursing, 37*(5), 56hn12–56hn14.

Dirks, F. (2008). Taking charge. *American Journal of Nursing, 108*(2), 72.

Doak, C. C., Doak, L. G., & Root, J. H. (1995). *Teaching patients with low literacy skills.* Philadelphia: J. B. Lippincott.

Donovan, H., Ward, S., Song, M., Heidrich, S., Gunnarsdottir, S., & Phillips, C. (2007). An update on the representational approach to patient education. *Journal of Nursing Scholarship, 39*(3), 259–265.

Gingerich, B. (2009). Client teaching guides for home health care. *Home Health Care Management & Practice, 21*(2), 145–146.

Graf, C. (2008). The lawton instrumental activities of daily living scale. *American Journal of Nursing, 108*(4), 52–62.

Knowles, M. S. (1990). *The adult learner: A neglected species* (4th ed.). Houston: Gulf Publishing.

Layne, L. (2008). Discharge planning. *Advance for Nursing, Pennsylvania, New Jersey, Delaware, 10*(1), 35–37.

Levensky, E., Forcehimes, A., O'Donohue, W. T., & Beitz, K. (2007). Motivational interviewing. *American Journal of Nursing, 107*(10), 50–59.

Lorenzen, B, Melby, C., & Earles, B. (2008). Using principles of health literacy to enhance the informed consent process. *AORN, 88*(1), 23–29.

Mauk, K. (2006). Reaching and teaching older adults. *Nursing, 36*(2), 17.

Nath, C. (2007). Literacy and diabetes self-management. *American Journal of Nursing, 107*(6), 43–49.

National Institute for Literacy. (2008). Fact sheet overview. Available at http://www.nifl.gov/nifl/facts/facts_overview.html

National Institute for Literacy. (2008). Health Literacy Facts. Available at http://www.nifl.gov/nifl/facts/health.html

North American Nursing Diagnosis Association–International (NANDA-I) (2009). *Nursing diagnoses: Definitions & classification 2009–20011.* West Sussex, UK: Wiley-Blackwell.

Partnership for Clear Health Communication at the National Patient Safety Foundation. (2006). What is health literacy? Available at http://www.npsf.org/pchc/health-literacy.php

Partnership for Clear Health Communication at the National Patient Safety Foundation (2007). Partnership for clear health communication joins forces with the national patient safety foundation. Available at http://www.npsf.org/pchc/chc-joins-npsf.php

Rankin, S. H., & Stallings, K. D. (2004). *Patient education in health and illness* (5th ed.). Philadelphia: Lippincott Williams & Wilkins.

Redman, B. K. (2007). *The practice of patient education* (10th ed.). St. Louis, MO: C. V. Mosby.

Rosenstock, I. (1974). Historical origins of the health belief model. *Health Education Monograph, 2*, 354.

Smith, L. (2007). Speaking up for medical language interpreters. *Nursing, 37*(12), 48–49.

The Joint Commission. (2007a). Joint Commission Conference Call on Health Literacy in America, February 7, 2007.

The Joint Commission. (2007b). "What did the doctor say?:" Improving health literacy to protect patient safety. Available at http://www.jointcommission.org/NR/rdonlyres/D5248B2E-E7E6-4121-8874-99C7B4888301/0/improving_health_literacy.pdf

Vesterlund, M. (2008). A right to understand. *American Journal of Nursing, 108*(2), 13.

Watson, J. (1985). *Nursing: The philosophy and science of caring.* Denver: Colorado University Press.

Nurse Leader and Manager

REHEMA KOHLS

Rehema is a college sophomore who comes to the healthcare center requesting information about sexually transmitted infections (STIs). During the visit, she says, "So many of my friends are concerned about STIs. They all say we should start a group on campus to discuss this problem, and they want me to set it up and be the leader. But I wouldn't know where to start or what to do!"

STEPHEN WALL

Stephen, a 65-year-old widower who lives alone, is admitted to the intensive care unit after an automobile accident in which he sustained trauma to the head, chest, abdomen, and lower extremities. He is being monitored continuously via numerous invasive devices and requires complex care. His closest family member, a 40-year-old son, lives approximately 75 miles away.

JACK CAMP

Jack, a middle-aged single man with a history of diabetes mellitus, is receiving care for a compound fracture of his left lower extremity being treated with an external fixator. Compliance with his diabetic therapy regimen is questionable; he states, "I really love my sweets!" The patient frequently voices loud complaints about his room, the food, and the hospital routine. He also uses his call light very frequently, stating, "I just want to see if it's working and if the nurses will come check on me."

After completing the chapter, you will be able to accomplish the following:

1. Identify the qualities, four skills, and differing styles of leaders.

2. List the four managerial functions.

3. Discuss the difference between leadership and management.

4. Summarize the steps in the process of change.

5. Describe areas in which beginning nurses can develop leadership skills.

6. Recognize the responsibilities associated with the delegation of nursing care.

7. Describe the role of a mentor.

KEY TERMS

autocratic leadership

change

decentralized decision-making process

delegation

democratic leadership

explicit power

implied power

laissez-faire leadership

leadership

management

planned change

power

quantum leadership

self-governance

situational leadership

transformational leadership

Today, healthcare providers are experiencing changes such as fiscal constraints, workforce shortages, sophisticated healthcare consumers, and technological/pharmacological advances. Never before has there been such a need for nurses to work competently and collaboratively with other healthcare professionals to secure cost-effective, high-quality healthcare for all. Although nurses might assume leadership roles by virtue of their positions, they only become effective leaders over time by understanding the complexities of coordinating care, remaining open to differing points of view, and understanding the interdependency of the entire healthcare team (See the accompanying Reflective Practice box). Leadership and management are intertwined, but leadership roles differ from management tasks or functions. In *The Seven Habits of Highly Effective People,* Stephen Covey (1999) clarified the difference, citing a quote from Peter Drucker: "Management is doing things right; leadership is doing the right things." This suggests that leadership involves philosophy, perception, and judgment whereas management tasks

are the core of the management role (Frankel, 2008). A supportive leader uses strategies that facilitate the delivery of safe, high-quality patient care in a positive environment.

Now, more than ever, it is important for nursing as a profession to be self-directed as it charts its future. To do all this successfully, nurses must be familiar with the healthcare organization in which they are employed, as well as the healthcare system at large.

LEADERSHIP

The concept of leadership is one of the most researched, studied, and debated fields of inquiry. Paradoxically, it is at the same time clear and vivid, and elusive and subtle. **Leadership** has been described as the ability to direct or motivate an individual or group to achieve set goals. Effective leaders in groups or systems do this by encouraging others to be their best selves as they work collaboratively in the pursuit of common organizational or unit goals. Leaders have power, whether it is explicit or implied. For example, an elected class leader has **explicit power** by virtue of his or her position. However, a student in the class who has no designated leadership position might, by force of his or her personality, have more power to influence the class than the designated leader. This is **implied power.**

> *Consider Jack Camp, the patient described in the Reflective Practice scenario. The patient assumed a position of "running things in his business," thus having the explicit power of his position. Based on this, the patient used "implied power" while hospitalized to exert control over his situation. The nurse's understanding of power would be important in developing a plan to deal with the patient's behavior.* ■

Power to influence a group depends on the person's leadership style and how the person fulfills leadership responsibilities. The dynamics of leadership involve applying that power for personal or organizational growth or change. Nurses who use leadership skills can become proficient in effecting desired changes in many areas, including their patients' health patterns, the healthcare agency, the community, the nursing profession, and the healthcare system in general.

Leadership Qualities

Most people admire a charismatic, dynamic, enthusiastic, visionary leader who is poised, confident, and self-directed. These characteristics define leaders such as Mother Teresa, John Kennedy, Martin Luther King, Gandhi, and others. Not everyone can be as dynamic and inspirational as these individuals were. Yet leaders do need to be comfortable with themselves (i.e., have a positive self-image) and present themselves as role models for followers. Ideally, they also have a vision that energizes the group and brings forth the best efforts of members. Critical thinkers and responsible decision makers commit high energy to achieving goals and are skilled in enlisting support and cooperation.

REFLECTIVE PRACTICE
Challenge to Ethical Skills

While in a clinical rotation my junior year, I was assigned the dreaded Jack Camp (I still remember his name). He was a middle-aged single man receiving care for a compound fracture of his left lower extremity being treated with an external fixator. He had a bad case of diabetes, and an even worse sweet tooth. Before I even met him, the nurses on the floor were saying things like "good luck," which made this junior nursing student extra paranoid (although I was grateful for the warning). The patient was known for voicing loud complaints about his room, the food, and the hospital routine. He also was using his call light very frequently. The nurses called him names and discussed their dislike of him in the nurses' station, which was in the center of the unit.

As the day progressed, I found out that all this patient wanted was some attention, because he was used to running things in his business. I actually found him entertaining.

Thinking Outside the Box: Possible Courses of Action

- Ignore the comments of the other nurses on the floor, hoping that no one else heard them.
- Report the nurses to my clinical instructor, possibly causing tension on the floor.
- Politely tell the nurses to keep it down and refrain from talking about the patient, risking my own comfort level; after all, I am only a visiting student—what do I know?

Evaluating a Good Outcome: How Do I Define Success?

- Act as a patient advocate despite my limited power, which means correcting unethical behaviors as cordially as possible.
- Have the courage to go to the next level if the nurses' behavior is not corrected.
- Inform the patient politely to modify his behavior.

Personal Learning: Here's to the Future!

My response was to ignore the nurses' comments and hope no one else heard them either. I was not courageous enough to be the patient advocate that we had been taught to be. I knew my response should have been to ask them to keep it down, which would allow them to maintain their personal opinions while at the same time keeping the comments from jeopardizing patient confidentiality. From this experience, I learned that you have to be a leader, speak up, and take the risk. Part of that means being able to go against the group, risking being ostracized. In doing so, others may follow your lead, but if they choose not to follow, at least you know you advocated for your patient. Since this experience, I have not been in a situation that has challenged my personal ethics, but I have the self-confidence to believe that I can be the leader that I spoke so passionately about.

Kim Gray, Georgetown University

Reflection

How do you think you would respond in a similar situation? Why? What does this tell you about yourself and about the adequacy of your skills for professional practice? Can you think of other ways to respond? What do you think the outcome might have been if the nursing student did speak up for the patient? Which type of leadership style might have been most effective with this group? What other skills (cognitive, interpersonal, technical, ethical/legal) would you need to respond well in this situation? Propose a plan that might effect a change in this situation. Do you agree with the criteria to evaluate a successful outcome? Would any other criteria be appropriate? If so, please explain.

Leaders value learning and must be knowledgeable. Nurse leaders and managers cannot be knowledgeable about all aspects of the profession. However, they must be creative in the development and use of scarce resources. For example, nurse leaders can use one another and other healthcare workers as resources, respecting each other's expertise. Contemporary nurse managers draw upon their own staff for clinical and organizational knowledge.

Political awareness is also important for nurse leaders. Knowing how to map the political terrain of the workplace is just as valuable as knowing how legislation at the local, state, and national levels affects the healthcare delivery system.

Flexibility is a must for all nursing leaders. All nursing functions and roles require flexibility. The needs of patients, families, and the nursing team can change from minute to minute. For example, a nurse coordinator might plan to involve staff in a discussion about how best to distribute new work responsibilities, but if there are three unexpected new admissions to the unit, the discussion may need to be postponed to a quieter time.

Leadership potential is present in all nurses. With education and practice, these qualities can be developed to the point at which a nurse is skilled in the many behaviors necessary for leadership. In 2004, the American Nurses Association (ANA) in *Nursing: Scope and Standards of Nursing Practice* defined specific professional performance guidelines for leadership (see Box 23-1). Professional nurses are accountable for these standards.

Box 23-1 **ANA STANDARDS OF NURSING PRACTICE**

Standard 15. Leadership
The registered nurse provides leadership in the professional practice setting and the profession.

Measurement Criteria
The registered nurse:
- Engages in teamwork as a team player and a team builder.
- Works to create and maintain healthy work environments in local, regional, national, or international communities.
- Displays the ability to define a clear vision, the associated goals, and a plan to implement and measure progress.
- Demonstrates a commitment to continuous, lifelong learning for self and others.
- Teaches others to succeed by mentoring and other strategies.

- Exhibits creativity and flexibility through times of change.
- Demonstrates energy, excitement, and a passion for quality work.
- Willingly accepts mistakes by self and others, thereby creating a culture in which risk taking is not only safe but also expected.
- Inspires loyalty through valuing of people as the most precious asset in an organization.
- Directs the coordination of care across settings and among caregivers, including oversight of licensed and unlicensed personnel in any assigned or delegated tasks.
- Serves in key roles in the work setting by participating on committees, councils, and administrative teams.
- Promotes advancement of the profession through participation in professional organizations.

American Nurses Association. (2004). *Nursing scope and standards of practice.* Washington, DC: Author.

Box 23-2 **CHECKLIST FOR THE BEGINNING NURSE WHO WISHES TO DEVELOP LEADERSHIP SKILLS**

Basic Attitudes and Skills
Read the statements on the right and circle the appropriate response: (1) rarely characterizes me, (2) sometimes characterizes me, and (3) often characterizes me.

1 2 3   1. I am self-directed. I know what I want and take the necessary steps to get it.

1 2 3   2. I know my strengths and limitations and feel confident with who I am and who I am becoming.

1 2 3   3. I get an idea ("vision") and energize others to help me "make it happen."

1 2 3   4. I coordinate or direct the activities of others, matching their abilities to the necessary task.

1 2 3   5. I think critically about a situation without letting my feelings or those of others bias my analysis.

1 2 3   6. Once I have identified a problem, I work at it until I resolve it—to the extent that this is within my power.

1 2 3   7. When I need help, I know where to find it and ask for it.

1 2 3   8. I recognize and encourage the talents of others and offer sincere compliments.

1 2 3   9. I accept responsibility for my decisions and behavior.

1 2 3   10. I accept compliments and enjoy my success.

1 2 3   11. I confront individuals who are abusing my rights or those of others in my group.

1 2 3   12. I use assertiveness techniques when defending rights.

1 2 3   13. I am flexible and can change direction once I see the value of another course of action.

1 2 3   14. I follow an appropriate chain of command when problem solving.

1 2 3   15. I question how nursing interventions might be improved.

The higher your score the better. Reread the statements where you checked "1" and see how you might plan to improve in these areas.

Beginning Execution of Leadership Role Responsibilities
Read the list of behaviors on the right and check the appropriate box—met or not met.

Met	Not Met	
☐	☐	1. Recognize some personal need you have been ignoring and take steps to ensure that it is met.
☐	☐	2. Think of some group you belong to (e.g., school, work, church, or social) whose members' needs are not being met and plan with other members to tackle the problem.
☐	☐	3. Recognize the special advocacy needs of a patient you believe is being underserved by the healthcare system. Become an advocate for this patient.
☐	☐	4. Find a nursing research study that recommends a specific type of care for one of your patients. Implement the recommendation and compare your findings with those of the researchers. Work collaboratively with the interdisciplinary team to implement needed changes.
☐	☐	5. Join a professional nursing organization and become an active member.
☐	☐	6. Analyze the media's portrayal of nurses in a specific television program, film, or book. Talk with a friend about how this portrayal of nursing influences your profession. Share your comments with the producer or author.
☐	☐	7. Contact your legislator to share your views about pending legislation.
☐	☐	8. Think about leaders you admire and respect; interview current nursing leaders; develop a plan for personal professional growth and development.
☐	☐	9. Develop a mentoring relationship with a nursing leader.

A full discussion of all these qualities is beyond the scope of this text, but Box 23-2 summarizes how one might approach the role of leader. Beginning nurses can monitor their progress by periodically reviewing the checklist provided.

> *Recall Rehema Kohls, the college sophomore considering starting a campus group on STIs. The nurse would apply knowledge of leadership qualities when helping Rehema to decide about leading the group. In addition, the nurse would demonstrate these qualities when interacting with Rehema.* ∎

Personal Leadership Skills

The four basic skills needed for nursing leadership listed below are not meant to be all-inclusive, but instead to serve as a basis for development:

- *Communication skills:* the ability to establish trusting interpersonal relationships with patients, peers, subordinates, and superiors to maximize goal achievement and enhance the personal growth of all participants
- *Problem-solving skills:* the ability to analyze all sides of a problem, to suspend judgment, to explore multiple options, and to work toward a creative solution (see the accompanying Nursing Advocacy in Action display)
- *Management skills:* the ability to direct others toward goal achievement; this ability involves the recognition and fostering of unique talents and skills of others and the ability to match these with necessary tasks, organizational skills, financial skills, and the ability to generate and use resources wisely
- *Self-evaluation skills:* the ability to assess honestly one's effectiveness and to accept both praise and criticism; the ability to direct personal professional growth and development

The last skill is critical, especially as you begin professional practice. The ability to know oneself is the cornerstone of success in either implicit or explicit leadership roles. In a *Harvard Business Review* article, Peter Drucker (1999), a scholar of leadership, wrote that to be successful in our current knowledge culture (of which nursing is a part), one must possess self-knowledge; by so doing, we can place ourselves in positions where we can make the greatest contribution. In terms of nursing leadership roles, this translates into formal authority of position, such as a unit coordinator or director or a clinical leader without a formal title. See Box 23-3: Personal Inquiries for Determining Complementary Leadership Roles and Working Environments.

> *Think back to Rehema Kohls, the college sophomore who is thinking about starting a campus discussion group on STIs. The nurse would incorporate knowledge of Drucker's identified need for self-knowledge and personal inquiries when helping Rehema in making her decision about starting and leading the group.* ∎

NURSING ADVOCACY IN ACTION

Patient Scenario

Everybody loves Sarah. Mature for her 9 years, Sarah has advanced leukemia and her only medical hope now is to transfer to a hospital 3,000 miles from home that has the bone marrow that she needs. There are, however, several problems.

1. Sarah's family is homeless and visits rarely. She makes excuses for them—saying how hard it is to be on the street and always trying to find shelter—but she couldn't hide her disappointment when no one visited on Christmas and her birthday. You have met the parents and were struck by their immaturity.
2. Sarah's physician is working passionately to get Sarah to the transplant center; the latest hurdle is ensuring that they will accept her given the fact that the family has no insurance or finances.
3. Many of Sarah's professional caregivers aren't sure that the bone marrow transplant is a good idea. It is doubtful the funds would be found to send any of her family with her, and the possibility exists that, if unsuccessful, she could die at the transplant center surrounded by strangers.

You mention these concerns to Sarah's doctor who replies, "But this is her only hope for cure!"

Implications for Nursing Advocacy

How will you respond if you are Sarah's nurse? Talk with your classmates and experienced nurses about the questions that follow.

- If you elect to advocate for Sarah, what practical steps can you take to ensure better health outcomes?
- What is it reasonable to expect of a student nurse, a graduate nurse, and an experienced nurse in this situation?
- What advocacy skills are needed to effectively respond to this challenge?

Leadership Styles

Many different styles of leadership are present in contemporary healthcare settings. The complexity and persistent, rapid change drive many of the leadership styles that you will observe. It is helpful to think of leadership as a behavior, as something one individual does to influence another. This influence takes many forms and requires much creativity, intellect, and savvy. Different styles are applicable in different contexts and with different levels of employees. A few of those styles are explained in the next section. New graduates

Box 23-3 PERSONAL INQUIRIES FOR DETERMINING COMPLEMENTARY LEADERSHIP ROLES AND WORKING ENVIRONMENTS

- *Identify your strengths:* Continually improve the things you do best; discover your "intellectual arrogance" (being bright is no substitute for knowledge); work on acquiring the skills and knowledge you need to fully realize your strengths; remedy your bad habits.
- *Evaluate how you accomplish work:* We all work in ways that yield the best results for us. Are you a visual or auditory learner? Do you learn best by reading or writing? Do you work more productively in teams or alone? Are you more productive as a decision maker or as an advisor?
- *Clarify your values:* Working in an organization or on a unit whose value system is unacceptable or incompatible

with yours will lead to frustration and poor performance. Identify your values and seek a work environment that is complementary, not adversarial.
- *Determine where you belong and what you can contribute:* In small or large organizations, as a decision maker or as an advisor, prepare for opportunities that emerge in response to these queries. In this dynamic industry, set reasonable short- to medium-range goals.
- *Assume responsibility for relationships:* Cultivate relationships and analyze the differences you may have with others. Know and understand the strengths, performance modes, and values of your coworkers and managers.

should carefully choose organizations that match their preferred leadership style.

Autocratic Leadership

Autocratic leadership, also called directive leadership or authoritarian leadership, involves the leader assuming complete control over the decisions and activities of the group. A nurse with an autocratic personality can be described as "firm, insistent, self-assured, and dominating with or without intent, and keeps at the center of attention" (Douglass, 1995). An extremely autocratic leader might make all decisions for workers or followers without considering the followers' ideas or feelings.

> *Consider Stephen Wall, the 65-year-old patient in the intensive care unit. The nurse would demonstrate autocratic leadership to perform specific care activities and to delegate responsibilities to appropriate personnel.* ■

Many nurses are used to working under autocratic leaders because this approach has been used in most hospitals until recently. It might have evolved from nursing's historical military and religious past, or from the industrial model of command and control prevalent in many organizations. This style of leadership is gradually being replaced by the democratic style of leadership as nurses demand and receive more say in decision making. However, there are many healthcare disciplines and different levels of professional maturity present in any situation. Some healthcare workers respond best to the directive approach.

In addition, some situations may require an autocratic leadership style. For example, Nurse A discovers that one of her patients is bleeding excessively from his surgical incision. She knows that he needs immediate attention, so she gives specific orders to another team member to attend to the other patients. She tells the registered nurse on her team to call the surgical resident to come as soon as possible. She implements a nursing plan of care to prevent further blood loss or complications. Nurse A assumed the autocratic style of leadership in this situation so that all of the necessary tasks

would be accomplished immediately. Although she rarely uses this style, she implemented it effectively in this emergency situation. This example supports the premise that leadership is context dependent.

Democratic Leadership

Democratic leadership, also called participative leadership, is characterized by a sense of equality among the leader and other participants. Decisions and activities are shared. Participants are encouraged to develop their skills and strengths within the group. The group and leader work together to accomplish mutually set goals and outcomes.

> *Recall Stephen Wall, the patient in the intensive care unit. The nurse would use democratic leadership to work collaboratively with other healthcare disciplines to plan the most effective care for the patient. For example, the nurse might need to work with the surgical and neurologic staff, respiratory therapy, physical therapy, and social services in developing the patient's plan of care.* ■

Most nurses currently use a democratic style of leadership. As professionals, nurses generally respond well to this style of leadership when they are the followers and feel more comfortable when they are the leaders of democratic groups. Group satisfaction and motivation are excellent benefits of this style.

In 1982, the American Academy of Nursing's Task Force on Nursing Practice in Hospitals conducted a study of 41 hospitals to identify and describe variables that created an environment that attracted and retained well-qualified nurses who promoted quality patient care through providing excellence in nursing services. These institutions were called "magnet" hospitals because they attracted and retained professional nurses who experienced a high degree of professional and personal satisfaction through their practice. These institutions used a decentralized decision-making process, **self-governance** at the unit level, and respect for and acknowledgment of professional autonomy. In 1990, the American Nurses Credentialing

Center (ANCC) developed a formal process to recognize excellence in nursing service and to confer "magnet" status. Magnet status is awarded for 4 years and organizations must reapply at the conclusion of this time frame. Originally, 14 characteristics were recognized that identified quality patient care, excellent nursing care, and innovations in professional nursing practice. These were defined as the Forces of Magnetism and are the current standards used for awarding of magnet status. A statistical analysis and review of evaluators' reports has resulted in the configuration of the original 14 attributes into 5 model components, effective in 2009 (Table 23-1). This new model includes the original 14 forces but reflects a greater focus on measuring outcomes and eliminated redundancy in documentation. Research and surveys support that magnet hospitals have better patient outcomes, shorter lengths of stay, higher patient satisfaction, and higher nurse job satisfaction and nurse retention than hospitals without this governance style of leadership (Marquis & Huston, 2009; ANCC, 2008; Huston, 2006a). Working in a magnet hospital can maximize the potential of new graduates who prefer democratic leadership. Additional information regarding magnet hospital status can be obtained from the American Nurses Credentialing Center at http://www.nursingworld.org/ancc/magnet.html.

An example of democratic leadership follows. Nurse B, a head nurse, observes that staff members have not been documenting patient teaching and learning in their progress notes. Nurse B is not sure why this has occurred but believes that this problem must be solved. He calls a staff meeting and leads a discussion to seek information on possible causes and solutions. Nurse B has decided that staff members need to be included in the problem-solving approach. He thinks the staff will be more motivated to document their teaching and the patients' learning if they have a say in what changes in practice are necessary and how the changes will be implemented. Nurse B has used the democratic style of leadership and **decentralized decision-making process** to resolve this issue.

Laissez-Faire Leadership

In **laissez-faire leadership,** also called nondirective leadership, the leader relinquishes power to the group, such that an outsider could not identify the leader in the group. This approach encourages independent activity by group members. This style depends on the strengths of followers to direct the group activities. It is most effective when all staff are clinical experts with a deep understanding of both clinical and administrative processes. This style is rarely useful because task achievement is difficult when each nurse is working independently, and the staffs on most units and departments have varying levels of clinical maturity. However, it can be used effectively when the leader wants a problem to be solved completely by expert staff group members.

> *Consider Stephen Wall, the patient with multiple trauma who is in the intensive care unit. The patient has multiple priority needs, requiring interdependent actions of many individuals. Use of laissez-faire leadership would not be effective in this situation.* ■

An example of laissez-faire leadership follows. Nurse C, a clinical coordinator, has read an interesting research study that supports a change in the current instructions being given to new mothers who are breastfeeding. She posts the article with a summary of findings in all the nurses' stations in the maternity unit.

Nurse C is using a laissez-faire leadership style. She is confident that individual staff members are capable professionals who are concerned with keeping up with current research findings that they will use to improve their nursing care.

Transformational Leadership

Transformational leadership can create revolutionary change. Often described as charismatic, these leaders are unique in their ability to inspire and motivate others. They create intellectually stimulating practice environments and challenge themselves and others to grow personally and professionally and to learn. Gifted in creating a common vision, they demonstrate passion for their vision and keep others similarly focused. One of the unique qualities of transformational leaders is their vulnerability. They communicate honestly and openly and can express emotions as well as ideas

TABLE 23-1	QUALITY STANDARDS AND INDICATORS FOR THE MAGNET RECOGNITION PROGRAM
Original "Forces of Magnetism" Attributes/Outcomes	2008 Magnet Model Components
1. Quality of Nursing Leadership 2. Organizational Structure 3. Management Style 4. Personnel Policies and Programs 5. Professional Models of Care 6. Quality of Care 7. Quality Improvement 8. Consultation and Resources 9. Autonomy 10. Community and Health 11. Nurses as Teachers 12. Image of Nursing 13. Interdisciplinary Relationships 14. Professional Development	1. Transformational Leadership 2. Structural Empowerment 3. Exemplary Professional Practice 4. New Knowledge, Innovation, and Improvements 5. Empirical Quality Results

as they share themselves with others. They show concern and care for others and are willing to take risks. They pay attention to process as well as outcomes.

An example of transformational leadership is as follows. Nurse D is troubled by the plight of women and children in the inner city where she lives. She unites with other nurses and healthcare professionals to design and implement strategies to meet their needs. Within 18 months, a nursing center is funded and running, improving maternal–child outcomes in the area. The founding group of healthcare professionals continues to meet monthly to dream about future strategies and to support each other in their work. They are proudest of the improved self-esteem and independence in many of the women they serve.

Situational Leadership

Generally speaking, nurses do best to use the leadership style with which they are most comfortable if that style is effective for the task at hand and for those they lead. The nurse's own personality, the group's personality, and the tasks or objectives to be accomplished should be considered in each leadership situation. **Situational leadership** theory considers the leader's style, the work group's maturity, and the situation at hand to form a comprehensive approach to management style.

For example, although all nurse managers in a healthcare agency might be charged with cutting costs, both the outcomes they target and the processes they use to achieve these outcomes might vary. The unique situations in each unit influence the management style used.

These leadership styles and their related similarities and differences have been used as models of skill development and maturation for most of the past century. Unfortunately, even the most creative of nursing leaders, who combine each of these styles to fit particular scenarios, frequently find they are lacking in depth and unresponsive to contemporary challenges.

Quantum Leadership

Porter-O'Grady and Malloch (2003), in *Quantum Leadership: A Textbook of New Leadership*, argued that leaders must move beyond the traditional modes used by all levels of workers. He, like Drucker (1999) and others, has begun to clarify the impact of the information age, identified at the turn of the last century, upon work and the worker. Vertical command and control structures that generated the leadership styles previously mentioned are no longer useful for managers and workers, nor are they able to yield productivity for organizations. The explosion of information and technology in healthcare, as in other industries, has spawned, by necessity, the "knowledge worker." This social transformation is affecting parts of all of our lives; perhaps most importantly, it is affecting how we lead and manage our organizations.

We are in a difficult transition period between the old and the new. In the old, change was viewed as an entity to be planned, carefully managed, and accepted. In the new "quan-

tum age," change is conceived as dynamic, ever-present, and continually unfolding. We are forced to experience the change at the same time as we perceive it, with little or no opportunity to definitively and laboriously plan and manage it.

Porter-O'Grady and Malloch (2003, p. 11) identified the following characteristics of **quantum leadership** and behaviors of healthcare leaders who must confront this dramatic social transformation:

1. Healthcare leaders must be able to communicate to others their vision of the future and bring energy and commitment to the reformation of the system.
2. They must be relentless communicators, challenging current ways of thinking and doing.
3. They must openly seek critiques of their work.
4. They must encourage all stakeholders to continually examine the appropriateness of current work rituals and routines and determine what should be retained and what should be left behind as no longer relevant.
5. They must raise questions about the efficacy and effectiveness of current work routines and whether they meet new and emerging expectations and reality.

Nursing leaders must model these new behaviors by combining these new attributes with the requisite technical skills.

MANAGEMENT

All nurses, to the extent that they work with others and influence others to be their best, can become leaders. However, some nurses hold positions in the healthcare system that also make them managers. The role of **management** is to plan, organize, direct, and control available human, material, and financial resources to deliver quality care to patients and families. The managerial role is frequently conceptualized as the technical dimension of formal leadership roles. These technical areas of expertise, particularly in the financial or clinical resource management dimension, are mandatory for contemporary nurse managers. A few of their direct responsibilities, identified in a previous section, can be conceptualized into these four traditionally broad areas:

- Planning: identifying problems and developing goals, objectives, and related strategies to meet the demands of the clinical arena
- Organizing: acquiring, managing, and mobilizing resources to meet both clinical and financial objectives
- Directing: leading others in achieving goals within the constraints of the current fiscal and workforce shortage scenarios. This is a demanding task for managers and staff alike.
- Controlling: implementing mechanisms for ongoing evaluation, particularly in areas of clinical quality and financial accountability

> *Remember Jack Camp, the patient with diabetes and an external fixator. One possible solution to the problem would be to enlist the aid of the nurse manager for this*

unit to address the problem of the staff's overt criticism of the patient. Using planning, organizing, directing, and controlling, the nurse manager could ultimately create an environment that is conducive to the patient's recovery and health and satisfying to staff caring for this patient. ■

It is increasingly challenging for the nurse manager to be both a clinical and a managerial expert; the explosion of clinical knowledge and expectations for managerial expertise place unrealistic demands on this role. Typical nurse managers are expected to manage their unit budget within prescribed constraints, deliver a high level of quality care to patients on the unit, develop and serve as mentors for junior staff, comply with regulatory requirements, and be experts at human resource management. Although the role might seem overwhelming, it can also be quite satisfying to the manager, the staff, and the organization. Collaboration and appropriate support from both superiors and subordinates can empower and motivate staff and facilitate a highly functioning team and best-practice clinical environment.

Gosling and Mintzberg (2003) and Marquis and Huston (2009) caution that management and leadership should be intertwined for each to be effective. Gosling and Mintzberg outline five ways that managers should act and reflect to accomplish effective change. These five managerial perspectives or mindsets are:

- The reflective mindset: allows managers to mentally digest experiences and reflect on them in a different way.
- The analytical mindset: encourages introspection so that one can recognize biases and see things in a unique way. This facilitates a change in course and movement toward resolution of problems.
- The worldly mindset: recognizes cultures and contexts or "seeing differently out to reflect differently in."
- The collaborative mindset: involves listening more than talking and allowing people to take initiative and control their own work.
- The action mindset: mobilizes energy to change while being sensitive about the capabilities of the team and the direction that is needed.

Effective managers have the ability to synthesize these mindsets into opportunities for better performance and effective change.

Nurse managers must be effective leaders to be successful. Nurse managers who cannot create a healthy group environment; who fail to resolve interpersonal issues that lower morale and result in numerous complaints from patients, nurses, and physicians; and who cannot develop a plan to resolve detrimental interpersonal issues lack leadership skills. The accompanying Research in Nursing display provides insights about effective leadership characteristics that nurse managers must exhibit.

RESEARCH IN NURSING
Bridging the Gap to Evidence-Based Practice

IDENTIFYING CHARACTERISTICS OF AN EFFECTIVE NURSE LEADER

Today's nurses face many challenges. Nurse leaders and managers have considerable responsibility for patient outcomes, use of resources, and productivity on their various units. They must also create a working environment that fosters group cohesion, nurse satisfaction, and commitment to the organization. When leadership is ineffective, morale suffers and productivity declines creating a negative impact on patient care and outcomes. Ultimately, an effective nurse leader shapes and influences nursing practice.

Related Research

Feltner, A., Mitchell, B., Norris, E., & Wolfe, C. (2008). Nurses' views on the characteristics of an effective leader. *AORN Journal*, 87(2), 363–372.

This descriptive study conducted at a magnet 316-bed acute care hospital in Florida involved interviews and surveys conducted with RNs in the Surgical Services Department. Initially, all 70 RNs in this department were sent a letter requesting their participation in this research and questioned regarding what constitutes an effective leader. Forty one-on-one interviews were conducted with special attention given to the characteristics identified as desirable in an effective leader. The four project leaders determined that the interview process added subjectivity to the final

rankings and developed an objective survey tool with a list of 15 leadership qualities gathered from the interview process. Thirty-seven participants completed the surveys and ranked each characteristic in order of importance. After scoring, the three most important leadership attributes were communication skills, fairness, and job knowledge. Based on all the information gathered, the team members also developed a definition of each of the 15 characteristics. An outcome of the survey was that many of the participants noted that one characteristic does not necessarily define a good leader nor do all 15 of the qualities have to be present. The situation and the people involved are also relevant factors.

Relevance to Nursing Practice

This study is one example of how nursing research can provide insight into those characteristics recognized as critical to successful leadership. Finding and encouraging RNs with potential leadership qualities contributes to everyone's growth and satisfaction. The characteristics viewed as leadership qualities can serve as standards for incorporation into daily practice. Nurses can use these leadership skills to become proficient in effecting change in many areas.

For additional research, visit thePoint.

Centralized and Decentralized Management Structures

In a centralized management structure, senior managers generally make decisions. Those further down in the hierarchy of the organization are often responsible for implementing decisions into which they had little input. In a decentralized management structure, on the other hand, decisions are made by those who are most knowledgeable about the issues being decided. Nurses are thus intimately involved in decisions concerning patient care. Nurse managers are accountable for what happens on their nursing unit, including patient census, staffing, supplies, and budget. A decentralized system invites greater accountability and responsibility because most nurses feel more responsible for decisions they have made themselves. However, you will most likely experience both modes of decision making, centralization and decentralization, in nursing units. Financial targets and other broad strategic directions are frequently established at executive levels of the organization. Clinical issues, processes of care delivery, clinical outcomes, and unit governance are usually resolved at the unit or department level.

Conflict Management

Nurse managers frequently encounter conflict between employees and between themselves and employees. Unresolved conflict can lower morale and threaten quality care.

Marquis and Huston (2009) described six styles for dealing with conflict—avoiding, accommodating, competing, compromising, collaborating, and smoothing—and noted that "the situation itself, the urgency of the decision, the power and status of the players, the importance of the issue, and the maturity of the people involved in the conflict" determine which strategy is most appropriate. Table 23-2 further defines these conflict resolution strategies. The problem is falling into a habitual style of conflict resolution that might not be the best for a particular situation. Effective nurses try out each style and learn to use the style best suited for each situation. This ability to determine the appropriate response to conflict and create a win–win solution for all parties is critical for a nurse to be an effective manager.

Managing Change

Change is the process of transforming or modifying something. It might be planned, unplanned, developmental, or, as Porter-O'Grady and Malloch suggested, quantum and ever-present. Nursing and the healthcare system are continually changing and evolving, and that momentum will only escalate in the years to come. Factors such as the increasing number of chronically ill and older people, the increasing role of government and industry in healthcare, the rising cost of healthcare, and the changing patterns of healthcare delivery have produced a need for innovation and change in healthcare. Once they have assessed the need for change, nurse

TABLE • 23-2	CONFLICT RESOLUTION STRATEGIES
Strategy	**Definition**
Avoiding	There is awareness of the conflict situation but the parties involved decide to either ignore the conflict or avoid/postpone its resolution. The conflict has not been resolved and may resurface later in an exaggerated format.
Collaborating	This is a joint effort to resolve the conflict with a win–win solution. All parties set aside previously determined goals, determine a priority common goal, and accept mutual responsibility for achieving this goal. This focus on problem solving is based on mutual respect, honest communication, and shared decision making.
Competing	This approach results in a win for one party at the expense of the other group/s. This win–lose confrontation can leave the loser frustrated with a desire to get even in the future. This strategy may be utilized when one party has more knowledge regarding the situation or when resistance is appropriate because of ethical concerns or unsafe patient care practices.
Compromising	For this technique to be effective, both parties must be willing to relinquish something of equal value. If that does not occur, then either or both parties may feel that they have lost the conflict and given up more than the other group.
Cooperating/Accommodating	One party makes a conscious decision to let the other group win, but frequently with this strategy, the accommodating party collects IOUs for use in the future. The original loss may result in a more positive outcome in the future.
Smoothing	Smoothing is an effort to complement the other party and focus on agreement rather than disagreement thus reducing the emotion in the conflict. The original conflict is rarely resolved with this technique.

Adapted from Marquis, B., & Huston, C. (2009). *Leadership roles and management functions in nursing* (pp. 493–495). Philadelphia: Lippincott Williams & Wilkins.

managers function as a visionary, assertive, and supportive role model in the implementation of the planned change.

Change Theory

There are many theories of change, most based on the classic theory of change proposed by Kurt Lewin (1951). Lewin identified the following three stages of change:

- Unfreezing: The need for change is recognized.
- Moving: Change is initiated after a careful process of planning.
- Refreezing: Change becomes operational.

These three rather simplistic stages do not fully reveal the very dynamic and personal nature of change of any kind. In healthcare, we can find numerous examples of using change theory to transform practice. Not so long ago, childbirth in the United States was routinely "medicalized." Women came to the hospital to deliver their babies; pain medications that interfered with the natural process of labor were routinely administered, necessitating forceps and assisted deliveries; and husbands, partners, and siblings were banished from the delivery room. Nurse midwives and others recognized the need for change (*unfreezing*) and set about researching childbirth and ways to improve infant and family outcomes. After a careful process of planning (*moving*), multiple natural childbirth options were made available to women and couples, and today they represent mainstream care (*refreezing*).

Similarly, someone who takes good health for granted might fail to develop healthy lifestyle practices until illness results in recognition of the need for change (*unfreezing*). A careful process of consultation and study might lead to the development of a well-developed fitness plan (*moving*), which ideally becomes part of the person's everyday life (*refreezing*). Effective nurses pay attention to their ability to influence the person's thinking and behavior in each stage of change.

Planned Change

Planned change is a purposeful, systematic effort to bring about change. Nurse managers most often implement planned change. The eight steps in the process of change, which are somewhat similar to the steps of the nursing process, are shown in Box 23-4. Kotter (1996) emphasized that for change to be successful, it is important to progress in sequence through each of the eight stages. Skipping any of the steps can result in the vision being sabotaged, momentum faltering, and frustration increasing for all involved in the process.

Before planning to make a change, a nurse manager should consider the following:

- What is amenable to change? Considering this question might reveal a behavior not amenable to change.
- How does the group function as a unit? Certain forces within a group may favor change, whereas other forces may resist it.
- Is the person or group ready for change and, if so, at what rate can that change be expected to be accepted? The pace of change must be consistent with the person's or group's readiness to assimilate change. Readiness involves both the ability and willingness to change. In contemporary healthcare organizations, change is dynamic, persistent, and very challenging. The concept of flexibility previously mentioned is put to a real test in any clinical or managerial arena.
- Are the changes major or minor? A series of small changes might be more easily accomplished than one large, dramatic change. The nursing leader/manager must support the staff during the difficult task of acquiring new skills and frequently new professional identities.

Resistance to Change

People might resist change for various reasons. The nurse manager/leader must identify whether any resistance is

---

Box 23-4 PLANNED CHANGE: AN EIGHT-STEP PROCESS

Planned change is a purposeful, systematic effort to alter or bring about change through the intervention of a change agent. The same steps apply whether dealing with individuals or groups.

1. *Recognize symptoms that indicate a change is needed and collect data.*
2. *Identify a problem to be solved through change.* Analyze the symptoms and reach a conclusion. Note resistance or barriers to change and factors that promote the desired change.
3. *Determine and analyze alternative solutions to the problem.* Consider the advantages, disadvantages, and consequences of each alternative. An analysis of various proposed solutions to a problem may result in using a combination of alternatives.
4. *Select a course of action from possible alternatives.* It is best to avoid initiating too many courses of action and thereby dissipating resources and energy.
5. *Plan for making a change.* This step is crucial to effect change successfully. Start by stating specific objectives, designing a

plan for change, developing timetables, selecting people to assist with making the change, and anticipating how to stabilize change and deal with resistance to change. Unless a plan is clearly designed, effecting change is likely to be a chaotic experience.

6. *Implement the selected course of action to effect change.* The plan for change is then put into effect. During this period, flexibility is important to adapt to unforeseen problems.
7. *Evaluate the effects of change by comparing them with objectives stated in the plan for change.* Adjustments can be made in the plan as necessary after evaluation. If the results of evaluation indicate that the course of action selected to solve a problem has been unsuccessful, an adjustment should be made or another course of action selected.
8. *Stabilize the change.* When a solution has been found, take measures to make the change permanent. Continue follow-up until the change is firmly established.

present, because this will determine the techniques that will be needed to overcome it. Change alters the balance of a group and resistance is an expected accompaniment to change.

THREAT TO SELF

People generally view change in terms of how they are affected personally. Personal threats might include a loss of self-esteem, a belief that more work will be required, or a belief that social relationships will be disrupted. For example, when hospitals began to use more unlicensed assistive personnel (UAP) for routine nursing care, many nurses resisted not only because of quality concerns but also because they found themselves legally and professionally responsible for supervising the care given by these new aides. There was also concern that some professional nurses would be replaced by unlicensed assistive personnel.

LACK OF UNDERSTANDING

Someone who does not understand the nature of change is likely to resist. The people who will be affected by the change must become involved and educated if resistance is to be overcome. For example, nurses who do not realize the effectiveness of using plans of care tend to resist preparing them because they believe they are not beneficial for providing patient care.

LIMITED TOLERANCE FOR CHANGE

Some people simply do not like to function in a state of flux or disequilibrium. A person might understand the need for change but might be unable to cope emotionally with it. For example, a nurse might resist change because of the temporary confusion the change is likely to cause.

DISAGREEMENTS ABOUT THE BENEFITS OF CHANGE

Resistance might occur when the change agent and those resisting change have different information. If the information known by the people resisting change is more accurate and relevant than the change agent's information, their resistance might be beneficial. For example, the supervisor of community health services proposes to implement, in a low-income neighborhood, a home healthcare plan that has been effective in a middle-class section of the city. The nurse in charge of the health program in the low-income area resists, believing that the plan will not be successful in a financially and educationally disadvantaged neighborhood.

FEAR OF INCREASED RESPONSIBILITY

Many people are worried about having to take on more complex responsibilities, especially if they feel unprepared for the planned changes. The changes might seem overwhelming, so they naturally resist them.

Overcoming Resistance to Change

Resistance can be subtle or distinct, gentle or aggressive. Responding to resistance is both a leadership responsibility and a challenge in which the leader uses leadership qualities,

leadership style, and knowledge of group dynamics to influence others toward a desired outcome. Nurses acting as change agents find the following guidelines helpful for overcoming resistance to change:

- Explain the proposed change to all affected people in simple, concise language.
- List the advantages of the proposed change, both for the individual and for members of the group.
- Relate the proposed change to the person's or group's existing beliefs and values.
- Help overcome resistance by providing opportunities for open communication and feedback.
- Indicate clearly how the change will be evaluated.
- If possible, introduce change gradually. Involve everyone affected by the change in the design and implementation of the process.
- Provide incentives for commitment to change, such as money, status, time off, or a better working environment.

> ➤ *Think back to Jack Camp, the patient described in the Reflective Practice display. The nurse could apply these guidelines when attempting to change staff behavior and the patient's behavior. Ultimately, a positive outcome for both could be achieved.* ■

Power

Nurses in leadership and managerial roles who wish to be effective change agents are sensitive to both the uses and abuses of power. **Power,** the ability to influence others to achieve a desired effect, has many sources. Nurses in management positions within an institution (e.g., director of nursing or nursing coordinator) have ascribed power associated with the role. A group might attribute power to different individuals because of their expertise, leadership, or charisma. When introducing change, it is helpful to recognize and enlist the support of key power players who can then encourage others to become involved. You can probably think of people in the groups to which you belong (school, church, civic groups) who are "natural leaders" because of their demonstrated ability to influence others. These are the "key power players" whose support is essential to effecting change. Nursing leaders recognize the strengths and limitations of their own power and encourage others to develop and use power constructively. This is done as part of "mapping the political terrain" of the unit or organization. Most change requires identification of the power brokers who will support the initiative.

> ➤ *Recall Rehema Kohls, the college sophomore considering starting a campus discussion group about STIs. The nurse at the healthcare center would identify that Rehema is considered by her peers to have power and to be a leader. The nurse would integrate this information in helping Rehema develop the group.* ■

Though power and gender issues are still recognized, many agree that this perspective has been changing over the last few decades. Women are accomplished professionals and occupy powerful leadership positions in corporations, healthcare organizations, and political arenas. The proverbial "glass ceiling" barrier has been broached and communication skills that promote group and team initiatives, long thought to be skills associated with females, are now valued by all. People are realizing that techniques for achieving and managing power vary and that the differences in the genders create unique approaches to increase effectiveness and promote positive outcomes (Marquis & Huston, 2009).

IMPLEMENTING LEADERSHIP AND MANAGEMENT SKILLS IN NURSING CARE

No one is born a leader. People develop leadership qualities through observation, knowledge, and experience. Nurses develop their leadership qualities in the same way, although they might enter nursing with some leadership experience. Nursing students and beginning practicing nurses have some leadership responsibilities, as described in the following sections, but they are still working at developing leadership skills and learning where and how to apply them. Fortunately, they have support systems for guidance.

Areas of Leadership

Leadership should be approached like any other new role or skill: slowly and carefully. Nursing students and beginning nurses should be prepared with all of the necessary tools or skills before attempting the new role. Initially, nurses develop leadership skills in well-defined clinical situations. With each experience, growth occurs and leadership is strengthened. It helps to remember that all nurse managers, nurse administrators, and nursing leaders also began as inexperienced nurses.

Patient Care Coordination

Even new graduate nurses have leadership responsibilities when they begin nursing. Nursing leadership begins with nursing care of the individual patient. Although patients are partners in their care planning, most do not have the knowledge base and skills to direct the plan. Through interpersonal skills and effective communication techniques, nurses lead their patients in acquiring new knowledge, solving problems, and changing behaviors. Managing care for even one patient can be an overwhelming responsibility for those new to nursing and its challenges. The student guide to organizing clinical responsibilities in Chapter 15 offers practical help.

An ongoing leadership challenge for all nurses is time management. Following are helpful steps for using your time effectively:

- Establish goals and priorities for each day. Identify what you need to accomplish each day, differentiating "need to do" from "nice to do" tasks. Be sure to include the patient

and/or the patient's family in establishing these priorities. Ask, "What is it important for you to accomplish today?"
- Evaluate your goals in terms of their ability to meet the needs of the patients entrusted to your care as well as your duties to yourself and your colleagues (other students and members of the team). If one student has a patient whose care requires assistance, other students can plan their day so that they will be able to help at a particular time. This sort of teamwork is an important element of care coordination.
- Establish a time line. Allocate priorities to hours in your workday so that you will recognize when you are falling behind schedule in time to correct it before the day is lost.
- Evaluate your success or failure in managing time. If you fail to accomplish your goals in the time at hand, you will need to determine whether your goals were overambitious, whether things happened beyond your control (e.g., your patient's condition worsened, requiring more care, or another student required your assistance), or whether you wasted time that could have been better spent (Fig. 23-1).
- Use the results of this evaluation to direct your next day's priorities and time line.

> *Remember Stephen Wall, the 65-year-old patient in the intensive care unit with multiple injuries. Due to his multiple and complex needs, time management for the nurse is crucial. Applying the steps identified above in this situation would be very helpful when planning and providing care.* ∎

Employee Responsibilities

Nurses have specific tasks or duties to perform. These tasks are determined by the plan and objective of the healthcare agency. It is important to read your job description carefully and to continue to evaluate how institutional factors influence your own practice of nursing. Factors that compromise quality care should be noted and addressed in consultation with experienced nurses.

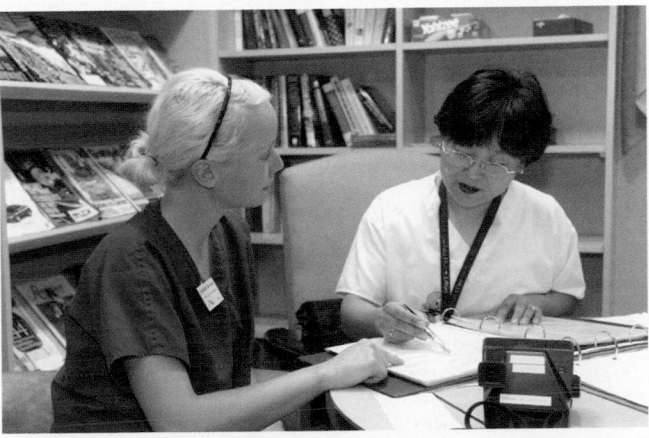

FIGURE 23-1. A student reviews her success in managing time with her clinical instructor. *(Photo by Joe Mitchell.)*

Nursing Care Delivery Models

Models of nursing care delivery systems are highlighted in Table 23-3. Over time, these have evolved from highly technical, industrial-based, assembly-line models to more professional, self-managed, cross-functional methods. According to Kerfoot (1995, p. 41), "As nurses have moved to accept more professional status and the responsibility of delegating and working through others, they have moved into advanced practice models in which there is less supervision, more opportunity for independent thought and creativity, and more accountability." The evolving models of patient care delivery demonstrate that professional nurses will increasingly be expected to have significant managerial competence. For certain, other models will evolve in this quantum age. Perhaps you will be the creator!

Guidelines for Delegating Nursing Care

New graduate nurses use leadership techniques when they direct the work of nonprofessional staff and volunteers and consider delegating tasks to nonprofessional staff. These individuals who are unlicensed and function in an assistive role to RNs are referred to as nursing assistive personnel (NAP) by the American Nurses Association (ANA) or unlicensed assistive personnel (UAP). The ANA (2008) released a position statement that supported the safe and effective use of delegation. **Delegation** involves the transfer of responsibility for the performance of an activity to another individual while retaining accountability for the outcome. It is a critical competency and essential skill for a registered nurse in today's healthcare

environment. Before delegating any nursing intervention, a number of factors should be considered: (1) the patient's condition, (2) the complexity of the activity, (3) the potential for harm, (4) the degree of problem solving and innovation necessary, (5) the level of interaction required with the patient, (6) capabilities of the NAP, and (7) the availability of professional staff to accomplish the unit workload. The ANA, which is committed to monitoring the regulation, education, and use of NAPs, recommends adherence to the following principles:

- It is the nursing profession that determines the scope of nursing practice.
- It is the nursing profession that defines and supervises the education, training, and use of any unlicensed assistant roles involved in providing direct nursing care.
- It is the registered nurse who is responsible and accountable for nursing practice.
- It is the registered nurse who supervises any assistant involved in providing direct patient care.
- It is the purpose of assistive personnel to work in a supportive role to the registered nurse, carrying out tasks to enable the professional nurse to concentrate on nursing care for the patient (ANA, 2008).

Nursing care or tasks that should never be delegated except to another RN include (Ayers & Montgomery, 2008):

- The initial and ongoing nursing assessment of the patient and his or her nursing care needs
- The determination of the nursing diagnosis, nursing care plan, evaluation of the patient's progress in relation to

TABLE • 23-3	EVOLVING MODELS OF NURSING CARE DELIVERY . . . EVOLVING ACCOUNTABILITY
Model	**Description**
Functional nursing	Nurses and other staff are assigned to specific tasks for a group of patients. Based on the assembly-line concept found in industry; specializing tasks increases efficiency but results in impersonal care.
Team nursing	A team made up of a registered nurse and other caregivers provides care to a designated group of patients on a given shift. Modified the depersonalized approach of functional nursing and focused on individual patient care.
Total care or case nursing	A nurse as caregiver provides total care to a group of patients for a designated shift. A patient-centered model; suffers from a lack of continuity between shifts and is expensive because highly paid nurses provide all aspects of care.
Primary nursing	A nurse is accountable for planning, evaluating, and directing the care of a patient 24 hours a day throughout the patient's stay. A method of providing comprehensive, individualized, and consistent care; expensive.
Case management	One nurse is responsible for overseeing the quality and financial outcomes of patient care; the nurse works collegially with physicians and other caregivers as well as with payers to manage patients along an agreed-on clinical pathway.
Patient-centered or patient-focused care	Cross-functional teams consisting of groups of professionals and assistive personnel from patient nursing and other departments work together as a unit-based team to provide care to a given group of patients. Care is designed around the needs of the patients and not the needs of the departments or professionals.
Collaborative practice model	Nurses and physicians work together in collaborative practice models.

care plan, and evaluation of the nursing care delivered to the patient

- The supervision and education of nursing personnel; patient teaching that requires an assessment of the patient and his or her education needs
- Any other nursing intervention that requires professional nursing knowledge, judgment, and/or skill.

In conclusion, the *Five Rights of Delegation* are:

- *Right Task*: One that is delegable for a specific patient
- *Right Circumstances*: Appropriate patient setting, available resources, and other relevant factors considered
- *Right Person*: Right person is delegating the right task to the right person to be performed on the right person (patient)
- *Right Direction/Communication*: Clear, concise description of the task, including its objective, limits, and expectations
- *Right Supervision*: Appropriate monitoring, evaluation, intervention as needed, and feedback (Steefel, 2007).

The Delegation Decision Tree distributed by the ANA is a helpful guide for nurses who are learning to delegate (Fig. 23-2). Refer to Chapter 15 for additional information on nursing delegation. Gradually, new nurses assume increased leadership responsibilities as they become primary nurses, case managers, or unit coordinators.

Nursing Department

The nursing team can also be viewed in the broader context of the entire nursing department of a healthcare institution or agency. Nurses should have an interest in the functioning of the department. Using this knowledge, nurses can seek information or change through appropriate channels. The more nurses understand how the nursing department runs, the better able they are to work constructively to meet the department's objectives.

Employing Institution or Agency

Nurses at all levels need to be knowledgeable about the administrative structure and functions of their employing institution or agency. When problems arise concerning professional, unit, departmental, or institutional or agency objectives, nurses must be able to use the proper channels of communication. For example, if a nurse believes that work assignments are routinely incompatible with basic patient safety and quality and gets no response after discussing this with an immediate nursing supervisor, he or she should take those complaints to the director of nursing. If the director of nursing fails to respond adequately, the nurse should determine to whom the director of nursing reports and should approach that individual. Similarly, a nurse concerned about medical care should first approach the medical attending; if he or she fails to respond, the nurse must then contact the nursing coordinator and in consult with him or her approach the medical director. The structure of these channels is shown in the agency's organization chart, which details the relationships among the various administrative positions,

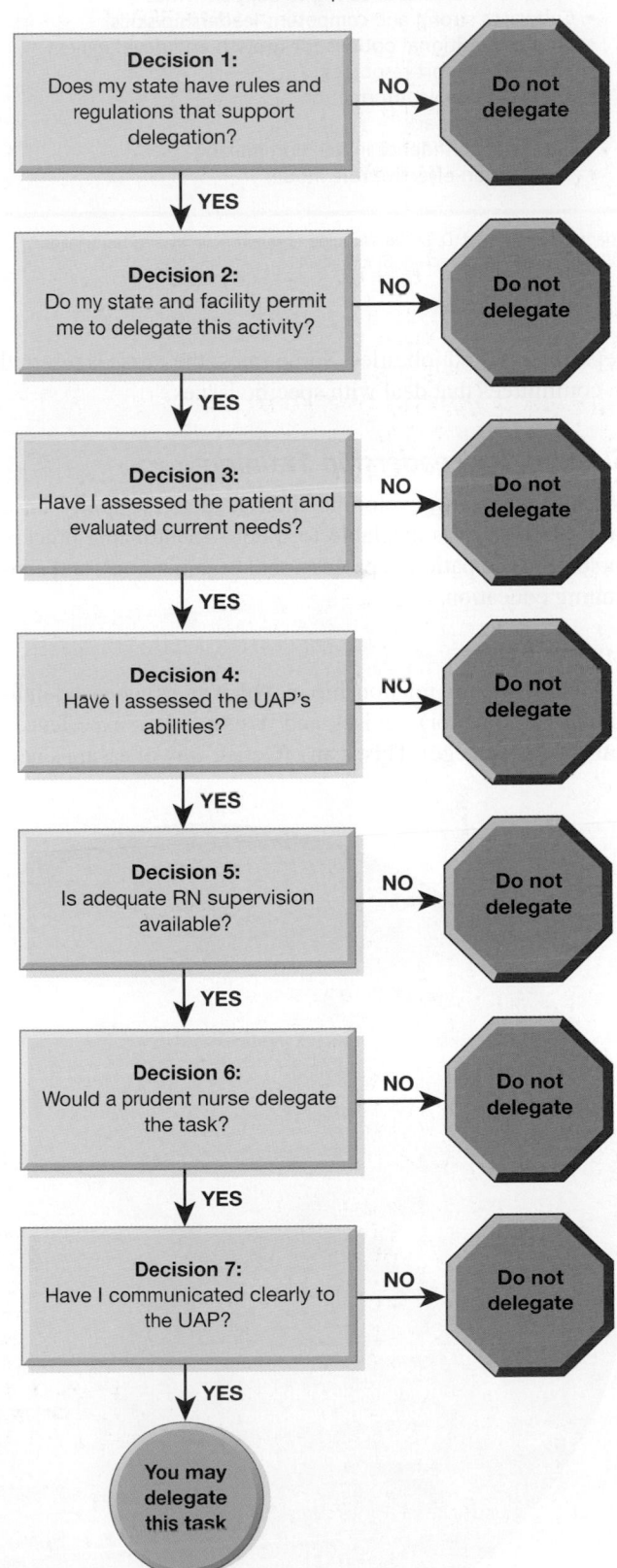

FIGURE 23-2. Sample delegation decision tree for delegated nursing responsibilities. (Used with permission from the *American Nurses Association.*)

FIGURE 23-3. The nurse preceptor advises and teaches nursing students by example. *(Photo by Joe Mitchell.)*

departments, and job titles. Sometimes, the nurse is referred to committees that deal with specific issues.

Support for Leadership Training

Nurses intent on developing their leadership ability have multiple resources available to them—mentorship, preceptorship, participation in professional organizations, and continuing education.

MENTORSHIP

Mentorship is a relationship in which an experienced individual (the mentor) advises and assists a less experienced individual (protégé). This is an effective way of easing a new nurse into leadership responsibilities. Mentors link with protégés by common interest and provide support, information, and network links. The relationship does not include financial reward. The advantages of having an effective mentor are highlighted in Box 23-5.

Mentorship is valuable in all types of nursing positions. As a nurse climbs the ladder of leadership responsibility, a mentor who is experienced in management and administrative functions might be of great assistance. A mentor can be key in helping a less experienced nurse assume added responsibilities and position changes. Many mentorship relationships also become lasting friendships.

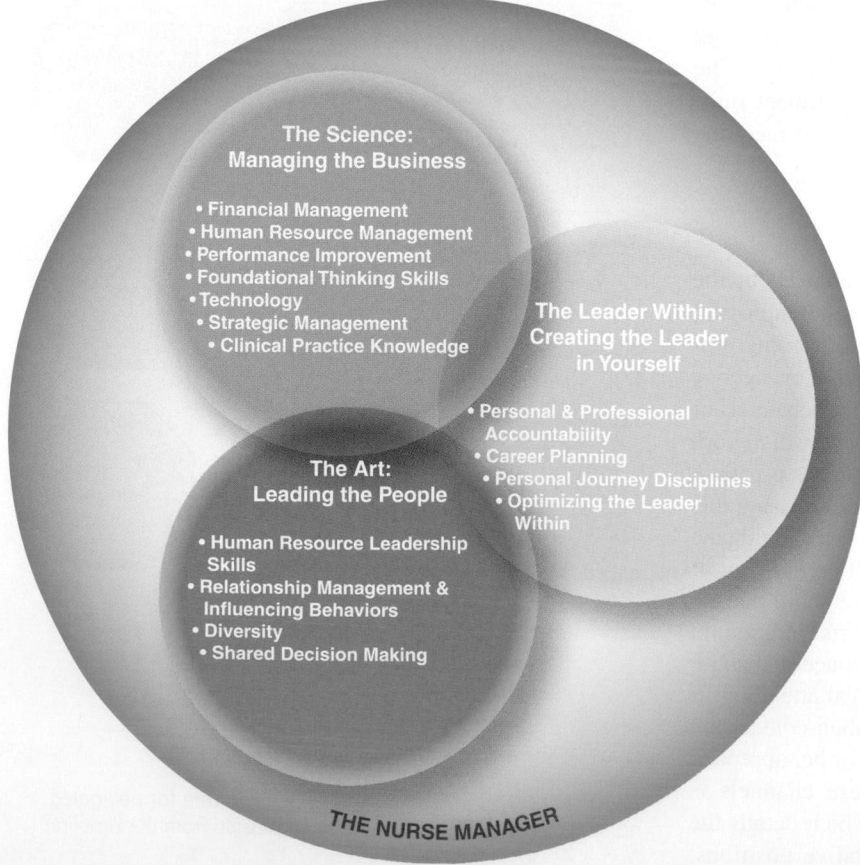

FIGURE 23-4. Nurse manager learning domain framework. (©2006 Nurse Manager Leadership Partnership. Used with permission. From American Association of Critical-Care Nurses [AACN]. [2009]. Nurse Manager Leadership Partnership. Available at http://www.aacn.org/WD/Practice/content/nursemanager inventorytool.pcms?menu=Practice.)

PRECEPTORSHIP

An alternative model is preceptorship. The preceptor (experienced nurse) is selected (and generally paid) to introduce an employee to new responsibilities through teaching and guidance. This orientation ensures that the new RN has the appropriate knowledge, skills, and support to care for patients safely and efficiently (Coll, 2007). The relationship is limited by the new employee's needs (Fig. 23-3).

PARTICIPATION IN NURSING AND OTHER PROFESSIONAL ORGANIZATIONS

The many nursing organizations at the international, national, state, district, and local levels were discussed in Chapter 1. They are major forces for nursing leadership and have active groups throughout the United States and abroad. The American Organization of Nurse Executives (AONE), recognizing the need for leadership development for nurse managers, has united with the American Association of Critical-Care Nurses (AACN) and the Association of PeriOperative Registered Nurses (AORN) and proposed a model that includes content on the science, the art, and the creation of the leader within oneself (AACN, 2008a) (see Figure 23-4). A Nurse Manager Inventory Tool is also available (AACN, 2008b). These are intended to engage nurses in exploring potential solutions to achieve their management goals. Nursing leadership can define what the future should look like and help make it happen. Participation in nursing and other professional organizations provides important opportunities for nurses to develop and exhibit leadership.

CONTINUING EDUCATION

Many programs for developing leadership, managerial, and administrative skills are available to nurses. Courses can also be taken by correspondence or over the Internet. Periodicals and books also provide continuing education for emerging leaders. Many continuing education programs are available to prepare nurses before they assume higher levels of leadership; some are geared to nurses already in such positions. Nurses should choose a program that matches their learning needs. Many State Boards of Nursing now require evidence of continuing education credits prior to renewal of RN licenses.

● Developing Critical Thinking Skills

1. Interview several experienced nurses and ask them what qualities make for the best nursing leaders. Reflect on your personal experience in groups (e.g., within your family, church, school, community). Identify the roles you characteristically assume and what qualities you bring to the group (e.g., enthusiasm, positive thinking, vision, self-direction). Consider whether those qualities will serve you well in professional nursing groups and situations. Are there new qualities you need to develop if you want to become an effective nurse leader? Why?

2. Identify a situation in your class or school that "cried out for change." Discuss with your classmates which

students emerged as leaders to address the need for change. Review and critique the steps they engaged in to bring about change. See if your group can reach consensus about the adequacy of their leadership behaviors.

● Practicing for NCLEX

1. When evaluating the leadership style of a particular nursing unit, which characteristic would lead the nurse to determine that an autocratic leadership style is being used?
   a. One person is responsible for all decision making.
   b. Activities are shared among all participants.
   c. Each staff member works independently of others.
   d. The leader shows concern for others, taking risks as necessary.

2. When developing a presentation about magnet hospitals, which characteristics would you include? (Select all that apply.)
   a. Are located in large, progressive, tertiary centers
   b. Demonstrate a decentralized decision-making process
   c. Exhibit better patient outcomes and staff retention
   d. Promote control of practice by medical personnel
   e. Allow staff self-scheduling

3. Which phrase best describes transformational leaders?
   a. Drive rapid organization-wide change
   b. Are frequently seen at senior or executive levels
   c. Are focused exclusively on outcomes
   d. Lack vision and vulnerability

4. When teaching a group of students about quantum leadership, which information would be most appropriate for the instructor to include? (Select all that apply.)
   a. Involves rapid leaps or departures from command-and-control structures
   b. Views change as something that is planned
   c. Requires openness to continual and consistent feedback
   d. Is responsive to persistent, unrelenting environmental change

5. A teaching plan about the differences between leadership and management would be considered effective if the students identified which as a difference?
   a. Formal titles differentiate the two constructs.
   b. Leadership is less tangible than management.
   c. Managerial skills are the technical side of leadership.
   d. Leadership and management are mutually exclusive.

6. There is evidence that planning for change can be beneficial for all. Which sequence would be best for the nurse to use when planning change?
   a. Planning, checking, implementing, evaluating
   b. Determining what to change, evaluating possible resistance, determining the appropriate rate and degree of change
   c. Unfreezing, freezing, and refreezing
   d. Communicating, problem solving, managing, and self-evaluating

7. Resistance to change is a part of organizational life. Which action(s) would be most effective in approaching this resistance? (Select all that apply.)
   a. Containing the anxiety in a small group and moving forward with the initiative
   b. Being sensitive to the personal dimensions that the change might affect
   c. Explaining the change and listing the advantages to the individual and the organization
   d. Reprimanding those who oppose the new initiative
   e. Seeking guidance from staff

8. A nurse is asked to act as a mentor. The nurse interprets this position as:
   a. A formal process for professional growth
   b. A paid responsibility of all nurses
   c. Limited to those with professional titles and rank
   d. A means for participation in a professional organization

9. The RN on a surgical unit is behind schedule administering her medications. Which of her other tasks can she safely delegate to a NAP?
   a. The assessment of a patient who has just arrived on the unit
   b. Documentation of a patient's I & O on the flow chart
   c. Teaching a patient with newly diagnosed diabetes about foot care
   d. Helping a patient who has recently undergone surgery out of bed for the first time

● Answers With Rationale

1. **a.** Autocratic leadership is traditionally viewed as one or a few individuals exercising decision-making power and control over others.

2. **b, c,** and **e.** Magnet hospitals offer shared decision making via self-governance structures and autonomous, accountable professional practice with nurses exerting control over the practice environment and participating in staff self-scheduling. Better patient outcomes in magnet hospitals have been empirically documented. Size and patient population characteristics have no relevance to magnet status. In nonmagnet hospitals, practice is dominated and in some instances controlled by physicians and others.

3. **a.** Transformational leaders might emerge from any level within the organization. Their focus is on both process and outcome. They are highly charismatic, are able to create a common vision, and take risks, thereby being vulnerable.

4. **a, c,** and **d.** Quantum leadership is dynamic and not dependent upon structured planned change.

5. **c.** Managerial skills are frequently defined as those relating to budgeting, the planning process, interviewing, adherence to employment law, and so forth, the technical side of leadership.

6. **b.** Planning for change involves a deliberate organizational assessment of what to change, how the change will be received, and the organization's ability to move forward with the change.

7. **b, c,** and **e.** Change is perceived to be ubiquitous, and so too is resistance to change. Individuals vary in their ability to understand and incorporate new learning and practice. In democratic, self-governance structures, staff can be instrumental in assisting with the process.

8. **a.** Mentoring is a deliberate, focused process leading to both personal and professional growth.

9. **b.** Nursing care that should never be delegated to a UAP includes the initial nursing assessment for a patient, patient teaching that requires an assessment, and any nursing intervention that requires professional nursing knowledge and judgment.

Taylor Suite Resources

The Taylor Suite offers these additional resources to enhance learning and facilitate understanding of this chapter:

- thePoint online resource, http://thepoint.lww.com/Taylor7E
- Student DVD-ROM included with the book
- Study Guide for Taylor's Fundamentals of Nursing

BIBLIOGRAPHY

American Association of Critical-Care Nurses (AACN). (2008a). Nurse manager leadership partnership. Available at http://www.aacn.org/WD/Practice/content/nursemanagerinventorytool.pcms?menu=Practice.

American Association of Critical-Care Nurses (AACN). (2008b). Nurse Manager Inventory Tool. Available at http://www.aacn.org/WD/Practice/Docs/12597_Inventory_Assesment_Inside.pdf

American Nurses Association (ANA). (2004). *Nursing: Scope and standards of practice.* Washington, DC: Author.

American Nurses Association (ANA). (2008). Safe staffing saves lives: ANA principles for delegation. Available at http://www.safestaffingsaveslives.org//WhatisSafeStaffing/SafeStaffingPrinciples/PrinciplesforDelegationhtml.aspx

American Nurses Credentialing Center (ANCC). (2008). A new model for ANCC's Magnet Recognition Program. Available at http://www.nursecredentialing.org/MagnetNewsArchive2008/NewMagnetModel.aspx

Ayers, D., & Montgomery, M. (2008). Delegating the "right" way. *Nursing, 38*(4), 56hn1–2.

Bernhard, L. A., & Walsh, M. (1994). *Leadership: The key to the professionalization of nursing* (3rd ed.). St. Louis, MO: C. V. Mosby.

Blyth, A. (2006). Team building: A daily task. *Pediatric Nursing, 18*(7), 44.

Candela, L., & Bowles, C. (2008). Recent RN graduates perceptions of educational preparation. *Nursing Education Perspectives, 29*(5), 266–271.

Casida, J., & Pinto-Zipp, G. (2008). Leadership-organizational culture relationship in nursing units of acute care hospitals. *Nursing Economics, 26*(1), 7–16.

Clements, J. (2003). Judi Clements training and development. Clifton Park, NY (speaker@nycap.rr.com).

Coll, R. (2007). Administrator preceptor. *Advance for Nurses, Pennsylvania, New Jersey, Delaware, 9*(1), 12.

Covey, S. (1999). *The seven habits of highly effective people.* London: Simon and Schuster.

Douglass, L. M. (1995). *The effective nurse: Leader and manager* (5th ed.). St. Louis: Mosby–Year Book.

Drucker, P. (1999). Managing oneself. *Harvard Business Review,* March–April, 65–74.

Dunn, R. (2002). *Haimann's healthcare management* (7th ed.). Chicago: Health Administration Press.

Edmonds, M., & Helms, S. (2008). At the edge of chaos: Building a resilient workforce helps prepare for managing the seemingly unmanageable. *Advance for Nurses, Pennsylvania, New Jersey, Delaware, 10*(15), 15.

Feltner, A., Mitchell, B., Norris, E., & Wolfe, C. (2008). Nurses' views on the characteristics of an effective leader. *AORN Journal, 87*(2), 363–372.

Frankel, A. (2008). What leadership styles should senior nurses develop? *Nursing Times.* Available at http://www.nursingtimes.net/whats-new-in-nursing/news-topics/nursing-leadership/what-leadership-styles-should-senior-nurses-develop/1811643.article

Gonzalez, C., & Rotman, S. (2008). Building blocks of teamwork. *Advance for Nurses, Pennsylvania, New Jersey, Delaware, 10*(5), 39–41.

Gosling, J., & Mintzberg, H. (2003). The five minds of a manager. *Harvard Business Review, 81*(11), 54–63.

Gurka, A. M. (1995). Transformational leadership: Qualities and strategies for the CNS. *Journal for Advanced Nursing Practice, 9*(3), 169–174.

Habel, M. (2009). Spread your wings: RNs have what it takes to be effective leaders. *Nursing Spectrum, 18*(2), 28–33.

Hersher, B. (2007). Developing future leaders. *Advance for Nurses, Pennsylvania, New Jersey, Delaware, 9*(20), 16.

Huston, C. (2006a). The current nursing shortage: Causes, consequences and solutions. In C. Huston (Ed.), *Professional issues in nursing.* Philadelphia: Lippincott Williams & Wilkins.

Huston, C. (2006b). The nursing profession's historic struggle to increase its power base. In C. Huston (Ed.), *Professional issues in nursing.* Philadelphia: Lippincott Williams & Wilkins.

Huston, C. (2009). 10 Tips for successful delegation. *Nursing, 39*(3), 54–56.

Kerfoot, K. (1995). Models of patient care delivery. In K. W. Vestal (Ed.), *Nursing management: Concepts and issues* (2nd ed., pp. 37–47). Philadelphia: J. B. Lippincott.

Kotter, J. (1996). *Leading change.* Boston: Harvard Business School Press.

Kramer, M., & Schmalenberg, C. (2004a). Essentials of a magnetic work environment: Part 1. *Nursing, 34*(6), 50–54.

Kramer, M., & Schmalenberg, C. (2004b). Essentials of a magnetic work environment: Part 2. *Nursing, 34*(7), 44–47.

Lewin, K. (1951). *Field theory in social science.* New York: Harper & Row.

Manion, J. (1995). Understanding the seven stages of change. *American Journal of Nursing, 95*(4), 41–43.

Marquis, B., & Huston, C. (2009). *Leadership roles and management functions in nursing.* Philadelphia: Lippincott Williams & Wilkins.

Marriner-Tomey, A. (1996). *Guide to nursing management and leadership.* St. Louis: Mosby–Year Book.

Porter-O'Grady, T., & Malloch, K. (2003). *Quantum leadership: A textbook of new leadership.* Boston: Jones & Bartlett.

Schmalenberg, C., & Kramer, M. (2008). Essentials of a productive work environment. *Nursing Research, 57*(1), 2–13.

Steefel, L. (2007). Safety in numbers. *Nursing Spectrum, 16*(8), 12–13.

Toofany, S. (2007). Team building and leadership: The key to recruitment and retention. *Nursing Management, 14*(1), 24–27.

Wood, D. (2008). A guide to mentorship by and for managers. *Fall 2008 Med/Surg Speciality Guide,* 40–41.

ACTIONS BASIC TO NURSING CARE

Unit VI focuses on the actions basic to practice—the nursing interventions planned, implemented, and evaluated to meet the healthcare needs of patients at any age, at any point along the health—illness continuum, and in all settings. The nursing interventions discussed in this unit are assessing vital signs, conducting a health history and physical assessment, maintaining safety, administering medications, and providing perioperative care.

Chapter 24 describes assessing vital signs, and Chapter 25 discusses conducting a health history and physical assessment. Nursing assessment is both an art and a science. The art of performing a skill is integrated into the science of nursing so that variations from normal are identified and evaluated and necessary nursing interventions are implemented. The findings from assessments provide a database necessary to maintain or restore health and promote wellness.

Nurses are responsible for meeting basic human needs for physical safety and security. Chapter 26 discusses promoting environmental safety (including threats from bioterrorism), identifying risk factors for patients at any age, and implementing teaching and other nursing actions to prevent accidents. Chapter 27 explains medical and surgical aseptic techniques necessary to prevent and to control the spread of microorganisms. Chapter 28 discusses complementary and alternative therapies, an ever-increasing component of healthcare.

Chapters 29 and 30 focus on collaborative and independent nursing interventions used to accurately and safely administer medications and provide perioperative care. In most instances, the physician prescribes the medications and performs the surgery while the nurse orders and implements nursing interventions to promote patient safety and knowledge and to facilitate optimal function or recovery in both hospital and home settings. Although institutional procedures and protocols are often used in these situations, nursing interventions are individualized to the unique needs of each person requiring care.

"*Our intent when we lay hands on the patient in bodily care is to comfort.*"

LYDIA HALL (1906–1969) • *an innovator in nursing practice, she developed the theory that the direct nurse-to-patient relationship is itself therapeutic and that nursing care is the chief therapy for critically ill patients.*

24 | Vital Signs

NOAH SHOOLIN

Noah is a 2-year-old who is brought to the emergency department by his mother. When the nurse attempts to obtain a tympanic temperature, the child begins to scream uncontrollably, crying and pushing the device away from his ear.

TOMAS ESPOSITO

Tomas is a middle-aged man admitted to the hospital. He is placed in a private room with specialized infection-control precautions, requiring staff to don a gown and gloves when entering the room each time. A morning assessment, including vital signs, is needed.

DORETHA RENFROW

Doretha brings her 65-year-old husband with high blood pressure to the clinic for evaluation. He is 5'10" and overweight. Mrs. Renfrow states, "I really would like to learn how to take my husband's blood pressure so that I can keep track of his progress. Can you teach me how to do it?"

After completing the chapter, you will be able to accomplish the following:

1. Explain the physiologic processes involved in homeostatic regulation of temperature, pulse, respirations, and blood pressure.

2. Compare and contrast factors that increase or decrease body temperature, pulse, respirations, and blood pressure.

3. Identify sites for assessing temperature, pulse, and blood pressure.

4. Assess temperature, pulse, respirations, and blood pressure accurately.

5. Demonstrate knowledge of the normal ranges for temperature, pulse, respirations, and blood pressure across the lifespan.

6. Provide information to patients about taking pulse and blood pressure at home.

KEY TERMS

afebrile	hypothermia
apnea	Korotkoff sounds
blood pressure	orthopnea
bradycardia	orthostatic
bradypnea	hypotension
diastolic pressure	pulse
dyspnea	pulse deficit
dysrhythmia	pulse pressure
eupnea	respiration
febrile	systolic pressure
fever	tachycardia
hypertension	tachypnea
hyperthermia	temperature
hypotension	vital signs

Vital signs are a person's temperature, pulse, respiration, and blood pressure (abbreviated as T, P, R, BP). Pain, often included as the fifth vital sign, is discussed in Chapter 35. The health status of an individual is reflected in these indicators of body functions, regulated through homeostatic mechanisms and falling within certain normal ranges. A change in vital signs might indicate a change in health. Assessing vital signs as part of a nursing assessment is a component of care in any setting. Institutional and agency policies govern when

and how frequently vital signs are assessed. For example, vital signs are assessed at least every 4 hours in hospitalized patients with elevated temperatures, with high or low blood pressures, with changes in pulse rate or rhythm, or with respiratory difficulty. In critical care settings, technologically advanced devices are used to continually monitor patients' vital signs. Regulations require monthly vital sign measurements in long-term care residents, but if the resident is classified as Medicare A (meaning they have been discharged from the hospital and now Medicare is paying for their stay to receive skilled nursing care) vital signs are taken daily. In the home and in some self-care and psychiatric units, assessments are made only as frequently as the nurse judges necessary.

Although vital sign assessment may be delegated to other healthcare personnel, it is the nurse's responsibility to ensure accuracy of data and to report abnormal findings. (See the accompanying Reflective Practice box for an example.) If a patient has abnormal or unusual physical signs or symptoms (e.g., chest pain or dizziness) or has unexpected changes in vital signs, the nurse should double-check the findings and further assess the patient. (Delegation is discussed in Chapters 15 and 23). The nurse should know the normal variations in vital signs that occur at various ages as listed in Table 24-1.

> *Recall Tomas Esposito, the patient requiring initial assessment described in the Reflective Practice display? The nurse's inability to auscultate heart and lung sounds would be an important finding that requires additional assessment. The nurse would need to evaluate these findings in conjunction with the patient's other vital signs.* ■

Vital signs are taken and compared with accepted normal values and the patient's usual patterns in a wide variety of instances, including screenings at health fairs and clinics, in the home, upon admission to a healthcare setting, when medications are given that affect cardiac rate and rhythm, before and after invasive diagnostic and surgical procedures, and in emergency situations (Box 24-1). Nurses take vital signs as often as a patient's condition requires such assessment. The skills of assessing each of the vital signs, with rationale for each action, and a discussion of normal and abnormal findings are presented in this chapter. See Chapter 25 for additional information about health assessment.

TEMPERATURE

Body **temperature** is the difference between the amount of heat produced by the body and the amount of heat lost to the environment measured in degrees. Heat is generated by metabolic processes in the core tissues of the body, transferred to the skin surface by the circulating blood, and then dissipated to the environment. Core body temperature is higher than surface body temperature and is normally maintained within a range of 36.0°C (97.0°F) to 37.5°C (99.5°F).

REFLECTIVE PRACTICE
Challenge to Ethical and Legal Skills

At clinical 2 weeks ago, I had four patients for the first time and I was very busy. One of my patients, Tomas Esposito, required specialized infection-control precautions, so every time I entered his room, I had to put on a gown and gloves. It was getting to be late in the morning and I still had not completed this patient's full assessment, including his vital signs. Upon entering the patient's room, I discovered that the separate stethoscope usually found in isolation rooms was not there. As a result, I had to remove my gown and gloves and go find the nurse to help me locate the stethoscope. Ultimately, the nurse had to get me a new isolation stethoscope set and put it together for me. Unfortunately, these stethoscopes are poor in quality.

   I went back to the patient's room and put on a new gown and gloves. By this time, Mr. Esposito was very irritable and just wanted me to do the assessment quickly and leave him alone. I attempted to listen to his heart sounds but I couldn't hear them. I played with the stethoscope for a few minutes and tried again, but I still couldn't hear his heart or lung sounds. My patient kept telling me to leave him alone. Being a 4th-year nursing student and self-sufficient in doing the basic patient assessment, I felt stupid going to get the nurse or my instructor and telling her I couldn't hear anything. I was really pressed for time and now was faced with a critical decision.

Thinking Outside the Box: Possible Courses of Action

- Remove my gown and gloves, get my instructor and the nurse and tell them that I was unable to hear heart and lung sounds, and request their assistance.
- Leave the patient alone as he requested, saving precious time, pretending that I completed the assessment, and charting the same findings as the previous shift's assessment.
- Explain to the nurse that the patient wasn't cooperating and ask her to do the assessment without my instructor knowing about it.
- Try to complete the assessment using my own stethoscope and risk passing the patient's infections on to my other patients.

Evaluating a Good Outcome: How Do I Define Success?

- Patient receives the highest quality of care.
- Professional integrity of all healthcare team members involved is maintained.
- All information charted is accurate.
- Ethical and legal principles are maintained.

Personal Learning: Here's to the Future!

Luckily, my conscience and my desire to always give the best care to my patients pushed me to the right decision. I took the time to remove my gown and gloves and went to find my instructor and the nurse. I told the nurse that I was having trouble hearing the patient's heart and lung sounds. She was very understanding and came to the room with me and tried herself. Upon further investigation, we found that the problem was a broken stethoscope, not my incompetence to complete an assessment. After assessing the patient with a properly functioning stethoscope, I found expiratory wheezing and documented it. This finding also provided a clue that I should probably keep a very close eye on this patient. Mr. Esposito ended up experiencing increasing difficulty breathing and his oxygen saturation levels began to drop into the 80% range. As a result, I realized just how important the initial assessment is when caring for a patient throughout the day. Hopefully, the lesson about how important it is to do the "right" thing for the patient will stick with me forever.

Catherine Barrell, Georgetown University

Reflection

How do you think you would respond in a similar situation? Why? What does this tell you about yourself and about the adequacy of your skills for professional practice? Can you think of other ways to respond? What might the nursing student have done to prevent the numerous trips in and out of the patient's room? To determine whether the stethoscope was functioning properly? How do you think the nursing student's time management and organizational skills affected the situation? What other skills (cognitive, interpersonal, technical, ethical/legal) would you need to respond well in this situation? What ethical principles did the nursing student incorporate into the response to the situation? What responses related to the patient's irritability would have been appropriate by the nursing student? Do you agree with the criteria to evaluate a successful outcome? Did the nursing student meet these criteria? Please explain.

There are individual variations of these temperatures as well as normal changes during the day, with core body temperatures being lowest in the early morning and highest in the late afternoon (Porth & Matfin, 2009).

   Core temperatures are measured by nurses at tympanic or rectal sites, but they may also be measured in the esophagus, pulmonary artery, or bladder by invasive monitoring devices.

Surface body temperatures are measured at oral (sublingual), axillary, and skin surface sites.

Physiology of Body Temperature

The core body temperature of a healthy person is maintained within a fairly constant range by the thermoregulatory set

TABLE • 24-1 AGE-RELATED VARIATIONS IN NORMAL VITAL SIGNS

Age	Temperature (°C)	Pulse (beats/min)	Respirations (breaths/min)	Blood Pressure (mm Hg)
Newborn	36.8 (Axillary)	80–180	30–80	73/55
1–3 yr	37.7 (Rectal)	80–140	20–40	90/55
6–8 yr	37 (Oral)	75–120	15–25	95/75
10 yr	37 (Oral)	75–110	15–25	102/62
Teens	37 (Oral)	60–100	15–20	102/80
Adults	37 (Oral)	60–100	12–20	120/80
>70 yr	36 (Oral)	60–100	15–20	120/80

point of the thermoregulatory center in the hypothalamus. This center receives messages from cold and warm thermal receptors located throughout the body, compares that information with its temperature set point, and initiates responses to either produce or conserve body heat or to increase heat loss.

Heat Production

The primary source of heat in the body is metabolism, with heat produced as a byproduct of metabolic activities that generate energy for cellular functions. Various mechanisms increase body metabolism, including hormones and exercise. When additional heat is required to maintain balance, epinephrine and norepinephrine (sympathetic neurotransmitters) are released to rapidly alter metabolism so that energy production decreases and heat production increases. Thyroid hormone, produced by the thyroid gland, also increases metabolism and heat production, but over a much longer time period. Shivering, a response that increases the production of heat, is initiated by the hypothalamus and results in muscle tremors. The contraction of pilomotor muscles of the skin, as occurs with shivering, causing piloerection, or "goose bumps" and reduces the size of the surface to minimize heat loss. Exercise increases heat production through muscle movements.

Box 24-1 WHEN TO ASSESS VITAL SIGNS

- On admission to any healthcare agency or institution
- Based on agency or institutional policy and procedures
- Any time there is a change in the patient's condition
- Any time there is a loss of consciousness
- Before and after any surgical or invasive diagnostic procedure
- Before and after activity that may increase risk, such as ambulation after surgery
- Before administering medications that affect cardiovascular and respiratory function

Heat Loss

The skin is the primary site of heat loss. The circulating blood brings heat to the skin's surface, where small connections between the arterioles and the venules lie directly below the skin surface. These connections, called arteriovenous shunts, may remain open to allow heat to dissipate (e.g., during exercise in hot environmental temperatures) to the skin and then to the external environment, or they may close and retain heat in the body (e.g., when the body is exposed to cold environmental temperatures). The sympathetic nervous system controls the opening and closing of the shunts in response to changes in core body temperature and in environmental temperature (Porth & Matfin, 2009).

Other heat losses occur through evaporation of sweat, through warming and humidifying of inspired air, and through elimination of urine and feces. Heat is transferred to the external environment through the physical processes of radiation, convection, evaporation, and conduction. These processes are defined and illustrated in Table 24-2.

Factors Affecting Body Temperature

A variety of factors affect body temperature. These factors include circadian rhythms, age, gender, stress, and environmental temperatures.

Circadian Rhythms

Many environmental and physiologic processes occur in repeated cycles of time. Some events in humans recur at 24-hour intervals, referred to as circadian (meaning nearly every 24 hours) rhythm. Predictable fluctuations in measurements of body temperature and blood pressure are examples of functions that have a circadian rhythm. For instance, body temperature is usually about 0.6°C (1° to 2°F) lower in the early morning than in the late afternoon and early evening. This variation tends to be somewhat greater in infants and children. The peak elevation of a person's temperature occurs in late afternoon, between 4 and 7 p.m.

TABLE • 24-2   MECHANISMS OF HEAT TRANSFER

	Radiation	Convection	Evaporation	Conduction
Definition	The diffusion or dissemination of heat by electromagnetic waves	The dissemination of heat by motion between areas of unequal density	The conversion of a liquid to a vapor	The transfer of heat to another object during direct contact
Example	The body gives off waves of heat from uncovered surfaces.	An oscillating fan blows currents of cool air across the surface of a warm body.	Body fluid in the form of perspiration and insensible loss is vaporized from the skin.	The body transfers heat to an ice pack, causing the ice to melt.

Radiation   Convection   Evaporation   Conduction

Age and Gender

Both the very old and the very young are more sensitive to changes in environmental temperature. Older adults lose some thermoregulatory control with aging and are at risk for harm from extremes of temperature. The body temperature of infants and children changes more rapidly in response to both hot and cold air temperatures.

> Consider Noah Shoolin, the 2-year-old brought to the emergency department by his mother. The nurse assessing the child's temperature would need to keep in mind the effect of environmental temperature changes on a child of this age. Efforts to prevent chilling and overheating would be incorporated into the child's plan of care. ■

Women tend to experience more fluctuations in body temperature than do men, probably the result of changes in hormones. The increase in progesterone secretion at ovulation increases body temperature as much as 0.3° to 0.6°C (0.5° to 1°F).

Environmental Temperature

Most of us respond to changes in environmental temperature by wearing clothing that either allows increased heat loss when it is hot or retains heat when it is cold. When one is exposed to extreme cold without adequate protective cloth-

ing, heat loss may be increased to the point of **hypothermia** (low body temperature). Similarly, if one is exposed to extremes of heat for long periods of time, **hyperthermia** (high body temperature) may result. Both hypothermia and hyperthermia may cause serious illness or death. Figure 24-1 illustrates the range of normal and abnormal body temperature when taken orally.

Normal Body Temperature

Body temperature varies among individuals, with a range of 0.3° to 0.6°C (0.5° to 1.0°F) from the average temperature considered to be within normal limits, although wider variations from the average temperature may be normal for some people. A person with a normal body temperature is referred to as **afebrile** ("without fever"). Table 24-3 shows the average normal temperature standards for healthy adults at various body sites.

Increased Body Temperature

Fever (pyrexia) is an increase above normal (considered to be 37°C or 98.6°F) in body temperature. A person with a fever is said to be **febrile.** Fever occurs in response to an upward displacement of the thermoregulatory set point from cytokines produced by pyrogens (microorganisms or substances that cause fever). Fever may also be the result of tissue injury, such as from myocardial infarction, pulmonary

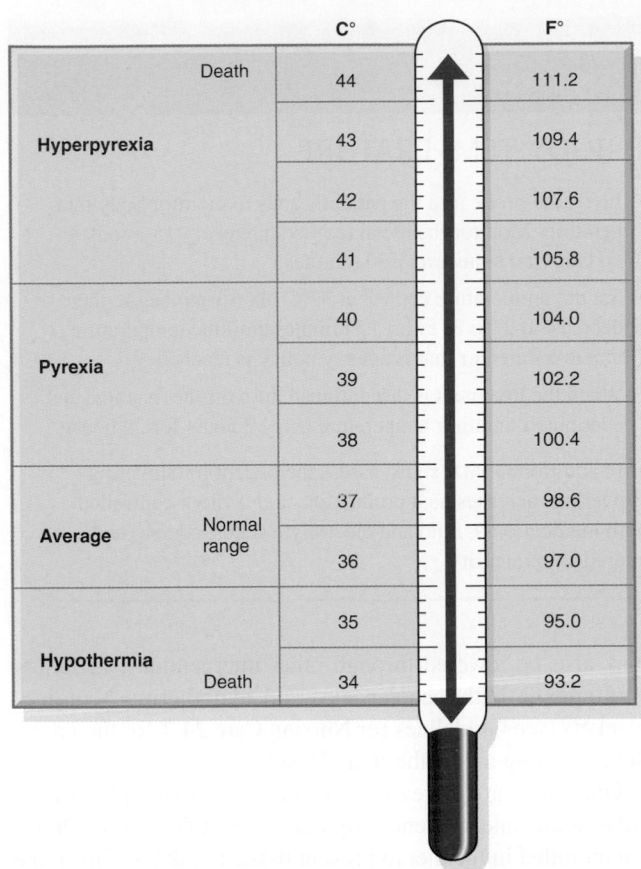

FIGURE 24-1. The range of human body temperature as measured orally, using a bulb thermometer as an example.

C°		F°
Death	44	111.2
Hyperpyrexia	43	109.4
	42	107.6
	41	105.8
	40	104.0
Pyrexia	39	102.2
	38	100.4
Average / Normal range	37	98.6
	36	97.0
	35	95.0
Hypothermia / Death	34	93.2

Box 24-2 TERMS AND DEFINITIONS FOR TYPES OF FEVER

Intermittent: The body temperature alternates regularly between a period of fever and a period of normal or subnormal temperature.

Remittent: The body temperature fluctuates several degrees more than 2°C (3.6°F) above normal but does not reach normal between fluctuations.

Constant: The body temperature remains consistently elevated and fluctuates less than 2°C (3.6°F).

Relapsing: The body temperature returns to normal for at least a day, but then the fever recurs.

Crisis: The fever returns to normal suddenly.

Lysis: The fever returns to normal gradually.

perature elevations of only slightly above normal, even in a serious infection.

When the set point is increased from a bacterial or viral infection, the hypothalamus initiates temperature-rising mechanisms: shivering, piloerection, vasoconstriction, and increased metabolism. After the body temperature rises to the new set point, heat-loss mechanisms (sweating, vasodilation, increased respirations) keep the body temperature from rising to dangerous levels. Most fevers are self-limiting, and the temperature returns to normal after the factors causing it are controlled. Box 24-2 lists terms used to describe types of fever. Hyperpyrexia is a high fever, usually above 41°C (105.8°F).

Other types of increased body temperature are hyperthermia, neurogenic fever, and fever of unknown origin (FUO). Hyperthermia differs from fever in that the hypothalamic set point is not changed, but in situations of extreme heat exposure or excessive heat production (e.g., during strenuous exercise), the mechanisms that control body temperature are ineffective. Neurogenic fever is the result of damage to the hypothalamus from pathologies such as intracranial trauma, intracranial bleeding, or increased intracranial pressure. This type of fever does not respond to antipyretic medications (Porth & Matfin, 2009). A fever of 38.3°C (101°F) or higher that lasts for 3 weeks or longer without an identified cause is diagnosed as an FUO.

emboli, cancer, trauma, and surgery. Although the purpose of fever is not fully understood, it signals infection and increases immune function (Porth & Matfin, 2009). However, fever, unless extremely high or low, is not harmful.

The onset and significance of a fever from an illness differs by one's age. The onset of a fever, which can be sudden or gradual, typically is more rapid in children than in adults. A mild elevation in temperature might indicate a serious infection in infants younger than 3 months of age who do not have well-developed temperature-control mechanisms. In older adults, who often have a lower baseline body temperature, fever may be one of the later signs of illness with tem-

TABLE · 24-3	AVERAGE NORMAL TEMPERATURES FOR HEALTHY ADULTS AT VARIOUS SITES			
Oral	**Rectal**	**Axillary**	**Tympanic**	**Forehead**
37.0°C	37.5°C	36.5°C	37.5°C*	34.4°C†
98.6°F	99.5°F	97.7°F	99.5°F	94.0°F

*The average normal tympanic temperature depends on the calibration and mode setting of the tympanic membrane thermometer.

†The manufacturer of Digitemp forehead thermometer (Hallcrest Products, 1820 Pickwick Lane, Glenview, IL 60025) says, "Most older children and adults have normal forehead temperatures between 93 and 95 degrees F."

Guidelines for Nursing Care • 24-1

USING A HYPOTHERMIA BLANKET TO LOWER BODY TEMPERATURE

Placing the patient on a special hypothermia blanket or pad may lower body temperature. This apparatus has coils through which a refrigerated solution circulates. It operates much like an Aqua-K heating unit (discussed in Chapter 32), except that the liquid is cooled instead of heated. When applying a hypothermia blanket, follow these steps:

- Place the hypothermia blanket on the bed and cover it with a sheet so the patient's skin does not come in direct contact with the cold blanket. Position the patient on the blanket.
- Connect the cooling blanket to the machine and select the cool temperature setting.

- Insert the probe into the patient's anus to monitor body temperature. Monitor the rectal temperature every 15 minutes and all vital signs every 30 minutes.
- Set the temperature control at 37°C (98.6°F) to begin, then decrease it 2° to 3° every 15 minutes until the temperature that is ordered or that is agency policy is reached.
- When the treatment is discontinued, turn off the machine and continue to monitor temperature every 2 hours for 24 hours.

In addition to vital signs, assess the patient for shivering (shivering increases heat production, and is often controlled with medications), fluid and electrolyte status, edema, and altered skin integrity.

Physical Effects of Fever

Patients with fever may experience loss of appetite; headache; hot, dry skin; flushed face; thirst; muscle aches; and fatigue. Respirations and pulse rate increase. Young children with high fevers may experience seizures and older adults may have periods of confusion and delirium. Fever blisters may develop in some people as the fever activates the type I herpes simplex virus. Fluid, electrolyte, and acid–base imbalances are potentially dangerous complications.

Methods of Reducing Fever

Determining the cause of the fever and treating its underlying cause is important. If the fever is the result of a bacterial infection, the appropriate antibiotic may be prescribed. Antipyretic (fever-reducing) drugs, such as aspirin or acetaminophen, may be administered in certain circumstances. These drugs reset the elevated set point regulated by the hypothalamus. Aspirin should not be given to children under 2 years of age unless prescribed. Aspirin also should not be given to children and teenagers with chickenpox or influenza because of a possible association with Reye's syndrome. Body temperature

may also be lowered through other interventions, including cool sponge baths, cool packs, and hypothermia (cooling) blankets (see Guidelines for Nursing Care 24-1 for the procedure for using a hypothermia blanket).

Oral fluids are increased to maintain cellular and intravascular status and prevent dehydration. Simple carbohydrates are included in the diet to prevent tissue breakdown from the hypermetabolic state. Nursing interventions and expected outcomes for the patient with a fever are outlined in the Examples of Nursing Interventions and Nursing Outcomes Classifications (NIC/NOC) box.

Decreased Body Temperature

Hypothermia is a body temperature below the lower limit of normal. Death may occur when the temperature falls below 34°C (93.2°F), but survival has been reported in isolated cases (such as in drowning in very cold water or burial in snow) when body temperatures have fallen in the range of severe hypothermia (28°C, or 82.4°F). Rates of chemical reactions in the body are slowed, thereby decreasing the metabolic demands for oxygen.

Examples of Nursing Interventions and Nursing Outcomes Classifications (NIC/NOC)

Fever Treatment

Nursing Interventions	Nursing Outcomes
- Monitor temperature as frequently as appropriate. - Monitor blood pressure, pulse, and respirations as appropriate. - Monitor intake and output. - Monitor for seizure activities. - Administer antipyretic medication as appropriate. - Administer IV fluids as appropriate. - Apply ice bag covered with a towel to groin and axilla.	- Vital Signs - Hydration - Thermoregulation - Risk Control: Hyperthermia

FIGURF 24-2. Types of thermometers used to assess body temperature. (**A**) Electronic thermometer. (**B**) Tympanic membrane thermometer. (**C**) Disposable paper thermometer for taking forehead temperature; the dots change color to indicate temperature. (**D**) Temporal artery thermometer.

Assessing Temperature

To accurately assess body temperature, the nurse must know what equipment to use, which site to choose, and what method is appropriate. Although the skill of taking a temperature may be delegated to assistive healthcare personnel, the nurse is responsible for assessing the effect of changes in body temperature and teaching the patient and caregivers about methods, normal values, and the need to report abnormal findings.

Equipment

Body temperature, measured in degrees, may be assessed with a variety of devices—electronic and digital thermometers, tympanic membrane thermometers, disposable single-use thermometers, temporal artery thermometers, and automated monitoring devices. Figure 24-2 illustrates the different types of thermometers.

Body temperature is documented in either Celsius or Fahrenheit degrees. Table 24-4 provides equivalent Celsius and Fahrenheit values as well as the method for conversion.

Glass thermometers with mercury-filled bulbs were once the standard equipment used to take a temperature, but most municipal regulations prohibit their use because mercury is a

TABLE • 24-4	EQUIVALENT CELSIUS AND FAHRENHEIT TEMPERATURES*
Celsius	**Fahrenheit**
34.0	93.2
35.0	95.0
36.0	96.8
36.5	97.6
37.0	98.6
37.5	99.5
38.0	100.4
38.5	101.3
39.0	102.2
40.0	104.0
41.0	105.8
42.0	107.6
43.0	109.4
44.0	111.2

*To convert Celsius to Fahrenheit, multiply by 9/5 and add 32. To change Fahrenheit to Celsius, subtract 32 and multiply by 5/9.

hazardous material. They may still be in use in some homes or in smaller long-term care facilities. Because glass thermometers are prone to break, they should never be used to take a temperature for a person who is unconscious or irrational, or in infants and young children. Information about the dangers of mercury, as well as how to handle a broken mercury thermometer, are important for nurses to know and teach. See Teaching Tips 24-1 for information. Bulb-type thermometers, containing liquids other than mercury (such as redyed petrolate), are available.

ELECTRONIC AND DIGITAL THERMOMETERS

Electronic and digital thermometers measure oral, rectal, or axillary body temperature over a time period from 1 to 60 seconds, depending on the site and product used. These battery-operated devices provide a numerical temperature display. The devices also have disposable probe covers to reduce the risk of infection transmission. Some models also provide the last measurement, a full 60-second pulse timer, and automatic conversion from the Fahrenheit to the Celsius scale. Assessing body temperature with an electronic thermometer is described in Skill 24-1.

TYMPANIC MEMBRANE THERMOMETERS

Tympanic membrane thermometers use infrared sensors to detect heat given off by the tympanic membrane. The probe is covered with a probe cover and inserted into the ear canal tightly enough to seal the opening (see Skill 24-1). The reading takes from 1 to 3 seconds, depending on the product.

➤ *Remember Noah Shoolin, the toddler described at the beginning of the chapter? Although a tympanic thermometer yields a quick reading, the nurse would need to verify the accuracy of the reading, especially in light of the child's current upset state, possibly by asking the mother if she had taken the child's temperature before coming to the emergency department or by using an alternative method.* ∎

Tips **TEACHING TIPS • 24-1**

MERCURY THERMOMETERS

Health Topic	Teaching Tip	Why Is This Important?
What is mercury?	• Mercury is a heavy, odorless, silver liquid. • Glass thermometers containing mercury are easily broken.	Mercury is a toxic and hazardous material that affects the central nervous system. The liquid and the vapors from the liquid are both considered dangerous. Mercury not only is hazardous to people, but also pollutes the environment (especially if it gets into water). Mercury poisoning can lead to problems with mental development and learning disabilities.
What to do if a mercury thermometer breaks	**What Not to Do** • Sweep the area. • Vacuum the area. • Pour mercury down the drain. • Wash mercury-contaminated clothes. • Use household cleaning agents to clean the spill. **What to Do** • Open windows and close off the room from the rest of the house. Use fans for at least an hour, if possible. • Use an eyedropper, a piece of heavy paper, or duct tape to scoop up the broken glass and beads of mercury. • Put the mercury, broken glass, and any materials used to scoop them up in a plastic zipper bag, and seal tightly with tape. Place this bag into a second bag and seal with tape, and then the second bag into a third bag, sealed with tape. Place the bags in a plastic wide-mouth sealable container. • Throw everything away that was exposed to the mercury (including linens, clothing, and towels). • Call your local health department to find out an approved disposal site. • Wash your hands with soap and water. Take a shower if you think any mercury touched other parts of the skin.	Sweeping breaks the mercury into smaller droplets. Mercury contaminates the vacuum. Mercury stays in the plumbing and contaminates the washing machine. Cleansing agents react with mercury, releasing a toxic gas.

DISPOSABLE SINGLE-USE THERMOMETERS

Disposable single-use thermometers are nonbreakable and register the temperature within seconds. Because they are used only once, they eliminate the danger of cross-infection and are used for patients in isolation.

Temperature-sensitive patches or tape, commonly applied to the abdomen or forehead, change color at different temperature ranges. These devices may be used to check the temperature of a toddler or young child. A thermometer should be used to reassess the temperature if the color on the tape or patch indicates that the temperature is out of the normal average range.

TEMPORAL ARTERY THERMOMETERS

Temporal artery thermometers measure body temperature by capturing the heat emitted by the skin over the temporal artery. These devices are battery operated and have a temperature display. Lawson et al. (2007) found oral and temporal artery measurements more accurate and precise than those taken by the axillary and ear routes.

AUTOMATED MONITORING DEVICES

Automated monitoring devices are used in various healthcare settings to measure body temperature, pulse, respirations, and blood pressure simultaneously. They require less of the nurse's time, especially when these assessments are required frequently.

Sites and Methods of Assessing Body Temperature

Health agency policies and procedures often specify the site to be used for assessing patients' temperatures; however, the nurse is expected to select and to use alternative sites when indicated. Factors affecting the site selection include the patient's age, state of consciousness, amount of pain, and other care or treatments (such as oxygen administration) being provided. It is customary to indicate the site used to assess the temperature when recording the measurement.

The sites most commonly used to assess body temperature are tympanic, oral (sublingual), anal, and axillary. An electronic probe is placed under the tongue (sublingual area) of a person's mouth to assess an oral temperature, in the anal canal to assess a rectal temperature, or in an axilla (armpit) to assess an axillary temperature. A probe is placed in the ear to assess a tympanic temperature. Single-use thermometers are placed over the skin, usually the forehead. Temporal artery thermometers are swiped over the skin covering the temporal artery. For most clinical purposes, it is satisfactory to assess a tympanic, an oral, a rectal, or an axillary temperature, provided proper technique is used, the site of the temperature is documented, and normal variations among the methods are considered. Comparing the recordings using two different sites is a method for double-checking the validity of an unusual measurement. The procedures for assessing body temperature at each site, with rationale for each step, are outlined in Skill 24-1.

ASSESSING A TYMPANIC MEMBRANE TEMPERATURE

The tympanic membrane temperature is considered a core body temperature. Infrared sensors in the thermometer sense heat from the body given off by the tympanic membrane. The thermometer does not touch the tympanic membrane. This site allows easy and safe measurement of temperature and is readily accessible. However, it should not be used for patients who have drainage from the ear or scars on the tympanic membrane. Temperature readings are not significantly altered by the presence of cerumen (earwax) or otitis media (infection of the middle ear).

ASSESSING AN ORAL TEMPERATURE

When selecting the oral site, the patient must be able to close his or her mouth around the probe. If a patient has had either hot or cold food or fluids or has been smoking or chewing gum, the general recommendation is to wait 15 to 30 minutes to allow the oral tissues to return to normal temperature. Oral temperatures should not be taken in people with diseases of the oral cavity and in those who have had surgery of the nose or mouth. In addition, oral temperatures should not be assessed in patients receiving oxygen by mask, because the time it takes to assess a reading is likely to result in a serious drop in the patient's blood oxygen level.

ASSESSING A RECTAL TEMPERATURE

The rectal temperature, a core temperature, is considered to be one of the most accurate routes. However, many patients are embarrassed at having their temperature taken rectally. The rectal site is an alternative when the oral site should not be used. The rectal site should not be used in newborns, children with diarrhea, and in patients who have undergone rectal surgery or have a disease of the rectum. Because the insertion of the thermometer into the rectum can slow the heart rate by stimulating the vagus nerve, assessing a rectal temperature for patients with heart disease or after cardiac surgery may not be allowed in some institutions. In addition, assessing a rectal temperature is contraindicated in clients who are neutropenic (have low white blood cell counts, such as in leukemia) and in clients who have certain neurologic disorders (e.g., spinal cord injuries).

ASSESSING AN AXILLARY TEMPERATURE

The axillary site may be used when both oral and rectal sites are contraindicated or when these sites are inaccessible. An axillary temperature is often assessed in healthy newborns to avoid the risk for perforating the wall of the rectum with the thermometer. Most authorities believe that when proper procedure is used, axillary temperatures are as accurate as oral or rectal temperatures.

Nursing Diagnoses

Examples of NANDA nursing diagnoses for alterations in body temperature are listed in the accompanying box.

Examples of NANDA Nursing Diagnoses
Altered Body Temperature

Nursing Diagnoses	Related Factors
Hyperthermia	Streptococcal upper respiratory infection Exposure to environmental heat without adequate cooling Surgery with general anesthesia
Hypothermia	Exposure to below freezing environmental temperature without adequate clothing
Risk for Imbalanced Body Temperature	Age (92 years) and head injury causing loss of consciousness
Ineffective Thermoregulation	Premature infant delivered at 30 weeks gestation

PULSE

The peripheral **pulse** is a throbbing sensation that can be palpated over a peripheral artery, such as the radial artery or the carotid artery. The peripheral pulses may be felt wherever an artery passes over a solid structure, such as bone or cartilage. An apical pulse may also be auscultated (listened to) over the apex of the heart as the heart beats.

Peripheral pulses are palpable when blood is ejected as the left ventricle contracts and pumps blood into the vascular system. As the heart contracts to eject blood into an already full aorta, smooth muscle in the arteries expands to compensate for the increase in pressure of the blood. This rhythmic distention of the arterial walls is the result of surges of blood as the heart beats. The distention of the arteries moves along the arterial system until it reaches the capillaries, where vessel walls lack elasticity and peripheral resistance to blood flow.

Characteristics of the pulse, including rate, quality (strong or weak), rhythm, and volume of blood ejected with each heartbeat (also referred to as stroke volume), are indicators of the effectiveness of the heart as a pump and the adequacy of peripheral blood flow. The heart rate affects the amount of blood ejected by the heart with each beat by determining the frequency with which the ventricle contracts. The quality and rhythm affect how much blood is ejected and if the beat is regular in rhythm. Further information about the control and mechanisms involved with blood flow and stroke volume is provided later with the discussion of blood pressure.

Physiology of the Pulse

The quantity of blood forced out of the left ventricle with each contraction is called the stroke volume (SV). The cardiac output (CO) is the amount of blood pumped per minute, and averages from 3.5 L/min to 8.0 L/min in a healthy adult (Porth & Matfin, 2009). This volume is determined by using the following formula: Cardiac Output = Stroke Volume × Heart Rate. Thus, the cardiac output of an adult with a stroke volume of 70 mL and a heart rate of 70 beats/min is 4.9 L/min. Cardiac output

increases during physical activity and decreases during sleep; it also varies depending on body size and metabolic needs.

The pulse is regulated by the autonomic nervous system through the sinoatrial (SA) node (the pacemaker) of the heart. Parasympathetic stimulation of the SA node via the vagus nerve decreases the heart rate, and sympathetic stimulation of the SA node increases the heart rate and force of contraction. The pulse rate is the number of pulsations felt over a peripheral artery or heard over the apex of the heart in 1 minute. This rate normally corresponds to the same rate at which the heart is beating.

Factors Affecting the Pulse

Many factors can affect both the heart rate and volume; however, compensatory mechanisms attempt to maintain a sufficient supply of blood to the cells at all times. For example, when the stroke volume decreases, such as when the blood volume is decreased because of hemorrhage, the heart rate increases to try to maintain the same cardiac output. Conversely, in a physically fit athlete whose heart pumps a maximum volume of blood per stroke, the heart rate may be at the low range or below the range of normal, yet the body cells remain adequately supplied.

Normal Pulse Rate

The normal pulse rate for adolescents and adults ranges from 60 to 100 beats/min. The pulse rate increases and decreases in response to a variety of physiologic mechanisms. It also might be altered by activity, medications, emotions, pain, heat and cold, and disease processes. Normal pulse rates change across the life span, gradually diminishing from birth to adulthood (see Table 24-1).

Increased Pulse Rate

As the heart rate increases, cardiac output usually also increases. However, a rapid rate (**tachycardia**) decreases cardiac filling time, which, in turn, decreases stroke volume

Box 24-3	FACTORS CONTRIBUTING TO TACHYCARDIA

- A decrease in blood pressure, such as occurs with blood loss, when the heart's compensatory mechanisms attempt to meet the need for increased cardiac output
- An elevated temperature, which usually causes an increase of about 7 to 10 beats/min for each 0.6°C (1°F) of elevation above normal
- Any condition resulting in poor oxygenation of blood, for example, chronic pulmonary disease or anemia
- Exercise, when the heart's compensatory ability attempts to meet the need for increased blood circulation
- Prolonged application of heat
- Pain
- Strong emotions, such as fear, anger, anxiety, and surprise
- Some medications (e.g., epinephrine [Adrenalin])

and cardiac output. An adult has tachycardia when the pulse rate is 100 to 180 beats/min. Box 24-3 lists the factors contributing to tachycardia.

Decreased Pulse Rate

Bradycardia is a pulse rate below 60 beats/min in an adult. The pulse rate is normally slower during sleep, in men, and in people who are thin. It slows during hypothermia as metabolic processes decrease. With aging, the pulse tends to become slower. Some medications specific to the work of the heart slow the heart rate while also strengthening the force of contraction to increase cardiac output.

Sinus bradycardia results when the SA node generates a slower-than-normal impulse rate. This type of bradycardia occurs at times when metabolic needs are decreased (e.g., during sleep, in hypothermia, in trained athletes at rest); from certain medications, such as beta blockers; from vagal stimulation (e.g., from bearing down to have a bowel movement), during suctioning of respiratory secretions, with severe pain, and in increased intracranial pressure and myocardial infarction. The nurse should immediately report bradycardia associated with difficult breathing, changes in level of consciousness, decreased blood pressure, ECG changes, and angina (heart pain). Emergency treatment consists of administering atropine intravenously to block vagal stimulation and to restore normal heart rate.

Pulse Amplitude and Quality

The pulse amplitude describes the quality of the pulse in terms of its fullness and reflects the strength of left ventricular contraction. It is assessed by the feel of the blood flow through the vessel. The amplitude of each pulse beat is normally strong at all areas where an artery can be palpated. Table 24-5 presents a scale often used to describe and document pulse amplitude.

In addition, the peripheral pulse may be described and documented as full and bounding when it is forceful, or weak and thready when it is feeble.

TABLE • 24-5	PULSE AMPLITUDE	
Number	**Definition**	**Description**
0	Absent pulse	No pulsation is felt despite extreme pressure.
1+	Thready pulse	Pulsation is not easily felt, and slight pressure causes it to disappear.
2+	Weak pulse	Stronger than a thready pulse; light pressure causes it to disappear.
3+	Normal pulse	Pulsation is easily felt, takes moderate pressure to cause it to disappear.
4+	Bounding pulse	The pulsation is strong and does not disappear with moderate pressure.

Pulse Rhythm

The pulse rhythm is the pattern of the pulsations and the pauses between them. This pattern is normally regular. An irregular pattern of heartbeats is called a **dysrhythmia.** Any irregularity in the heartbeat must be reported immediately. Common pulse rhythms are described and illustrated in Box 24-4.

Box 24-4	PULSE RHYTHMS

Regular Rhythms
The pulse rhythms and the pauses occur similarly.

Description	Pattern
Normal	
Weak	
Bounding	

Dysrhythmias
The pulsations or lengths of pauses occur with no pattern or predictability.

Description	Pattern
Bisferiens	
Pulsus alternans	
Bigeminal	

Premature contractions

Assessing the Pulse

The pulse may be assessed by palpating peripheral arteries or by auscultating the apical pulse with a stethoscope. The nurse needs to know how to use a stethoscope and which site and method are appropriate.

➤ *Remember Tomas Esposito, the middle-aged man requiring infection-control measures and assessment? Although the nurse had difficulty auscultating his heart and lung sounds, the nurse would need to assess both his radial and apical pulse. It is possible that by palpating his radial pulse and then attempting to auscultate his apical pulse and not hearing anything, the nurse might have a clue leading her to suspect that the stethoscope was not functioning properly.* ■

Equipment

The nurse most often assesses the pulse by using his or her fingers to palpate (feel) the radial artery. However, various types of equipment may be used to assess the pulse. For example, the stethoscope is used to auscultate the apical pulse, although a cardiac monitor may be used to assess the apical pulse in critical care or emergency department care. The monitor produces a graph or digital reading of the pulse rate and amplitude.

STETHOSCOPE

The acoustical stethoscope, the most common type used, has an amplifying mechanism connected to earpieces by tubing (Fig. 24-3).

The most common amplifying mechanisms of a stethoscope are the *diaphragm*, which is a large, flat disk, and the *bell*, which has a hollowed, upright, curved appearance. The diaphragm is more useful for hearing high-frequency sounds, such as respiratory sounds, because it screens out low-frequency sounds. The bell screens out high-frequency sounds and is more useful for hearing low-frequency sounds, such as those commonly made by the heart and the blood within the vessels.

The earpieces of the stethoscope should be selected to fit one's ear canals comfortably and snugly for the most effective

---

Guidelines for Nursing Care • 24-2

ASSESSING PERIPHERAL PULSE USING A PORTABLE DOPPLER ULTRASOUND DEVICE

- Determine the need to use a Doppler ultrasound device for pulse assessment.
- Bring necessary equipment to the bedside stand or overbed table.
- Perform hand hygiene and put on personal protective equipment (PPE), if indicated.
- Identify the patient.
- Explain the procedure to the patient.
- Put on gloves as appropriate. (Gloves are not usually worn to obtain a pulse measurement unless contact with blood or body fluids is anticipated.)
- Select the appropriate peripheral site based on assessment data.
- Move the patient's clothing to expose only the site chosen.
- Remove Doppler from charger and turn it on. Make sure that volume is set at low.
- Apply conducting gel to the site where you are auscultating the pulse.
- Hold the Doppler base in your nondominant hand. With your dominant hand, place the Doppler probe tip in the gel. Adjust the volume as needed. Move the Doppler tip around until the pulse is heard (see Figure).
- Using a watch with a second hand, count the heartbeat for 1 minute.
- Remove the Doppler tip and turn the Doppler off. Wipe excess gel off of the patient's skin with a tissue.
- Place a small X over the spot where the pulse is located with an indelible pen, depending on facility policy. Marking the

site allows for easier future assessment. It can also make palpating the pulse easier since the exact location of the pulse is known.
- Cover the patient and help him or her to a position of comfort.
- Wipe any gel remaining on the Doppler probe off with a tissue. Clean the Doppler probe per facility policy or manufacturer's recommendations.
- Remove PPE, if used. Perform hand hygiene.
- Return the Doppler to the charge base.
- Record pulse rate, rhythm, and site, and the fact that it was obtained with a Doppler.

FIGURE 24-3. A stethoscope. The two sides of the stethoscope amplifier are used for different purposes: the diaphragm is more useful for hearing high-frequency sounds, and the bell is more useful for hearing low-frequency sounds.

auscultation. The tips should be directed into the ear canal, not against the ear itself. They should be large enough to block out extraneous noises in the environment when the stethoscope is being used.

DOPPLER ULTRASOUND STETHOSCOPE

A Doppler ultrasound stethoscope may be used to assess pulses that are difficult to palpate or auscultate. The device has an earpiece or headset connected to an audio unit with an ultrasound transducer. Techniques for assessing pulses with a Doppler ultrasound device are outlined in Guidelines for Nursing Care 24-2.

Sites and Methods of Assessing the Pulse

Nurses must know the correct site and method for assessing the pulse. Although peripheral pulses are most commonly assessed, an apical pulse or an apical-radial pulse should be assessed in certain situations, described below.

ASSESSING PERIPHERAL ARTERIAL PULSES

Many peripheral artery sites might be used to assess the pulse by palpation. Figure 24-4 illustrates the most commonly used sites. Of these sites, the radial pulse site is assessed most often in children and adults. Skill 24-2 describes the steps for assessing a peripheral pulse via palpation.

Circulation to the legs and feet is assessed at the femoral, popliteal, posterior tibial, or dorsalis pedis sites. The carotid pulse site is used during emergency assessments, such as for patients who are in shock or have had a cardiac arrest. When taking a carotid pulse, lightly palpate only one side to prevent any decrease in cerebrovascular circulation. The brachial pulse site is used most often for infants.

ASSESSING THE APICAL PULSE

If a peripheral pulse is difficult to assess accurately because it is irregular, weak, or very rapid, the apical rate should be assessed using a stethoscope. An apical pulse is also assessed when giving medications that alter heart rate and rhythm. The contraction of the heart can be heard in the space between the fifth and the sixth ribs, about 8 cm (3 inches) to the left of the median line and slightly below the nipple

(Guidelines for Nursing Care 24-3). The apical rate of an infant can also be easily palpated with the fingertips as well as being auscultated.

ASSESSING THE APICAL-RADIAL PULSE

When the radial pulse is irregular, counting the pulse at the apex of the heart and at the radial artery simultaneously is used to assess the apical-radial pulse rate. Guidelines for Nursing Care 24-4 outlines the techniques for taking an apical-radial pulse.

A difference between the apical and radial pulse rates is called the **pulse deficit** and indicates that all of the heartbeats are not reaching the peripheral arteries or are too weak to be palpated.

Nursing Diagnoses

Examples of NANDA nursing diagnoses for alterations in the pulse are listed in the accompanying box.

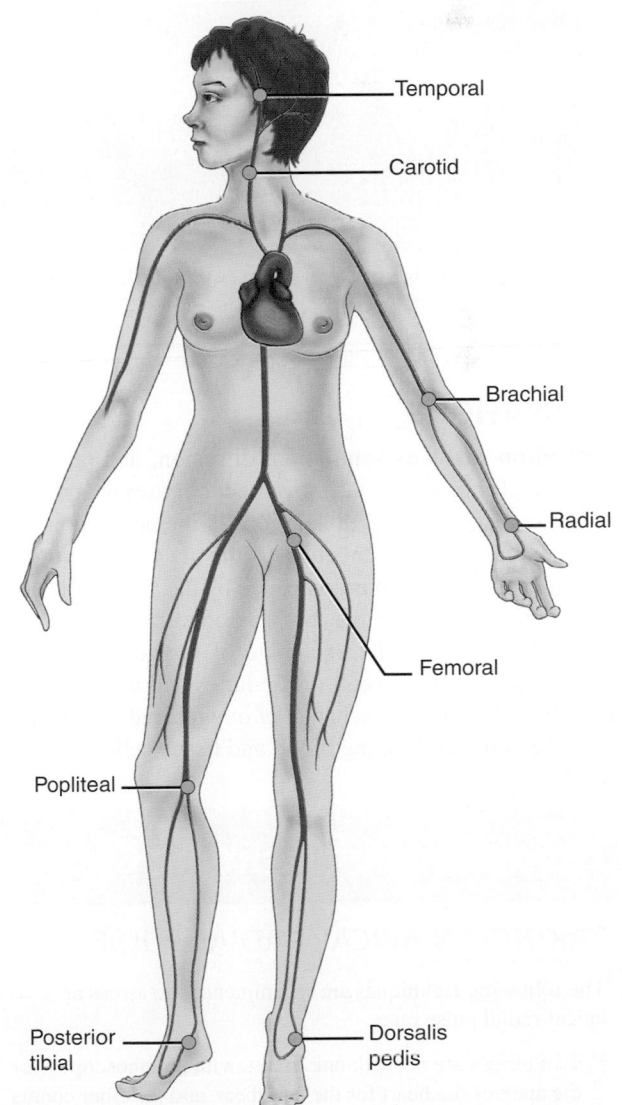

FIGURE 24-4. These arteries are located near the surface of the body. The pulse can be detected in any of these sites by light palpation.

Guidelines for Nursing Care • 24-3

ASSESSING THE APICAL PULSE

- Perform hand hygiene. Put on gloves as appropriate.
- Use alcohol swab to clean the diaphragm of the stethoscope. Use another swab to clean the earpieces if necessary.
- Assist patient to a sitting or reclining position and expose chest area; move the patient's clothing to expose only the apical site.
- Hold the stethoscope diaphragm against the palm of your hand for a few seconds (to warm it).

- Palpate the space between the fifth and sixth ribs (fifth intercostal space), and move to the left midclavicular line. Place the diaphragm over the apex of the heart (see Figure).
- Listen for heart sounds ("lub-dub"). Each "lub-dub" counts as one beat.
- Using a watch with a second hand, count the heartbeat for 1 minute.
- Cover the patient and help him or her to a position of comfort.
- Clean diaphragm of the stethoscope with an alcohol swab.
- Remove gloves, if necessary. Perform hand hygiene.

The apical pulse is usually found at (**A**) the fifth intercostal space just inside the midclavicular line and can be heard (**B**) over the apex of the heart.

RESPIRATIONS

Respiration involves ventilation, diffusion, and perfusion. Ventilation (or breathing) is movement of gases in and out of the lungs; inspiration (or inhalation) is the act of breathing in, and expiration (or exhalation) is the act of breathing out. Unlike heart rate, which is controlled by the autonomic nervous system, ventilation has both autonomic and voluntary control. Diffusion is the exchange of oxygen and carbon dioxide between the alveoli of the lungs and the circulating blood. Perfusion is the exchange of oxygen and carbon dioxide between the circulating blood and tissue cells.

Although nurses assess the manifestations of changes in all of these respiratory events, the component that is measured as a vital sign is ventilation, more commonly called respirations. Respiratory system assessment is described further in Chapter 25.

Physiology of Respirations

The rate and depth of breathing can change in response to tissue demands. These changes are brought about by the inhibition or stimulation of the respiratory muscles by the respiratory centers in the medulla and pons. Activation of

Guidelines for Nursing Care • 24-4

TAKING AN APICAL-RADIAL PULSE

The following techniques are recommended to assess an apical-radial pulse rate:

- Two nurses are needed; one listens with a stethoscope over the apex of the heart for the heartbeat, and the other counts the rate at the radial artery.
- The patient's chest wall is exposed so that the stethoscope can be placed directly on the skin of the chest wall.

- One watch with a sweep second hand is placed, so that both nurses can read it simultaneously.
- The nurses determine where they can best hear and feel the pulse and decide on a time to start counting, such as when the second hand on the watch is at a specified place (such as the number 12).
- Both nurses count for 1 full minute and record their counts.

Examples of NANDA Nursing Diagnoses

Altered Pulse

Nursing Diagnoses	Related Factors
Decreased Cardiac Output	History of congestive heart failure and dysrhythmias
	Traumatic injury with extensive blood loss
Ineffective Peripheral Tissue Perfusion	History of peripheral vascular disease with decreased popliteal pulses
Deficient Fluid Volume	Exposure to high environmental temperature, increased age, and tachycardia
Acute Pain	First postoperative day following major surgery, crying, and tachycardia

the respiratory centers occurs via impulses from chemoreceptors located in the aortic arch and carotid arteries, via stretch and irritant receptors in the lungs, and via receptors in muscles and joints. An increase in carbon dioxide is the most powerful respiratory stimulant, causing an increase in respiratory depth and rate. The cerebral cortex of the brain allows voluntary control of breathing, such as when singing or playing a musical instrument. See Chapter 39 for a further discussion of respiratory physiology.

The rate and depth of inhalation and exhalation are normally smooth, effortless, and without conscious effort. However, factors ranging from environmental changes to pathophysiologic alterations in various body systems may result in increases or decreases in respiratory rate and depth.

Factors Affecting Respirations

Many different factors affect respiratory rate and depth. These factors include exercise; respiratory and cardiovascular disease; alterations in fluid, electrolyte, and acid–base balances; medications; trauma; infection; pain; and emotions. Box 24-5 outlines the factors that affect respiratory rate, depth, and movements.

Normal Respiratory Rate

Under normal conditions, healthy adults breathe about 12 to 20 times each minute; infants and young children breathe more rapidly (see Table 24-1). Normal respiration is called **eupnea.** The relationship of one respiration to four heartbeats is fairly consistent in healthy people.

> ➤ *Think back to Noah Shoolin, the 2-year-old brought to the emergency department. The nurse would anticipate that the child's respiratory rate would be increased most likely as a result of his screaming and emotional upset.* ■

Increased Respiratory Rate

Tachypnea, an increased respiratory rate, may occur in response to an increased metabolic rate when a person has a

fever. Cells require more oxygen at this time and produce more carbon dioxide that must be removed. The rate increases as much as 4 breaths/min with every 0.6°C (1°F) that the temperature rises above normal. Any condition causing an

Box 24-5 FACTORS AFFECTING RESPIRATORY RATE, DEPTH, AND MOVEMENTS

- **Age:** The respiratory rate decreases with age, ranging from a normal range of 30–60 breaths/min in a newborn to 12–20 breaths/min in an adult.
- **Gender:** In males, respiratory movements are primarily diaphragmatic, whereas in women, there is greater intercostal muscle movement.
- **Exercise:** Exercise increases respiratory rate and depth.
- **Acid–base balance:** Alterations in acid–base balance (especially acidosis) commonly result in increased rate and depth of respirations (hyperventilation).
- **Brain lesions:** Lesions of the brain (such as hemorrhage or tumors) or brainstem can cause a change in both the depth and rate of respirations, most commonly manifested as Cheyne-Stokes respirations.
- **Increased altitude:** As an adaptation to higher altitudes, healthy people may exhibit Cheyne-Stokes respirations, especially when asleep. Higher altitudes also increase respiratory rate and depth prior to adaptation by increasing hemoglobin levels.
- **Respiratory diseases:** Any alterations in the normal respiratory structures may result in changes in respiratory rate, depth, and patterns, most often manifested as difficult breathing, using accessory muscles of respiration (such as the intercostal muscles), and increased rate. The depth may be shallower. Smoking can alter the pulmonary airways, resulting in an increase in respiratory rate at rest.
- **Anemia:** Anemia, a decrease in oxygen-carrying hemoglobin, may result in an increased rate of respirations.
- **Anxiety:** Anxiety can cause sighing type respirations (increased depth) and increased rate.
- **Medications:** Medications, such as narcotics, sedatives, and general anesthetics slow respiratory rate and depth. Other drugs, including amphetamines and cocaine, may increase rate and depth.
- **Acute pain:** Acute pain increases respiratory rate but may decrease respiratory depth.

increase in carbon dioxide and a decrease in oxygen in the blood, for example, respiratory diseases such as acute pneumonia or chronic obstructive respiratory disease, also tends to increase the rate and depth of respirations.

Decreased Respiratory Rate

Bradypnea, a decrease in respiratory rate, occurs in some pathologic conditions. An increase in intracranial pressure depresses the respiratory center, resulting in irregular or shallow breathing, slow breathing, or both. Certain drugs, such as narcotics (e.g., morphine, meperidine [Demerol]), depress the respiratory rate.

Respiratory Depth and Rhythm

The depth of respirations normally varies from shallow to deep. The depth of each respiration is about the same when resting or sleeping. Periodically, each person automatically inhales deeply (sighs), filling the lungs with more air than with the usual depth of respiration.

Certain terms are used to describe the nature and depth of respirations. **Apnea** refers to periods during which there is no breathing. If apnea lasts longer than 4 to 6 minutes, brain damage and death might occur. **Dyspnea** is difficult or labored breathing. A dyspneic patient usually has rapid, shallow respirations and appears anxious. Dyspneic people can often breathe more easily in an upright position, a condition known as **orthopnea.** While sitting or standing, gravity lowers organs in the abdominal cavity away from the diaphragm. This gives the lungs more room for expansion within the chest, allowing the intake of more air with each breath. Table 24-6 describes and illustrates various respiratory patterns.

Assessing Respirations

The nurse assesses respiratory rate (breaths per minute), depth (deep or shallow), and rhythm (regular or irregular) by inspection (observing and listening) or by listening with the stethoscope. Other methods of assessing respiratory effectiveness include monitoring arterial blood gas results and using a pulse oximeter to determine oxygenation of blood. A description of a pulse oximeter and a procedure for using it are found in Chapter 39. Skill 24-3 describes how to assess the respiratory rate. Further assessments of respirations are described in Chapter 25.

Nursing Diagnoses

Examples of NANDA nursing diagnoses for alterations in respirations are listed in the accompanying box.

BLOOD PRESSURE

Blood pressure refers to the force of the moving blood against arterial walls. Maximum blood pressure is exerted on the walls of arteries when the left ventricle of the heart contracts and pushes blood through the aortic valve into the aorta at the beginning of systole. The pressure rises as the ventricle contracts (systole) and falls as the heart relaxes (diastole). This continuous contraction and relaxation of the left ventricle creates a pressure wave that is transmitted through the arterial system (Porth, 2007). The highest pressure is the **systolic pressure.** When the heart rests between beats during diastole, the pressure drops. The lowest pressure present on arterial walls at this time is the **diastolic pressure.** The difference between the systolic and diastolic pressures is called the **pulse pressure.**

TABLE • 24-6	PATTERNS OF RESPIRATIONS		
	Description	**Pattern**	**Associated Features**
Normal	12–20 breaths/min Regular		Normal pattern
Tachypnea	>24 breaths/min Shallow		Fever, anxiety, exercise, respiratory disorders
Bradypnea	<10 breaths/min Regular		Depression of the respiratory center by medications, brain damage
Hyperventilation	Increased rate and depth		Extreme exercise, fear, diabetic ketoacidosis (Kussmaul's respirations), overdose of aspirin
Hypoventilation	Decreased rate and depth; irregular		Overdose of narcotics or anesthetics
Cheyne-Stokes respirations	Alternating periods of deep, rapid breathing followed by periods of apnea; regular		Drug overdose, heart failure, increased intracranial pressure, renal failure
Biot's respirations	Varying depth and rate of breathing, followed by periods of apnea; irregular		Meningitis, severe brain damage

Examples of NANDA Nursing Diagnoses	
Altered Respirations	
Nursing Diagnoses	**Related Factors**
Ineffective Breathing Pattern	Anxiety about diagnostic procedure for possible malignancy
	Increased intracranial pressure following head injury
	Infant delivered by cesarean delivery at 28 weeks gestation
Impaired Gas Exchange	Presence of acute respiratory distress following smoke inhalation
Risk for Activity Intolerance	History of smoking two packs of cigarettes a day for 20 years

Both systolic and diastolic pressure are determined by the cardiac output (discussed earlier with the pulse) and the peripheral resistance. Cardiac output is determined by the stroke volume and the heart rate. Peripheral resistance reflects the viscosity (thickness of the blood) and the changes in the radius of the arterioles.

Blood pressure is measured in millimeters of mercury (mm Hg) and is recorded as a fraction. The numerator is the systolic pressure; the denominator is the diastolic pressure. For example, if the blood pressure is 120/80 mm Hg, 120 represents the systolic pressure, and 80 represents the diastolic pressure. The pulse pressure, in this case, is 40 mm Hg.

Physiology of Blood Pressure

Arterial walls contain elastic tissue that allows them to stretch and distend (called compliance) as blood enters with each ventricular contraction. When the heart rests between each beat, the walls of the arteries return to their original position, although pressure in them does not drop to zero. The arterioles offer resistance to the pressure of the blood and keeps the blood entering the capillaries in a continuous flow rather than in spurts. Therefore, the elasticity of the arterial walls, in addition to the resistance of the arterioles, helps to maintain normal blood pressure. With increased age, the walls of arterioles become less elastic, which interferes with their ability to stretch and dilate. This can subsequently limit adequate blood flow and contribute to rising pressure within the vascular system.

Although blood moves through the circulatory system from areas of higher pressure to areas of lower pressure, blood pressure is controlled by various short-term and long-term mechanisms. These mechanisms regulate the blood pressure so that blood flow (and pressure) remains relatively constant.

Short-Term Regulation of Blood Pressure

The mechanisms for short-term blood pressure regulation (occurring over minutes or hours) are primarily neural (nerve) and humoral (pertaining to body fluids). These mechanisms correct temporary changes in pressure that occur during activities such as changing position or exercising, and are also responsible for maintaining blood pressure during life-threatening situations. In addition, increased cardiac output (from a stronger contraction and increased stroke volume) results in an increased blood pressure while a weak contraction of the heart with decreased cardiac output causes a decrease in blood pressure.

The neural centers for blood pressure regulation are located in lower pons and medulla in an area called the cardiovascular center. The cardiovascular center transmits parasympathetic impulses to the heart via the vagus nerve and sympathetic impulses to the heart and blood vessels via the spinal cord and peripheral sympathetic nerves. Stimulating the vagus nerve slows the heart rate; sympathetic stimulation increases the heart rate.

Pressure-sensitive receptors, called baroreceptors, are located in the heart and walls of arteries (such as the aortic arch and carotid). They are stimulated by changes in stretch of the blood vessel as blood pressure changes and send impulses to the cardiovascular center to initiate the appropriate changes in heart rate and vascular smooth muscle. For example, blood pressure normally decreases when rising from a lying to an upright position, resulting in decreased stretch of baroreceptors. In response, heart rate and peripheral vascular resistance increase in turn to increase blood pressure. During life-threatening situations, such as a serious hemorrhage, the same mechanisms are activated.

Many different humoral mechanisms along with hormones also help regulate blood pressure. Epinephrine, a sympathetic neurotransmitter, is released by the adrenal gland to increase heart rate and contractility, thereby increasing cardiac output. The renin-angiotensin-aldosterone system, through angiotensinogen II, causes vasoconstriction in the arterioles, which leads to increased peripheral vascular resistance as a short-term mechanism, and also increases sodium and water retention by the kidneys to increase circulatory fluid volume and thus increase blood pressure as a long-term mechanism (see discussion in next section). Vasopressin (antidiuretic hormone [ADH]) is released from the posterior pituitary when stimulated by decreased blood volume and blood pressure, or by an increased osmolality of body fluids. It has a direct vasoconstricting effect on blood vessels, increasing peripheral resistance.

Long-term Regulation of Blood Pressure

Long-term mechanisms are responsible for the on-going regulation of blood pressure. These mechanisms regulate extracellular fluid volume through the kidneys. They function by regulating blood pressure for an individual person's equilibrium point. Arterial pressure rises when the body contains too much extracellular fluid. In response, increased amounts of sodium and fluid are excreted by the kidneys to return the blood pressure to the individual's equilibrium point. When blood pressure decreases due to decreased extracellular fluid, the opposite effect occurs. Extracellular fluid volume regulates blood pressure directly by increasing cardiac output and renal blood flow and indirectly by autoregulation of blood flow, in which autoregulatory mechanisms redirect blood flow to various blood tissues.

Factors Affecting Blood Pressure

Because of the many factors that influence blood pressure, a single blood pressure measurement is not necessarily significant. Box 24-6 lists factors that commonly cause variations in blood pressure.

Normal Blood Pressure

Studies of healthy people indicate that blood pressure can be within a wide range and still be normal. Because of individual differences, it is important to know the normal blood pressure of a particular person. A rise or fall of 20 to 30 mm Hg

Box 24-6 FACTORS CONTRIBUTING TO BLOOD PRESSURE VARIATIONS IN HEALTHY PEOPLE

- **Age:** The older adult has decreased elasticity of the arteries, which increases peripheral resistance and, therefore, increases blood pressure.
- **Circadian rhythm:** Normal fluctuations occur during the day. The blood pressure is usually lowest on arising in the morning. The blood pressure has been noted to rise as much as 5 to 10 mm Hg by late afternoon, and it gradually falls again during sleep.
- **Gender:** Women usually have lower blood pressure than men of the same age until menopause.
- **Food intake:** Blood pressure increases after eating food.
- **Exercise:** Systolic blood pressure rises during periods of exercise and strenuous activity.
- **Weight:** Blood pressure is usually higher in people who are obese than in those who are thin.
- **Emotional state:** Emotions, such as anger, fear, excitement, and pain, generally cause the blood pressure to rise, but the pressure falls to normal when the situation passes.
- **Body position:** Blood pressure tends to be lower in a prone or supine position than when sitting or standing.
- **Race:** Race is a factor in increased blood pressure (hypertension), which is more prevalent and more severe in African American men and women.
- **Drugs/Medications:** Oral contraceptives cause a mild increase in blood pressure in many women.

TABLE · 24-7 CATEGORIES FOR BLOOD PRESSURE LEVELS IN ADULTS (AGES 18 AND OLDER)

Category	Blood Pressure Level (mm Hg)		
	Systolic		Diastolic
Normal*	<120	and	<80
Prehypertension	120–139	or	80–89
High Blood Pressure			
Stage 1	140–159	or	90–99
Stage 2	≥160	or	≥100

*In regard to risk of heart disease, optimal is defined as less than 120/80 mm Hg.
Source: Heart, Lung, and Blood Institute, National Institutes of Health. (2008). What is high blood pressure? Available at http://www.nhlbi.nih.gov/health/dci/Diseases/Hbp/HBP_WhatIs.html.

in a person's blood pressure is significant, even if it is within the generally accepted normal range. Although blood pressure varies constantly, sustained long-term changes are not considered normal. Table 24-7 lists the categories for blood pressure levels in adults.

The American Heart Association recommends that blood pressure readings be averaged on two or more subsequent occasions before determining if the blood pressure is outside acceptable parameters. Measurements should be taken after the patient rests for at least 5 minutes and has not consumed caffeine or smoked for 30 minutes before the measurement.

Increased Blood Pressure

Hypertension, one of the most common health problems, is blood pressure that is above normal for a sustained period. A diagnosis of hypertension is made when the systolic pressure is 140 mm Hg or higher or the diastolic pressure is 90 mm Hg or higher. The American Heart Association (2008) estimates that 73,000,000 American adults have hypertension. Of this number, the prevalence of hypertension is greater in blacks, American Indians, and Alaska natives than in whites. Its prevalence is also greater in older adults. In addition, as the epidemic of obesity continues in all age groups, the prevalence of hypertension in children and adolescents appears to also be increasing (Schwenk, 2007). This trend can be expected to continue with the aging of the "baby boomers," as the number of people with hypertension increases with aging.

Hypertension is a major risk factor for heart disease and is the most important risk factor associated with stroke. It is often called "the silent killer" because there are few symptoms beyond the increased blood pressure. The National Heart, Lung, and Blood Institute has outlined standards for diagnosing hypertension (see Table 24-7).

The two major classifications of hypertension are primary hypertension and secondary hypertension. Primary hypertension (also called essential hypertension) has no known cause. It is characterized by an increase above normal in both the systolic and diastolic pressures. Secondary hypertension, which is much less common than primary hypertension, is caused by another disease condition. Some of the common causes of secondary hypertension are kidney disease, disorders of the adrenal cortex, and disorders of the aorta.

The basis for hypertension is thought to be dysfunction of the neurohormonal system. Overactivation of both angiotensin and aldosterone result in an increase in blood pressure. Over time, this sustained increase results in a permanent remodeling and thickening of the blood vessels. As a result, there is increased peripheral resistance and a back-up of pressure to organs affected by the vascular system, such as the brain, heart, and kidneys. Disorders resulting from hypertension include thickening of the myocardium, enlargement of the ventricles, congestive heart failure, myocardial infarctions, stroke, and kidney damage.

There are many risk factors for the development of hypertension. Significant risks are a family history of hypertension, race, aging, and metabolic disorders such as type 2 diabetes mellitus, obesity, and high cholesterol. Lifestyle risk factors include a sedentary lifestyle; high dietary intake of salt, fats, and calories; use of oral contraceptives in women; and sleep apnea. Other high-risk factors include cigarette smoking and regular alcohol consumption.

➤ Remember Mrs. Renfrow, the wife of a man who is overweight and diagnosed with hypertension? The nurse would need to incorporate information about various risk factors for developing hypertension as well as information about risk related to hypertension in the teaching plan for Mrs. Renfrow. ∎

Hypertension can be controlled by medications and lifestyle changes. The categories of antihypertensive medications include diuretics (to decrease fluid volume), beta-adrenergic blockers (to block sympathetic stimulation and decrease cardiac output), vasodilators and calcium channel blockers (to relax smooth muscles of arterioles and decrease peripheral vascular resistance), and ACE inhibitors (to prevent vasoconstriction by angiotensin II and decrease circulatory fluid volume by reducing aldosterone production). Lifestyle changes include following a low-calorie, low-fat diet; losing excess weight and maintaining weight loss; limiting alcohol intake; eliminating smoking; reducing salt intake; and engaging in regular physical activity. Nurses can influence the health of the public through screenings, education, and referrals. See Promoting Health Literacy in Patients with Hypertension for more information.

Decreased Blood Pressure

Hypotension is below-normal blood pressure. A consistently low blood pressure (e.g., a systolic reading of 90–115 mm Hg) is normal in some adults, such as trained athletes. However, most cases of hypotension are the result of pathology. Pathologic hypotension might result from vasodilation

Promoting Health Literacy
IN PATIENTS WITH HYPERTENSION

Patient Scenario

Harry Miller, 66, went to his primary healthcare provider for his annual health assessment. He had gained 15 pounds in the past year. When the office nurse took his blood pressure, it was 166/92 mm Hg. The nurse took Mr. Miller's blood pressure again and then repeated it later after his health assessment was completed. Although the reading varied by a few points, it remained consistently high. Mr. Miller was obviously surprised at having hypertension because he said, "It has never been high before. There must be something wrong with your machine." His healthcare provider tried to discuss the need for changes in his lifestyle as well as the need to take the medication prescribed for his blood pressure, but Mr. Miller said he had no questions and rushed out of the examining room.

Nursing Considerations: *Tips for Improving Health Literacy*

Provide Mr. Miller with printed literature about high blood pressure, including causes and risks. Explain that it is important to control his high blood pressure to prevent serious risks, such as heart attack and stroke. Urge Mr. Miller and his wife to talk to a dietitian about a nutritious diet that would help him to lose weight; contains recommended servings of fiber, fruits, and vegetables; and contains less salt. Explain the action of the prescribed medication and the importance of taking the medication to reduce and control his blood pressure. Describe the importance of buying a home blood pressure monitor and keeping a record of his daily blood pressure. Encourage Mr. Miller to make an appointment to return to the office on a regular basis and to be prepared to ask his provider the following three questions:

- What is my main problem?
- What do I need to do?
- Why is it important for me to do this?

What additional measures can you take to help maintain health literacy in this patient and his wife? What other measures would be helpful for Mr. Miller if he did not speak English, could not read, or had other learning deficits?

Guidelines for Nursing Care • 24-5

ASSESSING ORTHOSTATIC HYPOTENSION

If orthostatic blood pressure measurements are ordered, use the following guidelines:

• Ask the patient to lie in a supine position for 3 to 10 minutes. At the end of this time, take initial blood pressure and pulse measurements.

• Assist the patient to sit on the side of the bed with legs dangling. After 1 to 3 minutes, take the blood pressure and pulse measurements.

• Assist the patient to stand (unless contraindicated). Wait 2 to 3 minutes and then take blood pressure and pulse measurements.

• Record the measurements for each position. An increase of 40 beats in the pulse rate or a decrease in blood pressure of 30 mm Hg is abnormal.

---

of the arterioles, failure of the heart to function as an effective pump, or loss of blood volume (such as with a hemorrhage). The nurse should immediately report assessments of hypotension, tachycardia, pallor, increased sweating, and confusion.

Orthostatic hypotension (postural hypotension) is a drop in systolic blood pressure of a number equal to or greater than 20 mm Hg or in diastolic blood pressure of a number equal to or greater than 10 mm Hg within 3 minutes of standing (Bickley, 2007). It is associated with weakness or fainting when one rises to an erect position (either supine to sitting, supine to standing, or sitting to standing) and is the result of peripheral vasodilation without a compensatory rise in cardiac output. Patients most at risk for postural hypotension are older adults, patients who have been on prolonged bed rest, and those who are dehydrated or have sustained a significant blood loss. Some drugs, such as meperidine hydrochloride (Demerol) cause hypotension.

Arising and moving about slowly, especially after a period of bed rest, might prevent orthostatic hypotension. When ambulating patients after surgery or prolonged bedrest, first raise the head of the bed, then assist the client to a sitting position on the side of bed (often called "dangling") for a few minutes to assess for dizziness or faintness, and then assist to a standing position. If the patient becomes dizzy or feels faint, return the patient to bed and place in a supine

position, which restores blood flow to the brain. Guidelines for Nursing Care 24-5 describes how to assess orthostatic hypotension.

Assessing Blood Pressure

To accurately assess blood pressure, the nurse must know the appropriate equipment to use, how to describe the sounds that are heard, and which site to choose.

Equipment

Blood pressure may be assessed with different types of devices. Most commonly, nurses assess blood pressure by using a stethoscope and sphygmomanometer. Blood pressure may also be estimated with a Doppler ultrasound stethoscope (described with the discussion of the pulse), estimated by palpation, and assessed with electronic or automated devices.

SPHYGMOMANOMETER

A sphygmomanometer is used to assess blood pressure. The sphygmomanometer consists of a cuff and the manometer (Fig. 24-5).

The cuff contains an airtight, flat rubber bladder covered with cloth. Selecting a cuff of the proper width (ranging from neonate to adult thigh) is essential to obtain an accurate

FIGURE 24-5. Parts of a sphygmomanometer. (**A**) Three cuff sizes: a small cuff for a child or a small or frail adult, a normal-sized cuff, and a large cuff, called a leg cuff, for measuring blood pressure on a leg, or for use on an obese adult. (**B**) An aneroid manometer.

TABLE • 24-8	RECOMMENDED BLOOD PRESSURE CUFF SIZES	
Cuff Size	**Cuff Measurements**	**Arm Circumference***
Newborn–premature infants	4 × 8 cm	
Infants	6 × 12 cm	
Older children	9 × 18 cm	
Small adult size	12 × 22 cm	22 to 26 cm
Adult size	16 × 30 cm	27 to 34 cm
Large adult size	16 × 36 cm	35 to 44 cm
Adult thigh size	16 × 42 cm	45 to 52 cm

*Select a blood pressure cuff that has a bladder width that is at least 40% of the arm circumference midway between the olecranon and the acromion.
From Pickering, T., Hall, J., Appel, L., et al. (2004). American Heart Association Scientific Statement. Recommendations for blood pressure measurement in humans and experimental animals. Part 1: Blood pressure measurement in humans: A statement for professionals from the subcommittee of professional and public education of the American Heart Association Council on High Blood Pressure Research. Available at http://hyper.ahajournals.org/cgi/content/full/45/1/142.

blood pressure reading. The width of the cuff should be about 40% of the circumference of the limb for which the measurement will be obtained. The bladder inside the cuff should enclose at least two thirds of the adult limb and all of a child's limb. If the cuff is too narrow, the reading could be erroneously high because the pressure is not evenly transmitted to the artery. This occurs, for example, when an average-sized cuff is used on an obese person.

▶ *Think back to Mrs. Renfrow, the wife of a patient with hypertension who is overweight. The nurse would need to caution Mrs. Renfrow to make sure that the device she uses to measure her husband's blood pressure is sized adequately. Otherwise, the readings may be erroneous, possibly leading to inappropriate management based on inaccurate readings or a false sense of security that the hypertension is being controlled.* ■

If a cuff is too wide (e.g., using an adult cuff on the arm of a child), the reading may be erroneously low because pressure is dispersed over a disproportionately large surface area. The American Heart Association recommends that the length of the cuff should be 80% of the arm circumference, and the width of the cuff should be 40% of the arm circumference. Recommendations by the American Health Association for the selection of an appropriately sized cuff are given in Table 24-8.

Depending on the product, cuffs may be disposable or reusable. They are closed around the limb with contact closures, such as nylon fabric that can be fastened to itself with Velcro or hooks. Some long cuffs are applied by encircling the arm several times. Two tubes are attached to the bladder within the cuff. One is connected to a manometer and the other is attached to a bulb used to inflate the bladder. The

bladder is inflated enough to obstruct the flow of blood through the artery. A needle valve on the bulb allows the cuff to be deflated while the pressure is being read.

AUTOMATED BLOOD PRESSURE MONITORS

Electronic blood pressure monitors sense pressure from blood flow within the artery wall, record the pressure readings, and display them in digital numbers (Fig. 24-6). They also may provide measurements of pulse rate, pulse oximetry, and/or temperature.

DOPPLER ULTRASOUND

The blood pressure may be taken with a Doppler ultrasound device, which amplifies sounds. This device is especially useful if the sounds are indistinct or are inaudible with a regular stethoscope. See Guidelines for Nursing Care 24-6 for assessment technique.

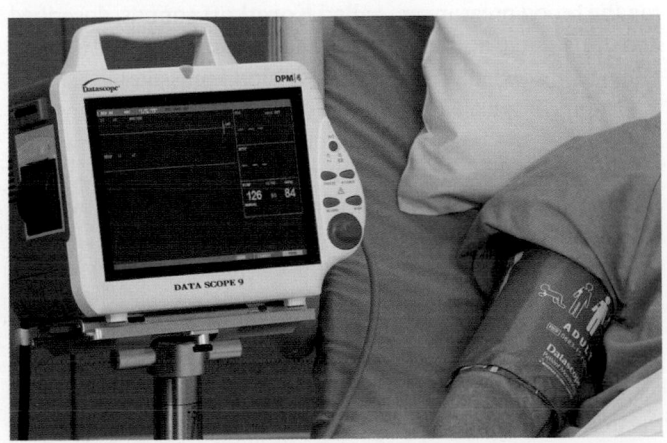

FIGURE 24-6. The automatic blood pressure monitor reports systolic, diastolic, and mean blood pressure. *(Photo by B. Proud)*

Guidelines for Nursing Care • 24-6

ASSESSING BLOOD PRESSURE USING A DOPPLER ULTRASOUND

- Determine the need to use a Doppler ultrasound device for blood pressure assessment.
- Perform hand hygiene and put on PPE, if indicated.
- Identify the patient.
- Explain the procedure to the patient.
- Select the appropriate limb for application of cuff.
- Have the patient assume a comfortable lying or sitting position with the appropriate limb exposed.
- Center the bladder of the cuff over the artery, lining the artery marker on the cuff up with the artery.
- Wrap the cuff around the limb smoothly and snugly, and fasten it. Do not allow any clothing to interfere with the proper placement of the cuff.
- Check that the needle on the aneroid gauge is within the zero mark. If using a mercury manometer, check to see that the manometer is in the vertical position and that the mercury is within the zero level with the gauge at eye level.
- Place a small amount of conducting gel over the artery.
- Hold the Doppler in your nondominant hand. Using your dominant hand, place the Doppler tip in the gel. Adjust the

- volume as needed. Move the Doppler tip around until you hear the pulse.
- Once the pulse is found using the Doppler, close the valve to the sphygmomanometer. Tighten the screw valve on the air pump.
- Inflate the cuff while continuing to use the Doppler on the artery. Note the point on the gauge where the pulse disappears.
- Open the valve on the manometer and allow air to escape quickly. Repeat any suspicious reading, but wait at least 1 minute between readings to allow normal circulation to return in the limb. Deflate the cuff completely between attempts to check the blood pressure.
- Remove the Doppler tip and turn the Doppler off. Wipe excess gel off of the patient's skin with tissue. Remove the cuff.
- Wipe any gel remaining on the Doppler probe off with a tissue. Clean the Doppler according to facility policy or manufacturer's recommendations.
- Return the Doppler to the charge base.
- Remove PPE, if used. Perform hand hygiene.
- Record the findings on paper, flow sheet, or computerized record. Identify arm used and site of assessment if other than brachial, and the fact that it was obtained with a Doppler.

DIRECT ELECTRONIC MEASUREMENT

It is possible to measure blood pressure directly through the insertion of a thin catheter into an artery (an arterial line). The tip of the catheter senses the pressure and transmits this information to a machine that displays the systolic and diastolic pressure in a waveform. This technique is used primarily in intensive care areas.

Korotkoff Sounds

The series of sounds for which the nurse listens when assessing the blood pressure are called **Korotkoff sounds,** described and illustrated in Table 24-9. These sounds are only heard when using a stethoscope to assess blood pressure.

In some adults, each of these sounds is distinct, whereas in others only the beginning and ending sounds are heard. It is important to determine institutional policy for recording blood pressure sounds and to be consistent in taking and documenting the readings.

The first sound heard through the stethoscope, which is the onset of phase I, represents the systolic pressure. It is recorded as the first number in the fraction—for example, if the blood pressure reading is 120/80 mm Hg, 120 is the systolic pressure. The second number, which represents the diastolic pressure (in this case, 80), notes the level at which either a change in or a cessation of the loud, distinct sounds took place. This occurs in either phase IV or phase V.

The blood pressure is most commonly recorded with two numbers written as a fraction, with the bottom number indicating either the change of the sound or the last sound heard. However, the American Heart Association recommends that in instances when both a change in the sounds and a cessation of the sounds are heard, all numbers should be recorded. In this case, the blood pressure would be recorded as 120/80/64. If the sounds were heard all the way down to zero, the blood pressure recording would be 120/80/0.

Sites and Methods of Assessing the Blood Pressure

Although various sites may be used to assess the blood pressure, the brachial artery and the popliteal artery are most commonly used.

ASSESSING A BRACHIAL ARTERY BLOOD PRESSURE

Skill 24-4 describes how to assess the blood pressure using the brachial artery. Table 24-10 describes the common causes associated with blood pressure assessment errors.

A brachial artery blood pressure assessment should not be taken on an arm with an intravenous line or with an arteriovenous fistula or shunt. Blood pressure assessment should also be avoided in the arm on the side of an axillary node

Phase	Description	Illustration
Phase I	Characterized by the first appearance of faint but clear tapping sounds that gradually increase in intensity; the first tapping sound is the systolic pressure	
Phase II	Characterized by muffled or swishing sounds; these sounds may temporarily disappear, especially in hypertensive people; the disappearance of the sound during the latter part of phase I and during phase II is called the *auscultatory gap* and may cover a range of as much as 40 mm Hg; failing to recognize this gap may cause serious errors of underestimating systolic pressure or overestimating diastolic pressure	
Phase III	Characterized by distinct, loud sounds as the blood flows relatively freely through an increasingly open artery	
Phase IV	Characterized by a distinct, abrupt, muffling sound with a soft, blowing quality; in adults, the onset of this phase is considered to be the first diastolic pressure	
Phase V	The last sound heard before a period of continuous silence; the pressure at which the last sound is heard is the second diastolic pressure	

TABLE • 24-9 KOROTKOFF SOUNDS

TABLE • 24-10 BLOOD PRESSURE ASSESSMENT ERRORS AND CONTRIBUTING CAUSES

Error	Contributing Causes
Falsely low assessments	• Hearing deficit • Noise in the environment • Viewing the meniscus from above eye level • Applying too wide a cuff • Inserting earpieces of stethoscope incorrectly • Using cracked or kinked tubing • Releasing the valve rapidly • Misplacing the bell beyond the direct area of the artery • Failing to pump the cuff 20 to 30 mm Hg above the disappearance of the pulse
Falsely high assessments	• Using a manometer not calibrated at the zero mark • Assessing the blood pressure immediately after exercise • Viewing the meniscus from below eye level • Applying a cuff that is too narrow • Releasing the valve too slowly • Reinflating the bladder during auscultation

Guidelines for Nursing Care • 24-7

ASSESSING BLOOD PRESSURE IN THE LEG

- Place the patient in the prone position, if possible. If that position is not possible, place the patient in the supine position with the knee slightly flexed.
- Use a cuff that is specifically made for this assessment, or one that is large enough to make an accurate assessment.
- Place the cuff 2.5 cm (1 inch) above the popliteal artery, with the bladder over the posterior of the midthigh (see Figure).
- Follow the same procedure for auscultation as for the brachial artery.

dissection or mastectomy because the pressure may increase the risk of lymphedema developing in the affected arm.

ASSESSING A POPLITEAL ARTERY BLOOD PRESSURE

When the patient's brachial artery is inaccessible, the nurse can assess the blood pressure using the popliteal artery in the leg. The systolic pressure is normally 10 to 40 mm Hg higher at this site, although the diastolic pressure is the same. The technique for assessment is outlined in Guidelines for Nursing Care 24-7.

PALPATING THE BLOOD PRESSURE

Assessing the blood pressure through palpation is sometimes referred to as the sensory detection method. It requires only the use of the sphygmomanometer. The cuff is inflated 30 mm Hg above the point at which the pulsation in the artery disappears. As the air in the cuff is released, the nurse feels for the return of the pulse. Usually, no diastolic pressure is recorded because the artery continues to pulsate as long as

blood flows through it. Some home patients assess their blood pressure this way. Instead of palpating the artery, however, the person notes the pressure on the manometer when experiencing the onset and disappearance of the throbbing sensation.

Nursing Diagnoses

Examples of NANDA nursing diagnoses for alterations in blood pressure are listed in the accompanying box.

TEACHING VITAL SIGNS FOR SELF-CARE AT HOME

Patients at home often need to check their own pulse or blood pressure. Guidelines for teaching self-assessment are presented in Teaching Tips 24-2.

Home blood pressure monitoring (HBPM) is being increasingly recommended (Pickering, Miller, Ogedegbe et al., 2008). Research has shown that readings at home are reliable, and are often lower than those taken in a healthcare

Examples of NANDA Nursing Diagnoses

Altered Blood Pressure

Nursing Diagnoses	Related Factors
Decreased Cardiac Output	Serious blood loss with hypovolemia Myocardial infarction with damage to cardiac pacemaker
Ineffective Health Maintenance	Lack of financial resources to seek medical care for hypertension
Readiness for Enhanced Self-Health Management	Blood pressure remains within normal limits for 6 months
Risk for Falls	History of falls, age (86 years), and presence of orthostatic hypotension

Tips   TEACHING TIPS · 24-2

SELF-CHECKING PULSE AND BLOOD PRESSURE

Health Topic	Teaching Tip	Why Is This Important?
Taking the Pulse	• The pulse is often taken before taking certain medications, such as those to make the heartbeat stronger. People who exercise and want to monitor the effect of the exercise on heart function also take their pulse. • It is necessary to be able to see a watch or a clock with a second hand when taking the pulse. • Place one arm on a firm surface so that the palm is upward. Using the middle three fingers of the other hand, gently feel the outside of the arm just below the wrist with the fingertips. Do not press hard. When pulsations are felt, watch the second hand of the watch or clock and begin to count when the second hand reaches 12 (any number is fine, but it is often easier to remember to always begin counting when the second hand is on 12). Count each pulsation (beat) for 1 minute (when the second hand again reaches 12), and write the number down.	If the pulse is very fast, very slow, or irregular, or if you have any concerns, contact your healthcare provider.
Taking the Blood Pressure	• The blood pressure is often taken to determine how well medications are working to control high blood pressure. The blood pressure is usually checked once a week. A record of blood pressure readings over time is more important than one reading. • The blood pressure can be measured at home with a blood pressure monitoring device or by using the mechanical devices found in many grocery or discount stores with a pharmacy. • If a home device is used, be sure the cuff is the proper size and that all parts of the device are working properly. The measurement should be taken while sitting comfortably, and the arm should be supported on a firm surface. Follow instructions that come with the home device.	If the blood pressure numbers increase or decrease by more than 10, or if you have any concerns, contact your healthcare provider. It is important to use the same device or machine each time and to write down the numbers.

provider setting. Recommended guidelines for HBPM follow:

• Advise patients to buy oscillometric BP monitors that measure BP on the upper arm with an appropriate cuff size.

• Explain that 2 to 3 readings should be taken while in a sitting position, both in the morning and at night. The readings should be recorded to show to the healthcare provider.

Skill · 24-1   Assessing Body Temperature

EQUIPMENT

• Digital, glass, or electronic thermometer, appropriate for site to be used
• Disposable probe covers
• Water-soluble lubricant for rectal temperature measurement

• Nonsterile gloves, if appropriate
• Additional personal protective equipment (PPE), as indicated

• Toilet tissue, if needed
• Pencil or pen, paper or flow sheet, computerized record

IMPLEMENTATION

ACTION

1. Check medical order or nursing care plan for frequency of measurement and route. More frequent temperature measurement may be appropriate based on nursing judgment.

   Bring necessary equipment to the bedside stand or overbed table.

RATIONALE

Assessment and measurement of vital signs at appropriate intervals provides important data about the patient's health status. Bringing everything to the bedside conserves time and energy. Arranging items nearby is convenient, saves time, and avoids unnecessary stretching and twisting of muscles on the part of the nurse.

Skill · 24-1 **Assessing Body Temperature** *continued*

ACTION	RATIONALE
2. Perform hand hygiene and put on PPE, if indicated.	Hand hygiene and PPE prevent the spread of microorganisms. PPE is required based on transmission precautions.
3. Identify the patient.	Identifying the patient ensures the right patient receives the intervention and helps prevent errors.
4. Close curtains around bed and close door to room if possible. Discuss procedure with patient and assess patient's ability to assist with the procedure.	This ensures the patient's privacy. Explanation relieves anxiety and facilitates cooperation. Dialogue encourages patient participation and allows for individualized nursing care.
5. Ensure the electronic or digital thermometer is in working condition.	Improperly functioning thermometer may not give an accurate reading.
6. Put on gloves if appropriate or indicated.	Gloves prevent contact with blood and body fluids. Gloves are usually not required for an oral, axillary, or tympanic temperature measurement, unless contact with blood or body fluids is anticipated. Gloves should be worn for rectal temperature measurement.
7. Select the appropriate site based on previous assessment data.	This ensures safety and accuracy of measurement.
8. Follow the steps as outlined below for the appropriate type of thermometer.	
9. When measurement is completed, remove gloves, if worn. Remove additional PPE, if used. Perform hand hygiene.	Removing PPE properly reduces the risk for infection transmission and contamination of other items. Hand hygiene prevents the spread of microorganisms.

Measuring a Tympanic Membrane Temperature

10. If necessary, push the "on" button and wait for the "ready" signal on the unit (Figure 1).	For proper function, thermometer must be turned on and warmed up.
11. Slide disposable cover onto the tympanic probe.	Use of a disposable cover deters the spread of microorganisms.
12. **Insert the probe snugly into the external ear using gentle but firm pressure, angling the thermometer toward the patient's jaw line (Figure 2). Pull pinna up and back to straighten the ear canal in an adult.**	If the probe is not inserted correctly, the patient's temperature may be noted as lower than normal.

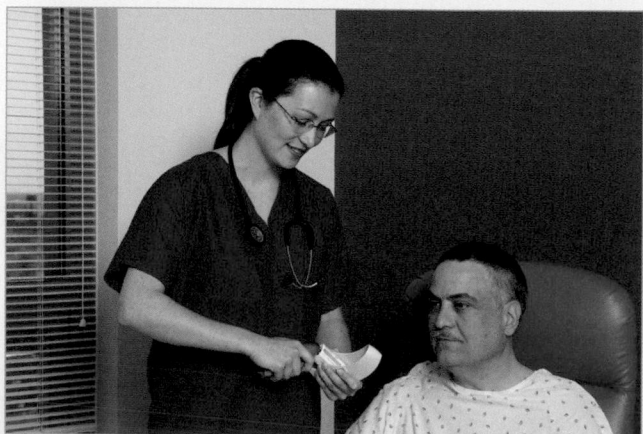

FIGURE 1. Turning unit on and awaiting the ready signal.

FIGURE 2. Thermometer in patient's ear canal with pinna pulled up and back.

13. Activate the unit by pushing the trigger button. The reading is immediate (usually within 2 seconds). Note the reading.	The digital thermometer must be activated to record the temperature.

ACTION

14. Discard the probe cover in an appropriate receptacle by pushing the probe-release button or use rim of cover to remove from probe (Figure 3). Replace the thermometer in its charger, if necessary.

FIGURE 3. Disposing of probe cover.

Assessing Oral Temperature

10. Remove the electronic unit from the charging unit, and remove the probe from within the recording unit.

11. Cover thermometer probe with disposable probe cover and slide it on until it snaps into place (Figure 4).

12. **Place the probe beneath the patient's tongue in the posterior sublingual pocket (Figure 5). Ask the patient to close his or her lips around the probe.**

FIGURE 4. Putting probe cover on the thermometer.

RATIONALE

Discarding the probe cover ensures that it will not be reused accidentally on another patient. Proper disposal prevents the spread of microorganisms. If necessary, the thermometer should stay on the charger so that it is ready to use at all times.

Electronic unit must be taken into the patient's room to assess the patient's temperature. On some models, by removing the probe, the machine is already turned on.

Using a cover prevents contamination of the thermometer probe.

When the probe rests deep in the posterior sublingual pocket, it is in contact with blood vessels lying close to the surface.

FIGURE 5. Inserting thermometer under the tongue in the posterior sublingual pocket.

(continued)

Skill · 24-1   Assessing Body Temperature   *continued*

ACTION

13. **Continue to hold the probe until you hear a beep (Figure 6). Note the temperature reading.**

14. Remove the probe from the patient's mouth. Dispose of the probe cover by holding the probe over an appropriate receptacle and pressing the probe release button (Figure 7).

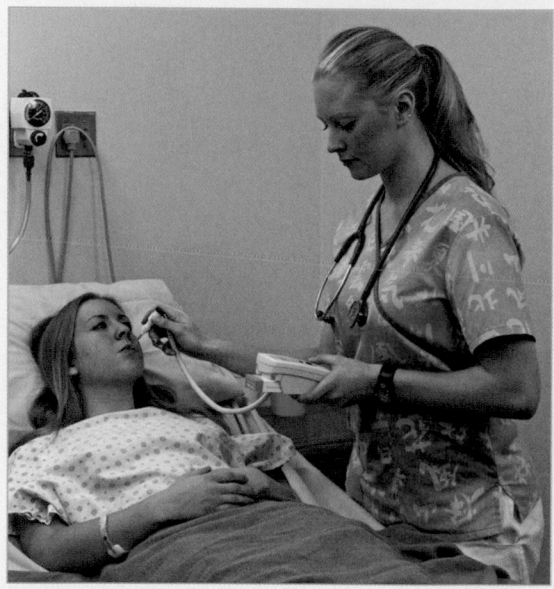

FIGURE 6. Holding probe in the patient's mouth.

15. Return the thermometer probe to the storage place within the unit. Return the electronic unit to the charging unit, if appropriate.

Assessing Rectal Temperature

10. Adjust the bed to a comfortable working height, usually elbow height of the caregiver (VISN 8, 2009). Put on nonsterile gloves.

11. Assist the patient to a side-lying position. Pull back the covers enough to expose only the buttocks.

12. Remove the rectal probe from within the recording unit of the electronic thermometer. Cover the probe with a disposable probe cover and slide it into place until it snaps in place (Figure 8).

13. **Lubricate about 1″ of the probe with a water-soluble lubricant (Figure 9).**

14. Reassure the patient. Separate the buttocks until the anal sphincter is clearly visible.

15. **Insert the thermometer probe into the anus about 1.5″ in an adult or 1″ in a child (Figure 10).**

RATIONALE

If left unsupported, the weight of the probe tends to pull it away from the correct location. The signal indicates the measurement is completed. The electronic thermometer provides a digital display of the measured temperature.

Disposing of the probe cover ensures that it will not be reused accidentally on another patient. Proper disposal prevents spread of microorganisms.

FIGURE 7. Pushing button to dispose of cover.

The thermometer needs to be recharged for future use. If necessary, the thermometer should stay on the charger so that it is ready to use at all times.

Having the bed at the proper height prevents back and muscle strain. Gloves prevent contact with contaminants and body fluids.

The side-lying position allows the nurse to visualize the buttocks. Exposing only the buttocks keeps the patient warm and maintains his or her dignity.

Using a cover prevents contamination of the thermometer.

Lubrication reduces friction and facilitates insertion, minimizing the risk of irritation or injury to the rectal mucous membranes.

If not placed directly into the anal opening, the thermometer probe may injure adjacent tissue or cause discomfort.

Depth of insertion must be adjusted based on the patient's age. Rectal temperatures are not normally taken in an infant, but may be indicted. Refer to the Special Considerations section at the end of the skill.

ACTION

RATIONALE

FIGURE 8. Removing appropriate probe and attaching disposable probe cover.

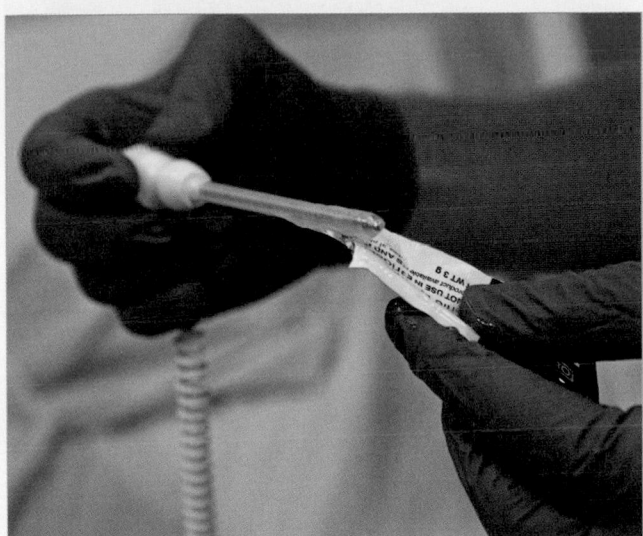

FIGURE 9. Lubricating thermometer tip.

FIGURE 10. Inserting thermometer into the anus.

16. Hold the probe in place until you hear a beep, then carefully remove the probe. Note the temperature reading on the display.

17. Dispose of the probe cover by holding the probe over an appropriate waste receptacle and pressing the release button.

18. Using toilet tissue, wipe the anus of any feces or excess lubricant. Dispose of the toilet tissue. Remove gloves and discard them.

19. Cover the patient and help him or her to a position of comfort.

20. Place the bed in the lowest position; elevate rails as needed.

21. Return the thermometer to the charging unit.

If left unsupported, movement of the probe in the rectum could cause injury and/or discomfort. The signal indicates the measurement is completed. The electronic thermometer provides a digital display of the measured temperature.

Proper probe cover disposal reduces risk of microorganism transmission.

Wiping promotes cleanliness. Disposing of the toilet tissue avoids transmission of microorganisms.

Ensures patient comfort.

These actions provide for the patient's safety.

The thermometer needs to be recharged for future use.

(continued)

Skill · 24-1 Assessing Body Temperature *continued*

ACTION

RATIONALE

Assessing Axillary Temperature

10. Move the patient's clothing to expose only the axilla (Figure 11).

11. Remove the probe from the recording unit of the electronic thermometer. Place a disposable probe cover on by sliding it on and snapping it securely.

12. **Place the end of the probe in the center of the axilla (Figure 12). Have the patient bring the arm down and close to the body.**

The axilla must be exposed for placement of the thermometer. Exposing only the axilla keeps the patient warm and maintains his or her dignity.

Using a cover prevents contamination of the thermometer probe.

The deepest area of the axilla provides the most accurate measurement; surrounding the bulb with skin surface provides a more reliable measurement.

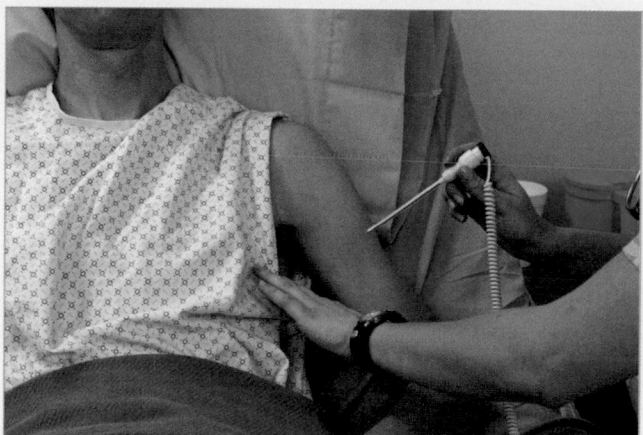

FIGURE 11. Exposing axilla to assess temperature.

FIGURE 12. Placing thermometer in center of axilla.

13. Hold the probe in place until you hear a beep, and then carefully remove the probe. Note the temperature reading.

14. Cover the patient and help him or her to a position of comfort.

15. Dispose of the probe cover by holding the probe over an appropriate waste receptacle and pushing the release button.

16. Place the bed in the lowest position and elevate rails as needed. Leave the patient clean and comfortable.

17. Return the electronic thermometer to the charging unit.

Axillary thermometers must be held in place to obtain an accurate temperature.

Ensures patient comfort.

Discarding the probe cover ensures that it will not be reused accidentally on another patient.

Low bed position and elevated side rails provide for patient safety.

Thermometer needs to be recharged for future use.

Assessing Temporal Artery Temperature

10. Brush the patient's hair aside if it is covering the temporal artery area.

11. Apply a probe cover.

12. Hold the thermometer like a remote, with your thumb on the red "ON" button. Place the probe flush on the center of the forehead, with the body of the instrument sideways (not straight up and down), so it is not in the patient's face (Figure 13).

13. Depress the "ON" button. Keep the button depressed throughout the measurement.

14. Slowly slide the probe straight across the forehead, midline, to the hairline (Figure 14). The thermometer will click; fast clicking indicates a rise to a higher temperature, slow clicking indicates the instrument is still scanning, but not finding any higher temperature.

Anything covering the area, such as a hat, hair, wigs, or bandages, would insulate the area, resulting in falsely high readings. Measure only the side of the head exposed to the environment.

Using a cover prevents contamination of the thermometer probe.

Allows for easy use of the device and reading of the display. Holding the instrument straight up and down could be intimidating for the patient, particularly young patients and/or those with alterations in mental status.

Midline on the forehead, the temporal artery is less than 2 millimeters below the skin; whereas at the side of the face, the temporal artery is much deeper. Measuring there would result in falsely low readings.

ACTION	RATIONALE

FIGURE 13. Placing the thermometer probe on the center of the forehead.

FIGURE 14. Sliding the probe across the forehead to the hairline.

15. Brush hair aside if it is covering the ear, exposing the area of the neck under the ear lobe. Lift the probe from the forehead and touch on the neck just behind the ear lobe, in the depression just below the mastoid (Figure 15).

Sweat causes evaporative cooling of the skin on the forehead, possibly leading to a falsely low reading. During diaphoresis, the area on the head behind the ear lobe exhibits high blood flow necessary for the arterial measurement; it is a double check for the thermometer (Exergen, 2007).

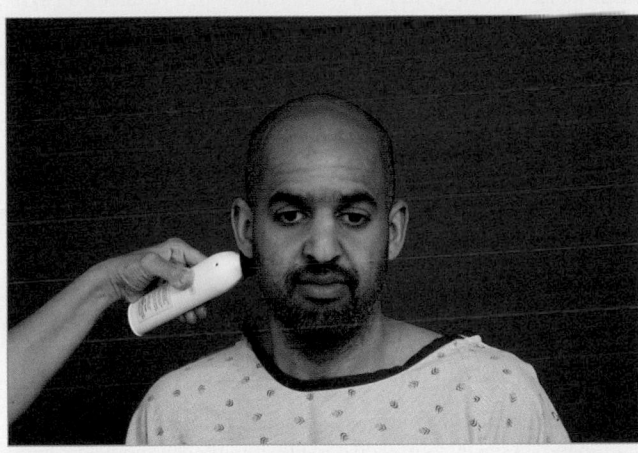

FIGURE 15. Touching the probe behind the ear.

16. Release the button and read the thermometer measurement.

17. Hold the thermometer over a waste receptacle. Gently push the probe cover with your thumb against the proximal edge to dispose of probe cover.

Discarding the probe cover ensures that it will not be reused accidentally on another patient.

18. Instrument will automatically turn off in 30 seconds, or press and release the power button.

Turns thermometer off.

DOCUMENTATION

Guidelines

Record temperature on paper, flow sheet, or computerized record. Report abnormal findings to the appropriate person. Identify the site of assessment if other than oral.

Sample Documentation

10/20/12 0800 Tympanic temperature assessed. Temperature 102.5°F. Patient states she has "a pounding" headache; denies chills, malaise. Physician notified. Received order to give 650 mg PO acetaminophen now. Incentive spirometer × 10 q 2 hours.
—*M. Evans, RN*

(continued)

Skill · 24-1   Assessing Body Temperature   *continued*

UNEXPECTED SITUATIONS AND ASSOCIATED INTERVENTIONS

- *Temperature reading is higher or lower than expected based upon the nurse's assessment:* Reassess temperature with a different thermometer. The thermometer may not be calibrated correctly. If using a tympanic thermometer, you will get lower readings if the probe is not inserted far enough into the ear.

- *During rectal temperature assessment, the patient reports feeling lightheaded or passes out:* Remove the thermometer immediately. Quickly assess the patient's blood pressure and heart rate. Notify the physician. Do not attempt to take another rectal temperature on this patient.

SPECIAL CONSIDERATIONS

General Considerations

- When using a tympanic thermometer, make sure to insert the probe into the ear canal tightly enough to seal the opening to ensure an accurate reading.

- Nonmercury glass thermometers used for oral readings commonly have long, thin bulbs. Those for rectal readings have a blunt bulb to prevent injury.

- Axillary temperatures are generally about 1 degree less than oral temperatures; rectal temperatures are generally about 1 degree higher.

- If the patient smoked, chewed gum, or consumed hot or cold food or fluids recently, wait 30 minutes before taking an oral temperature to allow the oral tissues to return to baseline temperature.

- Nasal oxygen is not thought to affect oral temperature readings. Do not assess oral temperatures in patients receiving oxygen by mask. Removal of the mask for the time period required for assessment could result in a serious drop in the patient's blood oxygen level.

- If the patient's axilla has been washed recently, wait 15 to 30 minutes before taking an axillary temperature to allow the skin to return to baseline temperature.

- A dirty probe lens and cone on the temporal artery thermometer can cause a falsely low reading. If the lens is not shiny in appearance, clean the lens and cone with an alcohol prep or swab moistened in alcohol.

Infant and Child Considerations

- Pull the pinna back and down when measuring tympanic temperature on a child younger than 3 years of age. For children older than 3 years of age, there is no need to manipulate the pinna (Kyle, 2008).

- Small children have a limited attention span and have difficulty keeping their lips closed long enough to obtain an accurate oral temperature reading. For children younger than 6 years, use the axillary or tympanic site or use a temperature-sensitive tape (although research is ongoing to determine the accuracy of the measurements).

- Chemical dot thermometers (liquid crystal skin contact thermometers) are sometimes used as alternatives in pediatric settings. These single-use, disposable, flexible thermometers have specific chemical mixtures in circles on the thermometer that change color to measure temperature increments of two tenths of a degree. Place the thermometer in the mouth with the dot side (sensor) down, into the posterior sublingual pocket. Keep this type of thermometer in the mouth for 1 minute, in the axilla 3 minutes, and the rectum 3 minutes. Read the color change 10 to 15 seconds after removing the thermometer. Read away from any heat source. Wearable, continuous-use chemical dot thermometers are available. These are placed under the axilla and must remain in place at least 2 to 3 minutes before taking the first reading; continuously thereafter. Replace thermometer and assess the underlying skin every 48 hours (Higgins, 2008; Hockenberry & Wilson, 2009).

- The Society of Pediatric Nurses (SPN) recognizes that temporal artery thermometry is accurate for infants less than 90 days old without fever, as well as for all patients greater than 90 days of age with or without fever, ill or well. The SPN recommends the temporal artery method should not be used in infants 90 days or younger who are ill, have a fever, or have an ill diagnosis. The rectal method should be used for these infants unless contraindicated by diagnosis in which case the axillary method should be used. In addition, in children 6 months of age or older, the tympanic or oral methods may be used with correct positioning of the ear (tympanic) and if the patient can cooperate (oral) (Asher & Northingon, 2008).

Home Care Considerations

- Teach patients using electronic or digital thermometers to clean the probe after use to prevent transmission of microorganisms between family members. Clean according to manufacturer's directions.
- Teach patients using nonmercury glass thermometers to clean the thermometer after use in lukewarm soapy water and rinse in cool water. Store in an appropriate place to prevent breakage and injury from the glass.
- Pacifier thermometers, which use the supra-lingual area, are available to screen for fever. These thermometers give an approximation to rectal temperature measurement in the home setting (Braun, 2006). This thermometer should be left in place for 3 to 6 minutes, based on manufacturer's recommendations.

Skill · 24-2 Assessing a Peripheral Pulse by Palpation

EQUIPMENT

- Watch with second hand or digital readout
- Pencil or pen, paper or flow sheet, computerized record
- Nonsterile gloves, if appropriate; additional PPE, as indicated

IMPLEMENTATION

ACTION	RATIONALE
1. Check medical order or nursing care plan for frequency of pulse assessment. More frequent pulse measurement may be appropriate based on nursing judgment.	Assessment and measurement of vital signs at appropriate intervals provides important data about the patient's health status.
2. Perform hand hygiene and put on PPE, if indicated.	Hand hygiene and PPE prevent the spread of microorganisms. PPE is required based on transmission precautions.
3. Identify the patient.	Identifying the patient ensures the right patient receives the intervention and helps prevent errors.
4. Close curtains around bed and close door to room if possible. Discuss procedure with patient and assess patient's ability to assist with the procedure.	This ensures the patient's privacy. Explanation relieves anxiety and facilitates cooperation.
5. Put on gloves as appropriate.	Gloves are not usually worn to obtain a pulse measurement unless contact with blood or body fluids is anticipated. Gloves prevent contact with blood and body fluids.
6. Select the appropriate peripheral site based on assessment data.	Ensures safety and accuracy of measurement.
7. Move the patient's clothing to expose only the site chosen.	The site must be exposed for pulse assessment. Exposing only the site keeps the patient warm and maintains his or her dignity.
8. Place your first, second, and third fingers over the artery (Figure 1). **Lightly compress the artery so pulsations can be felt and counted.**	The sensitive fingertips can feel the pulsation of the artery.
9. Using a watch with a second hand, count the number of pulsations felt for 30 seconds (Figure 2). Multiply this number by 2 to calculate the rate for 1 minute. **If the rate, rhythm, or amplitude of the pulse is abnormal in any way, palpate and count the pulse for 1 minute.**	Ensures accuracy of measurement and assessment.
10. Note the rhythm and amplitude of the pulse.	Provides additional assessment data regarding patient's cardiovascular status.
11. When measurement is completed, remove gloves, if worn. Cover the patient and help him or her to a position of comfort.	Removing PPE properly reduces the risk for infection transmission and contamination of other items. Ensures patient comfort.

(continued)

Skill · 24-2 Assessing a Peripheral Pulse by Palpation *continued*

ACTION	RATIONALE

FIGURE 1. Palpating the radial pulse.

12. Remove additional PPE, if used. Perform hand hygiene.

FIGURE 2. Counting the pulse.

Removing PPE properly reduces the risk for infection transmission and contamination of other items. Hand hygiene prevents the spread of microorganisms.

DOCUMENTATION

Guidelines

Record pulse rate, amplitude, and rhythm on paper, flow sheet, or computerized record. Identify site of assessment. Report abnormal findings to the appropriate person.

Sample Documentation

> 2/6/12 1000 Pulses regular, 2+ and equal in radial, popliteal, and dorsalis pedis sites.
> —M. Evans, RN

UNEXPECTED SITUATIONS AND ASSOCIATED INTERVENTIONS

- *The pulse is irregular:* Monitor the pulse for a full minute. If the pulse is difficult to assess, validate pulse measurement by taking the apical pulse for 1 minute. If this is a change for the patient, notify the physician.

- *The pulse is palpated easily, but then disappears:* Apply only moderate pressure to the pulse. Applying too much pressure may obliterate the pulse.

- *You cannot palpate a pulse:* Use a portable ultrasound Doppler to assess the pulse. If this is a change in assessment, notify the physician. If you cannot find the pulse using an ultrasound Doppler, notify the physician. If you can find the pulse using an ultrasound Doppler, place a small X over the spot where the pulse is located. This can make palpating the pulse easier since the exact location of the pulse is known.

SPECIAL CONSIDERATIONS

General Considerations

- The normal heart rate varies by age.

- When palpating a carotid pulse, lightly press only one side of the neck at a time. Never attempt to palpate both carotid arteries at the same time. Bilateral palpation could result in reduced cerebral blood flow (Weber & Kelley, 2007).

- If a peripheral pulse is difficult to assess accurately because it is irregular, feeble, or extremely rapid, assess the apical rate.

Infant and Child Considerations

- For children younger than 2 years of age, assess the apical pulse. Do not measure radial pulse because it is difficult to palpate accurately in this age group (Kyle, 2008).

- Measure the apical rate if the child has a cardiac problem or congenital heart defect.

Home Care Considerations

- Teach the patient and family members how to take the patient's pulse, if appropriate.

- Inform the patient and family about digital pulse monitoring devices.

- Teach family members how to locate and monitor peripheral pulse sites, if appropriate.

Skill · 24-3 Assessing Respiration

EQUIPMENT

- Watch with second hand or digital readout
- Pencil or pen, paper or flow sheet, computerized record
- PPE, as indicated

IMPLEMENTATION

ACTION	RATIONALE
1. **While your fingers are still in place for the pulse measurement, after counting the pulse rate, observe the patient's respirations (Figure 1).**	The patient may alter the rate of respirations if he or she is aware they are being counted.

FIGURE 1. Assessing respirations.

ACTION	RATIONALE
2. Note the rise and fall of the patient's chest.	A complete cycle of an inspiration and an expiration composes one respiration.
3. Using a watch with a second hand, count the number of respirations for 30 seconds. Multiply this number by 2 to calculate the respiratory rate per minute.	Sufficient time is necessary to observe the rate, depth, and other characteristics.
4. **If respirations are abnormal in any way, count the respirations for at least 1 full minute.**	Increased time allows the detection of unequal timing between respirations.
5. Note the depth and rhythm of the respirations.	Provides additional assessment data regarding patient's respiratory status.
6. When measurement is completed, remove gloves, if worn. Cover the patient and help him or her to a position of comfort.	Removing PPE properly reduces the risk for infection transmission and contamination of other items. Ensures patient comfort.
7. Remove additional PPE, if used. Perform hand hygiene.	Removing PPE properly reduces the risk for infection transmission and contamination of other items. Hand hygiene deters the spread of microorganisms.

DOCUMENTATION

Guidelines

Document respiratory rate, depth, and rhythm on paper, flow sheet, or computerized record. Report any abnormal findings to the appropriate person.

Sample Documentation

10/23/12 0830 Patient breathing at a rate of 16 respirations per minute. Respirations regular and unlabored.

—*M. Evans, RN*

(continued)

Skill · 24-3   Assessing Respiration   *continued*

UNEXPECTED SITUATIONS AND ASSOCIATED INTERVENTIONS

- *The patient is breathing with such shallow respirations that you cannot count the rate:* Sometimes it is easier to count respirations by auscultating the lung sounds. Auscultate lung sounds and count respirations for 30 seconds. Multiply by 2 to calculate the respiratory rate per minute. If the respiratory rate is irregular, count for a full minute. Notify the physician of the respiratory rate and the shallowness of the respirations.

SPECIAL CONSIDERATIONS

General Considerations

- If respiratory rate is irregular, count respirations for 1 minute.

Infant and Child Considerations

- For infants, count respirations for 1 full minute due to a normally irregular rhythm.
- Assess respirations in infants and children when the child is resting or sitting quietly, since respiratory rate often changes when infants or young children cry, feed, or become more active. The most accurate respiratory rate is obtained before disturbing the infant or child (Kyle, 2008).
- Infants' respirations are primarily diaphragmatic; count abdominal movements to measure respiratory rate. After 1 year of age, count thoracic movements (Kyle, 2008).

Skill · 24-4   Assessing a Brachial Artery Blood Pressure

EQUIPMENT

- Stethoscope
- Sphygmomanometer
- Blood pressure cuff of appropriate size
- Pencil or pen, paper or flow sheet
- Alcohol swab
- PPE, as indicated

IMPLEMENTATION

ACTION

1. Check physician's order or nursing care plan for frequency of blood pressure measurement. More frequent measurement may be appropriate based on nursing judgment.

2. Perform hand hygiene and put on PPE, if indicated.

3. Identify the patient.

4. Close curtains around bed and close door to room if possible. Discuss procedure with patient and assess patient's ability to assist with the procedure. Validate that the patient has relaxed for several minutes.

5. Put on gloves, if appropriate or indicated.

6. Select the appropriate arm for application of the cuff.

7. Have the patient assume a comfortable lying or sitting position with the forearm supported at the level of the heart and the palm of the hand upward (Figure 1). If the measurement is taken in the supine position, support the arm with a pillow. In the sitting position, support the arm yourself or by using the bedside table. If the patient is sitting, have the patient sit back

RATIONALE

Provides for patient safety.

Hand hygiene and PPE prevent the spread of microorganisms. PPE is required based on transmission precautions.

Identifying the patient ensures the right patient receives the intervention and helps prevent errors.

This ensures the patient's privacy. Explanation relieves anxiety and facilitates cooperation. Activity immediately prior to measurement can result in inaccurate results.

Gloves prevent contact with blood and body fluids. Gloves are usually not required for measurement of blood pressure, unless contact with blood or body fluids is anticipated.

Measurement of blood pressure may temporarily impede circulation to the extremity.

The position of the arm can have a major influence when the blood pressure is measured; if the upper arm is below the level of the right atrium, the readings will be too high. If the arm is above the level of the heart, the readings will be too low (Pickering et al., 2004). If the back is not supported, the diastolic pressure may be elevated falsely; if the legs are crossed, the

ACTION

in the chair so that the chair supports his or her back. In addition, make sure the patient keeps the legs uncrossed.

8. Expose the brachial artery by removing garments, or move a sleeve, if it is not too tight, above the area where the cuff will be placed.

9. Palpate the location of the brachial artery. **Center the bladder of the cuff over the brachial artery, about midway on the arm, so that the lower edge of the cuff is about 2.5 to 5 cm (1″–2″) above the inner aspect of the elbow. Line the artery marking on the cuff up with the patient's brachial artery.** The tubing should extend from the edge of the cuff nearer the patient's elbow (Figure 2).

FIGURE 1. Proper positioning for blood pressure assessment using brachial artery. *(Photo by B. Proud.)*

10. Wrap the cuff around the arm smoothly and snugly, and fasten it. Do not allow any clothing to interfere with the proper placement of the cuff.

11. Check that the needle on the aneroid gauge is within the zero mark (Figure 3). If using a mercury manometer, check to see that the manometer is in the vertical position and that the mercury is within the zero level with the gauge at eye level.

Estimating Systolic Pressure

12. Palpate the pulse at the brachial or radial artery by pressing gently with the fingertips (Figure 4).

13. Tighten the screw valve on the air pump.

14. **Inflate the cuff while continuing to palpate the artery. Note the point on the gauge where the pulse disappears.**

15. Deflate the cuff and wait 1 minute.

RATIONALE

systolic pressure may be elevated falsely (Pickering et al., 2004). This position places the brachial artery on the inner aspect of the elbow so that the bell or diaphragm of the stethoscope can rest on it easily. This sitting position ensures accuracy.

Clothing over the artery interferes with the ability to hear sounds and may cause inaccurate blood pressure readings. A tight sleeve would cause congestion of blood and possibly inaccurate readings.

Pressure in the cuff applied directly to the artery provides the most accurate readings. If the cuff gets in the way of the stethoscope, readings are likely to be inaccurate. A cuff placed upside down with the tubing toward the patient's head may give a false reading.

FIGURE 2. Placing the blood pressure cuff. *(Photo by B. Proud.)*

A smooth cuff and snug wrapping produce equal pressure and help promote an accurate measurement. A cuff wrapped too loosely results in an inaccurate reading.

If the needle is not in the zero area, the blood pressure may not be accurate. Tilting a mercury manometer, inaccurate calibration, or improper height for reading the gauge can lead to errors in determining the pressure measurements.

Palpation allows for measurement of the approximate systolic reading.

The bladder within the cuff will not inflate with the valve open.

The point where the pulse disappears provides an estimate of the systolic pressure. To identify the first Korotkoff sound accurately, the cuff must be inflated to a pressure above the point at which the pulse can no longer be felt.

Allowing a brief pause before continuing permits the blood to refill and circulate through the arm.

(continued)

Skill · 24-4   Assessing a Brachial Artery Blood Pressure   *continued*

ACTION

FIGURE 3. Ensuring gauge starts at zero. *(Photo by B. Proud.)*

Obtaining Blood Pressure Measurement

16. Assume a position that is no more than 3 feet away from the gauge.

17. Place the stethoscope earpieces in your ears. Direct the earpieces forward into the canal and not against the ear itself.

18. Place the bell or diaphragm of the stethoscope firmly but with as little pressure as possible over the brachial artery (Figure 5). Do not allow the stethoscope to touch clothing or the cuff.

RATIONALE

FIGURE 4. Palpating the brachial pulse. *(Photo by B. Proud.)*

A distance of more than about 3 feet can interfere with accurate readings of the numbers on the gauge.

Proper placement blocks extraneous noise and allows sound to travel more clearly.

Having the bell or diaphragm directly over the artery allows more accurate readings. Heavy pressure on the brachial artery distorts the shape of the artery and the sound. Placing the bell or diaphragm away from clothing and the cuff prevents noise, which would distract from the sounds made by blood flowing through the artery.

FIGURE 5. Proper placement of diaphragm of stethoscope. *(Photo by B. Proud.)*

ACTION

19. Pump the pressure 30-mm Hg above the point at which the systolic pressure was palpated and estimated. Open the valve on the manometer and allow air to escape slowly (allowing the gauge to drop 2–3 mm per second).

20. **Note the point on the gauge at which the first faint, but clear, sound appears that slowly increases in intensity. Note this number as the systolic pressure (Figure 6). Read the pressure to the closest 2 mm Hg.**

21. Do not reinflate the cuff once the air is being released to recheck the systolic pressure reading.

22. **Note the point at which the sound completely disappears (Figure 7).**

RATIONALE

Increasing the pressure above the point where the pulse disappeared ensures a period before hearing the first sound that corresponds with the systolic pressure. It prevents misinterpreting phase II sounds as phase I.

Systolic pressure is the point at which the blood in the artery is first able to force its way through the vessel at a similar pressure exerted by the air bladder in the cuff. The first sound is phase I of Korotkoff sounds.

Reinflating the cuff while obtaining the blood pressure is uncomfortable for the patient and may cause an inaccurate reading. Reinflating the cuff causes congestion of blood in the lower arm, which lessens the loudness of Korotkoff sounds.

The point at which the sound disappears corresponds to the beginning of phase V Korotkoff sounds and is generally considered the diastolic pressure reading (Pickering et al., 2004).

FIGURE 6. Measuring systolic blood pressure. *(Photo by B. Proud.)*

FIGURE 7. Measuring diastolic blood pressure. *(Photo by B. Proud.)*

23. Allow the remaining air to escape quickly. Repeat any suspicious reading, but wait at least 1 minute. Deflate the cuff completely between attempts to check the blood pressure.

24. When measurement is completed, remove the cuff. Remove gloves, if worn. Cover the patient and help him or her to a position of comfort.

25. Remove additional PPE, if used. Perform hand hygiene.

26. Clean the diaphragm of the stethoscope with the alcohol wipe. Clean and store the sphygmomanometer, according to facility policy.

False readings are likely to occur if there is congestion of blood in the limb while obtaining repeated readings.

Removing PPE properly reduces the risk for infection transmission and contamination of other items. Ensures patient comfort.

Removing PPE properly reduces the risk for infection transmission and contamination of other items. Hand hygiene deters the spread of microorganisms.

Appropriate cleaning deters the spread of microorganisms. Equipment should be left ready for use.

(continued)

Skill · 24-4   Assessing a Brachial Artery Blood Pressure   *continued*

DOCUMENTATION

Guidelines
Record the findings on paper, flow sheet, or computerized record. Report abnormal findings to the appropriate person. Identify arm used and site of assessment if other than brachial.

Sample Documentation

> 10/18/12   0945 Blood pressure taken in right arm 180/88. Physician notified. Ordered Captopril 25 PO mg BID. Blood pressure to be repeated 30 minutes after administering medication.
>
> —M. Evans, RN

SPECIAL CONSIDERATIONS

General Considerations

- If this is the initial nursing assessment of a patient, take the blood pressure on both arms. It is normal to have a 5- to 10-mm Hg difference in the systolic reading between arms. Use the arm with the higher reading for subsequent blood pressure measurements.

- If you have difficulty hearing the blood pressure sounds, raise the patient's arm, with cuff in place, over his or her head for 30 seconds before rechecking the blood pressure. Inflate the cuff while the arm is elevated, and then gently lower the arm while continuing to support it. Position the stethoscope and deflate the cuff at the usual rate while listening for Korotkoff sounds. Raising the arm over the head reduces vascular volume in the limb and improves blood flow to enhance the Korotkoff sounds (Pickering et al., 2004).

- Blood pressure may be assessed using an electronic device or Doppler ultrasound (see Guidelines for Nursing Care 24-2).

- Many electronic devices are not recommended for patients with irregular heart rates, tremors, or the inability to hold the extremity still. The machine will continue to inflate, causing pain for the patient.

- Monitors that measure blood pressure at the wrist are available. It is important for the wrist to be at heart level when readings are taken, to avoid error due to hydrostatic effect of differences in the position of the wrist relative to the heart. Some wrist monitors will only record a measurement when the monitor is held at heart level (Pickering et al., 2004).

- Diastolic pressure measured while the patient is sitting is approximately 5 mm Hg higher than when measured while the patient is supine; systolic pressure measured while the patient is supine is approximately 8 mm Hg higher than when measured in the patient who is sitting (Pickering et al., 2004).

Infant and Child Considerations

- In infants and small children, the lower extremities are commonly used for blood pressure monitoring. The more common sites are the popliteal, dorsalis pedis, and posterior tibial. Blood pressures obtained in the lower extremities are generally higher than if taken in the upper extremities. In children over 1 year old, the systolic pressure in the thigh tends to be 10 to 40 mm Hg higher than in the arm; the diastolic pressure remains the same (Kyle, 2008).

- Infants and children presenting with cardiac complaints should have blood pressures assessed in all four extremities (Kyle, 2008). Large differences among blood pressure readings can indicate heart defects.

- The fifth Korotkoff sound corresponds to diastolic BP in children. In some children, the Korotkoff sounds continue to 0 mm Hg. In this situation, the fourth Korotkoff sound, which is indicated by muffling of sound, is considered the diastolic reading (Schell, 2006).

Home Care Considerations

- Use a cuff size appropriate for limb circumference. Inform the patient that cuff sizes range from a pediatric cuff to a large thigh cuff and that a poorly fitting cuff may result in an inaccurate measurement.

- Inform patient about digital blood pressure monitoring equipment. Though more costly than manual cuffs, most provide an easy-to-read recording of systolic and diastolic measurements.

- Home monitoring devices should be checked for accuracy every 1 to 2 years (Pickering et al., 2004).

Developing Critical Thinking Skills

1. Take your own pulse several times a day, such as when you first get up, before and after meals, and before and after exercise. Write down the rate, rhythm, and quality of the pulse. What changes did you see? What are the physiologic rationales for these changes?

2. Describe differences you might expect to find in the vital signs of the following individuals, and include the physiologic reasons for these differences:
   - A teenager who has his first football practice in 95°F heat
   - An infant with a bacterial ear infection
   - A young woman arriving at the emergency department after an attempted assault
   - A middle-aged man who sustained serious trauma and bleeding in an automobile crash
   - A 92-year-old woman with a chronic respiratory disease

Practicing for NCLEX

1. A nurse assesses an oral temperature for a patient as 38.5°C (101.3°F). What term would the nurse use to report this temperature?
   a. Fever
   b. Hypothermia
   c. Hypertension
   d. Afebrile

2. A nurse is assessing vital signs on several hospitalized children. The nurse would plan to use the oral route to assess temperature for which patient?
   a. 6-month-old infant
   b. Patient receiving oxygen therapy by mask
   c. 15-year-old healthy adolescent
   d. Unconscious patient

3. When assessing a temperature rectally, the nurse would use extreme care when inserting the thermometer to prevent which of the following?
   a. An increase in heart rate
   b. A decrease in heart rate
   c. A decrease in blood pressure
   d. An increase in respirations

4. While taking an adult patient's pulse, a nurse finds the rate to be 140 beats/min. What should the nurse do next?
   a. Check the pulse again in 2 hours.
   b. Check the blood pressure.
   c. Record the information.
   d. Report the rate.

5. A patient complains of severe abdominal pain. When assessing the vital signs, the nurse would not be surprised to find what assessment?
   a. An increase in the pulse rate
   b. A decrease in body temperature
   c. A decrease in blood pressure
   d. An increase in respiratory depth

6. The nurse is taking an apical pulse. What equipment will he take into the patient's room?
   a. Sphygmomanometer
   b. Electronic thermometer
   c. Stethoscope
   d. Doppler apparatus

7. Two nurses are taking an apical-radial pulse and note a difference in pulse rate of 8 beats per minute. The nurse would document this difference as which of the following?
   a. Pulse deficit
   b. Pulse amplitude
   c. Ventricular rhythm
   d. Heart arrhythmia

8. Before assessing respirations, the nurse reviews normal rates for adults. Which rate would the nurse identify as normal?
   a. 1 to 6 breaths/min
   b. 12 to 20 breaths/min
   c. 60 to 80 breaths/min
   d. 100 to 120 breaths/min

9. A patient is having dyspnea. What would the nurse do first?
   a. Remove pillows from under the head
   b. Elevate the head of the bed
   c. Elevate the foot of the bed
   d. Take the blood pressure

10. A student nurse is learning to assess blood pressure. What does the blood pressure measure?
    a. Flow of blood through the circulation
    b. Force of blood against arterial walls
    c. Force of blood against venous walls
    d. Flow of blood through the heart

11. A nurse knows that the blood pressure is often higher in older adults based on the understanding that which of the following occurs with aging?
    a. Loss of muscle mass
    b. Changes in exercise level
    c. Decreased peripheral resistance
    d. Decreased elasticity in arterial walls

12. A patient has a blood pressure reading of 130/90 mm Hg when visiting a clinic. What would the nurse recommend to the patient?
    a. Follow-up measurements of blood pressure
    b. Immediate treatment by a physician
    c. Nothing, because the nurse considers this reading is due to anxiety
    d. A change in dietary intake

13. A nurse is documenting a blood pressure of 120/80 mm Hg. The nurse interprets the 120 to represent which of the following?
    a. Pulse rate
    b. Diastolic pressure
    c. Systolic pressure
    d. Pulse deficit

14. It is important to have the appropriate cuff size when taking the blood pressure. What error may result from a cuff that is too large or too small?
   a. An incorrect reading
   b. Injury to the patient
   c. Prolonged pressure on the arm
   d. Loss of Korotkoff sounds

15. A patient has intravenous fluids infusing in the right arm. When taking a blood pressure on this patient, what would the nurse do in this situation?
   a. Take the blood pressure in the right arm
   b. Take the blood pressure in the left arm
   c. Use the smallest possible cuff
   d. Report inability to take the blood pressure

● Answers With Rationales

1. *a.* Fever is an elevation of body temperature.

2. *c.* A healthy adolescent would be an appropriate patient for assessing temperature by the oral route.

3. *b.* Insertion of a rectal thermometer may stimulate the vagus nerve, which, in turn, would decrease heart rate. This may potentially be harmful for patients with cardiac problems.

4. *d.* A rate of 140 beats/min in an adult is an abnormal pulse and should be reported to the instructor or the nurse in charge of the patient.

5. *a.* The pulse often increases when an individual is experiencing pain. Pain does not affect body temperature and may increase (not decrease) blood pressure. Acute pain may increase respiratory rate but decrease respiratory depth.

6. *c.* The apical pulse can only be assessed by listening with a stethoscope.

7. *a.* The difference between the apical and radial pulse rate is called the pulse deficit.

8. *b.* The normal respiratory rate for adults is 12 to 20 breaths/min.

9. *b.* Elevating the head of the bed allows the abdominal organs to descend, giving the diaphragm greater room for expansion and facilitating lung expansion.

10. *b.* Blood pressure is the measurement of the force of blood against arterial walls.

11. *d.* With aging, elasticity in arterial walls is decreased, contributing to an elevated blood pressure reading.

12. *a.* A single blood pressure reading that is mildly elevated is not significant, but the measurement should be taken again over time to determine if hypertension is a problem. The nurse would recommend a return visit to the clinic for a recheck.

13. *c.* The systolic pressure is 120 mm Hg. The diastolic pressure is 80 mm HG.

14. *a.* A blood pressure cuff that is not the right size may cause an incorrect reading.

15. *b.* The blood pressure should be taken in the arm opposite the one with the infusion.

Taylor Suite Resources

The Taylor Suite offers these additional resources to enhance learning and facilitate understanding of this chapter:

- thePoint online resource, http://thepoint.lww.com/Taylor7E
- Student DVD-ROM included with the book
- Study Guide for Taylor's Fundamentals of Nursing
- Skill Checklists for Taylor's Fundamentals of Nursing
- Taylor's Clinical Nursing Skills: *Chapter 1, Vital Signs*
- Taylor's Video Guide to Clinical Nursing Skills: *Vital Signs*

BIBLIOGRAPHY

American Heart Association. (2008). Heart disease and stroke statistics. 2008 update: A report from the American Heart Association Statistics Committee and Stroke Statistics Subcommittee. *Circulation,117*, 4, e25–146.

Asher, C., & Northington, L. (2008). Society of Pediatric Nurses. Position statement for measurement of temperature/fever in children. *Journal of Pediatric Nursing, 23*(3), 234–236.

Ask these questions for children with fever. (2008). *ED Nursing, 11*(3), 32.

Ayoltt, M. (2007). Observing the sick child part 2B: Respiratory palpation. *Pediatric Nursing, 19*(1), 38–45.

Beard, R., & Day, M. (2008). Fever & hyperthermia: Learn to beat the heat. *Nursing, 38*(6), 28–31.

Bern, L., Brandt, M., Mbelu, N., Asonye, U., Fisher, T., Shever, Y., & Serrill, C. (2007). Differences in blood pressure values obtained with automated and manual methods in medical inpatients. *MEDSURG Nursing, 16*(6), 356–362.

Bickley, L. S. (2007). *Bates' guide to physical examination and history taking* (9th ed.). Philadelphia: Lippincott Williams & Wilkins.

Bradley, R. (2007). Improving respiratory assessment skills. *Journal for Nurse Practitioners, 3*(4), 276–277.

Braun, C. (2006). Accuracy of pacifier thermometers in young children. *Pediatric Nursing, 32*(5), 413–418.

Bulechek, G. M., Butcher, H. K., & Dochterman, J. M. (Eds). (2008). *Nursing interventions classification (NIC)* (5th ed.). St. Louis: Mosby Elsevier.

Cork, A. (2007). Theory and practice of manual blood pressure measurement. *Nursing Standard, 22*(14-15-16), 47–50.

Corwin, E. J. (2008). *Handbook of pathophysiology* (3rd ed.). Philadelphia: Lippincott Williams & Wilkins.

Exergen. (2007). Temporal scanner reference manual. Watertown, MA: Author. Available at www.exergen.com/medical/TAT/TAT5000Manual5.pdf. Accessed October 29, 2008.

Ferguson, A. (2007). Evaluation and treatment of fever in intensive care unit patients. *Critical Care Nursing Quarterly, 30*(4), 347–363.

Higgins, D. (2008). Patient assessment: Part 5—measuring pulse. *Nursing Times, 104*(11), 24–25.

Hockenberry, M., & Wilson, D. (2009). *Wong's essentials of pediatric nursing* (8th ed.). St. Louis: Elsevier Mosby.

Holzhauer, J., Reith, V., Malin, S., et al. (2007). Evaluation of a new method of thermometry for 3- to 36-month-old children. *Journal of Pediatric Nursing, 22*(2), 154.

Kyle, T. (2008). *Essentials of pediatric nursing.* Philadelphia: Wolters Kluwer Health/Lippincott Williams & Wilkins.

Lawson, L., Bridges, E., Ballou, I., Eraker, R., Greco, S., Shively, J., & Sochulak, V. (2007). Accuracy and precision of noninvasive temperature measurement in adult intensive care patients. *American Journal of Critical Care, 16,* 485–496.

Moorhead, S., Johnson, M., Maas, M., & Swanson, E. (Eds). (2008). *Nursing outcomes classification (NOC)* (4th ed.). St. Louis: Mosby Elsevier.

Moore, T. (2007). Respiratory assessment in adults. *Nursing Standard, 21*(49), 48–56.

NANDA International. (2009). *Nursing diagnoses: Definitions & classification 2009–2011.* West Sussex, UK: Wiley-Blackwell.

National Heart, Lung, and Blood Institute, National Institutes of Health. (2008). What is high blood pressure? Available at http://www.nhlbi.nih.gov/health/dci/Diseases/Hbp/HBP_WhatIs.html.

O'Riordan, M. (2008). Home is where the heart is: Call for greater use of home blood pressure monitoring. Medscape News. Available at http://www.medscape.com/viewarticle/575151.

Pickering, T., Miller, N., Ogedegbe, G., Krakoff, L., Artinian, N., & Goff, D. (2008). Call to action on use and reimbursement for home health pressure monitoring: Executive summary. *Hypertension, 52,* 1–9.

Porth, C. (2007). *Essentials of pathophysiology: Concepts of altered health states* (2nd ed.). Philadelphia: Lippincott Williams & Wilkins.

Porth, C., & Matfin, G. (2009). *Pathophysiology: Concepts of altered health states* (8th ed.). Philadelphia: Lippincott Williams & Wilkins.

Quatrana, B., Coffman, J., Kenkins, T., et al. (2007). The effects of respiratory rate and ingestion of hot and cold beverages on the accuracy of oral temperatures measured by electronic thermometers. *MEDSURG Nursing, 16*(2), 105–108, 100.

Rushing, J. (2005). Clinical do's & don'ts: Assessing for orthostatic hypotension. *Nursing, 35*(1), 30.

Schell, K. A. (2006). Evidence-based practice: Noninvasive blood pressure measurement in children. *Pediatric Nursing, 32*(3), 263–267.

Schwenk, T. L. (2007). Hypertension often undiagnosed in children. *Journal Watch, 6*(8), Massachusetts Medical Society. Available at http://www.medscape.com/viewarticle/562612

Understanding the Pathophysiology of fever. (2008). *Nursing, 38*(8), 56cc1–56cc2.

VISN 8 Patient Safety Center. (2009). *Safe patient handling and movement algorithms.* Tampa, FL: Author. Available at http://www.visn8.med.va.gov/patientsafetycenter/safePtHandling/default.asp.

Weber, J., & Kelley, J. (2007). *Health assessment in nursing* (3rd ed.). Philadelphia: Lippincott Williams & Wilkins.

Zeitz, K., & McCutcheon, H. (2006). Observations and vital signs: Ritual or vital for the monitoring of postoperative patients? *Applied Nursing Research, 19*(4), 204–211.

25 Health Assessment

BILLY COLLINS

Billy, a 9-year-old boy with a history of allergies, including an allergy to insect stings, is spending a week at summer camp. He reports to the camp counselor that he was just stung by a bee.

TAMMY BROWNING

Tammy, who is expecting her first child, has been on the obstetric unit for 1 week and is about to be moved to the delivery room. She and her partner, both in their late 20s, have a history of substance abuse, primarily alcohol and marijuana. A urine specimen is to be collected for routine evaluation and a drug screen. Tammy is unaware that drug testing will be done.

RAMONA LEWIS

Ramona, a 19-year-old college student, comes to the emergency department. She is upset and crying and reports that she was date raped.

LEARNING OBJECTIVES

After completing the chapter, you will be able to accomplish the following:

1. Explain the purposes and types of health assessment.

2. Follow guidelines for conducting a health history.

3. Prepare the patient and the environment for a health assessment.

4. Identify the equipment and positions used during a physical assessment.

5. Use the techniques of inspection, palpation, percussion, and auscultation appropriately during a physical assessment.

6. Conduct a physical assessment in a systematic manner.

7. Document health assessment findings in a concise, descriptive, and legally appropriate manner.

8. Describe nursing responsibilities before, during, and after diagnostic procedures.

KEY TERMS

adventitious breath sounds	focused assessment
auscultation	inspection
bronchial sounds	jaundice
bronchovesicular sounds	ongoing partial assessment
bruits	pallor
comprehensive assessment	palpation
cyanosis	percussion
ecchymosis	petechiae
edema	precordium
emergency assessment	turgor
erythema	vesicular breath sounds

onducting a health assessment involves collecting, validating, and analyzing subjective data (also called symptoms) and objective data (also called signs) to determine the overall level of physical, psychological, sociocultural, developmental, and spiritual health of a patient. Subjective data are experienced or known only by the patient (e.g., pain and nausea), and are gathered by verbal report during the health history. Objective data are directly observed or elicited through physical examination techniques.

Although most components of a health assessment are described in this chapter, some of the assessments (such as an internal eye examination, a vaginal examination, or a rectal examination) are usually carried out by healthcare providers with advanced education. However, nurses need to be familiar with all parts of a physical assessment so they can assist as necessary and also can explain the techniques and rationale for the assessment to patients.

HEALTH ASSESSMENT

A health assessment may be comprehensive, ongoing partial, focused, or emergency. A **comprehensive assessment** with a health history and complete physical examination is usually conducted when a patient first enters a healthcare setting, with information providing a baseline for comparing later assessments. An **ongoing partial assessment** is one that is conducted at regular intervals (e.g., at the beginning of each home health visit or each hospital shift) during care of the patient. This type of assessment concentrates on identified health problems to monitor positive or negative changes and evaluate the effectiveness of interventions. A **focused assessment** is conducted to assess a specific problem. For example, if a woman is having abdominal pain, the nurse asks questions about urinary problems, bowel problems, allergies, and menstrual history during the health history and then assesses vital signs and abdominal structures during the physical assessment. An **emergency assessment** is a type of rapid focused assessment conducted to determine potentially fatal situations. For example, assessing the airway, breathing, and circulation before beginning cardiopulmonary resuscitation is part of an emergency assessment.

▶ *Consider Billy Collins, the 9-year-old who was stung by a bee. In this situation, the nurse would conduct an emergency assessment to determine the immediate effects of the bee sting, assessing for indications of an allergic reaction such as respiratory difficulty. Once this emergency assessment is completed and any immediate treatments initiated, the nurse would complete a health history to identify the boy's history of any allergies.* ∎

A nursing health assessment differs from other types of health assessments (e.g., one performed by a physician) in that it is a holistic collection of information about factors that affect or are affected by one's level of health. Health assessment is an integral component of nursing care and is the foundation of the nursing process. The information from the nursing health assessment is used to formulate nursing diagnoses that require nursing care. Assessments are used to plan, implement, and evaluate teaching and care to promote an optimal level of health through interventions to prevent illness, restore health, and facilitate coping with disabilities or death. The information is also used to identify health problems that require interdisciplinary care or immediate referral to other healthcare providers. This chapter provides

REFLECTIVE PRACTICE

Challenge to Ethical and Legal Skills

I have always been interested in labor and delivery, so I was very excited to have the opportunity to follow a nurse in labor and delivery and assist and witness the beginning of life. I had no idea that the whole process could be so complicated.

It was here that I met Tammy Browning, who was expecting her first child. She and her partner were an interracial couple, in their late 20s or early 30s. They had been on the antepartum unit for approximately 1 week, and she was going to be moved to the delivery room shortly. Before entering the room, the nurse gave me a brief rundown of what we were expected to do throughout the morning.

On entering the patient's room for the first time, I was shocked at what I saw. The room was dark and extremely cluttered with food, candy wrappers, and trash overflowing onto the floor. The patient's partner had been sleeping in the room and both of their belongings were all over the place. I could not believe it! When we left the room, the nurse told me that both the patient and her partner had a history of drug use, mainly alcohol and marijuana. We had to get a urine sample from her to do a dipstick test. The specimen was also going to be used for a drug screen, but the patient was not going to be told about this. I was shocked and confused by this action. I thought that we had to tell the patient everything we were going to do—right?

Thinking Outside the Box: Possible Courses of Action

- Go along with what the nurse decided to do, and when we got out of the patient's room, ask why she decided to take this course of action.
- Inform myself of the legality of taking this route of action.

- Inform my instructor and head nurse about the case, asking if this was a usual occurrence and requesting that they tell or educate me on what basis they were allowed to do this.

Evaluating a Good Outcome: How Do I Define Success?

- Safety of patient and neonate is ensured.
- Patient and baby benefit from the decided-on course of action.
- No breach of duty or harm is done.

- Patient receives proper care and treatment regardless of her past drug use and results of the drug tests.
- Respect for patient is maintained.

Personal Learning: Here's to the Future!

I really had no idea what to do. Because I did not feel legally competent to challenge the nurse and suggest a different course of action, I followed her and went along with her story. Afterward, I asked her if we were allowed to do this. Her answer was that she was doing it because the patient had a history of drug use and she suspected that she had been smoking marijuana throughout her stay. The test was not going to harm the baby or the mother; if anything, the test was going to be beneficial in providing the most adequate care for her and her baby. It was also going to assist in preparing for any complications that may arise during the delivery.

When she gave me this explanation, I figured that her reasons were valid and it was all right to do this since no one was going to get hurt and it would be beneficial. However, I was left with the thought that we were violating the patient's privacy. I also spoke with my clinical instructor about the situation. Through this experience, I realized that I need to educate myself more on the legal aspects of nursing. I had never paid much attention to the fact that I am exposed to many legal situations every day as a healthcare provider. Therefore, I must be prepared to confront them. I think that it is vital to be skilled as well as to be competent medically and legally. By having this knowledge, many difficult situations may be avoided and/or resolved. With this knowledge, I will also be a better advocate for my patients.

Stephanie Cuellar, Georgetown University

Reflection

How would you respond in a similar situation? Why? What does this tell you about yourself and about the adequacy of your skills for professional practice? What do you think might have happened if the patient were told about the drug testing? Do you feel that the nurse's action of not telling the patient was based on appropriate ethical and legal principles? Why or why not? If so, what ethical and legal principles formed the basis for the action? If not, what ethical and legal principles were violated? Can you think of other ways to respond? What other skills (cognitive, interpersonal, technical, ethical/legal) would you need to respond well in this situation? Do you agree with the criteria to evaluate a successful outcome? Did the nursing student meet the criteria? Explain your answer.

information necessary to identify risks for or actual alterations in health, perform the skills of physical examination, and identify normal age-related variations in physical structures and functions. Health assessments are a part of nursing care for patients across the life span and may be conducted in any setting. (See the accompanying Reflective Practice box for an example). Additional information about assessment is found in Chapter 12.

Preparing the Patient

When conducting a nursing health assessment, it is important to consider and remain sensitive to the patient's physiologic needs (e.g., pain or decreased stamina because of age or illness) and psychological needs (e.g., anxiety about having the examination). Explain that the first part of the assessment will involve questions about the patient's health concerns, health habits, and lifestyle and that the information will only be shared with the patient's other healthcare providers (Fig. 25-1). Inform the patient that after the health history is completed, body structures will be examined.

The patient may be anxious for various reasons. Tell the patient that the assessments should not be painful. Explaining the assessment in general terms can help decrease the patient's embarrassment, fear of possible abnormal physical findings, or fear of "failing" a test. Be sure to then explain each assessment in greater detail as it is performed. Explain that drapes (covers) will be used during the examination, and only the area being assessed will be exposed. Answer the patient's questions directly and honestly.

> *Think back to Ramona Lewis, the college student who reported that she was a victim of date rape. The nurse would need to incorporate knowledge of the emotional and physical effects of rape when communicating with Ms. Lewis. In addition, the patient's anxiety is likely to be high; thus, using empathy, taking the time to explain things slowly, and establishing a trusting nurse–patient relationship are important.* ∎

FIGURE 25-1. A brief explanation of the examination before beginning and just before each stage alleviates patient fear and anxiety. *(Photo by B. Proud.)*

Preparing the Environment

The environment should be prepared before the health assessment is conducted. Clinics, offices, and hospitals may have a special examination room that provides a quiet, private space for assessment. If such a room is available, the examination table is prepared, a gown and drape for the patient are provided, and instruments and special supplies needed for the assessment are gathered. If the area is open to others, an enclosure with a curtain or screen is essential. The room should be warm enough to prevent chilling, and the area or room should be adequately lighted, either by sunlight or overhead lighting.

Direct the patient to a private dressing area or to a comfortable area in the home and ask the patient to change into a gown, if possible. If necessary, assist the patient with undressing. Ask the patient to empty the bladder before the examination to both promote patient comfort during the assessment and to facilitate assessment of the abdomen by the nurse.

Maintaining Cultural Sensitivity

Each person is a unique individual. Nurses must consider patients within the context of family, culture, and community (Weber & Kelley, 2009). Although the patient's culture does not affect how a health assessment is conducted, it is an integral component of the interactions between the nurse and the patient. Nurses should know risk factors for alterations in health that are based on racial inheritance and ethnic backgrounds, as well as normal variations that occur within races. Chapter 2 provides information about cultural diversity and the importance of providing culturally sensitive nursing care.

THE HEALTH HISTORY

A health history is a collection of subjective data that provides a detailed profile of the patient's health status. Nurses use therapeutic communication skills and interviewing techniques during the health history to establish an effective nurse–patient relationship and to gather data to identify actual and potential health problems as well as sources of strength. Effective interviewing skills are described in Chapters 12 and 21.

Information is collected during an interview with the patient, who is the primary source of data. Components of the health history, with examples of questions to ask, are outlined in Box 25-1. Nurses should know and be sensitive to cultural differences that influence how both verbal and nonverbal communications are interpreted.

The health history helps the nurse identify risk factors for alterations in health. Risk factors often relate specifically to the body system being assessed. Therefore, in this chapter, questions to ask regarding risk factors for altered health are provided in the health history section of the assessment for each body area or system. In addition, it is important to assess patients for warning signs of cancer (Box 25-2).

Box 25-1 COMPONENTS OF A HEALTH HISTORY

Biographical Data

Biographical information is often collected during admission to a healthcare facility or agency and documented on a specific form. Biographical data include:

- Name
- Address
- Gender
- Marital status
- Occupation
- Religious preference
- Healthcare financing
- Primary healthcare provider

Reason for Seeking Healthcare

The patient's reason for seeking care helps to focus the rest of the assessment. Ask an open-ended question, such as, "Tell me why you are here today." Be sure to document in the patient's own words. For example, if Nina Dunning comes into the clinic and states, "I am having trouble sleeping. At night, I can't seem to stop my thoughts. All I do is worry."

Incorrect documentation: Patient complains of insomnia and anxiety.

Correct documentation: "I am having trouble sleeping. At night, I can't seem to stop my thoughts. All I do is worry."

History of Present Health Concern

When taking the patient's history of present health concern, be sure to explore the symptoms thoroughly. Sample questions include:

- "When did you first begin having this problem?" "Did it happen suddenly or slowly?"
- "Show me exactly where you are having this problem."
- "What other symptoms have you had with this problem?"
- "How have you treated this problem?"

Medical History

A patient's medical history may provide insight to causes of current symptoms. It also alerts the nurse to certain risk factors. Medical history includes past illnesses, chronic health problems and treatment, and previous surgeries or hospitalizations. Sample questions include:

- "Tell me about the childhood illnesses, such as measles or mumps, that you had."
- "What are you allergic to?"
- "Describe any accidents, injuries, and surgeries you have had."
- "What prescribed or over-the-counter medications do you use? Do you take any herbal or dietary supplements?"

Family History

Certain disorders have genetic links. For example, a family history of cancer is a risk factor for cancer. Sample family history questions include:

- "How old are the members of your family?"
- "If any members of your family are not living, what caused their death?"
- "Is there any history of this health problem you have in other family members?"
- "Do any family members have chronic illnesses?"

Lifestyle

A patient's lifestyle contributes to his or her overall health and well-being. For example, smoking is related to many health problems. Sample lifestyle questions include:

- "Do you smoke, drink, or use drugs? If so, for how long and how much?"
- "Describe the foods you eat during a typical day."
- "Tell me about how well you sleep."
- "How much exercise do you get each day?"
- "Who in your family or community is available to help you with health problems if you need it?"

PHYSICAL ASSESSMENT

A physical assessment is the systematic collection of objective information. The physical assessment is usually conducted in a head-to-toe sequence or a system sequence but can be adapted to meet the needs of the patient. It is often necessary to modify the sequence, positions, and specific assessments based on the patient's age, energy level, cognitive and physical state, as well as time constraints. Even when modified, the physical assessment should be conducted in an organized and knowledgeable manner. Conducting an accurate physical assessment takes time and practice. Table 25-1 summarizes the components of a comprehensive physical assessment.

Equipment

The equipment used in a physical assessment should be readily accessible, clean or sterile, in proper working order, and organized for the correct sequence of use (Fig. 25-2). Equipment that will touch the patient should be warmed (by the examiner's hands or warm water) before use. Not all the instruments described below will be needed in every assessment and some equipment, such as a tongue blade and penlight, are not included in this discussion. Beginning students will not conduct all elements of a complete physical assessment, but the instruments and techniques are discussed here to promote understanding of what is being done by more advanced practitioners.

Box 25-2 RISK FACTORS FOR CANCER: AMERICAN CANCER SOCIETY CAUTION MODEL

Change in bowel or bladder habits
A sore that does not heal
Unusual bleeding or discharge
Thickening or lump in the breast or elsewhere
Indigestion or difficulty in swallowing
Obvious change in wart or mole
Nagging cough or hoarseness

From the American Cancer Society.

Stethoscope

The stethoscope, illustrated and described in Chapter 24, is used to auscultate heart, lung, abdomen, and cardiovascular

TABLE • 25-1	SUMMARY OF A COMPREHENSIVE PHYSICAL ASSESSMENT	
Component	**Equipment (as needed)**	**Assessment Parameters**
General survey	• Scales • Sphygmomanometer • Stethoscope	• Observe general appearance, hygiene, posture, gait, thought processes, and speech patterns. • Evaluate height and weight. • Take vital signs.
Integument	• Gloves	• Skin: Inspect for color and lesions; palpate for temperature, texture, and moisture. • Hair: Inspect for texture, loss, unusual growth, and infestations. • Nails: Inspect for color and condition.
Head and neck	• Gloves • Snellen chart • Ophthalmoscope • Otoscope • Tongue depressor	• Skull and face: Inspect for shape and symmetry. • Neck: Palpate trachea and thyroid gland. • Lymph nodes: Palpate for size, shape, consistency, and tenderness. • Eyes: Test visual acuity, extraocular movements, and peripheral vision; inspect for discharge, alignment, and internal structures. • Ears: Test hearing acuity; inspect position, external ear, tympanic membrane, and for cerumen. • Nose, mouth, and throat: Inspect for color, consistency, condition of teeth, exudate, and condition of tonsils; palpate for tenderness.
Thorax and lungs	• Gloves • Stethoscope • Tape measure	• Thorax: Inspect posture and respiratory rate; palpate for crepitus and expansion; percuss for tones; auscultate breath sounds. • Breasts: Inspect size, shape, symmetry, color, areolas, nipple (discharge), retraction, and dimpling; palpate for masses or tenderness. • Axillary lymph nodes: Palpate for size, shape, consistency, and tenderness.
Cardiovascular	• Stethoscope • Watch with a second hand	• Carotid arteries: Auscultate for bruit; palpate pulse strength. • Jugular vein: Inspect for pulsations and distention. • Precordium: Inspect for pulsations; palpate apical impulse, pulsations, and heart rate and rhythm; auscultate heart sounds and murmurs.
Peripheral vascular	• Stethoscope • Doppler (if needed)	• Peripheral pulses: Palpate for symmetry, character, strength, rate, and patency • Arms and legs: Inspect for color, hair pattern, veins, lesions, and edema; palpate for temperature.
Abdomen	• Stethoscope	• Abdomen: Inspect for size, shape, contour, lesions, distention, and hernia; percuss for tones; palpate for tenderness. • Bowel sounds: Auscultate for intensity, frequency, and pitch. • Liver: Percuss and palpate for location and consistency/size; palpate for tenderness. • Aorta: Auscultate for bruits; inspect for pulsations. **Remember: Sequence of techniques is different for the abdomen:** **inspection, auscultation, percussion, and then palpation.**
Male genitalia	• Gloves	• Penis: Inspect for inflammation, infestations, rashes, lesions, masses, and discharge. Palpate for masses. • Scrotum and testes: Inspect for inflammation, edema, and lesions; palpate for masses.
Female genitalia	• Gloves • Speculum • Lubricant • Applicators • Culture tubes • Pap test supplies	• External genitalia: Inspect for inflammation, infestations, rashes, lesions, masses, discharge (color, odor, amount), swelling, and bulging out of vagina. • Uterus: Palpate for size, position, shape, and consistency. • Ovaries: Palpate for size, shape, mobility, and tenderness.
Anus, rectum, prostate	• Gloves • Lubricant • Occult blood test	• Anus: Inspect and palpate for hemorrhoids, lumps, ulcers, and fissures. • Stool: Inspect for color; test for occult blood. • Prostate: Palpate for size, shape, consistency, and tenderness.

(continued)

TABLE • 25-1   SUMMARY OF A COMPREHENSIVE PHYSICAL ASSESSMENT *(continued)*

Component	Equipment (as needed)	Assessment Parameters
Musculoskeletal	None	• Gait: Inspect gait and posture. • Joints and muscles: Inspect for size, symmetry, color, and edema; palpate for nodules, crepitus, and strength. • Joints: Test range of motion.
Neurologic	• Reflex hammer • Sharp/dull objects • Aromatic scents	• Mental status: Assess level of awareness; level of consciousness; dress, grooming, and hygiene; speech; thought processes; and memory and abstract reasoning. • Cranial nerves: Test ability to smell, see, clench teeth, move eyes, have facial expressions, hear, taste, feel touch, swallow, shrug shoulders against resistance, and protrude tongue. • Fine motor movement: Test ability to repeatedly touch nose with hand, pat knees with palms and backs of hands, and run heel down opposite shin. • Sensory: Test ability to distinguish between sharp and dull touch. • Reflexes: Assess degree of response.

Not all assessments on this table are discussed in the narrative. Please consult an assessment textbook for additional information.

sounds (Fig. 25-3). The bell of the stethoscope is used to listen to low-pitched sounds (such as heart murmurs). Use gentle pressure against the body part being examined when assessing low-pitched sounds. The diaphragm of the stethoscope is used to listen to high-pitched sounds such as normal heart sounds, breath sounds, and bowel sounds. Use firm pressure against the body part being examined when assessing high-pitched sounds. When using the stethoscope, expose the body part to be auscultated and try to minimize environmental noises.

Ophthalmoscope

An ophthalmoscope is a lighted instrument used to visualize the interior structures of the eye. It consists of two parts: a body that contains the light source and a detachable head that contains lenses used to magnify the internal eye structures. The head, which is secured in the body, contains a dial, which when depressed and turned, turns on the illumination. The head also contains several lenses arranged on a wheel to control the focus for examining the structures in the eye. Each lens is labeled with a positive (black) or negative (red) number, with units of strength called diopters. Red numbers are used for near-sighted (myopic) patients, black numbers for far-sighted (hyperopic) patients. The zero lens is used when either the examiner or the patient has refractive (visual) errors.

Otoscope

An otoscope is a lighted instrument used to examine the external ear canal and the tympanic membrane. A speculum, which is attached to the body of the otoscope, directs the light in a narrow beam to improve visualization of ear structures. Specula come in various sizes; use the largest speculum that will extend into the patient's ear canal.

Snellen Chart

The Snellen chart, used as a screening test for distant vision, consists of characters arranged in 11 lines of different-sized type; the line of largest characters is at the top of the chart and the line of smallest characters is at the bottom. Scores ranging from 20/10 (the smallest line of characters) to 20/200 (the largest line of characters) are shown in the left-hand column, and distances are in the right-hand column next to the numbers.

Nasal Speculum

A nasal speculum is used to visualize the lower and middle turbinates of the nose. A penlight or flashlight is used for illumination. The blades of the speculum are inserted about 1 cm (1/2″) into each nostril and opened so that they do not press on the septum. Alternatively, the otoscope can be used to visualize the internal nares. The light is provided by the scope, and the shortest, widest speculum that will fit into the nostril is used.

Vaginal Speculum

A vaginal speculum is a two-bladed instrument used to examine the vaginal canal and cervix. The speculum is inserted into the vagina and the speculum blades are opened, allowing visualization and assessment of the vagina and cervix. The speculum must be warmed and lubricated with warm water or a water-soluble agent before insertion.

> *Remember Ramona Lewis, the college student who reported that she was a victim of date rape. A vaginal examination would be crucial for collecting data to confirm the rape. Warming and lubricating the speculum would be very important to provide patient comfort during this extremely upsetting time.* ■

Ophthalmoscope and otoscope set

Ophthalmoscope

Otoscope

Snellen chart

Percussion hammer

Tuning forks

Vaginal speculum

FIGURE 25-2. Instruments used in the physical assessment. *(Photos by Ken Kasper.)*

Tuning Fork

A tuning fork is a two-pronged metal instrument used to test auditory function and vibratory perception. The fork is activated to vibrate by holding the base and gently tapping the prongs against the palm of the examiner's hand. Once vibrating, the fork is held at the base to avoid diminishing the vibration.

Percussion Hammer

A percussion hammer (also called a reflex hammer) is an instrument with a triangular-shaped rubber head, used to test deep tendon reflexes. The handle of the hammer is held between the thumb and index finger to direct a brisk tap of the broad end of the head on the selected body area. The quick, firm tap is made with a rapid downward and backward

FIGURE 25-3. Stethoscope bell and diaphragm. Use the **bell** of the stethoscope to detect low-pitched sounds. The bell should be at least 1 inch wide. Hold the bell lightly against the body part being auscultated. Use the **diaphragm** of the stethoscope to detect high-pitched sounds. The diaphragm should be at least 1.5 inches wide for adults and smaller for children. Hold the diaphragm firmly against the body part being auscultated.

wrist action. The pointed end of the hammer is used for smaller areas.

Positioning

A variety of positions are used during a physical assessment (Box 25-3). During positioning, it is important to consider the patient's age, culture, health status, mobility, physical condition, energy level, and privacy. Positioning patients who are weak or have physical limitations may require assistance. Uncomfortable or embarrassing positions should not be maintained for long periods. The assessment should be organized so that several body systems can be assessed with the patient in one position, thus minimizing unneeded and possibly tiring movements.

Draping

Draping prevents unnecessary exposure, provides privacy, and keeps the patient warm during the physical assessment. Drapes may be paper, cloth, or bed linens. When conducting an assessment, expose only the body parts being assessed to maintain the patient's modesty and comfort.

Techniques of Physical Assessment

The four primary assessment techniques are inspection, palpation, percussion, and auscultation. These techniques are most often used in the sequence listed; variations are noted in the discussion of specific body areas later in the chapter. Bilateral body parts are always compared; for example, the assessment findings of one leg are compared with those of the other leg. Bilateral body parts are normally symmetric; that is, they have the same size and shape as well as the same characteristics, such as movement or pulses.

Inspection

Inspection is the process of performing deliberate, purposeful observations in a systematic manner. The nurse observes visually but also uses hearing and smell to gather data throughout the assessment. Inspection begins with the initial patient contact and continues through the entire assessment. Adequate natural or artificial lighting is essential for distinguishing the color, texture, and moisture of body surfaces. A quiet environment allows sounds to be heard.

Each area of the body is inspected for size, color, shape, position, and symmetry, noting normal findings and any deviations from normal. Inspection, followed by palpation, may sequentially be used during the assessment of each body part.

Palpation

Palpation uses the sense of touch. The hands and fingers are sensitive tools and can assess skin temperature, turgor (turgor is determined by various factors, such as the amount of fluids in the body and age), texture, and moisture, as well as vibrations within the body (such as the heart) and shape or structures within the body (e.g., the bones). Specific parts of the hand are more effective at assessing different qualities (Fig. 25-4). The dorsum (back) surfaces of the hand and fingers are used for gross measure of temperature. The palmar (front) surfaces of the fingers and finger pads are used to assess texture, shape, fluid, size, consistency, and pulsation. Vibration is palpated best with the palm of the hand.

The nurse's hands should be warm and the fingernails short. When conducting palpation, any area of tenderness is palpated last. Light (gentle), moderate, or deep palpation may be used, controlling the depth by the amount of pressure applied. For light palpation, apply pressure with the fingers

FIGURE 25-4. (*Left*) Palmar surfaces of the examiner's fingertips and finger pads are used for discriminatory sensation such as texture, vibration, presence of fluid, or size and consistency of a mass. (*Right*) The dorsum, or back of the hand, is used to assess surface temperature.

Box 25-3   POSITIONS USED IN PHYSICAL ASSESSMENT

Standing

The patient stands erect. This position should not be used for patients who are weak, dizzy, or prone to fall. It is used to assess posture, balance, and gait (while walking upright).

Standing

Sitting

The patient may sit in a chair or on the side of the bed or examining table, or remain in bed with the head elevated. It allows visualization of the upper body, facilitates full lung expansion, and is used to assess vital signs and the head, neck, anterior and posterior thorax, lungs, heart, breasts, and upper extremities.

Sitting

Supine

The patient lies flat on the back with legs extended and knees slightly flexed. It facilitates abdominal muscle relaxation and is used to assess vital signs and the head, neck, anterior thorax, lungs, heart, breasts, abdomen, extremities, and peripheral pulses.

Supine

Dorsal Recumbent

The patient lies on the back with legs separated, knees flexed, and soles of the feet on the bed. It is used to assess the head, neck, anterior thorax, lungs, heart, breasts, extremities, and peripheral pulses. It should not be used for abdominal assessment because it causes contraction of the abdominal muscles.

Dorsal recumbent

Sims Position

The patient lies on either side with the lower arm below the body and the upper arm flexed at the shoulder and elbow. Both knees are flexed, with the upper leg more acutely flexed. It is used to assess the rectum or vagina.

Sims

Prone

The patient lies flat on the abdomen with the head turned to one side. It is used to assess the hip joint and the posterior thorax.

Prone

Lithotomy

The patient is in the dorsal recumbent position with the buttocks at the edge of the examining table and the heels in stirrups. It is used to assess female genitalia and rectum.

Lithotomy

Knee-chest

The patient kneels, with the body at a 90-degree angle to the hips, back straight, arms above the head. It is used to assess the anus and rectum.

Knee-chest

together and depressing the skin and underlying structures less than 1 cm (0.5″) (Fig. 25-5A). Moderate palpation is conducted by depressing the skin surface 1 to 2 cm (0.5″ to 0.75″). For deep palpation, press inward about 2 cm (1″) (see Fig. 25-5B). Deep palpation, which carries a risk of internal injury, should be used cautiously and only by experienced practitioners.

Applying intermittent pressure to a specific area allows assessment of surface characteristics and underlying structures. Two hands are used for bimanual palpation (e.g., palpating breast tissue); one hand applies pressure and the other hand feels the tissue or structure. Characteristics of masses, as determined by palpation, are described in Table 25-2.

Percussion

Percussion is the act of striking one object against another to produce sound. The sound waves produced by the striking action over body tissues are known as percussion tones. Percussion is used to assess the location, shape, size, and density of tissues.

Both hands are used to produce sound waves. The nurse's nondominant hand is placed directly on the area to be percussed, with the fingers slightly separated and the middle finger placed firmly on the body surface (Fig. 25-6A). The other hand (dominant hand) provides the striking force, initiated

TABLE • 25-2	CHARACTERISTICS OF MASSES DETERMINED BY PALPATION
Quality	**Characteristics to Determine**
Shape	Round Ovoid Tubular Irregular
Size	Measured in centimeters
Consistency	Firm Edematous Spongy Cystic
Surface	Smooth Nodular Granular
Mobility	Fixed or nonmobile Mobile
Tenderness	Amount of tenderness to touch
Pulsatile	Pulsation can or cannot be felt in the mass

by a sharp downward wrist movement with the forearm stationary and the wrist relaxed. The tip of the middle finger of the dominant hand strikes the middle finger of the opposing hand (Fig. 25-6B). This action produces a vibration that allows discrimination among five different tones, described in Table 25-3.

Auscultation

Auscultation is the act of listening with a stethoscope to sounds produced within the body. Auscultation is performed by placing the stethoscope diaphragm or bell against the body part being assessed. When auscultating, the nurse should expose the part listened to, use the proper part of the stethoscope (diaphragm or bell) for specific sounds (see previous discussion of a stethoscope), and listen in a quiet environment.

Four characteristics of sound are assessed by auscultation: (1) pitch (ranging from high to low), (2) loudness (ranging from soft to loud), (3) quality (e.g., gurgling or swishing), and (4) duration (short, medium, or long).

GUIDELINES FOR CONDUCTING A PHYSICAL ASSESSMENT

Although there are various organizing structures for conducting a physical assessment, one often used proceeds from head to toe. Although each body system is discussed individually here, in reality, nurses usually combine several systems (e.g., while assessing the head and neck they also assess the cranial nerves, which are part of the neurological

FIGURE 25-5. Degrees of palpation. (**A**) In light palpation, light pressure is applied by placing the fingers together and depressing the skin and underlying structures about 1 cm (½″). (**B**) Deep palpation is used with caution. The skin and underlying structures are depressed about 2 cm (1″). *(Photos by B. Proud.)*

FIGURE 25-6. Percussion is used to assess the location, shape, size, and density of tissues. (**A**) The nondominant hand is placed directly on the area to be percussed, and the middle finger is placed firmly on the body surface. (**B**) The tip of the middle finger of the dominant hand strikes the joint of the middle finger of the opposite hand *(Photos by B. Proud.)*

system). The accompanying head-to-toe assessment video demonstrates proper technique.

Performing a General Survey

The general survey is the first component of the physical assessment. It includes observing the patient's overall appearance and behavior, taking vital signs, and measuring height and weight. Information from the general survey provides clues to the patient's overall health.

TABLE • 25-3	**PERCUSSION TONES**	
Tone	**Relative Intensity**	**Sample Location**
Flat	Soft	Thigh
Dull	Medium	Liver
Resonance	Loud	Normal lung
Hyperresonance	Very loud	Emphysematous lung
Tympany	Loud	Gastric air bubble or puffed-out cheek

Appearance and Behavior

Information about the patient's appearance and behavior provides information about various aspects of the patient's health. While collecting information during the health history, inspect the patient's body build, posture, and gait. Note proportion of height to weight, which provides insight into nutritional status. Observe whether the patient has an erect or slumped posture and evaluate movements and gait pattern for coordination. Uncoordinated or spontaneous movements may suggest neurologic problems. Note signs of illness, such as changes in posture, skin color, and respirations; nonverbal communication of pain or distress; and short attention span.

Observe hygiene and grooming (cleanliness, body odors) and note any deficits, which may indicate other problems. For example, patients with inappropriate dress (e.g., wrong for the season) or worn or dirty clothing may be experiencing feelings of depression or have inadequate financial resources. Assess cognitive processes (speech content and patterns; orientation to person, place, and time; appropriate verbal responses). As cognitive processes are controlled by the neurological system, these are discussed later in the chapter.

Clues to mood and mental health are provided by speech, facial expressions, ability to relax, eye contact, and behavior. If depression, anxiety, or other mental health disorders are suspected, use appropriate screening tools and refer as necessary. Box 25-4 presents the Geriatric Depression Scale, a useful tool in screening older adults for depression. The questionnaire is given to patients to complete.

Vital Signs

Vital signs are measured to establish a baseline for the database and to detect actual or potential health problems. Vital signs are discussed in detail in Chapter 24.

Height and Weight

The ratio of height to weight is an assessment of overall health and overnutrition or undernutrition. Height and weight should be measured using accurate scales and measuring devices. The patient should remove shoes and heavy clothing if the measurements are taken before undressing (Guidelines for Nursing Care 25-1). If the patient cannot stand erect, weight can be obtained using a chair or bed scale. The patient's actual height and weight can be compared with recommended average weights on a standardized reference chart (Table 25-4) as a general guideline for assessing nutritional status and health.

Children to 2 years of age should have their height measured in the recumbent position with the legs fully extended. Infants should be weighed without any clothing, and children should be weighed in their underwear.

Assessing the Integument

The integument is comprised of the skin, nails, hair, and scalp. Assessing the integumentary structures provides information about the patient's overall health status, as well as clues to

Box 25-4   GERIATRIC DEPRESSION SCALE (GDS)

Instructions: Circle the answer that best describes how you felt over the <u>past week</u>.

1. Are you basically satisfied with your life?	yes	no
2. Have you dropped many of your activities and interests?	yes	no
3. Do you feel that your life is empty?	yes	no
4. Do you often get bored?	yes	no
5. Are you in good spirits most of the time?	yes	no
6. Are you afraid that something bad is going to happen to you?	yes	no
7. Do you feel happy most of the time?	yes	no
8. Do you often feel helpless?	yes	no
9. Do you prefer to stay at home, rather than going out and doing things?	yes	no
10. Do you feel that you have more problems with memory than most?	yes	no
11. Do you think it is wonderful to be alive now?	yes	no
12. Do you feel worthless the way you are now?	yes	no
13. Do you feel full of energy?	yes	no
14. Do you feel that your situation is hopeless?	yes	no
15. Do you think that most people are better off than you are?	yes	no

Total Score _____

Scoring Instructions: Score 1 point for "no" to questions 1, 5, 7, 11, and 13. Score 1 point for "yes" to other questions. A total score of 5 or more suggests depression.

Ref. Yesavage: The use of Rating Depression Series in the Elderly, in Poon (Ed.). (1986). Clinical memory assessment of older adults. American Psychological Association.

Guidelines for Nursing Care • 25-1

OBTAINING HEIGHT AND WEIGHT WITH AN UPRIGHT BALANCE SCALE

Obtaining Height

- Ask the patient to remove shoes.
- Raise L-shaped sliding arm on the measuring device attached to the scale somewhat higher than the patient's approximate height.
- Ask the patient to step on the platform of the scale and stand erect with the back to the measuring device and the heels together.
- Lower the L-shaped sliding arm until it rests on top of the patient's head.
- Read the height in inches and record.
- Ask the patient to step down from the platform.

Obtaining Weight

- Balance the scale on zero.
- Ask the patient to remove shoes (and coat, if appropriate) and step onto the platform.
- Move the sliding indicator to the left until the scale balances.
- Read the weight in pounds and record.
- Ask the patient to step down from the platform.
- Return the scale weight indicator to zero.
- Considerations: Daily weights should be obtained at the same time each day (usually early morning), with the patient wearing the same clothing, and using the same scale.

Photo by B. Proud.

TABLE • 25-4 HEIGHT AND WEIGHT TABLE

Height Men	Weight (lb) Men*			Height Women	Weight (lb) Women†		
	Small Frame	Medium Frame	Large Frame		Small Frame	Medium Frame	Large Frame
5' 2"	128–134	131–141	138–150	4' 10"	102–111	109–121	118–131
5' 3"	130–136	133–143	140–153	4' 11"	103–113	111–123	120–134
5' 4"	132–138	135–145	142–156	5' 0"	104–115	113–126	122–137
5' 5"	134–140	137–148	144–160	5' 1"	106–118	115–129	125–140
5' 6"	136–142	139–151	146–164	5' 2"	108–121	118–132	128–143
5' 7"	138–145	142–154	149–168	5' 3"	111–124	121–135	131–147
5' 8"	140–148	145–157	152–172	5' 4"	114–127	124–138	134–151
5' 9"	142–151	148–160	155–176	5' 5"	117–130	127–141	137–155
5' 10"	144–154	151–163	158–180	5' 6"	120–133	130–144	140–159
5' 11"	146–157	154–166	161–184	5' 7"	123–136	133–147	143–163
6' 0"	149–160	157–170	164–188	5' 8"	126–139	136–150	146–167
6' 1"	152–164	160–174	168–192	5' 9"	129–142	139–153	149–170
6' 2"	155–168	164–178	172–197	5' 10"	132–145	142–156	152–173
6' 3"	158–172	167–182	176–202	5' 11"	135–148	145–159	155–176
6' 4"	162–176	171–187	181–207	6' 0"	138–151	148–162	158–179

*Weights at ages 25 to 59 years are based on lowest mortality. Weights in pounds are according to frame (in indoor clothing weighing 5 lb, shoes with 1-inch heels).

†Weights at ages 25 to 59 years are based on lowest mortality. Weights in pounds are according to frame (in indoor clothing weighing 3 lb, shoes with 1-inch heels).

local or systemic health problems. It also provides data about self-care activities to maintain health, hygiene, and nutrition. Assessing for skin cancer is essential and provides the base for teaching skin cancer prevention.

Health History

Identify risk factors for altered health during the health history by asking about the following:

- History of rashes, lesions, change in color, or itching
- History of bruising or bleeding in the skin
- History of allergies to medications, plants, foods, or other substances
- Exposure to the sun and sunburn history
- Presence of lesions (wounds, bruises, abrasions, or burns)
- Change in the color, size, or shape of a mole
- Recent chemotherapy or radiation therapy
- Exposure to chemicals that may be harmful to the skin, hair, or nails
- Degree of mobility
- Types of food eaten and liquids consumed each day

Physical Assessment

The skin, hair, and nails are assessed by inspection and palpation. Ask the patient to remove all clothing and put on an examination gown. Have the patient sit for most of the exam-

ination but anticipate the need for the patient to stand or lie on the side when the posterior part of the body is examined. Protect the patient's privacy by exposing only the body part being examined. If the patient has lesions of the skin (including the scalp) or an infestation of the hair with lice, wear gloves during palpation.

The skin is a general indicator of the patient's health status and provides information that might indicate an underlying disease. Begin the assessment with an overall inspection of the skin's condition. Assess specific areas of the skin during other body system assessments (e.g., you may assess the skin on the abdomen while performing other abdominal assessments). Ensure adequate lighting, which is essential for accurate assessments. Inspect the skin for color, vascularity, and lesions (Fig. 25-7), and palpate for temperature, moisture, turgor, and texture.

INSPECTING SKIN COLOR

Skin color varies among races and among individuals, ranging from a pinkish white to various shades of brown. Skin areas that are normally exposed, such as the face and hands, may have a somewhat different color from areas that are usually covered by clothing, but otherwise skin color is relatively constant. Take special care to detect color changes in dark-skinned patients, such as Blacks, Hispanics, Native Americans, people of Mediterranean descent, and Whites who are deeply suntanned. Some body areas of dark-skinned

FIGURE 25-7. The skin is inspected for color, vascularity, and lesions. *(Photo by B. Proud.)*

people, such as the palms of the hands and the soles of the feet, normally have less pigmentation than other body areas.

Changes in skin color include erythema, cyanosis, jaundice, and pallor (Table 25-5). These color changes are often easier to assess in light-skinned people. **Erythema** (redness of the skin) is more often seen in the face and the neck. It is associated with sunburn, inflammation, fever, trauma, and allergic reactions.

▶ *Think back to Billy Collins, the child who was stung by a bee. The nurse would use inspection skills to observe for erythema in the area of the sting.* ■

Cyanosis is a bluish or grayish discoloration of the skin in response to inadequate oxygenation. Cyanosis is assessed as a blue tinge in patients with white skin and as dullness in patients with dark skin. **Jaundice** is a yellow color of

the skin resulting from liver and gallbladder disease, some types of anemia, and excessive hemolysis (breakdown of red blood cells). It usually develops first in the sclera of the eyes and then in the skin and mucous membranes. Jaundice in dark-skinned people is more difficult to observe on the trunk of the body, but the sclera, oral mucous membranes, palms, and soles appear yellow to yellow-orange. **Pallor,** or paleness of the skin, often results from a decrease in the amount of circulating blood or hemoglobin, causing inadequate oxygenation of the body tissues. Depending on severity, pallor may be visible over the entire skin surface or only in the lips, nailbeds, mucous membranes, and conjunctiva. Pallor in dark-skinned people is seen as an ashen gray or yellow tinge.

INSPECTING SKIN VASCULARITY AND LESIONS

The skin is inspected for vascularity, bleeding, or bruising; these signs might relate to a cardiovascular, hematologic, or liver dysfunction. **Ecchymosis** is a collection of blood in the subcutaneous tissues, causing purplish discoloration. **Petechiae** are small hemorrhagic spots caused by capillary bleeding. If they are present, assess their location, color, and size.

▶ *Remember Ramona Lewis, the college student reporting a rape. The nurse would inspect the patient for signs and symptoms of trauma, including any ecchymosis. These findings would be important objective data to help substantiate the rape.* ■

Lesions are areas of diseased or injured tissue such as bruises, scratches, cuts, burns, insect bites, and wounds (breaks in the continuity of the skin). Lesions are categorized as primary or secondary. Primary lesions are those that may arise from previously normal skin (Table 25-6). Secondary

TABLE • 25-5	SKIN COLOR ASSESSMENT	
Color Variations	**Assessment Areas**	**Possible Causes**
Redness (erythema; flushing)	Facial area, localized area of skin on the body	Blushing, alcohol intake, fever, injury trauma, infection
Bluish (cyanosis)	Exposed areas, particularly the ears, lips, inside of the mouth, hands and feet, and nailbeds	Cold environment, cardiac or respiratory disease (decreased oxygenation)
Yellowish (jaundice)	Overall skin areas, mucous membranes, and sclera	Liver disease (increase in bilirubin levels)
Paleness (pallor)	Exposed areas, particularly the face and lips, conjunctivae, and mucous membranes	Anemia (decreased hemoglobin) Shock (decreased blood volume)
Vitiligo (whitish patchy areas on the skin)	Overall skin areas, lips, nailbeds, and conjunctivae	Depigmentation (congenital or autoimmune conditions)
Tanned or brown	Sun-exposed areas	Overexposure (increased melanin production), pregnancy (brown spots)

TABLE • 25-6	**PRIMARY SKIN LESIONS**		
Lesion Name	**Description**	**Example**	**Illustration**

Circumscribed, Flat, Nonpalpable Change in Skin Color

Macule	Lesion ≤1 cm	Petechiae, freckle	

Macule

Patch	Lesion >1 cm	Vitiligo	

Patch

Palpable, Elevated Solid Masses

Papule	Mass ≤0.5 cm	Mole	

Papule

Plaque	Mass >0.5 cm	Coalesced papules	

Plaque

Nodule	Mass 0.5–2 cm; firmer than a papule	Nevus (wart)	

Nodule

(continued)

TABLE • 25-6   PRIMARY SKIN LESIONS *(continued)*

Lesion Name	Description	Example	Illustration
Palpable, Elevated Solid Masses *(continued)*			
Tumor	Mass >2 cm	Lipoma	Tumor
Wheal	Irregular, superficial area of localized skin edema	Hives, mosquito bite	Wheal
Circumscribed, Superficial Skin Elevations Formed by Free Fluid in a Cavity Within the Skin Layers			
Vesicle	Filled with serous fluid, ≤0.5 cm	Herpes simplex	Vesicle
Bulla	Filled with serous fluid, >0.5 cm	2nd-degree burn	Bulla
Pustule	Filled with pus	Acne, impetigo	Pustule

Pustule

TABLE • 25-7	SECONDARY AND MISCELLANEOUS SKIN LESIONS	
Lesion Name	**Description**	**Example**
Secondary Lesions		
Loss of Skin Surface		
Erosion	Loss of superficial epidermis, moist, nonbleeding surface	Moist area after rupture of a vesicle, as in chickenpox
Ulcer	Loss of epidermis and dermis, may bleed and scar	Stasis ulcer
Fissure	Deep linear crack, extends into dermis	Athlete's foot
Material on the Skin Surface		
Crust	Dried residue of serum, pus, or blood	Impetigo
Scale	Thin flake of exfoliated dermis	Dandruff, dry skin
Miscellaneous Lesions		
Lichenification	Thickened and roughened epidermis, with increased visibility of skin furrows	Atrophic dermatitis
Atrophy	Thinning of the skin, loss of skin furrows, shiny appearance	Peripheral vascular disease
Excoriation	Scratch of the epidermis	
Scar	Fibrous tissue replaces tissue in the dermis or subcutaneous layer	
Keloid	Hypertrophied scar	
Other Common Skin Lesions, Not Technically Primary or Secondary		
Comedo	Plugged opening of a sebaceous gland, a hallmark of acne	Common blackhead
Telangiectasia	Small, dilated, red or bluish surface vessels; may be part of a basal cell carcinoma or skin injury from radiation	
Nevus	Flat to slightly elevated, round, evenly pigmented	Common mole

lesions result from changes in primary lesions (Table 25-7). Assess lesions and wounds for size, shape, depth, location, and presence of drainage or odor. (Wounds are discussed in Chapter 32.) Scars are healed wounds. Describe rashes (skin eruptions) in terms of their type, size, elevation, coloring, and presence of drainage or itching. Document the exact body surface areas involved.

PALPATING SKIN TEMPERATURE, TEXTURE, MOISTURE, AND TURGOR

The skin is normally warm and dry. An increase in skin temperature and moisture can indicate an elevated body temperature. The texture of the skin varies from smooth and soft to rough and dry. In the dehydrated patient, the texture is dry, loose, and wrinkled, and the mucous membranes are cracked and dry. An excessive amount of perspiration, such as when the entire skin is moist, is called diaphoresis.

Turgor is the fullness or elasticity of the skin. It is usually assessed on the sternum or under the clavicle by lifting a fold of skin with the thumb and first finger. Skin turgor is normal when the fold returns to its usual shape when released. When the patient is dehydrated, the skin's elasticity is decreased, and the skin fold returns slowly. However, this may be a normal finding in older patients (Fig. 25-8).

Difficulty in lifting a skin fold may indicate **edema** (excess fluid in the tissues). Edema is characterized by swelling, with taut and shiny skin over the edematous area. If the area of edema is palpated with the fingers, an indentation (measured in mm for depth of the indentation) may remain after the pressure is released; if the indentation is

very deep, it is called pitting edema. Edema may be graded as 0 (none), +1 (trace, 2 mm), +2 (moderate, 4 mm), +3 (deep, 6 mm), or +4 (very deep, 8 mm). Edema may be the result of overhydration, heart failure, kidney failure, trauma, or peripheral vascular disease.

INSPECTING THE NAILS

The nails are inspected for shape, angle, texture, and color. The nails should be somewhat convex and should follow the natural curve of the finger. The angle between the nail and its base should be about 160 degrees. The nails should be smooth, and the nail base, when palpated, should

FIGURE 25-8. To assess skin turgor, a small fold of skin is picked up and then released to return to its normal shape. Difficulty in lifting a skin fold may indicate presence of edema. *(Photo by B. Proud.)*

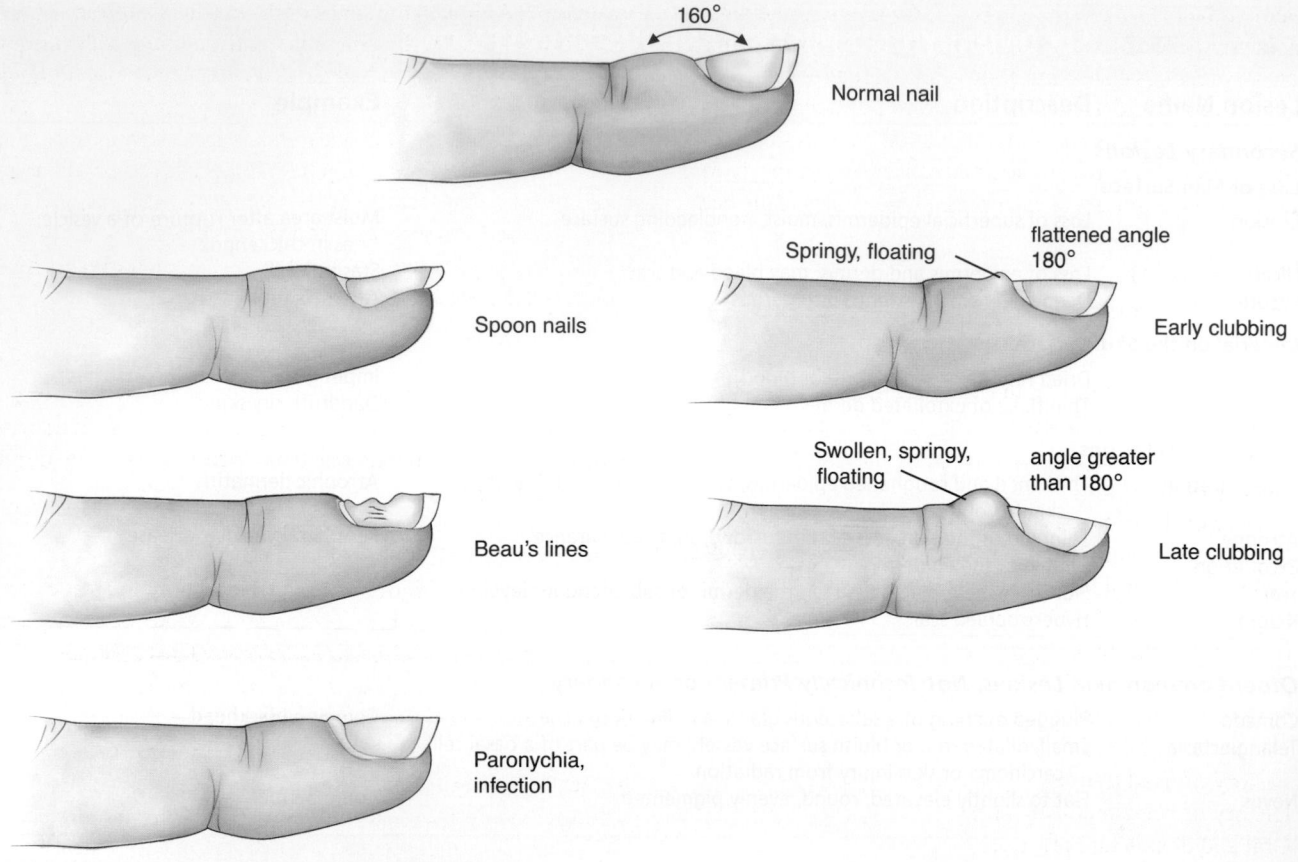

FIGURE 25-9. Examples of nail abnormalities.

be firm and nontender. Abnormal findings include indentations called Beau's lines (from acute illness), infection, painless separation of the nail plate from the nailbed (onycholysis) due to infection or trauma, increased brittleness or thickness and angulation (from anemia or iron deficiency anemia), and clubbing (from long-term lack of oxygenation). Figure 25-9 illustrates nail abnormalities.

INSPECTING THE HAIR AND SCALP

Hair is found on all body surfaces except the palms of the hands, the soles of the feet, and parts of the genitalia. Assess the hair for color, texture, and distribution. The hair is normally resilient, evenly distributed, and neither excessively dry nor oily. Abnormal findings include unusual balding (alopecia) and excessive amounts of hair on the face and body (hirsutism). Hair loss may be normal or may be the result of chemotherapy, radiation therapy, infection, hormonal disorders, or inadequate nutrition. Decreased oxygenation of peripheral tissues, especially of the lower extremities, may cause loss of hair. Excessive hair growth may occur in persons with hormonal disorders.

Separate the hair to inspect the scalp for color, dryness, scaliness, lumps, lesions, or lice. Nits, which are the white eggs of lice, can be differentiated from dandruff or lint because they are attached to the hair shaft. If any lumps or masses are palpated, note their location, size, tenderness, and mobility.

Normal Age-Related Variations

INFANT/CHILD

Common skin variations in newborns and children include:

- Jaundice and milia (whiteheads) in newborns
- Fine downy hair (lanugo) for the first 2 weeks of life
- Smooth, thin skin at birth
- Pubic hair development at the onset of puberty

OLDER ADULT

Common skin variations in the older adult include:

- Wrinkles, dryness, scaling, decreased turgor
- Raised dark areas (senile keratosis)
- Flat brown age spots (senile lentigines)
- Small round red spots (cherry angioma)
- Fine, brittle gray or white hair
- Hair loss
- Coarse facial hair in women, decreased body hair in men and women
- Thick, yellow toenails

Assessing the Head and Neck

Assessment of the head and neck includes the skull, face, eyes, ears, nose and sinuses, mouth and pharynx, trachea, thyroid gland, and lymph nodes. During the health history, note any health problems such as headaches or dizziness. If the patient smokes, include a discussion about ways to stop smoking in the plan of care. Physical examination of the structures of the head and neck provides data about the shape and structure of cranial bones, function of special senses (sight, hearing, taste, smell), nasal and oral structures, the size and consistency of the thyroid gland, and any swelling or pain in the lymph nodes in the neck.

Health History

Identify risk factors for altered health during the health history by asking about the following:

- Changes in vision or hearing with aging
- History of use of corrective lenses or hearing aids
- Loss of an eye (use of artificial eye)
- History of allergies
- History of disturbances in vision or hearing
- History of chronic illnesses such as hypertension, diabetes mellitus, or thyroid disease
- Exposure to harmful substances or loud noises
- Exposure to ultraviolet light
- History of smoking (how long, how many packs/day), chewing tobacco, or cocaine use
- History of eye or ear infections
- History of head trauma
- History of persistent hoarseness
- Oral and dental care practices

Physical Assessment

Assess the structures of the head and neck with the patient in a sitting position.

INSPECTING AND PALPATING THE HEAD AND FACE

Inspect and palpate the head for size and shape. The parts of the head and face should be in proportion to each other and symmetric. Although the shape of the normal skull varies considerably, generally the shape is gently curved with prominences at the frontal and parietal bones. Abnormal findings include lack of symmetry or unusual size or contour of the skull (either may be the result of trauma or diseases affecting the growth of bone) and tenderness. If the skull of a child or an adult appears disproportionately large or small, measure the circumference. Measuring head circumference is a normal part of infant assessment to the age of 2 years and should be conducted at each health-related visit.

Inspect the face for color, symmetry, and distribution of facial hair. Edema of the face, especially around the eye (periorbital edema), and involuntary facial movements (e.g., tics, fasciculations, tremors) are abnormal findings. If abnormalities are noted, document their location, amount, duration, and timing.

INSPECTING THE EYES

The structures (Fig. 25-10) and functions of the eyes are assessed by using a penlight, an ophthalmoscope, and an eye chart. Inspection is the primary assessment technique used. Assessment includes the external and internal eye structures, visual acuity, extraocular movements, and peripheral vision.

Inspecting External Eye Structures

The eyes, eyebrows, eyelids, eyelashes, lacrimal glands, pupils, and iris are inspected for position and alignment (Fig. 25-11). Asymmetry of position and alignment of the eyes may be caused by muscle weakness or a congenital abnormality. The eyebrows should be equally distributed; the eyelashes should curl outward.

Inspect the eyelids for color, edema, and equal coverage of the eyeball. Abnormal findings include drooping of the upper lids (ptosis), which may be attributable to damage to the oculomotor nerve, myasthenia gravis, or a congenital

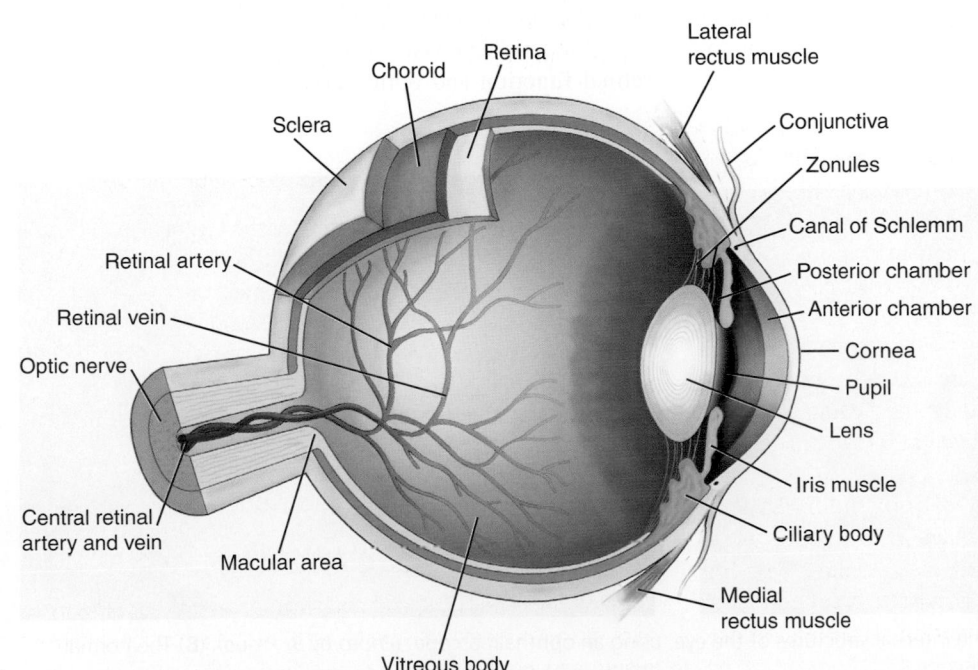

FIGURE 25-10. A cross-section of the eye.

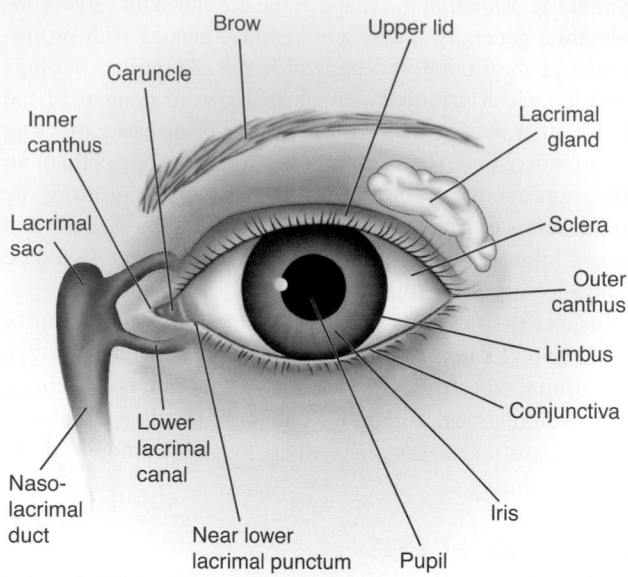

Brow
Upper lid
Caruncle
Inner canthus
Lacrimal gland
Lacrimal sac
Sclera
Outer canthus
Limbus
Conjunctiva
Lower lacrimal canal
Naso-lacrimal duct
Near lower lacrimal punctum
Iris
Pupil

FIGURE 25-11. The eye and surrounding structures.

disorder; inward turning of the lower lid and lashes (entropion); outward turning of the lower lid and lashes (ectropion); and redness or drainage (from infection of the lid margins, conjunctivae, or hair follicles). Inspect and palpate the lacrimal glands for edema and pain.

The pupils are normally black, equal in size, round, and smooth. The pupils may be pale and cloudy if the patient has cataracts (loss of opacity of the lens). Injury to the eye, glaucoma, and certain medications may cause the pupil to dilate (mydriasis); certain drugs can cause constriction (miosis), and unequal pupils may result from central nervous system injury or illness.

Assess the pupils for reaction to light and accommodation and for convergence (Guidelines for Nursing Care 25-2). Decreased or absent pupillary response indicates blindness or serious brain damage. Inability of the eyes to accommodate or converge is abnormal.

Inspecting Internal Eye Structures

The internal eye is examined with the ophthalmoscope (Fig. 25-12A) to assess the fundus, including the retina, optic nerve disc, macula, fovea centralis, and retinal vessels. Normal findings are a uniform red reflex; a clear, yellow optic nerve disc; a reddish retina; and light-red arteries and dark-red veins, the veins being about 1.5 times as large as the arteries (Fig. 25-12B). Abnormal findings include cloudiness of the lens (from cataracts), changes in the size and shape of blood vessels (from hypertension or arteriosclerosis), and changes in color and surface characteristics (from such health problems as diabetes mellitus, hypertension, trauma, inflammation, or a detached retina).

Using the ophthalmoscope is an advanced technique and takes practice. Guidelines for Nursing Care 25-3 highlights the key steps for assessing the internal eye.

Assessing Visual Acuity, Extraocular Movements, and Peripheral Vision

Visual acuity is assessed with the Snellen chart. Have the patient stand 20 feet from the chart and ask the patient to read the smallest line of letters possible, first with both eyes and then with one eye at a time (with the opposite eye covered). Note whether the patient's vision is being tested with or without corrective lenses.

Visual acuity is measured by using the standardized numbers listed on the side of the chart. The numerator is 20, representing the distance from which a person with normal vision (recorded as 20/20) can read the letters. The denominator represents the smallest line read accurately by the patient. Visual acuity is recorded as a fraction and is written as 20 over the smallest line read by the patient with no more than two inaccurate readings (such as "20/30–2 with glasses"). Thus, the larger the denominator, the poorer the vision.

Test extraocular movements by assessing the cardinal fields of vision for coordination and alignment. Normally both eyes move together, are coordinated, and are parallel. Tests for peripheral vision (or visual fields) are used to assess retinal function and optic nerve function. Full peripheral

FIGURE 25-12. (A) Examination of the internal structures of the eye, using an ophthalmoscope. *(Photo by B. Proud).* **(B)** The normal fundus as seen through an ophthalmoscope.

Guidelines for Nursing Care • 25-2

MEASURING PUPILLARY REACTION, SIZE, ACCOMMODATION, AND CONVERGENCE

Pupillary Reaction

- Ask the patient to look straight ahead.
- Bring the penlight from the side of the patient's face and briefly shine the light on the pupil (Figure A).
- Observe the pupil's reaction; it normally rapidly constricts (direct response) also pupil size (Figure B).
- Repeat the procedure and observe the other eye; it too normally will constrict (consensual reflex).
- Repeat the procedure with the other eye.

FIGURE A. Assessing pupillary reaction.

FIGURE B. Pupillary gauge measures pupils (dilation or constriction) in millimeters (mm).

Accommodation

- Hold the forefinger, a pencil, or other straight object about 10 to 15 cm (4″ to 6″) from the bridge of the patient's nose (Figure C).
- Ask the patient to first look at the object, then at a distant object, then back to the object being held. The pupil normally constricts when looking at a near object and dilates when looking at a distant object.

FIGURE C. Assessing accommodation.

(continued)

Guidelines for Nursing Care • 25-2

MEASURING PUPILLARY REACTION, SIZE, ACCOMMODATION, AND CONVERGENCE *continued*

Convergence

- Hold your finger about 6″ to 8″ from the bridge of the patient's nose.
- Move your finger toward the patient's nose to assess convergence (Figure D). The patient's eyes should normally converge (assume a cross-eyed appearance).

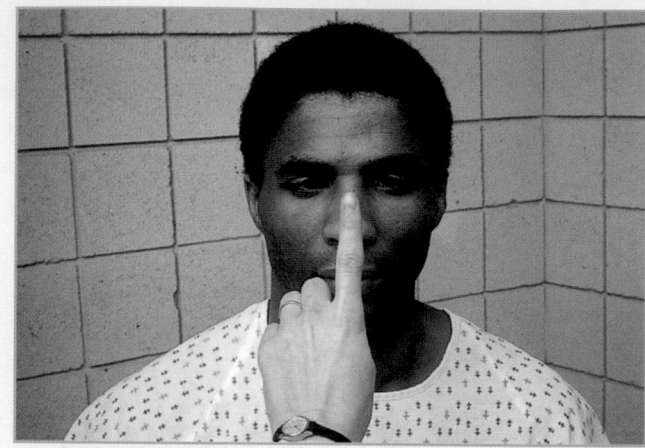

FIGURE D. Assessing convergence.

vision is normal. Guidelines for Nursing Care 25-4 describe how to assess extraocular movements and peripheral vision.

INSPECTING AND PALPATING THE EARS

The external ear is assessed by inspection and palpation. The middle ear and tympanic membrane are assessed by inspection (Fig. 25-13). An otoscope with the correct size of ear speculum is used to inspect the ear canal and tympanic membrane. A tuning fork and ticking watch are used to assess hearing acuity.

Inspecting and Palpating the External Ear

Inspect the external ear (Fig. 25-14) for shape, size, and lesions. The external surfaces of the ear should be smooth, and the shape and size of the ears should be symmetric and proportional to the head. Abnormal findings include unequal height and size, uneven color, and lesions. Gently palpate the external ear for pain, edema, or presence of lesions. Pain when manipulating the pinna is a symptom of an infection of the external ear.

Guidelines for Nursing Care • 25-3

ASSESSING THE INTERNAL EYE

- Assemble the ophthalmoscope. Begin with the light setting at the large white light and the lens wheel at 0 setting.
- Darken the room and have the patient remove glasses. Allow time for the patient's pupils to dilate. The patient should be sitting.
- Sit facing the patient and ask him or her to look straight ahead during the examination.
- Keep both eyes open while looking through the ophthalmoscope viewer.
- Use your right hand and eye to examine the patient's right eye, and your left hand and eye for the patient's left eye.
- Shine the light on the pupil and observe the round red or orange glow (the red reflex).

- Focusing on the red reflex, slowly move the ophthalmoscope toward the patient's eye.
- Rotate the lens wheel until internal eye structures are sharp and clear.
- Follow blood vessels toward the midline to locate the optic disc; note color, size, shape, margins, and central area (physiologic cup).
- Follow blood vessels outward to each of the four quadrants, assessing color, size, and pattern.
- Ask the patient to look up, down, and from side to side, assessing the characteristics of the retina.
- Locate the macula by first locating the optic disc and then looking toward the patient's temple for a small circular structure near the disc; note color, characteristics, and area of reflected light (fovea centralis).

Guidelines for Nursing Care • 25-4

ASSESSING EXTRAOCULAR MOVEMENTS AND PERIPHERAL VISION

Extraocular Movements

- Ask the patient to sit or stand about 2 feet away, facing you sitting or standing at eye level with the patient.
- Ask the patient to hold the head still and follow the movement of your forefinger or a penlight with the eyes.
- Keeping your finger or light about 1 foot from the patient's face, move it slowly through the cardinal positions: up and down, left and right, diagonally up and down to the left, diagonally up and down to the right (see Figure).

Peripheral Vision

- Have the patient stand or sit about 2 feet away, facing you at eye level.
- Ask the patient to cover one eye with a hand or an index card.
- Ask the patient to look directly at your nose and fix his or her eyes on that spot.
- Cover your own eye opposite the patient's closed eye.
- Hold one arm outstretched to one side (right or left) equidistant from you and the patient, and move your fingers into the visual fields from various peripheral points.
- Ask the patient to tell you when the fingers are first seen (both you and the patient should see the fingers at the same time).
- Repeat the procedure for the other eye.

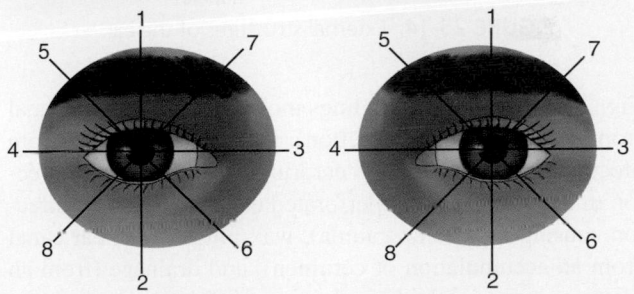

Testing extraocular movement of the eye.

Inspecting the Ear Canal and Tympanic Membrane

The otoscope is used to examine the ear canal and the tympanic membrane. Attach the largest speculum that will fit comfortably into the patient's ear to the otoscope. Insert the otoscope speculum as the patient's head is slightly tilted away from the examiner. To achieve better visualization, straighten the ear canal of the adult by gently pulling the pinna up and back. In children younger than 3 years of age, straighten the ear canal by pulling the pinna down and back.

The ear canal should be smooth and pink. Examine the canal for wax, discharge, and foreign bodies. The tympanic membrane should be intact, translucent, shiny, and gray

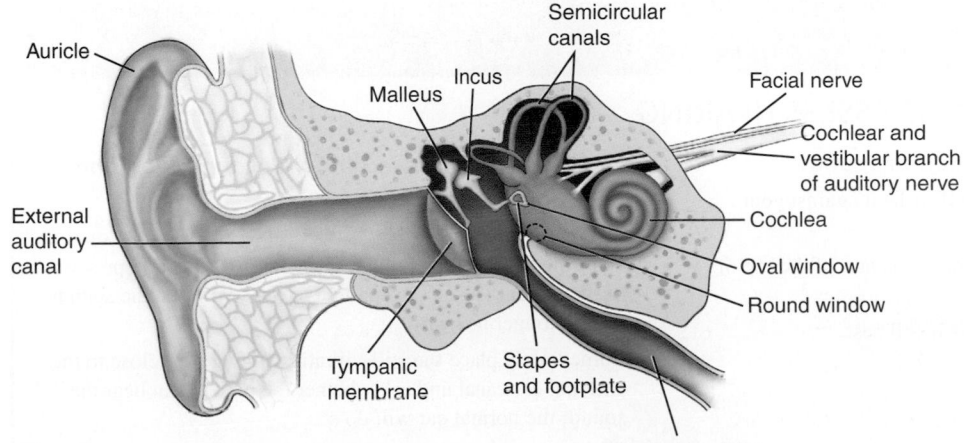

FIGURE 25-13. Internal structures of the ear.

FIGURE 25-14. External structures of the ear.

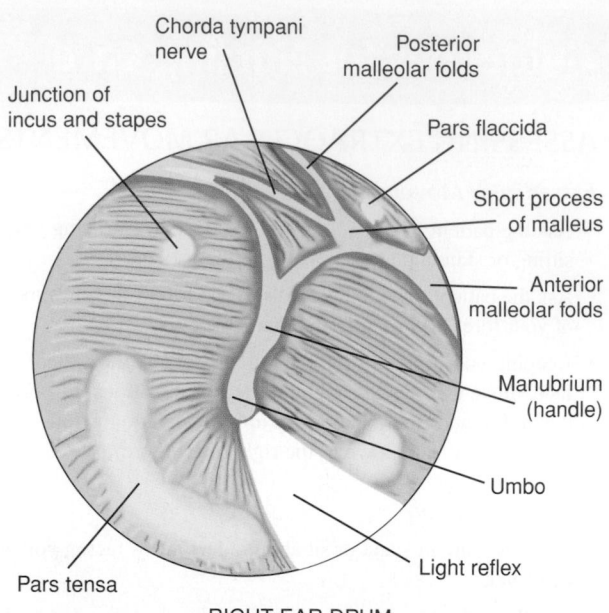

RIGHT EAR DRUM

FIGURE 25-15. Normal tympanic membrane, as seen through an otoscope.

(Fig. 25-15). Abnormal findings include redness of the canal (from inflammation or infection), mastoid tenderness (from infection), a red and swollen eardrum (symptoms of an infection in the middle ear), a perforated eardrum (from an infection causing rupture or trauma), wax plugs in the ear canal (from an accumulation of cerumen), and drainage (from an infection or foreign body in the ear canal).

Assessing Hearing and Sound Conduction

Hearing is assessed in one ear at a time by determining whether the patient can hear a whispered voice or a ticking watch from a distance of 1 to 2 feet. Assess hearing acuity out of the patient's line of vision (to prevent lip reading), with the opposite ear covered.

Tuning fork tests, such as the Weber and Rinne tests, help assess the type of hearing loss: conductive (the result of a problem with the transmission of sound waves through the outer and middle ear), sensorineural (from inner ear dam-

age), or a combination of both. Guidelines for Nursing Care 25-5 discusses how to assess hearing with a tuning fork.

The Weber test is used to assess for bone conduction of sound. With this test, the sound is normally heard in both ears or is localized at the center of the head. Patients with conductive hearing loss hear the sound better in the affected ear. If the sound is heard better in the ear without a problem, it indicates damage to the inner ear or a nerve disorder. The Rinne test is used to compare bone and air conduction of sound. With this test, hearing of air-conducted sound is normally greater than bone-conducted sound (documented as AC > BC). If the hearing loss is conductive, sound of bone conduction will be the same or greater than air conduction.

INSPECTING THE NOSE

Assessment of the nose involves examining the external nose, the nares, and the turbinates (Fig. 25-16). Inspect the

Guidelines for Nursing Care • 25-5

USING A TUNING FORK TO ASSESS HEARING

Weber's Test for Bone Conduction of Sound

- Hold the tuning fork at its base and strike it against your other palm so that the fork vibrates.
- Place the base of the tuning fork on the center of the top of the patient's head.
- Ask the patient where the sound is heard best.

Rinne's Test to Compare Air Conduction With Bone Conduction of Sound

- Strike the tuning fork as for Weber's test.
- Hold the base of the tuning fork against the mastoid process of the patient and ask the patient to tell you when the sound can no longer be heard.
- Immediately place the still-vibrating tuning fork close to the external ear canal and ask whether the patient can hear the sound; the normal ear will do so.
- Repeat the test with the other ear.

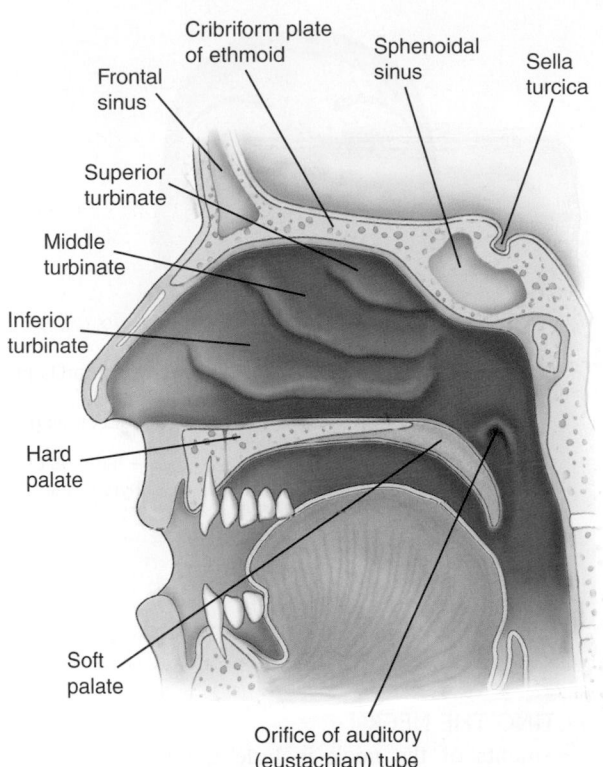

FIGURE 25-16. Cross-section of the nasal cavity.

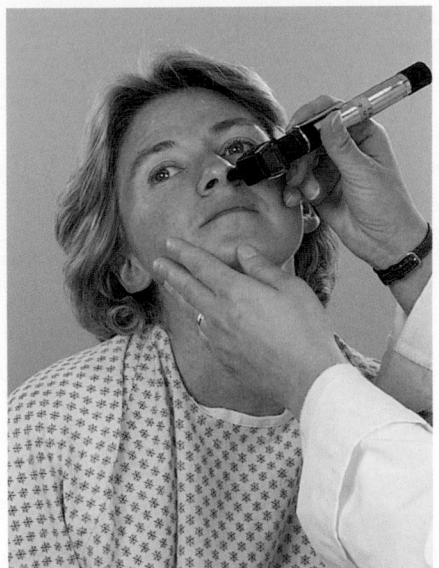

FIGURE 25-17. Examination of the nasal passages using an otoscope with a wide speculum. *(Photo by B. Proud.)*

nose and inspect and palpate the sinuses with the patient sitting and his or her head slightly tilted back.

Assess the nose for patency by occluding one nostril at a time and asking the patient to inhale and exhale through the nose. Inspect each nostril using an otoscope with a short, wide tip or using a nasal speculum and penlight (Fig. 25-17). It is not necessary to use a nasal speculum with a child; push the tip of the nose upward with your thumb and shine a light into the nares. Examine the mucous membranes for color and the presence of lesions, exudate, or growths. Also, inspect the nasal septum for intactness and deviation.

Normally, the nasal mucosa is moist and darker red than is the oral mucosa. Abnormal findings are swelling of the mucosa, bleeding or discharge (indicating allergies with inflammation or infection), perforation or deviation of the nasal septum (cocaine use may cause perforation; a deviated septum may be congenital or from trauma), and polyps (often seen with chronic allergies).

PALPATING THE SINUSES

The frontal and maxillary sinuses, located in the frontal and maxillary bones, respectively, are palpated for pain and edema. The frontal sinuses are palpated by gently pressing upward on the bony prominences located above each eye. The maxillary sinuses are palpated by gentle pressure on the bony prominences of the upper cheek (Fig. 25-18). Normally, the sinuses are not painful when

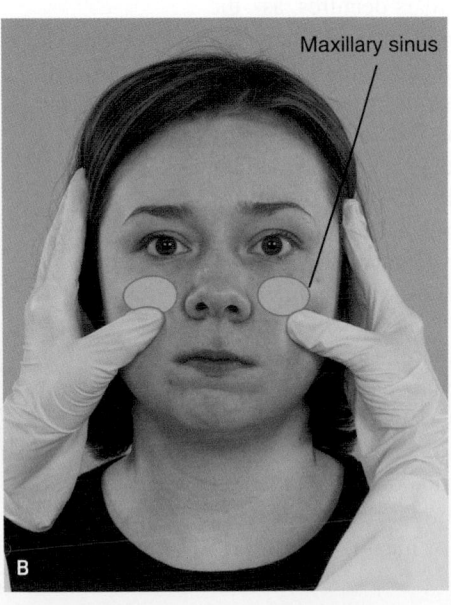

FIGURE 25-18. (**A**) The frontal sinuses are palpated by gently pressing upward on the bony prominences above each eye. (**B**) The maxillary sinuses are palpated by applying gentle pressure on the bony prominences of the upper cheek. *(Photos by B. Proud.)*

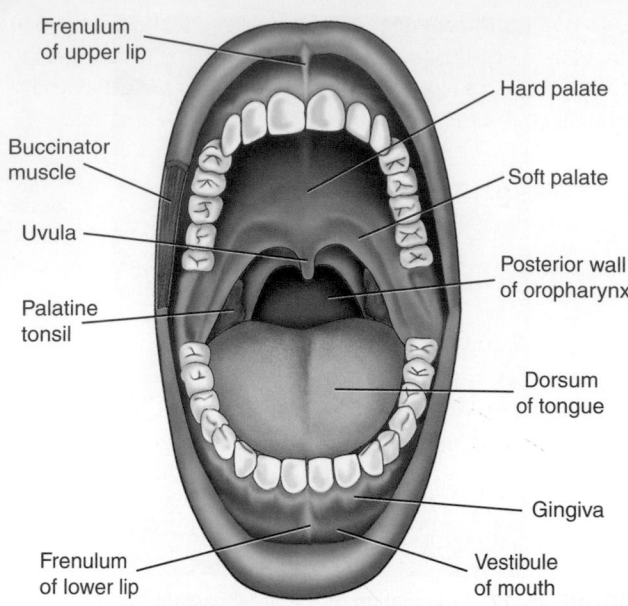

FIGURE 25-19. Structures of the mouth.

FIGURE 25-20. Structures of the neck.

palpated. Pain may be a finding if the sinuses are infected or obstructed.

INSPECTING THE MOUTH AND PHARYNX

The mouth and pharynx include the lips, tongue, teeth, gums, hard and soft palate, salivary gland, tonsillar pillars, and tonsils (Fig. 25-19). Equipment used to assess the mouth, pharynx, and neck includes a penlight, a tongue blade, a 4″ × 4″ gauze sponge, and gloves.

Assess the mouth and pharynx by inspecting the lips, gums and teeth, tongue, and hard and soft palates. Have the patient sit with the head tilted backward and the mouth opened wide. Use palpation if any abnormalities are noted during inspection. Wear gloves when assessing a patient's mouth and use 4″ × 4″ gauze to hold the tongue for palpation.

The lips should be pink, moist, and smooth. The tongue and mucous membranes are normally pink, moist, and free of swelling or lesions. If the patient wears dentures, ask the patient to remove them for inspection of the gums and roof of the mouth. The gums should be pink and smooth. With the patient's tongue relaxed on the floor of the mouth, examine the mucous membrane of the oropharynx while depressing the base of the tongue with a tongue depressor. The uvula is normally centered and freely movable. The tonsils, if present, are small, pink, and symmetric in size. The teeth should be regular and free of cavities or have dental restoration.

Abnormal findings are pallor, cyanosis, or redness and swelling of the mucous membranes; lesions of the mucosa and lips; swollen, red tonsils (indicating infection); swollen, red, and bleeding gums (from nutritional deficits, inflammation or infection, poorly fitted dentures, or poor oral hygiene); poorly aligned, missing, or carious teeth; a white coating on the tongue (from poor oral hygiene, irritation, or smoking); a fissured tongue (from dehydration); a bright-red tongue (seen in deficiencies of iron, vitamin B_{12}, or niacin); or a black, hairy tongue (from antibiotic use).

INSPECTING THE NECK

Assessments of the neck include the trachea, lymph nodes, and thyroid gland (Fig. 25-20). Assess the neck with the patient sitting and the neck slightly hyperextended. Ask the patient to tilt the head backward, forward, and side to side to assess range of motion. The neck should be symmetric, with full range of motion. Also assess the neck for venous distention. No neck vein distention (indicating heart problems) should be visible.

Palpating the Trachea and Lymph Nodes

The trachea, normally midline at the suprasternal notch, is palpated for alignment and position. An unequal space between the trachea and the sternocleidomastoid muscle on each side is an abnormal finding indicating tracheal displacement.

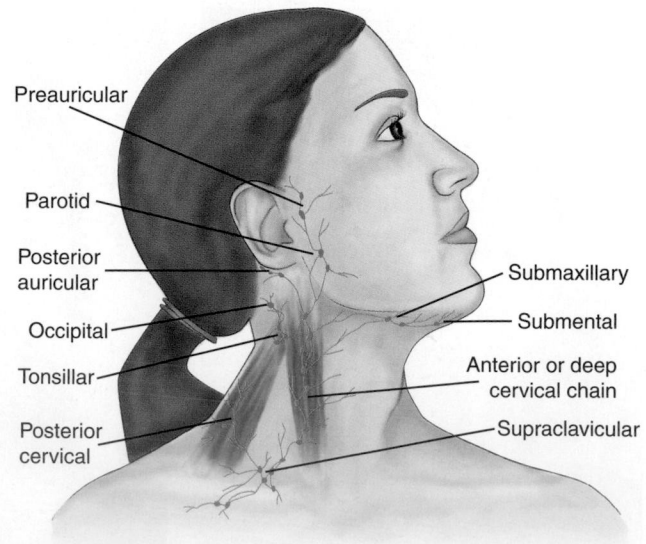

FIGURE 25-21. Location of the lymph nodes of the neck.

Palpate the lymph nodes (Fig. 25-21) with the pads of the fingers for enlargement, tenderness, and mobility. The nodes are generally not palpable; if palpable, they should be small, mobile, smooth, and nontender. If lymph nodes are palpable, assess location, size, consistency, mobility, and tenderness. Enlarged lymph nodes (lymphadenopathy) may indicate infection, autoimmune disorders, or metastasis of cancer.

Palpating the Thyroid Gland

Assess the thyroid gland using palpation, keeping in mind that the gland is not palpable in all patients. Use an anterior or posterior approach to palpate the thyroid gland with the patient in a sitting position (Guidelines for Nursing Care 25-6). Palpate for size, shape, symmetry, tenderness, and presence of any nodules. If palpable, the thyroid gland should feel soft but elastic. It should be nontender and should have no enlargement, masses, or nodules (which may indicate thyroid gland disease, infection of the thyroid, or cancer).

Normal Age-Related Variations

INFANT/CHILD

Common head and neck variations in newborns and children include:

- Closing of posterior fontanel at 8 weeks of age; soft anterior fontanel at about 18 months of age
- Gazing at and following bright objects by 1 month of age
- Focusing with both eyes by 6 months of age

Guidelines for Nursing Care • 25-6

PALPATING THE THYROID GLAND

Posterior Approach

- Standing behind the patient, place your hands around the patient's neck, with the fingertips over the lower half of the neck and trachea (see Figure A).
- Ask the patient to swallow, and feel for enlargement of the gland as it rises.
- Palpate each lobe of the thyroid by having the patient turn the head slightly toward the side to be examined; then gently displace the trachea with one hand.
- Ask the patient to swallow, and palpate the thyroid with the other hand.
- Repeat for the other side.

Anterior Approach

- Standing facing the patient, place the fingers of your left hand around the sternomastoid muscle (see Figure B).
- Ask the patient to swallow, and palpate (using the right hand) for enlargement.
- Repeat for the other side.

Palpating the thyroid (**A**) using a posterior approach. (**B**) Using an anterior approach. *(Photos by B. Proud.)*

- Pupils at the inner folds (pseudostrabismus)
- Startle reflex in newborns

OLDER ADULT

Common head and neck variations in the older adult include:

- Impaired near vision (presbyopia)
- Decreased color vision and peripheral vision
- Decreased adaptation to light and dark
- A white ring around the cornea (arcus senilis)
- Entropion and ectropion
- Hearing loss (presbycusis)
- Impaired conductive hearing
- Elongated ear lobes
- Prominent ear landmarks
- Decreased neck range of motion
- Nodular thyroid gland
- Smaller, more easily palpated lymph glands

Assessing the Thorax and Lungs

The thorax (Fig. 25-22) comprises the lungs, rib cage, cartilage, and intercostal muscles. Data from the health history may elicit a health problem, such as dyspnea or chest pain, as well as information about sleep patterns, cough, and sputum. A history of smoking indicates the need to include ways to stop smoking in the plan of care. Environmental exposure to certain inhalants (such as second-hand smoke, paint, air pollution, or asbestos fibers) in the home or workplace may increase the risk of respiratory diseases and cancer. Physical examination provides data about the bony structures of the thorax, respiratory effort, chest expansion, and breath sounds.

Health History

Identify risk factors for altered health during the health history by asking about the following:

- History of trauma to the ribs or lung surgery
- Number of pillows used when sleeping
- History of chest pain with deep breathing
- History of persistent cough with or without producing sputum
- History of allergies
- Environmental exposure to chemicals, asbestos, or smoke
- History of smoking (how long, how many packs/day)
- History of lung disease in family members or self
- History of frequent or chronic respiratory infections

Physical Assessment

Physical assessment of the thorax and lungs requires a stethoscope and a tape measure. The environment should be warm and adequately lit. The techniques for this assessment include inspection, palpation, percussion, and auscultation. The patient sits during the assessment. Percussion of the thorax is a more advanced procedure. Information about this assessment is included in nursing assessment texts.

FIGURE 25-22. Thoracic landmarks (**A**) Anterior. (**B**) Posterior.

INSPECTING THE THORAX

Begin inspection by observing the patient's chest for color, shape or contour, breathing patterns, and muscle development. The color should be even and consistent with the color of the patient's face. The shape or contour should have a downward equal slope at the rib cage. The chest should be symmetric, with the transverse diameter greater than the anteroposterior diameter. An increased anteroposterior diameter, as seen in chronic lung diseases, is described as barrel-chest (Fig. 25-23). Respirations should be smooth and even, ranging from 12 to 20 breaths/min.

Abnormal findings include an increase in chest size and contour, abnormal breathing patterns with use of accessory muscles (symptoms of respiratory disease, such as chronic obstructive pulmonary disease or asthma), unequal chest expansion (may occur in chest trauma or pneumonia), and abnormal respirations.

PALPATING THE THORAX

Palpation is used to detect areas of sensitivity, chest expansion during respirations, and vibrations (fremitus). Use the palmar surface of the hands to palpate the anterior and posterior thoracic landmarks (Fig. 25-24) in a sequential pattern for temperature, moisture, muscular development, and any tenderness or masses. The skin should be warm and dry, with symmetric muscular development, and no tenderness, masses, or vibrations. Abnormal findings may be cool or excessively dry or moist skin, muscle asymmetry, tenderness, masses, and vibrations.

Chest expansion is determined by placing the hands over the posterior chest wall, with the fingers at the level of T9 or T10. Ask the patient to take a deep breath, and observe the movement of your thumbs. The thorax should expand symmetrically (Fig. 25-25).

Normal adult chest   Barrel chest

FIGURE 25-23. Profile and anteroposterior diameter of normal adult chest and barrel chest.

AUSCULTATING BREATH SOUNDS

Auscultation is used to detect airflow within the respiratory tract. Ask the patient to breathe slowly and deeply through the mouth. Place the warmed diaphragm of the stethoscope over the thoracic landmarks and auscultate breath sounds in the same sequential pattern as used for palpation (see Fig. 25-24). Normally, breath sounds result from the free movement of air

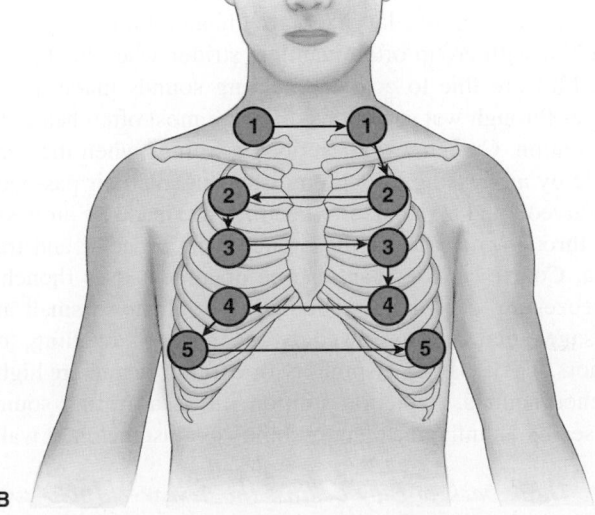

A   B

FIGURE 25-24. Posterior (**A**) and anterior (**B**) chest—landmarks and systematic sequence of assessment. The pattern is used for palpation, percussion, and auscultation of the chest.

FIGURE 25-25. Palpating the posterior thorax excursion. The examiner's hands are placed symmetrically on the patient's back (**A**). As the patient inhales, the examiner's hands should move apart symmetrically (**B**). *(Photos by B. Proud.)*

into and out of all parts of the bronchial tree. Listen for the duration, pitch, and intensity of the sounds.

Normal breath sounds (Table 25-8) vary over different parts of the lungs. **Bronchial sounds** heard over the trachea are high-pitched, harsh sounds, with expiration being longer than inspiration. **Bronchovesicular sounds** are heard over the mainstem bronchus and are moderate "blowing" sounds, with inspiration equal to expiration. **Vesicular breath sounds** are soft, low-pitched sounds, heard best over the base of the lungs during inspiration, which is longer than expiration.

Adventitious breath sounds are not normally heard in the lungs but, if present, may be auscultated (Table 25-9). Stertorous breathing is a general term used to refer to noisy, strenuous respirations. Stridor is a harsh, high-pitched sound heard on inspiration when there is a narrowing of the upper airway, such as the larynx or trachea. Infants or young children with croup often manifest stridor when breathing. Crackles are fine to coarse crackling sounds made as air moves through wet secretions; they are most often heard on inspiration. Crackles are described as "fine" when they are made by air passing through moisture in small air passages and alveoli and as "coarse" when they are made by air passing through moisture in the bronchioles, bronchi, and trachea. Coarse crackles can also be documented as rhonchi. Wheezes are continuous sounds that originate in small air passages that are narrowed by secretions, swelling, or tumors. They may be inspiratory or expiratory and are high-pitched sounds. A pleural friction rub is a grating sound caused by an inflamed pleura rubbing against the chest wall.

> *Think back to Billy Collins, the 9-year-old who was stung by a bee. Incorporating knowledge of the signs and symptoms of an allergic reaction, the nurse would inspect Billy's chest for accessory muscle use and auscultate his lungs, noting any evidence of wheezing, which is commonly noted with allergic reactions.* ■

Although stertorous respirations, stridor, and wheezes can be heard without amplification, crackles and pleural friction rubs are usually heard only by auscultation with a stethoscope. If a productive cough occurs during assessment of the thorax and lungs, the sputum should be assessed for color, consistency, and amount.

Normal Age-Related Variations

INFANT/CHILD

Common thorax and lung variations in newborns and children include:

- Louder breath sounds on auscultation
- More rapid respiratory rate (until 8 to 10 years of age)
- Use of abdominal muscles during respiration

OLDER ADULT

Common thorax and lung variations in older adults include:

- Increased anteroposterior chest diameter
- Increase in the dorsal spinal curve (kyphosis)
- Decreased thoracic expansion
- Use of accessory muscles to exhale

Assessing the Cardiovascular and Peripheral Vascular Systems

Cardiovascular and peripheral vascular assessment includes assessment of the heart and the extremities. Questions in the health history can identify supporting subjective data such as

TABLE • 25-8   NORMAL BREATH SOUNDS

Type, Description, and Location	Ratio of Inspiration to Expiration
Bronchial or Tubular Anterior Blowing, hollow sounds; auscultated over the trachea	Inspiration / Expiration Expiration is longer, lower, and higher-pitched than inspiration
Bronchovesicular First and second interspaces Anterior Posterior Medium-pitched, medium intensity, blowing sounds; auscultated over the first and second interspaces anteriorly and the scapula posteriorly	Inspiration Expiration Inspiration and expiration have similar pitch and duration
Vesicular Anterior Posterior Soft, low-pitched sounds; auscultated over the lung periphery	Expiration Inspiration Inspiration is longer, louder, and higher-pitched than expiration

leg pain, chest pain, or dyspnea on exertion. Data can also be used to identify activities of daily living and health behaviors that increase the risk of cardiovascular disease, including smoking, lack of exercise, and a diet high in calories, fats, and salt. If these risks are identified, the plan of care should include referral for additional diagnostic testing and teaching about health promotion activities. The physical examination is used to identify signs and symptoms of heart disease and peripheral vascular disease (most often found in the lower extremities).

Health History

Identify risk factors for altered health during the health history by asking about the following:

- History of chest pain, palpitations, or dizziness
- Swelling in the ankles and feet
- Number of pillows used to sleep
- Type and amount of medications taken daily
- History of heart defect, rheumatic fever, or chest or heart surgery
- Personal and family history of hypertension (high blood pressure), myocardial infarction (heart attack), coronary artery disease, high blood cholesterol levels, or diabetes mellitus
- History of smoking (how long, how many packs/day)
- History of alcohol use
- Type and amount of exercise
- Usual foods eaten each day

TABLE • 25-9	ABNORMAL BREATH SOUNDS
Type and Characteristics	**Illustration**
Wheeze (Sibilant) • Musical or squeaking • High-pitched, continuous sounds • Auscultated during inspiration and expiration • Occurs in small air passages	
Wheeze (Sonorous) • Sonorous or coarse • Low-pitched, continuous sounds • Auscultated during inspiration and expiration • Coughing may clear the sound	
Crackles • Bubbling, crackling, popping • Low- to high-pitched, discontinuous sounds • Auscultated during inspiration • Occurs in small air passages, alveoli, bronchioles, bronchi, and trachea	
Friction Rub • Rubbing or grating • Loudest over lower lateral anterior surface • Auscultated during inspiration and expiration	

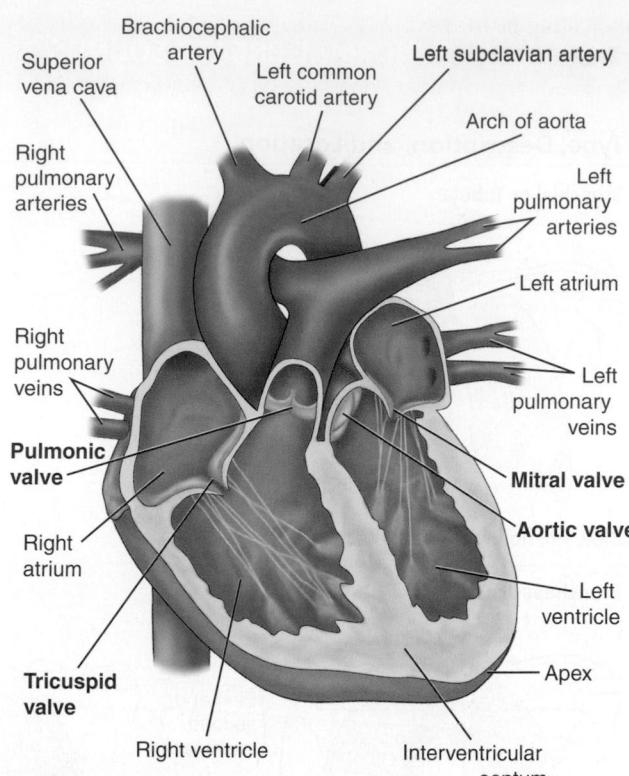

FIGURE 25-26. View of the interior of the heart showing the atrioventricular and semilunar valves responsible for normal heart sounds.

• Changes in color or temperature of the extremities
• History of pain in the legs when sleeping or pain that is worsened by walking
• History of blood clots or sores on the legs that do not heal

Physical Assessment

The techniques used for cardiovascular assessment are inspection, palpation, and auscultation. Necessary equipment includes a stethoscope with a bell and diaphragm and a sphygmomanometer. The patient may be in a sitting position or in a supine position with the head raised about 30 degrees. Adequate lighting is essential for inspection of color and for pulsations. A quiet environment is necessary for accurate auscultation of heart sounds. The nurse is usually positioned at the right side of the patient. Figure 25-26 provides a view of the heart, including the heart valves responsible for heart sounds.

Peripheral vascular assessment includes measuring the blood pressure and assessing the skin and perfusion of the extremities and the peripheral pulses. Assessments are made by inspection and palpation, with the patient sitting or supine. Peripheral vascular assessments may be combined with assessment of other body areas.

INSPECTING THE NECK AND PRECORDIUM

Observe the neck and **precordium** (the portion of the body over the heart and lower thorax, encompassing the

aortic, pulmonic, tricuspid, and apical areas, and Erb's point) (Fig. 25-27) for visible pulsations. Pulsations usually are absent except for the apical impulse, located at about the fourth or fifth intercostal space at the left midclavicular line. Inspect the epigastric area at the tip of the sternum for pulsation of the abdominal aorta. Findings of neck vein distention

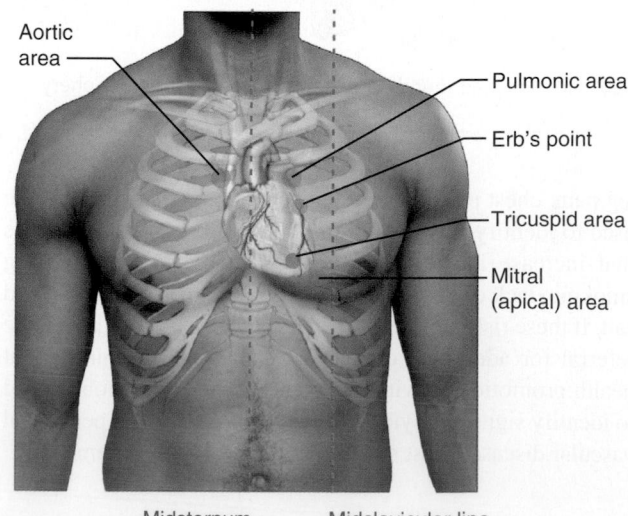

FIGURE 25-27. The precordium with the traditional cardiac landmarks and areas for auscultation.

(indicating heart disease) or visible pulsations in precordial areas other than the apical impulse (which may result from abnormalities of the ventricle) are considered abnormal.

PALPATING THE PRECORDIUM

Using the palmar surface of the hand with the four fingers held together, palpate the precordium gently for pulsations (Fig. 25-28). Remember to warm your hands. Palpate in a systematic manner, assessing specific cardiac landmarks—the aortic, pulmonic, tricuspid, and mitral areas and Erb's point.

FIGURE 25-28. Palpating areas of the precordium: (**A**) aortic area, (**B**) pulmonic area, and (**C**) apical (mitral) and tricuspid area. *(Photos by Ken Kasper.)*

Palpate the apical impulse in the mitral area. Note size, duration, force, and location in relationship to the midclavicular line. Normal findings include no pulsation palpable over the aortic and pulmonic areas, with a palpable apical impulse. Abnormal findings include precordial thrills, which are fine, palpable, rushing vibrations over the right or left second intercostal space, and lifts or heaves, which involve a rise along the border of the sternum with each heartbeat.

AUSCULTATING HEART SOUNDS

Auscultation is used to determine the heart sounds caused by closure of the heart valves. Ask the patient to breathe normally. Use systematic auscultation, beginning at the aortic area, moving to the pulmonic area, then to Erb's point, then to the tricuspid area, and finally to the mitral area (see Fig. 25-27). Use the diaphragm of the stethoscope first to listen to high-pitched sounds. Then use the bell to listen to low-pitched sounds. Focus on the overall rate and rhythm of the heart and the normal heart sounds (Box 25-5).

INSPECTING THE EXTREMITIES

Inspect the skin of the extremities for color, temperature, continuity, lesions (as described previously for assessment of the integument), venous patterns, and edema. Normally, venous patterns, varicosities, rashes, ulcers, or edema are absent on the lower extremities. However, if the patient has peripheral vascular disease (resulting in decreased blood flow and oxygenation of tissues), the skin of the lower extremities is typically pale and cool, shiny with brown discolorations, and hairless. The toenails are thickened. Phlebitis (inflammation of a vein) of the lower extremity is indicated by pain, redness, and swelling of the affected calf or thigh.

PALPATING PERIPHERAL PULSES

Use the pads of the index and middle fingers to palpate peripheral pulses for amplitude and symmetry. Palpate, carefully and one at a time, the carotid, brachial, radial, femoral, popliteal, dorsalis pedis, and posterior tibial pulses (see Fig. 24-4 in Chapter 24). These should be strong and equal bilaterally. The amplitude of the pulses may be documented as 0 (absent), 1+ (weak), 2+ (normal), 3+ (increased), or 4+ (bounding).

Abnormal findings include an absent, weak, thready pulse (which may indicate a decreased cardiac output), a forceful or bounding pulse (seen in hypertension and circulatory fluid overload), and an asymmetric pulse (related to impaired circulation). Other specific assessments to determine arterial blood flow include Allen's test, Buerger's test, and capillary refill (Guidelines for Nursing Care 25-7).

Normal Age-Related Variations
INFANT/CHILD

Common cardiovascular and peripheral vascular variations in newborns and children include:

* Visible cardiac pulsation if the chest wall is thin
* Sinus dysrhythmia (the rate increases with inspiration and decreases with expiration)

Box 25-5 HEART AND CARDIOVASCULAR SOUNDS

Normal Heart Sounds

During auscultation, the first heart sound, called S_1, is heard as the "lub" of "lub-dub." This sound occurs when the mitral and tricuspid valves close and corresponds to the onset of ventricular contraction (see figure). The sound, low-pitched and dull, is heard best at the apical area. The second heart sound, S_2, occurs at the termination of systole and corresponds to the onset of ventricular diastole. The "dub" of "lub-dub" represents the closure of the aortic and pulmonic valves. The sound of S_2 is higher pitched and shorter than S_1. The two sounds occur within 1 second or less, depending on the heart rate.

Normal findings include S_1 that is louder at the tricuspid and apical areas, with S_2 louder at the aortic and pulmonic areas.

Heart sounds in relation to the cardiac cycle and an electrocardiogram.

Abnormal Heart Sounds

Abnormal findings include extra heart sounds at any of the cardiac landmarks and abnormal rate or rhythm. Extra heart sounds are often heard when the patient has anemia or heart disease. A wide variety of conditions may alter the normal heart rate or rhythm, including serious infections, diseases of the heart muscle or conducting system, dehydration or overhydration, endocrine disorders, respiratory disorders, and head trauma. Extra heart sounds may be S_3, S_4, murmurs, or bruits.

S_3 and S_4

S_3, known as the third heart sound, is often represented by a "lub-dub-dee" pattern ("dee" being S_3); this sound is best heard with the stethoscope bell at the mitral area, with the patient lying on the left side. S_3 is considered normal in children and young adults and abnormal in middle-aged and older adults.

S_4 is the fourth heart sound, represented by "dee-lub-dub." S_4 is considered normal in older adults but abnormal in children and adults.

Murmurs

Heart murmurs are extra heart sounds caused by some disruption of blood flow through the heart. The characteristics of a murmur depend on the adequacy of valve function, rate of blood flow, and size of the valve opening. Grading of heart murmurs:

Grade	Description
I	A murmur so faint that it can be heard only with great effort
II	A faint murmur but one that can be easily detected
III	A moderately loud murmur
IV	A very loud murmur that is usually associated with a thrill sound
V	An extremely loud murmur
VI	An exceptionally loud murmur that can be heard while the stethoscope is lifted off the skin

Bruits

Bruits, which are abnormal sounds, are "swooshing" sounds similar to murmurs and are heard over major blood vessels. The sound indicates a partially blocked artery, causing blood to swirl, rather than flow normally. Bruits are most commonly heard over the carotid arteries, the abdominal aorta, and the femoral arteries.

- Presence of S_3 (in about one third of all children)
- More rapid heart rate (until about 8 years of age)

OLDER ADULT

Common cardiovascular and peripheral vascular variations in older adults include:

- Difficult-to-palpate apical pulse
- Difficult-to-palpate distal arteries
- Dilated proximal arteries
- More prominent and tortuous blood vessels; varicosities common
- Increased systolic and diastolic blood pressure
- Widening pulse pressure

Guidelines for Nursing Care • 25-7

ASSESSING PERIPHERAL CIRCULATION

Allen's Test

- Ask the patient to rest his or her hand on the examining table with the palm up and to make a fist.
- Use your thumbs to occlude the radial and ulnar arteries and ask the patient to open his or her hand (the palm will be pale).
- Release your thumb pressure and observe the return of color to the palm (this should normally take 3 to 5 seconds).

Buerger's Test

- Ask the patient to assume a supine position and then raise one arm or one leg about 1 foot (30 cm) above the level of his or her heart.

- Ask the patient to briskly move the leg or arm up and down for 1 minute, then to sit up and dangle the arm or leg downward.
- Observe the time it takes for the original color of the patient's skin to return and for the veins to fill. Normally, color returns in 10 seconds, and veins fill in 15 seconds.

Capillary Refill

- Using your thumb and forefinger, squeeze the patient's fingernail or toenail until it appears white.
- Release the pressure and observe the time it takes for normal color to return. Normally, color returns immediately.
- Assess capillary refill in children by pressing the skin lightly over the forehead or top of the hand. Release the pressure; observe the time for return of color.

Assessing the Breasts and Axillae

Each breast has a lymphatic network that drains into the underlying axilla (Fig. 25-29). Although the assessments and disorders described here focus on the female breast, men also are at risk for breast disease. The health history elicits risk factors for cancer of the breast, especially in females. Physical assessment of the breasts and axilla are primarily conducted to identify any lumps in the breasts and/or enlargement or pain in axillary lymph nodes; if assessed, the patient should have further diagnostic tests.

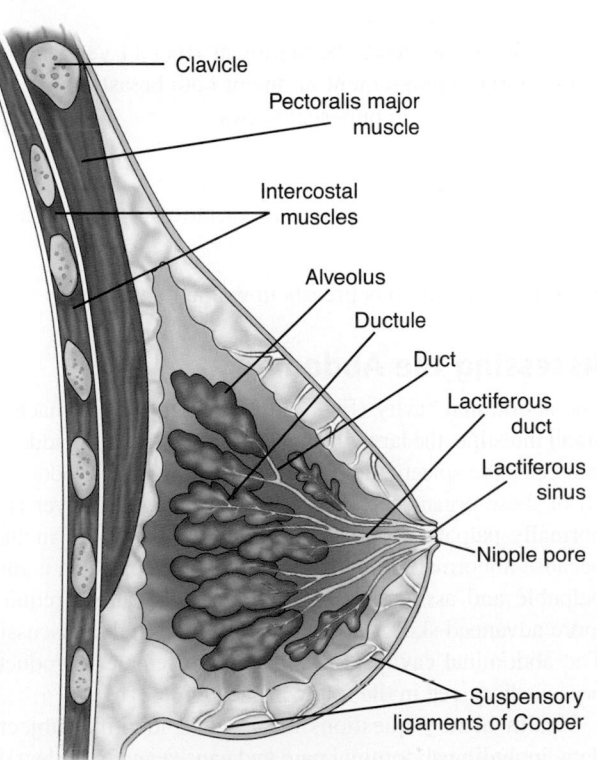

FIGURE 25-29. Lateral view of the female breast.

Clavicle
Pectoralis major muscle
Intercostal muscles
Alveolus
Ductule
Duct
Lactiferous duct
Lactiferous sinus
Nipple pore
Suspensory ligaments of Cooper

Health History

Identify risk factors for altered health during the health history by asking about the following:

- History of pain in one or both breasts, including relationship to menstrual period
- History of lumps or swelling, redness, change in size, or dimpling in the breasts
- History of discharge from the breast
- Family history of ovarian or breast cancer
- History of breast disease, biopsy, or surgery
- Menstrual and pregnancy history
- Use of hormones, oral contraceptives
- Exposure to radiation, benzene, or asbestos
- Usual dietary intake and alcohol consumption
- Knowledge and practice of breast self-examination
- Most recent clinical breast examination and mammogram

Physical Assessment

The breasts and axilla are assessed in both men and women using inspection and palpation. The patient can be sitting or lying supine. When sitting, the patient should sit erect, with arms at sides or raised overhead. When supine, the patient's hand on the side being examined is placed under the head.

INSPECTING THE BREASTS

Inspect the breasts for size, shape, symmetry, color, texture, and skin lesions. The breasts should be relatively symmetric, although variations are normal. The size varies among individuals. The shape of the breasts is round and smooth, and there should be no skin depressions (retraction) or puckering (dimpling). The color should be consistent with the rest of the skin, and the texture of the skin should be soft.

Inspect the areola and nipples for size and shape and the nipples for discharge, crusting, and inversion. The areolar and nipple areas should be equal in size, round or oval, with a smooth surface. Montgomery's tubercles (sebaceous glands on the areolae of the breasts) are a normal component of the areola. The nipples are normally everted. Discharge from the nipples is an abnormal finding except in pregnancy (leaking is normal during pregnancy and breastfeeding). Other abnormal findings include dimpling, lesions, and asymmetry.

PALPATING THE BREASTS AND AXILLAE

Palpate the breasts in each of the four quadrants (the upper outer quadrant, the lower outer quadrant, the upper inner quadrant, and the lower inner quadrant) to detect any abnormal lumps (Fig. 25-30). Guidelines for Nursing Care 25-8 provides instructions for palpation.

Palpate the nipple and areola and gently compress the nipple between the thumb and forefinger to assess for discharge. The breast tissue should be smooth and firm, with a granular consistency. If a mass is detected, carefully assess its location, size, shape, consistency, and tenderness. The breasts are normally tender during the week before menstruation.

An increase in the nodularity and tenderness of the breasts may be associated with the menstrual period or may indicate fibrocystic disease. Discharge, lumps, lesions, dimpling, asymmetry, and palpable lymph nodes may be indicative of breast cancer.

Palpate the axillary areas for lymph nodes (Fig. 25-31), which normally are nonpalpable and nontender. If any nodes are palpable, assess their location, size, shape, consistency, tenderness, and mobility. Palpable lymph nodes are an abnormal finding.

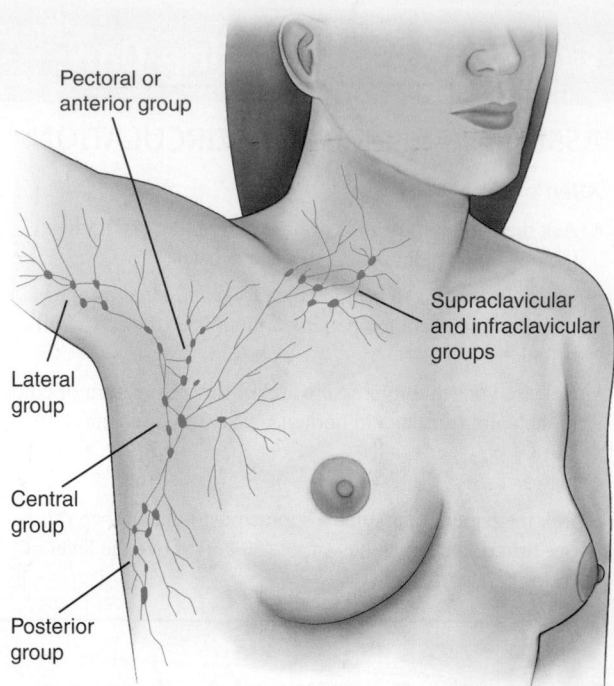

FIGURE 25-31. Location of the cervical, axillary, and mammary lymph nodes.

Normal Age-Related Variations

INFANT/CHILD

Common breast and axillae variations in newborns and children include:

- Breast enlargement and a white discharge from the nipples (up to 2 weeks of age)
- Female breast growth beginning at 10 or 11 years of age
- Temporary enlargement of one or both breasts (gynecomastia) in pubescent boys

OLDER ADULT

Common breast and axillae variations in older adults include:

- Granular, pendulous breasts in women

Assessing the Abdomen

The abdominal cavity (Fig. 25-32) contains the stomach, the small intestine, the large intestine, the liver, the gallbladder, the pancreas, the spleen, the kidneys, and the urinary bladder. Not all of these organs can be assessed. Although the liver is not normally palpable, the technique for assessing it is included because abnormal findings are important. The spleen is rarely palpable and assessment requires deep palpation (requiring more advanced skills), so it is not included in this discussion. The abdominal cavity also contains the female reproductive organs, discussed in the following section.

Health history questions are used to identify subjective data, including abdominal pain and nausea and to collect data about the patient's elimination patterns, fluid and nutritional

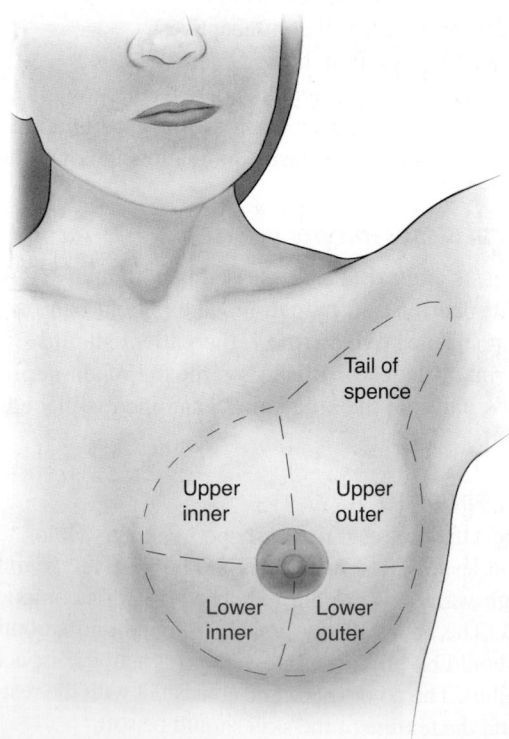

FIGURE 25-30. Location of assessment findings of the breast are identified by quadrant.

Guidelines for Nursing Care • 25-8

PALPATING THE BREASTS

Palpate each quadrant of each breast in a systematic method, either the circular, wedge, or vertical strip technique. The patient should be supine with a small pillow or towel beneath her back and the arm on the side of the breast to be examined raised above her head.

Circular

- Start at the tail of Spence and move in increasing smaller circles (Figure A).
- Use the pads of the first three fingers to gently compress the breast tissue against the chest wall.

FIGURE B. Wedge technique.

Vertical Strip

- Start at the outer edge of the breast and palpate up and down the breast (Figure C).
- Use the pads of the first three fingers to gently compress the breast tissue against the chest wall.

FIGURE A. Circular technique.

Wedge

- Work in a clockwise direction and palpate from the periphery toward the areola (Figure B).
- Use the pads of the first three fingers to gently compress the breast tissue against the chest wall.

FIGURE C. Vertical strip technique.

---

intake, and lifestyle. Physical examination is conducted to further assess problems with pain and to identify abdominal masses. Abdominal assessments are also used to assess the return of bowel sounds (e.g., after surgery) and retention of urine in the urinary bladder.

Health History

Identify risk factors for altered health during the health history by asking about the following:

- History of abdominal pain
- History of indigestion, nausea or vomiting, constipation or diarrhea
- History of food allergies or lactose intolerance
- Appetite and usual food and fluid intake
- Usual bowel and bladder elimination patterns
- History of gastrointestinal disorders, such as peptic ulcer disease, bowel disease, gallbladder disease, liver disease, or appendicitis

- History of urinary tract disorders such as infections, kidney stones, or kidney disease
- History of abdominal surgery or trauma
- Type and amount of prescribed and over-the-counter medications used
- Amount and type of alcohol ingestion
- For women, menstrual history

Physical Assessment

Use a warm stethoscope (it can be warmed with your hand) and ensure that lighting is adequate when assessing the abdomen. Also, make sure that your hands are warm and your fingernails are trimmed short. Ask the patient to empty the bladder. Position the patient in the supine position with the head slightly elevated and arms at the sides. Place small pillows under the head and knees for comfort. Make sure that the patient is warm and comfortable to help prevent contraction of the abdominal muscles, which makes palpation difficult.

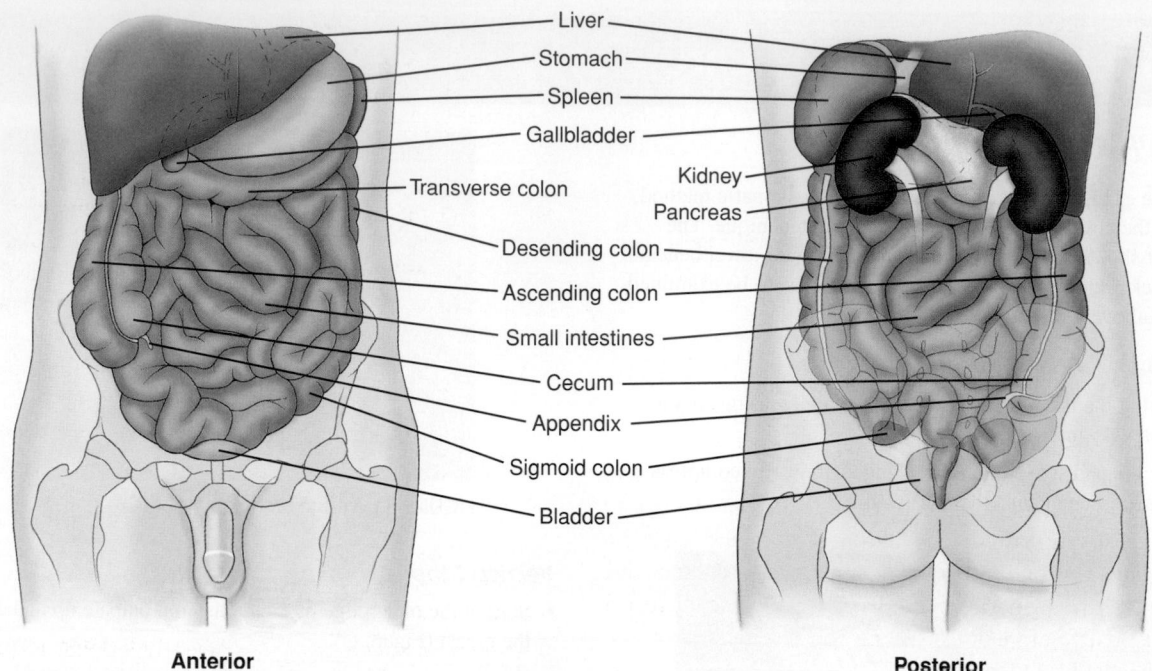

Anterior

Posterior

FIGURE 25-32. Organs of the abdominal cavity.

To locate organs more easily and to make documentation more specific, the abdomen can be divided into four quadrants: right upper, right lower, left upper, and left lower (Fig. 25-33). The sequence of techniques used to assess the abdomen is inspection, auscultation, percussion, and palpation. Percussion and palpation are done *after* auscultation because they stimulate bowel sounds. Ask the patient to breathe slowly and deeply through the mouth during the examination to promote relaxation. Ask the patient to iden-

tify painful areas of the abdomen and explain you will assess these at the end of the examination.

INSPECTING THE ABDOMEN

Sit at the side of the patient and look across the abdomen. A tangential view enhances shadows and contours. Inspect skin color and surface characteristics, including the umbilicus, contour, symmetry, peristalsis, pulsations, and visible masses. The skin color may be slightly lighter than exposed areas. Fine

Midline

Right Upper Quadrant

- Pylorous
- Duodenum
- Liver
- Right kidney and adrenal gland
- Hepatic flexure of colon
- Head of pancreas

Left Upper Quadrant

- Stomach
- Spleen
- Left kidney and adrenal gland
- Splenic flexure of colon
- Body of pancreas

Right Lower Quadrant

- Cecum
- Appendix
- Right ovary and fallopian tube (female)
- Right ureter and lower kidney pole
- Right spermatic cord (male)

Left Lower Quadrant

- Sigmoid colon
- Left ovary and fallopian tube (female)
- Left ureter and lower kidney pole
- Left spermatic cord (male)

Midline

- Urinary bladder
- Urethra (female)

FIGURE 25-33. Diagram of abdominal quadrants and outline of underlying organs.

white or silver lines (striae) may be visible, often the result of skin stretching from weight gain or pregnancy. The umbilicus should be centrally located and may be flat, rounded, or concave. The abdomen should be evenly rounded or symmetric, without visible peristalsis. In thin people, an upper midline pulsation may normally be visible. Abnormal findings include swelling of the abdomen (indicating fluid retention called ascites) and abdominal masses or unusual pulsations.

AUSCULTATING BOWEL SOUNDS AND VASCULAR SOUNDS

Auscultation is used to assess bowel sounds and vascular sounds.

Warm the stethoscope and using light pressure, place the flat diaphragm on the right lower quadrant of the abdomen. Because bowel sounds are transmitted through the entire abdomen, listening at one spot is usually sufficient (Bickley, 2007). Listen carefully for bowel sounds (gurgles and clicks, and note their frequency and character [usually occur every 5 to 34 seconds]). Before documenting bowel sounds as absent, the nurse must listen for 2 minutes or longer in each abdominal quadrant. Abnormal findings include increased bowel sounds (often heard with diarrhea or in early bowel obstruction), decreased bowel sounds (heard after abdominal surgery or late bowel obstruction), or absent bowel sounds (indicating peritonitis or paralytic ileus). Bowel sounds of high-pitched tinkling or rushes of high-pitched sounds indicate a bowel obstruction.

Using the bell of the stethoscope, auscultate over the abdominal aorta, femoral arteries, and iliac arteries for **bruits** (abnormal sounds heard over a blood vessel as blood passes an obstruction). A bruit may be heard if an occlusion or arterial insufficiency is present in an abdominal artery. Report and document changes in or absence of bowel and vascular sounds.

PERCUSSING THE ABDOMEN

Percussion is useful in assessing a full bladder or changes in abdominal contents. Percuss the abdomen in all four quadrants in a systematic, clockwise manner to identify fluid, masses, or air. Note the distribution of sounds. Normally, tympany, the dominant percussion tone, is heard over the abdomen while dullness is heard over the liver and a full bladder. Abnormal findings include decreased tympany and increased dullness, possibly caused by fluid or a mass.

PALPATING THE ABDOMEN

The pads of the fingers are used to palpate with a light, gentle, dipping motion. Watch the patient's face for nonverbal signs of pain during palpation. Palpate each quadrant in a systematic manner, noting muscular resistance, tenderness, enlargement of the organs, or masses. If the patient complains of abdominal pain, palpate the area of pain last. The abdomen should normally be soft, relaxed, and free of tenderness. Abnormal findings include involuntary rigidity, spasm, and pain (which may indicate trauma, peritonitis, infection, tumors, or enlarged or diseased abdominal organs).

PALPATING THE LIVER

The entire liver is not usually palpable, but the lower edge of the liver may be assessed with light palpation. To palpate bimanually, stand at the patient's right side and place your left hand under the patient's back at the level of the 11th to 12th ribs. With your fingertips pointing toward the patient's head, ask the patient to inhale and press up and in with your fingertips. The normal liver edge should feel firm and smooth and may be mildly tender. Abnormal findings include a hard and firm liver edge (found in cancer of the liver), nodularity (found with tumor, metastatic cancer, cirrhosis of the liver), and pain (from vascular engorgement as in congestive heart failure, hepatitis, or abscess). If the liver border is more than 1 to 3 cm below the costal margin, it is considered enlarged. Liver enlargement may result from hepatitis, liver tumors, cirrhosis, and vascular engorgement.

Normal Age-Related Variations

INFANT/CHILD

Common abdominal variations in newborns and children include:

- Umbilical cord in newborns; dries and falls off within the first few weeks of life
- A "pot-belly" (under 5 years of age)
- Visible peristaltic waves
- Easily palpated liver and spleen

OLDER ADULT

Common abdominal variations in older adults include:

- Decreased bowel sounds
- Decreased abdominal tone
- Liver border palpated more easily

Assessing Female Genitalia

The external female genitalia consist of the mons pubis, labia majora and minora, clitoris, vestibular glands, vaginal vestibule, vaginal orifice, and urethral opening (Fig. 25-34).

FIGURE 25-34. External female genitalia.

Information collected during the health history is especially helpful in identifying risk factors for cancer and health-related behaviors that may lead to sexually transmitted infections. During the physical assessment, the external genitalia may be examined. However, the internal pelvic examination is a skill most often performed by a physician or an advanced practice nurse. The female genitalia are assessed for lesions, discharge, masses, and enlargement of internal organs. The rectum and anus may be assessed during part of this examination if a total health assessment is being performed. Information about rectal examination is provided later in this chapter.

Health History

Identify risk factors for altered female health during the health history by asking about the following:

- Menstrual history (age of first and last period, length of flow, type of flow, pain)
- Sexual history (age at which sexual activity began, number and gender of partners)
- Pain with intercourse, difficulty achieving orgasm
- Number of pregnancies and live births
- History of sexually transmitted infection
- Use of contraceptives
- Frequency of pelvic examinations and Pap smears
- History of vaginal discharge, itching, or pain on urination
- History of smoking (how long, how many packs/day)
- Family history of reproductive or genital cancer

Physical Assessment

The genitalia are assessed by inspection and palpation. A description of an internal pelvic assessment of women is included in this chapter. This is an advanced assessment technique, but nurses often assist in performing vaginal examinations and need to be familiar with the procedure. In many instances, male healthcare providers will ask that a female be present in the room during the examination. Women from some cultures (e.g., Islam) may agree to a physical examination of the genitalia only by a female nurse or female physician. Equipment required includes a vaginal speculum (for the female examination), a good light source, and disposable gloves.

INSPECTING AND PALPATING THE EXTERNAL GENITALIA

Ask the patient to empty her bladder before the examination. Place (actually, the woman places herself) the woman in the lithotomy position on the examination table, with the legs in stirrups, and draped so that only the genitalia are exposed. Explain the procedure to her and help her to relax as it is performed. Be sure to wear gloves during this assessment.

Inspect the external genitalia for color, size of the labia majora and vaginal opening, lesions, and discharge. The vulva normally has more pigmentation than other skin areas, and the mucous membranes are dark pink and moist. The skin and mucosa should be smooth, without lesions or swelling. The labia should be symmetric without lesions or swelling. Lesions may be the result of infections (such as herpes or syphilis). There may normally be a small amount of clear or whitish vaginal discharge. The vaginal orifice varies in size, depending on the woman's age, sexual history, and having vaginal delivery. In children, loss of hymenal tissue between the 3 o'clock and 9 o'clock position indicates trauma (from digits, penis, or foreign objects). Palpate the labia for masses and the Bartholin's glands (located slightly below and to the left and right of the opening of the vagina) for swelling, pain, and discharge.

INSPECTING INTERNAL GENITALIA

A speculum is used to examine the internal genitalia. Guidelines for Nursing Care 25-9 lists the sequence of an internal vaginal examination.

Guidelines for Nursing Care • 25-9

EXAMINING THE VAGINA

- Explain the procedure to the patient.
- Warm the speculum under warm running water; if cytologic specimens are to be taken, the water serves as the lubricant; if no specimens are needed, a water-soluble lubricant may be used.
- Don gloves.
- Using two fingers placed just inside the vagina, press down gently on the posterior vaginal wall.
- Insert the speculum blades vertically into the vagina, the posterior portion pointed at a 45-degree angle. Ensure that no pubic hair is caught in the speculum.
- Turn the speculum so that the handle is down and the blades are in a horizontal position.

- Open the blades and close the screw that locks the blades open.
- Inspect the cervix and os for size, color, shape, lesions, and discharge.
- Obtain specimens, if needed.
- Withdraw the blades slowly, observing the vaginal walls.
- When the speculum blades are clear of the cervix, release the screw so that the blades close, and withdraw the speculum from the vagina.
- Provide the patient with tissues to remove the lubricating jelly (if used).

➤ *Think back to Ramona Lewis, the college student who arrived at the emergency department reporting that she was a victim of date rape. Examination of her external and internal genitalia is required to collect evidence indicating rape. The nurse would need to know the agency's policy and local and state legal requirements related to collection of rape evidence.* ■

Abnormal findings include redness, swelling of glands, discharge, lesions, and pain, which may indicate infection, an abscess, a polyp, or cancer. For related assessments of the urinary tract and sexually transmitted infections, see Chapters 37 and 45.

Normal Age-Related Variations

INFANT/CHILD

Common genitalia variations in newborns (resulting from exposure to maternal hormones in utero, normally seen in the first week after birth and subsiding by the second week after birth) and children include:

- Enlarged labia and clitoris in girls
- Breast enlargement in both boys and girls
- Vaginal discharge in girls, called pseudomenstruation
- Pubic hair and breast development occur at puberty and follow a regular sequence of development
- Menstruation begins about 2.5 years after puberty begins
- Irregular menstrual cycle for first 2 years

OLDER ADULT

Common genitalia variations in older women include:

- Decreased size of labia and clitoris
- Decreased amount of pubic hair
- Decreased vaginal secretions
- Shortened vaginal vault
- Pale, thin, and dry vaginal mucosa

Assessing Male Genitalia

The male genitalia (Fig. 25-35) include the penis, testicles, epididymis, scrotum, prostate gland, and seminal vesicles. In addition, the inguinal area may be assessed as part of this assessment. Information from the health history is helpful in identifying self-care and lifestyle factors that increase the risk of illnesses, such as testicular cancer or sexually transmitted infections. The physical examination is focused on detecting abnormal findings so that early diagnosis and treatment can be initiated.

Health History

Identify risk factors for altered male health during the health history by asking about the following:

- Frequency of digital rectal examinations
- Frequency of testicular self-examination (Fig. 25-36)

FIGURE 25-35. Organs of the male genital system.

- Use of contraceptives
- Occupational exposure to chemicals (tire and rubber manufacturing, farming, mechanics)
- History of sexually transmitted infection
- History of discharge from the penis
- Difficulty with urination (incontinence, hesitancy, frequency, voiding at night)
- History of erectile dysfunction

Physical Assessment

The patient may be standing or supine. Gloves are worn during this assessment.

INSPECTING AND PALPATING THE EXTERNAL GENITALIA

The external genitalia are inspected for size, placement, contour, appearance of the skin, redness, edema, and discharge. If the patient is uncircumcised, retract the foreskin for inspection of the glans penis. Assess the location of the urinary meatus. Inspect the scrotum for symmetry; it is not unusual for the left testicle to lie lower in the scrotal sac than the right testicle. The size, shape, and consistency of the scrotal contents (i.e., testes) should be similar bilaterally. Normal findings include skin that is free of lesions, and a foreskin (if present) that is intact, uniform in color, and easily retracted. The urinary meatus is normally located in the center of the glans penis and is free of discharge. The scrotum and testes should be free of masses and nontender.

Abnormal findings include lesions, redness, edema, pain, discharge, fluid-filled masses in the scrotum (symptoms of a hydrocele or varicocele), and displacement of the urinary meatus or difficulties with voiding. Edema, redness, discharge, or pain may indicate an infection. Voiding difficulties may result from scarring caused by infections or prostate enlargement. (See Chapters 37 and 45 for additional discussion of the male urinary tract and sexually transmitted infections.)

FIGURE 25-36. Testicular self-examination is to be performed once a month. A convenient time is after a warm bath or shower when the scrotum is relaxed. Both hands are used to palpate the testis; the normal testicle is smooth and uniform in consistency. (**A**) With the index and middle finger under the testis and the thumb on tip, roll the testis gently in a horizontal plane between the thumb and fingers, feeling for any evidence of a small lump or abnormality. (**B**) Follow the same procedure for palpation in a vertical plane. (**C**) Locate the epididymis (cord-like structure on the top and back of the testicle that stores and transports sperm). Repeat the examination for the other testis; it is normal to find one testis larger than the other. Any evidence of a small pea-sized lump should be checked by a physician. It may be due to an infection or a tumor growth.

INSPECTING AND PALPATING THE INGUINAL AREA

The inguinal area may be inspected at this time by asking the patient to bear down. Normally, the inguinal area is free of bulges. (Further assessment for inguinal hernia, inguinal lymph nodes, and femoral hernia are usually performed by a physician or an advanced practice nurse.)

Normal Age-Related Variations
INFANT/CHILD

Common genitalia variations in newborns and children include:

- Development of pubic hair and enlargement of the scrotum, testes, and penis occurs at puberty and follows a regular sequence to adult configuration.
- Spontaneous nocturnal emission of seminal fluid occurs at puberty.

OLDER ADULT

Common genitalia variations in older adults include:

- Decreased penis size
- Decreased pubic hair
- Decreased size and firmness of testes

Assessing the Rectum and Anus

Although the rectum and anus are not assessed in all patients, this assessment is a part of a total health assessment for both men and women. Information from the health history provides information about normal patterns of bowel elimination and identifies risks for illness (such as colon cancer) and health behaviors (such as frequency of digital rectal examinations [DRE] to assess for cancer or engaging in anal intercourse). Physical examination provides information to support teaching about risk for colon cancer and the risks of sexually transmitted infections (including AIDS) associated with unprotected anal sex. Physical assessments of the rectum and anus are primarily conducted by physicians or advanced practice nurses.

Health History

Identify risk factors for altered health during the health history by asking about the following:

- Bowel patterns, including constipation, diarrhea, or pain
- History of blood or mucus in the stool
- Family history of polyps, colon or rectal cancer, or prostate cancer
- History of hemorrhoids
- Frequency of DREs
- History of anal intercourse

Physical Assessment

Techniques used to assess the rectum and anus include inspection and palpation. Lubricant, gloves, and good lighting are necessary equipment. The patient may be in the Sims, knee–chest, or lithotomy position or may be standing and leaning over the examination table.

Inspection is used to assess the anal area, which normally has increased pigmentation and some hair growth. Palpation is used to assess the rectum, using a well-lubricated, gloved index finger. Sphincter tone at the anus should be firm and the mucosal lining smooth. (Fecal specimens may be taken at this time, if necessary.) Abnormal findings include relaxed sphincter tone; skin cracks, nodules, or hemorrhoids at the anal sphincter; bleeding (which may indicate hemorrhoids or colorectal cancer); and hard or abnormally colored (such as clay-colored or dark-black) stools.

If a rectal assessment is conducted in a woman, the cervix may be felt as a small, round mass when palpating the anterior rectal wall. Abnormal findings include changes in consistency. The prostate gland in men can be assessed for size, shape, and consistency by palpation through the anterior rectal wall; the gland is normally smooth, firm, and about 4 cm (1¾″) in size. Abnormal findings include enlargement or changes in consistency (which occur in benign prostatic enlargement or cancer).

Normal Age-Related Variations
INFANT/CHILD
Note: Normally physical examination of the rectum and anus is not performed in young children or adolescents.

OLDER ADULT
Common variations in older men include:

- Anus is darker in color
- Hemorrhoids are often present
- Prostate gland may be enlarged

Assessing the Musculoskeletal System
The primary structures of the musculoskeletal system are the bones, muscles, cartilage, ligaments, tendons, and joints. Health history information is used to evaluate the patient's ability to carry out activities of daily living and to collect data about areas such as pain, stiffness, and ability to move. Physical examination provides information about posture, gait, bone size and structure, joint range of motion (ROM), and muscle strength. Normally, the joints are bilaterally equal in size, shape, and color; are free of swelling, pain, nodules, or crepitus (grating sounds on movement); and can move through full ROM. Abnormal findings include deformity, crepitus, and limited ROM (indicating injury, inflammation and/or arthritis of the affected joints or bones, and muscle pain and/or weakness caused by injury or disease).

Health History
Identify risk factors for altered health during the health history by asking about the following:

- History of trauma, arthritis, or neurologic disorder
- History of pain or swelling in the muscles and/or joints
- Frequency and type of usual exercise
- Dietary intake of calcium
- History of any surgery on muscles or joints
- History of smoking (how long, how many packs/day)
- History of alcohol intake

Physical Assessment
The patient assumes a variety of positions, including standing, sitting, and supine. Assessments of the musculoskeletal system can be integrated into assessment of other body systems.

INSPECTING AND PALPATING THE MUSCLES
Examine the muscles by inspection and palpation of muscle groups and by testing muscle tone and strength. Muscle groups are observed for bilateral symmetry and palpated for tenderness. Normally, they are symmetric and nontender. Evaluate muscle tone (the normal condition of a muscle at rest) by putting each joint and extremity through passive range of motion. Assess muscle strength. Guidelines for Nursing Care 25-10 describes testing muscle strength.

Abnormal findings include atrophy (a decrease in size), tremors (involuntary movements), and flaccidity (without tone) of muscles. Other abnormal findings are loss of strength and tone, decreased range of motion, uncoordinated movements, swelling, and pain. Abnormal findings may indicate a musculoskeletal disease, trauma, or a neurologic disease.

PALPATING THE BONES
The bones are palpated for normal contour and prominence and for bilateral symmetry. Abnormal findings include pain, enlargement, asymmetry, and changes in contour. Abnormal findings may indicate trauma, degenerative joint disease, musculoskeletal disease, or a neurologic disease.

INSPECTING AND PALPATING THE JOINTS
Each joint is put through its full range of motion to assess the degree of movement. Joint movements include flexion, extension, hyperextension, abduction, adduction, supination, and pronation. Normally, each joint has full range of motion, is nontender, and moves smoothly. Palpate joints for the abnormal findings of pain, swelling, nodules, and crepitation (a grating sound heard or felt on movement).

INSPECTING SPINAL CURVES
With the patient standing, inspect the spine from the back and from the side. The spine normally has concave curves at the cervical and lumbar spine and convex curves at the thoracic and sacrococcygeal spine. The lumbar curve may be flattened with a herniated disk. Kyphosis (an increased thoracic spinal curve) is more often seen in older adults. An exaggerated lumbar curve (lordosis) is often seen during pregnancy or in obesity. Scoliosis is a lateral curvature of the spine with increased convexity on the side that is curved. School nurses often first identify scoliosis during screenings, which are recommended for girls in grades 5 and 7 and for boys in grades 8 or 9. Findings indicating scoliosis are illustrated in Figure 25-37.

Normal Age-Related Variations
INFANT/CHILD
Common musculoskeletal variations in newborns and children include:

- C-shaped curve of spine at birth; the anterior cervical curve develops at about 3 to 4 months of age, and the

(text continues on page 604)

Guidelines for Nursing Care • 25-10

ASSESSING MUSCLE STRENGTH

Assess muscle strength by asking the patient to move against resistance. Bilateral equal resistance should be present. Observe muscle contraction and determine muscle strength exerted. Muscle strength should be bilaterally equal, with a slight increase on the dominant side. Techniques for assessing the muscles include:

Shoulder Flexion

The patient flexes shoulder muscle against resistance of the examiner's hand (Figure A).

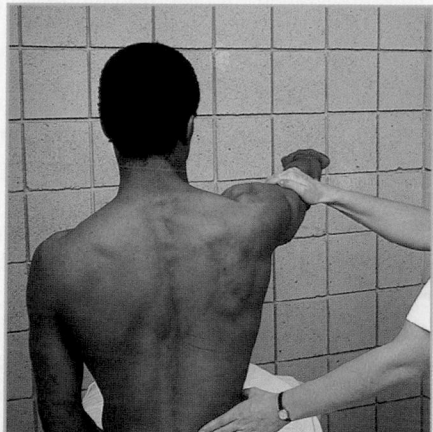

FIGURE A

Elbow Extension and Flexion

- The patient first extends the elbow against resistance by the examiner (Figure B).
- Then he flexes the elbow against resistance (Figure C).

FIGURE B

FIGURE C

Wrist Extension

The patient makes a fist and resists examiner's attempts to pull down wrist (Figure D).

FIGURE D

Grip

The patient squeezes the examiner's index and middle fingers (Figure E).

FIGURE E

(continued)

Guidelines for Nursing Care • 25-10

ASSESSING MUSCLE STRENGTH   *continued*

Hip Flexion

The patient attempts to raise his thigh against examiner's resistance (Figure F).

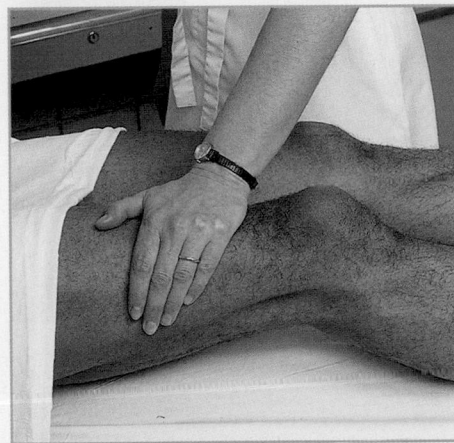

FIGURE F

Knee Flexion and Extension

- With the patient's knee bent and foot on the examining table, the patient attempts to keep foot down while the examiner attempts to straighten the patient's leg to test flexion (Figure G).

FIGURE G

- To test extension, the examiner supports the patient's knee and the patient attempts to straighten his leg against resistance at the ankle (Figure H).

Photos by Ken Casper.

FIGURE H

Ankle Plantar Flexion and Dorsiflexion

- The patient first pushes the balls of the feet against resistance of the examiner's hands (Figure I).
- Then, the patient attempts to pull against examiner's resistance (Figure J).

FIGURE I

FIGURE J

A

Is the head level and
centered over the trunk?

Are the shoulders the
same height?

B

Are the hips at the
same level?

When bent forward with arms
dropping toward feet, is rib cage
level on both sides?

FIGURE 25-37. Screening for scoliosis. (**A**) Normal position and spinal curves. (**B**) Scoliosis indicators.

anterior lumbar curve develops between 12 and 18 months of age

- Lordosis (an exaggerated lumbar curve)
- Pronation of the feet in children between 12 and 30 months of age
- Genu varum (bowleg) for 1 year after learning to walk

OLDER ADULT

Common musculoskeletal variations seen in older adults include:

- Loss of muscle mass and strength
- Decreased range of motion
- Kyphosis
- Decreased height
- Osteoarthritic changes in joints

Assessing the Neurologic System

Neurologic assessment includes cerebral function, cranial nerve function, cerebellar function, motor and sensory function, and reflexes. The health history is useful in obtaining information about activities of daily living and other pertinent data, such as dizziness, loss of sensation, headaches, and ability to see, hear, taste, and detect sensations. Physical examination is conducted to identify mental status and level of consciousness, cranial nerve function, muscle strength and coordination, and reflexes. Normally, the patient is alert and responsive, has full sensory function, and all muscle groups are bilaterally strong. Abnormal

findings are discussed with specific parts of the examination that follow.

Health History

Identify risk factors for altered health during the health history by asking about the following:

- History of numbness, tingling, or tremors
- History of seizures
- History of headaches
- History of dizziness
- History of trauma to the head or spine
- History of infections of the brain
- History of stroke
- Changes in the ability to hear, see, taste, or smell
- Loss of ability to control bladder and bowel
- History of high blood pressure
- History of smoking (how long, how many packs/day)
- History of chronic alcohol use
- History of diabetes mellitus or heart disease
- Use of prescription and over-the-counter medications
- Family history of high blood pressure, Alzheimer's disease, epilepsy, cancer, or Huntington's chorea
- Frequency of blood cholesterol tests and results
- Exposure to environmental hazards (e.g., lead, insecticides)

Physical Assessment

Evaluate cerebral function by observing the patient's behavior throughout the health history interview and physical assessment. Assess the patient's mental status, memory, emotional status, cognitive abilities, and behavior. Evaluate cerebellar function by assessing fine motor skills, coordination, and balance. Assess the sensory system by having the patient identify various sensory stimuli, and evaluate the reflexes by contraction of specific muscles.

Equipment for a neurologic assessment includes vials of aromatic substances (e.g., peppermint and vanilla), a visual acuity chart, a penlight, a sharp object (e.g., a large safety pin), cotton balls, vials of solution to test taste (e.g., salt or sugar), a tuning fork, a tongue depressor, a reflex hammer, and familiar objects, such as a key or coin. The patient should be sitting and the environment should be quiet.

ASSESSING MENTAL STATUS

Mental status assessment includes level of awareness, level of consciousness, behavior and appearance, memory, abstract reasoning, and language. On initial contact, begin to evaluate the patient's orientation to person, place, and time, as well as cognitive abilities and affect (whether the patient knows who he or she is, where he or she is, and the day or month or year). Observe the patient's appearance, general behavior, ability to speak clearly, and respond to questions. Note any variation in responses.

Assess the patients overall appearance. The patient should have a clean, neat appearance with erect posture; should be oriented to person, place, and time; should have memory recall (both short-term and long-term memory); and should be able to demonstrate coherent and logical thought processes. Abnormal findings include poor hygiene, inappropriate dress, disorientation, absent memory recall, and incoherent or illogical thought processes. These abnormal findings may indicate a mental health disorder, developmental delay, brain disease, cerebrovascular disorder, alcohol or drug intoxication, or a tumor.

> *Think back to Tammy Browning, the pregnant woman with a history of substance abuse. The nurse would assess the patient's mental status for clues suggesting recent drug use, incorporating knowledge of abnormal findings into the assessment.* ∎

The following discussion of each of the mental status components includes sample questions or specific assessments to use during the assessment.

Assessing Level of Awareness

Assess awareness by evaluating orientation to time, place, and person. The following questions may be used:

- *Time:* What is today's date? What day of the week is it? What season of the year is this? What was the last holiday?
- *Place:* Where are you now? What is the name of this city? What state are we in?
- *Person:* What is your name? How old are you? Who came to visit you this morning?

Although exceptions may occur, individuals who have impaired awareness first lose time orientation, followed by place orientation, and then person orientation. Remember that it is often difficult to know the exact date when one is ill, in pain, or in unfamiliar surroundings.

Assessing Level of Consciousness

Consciousness is the degree of wakefulness or the ability of a person to be aroused. This is not the same as orientation; a patient may be conscious but not oriented. Level of consciousness is described as follows:

- Awake and alert: fully awake; oriented to person, place, and time; responds to all stimuli, including verbal commands
- Lethargic: appears drowsy or asleep most of the time but makes spontaneous movements; can be aroused by gentle shaking and saying patient's name
- Stuporous: unconscious most of the time; has no spontaneous movement; must be shaken or shouted at to arouse; can make verbal responses, but these are less likely to be appropriate; responds to painful stimuli with purposeful movements
- Comatose: cannot be aroused, even with use of painful stimuli; may have some reflex activity (such as gag reflex); if no reflexes present, is in a deep coma

The Glasgow Coma Scale (Table 25-10) is a standardized assessment tool that assesses level of consciousness. Three parameters are evaluated: eye opening, motor response, and verbal response. Scores are given in each category, and a total score is recorded, with higher scores indicating a more normal level of functioning. A score of 7 or less defines coma. This is a more accurate evaluation of mental status over time.

TABLE • 25-10	GLASGOW COMA SCALE	
Component	**Response**	**Score**
Eye opening	Spontaneous	4
	To verbal command	3
	To pain	2
	No response	1
Motor response	To verbal command	6
	To localized pain	5
	Flexes/withdraws	4
	Flexes abnormally	3
	Extends abnormally	2
	No response	1
Verbal response	Oriented/talks	5
	Disoriented/talks	4
	Inappropriate words	3
	Incomprehensible sounds	2
	No response	1

Assessing Memory

Memory is assessed by asking questions that require answers demonstrating immediate recall and recall for past events. To assess immediate memory, ask the patient to repeat a series of numbers forward or backward (e.g., 3, 6, 9). Start with three numbers and gradually increase the digits until the patient cannot respond correctly. Most adults can repeat a series of five to eight numbers forward and four to six digits backward. You might also ask, "What did you eat for breakfast this morning?" To assess past memory, ask, "When is your birthday?" or "When is your wedding anniversary?"

Assessing Abstract Reasoning

Ask the patient to explain a proverb such as "the early bird catches the worm." If intellectual ability is impaired, the patient usually gives a literal explanation or repeats the phrase. Be sure that the phrase is not culture specific.

ASSESSING LANGUAGE

The cerebral cortex controls the ability to express self through writing, words, or gestures and to understand the spoken and written word. Some simple methods of assessing language capabilities include asking the patient to name items in the room (e.g., bed, flowers, gown, pajamas), to follow simple commands (such as "Point to your head"), to read a short sentence aloud, or to match printed and spoken words with appropriate pictures. Injury to the cortex can cause aphasia, which is a disorder of language ability. Aphasia may be expressive (the individual understands written and spoken words but cannot write or speak to communicate

TABLE • 25-11	**SUMMARY OF CRANIAL NERVES**		
Nerve (Number)	**Type**	**Functions**	**Methods for Examining Nerve**
Olfactory (I)	Sensory	Sense of smell	Test each nostril for smell reception with various agents and interpretation.
Optic (II)	Sensory	Sense of vision	Test vision for acuity and visual fields.
Oculomotor (III)	Motor	Pupil constriction Raise eyelids	Test pupillary reaction to light and ability to open and close eyelids.
Trochlear (IV)	Motor/ Proprioceptor	Downward inward eye movement	Test for downward and inward movement of the eye.
Trigeminal (V)	Motor Sensory	Jaw movements—chewing and mastication Sensation on the face and neck	Ask patient to open and clench jaws while you palpate the jaw muscles. Test face and neck for pain sensations, light touch, and temperature.
Abducens (VI)	Motor	Lateral movement of the eyes	Test ocular movement in all directions.
Facial (VII)	Motor Sensory	Muscles of the face Sense of taste on the anterior two thirds of the tongue	Ask the patient to raise eyebrows, smile, show teeth, and puff out cheeks. Test for the taste sensation with various agents.
Acoustic (VIII)	Sensory	Sense of hearing	Test hearing ability.
Glossopharyngeal (IX)	Motor Sensory	Pharyngeal movement and swallowing Sense of taste on the posterior one third of the tongue	Ask the patient to say "ah," and have patient yawn to observe upward movement of the soft palate; elicit gag response; note ability to swallow. Test for taste with various agents.
Vagus (X)	Motor/Sensory	Swallowing and speaking	Ask the patient to swallow and speak; note hoarseness.
Accessory (XI)	Motor/Sensory	Movement of shoulder muscles	Ask the patient to shrug shoulders against your resistance.
Hypoglossal (XII)	Motor	Movement of the tongue; strength of the tongue	Ask the patient to protrude tongue; ask patient to push tongue against cheek.

effectively) or receptive (the individual cannot understand written or spoken words). These aphasias may also be combined.

ASSESSING CRANIAL NERVE FUNCTION

The function of the 12 cranial nerves is assessed primarily during the neurologic assessment, although parts of cranial nerve function are assessed with other body systems (e.g., pupillary response during assessment of the face). Each nerve has a specific function and is evaluated individually. Table 25-11 outlines the cranial nerves, with their function and assessment methods.

ASSESSING MOTOR AND SENSORY FUNCTION

Motor ability is evaluated by assessing balance, gait, and coordination. Sensory function is assessed by testing sensory discrimination of pain, light touch, and vibrations.

Inspecting Balance and Gait

Evaluate balance and gait by having the patient walk across the room on the toes, on the heels, and heel to toe. Observe posture, balance, and arm and leg movements. The posture should be erect, with slight swaying in the standing position, and the gait even with simultaneous arm movements. Abnormal findings include loss of balance, shuffling, wide-based gait, and abnormal patterns of gait. These findings may indicate disorders of the motor, sensory, vestibular, and cerebellar systems.

Assessing Motor Function and Coordination

Evaluate motor function and coordination by having the patient rapidly touch each finger with the thumb, rapidly pat the hand on the thigh, and tap the foot on the floor (or against your hand, if the patient is supine). Repeat the sequence on the opposite limb. Normally, the movements are coordinated. If the patient is unable to perform these movements, it may indicate disease of the upper motor neurons or cerebellum.

Assessing Sensory Perception

Test sensory perception by evaluating the patient's response to pain, light touch, normal shapes, and vibration. With the patient's eyes closed, randomly touch the skin on the upper and lower extremities and the trunk with a sharp object and a soft object. The assessment proceeds from distal (hands, arms, feet, or legs) to proximal (the trunk). The patient should be able to distinguish between sharp (painful) and soft or dull touch. The same process is repeated by using the tuning fork to test for vibratory sensation by placing the activated fork on bony prominences. Sensory perception may also be assessed by asking the patient to close his or her eyes and identify familiar objects (such as a coin or key) by touching them. Abnormal findings include inability to perceive pain or light touch, inability to identify the location of touch, inability to identify familiar objects, and absence of vibratory sensation.

Assessing Deep Tendon Reflexes

Evaluate deep tendon reflexes to determine the functional ability of specific spinal segment levels. Use the reflex hammer to elicit muscle contraction and reflexes. The patient may be either sitting or supine. Table 25-12 illustrates selected reflexes, with normal responses and methods of assessment. Reflex responses are usually graded on a scale of 0 to 4, as listed in Table 25-12. A grade of 2 is considered a normal or active response.

Normal Age-Related Variations

INFANT/CHILD

Common neurologic variations for newborns and children include:

- Positive Babinski's reflex (normal in children between 12 and 24 months)
- Grasp reflex (present at birth)
- Motor control develops in head, neck, trunk, and extremities sequence

OLDER ADULT

Common neurologic variations for older adults include:

- Slower thought processes and verbal responses
- Decreased sensory ability (hearing, sight, smell, taste, temperature, pain)
- Slower coordination and voluntary movements
- Decreased reflex responses
- Appearance of confusion in unfamiliar surroundings
- Slower gait, with a wider base and flexed hips and knees
- Diminished deep tendon reflexes

DOCUMENTATION OF DATA

After completing the nursing history and assessment, organize all assessment data to identify actual and potential health problems, make nursing diagnoses, plan appropriate care, and evaluate the patient's responses to treatment. A pattern is often established that begins during the history and is confirmed during the physical assessment. For example, a health history of a woman diagnosed with multiple sclerosis (a neurologic disorder) might include data about fatigue and increased weakness and muscle spasms in the legs. Physical examination findings would include decreased muscle strength in the lower extremities. These data are used to support the nursing diagnosis of Activity Intolerance related to fatigue and lower extremity weakness. Document the data, with each system recorded individually. Box 25-6 illustrates an example of documentation.

THE NURSE'S ROLE IN DIAGNOSTIC PROCEDURES

Diagnostic procedures and tests provide crucial information about a patient's health, and their results become a part of the total health assessment. Nurse practitioners and physicians

(text continues on page 610)

TABLE • 25-12   NORMAL RESPONSES OF COMMONLY TESTED REFLEXES

How to Test Reflex	Normal Response
Biceps 	The contraction of the biceps can be seen and felt. To test the biceps reflex, the elbow is slightly bent and the palm faces downward. The examiner's thumb is placed on the biceps tendon at the bend in the elbow. The percussion hammer strikes the examiner's thumb.
Triceps 	The contraction of the triceps can be seen as the elbow extends. To test the triceps reflex, the patient's elbow is sharply bent; the forearm is placed across the chest wall with the palm turned toward the body. The triceps tendon is struck with the percussion hammer just above the elbow.
Knee 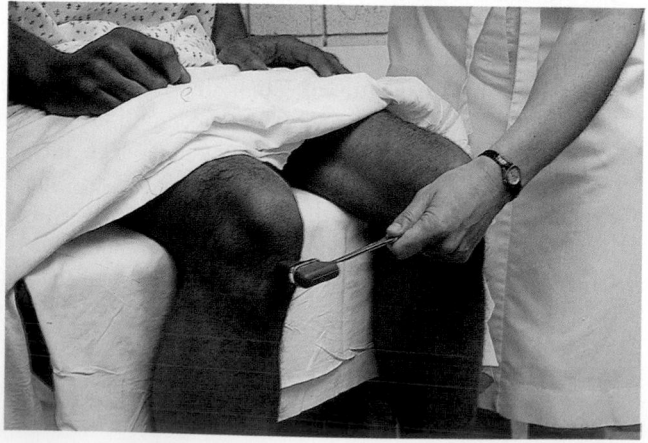	The contraction of the quadriceps causes the knee to extend. To test the knee reflex, the patient is in the sitting position. The patellar tendon just below the patella is struck with the percussion hammer. If the patient is lying down, the reflex is tested while the examiner's hands are placed under the knees to bend them.

(continued)

TABLE • 25-12 NORMAL RESPONSES OF COMMONLY TESTED REFLEXES *(continued)*	
How to Test Reflex	**Normal Response**
Ankle	The foot jerks and moves downward. To test the ankle reflex, the leg is bent at the knee and the foot is supported in a walking position. The Achilles tendon is struck with the percussion hammer.
Babinski	The toes bend or curl. The lateral aspect of the sole of the foot is stroked with an object, such as a key or a thumbnail, from the heel to the ball of the foot.

Grading of Reflexes on a 0 to 4+ Scale	Description
4+	Very brisk, hyperactive; often indicative of disease; often associated with clonus (rhythmic oscillations between flexion and extension)
3+	Brisker than average; possibly but not necessarily indicative of disease
2+	Average; normal
1+	Somewhat diminished; low normal
0	No response

Box 25-6 DOCUMENTING A HEALTH ASSESSMENT

Mrs. D. comes to a local community outpatient agency for her intolerance of eating fatty foods. She says, "I just started having a lot of gas and was sick to my stomach after eating fried foods." The nurse in charge of the agency makes the following assessments.

Health History

Mrs. D. is a 52-year-old woman who lives with her 54-year-old husband on a farm in a rural midwestern area. She graduated from high school and is employed as a secretary for a local insurance agency. Mrs. D. is well groomed, alert, and oriented. She occasionally takes over-the-counter medications for constipation and colds. She takes a prescription medication twice a day for "high blood pressure." She says she has about two mixed drinks a week and does not smoke. She has had five pregnancies, resulting in five living children.

Mrs. D. had her tonsils removed at 5 years of age, had an appendectomy at 22 years of age, and is allergic to penicillin (causes rash and difficulty breathing). She has had all her immunizations, but her last tetanus shot was 10 years ago. Her family history of illness is as follows:

Maternal grandfather, died of heart problems at 77 years of age

Maternal grandmother, died of diabetes complications at 69 years of age

Paternal grandfather, died of stroke at 82 years of age

Paternal grandmother, died of unknown causes at 56 years of age

Sister, 49 years of age, healthy

Brother, died at 22 years of age in a car accident

Physical Assessment

Vital signs: T = 98.8°F (orally), P = 82 beats/min,
    R = 16 breaths/min, BP = 150/88 mm Hg
Height/weight: 5 feet, 4 inches tall, 178 pounds

Integument: Skin warm and dry, normal turgor. Numerous freckles over face and arms. Old scar, RLQ (appendectomy). Nails convex and smooth. Hair dark brown, shiny, normal distribution.

Head and neck: Skull size and shape normal. Facial features symmetric. Can raise eyebrows, close eyes, smile, and puff out cheeks. External eye structures symmetric. Sclera white, con-

junctiva pink. Wears glasses to correct near-sightedness. Vision with glasses 20/30-2 on Snellen's chart. Pupils equal, round, and react to light bilaterally. Demonstrates accommodation, convergence, and peripheral vision. Lens clear. Hearing tested by use of a clock, which she heard clearly at 2 feet. External ears symmetric. Canals smooth and pink without excess cerumen. Tympanic membranes intact without redness or drainage. Right nostril clear, left nostril occluded with mucus. Left maxillary sinus slightly tender on palpation. Teeth in good repair with six fillings. Oral mucous membranes pink. Tonsils absent. Trachea midline, thyroid nonpalpable. No lymph nodes palpable.

Thorax/lungs/heart: Thorax symmetric with equal expansion. Respirations even and unlabored. Lung sounds clear. No visible pulsations noted in neck or precordium. S1 and S2 heard at pulmonic, aortic, tricuspid, and mitral areas. No extra heart sounds, murmurs, or bruits heard. Apical pulse 84 beats/min and regular.

Breasts and axilla: Skin pink. No dimpling or retraction noted. Areolae and nipples dark brown, no crusting or drainage. No masses palpated in breasts. Axillary lymph nodes are not palpable. To have mammogram at next visit.

Abdomen: Obese, rounded. Umbilicus midline. No pain on light palpation. Bowel sounds heard in all four quadrants. No bruits heard on auscultation.

Peripheral vascular: Pulses equal in both arms. Pulses equal in both legs. No edema present. Superficial varicose veins present on both lower extremities between ankle and knee. Toenails thick and yellow.

Genitalia: Will be assessed at next visit with pelvic and Papanicolaou's smear.

Rectum and anus: Inspected only. Small external hemorrhoids noted.

Musculoskeletal: Stands erect. Normal spinal curves. No joint deformities, tenderness, or crepitation. Full active range of motion in all joints. Muscle strength equal bilaterally, slightly stronger on the right (dominant side).

Neurologic: Alert and oriented to time, place, and person. Facial expressions appropriate. Speech clear and appropriate. Demonstrates long-term and short-term memory. All cranial nerves tests were intact. Fine motor movements intact. Gait even. Perceives pain or light touch appropriately. All reflexes = 2.

---

make decisions concerning which diagnostic tests to schedule when problems are noted during the health history or physical assessment or because of a problem stated by the patient. Table 25-13 presents an overview of different types of diagnostic procedures.

Nurses assist before, during, and after diagnostic tests. The nurse is also responsible for other activities associated with diagnostic tests, such as witnessing the patient's consent, scheduling the test, preparing the patient physically and emotionally for the test, providing care and teaching the patient and/or caregivers about the test, disposing of used equipment, and documenting the test.

> *Think back to Tammy Browning, the pregnant woman with a history of substance abuse. A urine specimen was to be obtained for routine testing. In addition, the specimen was to be used for drug testing without the patient's knowledge. Typically, a signed consent form is not necessary for urine specimens. However, the nurse would need to know the agency's policy and legal statutes of the area regarding consent for drug testing before obtaining the specimen.* ■

TABLE • 25-13	A GUIDE TO COMMON LABORATORY AND DIAGNOSTIC PROCEDURES	
Procedure	**Description**	**Examples**
Aspiration procedures	Studies in which a needle or similar instrument is inserted into a body organ or cavity. Fluid or tissue is aspirated, prepared, labeled, and sent to the laboratory for examination.	Liver biopsy Lumbar puncture Paracentesis Thoracentesis
Electrical impulse procedures	Studies that use a machine with electrodes attached to the body to monitor electric activity. Electric impulses are recorded on a graph and displayed on paper or an oscilloscope screen.	Electrocardiogram (EKG) Electroencephalogram (EEG)
Endoscopic procedures	Studies that allow for direct visual examination of various body cavities and organs by means of a hollow, lighted tube called an endoscope. The tube may be flexible or rigid. May be used to obtain tissue specimens for biopsy or microscopic examination.	Bronchoscopy Colonoscopy Gastroscopy Sigmoidoscopy Laparoscopy
Laboratory procedures	Studies in which body fluids, secretions, or tissues are sent to the laboratory for analysis	Blood studies Urine studies Sputum studies Fecal studies Biopsies
Radiography procedures	Because of the ability of x-rays to penetrate human tissues, x-ray studies provide a picture of body structures that looks like a negative of a photograph.	Chest x-ray Dye-enhanced cardiac catheterization
Magnetic resonance imaging (MRI)	The computer-based procedure provides physiologic information and detailed views of fluid-filled soft tissues.	MRI of the brain, spine, extremities, joints, heart, pelvis, and abdomen
Nuclear scanning	Studies that use the administration of a radionuclide and subsequent measurement of radiation from an organ to detect functional abnormalities	Brain scan Heart scan Lung scan Bone scan
Ultrasonography	Studies in which a harmless, high-frequency sound wave is emitted that penetrates the organ being studied. The sound waves bounce back to the sensor and are electronically converted into a picture of the organ or the contents of the organ.	Ultrasound of the pelvis, abdomen, heart, uterus

● Developing Critical Thinking Skills

1. Describe how you would explain a cardiovascular assessment to the following patients:
   - A healthy 5-year-old
   - A college student who has never been ill
   - A 50-year-old man who has never had a physical assessment
   - An 85-year-old woman with heart problems

2. When you are conducting a health history, your patient gives you strange answers. Later, during the mental status assessment, she gives you the wrong answers for the date and place. She also cannot remember what medica-

tions she takes. How would you document this information? What would you do next?

3. When you make a home visit to conduct an initial health history and physical assessment, the patient refuses to let you do more than assess vital signs. What would you do?

● Practicing for NCLEX

1. When assessing a patient's eyes, which instrument would the nurse use to visualize the retina?
   a. Otoscope
   b. Ophthalmoscope

c. Stethoscope

d. Tuning fork

2. Which of the following would be most important for a nurse to do to ensure the accuracy of inspection during assessment?

a. Compare bilateral body parts

b. Have 20/20 vision

c. Focus on selected body systems

d. Use touch judiciously

3. When palpating body structures, the nurse uses which sense?

a. Intuition

b. Vision

c. Hearing

d. Touch

4. Percussion over the stomach reveals a loud, drum-like sound. The nurse would document this finding as which of the following?

a. Dullness

b. Flatness

c. Tympany

d. Resonance

5. While conducting a physical assessment, the nurse uses the bell of the stethoscope to hear which type of sounds?

a. Tympanic sounds

b. Bowel sounds

c. Lung sounds

d. Heart sounds

6. Which technique would a nurse use to assess skin turgor?

a. Indent area with fingertips

b. Use a special type of lighting

c. Touch the area to detect moisture

d. Lightly pinch a fold of skin

7. A patient's visual acuity is assessed as 20/40 in both eyes using the Snellen chart. The nurse interprets this finding as which of the following?

a. The patient can see twice as well as normal

b. The patient has double vision

c. The patient has less than normal vision

d. The patient has normal vision

8. When using an otoscope to assess the tympanic membrane of an adult, the nurse straightens the ear canal by gently pulling the pinna in which direction?

a. Up and back

b. Down and forward

c. Away from the examiner

d. In any direction

9. Percussion of the thorax reveals a dull sound. The nurse interprets this to indicate which of the following?

a. An air-filled structure

b. A bony structure

c. Emphysematous tissue

d. Fluid or a solid mass

10. The nurse auscultates the thorax and lungs and hears coarse gurgling sounds on expiration. The nurse would describe these sounds as:

a. Adventitious breath sounds

b. Bronchovesicular breath sounds

c. Vesicular breath sounds

d. Bronchial sounds

11. When assessing heart sounds, the nurse understands that the sounds heard reflect which of the following?

a. Blood flow through the heart

b. Blood moving into the heart from the aorta

c. Closure of the heart valves

d. Contraction of the cardiac muscle

12. When palpating the breast of a woman during an assessment, the nurse would divide the breast into which of the following?

a. Quadrants

b. Halves

c. Entire breast tissue

d. Bilateral comparison

13. After inspecting a patient's abdomen, which technique would the nurse do next?

a. Percussion

b. Palpation

c. Auscultation

d. Whichever the patient agrees to

14. When assessing a patient's mental status, which of the following would the nurse be least likely to include when evaluating level of awareness?

a. Orientation to time

b. Ability to state where he is

c. Ability to state name

d. Level of consciousness

15. A nurse is conducting an assessment of a patient's cranial nerves. The nurse asks the patient to raise the eyebrows, smile, and show the teeth to assess which cranial nerve?

a. Olfactory

b. Optic

c. Facial

d. Vagus

● Answers With Rationale

1. *b.* Only the ophthalmoscope is used to assess the internal eye.

2. *a.* With inspection, a comparison of bilateral body parts is necessary for recognizing abnormal findings. Perfect vision is unnecessary; the nurse examines all body systems and uses touch during palpation.

3. *d.* Palpation is the technique that uses the sense of touch.

4. *b.* Tympany is a loud, drum-like sound, heard over an air-filled organ.

5. *d.* The bell of the stethoscope is used to hear low-pitched sounds, such as those produced by the heart and vascular system.

6. *d.* Skin turgor is assessed by lightly pinching a fold of skin and allowing it to return to its shape when released.

7. *c.* Normal vision is 20/20. A finding of 20/40 would mean that a patient has less than normal vision.

8. *a.* The ear canal of an adult is straightened by gently pulling the pinna of the ear up and back. In children younger than 3 years of age, the ear canal is straightened by pulling the pinna gently down and back.

9. *d.* A dull sound is heard when percussing over fluid or a solid mass.

10. *a.* Adventitious breath sounds are sounds not normally heard in the lungs.

11. *c.* Heart sounds result from closure of the heart valves.

12. *a.* The breast is divided into four quadrants—outer upper quadrant, outer lower quadrant, inner upper quadrant, and inner lower quadrant. Each quadrant is systematically palpated.

13. *c.* When assessing the abdomen, the sequence is inspection, auscultation, percussion, and palpation. Auscultation follows inspection because percussion and palpation stimulate bowel sounds.

14. *d.* Assessing consciousness is separate assessment and is not included in assessing a patient's level of awareness, which involves evaluating a patient's orientation to time, place (where the patient is), and person (who the patient is, such as his name or age).

15. *c.* Motor function of the facial nerve (cranial nerve VII) is assessed by asking the patient to raise the eyebrow, smile, and show the teeth.

Taylor Suite Resources

The Taylor Suite offers these additional resources to enhance learning and facilitate understanding of this chapter:

- thePoint online resource, http://thepoint.lww.com/Taylor7E
- Student DVD-ROM included with the book
- Study Guide for Taylor's Fundamentals of Nursing

- Taylor's Clinical Nursing Skills: *Chapter 2, Health Assessment*
- Taylor's Video Guide to Clinical Nursing Skills: *Physical Assessment*

BIBLIOGRAPHY

Adams, H., Corbett, J., & DeMyer, W. (2005). Save time with the 5-minute neurologic exam. *Patient Care, (39)*4, 41–47.

Armstrong, J., & Mitchell, E. (2008). Comprehensive nursing assessment in the care of older people. *Nursing Older People, (20)*1, 36–40.

Ayoltt, M. (2007). Observing the sick child Part 2B: Respiratory palpation. *Pediatric Nursing, 19*(1), 38–45.

Bald, H. (2006). The process of conducting a physical assessment: A nursing perspective. *British Journal of Nursing, 15*(13), 710–714.

Bickley, L. S. (2007). *Bates' guide to physical examination and history taking* (10th ed.). Philadelphia: Lippincott Williams & Wilkins.

Bolek, B. (2006). Strictly clinical: Facing cranial nerve assessment. *American Nurse Today, 1*(2), 21–22.

Bradley, R. (2007). Improving respiratory assessment skills. *Journal for Nurse Practitioners, 3*(4), 276–277.

Camillo, P. (2007). Should a rectal exam be a routine part of a pelvic examination? *Medscape Nurses.* Available at http://www.medscape.com/viewarticle/562990_print

Inott, T. (2007). Is it delirium, dementia, or depression? *Nursing, (37)*11, 65.

Jevon, P., & Cunningham, A. (2007). Inspection and palpation of the precordium. *Nursing Times, 103*(26), 26–27.

Keeping an eye on abnormalities. (2008). *Nursing, 38*(1), 48–49.

Lloyd, H., & Craig, S. (2007). A guide to taking a patient's history. *Nursing Standard, 22*(13), 42–48.

Lynn, P. (2008). *Taylor's clinical nursing skills: A nursing process approach* (2nd ed.). Philadelphia: Lippincott Williams & Wilkins.

McCarron, K. (2007). Jaundice: More than meets the eye. *Nursing Made Incredibly Easy! 5*(3), 25–27.

Moore, T. (2007). Respiratory assessment in adults. *Nursing Standard, 21*(49), 48–56.

Pullen, R. J. (2007). Assessing skin lesions. *Nursing, 37*(8), 44–45.

Weber, J., & Kelley, J. (2009). *Health assessment in nursing* (4th ed.). Philadelphia: Lippincott Williams & Wilkins.

Williams, M. D. (2007). Assessment of the neck and lymph nodes in the elderly patient. *Medscape.* Available at http://www.medscape.com/

26 | Safety, Security, and Emergency Preparedness

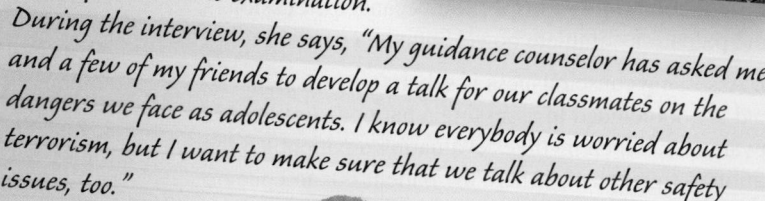

KARA GREENWOOD

Kara, a high school junior class representative and peer counselor, comes to the local community health center for a routine examination.
During the interview, she says, "My guidance counselor has asked me and a few of my friends to develop a talk for our classmates on the dangers we face as adolescents. I know everybody is worried about terrorism, but I want to make sure that we talk about other safety issues, too."

BESSIE WASHINGTON

Bessie, a 77-year-old woman, was recently discharged to her home after suffering a cerebrovascular accident (brain attack). She lives alone in a small one-bedroom apartment and uses a walker to ambulate. She says, "I have so much stuff crammed into this small apartment! I almost fell this morning going from my bedroom to the kitchen."

JUANITA AND INEZ FLORES

Juanita is a young mother of a 1-year-old girl, Inez, who is at the clinic for a well-child visit. While sitting on a cot with her daughter, whose legs are dangling at the edge of the cot about a foot above ground level, Juanita turns to get something out of her purse and the child falls to the floor and begins to cry loudly.

LEARNING OBJECTIVES

After completing the chapter, you will be able to accomplish the following:

1. Identify factors that affect safety in an individual's environment.
2. Identify patients at risk for injury.
3. Describe specific safety risk factors for each developmental stage.
4. Select nursing diagnoses for patients in unsafe situations.
5. Describe health-teaching interventions to promote safety for each developmental stage.
6. Describe strategies to decrease the risk for injury in the home.
7. Describe nursing interventions to prevent injury to patients in healthcare settings.
8. Identify alternatives to using restraints.
9. Explore resources for developing and evaluating an emergency management plan.
10. Evaluate the effectiveness of safety interventions.

KEY TERMS

asphyxiation
bioterrorism
chemical terrorism
disaster
ground
intimate partner
   violence (IPV)
nuclear terrorism
poison control center
restraint
safety event report
sentinel event

Safety and security are basic human needs. Safety, or freedom from danger, harm, or risk, is a paramount concern that underlies all nursing care, and patient safety is a responsibility of all healthcare providers. Safety is a focus in all healthcare facilities as well as in the home, workplace, and community. Many safety and security concerns are universal for all age groups, but there are unique considerations for each developmental stage.

Since the mass casualties that occurred in the terrorist attacks of September 11, 2001, as well as terrorist attacks in other parts of the world, the healthcare community has become increasingly aware of the need to be prepared should future incidents occur. Nurses are a vital part of any emer-

gency response team and need knowledge about biological, chemical, and radioactive agents as well as the skills and competencies required to respond safely and effectively.

This chapter provides practical information on safety and security and introduces concepts of emergency preparedness. The nursing process facilitates the nurse's ability to recognize, assess, diagnose, and plan nursing interventions to ensure safety for all ages in all environments. (See the accompanying Reflective Practice box.)

FACTORS AFFECTING SAFETY

Promoting safety and preventing injury are dual responsibilities of the nurse. Being aware of safety factors, such as developmental level and lifestyle, allows nurses to identify potential hazards and promote wellness. Injuries and deaths from motor vehicle accidents, falls, fire, suffocation, and poisoning occur with alarming regularity across the life span. Many of these injuries and deaths can be prevented with appropriate safety awareness and precautions. Violent behavior and its aftermath has also become a significant public safety concern.

Developmental Considerations

Each developmental level carries its own particular risks. Healthcare needs and safety risks change as individuals progress from infancy to the older adult stage. Physical and cognitive changes reflect these sequential stages. Ensuring that the environment is safe and secure requires an awareness of potential hazards for each developmental level. Studies have confirmed, for example, that pregnant women who use drugs, consume alcohol, or smoke expose their unborn children to substances that may adversely affect their normal growth and development. The nurse is often the initial healthcare provider in contact with an abused child or a battered woman. Prompt recognition of the potential or actual threat to safety is crucial, and the nursing assessment may play a vital role in identifying a harmful environment.

For children, potential hazards multiply as their motor skills develop and their environment expands, yet many childhood accidents are preventable. Adolescents face great dangers when they abuse drugs or alcohol or engage in high-risk sexual activity. The increasing number of adolescents who become pregnant or who are victims of alcohol-related motor vehicle accidents, sexually transmitted infections, and suicide are devastating outcomes of these unsafe behaviors.

Abuse of the elderly has increased dramatically and, given the expanding number of individuals over 65 years of age, the incidence of maltreatment in this vulnerable population is expected to escalate (College of American Pathologists, 2008). Nurses have first-hand experience with the specific hazards confronting each age group and situation.

Ideally, the nurse and the patient or family should work together to eliminate or reduce accident risks in the home, community, or healthcare setting. Nationally, community-based nurses and emergency nurses are establishing partnerships and venturing into the community to offer injury

REFLECTIVE PRACTICE

Challenge to Ethical and Legal Skill

I first met Juanita Flores while working at a children's hospital two summers ago in a nurse externship program. Juanita was the mother of a 1-year-old girl diagnosed with failure to thrive who had been on the rehabilitation unit for some time. The child was very small and had a feeding program prescribed. One day while I was in the room, Juanita was sitting on the cot with her daughter, whose legs were dangling at the edge of the cot, about 1 foot above ground level. I was taking the child's vital signs. As the mother turned her back for a minute to grab something from her bag, I turned away to wash my hands in the sink. All of a sudden, I heard a thud and crying as the child fell to the floor. Juanita tried to comfort her, picking her up and rocking and singing to her. Although I knew it was not completely my fault, I felt horrible about turning my back on the child for only the few seconds to wash my hands, the seconds that it took for the child to fall. Although Juanita was in the room, the child had been unsupervised for only a few seconds. However, I was not watching her at the moment the child fell. I wanted to tell my preceptor right away and knew I should in case anything had happened to the child, but I was nervous and afraid that I would get into trouble.

Thinking Outside the Box: Possible Courses of Action

- Tell my preceptor immediately that the child had fallen, and risk being asked why I had turned my back on the child.
- Report later that morning that the child had fallen earlier, and not make a big deal of it.
- Not mention it at all.

Evaluating a Good Outcome: How Do I Define Success?

- Patient is benefited by my actions, or at least is not harmed.
- My professional integrity is not compromised, nor is the personal integrity of the patient.
- A level of respect is maintained between the preceptor and student.
- Institutional policy for incident reporting is not violated.

Personal Learning: Here's to the Future!

Although I did tell my preceptor what had happened, I was not pleased by the way I handled the situation. Instead of reporting the incident right away, I waited until my preceptor was in the room with me, a half-hour or so later. I casually mentioned that the child had fallen earlier that morning but seemed to be fine. When my preceptor asked why I did not inform her earlier, I said that I couldn't find her and assumed that she was busy—plus, the child seemed fine and her mother was with her.

I was disappointed in how I dealt with this situation. Although I did not get reprimanded for the situation, an incident report was written documenting that the child had fallen. The physician also came to examine the child to ensure that the child was indeed okay. My preceptor stressed the importance of reporting incidents as soon as they happen, rather than delaying or ignoring them. This time the child was uninjured, but I learned that in the future I will report any problem immediately. A patient's fall could be detrimental. It is also very important to follow the institution's policy for reporting incidents to ensure both your professional integrity and the well-being of the patient.

Anne Hrynko, Georgetown University

Reflection

How do you think you would respond in a similar situation? Why? What does this tell you about yourself and about the adequacy of your skills for professional practice? Is the nurse extern's fear justification for the action? Please explain. What ethical and legal principles, if any, were violated in this situation? What liability would the nurse extern be required to assume? Can you think of other ways to respond? How might the nurse extern have interacted with the mother to promote the child's safety? What other skills (cognitive, interpersonal, technical, ethical/legal) would you need to respond well in this situation? Do you agree with the criteria to evaluate a successful outcome? How do you think this incident affected the relationship between the nurse extern and the preceptor? Please explain.

prevention activities to children and families. Nurses who role model good health behaviors are more effective teachers. Use Promoting Health 26-1 as a tool for self-evaluation of safety.

Education to promote awareness of potentially dangerous situations must begin as early as possible and continue throughout the life span. Assessment of specific risks for each developmental level and appropriate nursing interventions are discussed later in this chapter.

Lifestyle

Certain occupations, recreational activities, and environments place people in more hazardous situations.

Occupation

Occupation and work environment often contribute to a person's safety. Certain occupations have exposure to health hazards, such as excessive noise, pollution, toxic chemicals or

PROMOTING HEALTH • 26-1

Safety in the Community

Use the following assessment checklist to determine how well you are meeting your need for maintaining personal safety as you assist with healthcare delivery in the community. Then develop a prescription for self-care by choosing appropriate behaviors from the list of suggestions.

Assessment Checklist

❑ almost always ❑ sometimes ❑ almost never

❑ ❑ ❑   1. I wear a badge or clothing that identifies me as a healthcare worker.

❑ ❑ ❑   2. I dress in an unobtrusive, professional manner.

❑ ❑ ❑   3. I keep my car in good working order.

❑ ❑ ❑   4. I am aware of neighborhoods where personal safety and security may be a problem.

❑ ❑ ❑   5. I confirm directions to the patient's residence before the visit.

❑ ❑ ❑   6. I enter patients' homes only when invited in by a responsible adult.

Self-Care Behaviors

1. Call patients to schedule visits for an agreeable time.
2. Carry a map of the communities you plan to visit.
3. Avoid isolated areas.
4. Request that pets be secured before your visit.
5. Do not carry money, credit cards, or handbag on your person. If necessary, lock them in your trunk.
6. Avoid wearing expensive jewelry.
7. Carry a cell phone.
8. Request escort services as appropriate or make joint visits.
9. Keep your car locked when driving and when parked.
10. Make sure agency is aware of time/location of scheduled visits.

---

vapors, or infectious agents. For example, a worker who operates industrial machinery or works in a perilous setting or with chemicals has a greater risk for accidental injury. Nurses working in the operating room are regularly exposed to surgical smoke, a byproduct of laser and electrosurgery that contains chemicals that cause upper respiratory tract irritation (Association of periOperative Registered Nurses [AORN], 2008). Reproductive hazards may exist for women with long-term exposure to certain anesthetic agents. An antiviral preparation (ribavirin) used for respiratory infections in hospitalized infants and children and treatment of chronic hepatitis C may be harmful to a developing fetus (Pillitteri, 2010). Exposure to excessive noise (e.g., a construction site, extremely loud music) may lead to hearing loss.

Certain occupations also have increased risks of specific injuries. Nurses are frequently exposed to needlestick injuries and blood borne infections (American Nurses Association [ANA], 2008). The Occupational Safety and Health Administration (OSHA) identifies risks and develops standards to prevent serious injuries and illnesses caused by work-related musculoskeletal disorders resulting from repetitive motions. Back pain and carpal tunnel syndrome may occur from work-related repetitive motion.

Social Behavior

Some people by nature are more inclined to take risks and place themselves at jeopardy for injury. For example, failure to wear seat belts or to follow safety precautions is common behavior for some people. Others do not use appropriate protective equipment, such as wearing a helmet when riding a motorcycle. Such behaviors increase the risk for injury.

Stress may precipitate an unhealthful lifestyle that involves drug or alcohol abuse. For example, a high school student involved in multiple school activities and intent on maintaining his excellent grades may turn to an addictive substance such as methamphetamine as a stimulant. This drug temporarily allows the student to remain alert for more hours each day and complete required class assignments.

Nurses have always been strong patient advocates regarding safety concerns. Vulnerable populations such as individuals who have made poor lifestyle choices also need support and attention. See Nursing Advocacy in Action for an example of a nurse supporting a patient's safety and health.

Environment

Although much has been done to identify and control environmental pollutants, certain areas have proved to be more hazardous, and residents may be exposed to potentially unhealthy substances in the environment.

Living in an area where crime is prevalent can pose a threat to physical security and emotional well-being. Violence, acts of aggression, and terrorism are components of 21st-century life. Security measures such as locks, security systems, and exterior lighting can promote safety.

Mobility

Any limitation in mobility is potentially unsafe. An older patient with an unsteady gait is more prone to falling, and an

NURSING ADVOCACY IN ACTION

Patient Scenario

Ms. Jackson was admitted to the labor and delivery unit in active labor. She is in prison for killing her husband and is accompanied to the hospital by two armed guards. She is in shackles in the labor room "to prevent her escape." When you begin your shift, you find a woman in hysterics who has been in labor for 12 hours because of the position of the baby. You want to get her shackles off to try to make her more comfortable, but the guards aren't willing to help. They explain that it is policy to keep them on for felons like Ms. Jackson. You are horrified.

Implications for Nursing Advocacy

How will you respond if you are Ms. Jackson's nurse? Talk with your classmates and experienced nurses about the questions that follow.

- If you elect to advocate for Ms. Jackson and other women like her, what practical steps can you take to ensure better labor and delivery care?
- What is reasonable to expect of a student nurse, a graduate nurse, and an experienced nurse in this situation?
- What advocacy skills are needed to effectively respond to this challenge?

unfamiliar setting, such as a healthcare facility, may aggravate the problem. Someone with paralysis or a spinal cord injury may require assistance with even simple movements. Supportive devices, such as canes, walkers, and wheelchairs, may facilitate movement, but they require careful patient instruction and preparation for safe use. Recent surgery or a prolonged illness can temporarily affect a patient's mobility and necessitate special precautions to prevent falls or injuries. Nurses must assess a patient's risk for injury with a view toward maintaining independence and fostering self-esteem while providing a safe and predictable environment.

> *Think back to Bessie Washington, the 77-year-old woman with a cerebrovascular accident (brain attack) who lives alone in a small apartment and requires a walker to ambulate. To ensure that the patient remains safe, the nurse needs to assess the patient's home environment closely for hazards, especially based on the patient's statement that she almost fell.* ∎

Sensory Perception

Alterations in sensory perception can have a devastating effect on safety. Any impairment in sight, hearing, smell,

taste, or touch can reduce a person's sensitivity to the environment. Visual changes may cause a person to stumble, lose his or her balance, and fall. A patient with a hearing deficit may not be able to hear safety alarms, automobile horns, or sirens and may not hear healthcare instructions. A patient with a reduced ability to distinguish odors may fail to detect leaking gas or smoke. A patient with a loss of taste may have unsafe eating habits or may eat tainted food. A patient whose tactile sense is impaired may not perceive temperature extremes that are a threat to safety.

Knowledge

An awareness of safety and security precautions is crucial for promoting and maintaining wellness. A patient needs instructions, for example, to adhere to a medical regimen or to follow safety precautions when oxygen is in use. He or she requires a certain amount of knowledge to manage new equipment and unfamiliar procedures. Nursing assessment includes identifying and recognizing potentially threatening circumstances.

> *Recall Juanita Flores, the young mother of a 1-year-old who fell from a cot. The nurse's knowledge of potential threats to safety for infants, in conjunction with providing anticipatory guidance to the mother about safety issues for infants, would be essential to prevent injury.* ∎

Recommendations for specific safety and security precautions are included throughout this chapter.

Ability to Communicate

The ability to communicate is basic to many safety practices. The nurse must assess any factor that influences the patient's ability to receive and send messages. Fatigue, stress, medication, aphasia, and language barriers are examples of factors that can affect personal communication and prevent the patient from accurately perceiving events. For example, a medication side effect of drowsiness may interfere with a health teaching session between the nurse and the patient taking this drug. A valid assessment by the nurse not only identifies the patient's level of understanding, but also facilitates a positive communication experience.

Physical Health State

Anything that affects the patient's health state potentially can affect the safety of the environment. When a person is chronically ill or in a weakened state, the focus of healthcare includes preventing accidents as well as promoting wellness and restoring the individual to a healthy state. The nurse caring for a patient who is recovering from a stroke or brain attack, for example, identifies the patient's neuromuscular impairment, pays particular attention to health teaching concerning the person's ability to maintain a sense of balance, and carefully assists the patient with ambulation to prevent falls. Many patients who fall have a primary or secondary diagnosis of cardiovascular disease, such as a stroke. Prevention of complications and return to the optimal level of functioning require attention to safety and become primary concerns in a stroke rehabilitation program. The nurse strives to maximize the patient's potential by considering safety factors in all phases of the illness and recovery experience.

> ➤ *Consider Bessie Washington, the woman who is now at home after having a cerebrovascular accident. The nurse would incorporate knowledge of safety factors along with knowledge of the patient's mobility limitations to develop a plan of care that maximizes the patient's potential while maintaining patient safety.* ■

Psychosocial Health State

Stressful situations tend to narrow a person's attention span and make him or her more prone to accidents. Stress may occur over a long period, but the effects tend to be more devastating in the person's later years, when there is typically less adaptive and coping capacity. Depression may result in confusion and disorientation, accompanied by reduced awareness or concern about environmental hazards. Social isolation or lack of social contact may lead to a reduced level of concentration, errors in judgment, and a diminished awareness of external stimuli.

THE NURSING PROCESS FOR MAINTAINING SAFETY
Assessing

When performing a safety assessment, the nurse focuses on three categories: the individual, the environment, and specific risk factors.

Assessing the Individual

Assessment of the individual consists of a nursing history and a physical examination.

NURSING HISTORY

To help provide a safe environment, be alert to any history of falls or accidents, because a person with a history of falling is likely to fall again. Note any assistive devices that the patient uses (e.g., a cane or walker). Be alert to any history of drug or alcohol abuse. Family members and significant others are often valuable resources. Knowledge of family support systems and the home environment is crucial for the nurse to plan protective health measures. The initial assessment performed by the nurse upon admission to a healthcare facility summarizes all this information (refer to Nursing History in Chap. 12).

Some people seem more likely than others to have accidents. Some children, for example, are involved in multiple mishaps resulting in fractured bones or minor injuries requiring surgical repair. Adults at any age may also have this tendency. Experts disagree about the cause of accident-prone behavior, but most agree that a patient with a history of accidents is likely to have another one.

PHYSICAL EXAMINATION

Assess the patient's mobility status, ability to communicate, level of awareness or orientation, and sensory perception in the physical examination. Early identification of any potential safety hazards is essential. Recognize any manifestations that suggest domestic violence or neglect. Chapters 3 and 19 discuss families experiencing violence, neglect, or abuse.

Assessing the Environment

. Assessment of the environment requires the same attention to safety. Risks in the home, community, and healthcare agency may cause injury.

Environmental safety hazards can result in falls, fires, poisoning, suffocation, and accidents involving motor vehicles, equipment, and procedures. Nursing assessment includes identifying individuals at risk and recognizing unsafe situations. This requires knowledge of the factors that influence safety and predispose people to accidents. Recognizing these factors helps the nurse develop an individualized plan of care and nursing interventions for protecting the patient. Assessment includes an awareness of risk factors in both the home and the healthcare agency, with the focus on the patient's developmental level and health status.

As student nurses become increasingly involved in community and home care settings, they need also to assess their own environmental safety when visiting unfamiliar areas.

Performing a Specific Risk Factor Assessment

Be aware of the patients who are most at risk for injury as well as specific hazards. The following are common safety risks that nurses should assess.

FALLS

Falls can occur at any age, but among adults older than 65, they are the leading cause of injury fatality (Centers for Disease Control and Prevention [CDC], 2009b). A large portion of healthcare for the older adult is used to care for fall-related injuries. Medicare costs for the treatment of falls in this population continue to climb and are expected to rise to $54.9 billion by 2020 (CDC, 2009a). Falls occur in community settings, as well as in acute and long-term care facilities. Nearly one-third of older adults fall at home each year, and the most common injuries that result from a fall include hip or other fracture, head trauma, or soft-tissue injury (CDC, 2009b). Many falls at home go unreported because they do not cause injuries requiring medical attention. Also, the elderly fear activity restrictions, loss of independence, or placement in a nursing home. Fear of falling can also cause anxiety and panic and make an older adult more vulnerable to a fall.

Assessment of the risk for falling includes the use of nursing history and nursing examination. The nursing history and examination include inquiring about and inspecting for factors that contribute to falls. An individual is considered at high risk for a fall if he or she has any of the following characteristics:

- Age older than 65 years
- Documented history of falls
- Impaired vision or sense of balance
- Altered gait or posture
- A medication regimen that includes diuretics, tranquilizers, sedatives, hypnotics, or analgesics
- Postural hypotension
- Slowed reaction time
- Confusion or disorientation
- Impaired mobility
- Weakness and physical frailty
- Unfamiliar environment

Falls in the older adult can be prevented if they can be predicted, so continuous surveillance for environmental hazards is crucial in the healthcare facility and the home environment and of patients who are at risk for falls. Family members are an invaluable resource in assessing a patient's risk

for a fall. They can provide information regarding periods of weakness, confusion/disorientation, and a history of unreported falls.

> *Remember Bessie Washington, the older adult woman described at the beginning of the chapter. Based on the assessment of the patient, the nurse would identify Mrs. Washington's risk for falls as high. It would be crucial to incorporate this information into the patient's plan of care to ensure her safety.* ■

Most healthcare agencies have fall-prevention programs. See the accompanying PICO in Practice box. Nurses are responsible for identifying patients who are at high risk for falls, documenting pertinent assessments on the chart, and planning appropriate interventions to ensure their safety. A nurse whose behavior is reasonable and prudent and similar to the behavior that would be expected of another nurse in similar circumstances is unlikely to be found liable if a patient falls, even if an injury results. Checklists for preventing

PICO IN PRACTICE
Asking Clinical Questions

Scenario: You are the Nurse Manager of a neuroscience unit. You receive a report from your Nurse Administrator that the number of patients admitted to your unit this past quarter and who suffered falls with and without injuries are higher than expected. Your Nurse Administrator sits down with you to explain the meaning of these report findings. This type of report benchmarks trends in data from many similar-sized hospitals with units like yours across the nation and within your geographic region. Hospital units that have higher than average rates of patient falls as compared to other similar units are identified, with the aim that they find opportunities to improve their practices so that fewer patients suffer falls during their hospitalization. You wonder if there is a way to identify patients who are at high risk of falling when they are admitted to your unit, so that your staff may implement targeted fall prevention interventions.

- POPULATION: Patients admitted to a neuroscience unit
- INTERVENTION: Risk factor assessment for falling during hospitalization
- COMPARISON: None
- OUTCOME: Accurate identification of fall risk

PICO Question: Is there a focused assessment that can identify which patients on a neuroscience unit are at risk of falling during their hospitalization?

Finding: From a CINAHL database search: Rutledge, D. N., Donaldson, N. E., & Pravikoff, D. (1999). Fall risk assess-

ment and prevention in hospitalized patients. *Online Journal of Clinical Innovations, 1*(9), 1–33.
Rutledge, D. N., Donaldson, N. E., & Pravikoff, D. (2003). Update 2003: Fall risk assessment and prevention in hospitalized patients. *Online Journal of Clinical Innovations, 6*(5), 1–55.

There are multiple risk factors for patients' falls during hospitalization, many of which are commonly observed in patients with neurological diseases and neurological impairments. In addition, there are many environmental risk factors for patients' falls that could be modified by implementing modified nursing staffing patterns and by reorganizing the physical design of the hospital unit.

Strength of Evidence: Level I

Recommendation: You recommend to your Nurse Administrator that you lead the formation of a Quality Improvement project. You recommend that a multidisciplinary team of staff nurses, nurse educators, therapists, physicians, and environmental services personnel be tasked with identifying and implementing a valid and reliable fall risk assessment scale for patients admitted to your unit. You anticipate that after you accurately identify those patients at high risk of falls, the next step will be to identify and implement evidence-based strategies to prevent them from falling on your unit during their hospitalization.

falls at home and in healthcare facilities appear later in the chapter.

FIRES

Eighty percent (80%) of U.S. fire deaths occur in the home (CDC, 2008e). Many home fires are started because someone was smoking in bed or fell asleep while smoking on a sofa or chair. Kitchen stoves, candles, and electric heaters are other causes of home fires. Faulty wiring and unsafe electrical equipment cause fires in homes and healthcare facilities. Most fatal home fires occur while people are sleeping, and most people who die in house fires die of smoke inhalation rather than burns.

The risk for home fires can be determined by assessing the knowledge of family members and the presence of functioning smoke detectors. Approximately 50% of home fire deaths occur in a home without a smoke detector (CDC, 2008e).

People with limited financial resources should be asked about how they heat their house because the electricity or gas may have been turned off and space or kerosene heaters, wood stoves, or a fireplace may be the sole source of heat. Box 26-1 lists important fire safety issues as well as other safety issues that should be addressed when assessing for risk factors in the home.

Fire prevention and emergency response programs in healthcare facilities are sometimes viewed by staff as time-consuming or unnecessary exercises, but nurses must be prepared at all times to protect patients from injury. Hospitals are required by law to establish safety boards and to inspect the facility regularly for possible hazards. Equipment must be checked periodically, and escape routes must be kept open. Nurses, as part of their daily care procedures, must be aware of their agency's policies, review equipment and its proper functioning, and assess when and how often drills are performed.

POISONING

Although the incidence of childhood poisoning has been reduced drastically in the past 10 years, accidental poisoning remains a concern. According to the latest government statistics, more than 23,000 deaths resulted from accidental poisoning in 2005, with many more people suffering nonfatal effects of poisons (CDC, 2008f). Causes of unintentional poisoning in children are listed in Table 26-1. Substances most often ingested with lethal results include alcohol, tricyclic antidepressants, and theophylline while cosmetics, cleaning fluids, and analgesics are more commonly ingested by children with less toxic results. Three factors that put children most at risk for exposure to toxic substances include unsafe storage in the home, spending time in environments other than the home, and lack of attention on the part of the caregiver (Madden, 2008). In 2006, U.S. poison control centers reported approximately two million incident reports involving unintentional poison exposure (CDC, 2008f).

Consider the person's developmental stage when making a safety assessment. Younger children are more apt to ingest household chemicals, whereas older children may swallow medicines in a suicide attempt. Preschoolers are also at risk for ingestion of lead-containing substances in the home. Adolescents and young adults who experiment with drugs may experience accidental poisoning and death. The ready availability of inhalants on store shelves and in the home may provide the opportunity for children to sniff or "huff" these dangerous substances.

> ➤ *Recall Kara Greenwood, the adolescent asking for information about adolescent dangers. An important area to include in the discussion would be drug experimentation.* ■

An older person may inadvertently take an overdose of a medication because of confusion or forgetfulness. Poor vision is also a factor in accidental poisoning in older adults.

Most exposures to toxic fumes occur in the home. Poisoning may result from improper mixing of household substances, prolonged use of strong cleaning products, or malfunctioning household appliances (gas, oil, and kerosene heaters) that can release carbon monoxide. Carbon monoxide is a colorless, odorless, tasteless, and nonirritating gas, which makes it especially dangerous. Exposure can result in mild symptoms or progress to a life-threatening problem or long-term effects. Young children and older adults are more vulnerable to toxic fumes (U.S. Environmental Protection Agency [EPA], 2009).

Poison control centers provide checklists for "poison-proofing" a home and provide lists of toxic household items. Such lists are helpful when assessing and teaching the family about poisonous materials (see Box 26-1).

SUFFOCATION AND CHOKING

Suffocation, or **asphyxiation,** may occur at any age, but the incidence is greater in children. In suffocation, air does not reach the lungs and breathing stops. Common causes of suffocation are drowning, choking on a foreign substance inhaled into the trachea, and gas or smoke poisoning. An infant may suffocate when a pillow or a piece of plastic inadvertently covers the nose and mouth. Sixty percent (60%) of incidents of infant suffocation occur in the sleeping environment (Safe Kids USA, 2008). A young child may be strangled accidentally by the shoulder harness of a seat belt or become trapped while playing in a discarded refrigerator and suffocate.

Drowning is a form of suffocation. Nearly half of all drowning victims are children younger than 5 years of age. Most drowning deaths in young children occur because of inadequate supervision of a child in or near a bathtub or pool, even a small wading pool. Older children are more likely to drown while swimming or boating.

Educating the public about the causes of suffocation can save many lives. Assessing the knowledge level of individuals, especially parents, is vital. Nurses need to be alert to hazards that might cause a child to asphyxiate or choke (see Box 26-1).

Box 26-1   HOME SAFETY CHECKLIST

Fire and Burn Safety
- [ ] Have a list of emergency phone numbers posted near the phone.
- [ ] Install smoke detectors in each room (or at a minimum, on each floor).
- [ ] Replace smoke detector batteries when you reset your clock.
- [ ] Have a fire extinguisher available on each floor, and know how to use it.
- [ ] Practice a fire escape plan with your family.
- [ ] Teach all family members to stop, drop, and roll if clothing catches on fire.
- [ ] Keep matches and lighters out of reach of children.
- [ ] Keep lighted candles out of children's reach.
- [ ] Buy flame-resistant children's clothing, particularly sleepwear.
- [ ] Keep bedroom doors closed while sleeping (use monitor to listen for a child).
- [ ] Have ashtrays readily available if there is a smoker in the house.
- [ ] Enforce a strict "no smoking in bed" policy.
- [ ] After a party, check wastebaskets, ashtrays, furniture, and carpets for carelessly discarded cigarettes.
- [ ] Turn off a kerosene heater when no one is in the room and at bedtime.
- [ ] Operate your fireplace or wood-burning stove safely (flue open, fire screen covering the opening, annual chimney cleaning, proper disposal of ashes).
- [ ] Prevent trash or paint-saturated rags from accumulating in your garage.
- [ ] Store oily rags, gasoline, or other flammables away from heating sources or open flames, such as the pilot light of the water heater.
- [ ] Cook on back burners, and turn pot handles toward the back of the stove.
- [ ] Keep hot dishes away from the edges of tables and counters.
- [ ] Set water heater at a safe temperature (below 120°F).
- [ ] Check bath water temperature with the back of your wrist before placing a child in bath.
- [ ] Use sunscreen and protective clothing to minimize exposure to the sun and prevent sunburn.

Electrical Safety
- [ ] Maintain electrical cords in good condition.
- [ ] Protect unused electric outlets with safety covers.
- [ ] Use the proper replacement for a blown fuse.
- [ ] Keep an electric space heater away from curtains and flammable material.
- [ ] Turn off appliances before going to bed or leaving the house.
- [ ] Hire a professional to do electrical repairs.
- [ ] Never overload wall outlets or extension cords.
- [ ] Unplug appliances that are not in use.
- [ ] Do not permit children to use the microwave.

Preventing Poisoning
- [ ] Keep the phone number for the local poison control center next to the phone.
- [ ] Color-code medication bottles for those who are visually impaired.
- [ ] Syrup of ipecac is no longer recommended if poisoning should occur. Immediately contact the Poison Control Center (1-800-222-1222).
- [ ] Store all medicines in child-resistant containers in a locked medicine cabinet.
- [ ] Destroy old medicines (flush down the toilet).
- [ ] Keep all poisonous plants out of a child's reach.
- [ ] Avoid eating any fresh or prepared foods that look or smell spoiled.

- [ ] Store cleaning products, insecticides, and corrosives safely out of a child's reach.
- [ ] Avoid mixing caustic products with any other household product (dangerous chemical reactions may occur).
- [ ] Keep shampoos and cosmetics in a safe place.
- [ ] Use safety latches on cabinets.
- [ ] Store alcoholic beverages out of a child's reach.
- [ ] Check that paint or finish on furniture and toys is nontoxic.
- [ ] Install a carbon monoxide detector in your home.
- [ ] Have your furnace professionally inspected each year.
- [ ] Keep vents and chimneys clear of debris, and have them checked seasonally.
- [ ] Don't operate cars, motorized equipment, or charcoal or gas grills in enclosed spaces.

Preventing Falls and Other Injuries
- [ ] Keep stairways clear and uncluttered.
- [ ] Maintain walkways, stairs, and railings in good repair.
- [ ] Keep stairs, hallways, outside walkways, and working areas well lit.
- [ ] Install safety gates at tops and bottoms of stairways.
- [ ] Paint the bottom step of the stairs a different color.
- [ ] Apply nonslip adhesive strips to the bottom surface of the tub or shower.
- [ ] Have a raised toilet seat with support arms available if necessary.
- [ ] Provide grab bars next to the toilet and in the tub or shower area.
- [ ] Use sturdy chairs that have armrests.
- [ ] Eliminate scatter rugs, or secure them with adhesive strips on the underside.
- [ ] Use a handheld device, such as pincers, when reaching for inaccessible items.
- [ ] Buckle a child into an approved automobile safety seat even when making short trips.

Firearm Safety
- [ ] Keep guns and ammunition stored separately and locked up.
- [ ] Install trigger locks on all guns.
- [ ] Make certain that the key to the locked gun storage area is not available to a child or young person.
- [ ] Discuss the risk for injury from guns with your children.
- [ ] Instruct your child never to touch a gun or remain in a friend's house where a gun is accessible.

Preventing Asphyxiation or Choking
- [ ] Keep plastic bags out of a child's reach.
- [ ] Check that crib slats are no more than 2⅜ inches apart.
- [ ] Ensure that the mattress fits the sides of the crib snugly.
- [ ] Remove soft pillows or thick blankets from your infant's crib.
- [ ] Never place an infant on a waterbed to sleep.
- [ ] Cut food into small pieces before giving it to a young child.
- [ ] Supervise young children when eating and drinking.
- [ ] Avoid giving peanuts, hard candy, or other small treats to a young child.
- [ ] Keep small objects, such as jewelry, buttons, and safety pins, out of a child's reach.
- [ ] Use toys appropriate for the child's age.
- [ ] Always watch a child who is in the tub.
- [ ] Cover wading pools and sandboxes when not in use.
- [ ] Check that nearby swimming pools are enclosed with a fence that your child cannot easily climb over.
- [ ] Keep pool rescue equipment nearby.
- [ ] Supervise your child closely when near water.
- [ ] Know how to perform cardiopulmonary resuscitation and the Heimlich maneuver.

TABLE • 26-1	COMMON AGENTS IN CHILDHOOD POISONING		
Poisonous Agent	**Source**	**Common Clinical Manifestations**	**Treatment**
Acetaminophen	Products containing aceta- minophen (Tylenol)	Anorexia, nausea, vomiting, and liver toxicity	In the emergency department (ED), activated charcoal or acetylcysteine either orally or via NG tube
Hydrocarbons	Gasoline Kerosene Furniture polish Lamp oil	Gagging, coughing, choking, dyspnea, grunting, nausea, chills, fever, lethargy	*Never induce vomiting!* Contact physician or poison control center (PCC)
Caustics	Oven cleaner Drain openers Toilet bowl cleaners Battery contents Rust removers Hair perms	Burning pain in mouth and throat, drooling, edema of lips; oral, esophageal, gastric burns; vomiting, hemoptysis	*Never induce vomiting!* Never attempt to neutralize the caustic. Dilution with milk or water. Contact physician or PCC
Iron	Vitamin preparations (particularly pregnancy vitamins)	Nausea, vomiting, diarrhea, abdominal pain, melena, hematemesis, lethargy, coma	Contact PCC. In ED, stomach lavage (may remove unabsorbed pills); possible use of cathartic. If dose is toxic, use of chelating agent
Lead	Paint chips Paint dust Fumes from burning or swallowed batteries	May be asymptomatic, anorexia, abdom- inal pain, anemia, lead encephalitis, neurobehavioral deficits	Chelation therapy and monitoring of lead levels
Insecticides	Insecticide sprays	Nausea, vomiting, diarrhea, excessive salivation, confusion, depressed reflexes, seizures	Activated charcoal if swallowed. If clothing is contaminated, washing of skin and hair. IV atropine and a cholinesterase reactivator possible to ease symptoms.

Adapted from: Pillitteri, A. (2010). *Maternal & child health nursing* (6th ed.). Philadelphia: Lippincott Williams & Wilkins.

FIREARM INJURIES

Preventing injuries caused by firearms has become a major concern for health professionals. Intentional injuries caused by firearms are a leading cause of mortality in children. According to the CDC (2008g), 82% of homicide victims between the ages of 10 to 24 years of age are killed with a firearm. Some people believe that keeping a gun in the home provides protection for family and property, but if not stored properly, guns can be dangerous. The presence of a gun in the home is a huge risk factor. Young children are curious and like to explore their surroundings, and when they encounter a loaded gun, the outcome is often tragic. Also, having a gun in the house increases the risk for domestic homicide threefold.

Gun ownership is a sensitive issue, and nurses need to approach this topic in a nonjudgmental manner with the focus on injury prevention. The intent is to inform families about the risks of firearm injury and discuss appropriate safety measures (see Box 26-1).

Diagnosing

Unsafe situations and patients at risk are reflected in the nursing diagnosis and plan of care. The statement of the patient's actual or potential health status must be followed by the appropriate contributing factors or risk factors to individualize the nursing plan of care. Nursing diagnoses involving safety risks may include the following:

- Risk for Injury related to lack of awareness of environmental hazards; visual or auditory sensory deficits; history of falling; unsteady gait; substance abuse; refusal to use seat belt or child safety seat; effects of medication; age greater than 65 years; generalized weakness; biological, chemical, or nuclear exposure
- Risk for Poisoning related to impaired vision; medications stored in unlocked medicine cabinet that is accessible to a child; presence of poisonous plants; excess alcohol intake; use of illicit drugs; knowledge deficit; chemical contamination of food and water
- Risk for Suffocation related to a plastic bag that is accessible to a young child; child left unattended in bathtub; smoking in bed; placing an infant prone in a water bed; lack of safety precautions (door left on discarded refrigerator); unfamiliarity with fire prevention guidelines; household gas leaks
- Risk for Trauma related to history of previous falls; unsteady gait; presence of unsecured scatter rugs;

smoking in bed; inoperable smoke detector; history of substance abuse; lack of experience operating an automobile; presence of unsecured loaded gun in the home; high-crime neighborhood
- Impaired Home Maintenance related to insufficient finances; substance abuse; physical disability; inadequate support systems; lack of knowledge
- Risk for Disuse Syndrome related to use of physical restraints
- Risk for Contamination related to chemical contamination of food or water, exposure to bioterrorism, exposure to radiation, flaking or peeling paint in presence of young children, playing in outdoor areas where environmental contaminants are used, smoking

Outcome Identification and Planning

Many accidental injuries and deaths are preventable. Consider the various factors and the environment that affect the patient's safety and formulate expected outcomes uniquely suited to each situation and circumstance. Nursing interventions focus on meeting these safety needs. Some expected outcomes for patients that promote safety and prevent injury are as follows:

The patient will

- Identify unsafe situations in his or her environment
- Identify potential hazards in his or her environment
- Demonstrate safety measures to prevent falls and other accidents
- Establish safety priorities with family members or significant others
- Demonstrate familiarity with his or her environment
- Identify resources for safety information
- Remain free of injury during hospitalization

See additional examples of nursing outcomes and interventions in the NIC/NOC display.

Implementing

The patient's safety is integral to the nursing plan of care. It is important to intervene in order to control or modify the patient's environment. Safety recommendations in the following sections apply to health agency settings, the home, and the community. Nursing interventions are designed for each developmental level as well as for specific hazards in the environment. Adults who are developmentally disabled or who are experiencing dementia or delirium frequently need the same safety measures as those for children.

Preventing Injury

Injury control includes preventing injuries, providing acute care for injured patients, and rehabilitation services. Most importantly, injury prevention allows for the reduction of injuries through eliminating risky events, measuring the consequences of these events, and reducing the severity of injuries. There are many strategies for preventing injury. Interventions that include modification of the environment and education for individuals at risk have proved effective. Laws or regulations, such as those imposed by OSHA, also help to modify at-risk behavior.

Teaching to Promote Safety
PREVENTING ACCIDENTS

Teaching is an important intervention for accident prevention and health promotion. Many teaching opportunities concerning safety measures arise while the nurse performs regular patient care, and many resources are available to supplement health teaching (Fig. 26-1). Careful assessment, diagnosis, and planning prepare nurses to use these opportunities wisely.

Assessment data and statistical information often prove helpful to healthcare personnel who are developing a safety program for patients at risk. Safety education classes, in

---

Examples of Nursing Interventions and Nursing Outcomes Classifications (NIC/NOC)

Environmental Management: Safety

Nursing Interventions	Nursing Outcomes

• Identify safety hazards in the environment (i.e., physical, biological, and chemical).
• Modify the environment to minimize hazards and risks.
• Provide patient with emergency phone numbers (e.g., police, local health department, poison control center).
• Initiate and/or conduct screening programs for environmental hazards (e.g., lead and radon).
• Educate high-risk individuals and groups about environmental hazards.
	• Safe Home Environment:
	  • Space to move safely in environment.
	  • Carbon monoxide detector maintenance.
	  • Smoke detector maintenance.
	  • Safe storage of medications.
	  • Safe storage of firearms.
	  • Correction of lead hazard risks.
	  • Arrangement of furniture to reduce risks.

Bulechek, G., Butcher, H., & Dochterman, J. (2008). *Nursing interventions classification (NIC)* (5th ed., p. 326). St. Louis: Mosby, Inc. A full listing of nursing activities for each nursing intervention can be found in this book.
Moorhead, S., Johnson, M., Maas, M., & Swanson, E. (2008). *Nursing outcomes classification (NOC)* (4th ed., p. 614–615). St. Louis: Mosby, Inc. A full listing of indicators for each nursing outcome can be found in this book.

All-purpose fire
extinguishers
for the home

Toddler gates at
stairs and doors

Outlet covers
protect curious
tots from
electrical shock

Carbon monoxide detectors for the
home *(Photo courtesy of First Alert.)*

Car seats for infants
and children

FIGURE 26-1. The nurse's responsibilities in home safety are primarily that of education and counseling, including providing information about home safety devices and sources for additional information.

addition to situational health teaching, can be worthwhile for hospitalized patients and their family members. Studies have demonstrated that early assessment of vulnerable patients and preventive education programs can decrease the incidence of falls.

A school nurse has many opportunities and a ready audience for health teaching about safety, including screening programs (e.g., vision and hearing), fire prevention sessions, drug and alcohol prevention programs, firearm safety, and classes on various accident prevention techniques. Managing minor accidents at school often provides an opportunity

for additional preventive teaching. School nurses also interact with parents. In this setting, formal or informal health teaching can occur and should also include encouragement to do the following:

- Monitor the child's use of the Internet
- Get involved in school activities and ask pertinent questions
- Volunteer for safety committees that include staff and parents
- Ensure that the school's emergency preparedness plan is current

TEACHING TIPS • 26-1

PREVENTING ACCIDENTS AND PROMOTING SAFETY AT VARYING DEVELOPMENTAL STAGES

Developmental Stage/Safety Risks	Sample Teaching Tip	Why is This Important?
Fetus Abnormal growth & development	• Abstain from alcohol and caffeine while pregnant. • Stop smoking or reduce the number of cigarettes smoked per day. • Avoid all drugs, including OTC drugs, unless prescribed by a physician or midwife. • Avoid exposure to pesticides and certain environmental chemicals. • Avoid exposure to radiation.	Any factors, chemical or physical, can adversely affect the fertilized ovum, embryo, and developing fetus. A fetus is extremely vulnerable to environmental hazards.
Neonate (first 28 days of life) Infection Falls SIDS	• Wash hands frequently. • Never leave infant unsupervised on a raised surface without side rails. • Use appropriate infant car seat that is secured in the back seat facing the rear of the car. • Handle infant securely while supporting the head. • Place infant on back to sleep.	Physical care for the newborn includes maintaining a patent airway, protecting the baby from infection and injury, and providing optimal nutrition.
Infant Falls Injuries from toys Burns Suffocation or drowning Inhalation or ingestion of foreign bodies	• Supervise child closely to prevent injury. • Select toys appropriate for developmental level. • Use appropriate safety equipment in the home (e.g., locks for cabinets, gates, electrical outlet covers). • Never leave child alone in the bathtub. • Childproof the entire house.	Infants progress from rolling over to sitting, crawling, and pulling up to stand. They are very curious and will explore everything in their environment that they can.
Toddler Falls Cuts from sharp objects Burns Suffocation or drowning Inhalation or ingestion of foreign bodies/ poisons	• Have poison control center phone number in readily accessible location. • Use appropriate car seat for toddler. • Supervise child closely to prevent injury. • Childproof house to ensure that poisonous products, drugs, and small objects are out of toddler's reach. • Never leave child alone and unsupervised outside. • Keep all hot items on stove out of child's reach.	Toddlers accomplish a wide variety of developmental tasks and progress to walking and talking. They become more independent and continue to explore their environment.
Preschooler Falls Cuts Burns Drowning Inhalation or ingestion Guns and weapons	• Teach child to wear proper safety equipment when riding bicycles or scooters. • Ensure that playing areas are safe. • Begin to teach safety measures to child. • Do not leave child alone in the bathtub or near water. • Practice emergency evacuation measures. • Teach about fire safety.	Though more independent, preschoolers still have an immature understanding of dangerous behavior. They may strive to imitate adults and thus attempt dangerous behavior.
School-aged child Burns Drowning Broken bones Concussions (TBI) Inhalation or ingestion Guns and weapons Substance abuse	• Teach accident prevention at school and home. • Teach child to wear safety equipment when playing sports. • Reinforce teaching about symptoms that require immediate medical attention. • Continue immunizations as scheduled. • Provide drug, alcohol, and sexuality education. • Reinforce use of seat belts and pedestrian safety.	School-aged children have developed more refined muscular coordination, but increasing involvement in sports and play activities increases their risk for injury. TBI can cause disruption in brain function and death. Cognitive maturity improves their ability to understand safety instructions.

(continued)

TEACHING TIPS • 26-1

PREVENTING ACCIDENTS AND PROMOTING SAFETY AT VARYING DEVELOPMENTAL STAGES *(continued)*

Developmental Stage/Safety Risks	Sample Teaching Tip	Why is This Important?
Adolescent Drowning Motor vehicle accidents Guns and weapons Inhalation and ingestion	• Teach responsibilities of new freedoms that accompany being a teenager. • Enroll teen in safety courses (driver education, water safety, emergency care measures). • Emphasize gun safety. • Get physical examination before participating in sports. • Make time to listen to and talk with your adolescent (helps with stress reduction). • Follow healthy lifestyle (nutrition, rest, etc.). • Teach about sexuality, sexually transmitted infections, and birth control. • Encourage child to report any sexual harassment or abuse of any kind.	Adolescence is a critical period in growth and development. The adolescent needs increasing freedom and responsibility to prepare for adulthood. During this time, the mind has a great ability to acquire and use knowledge. The teen's peer group is a greater influence than parents during this stage.
Adult Stress Domestic violence Motor vehicle accidents Industrial accidents Drug and alcohol abuse	• Practice stress reduction techniques (e.g., meditation, exercise). • Enroll in a defensive driving course. • Evaluate the workplace for safety hazards and utilize safety equipment as prescribed. • Practice moderation when consuming alcohol. • Avoid use of illegal drugs. • Provide options and referrals to domestic violence victims.	As individuals progress through the adult years, visible signs of aging become apparent. Lifestyle behaviors and situational or family crises can also impact an adult's overall health and cause stress. Preventive health practices help adults improve the quality and duration of life
Older Adult Falls Motor vehicle accidents Elder abuse Sensorimotor changes Fires	• Identify safety hazards in the environment. • Modify the environment as necessary. • Attend defensive driving courses on courses designed for elderly drivers. • Encourage regular vision and hearing tests. • Ensure that eyeglasses and hearing aids are available if prescribed and functioning. • Wear appropriate footwear. • Have operational smoke detectors in place. • Objectively document and report any signs of neglect and abuse.	Accidental injuries occur more frequently in older adults because of decreased sensory abilities, slower reflexes and reaction times, changes in hearing and vision, and loss of strength and mobility. Collaboration between family and healthcare providers can ensure a safe, comfortable environment and promote healthy aging.

ADDRESSING DEVELOPMENTAL CONSIDERATIONS

Teaching Tips 26-1 lists common types of safety risks according to developmental age, along with sample teaching tips that should be discussed with parents and in the school. The following discussions of developmental stages are also applicable to teaching.

Neonate and Infant

Safety considerations begin with an awareness of behaviors that may harm the developing fetus. Newborns of mothers who smoke have a lower birth weight. Excessive alcohol consumption and use of drugs may cause adverse effects that are readily apparent at birth. Reinforce a pregnant woman's knowledge of the risks associated with excess alcohol consumption, smoking, drug use, and exposure to other dangers in the environment (see Teaching Tips 26-1). It is also important to stress the importance of regular doctor visits and the use of prenatal vitamins.

The nurse has many opportunities to educate parents about safety and accident prevention for infants. Young infants' lack of mobility limits opportunities for hazardous activity, but minimal safeguards are vital to prevent accidents. Safe care includes never leaving the infant unattended, using crib rails, and monitoring the setting for objects that the infant could place in the mouth and swallow. As the child becomes more active, parents and caregivers must be alert to hazards that a curious, mobile child may encounter. All items within reach must be carefully inspected and, if dangerous, kept in a safe place, out of the child's reach. Because infants frequently climb or pull up on objects, hot liquids and sharp instruments must be placed out of their reach. Also, remind parents that items that are small enough to fit through a standard toilet paper tube represent a potential choking hazard for young children.

All 50 states mandate the use of infant car seats and carriers when transporting a child in a motor vehicle. According to the Centers for Disease Control and Prevention, nearly 40% of all children who ride with an unbelted driver are not secured with child safety seats or seat belts (CDC, 2008d). A rear-facing safety seat placed in the back seat is recommended for infants who are younger than 1 year old and weigh less than 20 lb (9.1 kg). The high force of sudden air bag inflation can cause injury to an infant in a safety seat or a child in the front seat. One recent study found that 72% of parents in the 3,500 instances where car and booster seats were observed used car seats incorrectly (CDC, 2008d). Most parents do not secure the car seat tightly enough with the seat belt or fail to tighten the car seat's harness straps. These seemingly simple omissions can lead to tragic consequences. (See Teaching Tips 26-1 for additional safety counseling measures that focus on health teaching for this developmental level.)

Toddler and Preschooler

To prevent accidental injury and death in toddlers and preschoolers, parents need to childproof the home environment. Play areas should allow for exploration but still provide for safety. Vigilant supervision by parents and guardians should anticipate hazards in the environment and protect the child with precautionary devices. Childproofing products are available that help parents and children recognize dangerous items in the home and prevent injury.

> *Remember Juanita Flores, the mother of the child who fell off a cot. As part of the plan of care, the nurse would review safe infant care with Juanita and also provide anticipatory guidance related to toddler safety in preparation for the child's discharge home.* ∎

Ingestion of poisons or medications is a major threat for preschoolers. Their overconfidence and initiative also make them more likely to dart into the street while chasing a ball, climb into a discarded refrigerator, or play with matches. In addition, any child who is older than 1 year of age and between 20 and 40 lb should be placed in a forward-facing safety seat in the back seat of the vehicle.

Protecting a child also includes being alert to manifestations that indicate child maltreatment or abuse (Box 26-2). In 2006, approximately 900,000 children in the United States were victims of abuse or neglect and 75% of these children had no previous history of maltreatment (CDC, 2008c). Abuse can be physical, sexual, or emotional and may also be a result of neglect. All 50 states have laws that require healthcare personnel to report suspected child abuse. (See Teaching Tips 26-1 for health teaching topics that help safeguard toddlers and preschoolers.)

School-Aged Child

Although school-aged children are increasingly independent, they still need help avoiding activities that are potentially

---

Box 26-2   PHYSICAL AND BEHAVIORAL MANIFESTATIONS OF CHILD MALTREATMENT

History of unexplained or repeated injuries
Multiple or unexplained bruises
Multiple fractures (arms, legs, facial, ribs)
Thermal burns in a pattern
Scars or welts
Bite marks
Head injuries
Vaginal discharge
Urinary tract infection
Genital pain, itching, redness, or bruising
Sexually transmitted disease
Sleeping problems (nightmares)
Psychosomatic illnesses
Excessive sexual curiosity or play
Decreased attendance and performance in school
Reluctance to return home
Overly compliant, withdrawn, or passive
Fear of strangers

Adapted from Pullen, R. (2007). Screening for abuse and neglect. *Nursing, 37*(2), 69 and Child Welfare Information Gateway (2008). *Recognizing child abuse and neglect: Signs and symptoms.* Available at http://www.childwelfare.gov/pubs/factsheets/signs.cfm

---

dangerous. Accidents continue to be a leading cause of death. The nurse should counsel parents of school-aged children about specific interventions for safety at home, at school, and in the neighborhood.

All school-aged children need to be secured in safety seats, belt-positioning booster seats, or shoulder lap belts for their size. The National Highway Traffic Safety Administration recommends booster seats for children until they are 4'9" tall or at least 8 years of age and all children 12 years of age and younger should ride in the back seat, whenever possible, to eliminate the risk of injury from airbag deployment (National Highway Traffic Safety Administration [NHTSA], 2010). If no other arrangement is possible and an older child must ride in the front seat, move the vehicle seat as far back as possible away from the air bag and restrain the child properly based on his/her size.

Each year, a significant number of children younger than 10 years are injured in bicycle accidents. According to the most recent data, children 15 years and younger are involved in almost 60% of all bicycle-related injuries seen in U.S. emergency departments (CDC, 2009e). Many of these injuries involve the head or face. The protective effect of bicycle helmets among children is well documented. Studies indicate that legislation and injury prevention strategies have had a positive impact on increasing helmet use and decreasing the number and severity of bicycle accidents that result in a head injury in this very vulnerable population. However, their use is far from universal. Because of their multiple experiences with children and parents, nurses, whether in the emergency department or a well-child setting, have many opportunities for health teaching related to bicycle safety and helmet use. Points to include in any teaching session include the following:

- Children should wear helmets at all times when riding a bicycle.
- Young children who are secured in a child seat as a passenger on a bicycle should also wear a properly sized helmet.
- The helmet should rest flat on the top of the child's head (approximately 1″ above the eyebrows) and fit snugly.
- The chinstrap on the helmet should be adjusted so that it fits securely. If you can slide two fingers under the strap, the helmet is too loose.
- Any helmet that is involved or damaged in a crash should be discarded and replaced.
- Parents are effective role models for their children when they also wear helmets when riding a bicycle.

Sports or recreation-related activities can result in traumatic brain injury (TBI). A TBI usually results from a blow, bump, or jolt to the head that causes disruption in brain function (CDC, 2009g; Shields, 2007). Concussion is a milder form of TBI. It is estimated that over 2,600 deaths in children up to age 14 are caused by TBI (CDC, 2009g). Nurses in a variety of settings need to be alert for indications of TBI. Manifestations of TBI can be subtle, but the following are "concussion red flags" that parents, teachers, and nurses need to be aware of because they require a 911 call and immediate emergency room attention:

- Headaches that worsen
- Drowsy or difficult to awaken
- Unable to recognize people or places
- Unusual behavior
- Seizures
- Repeated vomiting
- Increasing confusion and/or irritability
- Neck pain
- Slurred speech (Shields, 2007).

The possibility of child abduction also needs to be addressed for this age group. Abduction occurs for a number of reasons and is a tragedy that devastates parents, families, and communities. Children may be kidnapped by unknown individuals or by someone they recognize. Some children suffer sexual assault or are murdered by their captors. Adults who prey on children often take advantage of the innocent and trusting nature of children to persuade the child to accompany them.

Children, even the very young, need basic instructions on how to recognize and respond to a potentially dangerous situation. Health teaching should also emphasize the need for parents to be alert and vigilant at all times regarding the whereabouts of their children.

The Amber Alert System can be activated when a child is missing and believed to be kidnapped. This critical response program uses the resources of law enforcement and the media to notify the public about an abduction. Identifying information is broadcast via radio, television, and highway bulletin boards. The Amber Alert is a powerful tool that helps recover kidnapped children and return them to their families.

Adolescent

Much of the adolescent's time is spent away from home, with his or her peer group, or in automobiles. Adolescents are particularly at risk for motor vehicle accidents, and the CDC (2009f) lists motor vehicle accidents as the number-one cause of death for school-aged children, adolescents, and young adults. Approximately 41% of all adolescent deaths from motor vehicle accidents involve the use of alcohol and/or other drugs (CDC, 2009f). Nurses and parents should collaborate to reinforce safety behaviors in adolescents. Education should focus on safe driving skills and the importance of wearing a seat belt. In addition, teaching should include discussions about drug and alcohol use.

Tobacco is an additional health problem for teenagers. According to the American Cancer Society (ACS), in 2007, 26% of high school students reported using some type of tobacco product (ACS, 2008). Federal law mandates a minimum age of 18 years to purchase tobacco products and bans billboard advertising within 1,000 feet of schools and playgrounds. Teenagers and younger children are influenced to use tobacco products via advertisements, TV, and movies. Most smokers start using tobacco as teenagers.

Educational programs and information can play a role in delaying or preventing smoking among young adults but concerned, involved parents have significant influence on their child's decision to smoke. Conversations regarding the risks of smoking can begin as early as 5 to 6 years of age because many children start using tobacco products at 11 years of age and may be addicted by age 14 (ACS, 2008).

Alcohol use among teenagers is more common than that of tobacco or illicit drugs (CDC, 2009d). According to statistics from the National Institute on Alcohol Abuse and Alcoholism [NIAAA] (2006), underage drinking claims the lives of approximately 5,000 individuals under the age of 21 each year. Almost 2,000 of these deaths occur from motor vehicle accidents. When young people drink alcohol, they are more likely to consume alcoholic drinks in significant number. "Binge drinking" involves the consumption of enough alcohol to elevate the blood alcohol concentration (BAC) to a level of 0.08% or more in 2 hours or less. This usually requires about five or more drinks for an adult male or four or more for a female (NIAAA, 2006). Approximately 20% of teenagers participate in binge drinking each month. Enforcement of zero-tolerance laws regarding drinking age and driving while under the influence of alcohol, prevention programs in schools, and family efforts to influence whether their children consume alcohol are all significant factors aimed at preventing underage drinking.

Teenagers abuse legally available drugs such as prescription medications and over-the-counter cough, cold, sleep, and diet medications. They also abuse illegal substances such as marijuana, stimulants including cocaine and methamphetamine, heroin, opiates, and designer drugs (Ecstasy). The use of illicit drugs among this age group has declined over the last 10 to 15 years but abuse of prescription medication and OTC drugs has remained at a high level. Abuse of these legal drugs can also have serious consequences progressing from mild effects on health to addiction and death (CDC, 2009d). Warning signs of alcohol and drug abuse during adolescence include physical fatigue, personality change, poor judgment, sudden mood changes, withdrawal from the family, a variety of school-related issues (negative attitude, drop in grades, failure), and social problems. Parents need to focus on open communication with their teenagers, role model appropriate behavior, and seek appropriate help and guidance once a problem with alcohol or drug abuse is recognized (American Academy of Child & Adolescent Psychiatry, 2008).

Body piercing has become increasingly popular with adolescents and young adults. Common sites for piercing include the ears, nose, eyebrows, lips, tongue, nipples, navel, and genitals. It is a quick procedure that does not require anesthesia, but the risk for infection, tissue trauma, and transmission of hepatitis B, C, and HIV is real.

Tattoos have also become increasingly popular. Tattoos are permanent markings on skin surfaces viewed as a form of body art. They carry similar risks as body piercings do. To prevent the spread of viruses and bacteria from one surface to another, the tattooist should: wear disposable gloves and change them when necessary, wash hands often, disinfect surfaces between procedures, clean reusable tools before sterilization, and use disposable supplies when possible (CDC, 2008b). Meticulous postpiercing and tattoo care reduce the risk for developing an infection. Nurses need to be informed about the health risks in order to be effective and well-informed health educators.

There are significant security issues related to adolescents and the use of guns. More than 2,600 deaths caused by firearms occurred in 15- to 19-year-olds in 2005. Homicide accounted for 66% of these deaths, 28% were suicides, and 4% were unintentional (U.S. Department of Health and Human Services [USDHHS], 2007). Adolescents need encouragement and education about ways to solve arguments without guns and violence, and guidance and direction for developing a healthful lifestyle while coping with the stresses of daily living. The accompanying Research in Nursing box describes the risk for suicide and use of sports and physical activity as possible deterrents.

> ➤ *Think back to Kara Greenwood, the adolescent who is to present a discussion on adolescent dangers. Numerous issues face adolescents today, and providing safety information is crucial to help adolescents make mature decisions about health hazards they are likely to encounter.* ∎

The use of the Internet has grown, particularly among teenagers. This has prompted legitimate safety concerns by parents. Certain individuals take advantage of the vulnerability of young children and teenagers by stalking them online and exploiting them sexually. According to the U.S.

Department of Justice Federal Bureau of Investigation, one in seven children in the 10 to 17 year old age group has received a sexual solicitation over the Internet (USAA Educational Foundation, 2009). Meeting someone with whom the person has communicated online poses the greatest safety risk for children. Safety guidelines for parents include addressing the following with their children:

- Discuss the dangers associated with the Internet with children. Review the family rules for online activity.
- Keep identifying information private (e.g., full name, address, telephone number). Children need to be reminded that anything posted on the Internet is available to the public at large. Use a screen name that does not contain any identifying information. Parents have the right to have an online site delete any personal information it has about their child.
- Investigate filtering software or methods of blocking out objectionable information.
- Be aware of the sites and services that your children access when online. Parents should be aware of their children's user names and passwords.
- Avoid public chat rooms and forums. Computer sex offenders often use chat rooms to contact potential victims.
- Never allow a child to arrange a meeting alone with someone they have met online. Parents should be involved if a meeting is planned and accompany their child.
- Never respond to e-mails or messages that are suggestive, obscene, threatening, or inappropriate in any way. If a parent becomes aware of the transmission or viewing of child pornography while online, report this immediately to your local FBI office and the CyberTipline at the National Center for Missing and Exploited Children (1-800-843-5678).
- Emphasize that everything said or anything read online may not be true.
- Monitor and set rules regarding the amount of time that children spend on the computer. Children are at the greatest risk when they are online in evening hours. Hours spent online late at night may indicate a potential problem.
- Be alert for downloaded files with suffixes that indicate images or pictures (e.g., .jpg, .gif, .bmp, .tif, or .pcx).
- Consider locating the computer in a central location in the house, rather than in a child's bedroom (USAA Educational Foundation, 2009).

Unfortunately, there are real dangers associated with online communication, and parents need to discuss these with their children. (See Teaching Tips 26-1 for additional safety topics.)

Adult

Young and middle-aged adults need to be reminded about the effects of stress on their lifestyle and health. Coping with the demands of raising a family and succeeding in a career

RESEARCH IN NURSING
Bridging the Gap to Evidence-Based Practice

EXPLORING PARTICIPATION IN SPORTS AND PHYSICAL ACTIVITY AS A DETERRENT TO AN ADOLESCENT'S RISK OF SUICIDE

According to data from the CDC, suicide is the third leading cause of death for adolescents. The rate of suicide for this age group increased 18% between 2003 and 2004. Females attempt suicide more frequently but males are more likely to complete it. The issue of adolescent suicide is even more troubling given the fact that for every successful suicide, there are at least 100 to 200 teenagers who have attempted suicide. Both the U.S. Department of Health and Human Services (USDHHS) in their Healthy People 2010 guidelines and the National Institute of Mental Health recognize the need to reduce the rate of completed suicides in adolescents and focus on specific risk factors. Nurses can assist in this effort by helping to promote safe behaviors for adolescents and understanding what troubled teenagers can do to be protected from feelings of hopelessness and depression.

Related Research

Taliaferro, L., Rienzo, B., Miller, D., Pigg, M., & Dodd, V. (2008). High school youth and suicide risk: Exploring protection afforded through physical activity and sport participation. *Journal of School Health, 78*(10), 545–553.

The goal of this research was to analyze data from the CDC's 2005 Youth Risk Behavior Survey comparing hopelessness and inclination to commit suicide in active and inactive students. There were almost 14,000 students in grades 9 through 12 who participated in this survey. Suicidal behavior was defined as whether students felt sad or hopeless everyday for 2 weeks and ever considered or attempted suicide. Students were directed to respond to questions about the time spent in physical activity for a 7-day period. Physical activity was defined as at least a 20-minute period that caused the student to sweat and breathe

hard while participating in an aerobic activity such as soccer, basketball, swimming, running, bicycling, or fast dancing. Their responses were categorized as either zero times a week, once or twice a week, three to five times a week, or six to seven times weekly. Sports participation consisted of either no involvement, participation on one or two high school or community teams, or highly involved athletes who are members of three or more teams.

Student responses to the survey confirmed findings from previous research that adolescents have a significant degree of hopelessness and suicidal behavior. Findings from this research demonstrated that hopelessness and suicidality were significantly lower among athletes than nonathletes. This was also true for male adolescents who were involved in frequent, vigorous activity. However, adolescent females who exercised and followed extreme dieting measures to lose weight were at increased risk of suicide. Future researchers need to also investigate gender and race differences when studying adolescent suicide.

Relevance to Nursing Practice

The results of this study give some direction to nurses and healthcare providers in their efforts to devise intervention strategies that interrupt feelings of hopelessness with intent to commit suicide in adolescents. Participation in sports may provide some degree of protection in addition to the social support and camaraderie that frequently exist in team activities. Familiarity with mechanisms that support adolescents is vital information for parents, school personnel, community agencies, and healthcare providers to prevent adolescent suicide.

For additional research, visit thePoint.

---

may lead to unsafe health habits and a reliance on drugs or alcohol.

Domestic violence is widespread in the United States. Studies indicate that each year, more than 2,000,000 adults in the United States are victims of **intimate partner violence (IPV),** which is domestic violence or battering between two people in a close relationship (CDC, 2006d). More than 85% of those abused are women (U.S. Department of Health & Human Services [USDHHS], 2009). Many men who batter their spouses also batter their children. Recent evidence suggests a relationship between childhood sexual abuse and certain physical symptoms in adulthood, such as gastrointestinal symptoms, eating disorders, and substance abuse. The nurse may be involved directly in health education and counseling measures or may suggest other resources to the family as additional support for safety and well-being and to interrupt the cycle of violence.

It is not always easy to confirm that a person has sustained injuries as a result of domestic abuse. Some studies have suggested that routine screening can prove effective, but

most experts agree that asking simple, specific questions in a private setting can also prove helpful. Box 26-3 is an example of an assessment tool that the nurse can use to identify victims of domestic violence.

It is vital that the caregiver follow the facility's protocol for addressing IPV. This will most likely include careful assessment of the victim's situation, the opportunity to speak with a trained victim advocate, information about safety options, and respect for the victim's right to self-determination without judging (CDC, 2006d).

Even if an abuse victim is not able or willing to take action when the question of domestic violence is addressed, information about making a safety plan is vital. These are critical steps that will provide a safety lifeline once the decision is made to break the cycle of violence. If in immediate danger, the abuse victim should call the police. Additional resources include the National Domestic Violence Hotline (1-800-799-SAFE) who will provide contact information regarding local domestic violence shelters and other resources.

Box 26-3   ABUSE ASSESSMENT SCREEN

1. WITHIN THE LAST YEAR, have you been hit, slapped, kicked, or otherwise physically hurt by someone?   YES   NO

   If YES, by whom? _____

   Total number of times _____

2. SINCE YOU'VE BEEN PREGNANT, have you been hit, slapped, kicked, or otherwise physically hurt by someone?   YES   NO

   If YES, by whom? _____

   Total number of times _____

MARK THE AREA OF INJURY ON THE BODY MAP. SCORE EACH INCIDENT ACCORDING TO THE FOLLOWING SCALE:

1 = Threats of abuse including use of a weapon

2 = Slapping, pushing: no injuries and/or lasting pain

3 = Punching, kicking, bruises, cuts and/or continuing pain

4 = Beating up, severe contusions, burns, broken bones

5 = Head injury, internal injury, permanent injury

6 = Use of weapon; wound from weapon

If any of the descriptions for the higher number apply, use the higher number.

SCORE
_____
_____
_____
_____
_____

3. WITHIN THE LAST YEAR, has anyone forced you to have sexual activities?   YES   NO

   If YES, who? _____

   Total number of times _____

Developed by the Nursing Research Consortium on Violence and Abuse. Readers are encouraged to reproduce and use this assessment tool.

A safety plan should include arrangements for a sudden departure and a list of actions and items the abuse victim will need to take during the escape. The following is a sample list:

- A place to stay if a sudden departure from home is necessary
- An escape route
- A person you can call in a crisis
- A signal to a neighbor that indicates you need immediate help
- Keys for the house and car
- Secure copies of important papers (e.g., birth certificates, Social Security cards, marriage and driver's licenses, passports, car title, insurance information, school and health records, bank account information)
- A packed bag with clothes, money, medications and prescriptions, credit cards
- Additional addresses and phone numbers for family, friends, a victim advocate, community resources, and legal assistance (USDHHS, 2009).

A safety plan is an initial step in the right direction toward a healthier, violence-free life.

Older Adult

Most accidents that involve older adults are preventable. Falls and motor vehicle accidents are significant hazards for this age group. Falls are the leading cause of injury-related deaths in adults 65 years and older (CDC, 2009b). Visual changes, slowed reaction time, and impaired thinking due to mental illness are realistic concerns that affect the older driver. Some become overly cautious, whereas others are prone to careless behavior. Teach the following interventions to help older adults drive safely: maintain the automobile in optimal driving condition, schedule regular eye examinations, wear corrective lenses when necessary, and keep noise from the radio and other equipment to a minimum. Some states require additional testing for older adults before they can renew their driver's license.

Fires also are a significant hazard for older adults. Factors such as confusion, forgetfulness, and diminished visual and olfactory senses place them at greater risk for burn injuries. Health teaching should include safety precautions if the older adult smokes in the home. Because it may be difficult to distinguish the intensity of temperatures, heating devices often used by older adults need to be carefully monitored and regulated. Smoke detectors indicate the presence of a fire that may not be recognized by an older person with a diminished sense of smell.

Accidental overdosing on medications is also a safety risk, possibly related to poor eyesight or confusion. Special devices such as medication trays can be prefilled to help prevent older patients from taking additional doses. (See Teaching Tips 26-1 for additional health teaching interventions directed at helping to promote a safe environment for older patients at home.)

Orienting the Person to Surroundings

A person who is familiar with his or her surroundings is less likely to experience an accidental injury. As part of the hospital admission routine, orient the patient to the safety features and equipment in the room. An explanation and demonstration of the adjustable bed and side rails, call system, telephone, television, and bathroom help the patient adjust to the new environment. The patient identification bracelet and a discussion of agency routine further ensure safety and assist the patient to adapt to the unfamiliar setting. Similarly, teach the importance of orienting an older person to new surroundings when the older person moves in with a family member or other caregiver.

Preventing Falls

PREVENTING FALLS IN THE HOME

Major causes of falls in the home include slippery surfaces, poor lighting, clutter, and improperly fitting clothing or slippers. Common traffic pathways in the home, the bathroom, and access areas to and from the home are hazardous areas for older adults. Measures as simple as installing hand rails in bathrooms and on stairs, ensuring good lighting, and discarding or repairing broken equipment around the home help prevent accidents (see Box 26-1). Safety assessments by the nurse can play a vital role in promoting safety in the home.

> ➤ *Consider Bessie Washington, the older woman who walks with a walker after suffering a cerebrovascular accident. Key to the patient's plan of care would be a thorough home safety assessment by the home care nurse. This assessment would be valuable in identifying areas that promote patient safety and hazards that need to be addressed.* ∎

Older adults can improve their balance and strengthen their lower extremities through regular physical activity. The martial art of tai chi is one exercise routine that has proved particularly effective. It involves slow, deliberate movements that can be practiced almost anywhere. Tai chi helps to prevent falls by developing balance control and stability in older adults.

PREVENTING FALLS IN THE HEALTHCARE FACILITY

Falls among older adults are the most common cause of hospital admissions for trauma (CDC, 2009b). The Joint Commission requires that hospitals implement fall prevention assessments and programs. Safety measures recommended to reduce the number of falls in acute and extended care facilities are given in Box 26-4.

One simple evaluation tool can help identify hospitalized patients at risk for falling. According to accreditation standards, The Hendrich II Fall Model, which can be administered quickly, evaluates eight independent risk factors (Figure 26-2). This tool also includes the Get Up and Go Test that measures a person's ability to rise from a seated position

| Box 26-4 | NURSING INTERVENTIONS TO PREVENT FALLS IN A HEALTHCARE FACILITY |

- Complete a risk assessment.
- Indicate risk for falling on patient's door and chart.
- Keep bed in low position.
- Keep wheels on bed and wheelchair locked.
- Leave call bell within patient's reach.
- Instruct patient regarding use of call bell.
- Answer call bells promptly.
- Leave a night light on.
- Eliminate all physical hazards in the room (clutter, wet areas on the floor).
- Provide nonskid footwear.
- Leave water, tissues, bedpan/urinal within patient's reach.
- Document and report any changes in patient's cognitive status to the physician and other nurses at the change of shift.
- Use alternative strategies when necessary instead of restraints.
- As a last resort, use the least restrictive restraint according to agency policy.
- If restraint is applied, assess patient at the required intervals.

(Hendrich, 2007). Performance on each physiologic factor merits a specific score and identifies individuals most at risk for falls.

Hendrich (2007) also addresses some misunderstandings about fall risk. Advanced age without the presence of other risk factors can no longer be viewed as a definite fall risk factor. Polypharmacy has long been listed as a risk factor but research has indicated that adverse effects related to the specific medication categories of antiepileptics and benzodiazepine drugs are more predictive of falling. A history of a previous fall has consistently been identified as a predictor of another fall. If a fall occurred as a direct result of a risk factor that has been resolved, one fall may not necessarily indicate that another fall is likely. One healthcare facility installed 24-hour camera surveillance in an effort to monitor patients at high risk for falls (Goodlett, Robinson, Carson, & Landry, 2009). Evaluation of this strategy is ongoing. Some common safety devices used in healthcare facilities are shown in Figure 26-3.

Using Restraints in Healthcare Facilities

Restraints are physical devices used to limit a patient's movement. Side rails, geriatric chairs with attached trays, and appliances tied at the wrist, ankle, or waist are types of physical restraints. Figure 26-4 shows examples of physical restraints that can be used for adults and children. Drugs that are used to control behavior and are not included in the person's normal medical regimen can be considered chemical restraints.

In the past, it was considered acceptable bedside care to restrain patients to protect them from harm, but recent studies have indicated that the use of restraints for this purpose is

Hendrich II Fall Risk Model © 2009

Risk Factor	Risk Points	
Confusion/Disorientation/Impulsivity	4	
Symptomatic Depression	2	
Altered Elimination	1	
Dizziness/Vertigo	1	
Gender (Male)	1	
Any Administered Antiepileptics (anticonvulsants): *(Carbamazepine, Divalproex Sodium, Ethotoin, Ethosuximide, Felbamate, Fosphenytoin, Gabapentin, Lamotrigine, Mephenytoin, Methsuximide, Phenobarbital, Phenytoin, Primidone, Topiramate, Trimethadione, Valproic Acid)*	2	
Any Administered Benzodiazepines: *(Alprazolam, Chlordiazepoxide, Clonazepam, Clorazepate Dipotassium, Diazepam, Flurazepam, Halazepam, Lorazepam, Midazolam, Oxazepam, Temazepam, Triazolam)*	1	
Get-up-and-go Test: "Rising from a Chair" *If unable to assess, monitor for change in activity level, assess other risk factors, document both on patient chart with date and time.*		
Ability to rise in single movement-No loss of balance with steps	0	
Pushes up, successful in one attempt	1	
Multiple attempts but successful	3	
Unable to rise without assistance during test *(OR if a medical order states the same and/or complete bed rest is ordered)* *If unable to assess, document this on the patient chart with the date and time*	4	
(A score of 5 or greater = High Risk) **TOTAL SCORE**		

FIGURE 26-2. Hendrich II Fall Risk Model™ *(© AHI of Indiana, Inc., 2009. Used with permission.)*

potentially dangerous. After 3 months of being restrained, nursing home residents were less able to perform activities of daily living, had lower cognitive abilities, and had difficulty walking independently (Agency for Healthcare Research and Quality [AHRQ], 2009). These adverse health consequences actually resulted in the need for additional staff because the

resident's condition had deteriorated. Additional negative outcomes of restraint use include skin breakdown and contractures, incontinence, depression, delirium, anxiety, aspiration and respiratory difficulties, and even death.

In the late 1970s, more than 25% of U.S. residents in nursing homes were restrained compared to a current average of

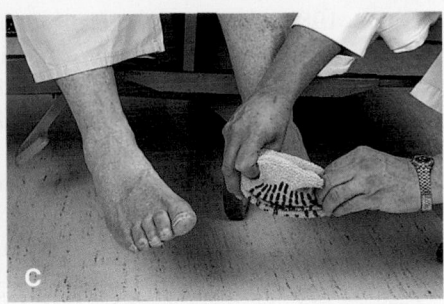

FIGURE 26-3. Some of the safety devices used in healthcare agencies and in the home to prevent falls. (**A**) Side rails on bed raised at patient's request; patient must be able to raise and lower the side rail himself. (**B**) Locking devices on wheeled equipment. (**C**) Nonskid slippers. *(Photos by B. Proud.)*

5% (Evans & Cotter, 2008). A recent study of metropolitan U.S. hospitals indicated that as many as 27,000 patients are restrained each day with most of the restraint use (56%) confined to ICUs. The main reason stated for use in this particular setting is to prevent the disruption of therapies such as ventilator use or intubation (Minnick, Mion, Johnson, Catrambone, & Leipzig, 2007). Older adults with dementia are most at risk of being restrained except for the ICU setting where younger adults are restrained at approximately the same percentage as older adults. The use of restraints is definitely declining as healthcare providers become more educated about the risks associated with their use.

Wrist restraint

Elbow restraint

Mummy restraint

FIGURE 26-4. A variety of restraints used for adults and children. The purpose of restraints is to help prevent the patient from being harmed. Restraints should not interfere with physiologic functioning such as impairing circulation, limiting muscular activity to the point of immobilization, or interfering with respiration. Restraints that can be adjusted to the desired activity limitation are most likely to be accepted by the patient and family.

Since 1987, the federal government and accrediting agencies have worked to reduce or eliminate the use of restraints. Initial guidelines formulated by the Health Care Financing Administration as part of the 1987 Omnibus Budget Reconciliation Act encouraged the limited use of restraints in long-term settings. Federal and state mandates, as well as The Joint Commission (TJC), recommend that acute care agencies use restraints only as a last resort. The current standard for long-term care facilities is to provide safe care without the use of physical or chemical restraints (Evans & Cotter, 2008).

Federal guidelines reinforce that in all settings the primary responsibility is to protect and promote patient's rights and that restraints may only be used to protect the patient, staff, or others. They must be discontinued at the earliest possible time. Any healthcare facility that accepts Medicare and Medicaid reimbursement must abide by the federal guidelines for the use of restraints. The Clinical Practice Committee of the American Geriatrics Society identifies certain principles that must be considered before the use of any restraints (Box 26-5).

Box 26-5 **AMERICAN GERIATRICS SOCIETY POSITION STATEMENT ON RESTRAINT USE**

Guidelines for restraint use include the following:
- Physical restraints should be used sparingly in non-emergency situations. Careful review, assessment, and documentation must indicate that alternatives have been attempted and that restraints are necessary at this time. The least restrictive device should be used.
- Investigation and treatment must be the first step when patient behavior suggests that restraints may be needed. Both patient and staff behavior should be reviewed and results of any treatment evaluated prior to making a decision about the use of restraints.
- The proper size and type of mechanical restraints must be applied according to manufacturer's recommendations to prevent alterations in skin integrity.
- On rare occasions, short-term use of restraints may be indicated if the patient is at significant risk of self-harm or injury. Restraints must be prescribed by a licensed practitioner and renewed according to state and federal guidelines.
- The patient and the restraint must be checked frequently. The restraining device must be removed periodically with attention given to ambulation (if appropriate), hydration, elimination, comfort, and social interaction.
- A restraint must be removed or discontinued at reasonable intervals to confirm the need for it.
- Ongoing staff education is necessary regarding the hazards of restraint use, the proper use and application of restraints, and alternative strategies to the use of restraints.
- Research into innovative alternatives to restraint use in acute and long-term care settings must be encouraged.

Adapted from: The American Geriatrics Society (2008). *AGS position statement: Restraint Use.* Available at http://www.americangeriatrics.org/products/positionpapers/restraintsupdate.shtml.

In 2002, the Sentinel Event Advisory Group was formed within TJC to develop patient safety goals. These help accredited agencies address specific areas of concern related to patient safety. According to TJC, a **sentinel event** is an unexpected occurrence involving death or serious physical or psychological injury, or the risk of death or injury (TJC, 2007). These signal the need for an immediate investigation and response. Patient death/injury while in restraints is responsible for 3.0% of reported sentinel events and listed among the 10 most frequent sentinel events as of December 31, 2009 (TJC, 2009).

USING SIDE RAILS AS RESTRAINTS

In the past, side rails were used to provide support and aid equilibrium, but it is now recognized that they can pose serious risks for a confused or agitated patient. A 1995 FDA Safety Alert informed healthcare agencies of the hazards associated with side rail use. A person of small stature has a greater risk for entrapment or injury. Death from asphyxiation has occurred when patients have become wedged between the mattress and the bed frame or side rail. Although patient entrapment is uncommon, it is often fatal (Todd, 2008). Most of the victims of side rail fatalities are frail, elderly, or confused, many with uncontrolled body movement. Most incidents of entrapment occur in a long-term care setting.

A side rail is not considered a restraint if the patient requests that it be raised to aid in getting in or out of bed. Some patients may request that side rails be used at night while they sleep so that they may feel more secure (see Fig. 26-3A). The patient must be able to raise and lower the side rail himself or herself. If a family member requests the use of side rails for a patient, it is the nurse's responsibility to review benefits and risks associated with their use and periodically evaluate the reason for their use. Side rails are not routinely recommended for all situations. It is the responsibility of healthcare facilities to evaluate existing bed systems for entrapment risks and investigate corrective actions that may be necessary to provide a safe environment for patients (Todd, 2008).

USING ALTERNATIVES TO RESTRAINTS

Careful nursing assessment is the key to identifying appropriate alternatives to restraint use and finding an individualized solution (Box 26-6). Figure 26-5 shows an example of a position-sensitive electronic device (Ambularm) that is an alternative to using restraints.

Nursing interventions may be used to reduce confusion or agitation and provide a safe environment. Using a restraint on an older patient who tends to wander is unjustified because a variety of alternative options can be used to keep such patients safe.

USING RESTRAINTS AS A LAST RESORT

Despite all efforts, restraints may be the only solution in some situations. The least restrictive restraint should be the first option. Restraints must never be applied for the convenience of the staff. The patient's family must be consulted and involved

Box 26-6 CHOOSING ALTERNATIVES TO RESTRAINTS

- Determine whether behavior pattern exists.
- Assess for pain and treat appropriately.
- Rule out causes for agitation. Assess respiratory status, vital signs, blood glucose level, fluid and electrolyte issues, and medications. Use standardized screening tools to evaluate change in function.
- Involve the family in patient's care.
- Ask family members or significant other to stay with the patient.
- Reduce stimulation, noise, and light.
- Distract and redirect, using a calming voice.
- Use simple, clear explanations and directions.
- Check environment for hazards.
- Use night light.
- Identify door of room (e.g., use of balloon, sign, patient's picture, ribbon).
- Use an electronic alarm system on a temporary basis (e.g., bed or position-sensitive alarms) to warn of unassisted activity.
- Allow restless patient to walk after ensuring that environment is safe.
- Use a large plant or piece of furniture as a barrier to limit wandering from designated area.
- Use low-height beds.
- Place floor mats on each side of the bed.
- Ensure the use of glasses and hearing aids, if necessary.
- Use pillows wedged against the side of the chair to keep patient positioned safely.
- Use full-length body pillows, a swimming pool noodle, or a rolled blanket to indicate the edge of the bed.
- Assist with toileting at frequent intervals.
- Arrange for a bedside commode.
- Make the environment as home like as possible; provide familiar objects.
- Provide a warm beverage.
- Provide comfortable rocking chairs.
- Use therapeutic touch.
- Play music or video selections of the patient's choice.
- Offer diversional activities, such as games and books.
- Encourage daily exercise/provide exercise and activities or relaxation techniques.
- Consider relocation of the patient to a room closer to the nursing station.
- Conceal tubing necessary for care. Anchor tubing securely. Conceal tubing with gauze wrap; unwrap regularly to assess site for complications.
- Investigate possibility of discontinuing bothersome treatment devices (e.g., intravenous line, catheter, feeding tube).

in the plan of care before applying restraints in a long-term care setting. They must be informed of the agency's policy regarding applying and removing restraints and may be asked to sign a release form to protect the agency from liability. Agency policy, TJC, and state and federal guidelines require an order from a physician or other healthcare professional licensed to prescribe in the state. The order should include the type of restraint, justification for the restraint, and criteria for removal. The order must never be written for p.r.n. use.

In an emergency, the physical restraint can be applied, but an order from a primary care provider must be obtained within 1 hour according to Joint Commission Standards. The order must state the intended duration of use. The patient must be monitored and assessed on a regular basis. Assessment must occur every 4 hours for an adult, at least every 2 hours for children ages 9 to 17 years, and at least

once every hour for children younger than 9 years. Documentation must reflect the date and time the restraint is applied, the type of restraint, alternatives that were attempted with their results, and notification of the patient's family and physician. Include the frequency of assessment, your findings, regular intervals when the restraint is removed, and nursing interventions. Constant re-evaluation of the need for the restraint is vital. Chapter 7 discusses the legal issues involved when restraints are used. Student nurses, from their earliest clinical experiences, need help to identify and assess the cause of a patient's behavior and not just the behavior itself. Careful patient assessment is needed to develop creative alternative strategies. Skill 26-1 demonstrates the proper method for applying restraints should they be necessary.

Preventing Fires and Maintaining Fire Safety

Careless smoking, faulty electrical equipment, and combustion of anesthetic agents are the most common causes of hospital fires. Orientations in healthcare agencies emphasize fire prevention information and the agency's smoking policy. Nurses are responsible for patients' safety and need to be familiar with the agency's fire safety plan, exits, the location and operation of fire extinguishers, and any special instructions for reporting a fire.

Most hospital procedures emphasize the following priorities and recommend that staff members remember the acronym RACE as a guide:

- Rescue anyone in immediate danger.
- Activate the fire code system and notify the appropriate person.

FIGURE 26-5. Ambularm device. *(Photo courtesy of AlertCare, Inc.)*

- Confine the fire by closing doors and windows.
- Evacuate patients and other people to a safe area.

Type ABC fire extinguishers, the most common kind used in healthcare agencies, contain a material similar to baking soda that can be used on any type of fire (Taschner, 2008).

In the home setting, cigarettes, grease, and electrical problems are most often responsible for fires. Educating parents about home fire safety includes having a plan of action similar to that used in healthcare settings. (See Box 26-1 for priorities and practical suggestions for fire and burn safety.)

Preventing Poisoning

Concerted efforts by individuals, communities, state governments, and the federal government have reduced the number of accidental deaths by poisoning. Childproof containers are primarily responsible for this reduction.

Nursing interventions involve health education aimed at preventing accidental poisoning in the home. Every household must have the telephone number of the nearest poison control center (PCC) readily available. Emphasize that parents should call the poison control center immediately, before attempting any home remedy. Parents may be instructed to bring the child immediately to an emergency facility for treatment. The focus of emergency treatment of poisoning is to stabilize vital body functions, prevent the absorption of the poison, and encourage excretion of the toxic substance.

Activated charcoal is considered the most effective agent for preventing absorption of the ingested toxin. It can bind with as much as 60% of a toxin when given 30 to 60 minutes after the ingestion. Activated charcoal is administered through a nasogastric tube in the emergency department

(Madden, 2008). Syrup of ipecac is no longer recommended because vomiting may be dangerous. A toxic substance may prove more hazardous coming up rather than when it was swallowed. Gastric lavage is no longer prescribed routinely for treatment of ingestion of a toxic substance because it may propel the poison into the small intestine, where absorption will occur. The amount of toxin removed by gastric lavage is relatively small.

Nursing education efforts can also change behaviors that place older adults at risk for medication-related poisoning. Although poisonings happen more frequently in children, poison control centers receive many calls from adults, particularly older adults, regarding accidental poisonings. Suggestions for preventing poisoning in older adults are included in the accompanying box, Focus on the Older Adult.

All healthcare providers should recommend that a carbon monoxide detector be installed to alert family members to toxic levels of the gas. Gas or oil companies and the local health authority can help identify and remove sources of contamination. Many communities are considering legislation requiring installation of carbon monoxide detectors by homeowners and landlords. (See Box 26-1 for additional tips for preventing poisoning).

Preventing Suffocation

As a result of suffocation, unconsciousness, respiratory failure, and cardiac arrest can occur. Emergency measures must start without delay, beginning with the removal of any obstruction and administration of cardiopulmonary resuscitation. When teaching parents, the nurse should emphasize careful supervision of children and should outline specific situations that place children at risk for suffocation. Health

FOCUS ON THE OLDER ADULT

NURSING STRATEGIES TO PREVENT MEDICATION-RELATED POISONING

Age Related Changes	Nursing Strategies
Confusion	• Do not hesitate to call the physician, nurse, or pharmacist with any questions. • Develop good communication with your physician, nurse, and pharmacist. • Use a medication calendar or diary to keep track of your dosing schedule. • Use a pill dispenser as a reminder tool.
Reduced vision	• Request large-print labels from your pharmacist.
Polypharmacy	• Report side effects from medications to your healthcare provider. • Do not share medications with others or take their pills. • When a drug is discontinued, throw away any remaining medication.
Effect of drugs in the aging body	• Keep the telephone numbers for your healthcare providers and the poison control center in a readily accessible place. • Do not stop taking any prescription drug or change the dose without first consulting the physician or nurse. • Avoid doubling a dose if you forget a medication. Check with the physician or nurse first. • Avoid mixing alcohol with medicines without first checking with the pharmacist.

education is a valuable preventive force (see Box 26-1 for specific interventions).

Preventing Injury From Firearms

Nurses are in a unique position to raise awareness and to help reduce high-risk behavior that may lead to firearm injuries and deaths. In homes, schools, and other healthcare settings, nurses can provide information on how parents can keep guns out of the hands of children. Parents may be unaware of how common gunshot injuries are or the dangers that can occur when a gun is accessible to children and young adults. As a prevention partner, the nurse can begin to have an impact on the epidemic of gun-related injuries and death (see Box 26-1 for measures to prevent injury from firearms).

Preventing Equipment-Related Accidents

With the marked increase in the use of highly sophisticated electronic equipment in healthcare settings, healthcare practitioners must learn to use the equipment properly and must recognize signs of malfunctioning equipment. Suction devices with inadequate vacuum and rate regulators or infusion equipment that delivers erratic amounts of solution have resulted in equipment-related accidents. Failure to use protective belts or side rails on stretchers and to lock wheelchair wheels can result in patient injury.

Electrical equipment can present a safety hazard to both the patient and healthcare practitioner when safety measures are ignored. Most electrical equipment used in hospitals is equipped with three-prong plugs. The third prong, when inserted into a properly wired wall outlet, provides a ground for the piece of equipment. A **ground** is a connection from an electricity source to the earth through which electric current leakage can be harmlessly conducted. Box 26-7 lists

FIGURE 26-6. An essential nursing responsibility is checking the patient's identification bracelet before any procedure. Here, the nurse checks the patient's identification before administering medications.

guidelines to help reduce the number of equipment-related accidents. Hospitals and long-term care facilities are required by federal law and FDA regulations to report to the FDA and the manufacturer of a device any suspected deaths or serious injuries related to use of the device (Rich, 2008).

Accidents in the home frequently result from careless use of equipment or from malfunctioning or poorly maintained equipment. Many injuries and deaths from electric shock can be prevented. Overloaded electric circuits, faulty appliances, frayed wires, careless use of electrical equipment, and handling of electrical devices and cords with wet hands or while wearing wet shoes can result in injury or death. (See Box 26-1 for specific guidelines to prevent electrical injury.)

Preventing Procedure-Related Accidents

The nurse must always be cautious and alert to prevent procedure-related accidents. Errors are possible when administering medications or intravenous solutions, transferring a patient, changing a dressing, or applying external heat to a patient's extremity. Therefore, nurses must follow correct procedures when administering care. Safeguards to prevent errors include making sure that the patient is identified correctly (Fig. 26-6). The nurse should use all available resources to answer any questions about correct procedure.

In an effort to promote a culture of safety, The Joint Commission publishes an annual list of National Patient Safety Goals. These are established based on sentinel events that have been reported and include the corrective actions recommended as a response to these sentinel events. Some goals are ongoing while others may get removed from the annual list once the hospitals have incorporated the recommended practices to meet a particular safety goal into their standards of operation (Kirkpatrick, 2009). The goals and related requirements are specific to each accreditation program (e.g., ambulatory care, assisted living, long-term care). Accreditation by TJC requires that a healthcare organization provide evidence

---

Box 26-7 DECREASING EQUIPMENT-RELATED ACCIDENTS

- Use equipment only for the use for which it was intended.
- Do not operate equipment with which you are unfamiliar.
- Handle equipment with care to prevent damaging it.
- Use three-prong electric plugs whenever possible.
- Do not twist or bend electric cords. The wires inside the cord may break.
- Be alert to signs that indicate equipment is faulty such as breaks in electric cords, sparks, smoke, electric shocks, loose or missing parts, and unusual noises or odors. Report signs of trouble immediately.
- Make certain that electric cords are not in a position to be trapped as beds are raised or lowered. This can strip insulation covering the electric wires.
- Be alert for wet surfaces on areas where electric cords or connections are present.
- Make certain when charging defibrillator batteries that "charging" indicator light is on.
- Implement a process for reporting and addressing problems with equipment.

Box 26-8 THE UNIVERSAL PATIENT COMPACT™: PRINCIPLES FOR PARTNERSHIP

As your healthcare partner, we pledge to:
- Include you as a member of the team
- Treat you with respect, honesty, and compassion
- Always tell you the truth
- Include your family or advocate when you would like us to
- Hold ourselves to the highest quality and safety standards
- Be responsive and timely with our care and information to you
- Help you to set goals for your healthcare and treatment plans
- Listen to you and answer your questions
- Provide information to you in a way you can understand
- Respect your right to your own medical information
- Respect your privacy and the privacy of your medical information
- Communicate openly about benefits and risks associated with any treatments
- Provide you with information to help you make informed decisions about your care and treatment options
- Work with you, and other partners who treat you, in the coordination of your care

As a patient, I pledge to:
- Be a responsible and active member of my healthcare team
- Treat you with respect, honesty, and consideration
- Always tell you the truth
- Respect the commitment you have made to healthcare and healing
- Give you the information that you need to treat me
- Learn all that I can about my condition
- Participate in decisions about my care
- Understand my care plan to the best of my ability
- Tell you what medications I am taking
- Ask questions when I do not understand and until I do understand
- Communicate any problems I have with the plan for my care
- Tell you if something about my health changes
- Tell you if I have trouble reading
- Let you know if I have family, friends, or an advocate to help me with my healthcare

that these goals have been addressed and requirements have been met. Effective alternatives may be acceptable, depending on the services provided by the particular healthcare organization. National Patient Safety Goals are available on The Joint Commission Web site at: http://www.jointcommission.org/PatientSafety/NationalPatientSafetyGoals/

Filing a Safety Event Report

An accident or incident that compromises safety in a healthcare agency requires the completion of a **safety event report.** This is a confidential document, formerly referred to as an incident report, that objectively describes the circumstances of the accident or incident. The report also details the patient's response and the examination and treatment of the patient after the incident. The nurse completes the event report immediately after the incident and is responsible for recording the circumstances and the effect on the patient in the medical record. The safety event report is not a part of the medical record and should not be mentioned in the documentation. Because laws vary in different states, nurses must know their own state law regarding safety event reports.

> *Recall Juanita Flores, the young mother whose child fell off the cot. As a result of the fall, a safety event report was completed.* ∎

All safety event reports are reviewed carefully to detect any potentially threatening situation or pattern. These reports are discussed in more detail in Chapter 7.

When an incident results in a patient injury, the nurse has a responsibility to speak openly and honestly with the

patient and family. The Joint Commission includes a standard that requires disclosure of unanticipated outcomes to patients. Rothrock (2008) emphasizes that disclosure accompanied by an apology is "critical to advancing patient trust and a culture of safety in healthcare organizations." The National Patient Safety Foundation (2008), in an effort to focus on safe delivery of high-quality care, has developed a framework outlining a true partnership between patients and providers. The Universal Patient Compact: Principles for Partnership (Box 26-8) describes a patient-/family-centered process that "creates an understanding between the parties about how they will work together." The National Patient Safety Foundation's Principles for Partnership represent a concerted effort to demonstrate a healthcare organization's commitment to respect the rights of patients and incorporate these beliefs into their mission.

Maintaining Emergency Preparedness

Emergency preparedness has always been a concern for healthcare workers. Nurses, as members of emergency response teams, need to be aware of their role when an emergency or disaster occurs. Existing community resources are usually sufficient to respond to an emergency situation, such as a multiple vehicle collision, a fire in an apartment complex involving a significant number of burn injuries, or an explosion or plane crash. Since the September 11, 2001, terrorist attacks in New York, Washington, D.C., and Pennsylvania and the subsequent anthrax attacks, attention has been focused on national security and strategies for sustaining emergency preparedness levels, as well as the need for communities to step up the level of their involvement in emergency preparedness for any disaster.

A **disaster** is broadly defined as a tragic event of great magnitude that requires the response of people outside the involved community. Disasters can be categorized as natural (e.g., massive flooding following a hurricane or an earthquake) or man-made (e.g., a toxic spill, war, or a terrorist event). In any disaster, the lives of the victims, their families, and the community and nation are affected in incalculable ways.

> ➤ *Think back to Kara Greenwood, the adolescent described in the beginning of the chapter. Her statement revealed her peer group's awareness of terrorism. Kara would need to obtain additional information about terrorism from community sources when preparing the discussion.* ■

Based on national and world events, the efforts of government agencies, in conjunction with accreditation bodies such as The Joint Commission, have contributed to the considerable progress that hospitals have made in disaster preparedness (USDHHS, 2009). Disaster training is more rigorous and standardized and encompasses the entire community and its resources. These healthcare coalitions provide the foundation for improved response capacity.

The CDC is also committed to responding rapidly to mass trauma events and chemical, biological, radiological, and nuclear agents. The CDC's Health Alert Network has upgraded the capacity of state and local health agencies to detect and communicate varying health threats (CDC, 2009c). The CDC has also collaborated with pharmaceutical companies and other partners to create regional stockpiles of the drugs that would be needed to treat man-made outbreaks of disease, such as anthrax, plague, and other diseases quickly. It is a prescription for great danger if the United States does not continue to develop the optimal emergency preparedness capabilities that it needs to protect its communities.

ADDRESSING BIOLOGICAL THREATS

Bioterrorism involves the deliberate spread of pathogenic organisms into a community to cause widespread illness, fear, and panic (Haag, 2007). The organisms used in a mass attack may not be routine, and the clinical manifestations may be vague and nonspecific. Table 26-2 outlines some of the more common biological agents, including symptoms and interventions. If an unusual number of people suddenly experience similar signs and symptoms, healthcare personnel should consider whether they may have been exposed to a biological agent.

Healthcare personnel must adhere to the Standard Precautions recommended by the CDC. For certain diseases, additional safeguards may be necessary. If a contagious disease is suspected, the patient should be isolated accordingly. Although not usually required with biological agents, decontamination may be necessary if a patient's exposure status is uncertain. The patient may need to bathe or shower with soap and place his or her clothing in sealed plastic bags.

ADDRESSING CHEMICAL THREATS

The use of chemical agents as a terrorist weapon is a growing concern. **Chemical terrorism** involves the deliberate release of a chemical compound that has the potential for harming people's health (CDC, 2006a). The chemical would probably be dispersed in an enclosed space, such as a subway or a closed sports arena, to cause the maximum effect. Chemical agents act rapidly, and immediate decontamination is crucial before patients are transported to a hospital. Emergency preparedness requires the swift transfer of portable decontamination units, equipment, and trained personnel to the site of the chemical attack.

Several categories of chemicals can be used as weapons of mass destruction:

- Choking/Lung/Pulmonary agents
- Blood Agents
- Vesicants/Blister Agents
- Nerve agents
- Incapacitating agents

Box 26-9 summarizes the effects of the various chemical agents.

ADDRESSING NUCLEAR THREATS

Nuclear terrorism involves intentional introduction of radioactive materials into the environment for the purpose of causing injury and death (CDC, 2006b). The attack might involve use of a radiation dispersal device ("dirty bomb"), a planned assault at a nuclear power station or weapons facility, or dispersal of radioactive material into the food or water

---

Box 26-9 CATEGORIES OF CHEMICAL AGENTS

Choking Lung/Pulmonary Agents
Examples: phosgene (CG), diphosgene (DP), chlorine (CL)
Effects: dyspnea, cough, pulmonary edema

Blood Agents
Examples: hydrogen cyanide (AC), cyanogen chloride (CK)
Effects: loss of consciousness, convulsions, respiratory arrest

Vesicants/Blister Agents
Examples: sulfur mustard (H or HD), lewisite (L)
Effects: skin erythema and blisters, eye irritation, progressively severe respiratory symptoms, damage to bone marrow

Nerve Agents
Examples: tabun (GA), sarin (GB), soman (GD)
Effects: constricted pupils, reddened eyes, loss of consciousness, convulsions, respiratory arrest

Incapacitating Agents
Examples: glycolate anticholinergic compound (BZ), Agent 15
Effects: hyperthermia, bizarre behavior, delirium

Adapted from Centers for Disease Control and Prevention (CDC). (2006). *Emergency preparedness: Chemical categories.* Available at http://www.bt.cdc.gov/agent/agentlistchem-category.asp.

TABLE • 26-2   BIOLOGICAL AGENTS OF CONCERN

Agents	Clinical Manifestations	Treatment/Protection
Anthrax (*Bacillus anthrax*)	Symptoms variable based on form of anthrax: • Cutaneous: skin lesion with local edema that progresses, enlarges, ulcerates, and becomes necrotic • Gastrointestinal: nausea, vomiting, fever, abdominal pain, hematemesis, severe diarrhea • Inhalational: fever, fatigue, cough, dyspnea, pain, may progress to meningitis, septicemia, shock, and death	Standard precautions Decontamination possibly required for recent exposure Rapid administration of antimicrobial therapy Supportive therapy for shock, fluid volume deficit, and airway management Vaccine available; currently recommended only for high-risk populations
Plague or "black death" (*Yersinia pestis*)	Expected attack most likely airborne (inhalation of bacilli) with sudden appearance in ED of multiple patients with respiratory symptoms Symptoms similar to a severe respiratory infection Progresses rapidly to severe pneumonia, sepsis, and death	Standard precautions with droplet precautions until 48 hours after initiation of antibiotic therapy Antibiotic of choice: streptomycin (IM) or gentamicin sulfate (IM or IV). Possible use of oral antibiotics (effective when mass numbers of people are ill) Fatality rate of 100% for those not receiving treatment within 24 hours of onset of symptoms
Smallpox (*Variola major*, viral agent)	Spread via direct contact or inhalation of respiratory droplets; most likely to be spread via aerosol route Flu-like symptoms Characteristic rash that progresses to crusted scabs in 5 days, most prominent on face and extremities	Strict contact and airborne precautions for duration of illness—vaccination for those exposed No proven treatment Supportive care including possible antibiotics if secondary infections develop Use of antiviral agents under investigation Vaccine available; currently recommended only for high-risk populations
Botulism (*Clostridium botulinum*)	Possible release via airborne method, or contaminated food supplies Ocular symptoms such as blurred vision Skeletal muscle paralysis that progresses symmetrically and in a descending manner Muscle weakness that can result abruptly in respiratory failure	Standard precautions Passive immunization with botulinum antitoxin Supportive respiratory care
Tularemia (*Francisella tularensis*)	Transmission via contaminated water, food, and soil; most likely aerosolization of bacteria for use as a biological weapon Fever Nonproductive or productive cough Possible progression to respiratory failure	Standard precautions Drug therapy such as streptomycin or gentamicin sulfate Fluid and respiratory support measures Vaccine under investigation
Viral hemorrhagic fevers (e.g., Lassa, Ebola, Marburg, yellow, and dengue fevers)	Possible spread via aerosol infection Fever Myalgias Conjunctival symptoms Mild hypotension Petechial hemorrhages Progresses to shock and hemorrhage	Standard, droplet, and contact precautions for the duration of illness; additional precautions, including use of negative-pressure room, N95 or higher respirator Use of personal protective equipment (PPE) (see Chap. 27) No proven treatment other than supportive care Avoidance of aspirin or other anticlotting drugs

Adapted from: Centers for Disease Control and Prevention (CDC). (2006). *General fact sheets on specific bioterrorism agents.* Available at http://emergency.cdc.gov/bioterrorism/factsheets.asp.

supply. Even a small amount of radioactive material can have devastating effects.

Radiation burns occur as a result of exposure to a radioactive source. The severity of injury depends on a variety of factors, including the duration of the exposure and the distance between the source and the person. A higher dose increases the likelihood of developing later effects such as bone marrow depression and cancer. Although the likelihood of a nuclear attack may be small, nurses need to be well informed, familiar with their agency's emergency response plan, and prepared to deal with a nuclear emergency.

Nurses serving on a radiological emergency response team must protect themselves and wear the necessary equipment, including a radiation detection device. They will

TABLE • 26-3 EMERGENCY PREPAREDNESS RESOURCES	
Organization	**Activities**
National Disaster Medical System (NDMS) http://www.hhs.gov/aspr/opeo/ndms/index.html	Has responsibility for managing and coordinating the federal medical response to major emergencies and federally declared disasters
Federal Emergency Management Agency (FEMA) http://www.fema.gov	Works to build and support the national emergency management system
Centers for Disease Control and Prevention (CDC) http://www.cdc.gov	Acts as the lead federal agency for disease prevention and control activities; provides backup support to state and local health departments
The Joint Commission (TJC) http://www.jointcommission.org	Accredits facilities according to established safety and quality standards; revises the emergency management standards for healthcare facilities
American Red Cross http://www.redcross.org	Acts as the lead nongovernmental agency that provides safety information and disaster response
American Hospital Association http://www.aha.org (For disaster readiness, see http://www.aha.org/aha_app/issues/Emergency-Readiness/advocacy-emergency-readiness.jsp)	American Hospital Association connection to disaster readiness resources
Department of Homeland Security http://www.dhs.gov/index.shtm	Protects the nation against further terrorist attacks and coordinates the response for future emergencies

assess patients in a radiation emergency area (REA) designated by the hospital's emergency response plan. If patients have not been decontaminated at the scene of the attack, decontamination will occur at the medical facility.

PREPARING FOR MASS TRAUMA TERRORISM

Terrorists have used bombs and other explosives in a variety of ways (e.g., roadside devices, on public transportation) to inflict mass trauma injuries and cause multiple fatalities. Proximity to the detonation determines the severity of injuries and mortality rates. Blast lung injury (BLI) has recently been recognized as a direct consequence of the blast wave from a high explosive detonation (CDC, 2008a). Once the condition is diagnosed, the patient may require complex care and should be admitted to an intensive care unit. Few emergency healthcare providers in the United States have experience treating patients with explosion-related injuries.

IDENTIFYING DISASTER RESOURCES

Each healthcare facility should determine in advance how to deliver care should an emergency or disaster occur. This involves collaboration with internal committees and external agencies. Organizations that serve as resources for recommendations and updated information are listed in Table 26-3.

ADDRESSING PSYCHOLOGICAL ASPECTS OF DISASTERS

Disasters affect the lives of victims, family members, and healthcare personnel in many ways. Fear and panic can be expected, as well as anger, horror, and real and exaggerated concerns about possible future events. Nurses and other healthcare providers, as first responders, rescue and recovery workers, or staff at a medical facility, can help to minimize panic by addressing risks and providing careful explanations. Anxiety can be treated with reassurance. The impact of a disaster on each person varies, and it can have lingering effects. Most disaster survivors experience normal stress reactions, but some may exhibit acute stress disorder or posttraumatic stress disorders that require treatment. Emergency preparedness education and planning must also address mental health issues.

Evaluating

Evaluation is the final step of the nursing process. The accompanying concept map illustrates the nursing process for the care of Bessie Washington. Nurses must evaluate the effectiveness of their interventions to promote environmental safety, prevent injury, and promote emergency preparedness. If the expected patient outcomes have been met and evaluative criteria have been satisfied, the patient should be able to accomplish the following:

- Correctly identify real and potential unsafe environmental situations
- Implement safety measures in the environment
- Use available resources to obtain safety information
- Incorporate accident prevention practices into activities of daily living
- Remain free of injury.

Bessie Washington, age 77, has been discharged to home after sustaining a cerebral vascular accident (CVA). She is experiencing residual weakness in her right arm and leg and she has a right visual field cut that affects her ability to see things in her right field of vision. She is taking metoprolol for hypertension and an anticoagulant to prevent further CVAs. In the hospital, Ms. Washington's blood pressure was 110/60mm Hg and her heart rate was 62 beats per minute and irregular. She was discharged with a referral to visiting nurse and home physical therapy. The visiting nurse finds that she lives alone in a first floor apartment and uses a walker to ambulate. She tells the visiting nurse, "I have so much stuff crammed into this small apartment. I almost fell going from my bedroom to the kitchen." The nurse notes that Ms. Washington drags her right leg when ambulating and drifts to her weak side when sitting. When asked about activities of daily living, Ms. Washington says that she has been unable to perform chores.

Priority 1

Nursing Diagnosis: Risk for Fall related to physical disability and environmental conditions.
Supporting Data:
• Experiencing right-sided weakness
• Uses walker to ambulate
• Experiencing right visual field cut
• Takes multiple medications
• BP 110/60mm Hg; HR 62 bpm, irregular
• Lives in a cluttered environment

Priority 2

Nursing Diagnosis: Impaired Mobility related to recent CVA.
Supporting Data:
• Experiencing right-sided weakness
• Drags rt. leg when ambulating
• Uses walker to ambulate
• Drifts to weak side when sitting or ambulating

Priority 3

Nursing Diagnosis: Impaired Home Maintenance related to acute illness.
Supporting Data:
• "I almost fell going from my bedroom to the kitchen."
• Unable to perform house chores
• Lives alone in first-floor apartment
• Recent CVA

Outcome:
Patient will demonstrate safety measures to prevent falls.

Outcome:
Patient will demonstrate safe ambulation techniques, participate in physical therapy and prescribed treatment, and increase strength.

Outcome:
Patient will maintain her environment, utilize resources to assist with house chores, and incorporate adaptive strategies to assist with activities of daily living.

Nursing Interventions:
• Encourage patient to turn head from side to side to see all of environment.
• Teach patient to sit upright at first and then rise slowly to prevent orthostatic hypotension.
• Remove any throw rugs or obstacles.
• Obtain assistive equipment such as raised toilet seat, grab bars, shower chair, etc.
• Reinforce importance of having prescribed lab work to maintain therapeutic anticoagulant levels.
• Identify resources to assist in clearing cluttered environment.

Nursing Interventions:
• Assess level of mobility and strength.
• Assess patient's insight into own motor deficit.
• Reinforce proper techniques for use of walker as taught by physical therapy.
• Encourage patient to perform prescribed exercises throughout the day
• Encourage frequent rest periods.

Nursing Interventions:
• Perform home evaluation.
• Request referral to occupational therapy to assist with adaptive strategies to perform activities of daily living.
• Identify family and community resources to assist with chores around house within financial constraints.

Evaluation: Ms. Washington demonstrated proper techniques while ambulating. Her children have offered to straighten up her apartment. Throw rugs were removed. She has had her lab work drawn and her anticoagulant medication was adjusted. Continue home visits for reinforcement.

Evaluation: Ms. Washington is performing exercises as prescribed. Her strength is rated a +2 on the right side and a +4 on the left side. She does more than the prescribed exercise and needs to be reminded to rest. She is attempting to ambulate too quickly. Instructed to slow down.

Evaluation: OT is working with Ms. Washington. Adaptive strategies were devised and she has demonstrated these strategies. Church resources were identified to assist with chores during the recovery period. Continue visiting nurse to monitor home maintenance.

- - - - - **Relationship**   **Assessment**   **Nursing Diagnosis**   **Outcome Identification**   **Interventions**   **Evaluation**

Concept map displaying the nursing process for Bessie Washington.

Skill · 26-1   Applying an Extremity Restraint

EQUIPMENT

- Appropriate cloth restraint for the extremity that is to be immobilized
- Padding, if necessary, for bony prominences
- PPE, as indicated

IMPLEMENTATION

ACTION

1. Determine need for restraints. Assess patient's physical condition, behavior, and mental status.

2. Confirm agency policy for application of restraints. **Secure an order from the primary care provider, or validate that the order has been obtained within the past 24 hours.**

3. Perform hand hygiene and put on PPE, if indicated.

4. Identify the patient.

5. Explain reason for use to patient and family. Clarify how care will be given and how needs will be met. Explain that restraint is a temporary measure.

6. Include the patient's family and/or significant others in the plan of care.

7. Apply restraint according to manufacturer's directions:

   a. Choose the least restrictive type of device that allows the greatest possible degree of mobility.

   b. Pad bony prominences.

   c. Wrap the restraint around the extremity with the soft part in contact with the skin. If hand mitt is being used, pull over hand with cushion to the palmar aspect of hand (Figure 1). Secure in place with the Velcro® straps.

8. **Ensure that two fingers can be inserted between the restraint and patient's wrist or ankle (Figure 2).**

RATIONALE

Restraints should be used only as a last resort when alternative measures have failed and the patient is at increased risk for harming himself or others.

Policy protects the patient and the nurse and specifies guidelines for application as well as type of restraint and duration. **The Joint Commission (TJC) standards require that a new order for restraints must be written every 24 hours.**

Hand hygiene and PPE prevent the spread of microorganisms. PPE is required based on transmission precautions.

Identifying the patient ensures the right patient receives the intervention and helps prevent errors.

Explanation to patient and family may lessen confusion and anger and provide reassurance. A clearly stated agency policy on application of restraints should be available for patient and family to read. In a long-term care facility, the family must give consent before a restraint is applied.

This promotes continuity of care and cooperation.

Proper application prevents injury.

This provides minimal restriction.

Padding helps prevent skin injury.

This prevents excess pressure on extremity.

Proper application ensures that there is no interference with the patient's circulation and potential alteration in neurovascular status.

FIGURE 1. Using a hand mitt.

FIGURE 2. Ensuring that two fingers can be inserted between the restraint and the patient's wrist.

(continued)

Skill · 26-1 Applying an Extremity Restraint *continued*

ACTION	RATIONALE

ACTION

9. Maintain restrained extremity in normal anatomic position. **Use a quick-release knot (Figure 3) to tie the restraint to the bed frame, not side rail (Figure 4). The restraint may also be attached to chair frame.** The site should not be readily accessible to patient.

RATIONALE

Maintaining a normal position lessens possibility of injury. A quick-release knot ensures that the restraint will not tighten when pulled and can be removed quickly in an emergency. Securing the restraint to a side rail may injure the patient when the side rail is lowered. Tying the restraint out of the patient's reach promotes security.

Magnus hitch

Clove hitch

Loop

FIGURE 3. Quick-release knots for securing restraint to bed frame.

FIGURE 4. Securing restraint to bed frame.

10. Remove PPE, if used. Perform hand hygiene.

Removing PPE properly reduces the risk for infection transmission and contamination of other items. Hand hygiene prevents transmission of microorganisms.

11. Assess the patient at least every hour or according to facility policy. Assessment should include: the placement of the restraint, neurovascular assessment of the affected extremity, and skin integrity. In addition, assess for signs of sensory deprivation such as increased sleeping, daydreaming, anxiety, panic, and hallucinations.

Improperly applied restraints may cause skin tears, abrasions, or bruises. Decreased circulation may result in paleness, coolness, decreased sensation, tingling, numbness, or pain in extremity. Use of restraints may decrease environmental stimulation and result in sensory deprivation.

12. **Remove restraint at least every 2 hours, or according to agency policy and patient need.** Perform range-of-motion exercises.

Removal allows nurse to assess patient and reevaluate need for restraint. It also allows interventions for toileting, provision of nutrition and liquids, exercise, and change of position. Exercise increases circulation in restrained extremity.

13. Evaluate patient for continued need of restraint. Reapply restraint only if continued need is evident and order is still valid.

Continued need must be documented for reapplication.

14. Reassure patient at regular intervals. Provide continued explanation of rationale for interventions, reorientation if necessary, and plan of care. **Keep call bell within easy reach.**

Reassurance demonstrates caring and provides opportunity for sensory situation as well as ongoing assessment and evaluation. Patient can use call bell to summon assistance quickly.

DOCUMENTATION

Guidelines

Document alternative measures attempted before applying restraint. Document patient assessment before application. Record patient and family education and understanding regarding restraint use. Document family consent if necessary, according to facility policy. Document reason for restraining patient, date and time of application, type of restraint, times when removed, and result and frequency of nursing assessment. Obtain a new order after 24 hours if restraints are still necessary.

Sample Documentation

7/10/12 0830 Patient disoriented and combative. Attempting to remove tracheostomy and indwelling urinary catheter. Sitting at bedside, patient continued to tug at catheter and pull on tracheostomy. Family unwilling to sit with patient. Wrist restraints applied bilaterally as ordered.

—K. Urhahn, RN

7/10/12 1030 Patient continues to be disoriented and combative. Wrist restraints removed for 30 minutes during patient's bath; skin intact, hands warm, even skin tone, + radial pulses, + movement; passive and active range of motion completed. Wrist restraints reapplied.

—K. Urhahn, RN

UNEXPECTED SITUATIONS AND ASSOCIATED INTERVENTIONS

- *Patient has an IV catheter in the right wrist and is trying to remove drain from wound:* The left wrist may have a cloth restraint applied. Due to the IV in the right wrist, alternative forms of restraints should be tried, such as a cloth mitt or an elbow restraint.
- *Patient cannot move left arm:* Do not apply restraint to an extremity that is immobile. If patient cannot move the extremity, there is no need to apply a restraint. Restraint may be applied to right arm after obtaining an order from the primary care provider.

SPECIAL CONSIDERATIONS

- Do not position patient flat in a supine position with wrist restraints. If patient vomits, aspiration may occur.
- Check restraint for correct size before applying. Extremity restraints are available in different sizes. If restraint is too large, patient may free the extremity. If restraint is too small, circulation may be affected.
- Consider keeping a pair of scissors with emergency supplies in case the restraints cannot be untied quickly.

● Developing Critical Thinking Skills

1. You are the visiting nurse for a frail older patient who lives alone in her own home and prizes her independence. You assess her to be at high risk for falls because of her general weakness, the medication she takes, and a long history of indifference to safety counseling. What nursing interventions are likely to be most effective in ensuring her safety?

2. Identify the safety hazards and threats to security for which you and family members of different ages are most at risk. What anticipatory planning and teaching could be done to prevent these hazards? Note your willingness and that of your family to make the necessary changes, and identify the nursing strategies that would be most likely to secure patient cooperation in making the needed changes.

● Practicing for NCLEX

1. A school nurse is preparing a talk on healthcare topics for adolescents. Which of the following would be important for the nurse to include?
   a. Less than 10% of students report regular tobacco use
   b. Reaching a BAL of 0.08 within 2 hours constitutes binge drinking.
   c. Teenagers are more likely to drink and drive
   d. Peer pressure has an insignificant effect on adolescent substance use

2. The nurse is teaching parents of a toddler about the use of car seats. The nurse demonstrates an understanding of this measure by stating that car seats are mandatory in which of the following conditions?
   a. In all 50 states
   b. In 36 of the 50 states
   c. If a seat belt is not available
   d. On interstate highways

3. A nurse is assessing the following children. Which child would the nurse identify as having the greatest risk for choking and suffocating?
   a. A toddler playing with his 9-year-old brother's construction set
   b. A 4-year-old eating yogurt for lunch
   c. An infant covered with a small blanket and asleep in the crib
   d. A 3-year-old drinking a glass of juice

4. Which of the following would be most important for the nurse to keep in mind regarding the use of side rails for a confused patient?
   a. They prevent confused patients from wandering
   b. A history of a previous fall from a bed with raised side rails is insignificant
   c. Alternative measures are ineffective to prevent wandering
   d. A person of small stature is at increased risk for injury from entrapment

5. When describing safety issues and related mortality to a local senior citizens group, which of the following would the nurse identify as the leading cause of accidental death for people 79 years of age and older?
   a. Fires
   b. Exposure to temperature extremes
   c. Drug overdose
   d. Falls

6. Nursing education efforts that focus on prevention of firearm injuries are important for which of the following reasons?
   a. The elderly population is particularly at risk for firearm injuries.
   b. Most homicide victims, 10 to 24 years of age, are killed with a gun.
   c. The National Safety Council recommends a gun in every household to protect its members.
   d. They have contributed to a decrease in injuries and deaths from guns.

7. When discussing emergency preparedness with a group of first responders, which of the following would be important to include about preparation for a terrorist attack?
   a. Posttraumatic stress disorders can be expected in most survivors of a terrorist attack
   b. The FDA has collaborated with drug companies to create stockpiles of emergency drugs
   c. Even small doses of radiation result in bone marrow depression and cancer

   d. Blast lung injury is a serious consequence following detonation of an explosive device

8. An older resident who is disoriented likes to wander the halls of his long-term care facility. Which of the following would be most appropriate for the nurse to use as an alternative to restraints?
   a. Sitting him in a geriatric chair near the nurses' station
   b. Using the sheets to secure him snugly in his bed
   c. Keeping the bed in the high position
   d. Identifying his door with his picture and a balloon

9. While discussing home safety with the nurse, a patient admits that she always smokes a cigarette in bed before falling asleep at night. Which nursing diagnosis would be the priority for this patient?
   a. Impaired Gas Exchange related to cigarette smoking
   b. Anxiety related to inability to stop smoking
   c. Risk for Suffocation related to unfamiliarity with fire prevention guidelines
   d. Deficient knowledge related to lack of follow-through of recommendation to stop smoking

10. A male patient has weakened knees due to arthritis. The home healthcare nurse determines that he understands the need for safety modifications at home by which of the following?
    a. Using the towel bar for support to stand up from the commode
    b. Leaning on the pedestal table in his bedroom when he dresses
    c. Sitting primarily in chairs with armrests
    d. Using a small stepladder to reach an item on an upper shelf

11. When a fire occurs in a patient's room, which of the following would be the nurse's priority?
    a. Rescue the patient
    b. Extinguish the fire
    c. Sound the alarm
    d. Run for help

12. The nurse is planning a health teaching session for new parents about poisoning emergencies. Which of the following would the nurse emphasize that the parents do first?
    a. Use salt water to induce vomiting
    b. Rush the child to the emergency department
    c. Call the poison control center
    d. Routinely administer syrup of ipecac for any poison ingestion

13. Joint Commission guidelines regarding the use of restraints recommend which of the following?
    a. Vest restraints be used because they are the least restrictive type
    b. Restraints should be used for 48 hours in nonpsychiatric patients
    c. Restraints should be applied to prevent wandering behavior
    d. Alternative measures must be attempted first

14. The nurse orients an older patient to the safety features in her hospital room. Which of the following is a vital component of this admission routine?
    a. Explain how to use the telephone
    b. Introduce the patient to her roommate
    c. Review the hospital policy on visiting hours
    d. Explain how to operate the call bell

15. When completing a safety event report, the nurse should do which of the following?
    a. Include suggestions on how to prevent the incident from recurring
    b. Provide minimal information about the incident
    c. Discuss the details with the patient before documenting them
    d. Objectively describe the incident in detail

● Answers With Rationale

1. **b.** Raising the BAC to 0.08 or greater in a 2-hour period constitutes binge drinking. For this age group, 26% report using a tobacco product. Teenagers are less likely to drink and drive but more likely to have an accident if they do combine both behaviors. Much of adolescents' spare time is spent away from home and with peers, and peers are most influential in their decision making.

2. **a.** All 50 states require the use of safety seats for infants and toddlers at all times.

3. **a.** A young child may place small or loose parts in his or her mouth; a toy that is safe for a 9-year-old could kill a toddler. An infant sleeping in a crib without a pillow or large blanket and a 3-year-old and a 4-year-old drinking juice and eating yogurt are not particular safety risks.

4. **d.** Studies of restraint-related deaths have shown that people of small stature are more likely to slip through or between the side rails. The desire to prevent a patient from wandering is not sufficient reason for the use of side rails. Creative use of alternative measures indicates respect for the patient's dignity and may in fact prevent more serious fall-related injuries. A history of falls from a bed with raised side rails carries a significant risk for a future serious incident.

5. **d.** Falls are the leading cause of accidental death in the population 79 years of age and older. Fires, exposure to temperature extremes, and drug overdoses are significant causes of accidental death, but not in this age group.

6. **b.** Guns are responsible for over 80% of homicides for 10- to 24-year-old individuals. Keeping a gun in the home can have dangerous consequences and increases the risk for domestic violence. Young children may also be unintentionally injured or killed. Recent efforts to prevent injuries from guns have become more serious because violent behavior has increased in our society.

7. **d.** Blast lung injury is a recognized consequence following exposure to an explosive device. The CDC is the federal agency that has collaborated with the pharmaceutical companies to stockpile drugs for an emergency. A high dose of radiation exposure can result in bone marrow depression and cancer. Most survivors of a terrorist event will experience stress and some (possibly one-third of survivors) may exhibit posttraumatic stress disorder.

8. **d.** This allows the resident to be on the move and be more likely to find his room when he wants to return. The alternative would be to not allow him to wander. Many facilities use this kind of approach. Identifying his door with his picture and a balloon may work as an alternative to restraints. Using the geriatric chair and sheets are forms of physical restraint. Leaving the bed in the high position is a safety risk and would probably result in a fall.

9. **c.** Because Mrs. Fuller is not aware that smoking in bed is extremely dangerous, she is at risk for suffocation from fire. The other three nursing diagnoses are correctly stated but are not a priority in this situation.

10. **c.** Chairs with armrests can be used to increase the patient's leverage as he attempts to rise. Towel bars are not designed to provide support, the pedestal table is unsteady and unsafe, and standing on a stool and reaching puts the patient at risk for falling.

11. **a.** The patient's safety is always the priority. Sounding the alarm and extinguishing the fire are important after the patient is safe. Calling for help, rather than running for assistance, allows you to remain with your patient and is more appropriate, if possible.

12. **c.** Always call the poison control center before attempting any home remedies. Answers *a* and *d* can have serious consequences for the child and should not be attempted. The poison control center can supply the doctor or emergency department with specific information to assist in the victim's care.

13. **d.** Careful assessment and attempts to find effective alternative measures are required before applying a restraint. Wandering behavior is not an indication for restraints. Less restrictive restraints may include side rails, a geriatric chair, or wrist restraints instead of a vest. TJC recommends not using restraints for more than 24 hours on nonpsychiatric patients.

14. **d.** Knowing how to use the call bell is a safety priority; knowing how to use the phone, meeting the roommate, and knowledge of visiting hours will not necessarily prevent an accidental injury.

15. **d.** A safety event report is a legal document and must be as objective and complete as possible. It is not a collaborative effort with the patient, and any suggestions to prevent this from happening again should be discussed at a postincident conference.

Taylor Suite Resources

The Taylor Suite offers these additional resources to enhance learning and facilitate understanding of this chapter:

- thePoint online resource, http://thepoint.lww.com/Taylor7E
- Student DVD-ROM included with the book
- Study Guide for Taylor's Fundamentals of Nursing
- Skill Checklists for Taylor's Fundamentals of Nursing
- Taylor's Clinical Nursing Skills: *Chapter 3, Safety*

BIBLIOGRAPHY

Agency for Healthcare Research and Quality. (2009). Elderly/long-term care: Use of physical restraints in nursing homes creates substantial adverse consequences for residents. Available at http://www.ahrq.gov/research/mar09/0309RA9.htm.

American Academy of Child & Adolescent Psychiatry. (2008). *Teens: Alcohol and other drugs.* Available at http://www.aacap.org/cs/root/facts_for_families/teens_alcohol_and_other_drugs

American Cancer Society (ACS). (2008). *Child and teen tobacco use: Understanding the problem.* Available at http://www.cancer.org/docroot/PED/content/PED_10_2X_Child_and_Teen_Tobacco_Use.asp?sitearea=PED.

American Nurses Association (ANA). (2008). *Workplace safety and needlestick injuries are top concerns for nurses.* Available at http://www.nursingworld.org/MainMenuCategories/OccupationalandEnvironmental/occupationalhealth/SafeNeedles/WorkplaceSafetyTopConcerns.aspx

American Safety and Health Institute. (2003a). *Basic first aid for the community and workplace* (3rd ed.). Holiday, FL: Author.

American Safety and Health Institute. (2003b). *Essentials in basic emergency care.* Holiday, FL: Author.

Association of periOperative Registered Nurses (AORN). (2008). *AORN position statement on surgical smoke and bio-aerosols.* Available at http://www.aorn.org/PracticeResources/AORNPositionStatements/SurgicalSmokeAndBioAerosols/

Bulechek, G., Butcher, H., & Dochterman, J. (2008). *Nursing interventions classification (NIC)* (5th ed.). St. Louis: Mosby, Inc.

Centers for Disease Control and Prevention (CDC). (2006a). *Emergency preparedness: Chemical categories.* Available at http://www.bt.cdc.gov/agent/agentlistchem-category.asp

Centers for Disease Control and Prevention (CDC). (2006b). *Frequently asked questions about a radiation emergency.* Available at http://www.bt.cdc.gov/radiation/emergencyfaq.asp

Centers for Disease Control and Prevention (CDC). (2006c). *General fact sheets on specific bioterrorism agents.* Available at http://emergency.cdc.gov/bioterrorism/factsheets.asp

Centers for Disease Control and Prevention (CDC). (2006d). *Understanding intimate partner violence.* Available at http://www.cdc.gov/violenceprevention/pdf/IPV_factsheet-a.pdf

Centers for Disease Control and Prevention (CDC). (2008a). *Blast lung injury: Prehospital care.* Available at http://emergency.cdc.gov/masscasualties/blastlunginjury_prehospital.asp

Centers for Disease Control and Prevention (CDC). (2008b). *Body art.* Available at http://www.cdc.gov/niosh/topics/bbp/bodyart/default.html

Centers for Disease Control and Prevention (CDC). (2008c). *Child maltreatment.* Available at http://www.cdc.gov/ViolencePrevention/childmaltreatment/index.html

Centers for Disease Control and Prevention (CDC). (2008d). *Child passenger safety: Fact sheet.* Available at http://www.cdc.gov/ncipc/factsheets/childpas.htm

Centers for Disease Control and Prevention (CDC). (2008e). *Fire deaths and injuries: Fact sheet.* Available at http://www.cdc.gov/HomeandRecreationalSafety/Fire-Prevention/fires-factsheet.html

Centers for Disease Control and Prevention (CDC). (2008f). *Poisoning in the United States: Fact sheet.* Available at http://www.cdc.gov/ncipc/factsheets/poisoning.htm

Centers for Disease Control and Prevention (CDC). (2008g). *Youth violence.* Available at http://www.cdc.gov/ViolencePrevention/youthviolence/

Centers for Disease Control and Prevention (CDC). (2009a). *Costs of falls among older adults.* Available at http://www.cdc.gov/HomeandRecreationalSafety/Falls/fallcost.html

Centers for Disease Control and Prevention (CDC). (2009b). *Falls among older adults: An overview.* Available at http://cdc.gov/HomeandRecreationalSafety/Falls/adultfalls.html

Centers for Disease Control and Prevention (CDC). (2009c). *Health alert network.* Available at http://www2a.cdc.gov/han/Index.asp

Centers for Disease Control and Prevention (CDC). (2009d). *Healthy youth: Alcohol & drug use.* Available at http://www.cdc.gov/HealthyYouth/alcoholdrug/index.htm

Centers for Disease Control and Prevention (CDC). (2009e). *Home & Recreational Safety: Bicycle related injuries.* Available at http://www.cdc.gov/HomeandRecreationalSafety/bikeinjuries.html

Centers for Disease Control and Prevention (CDC). (2009f). *Teen drivers: Fact sheet.* Available at http://www.cdc.gov/MotorVehicleSafety/Teen_Drivers/teendrivers_factsheet.html

Centers for Disease Control and Prevention (CDC). (2009g). National Center for Injury Prevention and Control. *What is traumatic brain injury?* Available at http://www.cdc.gov/ncipc/tbi/TBI.htm

Child Welfare Information Gateway. (2008). *Recognizing child abuse and neglect: Signs and symptoms.* Available at http://www.childwelfare.gov/pubs/factsheets/signs.cfm

College of American Pathologists (CAP). (2008). *Elder maltreatment.* Available at http://www.cap.org/apps/cap.portal?_nfpb=true&cntvwrPtlt_actionOverride=%2Fportlets%2FcontentViewer%2Fshow&_windowLabel=cntvwrPtlt&cntvwrPtlt%7BactionForm.contentReference%7D=statements%2Felder_maltreatment_08.html&_state=maximized&_pageLabel=cntvwr

Cowles, L., & Carter, S. (2007). At the ready. *Advance for Nurses, 9*(22), 35–36.

Eliopoulos, C. (2003). *Gerontological nursing* (5th ed.). Philadelphia: Lippincott Williams & Wilkins.

Evans, L., & Cotter, V. (2008). Avoiding restraints in patients with dementia. *American Journal of Nursing, 108*(3), 40–50.

Goodlett, D., Robinson, C., Carson, P., Landry, L. (2009). Focusing on video surveillance to reduce falls. *Nursing, 39*(2), 20–21.

Haag, R. (2007). The basics of bioterrorism preparedness. *Advance for Nurses, 9*(21), 37–39.

Hendrich, A. (2007). Predicting patient falls: Using the Hendrich II Fall Risk Model in clinical practice. *American Journal of Nursing, 107*(11), 50–59.

Kirkpatrick, C. (2009). Safety first: The Joint Commission's national patient safety goals for 2009. *Spring 2009 Med/Surg Specialty Guide,* 24–30.

Madden, M. (2008). Responding to pediatric poisoning. *Nursing, 38*(8), 52–55.

Minnick, A., Mion, L., Johnson, M., Catrambone, C., & Leipzig, R. (2007). Prevalence and variation of physical restraint use in acute care settings in the U.S. *Journal of Nursing Scholarship, 39*(1), 30–37.

Moorhead, S., Johnson, M., Maas, M., & Swanson, E. (2008). *Nursing outcomes classification (NOC)* (4th ed.). St. Louis: Mosby, Inc.

National Highway Traffic Safety Administration (NHTSA). 2010. *Securing our most precious cargo.* Available at http://www.nhtsa.dot.gov/staticfiles/DOT/NHTSA/Traffic%20Injury%20Control/Articles/Associated%20Files/LATCH-factsheet.pdf

National Institute on Alcohol and Alcoholism (NIAAA). (2006). *Alcohol alert: Underage drinking.* Available at http://pubs.niaaa.nih.gov/publications/AA67/AA67.htm

National Patient Safety Foundation. (2008). *The universal patient compact: Principles for partnership.* Available at http://www.npsf.org/paf/compact.php

North American Nursing Diagnosis Association (NANDA) International. (2009). *Nursing diagnoses: Definitions & classifications 2009–2011.* Oxford, UK: Wiley-Blackwell.

Pillitteri, A. (2010). *Maternal & child nursing: Care of the childbearing and childrearing family* (6th ed.). Philadelphia: Lippincott Williams & Wilkins.

Pullen, R. (2007). Screening for abuse and neglect. *Nursing, 37*(2), 69.

Rich, S. (2008). How human factors lead to medical device adverse events. *Nursing, 38*(6), 62–63.

Rothrock, J. (2008). Trends & issues: Those three little words, "We're very sorry." *Advance for Nurses, 10*(10), 13.

Safe Kids USA. (2008). Seasonal safety: Protecting kids from choking, suffocation and strangulation. Available at http://www.usa.safekids.org/tier3_cd.cfm?folder_id=301&content_item_id=26551

Schooley, C., & Kelly, A. (2008). Home hazards: Can children recognize the dangers? *Journal of Trauma Nursing, 15*(3), 131–135.

Sharaf, A., & Ibrahim, H. (2008). Physical and psychosocial correlates of fear of falling. *Journal of Gerontological Nursing, 34*(12), 27–35.

Shields, J. (2007). Fall lesson plan: Evaluating children for concussion. *Nursing Spectrum, 16*(19), 8–9.

Spader, C. (2006). RNs ready for disaster. *Nursing Spectrum, 15*(18), 8–11.

Steinhauer, R., & Bauer, J. (2002). A readied answer: The emergency management plan. *RN, 65*(6), 40–46.

Taliaferro, L., Rienzo, B., Miller, D., Pigg, M., & Dodd, V. (2008). High school youth and suicide risk: Exploring protection afforded through physical activity and sport participation. *Journal of School Health, 78*(10), 545–553.

Taschner, M. (2008). Responding to a fire emergency. *Nursing, 38*(5), 44–47.

The American Geriatrics Society. (2008). *AGS position statement: Restraint use.* Available at http://www.americangeriatrics.org/products/positionpapers/restraintsupdate.shtml

The Joint Commission. (2010). *Sentinel event statistics.* Available at http://www.jointcommission.org/NR/rdonlyres/377FF7E7-F565-4D61-9FD2-593CA688135B/0/SE_Stats_31_Dec_2009.pdf

The Joint Commission. (2009). *Sentinel event statistics.* Available at http://www.jointcommission.org/NR/rdonlyers/241CD6F3-6EF0-439C-90AD-7FEAE5EDCEA5/0/SE_Stats12_08.pdf

Todd, J. (2008). Waking up to hospital bed entrapment risks. *Nursing, 38*(1), 14–15.

USAA Educational Foundation. (2009). *Internet safety for teens.* Available at http://www.usaaedfoundation.org/family/it01.asp

U.S. Department of Health and Human Services. (2007). Child Health USA 2007. *Adolescent mortality from traffic and firearm injuries.* Available at: http://mchb.hrsa.gov/chusa07/hstat/hsa/pages/225amtfi.html

U.S. Department of Health and Human Services. (2009). *Hospitals rising to the challenge: The first five years of the U.S. hospital preparedness program and priorities going forward.* Available at http://www.upmc-biosecurity.org/website/resources/publications/2009/2009-04-16-hppreport.html

U.S. Department of Health and Human Services. (2009). *Violence against women: Domestic and intimate partner violence.* Available at http://www.womenshealth.gov/violence/types/domestic.cfm

U.S. Environmental Protection Agency. (2008). *Avoiding CO poisoning.* Available at http://www.epa.gov/iaq/pubs/coftsht.html

U.S. Environmental Protection Agency. (2009). *Carbon monoxide poisoning prevention.* Available at http://www.epa.gov/aging/resources/factsheets/pcmp/index.htm

Veenema, T. G. (2003). *Disaster nursing and emergency preparedness for chemical, biological, radiological terrorism, and other hazards.* New York: Springer Publishing Co.

Walker-Cillo, G. (2006). Bioterrorism: We put our plan to the test. *RN, 69*(4), 36–41.

Wiseman, R. (2007). Responding to disaster emergencies. *Advance for Nurses, 9*(20), 33–35.

27 Asepsis and Infection Control

JACKSON RAY IVERS

Jackson Ray comes to visit his mother, who has been hospitalized for tuberculosis. He notices a sign on the door to check at the nurse's desk before entering. He asks, "What's going on? Why do I have to wash my hands and wear a mask?"

ESTHER BAILEY

Esther, a 72-year-old female patient on the unit recovering from abdominal surgery and receiving antibiotic therapy for a wound infection, requires insertion of an indwelling urinary catheter due to the development of postoperative urinary retention and an inability to void.

GISELLE TURHEIS

Giselle, a 38-year-old woman undergoing chemotherapy treatment for leukemia, states "I know that my risk for infection is really high because of my poor immune status. But how do I respond to my Sunday school class, who are used to greeting me with a big hug. I want to be safe, but I know that I need these hugs too!"

LEARNING OBJECTIVES

After completing the chapter, you will be able to accomplish the following:

1. Explain the infection cycle.
2. Describe nursing interventions used to break the chain of infection.
3. List the stages of an infection.
4. Identify patients at risk for developing an infection.
5. Identify factors that reduce the incidence of healthcare-associated infection.
6. Identify situations in which hand hygiene is indicated.
7. List nursing diagnoses for a patient who has or is at risk for infection.
8. Describe strategies for implementing CDC guidelines for standard and transmission-based precautions when caring for patients.
9. Implement recommended techniques for medical and surgical asepsis.

KEY TERMS

aerobic
anaerobic
antibody
antigen
antimicrobial
asepsis
bacteria
disinfection
endemic
endogenous
exogenous
fungi
healthcare-associated infection (HAI)
host
iatrogenic

infection
isolation
medical asepsis
nosocomial
pathogens
personal protective equipment (PPE)
reservoir
standard precautions
sterilization
surgical asepsis
transmission-based precautions
vector
virulence
virus

A major concern for health practitioners is the danger of spreading microorganisms from person to person and from place to place. Microorganisms are naturally present in almost all environments. Some are beneficial; some are not. Some are harmless to most people, and others are harmful to many people. Still others are harmless except in certain circumstances.

Government agencies at the international, national, state, and local levels; health personnel; and individuals recognize the need for an organized, systematic approach to the control of infections. Such efforts include mass immunization programs, laws concerning safe sewage disposal, regulations for the control of communicable diseases, and hospital infection-surveillance programs. Medical science continues to grapple with problems caused by increasingly virulent organisms that have become drug resistant and with problems related to patients who are immunologically compromised.

Prevention of infection is a major focus for nurses. As primary caregivers, nurses are involved in identifying, preventing, controlling, and teaching the patient about infection (see the Reflective Practice box for an example). Use of the nursing process can prove critical in breaking the cycle of infection.

INFECTION
Infection Cycle

An **infection** is a disease state that results from the presence of **pathogens** (disease-producing microorganisms) in or on the body. An infection occurs as a result of a cyclic process, consisting of six components, as shown in Figure 27-1. These components are:

- Infectious agent
- Reservoir
- Portal of exit
- Means of transmission
- Portals of entry
- Susceptible host

Infectious Agent

Some of the more prevalent agents that cause infection are bacteria, viruses, and fungi. **Bacteria,** the most significant and most commonly observed infection-causing agents in healthcare institutions, can be categorized in various ways. They are categorized by shape as spherical (cocci), rod shaped (bacilli), or corkscrew shaped (spirochetes). Bacteria can be categorized as either gram positive or gram negative, based on their reaction to the Gram stain. For example, gram-positive bacteria have a thick cell wall that resists decolorization (loss of color) and are stained violet. However, gram-negative bacteria have chemically more complex cell walls and can be decolorized by alcohol. Thus, gram-negative bacteria do not stain. This information is crucial for physicians when prescribing the most appropriate antibiotic therapy because antibiotics are classified as specifically effective against only gram-positive organisms or as broad spectrum and effective against several groups of microorganisms. Another distinguishing characteristic of (or way of categorizing) bacteria is their need for oxygen. Most bacteria

REFLECTIVE PRACTICE

Challenge to Ethical and Legal Skills

This is my last clinical rotation before graduation and it has been a difficult year. My focus has been somewhat off for a while, and I haven't been as prepared as I should have been for my clinical and classroom experiences. My clinical instructor has been on my case for the last few weeks. I'm also realizing that in no time at all I will be out of school and on my own when it comes to patient care. So, all of a sudden, I'm eager for as many clinical experiences as I can get. To make a long story short, I'm thrilled when offered the opportunity to catheterize Esther Bailey, a 72-year-old female patient on my unit. I quickly review the procedure and go to the patient's room, with the catheterization supplies in hand, feeling semiconfident. After introducing myself and my clinical instructor and explaining what I'm about to do, I open the sterile package, prepare the sterile field, and cleanse the meatus. In one quick moment, as the patient asks a question and diverts my instructor's gaze, I realize to my horror that I've contaminated the catheter. I've got a split second to decide what to do. I can tell my instructor what happened, obtain a new kit, and proceed anew, or pretend nothing happened and continue. I don't like that I'm even considering not admitting the mistake, after everything that has been drilled into us about the importance of sterility and the consequences of nosocomial infections. But I'm also prudent enough to realize that it is time to leave the unit because the rest of the group is waiting for postconference. Plus, after all, there are financial costs to ordering another tray. But what if I do not admit the error and by chance the instructor did see me contaminate the catheter? Then my goose is really cooked!

Thinking Outside the Box: Possible Courses of Action

- Obviously the simplest solution: admit my error and accept the consequences.
- Request a new catheter and inform my instructor later that the patient moved just as I was preparing to enter the meatus (a bit of deception but this makes the error not my fault).
- Alternatively, pretend that nothing happened and pray that no harm comes to the patient (after all,

how much bacteria do you need to contaminate a catheter? . . . and the patient is receiving antibiotic therapy anyway).
- Continue and not even be bothered by the contamination (Life is one big risk for everyone, right? All that matters is that you take care of #1).

Evaluating a Good Outcome: How Do I Define Success?

- Patient benefited from my actions or, at the very least, was not harmed.
- No one's integrity is compromised or sacrificed.

- No violations of the standards of practice or the American Nurses Association's Code of Ethics occurred.

Personal Learning: Here's to the Future!

At least I can say there was a happy ending to this story. I did stop, explain what happened, and waited while someone ran for a new catheterization tray. Amazingly, my instructor told me later that she valued my maturity and honesty and ability to put the needs of the patient

ahead of my own needs, stating that I "might just have what it takes after all!" I'm not sure how often I'll be called upon to put the needs of a patient ahead of my own needs but hopefully I'll be ready to respond selflessly each time.

Reflection

How do you think you would respond in a similar situation? Why? What does this tell you about yourself and about the adequacy of your skills for professional practice? Can you think of other ways to respond? Did the nursing student perform legally, adhering to the standards of practice? If not, what violations occurred? What ethical principles might have been violated had the nursing student not reported the catheter contamination? How did the nursing student adhere to principles of medical and surgical asepsis? What other skills (cognitive, interpersonal, technical, ethical/legal) would you need to respond well in this situation? Do you agree with the criteria to evaluate a successful outcome? Were the criteria met? If not, what else might the nursing student have done to ensure a successful outcome?

require oxygen to live and grow and are, therefore, referred to as **aerobic.** Those that can live without oxygen are **anaerobic** bacteria.

A **virus** is the smallest of all microorganisms, visible only with an electron microscope. Many infections are caused by viruses, including the common cold and the deadly disease, acquired immunodeficiency syndrome (AIDS). Antibiotics have no effect on viruses; however, there are some antiviral medications available that seem to be effective with some

viral infections. When given in the prodromal stage of certain viruses, these medications can shorten the full stage of the illness.

Fungi, plant-like organisms (molds and yeasts) that also can cause infection, are present in the air, soil, and water. Some examples of infections caused by fungi include athlete's foot, ringworm, and yeast infections. These infections are treated with antifungal medications; however, many infections due to fungi are resistant to treatment.

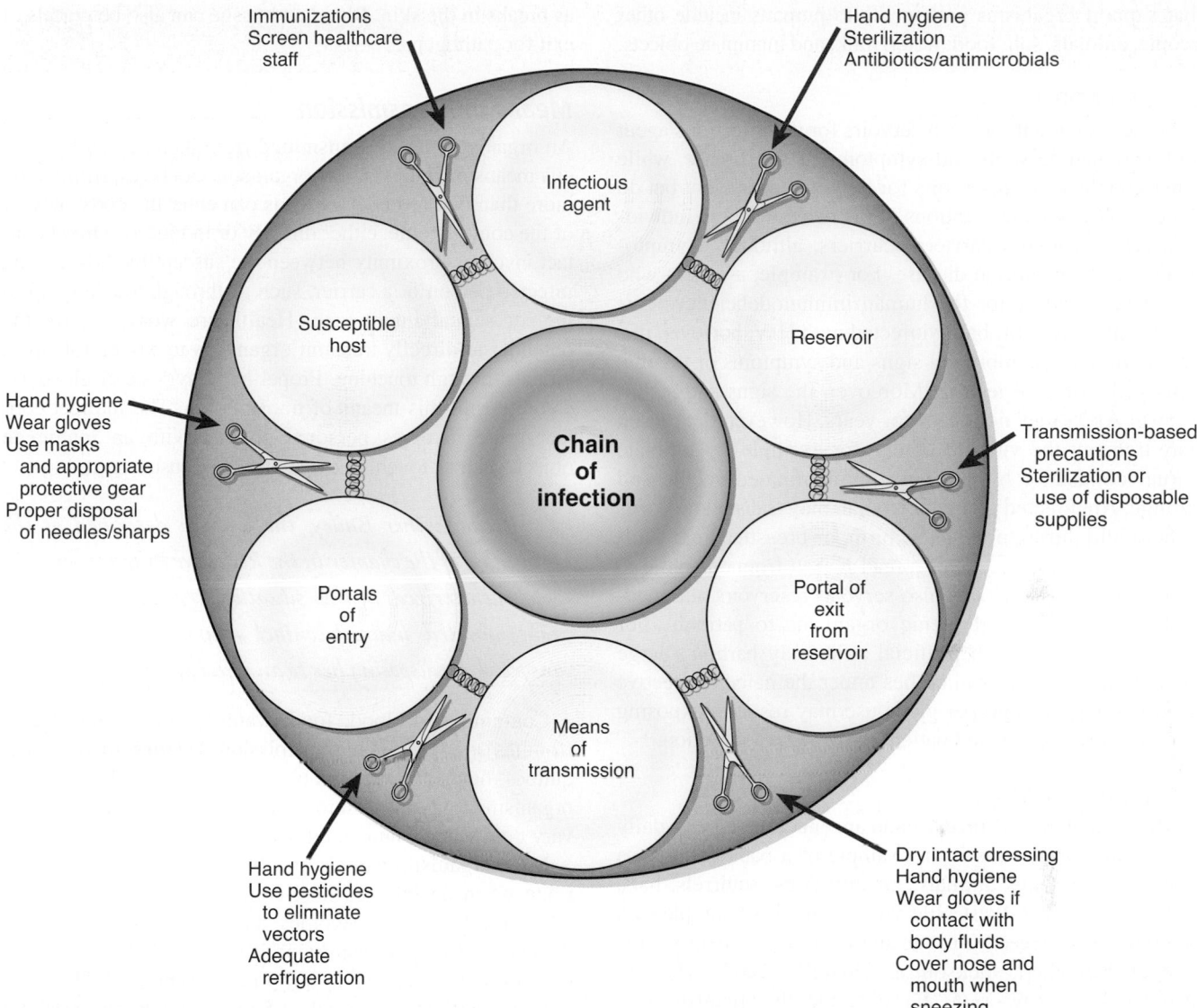

FIGURE 27-1. The infection cycle is demonstrated as a chain. The goal is to break the links of the chain to end the cycle. *(Adapted from Murphy, D. [1998]. Infectious microbes and disease: General principles. Nursing Spectrum, 7[2], 12–14.)*

Not all organisms to which a person is exposed cause disease. An organism's potential to produce disease in a person depends on a variety of factors, including:

- Number of organisms
- **Virulence** of the organism, or its ability to cause disease
- Competence of the person's immune system
- Length and intimacy of the contact between the person and the microorganism

Identifying the type of infection and infectious agent is not always an easy process. Sometimes new diseases appear and healthcare workers race to identify them so that treatment can begin. This is the process that occurred with AIDS and with severe acute respiratory syndrome (SARS). Other times, a disease that is **endemic** or occurs with predictability in one specific region or population can appear in a different geographical location. For example, dengue fever that is endemic in Southeast Asia has the potential to emerge in the United

States and pose a major public health problem (Leung-Chen, 2008a). In cases like these, countries draw information from one another to learn about treatment options.

Under normal conditions, some organisms may not produce disease. Microorganisms that commonly inhabit various body sites and are part of the body's natural defense system are referred to as normal flora. Other factors may intervene, causing this usually harmless organism to generate an infection. Bacteria that normally cause no problem but, with certain factors, may potentially be harmful are referred to as opportunists. For example, one type of *Escherichia coli* normally resides in the intestinal tract and causes no harm. However, if it migrates to the urinary tract, it can lead to urinary tract infection.

Reservoir

The **reservoir** for growth and multiplication of microorganisms is the natural habitat of the organism. Possible reservoirs that support organisms pathogenic to humans include other people, animals, soil, food, water, milk, and inanimate objects.

OTHER PEOPLE

Some individuals act as reservoirs for the infectious agent and demonstrate signs and symptoms of the disease, while other people act as reservoirs for the infectious agent but do not exhibit any manifestations of the disease. These individuals are considered carriers. Carriers, although asymptomatic, can transmit the disease. For example, a person who has tested positive for the human immunodeficiency virus (HIV) antibody is probably infected with HIV; however, this person may not exhibit any signs and symptoms of the disease at the time of testing. Moreover, the signs and symptoms of AIDS may not occur for years. However, the person may transmit the virus to others, for example, by intimate sexual contact or by sharing a contaminated needle and syringe. An infected pregnant woman may transmit the virus to her child during pregnancy, birth, or breastfeeding. Children in daycare centers can spread *E. coli* from one child to another child. Nurses can also serve as reservoirs and inadvertently transfer pathogenic organisms to patients. For example, a nurse with artificial nails may harbor a large number and variety of microbes under the nails. Ineffective handwashing or improper glove use may result in exposing an immunocompromised patient to the risk of infection.

OTHER RESERVOIRS

Many other reservoirs exist and are encountered on a daily basis. The rabies virus is an example of a pathogen whose reservoir is various animals, notably dogs, squirrels, bats, and raccoons. The West Nile virus is another example of a pathogen whose reservoir is an animal, most frequently birds (Siegel, Rhinehart, Jackson, & Chiarello, 2007). The soil also can act as a reservoir. For example, the organisms that cause gas gangrene and tetanus are examples of pathogens whose reservoir is soil.

Water can harbor *Giardia, E. coli* 0157-H7, and *Shigella*. Drinking or swimming in contaminated water can begin the infectious cycle in a person. Undercooked ground beef, tomatoes, and bagged spinach are reservoirs that have been identified as responsible for recent outbreaks of *E. coli* infections. The Centers for Disease Control and Prevention (CDC) recommends that all ground beef be cooked until well done and new laws keep fruits and vegetables safer when they are grown, picked, and washed. Milk can contain *Listeria* unless it is pasteurized. Inanimate objects can harbor organisms, such as influenza, which may be spread if a person touches a contaminated article and then touches his or her nose or eyes.

Portal of Exit

The portal of exit is the point of escape for the organism from the reservoir. The organism cannot extend its influence unless it moves away from its original reservoir. Usually, each type of microorganism has a primary exit route. In humans, common portals of exit or escape routes include the respiratory, gastrointestinal, and genitourinary tracts, as well

as breaks in the skin. Blood and tissue can also be portals of exit for pathogens.

Means of Transmission

An organism may be transmitted from its reservoir by various means or routes. Some organisms can be transmitted by more than one route. Organisms can enter the body by way of the contact route, either directly or indirectly. Direct contact involves proximity between the susceptible host and an infected person or a carrier, such as through touching, kissing, or sexual intercourse. Healthcare workers have the potential to directly transmit organisms to susceptible individuals through touching. Proper hand hygiene or glove use can interrupt this means of transmission. The indirect contact route involves personal contact with an inanimate object, such as touching a contaminated instrument.

> ➤ *Recall Esther Bailey, the woman described at the beginning of the chapter in the Reflective Practice box, who was catheterized. In this situation, the catheter becomes contaminated. Indirect contact occurs if this catheter is inserted, predisposing her to an infection.* ∎

Contaminated blood, food, water, or inanimate objects (fomites) are vehicles of transmission. **Vectors,** such as mosquitoes, ticks, and lice, are nonhuman carriers that transmit organisms from one host to another, that is, by injecting salivary fluid when a human bite occurs.

Microorganisms can also be spread through the airborne route when an infected host coughs, sneezes, or talks, or when the organism becomes attached to dust particles. Another means of transmission is through droplets. Droplet transmission is similar to airborne transmission. However, airborne particles are less than 5 mcm, and droplet particles are greater than 5 mcm. Table 27-1 summarizes the means of transmission for several organisms, their reservoirs, and examples of diseases they transmit.

Portal of Entry

The portal of entry is the point at which organisms enter a new host. The organism must find a portal of entry to a host or it may die. The entry route into the new host often is the same as the exit route from the prior reservoir. The urinary, respiratory, and gastrointestinal tracts and the skin are common portals of entry.

Susceptible Host

Microorganisms can continue to exist only in a source that is acceptable (a **host**) and only if they overcome any resistance mounted by the host's defenses. Susceptibility is the degree of resistance the potential host has to the pathogen. Hospital patients are often in a weakened state of health because of illness and have less resistance. Thus, they are more susceptible for infection. Many factors influence a host's susceptibility; these are discussed later in the chapter.

TABLE • 27-1   ORGANISMS CAPABLE OF CAUSING DISEASE

Organism	Reservoir	Means of Transmission	Disease Transmitted
Staphylococcus aureus	Skin surface Mouth Nose Throat	Contact (direct)	Wound infection Abscess Carbuncle Boil
Hepatitis B virus	Blood Feces Body fluids and excretions	Contact (indirect)	Hepatitis B
Human immunodeficiency virus	Blood Semen Vaginal secretions Breast milk	Contact (direct) Contact (ingestion)	Acquired immunodeficiency syndrome
Mycobacterium tuberculosis *Borrelia burgdorferi*	Sputum (respiratory tract) Ticks (sheep, cattle, deer, mice)	Airborne Vectors Contact (direct)	Tuberculosis Lyme disease *E. coli* infection
Escherichia coli	Feces Undercooked meat (beef) Unpasteurized apple juice Tomatoes, peppers, spinach	Contact (ingestion)	
Salmonella	Intestinal tracts of humans and other animals, including birds	Contact (ingestion)	Diarrheal illness

> *Remember Giselle Turheis, the woman with leukemia and a compromised immune status. Her susceptibility to infection is increased because of the lack of an adequate functioning immune system.* ■

Stages of Infection

An understanding of the stages in the development of an infection is necessary to intervene and disrupt the infection cycle. An infection progresses through the following phases:

- Incubation period
- Prodromal stage
- Full stage of illness
- Convalescent period

The course and severity of the infection, as well as the patient's response, influence the type and extent of nursing care provided.

Incubation Period

The incubation period is the interval between the pathogen's invasion of the body and the appearance of symptoms of infection. During this stage, the organisms arc growing and multiplying. The length of incubation may vary. For example, the common cold has an incubation period of 1 to 2 days, whereas tetanus has an incubation period ranging from 2 to 21 days.

Prodromal Stage

A person is most infectious during the prodromal stage. Early signs and symptoms of disease are present, but these are often vague and nonspecific, ranging from fatigue and malaise to a low-grade fever. This period lasts from several hours to several days. During this phase, the patient often does not realize that he or she is contagious. As a result, the infection spreads.

Full Stage of Illness

The presence of specific signs and symptoms indicates the full stage of illness. The type of infection determines the length of the illness and the severity of the manifestations. Symptoms that are limited or occur in only one body area are referred to as localized symptoms, whereas symptoms manifested throughout the entire body are referred to as systemic symptoms.

Convalescent Period

The convalescent period is the recovery period from the infection. Convalescence may vary according to the severity of the infection and the patient's general condition. The signs and symptoms disappear, and the person returns to a healthy state. However, depending on the type of infection, the person may have a temporary or permanent change to his or her previous health state even after the convalescent period.

A person may continually pass through the four phases with the same infectious process, such as with herpes simplex. Although there may have been only one infectious exposure, the infection may continue to cycle through the phases.

The Body's Defense Against Infection

One of the first lines of defense against infection is the body's normal flora. Flora helps to keep potentially harmful bacteria from invading the body. In addition to the normal flora that inhabit various body sites, other defense systems help a person combat infection. These include the inflammatory response and immune response.

Inflammatory Response

The inflammatory response is a protective mechanism that eliminates the invading pathogen and allows for tissue repair to occur. Inflammation helps the body to neutralize, control, or eliminate the offending agent and to prepare the site for repair (Smeltzer, Bare, Hinkle, & Cheever, 2010). In addition to infection, the inflammatory response also occurs in response to injury. It is either an acute or chronic process.

The cardinal signs of acute infection are redness, heat, swelling, pain, and loss of function and usually appear at the site of the injury or inflammation. The vascular and cellular stages are the main components of the inflammatory process and these physiological processes are responsible for the appearance of the cardinal signs. Initially, in the vascular stage, small blood vessels constrict in the area followed by vasodilatation of arterioles and venules that supply the area. This increase in blood flow results in redness and heat in the area. Histamine also is released leading to an increased permeability of vessels, which allows protein-rich fluid to pour into the area. At this point, swelling, pain, and loss of function can occur.

During the cellular stage, white blood cells (leukocytes) move quickly into the area. Neutrophils, the primary phagocytes, engulf the organism and consume cell debris and foreign material. Exudate composed of fluid, cells, and inflammatory byproducts is released from the wound. The exudate may be clear (serous), contain red blood cells (sanguinous), or contain pus (purulent). The amount of exudate depends on the size and location of the wound. The damaged cells then are repaired by either regeneration (replacement with identical cells) or the formation of scar tissue (Porth, 2007). Refer to Chapters 32 and 42 for additional discussion of the inflammatory response.

Immune Response

Another defense system is the immune response. The immune response involves specific body responses to an invading foreign protein, such as bacteria, or in some cases, to the body's own proteins. The complex mechanisms that constitute the immune response occur as the body attempts to protect and defend itself. The foreign material is called an **antigen,** and the body commonly responds to the antigen by producing an **antibody.** This antigen–antibody reaction, also known as humoral immunity, is one component of the overall immune response. The other component that also helps the body defend against

invaders is a cell-mediated defense, or cellular immunity. It involves an increase in the number of lymphocytes (white blood cells) that destroy or react with cells the body recognizes as harmful. Although these complicated chemical and mechanical responses are not completely understood, it is known that they help to defend the body specifically against bacterial, viral, and fungal infections, as well as malignant cells.

Factors Affecting the Risk for Infection

The susceptibility of the host depends on various factors:

- Integrity of skin and mucous membranes, which protect the body against microbial invasion
- pH levels of the gastrointestinal and genitourinary tracts, as well as the skin, which help to ward off microbial invasion
- Integrity and number of the body's white blood cells, which provide resistance to certain pathogens
- Age, sex, race, and hereditary, which influence susceptibility. Neonates and older adults appear to be more vulnerable to infection. (See the accompanying box, Focus on the Older Adult.)
- Immunizations, natural or acquired, which act to resist infection
- Level of fatigue, nutritional and general health status, the presence of preexisting illnesses, previous or current treatments, and certain medications, which play a part in the susceptibility of a potential host
- Stress level, which if increased, may adversely affect the body's normal defense mechanisms
- Use of invasive or indwelling medical devices, which provide exposure to and entry for more potential sources of disease-producing organisms, particularly in a patient whose defenses are already weakened by disease

▶ *Think back to Esther Bailey, the woman being catheterized who also has developed a postoperative wound infection. Undergoing abdominal surgery disrupts the integrity of the skin and mucous membranes, thereby increasing her risk for a wound infection.* ■

Health habits that promote wellness can reduce potential risk factors, thus decreasing the susceptibility of a host. Sensible nutrition, adequate rest and exercise, stress-reduction techniques, and good personal hygiene habits can help maintain optimum bodily function and immune response. Unsafe sex practices and sharing intravenous (IV) needles are potentially dangerous and provide an opportunity for pathogens to enter a host and cause an infection.

THE NURSING PROCESS FOR INFECTION PREVENTION AND CONTROL

It is imperative that healthcare practitioners safeguard the individuals entrusted to their care by controlling diseases and preventing the spread of infection. Vigilant preventive care can limit exposure to potentially harmful infectious organisms and reduce the occurrence of infection.

FOCUS ON THE OLDER ADULT

AGE-RELATED CHANGES PREDISPOSING TO INFECTION

Infection Risk	Age-related Changes	Nursing Strategies
Pulmonary infections	• Decreased cough reflex • Decreased elastic recoil of lungs • Decreased activity of cilia • Abnormal swallowing reflexes	• Place patient in sitting position to eat and drink • Encourage patient to drink plenty of fluids unless contraindicated • Encourage patient to cough and deep breathe or use incentive spirometer as ordered • Recommend pneumococcal vaccination once in a lifetime and influenza vaccination annually
Urinary tract infections	• Incomplete emptying of bladder • Decreased sphincter control • Bladder-outlet obstruction due to enlarged prostate gland • Pelvic floor relaxation due to estrogen depletion • Reduced renal blood flow	• Discuss with patient need to void at regular intervals • Encourage patient to drink plenty of fluids unless contraindicated • Administer medications for enlarged prostate (benign prostate hypertrophy) and estrogen depletion as ordered • If patient wears absorbent product such as incontinence pad, instruct patient to change pad frequently and perform good "pericare" • Assess for UTIs (may be atypical in elderly patient) • Discuss the need for patient to void immediately after sexual intercourse
Skin infections	• Loss of elasticity • Increased dryness • Thinning of epidermis • Slowing of cell replacement • Decreased vascular supply	• Encourage patient to drink plenty of fluids, unless contraindicated • Help patient to perform good hygiene practices daily • Apply lotion to skin as needed • Assess frequently for any breaks in skin integrity, rashes, or changes in skin

*Atypical clinical manifestations of infection in an older adult include confusion, disorientation, lethargy, anorexia, delayed fever response, falls, incontinence, and failure to thrive.

Assessing

The nurse plays a critical role in preventing and controlling infection. This role begins with early detection and surveillance techniques. The extent of nursing interventions depends on the susceptibility of the host, the virulence of the organism, and the patient's signs and symptoms.

Inquire about the patient's immunization status and previous or recurring infections. Observe nonverbal cues and gather information about the history of the current disease. Nursing assessments include observing for signs and symptoms of a local or systemic infection. A localized infection can result in redness, swelling, warmth in the involved area, pain or tenderness, and loss of function of the affected part. Manifestations of a systemic infection include fever, often accompanied by an increase in pulse and respiratory rate, lethargy, anorexia, and tenderness and enlargement of lymph nodes that drain the area when an infection is present. Laboratory data can provide further insight into the presence of an infectious process. Any of the laboratory test results outlined in Box 27-1 may indicate the presence of an infection.

Box 27-1   LABORATORY DATA INDICATING AN INFECTION

• Elevated white blood cell (leukocyte) count—normal value is 5,000 to 10,000/mm^3
• Increase in specific types of white blood cells (differential count or percentage of each cell type)

Neutrophils	Normal = 60%–70%	Increased in acute infections that produce pus; increased risk for acute bacterial infection if decreased; may also be increased in response to stress.
Lymphocytes	Normal = 20%–40%	Increased in chronic bacterial and viral infections
Monocytes	Normal = 2%–8%	Increased in severe infections and function as a scavenger or phagocyte
Eosinophil	Normal = 1%–4%	May be increased in allergic reaction and parasitic infection
Basophil	Normal = 0.5%–1%	Usually unaffected by infections

• Elevated erythrocyte sedimentation rate—red blood cells settle more rapidly to the bottom of a tube of whole blood when an inflammation is present
• Presence of pathogen in urine, blood, sputum, or other draining cultures

Examples of NANDA Nursing Diagnoses

Asepsis and Infection Control

Nursing Diagnoses	Related Factors	Sample Defining Characteristics
Anxiety	Social isolation High risk for infection	"I'm afraid I won't see the nurses very much because they have to put on all this equipment whenever they come into my room." "You don't get many visitors when you're isolated like this. Everyone's afraid they'll get what I have." "In class, I sit next to the girl who was rushed to the hospital with meningitis. I'm so nervous that I'll get it, too. She's really sick!"
Risk for Latex Allergy Response	Occupational exposure History of multiple surgical procedures	"The last time I ate a banana, I broke out in hives. The same thing happens to me when I eat avocado." "I've been a dental hygienist for 8 years now, but this past month, I've noticed that several hours after I remove my gloves, I get a raised, red rash on my hands and up my arms." "I'm able to get around pretty good now in my wheelchair, but I've had many, many surgeries because I was born with spina bifida. They tell me I need to be very careful about any reactions to latex products."
Activity Intolerance	Effects of infectious process Generalized weakness	"I knew I should have gotten the flu shot. I've been so sick with it and feel so weak that I can hardly get out of bed." Patient admitted with probable diagnosis of tuberculosis. Awaiting results of AFB smears. He is acutely ill, has extreme fatigue, productive cough, low-grade fever, and chills and sweats at night. Isolation is standard precaution with additional airborne precautions. Required assistance with all ADLs.

Compilation of this assessment data constitutes a unique nursing database that suggests nursing interventions for patients at risk for infection or those in whom an infection is already present.

Diagnosing

The potential for infection or the presence of an infection in a patient suggests possible nursing diagnoses. The focus of nursing care depends on a nursing diagnosis that accurately reflects the patient's condition. The following are examples of nursing diagnoses related to an infectious process:

- Risk for Infection related to presence of chronic disease; altered immune response; effects of medication; altered skin integrity; malnutrition; presence of invasive or indwelling medical device; lack of proper immunization
- Social Isolation related to presence of communicable disease (AIDS)
- Impaired Oral Mucous Membrane related to ineffective dental hygiene; trauma; side effect of medication; presence of invasive medical device

- Deficient Diversional Activity related to lack of visitors; restrictions imposed by airborne precautions
- Risk for Imbalanced Body Temperature related to infectious process; dehydration
- Anxiety related to high risk for infection; social isolation

See additional examples of nursing diagnoses with defining characteristics in the accompanying NANDA box.

Outcome Identification and Planning

The nurse develops appropriate patient outcomes after reviewing the assessment data, considering the cycle of events resulting in an infection, and incorporating the principles of infection control. Planning outcomes that prevent infection or interfere with the infection cycle is an exciting challenge, providing an opportunity to see the positive results from one's efforts, that is, effective nursing interventions aimed at controlling or preventing infection. The following examples of expected patient outcomes are appropriate for preventing infection and using infection-control techniques. The patient will:

Box 27-2 PRACTICING BASIC PRINCIPLES OF MEDICAL ASEPSIS IN PATIENT CARE

- Practice good hand hygiene.
- Keep soiled items and equipment from touching the clothing. Carry soiled linens or other used articles so that they do not touch your clothing.
- Do not place soiled bed linen or any other items on the floor, which is grossly contaminated. It increases contamination of both surfaces.
- Avoid having patient cough, sneeze, or breathe directly on others. Provide them with disposable tissues, and instruct them, as indicated, to cover their mouth and nose to prevent spread by airborne droplets.
- Move equipment away from you when brushing, dusting, or scrubbing articles. This helps prevent contaminated particles from settling on the hair, face, and clothing.
- Avoid raising dust. Use a specially treated cloth or a dampened cloth. Do not shake linens. Dust and lint particles constitute a vehicle by which organisms may be transported from one area to another.
- Clean the least soiled areas first and then the more soiled ones. This helps prevent having the cleaner areas soiled by the dirtier areas.

- Dispose of soiled or used items directly into appropriate containers. Wrap items that are moist from body discharge or drainage in waterproof containers, such as plastic bags, before discarding into the refuse holder so that handlers will not come in contact with them.
- Pour liquids that are to be discarded, such as bath water, mouth rinse, and the like, directly into the drain to avoid splattering in the sink and onto you.
- Sterilize items that are suspected of containing pathogens. After sterilization, they can be managed as clean items, if appropriate.
- Use practices of personal grooming that help prevent spreading microorganisms. Examples include shampooing the hair regularly, keeping it short or pinned up to limit the possibility of carrying microorganisms on hair shafts, keeping the fingernails short and free of broken cuticles and ragged nail edges, and avoiding wearing rings with grooves and stones that may harbor microorganisms.
- Follow guidelines conscientiously for standard and transmission-based precautions as prescribed by agency.

- Demonstrate effective hand hygiene and good personal hygiene practices
- Identify the signs of an infection
- Maintain adequate nutritional intake
- Demonstrate proper disposal of soiled articles
- Use appropriate cleansing and disinfecting techniques
- Demonstrate an awareness of the necessity of proper immunizations
- Demonstrate stress-reduction techniques
- Verbalize an understanding of health risks associated with a latex allergy

Implementing

The practice of **asepsis** includes all activities to prevent infection or break the chain of infection. The nurse uses aseptic techniques to halt the spread of microorganisms and minimize the threat of infection. There are two asepsis categories: medical asepsis and surgical asepsis. **Medical asepsis,** or clean technique, involves procedures and practices that reduce the number and transfer of pathogens. Medical asepsis procedures, for example, include performing hand hygiene and wearing gloves. **Surgical asepsis,** or sterile technique, includes practices used to render and keep objects and areas free from microorganisms. Surgical asepsis procedures could include inserting an indwelling urinary catheter or inserting an IV catheter.

Using Medical Asepsis

Medical asepsis techniques are used continuously both within and outside health agencies, based on the assumption that pathogens are likely to be present. For example, shared drinking cups are considered unsanitary because a person harboring pathogens may transfer them to the cup when used. In a

healthcare facility, if a specific pathogen is known to be present, special methods of medical asepsis are used to prevent further spread of the organism. Nearly every nursing activity includes practices of medical asepsis. Therefore, the nurse assumes a major responsibility for breaking the cycle of infection by providing safe patient care and protecting the patient, as well as the nurse, from microorganisms that may cause disease. Box 27-2 highlights the basic practices of medical asepsis for nurses to use when giving care to patients.

The transfer of pathogens from person to person can be decreased by limiting the dissemination of pathogens. The most practical way to accomplish this is through the use of barriers that prevent common vehicles from transmitting the pathogens. Barriers are ways to decrease the spread of pathogens and include hand hygiene, personal protective equipment (discussed later), and other barrier techniques. Figure 27-2 shows how barriers break the infection cycle. Nurses must understand the various precautions or barrier techniques if they are to use them correctly and minimize infection risks to patients as well as to themselves (see Promoting Health 27-1: Infection Control Precautions and Barrier Techniques).

PERFORMING HAND HYGIENE

Hand hygiene is the most effective way to help prevent the spread of infectious agents. The CDC, the government agency responsible for investigating, preventing, and controlling disease, issued guidelines for hand hygiene in healthcare settings (CDC, 2002). According to the CDC, the term hand hygiene applies to either handwashing with plain soap and water, use of antiseptic handrubs including waterless alcohol-based products, or surgical hand antisepsis (CDC, 2002). Although there is agreement that hand hygiene is the most important procedure for preventing infections,

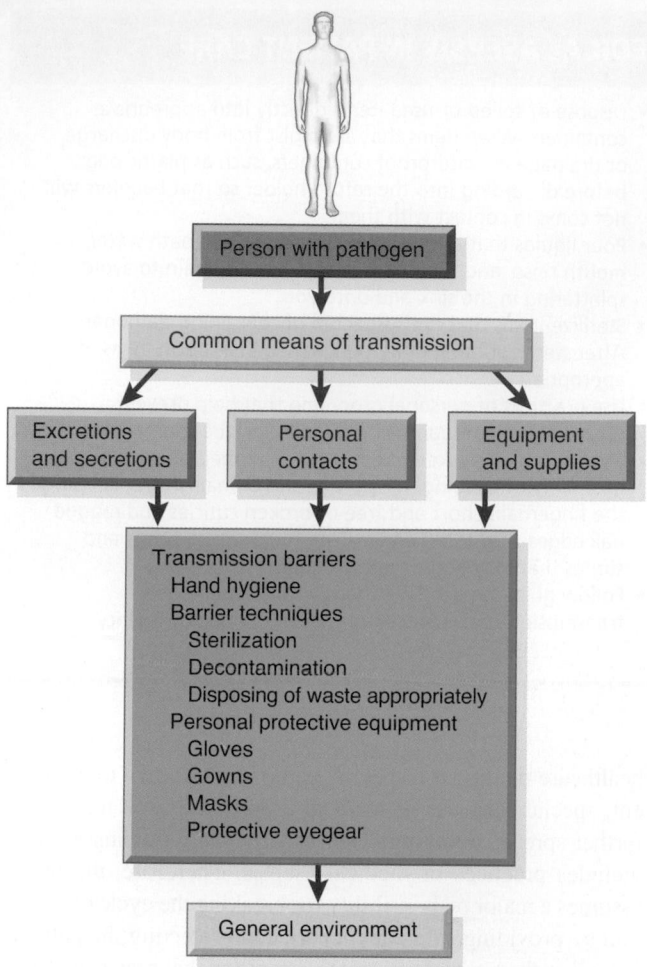

FIGURE 27-2. Transmission barriers help prevent the transporting of pathogens from the infected person to the general environment.

this procedure is still not performed consistently in healthcare settings with compliance rates generally below 50% (Institute for Healthcare Improvement (IHI), 2006a). Haas and Larson (2008) cite the following as contributing factors to poor compliance with hand hygiene practices:

- Lack of access to sinks
- Lack of time
- Skin irritation
- Ignorance about the importance of hand hygiene
- Individual preferences and habits
- Insufficient institutional commitment to appropriate hand hygiene procedures.

They also summarize recommendations to improve compliance with hand hygiene. These include collaboration and leadership in the healthcare environment, ensuring the availability of hand hygiene products, collecting data on compliance and infection rates, and focusing on individual accountability.

The Joint Commission (previously referred to as the Joint Commission on Accreditation of Hospitals), in their 2010 Patient Safety Goal to "prevent infection," includes a recommendation to use the hand hygiene guidelines published by CDC or the World Health Organization (2009). Also, as part

of their "Speak Up" program, the Joint Commission encourages consumers to insist on hand hygiene measures from all healthcare staff involved in their care. Nurses need to focus on this simple, yet essential, procedure that can interrupt the cycle of infection.

Bacteria

Two types of bacterial flora are normally found on the hands: transient bacteria and resident bacteria (Table 27-2). Transient bacteria, although usually easily removed by thorough handwashing, have the potential to adjust to the environment of the skin when they are present in large numbers over a long period and become resident bacteria. If pathogenic organisms become resident bacteria on the skin, the hands then become carriers of the particular organism. Therefore, to help prevent transient bacteria from becoming resident bacteria, it is important to clean the hands promptly when they are visibly soiled, after each contact with contaminated materials, and after removing gloves. (See the accompanying PICO in Practice box.)

Cleansing Agents

Various hand hygiene products are available. Soaps and detergents, also referred to as nonantimicrobial agents, are considered adequate for routine mechanical cleansing of the hands and removal of most transient microorganisms. They help remove soil because they lower surface tension and act as emulsifying agents. Bar, liquid, leaflet, and powdered soaps are all effective. Use of a particular type in a healthcare agency often depends on personnel or agency preference.

Using handwashing products that contain an **antimicrobial** or antibacterial ingredient is recommended in any setting where the risk for infection is high. When present in certain concentrations, these agents can kill bacteria or suppress their growth. Numerous studies have documented that alcohol-based handrubs more effectively reduce bacterial counts on the hands of healthcare personnel than antimicrobial soap does. Alcohol-based handrubs have an alcohol concentration between 60% and 95% and are available as foam, gel, or lotions. When the alcohol-based handrubs were initially recommended for hand hygiene, there was concern that they posed a fire hazard. The National Fire Protection Association (NFPA) fire codes initially prohibited their installation in exit corridors but has since approved the use of alcohol handrub dispensers provided that certain conditions for installation are satisfied (Joint Commission, 2008).

Techniques

If the healthcare worker's hands are not visibly soiled, alcohol-based handrubs are recommended because they save time, do not require a sink, are easy to use, reduce bacterial count, and efficiently kill many fungi and viruses on the hands. In these situations, an alcohol-based handrub can be used to decontaminate hands in the following clinical situations:

- Before and after direct contact with patients
- Before and after using gloves

PROMOTING HEALTH • 27-1

Infection Control Precautions and Barrier Techniques

Use the assessment checklist to determine how well you are observing infection control or barrier precautions as you care for patients in a healthcare facility or in a community setting. Then develop a prescription for self-care by choosing appropriate behaviors from the list of suggestions.

Assessment Checklist

| ☐ almost always ☐ sometimes ☐ almost never |

☐ ☐ ☐ 1. Perform hand hygiene before and after contact with a patient.

☐ ☐ ☐ 2. I wear PPE if contact with blood or body fluids is a possibility.

☐ ☐ ☐ 3. I cover my nose and mouth when coughing and sneezing and properly dispose of tissues.

☐ ☐ ☐ 4. I use additional protective equipment (gowns, masks, goggles) when necessary.

☐ ☐ ☐ 5. I avoid recapping any needles.

☐ ☐ ☐ 6. I place needles or other sharp objects in a puncture-proof disposable container.

☐ ☐ ☐ 7. I dispose of used or contaminated objects and equipment in a leak-resistant plastic trash bag.

Self-Care Behaviors

1. Read infection control standards published by OSHA and CDC.
2. Attend programs that provide updates on current CDC/OSHA policies.
3. Maintain strict personal hygiene habits.
4. Obtain immunizations when available.
5. Assess for any signs and symptoms of an infection.
6. Perform hand hygiene frequently.
7. Perform hand hygiene immediately after removing gloves.
8. Practice cough etiquette to prevent transmission of respiratory infections.
9. Protect myself with the barriers necessary to prevent exposure to blood, body fluids, or secretions.
10. Follow agency policy if any exposure to blood or body substance occurs.
11. Never eat, drink, smoke, apply cosmetics or lip moistener, or handle contact lenses in an area where occupational exposure is possible.

• Before inserting urinary catheters, peripheral vascular catheters, or invasive devices that do not require surgical placement
• If moving from a contaminated body site to a clean body site during patient care
• After contact with objects (including equipment) located in the patient's environment.

When used repeatedly, alcohol-based handrubs cause less dryness and skin irritation than soap products do. Those who have sensitive skin may benefit from use of an alcohol-based product that contains lotion. See Guidelines for Nursing Care 27-1 for directions on how to use an alcohol-based handrub.

Controversy does exist regarding the use of alcohol-based handrubs when *Clostridium difficile* organisms have been

TABLE • 27-2   BACTERIAL FLORA ON THE HANDS

Types of Bacterial Flora	Characteristics	Effective Hand Hygiene Measures
Transient	• Occur on hands with activities of daily living • Relatively few in number on clean and exposed areas of the skin • Attached loosely on skin usually in grease, fats, and dirt • Found in greatest number under the fingernails • Can be pathogenic or nonpathogenic	Can be removed relatively easily by frequent and thorough handwashing.
Resident	• Normally found in creases in the skin • Usually stable in number and type • Cling tenaciously to skin by adhesion and absorption	Considerable friction with a brush is required to remove them. Less susceptible to antiseptics than are transient bacteria.

PICO IN PRACTICE
Asking Clinical Questions

Scenario: You are a staff nurse newly hired to a general medicine unit. Your assigned preceptor calls in sick one day. Another seasoned nurse assigned to the unit, Donna, agrees to serve as your substitute preceptor for that shift. One of your assigned patients must have a nasogastric tube placed. You ask Donna to observe you perform this procedure and you do so without incident, following the hospital's Nursing Policies and Procedures for inserting nasogastric tubes. You washed your hands and donned nonsterile gloves to prepare for the procedure, and Donna had done the same, anticipating that you might require some assistance. However, when you both take off your gloves, only you perform hand hygiene with an alcohol-based handrub. After you leave the patient's room, you ask Donna why she hadn't performed hand hygiene when she removed her gloves. She shrugs at you, visibly annoyed, and retorts "Well, my hands were clean when I put my gloves on and the gloves weren't dirty, so why should I?" You wonder whether or not this is appropriate hand hygiene policy to follow on your unit, and whether performing hand hygiene on nonsoiled hands after removing gloves could reduce rates of hospital-associated infections.

The next day, your preceptor, Lisa, returns to work. You have developed excellent rapport with Lisa, and discretely ask her about the appropriateness of Donna's actions. Lisa notes that the current hospital hand hygiene policy does not specify whether hand hygiene should be performed on nonsoiled hands after gloves are removed. She tasks you with developing an evidence-based recommendation that you and she will then take to your unit-based council and Nurse Manager.

- POPULATION: Direct-care gloved nurses without soiled hands
- INTERVENTION: Hand hygiene after removal of gloves

- COMPARISON: Removal of gloves only without hand hygiene
- OUTCOME: Lower rates of hospital-associated infections on the unit

PICO Question: Among direct-care gloved nurses who have not soiled their hands, is performing hand hygiene after removal of gloves associated with lower rates of hospital-associated infections on the unit than removal of gloves without hand hygiene?

Finding: From the National Guidelines Clearinghouse: Hand hygiene recommendations. (2008). In Betsy Lehman Center for Patient Safety and Medical Error Reduction, JSI Research and Training Institute, Inc. Prevention and control of healthcare-associated infections in Massachusetts. Part 1: Final recommendations of the Expert Panel. Boston, MA: Massachusetts Department of Public Health, p. 36–41.

This expert panel strongly recommends that all healthcare providers that come in contact with patients decontaminate their hands after gloves are removed. The panel specifies that decontamination of hands may include handwashing, using either a nonantimicrobial soap and water or an antimicrobial soap and water, or using an alcohol-based handrub.

Level of Evidence: Level I

Recommendation: You and Lisa propose to your Nurse Manager and your unit-based council that steps be taken to revise the existing hand hygiene policy so that nurses are advised to decontaminate their hands after removal of gloves, regardless of whether or not their hands are soiled.

Guidelines for Nursing Care • 27-1

HAND HYGIENE: USING AN ALCOHOL-BASED HANDRUB

- Apply product to the palm of one hand, using the amount of product recommended on the package (it will vary according to the manufacturer but usually is 1 to 3 mL).
- Rub hands together, making sure to cover all surfaces of the hands, fingers, and in between the fingers. Also, clean the fingertips and the area beneath the fingernails.

- Continue rubbing until the hands are dry (at least 15 seconds).

identified. *C. difficile* is a gram-positive, anaerobic, spore-forming bacterium that is normally found in the intestines of many adults (Austin, 2007; Valente, 2007). It is responsible for 75% of the healthcare-associated diarrhea diagnosed particularly in elderly patients and long-term care residents. Antibiotic therapy is frequently identified as the underlying cause of *C. difficile* because it changes the normal intestinal flora, decreases resistance, and allows *C. difficile* to colonize the large intestine (Valente, 2007). This organism is found in the feces of an infected person and can be transmitted to other people if they touch their mouth after they have come in contact with items or surfaces that are contaminated with the bacteria (CDC, 2007). Since healthcare workers are most frequently responsible for the spread of *C. difficile*, handwashing is the most important preventive measure. If C. *difficile* is in the spore state, alcohol handrubs may be ineffective against it. Many healthcare facilities recommend handwashing with soap and water to rid hands of the organisms and use of special disinfectants instead of the routine hospital cleaning products to decontaminate patient care items and the patient's room. The CDC has not addressed the use of alcohol-based rubs versus handwashing with soap and water to eradicate *C. difficile* bacteria.

A recent research study questioned the effectiveness of using alcohol-based hand gel to prevent infections in an ICU setting (Rupp, Fitzgerald, Puumala, Anderson, Craig, Iwen et al., 2008). Even though the nurses and doctors surveyed in this study had nearly doubled their use of the gel, it did not curb the infection rates in their patients. The researchers indicated that other factors such as the availability of the gel, presence of rings and longer fingernails on the healthcare staff, poor handling of catheters, and patient treatment areas that weren't optimally clean may have affected the results of this study. The CDC Guideline for Hand Hygiene in Health-Care Settings (2002) specifies that healthcare personnel involved in patient care should not wear artificial nails because they are more likely to be associated with higher bacterial counts. Natural nails should be less than one quarter (1/4) of an inch long. Wearing artificial nails in the operating room (OR) is a citable offense during the Joint Commission accreditation process.

If a healthcare worker's hands are visibly soiled or contaminated with blood or body fluids, washing the hands with either antimicrobial soap or nonantimicrobial soap and water is required. Handwashing is also required before eating and after using the restroom.

Effective handwashing requires at least a 15-second scrub with plain soap or disinfectant and warm water. Hands that are visibly soiled need a longer scrub. Recommended handwashing techniques for medical asepsis are listed in Skill 27-1 at the end of this chapter.

Hand antisepsis before assisting with a surgical procedure involves a more lengthy scrub, reducing resident and transient flora from the forearms and hands. This procedure, known as surgical hand scrub, incorporates surgical asepsis and is described in texts that deal with operating and delivery room procedures. The CDC guideline recommends using an antimicrobial soap or alcohol-based surgical hand scrub product with persistent activity for surgical hand antisepsis. Scrub time is also reduced significantly when alcohol-based scrub agents are used.

Preventing Healthcare-Associated Infections

For various reasons and sometimes despite best efforts, certain patients in health agencies develop **healthcare-associated infections (HAIs)** during the course of treatment for other infections. These conditions were not noted as being present on admission. The term **nosocomial** is used specifically to indicate something originating or taking place in a hospital. The source of infection may be either exogenous or endogenous. An infection is referred to as **exogenous** when the causative organism is acquired from other people. An **endogenous** infection occurs when the causative organism comes from microbial life harbored in the person. An infection is referred to as **iatrogenic** when it results from a treatment or diagnostic procedure. Not all nosocomial infections are iatrogenic.

Prevention of HAI is a major challenge for healthcare providers. In the United States, HAIs account for approximately 2 million infections, 99,000 deaths, and approximately $30.5 billion dollars in excess healthcare costs annually (Klevens, Edwards, Richards, Horan, Gaynes, Pollock et al., 2007). The cost of the additional hospital care days necessary to treat a HAI is staggering, particularly in light of the efforts to control spiraling healthcare expenses. With its focus on patient safety, the Joint Commission mandates that death or serious injury caused by an infection-related event must be reported as a sentinel event (see Chapter 26 for a discussion of sentinel event; Joint Commission, 2008).

Effective October 1, 2008, the Centers for Medicare and Medicaid Services (CMS) will no longer reimburse hospitals for eight preventable hospital-acquired conditions. Urinary tract infections from improper use of catheters, vascular catheter-associated infections, and certain surgical site infections are included on the list. Nine other HAIs are also being considered for addition to the list. In order to comply with this ruling, hospitals will need to report whether these conditions existed when the patients were admitted to their facility (Kurtzman & Buerhaus, 2008). At this time, it is unknown how this effort by the government to improve the quality of care will affect nurses. It is an evolving process and there is the potential that the critical impact that nurses can have on decreasing the number of HAIs will be recognized and more easily verified. The risk for nurses is that if hospital revenues decline, nursing may be viewed as part of the reason for this outcome.

HAIs are specifically addressed in The Institute for Healthcare Improvement (IHI) "5 Million Lives Campaign," instituted as a collaborative effort to save lives and reduce patient injuries (IHI, 2006b). This is a voluntary initiative that aims to protect patients from five million incidents of medical harm over a 2-year period. The IHI promotes the use of "care bundles" or evidence-based protocols that reduce the incidence of catheter-related infections and ventilator-associated pneumonia. Their belief is that 100% compliance with these bundles will significantly reduce the occurrence of both of these infections.

To address HAIs, healthcare agencies have found the following measures to be successful in reducing their incidence:

- Instituting constant surveillance by infection-control committees and nurse epidemiologists. Their work can reduce infections significantly when aggressive control measures are initiated based on their findings.
- Having written infection-prevention practices for all agency personnel. Adherence to hand hygiene recommendations and infection-control precaution techniques can prevent many HAIs.
- Using practices to promote and keep patients in the best possible physical condition. Measures include meeting the patient's needs for nutrition, fluids, rest, oxygen, and physical and psychological comfort and security.

Research has also indicated that staffing issues may have an impact on healthcare-acquired infections. Staffing takes into account registered nurse-to-patient ratios, level of RN experience, and the use of temporary workers. Many times, nurses have a heavy patient load and do not take the time to use proper hand hygiene. This may also happen if the nurse is new and is overwhelmed with his or her assignment and fails to perform appropriate hand hygiene. Stone & Gershon (2007) concluded that ICUs with higher RN staffing rates had a lower incidence of certain HAIs and that there was evidence that, when nurses worked overtime, there was an increase in catheter-associated urinary tract infections.

Mandatory public reporting of healthcare-associated infection rates is required in a large number of states (Association for Professionals in Infection Control and Epidemiology [APIC], 2008a). Advocates of mandatory reporting believe that all agencies should report HAI rates and that this public disclosure will allow consumers to make more informed choices regarding the selection of a healthcare facility. The difficulty in creating a central database of HAIs is that agencies treat different types of patients with varying levels of complexity, and the HAIs that they identify and monitor are unique to their particular population. If HAI rates are to be compared, all agencies must monitor the same infections and collect and report data using the same methods.

USING INVASIVE MEDICAL DEVICES

Most healthcare-associated infections are caused by bacteria, such as *E. coli*, *Staphylococcus aureus*, *Streptococcus faecalis*, *Pseudomonas aeruginosa*, and *Klebsiella* species. Many of the HAIs can be traced to an invasive device, such as a urinary catheter or venous access catheter. For example, urinary tract infections account for 32% of HAIs annually followed by surgical-site infections, pneumonia, and blood-stream infections. The latter two HAIs have the highest mortality rates (Vrtis, 2008).

> *Consider Esther Bailey, the 72-year-old woman who has had abdominal surgery and developed a wound infection. The patient already has one infection. However, insertion of the catheter increases her risk for an additional infection, directly related to the use of the catheter.* ■

The increasing use of biomedical equipment is often cited as a causative factor. In addition to indwelling catheters and venous access catheters, other devices associated with causing infection include hemodynamic monitoring lines, hemodialysis equipment, and respiratory equipment. Patients receiving mechanical ventilation are especially at risk for healthcare-associated pneumonia. Often, it is the hands of the healthcare worker using the instruments or equipment that are the most significant means for the transmission of the pathogens.

DEALING WITH ANTIBIOTIC-RESISTANT ORGANISMS

A significant and disturbing trend continues to be the development of healthcare-associated pathogens resistant to antibiotics. The indiscriminate use of broad-spectrum antibiotics has allowed once-susceptible bacteria to develop defenses against antibiotics. As a result, resistant organisms, such as methicillin-resistant *S. aureus* (MRSA), vancomycin-intermediate *S. aureus* (VISA), vancomycin-resistant *S. aureus* (VRSA), and vancomycin-resistant enterococci (VRE) have emerged.

MRSA

Staphylococcus aureus bacteria are normally found in the nasal mucous membranes, on the skin, and in the respiratory and gastrointestinal tracts. Approximately one-third of the people in the United States are colonized with "staph," meaning that the organism is present in these locations but the individual does not have symptoms and remains healthy and uninfected. They can, however, pass the organism on to others. In the 1960s, a strain of this bacteria emerged that was resistant to the broad-spectrum antibiotic (methicillin), normally the drug of choice used to treat these infections. The very powerful antibiotic, vancomycin, had to be used to treat the MRSA infections that primarily occurred in healthcare settings. In the 1980s, a type of MRSA appeared in the wider community. Community-associated MRSA (CA-MRSA), a common cause of skin infections in the United States, has been rapidly spreading into hospitals (Klein, Smith, & Laxminaray, 2007). Those most at risk are young children, older adults, and patients diagnosed with HIV or AIDS. Contact sports and sharing personal items also increase the risk. (Refer to the accompanying Research in Nursing box for a discussion of MRSA organisms in the home environment.)

Treatment guidelines for community-acquired MRSA include the following:

- Incision and drainage of abscesses in patients with mild to moderate infections. Antimicrobial therapy may not be required.

RESEARCH IN NURSING
Bridging the Gap to Evidence-Based Practice

MRSA OCCURRENCE IN THE HOME ENVIRONMENT

Nurses play a vital role in the efforts to prevent community-associated MRSA (CA-MRSA), but the extent of MRSA in the home setting on inanimate objects has been reported but not well documented. Community-associated MRSA usually does not cause serious problems and most often results in skin manifestations. It also tends to be less drug resistant than the healthcare-associated version. Healthy people can be colonized with MRSA and have no ill effects; however, they can readily transmit the organism to others. MRSA has been cultured from inanimate objects in the home but this has not been well documented. It is generally recognized that sensible hygiene practices can reduce the risk of MRSA in the home but questions arise regarding the specific preventive measures needed if MRSA is found on surfaces in the home.

Related Research

Scott, E., Duty, S., & Callahan, M. (2008). A pilot study to isolate *Staphylococcus aureus* and methicillin-resistant *S. aureus* from environmental surfaces in the home. *American Journal of Infection Control, 36*(3), 190–197.

The objective of this study was to verify the presence of *S. aureus* and MRSA on surfaces in homes with healthy individuals and pets and identify risk factors associated with the presence of MRSA on inanimate objects in the home. Thirty-five participants met the criteria for entry into this study. These included having a child in diapers and a dog or cat in the home, and location

within a 30-mile radius of Boston, MA. Once demographic and health information was collected, cultures were taken from 32 hand-contact surfaces in the kitchen, bathroom, office, infant room, and pet areas in each home. *S. aureus* was isolated in 34 of the 35 homes. MRSA was found on a variety of household surfaces in 9 of the 35 homes and 7 of these 9 homes had a cat. Previous studies had also indicated a positive correlation between cats and MRSA. Known risk factors for MRSA (frequent antibiotic use, recent hospitalization, and MRSA infections in family members) were not a factor in any of the households. Forty-four percent (44%) of the nine homes with MRSA had children in childcare but this was not statistically significant. The presence of MRSA on inanimate surfaces confirmed the potential for transmission of infection via these hand-contact surfaces in the home.

Relevance to Nursing Practice

This study implied that it is important for healthcare providers to educate the public about appropriate hygiene measures in the home in order to avoid spreading MRSA among family members or to other people. Additional studies are necessary to investigate the potential for transmission of bacteria from human to cat and cat to human since a cat in the home was a positive correlation. Hand-contact sites where MRSA was found in the home need further investigation. Hand hygiene practices in the home need reinforcement since this is the best protection against MRSA.

For additional research, visit the**Point.**

- If incision and drainage are not effective and systemic or serious infection results, antimicrobial therapy may be necessary.
- Antimicrobial therapy may be prescribed for 7 to 10 days depending on the severity of the infection. Medications may include trimethoprim-sulfamethoxazole (Bactrim and others), minocycline (Minocin), doxycycline (Vibramycin and others), and clindamycin (Cleocin and others).
- Tetracycline hydrochloride (Achromycin) is not recommended for any pregnant patient or children under the age of 8 (Leung-Chen, 2008a).

The healthcare-associated MRSA strain, on the other hand, has more serious implications and accounts for more than 60% of the infections that occur in hospitals. It can be responsible for bloodstream infections, wound infections, ventilator-associated pneumonia, and multidrug resistance (Leung-Chen, 2008b). Intravenous vancomycin is the drug of choice for healthcare-associated MRSA, but if the bacteria develop resistance to vancomycin, then the infection can be treated with a synthetic antibiotic, such as linezolid (Zyvox). In a healthcare setting, the main mode of transmission is through contact with the contaminated hands of healthcare personnel or contact with equipment (CDC, 2007). Basic infection control practices are the key to the prevention and control of MRSA and guidelines are outlined in Box 27-3.

VISA, VRSA, and VRE

Vancomycin intermediate-resistant *S. aureus* (VISA) emerged in 2002 in the United States closely followed by vancomycin-resistant *S. aureus* (VRSA) that was totally resistant to vancomycin. Once bacteria develop drug resistance, they progress from being sensitive to an antibiotic to an intermediate resistance followed by complete resistance to the antibiotic (Kjonegaard & Myers, 2005). Treating these two organisms has provided a formidable challenge because antibiotics that are available and able to treat this organism are limited. Linezolid (Zyvox) and quinupristin-dalfopristin (Synercid) are alternative antibiotics that can be used in place of vancomycin. They are very expensive and resistance to linezolid has been reported. Patients at risk of developing VISA and VRSA are individuals with a history of renal failure requiring either hemodialysis or peritoneal dialysis, a previous MRSA infection, or a history of prior and possibly prolonged use of vancomycin (Todd, 2006a). Effective infection control measures are imperative to control the spread of VISA and VRSA and prudent use of vancomycin is an important preventive measure.

Vancomycin-resistant enterococci (VRE) is another serious pathogen in hospitals. Enterococci, a species of *streptococcus* often found in normal intestinal and female genital tracts, can cause healthcare-associated infections with a high mortality rate if the organism is vancomycin resistant.

Box 27-3   CONTROLLING MRSA IN A HEALTHCARE SETTING

The following guidelines are effective measures to prevent and control the spread of MRSA:

- Practice recommended hand hygiene techniques.
- Ensure that cleaning and disinfection of the patient care environment is a priority.
- Consider performing cultures when patients are admitted to the hospital to determine if an individual is colonized or infected with MRSA. This involves swabbing likely sites for colonization and sending the samples to be cultured. Certain patient groups may be cultured such as ICU patients or individuals admitted from a long-term care facility.

- The infection control program at each facility would be responsible for evaluating the benefit of active surveillance.
- Follow contact isolation protocols for any patient colonized or infected with MRSA. A private room is preferable but patients who both have MRSA can share a room.
- Adhere to best practice interventions or "bundles" when they are available for patients most vulnerable to MRSA. These include patients with a central line catheter and those requiring mechanical ventilation.

Adapted from: Yamamoto, L., & Marten, M. (2007). Listen up MRSA: The bug stops here. *Nursing, 37*(12), 50–55.

Originally treated with penicillin, ampicillin, and then gentamicin, the enterococci became resistant to each drug. Subsequently, physicians again prescribed vancomycin as the drug of choice. However, resistance has developed to this and treatment options are limited to the two newer antibiotics previously mentioned for VISA and VRSA—linezolid and quinupristin-dalfopristin. Risk factors for VRE include:

- Compromised immune systems
- Recent abdominal or chest surgery
- Presence of urinary or central IV catheter
- Prolonged antibiotic use, especially with vancomycin
- Lengthy hospital stay especially in an ICU (Cooper, 2008).

VRE is spread via contact with the feces, urine, or blood of an infected or colonized person. Healthcare providers have the potential to spread VRE on their hands from one patient to another. Medical equipment and environmental surfaces can also harbor this organism. Appropriate hand hygiene and contact precautions can halt the spread of VRE. Careful assessment, intervention, and evaluation of high-risk patients and situations by nurses helps to minimize infection and reduce the unnecessary suffering imposed on patients.

STERILIZING AND DISINFECTING

Cleansing, disinfection, and sterilization help to break the cycle of infection and prevent disease. Most healthcare agencies provide patient-care items that are sterile when purchased and disposed of after use. Some items, such as pitchers, water glasses, and plastic basins, may be used repeatedly but by one patient only. On discharge, they are then discarded or sent home with the patient.

Healthcare agencies usually maintain a central supply unit where most reusable equipment is cleaned, kept in good working order, and sterilized as indicated. In the home and in some small health agencies, the nurse sometimes must make decisions about how to prepare equipment and supplies that are safe for patient use. Although nurses may not be directly involved in the actual process, they must be aware of the critical role that nurses play in preventing infection.

Several processes are used to destroy microorganisms. **Disinfection** destroys all pathogenic organisms except spores; **sterilization** destroys all microorganisms, including spores. Disinfection can be used when preparing the skin for a procedure or cleaning a piece of equipment that does not enter a sterile body part. Sterilization is usually performed on equipment that is entering a sterile portion of the body. Disinfection and sterilization of contaminated or infected objects and good hand hygiene diminish and often eliminate microorganisms as potential sources of infection.

Method Selection

Various factors influence the choice of sterilization and disinfection methods, including the following:

- Nature of organisms present: The CDC recommends that all supplies, linens, and equipment in a healthcare setting should be treated as if the patient were infectious. Some organisms are easily destroyed, whereas others can withstand certain common sterilization and disinfection methods.
- Number of organisms present: The more organisms present on an item, the longer it takes to destroy them.
- Type of equipment: Equipment with small lumens, crevices, or joints requires special care. Certain articles that may be damaged by various sterilization and disinfection methods require special handling.
- Intended use of equipment: The need for medical or surgical asepsis influences the preparation and cleaning of equipment. In the home, it may be safe to use equipment and supplies that are clean, but most healthcare agencies prefer to use sterilized articles for patient care.
- Available means for sterilization and disinfection: The choice of chemical or physical means of sterilization and disinfection depends on the nature and number of organisms, the type and intended use of the equipment, and the availability and practicality of the means. (Table 27-3 lists the types of methods for sterilization and disinfection.)
- Time: Time is a key factor when sterilizing or disinfecting articles. Failure to follow the recommended time periods is grossly negligent.

TABLE • 27-3	METHODS OF STERILIZATION AND DISINFECTION	
Method	**Discussion**	**Caution**
Physical		
Steam	Higher temperature caused by higher pressure destroys organisms (e.g., autoclaving)	Most plastic and rubber devices are damaged by autoclaving.
Boiling water	Frequently used in the home—simple and inexpensive; boil item for at least 10 minutes	Spores and some viruses are not destroyed by boiling.
Dry heat	Alternative sterilization method for home. Used for metal items. Heat oven to 350°F for 2 or more hours.	Insufficient to destroy all microorganisms. Not used in healthcare agencies.
Radiation	Used for pharmaceuticals, foods, plastics, and other heat-sensitive items	Object must be directly exposed to ultraviolet radiation on all surfaces. Poses risk to personnel.
Chemical		
Ethylene oxide gas	Destroys microorganisms and spores by interfering with metabolic processes in cells. Gas is released while items (oxygen and suction gauges, blood pressure equipment) are contained in autoclave.	Precautions necessary because gas is toxic to humans.
Chemical solutions	Generally used for instrument and equipment disinfection and for housekeeping disinfection. Chlorines are useful for disinfecting water and for housekeeping purposes. A solution of sodium hypochlorite (household bleach) in a 1:100 dilution effectively inactivates human immunodeficiency virus. Betadine and alcohol are also used as disinfectants.	Method does not destroy all spores and may cause corrosion on metal surfaces.

Techniques

Proper cleaning of items used in healthcare before they are sterilized or disinfected is essential to reduce the number of organisms and to dislodge them from crevices and from under layers of contaminating substances. The following techniques are recommended for cleaning equipment:

- Wear waterproof gloves at all times.
- Rinse the articles first with cold running water to remove organic material. Heat coagulates certain organic material, which makes removal more difficult.
- Wash the articles, after rinsing them, in warm water that contains detergent or soap. The combination of warm water and soap facilitates emulsification and removal of dirt and debris.
- Use a brush with stiff bristles, as indicated, to clean the articles thoroughly. Friction aids in the removal of organisms and debris from difficult-to-reach areas.
- Rinse and dry the article thoroughly.
- Prepare the cleaned equipment for sterilization or disinfection.
- Consider the brush, gloves, and the sink or basin in which the articles were cleaned as highly contaminated, and treat or discard them accordingly.

USING PERSONAL PROTECTIVE EQUIPMENT AND SUPPLIES

According to the 1992 Occupational Safety and Health Administration (OSHA) ruling, healthcare agencies must provide employees with the equipment and supplies necessary to minimize or prevent exposure to infectious material. This **personal protective equipment (PPE)** includes gloves, gowns, masks, and protective eye gear. Skill 27-2 illustrates the proper use of this equipment.

Gloves

Gloves, not a substitute for good hand hygiene, are worn only once and discarded appropriately according to agency policy. Then hands are thoroughly decontaminated with meticulous hand hygiene. Each patient interaction requires a clean pair of gloves, and some care activities for an individual patient may necessitate changing gloves more than once. Gloves should always be changed prior to moving from a contaminated task to a clean one. When care activities do not involve the possibility of soilage of hands with body fluids, gloves are not necessary. Activities such as turning a patient, feeding a patient, taking vital signs, and changing IV fluid bags do not require the use of gloves as long as the potential contact with body fluids is not present.

While wearing gloves, never do the following: leave the patient's room (unless transporting a contaminated item or a patient requiring transmission-based precautions), write in the patient's chart, or use the computer keyboard or telephone in the nurses' station. Also, healthcare workers should not touch their pagers or cell phones without performing good hand hygiene first.

Wearing gloves does not eliminate the need for proper hand hygiene. In reality, the warmth and moisture inside gloves create an ideal environment for bacteria to multiply, making it even more important to perform good hand hygiene before and after using gloves. Research also indicates that gloving does not guarantee complete protection from infectious organisms. Gloves provide a barrier but are not impenetrable. It has been shown that many times glove-barrier failure goes undetected by the healthcare worker. Double gloving (putting on two gloves) is recommended if the healthcare worker is going to be exposed to blood or body fluids.

As mentioned, gloves are not always an impenetrable barrier. In high-risk settings, such as the operating room, glove failure is common. Reports indicate that during surgery, particularly operative procedures longer than 3 hours, gloves fail more than 50% of the time (Graves & Twomey, 2002). Being exposed to body fluids and blood and handling many surgical instruments are both factors contributing to glove failure. For example, tiny tears or cuts that occur in the gloves often are not observed until the gloves are removed after surgery and blood is visible on the hands. In an effort to provide a safer working environment, electronic glove-monitoring devices combined with ongoing education about safe gloving technique and injury prevention are being used. In addition, double gloving with a colored glove under a translucent outer glove is an alternative solution to detect a breach in glove integrity (Graves & Twomey, 2002).

Approximately 3% to 22% of healthcare workers are sensitized to traditional latex, with reactions ranging from local skin reactions to urticaria (hives) to systemic anaphylaxis, an exaggerated allergic reaction that can result in death (U.S. Food and Drug Administration, 2008). The cornstarch powder or talc used to make gloves easier to put on is a major causative factor in any latex allergy. The powder binds with the latex protein and becomes airborne, where it can remain for 5 to 12 hours after healthcare workers don or remove gloves. Powder particles may be inhaled or absorbed into skin or mucous membranes or enter the bloodstream. Repeated exposures have been shown to lead to a latex sensitivity. If the person continues to be exposed to latex after a sensitivity has developed, the person may demonstrate signs of a latex allergy. At present, there is no cure for a latex allergy.

The National Institute for Occupational Safety and Health (NIOSH) recommends that nonlatex gloves or powder-free, low-allergen latex gloves (if latex gloves are used) be available for employees. An employer must provide alternative gloves, if needed, according to the OSHA Blood-borne Pathogens Standard (OSHA, 2005). A new latex glove has recently become available that may prove to be a safer alternative to individuals sensitive to traditional latex. The Yulex Patient Examination Glove is derived from the guayule bush that is native to the Southwestern United States and does not contain the protein found in the sap of a rubber tree used in traditional latex gloves (U.S. Food and Drug Administration, 2008). Because a totally "latex-free" environment is considered unattainable given the ubiquitous nature of latex, a "latex-safe" healthcare environment is essential for patients with a latex allergy. All healthcare facilities are required to

have a written policy that identifies how to deal with latex-sensitive employees and patients. Awareness of an allergy to latex is also important for safe home care. Nurses need to ask whether patients have experienced any unusual signs or symptoms when blowing up balloons, using latex condoms, or wearing rubber gloves for dishwashing or cleaning. Box 27-4 summarizes information on latex allergy for healthcare personnel and patients.

GOWNS

Gowns are usually worn to prevent soiling of the healthcare worker's clothing by the patient's blood and body fluids. They provide barrier protection and are donned immediately before entering the patient's room. Individual gown technique is recommended; this means that a gown is worn only once and is then discarded appropriately according to agency policy. A waterproof or impervious gown is used if there is an increased likelihood of contact with the patient's blood or body fluids. If a gown becomes heavily soiled or moistened with blood or body fluids when caring for a patient, remove it, perform thorough hand hygiene, and put on a clean gown. There is no one special technique for applying a gown used as a barrier, but recommended practices for removing a soiled gown are described in Skill 27-2.

Masks

Masks help prevent the wearer from inhaling large-particle aerosols, which usually travel short distances (about 3 feet), and small-particle droplet nuclei, which can remain suspended in the air and travel longer distances. Masks also discourage the wearer from touching the eyes, nose, and mouth, thus limiting contact of organisms with mucous membranes.

Various mask practices are used. In some instances, all personnel and all the patient's visitors wear masks; in other situations, a patient requiring specific precautions wears the mask when transported outside his or her room to protect healthcare personnel and other patients from any exposure to pathogens.

A mask is worn only once and never lowered around the neck and then brought back over the mouth and nose for reuse. How long one can wear one mask while caring for one patient is the subject of debate. Regardless of the time worn, a mask must be changed before it becomes damp from the wearer's exhalations. (See Skill 27-2 for the recommended practice for applying and removing a mask.)

The serious increase in the number of multidrug-resistant tuberculosis cases prompted new guidelines to prevent the transmission of this disease. According to CDC guidelines, either a high-efficiency particulate air (HEPA) filter respirator or N95 respirator certified by NIOSH must be worn when entering the room of a patient with known or suspected tuberculosis.

The respirators filter inspired air, whereas surgical masks filter only expired air. Caregivers have expressed difficulty wearing the HEPA-style respirator for extended periods of time, but the N95 respirator, which is designed to filter out particles as small as 1 mcm with 95% efficiency, fits more

Box 27-4 LATEX ALLERGY SUMMARY

Risk Factors
- Healthcare workers who wear latex gloves
- People with allergic tendencies
- People with food allergies, specifically banana, papaya, avocado, potatoes, kiwi fruit, chestnuts, and pineapples
- Latex-industry workers
- People with asthma, spina bifida, or a history of multiple surgical procedures or exposures to latex

Types of Reactions
- *Irritant contact dermatitis:* nonallergic dermatitis, restricted to area that has made contact with the latex. Gloves may cause erythematous and pruritic hands. This is not a true allergy.
- *Chemical sensitivity dermatitis or delayed hypersensitivity:* allergic contact dermatitis, displayed as dry, crusty bumps, erythema, pruritus, scaling vesicles, papular lesions at site of contact, including the palms; not a life-threatening reaction, however, person should be aware of latex contact.
- *Latex allergy or Type I hypersensitivity:* systemic reactions, displayed as rhinitis, conjunctivitis, angioedema, bronchospasm, shock, and/or systemic anaphylactic reactions; this is a life-threatening sensitivity.

Diagnosis
- RAST: blood test for IgE antibodies to latex
- Skin prick: small amount of serum derived from latex placed on small prick in skin
- Glove challenge: patient wearing a latex glove for period of time, with periodic checking for any signs of latex reactions listed above

CAUTION: Any time a person with suspected latex allergies is exposed to latex, emergency equipment should be available.

Treatment
- Avoidance of latex-containing products
- Localized reaction treated with oral diphenhydramine, cool compresses, and hydrocortisone 1% cream
- Systemic reaction possibly treated with epinephrine subcutaneously, systemic steroids, antihistamines, with transport to the emergency department

Protocols for Patients With Latex Allergies
- Assess patient for allergy to latex products.
- Place allergy sticker on chart, a Caution sign on door, and an allergy band on the patient's wrist.
- Remove all latex-containing articles from room.
- Place three-way stopcocks in IV lines for medication administration. Place tape over any injection ports on IV tubing.
- Remove rubber stoppers from vials before drawing up medications.
- If available, place a cart containing all latex-free supplies in or outside of patient's room.
- Use glass syringes if no latex-free alternative is available.
- Cover latex portion of blood pressure cuff or stethoscope before using on patient.
- Wear vinyl or synthetic gloves when caring for patient.

Frequently Used Products That Contain Latex
Blood pressure cuffs	Stethoscopes
Electrode pads	Tourniquets
IV tubing	Syringes
Foley catheters	Surgical masks
Baby bottle nipples	Pacifiers

Adapted from: Girard, N. (Ed.). (2004). AORN latex guideline. *AORN Journal, 79*(3), 653–672; and Bean, K. (Ed.). (2004). SGNA guidelines: Guidelines for preventing sensitivity and allergic reactions to natural rubber latex in the workplace. *Gastroenterology Nursing, 27*(4), 191–196.

comfortably against the face (Fig. 27-3). The N95 mask also costs considerably less than the HEPA filter respirators. The elastic straps on these respirators provide more protection and a better fit than the ties on regular surgical masks.

> *Think back to Jackson Ray Ivers, the son coming to visit his mother who is hospitalized with tuberculosis. The nurse would incorporate knowledge of tuberculosis transmission and appropriate barriers to explain to Mr. Ivers about the need for wearing a mask, or, in this case, a respirator.* ∎

Protective Eyewear
Protective eyewear, such as goggles or a face shield, must be available whenever there is a risk of contaminating the mucous membranes of the eyes. For example, suctioning a tracheostomy or assisting with an invasive procedure that may result in splattering of blood or other body fluids requires protection for the caregiver. Plain glasses are unacceptable because side shields are required.

FIGURE 27-3. The Type N95 healthcare particulate respirator is NIOSH approved. It meets CDC guidelines for tuberculosis exposure control and is designed specifically for use in a healthcare setting. *(Courtesy of 3M Health Care.)*

HANDLING AND DISPOSING OF SUPPLIES

Used equipment may be disposed of after use or, if reusable, bagged according to agency policy, sent to a central cleaning area, and sterilized or disinfected. Double bagging may be required if the single bag is not secure or is soiled on the outside. A contaminated item must never be used for another patient.

Double bagging of trash and linen is usually needed only if the outside of the bag is visibly soiled. Some linen bags are water soluble and dissolve in hot water, making it unnecessary for workers to handle the contaminated linen. The use of paper trays and plastic eating utensils does not prevent transmission of organisms and is no longer recommended. The combined hot water and detergent used in commercial dishwashers sufficiently decontaminates dishes, glasses, and utensils. All spills of body fluids or substances must be immediately cleaned with the appropriate chemical germicide or disinfectant.

When collecting a specimen, take care to prevent the outside of the container from becoming contaminated with any secretions or body fluids. Place all laboratory specimens in plastic bags and seal the bags to prevent leakage during transportation. A bag marked "BIOHAZARDS" is used to dispose of trash that contains liquid or semiliquid blood or other potentially infective material (OPIM), trash contaminated with blood or OPIM that would release these substances if compressed, and trash that is caked with dried blood or OPIM and is capable of releasing these materials during handling.

USING ISOLATION PRECAUTIONS

In addition to barriers, specific precautions have been established to prevent the transmission of infection. Historically, the term **isolation,** a protective procedure that limits the spread of infectious diseases among hospitalized patients, hospital personnel, and visitors, has been used. In 2007, the CDC updated its specific guidelines for transmission-based precautions (see discussion later in this chapter).

Historical Perspective

Early practices involved isolating or quarantining infected patients together in a separate facility where few, if any, aseptic techniques were employed. At the beginning of the 20th century, efforts at isolation moved toward placing infected individuals together in one hospital (infectious disease hospitals) or a hospital ward where caregivers used gowns and antiseptic solutions for handwashing as barriers to disease transmission. Eventually, infectious disease hospitals closed, including those set aside for people with tuberculosis. Patients who were considered infectious were routinely placed on general hospital units in separate rooms or in multiple-patient rooms with other patients who had the same infection.

By 1970, the CDC was actively involved in developing and recommending infection-control practices and procedures for hospitals.

Occupational Safety and Health Administration (OSHA) Regulations

OSHA, a government agency that administers the Occupational Safety and Health Act of 1970, establishes minimum health and safety standards for workers. In 1991, OSHA issued regulations for use of universal precautions in all situations and settings in which occupational exposures to blood and other potentially infectious materials were possible. This ruling reinforced CDC guidelines for universal precautions and made violations punishable with severe fines. Recognizing that hepatitis B virus (HBV) poses the greatest bloodborne risk to healthcare workers, OSHA also required that employers offer HBV vaccine free of charge to employees to prevent its transmission. The American Nurses Association continues to urge OSHA to extend this directive to provide immunization and mandate protection against bloodborne diseases for nursing students who practice in these healthcare facilities.

OSHA has also fined hospitals that fail to use equipment or devices that reduce the risk for needlestick injuries for employees.

Current CDC Guidelines

The 2007 CDC guidelines update previous recommendations from the 1996 Guidelines for Isolation Precautions in Hospitals (Siegel, Rhinehart, Jackson, & Chiarello, 2007). These newer guidelines recognize that healthcare delivery occurs in other settings beside acute care hospitals. They reflect the emergence of new pathogens (e.g., SARS, *C. difficile*, MRSA), methods to prevent transmission of multidrug resistant organisms, and the CDC's concern regarding biological terrorism. In this recent guideline, the term "nosocomial infection" has been replaced with "healthcare-associated infection." Nurses must understand the various precautions or barrier techniques if they are to use them correctly and minimize infection risks to patients as well as to themselves (see Promoting Health 27-1: Infection-Control Precautions and Barrier Techniques earlier in the chapter).

The revised guideline continues the designation of two tiers of precautions:

- **Standard precautions:** precautions used in the care of all hospitalized individuals regardless of their diagnosis or possible infection status. These precautions apply to blood, all body fluids, secretions, and excretions except sweat (whether or not blood is present or visible), nonintact skin, and mucous membranes. New additions here are Respiratory Hygiene/Cough Etiquette, safe injection practices, and directions to use a mask when performing high-risk prolonged procedures involving spinal canal punctures.
- **Transmission-based precautions:** precautions used in addition to standard precautions for patients in hospitals with suspected infection with pathogens that can be transmitted by airborne, droplet, or contact routes. New to the 2007 guidelines is a directive to don personal protective equipment (PPE) when entering the room of a

patient on contact or droplet precautions. Previously, PPE was only required when the nurse was delivering care within 3 feet of the patient. These categories recognize that a disease may have multiple routes of transmission.

▶ *Recall Jackson Ray Ivers, the son of a patient with tuberculosis. Based on the nurse's knowledge of disease transmission, the nurse institutes airborne precautions for the patient and instructs Mr. Ivers in the need for proper hand hygiene and the use of a mask.* ■

The three types of transmission-based precautions (airborne, droplet, or contact) may be used alone or in combination, but always in addition to standard precautions. Box 27-5 summarizes the revised CDC guidelines along with a listing of specific recommendations for both tiers of precautions. Hospitals are encouraged to modify these recommendations as needed for implementation of their infection-control strategy.

The CDC continues to recommend the use of puncture-resistant containers for disposal of all needles and sharps. Since most needlestick injuries occur during recapping, never recap needles. The most serious risk associated with needlestick injury is the possible exposure to bloodborne

---

Box 27-5 SUMMARY OF CDC GUIDELINES FOR ISOLATION PRECAUTIONS IN HEALTHCARE SETTINGS 2007

Standard Precautions (Tier 1)
- Follow hand hygiene techniques.
- *Wear clean nonsterile gloves* when touching blood, body fluids, excretions or secretions, contaminated items, mucous membranes, and nonintact skin. Change gloves between tasks on the same patient as necessary and remove gloves promptly after use.
- *Wear personal protective equipment* such as mask, eye protection, face shield, or fluid-repellent gown during procedures and care activities that are likely to generate splashes or sprays of blood or body fluids. Use gown to protect skin and prevent soiling of clothing.
- *Follow Respiratory Hygiene/Cough Etiquette.* Any patients, family members, and visitors with undiagnosed, transmissible respiratory infections require education to cover their mouth and nose with a tissue when coughing and promptly dispose of the tissue. During periods of increased occurrence of respiratory infections, offer a surgical mask to coughing patients and other symptomatic persons upon entry to the healthcare facility or office. Encourage the coughing patient to maintain more than a 3-foot separation from other persons in the healthcare facility or office.
- *Avoid recapping used needles.* If you must recap, never use two hands. Use a needle-recapping device or the one-handed scoop technique. Place needles, sharps, and scalpels in appropriate puncture-resistant containers after use.
- *Use Safe Injection Practices* including single dose vials when possible; use disposable needles and syringes for each injection, and prevent contamination of injection equipment and medication.
- *Wear face mask* if placing a catheter or injecting material into the spinal or epidural space.
- *Handle used patient care equipment that is soiled with blood or identified body fluids, secretions, and excretions carefully* to prevent transfer of microorganisms. Clean and reprocess items appropriately if used for another patient.
- *Use adequate environmental controls* to ensure that routine care, cleaning, and disinfection procedures are followed.
- *Review room assignments carefully.* Place patients who may contaminate the environment in private rooms (such as an incontinent patient).

Transmission-Based Precautions (Tier 2)
The following precautions are recommended in addition to standard precautions:

Airborne Precautions
- Use these for patients who have infections that spread through the air such as tuberculosis, varicella (chicken pox), rubeola (measles), and possibly SARS.
- Place patient in private room that has monitored negative air pressure in relation to surrounding areas, 6 to 12 air changes per hour, and appropriate discharge of air outside or monitored filtration if air is recirculated. Keep door closed and patient in room.
- Wear a mask or respirator when entering room of patient with known or suspected tuberculosis. If patient has known or suspected rubeola (measles) or varicella (chicken pox), respiratory protection should be worn unless person entering room is immune to these diseases.
- Transport patient out of room only when necessary and place a surgical mask on the patient if possible.
- Consult CDC Guidelines for additional prevention strategies for tuberculosis.

Droplet Precautions
- Use these for patients with an infection that is spread by large-particle droplets such as rubella, mumps, diphtheria, and the adenovirus infection in infants and young children.
- Use a private room, if available. Door may remain open.
- Wear PPE upon entry into the room for all interactions that may involve contact with the patient and potentially contaminated areas in the patient's environment.
- Transport patient out of room only when necessary and place a surgical mask on the patient if possible.
- Keep visitors 3 feet from the infected person.

Contact Precautions
- Use these for patients who are infected or colonized by a Multidrug-resistant organism (MDRO).
- Place the patient in a private room, if available.
- Wear PPE whenever you enter the room for all interactions that may involve contact with the patient and potentially contaminated areas in the patient's environment. Change gloves after having contact with infective material. Remove PPE before leaving the patient environment, and wash hands with an antimicrobial or waterless antiseptic agent.
- Limit movement of the patient out of the room.
- Avoid sharing patient-care equipment.

pathogens such as HBV, hepatitis C virus (HCV), and HIV. Hospitals now purchase needleless, protected, or recessed IV systems. Although this equipment is more expensive, studies have determined that its higher costs may be almost totally offset by lower costs of treatment and follow-up of needlestick injuries to employees. The safe injection practices included in the latest guidelines are a response to outbreaks of HBV and hepatitis C virus (HCV) in patients in ambulatory care settings. They list recommendations to use single dose vials when possible and use sterile, single-use disposable needles and a new sterile syringe for each injection. Efforts should focus on preventing contamination of injection equipment and medication. Nurses must still be accountable for their own safe work practices.

PROVIDING CARE IN SPECIAL SITUATIONS

Occasionally, nurses need to use neutropenic precautions for a patient whose immune system is compromised (e.g., one recovering from transplantation surgery or receiving chemotherapy). Those who are immunosuppressed more often than not become infected by organisms harbored in their own bodies, rather than by pathogens present in the environment or transmitted from other people. As with all patients, standard precautions are required, but some additional measures are helpful when a patient's ability to withstand any bacterial invasion is compromised.

Recommendations in this situation include the following:

- Ensure that caregiver is healthy.
- Restrict visits from friends and family members who have colds or contagious illnesses.
- Avoid collection of standing water in the room (e.g., with flowers or in humidifiers) to prevent bacteria typically found in this water.

The latest CDC isolation guidelines also address environmental controls that foster a "protective environment" to decrease the risk of infection in the MOST severely immunocompromised patients.

The increasing number of individuals who are ill or immunocompromised, coupled with increasingly virulent organisms, poses sterilization and disinfection concerns for home environments. Common measures that reduce the risk of infection at home include the following:

- Wash hands frequently—before preparing food, before eating, and after using the restroom
- Keep immunizations up to date
- Clean and disinfect kitchen surfaces, especially when preparing meat, chicken, and fish
- Avoid sharing personal items
- Cook food to the proper internal temperature
- Promptly refrigerate or freeze perishables, prepared foods, and leftovers

After thorough cleaning, some contaminated items may be disinfected by placing them in boiling water or using common household disinfectants such as bleach, isopropyl alcohol (70%), or acetic acid (white vinegar). Controlling disease

and preventing infections from spreading is a vital home care consideration for everyone.

Using Surgical Asepsis

Surgical asepsis techniques, used regularly in the operating room, labor and delivery areas, and certain diagnostic testing areas, are also used by the nurse at the patient's bedside. Procedures that involve the insertion of a urinary catheter, sterile dressing changes, or preparing an injectable medication are examples of surgical asepsis techniques. An object is considered sterile when all microorganisms, including pathogens and spores, have been destroyed. For example, the needle for an injection must be handled so that it is sterile when inserted into a patient. Sterile forceps or gloves are used to handle sterile dressings to protect against contamination. The basic principles of surgical asepsis are listed in Box 27-6.

When observing *medical asepsis,* areas are considered contaminated if they bear or are suspected of bearing pathogens; whereas when following *surgical asepsis,* areas are considered contaminated if they are touched by any object that is not also sterile. One of the most important aspects of surgical and medical asepsis is that the effectiveness of both depends on faithful and conscientious practice by those carrying them out. It is far better to err on the side of safety when using surgical asepsis than to take the slightest chance of possible contamination. Being a patient advocate requires vigilant aseptic technique and a willingness to speak up if the patient's safety has been compromised by improper procedures.

> ➤ *Think back to Esther Bailey, the woman described in the Reflective Practice box. The nurse acted appropriately by speaking up about the possible contamination of the catheter. Had this catheter been used, the patient's safety would have been compromised.* ∎

Explaining the surgical asepsis procedure to patients facilitates their cooperation. Inform the patient about which objects and areas may not be touched, and direct the patient to avoid sudden movements that might contaminate the equipment. This helps the patient assist in maintaining the sterility of the procedure.

OPENING A STERILE PACKAGE AND PREPARING A STERILE FIELD

Commercially prepared sterile items may be sealed in paper or packaged in plastic containers. Sterile packages may be opened on a flat surface or while held in the hands. Skill 27-3 illustrates how to open a sterile package and prepare a sterile field. A sterile item should be covered if it is not used immediately. Reapply the cover by touching only the outside of the wrapper and reversing the opening order.

POURING STERILE SOLUTIONS

Care is necessary when pouring sterile liquids onto a sterile dressing or into a sterile basin. The outer surfaces of the

Box 27-6   PRACTICING BASIC PRINCIPLES OF SURGICAL ASEPSIS

- Allow only a sterile object to touch another sterile object. Unsterile touching sterile means contamination has occurred.
- Open sterile packages so that the first edge of the wrapper is directed away from the worker to avoid the possibility of a sterile surface touching unsterile clothing. The outside of the sterile package is considered contaminated. Opening a sterile package is shown and described in Skill 27-3.
- Avoid spilling any solution on a cloth or paper used as a field for a sterile setup. The moisture penetrates through the sterile cloth or paper and carries organisms by capillary action to contaminate the field. A wet field is considered contaminated if the surface immediately below it is not sterile.
- Hold sterile objects above the level of the waist. This will ensure keeping the object within sight and preventing accidental contamination.
- Avoid talking, coughing, sneezing, or reaching over a sterile field or object. This helps to prevent contamination by

droplets from the nose and the mouth or by particles dropping from the worker's arm.
- Never walk away from or turn your back on a sterile field. This prevents possible contamination while the field is out of the worker's view.
- Keep all items sterile that are brought into contact with broken skin, or used to penetrate the skin to inject substances into the body, or to enter normally sterile body cavities. These items include dressings used to cover wounds and incisions, needles for injection, and tubes (catheters) used to drain urine from the bladder.
- Use dry, sterile forceps when necessary. Forceps soaked in disinfectant are not considered sterile.
- Consider the edge (outer 1 inch) of a sterile field to be contaminated.
- Consider an object contaminated if you have any doubt as to its sterility.

---

bottle and cap are considered unsterile, whereas the inside areas and the solution are considered sterile. After a solution has been opened, the outer bottle should be labeled and dated if it is to be reused. Most solutions are considered sterile for 24 hours after they are opened. When pouring from a bottle, grasp the bottle so that the label is in the palm of your hand. This action prevents any of the liquid from running over the label and making it illegible. Avoid splashing the liquid since this would contaminate the sterile field (see Skill 27-3).

ADDING STERILE SUPPLIES TO A STERILE FIELD

After establishing a sterile field, it may be necessary to add items such as instruments or additional supplies to the sterile field. Item 6 in Skill 27-3 demonstrates this technique. Once a sterile field is established, objects on a field may be handled only by using sterile forceps or with hands wearing sterile gloves.

PUTTING ON STERILE GLOVES

Sterile gloves are donned in a way that allows only the inside of the gloves to come in contact with the hands. Skill 27-4 describes the proper technique for putting on sterile gloves.

After the gloves are on, only sterile items may be handled with the sterile-gloved hands. Careful removal of the gloves reduces any hand contact with contaminated materials. Good hand hygiene technique before and after putting on sterile gloves is imperative.

POSITIONING A STERILE DRAPE

The sterile drape, which ideally is waterproof, may be used to extend the sterile working area. Using sterile gloves allows the nurse to handle the entire drape surface. For protection when positioning, fold the upper edges of the drape over the sterile-gloved hands (Fig. 27-4). When sterile

gloves are not worn, the nurse can touch only the outer 1 inch (2.5 cm) of the drape. Use caution when gently shaking the drape open so as not to touch one's clothing or an unsterile object. Hold the drape by the 1-inch upper edge and position the drape over the desired area. Do not reach over the drape because this would contaminate a sterile area.

Meeting Needs of Patients Requiring Infection-Control Precautions

The psychological implications of infection-control precautions are usually great, whether the patient is strictly separated from others or needs only to observe relatively simple precautions (see the accompanying box, Through the Eyes of a Student).

The current standard precautions of the CDC treat all people in a similar manner and greatly minimize the psychological trauma of feeling unclean and undesirable that often occurred with earlier measures. Sensory deprivation and loss of self-esteem may occur, however, with transmission-based precautions. Friends and relatives, as well as healthcare personnel, may be inclined to spend less time with the patient because they are afraid that they will contract the disease or because of the inconvenience of coping with specific transmission precaution procedures. This may lead to inconsistent recording of vital signs, irregular documentation, and less patient monitoring on the part of caregivers. Research has also verified that patients placed in isolation because of the presence of a communicable disease may suffer unintended consequences such as an increase in incidents of depression, fewer visits from healthcare staff, and an increase in the number of medication errors (Delahanty & Myers, 2007). Nursing measures to help prevent the sensory deprivation and loss of self-esteem associated with isolation precautions are discussed in Chapters 41 and 44.

Health teaching about transmission-based precautions can ease the fears of patients and family members. Both must

FIGURE 27-4. Techniques of cuffing a sterile drape over gloved hands.

understand the pertinent epidemiologic facts and how to carry out the specific precautions. It is helpful to emphasize the following:

- Precautions are temporary.
- The precautions and protective equipment worn by the staff protect the patient, the caregiver, and other patients.
- Proper hand hygiene before and after visiting the patient is the most effective measure to prevent spread of the disease.
- Continued explanations about procedures and continued updates on progress help to minimize anxiety.

Nurses must document their health teaching about barrier precautions in the patient's plan of care. A well-informed

nurse who understands how to protect both self and patients and a well-informed patient who is cooperating in his or her care represent superior communicable disease precautions.

Raising Ethical Concerns About Infection Risks

Infection control and precautions minimize infection risks for patients as well as healthcare workers. However, the increasing numbers of people infected with HIV, HBV, and HCV have led to serious ethical concerns and controversy related to the risk for transmitting these diseases. At issue are the rights of the patient versus the rights of the healthcare worker and the healthcare agency. Refer to the accompanying box, Nursing Advocacy in Action, for an example of a

Through the Eyes of a Student

She was the cutest little girl I have ever known. She was infected with HIV from birth. Her mother was an IV drug user and engaged in unprotected sex with multiple partners. This little girl, who came into the world with an innocent, fresh, new face full of unconditional love, could not walk, could not talk, could not chew, could not control her urine or bowel movements—but boy could she smile! In the beginning, I was so terrified of contracting AIDS that I couldn't walk into her room without a mask, gown, gloves, protective eyewear, and basically a full protective body spacesuit. At the end, I wanted to take her into my home and give her all the love, support, and care she needed. I am not saying that I didn't wear gloves when I changed her diapers or when I flushed her heparin lock because I did . . . I was very careful. But I realized that she is a

person, a person full of feelings, a person who needed me, and from whom I could learn. People with AIDS virus are just that—people. We need to learn to treat them as such.

I also learned not to fear the person who is diagnosed with HIV infection or AIDS. I know that I will take the proper safety precautions with this person. The person I need to fear is the cute little old man who would never have AIDS because "he's not the type." If I don't use precautions, it is possible that one day I'll become infected through contact with someone who is "not the type." If that should ever happen, I hope everyone who cares for me will treat me as a real person and not be afraid.

—*Karmi N. Soder*
Georgetown University, Washington, DC

NURSING ADVOCACY IN ACTION

Patient Scenario

Ms. Samol is a 38-year-old patient in the medical intensive care unit who is dying of AIDS-related complications. Since being diagnosed with AIDS, she has refused to inform her husband and family of her AIDS status. She even has an advance directive, which forbids the disclosure of her diagnosis when she can no longer advocate for herself. Her husband and mother cannot understand why the doctors and nurses cannot treat her "pneumonia"—the only diagnosis she gave them. The doctors and nurses caring for Ms. Samol believe that her husband has the right to know his wife's diagnosis so that he can make decisions in his own best interest about being tested, having their children tested, etc.

Implications for Nursing Advocacy

What would you do if you were Ms. Samol's nurse? Talk with your classmates and experienced nurses about the questions that follow.

- If you elect to advocate for the Samols, what practical steps can you take to ensure better health outcomes? Are there any legal guidelines for what you can and cannot do?
- What is reasonable to expect of a student nurse, a graduate nurse, and an experienced nurse in this situation?
- What advocacy skills are needed to effectively respond to this challenge?

scientiously adhere to appropriate infection-control precautions seriously reduce the risk for infection for patients and themselves.

Reporting Accidental Exposure

Nurses are accountable for their own safety. Any needlestick injury or accidental exposure to blood or body fluids must be reported immediately so that appropriate interventions can be used. Failure to notify an employer of an exposure may result in personal jeopardy as well as loss of compensation if an infection develops. An agency's plan for this type of exposure typically includes the following:

- Washing the exposed area immediately with warm water and soap
- Reporting the incident to the appropriate person and completing an incident or injury report if required by the agency
- Informing the agency of the source (patient's name) and nature of the exposure
- Consenting to an initial baseline blood test, if agreeable, to determine personal HIV and HBV status, with repeat blood testing 6 weeks after exposure and at 3-month, 6-month, and 1-year intervals
- Consenting to postexposure prophylaxis, if recommended, at the appropriate time
- Awaiting blood test results of the involved patient (with his or her consent) to determine HIV, HBV, and HCV status. State laws may vary concerning this practice.
- Attending counseling session regarding safe practices to protect self and others

Working With the Infection Preventionist

In the hospital, the nurse is responsible for educating patients and staff about effective infection-control techniques and for collecting statistics about infections. Many hospitals rely on this specialized practitioner, referred to as the infection preventionist, to survey laboratory reports and review records for patients at risk, as well as suggest approaches to potentially dangerous situations (APIC, 2008b). Other responsibilities include:

- Developing a plan to reduce the occurrence of healthcare-associated infections
- Collaborating with state and local health departments regarding recommended or mandatory reporting of healthcare-associated infections
- Developing a plan to respond to an act of bioterrorism
- Evaluating new products
- Providing routine consultations to staff and patients regarding infection control issues (APIC, 2008b).

situation where the nurse must reconcile the patient's right to make choices versus the well-being of family members.

Questions such as the following are being debated:

- Should all hospital patients be routinely tested for HIV infection?
- Should HIV testing be mandatory for all healthcare workers?
- Should healthcare workers infected with HIV be permitted to perform exposure-prone invasive procedures?
- What procedures should be considered exposure-prone?
- Will healthcare facilities be liable if they allow HIV-positive staff to care for patients?
- Should pregnant healthcare providers be expected to care for patients with infectious diseases?

The CDC and various medical and nursing groups are seeking consensus on these issues, based on scientific information and valid statistical evidence. Although the CDC has issued guidelines related to these topics, not all states have adopted the guidelines. Additionally, some states have revised them. All agree, however, that healthcare workers who con-

Intensive investigative strategies create a positive environment that significantly reduces the incidence of healthcare-associated infections in healthcare facilities. The infection preventionist knows the devastating effects of infection and is intent on promoting health and fostering a systematic approach to infection control.

In the home, the infection preventionist's duties include surveillance for agency-associated infections, education, consultation, epidemiologic investigation, quality-improvement activities, and policy and procedure development. OSHA regulations state that home care agencies must have an infection-control program and that OSHA infection-control standards and policies must be available to all staff for reference.

Teaching About Infection Control

Teaching about medical asepsis and infection control is a challenging nursing responsibility. Patients need to be aware of techniques that prevent the spread of infection. Use of the nursing process in infection control protects both the patient and the nurse.

Medical asepsis techniques are appropriate for most procedures in the home, except for self-injection technique and venous catheter care, which require surgical asepsis. The patient frequently must make adjustments and improvise with the resources and supplies available for his or her use. In addition, the nurse emphasizes effective hand hygiene and other hygiene practices that interrupt the infection cycle. To satisfy OSHA requirements, many home care agencies have either a full-time or part-time infection preventionist.

Patients should be taught to use basic principles of asepsis at home and in public facilities. These involve the activities of daily living (see Chapter 31 for a discussion of personal hygiene). Following are examples of medical asepsis practices recommended in the home:

- Washing hands before preparing food and before eating
- Preparing foods at temperatures high enough to ensure that they are safe to eat, the most common example being the preparation of fresh meat
- Washing hands, cutting boards, and utensils with hot, soapy water before and after handling raw poultry and meat
- Keeping foods refrigerated, especially those containing mayonnaise
- Washing raw fruits and vegetables before serving them
- Using pasteurized milk and fruit juices
- Washing hands after using the bathroom
- Using individual personal care items, such as washcloths, towels, and toothbrushes, rather than sharing

> ➤ *Think back to Giselle Turheis, the woman with leukemia and a compromised immune system. When teaching the patient about measures to prevent infection, the nurse would stress the use of proper practices in the home to reduce the patient's risk for infection.* ∎

Patients also may need teaching about ways to prevent infection in public facilities, such as with the following:

- Wash hands after using any public bathroom.
- Use paper towels or hot-air dryers in restrooms.
- Use individually wrapped drinking straws.
- Use tongs to lift food from common service trays in cafeterias, food stores, and salad bars.

The community reinforces medical asepsis practices in various ways, including the following:

- Using sterilized combs and brushes in barber and beauty shops
- Performing examination of food handlers for evidence of disease
- Encouraging food handlers to receive the hepatitis A vaccination
- Enforcing frequent handwashing by food handlers

Evaluating

Nurses as primary caregivers can intervene in and positively affect a patient's outcome. By assessing the person at risk, selecting appropriate nursing diagnoses, planning, and intervening to maintain a safe environment, the nurse can reduce a patient's potential for developing an infection (see the accompanying concept map for an example).

Evaluation of the plan of care determines whether the individual's need for safety is being met effectively. Ongoing systematic evaluation is crucial for nurses who strive to maintain a secure environment for their patients as well as themselves. If patient goals have been met and evaluative criteria have been satisfied, the patient will accomplish the following:

- Correctly use techniques of medical asepsis
- Identify health habits and lifestyle patterns that promote health
- State the signs and symptoms of an infection
- Identify unsafe situations in the home environment

Esther Bailey, age 72, is 4 days postoperative abdominal surgery and has a wound infection. She is receiving continuous intravenous (IV) fluids of 5% dextrose and 0.45% normal saline with 20 mEq potassium chloride at 75 mL/hour and an IV antibiotic once a day. She has a nasogastric tube connected to suction. Upon assessment, you find bowel sounds are absent and the abdomen is slightly distended. The midline incision is draining small amount of tan purulent material and has a gauze dressing in place. During the dressing change, you note the skin edges are reddened and edematous. Wound cultures reveal heavy growth of *S. aureus*. Her temperature has been as high as 101°F in the past 24 hours. Lab work is significant for an elevated white blood cell count (WBC). Esther has been using the incentive spirometer but has poor inspiratory effort due to incisional pain. You find her lung sounds are clear but diminished in the bases. Her urinary catheter was removed 8 hours ago. Since then, she has been unable to void, so the catheter is going to be reinserted.

Priority 1

Risk for Infection, actual and potential, related to documented wound infection and an increased risk of infection due to invasive therapy
Supporting Data:
- Abdominal incision reddened and edematous with tan purulent drainage
- Wound culture shows *S. aureus*
- Receiving IV antibiotics
- Temperature max 101°F
- Elevated WBC
- IV catheter and parenteral therapy
- Indwelling urinary catheter insertion

Outcome:
Patient will demonstrate signs of wound healing and no further signs of infection; WBC and temperature will return to normal.

Nursing Interventions:
- Assess temperature every 4 hours
- Monitor WBC count
- Administer antibiotics as prescribed
- Maintain aseptic technique with indwelling urinary catheter insertion and parenteral therapy
- Change abdominal dressing using sterile technique once a day and prn
- Dispose of soiled dressings appropriately
- Utilize proper handwashing technique
- Note appearance of incision
- Monitor characteristics of urine

Evaluation: Catheter was inserted using aseptic technique. Catheter draining clear yellow urine. Temperature returned to normal. WBC count remains elevated. No significant change noted in incision. Continue interventions.

Priority 2

Ineffective Breathing Pattern related to postoperative incisional pain, increasing risk of atelectasis
Supporting Data:
- Poor effort with use of incentive spirometer
- Experiencing incisional pain
- Elevated WBC
- Temperature max 101°F
- Lung sounds clear but diminished in bases

Outcome:
Patient will perform coughing and deep breathing exercises; inspiratory effort will improve; and patient will remain free from a pulmonary infection.

Nursing Interventions:
- Encourage coughing and deep breathing exercises every 2 hours; assist to splint incision
- Assess pain level (scale of 0–10)
- Administer pain medication as prescribed
- Encourage use of incentive spirometer every hour as prescribed
- Auscultate lungs for presence of abnormal sounds
- Note characteristics of any sputum produced
- OOB to chair/reposition every 2 hours

Evaluation: Patient is performing coughing and deep breathing exercises effectively after adequate pain control. Occasional cough is nonproductive. Lungs are now clear with equal bilateral breath sounds. Continue interventions.

Priority 3

Imbalanced Body Temperature related to an infectious process
Supporting Data:
- Temperature max 101°F
- Wound culture shows *S. aureus*
- Elevated WBC
- Abdominal incision reddened and edematous with tan purulent drainage

Outcome:
Patient will maintain body temperature within normal limits.

Nursing Interventions:
- Assess temperature every 4 hours
- Administer antibiotics as prescribed
- Administer antipyretics as prescribed
- Remove excessive blankets when febrile
- If diaphoretic with fever, bathe and change linens as needed

Evaluation: Esther's temperature has returned to normal. Continue to monitor.

- - - - - Relationship ▪ Assessment ▪ Nursing Diagnosis ▪ Outcome Identification ▪ Interventions ▪ Evaluation

Concept map displaying the nursing process for Esther Bailey.

Skill · 27-1 Performing Hand Hygiene Using Soap and Water (Handwashing)

EQUIPMENT

- Antimicrobial or nonantimicrobial soap (if in bar form, soap must be placed on a soap rack)
- Paper towels
- Oil-free lotion (optional)

IMPLEMENTATION

ACTION	RATIONALE
1. Gather the necessary supplies. Stand in front of the sink. Do not allow your clothing to touch the sink during the washing procedure (Figure 1).	The sink is considered contaminated. Clothing may carry organisms from place to place.
2. Remove jewelry, if possible, and secure in a safe place. A plain wedding band may remain in place.	Removal of jewelry facilitates proper cleansing. Microorganisms may accumulate in settings of jewelry. If jewelry was worn during care, it should be left on during handwashing.
3. Turn on water and adjust force (Figure 2). Regulate the temperature until the water is warm.	Water splashed from the contaminated sink will contaminate clothing. Warm water is more comfortable and is less likely to open pores and remove oils from the skin. Organisms can lodge in roughened and broken areas of chapped skin.

FIGURE 1. Standing in front of sink.

FIGURE 2. Turning on the water at the sink.

ACTION	RATIONALE
4. Wet the hands and wrist area. Keep hands lower than elbows to allow water to flow toward fingertips (Figure 3).	Water should flow from the cleaner area toward the more contaminated area. Hands are more contaminated than forearms.
5. Use about 1 teaspoon of liquid soap from dispenser or rinse bar of soap and lather thoroughly (Figure 4). Cover all areas of hands with the soap product. Rinse soap bar again and return to soap rack.	Rinsing the soap before and after use removes the lather, which may contain microorganisms.
6. With firm rubbing and circular motions, wash the palms and backs of the hands, each finger, the areas between the fingers (Figure 5), and the knuckles, wrists, and forearms. **Wash at least 1 inch above area of contamination.** If hands are not visibly soiled, wash to 1 inch above the wrists (Figure 6).	Friction caused by firm rubbing and circular motions helps to loosen dirt and organisms that can lodge between the fingers, in skin crevices of knuckles, on the palms and backs of the hands, and on the wrists and forearms. Cleaning less contaminated areas (forearms and wrists) after hands are clean prevents spreading microorganisms from the hands to the forearms and wrists.
7. Continue this friction motion for at least 15 seconds.	Length of handwashing is determined by degree of contamination.
8. Use fingernails of the opposite hand or a clean orangewood stick to clean under fingernails (Figure 7).	Area under nails has a high microorganism count, and organisms may remain under the nails, where the organisms can grow and be spread to other persons.
9. Rinse thoroughly with water flowing toward fingertips (Figure 8).	Running water rinses microorganisms and dirt into the sink.

FIGURE 3. Wetting hands to the wrist.

FIGURE 4. Lathering hands with soap and rubbing with firm circular motion.

FIGURE 5. Washing areas between fingers.

FIGURE 6. Washing to 1 inch above the wrist.

FIGURE 7. Using fingernails to clean under nails of opposite hand.

FIGURE 8. Rinsing hands under running water with water flowing toward fingertips.

(continued)

Skill · 27-1 Performing Hand Hygiene Using Soap and Water (Handwashing) *continued*

ACTION	RATIONALE
10. Pat hands dry with a paper towel, beginning with the fingers and moving upward toward forearms, and discard it immediately. Use another clean towel to turn off the faucet. Discard towel immediately without touching other clean hand.	Patting the skin dry prevents chapping. Dry hands first because they are considered the cleanest and least contaminated area. Turning the faucet off with a clean paper towel protects the clean hands from contact with a soiled surface.
11. Use oil-free lotion on hands, if desired.	Oil-free lotion helps to keep the skin soft and prevents chapping. It is best applied after patient care is complete and from small, personal containers. Oil-based lotions should be avoided because they can cause deterioration of gloves.

DOCUMENTATION

The performance of handwashing is not generally documented.

SPECIAL CONSIDERATIONS

General Considerations

- An antimicrobial soap product is recommended for use with handwashing before participating in an invasive procedure and after exposure to blood or body fluids. The length of the scrub will vary based on need.
- Liquid or bar soap, granules, or leaflets are all acceptable forms of nonantimicrobial soap.

Home Care Considerations

- Home care providers should consider bringing their own liquid soap and disposable paper towels into the home for washing and drying their hands instead of using potentially contaminated bar soap and towels in the patient's home (Grossman et al., 2008).
- Proper hand hygiene before leaving a home and immediately upon entering another home is imperative (McGoldrick & Rhinehart, 2007).

Skill · 27-2 Using Personal Protective Equipment

EQUIPMENT

- Gloves
- Mask (surgical or particulate respirator)
- Impervious gown
- Protective eyewear (does not include eyeglasses)
- Equipment for PPE may vary depending on facility policy.

IMPLEMENTATION

ACTION	RATIONALE
1. Check medical record and nursing plan of care for type of precautions and review precautions in infection-control manual.	Mode of transmission of organism determines type of precautions required.
2. Plan nursing activities before entering patient's room.	Organization facilitates performance of task and adherence to precautions.
3. Perform hand hygiene.	Hand hygiene prevents the spread of microorganisms.
4. Provide instruction about precautions to patient, family members, and visitors.	Explanation encourages cooperation of patient and family and reduces apprehension about precaution procedures.
5. Put on gown, gloves, mask, and protective eyewear, based on the type of exposure anticipated and category of isolation precautions.	Use of PPE interrupts chain of infection and protects patient and nurse. Gown should protect entire uniform. Gloves protect hands and wrists from microorganisms. Masks protect nurse or patient from droplet nuclei and large-particle aerosols. Eyewear protects mucous membranes in the eye from splashes.

ACTION

a. Put on the gown, with the opening in the back. Tie gown securely at neck and waist (Figure 1).

b. Put on the mask or respirator over your nose, mouth, and chin (Figure 2). Secure ties or elastic bands at the middle of the head and neck. If respirator is used, perform a fit check. Inhale; the respirator should collapse. Exhale; air should not leak out.

c. Put on goggles (Figure 3). Place over eyes and adjust to fit. Alternately, a face shield could be used to take the place of the mask and goggles (Figure 4).

d. Put on clean disposable gloves. Extend gloves to cover the cuffs of the gown (Figure 5).

RATIONALE

Gown should fully cover the torso from the neck to knees, arms to the end of wrists, and wrap around the back.

Masks protect nurse or patient from droplet nuclei and large-particle aerosols. A mask must fit securely to provide protection.

Eyewear protects mucous membranes in the eye from splashes. Must fit securely to provide protection.

Gloves protect hands and wrists from microorganisms.

FIGURE 1. Tying gown at neck and waist.

FIGURE 2. Applying mask applied over nose, mouth, and chin.

FIGURE 3. Putting on goggles.

FIGURE 4. Putting on face shield.

FIGURE 5. Putting on gloves, ensuring gloves cover gown cuffs.

(continued)

Skill · 27-2 Using Personal Protective Equipment *continued*

ACTION	RATIONALE
6. Identify the patient. Explain the procedure to the patient. Continue with patient care as appropriate.	Patient identification validates the correct patient and correct procedure. Discussion and explanation help allay anxiety and prepare the patient for what to expect.

Remove PPE

7. Remove PPE: Except for respirator, remove PPE at the doorway or in anteroom. Remove respirator after leaving the patient room and closing door.	Proper removal prevents contact with and the spread of microorganisms. Outside front of equipment is considered contaminated. The inside, outside back, ties on head and back, are considered clean; areas of PPE that are not likely to have been in contact with infectious organisms.
a. If impervious gown has been tied in front of the body at the waistline, untie waist strings before removing gloves.	Front of gown, including waist strings, are contaminated. If tied in front of body, the ties must be untied prior to removing gloves.
b. Grasp the outside of one glove with the opposite gloved hand and peel off, turning the glove inside out as you pull it off (Figure 6). Hold the removed glove in the remaining gloved hand.	Outside of gloves are contaminated.
c. Slide fingers of ungloved hand under the remaining glove at the wrist, taking care not to touch the outer surface of the glove (Figure 7).	Ungloved hand is clean and should not touch contaminated areas.
d. Peel off the glove over the first glove, containing the one glove inside the other (Figure 8). Discard in appropriate container.	Proper disposal prevents transmission of microorganisms.
e. To remove the goggles or face shield: Handle by the headband or ear pieces (Figure 9). Lift away from the face. Place in designated receptacle for reprocessing or in an appropriate waste container.	Outside of goggles or face shield is contaminated. Handling by headband or ear pieces and lifting away from face prevents transmission of microorganisms. Proper disposal prevents transmission of microorganisms.
f. To remove gown: Unfasten ties, if at the neck and back. Allow the gown to fall away from shoulders. Touching only the inside of the gown, pull away from the torso. Keeping hands on the inner surface of the gown, pull from arms. Turn gown inside out. Fold or roll into a bundle and discard.	Gown front and sleeves are contaminated. Touching only the inside of the gown and pulling it away from the torso prevents transmission of microorganisms. Proper disposal prevents transmission of microorganisms.

FIGURE 6. Grasping the outside of one glove and peeling off.

FIGURE 7. Sliding fingers of ungloved hand under the remaining glove at the wrist.

FIGURE 8. Pulling glove off the hand and over the other glove.

ACTION

RATIONALE

FIGURE 9. Removing goggles by grasping ear pieces.

g. To remove mask or respirator: Grasp the neck ties or elastic, then top ties or elastic and remove. Take care to avoid touching front of mask or respirator. Discard in waste container. If using a respirator, save for future use in the designated area.

Front of mask or respirator is contaminated; **Do Not Touch.** Not touching the front and proper disposal prevent transmission of microorganisms.

8. Perform hand hygiene immediately after removing all PPE.

Hand hygiene prevents spread of microorganisms.

DOCUMENTATION

It is not usually necessary to document the use of specific articles of PPE or each application of PPE. However, documentation should be recorded regarding the implementation and continuation of specific transmission-based precautions as part of the patient's care.

UNEXPECTED SITUATIONS AND ASSOCIATED INTERVENTIONS

• *The nurse did not realize the need for protective equipment at beginning of task:* Stop task and obtain appropriate protective wear.

• *The nurse is accidentally exposed to blood and body fluids:* Stop task and immediately follow agency protocol for exposure, including reporting the exposure.

Skill · 27-3 Preparing a Sterile Field and Adding Sterile Items to a Sterile Field

EQUIPMENT

• Sterile wrapped drape or commercially prepared sterile package
• Additional sterile supplies, such as dressings, containers, or solution, as needed
• PPE, as indicated

IMPLEMENTATION

ACTION

RATIONALE

1. Perform hand hygiene and put on PPE, if indicated.

Hand hygiene and PPE prevent the spread of microorganisms. PPE is required, based on transmission precautions.

2. Identify the patient. Explain the procedure to the patient.

Patient identification validates the correct patient and correct procedure. Discussion and explanation help allay anxiety and prepare the patient for what to expect.

(continued)

Skill · 27-3 Preparing a Sterile Field and Adding Sterile Items to a Sterile Field *continued*

ACTION	RATIONALE
Preparing a Sterile Field	
3. Check that packaged sterile drape is dry and unopened. Also, note expiration date, making sure that the date is still valid.	Moisture contaminates a sterile package. Expiration date indicates period that package remains sterile.
4. Select a work area that is waist level or higher.	Work area is within sight. Bacteria tend to settle, so there is less contamination above the waist.
5. Open sterile wrapped drape or commercially prepared kit.	
For a Prepackaged Sterile Drape	
a. Open the outer covering of the drape. Remove sterile drape, lifting it carefully by its corners. Hold away from body and above the waist and work surface.	Outer 1 inch (2.5 cm) of drape is considered contaminated. Any item touching this area is also considered contaminated.
b. Continue to hold only by the corners. Allow the drape to unfold, away from your body and any other surface (Figure 1).	Touching outer side of wrapper maintains sterile field. Contact with any surface would contaminate the field.
c. Position the drape on the work surface with the moisture-proof side down (Figure 2). This would be the shiny or blue side. Avoid touching any other surface or object with the drape. If any portion of the drape hangs off the work surface, that part of the drape is considered contaminated.	Moisture-proof side prevents contamination of the field if it becomes wet. The moisture penetrates the sterile cloth or paper and carries organisms by capillary action to contaminate the field. A wet field is considered contaminated if the surface immediately below it is not sterile.
For a Commercially Prepared Kit or Tray	
a. Open the outside cover of the package and remove the kit or tray (Figure 3). Place in the center of the work surface, with the topmost flap positioned on the far side of the package.	This allows sufficient room for sterile field.
b. Reach around the package and grasp the outer surface of the end of the topmost flap, holding no more than 1 inch from the border of the flap. Pull open away from the body, keeping the arm outstretched and away from the inside of the wrapper (Figure 4). Allow the wrapper to lie flat on the work surface.	This maintains sterility of inside of wrapper, which is to become the sterile field. Outer surface of the wrapper is considered unsterile. Outer 1-inch border of the wrapper is considered contaminated.
c. Reach around the package and grasp the outer surface of the first side flap, holding no more than 1 inch from the border of the flap. Pull open to the side of the package, keeping the arm outstretched and away from the inside of the wrapper (Figure 5). Allow the wrapper to lie flat on the work surface.	This maintains sterility of inside of wrapper, which is to become the sterile field. Outer surface of the wrapper is considered unsterile. Outer 1-inch border of the wrapper is considered contaminated.
d. Reach around the package and grasp the outer surface of the remaining side flap, holding no more than 1 inch from the border of the flap. Pull open to the side of the package, keeping the arm outstretched and away from the inside of the wrapper (Figure 6). Allow the wrapper to lie flat on the work surface.	This maintains sterility of inside of wrapper, which is to become the sterile field. Outer surface of the wrapper is considered unsterile. Outer 1-inch of border of the wrapper is considered contaminated.
e. Stand away from the package and work surface. Grasp the outer surface of the remaining flap closest to the body, holding not more than 1 inch from the border of the flap. Pull the flap back toward the body, keeping arm outstretched and away from the inside of the wrapper (Figure 7). Keep this hand in place. Use other hand to grasp the wrapper on the underside (the side that is down to the work surface). Position the wrapper so that when flat, edges are on the work surface, and do not hang down over sides of work surface (Figure 8). Allow the wrapper to lie flat on the work surface.	This maintains sterility of inside of wrapper, which is to become the sterile field. Outer surface of the wrapper is considered unsterile. Outer 1-inch border of the wrapper is considered contaminated.
f. The outer wrapper of the package has become a sterile field with the packaged supplies in the center (Figure 9). Do not touch or reach over the sterile field.	Sterility of the field and contents are maintained.
Adding Items to a Sterile Field	
6. Place additional sterile items on field as needed.	Sterility of the field is maintained.

FIGURE 1. Holding drape by corners and allowing it to unfold away from body and surfaces.

FIGURE 2. Positioning drape on work surface with the moisture-proof side down.

FIGURE 3. Opening outside cover of package.

FIGURE 4. Pulling top flap open, away from body.

FIGURE 5. Pulling open the first side flap.

FIGURE 6. Pulling open the remaining side flap.

(continued)

Skill · 27-3   Preparing a Sterile Field and Adding Sterile Items to a Sterile Field *continued*

ACTION

FIGURE 7. Pulling open flap closest to body.

RATIONALE

FIGURE 8. Positioning wrapper on work surface.

FIGURE 9. Outside wrapper of package is now sterile field.

To Add an Agency-Wrapped and Sterilized Item

a. Hold agency-wrapped item in the dominant hand, with top flap opening away from the body. With other hand, reach around the package and unfold top flap and both sides.

b. Keep a secure hold on item through the wrapper with the dominant hand. Grasp the remaining flap of the wrapper closest to the body, taking care not to touch the inner surface of the wrapper or the item. Pull the flap back toward the wrist, so the wrapper covers the hand and wrist.

c. Grasp all the corners of the wrapper together with the nondominant hand and pull back toward wrist, covering hand and wrist. Hold in place.

d. Hold the item 6 inches above the surface of the sterile field and drop onto the field. Be careful to avoid touching the surface or other items or dropping onto the 1-inch border.

To Add a Commercially Wrapped and Sterilized Item

a. Hold package in one hand. Pull back top cover with other hand. Alternately, carefully peel the edges apart using both hands (Figure 10).

Only sterile surface and item are exposed before dropping onto sterile field.

Only sterile surface and item are exposed before dropping onto sterile field.

Only sterile surface and item are exposed before dropping onto sterile field.

This prevents contamination of the field and inadvertent dropping of the sterile item too close to the edge or off the field. Any items landing on 1-inch border are considered contaminated.

Contents remain uncontaminated by hands.

ACTION	RATIONALE

b. After top cover or edges are partially separated, hold the item 6 inches above the surface of the sterile field. Continue opening the package and drop the item onto the field (Figure 11). Be careful to avoid touching the surface or other items or dropping onto the 1-inch border.

This prevents contamination of the field and inadvertent dropping of the sterile item too close to the edge or off the field. Any items landing on 1-inch border are considered contaminated.

c. Discard wrapper.

A neat work area promotes proper technique and inadvertent contamination of the field.

FIGURE 10. Carefully peeling edges apart.

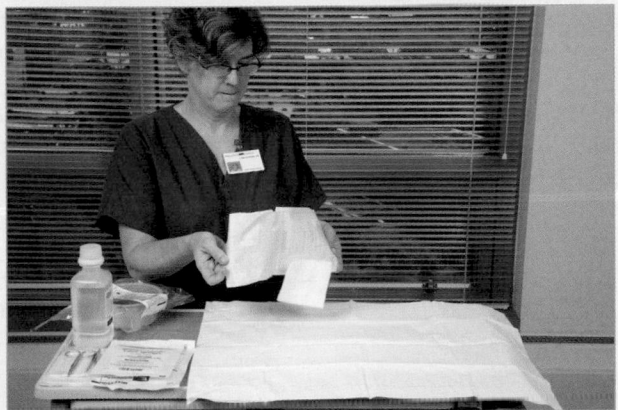

FIGURE 11. Dropping sterile item onto sterile field.

To Add a Sterile Solution

a. Obtain appropriate solution and check expiration date.

Once opened, a bottle should be labeled with date and time. Solution remains sterile for 24 hours once opened.

b. Open solution container according to directions and **place cap on table away from the field with edges up (Figure 12).**

Sterility of inside cap is maintained.

c. Hold bottle outside the edge of the sterile field with the label side facing the palm of your hand and prepare to pour from a height of 4 to 6 inches (10 to 15 cm). The tip of the bottle should never touch a sterile container or field.

Label remains dry, and solution may be poured without reaching across sterile field. Minimal splashing occurs from that height. Accidentally touching the tip of the bottle to a container or dressing contaminates them both.

d. Pour required amount of solution steadily into sterile container previously added to sterile field and positioned at side of sterile field or onto dressings (Figure 13). **Avoid splashing any liquid.**

A steady stream minimizes the risk of splashing; moisture contaminates sterile field.

FIGURE 12. Opening bottle of sterile solution and placing cap on table with edges up.

FIGURE 13. Pouring solution into sterile container.

(continued)

Skill · 27-3 Preparing a Sterile Field and Adding Sterile Items to a Sterile Field *continued*

ACTION	RATIONALE
e. Touch only the outside of the lid when recapping. Label solution with date and time of opening.	Solution remains uncontaminated and available for future use.
7. Continue with the procedure as indicated.	
8. When procedure is completed, remove PPE, if used. Perform hand hygiene.	Removing PPE properly reduces the risk for infection transmission and contamination of other items. Hand hygiene prevents the spread of microorganisms.

DOCUMENTATION

It is not usually necessary to document the preparation of a sterile field. However, documentation should be recorded regarding the use of sterile technique for any procedure performed using sterile technique.

UNEXPECTED SITUATIONS AND ASSOCIATED INTERVENTIONS

- *A part of the sterile field becomes contaminated:* When any portion of the sterile field becomes contaminated, discard all portions of the sterile field and start over.
- *The nurse realizes a supply is missing after setting up the sterile field:* Call for help. Do not leave the sterile field unattended. If the nurse is not able to visualize the sterile field at all times, it is considered contaminated.
- *The patient touches the sterile field:* If the patient touches the sterile field, discard the supplies and prepare a new sterile field. If the patient is confused, it is a good idea to have someone assist by holding the patient's hands and/or reinforcing what is happening.

Skill · 27-4 Putting on Sterile Gloves and Removing Soiled Gloves

EQUIPMENT

- Sterile gloves of the appropriate size
- PPE, as indicated

IMPLEMENTATION

ACTION	RATIONALE
1. Perform hand hygiene and put on PPE, if indicated.	Hand hygiene and PPE prevent the spread of microorganisms. PPE is required based on transmission precautions.
2. Identify the patient. Explain the procedure to the patient.	Patient identification validates the correct patient and correct procedure. Discussion and explanation help allay anxiety and prepare the patient for what to expect.

Putting on Sterile Gloves

ACTION	RATIONALE
3. Check that the sterile glove package is dry and unopened. Also, note expiration date, making sure that the date is still valid.	Moisture contaminates a sterile package. Expiration date indicates period that package remains sterile.
4. Place sterile glove package on clean, dry surface at or above your waist.	Moisture could contaminate the sterile gloves. Any sterile object held below the waist is considered contaminated.
5. Open the outside wrapper by carefully peeling the top layer back (Figure 1). Remove inner package, handling only the outside of it.	This maintains sterility of gloves in inner packet.
6. Place the inner package on the work surface with the side labeled "cuff end" closest to the body.	Allows for ease of glove application.
7. Carefully open the inner package. Fold open the top flap, then the bottom and sides (Figure 2). Take care not to touch the inner surface of the package or the gloves.	The inner surface of the package is considered sterile. The outer 1-inch border of the inner package is considered contaminated. The sterile gloves are exposed with the cuff end closest to the nurse.

FIGURE 1. Pulling top layer of outside wrapper back.

FIGURE 2. Folding back side flaps.

8. With the thumb and forefinger of the nondominant hand, grasp the folded cuff of the glove for dominant hand, touching only the exposed inside of the glove (Figure 3).

9. Keeping the hands above the waistline, lift and hold the glove up and off the inner package with fingers down (Figure 4). **Be careful it does not touch any unsterile object.**

Unsterile hand touches only inside of glove. Outside remains sterile.

Glove is contaminated if it touches any unsterile objects.

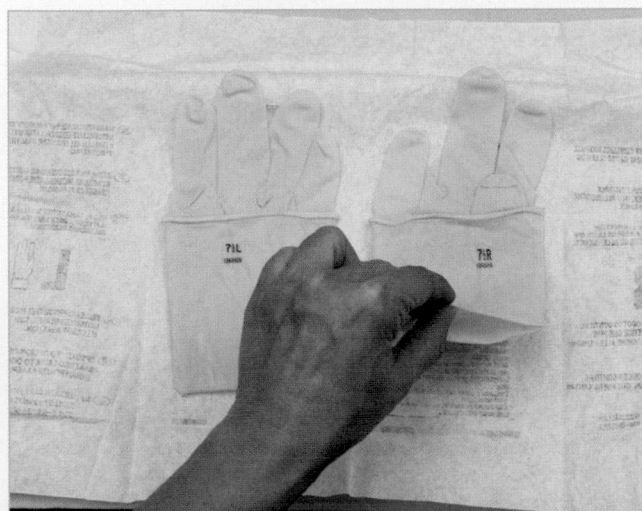

FIGURE 3. Grasping cuff of glove for dominant hand.

FIGURE 4. Lifting glove from package.

10. Carefully insert dominant hand palm up into glove (Figure 5) and pull glove on. Leave the cuff folded until the opposite hand is gloved.

11. Hold the thumb of the gloved hand outward. Place the fingers of the gloved hand inside the cuff of the remaining glove (Figure 6). Lift it from the wrapper, taking care not to touch anything with the gloves or hands.

Attempting to turn upward with unsterile hand may result in contamination of sterile glove.

Thumb is less likely to become contaminated if held outward. Sterile surface touching sterile surface prevents contamination.

(continued)

Skill · 27-4   Putting on Sterile Gloves and Removing Soiled Gloves   *continued*

ACTION

FIGURE 5. Inserting dominant hand into glove.

12. Carefully insert nondominant hand into glove. Pull the glove on, taking care that the skin does not touch any of the outer surfaces of the gloves.

13. **Slide the fingers of one hand under the cuff of the other and fully extend the cuff down the arm, touching only the sterile outside of the glove (Figure 7). Repeat for the remaining hand.**

14. **Adjust gloves on both hands if necessary, touching only sterile areas with other sterile areas (Figure 8).**

FIGURE 7. Sliding fingers of one hand under cuff of other hand and extending cuff down the arm.

15. Continue with procedure as indicated.

Removing Soiled Gloves

16. Use dominant hand to grasp the opposite glove near cuff end on the outside exposed area. Remove it by pulling it off, inverting it as it is pulled, keeping the contaminated area on the inside (Figure 9). Hold the removed glove in the remaining gloved hand.

RATIONALE

FIGURE 6. Sliding fingers under cuff of glove for nondominant hand.

Sterile surface touching sterile surface prevents contamination.

Sterile surface touching sterile surface prevents contamination.

Sterile surface touching sterile surface prevents contamination.

FIGURE 8. Adjusting gloves as necessary.

Contaminated area does not come in contact with hands or wrists.

ACTION

RATIONALE

FIGURE 9. Inverting glove as it is removed.

17. Slide fingers of ungloved hand between the remaining glove and the wrist (Figure 10). **Take care to avoid touching the outside surface of the glove.** Remove it by pulling it off, inverting it as it is pulled, keeping the contaminated area on the inside, and securing the first glove inside the second (Figure 11).

Contaminated area does not come in contact with hands or wrists.

FIGURE 10. Sliding fingers of ungloved hand inside remaining glove.

FIGURE 11. Inverting glove as it is removed, securing first glove inside it.

18. Discard gloves in appropriate container. Remove additional PPE, if used. Perform hand hygiene.

Proper disposal and removal of PPE reduces the risk for infection transmission and contamination of other items. Hand hygiene prevents the spread of microorganisms.

DOCUMENTATION

It is not usually necessary to document the addition of sterile items to a sterile field. However, documentation should be recorded regarding the use of sterile technique for any procedure performed using sterile technique.

UNEXPECTED SITUATIONS AND ASSOCIATED INTERVENTIONS

• *Contamination occurs during application of the sterile gloves:* Discard gloves and open new package of sterile gloves.

• *A hole or tear is noticed in one of the gloves:* Discard gloves and open new package of sterile gloves.

• *A hole or tear is noticed in one of the gloves during the procedure:* Stop procedure. Remove damaged gloves. Wash hands or perform hand hygiene (depending on whether soiled or not) and put on new sterile gloves.

(continued)

Skill · 27-4   Putting on Sterile Gloves and Removing Soiled Gloves   *continued*

- *The patient touches the nurse's hands or the sterile field:* If the patient touches the nurse's hands and nothing else, the nurse may remove the contaminated gloves and put on new, sterile gloves. It is always a good idea to bring two pairs of sterile gloves into the room, depending on facility policy. If the patient touches the sterile field, discard the supplies and prepare a new sterile field. If the patient is confused, it is a good idea to have someone assist you by holding the patient's hands or reinforcing what is happening.

- *Patient has a latex allergy:* Obtain latex-free sterile gloves.

● Developing Critical Thinking Skills

1. A nurse cannot help but notice that whenever a particular surgeon makes rounds, he ignores basic principles of asepsis. He will move from one patient to another, touching dressings without washing his hands between patients. He is also inconsistent in his practice of sterile technique. You suspect that there is a higher rate of postoperative infection among his patients. What do you do?

2. A friend who is a nursing student always wears gloves when doing anything for ill patients. You are more selective in your use of gloves. She tells you that you are a fool for "taking chances" because you never know what you may pick up and bring home. Should this be a matter of personal preference? Is one position more consistent with good nursing? Are your instructors consistent in how they would respond to the above question?

● Practicing for NCLEX

1. What are the smallest infectious agents capable of causing an infection?
   a. Bacteria
   b. Viruses
   c. Molds
   d. Yeasts

2. Your patient has developed a low-grade fever and states that she has felt very tired lately. You interpret these findings as indicating which stage of infection?
   a. Incubation period
   b. Prodromal stage
   c. Full stage of illness
   d. Convalescent period

3. Efforts by healthcare facilities to reduce the incidence of HAIs include an awareness of which of the following?
   a. The CDC requires all states to report HAI rates from each hospital.
   b. The gastrointestinal tract is a common site for HAIs.
   c. Joint Commission considers death or serious injury from HAIs a sentinel event
   d. The causal agent for most HAIs is viral.

4. A patient develops a urinary tract infection after an indwelling urinary catheter has been inserted. This would most accurately be termed as which type of infection?
   a. A viral infection
   b. A chronic infection
   c. An iatrogenic infection
   d. An opportunistic infection

5. The nurse has opened the sterile supplies and donned two sterile gloves to complete a sterile dressing change, a procedure that requires surgical asepsis. The nurse must do which of the following?
   a. Keep splashes on the sterile field to a minimum
   b. Cover the nose and mouth with gloved hands if a sneeze is imminent
   c. Use forceps soaked in a disinfectant
   d. Consider the outer 1 inch of the sterile field as contaminated

6. The CDC standard precaution recommendations apply to which of the following?
   a. Only patients with diagnosed infections
   b. Only blood and body fluids with visible blood
   c. All body fluids including sweat
   d. All patients receiving care in hospitals

7. In addition to standard precautions, the nurse caring for a patient with rubella would plan to implement what type of precautions?
   a. Droplet precautions
   b. Airborne precautions
   c. Contact precautions
   d. Universal precautions

8. When caring for a patient with latex allergy, the nurse creates a latex-safe environment by doing which of the following?
   a. Carefully cleaning the wall-mounted blood pressure device before using it
   b. Donning latex gloves outside the room to limit powder dispersal
   c. Using a latex-free pharmacy protocol
   d. Placing the patient in a semiprivate room

9. Which organization(s) initially developed the guidelines for minimum protection standards for infection prevention and control?
   a. OSHA
   b. Individual healthcare facilities
   c. The state governing body
   d. The CDC

10. Which of the following lists the recommended sequence for removing soiled personal protective equipment when the nurse prepares to leave the patient's room?
    a. Gown, goggles, mask, gloves, and exit the room
    b. Gloves, wash hands, remove gown, mask, and goggles
    c. Gloves, goggles, gown, mask, and wash hands
    d. Goggles, mask, gloves, gown, and wash hands

11. For a nurse under normal conditions with unsoiled hands, effective hand hygiene between patients requires which of the following?
    a. At least a 15-second scrub with plain soap and water
    b. At least a 23-minute scrub with an antimicrobial soap
    c. Use of an alcohol-based antiseptic handrub
    d. That a mask be worn when scrubbing

12. Which hospitalized patient is most at risk for developing a healthcare-associated infection?
    a. Mr. Y, a 60-year-old patient who smokes two packs of cigarettes daily
    b. Mrs. J, a 40-year-old patient who has a white blood cell count of 6,000/mm^3
    c. Mr. L, a 65-year-old patient who has an indwelling urinary catheter in place
    d. Mrs. M, a 60-year-old patient who is a vegetarian and slightly underweight

13. A patient develops food poisoning from contaminated potato salad. What is the means of transmission for the infecting organism?
    a. Direct contact
    b. Vector
    c. Vehicle
    d. Airborne

14. A nurse is caring for an obese 62-year-old patient with arthritis who has developed an open reddened area over his sacrum. Which of the following is a priority nursing diagnosis?
    a. Imbalanced Nutrition: More Than Body Requirements related to immobility
    b. Impaired Physical Mobility related to pain and discomfort
    c. Chronic Pain related to immobility
    d. Risk for Infection related to altered skin integrity

15. The nurse teaches a patient at home to use clean technique when changing a wound dressing. This is which of the following?
    a. The nurse's preference
    b. Safe for the home setting
    c. Unethical behavior
    d. Grossly negligent

● Answers With Rationale

1. **b.** A virus is the smallest of all microorganisms and can be seen only with a special microscope. Molds and yeasts (fungi) and bacteria are larger infectious agents.

2. **b.** During the prodromal stage, the person has vague signs and symptoms, such as fatigue and a low-grade fever. There are no obvious symptoms of infection during the incubation period, and they are more specific during the full stage of illness, before disappearing by the convalescent period.

3. **c.** According to the Joint Commission, death or serious injury caused by an infection-related event is considered a sentinel event and must be reported. Currently, more than twenty states have legislation requiring that HAI rates be reported to the CDC. The gastrointestinal tract is not particularly prone to HAIs. Bacteria cause most HAIs.

4. **c.** An infection that develops as a result of the insertion of an indwelling catheter is termed iatrogenic. Because this infection just developed, it is not chronic, nor did it occur because of any altered physiology that may give an opportunistic organism a chance to cause infection. Urinary infections are bacterial, not viral.

5. **d.** Considering the outer inch of a sterile field as contaminated is a principle of surgical asepsis. Moisture such as from splashes contaminates the sterile field, and sneezing would contaminate the sterile gloves. Forceps soaked in disinfectant are not considered sterile.

6. **d.** Standard precautions apply to all patients receiving care in hospitals, regardless of their diagnosis or possible infection status. These recommendations include blood, all body fluids, secretions, and excretions except sweat, nonintact skin, and mucous membranes.

7. **a.** Rubella is an illness transmitted by large-particle droplets and requires droplet precautions in addition to standard precautions. Airborne precautions are used for patients who have infections spread through the air with small particles, for example, tuberculosis, varicella, and rubeola. Universal precautions and body-substance isolation are incorporated into the new CDC standard precautions recommendations.

8. **c.** A latex-free pharmacy protocol is a vital component when creating a safe environment for this patient. Wall-mounted blood pressure devices have latex tubing and should not be touched or used on the patient. Latex gloves could cause a serious allergic response; only synthetic gloves are allowed in a latex-free environment. A private room is best to minimize the possibility of latex exposure from something used for the other patient.

9. *d.* The CDC established the initial minimum requirements for infection prevention and control. OSHA has issued and monitors regulations for use of infection control precautions in situations and settings in which exposure to blood and other infectious materials is possible.

10. *c.* Gloves are always removed first because they are most likely to be contaminated, and hands should be washed thoroughly after the equipment has been removed and before leaving the room.

11. *c.* Hands that are not visibly soiled can be effectively cleaned with an alcohol-based handrub. Neither a mask nor an antimicrobial soap is required in this situation or setting. Hands that are visibly soiled require a wash with either a nonantimicrobial soap and water or an antimicrobial soap and water.

12. *c.* Indwelling urinary catheters have been implicated in most healthcare-associated infections. Cigarette smoking, a normal white blood cell count, and a vegetarian diet have not been implicated as risk factors for HAIs.

13. *c.* Contaminated food is a vehicle for transmitting an infection. Direct contact requires proximity between the susceptible host and an infected person. A vector is a nonhuman carrier, such as an insect, and the airborne means of transmission carries the organism in droplet nuclei or with dust.

14. *d.* The priority diagnosis in this situation is the possibility of an infection developing in the open skin area. The others may be potential or probable diagnoses for this patient and may also require nursing interventions after the first diagnosis is addressed.

15. *b.* In the home setting, where the patient's environment is more controlled, medical asepsis is usually recommended, with the exception of self-injection. This is the appropriate procedure for the home and is neither unethical nor grossly negligent.

Taylor Suite Resources

The Taylor Suite offers these additional resources to enhance learning and facilitate understanding of this chapter:

- thePoint online resource, http://thepoint.lww.com/Taylor7E
- Student DVD-ROM included with the book
- Study Guide for Taylor's Fundamentals of Nursing
- Skill Checklists for Taylor's Fundamentals of Nursing
- Taylor's Clinical Nursing Skills: *Chapter 4, Asepsis and Infection Control*
- Taylor's Video Guide to Clinical Nursing Skills: *Asepsis*

BIBLIOGRAPHY

Association for Professionals in Infection Control and Epidemiology (APIC). (2005). *Hand hygiene for healthcare workers.* Available at http://www.apic.org/AM/Template.cfm?Section=Search&section=Brochures&template=/CM/ContentDisplay.cfm&ContentFileID=297.

Association for Professionals in Infection Control and Epidemiology (APIC). (2008a). *Healthcare-associated reporting laws and regulation.* Available at: http://www.apic.org/am/images/maps/mandrpt_map.gif

Association for Professionals in Infection Control and Epidemiology (APIC). (2008b). *New name for infection control profession.* Available at http://www.apic.org/AM/Template.cfm?Section&Search&section=News_Release&template=CM/ContentDisplay.cfm&ContentFileID=10729

Austin, N. (2007). A nurse's battle with *C. diff. RN, 70*(3), 39–43.

Centers for Disease Control and Prevention (CDC). (2002). Guideline for hand hygiene in health-care settings. *Morbidity and Mortality Weekly Report 2002, 51*(RR16), 1–45.

Centers for Disease Control and Prevention (CDC). (2007). *MRSA in healthcare settings.* Available at http:www.cdc.gov/ncidod/dhqp/ar_MRSA_spotlight_2006.html

Centers for Disease Control and Prevention (CDC), Healthcare Infection Control Practices Advisory Committee (HICPAC). (2005). *Guidance on reporting of healthcare-associated infections.* Available at http://www.cdc.gov/ncidod/hip/PublicReportingGuide.pdf.

Cooper, E. (2008). VRE: How you can stop the spread of this drug-resistant organism. *RN, 71*(2), 27–31.

Delahanty, K., & Myers, F. (2007). Infection control survey report. *Nursing, 37*(6), 28–36.

Girard, N. (2004). AORN latex guideline. *AORN Journal, 79*(3), 653–656.

Graves, P., & Twomey, C. (2002). The changing face of hand protection. *AORN Journal, 76*(2), 248–264.

Grossman, S., & DeBartolomeo Mager, D. (2008). Managing the threat of methicillin-resistant Staphylococcus aureus in home care. *Home Healthcare Nurse, 26*(6), 356–366.

Haas, J., & Larsen, E. (2008). Compliance with hand hygiene guidelines: Where are we in 2008? *American Journal of Nursing, 108*(8), 40–45.

Hilburn, J., Hammond, B., Fendler, E., & Groziak, P. (2003). Use of alcohol hand sanitizer as an infection control strategy in an acute care facility. *American Journal of Infection Control, 31*(2), 109–116.

Holcomb, S. (2008). MRSA infections. *Nursing, 38*(6), 33.

Institute for Healthcare Improvement (IHI). (2006a). *How to guide: Improving hand hygiene, A guide for improving practices among health care workers.* Cambridge, MA.

Institute for Healthcare Improvement (IHI). (2006b). *Protecting 5 million lives from harm.* Available at http://www.ihi.org/IHI/Programs/Campaign/Campaign.htm?TabID=1

Jackson, M., Chiarello, L., & Gaynes, R. (2002). Nurse staffing and health care-associated infections: Proceedings from a working group meeting. *American Journal of Infection Control, 30*(4), 199–206.

Kjonegaard, R., & Myers, F. (2005). Arresting drug-resistant organisms. *Nursing, 35*(6), 48–50.

Klein, E., Smith, D., & Laxminaray, R. (2007). Hospitalizations and deaths caused by methicillin-resistant *Staphylococcus aureus* United States, 1999–2005. Emerging *Infectious Diseases, 13*(12), 1840–1846.

Klevens, R., Edwards, J., Richards, C., Horan, T., Gaynes, R., Pollock, D., & Cardo, D. (2007). Estimating health care-associated infections and deaths in U.S. hospitals, 2002. *Public Health Reports, 122*, 160–166.

Kurtzman, E., & Buerhaus, P. (2008). New Medicare payment rules: Danger or opportunity for nursing? *American Journal of Nursing, 108*(6), 30–35.

Leung-Chen, P. (2008a). Dengue fever: Coming soon to a hospital near you? *American Journal of Nursing, 108*(4), 26–28.

Leung-Chen, P. (2008b). Everybody's crying MRSA. *American Journal of Nursing, 108*(8), 29–31.

McCaughey, B. (2008). *Unnecessary deaths: The human and financial cost of hospital infections* (3rd ed.). Committee to Reduce Infection Deaths (rid). Available at http://www.hospitalinfection.org.

McGoldrick, M., & Rhinehart, E. (2007). Managing multidrugresistant organisms in home care and hospice: Surveillance, prevention, and control. *Home Healthcare Nurse, 25*(9), 580–588.

North American Nursing Diagnosis Association (NANDA) International. (2009). *Nursing diagnoses: Definitions & classifications 2009–2011*. West Sussex, UK: Wiley-Blackwell.

Occupational Safety & Health Administration (OSHA). (2005). *Latex allergy OSHA standards.* Available at http://www.osha.gov/SLTC/latexallergy/standards.html.

Oriolo, S. (2006). *C. difficile*: A menace in hospitals and homes alike. *Nursing, 36*(8), 14–15.

Porth, C. (2007). *Essentials of pathophysiology: Concepts of altered health states (2nd ed.).* Philadelphia: Lippincott Williams & Wilkins.

Rupp, M., Fitzgerald, T., Puumala, M., Anderson, J. R., Craig, R., Iwen, P. C., Jourdan, D., et al. (2008). Prospective, controlled, cross-over trial of alcohol-based hand gel in critical care units. *Infection Control & Hospital Epidemiology, 29*, 8–15.

Scott, E., Duty, S., & Callahan, M. (2008). A pilot study to isolate *Staphylococcus aureus* and methicillin-resistant *S. aureus* from environmental surfaces in the home. *American Journal of Infection Control, 36*(6), 458–60.

Siegel, J., Rhinehart, E., Jackson, M., & Chiarello, L. (2006). *Management of Multidrug-Resistant Organisms in Healthcare Settings, 2006.* Available at http://www.cdc.gov/hicpac/pdf/isolation/Isolation2007.pdf

Siegel, J., Rhinehart, E., Jackson, M., & Chiarello, L. (June 2007). *Guideline for isolation precautions: Preventing transmission of infectious agents in healthcare settings 2007.* Available at http://www.cdc.gov/ncidod/dhqp/pdf/guidelines/Isolation2007.pdf

Smeltzer, S., Bare, B., Hinkle, J. H., Cheever, K. H. (2010). *Brunner & Suddarth's textbook of medical-surgical nursing* (12th ed.). Philadelphia: Lippincott Williams & Wilkins.

Stone, P., & Gershon, R. (2007). Nurse work environments and occupational safety in intensive care units. *Medical Care, 45*(6), 571–578.

The Joint Commission. (2010). 2010 Hospital National Patient Safety Goals. Available at http://www.jointcommission.org/NR/rdonlyres/E4ADEAB0-10C6-494A-9EE4-FDBC28337D65/0/HAP_2010_NPSG.pdf

Todd, B. (2006a). Beyond MRSA: VISA and VRSA. *American Journal of Nursing, 106*(4), 28–30.

Todd, B. (2006b). *Clostridium difficile*: Familiar pathogen, changing epidemiology. *American Journal of Nursing, 106*(5), 33–36.

Valente, S. (2007). Keep *C. difficile* at bay. *Nursing, 37*(10), 56hn1.

Vrtis, M. (2008). Is your patient taking the right antimicrobial? *American Journal of Nursing, 108*(6), 49–55.

U.S. Food and Drug Administration (FDA). (2008). *FDA clears glove made from new type of latex.* Available at http://www.fda.gov/bbs/topics/NEWS/2008/NEW01822.html

Walker, B. (2007). New guidelines for fighting multidrug-resistant organisms. *Nursing, 37*(5), 20.

World Health Organization. (2009). WHO guidelines on hand hygiene in health care. Available at http://whqlibdoc.who.int/publications/2009/9789241597906_eng.pdf

Yamamoto, L., & Marten, M. (2007). Listen up MRSA: The bug stops here. *Nursing, 37*(12), 50–55.

28 Complementary and Alternative Therapies

BRIAN LEGETT

Brian, a 30-year-old man with a long history of back problems due to a work injury, comes to the clinic for evaluation. He states, "I've had so many kinds of treatment, and nothing seems to work. Maybe I should see a chiropractor?"

SYLVIA PUENTES

Sylvia, a middle-aged woman, is scheduled for abdominal surgery next week. She comes to the outpatient clinic for preoperative evaluation and laboratory testing and says, "I'm really anxious about the surgery, but I don't want to take any medicines. Is there anything I can do to help me relax?"

LEE CHEN

Lee, a 65-year-old man dying of lung cancer, was brought to the United States from China by his two daughters, who believed that U.S. medicine would cure him. Mr. Chen did not respond to any of the therapies that were attempted, and the team wants to transition to palliative care. The daughters are unwilling to authorize removal of ventilatory support or sign a do-not-resuscitate order. They request an acupuncturist, but the physician refuses their request.

LEARNING OBJECTIVES

After completing the chapter, you will be able to accomplish the following:

1. Differentiate complementary and alternative medicine from allopathic medicine.

2. Compare and contrast the beliefs about the origin of disease and ways to promote health of each of the five main categories of CAM/CAT.

3. Describe ways in which nurses can use knowledge of complementary and alternative modalities in providing patient care.

4. Identify the knowledge the public should possess about CAT if they wish to be informed consumers.

5. Describe ways in which nurses can use selected complementary and alternative modalities for self-care and health promotion.

KEY TERMS

acupuncture	imagery
allopathic medicine	integrative care
alternative modalities	intercessory prayer
aromatherapy	meridian
aura	naturopathic medicine
Ayurveda	qi
chakra	qi gong
chiropractic medicine	relaxation response
complementary therapies	shamanism
	Therapeutic Touch (TT)
dosha	Traditional Chinese Medicine (TCM)
Healing Touch (HT)	
holism	Yin
holistic nursing	Yang
homeopathy	

Many people in the United States are using complementary and alternative therapies (CAT) to promote health and assist with healing from illness. The term "complementary and alternative therapies" refers to interventions that are **complementary therapies** (they can be used with traditional medical interventions and thus complement them) as well as **alternative modalities** (not included in the scope of conventional medical care). However, CAT are neither standardized nor part of an existing system, as is conventional medical care. The term "complementary and alternative medicine" (CAM) is widely used; however, many nurses use CAT instead,

because people without medical degrees practice CAM/CAT. This chapter discusses basic CAT that a practicing nurse needs to understand to provide safe nursing care.

Nurses need to be knowledgeable about CAT primarily for three reasons. First, patients, families, physicians, and institutions increasingly expect practicing nurses to be knowledgeable about CAT. Many patients use these types of therapies as outpatients and want to continue their use as inpatients. They or family members may expect nurses to administer herbal preparations or nutritional supplements. It is not uncommon for individuals to retain ethnic healthcare practices although they reside in the United States. In this situation, nurses can assist patients by accommodating special healing practices as much as possible. Also, as evidence grows demonstrating the effectiveness of selected CAT, many institutions now provide complementary therapies to inpatients as part of total patient care. See the accompanying Reflective Practice display.

Second, many nurses are expanding their clinical practice by incorporating CAT. Many state Boards of Nursing recognize select alternative/complementary modalities as part of nursing practice and have provisions for the safe practice of these modalities by registered nurses.

Finally, although CAT may seem totally safe, some therapies have led to harmful and at times lethal outcomes. Nurses play an important role in educating the public about how these therapies can be used safely and effectively. This chapter will provide helpful resources for education.

INTRODUCTION TO COMPLEMENTARY AND ALTERNATIVE THERAPIES

Although the use of most complementary and alternative therapies predates modern medicine, it was not until recently that nursing and medical schools began to teach about their use. The sharp divide between traditional medicine and CAT has now softened, and successful practitioners know how to combine the two.

Traditional Medicine and CAT

Allopathic medicine (or biomedicine) has been dominant for about 100 years and has spearheaded remarkable advances in biotechnology, surgical interventions, pharmaceutical approaches, and diagnostic tools. Allopathic medical care is particularly effective when aggressive treatment is needed in emergency or acute situations.

However, allopathic medical care has not been totally effective in dealing with chronic illness, a persistent problem. Increasingly, CAT are being used as an "answer" to the problem of chronic illness. The CAT and allopathic systems differ fundamentally in several ways (Table 28-1). Until recently, the majority of decision making in CAT has been based on observation, experience, and traditional healing manuscripts in contrast to allopathic medicine, which has moved away from these methodologies to evidence-based practice.

Many CAT are based on a theory and philosophy of holism upon which holistic nursing also is based. Many practitioners and consumers of healthcare choose to combine allopathic

REFLECTIVE PRACTICE

Challenge to Cognitive Skills

This spring, while working on an oncology floor, I was caring for Lee Chen, a 65-year-old man dying of lung cancer. His two daughters, who were living in the United States, had brought him from China to the United States, believing that U.S. medicine would cure him. Unfortunately, Mr. Chen had not responded to any of the therapies that were attempted, and all of his professional caregivers believed that the goal of treatment should now be preparation for a comfortable and dignified death using compassionate palliative care. His daughters, however, were unwilling to accept this goal and would not authorize removing him from ventilatory support or issuing a do-not-resuscitate order. Mr. Chen could no longer speak on his own behalf. One afternoon, one of his daughters informed Mr. Chen's physician that she was going to bring an acupuncturist in to work on her father. The physician told her in no uncertain terms that he would not allow "voodoo medicine" on his unit. I wasn't sure what to do, because both daughters were growing more and more upset, and this answer seemed like the "last straw."

Thinking Outside the Box: Possible Courses of Action

- Accept the status quo and try to comfort the daughters.
- Support the physician's judgment and try to get the daughters to see things his way.
- Learn more about acupuncture and related benefits and harms (I have never seen it done and know very little about what to expect).
- Find out if the physician really had the authority to forbid acupuncture on this patient.
- Advocate for the patient and his family if there is a possibility that acupuncture will benefit him.

Evaluating a Good Outcome: How Do I Define Success?

- Patient receives culturally appropriate care consistent with the goals of compassionate palliative care.
- The patient is not harmed.
- Mr. Chen's daughters feel supported as they struggle with decisions and anticipatory grieving.
- All healthcare team members (including Mr. Chen's physician) learn about acupuncture and other comple-
- mentary and alternative therapies, as well as about the hospital's policies regarding their use.
- The physician is confronted in a professional manner about the behavior as increasing the stress on the family caregivers.
- I grow in my knowledge of how to incorporate CAM into my care.

Personal Learning: Here's to the Future!

I was so upset by the daughters' distress that I decided to learn more about acupuncture. After searching the Internet and talking with a nurse who was receiving acupuncture treatments, I decided that acupuncture treatments were unlikely to harm the patient; in fact, the treatments just might help to increase his comfort level. At the very least, Mr. Chen's daughters would believe that we respected and supported their efforts to help their father. I was also hopeful that the professional caregiving team would learn more about culturally competent care. When I spoke with the head nurse, she was understanding about my goals and actually confronted Mr. Chen's doctor and secured his approval for having the acupuncturist visit. I learned that the acupuncturist had to be credentialed by our hospital. While Mr. Chen's cancer did not respond to the acupuncture treatment, he did seem more comfortable, and his daughters couldn't thank me enough. I talked with them about how impressive their devotion to their father was and also mentioned that they may need to give him one last gift, the gift of "letting go." Unfortunately, I never saw this family again because this was my last week on this unit.

Melinda Ventura, Georgetown University

Reflection

How do you think you would respond in a similar situation? Why? What does this tell you about yourself and about the adequacy of your skills for professional practice? Can you think of other ways to respond? What factors do you think may have played a role in the physician's answer? How did the nursing student promote culturally competent care? Imagine if the nursing student (rather than the head nurse) had approached the physician to allow the acupuncturist to visit. Do you think that the physician's answer would have been the same as it was when the head nurse confronted him? Please explain why or why not. What other skills (cognitive, interpersonal, technical, ethical/legal) would you need to respond well in this situation? Do you agree with the criteria to evaluate a successful outcome? Did the nursing student meet the criteria? Please explain.

Table • 28-1	BELIEFS UNDERLYING COMPLEMENTARY AND ALTERNATIVE THERAPIES AND THE ALLOPATHIC THERAPIES	
Complementary and Alternative Therapies	**Allopathic Therapies**
Mind, body, and spirit are integrated and together influence health and illness.	Illness occurs in either the mind or the body, which are separate entities.
Health is a balance of body systems: mental, social and spiritual, as well as physical.	Health is the absence of disease.
Illness is a manifestation of imbalance or disharmony.	The main causes of illness are considered to be pathogens (bacteria or viruses) or biochemical imbalances.
Symptoms are a sign or reflection of a deeper instability within the person; restoring physical and mental harmony will alleviate the symptoms. Healing is a slow process that involves the whole person.	Curing seeks to destroy the invading organism or repair the affected part.
Emphasis is on health. Healing is done by the patient; care is individualized.	Emphasis is on disease and high technology. Drugs, surgery, and radiation are among the key tools for dealing with the medical problems.

modalities and CAT using an integrative approach. These concepts are discussed below.

Holism

Holism is a theory and philosophy that focuses on connections and interactions between parts of the whole. In contrast, the prevailing scientific approach has focused on reductionism, the goal of which is to reduce all phenomena to the smallest possible atom, particle, or interaction. Using a holistic perspective, all living organisms, including humans, are continuously connecting and interacting with their environment. Further, parts of the organism, whether they are systems, subsystems, or cells, are also continuously interacting and changing. This continual interaction and change means that the body is not the sum of its parts (as in reductionism), but that it is a unified, dynamic whole.

Although one might view holism as a recently developed belief system, holism in fact was the predominant belief throughout history until sometime before René Descartes, a French philosopher who lived in the early part of the 17th century. He and other influential thinkers asserted that the mind and body were separate from each other. That belief lasted until the early 20th century, when researchers began to prove that there was a connection between the mind and the body.

One of the 20th-century researchers, Hans Selye, developed the term "general adaptation syndrome" (GAS) to describe the general holistic pattern that emerges when people experience stress/illness. The GAS reflects a general response that occurs in various parts of the body. This theory holds that when a person is sick, he or she is "sick all over," not just where symptoms manifest. Selye also demonstrated that adrenal exhaustion can be caused by emotional tension, such as suppressed rage or frustration. (For more on the GAS, see Chapter 42.)

A holistic philosophy underlies many CAT. People have a mind, body, emotions, and spirit that are connected and function as a unified whole. A change in any part of the organism will be reflected in other parts. When someone feels the emotion of sadness, he or she may have a physical response of crying. In addition, when a person feels stressed and overwhelmed, the face and body language frequently reflect these conditions.

Holistic nursing is nursing practice built on a holistic philosophy. Since holism is a philosophy and not a specific nursing role, holistic nurses can be found in all varieties of healthcare settings as well as in independent practice settings. In addition, holistic nurses frequently add CAT to their practice. Most holistic nurses use CAT for self-care, an essential component of holistic practice. The American Holistic Nurse Association (AHNA) promotes the education of nurses, other healthcare professionals, and the public in all aspects of holistic caring and healing. The efforts of AHNA recently resulted in the recognition of holistic nursing as an "official nursing specialty" by the American Nurses Association. In 2000, the American Holistic Nursing Association published standards for holistic nursing practice (Frisch, Dossey, Guzzetta, & Quinn, 2000). Registered nurses can become certified in basic and advanced holistic nursing through the American Holistic Nurses' Certification Corporation (AHNCC).

Integrative Care

A person who uses **integrative care** uses some combination of allopathic medicine and CAT (Table 28-2). There are several types of integrative care models used throughout the United States, and they can be housed in virtually all healthcare delivery structures. Optimally, these models include sensitive and knowledgeable healthcare providers who work with patients to design a plan of care that combines the best

TABLE • 28-2	INTEGRATIVE CARE OF THE COMMON COLD*
Complementary and Alternative Therapies	**Allopathic Approaches**
Acupuncture to appropriate areas to reduce sinus congestion	Decongestant over-the-counter medications
Rest and fluids	Rest and fluids
Herbs, vitamin C to stimulate immune system	Vitamin C to stimulate immune system

*In this example, adding herbs and/or acupuncture to a typical allopathic approach would represent integrative care.

of allopathic medicine and CAT while avoiding harmful interactions and which is responsive to the patient's preferences.

CAT and Nursing

CAT consists of a large variety of therapies that are based on a set of beliefs different from those of allopathic medicine. Some of these modalities have developed fairly recently (e.g., guided imagery), while others have been used for thousands of years as components of ancient healing systems (e.g., Ayurveda or traditional Chinese medicine). Some therapies can be used effectively without assistance (e.g., nutritional approaches, deep breathing exercises), while others (e.g., naturopathy, acupuncture) are more effective when used with guidance from practitioners who have particular knowledge and expertise.

Many people use CAT for stress management/reduction. Techniques such as relaxation with focused breathing, meditation, imagery, biofeedback, and massage are used in all stages of health and illness to promote healing and/or manage symptoms. Because stress can contribute to illness, CAT can sometimes be effective in reducing symptoms and enhancing quality of life, and nurses can assist clients—and themselves—with these therapies.

> *Recall Sylvia Puentes, the anxious patient scheduled for surgery. The nurse's knowledge of CAT would be important in helping this patient to reduce her preoperative anxiety. The nurse could discuss various methods available, allowing the patient to select the one that seems best for her. Such actions help develop a trusting nurse–patient relationship and foster a sense of self-esteem in the patient by allowing her to participate in the plan of care and decision making.* ∎

Use of CAT in the United States

The most comprehensive and reliable findings to date on Americans' use of CAT are released by the National Center

for Complementary and Alternative Medicine (NCCAM) and the National Center for Health Statistics (NCHS), part of the Centers for Disease Control and Prevention). The findings below are based on the 2008 edition of the NCHS's National Health Interview Survey (NHIS), an annual study in which tens of thousands of Americans are interviewed about their health- and illness-related experiences (Barnes, Bloom, & Nahin, 2008). The report is available, along with a press release and graphics, at nccam.nih.gov/news/camstats/.

Prevalence of CAT

The 2007 survey found that in the United States, approximately 38% of adults (about 4 in 10) and approximately 12% of children (about 1 in 9) were using some form of CAT in the 12 months before the survey. Consistent with results from the 2002 NHIS, in 2007, CAT use was more prevalent among women, adults aged 30 to 69, adults with higher levels of education, adults who were not poor, adults living in the West, former smokers, and adults who were hospitalized in the last year. For adults younger than 65 years of age, in 2002 and 2007, those with private health insurance were more likely than those with public health insurance or uninsured adults to use CAT.

There also are cultural variations. The breakdown of CAT use by race or ethnicity among adults is as follows: American Indian/Alaska Native 50.3%, White 43.1%, Asian 39.9%, Black 25.5%, and Hispanic 23.7%.

Reasons for Using CAT

People use CAT for an array of diseases and conditions. Generally, persons who choose CAT approaches are seeking ways to improve their health and well-being or to relieve symptoms associated with chronic, even terminal, illnesses or the side effects of conventional treatments for them. Other reasons for choosing to use CAT include having a holistic health philosophy or a transformational experience that changes one's worldview and wanting greater control over one's own health. For example, American adults are most likely to use CAT for musculoskeletal problems such as back, neck, or joint pain. However, the use of CAT for head or chest colds decreased from 2002 to 2007.

Most Frequently Used CAT

In 2007, the CAT most commonly used by U.S. adults in the past 12 months were nonvitamin, nonmineral, natural products (17.7%); deep breathing exercises (12.7%); meditation (9.4%); chiropractic or osteopathic manipulation (8.6%); massage (8.3%); and yoga (6.1%). Among U.S. adults, the use of some mind–body therapies, specifically deep breathing exercises, meditation, and yoga, increased between 2002 and 2007. Between 2002 and 2007, increased use was also seen for acupuncture, massage therapy, and naturopathy. Between 2002 and 2007, there was a significant decrease in the use of the Atkins diet.

Use of CAT with Children

In 2007, the CAT most commonly used by U.S. children in the past 12 months included nonvitamin, nonmineral, natural products (3.9%); chiropractic or osteopathic manipulation (2.8%); deep breathing exercises (2.2%); yoga (2.1%); and homeopathic treatment (1.3%). Children whose parents used CAT were about twice as likely as all U.S. children to have used nonvitamin, nonmineral, natural products (9.2% and 3.9%); chiropractic or osteopathic manipulation (5.7% and 2.8%); deep breathing exercises (5.4% and 2.2%); yoga (4.7% and 2.1%); and homeopathic treatment (2.8% and 1.3%) in the past 12 months.

Growth of CAT Industry

The 2004 study of CAT use (Barnes Powell-Griner, McFann, & Nahin, 2004) reported that an *estimated* $36 billion to $47 billion were spent on CAT in 1997. Eighty-five percent of schools of nursing responding to a survey reported that CAT was included in their curricula (Fenton & Morris, 2003). Approximately two thirds of medical schools in the United States offer courses in CAT, either as elective or required courses. Insurers increasingly pay for selected CAT for particular identified conditions. Scores of private organizations provide classes and workshops for consumers as well as education and practical experience for healthcare providers.

Many private and governmental organizations have been developed to deal with CAT. The National Center for Complementary and Alternative Medicine (NCCAM) in the National Institutes of Health (NIH) funds research on CAT and is a great first resource for professionals and the pubic seeking information about CAT. See Box 28-1 for NCCAM's advice to the public about being an informed consumer. The special White House Commission on Complementary and Alternative Medicine Policy (WHCCAMP)

issued an extensive report in March 2002, addressing policy issues specific to CAT. The following are the 10 guiding principles they used before issuing recommendations (www.whccamp.hhs.gov/es.html, retrieved February 4, 2009):

1. A wholeness orientation in healthcare delivery.
2. Evidence of safety and efficacy.
3. The healing capacity of the person.
4. Respect for individuality.
5. The right to choose treatment.
6. An emphasis on health promotion and self-care.
7. Partnerships as essential to integrated healthcare.
8. Education as a fundamental healthcare service.
9. Dissemination of comprehensive and timely information.
10. Integral public involvement.

The U.S. Food & Drug Administration (FDA) is seeking to increase regulations for dietary supplements. Lastly, the Foundation for Alternative Medicine (NFAM) is engaged in international research to determine "best practices" for cancer treatment.

CAT CATEGORIES

NCCAM classifies the major CAT into five categories (or domains): whole medical systems, mind–body therapies, energy medicine, biologically based practices, and manipulative and body-based practices. Each category contains several therapies. For example, meditation is a therapy included in the mind–body category. Box 28-2 describes each of the categories. Table 28-3 lists examples of alternative treatments from these categories that work on pain, describing what they help and how they work. This chapter includes information on some of the most widely used CAT of interest to practicing nurses.

Box 28-1 **COMPLEMENTARY AND ALTERNATIVE MEDICINE (CAM): BE AN INFORMED CONSUMER**

- Take charge of your health by being an informed consumer.
- Talk with your healthcare providers when making any decisions about using complementary and alternative medicine (CAM). Your healthcare providers can give you advice based on your medical needs.
- If you are thinking about using a CAM therapy, learn the facts. Is it safe? Does it work?
- Find out what scientific studies have been done. It is not a good idea to use a CAM therapy simply because you have seen it in an advertisement or on a Web site or because people have told you that it worked for them.
- Keep in mind that the number of Web sites offering health-related resources grows every day. Many sites provide valuable information, while others may have information that is unreliable or misleading. To evaluate the quality of a Web site, take a look at who runs the site, who pays for

it, and the purpose of the site. Also, check out where the information comes from, how it is selected, and how current it is.
- Scientific research on many CAM therapies is relatively new, so information about safety and effectiveness may not be available for every therapy. However, many studies of CAM treatments are underway, and researchers are always learning more about CAM.
- You can find reliable information on CAM through the National Institutes of Health's National Center for Complementary and Alternative Medicine (NCCAM). The NCCAM Web site (http://nccam.nih.gov/) provides a variety of useful information as well as links to other trustworthy sources. You can also contact the NCCAM Clearinghouse staff (call toll-free at: 1-888-644-6226 or e-mail info@nccam.nih.gov for help).

From National Institutes of Health. http://nihseniorhealth.gov/cam/beaninformedconsumer/.

Box 28-2 CAT DOMAINS

Whole (or alternative) medical systems are similar to the Western, allopathic model in that they are complete systems of theory and practice. They consist of a set of beliefs about the origin of diseases, ways to promote health, and types of treatment.

Mind–body medicine uses a variety of techniques designed to enhance the mind's ability to affect bodily function and symptoms.

Energy medicine involves the use of energy fields, such as magnetic fields or biofields (energy fields that some believe surround and penetrate the human body).

Manipulative and body-based practices work with the structures and systems of the body, including bones and joints, soft tissues, and circulatory and lymphatic systems.

Biologically based practices include the use of botanicals (herbs), animal-derived extracts, vitamins, minerals, fatty acids, amino acids, proteins, prebiotics and probiotics, whole diets, and functional foods.

Source: National Center for Complementary and Alternative Medicine, http://www.nccam.nih.gov.

TABLE • 28-3 ALTERNATIVE TREATMENTS THAT WORK ON PAIN

Type	What They Help	How They Help	Examples
Movement-Based Therapies: Physical exercises and practices	Musculoskeletal pain, joint pain, and lower-back pain	By strengthening muscles supporting joints, improving alignment, and releasing endorphins	• **Physical therapy:** Specialized movements to strengthen weak areas of the body, often through resistance training • **Yoga:** An Indian practice of meditative stretching and posing • **Pilates:** A resistance regimen that strengthens core muscles • **Tai chi:** A slow, flowing Chinese practice that improves balance • **Feldenkrais:** A therapy that builds efficiency of movement
Nutritional and Herbal Remedies: Food choices and dietary supplements (ask your doctor before using supplements)	All chronic pain but especially abdominal discomfort, headaches, and inflammatory conditions, such as rheumatoid arthritis	By boosting the body's natural immunity, reducing pain-causing inflammation, soothing pain, and decreasing insomnia	• **Anti-inflammatory diet:** A Mediterranean eating pattern high in whole grains, fresh fruits, leafy vegetables, fish, and olive oil • **Omega-3 fatty acids:** Nutrients abundant in fish oil and flaxseed that reduce inflammation in the body • **Ginger:** A root that inhibits pain-causing molecules • **Turmeric:** A spice that reduces inflammation • **MSM:** Methylsulfonylmethane, a naturally occurring nutrient that helps build bone and cartilage
Mind–Body Medicine: Using the powers of the mind to produce changes in the body	All types of chronic pain	By reducing stressful (and, hence, pain-inducing) emotions such as panic and fear, and by refocusing attention on subjects other than pain	• **Meditation:** Focusing the mind on something specific (such as breathing or repeating a word or phrase) to quiet it • **Guided imagery:** Visualizing a particular outcome or scenario with the goal of mentally changing one's physical reality • **Biofeedback:** With a special machine, becoming alert to body processes, such as muscle tightening, to learn to control them • **Relaxation:** Releasing tension in the body through exercises such as controlled breathing

(continued)

TABLE • 28-3	**ALTERNATIVE TREATMENTS THAT WORK ON PAIN** *(continued)*		
Type	**What They Help**	**How They Help**	**Examples**
Energy Healing: Manipulating the electrical energy—called chi in Chinese medicine—emitted by the body's nervous system	Pain that lingers after an injury heals, as well as pain complicated by trauma, anxiety, or depression	By relaxing the body and the mind, distracting the nervous system, producing natural painkillers, activating natural pleasure centers, and manipulating chi	• **Acupuncture:** The insertion of hair-thin needles into points along the body's meridians, or energetic pathways, to stimulate the flow of energy throughout the body; proven helpful for postsurgical pain and dental pain, among other types • **Acupressure:** Finger pressure applied to points along the meridians, to balance and increase the flow of energy • **Chi gong:** Very slow, gentle physical movements, similar to tai chi, that cleanse the body and circulate chi • **Reiki:** Moving a practitioner's hands over the energy fields of the client's body to increase energy flow and restore balance
Physical Manipulation: Hands-on massage or movement of painful areas	Musculoskeletal pain, especially lower-back and neck pain; pain from muscle underuse or overuse; and pain from adhesions or scars	By restoring mobility, improving circulation, decreasing blood pressure, and relieving stress	• **Massage:** The manipulation of tissue to relax clumps of knotted muscle fiber, increase circulation, and release patterns of chronic tension • **Chiropractic:** Physically moving vertebrae or other joints into proper alignment, to relieve stress • **Osteopathy:** Realigning vertebrae, ribs, and other joints, as with chiropractic; osteopaths have training equivalent to that of medical doctors
Lifestyle Changes: Developing healthy habits at home and work	All types of chronic pain	By strengthening the immune system and enhancing well-being, and by reframing one's relationship to (and, thus, experience of) chronic pain	• **Sleep hygiene:** Creating an optimal sleep environment to get deep, restorative rest; strategies include establishing a regular sleep–wake schedule and minimizing light and noise. • **Positive work environment:** Having a comfortable workspace and control over one's activities to reduce stress and contribute to the sense of mastery over pain. • **Healthy relationships:** Nurturing honest and supportive friendships and family ties to ease anxiety that exacerbate pain. • **Exercise:** Regular activity to build strength and lower stress

Research shows these therapies can ease discomfort. For more information, visit the Web site of the National Center for Complementary and Alternative Medicine (www.nccam.nih.gov).
Used with permission. From Khazzoom, L. (2009, January & February). Drug free remedies for chronic pain. *AARP the Magazine,* p. 30.

Whole Medical Systems

A whole medical system (or alternative medical system) consists of a philosophy and theory about health and illness along with specific types of treatment. These systems have developed independently from allopathic medicine and are generally culturally based. Ayurveda, traditional Chinese medicine, shamanism (which includes native traditions), homeopathy, naturopathy, and chiropractic medicine are examples of whole medical systems.

Ayurveda

Ayurveda originated in the Vedic civilization of India about 4,000 years ago. "It is a science of life that delineates the diet, medicines, and behaviors that are beneficial or harmful for life. Ayurveda considers that balance among people, the

environment, and the larger cosmos is integral to human health" (Bright, 2002, p. 273).

Central to Ayurvedic medicine is understanding the patient's basic constitution, or **dosha.** The three doshas in Ayurvedic medicine are *vata* (changeable), *pitta* (intense), and *kapha* (relaxed). People can display one dosha predominately or can be a combination of two or three doshas. One's dosha can be equated with one's genetic make-up. A person whose doshas are balanced experiences, health, and well-being in mind, body, and spirit. Since each dosha has particular characteristics, when a dosha is out of balance, an individual typically displays signs and symptoms (including disease) characteristic of the imbalance. Imbalance in the doshas can be caused by a number of factors, including stress, lifestyle, and improper diet.

Diagnosis is made by information obtained in a detailed holistic history, review of symptoms, and selected physical observations. Ayurveda includes mind–body medicine and biologically based practices. Many treatment modalities are specific for each dosha and may include nutrition, exercise, herbs, breathing, meditation, massage, aromatherapy, and purification. The quality of care received from an Ayurvedic practitioner can vary considerably based on the practitioner's educational preparation. An individual can be certified as an Ayurvedic practitioner after attending a qualified 2-year program. In addition, there are prerequisites for background preparation.

YOGA

Yoga "has been practiced for thousands of years in India, where it is a way of life that includes ethical models for behavior and mental and physical exercises aimed at producing spiritual enlightenment" (Fontaine, 2005, p. 265). Yoga has developed as a component of Ayurveda. In the United States, yoga is practiced independently or paired with other health-promoting activities that assist people to achieve unity and wholeness.

Gate pose

Down dog pose

Tree pose

Virabhadrasana I pose
(Warrior I pose)

Parivrtta trikonasana
(Revolved triangle pose)

FIGURE 28-1. Sample yoga poses.

Generally, yoga consists of various physical postures that are practiced to promote strength and flexibility, increase endurance, promote relaxation, and reduce one's response to stress. Breathing exercises, posture awareness, spiritual practices, and mind–body centering can be added to the basic postures. Basic yoga postures are illustrated in Figure 28-1. Common types of yoga include:

- Ashtanga, which focuses on synchronizing breath with a fast-paced series of postures.
- Bikram, which is done in a 105-degree studio with 26 set postures.
- Iyengar, which focuses on proper alignment and holding poses for a relatively longer time.
- Kripaula, or "gentle yoga," which focuses on relaxation and coming into balance.

Special considerations may be necessary for patients who want to continue their Ayurvedic program. For example, some may have special dietary (e.g., vegetarian) needs, some may need time set aside for self-care such as meditation, and some may desire to continue taking an herbal/supplement. All precautions related to herbal and pharmaceutical interactions should be followed with Ayurvedic herbal preparations.

Yoga can be used throughout the life span. Some postures are contraindicated during menstruation, after surgery, and in the presence of disease. Consumers can buy yoga tapes or DVDs or attend yoga classes. Yoga instructors come from a variety of backgrounds and usually are happy to discuss their preparation and knowledge with potential students. Encourage patients to find a type of yoga that is compatible with their physical condition and goals.

Traditional Chinese Medicine

Traditional Chinese medicine (TCM) is similar to Ayurveda in at least two ways. First, TCM as a healing system is thousands of years old. Second, a principle of TCM is that the interaction of people with their environment is most significant in creating health.

"The concept most central to TCM is **qi** or chi (pronounced *chee*), which is translated as energy. Qi represents an invisible flow of energy that circulates through plants, animals, and people as well as the earth and sky" (Fontaine, 2005, p. 51).

Qi is further viewed as either yin or yang energy. **Yin** (cool, moist, dark) and **yang** (hot, dry, light) are opposites and complementary, and health is present when they are in balance in a person and his or her total environment. Conversely, an imbalance of yin and yang is considered to be the cause of illness.

The goal of the TCM diagnostic process is to arrive at the pattern of disharmony that is being manifested by the person. TCM practitioners obtain a holistic history; observe particular parts of the body, such as the tongue; and palpate pulses. TCM includes energy medicine and biology-based practices; treatment may consist of acupuncture, with or without moxibustion (burning an herb above the acupuncture needle), dietary prescriptions, herbs, massage, and energy exercises, such as qi gong. Accredited schools that provide TCM education require extensive college-level coursework followed by an educational program of about 4 years.

ACUPUNCTURE

Although records document the existence of traditional acupuncture treatments in China dating back 5,000 years, **acupuncture** has been prevalent in the United States only since the 1970s. Acupuncture gained national media attention in 1971 when James Reston, a correspondent for the *New York Times,* had an appendectomy in Beijing using acupuncture instead of general anesthesia and postoperative analgesia. Reston's reports of his experience stimulated significant interest in acupuncture and TCM.

> *Remember Lee Chen, the terminally ill patient whose daughters asked for an acupuncturist. When developing the plan of care, the nurse would need to investigate Mr. Chen's culture and examine the beliefs associated with acupuncture. Based on an understanding of this information, the nurse would be better prepared to advocate for the patient and daughters.* ■

Acupuncture addresses a person's qi. Qi is believed to flow vertically in the body through an intricate structure of 12 major **meridians,** energy circuits that nourish and support all cells and organs of the body (Bright, 2002) (Fig. 28-2). Acupuncture consists of placing very thin, short, sterile needles at particular acupoints, believed to be centers of nerve and vascular tissue, along a meridian

FIGURE 28-2. Acupuncture meridians.

FIGURE 28-3. Placement of acupuncture needles.

(Fig. 28-3). Acupuncture either increases or decreases the flow of qi (chi) along the meridian, restoring the balance of yin and yang. This change in the flow of energy contributes to healing.

> *Consider Mr. Chen, the terminally ill patient whose daughters requested that he receive acupuncture. Applying the theory underlying acupuncture's mechanism of action, the nurse would understand that the daughters' request is based on their belief and desire for their father's condition to improve. The nurse would incorporate this understanding in discussions with the daughters about their father's condition. In addition, the nurse would also begin assisting the daughters to "let go" and begin the grieving process should the patient's condition remain unchanged, even after the acupuncture.* ■

Acupuncture is used for a variety of reasons, including reducing pain, promoting adherence to substance abuse programs, and minimizing nausea and vomiting due to chemotherapy and pregnancy. Licensed acupuncturists have graduated from an accredited acupuncture school after significant college-level coursework. In addition, they have passed a licensure examination.

Acupuncture is generally provided in clinics or private offices, although it is possible for acupuncturists to provide acupuncture on inpatients. In this situation, patients may need up to 1 hour of uninterrupted time in bed while the needles are in place.

QI GONG

Qi gong is a system of postures, exercises (both gentle and dynamic), breathing techniques, and visualization that regulates the qi. "The majority of qi gong exercises or meditations enhance systemic health. They are designed to restore the healing system, the body's innate intelligence, so it knows how to correct and heal itself" (Horrigan, 2003, p. 86). Qi gong postures are illustrated in Figure 28-4. For techniques specific to particular diseases, a patient can consult a qi gong teacher. Tai chi, which many say developed from qi gong, has been used successfully in patients in long-term care facilities to promote balance and coordination.

As with yoga, qi gong can be learned through the use of videos/DVDs or in a class. Encourage those interested to ask potential instructors about their background and knowledge.

Shamanism

Shamanism has been the most widely practiced medical system on our planet. Shamanism originated with indigenous people in many geographic areas of the world, including Hawaii, Ecuador, Tibet, West Africa, Israel, Peru, Colombia, and East Asia. The Celtic and Hmong traditions also have established shamanic practices (Webb, 2004).

In shamanism, illness and other forms of distress are thought to originate in the spirit world. The shaman or medicine man/woman possesses the ability to access the spirit world, which is done on behalf of individuals or the community, and return to "ordinary reality" with information on the proper treatment. Treatment may consist of retrieving lost soul energy, restoring the individual to right relationship with the spirit world, and treating symptoms. General healing techniques involve native plants and herbs, animals, rituals, ceremonies, and purification techniques (Webb, 2004).

In the United States, many ethnic cultures commonly practice some form of shamanism, so the nurse needs to have an awareness of and tolerance for shamanic practice.

FIGURE 28-4. Qi gong postures.

For example, in the United States, traditional Hmong and Native American populations may have particular beliefs related to health and illness and practice specific ceremonies and rituals to properly care for the spirit of the deceased.

The American Cancer Society has a Web site that includes information about how different groups of individuals make treatment decisions. The Web site reports that the most common aspects of Native American healing include the use of herbal remedies, purifying rituals, shamanism, healing myths, and spiritual healing to treat illnesses of both the body and spirit. Traditional healers aim to "make whole" by restoring well-being and harmonious relationships with the community and the spirit of nature.

Nurses need to be aware of the beliefs of various ethnic groups. For example, Native American beliefs about healing include the following:

- Illness stems from spiritual problems
- Diseases are more likely to invade the body of a person who is imbalanced, has negative thinking, and lives an unhealthy lifestyle
- Spirit is an inseparable element of healing, and medicine is part of spirit
- Healing takes time
- The distractions of modern life interfere with potential healing agents
- Modern culture encourages us to maintain a low level of emotional awareness
- Ceremony is important to receive guidance and assistance from the spiritual dimension

Homeopathy

Samuel Hahnemann, a German physician, developed **homeopathy** approximately 200 years ago. Homeopathy is based on the belief of supporting the body while the symptoms are allowed to "run their course." Homeopaths believe that this process stimulates and strengthens the immune system and promotes healing (Bright, 2002).

The allopathic approach to dealing with illness is frequently to suppress symptoms; for example, acetaminophen can be given to reduce a fever. In contrast, homeopaths believe that when symptoms are suppressed in this manner, the condition "goes deeper" into the body, making it ultimately more difficult to cure.

Homeopathic practice is based on two fundamental laws. The Law of Similars states that a natural substance that produces a given symptom in a healthy person will cure it in a sick person. The Law of Infinitesimals states that the smallest dose possible will have the desired effect. Although these concepts may seem unusual, they are the same concepts that underlie contemporary immunization practice (Bright, 2002).

Classical homeopathy looks for individual patterns. "Homeopaths believe people get sick in individual ways, showing distinctive patterns of symptoms. . . . Homeopaths do not believe in the existence of 'disease entities' . . . Rather, they concern themselves only with identifying the particular pattern of symptoms of an individual patient" (Weil, 1988, pp. 8–9). Health is viewed as a condition of well-being and vitality.

Diagnosis is based on a thorough, holistic history and a determination of the pattern of the individual. Treatment (applying the Law of Similars) consists of matching the pattern the patient is exhibiting with a remedy that would create the same symptom pattern in a healthy person. Remedies in the proper dosages are prepared by clinicians.

Hahnemann himself took many of the remedies to establish what symptoms the remedies produced (Bright, 2002). Homeopathic remedies were effective against the epidemics of cholera, typhus, and scarlet fever in the 19th century in the United States and other countries. Today, homeopathy is practiced widely and is a part of the healthcare system in countries such as France, Great Britain, and Brazil. It is becoming more available in the United States (Bright, 2002).

According to the National Center for Homeopathy, homeopathy is practiced by a wide variety of healthcare practitioners, including medical doctors, osteopaths, naturopathic physicians, nurse practitioners, physician assistants, dentists, veterinarians, chiropractors, acupuncturists, nurse midwives, and podiatrists, as well as by professional homeopaths, who practice only homeopathy and are unlicensed in any other discipline.

The problem for the consumer is that the practitioner's level of competence in homeopathy often has little to do with his or her type of licensure. The best test of qualifications is whether they have been certified in homeopathy. The following are widely recognized credentials in classical homeopathy: CCH (Certified Classical Homeopath), DHt (Diplomate in Homeotherapeutics, available for MDs and DOs), and DHANP (Diplomate of the Homeopathic Academy of Naturopathic Physicians, available for naturopathic physicians). Another recognized certification is the Diplomate of the National Board of Homeopathic Examiners (DNBHE) (http://nationalcenterforhomeopathy.org/resources/find_homeopath.jsp).

Clinical homeopathy is a newer branch of homeopathy that treats particular constellations of symptoms. These remedies are available over the counter in health-food stores and some drugstores. Examples of these remedies include:

- Arnica, a topical cream or oral pellets used for muscle soreness or bruising, joint sprains or strains
- Calendula, an ointment applied to cuts, scrapes, burns, sores, and nonfungal eruptions
- Nux vomica, a remedy for stress, overwork, impatience, and irritability
- Ignatia, a remedy immediately following grief or loss, extreme sadness

Remedies can be counteracted by things such as strong chemicals, herbs, and pharmaceuticals. If a patient is using homeopathy for postoperative recovery, the remedy may be repeated several times because of all the potential antidotes in the environment. Because homeopathic practitioners want the illness to "run its course," it is not uncommon for symptoms to get worse before they get better. Both nurses and patients using homeopathic remedies need to know what is reasonable to expect.

Naturopathy

Naturopathy is a relatively new system of medicine that began in the early 1900s in the United States. "**Naturopathic medicine** is not only a system of medicine but also a way of life, with emphasis on client responsibility, client education, health maintenance, and disease prevention. It may be the model health system of the future with the movement toward healthy lifestyles, healthy diets, and preventive health care" (Fontaine, 2005, p. 173).

Naturopathic physicians engage in a rigorous educational program similar to that of allopathic physicians. They practice as primary care providers and use a scientific method for diagnosis and treatment. Naturopaths believe in the "vitalist doctrine," which maintains that "the organism's vitality and susceptibility are just as important as, or more important than, the causes of disease" (Bright, 2002, p. 187).

Naturopaths believe that health is a dynamic state of being that provides abundant energy for people to deal with life in our complex society. Much of illness can be attributed, at least in part, to ignoring "natural laws," such as engaging in a sedentary lifestyle without adequate time for exercise; exposing oneself to environmental toxins; eating processed, overcooked foods; engaging in negativity or harboring negative thoughts; and not getting adequate rest or relaxation.

Therapies strive to support the self-healing mechanism of the body. Naturopaths employ an eclectic group of modalities, including acupuncture, clinical nutrition, herbal medicine, hydrotherapy (therapeutic use of water), osteopathy (massage and manipulation), and TCM. Licensed naturopathic physicians (ND) complete a 4-year graduate-level medical school after 3 years of standard premedical courses.

Naturopathic physicians may have responsibility for their patients while they receive inpatient care. Patients who are being treated by a naturopathic physician will probably have a different plan of care than those being treated by allopathic physicians.

Chiropractic Medicine

Chiropractic medicine is the relationship between the structure (the spine) and function (mainly the nervous system) of the human body to restore and preserve health.

The underlying principle is that the functions of the body are controlled by the nervous system, mainly 31 pairs of spinal nerves that feed all organs of the body after branching off the spinal column. Since these nerves are surrounded by vertebrae and other musculoskeletal components, any distortion of the structure of the musculoskeletal system affects the nervous system (Bright, 2002).

The nervous system problem is sometimes caused by a subluxation, which occurs when a joint such as a vertebral bone is out of alignment. By adjusting the spine, the joint is brought into proper alignment and the pressure on the nerve is released.

Diagnosis can be made by health history, physical examination, and x-rays if needed. Treatments consist of manipulation and other modalities to decrease discomfort and aid the healing process, including ice, heat, ultrasound, electrical muscle stimulation, massage, herbs, and nutritional supplements (Bright, 2002).

Doctors of chiropractic medicine (DC) are licensed and attend 4 years of chiropractic school after prerequisite coursework. At this time, most chiropractic treatment is conducted on outpatients.

A good understanding of chiropractic medicine allows the nurse to answer patients' questions and ask questions about a patient's current treatments. This knowledge also helps to allow nurses to be able to refer patients asking questions about chiropractic medicine to reliable sources of information.

➤ *Recall Brian Legett, the patient with chronic back problems who has experienced little relief and is asking about seeing a chiropractor. When responding to Mr. Legett, the nurse would need to explain the underlying principles of chiropractic science. In addition, the nurse, in conjunction with other healthcare team members involved in the patient's plan of care, would need to review the patient's history thoroughly to identify (if possible) the underlying cause of his back problems and the various treatments attempted. This review would be important in determining if a referral to a chiropractor would be appropriate.* ■

Mind–Body Modalities

Most people acknowledge that there is a mind–body connection. Situations such as insomnia related to anxiety the night before a major examination or a migraine headache triggered by a fight with a spouse or good friend indicate that some connection does indeed exist. Recent research has expanded our knowledge of how the mind and body communicate with each other.

Knowing how this communication occurs assists in the understanding of the mind–body modalities of relaxation, meditation, and imagery. These three therapies can be useful for patients as well as self-care for nurses.

➤ *Think back to Sylvia Puentes, the anxious preoperative patient. The nurse would need to incorporate an understanding of the mind–body connection when discussing possible suggestions for anxiety relief.* ■

The scientific field of psychoneuroimmunology (PNI) studies neurochemicals such as neuropeptides that are now believed to be the messenger molecules that connect the body and mind. Neuropeptides have properties that allow them to affect neurologic and physiologic tissue receptors. Many neuropeptide receptor sites lie along the gastrointestinal tract; this explains why people can experience a large variety of gastrointestinal symptoms in response to emotional situations. Neuropeptides are produced as needed and travel through all spaces of the body in blood as well as other body fluids. Because they frequently travel and act quickly and are produced only as needed, there is as yet no way to measure them in the body.

Benson (1975) studied the **relaxation response** extensively. Dossey and Keegan (2009) described this response as "an alert, hypokinetic process of decreased sympathetic nervous system arousal" (p. 260). The response can also be viewed as the opposite of Selye's GAS response. Relaxation, which included meditation, was the most popular CAT therapy reported in the Eisenberg studies (Eisenberg et al., 1993, 1998).

Relaxation

Relaxation techniques promote parasympathetic activity, helping to reduce sympathetic activity and restore the balance of the two systems.

Sympathetic system dominance, characterized by increased epinephrine levels in the body, can contribute to symptoms such as hypertension, cool hands and feet, tight muscles, increased heart rate, and increased respiratory rate (Dossey & Keegan, 2009). The ultimate goal is to increase the parasympathetic system influence in the mind–body and thus reduce the effect of stress and stress-related illness on the body.

Relaxation can be useful whether a patient is experiencing a single stressful event, such as surgery, or chronic stress. Patient benefits include reduced anxiety, muscle tension and pain, improved functioning of the immune system, enhanced sleep and rest, and an improved overall sense of well-being.

Dossey and Keegan (2009) discussed several relaxation techniques, including meditation, and modern relations methods such as progressive muscle relaxation, autogenic training, biofeedback, body scanning, and hypnosis. Because these modalities are quite different, the type of relaxation modality chosen needs to be individually suited to the patient.

> *Recall Mr. Chen, the terminally ill patient described in the Reflective Practice display. When developing the plan of care, the nurse needs to include the patient's daughters. Therefore, when interacting with the patient's daughters, the nurse would also assess their stress level as they cope with their father's deteriorating condition. This assessment could provide valuable information about the cultural beliefs and values of each daughter, leading the nurse to suggest possible culturally appropriate methods for relaxation.* ∎

Nurses can assist patients to begin to achieve a relaxation response by focusing on their breathing. Patients can breathe into a stressful or painful area, lengthen their breathing, or focus on abdominal or diaphragmatic breathing. Benson (1975) found it helpful to use a mental device such as a repetitive phrase to remind the body to relax.

Nurses can also practice relaxation as part of their self-care, enabling them to better deal with personal and work-related stress. Relaxation exercises can be done anywhere, at any time, and without cost. Numerous relaxation guides and CDs are available online.

Meditation

Meditation has been part of many spiritual and healing traditions for hundreds of years.

It seeks to change one's physiology to a more relaxed state and alter one's perception to an increased acceptance of reality. Mindfulness-based stress reduction (MBSR), a form of meditation, was developed by Kabat-Zinn (1990). He established the first program in 1979 at the University of Massachusetts Medical Center. More than 200 MBSR programs modeled on the original program have been offered at healthcare settings in the United States (Roth & Stanley, 2002). Although mindfulness meditation comes from the Buddhist tradition, it can be practiced in any context. According to Kabat-Zinn (1990), "Mindfulness is basically just a particular way of paying attention" (p. 12). Participants learn sitting and walking meditation, techniques such as body scanning and breathing techniques, and methods of handling physical and emotional pain. Outcomes include more patience, less anger and fewer temper bursts, better interpersonal communication, greater harmony in interpersonal relations, decreased use of medications for sleep and anxiety, decreased/ceased smoking, weight loss, greater acceptance of aspects of life over which one has no control, and marked improvement in overall sense of well-being (Roth & Stanley, 2002).

Patients seeking inpatient care might have a meditation practice they want to continue. Nurses can provide the time necessary for this. Nurses too could benefit from a meditation practice and could experience a brief meditation during breaks from patient care activities.

Guided Imagery

Guided imagery was first used in the 1970s by children with leukemia as an adjunct to chemotherapy. These children imagined their white blood cells "gobbling up" the cancer cells.

Imagery involves using all five senses to imagine an event or body process unfolding according to a plan. When all senses are involved in the experience, the imaginary situation is more fully encoded in the body and more likely to take place. A relaxation technique is frequently used to prepare the mind and body before beginning an imagery session.

According to Rossman (2000), "The ultimate mechanisms of imagery are still a mystery" (p. 18). He believes differences in left and right brain processing help to explain imagery. The left brain processes information in a linear fashion, while the right brain processes information simultaneously. "The imagery it [right brain] produces often lets you see the big picture and experience the way an illness is related to events and feelings you might not have considered important" (p. 19).

Research studies have demonstrated that imagery assists patients with AIDS and cancer to extend their lives, as well as enhance their quality of life. People experiencing migraine headaches and fibromyalgia have received symptomatic relief (Bright, 2002).

You can assist clients with imagery in several ways:

- Many kinds of imagery tapes with scripts are available that patients can use independently. If some of these are available on the nursing unit, patients can determine what types of tapes they would like to use or purchase. Patients can also be assisted to write a script and record it for their own use.
- Nurses can work with patients using "outcome imagery," which might consist of using a picture or photograph to visualize the desired outcome in a body part or in a situation. Patients can add to the visual cue and develop a total image.
- During a painful or stressful event, such as an intravenous line being started, the patient can "go to a favorite place" and imagine being there with all the pleasant experiences related to that space.

> *Think back to Sylvia Puentes, the anxious patient scheduled for surgery. Any of these types of imagery techniques would be appropriate suggestions for the patient. However, the nurse needs to assess the patient's preferences, beliefs, and ability to participate in these techniques to determine the best recommendation.* ∎

The Nurses Certificate Program in Imagery is endorsed by the American Holistic Nurses Association (AHNA). See the Web site at the end of the chapter for information.

Prayer

According the NCCAM, when prayer is included in the definition of CAT, the domain of mind–body medicine is the most commonly used domain (53%). **Intercessory prayer** involves praying for the benefit of another person to the Judeo-Christian God. Dossey (1993) thoroughly explored this subject, exploring areas such as beliefs about prayer, the process of praying, and whether a physician's beliefs are important in the healing relationship. This area can be controversial and needs to be explored with patients using sensitivity and cultural knowledge.

Although the effectiveness of prayer is considered difficult to measure, a classic study on intercessory prayer done in 1988 has withstood many critiques and is widely accepted as a valid study. It is known that people pray for their own healing, but this area has not been studied in a research format. Additional information and nursing considerations are covered in Chapter 46, Spirituality.

Humor Therapy

Norman Cousins was a well-known editor of the *Saturday Review* when he contracted ankylosing spondylitis in 1964. He wrote about using humor in his therapy program to treat his acute and debilitating illness. He found that after watching 10 minutes of Marx Brothers (comedians) tapes and "belly-laughing," his sedimentation rate (a measure of inflammation in the body) decreased by at least five points permanently (Cousins, 1979). More recent research (Bennett et al., 2003) found that improved immune response was correlated with experiences of "mirthful laughter."

Wooten (2005) discusses suggestions for a "humor program" on a nursing unit, which may include establishing a unit "laughter library," setting up a "humor room" where patients and families can play games, setting up a "comedy cart" with funny masks and games, or enlisting clown volunteers to visit on a regular basis.

Aromatherapy

Aromatherapy using essential oils was practiced in ancient Egypt and India more than 6,000 years ago. Oils were used in religious ceremonies, for medicinal purposes, and in perfumes and cosmetics. Today, one cannot go to a shopping mall without seeing scented candles and various other "aromatherapy" products.

Medicinally, aromatherapy is the "use of essential oils of plants to treat symptoms and as such has no theory of health and illness nor a system of diagnosis" (Fontaine, 2005, p. 143). The fragrance of these oils is believed to ultimately affect the very sensitive amygdala of the limbic system in the brain, where emotional memories are stored and released. "Thus, the sense of smell can evoke powerful memories in a split second and change people's perceptions and behaviors" (Fontaine, 2005, p. 148).

Commonly used essential oils in a healthcare setting are ginger or peppermint for nausea and lavender or chamomile for insomnia (Fontaine, 2005). Essential oils vary in quality and potency depending upon the manufacturing processes. If specific essential oils are approved for use in an inpatient setting, education on these oils should be provided. In addition, some people are highly sensitive to strong fragrances, particularly concentrated essential oils. This might preclude their use in some patient settings.

Certification in Aromatherapy for Health Professionals is available. This course is endorsed by AHNA, and information is available on the Web site listed at the end of the chapter.

Energy Medicine Modalities

Without realizing it, you may have heard a person talk about energy. The terms "resonance" ("I really resonate with you") and "wavelength" ("We are on the same wavelength") were used in Einstein's theory of physics. Today, Einstein's theory of physics, or energy theory, has been added to the sciences of biology and chemistry to express ideas about health and illness as well as to explain the human organism (Gerber, 2001).

All organisms are dependent on a subtle vital force that creates order in the system (Gerber, 2001). This vital force has been known to healing systems and people in various cultures for centuries and has been called a variety of names throughout history, such as vital life force (general usage), *pneuma* (ancient Greece), *qi* or *chi* (China and Japan), and *pran* (India) (Hover-Kramer, 2002). Many traditions consider this subtle energy to reflect the spiritual nature of people and to refer to individuals as mind, body, and spirit.

This life force feeds and nourishes the organism and is carried via two energetic structures that interact with each other: chakras and the etheric body. **Chakras** are concentrated areas of energy aligned vertically in the body that relate to each other as well as to specific areas of the body, mind, and spirit (Fig. 28-5). The etheric body (**aura**) consists of at least seven layers of energy that surround the body and relate to the chakras (Fig. 28-6). There is scientific evidence that following conception, energetic structures are the first to develop and, in some cases, serve as templates for cellular and organ development (Gerber, 2001). This finding supports the expression, "We are energy first." Energy therapies used for healing are based on the belief that they can

FIGURE 28-6. First four layers of the human aura.

affect this primary life force and thus contribute to physiologic healing.

The North American Nursing Diagnosis Association (NANDA) recognizes disturbed energy field as a nursing diagnosis. Defining characteristics of the disturbed field relate to movement, sounds, temperature change, visual changes, and disruption. There are many forms of energy work that seek to reduce disturbance in the energy field. Qi gong and acupuncture were discussed earlier in the chapter; additional therapies are discussed below.

Therapeutic Touch

Therapeutic Touch (TT), founded by Delores Krieger in the 1970s, is the use of the hands on or near the body with the intent to help or heal. The TT process consists of centering, assessing the energy field, and rebalancing the field using modulation, "unruffling," and other techniques (Krieger, 1993).

TT uses four primary scientific premises:

1. All the life sciences agree that, physically, a human being is an open energy system.
2. Anatomically, a human being is bilaterally symmetrical.
3. Illness is an imbalance in an individual's energy field.
4. Human beings have natural abilities to transform and transcend their conditions of living (Krieger, 1993, pp. 12–13).

Workshops and other learning opportunities are available for nurses to learn energy healing techniques. Energy work

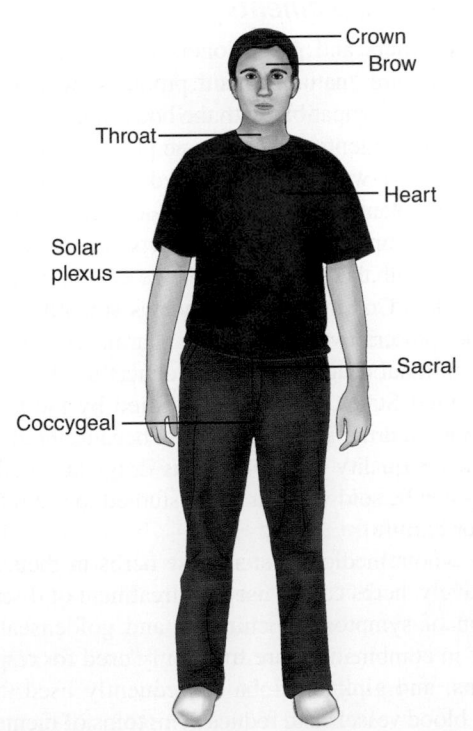

FIGURE 28-5. Location of the seven major chakras.

can assist patients in virtually all settings and all age groups, although advanced knowledge is necessary to work with babies and other vulnerable populations.

Registered nurses can become credentialed in TT. Details are available on the Nurse Healers Web site.

Healing Touch

Healing Touch (HT), founded by Janet Mengten in the 1980s, uses a collection of energy techniques to assess and treat the human energy system, thus affecting physical, emotional, mental, and spiritual health and healing. The current HT textbook contains about 20 specific energy techniques to be used in particular patient situations. The goal of HT is to restore wholeness through harmony and balance (Hover-Kramer, 2002).

HT energy techniques have been collected from well-known healers as well as shamanic and aborigine traditions. These techniques are taught in three or more leveled workshops by instructors certified by Healing Touch International.

Box 28-3 describes when HT can be used. Certification in HT for people from various backgrounds is available through Healing Touch International after completion of a series of classes and experiences. The program is endorsed by AHNA, and class information is available on the Web site.

Sound Healing

Music is another modality that has been viewed as therapeutic for thousands of years. Today, music has demonstrated effectiveness in reducing pain, decreasing anxiety, promoting relaxation, and in distracting persons from unpleasant sensations so they are empowered to heal (McCaffrey & Locsin, 2002).

Music consists of sound waves that vibrate at particular frequencies. When these frequencies are harmonious with our bodies, we experience the music as pleasant. Mozart's music has been found to be particularly healing because of its musical qualities (Campbell, 1997). Some music (e.g., "grunge rock") could be perceived to be detrimental to healing because it was found to increase hostility, sadness, ten-

sion, and fatigue and decrease relaxation and mental clarity (McCraty et al., 1998).

Music can be used to promote healing in several ways. Patients can use their selected CDs for listening prior to surgery or other stressful events, during imagery, and while relaxing. Music is frequently played in operating rooms and harp or piano music is played in patient lounges and lobbies.

> ▶ *Remember Sylvia Puentes, the anxious preoperative patient described at the beginning of the chapter. Based on an assessment of the patient's likes and dislikes, the nurse might suggest music therapy as a means to reduce the patient's preoperative anxiety.* ■

Biologically Based Practices

Botanical agents (herbs) and nutritional supplements are chemical compounds that are ingested with the hope of achieving a therapeutic goal. They are becoming increasingly popular with consumers, who can buy many of these preparations over the counter or from company distributors. Currently, dietary supplements (which include herbs and nutritional supplements) are considered foods and manufacturers need to follow FDA labeling requirements. Some product sample analyses have revealed inconsistencies in the amount of active ingredients. Because of these inconsistencies as well as for other reasons, in 2004 the Institute of Medicine issued a report recommending a framework for cost-effective and science-based evaluation of dietary supplements by the FDA.

Botanicals (Herbal Products) and Nutritional Supplements

Some consumers and practitioners are attracted to herbs because they are "natural" plant products, which are perceived as more compatible with the body than manufactured pharmaceutical agents. In fact, some pharmaceutical agents (e.g., Digitalis) were first produced as natural products derived from plants and now are produced chemically.

In many countries, herbal products are regulated and available through the primary healthcare system. In Germany, for example, "Commission E" reviews scientific data and establishes prescriptive standards for pharmaceuticals, including conventional drugs and plant products used for healing. In the United States, herbs are classified by the FDA as a food and not a drug. This is important because herbs are not regulated for quality and potency as drugs are, and herbal formulas can be sold without being studied to see if they are helpful or harmful.

Many whole medical systems use herbs in their system. Alternatively, herbs can be used for treatment of disease and reduction of symptoms. Echinacea and goldenseal (separately or in combination) are frequently used for respiratory infections, and ginkgo biloba is frequently used to dilate cerebral blood vessels and reduce symptoms of memory loss and mental confusion.

Box 28-3	**WHEN HEALING TOUCH CAN BE USED**

- Stimulate wound healing
- Relieve pain
- Reduce anxiety and stress
- Energize the auric field
- Promote health
- Assist patients before and after medical treatments and procedures such as surgery
- Support the dying process

Modified from Bulbrook, M. J., & Mentgen, J. (2002). *Healing Touch level I notebook* (4th ed.). Carrboro, NC: North Carolina Center for Healing Touch, p. 21.

Tips **TEACHING TIPS • 28-1**

USING HERBS AND SUPPLEMENTS

Teaching Tip	Why Is This Important?
Get information from knowledgeable and reliable sources.	Advertising media and many sources on the Internet frequently seek primarily to sell the product, not educate the consumer.
Buy name-brand products that are produced by reputable companies to increase your chances of getting a high-quality product.	Since this industry is not regulated, contamination and inconsistency in the amount of product sometimes occur.
The word "standardized" on an herbal product means that it consistently contains the percentage of the herb stated on the label.	A standardized product means that it contains a certain amount of active ingredient.
Whenever possible, buy single products.	If the product contains several ingredients and you have a reaction or positive response, you won't know which ingredient was the causative agent.
Take the proper dose and monitor side effects.	Herbal remedies are natural medicines and can be toxic in higher-than-recommended doses.
Give the product adequate time to work.	Herbs frequently take longer to produce a therapeutic effect than allopathic preparations.
Become knowledgeable about the product and your reason for using it.	Consumers who initiate any type of self-care tend to make better decisions if they are well informed.

Modified from Fontaine, K. L. (2005). *Healing practices* (2nd ed., pp. 136–137). Upper Saddle River, NJ: Prentice-Hall.

Nutritional supplements are chemical compounds that contain ingredients (vitamins, minerals, enzymes, amino acids, essential fatty acids) believed to promote health. These products have a wide range of safety and effectiveness.

Increasing numbers of patients are using herbs and supplements. Nurses need to be aware of the various products available and provide education to patients to ensure safety with their use (Teaching Tips 28-1).

Extensive specialized education is required before a nurse can be competent to advise patients on the use of herbs and supplements. However, nurses are finding that information about certain herbs adds an aspect of safety to their practice. For example, some herbs and/or supplements may interact with prescribed medications patients are taking. Ginkgo biloba, the most widely sold herb in Europe and used by many to improve memory, affects platelet function and thus should not be used concurrently with warfarin or aspirin. Some nursing pharmacology courses include information on commonly used herbs. Women who are pregnant or nursing and children should be especially cautious about using herbal supplements either alone or in mixtures, since these products can act like drugs.

"Natural" does not mean safe. For example, the herbs kava and comfrey have been linked to serious liver damage.

Nutritional Therapy

The eating habits of people in the United States are being scrutinized because of the alarming increase in obesity,

particularly in children, and chronic illnesses in all age groups. The so-called typical diet consisting of prepared and processed foods and large amounts of meat, dairy products, and sugar is highly suspect.

Many popular eating plans that purport to address these health problems have been endorsed by people with a variety of credentials. The diversity of these approaches is understandably very confusing to the consumer. Although an examination of these popular diets is beyond the scope of this book, it does appear that people have individual needs and preferences with respect to foods. In fact, this belief has been a cornerstone of holistic nutritional approaches for centuries in the TCM and Ayurvedic systems (see also Chapter 36). Teaching Tips 28-2 provides guidelines for teaching about holistic approaches to food choices. It is common to find many of these approaches endorsed by naturopathic practitioners.

Manipulative and Body-Based Practices

This group of therapies includes therapeutic massage—an assortment of techniques that involve manipulation of soft tissues of the body through pressure and movement, as well as a variety of techniques such as Rolfing, shiatsu, Feldenkrais, Alexander, myofascial release, and others. The goal is to break up tension held in body structures, promote communication between mind–body structures, promote detoxification, and generally improve body functioning. Some of these therapies can be painful while they work to

TEACHING TIPS • 28-2

HOLISTIC APPROACHES TO FOOD CHOICES

Teaching Tip	Why Is This Important?
Reduce amounts of processed foods.	Processing frequently reduces the nutrients available for absorption. For example, canned foods frequently have lower nutritional values than frozen foods.
Reduce/eliminate soft drinks (colas).	They are "fake food" and have no nutritional value.
Avoid eating foods with preservatives.	Preservatives are artificial substances that the body ultimately needs to excrete, usually through the urine or feces. This excretion process uses energy the body could use for other processes.
Reduce intake of refined and natural sugars.	The "average" individual in the United States consumes an unhealthy amount of glucose. Among other things, excess glucose places an increased demand on the pancreas, kills the natural bacterial flora found in the gastrointestinal tract that is necessary for absorption, and interferes with cellular absorption of nutrients.
Reduce intake of artificial sweeteners, including aspartame.	Since aspartame is not a food, it needs to be excreted, and there is some evidence that it is toxic to humans. In some countries (Japan), aspartame is extensively regulated. Replace aspartame with stevia, a natural sweetener available in liquid or granulated form.
Eat organically grown foods.	If grown according to rigorous organic regulations, these foods contain no pesticides or chemical byproducts, which are toxins in the body.
Reduce intake of dairy products.	Many dairy cows are regularly given antibiotics and, in some cases, hormones. Breakdown products from these substances may be found in milk.
Consider adopting a vegetarian diet.	Animals are increasingly fed antibiotics and potentially contaminated foods. Increasingly, fish are being contaminated with mercury and other pollutants.
Eat foods in season.	Foods produced "out of season" are treated with chemicals to ripen them since they are picked before ripening.
Be aware of genetically engineered, radiated food.	Become informed about these processes before you make a decision as to whether you want to eat these foods.

oxygenate tissues, break up lymphatic congestion, release muscle tightness, and promote circulation. These therapies require specialized preparation and are typically useful in rehabilitation or health-promotion types of settings.

NURSING IMPLICATIONS OF CAT

The development of CAT continues to be a market-driven and, in some respects, a patient-driven phenomenon. Many patients/consumers are unsatisfied with allopathic treatments and are turning to CAT for relief of symptoms and healing. Since healthcare currently operates on a business model, it is probable that more CAT will become available to deal with real or perceived market needs. Many of these therapies are not covered by third-party payers, which means that consumers must pay out of pocket for them. In addition, government and professional groups do not regulate most of the therapies. Because of this lack of regulation, there can be inconsistencies among the preparation and care provided by practitioners.

There is a great opportunity here for nurses to expand their practice to meet existing patient needs, as well as to promote health. See Focused Assessment Guide 28-1: Holistic Care for an identification of areas in which a holistic nurse can improve patient care. As new therapies demonstrate their effectiveness, they can be added to the assessment.

Nursing is expanding its knowledge base to include information that explains selected CAT. For example, pharmacology courses in schools of nursing frequently include information on herbs. Certifications in basic holistic nursing for nurses with a baccalaureate degree and in advanced Holistic Nursing for nurses with a master's degree are available through the American Holistic Nurses' Certification Corporation (AHNCC). It is expected that CAT will become a larger part of the practice for some nurses. See the accompanying Research in Nursing and PICO in Practice boxes.

Patient education about CAT is essential. Patients and the public need to know about the safe and effective use of CAT.

FOCUSED ASSESSMENT GUIDE • 28-1

HOLISTIC CARE

Factors to Assess	Questions and Approaches
Stress	What measures does the patient use to reduce stress? If the patient wants to continue a meditation, relaxation, or imagery practice while receiving care, explore ways in which that can be accomplished.
Music/sound preferences	What preferences does the patient have for music or environmental sounds (e.g., ocean waves, birds) either while meditating or relaxing? The patient could provide his or her own music if preferred music is not available.
Diet	What dietary preferences does the patient have (e.g., vegetarian, no processed foods)? Communicate these preferences to nutritional services.
Environmental sensitivity	Is the patient sensitive to environmental odors or fragrances? If so, can an air purifier be brought to the room?
Use of herbs and supplements	Is the patient taking any herbs or supplements as directed by a CAT practitioner or purchased over the counter? If so, obtain the names of the herbs/supplements, dosages, and reasons for their use. If the patient has these substances in his or her possession, follow applicable institutional policies.
Use of CAT healthcare provider	Is the patient planning to use a primary CAT provider while receiving allopathic care? If so, convey appropriate information to the primary allopathic provider.

RESEARCH IN NURSING
Bridging the Gap to Evidence-Based Practice

MASSAGE THERAPY AND THERAPEUTIC TOUCH

Massage therapy and Therapeutic Touch (TT) are *complementary* healing modalities used by healthcare providers to reduce anxiety, accelerate relaxation, decrease pain, and enhance immunity. Research studies continue to report on the effects of these therapies.

Massage Therapy: Related Research

Hughes, D., Ladas, E., Rooney, D., & Kelly, K. (2008). Massage therapy as a supportive care intervention for children with cancer. *Oncology Nursing Forum, 35*(3), 431–442.

This study reviewed relevant literature about massage therapy to assess the feasibility of integrating the body-based *complementary* and alternative medicine (CAM) practice as a supportive care intervention for children with cancer. Data was compiled from PubMed®, online references, published government reports, and the bibliographies of retrieved articles, reviews, and books on massage and massage and cancer. More than 70 citations were reviewed.

Findings revealed that massage therapy may help mitigate pain, anxiety, depression, constipation, and high blood pressure and may be beneficial during periods of profound immune suppression. Massage techniques light to medium in pressure are appropriate in the pediatric oncology setting. The researchers concluded that massage is an applicable, noninvasive, therapeutic modality that can be integrated safely as an adjunct intervention for managing side effects and psychological conditions associated with anticancer treatment in children. Massage may support immune function during periods of immunosuppression.

For additional research, visit thePoint.

Therapeutic Touch: Related Research

Coppa, D. (2008). The internal process of therapeutic touch. *Journal of Holistic Nursing, 26*(1), 17–24.

This qualitative research study was conducted to describe the nature of the core process of TT in adults and full-term infants as practiced by five professional nurses, each treating one adult and one infant. Analysis of data obtained from interviews and focused participant observations was conducted. Findings provide empirical data to depict an overall process divided into three phases: (a) preparation, (b) treatment, and (c) termination, that adheres to the standard process as described by Krieger. It expands on the description of each phase, including two new subcomponents, orienting and disengagement, not previously seen in the literature. Lastly, the study describes the modification of the TT process with infants compared to adults.

Implications for Nursing

Based on the findings of the study on massage therapy, nurses, especially pediatric oncology nurses, are vital in helping patients safely integrate CAT, such as massage therapy, into conventional treatment. Pediatric oncology nurses can help maximize patient outcomes by assessing, advocating, and coordinating massage therapy services as a supportive care intervention. Additionally, nurses can use the information from the study on TT to plan accordingly to ensure that adequate time is available for preparing, actual treatment, and termination.

PICO IN PRACTICE
Asking Clinical Questions

Scenario: You are a staff nurse who works in an outpatient oncology clinic, a position that you have held for the past 8 months. You are also a licensed massage therapist, and practiced massage therapy at a health spa for several years before going back to school to study nursing. Over the course of the past several months, you note that many of the patients who come to the clinic for chemotherapy complain of stress and sleep disorders. You believe that implementing massage techniques with some of these patients could help improve their sleep patterns.

* Population: Patients with cancer who receive chemotherapy in a clinic
* Intervention: Therapeutic massage
* Comparison: None
* Outcome: Improved sleep patterns

PICO Question: Can therapeutic massage result in improved sleep patterns in patients with cancer who receive chemotherapy in an oncology clinic?

Finding: From the Oncology Nursing Society: Oncology Nursing Society Putting Evidence into Practice (PEP) (2008). *Sleep/wake disturbances evidence table.* Available at www.ons.org/research/.

Evidence from this table notes multiple limitations of two studies conducted with cancer outpatients who received therapeutic massage. Results from these studies do not clearly advocate that therapeutic massage improves sleep in patients with cancer, though it apparently does not cause any undue effects or harm to them.

Level of Evidence: Level III

Recommendation: You make an appointment to meet with your facility's Nurse Researcher, to ask her whether it is advisable to conduct a pilot study with a small group of patients treated at your clinic to find whether therapeutic massage improves their sleep patterns.

Numerous resources exist to educate healthcare professionals and the public, such as those listed in the accompanying boxes and at the end of the bibliography. Box 28-4 provides guidelines for evaluating Internet medical resources. The National Center for Complementary and Alternative Medicine supports a Web site called "Time to Talk" to encourage patients to discuss use of CAT with their healthcare providers (nccam.nih.gov/timetotalk/).

Box 28-4 10 THINGS TO KNOW ABOUT EVALUATING MEDICAL RESOURCES ON THE WEB

The number of Web sites offering health-related resources grows every day. Many sites provide valuable information, while others may have information that is unreliable or misleading. This short guide contains important questions you should consider as you look for health information online. Answering these questions when you visit a new site will help you evaluate the information you find.

Questions to Ask
1. Who runs this site?
2. Who pays for the site?
3. What is the purpose of the site?
4. Where does the information come from?
5. What is the basis of the information?
6. How is the information selected?
7. How current is the information?
8. How does the site choose links to other sites?
9. What information about you does the site collect, and why?
10. How does the site manage interactions with visitors?

See NCCAM (http://nccam.nih.gov/) for answers to these questions.

● Developing Critical Thinking Skills

1. You are caring for a culturally diverse population. How would you appropriately assess for and implement CAT into your nursing care simultaneously demonstrating respect for your patients' beliefs and preferences with your commitment to evidence-based nursing/medicine?

2. The family of a woman dying of cancer approaches you with a brown paper bag of ground herbs and asks you to mix them with the patient's next tube feeding. They are very upset that she isn't healing and believe the herbs might help. How do you respond and what is the basis for your response? Talk with other students about what they would do and compare your responses.

3. A nurse who practices Therapeutic Touch tells you that she finds it very helpful for all sorts of patients. When you press her for details, you learn that she even practices this technique on patients who are sleeping without their consent. Are you troubled by this? Is patient consent needed for CAT in the same way it is needed for allopathic treatments?

● Preparing for NCLEX

1. A nurse is describing which type of CAT as involving the use of meridian energy circuits to nourish and support all cells and organs of the body?
   a. Energy healing approaches
   b. Acupuncture
   c. Chiropractic science
   d. Therapeutic Touch

2. After reviewing the different complementary and alternative therapies, a group of students demonstrate understanding when they identify which of the following as reflecting CAT?
   a. Safe interventions to supplement traditional care
   b. Used by a minority of inpatients
   c. Recognized by half of the state Boards of Nursing
   d. Relatively new

3. What is a combination of traditional medical care and CAT called?
   a. Integrative care
   b. Holism
   c. Allopathy
   d. Traditional Chinese medicine

4. Which CAT uses the Law of Similars and the Law of Infinitesimals?
   a. Energy healing approaches
   b. Ayurveda
   c. Allopathy
   d. Homeopathy

5. Which CAT is most similar to the current health-promotion/disease-prevention models?
   a. Naturopathic medicine
   b. Chiropractic science
   c. Nutritional supplements
   d. Acupuncture

6. Neuropeptides are messenger molecules for which type of CAT?
   a. Holism
   b. Mind–body modalities
   c. Energy healing approaches
   d. Botanical supplements

7. Which of the following is a CAT that involves active participation by the patient and is often used in pre- and postoperative pain control?
   a. Acupuncture
   b. Therapeutic Touch
   c. Botanical supplements
   d. Guided imagery

8. The relaxation response is opposite of which person's ideas?
   a. Einstein
   b. Selye
   c. Descartes
   d. Kabot-Zinn

9. Which of the following is true of energy healing approaches?
   a. They have a North American Nursing Diagnosis Association (NANDA)-recognized nursing diagnosis.
   b. They have an American Holistic Nurses Association certification in energy imagery.
   c. They are a result of the concepts from Albert Einstein's theory of relativity.
   d. They have an underlying principle that body functions are controlled by the nervous system.

● Answers With Rationale

1. *b.* Acupuncture consists of placing very thin, short, sterile needles at particular acupoints, believed to be centers of nerve and vascular tissue, along a meridian. Energy healing uses the chakras. Chiropractic science uses the spine and nervous system. Therapeutic Touch uses energy fields.

2. *c.* These modalities are not always safe. You may not be aware of who uses CAT, so assessment is imperative. Some of these modalities are thousands of years old.

3. *a.* Holism is interaction between parts of a whole. Allopathy is traditional medical care. Traditional Chinese medicine involves an interaction of people and their environment.

4. *d.* The Law of Similars states that a natural substance that produces a given symptom in a healthy person will cure it in a sick person. The Law of Infinitesimals states that the smallest dose possible will have the desired effect. Although these concepts may seem unusual, they are the concepts that underlie contemporary immunization practice.

5. *a.* Naturopathic medicine is not only a system of medicine, but also a way of life, with emphasis on client responsibility, client education, health maintenance, and disease prevention. It may be the model health system of the future with the movement toward healthy lifestyles, healthy diets, and preventive healthcare. The other modalities have received recent re-acceptance.

6. *b.* The scientific field of psychoneuroimmunology (PNI) studies neurochemicals, including neuropeptides, which are now believed to be the messenger molecules that connect the body and mind. Neuropeptides have properties that allow them to affect neurologic and physiologic tissue receptors.

7. *d.* Imagery involves using all five senses to imagine an event or body process unfolding according to a plan. A patient can be encouraged to "go to a favorite place." With the other modalities, the patient is more passive.

8. *b.* Hans Selye developed the term "general adaptation syndrome" (GAS) to describe the general holistic pattern that emerges when people experience stress or illness. The relaxation answer is an alert, hypometabolic state of decreased sympathetic nervous system arousal. Einstein developed the theory of energy. Descartes "separated" mind and body. Kabot-Zinn developed the mindfulness-based stress reduction concept.

9. *a.* Disturbed energy field is an accepted nursing diagnosis. AHNA has certificate programs in Healing Touch, a type of energy modality. Einstein's related theory was the "theory of energy." An underlying principle that body functions are controlled by the nervous system relates to chiropractic science.

Taylor Suite Resources

The Taylor Suite offers these additional resources to enhance learning and facilitate understanding of this chapter:

- thePoint online resource, http://thepoint.lww.com/Taylor7E
- Student DVD-ROM included with the book
- Study Guide for Taylor's Fundamentals of Nursing

BIBLIOGRAPHY

Achterberg, J. (1985). *Imagery in healing: Shamanism and modern medicine.* Boston: Shambhala.

Adams, J., & Tovey, P. (2007). *Complementary and alternative medicine in nursing and midwifery: Towards a critical social science.* New York: Routledge.

American Cancer Society. Native American Healing. Retrieved April 22, 2010 http://www.cancer.org/docroot/ETO/content/ETO_5_3X_Native_American_Healing.asp?sitearea=ETO

Antall, G. F., & Kresevic, D. (2004). The use of guided imagery to manage pain in an elderly orthopaedic population. *Orthopaedic Nursing, 23*(5), 335–340.

Barnes, P. M., Powell-Griner, E., McFann, K., & Nahin, R. L. (2004). Complementary and alternative medicine use among adults: United States, 2002. Advance data from vital and health statistics; no. 343. Hyattsville, MD: National Center for Health Statistics.

Barnes, P. M., Bloom, B., & Nahin, R. (2008). *CDC National Health Statistics Report #12.* Complementary and Alternative Medicine Use Among Adults and Children: United States, 2007. Available at nccam.nih.gov/news/camstats/.

Bennett, M. P., Zeller, J. M., Rosenberg, L., & McCann, J. (2003). The effect of mirthful laughter on stress and natural killer cell activity. *Alternative Therapies, 9*(2), 38–43.

Benson, H. (1975). *The relaxation response.* New York: William Morrow & Co.

Benson, H. (1984). *Beyond the relaxation response.* New York: Times Books.

Bright, M. A. (2002). *Holistic health and healing.* Philadelphia: F. A. Davis.

Bulbrook, M. J., & Mentgen, J. (2002). *Healing Touch level 1 notebook* (4th ed.). Carrboro, NC: North Carolina Center for Healing Touch.

Campbell, D. (1997). *The Mozart effect.* New York: Avon Books.

Chopra, D. (2000). *Perfect health.* New York: Three Rivers Press.

Complementary alternative modalities. (2004). *Home health care management & practice, 16*(6), 449–520.

Cousins, N. (1979). *Anatomy of an illness.* New York: Bantam Books.

Denner, S. S. (2008). The evolving doctrine of informed consent for complementary and integrative therapy. *Holistic Nursing Practice, 22*(1), 37–43.

Dossey, B. M., & Keegan, L. (2009). *Holistic nursing. A handbook for practice* (5th ed.). Sudbury, MA: Jones and Bartlett Publishers.

Dossey, L. (1993). *Healing words.* New York: HarperCollins.

Eisenberg, D. M., Kessler, R. C., Foster, C., Norlock, F. E., Calkins, D. R., & Delbanco, T. L. (1993). Unconventional medicine in the United States. *New England Journal of Medicine, 328*(4), 246–252.

Eisenberg, D. M., Davis, R. B., Ettner, S. L., Appel, S., Wilkey, S., Van Rompay, M., et al. (1998). Trends in alternative medicine use in the United States, 1990–1997. *New England Journal of Medicine, 280*(18), 1569–1575.

Ernst, E. (2006). Acupuncture—a critical analysis. *Journal of Internal Medicine, 259*(2), 125–137.

Fenton, M. V., & Morris, D. L. (2003). The integration of holistic nursing practices and complementary and alternative modalities into curricula of schools of nursing. *Alternative Therapies in Health and Medicine, 9*(4), 62–67.

Ferguson, M. (1987). *Aquarian conspiracy: Personal and social transformation in our time.* New York: J. P. Tarcher.

Fontaine, K. L. (2005). *Healing practices* (2nd ed.). Upper Saddle River, NJ: Pearson Education.

Freeman, L. (2004). *Mosby's complementary & alternative medicine.* St. Louis: Mosby.

Frisch, N., Dossey, B., Guzzetta, C., & Quinn, J. (2000). *AHNA standards of holistic nursing practice: Guidelines for caring and healing.* Gaithersburg, MD: Aspen Publishers.

Frisch, N. (2001, May 31). Standards for holistic nursing practice: A way to think about our care that includes complementary and alternative modalities. *Online Journal of Issues in Nursing, 6*(2), Manuscript 4.

Gerber, R. (2000). *Vibrational medicine for the 21st century.* New York: HarperCollins.

Gerber, R. (2001). *Vibrational medicine* (3rd ed.). Rochester, VT: Bear & Company.

Horrigan, B. (1996). Janet Quinn, RN, PhD: Therapeutic Touch and a healing way. *Alternative Therapies in Health and Medicine, 2*(4), 69–75.

Horrigan, B. (1999). Michael Murray, ND: A natural approach to health. *Alternative Therapies in Health and Medicine, 5*(2), 77–84.

Horrigan, B. (2003). Ken Cohen, MA, MSTH: Healing through ancient traditions: Qigong and Native American medicine. *Alternative Therapies in Health and Medicine, 9*(3), 83–91.

Hover-Kramer, D. (2002). *Healing Touch. A guidebook for practitioners.* Albany, NY: Delmar.

Institute of Medicine, Committee on the Use of Complementary and Alternative Medicine by the American Public. (2005). Complementary and alternative medicine (CAM) in the United States. Washington, DC: National Academy Press.

Jackson, C. (2004). Healing ourselves, healing others. *Holistic Nursing Practice, 18*(3), 127–141.

Kabat-Zinn, J. (1990). *Full catastrophe living.* New York: Delacorte Press.

Krieger, D. (1993). *Accepting your power to heal.* Santa Fe, NM: Bear & Company.

Lindquist, R., Tracy, M. F., Savik, K., & Watanuki, S. (2005). Regional use of complementary and alternative therapies by critical care nurses. *Critical Care Nurse, 25*(2), 63–64, 66–68, 70–72.

Maddocks-Jennings, W., & Wilkinson, J. M. (2004). Aromatherapy practice in nursing: Literature review. *Journal of Advanced Nursing, 48*(1), 93–103.

Mao, J. J., Farrar, J. T., Xie, S. X., Bowman, M. A., & Armstrong, K. (2007). Use of complementary and alternative medicine and prayer among a national sample of cancer survivors compared to other populations without cancer. *Complement Ther Med, 15*(1), 21–9.

McCaffrey, R., & Locsin, R. C. (2002). Music listening as a nursing intervention: A symphony of practice. *Holistic Nursing Practice, 16*(3), 70–77.

McCraty, R., Barrios-Choplin, B., Atkinson, M., Tomasino, D. (1998). The effects of different types of music on mood, tension, and mental clarity. *Alternative Therapies, 4*(1), 75–84.

Meghani, N., Lindquist, R., & Tracy, M. F. (2003). Critical care nurses' desire to use complementary alternative modalities (CAM) in critical care and barriers to CAM use. *DCCN: Dimensions of Critical Care Nursing, 22*(3), 138–144.

Mehl-Madrona, L. E. (1999). Native American medicine in the treatment of chronic illness: Developing an integrated program and evaluating its effectiveness. *Alternative Therapies, 5*(1), 36–44.

Morris, D. L., Fenton, M. V., & Mercer, Z. B. (2004). Identification of national trends in nursing education through the use of an online survey. *Nursing Outlook, 52*(5), 248–254.

Nahin, R. L., Dahlhamer, J. M., Taylor, B. L., Barnes, P. M., Stussman, B. J., Simile, C.M., et al. (2007). Health behaviors and risk factors in those who use complementary and alternative medicine. *BMC Public Health, 7*(147), 217.

National Cancer Institute. (2010). *Acupuncture (PDQ)*. National Cancer Institute Web site. Available at http://www.cancer.gov/cancertopics/pdq/cam/acupuncture.

National Center for Complementary and Alternative Medicine. (2005). Expanding horizons of health care: Strategic plan 2005–2009. Available at http://nccam.nih.gov/about/plans/2005.

National Center for Health Statistics. (2007). National health interview survey (NHIS): 2007 data release [online]. Available at http://www.cdc.gov/nchs/about/major/nhis/nhis_2007_data_release.htm.

National Center for Health Statistics. (2008). National Health Interview Survey (NHIS): Public-use data release. NHIS survey description [online]. Available at ftp://ftp.cdc.gov/pub/Health_Statistics/NCHS/Dataset_Documentation/NHIS/2007/srvydesc.pdf.

NCCAM educational campaign. (2009). *Time to talk. National center for complementary and alternative medicine (online)*. Available at http://nccam.nih.gov/timetotalk/.

Pert, C. (1999). *Molecules of emotion: The science behind mind–body medicine*. New York: Simon & Schuster.

Ross, S. M. (2009). Integrative therapeutic considerations in alcohol abuse. *Holistic Nursing Practice, 23*(1), 69–72,

Rossman, M. L. (2000). *Guided imagery for self-healing*. Tiburon, CA: H. J. Kramer.

Roth, B., & Stanley, T-W. (2002). Mindfulness-based stress reduction and healthcare utilization in the inner city: Preliminary findings. *Alternative Therapies, 8*(1), 60–66.

Sand-Jecklin, K., Hoggatt, B., & Badzek, L. (2004). Know the benefits and risks of using common herbal therapies. *Holistic Nursing Practice, 18*(4), 192–198.

Seskevich, J. E., Crater, S. W., Lane, J. D., & Krucof, M. W. (2004). Beneficial effects of noetic therapies on mood before percutaneous intervention for unstable coronary syndromes. *Nursing Research, 53*(2), 116–121.

Shames, K. H. (1996). *Creative imagery in nursing*. Albany, NY: Delmar.

Snyder, M., & Lindquist, R. (2006). Complementary/alternative therapies in nursing (5th ed.). New York: Springer Publishing Company.

Sparber, A. (2001). State boards of nursing and scope of practice of registered nurses performing complementary therapies. *Online Journal of Issues in Nursing, 6*(2), 6–7.

Taylor-Piliae, R. E., & Forelicher, E. S. (2004). The effectiveness of Tai Chi exercise in improving aerobic capacity: A meta-analysis. *Holistic Nursing Practice, 18*(5), 254–263.

Ullman, R., & Reichenberg-Ullman, J. (1997). *Homeopathic self-care*. New York: Three Rivers Press.

Vitale, A. (2007, July-August). An integrated review of Reiki touch therapy research. *Holistic Nursing Practice,* 167–179.

Webb, H. S. (2004). *Traveling between the worlds: Conversations with contemporary shamans*. Charlottesville, VA: Hampton Roads.

Weil, A. (1988). *Health and healing*. Boston: Houghton Mifflin.

Wooten, P. (2005). Humor, laughter, and play: Maintaining balance in a serious world. In B. M. Dossey, L. Keegan, & C. Guzzetta (Eds.), *Holistic nursing* (4th ed., pp. 497–520). Sudbury, MA: Jones and Bartlett.

Wright, L. D. (2001). Meditation: Myths and misconceptions. *Alternative Therapies, 7*(2), 96–97.

29 | Medications

REGINA SAUDER

Regina, a 73-year-old woman with a history of lymphoma, has presented to the emergency room with pain, swelling, and erythema of her left calf. She has been diagnosed with a left leg deep vein thrombosis (DVT). She is receiving intravenous heparin and oral warfarin. When she is discharged, she will need to have weekly blood testing to ensure therapeutic levels of the warfarin.

MILDRED CAMPBELL

Mildred, a 65-year-old woman with a history of arthritis and hypertension (high blood pressure), comes to the clinic for evaluation of her painful joints. She states, "I just saw this new medicine advertised on television that is supposed to be really helpful in relieving joint pain. What do you think? Is it something I should try?"

FRANÇOIS BAPTISTE

François is an elderly man with a wound infection requiring intravenous antibiotic therapy. He is scheduled to receive his next dose at 10 a.m. The medication delivered by the pharmacy is labeled with the correct drug and dose, but with another patient's name.

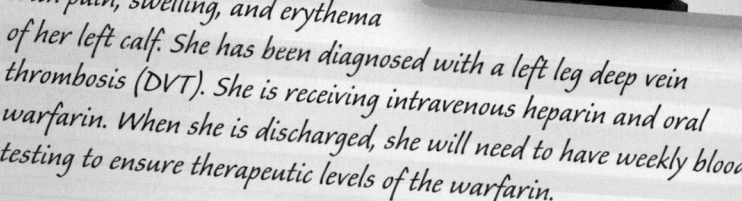

LEARNING OBJECTIVES

After completing the chapter, you will be able to accomplish the following:

1. Discuss drug legislation in the United States.

2. Describe drug names, types of preparations, and types of drug orders.

3. Identify drug classifications and actions.

4. Discuss adverse effects of drugs, including allergy, drug tolerance, toxic effect, idiosyncratic effect, and interactions.

5. Calculate drug dosages, using the various systems of equivalents.

6. Obtain patient information necessary to establish a medication history.

7. Describe principles used to prepare and administer medications safely by the oral, parenteral, topical, and inhalation routes.

8. Develop teaching plans to meet patient needs specific to medication administration.

KEY TERMS

absorption	peak level
adverse drug effect	pharmacodynamic
allergic effect	pharmacokinetic
ampule	pharmacology
anaphylactic reaction	pharmacotherapeutic
anaphylaxis	piggyback delivery
antagonist effect	system
cumulative effect	placebo
distribution	p.r.n. order
drug tolerance	stat order
excretion	subcutaneous injection
generic name	synergistic effect
half-life	teratogenic
idiosyncratic effect	therapeutic range
inhalation	topical application
intradermal injection	toxic effect
intramuscular injection	trade name
intravenous route	trough level
metabolism	vial
mini-infusion pump	volume-control
official name	administration set
parenteral	Z-track technique

Medication administration is a basic nursing function that involves skillful technique and consideration of the patient's development, health status, and safety. The nurse administering medications needs a knowledge base about drugs, including drug names, preparations, classifications, adverse effects, and physiologic factors that affect drug action.

The nursing process can be applied to medication administration. Assessment includes a comprehensive medication history, awareness of the patient's allergies, and patient assessment, as well as ongoing assessments of the patient's response during and after medication administration. Nursing diagnoses are developed from the assessment data. Patient-centered outcomes are evaluated after implementation of the plan of care and are tailored to the patient's needs.

A drug or medication is any substance that modifies body functions when taken into the body. The study that deals with chemicals that affect the body's functioning is called **pharmacology.** A pharmacist is a person licensed to prepare and dispense drugs. Physicians, dentists, psychiatrists, podiatrists, physician assistants, and advance practice nurses have prescriptive authority. Prescriptive authority for advance practice nurses (clinical nurse specialists, nurse practitioners, certified nurse anesthetists, nurse midwives) and physician assistants varies in the degree of independence and the medications that may be prescribed from state to state. Nurses must be familiar with the laws relative to prescriptive authority in their state of practice. The prescriber conveys medication plans to others by an order called a prescription. After the pharmacist prepares the medication, the nurse administers the medication to the patient. This chain provides a check-and-balance system for medication administration. If an error is made when the order is written, the pharmacist or nurse administering the medication has the opportunity to note the discrepancy. If an error occurs when the pharmacy dispenses the medication, the administering nurse has the opportunity to note this discrepancy. See the accompanying Reflective Practice box for an example.

Information about specific drugs is available in pharmacology texts and drug reference books. Computer programs and electronic databases are available for up-to-date medication information. Nurses must have sufficient knowledge about the drugs being administered to safely care for their patients. The Joint Commission has made several recommendations with regards to safe practice when administering medications. Up-to-date information about these recommendations can be found at http://www.jointcommission.org/PatientSafety/NationalPatientSafetyGoals/.

PRINCIPLES OF PHARMACOLOGY

An overview of basic pharmacology includes drug nomenclature, types of drug preparations, drug classification, mechanisms of drug action, adverse drug effects, and factors affecting drug action, as well as drug blood level monitoring and pertinent U.S. drug legislation.

REFLECTIVE PRACTICE
Challenge to Ethical and Legal Skills

During my clinical rotation for complex care a few weeks ago, I met François Baptiste, an elderly man with a wound infection requiring intravenous antibiotic therapy. He was due for a certain IV antibiotic to be hung at 1000. When I checked his drawer at 0800 and 0900, the antibiotic was not there. However, the nurse I was working with told me not to call pharmacy about it yet since the pharmacy staff often comes and replaces the drawers in the medication carts before 1000 anyway. So, I didn't call pharmacy. Sure enough, a pharmacy representative came up that hour and changed the medication drawers. At 1000, I went to look in my patient's drawer. What I found confused me a great deal! Yes, the bag of medication was in there. Yes, it was the right drug and the right dose. However, it was the wrong patient! The label on the bag in my patient's drawer had another patient's name on it. I looked up information on that other patient, and it turned out he was also a patient on the unit. This patient was also receiving the same drug at the same dose but at a different time. I wondered if I should hang this bag for my patient because he was due for it, even though it had someone else's name and medical record number on the label. It was, after all, the same drug and the same dose.

Thinking Outside the Box: Possible Courses of Action

- Change the patient's name on the label and hang the bag.
- Call pharmacy to ask about the mix-up. If the bag did, indeed, contain the same medication at the same dose, then change the patient's name on the label and hang it for my patient.
- Check the other patient's medication administration record (MAR) to confirm that he is, indeed, receiving the same drug at the same dose as my patient, and if so, use this bag for my patient (since it is in my patient's drawer and my patient is due for it).

- Ask my nurse and/or preceptor what to do. Is it okay, safe, and legal to use this bag if someone else's name is on the label? If they say yes, check with the nurse caring for the patient whose name is on the label to make sure she does not need the medication right now.
- Send the bag back to pharmacy, requesting they send up a new one with an accurate label.
- Call pharmacy, ask them to send up a new bag with an accurate label, and tell them I am giving the other bag to the other patient's nurse.

Evaluating a Good Outcome: How Do I Define Success?

- The right patient receives the right drug, at the right dose, at the right time, via the right route, with the right documentation, understanding the right rationale.
- The patient feels comfortable and safe with the drug being administered to him.
- The needs of my patient and those of the patient whose name was on the bag are assessed and met.

- Both patients have the medication available to them when they need it and are due for it.
- My education and my license, along with that of my nurse and preceptor, are not put at risk by an avoidable medication error.
- My legal skills are sharpened by thinking through and working through the situation.

Personal Learning: Here's to the Future!

Ultimately, I addressed the situation step by step to make sure all the bases were covered. First, I checked the other patient's drawer to see if he had a bag of this IV antibiotic. He did not, which led me to believe that either his bag was placed in my drawer by accident, or his bag had not been made yet (that the bag in my patient's drawer was intended for my patient but had the wrong label on it). Then I checked my patient's MAR and that of the other patient. Indeed, both were ordered to receive the same drug at the same dose via the same route. However, my patient was due for it at 1000, the other patient was due for it at 1400. Next, I brought the medication bag, the MARs, and my other paperwork to my clinical preceptor and to the nurses caring for my patient and the other patient. They all agreed that the bag that was in my drawer was the right drug at the right dose, even though it had the wrong name on the label. However, it is not the nurse's responsibility or legal right to dispense medication. For this reason, the bag of medication needs to be returned to the pharmacy because it was labeled with the wrong name. The pharmacist must relabel the medication, preparing and dispensing a correctly labeled dose for each patient. I called the pharmacy, explained what I had found, and told them I would be returning the

dose that had been delivered to my patient. I requested a correct dose for 1000 for my patient. The pharmacy delivered a new bag of medication, correctly labeled, in time for the patient's 1000 dose. After checking everything again, I administered the medication to my patient. My patient did not have an adverse reaction, the other patient got his medication when it was due, and no mistakes were made by any of the nurses. The only mistake that was made was by pharmacy, which put the wrong label on the bag and then put the bag in the drawer.

I learned that checking and double-checking medication labels is extremely important. After a while, we all have a tendency to get into the habit of glancing at things when we are in a hurry, especially when it involves labels we look at all the time, feeling confident that we would recognize a problem. This is not the first time I could have missed a change on the label—there have been several times when I did not think to check every single thing on a label. That's because after giving it so many times, I felt it had become routine. But every time I am tempted not to double-check a label, I am reminded of this situation. As a result, I triple-check things, because those are the times when I may not paying as close attention as I need to be.

(continued)

Drug Nomenclature

Drugs have several names, including chemical, generic, official, and trade. The chemical name is a precise description of the drug's chemical composition. The chemical name identifies the drug's atomic and molecular structure using exact chemical language and terminology. The **generic name,** which identifies the drug's active ingredient, is the name assigned by the manufacturer that first develops the drug. Often, the generic name is derived from the chemical name. The **official name** is the name by which the drug is identified in the official publications, United States Pharmacopeia and National Formulary (USP and NF). The official name is often the generic name. The **trade name,** also referred to as the brand name or proprietary name, is selected by the drug company that sells the drug and is protected by trademark. A drug can have several trade names when produced by different manufacturers.

Nurses should be familiar with a drug's generic and trade names. For example, acetaminophen (generic name) has trade names such as Tylenol, Tempra, and Liquiprin. Recognizing a drug's name is an important part of the nurse's responsibilities when transcribing orders and administering medication therapies.

Types of Drug Preparations

Drugs are available in many forms, or preparations. The form in which the drug is prepared may determine the route of administration. Drug preparations are available for oral, topical, and parenteral administration. Some drugs may be prepared in only one form to be administered by a certain route. Others may be supplied in several preparations, allowing them to be given through various routes. One type of preparation may be desirable in a given situation. For example, a liquid preparation of a medication would be indicated for a young child who cannot swallow solid preparations, such as tablets. A suppository may be indicated to deliver a medication for a patient who cannot take anything by mouth. Table 29-1 describes drug preparations commonly used by nurses.

Drug Classifications

Drug classifications, or drug classes, are groups of drugs that share similar characteristics. Drugs are classified in several ways. For example, drugs may be classified by effect on body systems (e.g., drugs that affect the respiratory system, drugs that affect the cardiovascular system), by chemical composition, or by the clinical indication for the drug or therapeutic action (e.g., analgesic, antibiotic). Knowledge related to the class of drug can be applied to individual drugs in that class.

Mechanisms of Drug Action
Pharmacokinetics

Pharmacokinetics is the effect of the body on the drug. It is the movement of drug molecules in the body in relation to the drug's absorption, distribution, metabolism, and excretion.

ABSORPTION

Absorption is the process by which a drug is transferred from its site of entry into the body to the bloodstream. Absorption of a drug is influenced by several factors, which are discussed below.

TABLE • 29-1	COMMON TYPES OF DRUG PREPARATIONS
Preparation	**Description**
Capsule	Powder or gel form of an active drug enclosed in a gelatinous container; may also be called liquigel
Elixir	Medication in a clear liquid containing water, alcohol, sweeteners, and flavor
Enteric coated	A tablet or pill coated to prevent stomach irritation
Extended release	Preparation of a medication that allows for slow and continuous release over a predetermined period; may also be referred to as CR or CRT (controlled release), SR (sustained or slow release), SA (sustained action), LA (long acting), or TR (timed release)
Liniment	Medication mixed with alcohol, oil, or soap, which is rubbed on the skin
Lotion	Drug particles in a solution for topical use
Lozenge	Small oval, round, or oblong preparation containing a drug in a flavored or sweetened base, which dissolves in the mouth and releases the medication; also called *troche*
Ointment	Semisolid preparation containing a drug to be applied externally; also called an *unction*
Pill	Mixture of a powdered drug with a cohesive material; may be round or oval
Powder	Single or mixture of finely ground drugs
Solution	A drug dissolved in another substance (e.g., in an aqueous solution)
Suppository	An easily melted medication preparation in a firm base such as gelatin that is inserted into the body (rectum, vagina, urethra)
Suspension	Finely divided, undissolved particles in a liquid medium; should be shaken before use
Syrup	Medication combined in a water and sugar solution
Tablet	Small, solid dose of medication, compressed or molded; may be any color, size, or shape; *enteric-coated tablets* are coated with a substance that is insoluble in gastric acids to reduce gastric irritation by the drug
Transdermal patch	Unit dose of medication applied directly to skin for diffusion through skin and absorption into the bloodstream

Route of Administration

The rate of absorption depends on the route of administration. Drugs given orally usually take the longest to be absorbed. Injected medications are usually absorbed more rapidly than oral medications. Drugs administered intravenously are placed directly into the bloodstream and thus technically are not absorbed and take effect quickly (Aschenbrenner & Venable, 2009).

Lipid Solubility

Cell membranes have a fatty acid layer. A drug that is more lipid soluble can be absorbed more readily and pass more easily through the cell membrane.

pH

Acidic drugs are well absorbed in the stomach. Drugs that are basic remain ionized or insoluble in an acid environment. These drugs are not absorbed before reaching the small intestine. The concept of acid–base balance is further discussed in Chapter 40.

Blood Flow

Absorption is increased with increased blood flow. Patients with impaired circulatory function absorb drugs less rapidly than do patients with normal circulatory function.

Local Conditions at the Site of Administration

The more extensive the absorbing surface, the greater the absorption of the drug and the more rapid the effect. For example, a patient with burns would have poor absorption from an intramuscular injection. Food in the stomach can delay the absorption of some medications or enhance the rate of absorption of other drugs. Drug absorption can be manipulated with sustained-release preparations or enteric-coated preparations. Enteric-coated preparations are resistant to the digestive action of the stomach.

Drug Dosage

A loading dose, or a larger than normal dose, is usually given when a patient is in acute distress and the maximum therapeutic effect is desired as quickly as possible. If drug toxicity occurs, it can be detected quickly and treated in the controlled hospital environment. A maintenance dose is a lower dosage that becomes the usual or daily dosage. Patients who receive digoxin or phenobarbital, for example, may receive loading doses when therapy is initiated. The goal of drug dosing is to give a dose that achieves the desired therapeutic effect of the drug (**pharmacotherapeutics**) without causing other undesirable effects (*adverse effects*, discussed later) (Aschenbrenner & Venable, 2009).

DISTRIBUTION

After a drug has been absorbed into the bloodstream, it is distributed throughout the body. **Distribution** depends on blood flow to the tissues, the drug's ability to leave the bloodstream, and the drug's ability to enter the cells (Aschenbrenner & Venable, 2009). Certain other factors may also influence distribution. The drug may bind to plasma proteins, which causes unequal distribution and prevents the drug from reaching its intended site of action. Another factor affecting distribution is the blood–brain barrier. The blood–brain barrier is a structure made up of tightly packed capillary walls that supply blood to the brain. It prevents toxins and poisons from reaching the brain. Unfortunately, many drugs cannot penetrate the barrier, obviously influencing distribution. Some drugs fail to penetrate the tissues of the central nervous system as readily as others. The placenta, on the other hand, is not a barrier like the blood–brain barrier. Drugs readily move across the placenta, and many drugs produce harmful effects in the fetus. These factors must be considered when planning and implementing drug therapies. Any concern about the safe use of a medication during pregnancy can be identified in a pharmacology text, through consultation with a pharmacist, or from a computer resource.

METABOLISM

Metabolism, or biotransformation, is the change of a drug from its original form to a new form. The liver is the primary site for drug metabolism. Various processes and enzymes are involved in metabolism. Physiologic changes associated with aging, the presence of liver disease, or other factors that impair the functioning of the liver decrease the ability of the liver to metabolize drugs. Other tissues, such as those of the gastrointestinal tract, lungs, kidney, and skin, have a role in drug metabolism (Aschenbrenner & Venable, 2009). Pharmacology texts provide more detailed explanations of metabolism.

EXCRETION

After the drug is broken down to an inactive form, **excretion** of the drug occurs. Excretion is the process of removing a drug, or its metabolites (products of metabolism), from the body. The kidneys excrete most drugs. The lungs are the primary route for the excretion of gaseous substances, such as inhalation anesthetics. Many drugs are excreted through bile in the gastrointestinal tract. The sweat, salivary, and mammary glands are also routes of drug excretion.

Some medications may be contraindicated, or dosages may need to be adjusted, if renal excretion is impaired. Changes associated with aging, disease, or the presence of other factors that impair the functioning of the kidneys can decrease their ability to excrete drugs. Manufacturers are required by law to include specific information regarding implications for geriatric patients on the package inserts of certain drugs. Of particular concern are details concerning the excretion of these drugs in older adults whose renal function has declined. This law affects psychotropic drugs, nonsteroidal anti-inflammatory agents, oral hypoglycemic agents, anticoagulants, certain broad-spectrum antibiotics, and cardiac drugs.

Pharmacodynamics

Drugs act at the cellular level to achieve the desired effects. The process by which drugs alter cell physiology and affect the body is called **pharmacodynamics** (Aschenbrenner & Venable, 2009). Drugs turn on, turn off, promote, or block responses that are part of the body's processes. One mechanism of drug action is a drug–receptor interaction, in which the drug interacts with one or more cellular structures to alter cell function. These specialized structures are called receptor sites. The drug fits the receptor as a key fits a lock. Drugs may also combine with other molecules in the body to achieve their effect. For example, a drug may combine with an enzyme to achieve the desired effect, which is referred to as a drug–enzyme interaction. Other drugs act on the cell membrane or alter the cellular environment to achieve their effect.

Adverse Drug Effects

Although therapeutic effect is the desired outcome in medication administration, sometimes secondary undesirable effects occur. Undesirable effects other than the intended therapeutic effect of a drug are known as **adverse drug effects** (Aschenbrenner & Venable, 2009). Some adverse effects are predictable and may be tolerated as part of the therapy. For example, morphine, a narcotic agonist, is used to treat moderate to severe and chronic pain. A known adverse effect with morphine use is constipation. However, the benefit of pain relief usually outweighs the adverse effect of constipation, so that often, the adverse effect is accepted and managed with stool softeners and laxatives. On the other hand, adverse effects can be severe and may require discontinuation of the drug, depending on whether the benefit of the drug outweighs the harm from the adverse effect. For example, another common adverse effect of morphine is nausea and vomiting. If uncontrollable and severe, persistent nausea and vomiting will result in discontinuation of the morphine and a switch to another type of pain medication. Another example of an adverse drug effect is the development of an iatrogenic disorder caused unintentionally by drug therapy. Neutropenia caused by chemotherapy is an example of this. Other types of adverse effects discussed below include allergic effects, drug tolerance, toxic effects, idiosyncratic effects, and drug interactions.

It is important to monitor for adverse effects from drug therapy. Serious adverse reactions must be documented according to agency policy and should be reported to a national database, such as MedWatch. MedWatch is a safety information and voluntary adverse events reporting program, sponsored by the U.S. Food and Drug Administration (FDA), which also provides up-to-date information about medication errors and potential or actual medical product problems and errors (Aschenbrenner & Venable, 2009). According to FDA criteria, a serious adverse drug event is defined as an action that is life threatening, requires intervention to prevent death or permanent impairment, and/or leads to death, hospitalization, disability, or congenital anomaly. Nurses and healthcare professionals are encouraged to complete a form that provides information on a medication or medical product that they suspect either has caused harm or has the potential to cause harm and submit the form to the MEDWATCH program. This provides a national tracking of all serious adverse drug reactions. Reporting of serious adverse effects is necessary for corrective action to take place to protect patients. This information is used to revise drug labels, add warnings for healthcare providers, create patient medication guides, or withdraw a drug from the market (U.S. FDA, 2009c). Additional information regarding reporting adverse events is discussed at the end of the chapter, in the section on Preventing and Responding to Medication Errors.

Allergic Effect

An **allergic effect** is an immune system response that occurs when the body interprets the administered drug as a foreign substance and forms antibodies against the drug. Drug allergies can be manifested in a variety of symptoms ranging from minor to serious. The reaction can occur immediately after the patient receives the medication or be delayed for hours to days. Symptoms may become more severe each time the drug is introduced into the body. Some of the signs and symptoms of a drug allergy are rash, urticaria, fever, diarrhea, nausea, and vomiting. The most serious allergic effect is called an **anaphylactic reaction (anaphylaxis).** Anaphylaxis is life threatening and results in respiratory distress, sudden severe bronchospasm, and cardiovascular collapse. This reaction is treated with vasopressors, bronchodilators, corticosteroids, oxygen therapy, intravenous fluids, and antihistamines.

Drug Tolerance

Drug tolerance occurs when the body becomes accustomed to the effects of a particular drug over a period of time. Larger doses of the drug must be taken to produce the desired effect. For example, patients using morphine for an extended period of time become tolerant to the drug's therapeutic effects and eventually need higher and higher doses to control their pain.

Toxic Effect

Toxic effects (toxicities) are specific groups of symptoms related to drug therapy that carry risk for permanent damage or death (Aschenbrenner & Venable, 2006). The organ or system affected by the toxicity is used to name the toxicity, as in hepatotoxicity, or damage to the liver. Toxicities can

occur from a **cumulative effect.** A cumulative effect occurs when the body cannot metabolize one dose of a drug before another dose is administered. The drug is taken in more frequently than it is excreted, and each new dose increases the total quantity in the body.

Idiosyncratic Effect

An **idiosyncratic effect** (sometimes called paradoxical effect) is any unusual or peculiar response to a drug that may manifest itself by over response, under response, or even the opposite of the expected response. Idiosyncratic effects are related to a patient's unique response to a drug and are thought to be the result of genetic enzyme deficiencies that lead to an abnormal mechanism of drug breakdown. Older patients often have unpredictable or erratic responses to medications.

Drug Interactions

Drug interactions occur when one drug is affected in some way by another drug, a food, or another substance that is taken at the same time. Drug interactions may be advantageous when, for example, a medication is given to decrease the adverse effects of a drug or increase its therapeutic effects. Other drug interactions are not beneficial: for example, interactions that decrease the therapeutic effect and/or increase the adverse effects. In a drug–drug interaction, the combined effect of two or more drugs acting simultaneously produces an effect either less than that of each drug alone (**antagonist effect**) or greater than that of each drug alone (**synergistic effect**). Alcohol and barbiturates, for example, when taken together create an unbeneficial synergistic effect with the potential for significantly increased central nervous system depression. It is important to be knowledgeable about, and alert for, drug interactions and the effects of drug therapy.

Drug interactions in older adults are a very real and dangerous problem because older adults are more likely to take more than one drug (Bushardt & Jones, 2005; Greenawalt, 2009). Elderly patients often see more than one physician and do not always remember to bring the medications that they are taking to each physician they see. This leads to polypharmacy (the taking of more than two medications at a time), which can result in serious drug interactions.

> *Think back to Mildred Campbell, the 65-year-old woman with arthritis and hypertension (high blood pressure) asking about a recently advertised medication for joint pain relief. The nurse should assess the patient's medication history to determine her current medication regimen. This information is crucial to obtain so that the nurse can evaluate for possible polypharmacy and potential risks for drug interactions, even before discussing whether the advertised medication would be appropriate.* ■

Dietary supplements and herbal and "natural" remedies are another potential problem area for drug interactions. Many patients do not consider dietary supplements, herbal, and natural remedies to be medications because they can purchase these items at a nutrition store and consider them safe to use. However, many of these products have recognized pharmacological effects, unexpected allergic reactions, and problematic drug–supplement interactions (Heyneman, 2003). When asking patients if they are taking any medications, specifically ask if they are taking any herbal or natural supplements. Healthcare providers need to be aware of the intended benefits, possible adverse effects, potential drug interactions, and perioperative implications related to these types of supplements (Capriotti, 2004a). Further information related to dietary supplements and natural and herbal products can be found at the U.S. Food and Drug Administration's Web site (www.fda.gov/Food/DietarySupplements/default.htm) and the National Center for Complementary and Alternative Medicine (NCCAM) (http://nccam.nih.gov/).

Factors Affecting Drug Action

Certain variables can influence the action or effect of a medication. These variables include developmental considerations, patient's body weight, patient's gender, genetic and cultural factors, psychological factors, pathology, environment, and timing of medication administration.

Developmental Considerations

During pregnancy, many drugs are contraindicated because of their possible adverse effects on the fetus. Certain drugs, referred to as **teratogenic,** are known to have the potential to cause developmental defects in the embryo or fetus and are definitely contraindicated. Examples of teratogenic drugs include cocaine, alcohol, phenytoin (Dilantin, an anticonvulsant), and isotretinoin (Accutane, a medication used to treat severe acne). Some drugs cross into breast milk, so breastfed infants are also at risk for adverse effects from drugs in the mother's circulation. Small body size, reduced weight, and reduced body water also alter distribution, as do decreases in cardiac output and organ perfusion. Therefore, a child's medication dose is smaller than an adult's dose. Infants are especially sensitive to medications because of the immaturity of their organs and immaturity of the blood–brain barrier. Older people are sensitive to medications because their bodies have experienced physiologic changes associated with the aging process, including decreased gastric motility, muscle mass, acid production, and blood flow, which affect drug absorption. They may also be more susceptible to certain adverse effects. Liver function declines with advancing age, and changes occur in the hepatic enzymes involved in drug metabolism. Blood flow to the liver decreases secondary to a decrease in cardiac output. Drugs are excreted more slowly from the body as a result of changes in kidney function. Receptor sensitivity is altered in older people, and their sensitivity to certain drugs increases. The physiologic changes in older people that increase drug susceptibility are summarized in the accompanying display, Focus on the Older Adult.

> Recall Mr. Baptiste, the elderly patient receiving intravenous antibiotics for a wound infection. The nurse would need to consider age-related changes that might interfere with the drug action, being especially alert for signs and symptoms of drug toxicity. ■

Weight

Expected responses to drugs are based largely on the reactions that occur when the drugs are given to healthy adults (18 to 65 years of age, 150 lb [68 kg]). It is important to know the usual dose for a medication before administering it. Drug doses for children are calculated by weight or body surface area (BSA).

Gender

The difference in the distribution of body fat and fluids in men and women is a minor factor affecting the action of some drugs. To date, most research on drugs and their actions and effects has been conducted on men. Future clinical drug trials are expected to include more women to document the effects of hormonal fluctuations.

Cultural and Genetic Factors

Religious restrictions and beliefs or cultural practices may affect the patient's acceptance of, response to, and compliance with certain drug therapies. Healthcare providers need an understanding of a patient's cultural values, beliefs, and practices to provide culturally acceptable care (Purnell, 2009). For example, Christian Scientists place their faith in spiritual healing; therefore, they do not take medicine. A Christian Scientist would not participate in a childhood vaccination program or pharmaceutical therapy to manage disease (Ward, 1988). Herbal treatments that are popular in some cultures may interfere with or counteract the action of prescribed medication.

Ethnopharmacology is the study of the effect of ethnicity on responses to prescribed medication, especially drug absorption, metabolism, distribution, and excretion. It includes pharmacogenetics, the study of genetic variations in response to drugs. Differences in the responses of patients receiving the same medication may result from genetic differences, such as genetic variations in certain enzymes that may cause differing drug response. Ethnicity influences response to certain medications. Certain ethnic groups have more of these variations than do others (Muñoz & Hilgenberg, 2005). Nurses need to know about medications that may produce varied responses in patients from different ethnic groups. Specifically, there may be important variations in the therapeutic dose and/or incidence of adverse effects; some patients in certain ethnic groups obtain therapeutic responses at lower doses than those usually prescribed, while other patient groups experience less effect or more effect from prescribed medications than expected. For example, certain angiotensin-converting enzyme inhibitors have been found to be less

FOCUS ON THE OLDER ADULT

AGING AND DRUG RESPONSE

Age-Related Changes	Implication or Response	Nursing Interventions
Decreased gastric motility; increased gastric pH	Stomach irritation; nausea; vomiting; gastric ulceration	• Assess for symptoms of gastrointestinal discomfort • Assess stools for blood
Decreased lean body mass; decreased total body water	Decreased distribution water-soluble drugs and higher plasma concentrations, leading to increased possibility of drug toxicity	• Assess for signs of drug interactions or toxicity • Monitor blood levels of drugs • Monitor fluid balance; intake and output
Increased adipose tissue	Accumulation of fat-soluble drugs; delay in elimination from and accumulation of drug in the body, leading to prolonged action and increased possibility of toxicity	• Assess for signs of drug interactions or toxicity • Monitor blood levels of drugs
Decreased number of protein-binding sites	Higher drug plasma concentrations, leading to increased possibility of drug toxicity	• Assess for signs of drug interactions or toxicity • Monitor blood levels of drugs • Monitor laboratory values—albumin and prealbumin
Decreased liver function; decreased enzyme production for drug metabolism; decreased hepatic perfusion	Decreased rate of drug metabolism; higher drug plasma concentrations, leading to prolonged action and increased possibility of drug toxicity	• Assess for signs of drug interactions or toxicity • Monitor blood levels of drugs • Monitor laboratory values—hepatic enzymes
Decreased kidney function, renal mass, and blood flow	Decreased excretion of drugs, leading to possible increased serum levels/toxicity	• Assess for signs of drug interactions or toxicity • Particularly monitor NSAID use; may decrease renal blood flow and function • Monitor blood levels of drugs • Monitor laboratory values—creatinine clearance, blood urea nitrogen, serum creatinine
Alterations in normal homeostatic responses; altered peripheral venous tone	Exacerbated response to cardiovascular drugs; more pronounced hypotensive effects from medications	• Assess for signs of drug interactions or toxicity • Monitor blood levels of drugs • Monitor vital signs • Orthostatic hypotension precautions
Alterations in blood–brain barrier	Enhanced central nervous system penetration of fat-soluble drugs; increased possibility for alterations in mental status, dizziness, gait disturbances	• Assess for signs of drug interactions or toxicity • Assess for dizziness and light-headedness • Fall safety precautions
Decreased central nervous system efficiency	Prolonged effect of drugs on the central nervous system; exacerbated response to analgesics and sedatives	• Assess for signs of drug interactions or toxicity • Assess for alterations in neurological status • Monitor vital signs and pulse oximetry
Decreased production of oral secretions; dry mouth	Difficulty swallowing oral medications	• Monitor ability to swallow medications, especially tablets and capsules • Discuss changing medications to forms that can be crushed and/or liquid forms with prescribing practitioner
Decreased lipid content in skin	Possible decrease in absorption of transdermal medications	• Monitor effectiveness of transdermal preparations

Adapted from Aschenbrenner, D., & Venable, S. (2009). *Drug therapy in nursing* (3rd ed.). Philadelphia: Wolters Kluwer Health/Lippincott Williams & Wilkins; Tabloski, P. (2010). *Gerontological nursing* (2nd ed.). Upper Saddle River, NJ: Pearson Prentice Hall; Porth, C., & Matfin, G. (2009). *Pathophysiology: Concepts of altered health states* (8th ed.). Philadelphia: Wolters Kluwer Health/Lippincott Williams & Wilkins; and Smeltzer, S., Bare, B., Hinkle, J. H., & Cheever, K. H. (2010). *Brunner & Suddarth's textbook of medical-surgical nursing* (12th ed.). Philadelphia: Lippincott Williams & Wilkins.

Box 29-1 TIPS FOR COMMUNICATING EFFECTIVELY ABOUT MEDICATION WITH CULTURALLY DIVERSE PATIENTS

- Acquire basic information about health beliefs and practices of various cultural groups in your healthcare setting. This provides a basis for assessing patient's beliefs and practices. Recognize, however, that within all cultures and ethnic groups, there are members who do not hold all the values of the group.
- Be alert to atypical drug responses or unexpected adverse effects that may occur in certain ethnic groups. This knowledge helps you direct assessment questions as appropriate.
- Ask specifically about the use of folk or home remedies prescribed by a nontraditional healer.
- Ask specific questions about possible adverse effects, rather than asking general questions or waiting for the patient to voice concerns. For example, do not ask, "Are you having any problems with your medicine?" Instead, ask, "Have you noticed any unusual, involuntary movements?"
- Consider culture when teaching patients and families. Ask, "What do you think caused your health problem?" and "What treatment do you think will help?" Include culturally sensitive information in all basic health teaching.
- Determine the patient's language preferences for spoken and written communication.
- Use printed or audiovisual information that is in the language spoken by your patients.
- Encourage cultural sensitivity in healthcare workers in your particular setting.
- Recognize that diversity exists within cultural groups. For example, the Hispanic population includes Mexicans, Cubans, Puerto Ricans, and other Latino groups.
- Emphasize threads or messages in health teaching that are common to all cultures (e.g., concern about family, faith, and home).
- Help culturally diverse patients to value and understand the importance of communicating concerns and asking questions about prescribed medications. Patients and families need to know how to identify major adverse effects of the medications they are taking and the appropriate person(s) to contact if these effects are noted.

Adapted from Muñoz, C., & Hilgenberg, C. (2005). Ethnopharmacology. *American Journal of Nursing, 105*(8), 40–47; and Purnell, L. (2009). *Guide to culturally competent health care* (2nd ed.). Philadelphia: F. A. Davis.

---

effective in members of the African American population. Alternately, certain thiazide diuretics appear to be better for controlling hypertension in African Americans. African American, Japanese, and Taiwanese patients may experience elevated serum drug levels when lithium is prescribed in the usual dosages, thus experiencing symptoms of drug toxicity. Care must be taken, however, to avoid making sweeping generalizations and assumptions. Ethnicity influences responses to certain medications, but no two individuals are alike.

General and specific cultural knowledge allows the healthcare provider to ask the right questions when interacting with patients of varying backgrounds. Nurses who are aware of the specific needs and beliefs of culturally diverse patient populations are better able to communicate effectively and provide optimal care. Box 29-1 gives guidelines for effective communication about medication with culturally diverse patients.

Psychological Factors

The patient's expectations of the medication may affect the response to the medication, as, for instance, in studies of drug effects in which some patients receive a placebo. A **placebo** is a pharmacologically inactive substance. In clinical drug trials, one group of patients receives the active drug, whereas another group receives a placebo to study the drug's effects. Some patients appear to have the same response with the placebo as with the active drug.

Pathology

The presence of disease can affect drug action. For example, the liver is the primary organ for drug breakdown, so pathologic conditions that involve the liver may slow metabolism and alter the dosage of the drug needed to reach a therapeutic level. The kidneys excrete most drugs and their byproducts from the body. Pathologic conditions that involve the kidneys would change excretion and alter the dosage of the drug required to obtain a therapeutic level. These types of conditions also influence the presence of adverse effects, such as toxicities.

Environment

The patient's environment may influence his or her response to medications. Sensory deprivation and overload may affect drug responses. The patient who receives pain medication or a sedative in an active, noisy environment may not be able to benefit fully from the medication's effects, whereas those receiving pain medication in a quiet environment and using an additional relaxation method, such as guided imagery, may have a longer benefit from the pain medication. The relative oxygen deprivation at high altitudes may increase sensitivity to some drugs.

In addition, nutritional state can also affect the body's reaction to certain drugs. When dietary factors are altered, drug therapy may produce different effects in the body than would normally occur. For example, many drugs normally bind to proteins in the plasma. Lowered protein levels in the body means less drug bound to plasma proteins, leading to a higher concentration of free drug in the body. A higher drug concentration increases the drug's effect in the body and the risk for adverse effects (Aschenbrenner & Venable, 2009).

Timing of Administration

The presence of food in the stomach can delay the absorption of orally administered medications. Alternately, some medications should be given with food to prevent gastric irritation, and the nurse should consider this when establishing a patient's medication schedule. Other medications may have enhanced absorption if taken with certain foods. Circadian rhythms and cycles may also influence drug action.

Drug Dose and Serum Drug Levels

Blood levels of a drug are often measured to help evaluate whether a drug's dose is at a level to achieve the desired effect and below the level at which adverse effects occur (Aschenbrenner & Venable, 2009).

After a drug has been absorbed, its serum level can be monitored by drawing a blood specimen and measuring the level of the drug in the serum. This is recommended for certain medications (e.g., aminoglycoside antibiotics, digoxin, warfarin) to ensure that a therapeutic range is maintained. A drug's **therapeutic range** is the concentration of drug in the blood serum that produces the desired effect without causing toxicity. The **peak level,** or highest plasma concentration, of the drug should be measured when absorption is complete. The peak level may be affected by factors that affect drug absorption as well as the route of administration. The **trough level** is the point when the drug is at its lowest concentration, and this specimen is usually drawn in the 30-minute interval before the next dose. The dosage schedule, as well as the half-life of the drug, can modify the trough level. A drug's **half-life** is the amount of time it takes for 50% of the blood concentration of a drug to be eliminated from the body. Monitoring these levels ensures that therapeutic ranges are obtained without reaching toxic levels.

> ➤ *Consider Regina Sauder, the woman admitted to the hospital with a deep vein thrombosis. She is receiving intravenous heparin and oral warfarin, both of which are monitored using blood tests. Her dose of each drug is adjusted based on the results to ensure the appropriate therapeutic effect.* ■

Drug Legislation

In 1906, the Pure Food and Drug Act designated the United States Pharmacopeia and the National Formulary as the official drug standards in the United States, which set national standards for drug quality. This act also empowered the federal government to enforce these standards. This legislation was updated in 1938 by the Federal Food, Drug and Cosmetic Act, prohibiting adulterated or mislabeled drugs from being made available. The Food and Drug Administration (FDA) enforces this law. Extensive testing of new drugs is required before they may be marketed for use. An amendment to the Federal Food, Drug and Cosmetic Act in 1952 distinguished prescription drugs from nonprescription (over-the-counter) drugs and provided directions for dispensing prescription drugs. An additional amendment in 1962 increased controls on drug safety, requiring tighter testing of drugs and written inclusion of adverse reactions and contraindications for approved drugs.

The Kefauver-Harris Amendment of 1962 required adverse reactions and contraindications to be included in drug literature. The Comprehensive Drug Abuse Prevention and Control Act, also known as the Controlled Substances Act, was passed in 1970. This law regulates the distribution of narcotics and other drugs of abuse. Such drugs have been categorized according to their therapeutic usefulness and potential for abuse. Government programs for the prevention and treatment of drug abuse were established.

PRINCIPLES OF MEDICATION ADMINISTRATION
Medication Orders

No medication may be given to a patient without a medication order from a licensed practitioner. Each health agency has a policy specifying the manner in which the practitioner writes an order. In some instances, orders are written on a form designed specifically for a primary care provider's order. This becomes part of a patient's permanent record. Many healthcare facilities use a computer-generated pharmacy order system and can receive a medication order by fax from the physician. Some facilities are beginning to use computer prescriber order-entry systems (CPOE). CPOE systems allow the prescriber to enter medication orders in a standard format. CPOEs guide the prescriber in complete, accurate, and appropriate ordering. The computer sends the order directly to the pharmacy and enters the order into the patient's permanent record. This prevents any guessing when handwriting is illegible or drug names are similar. Some of the information this system provides includes recommended dosing of medications, drug-specific information, current patient information, laboratory tests that monitor the action of the drug, and potential interactions that may occur with other medications or food (Carroll, 2003; Grissinger & Globus, 2004; Hughes & Ortiz, 2005; McIntyre & Courey, 2007). A computerized order-entry system can make medication administration safer and reduce adverse drug events.

Safe practice dictates that a nurse follows only a written or typed order, or an order entered into a computer order-entry system because these types of orders are less likely to result in error or misunderstanding. Under certain circumstances, such as in an emergency, a verbal order from the physician may be given to a registered nurse or a pharmacist. In most settings, a student nurse is not permitted to accept a verbal order from a physician. The legal implications for dispensing and administering an agent without a written order vary, and nurses must be familiar with the exact agency policy whenever called on to administer therapeutic agents. The legal implications of verbal orders are discussed in Chapter 7.

Usual hospital policy dictates that when a patient is admitted, unless specific orders to the contrary are written, all drugs that the physician may have ordered while the patient was at home are discontinued. This can be a problem when a patient brings medications from home to the hospital. To avoid the possibility of having the patient continue to take the home medications while receiving the same ones or others under new orders, all medications should be sent home with the family or removed from the patient's unit and placed in safekeeping. This requires an explanation to the patient and the family of how the patient's drug plan is to be implemented.

However, in some inpatient facilities, patients keep their medications at their bedside and learn, or continue, to administer them as they would at home. It is believed that this approach helps to promote patients' independence. Be aware when patients are allowed to take their own medications while hospitalized and know each medication's purpose and possible adverse effects. Also, make a notation on the patient's plan of care so that everyone knows the patient has medications at the bedside.

When a patient has had surgery, is transferred to another clinical service, or is transferred to another health agency, it is general practice that all orders related to drugs are discontinued and new orders are written in the new setting. It is important to carefully check that all medications that are appropriate are reordered. Medication reconciliation, the process of specifying medications and maintaining a current, accurate list of medications the patient is receiving, has been shown to decrease the incidence of medication errors that occur during care at points of transition (Barnsteiner, 2005). The accuracy of the list is validated, reviewed, and amended; the Joint Commission includes medications reconciliation as part of the 2010 National Patient Safety Goals. Goal 8 identifies accurate and complete reconciliation of medications across the continuum of care (Joint Commission, 2010). Medication reconciliation should also occur at the time of patient discharge from a facility, with the primary care provider identifying those drugs to be continued and those to be discontinued (Barnsteiner, 2005).

Types of Orders

There are several types of orders that a prescriber may write. A standing order is carried out as specified until it is canceled by another order. Many practitioners whose practices are limited to a particular clinical area have a specified set of written orders for all their hospitalized patients. These are also referred to as standing orders. A practitioner may write a standing order with specified limitations; that is, the prescriber specifies that a certain order is to be carried out for a stated number of days or times. After the stated period has passed, the order is canceled automatically.

The prescriber may write a **p.r.n. order** ("as needed") for medication. The patient receives medication when it is requested or required. P.r.n. orders are commonly written for treatment of symptoms. For example, medications used for pain relief, to relieve nausea, and for sleep aids are often written as a p.r.n. or as needed order.

Another type of order is the single, or one time, order. With this type of order, the directive is carried out only once, at a time specified by the prescriber. Medication to be administered immediately before surgery is an example of a single order. A **stat order** also is a single order, but it is carried out immediately. A stat order for a bronchodilator or an antihistamine would be carried out immediately for a patient who is experiencing an anaphylactic drug reaction.

Parts of the Medication Order

The medication order consists of seven parts:

1. Patient's name
2. Date and time the order is written
3. Name of drug to be administered
4. Dosage of the drug
5. Route by which the drug is to be administered
6. Frequency of administration of the drug
7. Signature of person writing the order

Medication orders require the drug, dose, rate, route, frequency, and, when appropriate, duration to be explicit and specific to the needs of the patient in order to achieve the desired outcome (Shane, 2009). In effect, medication orders are sentences where an error or lack of precision in any of the elements of the order can result in unintended consequences (Shane, 2009).

PATIENT'S NAME

The patient's full name is used. The middle name or initial should be included to avoid confusion with other patients. In many agencies, the patient's full name and identification number and the primary care provider's name are labeled on all sheets on the patient's chart, including the medical order sheet. Be extremely careful when administering medications when there is more than one patient on the unit with the same last name. Not only can the nurse give the wrong patient the wrong medication, but also a prescriber may write an order in the wrong patient's chart.

DATE AND TIME THE ORDER IS WRITTEN

The date the order is written is given, sometimes including the time as well. Because the nursing staff in inpatient agencies changes several times during each 24-hour period, the date and time help to prevent errors of oversight as different nurses take charge of the patient's care. When an order is to be followed for a specified number of days, the date and time are important so that the discontinuation date and time can be determined accurately. State law determines the length of time an order for a narcotic remains valid. Therefore, the date and time the order is written are essential for determining when the order for a narcotic becomes invalid. Hospitals are utilizing many computer applications in patient care. Examples of such technology include a computer-generated database, computer-generated medication administration orders, and computer-generated flow sheets. This technology is helping to improve patient safety, but it also requires that nurses check patient information frequently for changes in the patient's status as well as implementation of new medication orders.

NAME OF DRUG TO BE ADMINISTERED

The name of the drug is stated in the order, either by the brand name or by the generic name. Certain brand names are well known, but the practice of using the generic name is considered safest and is required by some healthcare agencies.

A nurse unfamiliar with a drug can use several sources to obtain information. The United States Pharmacopeia-National Formulary (USP-NF) is the official source in the United States. Most other countries have similar references that describe official therapeutic agents. Most facilities also provide their own formulary, listing the drugs stocked by the facility. Healthcare agencies are also providing access to online medication information sites. The *Physicians' Desk Reference* (PDR) is another source of information that is supplied by pharmaceutical companies. In addition, information about drugs can be obtained from the hospital pharmacist, the physician, and any of several texts written specifically for the nursing role in the management of drug therapy. Many of these nursing-specific texts are available as software and can be loaded onto handheld devices such as PDAs and Smartphones.

DOSAGE OF THE DRUG

The dosage of a drug can be stated in either the metric or the apothecary system. These systems are described below in the section Dosage Calculations. The metric system has been adopted internationally, is the most widely used, and is the safest measurement system for drug dosages. Apothecary measurements are used less frequently. A medication error may occur if nurses are unfamiliar with the apothecary system, if the physician's handwriting is illegible, or if administration equipment, such as syringes, cups, or reference sources, uses only metric measurement. Self-administered drugs are commonly labeled in household measurements to facilitate administration. Most agencies post a table of common equivalent dosages for people who have learned to use one system and find that the agency for which they work uses the other system. Although these tables are convenient and useful, the nurse should be prepared to convert from one system to the other because such tables are not available in every situation.

It is important to be familiar with common equivalent measurements when using household equipment, such as teaspoons and tablespoons, because the home is usually not equipped with special measuring devices; however, instruct patients to use measuring spoons and not silverware if administration equipment is not available due to the variability of the amount silverware can hold. The most common equivalents can be found in Appendix A.

Certain standard abbreviations are used to indicate drug amounts, and it is important to know the common abbreviations before administering drugs. See Box 17-3 in Chapter 17 for common abbreviations used in drug orders. Several abbreviations used in the past have been identified as having the potential to cause errors. The Joint Commission has identified an official "do not use" list of abbreviations. See Table 17-2 in Chapter 17 for this list.

ROUTE BY WHICH THE DRUG IS TO BE ADMINISTERED

The route to be used when administering a medication is stated clearly because some drugs can be given in more than one way and others may be used safely through only one route. Table 29-2 describes common routes by which medications are administered. See "The Nursing Process for Administering Medications" for guidelines on administering drugs by these routes.

FREQUENCY OF ADMINISTRATION OF THE DRUG

The time and frequency with which a drug is to be administered are usually stated in standard abbreviations in the medication order, although many abbreviations used in the past have been phased out due to error and safety concerns. Common abbreviations used in writing prescriptions, including time and frequency, are listed in Chapter 17, Box 17-3.

The nursing service, facility policy, and pharmacy departments of inpatient facilities usually determine the hours at which routine drugs are given. For example, an every–4-hour drug administration may be at the times of noon, 4 p.m., 8 p.m., midnight, 4 a.m., and 8 a.m. Another agency may use the hours 1 p.m., 5 p.m., 9 p.m., 1 a.m., 5 a.m., and 9 a.m. To lessen the risk for error, many healthcare facilities use the 24-hour clock (or military time), which designates midnight as 0000 hours and runs until 2400 hours. If an administration order states that the drug is to be given before or after meals, the time of administration depends on the hours at which meals are served. It is a nursing and pharmacy responsibility to check that times for medication administration correspond to safe practice for that drug.

If a drug is to be given only once or twice a day, the decision about which hours to use depends on the nature of the drug and the patient's plan of care, as well as the standard facility administration times. Whenever possible, the patient's choice of time should be considered.

Drugs should be administered punctually as ordered. A nurse administering drugs to several patients, however, cannot give all of the drugs exactly on the hour indicated. Agency policies vary, but a common one is that drugs should be administered within a half-hour before or after the indicated hour. Thus, a drug to be administered at 9 a.m. can be administered any time between 8:30 a.m. and 9:30 a.m. using this policy. However, this policy does not apply to all drugs. A preoperative medication ordered to be given at 7:30 a.m. should be administered at that hour because the time was planned in relation to the time surgery is to begin. Preoperative medications may also be given when the nursing unit receives a call from the operating room to premedicate the surgical patient. This also holds true when patients are given drugs before certain diagnostic procedures and with stat orders.

SIGNATURE OF PERSON WRITING THE ORDER

The signature, with title, of the person writing the order follows the order. The signature, with title, is important for legal reasons because the authority to prescribe drugs is defined by state laws. Also, if there is a question about the order, the

TABLE • 29-2 ROUTES FOR ADMINISTERING DRUGS	
Terms Used to Describe Route	**How Drug Is Administered**
Oral route	Having patient swallow drug
Enteral route	Administering drug through an enteral tube
Sublingual administration	Placing drug under tongue
Buccal administration	Placing drug between cheek and gum
Parenteral route	Injecting drug into
Subcutaneous injection	Subcutaneous tissue
Intramuscular injection	Muscle tissue
Intradermal injection	Corium (under epidermis)
Intravenous injection	Vein
Intraarterial injection	Artery
Intracardial injection	Heart tissue
Intraperitoneal injection	Peritoneal cavity
Intraspinal injection	Spinal canal
Intraosseous injection	Bone
Topical route	Applying drug onto skin or mucous membrane
Vaginal administration	Vagina
Rectal administration	Rectum
Inunction	Rubbing drug into skin
Instillation	Placing drug into direct contact with mucous membrane
Irrigation	Flushing mucous membrane with drug in solution
Skin application	Applying transdermal patch
Pulmonary route	Having patient inhale drug

signature indicates who should be contacted. Many facilities require the prescriber to also print his/her name with the signature, to facilitate reading of the prescriber's name.

Checking the Medication Order

Agency policy specifies the manner in which the medication order is checked. Various systems are used, and nurses should be familiar with the system used in the agency where they work and should implement it correctly to minimize errors.

In many institutions, the order is copied onto the patient's medication record, often called a MAR (medication administration record). Increasing numbers of healthcare facilities are computerizing patient records, including medication records (CMAR [computerized medication administration record]). The nurse is responsible for checking that the medication order was transcribed correctly by comparing it with the original order. The nurse is also responsible for double-checking the dosage and appropriateness of the medication.

Questioning the Medication Order

Nurses are legally responsible for the drugs they administer. Any drug order suspected to be in error should be questioned. The suspected error may be in any part of the order. When preparing to administer a medication, ask: Do the patient's condition, symptoms, and health status warrant receiving this medication? Does it make sense for the patient to have this medication? Is the correct dose and preparation ordered (Hughes & Ortiz, 2005)? The legal implications are

serious in a situation in which there is an error in a drug order and the nurse could be expected, based on knowledge and experience, to have noted and reported the error.

On occasion, the nurse may not think that there is an error in the order but may not understand why the medication has been prescribed. In such instances, ask the prescriber how the order relates to the patient's plan of care. This may prevent a medication error if the wrong medication has been ordered.

Confusion over the placement of a decimal point can lead to a medication error. A zero should always precede a decimal point (e.g., 0.1 mg) for clarity. The use of a trailing zero (e.g., 1.0) is not considered good practice and has been included in the Joint Commission's "Do not use" list. See Table 17-2 in Chapter 17 for additional abbreviations included in this list.

A drug to which the patient is allergic may be prescribed inadvertently. Best practice is to question the patient if they have ever received the medication and if they are aware of any reaction to the medication. The patient may describe past adverse reactions with the drug. It is general practice to indicate clearly on the patient's chart any drug allergies. The drug should not be given and the order should be questioned when, in the nurse's judgment, the patient is allergic to a drug. In many healthcare facilities, the patient may also wear a wristband that indicates specific allergies. An allergic reaction can be life threatening to the patient.

In addition, a drug may be ordered that would potentially interact with another medication the patient is taking. All medications that a nurse is unfamiliar with should be verified before administration to avoid possible drug interactions. If a nurse has difficulty reading an order, guessing is gross carelessness; checking with the person who wrote the order is the only safe procedure.

Nurses have the right to refuse to administer any medication that, based on their knowledge and experience, may be harmful to the patient. Although this situation seldom occurs, it is important to understand that the patient's safety is a primary objective in the administration of medications. Always notify the primary care provider of the refusal to administer any medication. Document any concerns regarding medication orders in the patient's medical record, and note the contact of the primary care provider, the response of the primary care provider, and any related interventions.

Medication Supply Systems

Medications are supplied in a number of ways. Many facilities make use of one or more systems in conjunction with each other, or variations of systems. A change to unit dose dispensing on a patient-specific basis is now the standard of practice for most hospitals. Pharmaceutical manufacturers should also provide all medications in health systems in unit dose packages (American Society of Health-System Pharmacists [ASHP], 2009). Computerized automated dispensing cabinets (ADCs) are a new technology based on stock supply of unit dose medications. A large cabinet containing stock medications for the unit is used. The nurse accesses the system with a user name and password, calling up a medication list for a specific patient or a list of available medications. In many systems, only medications entered for a specific patient are available for withdrawal at any one time. A computerized medication dispensing system is shown in Figure 29-1. With an individual unit dose supply system, each patient is sup-

plied with the medication needed for a period of time. The nurse is responsible for accurately obtaining the prescribed medications from the patient's supply. In the unit dose system, the pharmacist simplifies medication preparation by packaging and labeling each dosage for a 24-hour period.

Some nursing units use a medication cart for the administration of medications. The standard cart contains individual drawers into which the medications for each patient are placed. The drawer is labeled with the patient's name. The nurse moves the cart from room to room when dispensing medications.

Another medication delivery system uses bar-code–enabled medication administration (BCMA). BCMA prevents one "wrong-patient" error and almost five "wrong-time" errors each day (Shane, 2009). Just as a CPOE has improved the safe prescribing of medications, the use of BCMA technology can improve patient safety and the accuracy of medication administration and documentation (ASHP, 2009). When using a computerized bar-coded administration system, each patient and each nurse wear identification with a unique bar code to identify the individual. Each drug is packaged with a bar code that includes its unique National Drug Code number to identify the form and dosage. The nurse scans his or her own ID, the patient's ID, and each package of medication to be administered. The system confirms the nurse's dispensing authority and the patient's ID, matching the patient with his medication profile. If any of the information is incorrect or does not match, an alert message will appear on the screen notifying the nurse of the discrepancy. The system also records the medication administration and stores the information (ASHP, 2009; Carroll, 2003; Grissinger & Globus, 2004).

Dosage Calculations
Systems of Measurement

Nurses need to be proficient in the use of weights and measures as well as systems of measurement to calculate drug dosages and prepare medications for administration. Three systems of measurement are used for administering medications: the metric system, the apothecary system, and the household system. All three systems of measurement are in use in the United States. The nurse may be called on to convert dosages from one system to another. It is extremely important to be able to calculate commonly used equivalents, as listed in Appendix A. Practice the Medication Calculation Problems at the end of this chapter to develop your dose calculation skills.

METRIC SYSTEM

The metric system is the most widely accepted and convenient system. The basic units of measurement are the meter (linear), the liter (volume), and the gram (weight). The metric system is a decimal system, in which each unit can be divided into multiples of 10 (10, 100, 1,000). Calculations in the metric system often involve moving the decimal point to the right or left. In the preparation of medications, the following metric units are typically used:

FIGURE 29-1. Computerized medication dispensing system.

Weight

- 1 kilogram = 1,000 grams
- 1 gram = 1,000 milligrams
- 1 milligram = 1,000 micrograms

Volume

- 1 liter = 1,000 milliliters or cubic centimeters

It may be necessary to convert drug dosages to a different unit in the metric system. To convert a larger unit into a smaller unit, move the decimal point to the right (the new number is larger than the original). To convert a smaller unit into a larger unit, move the decimal point to the left (the new number is smaller than the original). *Example 1:* 0.5 g equals how many milligrams? Move the decimal point three places to right; the answer is 500 mg. *Example 2:* 900 mg equals how many grams? Move the decimal point three places to the left; the answer is 0.9 g.

APOTHECARY SYSTEM

The apothecary system is less convenient and precise than the metric system and is infrequently used. The basic unit of weight is the grain. The minim, dram, ounce, pint, and quart are used for volume. In the apothecary system, Roman numerals are used to express numbers (grains X), and quantities less than 1 are written in fraction form (grains 1/4).

HOUSEHOLD SYSTEM

The household system is the least accurate system of measurement and is not widely used except in home settings. Teaspoon, tablespoon, teacup, and glass are commonly used household measures. As discussed previously, teaspoon and tablespoon refer to measuring spoons, not silverware.

Methods for Computing Drug Dosages

Drugs are sometimes prepared and supplied in the amount ordered by the prescriber, and the nurse can see when checking the medication label that no calculation is necessary. At other times, drugs are not prepared and supplied in the exact quantities called for in the medication order, and the nurse must do a dosage calculation to determine what quantity of medication the patient is to receive.

FORMULA METHODS

Several formulas can be used to calculate drug dosages. One such formula consists of ratios to set up a proportion and can be used to calculate dosages for both solid and liquid preparations. A ratio shows the relation between numbers. A proportion contains two ratios. The nurse is usually seeking the quantity of on-hand medication that is equal to the desired dosage (the dosage ordered). The formula is as follows:

$$\frac{\text{dose on hand}}{\text{quantity on hand}} = \frac{\text{dose desired}}{X(\text{quantity desired})}$$

The dosage must be in the same unit of measurement. This applies to the quantity as well. Dosages are on the top line of the proportion, quantities on the bottom line. After the numbers are placed in the proportion, cross-multiply to find the desired quantity.

Example: Amoxicillin, 625 mg PO, is ordered. It is supplied as a liquid preparation containing 250 mg in 5 mL. How much does the nurse administer?

$$\frac{250 \text{ mg}}{5 \text{ mL}} = \frac{625 \text{ mg}}{X \text{ mL}}$$

Cross-multiply:

$$3,125 = 250X$$
$$X = 12.5 \text{ mL}$$

Example: Phenobarbital, gr i PO, is ordered. It is available in 30-mg tablets. How many tablets does the nurse administer? There are two systems of measurement in this problem. The nurse checks the list of equivalents to learn that 60 mg is equivalent to grains i.

$$\frac{30 \text{ mg}}{1 \text{ tablet}} = \frac{60 \text{ mg}}{X \text{ tablets}}$$
$$60 = 30X$$
$$X = 2 \text{ tablets}$$

Another formula that can be used to calculate drug dosages is as follows:

$$\frac{\text{dose desired}}{\text{dose on hand}} \times \text{quantity on hand} = \text{desired quantity}$$

This formula can be used for both liquid dosages and fractions of tablets.

DIMENSIONAL ANALYSIS

Another method that is used to compute medication dosages is dimensional analysis. Dimensional analysis, also known as factor-labeled method or conversion-factor method, is a systematic, straightforward approach to setting up and solving problems that require conversions. It is a way of thinking about problems that can be used when two quantities are directly proportional to each other, but one needs to be converted using a conversion factor in order for the problem to be solved (Craig, 2009). When using dimensional analysis, the first numerator must be what you are solving for. For instance, in the amoxicillin example, you would set up the equation like this:

$$\text{mL} = (5 \text{ mL}/250 \text{ mg}) \times 625 \text{ mg} = 12.5 \text{ mL}$$

Dimensional analysis can also encompass conversion factors all in the same formula. For instance, the nurse is to administer 50 mcg fentanyl. The pharmacy supplies the nurse with an ampule of fentanyl 0.1 mg/2 mL. How much should the nurse administer? To solve the problem, the mg needs to be converted to mcg. This can all be done in the same calculation.

$$\text{mL} = (2 \text{ mL}/0.1 \text{ mg}) \times (1 \text{ mg}/1,000 \text{ mcg}) \times 50 \text{ mcg}$$
$$= 1 \text{ mL}$$

Pediatric Calculations

According to Kyle (2008), the most common method for calculating pediatric medication doses is based on body weight, due to the wide range of size differences from infants to toddlers to school-aged children. The recommended dosage is usually expressed as the amount of drug to be given over a 24-hour period (mg/kg/day) or as a single dose (mg/kg/dose). When calculating pediatric drug dosages, check whether the prescribed amount is per dose or per 24-hour period. A medication overdose can occur if the nurse does not note that the calculation is per 24 hours and gives the total amount of medication in one dose. Weigh the child and, if necessary, convert the weight into kilograms by dividing the child's weight in pounds by 2.2 to compute the equivalent kilograms of weight. Then multiply the child's weight in kilograms by the prescribed dose to obtain the appropriate dose for the child. A drug reference book will identify the safe dose range for pediatric drug dosages based on weight.

Using Safety Measures While Preparing Drugs

Medication errors are defined as the preventable inappropriate use of medications. These errors occur when medications are ordered, transcribed, dispensed, administered, and monitored. Medication errors may or may not have serious consequences (Hughes & Ortiz, 2005). Medication errors can occur with almost any type of drug. Errors are more common with certain classes of medications, such as analgesics, antibiotics, anticoagulants, chemotherapeutic agents, diabetic medications, and cardiovascular agents. This is thought to possibly be due to the pharmacologic properties of the drugs that result in more adverse effects, toxicities, and interactions. Medication errors are also common in drugs with narrow therapeutic levels and in drugs prescribed frequently (Hughes & Ortiz, 2005). Safety is of the utmost importance in preparing and implementing drug administration. There are many interventions that can minimize the risk for medication errors. The following is a discussion of those interventions.

Three Checks and the Rights of Medication Administration

Observe the three checks and the rights of medication administration when administering medications to ensure medications are being administered safely. The use of the previously discussed technology, such as bar-code labeling and medication administration, does not remove from the nurse the primary responsibility for assuring safe medication administration. Check the label on the medication package or container three times during medication preparation and administration. The label should be read:

1. **When the nurse reaches for the container or unit dose package;**

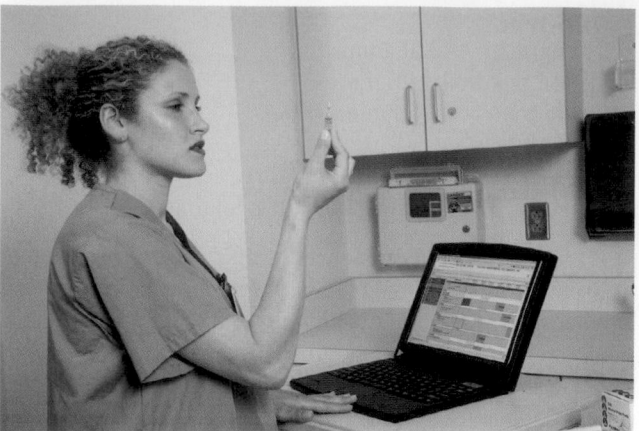

FIGURE 29-2. Comparing medication label with CMAR.

2. **After retrieval from the drawer and compared with the CMAR, or compared with the CMAR immediately before pouring from a multidose container; and**
3. **When replacing the container to the drawer or shelf or before giving the unit dose medication to the patient.**

Figure 29-2 illustrates the comparison of a medication label with the CMAR (second label check) to ensure accuracy.

The rights of medication administration can help to ensure accuracy when administering medications. Ensure that the (1) **right medication** is given to the (2) **right patient** in the (3) **right dosage** through the (4) **right route** at the (5) **right time.** Additional rights have been suggested to include ensuring (6) the *right reason* and (7) the *right documentation* (Balas et al., 2004; Pape, 2003). Validating the right reason requires the nurse to understand the rationale for administration and answer the question, "Does it make sense?" The right documentation refers to accurate and timely documentation of administration.

The importance of the three checks and the rights of medication administration cannot be overemphasized. The rights of medication administration (right patient, right drug, right dose, right route, right time, right reason, right documentation) are principles that nurses have been taught as part of their nursing education; however, nurses may not always adhere to the rights and may also lack knowledge about the medication, including the indication, usual dose, route, actions, adverse effects, contraindications, and drug–drug or food–drug interactions (Shane, 2009). The safe nurse does not allow automatic habits of preparing medications or technology to replace constant thinking, purposeful action, and repeated checking for accuracy.

▶ *Think back to Mr. Baptiste, the patient described in the beginning of the chapter and the Reflective Practice display. By adhering to the rights of medication administration, the nurse would be able to determine that the medication delivered by the pharmacy was labeled incorrectly.* ▪

Maintaining a Safe Environment

An environment that promotes safety and good working habits contributes to accuracy in the preparation of drugs for administration. Simmons et al. (2009) discuss physical working conditions that can influence the nurse's ability to perform safely. Good lighting must be present when preparing drugs. Increased noise and noise disruptions decrease the ability to concentrate. As a result, medications should be prepared in a relatively quiet location. The nurse who is preparing drugs should work alone. This practice helps to avoid distractions and interruptions, which may lead to errors.

After beginning to prepare drugs for administration, do not leave them unattended. If it is imperative to leave for a short time, place the drugs that have been prepared in a locked area, such as in the medication cart. The nurse who prepares the medication also administers the drug and records the drug administration. When not working at the medication cart, it should be locked. The locking of the medication cart is a requirement of the certifying bodies of hospitals.

Handling Controlled Substances Safely

Medication dispensing rooms should be locked. In addition, controlled substances are kept in a locked drawer or container as an added safety measure, providing for a "double locked" system. Narcotics or controlled substances may be ordered only by physicians, and in some states nurse practitioners, who are registered with the Department of Justice, Bureau of Narcotics, and Dangerous Drugs. According to federal law, a record must be kept for each narcotic that is administered. Healthcare agencies provide forms for keeping such records, and these forms are kept with the narcotics. Although the forms differ, the following information usually is required:

- Name of the patient receiving the narcotic
- Amount of the narcotic used
- Hour the narcotic was given
- Name of the physician who prescribed the narcotic
- Name of the nurse who administered the narcotic

It is common practice to check narcotics daily at specified intervals. In hospitals, checking is usually performed at each shift change. The amount of narcotics on hand is counted, and each used narcotic must be accounted for on the narcotic record. Many facilities use a computerized system for dispensing narcotics. The nurse has a secure identification code that provides access into the system, identifies the patient by name or identification number, and verifies the count for each drug as it is removed. Because this secure identification code is equivalent to the nurse's signature, it should never be given out to other staff members. Unless the narcotic count is incorrect, this eliminates the need to check the narcotic count at specific intervals each day. A narcotic count that does not check properly must be reported immediately. The law requires these special precautions to aid in the control of drug abuse by patients and healthcare workers.

The nurse administering narcotics has an important responsibility to see that the federal law is observed. If for any reason a narcotic prepared for administration has to be discarded, a second nurse should act as a witness, and that person should also sign the narcotic sheet. Document with a witness any time a full dosage is not given and some of the narcotic needs to be disposed of. For instance, if 3 mg of a narcotic has been ordered and the nurse uses a 4-mg syringe, the remaining 1 mg should be disposed of while a witness is watching, and both nurses should sign the documentation.

Identifying the Patient

Positive identification of the patient is essential to safe drug administration. Before administering the drug, check carefully to see that the right drug is being given to the right patient. Patients in inpatient healthcare agencies usually wear identification bracelets. Identify the patient by checking the identification bracelet, as shown in Figure 29-3. Validate the patient's name (first identifier) and identification number, medical record number, and/or birth date (second identifier), comparing with the CMAR or MAR. Specific identifiers used depend on facility policy. Also, ask the patient to state his or her name if possible. It is considered unsafe to call the patient by name because the patient may respond even if the nurse uses the wrong name. If using a bar-code system, the nurse will also scan the patient's bracelet. The computer system will validate the patient's identification. In some long-term care facilities a current photograph of the resident, displayed above the resident's bed, can also be used for identification. The 2010 National Patient Safety Goals established by the Joint Commission state that whenever administering patient medications, at least two patient identifiers should be used (Joint Commission, 2010). The patient's room number or physical location may not be used to validate patient identification (Joint Commission, 2010).

FIGURE 29-3. Checking patient's identity.

FOCUSED ASSESSMENT GUIDE • 29-1

MEDICATIONS

Factors to Assess	Questions and Approaches
Previous and current drug use	What medications are you taking that the primary care provider prescribed for you?
	What over-the-counter medications, natural, or herbal supplements are you taking on a regular basis?
	Do you use nonmedicinal drugs (e.g., alcohol, caffeine, home remedies)?
	How often do you use them?
	What is the reason for taking the medication?
	What medications have you taken during the past year and for what reasons?
	Is there anything else you have tried to alleviate your symptoms?
Medication schedule	At what times do you take your medications?
	Is there any special way your medication has to be prepared (e.g., crushing and mixing with applesauce)?
	Do you have any special method for remembering to take your medications?
Response to medications	Have the medications had the expected effects?
	Have you ever experienced any adverse or unexpected reactions to the medications?
	Is there a family history of this type of reaction to medication?
	Do you have any allergies to medications?
	What happens when you take this medication?
Attitude toward drugs and use of drugs	How do you feel about taking medications?
	Why do you take the medications?
Compliance with regimen	Can you tell me your understanding of the reason for taking the medications?
	Can you describe how you follow the medication schedule?
	Are there any problems that prevent you from following the medication regimen?
Storage	Where are your medications stored at home?
	How long do you keep medications in the home?
	Can you show me any medications you have on hand?

THE NURSING PROCESS FOR ADMINISTERING MEDICATIONS

Assessing

Assessment of the patient receiving medications begins during a nursing history. One component of this is the medication history. During the interview, the nurse can adapt questions to meet the patient's needs and level of understanding. Avoid using medical jargon that the patient may not understand, but instead you should use familiar terms. For instance, the patient may refer to a diuretic as the "water pill" or to an anticoagulant as a "blood thinner." Areas to be included in the medication history are listed in the accompanying Focused Assessment Guide.

> ➤ *The nurse caring for Mildred Campbell would need to incorporate this information when assessing the patient.*

This information is extremely important to prevent possible drug interactions should the patient decide to use the medication advertised on television. ∎

Additional information to be assessed includes the patient's health status, current and past illnesses, laboratory test results, and known drug allergies. Assess the patient with regard to medications during the nursing history and continue the assessment during and after medication administration.

Diagnosing

Data that the nurse collects may lead to the development of several nursing diagnoses related to medication administration. Each nursing diagnosis statement identifies a patient problem and suggests expected patient outcomes. The etiology of the problem directs nursing interventions. The following are examples of appropriate nursing diagnoses:

- Ineffective Health Maintenance related to lack of knowledge about anticoagulant medication regimen
- Anxiety related to daily self-injection of insulin
- Disturbed Body Image related to effects of chemotherapy
- Constipation related to use of narcotics
- Risk for Aspiration related to impaired swallowing of oral medications
- Risk for Poisoning related to confusion about medication dosages
- Deficient Knowledge related to interactions between herbal remedies and prescribed medications
- Noncompliance with Medication Regimen related to adverse drug effects, cost of medications, confusion, lack of motivation, visual impairment, complexity of regimen
- Disturbed Sleep Pattern related to consistent use of sedative-hypnotics

Additional examples of diagnoses with related etiologic factors and defining characteristics appear in Examples of NANDA Nursing Diagnoses: Medications.

Outcome Identification and Planning

Nursing measures for patients receiving medication are directed toward the patient's achievement of the following goals:

- Expected therapeutic effects will be demonstrated within a specified timeframe
- Expected change in symptoms. For example, the patient's pain will be relieved, or vital signs will return to baseline.
- Maintenance of therapeutic blood levels of medication.
- The patient will demonstrate knowledge regarding his or her medication.

Implementing

Remain with the patient and make sure that the medication is taken. If the patient receives several drugs, offer them separately so that if one is refused or dropped, positive identification can be made and the drug can be recorded or replaced. Never leave medications at the bedside for the patient to take later. This is an unsafe practice because the patient may forget to take the medication, or someone else may take the medication. Record medication administration as soon as possible after the patient takes the medication. Some agencies allow patients to self-administer certain drugs to promote the patient's independence. Be familiar with agency policy on this matter.

Table 29-3 summarizes questions to ask and actions to take when administering drugs by any route to ensure the correct administration of medications, as well as examples of nursing interventions to promote safe medication administration and appropriate outcomes. The accompanying Examples of Nursing Interventions and Nursing Outcomes Classifications (NIC/NOC) box lists standardized nursing interventions and corresponding outcomes related to promoting safe and effective medication administration.

Administering Oral Medications

Drugs given orally are intended for absorption in the stomach and small intestine. The oral route is the most commonly used route of administration. It is usually the most convenient and comfortable for the patient. Drug action has a slower onset and a more prolonged, but less potent, effect with oral administration of drugs compared to administration via other routes. There are certain situations in which oral medications

Examples of NANDA Nursing Diagnoses

Medications

Nursing Diagnoses	Related Factors	Sample Defining Characteristics
Constipation	Dehydration, opiate use, irregular defecation habits, anesthesia, decreased physical activity	*"I feel bloated."* Seventy-year-old man 5 days after a left thoracotomy. Abdomen slightly distended with hypoactive bowel sounds. Severe flatus. Last bowel movement day of surgery.
Deficient Knowledge	Lack of interest in learning, information misinterpretation, lack of recall	Fifty-year-old woman with recently diagnosed diabetes. "I don't see why all this is necessary. I don't have time for all this!" Asking friends and family to provide snacks and food from home in addition to her meal trays. Unable to verbalize information regarding new oral hypoglycemic agent she is taking, unable to demonstrate finger stick blood sugar procedure.
Sexual Dysfunction related to adverse effects of anti-hypertensive drug	New medication regimen, including anti-hypertensive agent	"I hate the way I feel. My wife doesn't understand. I think I should stop taking that blood pressure pill." Patient and wife verbalize dissatisfaction with sexual function and inability to achieve desired satisfaction since beginning oral antihypertensive therapy.

TABLE • 29-3   ENSURING CORRECT ADMINISTRATION OF MEDICATIONS

"Right" to Ensure	Questions to Ask	Actions to Take
When Preparing to Give Medication		
Right drug	• Has the patient been given this medication before? • Given the patient's symptoms and diagnosis, does it make sense for the patient to have this medication?	• Determine if the patient has any known drug allergies or sensitivities. • Assess the patient's other medications to detect possible contraindications. • Make sure it is the right medication; packaging, labeling, and spelling of some drugs look alike. • Have another person double check all medications and mathematical calculations.
Right reason	• Do the patient's condition, symptoms, and health status warrant receiving this medication?	• Determine if the patient has the condition the medication is used for.
Right dose and preparation	• Is the correct dose being administered? • How is the medication administered?	• Ensure labeling is legible and clearly understood.
Immediately before Administering the Medication		
Right patient	• Is this the right patient to receive this medication?	• Verify the identity of the patient using at least two identifiers name and date of birth (check wristband, ask patient his name).
Right time	• Is this the correct time for the medication to be administered?	• Check when the medication was last administered. If the drug is new, document when it is first given.
Right route	• Is it appropriate to administer the medication orally, intravenously, by injection, or other route?	• Check the original orders to verify the route of administration.
After the Medication has been Administered		
Right drug, right dose, and right rate	• How is the patient responding to the medication?	• Monitor the patient to: —determine the efficacy of the drug. —detect and prevent complication. —evaluate and document changes in health status. • When applicable, assess the patient's laboratory values to detect changes. • Provide patient education, when possible, so patient is alert to adverse effects and changes in how he feels.
Right documentation	• Has the correct documentation been completed according to facility policy?	• Complete documentation according to facility policy immediately after administering any medication. • Document and communicate to the appropriate healthcare provider any signs and symptoms indicative of any adverse effects.

Modified from Abrams, A., Lammon, C., Pennington, S., & Goldsmith, T. (2008). *Clinical drug therapy. Rationales for nursing practice* (9th ed.). Philadelphia: Wolters Kluwer Health/Lippincott Williams & Wilkins; and Hughes, R., & Ortiz, E. (2005). Medication errors. *American Journal of Nursing, 105*(Suppl 35), 14–24.

should not be administered, such as when the patient has difficulty swallowing, is unconscious, is to receive nothing by mouth, or is vomiting. Occasionally, a patient may unintentionally or intentionally hide a medication in the mouth, or "cheek" it. Check that the medication was actually swallowed before recording that it has been taken.

Oral medications are available in solid and liquid form. Solid preparations include tablets, capsules, and pills. Some tablets are scored for easy breaking if a partial quantity is needed. Unless a tablet is scored, do not break it because doing so could result in an inaccurate dose. Enteric-coated

tablets are covered with a hard surface that impedes absorption until the tablet has left the stomach; thus, the medication is released in the small intestine. Enteric-coated tablets are used when the active ingredient of the drug is irritating to the stomach mucosa. As a result, less GI irritation occurs, and the medication is protected from destruction by gastric acid. Enteric-coated tablets should not be chewed or crushed because crushing the medication destroys the action of the coating. Other forms of oral medications that should not be chewed or crushed without checking with the prescriber include any of the extended-release forms of medications,

---

Examples of Nursing Interventions and Nursing Outcomes Classifications (NIC/NOC)

Medications

Nursing Interventions	Nursing Outcomes
• Medication Administration	• Knowledge: Medication
• Teaching: Prescribed Medication	• Medication Response
• Medication Reconciliation	• Client Satisfaction: Teaching
• Medication Management	• Knowledge: Treatment Regimen
• Analgesic Administration	• Safe Home Environment
	• Pain Control

From: Bulechek, G., Butcher, H. & McCloskey Dochterman, J. (Eds.). (2008). *Nursing interventions classification (NIC)*. (5th ed., p. 153). St. Louis, MO: Mosby Elsevier; and Moorhead, S., Johnson, M., Maas, M., & Swanson, E. (Eds.). (2008). *Nursing outcomes classification (NOC)*. (5th ed., p. 806). A full listing of nursing activities for each nursing intervention and outcomes can be found in these books.

---

such as SR (sustained release), XL (extended release), CR or CRT (controlled release), SA (sustained action), or LA (long acting). Chewing and/or crushing these medications destroys their extended-release delivery mechanism and may result in potentially toxic peaks and low troughs (Toedter Williams, 2008). Certain narcotics that were previously administered parenterally can now also be administered in a lollipop or oral-transmucosal form.

Liquid preparations include elixirs, spirits, suspensions, and syrups. Some are water-based solutions, and others are alcohol-based solutions. If the patient has had a previous drug or alcohol addiction, medications containing alcohol should be avoided. Disposable, calibrated cups are available for the administration of liquid medications. For patients who find it difficult to take liquids from a cup, the medication can be placed in the mouth directly using a plastic oral syringe without a needle. The syringe should be placed between the gum and cheek and the liquid given to the patient slowly. This technique, in addition to having the patient in an upright or side-lying position, helps prevent the patient from choking and aspirating the medication. When administering a drug with a syringe, do not place the safety cap back over the syringe after drawing up the medication. This could pose an aspiration risk if the safety cap was not removed before administering the dose and the cap was accidentally injected into a patient's mouth. Shake emulsions and suspensions well and administer them promptly to ensure accurate dosage.

Liquids are available in multidose bottles and single-dose containers. If a label becomes difficult to read or accidentally comes off the container, return the container to the pharmacy. Never give a medication from a bottle without a label or with a label that cannot be read with accuracy. Because of the danger of error, do not return unused medications to their bottles. Exercise care in pouring to prevent unnecessary loss. Do not transfer medications from one pharmacy container to another. Many medication bottles now have an identification code number on them. If similar medications were mixed and a patient had a reaction, it would be difficult to identify which drug was responsible.

Do not use a medication with an unexpected precipitate, or one that has changed color. Skill 29-1 describes the techniques for preparing and administering oral medications.

SPECIAL TECHNIQUES

Certain drugs that are given orally can discolor the teeth or damage the enamel. The administration technique for this medication is to mix it well with water or some other liquid, have the patient take the medication mixed with liquid through a drinking straw, and encourage the patient to drink water after administration. This practice reduces the strength of the drug that comes in contact with the teeth.

Some patients object to the taste of certain medications. The following techniques help disguise or mask an objectionable taste:

- Crush the medication and add it to food or a drink so that the patient can swallow it. Many times the food or drink will mask the flavor of the medication. However, as previously discussed, some drugs cannot be crushed (e.g., enteric-coated and sustained-release capsules). Check with the pharmacist or a pharmacology reference if you are uncertain about crushing a medication.
- Allow the patient to suck on a small piece of ice for a few minutes before taking the medication. The ice numbs the taste buds, and the objectionable taste is less discernible.
- Store oily medications in the refrigerator. Cold oil is less aromatic than oil at room temperature.
- Place the medication in a syringe, and place the syringe well back on the tongue, being careful not to trigger the patient's gag reflex. This places the medication on the part of the tongue with few taste buds.
- Offer oral hygiene immediately after giving the medication.
- Give the medication with generous amounts of water or other liquids, if permitted, to dilute the taste.

Children

It can be challenging and frustrating to administer medications to infants and children. Children younger than 5 years have difficulty swallowing tablets and capsules. Therefore, most medications are available in liquid form. Nursing responsibility includes teaching and preparing family members to administer medications to a child at home. In addition to understanding the medication order and the reason for the medication, the caregiver should be able to demonstrate any special techniques involved in administering the prescribed drugs. Actions to take to prevent errors when parents or other caregivers need to administer medications include asking, demonstrating, and planning. Question caregivers about their experiences giving medications to their children, about access to proper dosing devices, and previous use of the devices. Demonstrate how to use the appropriate dosing device that will be used at home. Ensure the caregivers give a correct return demonstration. Help caregivers plan for the times of the day to give the medication. In addition, provide written instructions that clearly state the dose and times of the day for administration. Helpful strategies for administering oral medications to children include the following:

- Use a dropper to give infants or very young children liquid medications while holding them in a sitting or semisitting position. Place the medication between the gum and cheek to prevent aspiration.
- Crush uncoated tablets or empty a soft capsule and mix the medication with soft foods, such as potatoes, pudding, ice cream, or cooked or hot cereal, for patients who are likely to aspirate liquids. Proper absorption may not occur if coated tablets or hard capsules are added to food.
  - Take care when selecting the food to be mixed with the medication. The item should not be an essential part of the child's diet, such as formula or the child's favorite food. The child may refuse to eat a food associated with medications.
  - If a medication has an objectionable taste, warn the child if he or she is old enough to understand. Failing to warn the child is likely to decrease the child's trust in the nurse.
- Offer the child a flavored ice pop or frozen fruit bar immediately before taking the medication. It numbs the tongue, making the taste of the medication less evident.
- Praise the child for a job well done after he or she swallows the medication.

Older Adults

Techniques for administering medications to older people include the following:

- Allow extra time to administer medications to older patients because their reflexes may be slowed and their understanding of the treatment decreased.
- Older patients may have difficulty swallowing medications and may find it easier to take their medications when crushed or given in liquid form. Initiate swallowing by massaging the laryngeal prominence or the area just below the chin prominence. The pressure from the gentle massage creates the desire to swallow. A speech therapist may offer additional suggestions for patients who have difficulty swallowing.

- Reevaluation of the drug dosage is necessary with the older patient. Weight and age should be used as criteria for determining the dosage.
- Assist the older patient to set up a schedule as a reminder to take medications as scheduled at home.
- Monitor the patient carefully for adverse effects that may result from the drug regimen. These may be magnified in older individuals.
- Teach patients the names of drugs, rather than distinguishing them by color. Manufacturers may vary the colors of generic drugs, and the visual changes associated with aging may make it more difficult to identify medications by their color.

In older adults, successful self-management of medication may be promoted by establishing habits, adjusting routines, tracking medications, simplifying medication practices, and improving patient education related to the relationship of medications to maintaining health (Swanlund, Scherck, Metcalfe, & Jesek-Hale, 2008). See the accompanying Research in Nursing box, Self-Management of Medications.

ADMINISTERING MEDICATIONS THROUGH AN ENTERAL FEEDING TUBE

Patients with a gastrointestinal tube (nasogastric, nasointestinal, percutaneous endoscopic gastrostomy [PEG], or jejunostomy [J] tube) often receive medication through the tube. The insertion of the tube and care of the patient with an enteral feeding tube are described in Chapter 36. The following are suggestions for giving medications through the tube:

- Use liquid medications when possible because they are absorbed readily and less likely to cause tube occlusions (Toedter Williams, 2008).
- Certain solid dosage medications can be crushed and combined with liquid. Medications should be crushed to a fine powder and mixed with 15 to 30 mL of water before delivery through the tube (Toedter Williams, 2008).
- Certain capsules may be opened, emptied into liquid, and administered through the tube (Toedter Williams, 2008). Check manufacturer recommendations and/or with a pharmacist to verify.
- Bring the liquid medication to room temperature. Cold liquids may cause patient discomfort.
- Elevate the head of the bed to prevent reflux.
- Remove the clamp from the tube and use the recommended procedure for checking tube placement in the stomach or intestine before administering the drug.
- Flush the tube with 15 to 30 mL water (5 to 10 mL for children) before giving the medication and immediately after giving the medication. Flushing helps to maintain tube patency.
- Give medications separately and flush with water between each drug. Some medications may interact with each other or become less effective if mixed with other drugs.

- If the tube is connected to suction, keep it disconnected from the suction and clamped for 20 to 30 minutes after administration of the medication to allow absorption.
- If the patient is receiving tube feedings, review information about the drugs to be administered. Absorption of some drugs, such as phenytoin (Dilantin) is affected by tube feeding formulas. Discontinue a continuous tube feeding and leave the tube clamped for the required period of time before and after the medication has been given, according to the reference and facility protocol.
- Document the water intake and liquid medication by tube on the intake and output record. Adjust the amount of water used if the patient's fluid intake is restricted.

ADMINISTERING SUBLINGUAL AND BUCCAL MEDICATIONS

Certain drugs, such as nitroglycerin, are administered sublingually; that is, a tablet is placed under the patient's tongue. Another method is to administer the medication between the cheek and gum, known as buccal administration. These areas are rich in superficial blood vessels, which allow the drug to be absorbed relatively rapidly into the bloodstream for quick systemic effects. Sublingual and buccal medications should not be swallowed, but rather held in place so that complete absorption can occur. Before administering a sublingual or buccal drug, offer the patient a drink of water (if the patient is permitted to have fluids) or oral care (if the patient is NPO). This ensures that the tablet will dissolve appropriately.

Administering Parenteral Medications

The word **parenteral** means outside the intestines or alimentary canal. Several methods to administer a medication by the parenteral route involve injecting the medication into those body tissues outside of the intestines or alimentary canal and into the circulatory system. Table 29-2 defines terms used to describe various types of injections. Advanced injection techniques consist of injecting medications into an artery, the peritoneum, heart tissues, the spinal canal, and bones. Techniques for injecting medications into these areas are discussed in clinical texts. In most instances, physicians or specialized practitioners are responsible for these procedures.

EQUIPMENT
Needles and Syringes

Needles are available in various lengths and gauges, with different sizes of bevels. The needle length used depends on the route of administration. The gauge refers to the diameter of the needle. Needle gauges are numbered 18 through 30. As the diameter of the needle increases, the gauge number decreases. For example, an 18-gauge needle is larger in diameter than a 30-gauge needle. The bevel of the needle is its sloped edge, designed to make a narrow, slit-like opening that closes quickly.

Syringes are supplied in various sizes. Most syringes are plastic and disposable. Some syringes are supplied with the needle attached; others are not, in which case you should select an appropriate needle. Figure 29-4 shows the parts of a needle and the parts of a syringe.

Choose the equipment needed for an injection based on the following criteria:

- Route of administration: A longer needle is required for an intramuscular injection than for an intradermal or a subcutaneous injection. See each individual route for specific guidelines regarding needle length and gauge.

FIGURE 29-4. Parts of a needle and syringe.

Plunger

Barrel

Threads for Luer lock

Needle hub

Needle

Safety guard

Shaft

Lumen

Bevel

prevent a needlestick injury. If recapping is absolutely unavoidable, use the one-handed technique. This technique and additional measures to protect healthcare workers from accidental transmission of infectious diseases are discussed in Chapter 27, Asepsis and Infection Control.

When administering parenteral injections, it is imperative that surgical asepsis and sterile technique must be followed strictly to avoid introducing organisms into the body. The parts of the syringe and needle that must be kept sterile during the procedure of preparing and administering an injection include the inside of the barrel, the part of the plunger that enters the barrel, the tip of the barrel, and the needle, except for the exterior of the needle hub. Surgical asepsis also applies to cleaning the skin for an injection. The skin is cleaned with alcohol or another antimicrobial in a circular motion, working from the center of the designated site outward.

Needleless Systems

The risk for accidental needle sticks and exposure to blood borne pathogens is reduced significantly with the use of needleless devices or protected needles. Chapter 27, Asepsis and Infection Control, describes the rationale for these systems of protection for healthcare workers. Needleless systems are available for intravenous use, including recessed and shielded intravenous needle connectors, as well as blunt cannulas that are inserted into special receptor sites on tubing or lock setups. Discard all needleless devices or blunt cannulas in special containers that are puncture-proof, leak-proof, and labeled clearly. Figure 29-5 shows an example of a needleless administration device.

PREPARING MEDICATIONS FOR ADMINISTRATION BY INJECTION

Drugs that are administered by injection are packaged in several ways. Those that deteriorate in solution are usually dispensed as powders and are reconstituted immediately before injection. Drugs that remain stable in solution are usually dispensed in ampules, bottles, prefilled cartridges, or vials in an aqueous or oily solution or suspension. Drugs may be dispensed in single-dose glass ampules, single-dose rubber-capped vials, multidose rubber-capped vials, and prefilled cartridges.

Removing Medication From an Ampule

An **ampule** is a glass flask that contains a single dose of medication for parenteral administration. Figure 29-6 shows an example of an ampule. There is no way to prevent airborne contamination of any unused portion of medication after the ampule is opened, so if not all the medication is used, discard the remainder. Medication is removed from an ampule after its thin neck is broken. Take special care when breaking the ampule so you do not get cut. If you cut yourself on the ampule, discard the ampule and medication. Because of the risk of small glass shards falling into the ampule, use a filter needle to remove the medication from the vial and then discard it appropriately. Place an unfiltered

- Viscosity of the solution: Some medications are more viscous than others and require a large-lumen needle to inject the drug.
- Quantity to be administered: The larger the amount of medication to be injected, the greater the capacity of the syringe.
- Body size: An obese person requires a longer needle to reach muscle tissue than does a thin person. A thin person or an older adult with decreased muscle mass requires a shorter needle.
- Type of medication: There are special syringes for certain uses. An example is the insulin syringe used to inject insulin.

Once used, do not recap needles. After use, place needles and syringes in puncture-resistant containers without being recapped because most needlestick injuries occur during recapping. Acute care facilities are required to provide needles with needle guards to prevent accidental injury. After the injection is given, push the needle guard into place, preventing injury. Other needle and syringe combinations have a retractable needle that locks and seals inside the syringe barrel. Prefilled syringes are manufactured with retractable needle sheath covers. With these syringes, once the needle is contaminated, the top slides forward and over the needle to

FIGURE 29-5. (**A**) Needleless administration devices. (**B**) Syringe attached to needleless administration device. *(Photos by B. Proud.)*

needle of appropriate size on the syringe before administering the medication. Invert the ampule or place it on a flat surface to draw the solution into the syringe. Care must be taken not to contaminate the needle by touching the rim of the ampule. Skill 29-2 shows how to remove medication from an ampule.

Removing Medication From a Vial

A **vial** is a glass bottle with a self-sealing stopper through which the medication is removed (Fig. 29-7). For safety in transporting and storing, the vial is usually covered with a soft metal cap that can be removed easily. The rubber stopper that is then exposed is the means of entrance into the vial.

Some drugs are dispensed in vials that contain several doses. This means that the nurse can remove several doses from the same container. To prevent microbial growth in the vial, each multidose vial is usually good for only 24 hours. Label the vial with the time and date when first used. After the initial use of the multidose vial, wipe the rubber stopper with alcohol each time the medication is removed from the vial. To facilitate removal of medication, inject air into the vial. The amount of air injected into the vial is the same

amount as the desired quantity of solution. The Centers for Disease Control and Prevention (CDC) recommends that medications packaged as multiuse vials be assigned to a single patient whenever possible. In addition, it is recommended that the top of the vial be cleaned prior to each entry and that a new sterile needle and syringe is used with each entry (CDC, 2008a; CDC, 2008b). Skill 29-3 details how to remove medication from a vial.

Using a Prefilled Cartridge or Syringe

Prefilled cartridges provide a single dose of medication. Insert the cartridge into a reusable holder or injection device. Before giving the injection, check the dosage in the cartridge and clear the cartridge of excess air. Most prefilled cartridges are overfilled; therefore, eject any excess medication to give an exact dose and avoid a medication error. Tubex and Carpuject are two types of prefilled cartridges. Figure 29-8 shows examples of prefilled cartridges and injector devices.

Similar to prefilled cartridges are prefilled syringes. These are syringes that are already filled with a medication and usually have their own needle attached. Like prefilled cartridges,

FIGURE 29-6. Ampule. *(Photo by B. Proud.)*

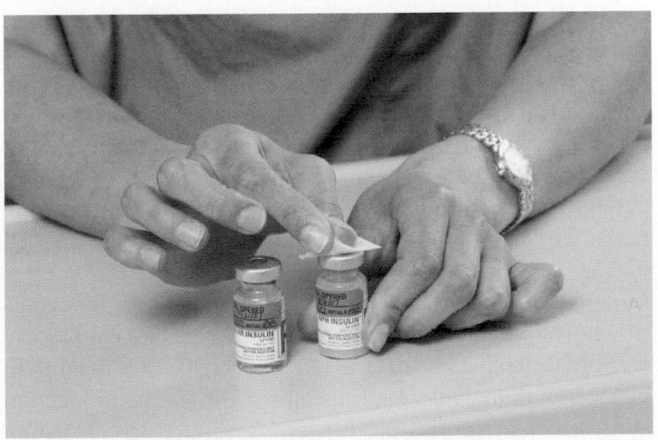

FIGURE 29-7. Vials. *(Photo by B. Proud.)*

FIGURE 29-8. Prefilled cartridge and injector device. *(Photo by B. Proud.)*

these syringes also come with excess air. In some cases, this air should not be expelled before administering the medication. Enoxaparin (Lovenox) is an example of a syringe where the air should not be expelled before administering.

Mixing Medications in One Syringe

When considering mixing two medications in one syringe, first ensure that the two drugs are compatible. Certain medications, such as diazepam (Valium), are incompatible with other drugs in the same syringe. Other drugs have limited compatibility and should be administered within 15 minutes of preparation. Incompatible drugs may become cloudy or form a precipitate in the syringe. Discard these medications and reprepare the drugs in separate syringes. Mixing more than two drugs in one syringe is not recommended. If it must be done, contact the pharmacist to determine the compatibility of the three drugs, as well as the compatibility of their pH values and the preservatives that may be present in each drug. A drug compatibility table should be available to nurses who are preparing medications.

Preparation of medications in one syringe depends on how the medication is supplied. When using a single-dose vial and a multidose vial, inject air into both vials and draw the medication in the multidose vial into the syringe first. This prevents the contents of the multidose vial from being contaminated with the medication in the single-dose vial. The steps to follow when preparing medications from two multidose vials in one syringe are illustrated in Figure 29-9. When preparing medications from an ampule and a vial, prepare the medication in the vial first. Draw up the medication in the ampule after the medication in the vial.

Mixing Insulins in One Syringe. Insulin, a naturally occurring hormone produced by the pancreas, enables cells to use carbohydrates. Two of the issues relative to insulin in patients with diabetes mellitus include no insulin production or insufficient insulin production. Several types of insulin are available for use by patients with diabetes mellitus.

FIGURE 29-9. Mixing medications (insulin) in one syringe.

Insulins vary in their onset and duration of action and are classified as rapid acting, short acting, intermediate acting, and long acting (Aschenbrenner & Venable, 2009). A patient may receive more than one type of insulin. A patient may be treated with a basal insulin, such as insulin glargine (Lantus), insulin detemir (Levemir), or NPH insulin to cover the body's basal metabolic needs. In addition, the patient will probably also be treated with a prandial (with a meal) or preprandial (before a meal) insulin, such as insulin lispro (Humalog) or insulin aspart (NovoLog), to prevent postprandial (after meal) hyperglycemia (high blood glucose). Lantus and Levemir cannot be mixed with other insulins. Patients treated with other insulins may require the mixing of the two insulins in one syringe. Before administering any insulin, be aware of the onset time, peak, and duration of effects and ensure that proper food is available. Refer to a drug reference for a listing of the different types of insulin and action specific to each type.

Insulin dosages are calculated in units. The scale commonly used is U100, which is based on 100 units of insulin contained in 1 mL of solution. An insulin syringe is also calibrated in units. Insulin is also available in "insulin pens." Before administering insulin, check the dosage with the medical orders. Skill 29-4 gives the steps for mixing two types of insulins in the same syringe. Insulin administration is discussed further later in the chapter in the section, "Administering Medications Subcutaneously."

Reconstituting Powdered Medications

Occasionally, a drug is supplied as a powder in a vial. A liquid, or diluent, must be added to the powder before it is administered as a solution. The technique of adding a diluent to a powdered drug is called reconstitution. Information needed for reconstitution, such as the specific solution to use for the diluent and dosage calculation, is usually found on the vial label. Additional sources of information about reconstitution of medications are package inserts and the pharmacist.

Another form that powdered medications may come in is an Act-O-Vial (Pfizer). Act-O-Vials have the diluent and powder in the same vial but separated by a rubber stopper. When the nurse is ready to administer the medication, the rubber stopper is deployed, and the Act-O-Vial is agitated gently to mix the diluent and powder.

ADMINISTERING MEDICATIONS INTRADERMALLY

Intradermal injections are administered into the dermis, just below the epidermis. The intradermal route has the longest absorption time of all the parenteral routes. For this reason, intradermal injections are used for sensitivity tests, such as tuberculin and allergy tests, and local anesthesia. The advantage of the intradermal route for these tests is that the body's reaction to substances is easily visible, and degrees of reaction are discernible by comparative study.

Sites commonly used are the inner surface of the forearm and the upper back, under the scapula. Equipment used for an intradermal injection includes a tuberculin syringe calibrated in tenths and hundredths of a milliliter. A 1/4" to 1/2", 26- or 27-gauge needle is used. The dosage given intradermally is small, usually less than 0.5 mL. The angle of administration for an intradermal injection is 5 to 15 degrees. Skill 29-5 demonstrates how to administer an intradermal injection.

ADMINISTERING MEDICATIONS SUBCUTANEOUSLY

Subcutaneous injections are administered into the adipose tissue layer just below the epidermis and dermis. This tissue has few blood vessels, so drugs administered here have

FIGURE 29-10. Sites on the body where subcutaneous injections can be given.

a slow, sustained rate of absorption into the capillaries. This route is used to administer drugs such as insulin and heparin.

Subcutaneous Injection Sites

Various sites may be used for subcutaneous injections, including the outer aspect of the upper arm, the abdomen (from below the costal margin to the iliac crests), the anterior aspects of the thigh, the upper back, and the upper ventral or dorsogluteal area (Fig. 29-10). Avoid sites that are bruised, tender, hard, swollen, inflamed, or scarred. These conditions could affect absorption or cause discomfort and injury (Hunter, 2008). Absorption rates differ among the various sites. Injections in the abdomen are absorbed most rapidly; ones in the arms are absorbed somewhat more slowly; those in the thighs, even more slowly; and those in the upper ventral or dorsogluteal areas have the slowest absorption (American Diabetes Association [ADA], 2004; Caffrey, 2003).

Equipment

It is important to choose the right equipment to ensure depositing the medication into the intended tissue layer and not the underlying muscle. Equipment used for a subcutaneous injection includes a syringe of appropriate volume for the amount of drug being administered. A 25- to 30-gauge, 3/8" to 1" needle can be used. The 3/8" and 5/8" needles are most commonly used. Choose the needle length based on the amount of subcutaneous tissue present, which is based on the patient's body weight and build (Annersten & Willman, 2005). Usually, no more than 1 mL of solution is given subcutaneously. Giving larger amounts adds to the patient's discomfort and may predispose to poor absorption. Some medications are packaged in prefilled cartridges with a needle attached. Enoxaparin (Lovenox), for example, is provided this way. Confirm that the provided needle is appropriate for the patient before use. If not, the medication will have to be transferred to another syringe and the appropriate needle attached.

Procedure

Subcutaneous injections are administered at a 45- to 90-degree angle. Choose the angle of needle insertion based on the amount of subcutaneous tissue present and the length of the needle. Generally, the shorter, 3/8″ needle should be inserted at a 90-degree angle, and the longer, 5/8″ needle is inserted at a 45-degree angle. Recommendations differ regarding pinching or bunching of a skin fold for administration. Pinching is advised for thinner patients and when a longer needle is used to lift the adipose tissue away from underlying muscle and tissue. If pinching is used, once the needle is inserted, release the skin to avoid injecting into compressed tissue (Rushing, 2004).

Aspiration, or pulling back on the plunger to check that a blood vessel has been entered, is not necessary and has not proved to be a reliable indicator of needle placement. The likelihood of injecting into a blood vessel is small (Rushing, 2004; Stephens, 2003). Aspiration is definitely contraindicated with administration of heparin because this action can result in hematoma formation. The American Diabetes Association (ADA) (2004) has stated that routine aspiration is not necessary when injecting insulin.

If blood or clear fluid appears at the site after withdrawing the needle, apply gentle pressure. Massaging the site is not necessary and can damage underlying tissue and increase the absorption of the medication. Massaging after heparin administration can contribute to hematoma formation.

It is necessary to rotate sites or areas for injection if the patient is to receive frequent injections. This helps to prevent buildup of fibrous tissue and permits complete absorption of the medication. Because absorption rates vary from site to site, it is recommended that patients administering their own insulin use the same area of the body at the same time every day to ensure more consistent absorption and prevent tissue changes from repeated use of the same site (ADA, 2004; Caffrey, 2003). For instance, every morning the patient may use the abdomen for insulin injection, and every evening before dinner, the patient may inject the insulin into the arms or thighs. In each case, the injections should be given an inch away from the previous injection site so that the same area will not be used again in the same month. A small spot bandage or piece of tape can be used to mark the first injection site, with subsequent injections rotated in a circle around that site. After this area has been used, an adjacent site, an inch away, can be selected, using the same rotation format. A marked diagram incorporated into the patient's plan of care is also helpful for noting alternative sites. Do not rely on memory. The patient cannot always recall the site of the previous injection, so the site of administration is recorded in the patient's record.

Skill 29-6 shows the procedure for administering medications subcutaneously. Techniques for reducing discomfort in subcutaneous administrations are listed after the section "Administering Medications Intramuscularly."

Drug-Specific Equipment and Techniques

Various drugs require very specific equipment and/or techniques. Insulin is prepared using an insulin syringe. Other drugs are never administered with an insulin syringe. Insulin syringes are available with 28- to 30-gauge, 5/16″ and 1/2″ length needles, and in 3/10-mL to 1-mL sizes. The shorter needles (5/16″) are becoming the more common length used. Shorter needles are less painful, and there is less risk for inadvertent injection into muscle tissue. Insulin pens are also available for insulin administration. Insulin pens are prefilled devices that combine the insulin container and syringe. Patients attach a needle for each administration, dial a dose of insulin, and depress a plunger to administer the dose. See Guidelines for Nursing Care 29-1: Using an Insulin Pen.

Heparin is also administered subcutaneously. The abdomen is the most commonly used site. Avoid the area 2″ around the umbilicus and the belt line. The manufacturer's directions for subcutaneous administration of low-molecular-weight heparin preparations, such as enoxaparin (Lovenox), include specific instructions regarding administration site and technique (Sanofi Aventis, 2008). Administer enoxaparin in an area on the abdomen between the left or right anterolateral and left or right posterolateral abdominal wall (Fig. 29-11). To administer the medication, pinch the tissue gently and insert the needle at a 90-degree angle. In addition, enoxaparin is packaged in a prefilled syringe with an air bubble. Do not expel the air bubble before administration.

Some medications, such as insulin and morphine, may be administered continuously via the subcutaneous route. Continuous subcutaneous insulin infusion (CSII or insulin pump) allows for multiple preset rates of insulin delivery. This system uses a small computerized reservoir that delivers insulin via tubing through a needle inserted into the subcutaneous tissue. The pump is programmed to deliver multiple preset rates of insulin delivery. The settings can be adjusted for exercise and illness, and bolus doses can be delivered related to meals. Sites are changed every 2 to 3 days. Figure 29-12 shows a patient wearing an insulin pump. Another example of a medication given via continuous subcutaneous infusion is morphine. Subcutaneous morphine infusion can

Anterior view   Posterior view
FIGURE 29-11. Sites for administration of enoxaparin.

Guidelines for Nursing Care • 29-1

USING AN INSULIN PEN

- Perform hand hygiene.
- Identify the patient.
- Explain procedure to patient.
- Remove the pen cap.
- Insert an insulin cartridge into the pen, following the manufacturer's directions.
- Clean the tip of the reservoir with alcohol.
- Invert the pen 20 times to mix if using an insulin suspension.
- Remove the protective tab from the needle.
- Screw the needle onto the reservoir.
- Remove the outer and inner needle caps.
- Hold the pen upright and tap to force any air bubbles to the top.
- Dial the dose selector to 2 units to perform an "air shot" to get rid of bubbles.
- Hold the pen upright and press the plunger firmly. Watch for a drop of insulin at the needle tip.
- Check the drug reservoir to make sure enough insulin is available for the dose.
- Check that the dose selector is at "0," then dial the units of insulin for the dose.
- Put on gloves.
- Clean the injection site and administer the subcutaneous injection, holding the pen like a dart. Push the button on the pen all the way in.

- Keep the button depressed and count to 6 before removing from the skin.
- Remove the needle from the pen and dispose in a sharps container.
- Remove gloves and additional PPE, if used. Perform hand hygiene.
- Document administration on the CMAR/MAR, including the injection site.

Patient using an insulin pen. *(Photo by B. Proud.)*

Adapted from Moshang, J. (2005). Making a point about insulin pens. *Nursing, 35*(2), 46–47.

be used for palliative dyspnea and pain management (Ben-Aharon, Gafter-Gvili, Paul, Leibovici, & Stemmer, 2008; Elsner, Radbruch, Loick, Gärtner, & Sabatowski, 2005). Advantages of continuous subcutaneous medication infusion include the longer rate of absorption via the subcutaneous route and convenience for the patient.

FIGURE 29-12. Patient wearing an insulin pump. *(Photo by B. Proud.)*

ADMINISTERING MEDICATIONS INTRAMUSCULARLY

Intramuscular injections deliver medication through the skin and subcutaneous tissues into certain muscles. Muscles have larger and a greater number of blood vessels than does subcutaneous tissue, allowing faster onset of action than with subcutaneous injections. Some medications administered intramuscularly are formulated to have a longer duration of effect. The deposit of medication creates a depot at the site of injection, designed to deliver slow, sustained release over hours, days, or weeks. This route is used to administer drugs such as antibiotics, hormones, and vaccines, such as the pneumococcal and hepatitis vaccines. The accompanying box, Through the Eyes of a Student, relates one student's experience administering an intramuscular injection.

Intramuscular Injection Sites

Various sites may be used for intramuscular injections. To avoid complications, it is important to be able to identify anatomic landmarks and site boundaries and to use an accurate, careful technique when administering intramuscular injections. If care is not taken, possible complications include

Through the Eyes of a Student

I entered my patient's room, knowing that she had had surgery less than 12 hours before my arrival, and introduced myself. I asked how she was feeling, to which she immediately responded, "I feel really sick. I think I'm going to throw up. I need something—*now!*" I told her that I would check the medication orders and be back as soon as possible. I walked quickly to the medication administration record, and there it was glaring at me in black and white on the CMAR: "Prochlorperazine (Compazine), 10 mg IM q 6 hr p.r.n. nausea or vomiting." My mind raced as I thought, "I have never given an IM injection. There has to be something else ordered." I knew there wasn't. I found my clinical instructor and announced, "My patient needs an IM injection." Given the anxiety I was feeling, everything went surprisingly well as we prepared the medication. I went over the procedure one last time before entering the patient's room.

We approached the patient just in time for her to look at us in sheer terror and cry, "I hope that shot isn't for me; I hate them," which did nothing for my already shaking hands. I explained that she couldn't take a pill because she could not have anything by mouth because of the nature of her surgery and that this would help. She was agreeable after hearing the rationale. My instructor and I positioned the patient on her side—a feat in itself—so that I could give her the shot in the ventrogluteal area.

I marked the landmarks at least half a dozen times, wiped the area with alcohol, and asked her if she was ready for the injection. *Big mistake!* She swiftly replied, "No, but get it over with." I took a minute to reassure her (and silently, me) again.

A little voice in my head repeated the words my *technologies* professor had said a million times, "Darting action is the key to a successful injection." So, I aimed at the bull's-eye that appeared in front of my eyes. My hand, which seemed to be moving in slow motion, propelled downward at a 90-degree angle. Secretly, I prayed that I would not hit my own hand. I looked down and it was a bull's-eye, thank goodness, but the needle had not penetrated the muscle! The patient successfully tensed her muscle tight enough to intercept the needle midflight. At that moment, she relaxed, probably because she thought the worst was over, and I pushed the needle into place. I slowly drew back the plunger to make sure no blood appeared in the syringe. I began injecting the prochlorperazine slowly, watching my hands shake. Then I withdrew the needle and gently applied pressure over the site. It was over and I wanted to scream, "I did it!" but I kept my composure to feign the experience I lacked. Giving my first IM injection was not as bad as I thought it would be!

—Alison L. Moriarty
Georgetown University, Washington, DC

---

abscesses; cellulitis; injury to blood vessels, bones, and nerves; lingering pain; tissue necrosis; and periostitis (inflammation of the membrane covering a bone). Avoid any site that is bruised, tender, hard, swollen, inflamed, or scarred.

Consider the age of the patient, medication type, and medication volume when selecting a site for intramuscular injection. See Table 29-4 for information related to intramuscular site selection. Rotate the sites used to administer intramuscular medications when therapy requires repeated injections. Whatever pattern of rotating sites is used, provide a description of it in the patient's plan of nursing care.

The *ventrogluteal site* (see Fig. 29-13A) involves the gluteus medius and gluteus minimus muscles in the hip area. This site offers a large muscle mass that is relatively free from major nerves and blood vessels, the area is clean (fecal contamination is rare at this site), and the patient can be on the back, abdomen, or side for the injection. To relax the gluteal muscle, the patient may flex the knees while lying on the back, point the toes inward while lying in the prone position, and flex the upper leg in front of the lower leg in the side-lying position. Although any of the three positions just described may be used when injecting into the ventrogluteal site, nurses increasingly prefer the side-lying position.

To locate the ventrogluteal site, place the palm of your hand over the greater trochanter, with your fingers facing the patient's head. The right hand is used for the patient's left hip, or the left hand for the right hip, to identify landmarks. Place the index finger on the anterosuperior iliac spine and

TABLE • 29-4	INTRAMUSCULAR SITE SELECTION
Criteria	**Recommended Site**
Age of Patient	
Infants	Vastus lateralis
Toddlers and children	Vastus lateralis or deltoid
Adults	Ventrogluteal or deltoid
Medication Type	
Biologicals (infants and young children)	Vastus lateralis
Biologicals (older children and adults)	Deltoid
Hepatitis B/Rabies	Deltoid
Medications that are known to be irritating, viscous or oily solutions	Ventrogluteal

Adapted from Centers for Disease Control and Prevention (CDC). (2009). The pink book: Appendices. Epidemiology and prevention of vaccine preventable diseases (11th ed.). Appendix D. Vaccine administration. Vaccine administration guidelines. Available www.cdc.gov/vaccines/pubs/pinkbook/pink-appendx.htm#appd;download/slides/admin-images.ppt; and Nicoll, L., & Hesby, A. (2002). Intramuscular injection: An integrative research review and guideline for evidence-based practice. *Applied Nursing Research, 16*(2), 149–162.

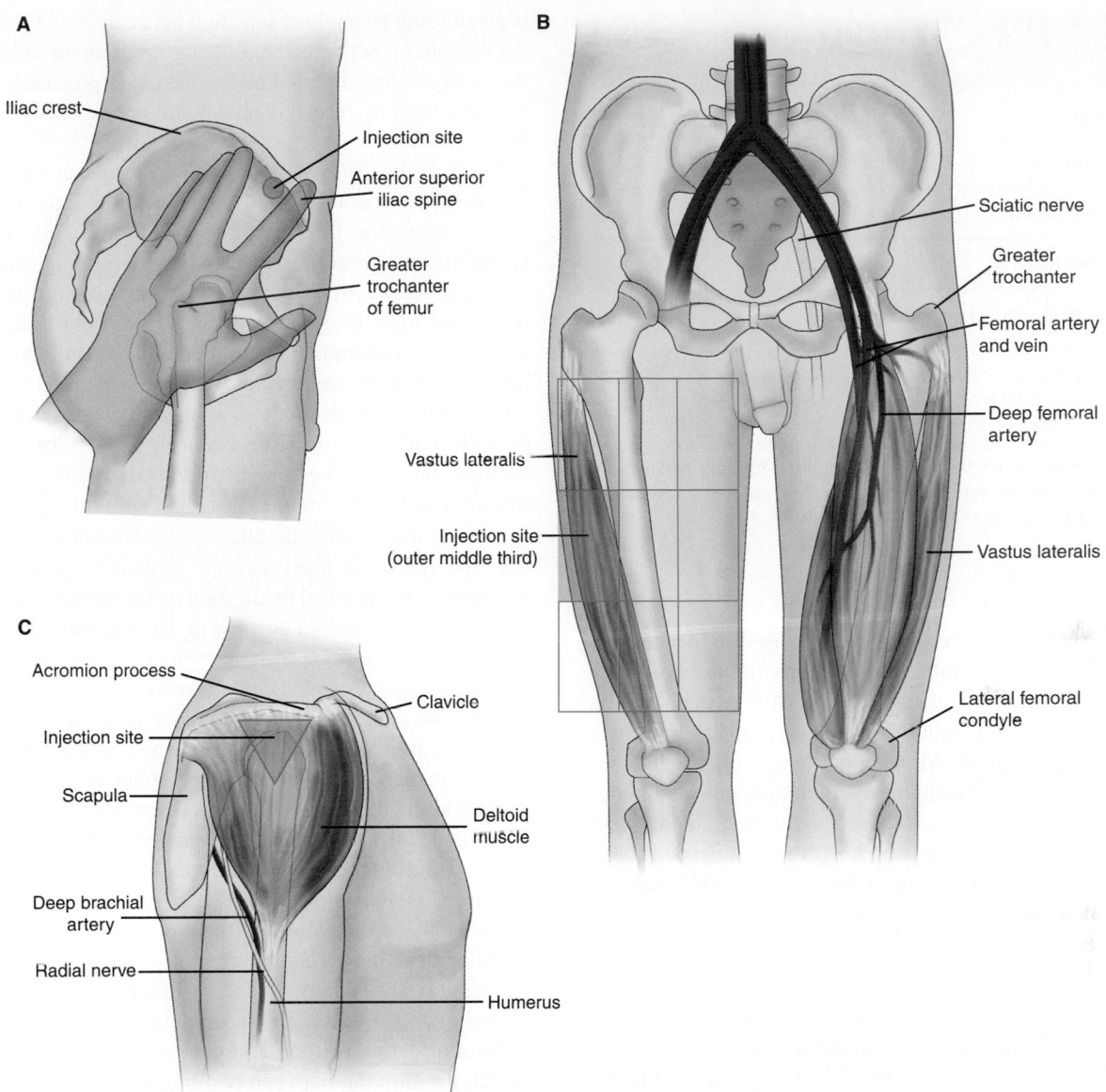

FIGURE 29-13. Sites for intramuscular injections. Descriptions for locating the sites are given in the text. (**A**) The ventro-gluteal site is located by placing the palm on the greater trochanter and the index finger toward the anterosuperior iliac spine. (**B**) The vastus lateralis site is identified by dividing the thigh into thirds, horizontally and vertically. (**C**) The deltoid muscle site is located by palpating the lower edge of the acromion process.

extend the middle finger dorsally, palpating the iliac crest. A triangle is formed, and the injection is given in the center of the triangle.

The *vastus lateralis* (see Fig. 29-13B) involves the quadriceps femoris muscle and is located along the anterolateral aspect of the thigh. There are no large nerves or vessels in its proximity, and it does not cover a joint. To locate the site, divide the thigh into thirds horizontally and vertically and administer the injection in the outer middle third. This space provides a large number of injection sites. The vastus lateralis site is particularly desirable for infants and children, whose gluteal muscles are developed poorly. Restrain infants between the nurse's arm and body to safely administer an injection here.

The *deltoid muscle* is located in the lateral aspect of the upper arm (see Fig. 29-13C). It is the recommended site for

vaccines for adults and may be used for children between 1 and 18 years of age for vaccine administration (CDC, 2008c). The deltoid muscle is not developed enough in infants to absorb medication adequately.

Damage to the radial nerve and artery is a risk with use of the deltoid site. Intramuscular injections into the deltoid muscle should be limited to 1 mL of solution. Locate the deltoid muscle by palpating the lower edge of the acromion process. A triangle is formed at the midpoint in line with the axilla on the lateral aspect of the upper arm, with the base of the triangle at the acromion process. Hepatitis B virus vaccine is one medication that should be given in the deltoid muscle in adults to induce adequate levels of the antibody.

The dorsogluteal site has been previously identified as a possible site to be used for intramuscular medication

TABLE · 29-5	INTRAMUSCULAR INJECTION NEEDLE LENGTH
Site/Age	Needle Length
Vastus lateralis	5/8" to 1"
Deltoid (children)	5/8" to 1¼"
Deltoid (adults)	5/8" to 1½"
Ventrogluteal (adults)	1½"

Adapted from Centers for Disease Control and Prevention (CDC). (2009). The pink book: Appendices. Epidemiology and prevention of vaccine preventable diseases (11th ed.). Appendix D. Vaccine administration. Vaccine administration guidelines. Available www.cdc.gov/vaccines/pubs/pinkbook/pink-appendx.htm#appd.; and Nicoll, L., & Hesby, A. (2002). Intramuscular injection: An integrative research review and guideline for evidence-based practice. *Applied Nursing Research, 16*(2), 149–162.

administration. However, this site has been associated with inadvertent injection into subcutaneous tissue because the area is covered with subcutaneous tissue in many people; injection into subcutaneous tissue alters drug absorption and causes tissue irritation. More importantly, this site has been associated with significant injury, including pain and temporary or permanent paralysis, caused by damage to the sciatic nerve. Therefore, this site is no longer recommended for use for intramuscular injections (Greenway, 2004; Nicoll & Hesby, 2002; Small, 2004).

Equipment

It is important to choose the right equipment for a particular intramuscular injection. Needle length should be based on the site for injection and the patient's age (see Table 29-5 for intramuscular needle length recommendations). Patients who are obese may require a longer needle and those who are emaciated may require a shorter needle. Appropriate gauge is determined by the medication being administered. Generally, biological agents and medications in aqueous solutions should be administered with a 20- to 25-gauge needle. Medications in oil-based solutions should be administered with an 18- to 25-gauge needle. Many medications come in prefilled syringe units. If a needle is provided on the prefilled unit, ensure that the needle on the unit is the appropriate length for the patient and situation.

Procedure

The volume of medication that can be administered intramuscularly varies based on the intended site. Generally, 1 to 4 mL is the accepted volume range, with no more than 1 mL given at the deltoid site. The less-developed muscles of children and elderly people limit the intramuscular injection to 1 to 2 mL.

Administer the intramuscular injection so that the needle is perpendicular to the patient's body. This should ensure that it

is given using an angle of injection between 72 to 90 degrees. An outdated practice is the drawing up of an air bubble into the syringe after the medication has been prepared. This is not supported by research and should not be used (Nicoll & Hesby, 2002).

Many of the drugs given intramuscularly can cause irritation to subcutaneous tissues when backflow into the tissues occurs along the injection track. Therefore, the **Z-track technique** is recommended for all intramuscular injections to ensure medication does not leak back along the needle track and into the subcutaneous tissue (Nicoll & Hesby, 2002). This technique reduces pain and discomfort, particularly for patients receiving injections over an extended period. The Z-track method is also suggested for elderly patients who have decreased muscle mass. Some agents, such as iron, are best given via the Z-track method due to the irritation and discoloration associated with this agent.

In the Z-track technique, attach a clean needle to the syringe after the syringe is filled with the medication to prevent the injection of any residual medication on the needle into superficial tissues. Pull the skin down or to one side about 1" (2.5 cm) and hold in this position with the nondominant hand. Insert the needle and inject the medication slowly. Withdraw the needle steadily and release the displaced tissue to allow it to return to its normal position. Massage of the site is not recommended because it may cause irritation by forcing the medication to leak back into the needle track. However, gentle pressure may be applied with a dry sponge. The procedure for administering a Z-track injection is outlined in Skill 29-7.

A previously included practice in intramuscular injection is the inclusion of aspiration (the process of pulling back on the plunger of the syringe before injection to ensure that the medication is not injected into a blood vessel). However, according to the CDC (2009), aspiration is not required.

An alternative method for intramuscular injection is to stretch the skin flat between two fingers and hold it taut for needle insertion. This technique for administering an intramuscular injection is illustrated in Figure 29-14. Figure 29-15

FIGURE 29-14. Spreading the skin taut at ventrogluteal site. *(Photo by Rick Brady.)*

FIGURE 29-15. Comparison of the angles of insertion for intramuscular, subcutaneous, and intradermal injections.

compares the angles for needle insertion for different forms of injections. Box 29-2 provides techniques for reducing discomfort when injecting medications subcutaneously or intramuscularly.

ADMINISTERING MEDICATIONS INTRAVENOUSLY

Intravenous administration of medications delivers the drug directly into the bloodstream. Medications administered intravenously have an immediate effect. The **intravenous route** is the most dangerous route of administration because the drug is placed directly into the bloodstream, it cannot be recalled, and its actions cannot be slowed. Intravenous administration is the route used in most emergency situations when immediate absorption is required. There also are many nonemergency clinical situations in which drugs are administered intravenously. Patient-controlled analgesia (PCA) allows the patient to control administration of an intravenous analgesic for pain management (refer to Chapter 35). Skill 40-1 in Chapter 40 describes the basic technique for administering an intravenous infusion. There are several ways to administer

---

Box 29-2   REDUCING DISCOMFORT IN SUBCUTANEOUS AND INTRAMUSCULAR ADMINISTRATIONS

The following are recommended techniques for reducing discomfort when injecting medications subcutaneously or intramuscularly:

- Select a needle of the smallest gauge that is appropriate for the site and solution to be injected, and select the correct needle length.
- Be sure the needle is free of medication that may irritate superficial tissues as the needle is inserted. The recommended procedure is to use two needles—one to remove the medication from the vial or ampule and a second one to inject the medication. If medication is in a prefilled syringe with a nonremovable needle and has dripped back on the needle during preparation, gently tap the barrel to remove the excess solution.
- Use the Z-track technique for intramuscular injections to prevent leakage of medication into the needle track, thus minimizing discomfort.
- Inject the medication into relaxed muscles. There is more pressure and discomfort when the medication is injected into a contracted muscle.
- Do not inject areas that feel hard on palpation or tender to the patient.

- Insert the needle with a dart-like motion without hesitation, and remove it quickly at the same angle at which it was inserted. These techniques reduce discomfort and tissue irritation.
- Do not administer more solution in one injection than is recommended for the site. Injecting more solution creates excess pressure in the area and increases discomfort.
- Inject the solution slowly so that it may be dispersed more easily into the surrounding tissue (10 seconds per 1 mL).
- Apply gentle pressure after injection, unless this technique is contraindicated.
- Allow the patient who is fearful of injections to talk about his or her fears. Answer the patient's questions truthfully, and explain the nature and purpose of the injection. Taking the time to offer support often allays fears and decreases discomfort.
- Rotate sites when the patient is to receive repeated injections. Injections in the same site may cause undue discomfort, irritation, or abscesses in tissues.

medications intravenously. Observe aseptic technique when administering medications intravenously to prevent introduction of microorganisms.

Medications via Intravenous Solution

Medications may be added to the patient's infusion solution. In most facilities, the pharmacist adds the prescribed drug to a large volume of intravenous solution.

When medication is administered by continuous infusion, the patient receives it slowly and over a long period. Although this can be an advantage when it is desirable to give the medication slowly, it is a disadvantage when the patient needs to receive the drug more quickly. Also, if for some reason not all of the solution can be infused, the patient will not receive the prescribed amount of the medication. Check the patient receiving medication by a continuous intravenous infusion for possible adverse effects at least every hour.

Medications via an Intravenous Bolus or Push

A medication can be administered as an intravenous bolus or push. This involves a single injection of a concentrated solution directly into an intravenous line (Skill 29-8). The drug is administered very slowly over at least 1 minute. Confirm exact administration times by consulting a pharmacist or drug reference.

Medications via Intermittent Intravenous Infusion

Medications can be administered by intermittent intravenous infusion. The drug is mixed with a small amount of the intravenous solution, such as 50 to 100 mL, and administered over a short period at the prescribed interval (e.g., every 4 hours). The administration is most often performed using an intravenous infusion pump, which requires the nurse to program the infusion rate into the pump. "Smart (computerized) pumps" are being used by many facilities for intravenous infusions, including intermittent infusions. Smart pumps also require programming of infusion rates by the nurse, but also are able to identify dosing limits and practice guidelines to aid in safe administration. Refer to the accompanying Research in Nursing box regarding the use of "Smart Pumps." More information about intravenous infusions and smart pumps is provided in Chapter 40, Fluid, Electrolyte, and Acid-Base Balance. Administration may be achieved by gravity infusion, which requires the nurse to calculate the infusion rate in drops per minute. The best practice however, is to use an intravenous infusion pump. The calculated flow rate of a medication administered via gravity can be altered when the patient bends their extremity proximal to the intravenous insertion site, lifts their extremity, or has an infiltration at the insertion site.

As mentioned, needleless devices are recommended by the CDC and the Occupational Safety and Health Administration. Needleless devices prevent needlesticks and provide access to the primary venous line. Access or connection ports are used to connect intermittent intravenous infusions. A patient with an intravenous line in place can receive the solution containing the medication by way of a piggyback setup, a volume-control administration set (e.g., Pediatrol or Volutrol), or a mini-infusion pump (syringe pump).

The intravenous **piggyback delivery system** requires the intermittent or additive solution to be placed higher than the primary solution container. An extension hook provided by the manufacturer provides for easy lowering of the main intravenous container. The port on the primary intravenous line has a back-check valve that automatically stops the flow

RESEARCH IN NURSING
Bridging the Gap to Evidence-Based Practice

"SMART PUMPS"

Medication errors occur frequently and are a serious problem in healthcare. Medication errors may have serious consequences. Healthcare institutions and healthcare providers have a responsibility to prevent medication errors. "Smart pump" technology is one intervention to use to reduce errors.

Related Research

Rosenkoetter, M., Bowcutt, M., Khasanshina, E., Chernecky, C., & Wall, J. (2008). Perceptions of the impact of "Smart Pumps" on nurses and nursing care provided. *Journal of the Association for Vascular Access, 13*(2), 60–69.

This study focused on the perceptions of nurses regarding the impact of the implementation of "smart pump" technology and its impact on nursing care provided, medication errors, and job satisfaction. Results indicate that the nurses perceived the use of the pumps increased safe medication administration, did not decrease the perception of the punitive nature of reporting

medication errors, and did not increase the nurses' workload. The participants also reported that the use of the pumps made daily routines easier. The pump was perceived to increase self-confidence, but had no effect on the use of pharmacy staff. The pump also increased patient/family confidence in care received. There was no relationship with age, years of nursing experience, and staff nursing degree earned.

Relevance to Nursing Practice

Nurses should welcome the adoption of new technologies to improve nursing practice and decrease medication errors. This study reinforces that technology is easy to use, should not be feared, the use of smart pumps can increase job satisfaction, increase self-confidence, and decrease anxiety of making IV medication errors. The importance of the perceptions of the nursing staff in the implementation of new technology should be considered by a facility that is planning a major technological change.

For additional research, visit thePoint.

of the primary solution, allowing the secondary or piggyback solution to flow when connected. A tandem delivery setup is similar, except that both solutions remain at the same height and there is no back-check valve at the secondary port on the primary line. This type of setup is used infrequently because the solution from the primary intravenous line will back up into the tandem line if this intermittent infusion is not clamped immediately after it is infused. Because manufacturers' designs vary, check the directions carefully for the systems used in the agency. Intravenous administration of medications using a piggyback setup is explained in Skill 29-9.

Medications can also be placed in a **volume-control administration set** for intermittent intravenous infusion. The medication is diluted with a small amount of solution and administered through the patient's intravenous line (see Skill 29-9). This type of equipment is commonly used for infusing solutions into children, critically ill, and older patients when the volume of fluid infused is a concern.

The **mini-infusion pump** (syringe pump) for intermittent infusion is battery operated and allows medication mixed in a syringe to be connected to the primary line and delivered by mechanical pressure applied to the syringe plunger (see Skill 29-9).

A medication or drug infusion lock, also known as an intermittent peripheral venous access device, is used for patients who require intermittent intravenous medication, but not a continuous intravenous infusion. This device consists of a needle or catheter connected to a short length of tubing capped with a sealed injection port. A peripheral venous access device is shown in Skill 29-10. After the catheter is in place in the patient's vein, anchor the catheter and tubing to the patient's arm so that the catheter remains in place until the patient no longer requires the repeated medication intravenously.

A peripheral venous access device allows the patient more freedom than a continuous intravenous infusion. The patient is connected to the intravenous line when it is time to receive the medication and disconnected when the medication is completed. It is important to keep the device patent (working) by flushing with small amounts of saline pushed through the device on a routine basis. Do not start intermittent infusion until intravenous placement is confirmed. Flush the peripheral venous access device before the infusion is begun and after the infusion is completed to clear the vein of any medication and to prevent clot formation in the needle. The procedure for flushing this device with saline is discussed in Skill 29-10. Assess the intravenous site for complications (see Chapter 40). If infiltration or phlebitis occurs, remove the device and replace in a new site.

In addition to a peripheral intravenous line, intermittent intravenous medication may be administered through a central venous access device (CVAD). Many of these devices have particular specifications to be followed when using for administration of fluids or medication. It is important to be aware of the specifics for the device being used. Facilities have specific policies in place for reference. CVADs are discussed in more detail in Chapter 40.

Administering Topical Medications

Medications delivered via the topical route are applied to the skin or mucous membranes, including the eyes, ears, nose, rectum, vagina, and lungs. **Topical applications** are usually intended for direct action at a particular site, although some can have systemic effects and are given for systemic effect. The action depends on the type of tissue and the nature of the agent.

If the site of application is readily accessible, such as the skin, an agent can easily be placed onto it. If it is a cavity, such as the nose, or is enclosed, such as the eye, a mechanical applicator may be needed to introduce the drug.

SKIN APPLICATIONS

The skin is a mechanical and chemical barrier that protects the underlying tissues. It is a sense organ, with receptors that respond to touch, pain, pressure, and temperature. The skin helps in excretion, in regulating body temperature, and in storing essentials to the body such as water, salts, and glucose.

When a drug is incorporated in an agent such as an ointment and rubbed into the skin for absorption, the procedure is referred to as an inunction. On normal skin, drugs are absorbed into the lining of the sebaceous glands. Absorption is hindered because of the protective outer layer of the skin, which makes penetration difficult and because of the fatty substances that protect the lining of the glands. Cleaning the skin thoroughly with soap or detergent and water before administration and then rubbing the medicated preparation into the skin can enhance absorption. Absorption can also be improved by using a drug mixed in an ointment or added to a liniment that will mix with the fat in the gland lining. When indicated, local heat applied to the application area can improve blood circulation and promote absorption. To prevent any absorption by the nurse's skin, gloves should be worn during the application of topical medications. The following are typical preparations applied to skin areas:

- Powders are used to promote drying of the skin and prevent friction on the skin. Use caution when applying to prevent inhalation of the powder. Apply the powder to a gauze square and then apply to the desired site to minimize inhalation of airborne particles.
- Ointments provide prolonged contact of a medication with the skin and soften the skin. They are usually thoroughly massaged into intact skin.
- Creams and oils lubricate and soften the skin and prevent drying of the skin. If a large part of the body is to be covered, warm the preparation in the hands or fingers to prevent chilling.
- Lotions protect and soothe the skin. Shake lotions thoroughly before using, and apply with cotton balls or gauze.
- Transdermal delivery systems utilize reservoirs, micro reservoirs, adhesives, or matrices. These systems are a "sandwich" of layers, each with a specific job. An impermeable backing prevents drug diffusion from the exposed portion. The drug layer of the system contains drug, with a rate-controlling layer to slow the release of

the drug over time, ending with an adhesive layer to enhance the attachment of the system to the patient's skin (Ball & Smith, 2008).

The transdermal route is being used more frequently to deliver medication. This involves applying to the skin a disk or patch that contains medication intended for daily use or for longer intervals. Transdermal patches are commonly used to deliver hormones, narcotic analgesics, cardiac medications, and nicotine. Transdermal patches that contain estrogen should not be applied to breast tissue due to the associated risks of breast cancer. Medication errors have occurred when patients applied multiple patches at once or failed to remove the overlay on the patch that exposes the skin to the medication. Narcotic analgesic patches are associated with the most adverse drug effects. Clear patches have a cosmetic advantage but can be difficult to find on the patient's skin when they need to be removed or replaced. Despite a slow onset of action, transdermal drug patches maintain consistent serum drug levels. See Guidelines for Nursing Care 29-2: Applying Transdermal Patches.

EYE INSTILLATIONS AND IRRIGATIONS

The receptors for the sense of sight are located in the eye. The outer layer of the eyeball is called the sclera. The cornea is the transparent part of the sclera in front of the eyeball. The sclera is fibrous and tough, but the cornea is injured easily by trauma. For this reason, applications to the eye seldom are placed directly onto the eyeball. Because direct application cannot be made onto the sensitive cornea, applications intended to act on the eye or the lids are placed onto, or instilled or irrigated into, the lower conjunctival sac.

The eye is a delicate organ, highly susceptible to infection and injury. Although the eye is never free of microorganisms, the secretions of the conjunctiva have a protective action against many pathogens. For maximum safety for the patient, the equipment, solutions, and ointments introduced into the conjunctival sac should be sterile. If this is not possible, follow the most careful guidelines for medical asepsis.

Eyedrops

Eyedrops are instilled for their local effects, such as for pupil dilation or constriction when examining the eye, for treating an infection, or for controlling intraocular pressure in patients with glaucoma. The type and amount of solution depend on the purpose of the instillation. See Guidelines for Nursing Care 29-3: Instilling Eyedrops.

Ointments

Various types of medication in ointment form may be prescribed for the eye. These ointments are usually used for a local infection or irritation. Eye ointments are dispensed in a tube. A small amount of ointment is distributed along the exposed lower conjunctival sac after the eyelids and eyelashes have been cleansed. About 1/2" of ointment is squeezed from the tube along the exposed sac moving from the inner canthus to the outer canthus of the eye. After the application, the eyes should be closed. The warmth helps to liquefy the ointment. Instruct the patient to move the eye because this helps to spread the ointment under the lids and over the surface of the eyeball. Explain that the ointment may temporarily blur vision; encourage the patient not to rub the eye.

Guidelines for Nursing Care • 29-2

APPLYING TRANSDERMAL PATCHES

- Perform hand hygiene.
- Identify the patient.
- Explain procedure to patient.
- Put on gloves.
- Assess patient's skin where patch is to be placed, looking for any signs of irritation or breakdown. Site should be clean, dry, and free of hair. Rotate application sites.
- Remove the old patch before applying the new one. Fold patch in half with adhesive sides sticking together and discard according to facility policy.
- Gently wash the area where the old patch was with soap and water.
- Remove the patch from its protective covering. Write your initials and the date and time of administration on the label side of the patch.
- Remove the covering without touching the medication surface. Apply the patch to the patient's skin. Use the palm of your hand to press firmly for about 10 seconds. Do not massage.
- Remove gloves and perform hand hygiene.
- Apply the patch at the same time of the day, according to the order and medication specifications.
- Document site of application on the MAR.
- Evaluate patient's response to medication within appropriate time frame.
- Check for dislodgement of the patch if the patient is active. Read information about the patch or consult with the prescriber or pharmacist to determine reapplication schedule and procedure.
- Assess for any skin irritation at application site. If necessary, remove the patch, wash the area carefully with soap and water, and allow skin to air dry. Apply a new patch at a different site. Assess the potential for adverse reaction.
- Aluminum backing on a patch necessitates precautions if defibrillation is required. Burns and smoke may result.

Guidelines for Nursing Care • 29-3

INSTILLING EYEDROPS

- Perform hand hygiene.
- Identify the patient.
- Explain procedure to patient.
- Put on gloves.
- Offer the patient paper tissues to remove solution and tears that may spill from the eye during the procedure.
- Clean the eyelids and eyelashes of any drainage with cotton balls or gauze squares moistened with normal saline solution. Debris can be carried into the eye when the conjunctival sac is exposed. Use each area of the cleaning surface once, moving from the inner toward the outer canthus to prevent carrying debris to the lacrimal ducts.
- Tilt the patient's head back slightly if sitting, or place the patient's head over a pillow if lying down. The head may be turned slightly to the affected side to prevent solution or tears from flowing toward the opposite eye.
- Remove the cap from the medication bottle, being careful not to touch the inner side of the cap.
- Invert the monodrip plastic container that is commonly used to instill eyedrops.
- Have the patient look up while focusing on something on the ceiling.
- Place the thumb or two fingers near the margin of the lower eyelid immediately below the eyelashes, and exert pressure downward over the bony prominence of the cheek. The lower conjunctival sac is exposed as the lower lid is pulled down.
- Hold the dropper close to the eye but avoid touching the eyelids or lashes. Touching the eye, eyelids, or lashes can contaminate the medication in the bottle; startle the patient, causing blinking; or injure the eye.
- Squeeze the container and allow the prescribed number of drops to fall in the lower conjunctival sac. Do not allow

medication to fall onto cornea. This may injure the cornea or cause the patient to have an unpleasant sensation.

- Release the lower lid after the eyedrops are instilled. Ask the patient to close the eyes gently.
- Apply gentle pressure with your gloved finger over the inner canthus to prevent the eyedrops from flowing into the tear duct. This minimizes the risk of systemic effects from the medication.
- Instruct the patient not to rub the affected eye.
- Remove gloves and perform hand hygiene.
- Chart the administration of medication on the MAR after the drops have been administered.
- Evaluate the patient's response to the medication within the appropriate time frame.

With the lower lid pulled down, the nurse prepares to administer the eyedrops on the lower conjunctival sac.

Eye Irrigation

Eye irrigation is performed to remove secretions or foreign bodies or to cleanse and soothe the eye. In an emergency, eye irrigation can be used to remove chemicals that may burn the eye. Copious amounts of tap water should be used to remove chemicals such as acid. The irrigation should continue for at least 15 minutes, and then professional help should be sought. Many emergency rooms have eye flush stations to help with eye irrigations. Care should be taken so that the overflowing irrigation fluid does not contaminate the other eye. See Guidelines for Nursing Care 29-4: Irrigating the Eye.

Eye Medication Disks

An eye medication disk is flexible and resembles a contact lens. These disks contain medication that is released gradually into the conjunctival sac. Once applied, the disk remains in place for as long as a week before being removed and discarded. When properly placed, the disk is completely covered

by the lower eyelid, allowing the patient to wear contact lenses, swim, and sleep with the disk in place. Eye medication disks are usually applied at bedtime because they initially cause blurring of vision. See Guidelines for Nursing Care 29-5: Applying an Eye Medication Disk.

EAR INSTILLATIONS AND IRRIGATIONS

The ear contains the receptors for hearing and equilibrium. It consists of the external ear, the middle ear, and the inner ear. The external ear consists of the auricle or pinna and the exterior auditory canal. The auditory canal serves as a passageway for sound waves. Drugs or irrigations are instilled into the auditory canal for their local effect. They are used to soften wax, relieve pain, apply local anesthesia, destroy organisms, or destroy an insect lodged in the canal, which can cause almost intolerable discomfort. If the ear canal has swollen to the point that medication cannot pass, a long piece of cotton material called a wick is inserted so that one end is

Guidelines for Nursing Care • 29-4

PERFORMING AN IRRIGATION OF THE EYE

- Warm the solution to be instilled to body temperature to minimize discomfort for the patient.
- Perform hand hygiene.
- Identify the patient.
- Explain the procedure to the patient.
- Position the patient, sitting or lying, with head tilted toward side of affected eye. Protect patient and bed with a waterproof pad.
- Put on gloves.
- Clean the patient's eye with a moistened washcloth, wiping from the inner canthus to outer canthus. Use a different part of the washcloth for each stroke.
- Place curved basin at cheek on side of affected eye to receive irrigating solution.
- Fill irrigation syringe with prescribed solution.

- Gently pull down on lower eyelid to expose conjunctival sac. Hold upper lid open.
- Hold syringe about 1 inch from eye. Direct flow of solution from inner to outer canthus along conjunctival sac. Avoid touching any part of the eye with the syringe.
- Pause irrigation periodically. Have patient close eye for a moment. Irrigate until solution is clear or all solution has been used.
- Dry periorbital area after irrigation.
- Remove gloves and perform hand hygiene.
- Evaluate the patient's response to the procedure.
- Document the administration of irrigation on the MAR. Document the procedure, assessments, and patient response.

near the middle ear and the other end is external. This cotton then acts as a wick to help medication get into the canal.

The tympanic membrane separates the external ear from the middle ear. Normally, it is intact and closes the entrance to the middle ear completely. If it is ruptured or has been opened by surgical intervention, the middle ear and the inner ear have a direct passage to the external ear. When this occurs, installations and irrigations should be performed with the greatest of care to prevent forcing materials from the outer ear into the middle ear and the inner ear. Sterile technique is used to prevent infection.

Ear Drops

Follow the techniques listed in Guidelines for Nursing Care 29-6: Instilling Ear Drops when placing drops in the external auditory canal.

Ear Irrigations

Irrigations of the external auditory canal are ordinarily done for cleaning purposes or for applying heat to the area. Typically, normal saline solution is used, although an antiseptic solution may be indicated for local action. To prevent pain, the irrigation solution should be at least at room temperature. An irrigation syringe is used in most instances. An irrigating container with tubing and an ear tip may also be used, especially if the purpose of the irrigation is to apply heat to the area. See Guidelines for Nursing Care 29-7: Irrigating the Ear.

NASAL INSTILLATIONS

Besides serving as the olfactory organ, the nose functions as an airway to the lower respiratory tract and protects the tract by cleaning and warming the air taken in by inspiration.

Guidelines for Nursing Care • 29-5

APPLYING AN EYE MEDICATION DISK

- Perform hand hygiene.
- Identify the patient.
- Explain the procedure to the patient.
- Put on gloves.
- Open disc package. Position the disk with the convex side adhering to your fingertip.
- Ask the patient to look up, and use the other hand to pull the patient's lower eyelid down gently.
- Place the disk in the conjunctival sac and lift the lower eyelid up and over the disk. If properly positioned, the disk should not be visible at this time.

- Remove gloves and perform hand hygiene.
- Document the medication administration on the MAR. Document the procedure, assessments, and patient response.
- For removal, perform hand hygiene and put on gloves.
- Expose the disk by gently pulling down on the patient's lower eyelid.
- Use the forefinger and thumb of the other hand to gently pinch the disk and lift it out of the patient's eye.
- Remove gloves and perform hand hygiene.

Guidelines for Nursing Care • 29-6

INSTILLING EAR DROPS

- Warm the solution to be instilled to body temperature to minimize discomfort for the patient.
- Perform hand hygiene.
- Identify the patient.
- Explain the procedure to the patient.
- Put on gloves.
- Offer a tissue to the patient.
- Clean the external ear of drainage with cotton balls moistened with normal saline solution, as necessary.
- Place the patient on the unaffected side in bed, or if ambulatory, have the patient sit with the head well tilted to the side so that the affected ear is uppermost. This positioning prevents the drops from escaping from the ear.
- Draw up the amount of solution needed in the dropper. Excess medication should not be returned to a stock bottle. A monodrip plastic container may also be used.
- Straighten the auditory canal by pulling the cartilaginous portion of the pinna up and back in an adult (Fig. A), straight back for a school-aged child (Fig. B), and down and back in an infant or a child under age 3 years (Fig. C). Pulling on the

pinna as described helps to straighten the canal properly for ear instillation.

- Hold the dropper in the ear with its tip above the auditory canal. For an infant or an irrational or restless patient, protect the dropper with a piece of soft tubing to help prevent injury to the ear.
- Allow the drops to fall on the side of the canal. It is uncomfortable for the patient if drops fall directly onto the tympanic membrane.
- Release the pinna after instilling the drops, and have the patient maintain the position to prevent the medication from escaping.
- Gently press on the tragus a few times to help move the medication from the canal toward the tympanic membrane.
- If ordered, loosely insert a cotton ball to prevent medication from leaking out.
- Wait 5 minutes before instilling drops in the second ear, if ordered.
- Remove gloves and perform hand hygiene.
- Document the medication administration on the MAR. Document the procedure, assessments, and patient response.

(**A**) Adult patient positioned for eardrop instillation; nurse straightens the auditory canal by pulling the cartilaginous portion of the pinna up and back. (**B**) School-aged child positioned for eardrop instillation; nurse straightens the auditory canal by pulling the cartilaginous portion of the pinna straight back. (**C**) Child under 3 years of age ready for eardrop instillation; nurse straightens the auditory canal by pulling the cartilaginous portion of the pinna down and back. Child can be held by parent.

Guidelines for Nursing Care • 29-7

IRRIGATING THE EAR

- Warm the solution to be instilled to body temperature to minimize discomfort for the patient.
- Perform hand hygiene.
- Identify the patient.
- Explain the procedure to the patient.
- Put on gloves.
- Position patient, sitting or lying, with head tilted toward side of affected ear. Protect patient and bed with waterproof pad. Position basin under ear to receive irrigating solution.
- Clean pinna and meatus of auditory canal as necessary with cotton-tipped applicators moistened with tap water.
- Fill syringe with warm solution. If irrigating container is used, prime the tubing.

- Straighten auditory canal by pulling cartilaginous portion of pinna up and back for an adult.
- Direct a steady, slow stream of solution against the roof of the auditory canal, using only enough force to remove secretions. Do not occlude the auditory canal with the irrigating nozzle. Allow solution to flow out unimpeded.
- When irrigation is complete, place cotton ball loosely in auditory meatus. Position patient on the same side as the affected ear, with towel or absorbent pad under ear.
- Remove gloves and perform hand hygiene.
- Document the medication administration on the MAR. Document the procedure, assessments, and patient response.
- Evaluate the patient's response. Remove cotton ball after 10 to 15 minutes, or per order. Assess drainage.

Cilia project on most of the surfaces of the nasal mucous membrane and help remove particles of dirt and dust from the inspired air. The nose also serves as a resonator when speaking and singing.

Nasal instillations are used to treat allergies, sinus infections, and nasal congestion. Medications with a systemic effect, such as vasopressin, may also be prepared as a nasal instillation. The nose is normally not a sterile cavity, but, because of its connection with the sinuses, it is important to observe medical asepsis carefully when using nasal instillations. See Guidelines for Nursing Care 29-8: Instilling Nose Drops.

Medications may also be applied to the nasal mucous membrane in a spray using a small atomizer. Hold the end of the nose up, and place the tip of the nozzle just inside the naris and directed backward. Use only enough force to bring

the spray into contact with the membrane; too much force may drive the solution and contamination into the sinuses and eustachian tubes.

VAGINAL APPLICATIONS

A healthy vagina contains few pathogens, but many nonpathogenic organisms. The nonpathogens are important because they protect the vagina from the invasion of pathogens. The normal secretions in the vagina are acidic and further serve to protect the vagina from microbial invasion. Therefore, the normal mucous membrane is its own best protection.

Creams, foams, and tablets can be applied intravaginally using a narrow, tubular applicator with an attached plunger. Suppositories that melt when exposed to body heat are also administered by vaginal insertion. Refrigerate suppositories for storage.

Guidelines for Nursing Care • 29-8

INSTILLING NOSE DROPS

- Perform hand hygiene.
- Identify the patient.
- Explain the procedure to the patient.
- Put on gloves.
- Provide the patient with paper tissues and ask that the patient blow his or her nose before instilling the nose drops.
- Have the patient sit up with head tilted well back. If the patient is lying down, tilt the head back over a pillow. These positions allow the solution to flow well back into the naris.
- Draw sufficient solution into the dropper for both nares. Excess solution should not be returned to a stock bottle.

- Hold up the tip of the nose and place the dropper just inside the naris about one third of an inch without touching the nare. Instill the prescribed number of drops in one naris and then into the other. Protect the dropper with a piece of soft tubing if the patient is an infant or young child. Touching the nares with the dropper may cause the patient to sneeze and contaminate the dropper.
- Have the patient remain in position with the head tilted back for a few minutes to prevent the solution from escaping.
- Remove gloves and perform hand hygiene.
- Document the medication administration on the MAR. Document the procedure, assessments, and patient response.

Guidelines for Nursing Care • 29-9

INSERTING VAGINAL SUPPOSITORY OR CREAM

- Perform hand hygiene.
- Identify the patient.
- Explain the procedure to the patient.
- Put on gloves.
- Fill a vaginal applicator with the prescribed amount of cream, or have a suppository ready.
- Lubricate the applicator with water, as necessary. A suppository may be lubricated with a water-soluble gel.
- Ask patient to void before inserting medication.
- Use lithotomy position and provide draping.
- Spread the labia well with the fingers, and clean the area at the vaginal orifice with a washcloth and warm water to remove discharge. Use a different corner of the washcloth with each stroke, moving downward.

- Introduce the applicator gently in a rolling manner while directing it downward and backward to follow the normal contour of the vagina for its full length. Push the plunger to its full length, and then gently remove the applicator with the plunger depressed. Insert a suppository with gloved fingers well into the vagina.
- Ask the patient to remain in the supine position for 5 to 10 minutes after insertion.
- Offer the patient a perineal pad to collect excess drainage.
- Remove gloves and perform hand hygiene.
- Document the medication administration on the MAR. Document the procedure, assessments, and patient response.

 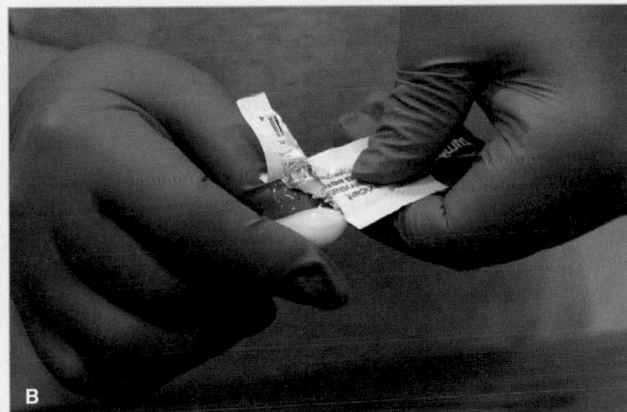

(**A**) Filling vaginal applicator with cream. (**B**) Lubricating vaginal suppository.

Ask the patient to void before inserting the medication. Position the patient so that she is lying on her back with the knees flexed. Maintain privacy with draping. Provide adequate light to visualize the vaginal opening. See Guidelines for Nursing Care 29-9: Inserting Vaginal Suppository or Cream.

RECTAL INSTILLATIONS

Rectal suppositories are used primarily for their local action, such as laxatives and fecal softeners. Systemic effects are also achieved with rectal suppositories. Acetaminophen suppositories are used for an antipyretic effect, and many antiemetics are available in suppository form to relieve nausea and vomiting.

Use clean disposable gloves to prevent contamination with feces and microorganisms. Refer to Guidelines for Nursing Care 29-10: Inserting a Rectal Suppository. After the suppository is inserted, the patient should remain in that position for 5 minutes. If the suppository is for laxative pur-

poses, it must remain in position for 35 to 45 minutes, or until the patient feels the urge to defecate.

Administering Medications by Inhalation

Drugs for **inhalation** are aerosolized, delivered in small particles, and breathed in by the patient. The lungs are supplied richly with blood and have a large surface area. These characteristics allow drugs to be absorbed easily from the lower respiratory tract. Inhalation may be used to administer several different classes of drugs with varying properties and indications (Lannefors, 2006). The smaller the particles of inhaled medication, the lower in the respiratory tract the medication tends to travel. A disadvantage of using this route is that the drug dosage is difficult to establish.

Drugs classified as bronchodilators are an example of a medication administered by inhalation. Bronchodilators act to decrease resistance to airflow by enlarging air passageways. Bronchodilators promote relaxation of musculature in the tracheobronchial tree. The relaxed passages produce less

Guidelines for Nursing Care • 29-10

INSERTING A RECTAL SUPPOSITORY

- Perform hand hygiene.
- Identify the patient.
- Explain the procedure to the patient.
- Put on gloves.
- Assist the patient to his left side in a Sims position. Drape accordingly to expose only the buttocks.
- Remove the suppository from its wrapper. Apply lubricant to the rounded end. Lubricate the index finger of your dominant hand.
- Separate the buttocks with your nondominant hand and instruct the patient to breathe slowly and deeply through the mouth while the suppository is being inserted.

- Using your index finger, insert the suppository, round end first, along the rectal wall. Insert about 3 to 4 inches.
- Use toilet tissue to clean any stool or lubricant from around the anus. Release the buttocks. Encourage the patient to remain on his side for at least 5 minutes and retain the suppository for the appropriate amount of time for the specific medication.
- Remove gloves and perform hand hygiene.
- Document the medication administration on the MAR. Document the procedure, assessments, and patient response.

resistance to airflow and provide an opened respiratory passageway. Bronchodilators are further discussed in Chapter 39.

Drugs for inhalation may be administered by a hand atomizer or a nebulizer. These devices break up the medication into a mist for more efficient inhalation. The hand-held, metered-dose inhaler (MDI) is often used incorrectly, and the correct dose of medication is not delivered. For better medication delivery, a spacer should be used whenever using an MDI, particularly with a child. Refer to Guidelines for Nursing Care 29-11: Using an Inhaled Medication Device.

Nebulization may also result from the force of an oxygen stream or compressed air passed through the fluid in a nebulizer or an atomizer. This method is valuable for patients who require inhalation of a drug several times a day when the hand atomizer is fatiguing. Infants and toddlers can also benefit from nebulized medications. With the use of an oxygen mask, a child can receive medications with minimal interruption of his or her activities. Oxygen masks for the pediatric population come in a variety of sizes and also have dinosaurs or turtles to make the mask less intimidating for the child. The oxygen stream is also useful in the production of vapors when high humidity is needed continuously for long periods. (See Guidelines for Nursing Care 29-11.)

Dry powder inhalers (DPI) are another type of delivery method for inhaled medications. DPIs are breath activated. The drug output and size distribution of the aerosol from a DPI is more or less dependent on the flow rate through the device, requiring a powerful, deep inspiration (Lannefors, 2006). (See Guidelines for Nursing Care 29-11.)

Documenting Medication Administration

The medication record is a legal document. Recording each dose of medication as soon as possible after it is given provides a documented record that can be consulted if there are any questions about whether the patient received the med-

ication. Do not record medications before they are given. If the medication were then not given, the medication record would show falsely that the patient received the medication. Different forms are used for recording medications; an example of a computerized medication administration record (CMAR) is given in Figure 29-16.

The name of the medication, dosage, route of administration, time given, and nurse's initials are noted in the record. Record the site used for an injection. The identity of the nurse completing the documentation is recorded based on the unique user ID and password assigned to each nurse when a CMAR is used. Other specific patient information may be required. For instance, record the pulse rate when administering some cardiac drugs or record a description of the effects on the patient's pain when administering analgesics.

OMITTED DRUGS

Drugs may be omitted intentionally or inadvertently. The omission and the reason for it are documented on the

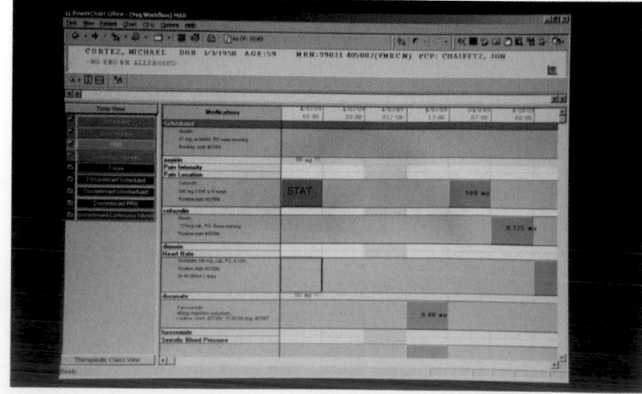

FIGURE 29-16. Example of a computerized medication administration record. (Photo by B. Proud.)

Guidelines for Nursing Care • 29-11

USING AN INHALED MEDICATION DEVICE

- Assess the patient's ability to manage a small-volume nebulizer, metered-dose inhaler, or dry powder inhaler.
- Explain, demonstrate, and encourage the patient to manipulate the inhaler or nebulizer apparatus.
- Encourage the patient to wash hands thoroughly before using device.

The Small-Volume Nebulizer

- Perform hand hygiene.
- Identify the patient.
- Explain the procedure to the patient.
- Remove the nebulizer cup from the device, open it, and place it on a flat working surface.
- Place premeasured unit dose medication in the bottom section of the cup or use a dropper to place concentrated dose of medication in cup and add prescribed fluid to dilute it.
- Screw the top portion of nebulizer cup back in place and attach the cup to the nebulizer.
- Attach one end of tubing to the stem on the bottom of the nebulizer cuff and the other end to the air compressor or oxygen source (if valve to control airflow is not available, a Y tube can be added to the tubing so that one branch of the Y tube connects to the nebulizer cup and the other branch is left open).
- Turn on the air compressor or oxygen.
- Check that a fine medication mist is produced by opening valve or placing thumb over open branch of Y tube.
- Place mouthpiece into mouth and grasp securely with teeth and lips.
- Inhale slowly through the mouth (a nose clip may be necessary if patient is also breathing through the nose).
- Hold each breath for 5 to 10 seconds or as long as possible before exhaling.
- Continue this inhalation technique until all medication in the nebulizer cup has been aerosolized (usually about 15 minutes).
- If desired, gargle with tap water after using nebulizer.
- Rinse the equipment in warm water and allow to air dry on a clean towel.

The Metered-Dose Inhaler

- Perform hand hygiene.
- Identify the patient.
- Explain the procedure to the patient.
- Remove the mouthpiece cover and shake inhaler well.
- Follow caregiver's or manufacturer's recommendations for placement of the mouthpiece. Two methods are possible:
  - Hold the inhaler 1 to 2 inches in front of open mouth; or

Small-volume nebulizer.

- Place mouthpiece into mouth grasping securely with teeth and lips (an MDI coupled with a spacer or extender is always placed in the mouth).
- Take a deep breath and exhale.
- Inhale slowly and deeply through the mouth. Press down on the medication canister while continuing to inhale a full breath (when using a spacer or extender, depress the canister about one fourth or one third through the inspiration).

Patient using a metered-dose inhaler with a spacer. *(Photo by Rick Brady.)*

(continued)

Guidelines for Nursing Care • 29-11

USING AN INHALED MEDICATION DEVICE *continued*

- Hold your breath for 5 to 10 seconds or as long as possible.
- Exhale slowly through pursed lips.
- If another puff is prescribed, wait 1 to 5 minutes before the next inhalation.
- If desired, gargle with tap water and blow nose into a tissue to remove any remaining trace of medication. If MDI is a steroid, this must be done to prevent oral fungal infection.
- Use mild soap and water to clean the mouthpiece, rinse it, and let it dry before replacing it.
- Follow physician's order regarding frequency of inhaler use.

The Dry Powder Inhaler (DPI)

- Understand the specific instructions for your DPI.
- Perform hand hygiene.
- Identify the patient.
- Explain the procedure to the patient.
- Remove the cap and load a dose if necessary.
- Seal your lips around the mouthpiece.
- Do not block the opening with your tongue or teeth.
- Breathe in quickly and deeply, over 2 to 3 seconds.
- Remove the DPI from your mouth.
- Hold your breath for 5 to 10 seconds, or as long as possible.
- If a second dose is necessary, wait 1 to 5 minutes.
- Rinse your mouth or brush your teeth after using.
- Never exhale into the mouthpiece.
- If mist can be seen from the mouth or nose, the DPI is being used incorrectly.
- Keep the cap in place to prevent dirt from entering the DPI.
- Follow the manufacturer's directions to clean the DPI.

Special Considerations

- Teach patients how to tell when their inhaler is empty. Keep a diary or record of inhaler use and discard the inhaler on reaching the labeled number of doses (usually 200 to 400). This method is cumbersome and impractical for some patients, but it is the only reliable way to determine how much medication remains in a metered-dose inhaler (Sander et al., 2006). Floating the canister in water is not reliable and is contraindicated. Immersion in water can cause valve obstruction and threatens product integrity (Sander et al., 2006; Rubin & Durotoye, 2004).

Home Considerations

- Once a week, MDI mouthpiece, spacer or extender, or nebulizer parts should be soaked in a vinegar solution (1 pint of water to 2 oz of vinegar) for 20 minutes. Rinse with clean water and allow to air dry.

Holding chamber (a type of spacer) with mask

Metered dose inhalers

Dry powder inhaler

Examples of metered dose inhalers, spacer, and dry powder inhaler.

---

patient's record. Drugs may be omitted intentionally for the following reasons:

- The patient is to have a diagnostic test and is to fast before the test. Oral drugs are usually omitted, or their administration is delayed, depending on the primary care provider's orders.
- The problem for which the medication is intended no longer exists. For example, a laxative has been ordered for a patient. The patient has had a bowel movement and no longer needs the laxative. The laxative is then omitted.

- The patient is suspected of having an allergy to the medication. Any suspected allergy should be reported to the primary care provider.

To reduce the incidence of medication errors and enhance patient safety, many healthcare facilities are using computerized medication administration record systems. These automated records give the pharmacy the ability to track statistical information, maintain inventory control of drugs, and integrate this information with the central billing system.

REFUSED DRUGS

If the patient refuses to take a drug that is considered essential to the therapeutic regimen, report this promptly. It is important to determine the reason for the refusal and to help the patient accept needed drugs. If the patient is not persuaded by reasonable efforts and adamantly refuses to take a medication, it is unwise to continue urging the patient. Patients have the right to refuse therapy; recognize and respect that right. Describe the refusal to take prescribed drugs and the manner in which the situation was managed on the patient's record and report the refusal according to facility policy.

Preventing and Responding to Medication Errors

Nurses should take every precaution to avoid errors when administering therapeutic agents. The importance of the three checks and the rights of medication administration cannot be overemphasized. Utilization of these steps aids nurses in the prevention of medication errors. Common types of medication errors include the following:

- Inappropriate prescribing of the drug (e.g., incorrect dose, quantity, or route, or inadequate instruction)
- Extra, omitted, or wrong doses
- Administration of a medication to a patient that was not ordered for him or her (see Focused Critical Thinking Guide 29-1)
- Administration of a drug by an incorrect route or at an incorrect rate
- Failure to give a medication within the prescribed time interval
- Incorrect preparation of a drug before administration
- Improper technique when administering a drug
- Giving a drug that has deteriorated

Medication errors occur most often at points of transition in care: on admission to a hospital, at transfer from one department to another, and at discharge home or to another facility. The principal cause of medication error at these times is the incorrect or incomplete transfer of medication information (Barnsteiner, 2005). Nurses and other healthcare providers must be vigilant in order to minimize the high risk for harm from adverse drug events when communication about medications is not clear and in carefully checking that all medications that are appropriate are reordered. A medication reconciliation process that maintains a current, accurate list of medications a patient has received has been shown to decrease the incidence of medication errors that occur at these points of transition in patient care (Barnsteiner, 2005). Nurses are often responsible for management of these lists and need to be on heightened alert to watch for errors at these points of transition.

Prompt acknowledgment of errors may minimize their possible detrimental effect. The immediate priority is the safety of the patient. The following steps are recommended when a medication error occurs:

1. Check the patient's condition immediately when the error is noted. Observe for the development of adverse effects related to the error.
2. Notify the nurse manager and the primary care provider to discuss possible courses of action, depending on the patient's condition.
3. Write a description of the error on the patient's medical record, including remedial steps that are taken.
4. Complete the form used for reporting errors, as dictated by facility policy. These forms, called special event, event, or unusual occurrence reports, require an objective, complete account of the medication error. Include the steps taken after the error was recognized. For legal reasons, describe the error fully and accurately. Medication errors are a common allegation in nursing liability cases. Do not document in the patient's record the fact that an incident report was filed.

There are several voluntary external reporting programs that track medication errors. Nurses and other healthcare providers are encouraged to report medication errors to these organizations. Reporting errors to one of these programs assists in learning more about patient safety, enhancing patient safety standards, and implementing practices to reduce errors. MEDWATCH (www.fda.gov/Safety/MedWatch/default.htm) is administered by the FDA. The National Coordinating Council for Medication Error Reporting and Prevention (www.nccmerp.org) is a cooperative effort supported by organizations from a wide variety of backgrounds, including consumer, health system, trade and manufacturer, nursing, pharmacy, and medicine organizations, as well as government, licensing, and risk management agencies. MEDMARX (www.medmarx.com) is a subscription database operated by the U.S. Pharmacopeia (USP) used by hospitals and healthcare systems to track and trend adverse drug reactions and medication errors.

Although event reports often have a negative connotation for many nurses, they can provide vital information that can be used to prevent the error from being repeated in the future. These tools can provide tracking of errors throughout the institution, providing information that may prevent future medication errors. The emphasis should be on the collaborative efforts necessary to provide safe patient care and decrease the incidence of errors. Peer review committees have proved effective in some healthcare settings.

Another effort to prevent medication errors involves the assignment of pharmacists to patient care areas in the hospital. The pharmacists spend time on the units and interact directly with the nurses, physicians, and other healthcare providers to ensure safe medication delivery. They review patient profiles, discuss adverse effects of drugs and potential drug interactions, and ensure that medications are administered at appropriate times across nursing shifts. This team approach has the potential to reduce medication errors significantly.

The health information technologies discussed previously, including computerized health records, computerized

FOCUSED CRITICAL THINKING GUIDE • 29-1

Medications

You are caring for two residents in a long-term care facility. One of your residents is scheduled to receive a B$_{12}$ injection, and because it will be your first intramuscular injection, it has you more than a little apprehensive. You are eagerly waiting for the moment when your instructor will be free to supervise your injection. Meanwhile, she has cleared you to administer the 10 a.m. meds, and you bring a multivitamin, a diuretic, and an anti-inflammatory agent to one of your assigned residents. When you go to record the medications you administered, you suddenly realize to your horror that you brought them to the wrong resident. When you grab your buddy and confide your error, she says, "Whatever you do, don't tell Miss McMullen [the clinical instructor]. She gets spastic about med errors and has a reputation for gleefully failing students!" You remember that the resident who received the wrong medications has no known drug allergies and you think that she probably wouldn't suffer any adverse effects from the meds she received. What should you do?

1. Identify Goal of Thinking

Determine how you ought to respond to the realization that you administered medications to the wrong resident.

2. Assess Adequacy of Knowledge

Pertinent circumstances: A resident has received three medications that were not ordered for her. *You are a nursing student in your first clinical rotation* and fear your clinical instructor's response should you inform her about your error. You are unsure of the harm that might result from the resident receiving the wrong medication.

Prerequisite knowledge: To decide how you should respond in this situation, you need to understand your professional obligations, which include your moral and legal accountability for having committed a medication error. You will need knowledge of the pharmacologic action of each of the medications you administered and their potential adverse effects on the resident who received them (possible interactions with other medications she is receiving, contraindications with related adverse effects, etc.). You recognize that there is no way for you to get the knowledge you need to make a morally and legally defensible response unless you admit your error to a responsible party.

Room for error/Time constraints: Because you do not know the effects of these medications, you are not in a position to judge how much room there is for error, nor are you able to make a prudent decision about how much time you have to act. The only defensible response is to seek help to clarify your position immediately because a resident's well-being is potentially at stake. No imagined personal costs would justify a delay in your admission of your error.

3. Address Potential Problems

The most serious obstacle to critical thinking in this situation would be an inability to think rationally about your obligation to report the error because of your fear of being censured by your clinical instructor. You will want to examine critically your friend's claim that your instructor will respond harshly because this may, in fact, not be the case. You will also want to test your friend's unstated assumption that your primary obligation in this sort of situation is to take care of yourself—even if this course of action results in harm to a patient. It would be helpful to think through the consequences of every healthcare professional behaving in this manner.

4. Consult Helpful Resources

Given that you are new to medication administration and are unable to assess the potential harm caused to the resident who received the wrong medications, you will find that your most helpful resource is your instructor, and you will need to enlist her assistance immediately. She will probably want to contact the resident's physician to determine whether there are any contraindications to this resident's receiving the medications you administered or possible interactions with other medications. A pharmacist may also need to be consulted. You will want to be familiar with the institution's policy on medication errors and will need to know how to complete an incident report. If the nursing home has a risk manager, you may want to consult him or her.

5. Critique Judgment/Decision

You have two options here: Admit your error and initiate appropriate follow-up, or attempt to cover up your error and "hope for the best." Your decision will basically be made on the strength of your moral conviction that your primary obligation is to safeguard patient well-being, even should this involve some self-sacrifice. Once you recognize the potentially disastrous consequences of patients not being able to trust healthcare professionals to act in their best interests, you decide that there really is only one professionally acceptable response in this situation, and you inform your instructor. It turns out that the resident who received the wrong medications suffered no adverse reactions. You, on the other hand, spend an awful morning following up on your error and even have to delegate your B$_{12}$ injection to another student while you are admitting your error to the resident, her attending, and the charge nurse and completing the special event report. At the end of the day, your instructor compliments you for your honesty and sense of responsibility and cautions you not to repeat the mistake. You are grateful that your worst fears (*failing*) weren't confirmed and leave the unit having learned a powerful lesson about the costs of being accountable.

provider order entry, bar coding, automated drug-dispensing systems, and unit dosing, can potentially contribute to reducing medication errors. However, the person administering the medication, the nurse, needs to remain vigilant in preventing errors.

Teaching About Medications and Abuse

Teaching about medications is an ongoing process and should begin as soon as the patient is admitted to the healthcare facility. Developing a plan of care related to medications is an important part of nursing care. See the Nursing Plan of Care for Regina Sauder included at the end of the chapter. In many cases, patients continue a prescribed medication regimen at home after discharge from the hospital. A factor that affects the patient's compliance with the medication regimen at home is education about the prescribed medications. Teaching should be tailored to the patient's level of understanding. Written instructions can be used as a reference for the patient. See Teaching Tips 29-1: Medications.

Explain the techniques of medication administration to the patient and family. Before being discharged from a healthcare facility, the patient should practice the necessary techniques under the supervision of a nurse to acquire sufficient skill for safe administration. Many patients have learned to give themselves injections, as well as many other medications, when the teaching was planned well and the patient was able and willing to learn.

Emphasize the importance of taking medications as prescribed and for as long as prescribed. A common error made by patients is simply omitting a drug, either through carelessness or because they believe that missing a dose is not important. Various aids are available to remind the patient to take his or her medication on schedule. Medication containers that beep when a dose is due to be taken, scratch-off dots on a medication label, and an electronic cap that signals dosage time and records each time the cap is removed are available. Advise patients to keep their medications with them when they travel. If luggage is lost or misplaced, refilling the prescription may be difficult.

Instruct the patient not to alter the dosage without consulting the primary care provider. Also, teach the patient not to discontinue medications when symptoms disappear. Drugs used to maintain health, such as those used to control high blood pressure, need to be continued as ordered to avoid recurrence of symptoms.

TEACHING TIPS • 29-1

MEDICATIONS

Health Topic	Teaching Tip	Why Is This Important?
General information	• Medication name and dosage • Intended effects of medication • Expected adverse effects of medication	Patients should know the names and reasons for medications in case of medical emergencies. Patients should also know expected adverse effects of the medication so they do not stop taking the medication.
Taking the medication	• Medications should be taken at the same time every day. • Teach whether food, beverages, or other medications have any effect on the medication. • Teach what patient should do if a dose is missed. • Teach patient to take medications as prescribed for as long as prescribed. • Teach not to alter drug dosage without consulting healthcare provider.	If patients make taking medications a part of their daily routine, they are less likely to miss a dose. Some medications require food to prevent stomach irritation; absorption of other medications is impeded by food in the stomach. Patients are likely to miss a dose of medication and need to know what to do if this happens. Some medications have severe consequences if stopped abruptly; others need to be taken for a set period of time and at a recommended dosage to be effective.
Special instructions	• Teach what to do when adverse effects occur. • Keep medications with them when traveling. • Do not share medications with other people. • Proper storage • Keep a list of all medications, including OTC drugs, dietary supplements, herbs, and natural supplements.	Patients need to know whom to contact if any adverse effects occur. Luggage can be lost or misplaced. Teach patients that just because someone else has similar symptoms, it does not mean that the same medication should be taken. Medication should be kept out of the reach of children and pets. For labeling purposes, medications should be kept in the container in which they were dispensed. Some medications are sensitive to humidity and light; keep medications in a cool, dry place. Keep your healthcare providers up to date about your list.

NURSING ADVOCACY IN ACTION

Substance abuse during pregnancy results in significant health problems for the mother, the fetus, and the newborn. Recently, OxyContin has become a popular alternative to other street drugs such as heroin. In utero exposure to opiates is associated with neonatal abstinence syndrome in as many as 55% to 94% of exposed infants. The onset and severity of the infant's withdrawal from the drug varies with the type and duration of the drug taken by the mother.

Patient Scenario

Jasmine is a 24-year-old single mother who is homeless. She has a history of injecting OxyContin (120 to 500 mg/day) intravenously for the past 2 years due to pain in her back. She has a history of barbiturate abuse during her last pregnancy. She has delivered two other infants prematurely at 32 weeks and 36 weeks. Both of these children are in foster care.

Implications for Nursing Advocacy

How will you respond if you are Jasmine's clinic nurse? Talk with your classmates and experienced nurses about the questions that follow.

- If you elect to advocate for Jasmine and her baby what practical steps can you take to ensure better health outcomes?
- What is reasonable to expect of a student nurse, a graduate nurse, and an experienced nurse in this situation?
- What advocacy skills are needed to effectively respond to this challenge?

PROMOTING HEALTH • 29-1

Medications

Use the following assessment checklist to determine how well you are meeting your need for safe medication practices. Then develop a prescription for self-care by choosing appropriate behaviors from the list of suggestions.

Assessment Checklist

❏ almost always	❏ sometimes	❏ almost never

❏ ❏ ❏ 1. I store medications in a safe place (e.g., a cool, dry place, away from direct sunlight, out of the reach of children).

❏ ❏ ❏ 2. I discard medications that have passed their expiration date.

❏ ❏ ❏ 3. I wear a Medic-Alert tag or carry information that identifies a drug allergy or required medication.

❏ ❏ ❏ 4. I am cautious about combining prescribed medication with OTC drugs, herbal supplements, alcohol, or foods that can interact with the drug.

Self-Care Behaviors

1. Finish all prescriptions as ordered by physician or nurse practitioner.
2. Avoid foods, alcohol, or over-the-counter drugs and herbal supplements that may interact with a prescribed drug.
3. Use available resources (textbooks, pharmacist, physician) to verify the potential for drug interactions or possible adverse effects of a medication.
4. Use a reminder system to maintain medication schedule.
5. Avoid sharing medications or taking someone else's prescribed pills.
6. Complete any laboratory tests necessary for maintenance or adjustment of a medication regimen.
7. Practice safe behaviors when storing medications.
8. Purchase drugs from the same pharmacy as an additional safeguard with multiple medication regimens.

Information to promote safe medication practices, such as information about prescription and over-the-counter medications, medication safety, medication administration, and alternative medications is available online. Check out these sites: MedlinePlus at www.nlm.nih.gov/medlineplus and Safe Medication at www.safemedication.com (provided by the American Society of Health System Pharmacists).

Caution the patient not to share prescribed medications with other family members or with friends and neighbors. Inappropriate use of another person's drugs can have serious consequences.

The patient should be able to verbalize the following:

- How and when to administer the medication
- When to notify the healthcare provider
- Expected adverse effects and adverse effects

Nurses have a responsibility to teach about drug abuse. Teaching may take place on an individual basis or on a family or community level. Drug abuse is a major public health concern worldwide, especially among teenagers and young adults. (Refer to the Nursing Advocacy in Action box.) Continued public and individual education is indicated, and nurses are also expected to set high standards for their own behavior and the use of drugs. Because drug abuse is increasingly common in healthcare providers, nurses who suspect that a colleague is abusing drugs must observe, document, and intervene for the patients' safety.

Nurses working with patients to promote appropriate behaviors related to medication administration should examine their own behaviors as factors in the success of the plan. Nurses who role model good health behaviors are more effective teachers. Use the display, Promoting Health 29-1: Medications, for yourself before using it with others.

Evaluating

Assess the effectiveness of drugs in several ways. Clinical observation is the first method. Collect subjective data from the patient (e.g., "My pain has disappeared") and collect objective data (e.g., the patient's vital signs) to evaluate effectiveness of the medication. It is also important to assess the patient for adverse drug effects.

Measurement of drug levels in body fluids provides data about the patient's response to a particular medication. For many drugs, including digoxin, warfarin, anticonvulsants, and aminoglycoside antibiotics, monitoring blood levels is an important component of therapy. Test the patient to determine whether the drug level in the blood is within the therapeutic range. Drug dosages may be adjusted based on the serum drug level. Monitoring systems can also assist the nurse in evaluating drug effectiveness. For the patient with an arrhythmia, for example, a cardiac monitor can show a change in heart rhythm.

See the accompanying Nursing Plan of Care for Regina Sauder for an example of the nursing process for medication administration.

NURSING PLAN OF CARE · 29-1

For Regina Sauder

Regina Sauder, 73 years old, presented to the emergency room with pain, swelling, and erythema of her left calf. She has a history of lymphoma. Vascular studies of the lower extremities showed a left leg deep vein thrombosis. She was admitted to the hospital and started on intravenous heparin. After 3 days of heparin therapy, she was started on warfarin, in addition to the heparin. Her warfarin dose is being adjusted based on her daily INR level. Daily assessment of her INR level will continue in the hospital until her level is therapeutic. Initially, weekly monitoring of the INR level will continue after discharge.

ASSESSMENT FINDINGS
- PTT is 60 seconds; within expected parameters for adequate hypercoagulation with heparin therapy.
- INR is 1.2; in the low end of expected parameter for adequate hypercoagulation with warfarin therapy.
- Patient's left lower leg without swelling, tenderness, and erythema.
- Patient states, "It feels so much better. I had so much pain, but not now. But, why am I taking two different medications? Am I going to have to go home with this tube in my arm?" Mrs. Sauder appears anxious, is fidgeting, and becomes tearful during the conversation with the nurse. She states, "I think this new pill sounds scary." Her husband reports unease about his wife's ability "to keep track of everything."
- Patient and husband unable to verbalize knowledge regarding signs of bleeding, dosage, timing of administration, dietary guidelines, or need for scheduled follow-up blood work.
- Patient and her husband live in a two-story home, with the bathroom on the second floor.

NURSING DIAGNOSIS	Risk for Injury, bleeding, related to adverse effects of warfarin and falls
EXPECTED OUTCOME	By 3/20/12, the patient and her husband will:

- Be able to identify signs and symptoms of bleeding

(continued)

NURSING PLAN OF CARE · 29-1

For Regina Sauder *(continued)*

Nursing Interventions	Rationale	Evaluative Statement
Provide instruction identifying signs and symptoms of bleeding	Focuses teaching session on a single idea, allowing the patient to concentrate more completely on the material. Older patients and highly anxious patients have reduced short-term memory and benefit from mastery of one concept at a time.	3/19/12 Outcome met. Mrs. Sauder and her husband are able to identify signs and symptoms of bleeding to report to their physician. *B. Huber, RN*
Give patient and husband written pamphlet from drug manufacturer	Provide information using various mediums because different people take in information in different ways. Provides concrete reinforcement.	
Encourage questions	Patients and family members often feel shy or embarrassed about asking questions. Gives permission to ask.	

EXPECTED OUTCOME By 3/20/12, the patient's husband will:

• Remove from their home potential hazards that could lead to falls.

Nursing Interventions	Rationale	Evaluative Statement
Review with patient and husband potential causes of falls at home	Falls may cause internal bleeding.	3/18/12 Outcome met. Husband removed several loose rugs, repaired loose stairs, and improved the lighting at the stairs to the bathroom. *B. Clapp, RN*
Assist the patient and husband in evaluating their home environment to identify potential hazards	Remove potential hazards to prevent falls and injury	
Encourage the use of proper lighting, handrails on stairways, removal of scatter rugs, fastening loose carpet edges	Remove potential hazards to prevent falls and injury	

SAMPLE DOCUMENTATION

3/17/12 Nursing
Patient, husband, and nurse met to discuss potential effects of warfarin therapy and risk for injury. Discussion centered on importance of preventing injury while on warfarin at home. See plan of care. Patient progress will be evaluated in 4 days, 3/21/12.

B. Clapp, RN

Skill · 29-1   Administering Oral Medications

EQUIPMENT

- Medication in disposable cup or oral syringe
- Liquid (water, juice, etc.) with straw if not contraindicated
- Medication cart or tray
- Computer-generated Medication Administration Record (CMAR) or Medication Administration Record (MAR)
- PPE, as indicated

IMPLEMENTATION

ACTION	RATIONALE
1. Gather equipment. Check each medication order against the original in the medical record, according to facility policy. Clarify any inconsistencies. Check the patient's chart for allergies.	This comparison helps to identify errors that may have occurred when orders were transcribed. The primary care provider's order is the legal record of medication orders for each facility.
2. Know the actions, special nursing considerations, safe dose ranges, purpose of administration, and adverse effects of the medications to be administered. Consider the appropriateness of the medication for this patient.	This knowledge aids the nurse in evaluating the therapeutic effect of the medication in relation to the patient's disorder and can also be used to educate the patient about the medication.
3. Perform hand hygiene.	Hand hygiene prevents the spread of microorganisms.
4. Move the medication cart to the outside of the patient's room or prepare for administration in the medication area.	Organization facilitates error-free administration and saves time.
5. Unlock the medication cart or drawer. Enter pass code into computer and scan employee identification, if required.	Locking of the cart or drawer safeguards each patient's medication supply. Hospital accrediting organizations require medication carts to be locked when not in use. Entering pass code and scanning ID allows only authorized users into the computer system and identifies user for documentation by the computer.
6. **Prepare medications for one patient at a time.**	This prevents errors in medication administration.
7. Read the CMAR/MAR and select the proper medication from the patient's medication drawer or unit stock.	This is the first check of the label.
8. Compare the label with the CMAR/MAR (Figure 1). Check expiration dates and perform calculations, if necessary. Scan the bar code on the package, if required.	This is the second check of the label. Verify calculations with another nurse to ensure safety, if necessary.
9. Prepare the required medications:	
a. *Unit dose packages:* Place unit dose-packaged medications in a disposable cup. **Do not open the wrapper until at the bedside.** Keep narcotics and medications that require special nursing assessments in a separate container.	Wrapper is kept intact because the label is needed for an additional safety check. Special assessments may be required before giving certain medications. These may include assessing vital signs and checking laboratory test results.
b. *Multidose containers:* When removing tablets or capsules from a multidose bottle, pour the necessary number into the bottle cap and then place the tablets or capsules in a medication cup. Break only scored tablets, if necessary, to obtain the proper dosage. Do not touch tablets or capsules with hands.	Pouring medication into the cap allows for easy return of excess medication to bottle. Pouring tablets or capsules into the nurse's hand is unsanitary.
c. *Liquid medication in multidose bottle:* When pouring liquid medications out of a multidose bottle, hold the bottle so the label is against the palm. Use the appropriate measuring device when pouring liquids, and read the amount of medication at the bottom of the meniscus at eye level (Figure 2). Wipe the lip of the bottle with a paper towel.	Liquid that may drip onto the label makes the label difficult to read. Accuracy is possible when the appropriate measuring device is used and then read accurately.
10. **When all medications for one patient have been prepared, recheck the labels with the CMAR/MAR before taking them to the patient. Replace any multidose containers in the patient's drawer or unit stock. Lock the medication cart before leaving it.**	This is a *third* check to ensure accuracy and to prevent errors. Locking the cart or drawer safeguards the patient's medication supply. Hospital accrediting organizations require medication carts to be locked when not in use. Some facilities require the third check to occur at the bedside, after identifying the patient and before administration.

(continued)

Skill · 29-1 **Administering Oral Medications** *continued*

ACTION

FIGURE 1. Comparing medication label with the CMAR.

11. Transport medications to the patient's bedside carefully, and keep the medications in sight at all times.

12. **Ensure that the patient receives the medications at the correct time.**

13. Perform hand hygiene and put on PPE, if indicated.

14. Identify the patient. Usually, the patient should be identified using two methods. Compare the information with the CMAR or MAR.

    a. Check the name and identification number on the patient's identification band (Figure 3).

    b. Ask the patient to state his-or her name and birth date, based on facility policy.

    c. If the patient cannot identify him- or herself, verify the patient's identification with a staff member who knows the patient for the second source.

15. **Scan the patient's bar code on the identification band, if required** (Figure 4).

FIGURE 3. Checking patient's name and ID number with the CMAR.

RATIONALE

FIGURE 2. Measuring at eye level. *(Photo by B. Proud.)*

Careful handling and close observation prevent accidental or deliberate disarrangement of medications.

Check agency policy, which may allow for administration within a period of 30 minutes before or 30 minutes after the designated time.

Hand hygiene and PPE prevent the spread of microorganisms. PPE is required based on transmission precautions.

Identifying the patient ensures that the right patient receives the medications and helps prevent errors.

This is the most reliable method. Replace the identification band if it is missing or inaccurate in any way.

This requires a response from the patient, but illness and strange surroundings often cause patients to be confused.

This is another way to double check identity. Do not use the name on the door or over the bed, because these may be inaccurate.

The bar code provides an additional check to ensure that the medication is given to the right patient.

FIGURE 4. Scanning the bar code on the patient's identification bracelet. *(Photo by B. Proud.)*

ACTION

16. **Complete necessary assessments before administering medications. Check the patient's allergy bracelet or ask the patient about allergies. Explain the purpose and action of each medication to the patient.**

17. Assist the patient to an upright or lateral position.

18. Administer medications:

a. Offer water or other permitted fluids with pills, capsules, tablets, and some liquid medications.

b. Ask whether the patient prefers to take the medications by hand or in a cup.

19. **Remain with the patient until each medication is swallowed. Never leave medication at the patient's bedside (Figure 5).**

RATIONALE

Assessment is a prerequisite to administration of medications.

Swallowing is facilitated by proper positioning. An upright or side-lying position protects the patient from aspiration.

Liquids facilitate swallowing of solid drugs. Some liquid drugs are intended to adhere to the pharyngeal area, in which case liquid is not offered with the medication.

This encourages the patient's participation in taking the medications.

Unless the nurse has seen the patient swallow the drug, the drug cannot be recorded as administered. The patient's chart is a legal record. Only with a physician's order can medications be left at the bedside.

FIGURE 5. Remaining with the patient until each medication is swallowed.

20. Assist the patient to a comfortable position. Remove PPE, if used. Perform hand hygiene.

21. Document the administration of the medication immediately after administration. See Documentation section below.

22. Evaluate patient's response to medication within appropriate time frame.

Promotes patient comfort. Proper removal of PPE prevents transmission of microorganisms. Hand hygiene deters the spread of microorganisms.

Timely documentation helps to ensure patient safety.

The patient needs to be evaluated for therapeutic and adverse effects from the medication.

DOCUMENTATION

Guidelines

Record each medication administered on the CMAR/MAR or record using the required format immediately after it is administered, including date and time of administration (Figure 6). If using a bar-code system, medication administration is automatically recorded when scanned. PRN medications require documentation of the reason for administration. Prompt recording avoids the possibility of accidentally repeating the administration of the drug. If the drug was refused or omitted, record this in the appropriate area on the medication record and notify the primary care provider. This verifies the reason medication was omitted and ensures that the primary care provider is aware of the patient's condition. Recording of administration of a narcotic may require additional documentation on a narcotic record, stating drug count and other specific information. Record fluid intake if intake and output measurement is required.

(continued)

Skill · 29-1 **Administering Oral Medications** *continued*

FIGURE 6. Recording each medication administered on the CMAR.

Sample Documentation

8/6/12 0835 Patient states he is having constant stabbing leg pains. Rates pain as an 8/10. Percocet 2 tabs administered.

—*K. Sanders, RN*

8/6/12 0905 Patient resting comfortably. Rates leg pain as a 1/10.

—*K. Sanders, RN*

8/6/12 1300 Patient states he does not want pain medication, despite return of leg pain. States, "It made me feel woozy last time." Feelings discussed with patient. Patient agrees to take Percocet 1 tab at this time.

—*K. Sanders, RN*

8/6/12 1320 Percocet, 1 tablet given PO.

—*K. Sanders, RN*

UNEXPECTED SITUATIONS AND ASSOCIATED INTERVENTIONS

- *Patient states that it feels like medication is lodged in throat:* Offer patient more fluids to drink. If allowed, offer the patient bread or crackers to help move the medication to the stomach.

- *It is unclear whether the patient swallowed the medication:* Check in the patient's mouth, under tongue, and between cheek and gum. Patients with altered mental status may not be aware that the medication was not swallowed. Also, patients may "cheek" medications to avoid taking the medication or to save it for later use. Watch patients requiring suicide precautions closely to ensure that they are not "cheeking" the medication or hiding it in the mouth. These patients may be trying to accumulate a large amount of medication to take all at once in a suicide attempt. Substance abusers may cheek medication to accumulate a large amount to take all at once so that they may feel a high from medication.

- *Patient vomits immediately or shortly after receiving oral medication:* Assess vomit, looking for pills or fragments. Do not readminister medication without notifying primary care provider. If a whole pill is seen and can be identified, the primary care provider may ask that the medication be administered again. If a pill is not seen or medications cannot be identified, do not readminister the medication in order to prevent the patient from receiving too large a dose.

- *Child refuses to take oral medications:* Some medications may be mixed in a small amount of food, such as pudding or ice cream. Do not add the medication to liquids because the medication may alter the taste of liquids; if child then refuses to drink the rest of the liquid, you will not know how much of the medication was ingested. Use creativity when devising ways to administer medications to a child. See the section below, "Infant and Child Considerations," for suggestions.

- *The capsule or tablet falls to the floor during administration.* Discard and obtain a new dose for administration. This prevents contamination and transmission of microorganisms.
- *Patient refuses medication.* Explore the reason for the patient's refusal. Review the rationale for using the drug and any other information that may be appropriate. If you are unable to administer the medication despite education and discussion, document the omission according to facility policy and notify the primary care provider.

SPECIAL CONSIDERATIONS

General Considerations

- Some liquid medication preparations, such as suspensions, require agitation to ensure even distribution of medication in the solution. Be familiar with the specific requirements for medications you are administering.
- Place medications intended for sublingual absorption under the patient's tongue. Instruct the patient to allow the medication to dissolve completely. Reinforce the importance of not swallowing the medication tablet.
- Some oral medications are provided in powdered forms. Verify the correct liquid to dissolve the medication in for administration. This information is usually included on the package; verify any unclear instructions with a pharmacist or medication reference. If there is more than one possible liquid to dissolve the medication in, include the patient in the decision process; patients may find one choice more palatable than another.
- Ongoing assessment is an important part of nursing care to evaluate patient response to administered medications and early detection of adverse effects. If an adverse effect is suspected, withhold further medication doses and notify the patient's primary care provider. Additional intervention is based on type of reaction and patient assessment
- If the patient questions a medication order or states the medication is different from the usual dose, always recheck and clarify with the original order and/or primary care provider before giving the medication.
- If the patient's level of consciousness is altered or his or her swallowing is impaired, check with the primary care provider to clarify the route of administration or alternative forms of medication. This may also be a solution for a pediatric or a confused patient who is refusing to take a medication.
- Patients with poor vision can request large-type labels on medication containers. A magnifying lens also may be helpful.
- Provide written medication information to reinforce discussion and education in the appropriate language if the patient is literate. If the patient is unable to read, provide written information to family or significant other, if appropriate. Written information should be at a 5th-grade level to ensure ease of understanding.
- If the patient has difficulty swallowing tablets, it may be appropriate to crush the medication to facilitate administration. However, not all medications can be crushed or altered; long-acting and slow-release drugs are examples of medications that cannot be crushed. Therefore, it is important to consult a medication reference and/or pharmacist. If the medication can be crushed, use a pill crusher or mortar and pestle to grind the tablet into a powder. Crush each pill one at a time. Dissolve the powder with water or other recommended liquid in a liquid medication cup, keeping each medication separate from the others. Keep the package label with the medication cup for future comparison of information. Combine the crushed medication with a small amount of soft food, such as applesauce or pudding, to facilitate administration.

Infant and Child Considerations

- Special devices, such as oral syringes and calibrated nipples, are available in a pharmacy to ensure accurate dose calculations for young children and infants.
- Some creative ways to administer medications to children include: have a "tea party" with medicine cups, place oral syringe (without needle) or dropper in the space between the cheek and gum and slowly administer the medication, or save a special treat for after the medication administration (e.g., movie, playroom time, or a special food if allowed).

(continued)

Skill · 29-1   Administering Oral Medications *continued*

- The FDA has received reports of infants choking on the plastic caps that fit on the end of syringes when used to administer oral medications. They recommend the following: remove and dispose of caps before giving syringes to patients or families, caution family caregivers to dispose of caps on syringes they buy over the counter, and report any problems with syringe caps to the FDA. Companies manufacture syringes labeled "oral use" without the caps on them.

Older Adult Considerations

- Elderly patients with arthritis may have difficulty opening childproof caps. On request, the pharmacist can substitute a cap that is easier to open. A rubber band twisted around the cap may provide a more secure grip for older patients.
- Consider large-print written information when appropriate.
- Physiologic changes associated with the aging process, including decreased gastric motility, muscle mass, acid production, and blood flow, can affect patient's response to medication, including drug absorption and increased risk of adverse effects. Older adults are more likely to take multiple drugs, so drug interactions in the older adult are a very real and dangerous problem. Refer to Focus on the Older Adult: Aging and Drug Response.

Home Care Considerations

- Encourage the patient to discard expired prescription medications.
- Discuss safe storage of medications when there are children and pets in the environment.
- Discuss with parents the difference in over-the-counter medications made for infants and medications made for children. Many times parents do not realize that there are different strengths to the actual medications, leading to under- or overdosing.
- Encourage patients to carry a card listing all medications, dosage, and frequency in case of an emergency.
- Discuss the importance of using an appropriate measuring device for liquid medications. Caution patients not to use eating utensils for measuring medications; use a liquid medication cup, oral syringe, or measuring spoon to provide accurate dosing.

Skill · 29-2   Removing Medication from an Ampule

EQUIPMENT

- Sterile syringe and filter needle
- Ampule of medication
- Small gauze pad
- Computer-generated Medication Administration Record (CMAR) or Medication Administration Record (MAR)

IMPLEMENTATION

ACTION	RATIONALE
1. Gather equipment. Check the medication order against the original order in the medical record, according to facility policy. Clarify any inconsistencies. Check the patient's chart for allergies.	This comparison helps to identify errors that may have occurred when orders were transcribed. The primary care provider's order is the legal record of medication orders for each facility.
2. Know the actions, special nursing considerations, safe dose ranges, purpose of administration, and adverse effects of the medications to be administered. Consider the appropriateness of the medication for this patient.	This knowledge aids the nurse in evaluating the therapeutic effect of the medication in relation to the patient's disorder and can also be used to educate the patient about the medication.
3. Perform hand hygiene.	Hand hygiene deters the spread of microorganisms.
4. Move the medication cart to the outside of the patient's room or prepare for administration in the medication area.	Organization facilitates error-free administration and saves time.

ACTION

5. Unlock the medication cart or drawer. Enter pass code and scan employee identification, if required.

6. **Prepare medications for one patient at a time.**

7. Read the CMAR/MAR and select the proper medication from the patient's medication drawer or unit stock.

8. Compare the label with the CMAR/MAR. Check expiration dates and perform calculations, if necessary. Scan the bar code on the package, if required.

9. Tap the stem of the ampule (Figure 1) or twist your wrist quickly (Figure 2) while holding the ampule vertically.

RATIONALE

Locking of the cart or drawer safeguards each patient's medication supply. Hospital accrediting organizations require medication carts to be locked when not in use. Entering pass code and scanning ID allows only authorized users into the system and identifies user for documentation by the computer.

This prevents errors in medication administration.

This is the first check of the label.

This is the second check of the label. Verify calculations with another nurse to ensure safety, if necessary.

This facilitates movement of medication in the stem to the body of the ampule.

FIGURE 1. Tapping stem of the ampule.

FIGURE 2. Twisting wrist quickly while holding the ampule vertically.

10. Wrap a small gauze pad around the neck of the ampule.

11. Use a snapping motion to break off the top of the ampule along the scored line at its neck (Figure 3). **Always break away from your body.**

12. Attach filter needle to syringe. Remove the cap from the filter needle by pulling it straight off.

This protects the nurse's fingers from the glass as the ampule is broken.

This protects the nurse's face and fingers from any shattered glass fragments.

Use of a filter needle prevents the accidental withdrawing of small glass particles with the medication. Pulling cap off in a straight manner prevents accidental needlestick.

(continued)

Skill · 29-2   Removing Medication from an Ampule   *continued*

FIGURE 3. Using a snapping motion to break top of the ampule.

13. Withdraw medication in the amount ordered plus a small amount more (approximately 30% more). **Do not inject air into the solution.** Use either of the following methods. **While inserting the filter needle into the ampule, be careful not to touch the rim.**

By withdrawing an additional small amount of medication, any air bubbles in the syringe can be displaced once the syringe is removed and there will still be ample medication in the syringe. The contents of the ampule are not under pressure; therefore, air is unnecessary and will cause the contents to overflow. The rim of the ampule is considered contaminated.

a. Insert the tip of the needle into the ampule, which is upright on a flat surface, and withdraw fluid into the syringe (Figure 4). **Touch the plunger at the knob only.**

Handling the plunger at the knob only will keep the shaft of the plunger sterile.

b. Insert the tip of the needle into the ampule and invert the ampule (Figure 5). Keep the needle centered and not touching the sides of the ampule. Withdraw fluid into syringe. **Touch the plunger at the knob only.**

Surface tension holds the fluids in the ampule when inverted. If the needle touches the sides or is removed and then reinserted into the ampule, surface tension is broken, and fluid runs out. Handling the plunger at the knob only will keep the shaft of the plunger sterile.

FIGURE 4. Withdrawing medication from upright ampule. *(Photo by B. Proud.)*

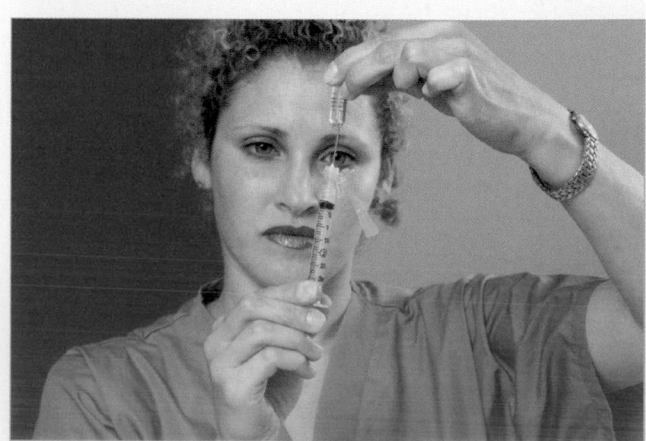

FIGURE 5. Withdrawing medication from inverted ampule. *(Photo by B. Proud.)*

ACTION

RATIONALE

14. Wait until the needle has been withdrawn to tap the syringe and expel the air carefully by pushing on the plunger. **Check the amount of medication in the syringe with the medication dose and discard any surplus according to facility policy.**

Ejecting air into the solution increases pressure in the ampule and can force the medication to spill out over the ampule. Ampules may have overfill. Careful measurement ensures that the correct dose is withdrawn.

15. **Recheck the label with the CMAR/MAR.**

This is the *third* check to ensure accuracy and to prevent errors. Some facilities require the third check to occur at the bedside, after identifying the patient and before administration.

16. **Engage safety guard on filter needle and remove the needle. Discard the filter needle in a suitable container. Attach appropriate administration device to syringe.**

Filter needle used to draw up medication should not be used to administer the medication, to prevent any glass shards from entering the patient.

17. Discard the ampule in a suitable container.

Any medication that has not been removed from the ampule must be discarded because there is no way to maintain sterility of contents in an opened ampule.

18. Lock the medication cart before leaving it.

Locking the cart or drawer safeguards the patient's medication supply. Hospital accrediting organizations require medication carts to be locked when not in use.

19. Perform hand hygiene.

Hand hygiene deters the spread of microorganisms.

20. Proceed with administration, based on prescribed route.

See appropriate skill for prescribed route.

DOCUMENTATION

It is not necessary to record the removal of the medication from the ampule. Record each medication administered on the CMAR/MAR or record using the required format immediately after it is administered, including date and time of administration. If using a bar-code system, medication administration is automatically recorded when scanned. PRN medications require documentation of the reason for administration. Prompt recording avoids the possibility of accidentally repeating the administration of the drug. If the drug was refused or omitted, record this in the appropriate area on the medication record and notify the primary care provider. This verifies the reason medication was omitted and ensures that the primary care provider is aware of the patient's condition. Recording of administration of a narcotic may require additional documentation on a narcotic record, stating drug count and other specific information. Record fluid intake if intake and output measurement is required.

UNEXPECTED SITUATIONS AND ASSOCIATED INTERVENTIONS

- *Nurse cuts self while trying to open ampule:* Discard ampule in case contamination has occurred. Bandage wound and obtain a new ampule. Report according to facility policy.
- *All of medication was not removed from the stem and there is not enough medication left in body of ampule for dose:* Discard ampule and drawn medication. Obtain a new ampule and start over. Medication in original ampule stem is considered contaminated once neck of ampule has been placed on a nonsterile surface.
- *Nurse injects air into inverted ampule, spraying medication:* Wash hands to remove any medication. If any medication has gotten into eyes, perform eye irrigation. Obtain a new ampule for medication dose. Report injury, if appropriate, according to facility policy.
- *Medication is drawn up without using a filter needle:* Replace needle with a filter needle. Inject the medication through the filter needle into a new syringe and then administer to patient.
- *Plunger becomes contaminated before inserted into ampule:* Discard needle and syringe and start over. If plunger is contaminated after medication is drawn into the syringe, it is not necessary to discard and start over. The contaminated plunger will enter the barrel of the syringe when pushing the medication out and will not contaminate the medication.

Skill · 29-3 Removing Medication From a Vial

EQUIPMENT

- Sterile syringe and needle or blunt cannula (size depends on medication being administered and patient)
- Vial of medication
- Antimicrobial swab
- Second needle (optional)
- Filter needle (optional)
- Computer-generated Medication Administration Record (CMAR) or Medication Administration Record (MAR)

IMPLEMENTATION

ACTION	RATIONALE
1. Gather equipment. Check the medication order against the original order in the medical record, according to facility policy.	This comparison helps to identify errors that may have occurred when orders were transcribed. The primary care provider's order is the legal record of medication orders for each facility.
2. Know the actions, special nursing considerations, safe dose ranges, purpose of administration, and adverse effects of the medications to be administered. Consider the appropriateness of the medication for this patient.	This knowledge aids the nurse in evaluating the therapeutic effect of the medication in relation to the patient's disorder and can also be used to educate the patient about the medication.
3. Perform hand hygiene.	Hand hygiene deters the spread of microorganisms.
4. Move the medication cart to the outside of the patient's room or prepare for administration in the medication area.	Organization facilitates error-free administration and saves time.
5. Unlock the medication cart or drawer. Enter pass code and scan employee identification, if required.	Locking of the cart or drawer safeguards each patient's medication supply. Hospital accrediting organizations require medication carts to be locked when not in use. Entering pass code and scanning ID allows only authorized users into the system and identifies user for documentation by the computer.
6. **Prepare medications for one patient at a time.**	This prevents errors in medication administration.
7. Read the CMAR/MAR and select the proper medication from the patient's medication drawer or unit stock.	This is the *first* check of the label.
8. Compare the label with the CMAR/MAR. Check expiration dates and perform calculations, if necessary. Scan the bar code on the package, if required.	This is the *second* check of the label. Verify calculations with another nurse to ensure safety, if necessary.
9. Remove the metal or plastic cap on the vial that protects the rubber stopper.	Needs to be removed to access medication in vial.
10. **Swab the rubber top with the antimicrobial swab and allow to dry.**	Antimicrobial swab removes surface bacteria contamination. Allowing the alcohol to dry prevents it from entering the vial on the needle.
11. Remove the cap from the needle or blunt cannula by pulling it straight off. Touch the plunger at the knob only. Draw back an amount of air into the syringe that is equal to the specific dose of medication to be withdrawn. Some facilities require use of a filter needle when withdrawing premixed medication from multidose vials.	Pulling cap off in a straight manner prevents accidental needlestick injury. Handling the plunger at the knob only will keep the shaft of the plunger sterile. Because a vial is a sealed container, before fluid is removed, injection of an equal amount of air is required to prevent the formation of a partial vacuum. If not enough air is injected, the negative pressure makes it difficult to withdraw the medication. Using a filter needle prevents any solid material from being withdrawn through the needle.
12. Hold the vial on a flat surface. Pierce the rubber stopper in the center with the needle tip and inject the measured air into the space above the solution (Figure 1). Do not inject air into the solution.	Air bubbled through the solution could result in withdrawal of an inaccurate amount of medication.
13. **Invert the vial. Keep the tip of the needle or blunt cannula below the fluid level (Figure 2).**	This prevents air from being aspirated into the syringe.
14. Hold the vial in one hand and use the other to withdraw the medication. Touch the plunger at the knob only. **Draw up the prescribed amount of medication while holding the syringe vertically and at eye level (Figure 3).**	Handling the plunger at the knob only will keep the shaft of the plunger sterile. Holding the syringe at eye level facilitates accurate reading, and the vertical position makes removal of air bubbles from the syringe easy.

ACTION

RATIONALE

FIGURE 1. Injecting air with vial upright.

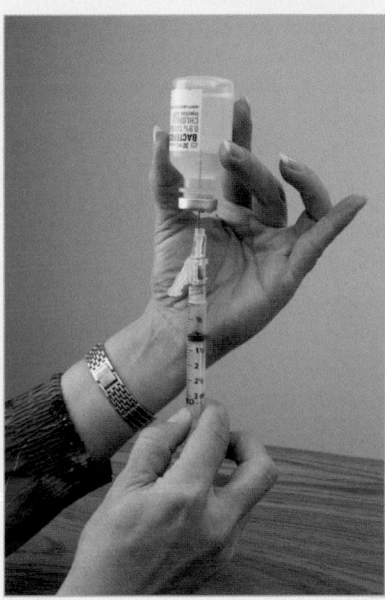

FIGURE 2. Positioning needle tip in solution.

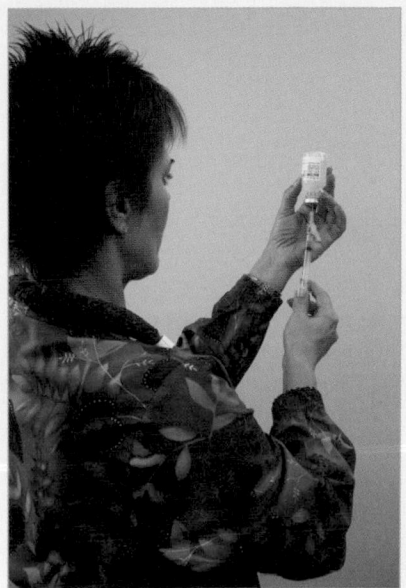

FIGURE 3. Withdrawing medication at eye level.

15. If any air bubbles accumulate in the syringe, tap the barrel of the syringe sharply and move the needle past the fluid into the air space to re-inject the air bubble into the vial. Return the needle tip to the solution and continue withdrawal of the medication.

Removal of air bubbles is necessary to ensure accurate dose of medication.

16. After the correct dose is withdrawn, remove the needle from the vial and carefully replace the cap over the needle. **If a filter needle has been used to draw up the medication, remove it and attach the appropriate administration device.** Some facilities require changing the needle, if one was used to withdraw the medication, before administering the medication.

This prevents contamination of the needle and protects the nurse against accidental needlesticks. A one-handed recap method may be used as long as care is taken not to contaminate the needle during the process. Filter needle used to draw up medication should not be used to administer the medication to prevent any solid material from entering the patient. Changing the needle may be necessary because passing the needle through the stopper on the vial may dull the needle.

17. **Check the amount of medication in the syringe with the medication dose and discard any surplus.**

Careful measurement ensures that correct dose is withdrawn.

18. **Recheck the label with the CMAR/MAR.**

This is the *third* check to ensure accuracy and to prevent errors. Some facilities require the third check to occur at the bedside, after identifying the patient and before administration.

19. **If a multidose vial is being used, label the vial with the date and time opened, and store the vial containing the remaining medication according to facility policy.**

Because the vial is sealed, the medication inside remains sterile and can be used for future injections. Labeling the opened vials with a date and time limits its use after a specific time period.

20. Lock the medication cart before leaving it.

Locking the cart or drawer safeguards the patient's medication supply. Hospital accrediting organizations require medication carts to be locked when not in use.

21. Perform hand hygiene.

Hand hygiene deters the spread of microorganisms.

22. Proceed with administration, based on prescribed route.

See appropriate skill for prescribed route.

(continued)

Skill · 29-3   Removing Medication From a Vial   *continued*

DOCUMENTATION

It is not necessary to record the removal of the medication from the vial. Record each medication administered on the CMAR/MAR or record using the required format immediately after it is administered, including date and time of administration. If using a bar code system, medication administration is automatically recorded when scanned. PRN medications require documentation of the reason for administration. Prompt recording avoids the possibility of accidentally repeating the administration of the drug. If the drug was refused or omitted, record this in the appropriate area on the medication record and notify the primary care provider. This verifies the reason medication was omitted and ensures that the primary care provider is aware of the patient's condition. Recording of administration of a narcotic may require additional documentation on a narcotic record, stating drug count and other specific information. Record fluid intake if intake and output measurement is required.

UNEXPECTED SITUATIONS AND ASSOCIATED INTERVENTIONS

- *A piece of rubber stopper is noticed floating in medication in syringe:* Discard the syringe, needle, and vial. Obtain a new vial, syringe, and needle and prepare dose as ordered.

- *As needle attached to syringe filled with air is inserted into vial, the plunger is immediately pulled down:* If possible to withdraw medication, continue steps as explained above. If such a vacuum has formed that this is impossible, remove syringe and inject more air into the vial. This is caused by previous withdrawal of medication without the addition of air into the vial.

- *Plunger is contaminated before injecting air into vial:* Discard needle and syringe and start over. If plunger is contaminated after medication is drawn into syringe, it is not necessary to discard and start over. The contaminated plunger will enter the barrel of the syringe when pushing the medication out and will not contaminate the medication.

Skill · 29-4   Mixing Medications From Two Vials in One Syringe

EQUIPMENT

- Two vials of medication (insulin in this example)
- Sterile syringe (insulin syringe in this example)
- Antimicrobial swabs
- Computer-generated Medication Administration Record (CMAR) or Medication Administration Record (MAR)

IMPLEMENTATION

ACTION	RATIONALE
1. Gather equipment. Check medication order against the original order in the medical record, according to facility policy.	This comparison helps to identify errors that may have occurred when orders were transcribed. The primary care provider's order is the legal record of medication orders for each facility.
2. Know the actions, special nursing considerations, safe dose ranges, purpose of administration, and adverse effects of the medications to be administered. Consider the appropriateness of the medication for this patient.	This knowledge aids the nurse in evaluating the therapeutic effect of the medication in relation to the patient's disorder and can also be used to educate the patient about the medication.
3. Perform hand hygiene.	Hand hygiene deters the spread of microorganisms.
4. Move the medication cart to the outside of the patient's room or prepare for administration in the medication area.	Organization facilitates error-free administration and saves time.
5. Unlock the medication cart or drawer. Enter pass code and scan employee identification, if required.	Locking of the cart or drawer safeguards each patient's medication supply. Hospital accrediting organizations require medication carts to be locked when not in use. Entering pass code and scanning ID allows only authorized users into the system and identifies user for documentation by the computer.

ACTION	RATIONALE
6. **Prepare medications for one patient at a time.**	This prevents errors in medication administration.
7. Read the CMAR/MAR and select the proper medications from the patient's medication drawer or unit stock.	This is the *first* check of the labels.
8. Compare the labels with the CMAR/MAR. Check expiration dates and perform calculations, if necessary. Scan the bar code on the package, if required.	This is the *second* check of the labels. Verify calculations with another nurse to ensure safety, if necessary.
9. If necessary, remove the cap that protects the rubber stopper on each vial.	The cap protects the rubber top.
10. **If medication is a suspension (e.g., NPH insulin), roll and agitate the vial to mix it well.**	There is controversy regarding how to mix insulins in suspension. Some sources advise rolling the vial and others advise shaking the vial. Consult facility policy. Regardless of the method used, it is essential that the suspension be mixed well to avoid administering an inconsistent dose. Regular insulin, which is clear, does not need to be mixed before withdrawal.
11. Cleanse the rubber tops with antimicrobial swabs.	Antimicrobial swab removes surface contamination. Some sources question whether cleaning with alcohol actually disinfects or instead transfers resident bacteria from the hands to another surface.
12. Remove cap from needle by pulling it straight off. Touch the plunger at the knob only. Draw back an amount of air into the syringe that is equal to the dose of modified insulin to be withdrawn.	Pulling cap off in a straight manner prevents accidental needlestick. Handling the plunger by the knob only ensures sterility of the shaft of the plunger. Before fluid is removed, injection of an equal amount of air is required to prevent the formation of a partial vacuum, because a vial is a sealed container. If not enough air is injected, the negative pressure makes it difficult to withdraw the medication.
13. Hold the modified vial on a flat surface. Pierce the rubber stopper in the center with the needle tip and inject the measured air into the space above the solution (Figure 1). Do not inject air into the solution. Withdraw the needle.	Unmodified insulin should never be contaminated with modified insulin. Placing air in the modified insulin first without allowing the needle to contact the insulin ensures that the second vial entered (unmodified) is not contaminated by the medication in the other vial. Air bubbled through the solution could result in withdrawal of an inaccurate amount of medication.
14. Draw back an amount of air into the syringe that is equal to the dose of unmodified insulin to be withdrawn.	Before fluid is removed, injection of an equal amount of air is required to prevent the formation of a partial vacuum, because a vial is a sealed container. If not enough air is injected, the negative pressure makes it difficult to withdraw the medication.
15. Hold the unmodified vial on a flat surface. Pierce the rubber stopper in the center with the needle tip and inject the measured air into the space above the solution (Figure 2). Do not inject air into the solution. Keep the needle in the vial.	Air bubbled through the solution could result in withdrawal of an inaccurate amount of medication.
16. Invert vial of unmodified insulin. Hold the vial in one hand and use the other to withdraw the medication. Touch the plunger at the knob only. **Draw up the prescribed amount of medication while holding the syringe at eye level and vertically (Figure 3).** Turn the vial over and then remove needle from vial.	Holding the syringe at eye level facilitates accurate reading, and the vertical position makes removal of air bubbles from the syringe easy. First dose is prepared and is not contaminated by insulin that contains modifiers.
17. Check that there are no air bubbles in the syringe.	The presence of air in the syringe would result in an inaccurate dose of medication.
18. **Check the amount of medication in the syringe with the medication dose and discard any surplus.**	Careful measurement ensures that correct dose is withdrawn.
19. **Recheck the vial label with the CMAR/MAR.**	This is the *third* check to ensure accuracy and to prevent errors. Some facilities require the third check to occur at the bedside, after identifying the patient and before administration.
20. Calculate the endpoint on the syringe for the combined insulin amount by adding the number of units for each dose together.	Allows for accurate withdrawal of second dose.

(continued)

Skill · 29-4   Mixing Medications From Two Vials in One Syringe *continued*

ACTION

FIGURE 1. Injecting air into modified insulin preparation.

21. Insert the needle into the modified vial and invert it, taking care not to push the plunger and inject medication from the syringe into the vial. Invert vial of modified insulin. Hold the vial in one hand and use the other to withdraw the medication. Touch the plunger at the knob only. **Draw up the prescribed amount of medication while holding the syringe at eye level and vertically (Figure 4). Take care to only withdraw the prescribed amount.** Turn the vial over and then remove needle from vial. Carefully recap the needle. Carefully replace the cap over the needle.

FIGURE 3. Withdrawing the prescribed amount of unmodified insulin.

RATIONALE

FIGURE 2. Injecting air into the unmodified insulin vial.

Previous addition of air eliminates need to create positive pressure. Holding the syringe at eye level facilitates accurate reading. Capping the needle prevents contamination and protects the nurse against accidental needlesticks. A one-handed recap method may be used as long as care is taken to ensure that the needle remains sterile.

FIGURE 4. Withdrawing modified insulin.

ACTION

22. **Check the amount of medication in the syringe with the medication dose.**

23. **Recheck the vial label with the CMAR/MAR.**

24. **Label the vials with the date and time opened, and store the vials containing the remaining medication according to facility policy.**

25. Lock medication cart before leaving it.

26. Perform hand hygiene.

27. Proceed with administration, based on prescribed route.

RATIONALE

Careful measurement ensures that correct dose is withdrawn.

This is the *third* check to ensure accuracy and to prevent errors. Some facilities require the third check to occur at the bedside, after identifying the patient and before administration.

Because the vial is sealed, the medication inside remains sterile and can be used for future injections. Labeling the opened vials with a date and time limits its use after a specific time period. The Centers for Disease Control and Prevention (CDC) recommends that medications packaged as multiuse vials be assigned to a single patient whenever possible (CDC, 2008a; CDC, 2008b).

Locking the cart or drawer safeguards the patient's medication supply. Hospital accrediting organizations require medication carts to be locked when not in use.

Hand hygiene deters the spread of microorganisms.

See appropriate skill for prescribed route.

DOCUMENTATION

It is not necessary to record the removal of the medication from the vials. Record each medication administered on the CMAR/MAR or record using the required format immediately after it is administered, including date and time of administration. If using a bar code system, medication administration is automatically recorded when scanned. PRN medications require documentation of the reason for administration. Prompt recording avoids the possibility of accidentally repeating the administration of the drug. If the drug was refused or omitted, record this in the appropriate area on the medication record and notify the primary care provider. This verifies the reason medication was omitted and ensures that the primary care provider is aware of the patient's condition. Recording of administration of a narcotic may require additional documentation on a narcotic record, stating drug count and other specific information.

UNEXPECTED SITUATIONS AND ASSOCIATED INTERVENTIONS

- *Nurse contaminates plunger before injecting air into insulin vial:* Discard needle and syringe and start over. If plunger is contaminated after medication is drawn into the syringe, it is not necessary to discard and start over. The contaminated plunger will enter the barrel of the syringe when pushing the medication out and will not contaminate the medication.

- *Nurse allows modified insulin to come in contact with the needle before entering the unmodified insulin vial:* Discard needle and syringe and start over.

- *Nurse notices that the combined amount is not the ordered amount (e.g., nurse has less or more units in combined syringe than ordered):* Discard syringe and start over. There is no way to know for sure which dosage is wrong or which medication should be expelled.

- *Nurse injects medication from first vial (in syringe) into second vial:* Discard vial and syringe and start over.

SPECIAL CONSIDERATIONS

General Considerations

- A patient with diabetes who is visually impaired may find it helpful to use a magnifying apparatus that fits around the syringe.

- Before attempting to explain or demonstrate devices that help low-vision diabetic patients to prepare their medication, attempt to use the device yourself under similar circumstances. To detect any difficulties the patient may experience, practice using the aid with your eyes closed or in a poorly lit room.

Infant and Child Considerations

- School-aged children are generally able to prepare and administer their own injections, such as insulin, with supervision (Kyle, 2008). Parents/significant others and the child should be involved in teaching.

Skill · 29-5   Administering an Intradermal Injection

EQUIPMENT

- Prescribed medication
- Sterile syringe, usually a tuberculin syringe calibrated in tenths and hundredths, and needle, ¼″ to ½″, 26- or 27-gauge

- Antimicrobial swab
- Disposable gloves
- Small gauze square

- Computer-generated Medication Administration Record (CMAR) or Medication Administration Record (MAR)
- PPE, as indicated

IMPLEMENTATION

ACTION	RATIONALE
1. Gather equipment. Check each medication order against the original order in the medical record according to facility policy. Clarify any inconsistencies. Check the patient's chart for allergies.	This comparison helps to identify errors that may have occurred when orders were transcribed. The primary care provider's order is the legal record of medication orders for each facility.
2. Know the actions, special nursing considerations, safe dose ranges, purpose of administration, and adverse effects of the medications to be administered. Consider the appropriateness of the medication for this patient.	This knowledge aids the nurse in evaluating the therapeutic effect of the medication in relation to the patient's disorder and can also be used to educate the patient about the medication.
3. Perform hand hygiene.	Hand hygiene prevents the spread of microorganisms.
4. Move the medication cart to the outside of the patient's room or prepare for administration in the medication area.	Organization facilitates error-free administration and saves time.
5. Unlock the medication cart or drawer. Enter pass code and scan employee identification, if required.	Locking of the cart or drawer safeguards each patient's medication supply. Hospital accrediting organizations require medication carts to be locked when not in use. Entering pass code and scanning ID allows only authorized users into the system and identifies user for documentation by the computer.
6. **Prepare medications for one patient at a time.**	This prevents errors in medication administration.
7. Read the CMAR/MAR and select the proper medication from the patient's medication drawer or unit stock.	This is the *first* check of the label.
8. Compare the label with the CMAR/MAR. Check expiration dates and perform calculations, if necessary. Scan the bar code on the package, if required.	This is the *second* check of the label. Verify calculations with another nurse to ensure safety.
9. If necessary, withdraw medication from an ampule or vial, as described in Skills 29-2 and 29-3.	
10. **When all medications for one patient have been prepared, recheck the label with the CMAR/MAR before taking them to the patient.**	This is a *third* check to ensure accuracy and to prevent errors. Some facilities require the third check to occur at the bedside, after identifying the patient and before administration.
11. Lock the medication cart before leaving it.	Locking the cart or drawer safeguards the patient's medication supply. Hospital accrediting organizations require medication carts to be locked when not in use.
12. Transport medications to the patient's bedside carefully, and keep the medications in sight at all times.	Careful handling and close observation prevent accidental or deliberate disarrangement of medications.
13. **Ensure that the patient receives the medications at the correct time.**	Check agency policy, which may allow for administration within a period of 30 minutes before or 30 minutes after the designated time.
14. Perform hand hygiene and put on PPE, if indicated.	Hand hygiene and PPE prevent the spread of microorganisms. PPE is required based on transmission precautions.
15. Identify the patient. Usually, the patient should be identified using two methods. Compare information with the CMAR or MAR.	Identifying the patient ensures the right patient receives the medications and helps prevent errors.
a. Check the name and identification number on the patient's identification band.	This is the most reliable method. Replace the identification band if it is missing or inaccurate in any way.

ACTION

b. Ask the patient to state his or her name and birth date, based on facility policy.

c. If the patient cannot identify him- or herself, verify the patient's identification with a staff member who knows the patient for the second source.

16. Close the door to the room or pull the bedside curtain.

17. Complete necessary assessments before administering medications. Check allergy bracelet or ask the patient about allergies. Explain the purpose and action of the medication to the patient.

18. Scan the patient's bar code on the identification band, if required.

19. Put on clean gloves.

20. Select an appropriate administration site. Assist the patient to the appropriate position for the site chosen. Drape as needed to expose only area of site to be used.

21. Cleanse the site with an antimicrobial swab while wiping with a firm, circular motion and moving outward from the injection site. Allow the skin to dry.

22. Remove the needle cap with the nondominant hand by pulling it straight off.

23. Use the nondominant hand to spread the skin taut over the injection site (Figure 1).

RATIONALE

This requires a response from the patient, but illness and strange surroundings often cause patients to be confused.

This is another way to double-check identity. Do not use the name on the door or over the bed because these may be inaccurate.

This provides patient privacy.

Assessment is a prerequisite to administration of medications. Explanation provides rationale, increases knowledge, and reduces anxiety.

Provides additional check to ensure that the medication is given to the right patient.

Gloves help prevent exposure to contaminants.

Appropriate site prevents injury and allows for accurate reading of the test site at the appropriate time. Draping provides privacy and warmth.

Pathogens on the skin can be forced into the tissues by the needle. Moving from the center outward prevents contamination of the site. Allowing skin to dry prevents introducing alcohol into the tissue, which can be irritating and uncomfortable.

This technique lessens the risk of an accidental needlestick.

Taut skin provides an easy entrance into intradermal tissue.

FIGURE 1. Spreading the skin taut over the injection site.

24. Hold the syringe in the dominant hand, between the thumb and forefinger with the bevel of the needle up.

Using the dominant hand allows for easy, appropriate handling of syringe. Having the bevel up allows for smooth piercing of the skin and introduction of medication into the dermis.

25. Hold the syringe at a 5- to 15- degree angle from the site. **Place the needle almost flat against the patient's skin (Figure 2), bevel side up, and insert the needle into the skin. Insert the needle only about ¹/₈″ with entire bevel under the skin.**

The dermis is entered when the needle is held as nearly parallel to the skin as possible and is inserted about ¹/₈″.

26. Once the needle is in place, steady the lower end of the syringe. Slide your dominant hand to the end of the plunger.

Prevents injury and inadvertent advancement or withdrawal of needle.

27. Slowly inject the agent while watching for a small wheal or blister to appear (Figure 3).

The appearance of a wheal indicates the medication is in the dermis.

(continued)

Skill · 29-5 Administering an Intradermal Injection *continued*

ACTION

FIGURE 2. Inserting the needle almost level with the skin.

28. Withdraw the needle quickly at the same angle that it was inserted. Do not recap the used needle. Engage the safety shield or needle guard.

29. **Do not massage the area after removing needle. Tell patient not to rub or scratch the site. If necessary, gently blot the site with a dry gauze square. Do not apply pressure or rub the site.**

30. Assist the patient to a position of comfort.

31. Discard the needle and syringe in the appropriate receptacle.

32. Remove gloves and additional PPE, if used. Perform hand hygiene.

33. Document the administration of the medication immediately after administration. See Documentation section below.

34. Evaluate patient's response to medication within appropriate time frame.

35. Observe the area for signs of a reaction at determined intervals after administration. Inform the patient of the need for inspection.

RATIONALE

FIGURE 3. Observing for wheal while injecting medication.

Withdrawing the needle quickly and at the angle at which it entered the skin minimizes tissue damage and discomfort for the patient. Safety shield or needle guard prevents accidental needlestick injury.

Massaging the area where an intradermal injection is given may spread the medication to underlying subcutaneous tissue.

This provides for the well-being of the patient.

Proper disposal of the needle prevents injury.

Removing PPE properly reduces the risk for infection transmission and contamination of other items. Hand hygiene prevents the spread of microorganisms.

Timely documentation helps to ensure patient safety.

The patient needs to be evaluated for therapeutic and adverse effects from the medication.

With many intradermal injections, the nurse will need to look for a localized reaction in the area of the injection at the appropriate interval(s) determined by the type of medication and purpose. Explaining this to the patient increases compliance.

DOCUMENTATION

Record each medication administered on the CMAR/MAR or record using the required format, including date, time, and the site of administration, immediately after administration. Some facilities recommend circling the injection site with ink. Circling the injection site easily identifies the site of the intradermal injection and allows for future careful observation of the exact area. If using a bar code system, medication administration is automatically recorded when scanned. PRN medications require documentation of the reason for administration. Prompt recording avoids the possibility of accidentally repeating the administration of the drug. If the drug was refused or omitted, record this in the appropriate area on the medication record and notify the primary care provider. This verifies the reason medication was omitted and ensures that the primary care provider is aware of the patient's condition.

UNEXPECTED SITUATIONS AND ASSOCIATED INTERVENTIONS

- *Nurse does not note wheal or blister at site of injection:* Medication has been injected subcutaneously. Document according to facility policy and inform the primary care provider. Nurse may need to obtain an order to repeat the procedure.

- *Medication leaks out of injection site before needle is withdrawn:* Needle was inserted less than ⅛″. Document according to facility policy and inform the primary care provider. Nurse may need to obtain an order to repeat the procedure.

- *Nurse sticks self with needle before injection:* Discard needle and syringe appropriately. Follow facility policy regarding needlestick injury. Prepare new syringe with medication and administer to patient. Complete appropriate paperwork and follow facility's policy regarding accidental needlestick injuries.

- *Nurse sticks self with needle after injection:* Discard needle and syringe appropriately. Follow facility policy regarding needlestick injury. Complete appropriate paperwork and follow facility's policy regarding accidental needlesticks.

SPECIAL CONSIDERATIONS

- Ongoing assessment is an important part of nursing care to evaluate patient response to administered medications and early detection of adverse effects. If an adverse effect is suspected, withhold further medication doses and notify the patient's primary healthcare provider. Additional intervention is based on type of reaction and patient assessment.

- Aspiration, pulling back on the plunger after insertion and before administration, is not recommended for an intradermal injection. The dermis does not contain large blood vessels.

- Some agencies recommend administering intradermal injections with the bevel down instead of the bevel up. Check facility policy.

Skill · 29-6   Administering a Subcutaneous Injection

EQUIPMENT

- Prescribed medication
- Sterile syringe and needle. Needle size depends on the medication administered and patient body type (see previous discussion).
- Antimicrobial swab
- Disposable gloves
- Small gauze square
- Computer-generated Medication Administration Record (CMAR) or Medication Administration Record (MAR)
- PPE, as indicated

IMPLEMENTATION

ACTION

1. Gather equipment. Check each medication order against the original order in the medical record, according to facility policy. Clarify any inconsistencies. Check the patient's chart for allergies.

2. Know the actions, special nursing considerations, safe dose ranges, purpose of administration, and adverse effects of the medications to be administered. Consider the appropriateness of the medication for this patient.

3. Perform hand hygiene.

4. Move the medication cart to the outside of the patient's room or prepare for administration in the medication area.

RATIONALE

This comparison helps to identify errors that may have occurred when orders were transcribed. The primary care provider's order is the legal record of medication orders for each facility.

This knowledge aids the nurse in evaluating the therapeutic effect of the medication in relation to the patient's disorder and can also be used to educate the patient about the medication.

Hand hygiene prevents the spread of microorganisms.

Organization facilitates error-free administration and saves time.

(continued)

Skill · 29-6   Administering a Subcutaneous Injection   *continued*

ACTION	RATIONALE
5. Unlock the medication cart or drawer. Enter pass code and scan employee identification, if required.	Locking of the cart or drawer safeguards each patient's medication supply. Hospital accrediting organizations require medication carts to be locked when not in use. Entering pass code and scanning ID allows only authorized users into the system and identifies user for documentation by the computer.
6. **Prepare medications for one patient at a time.**	This prevents errors in medication administration.
7. Read the CMAR/MAR and select the proper medication from the patient's medication drawer or unit stock.	This is the *first* check of the label.
8. Compare the label with the CMAR/MAR. Check expiration dates and perform calculations, if necessary. Scan the bar code on the package, if required.	This is the *second* check of the label. Verify calculations with another nurse to ensure safety, if necessary.
9. If necessary, withdraw medication from an ampule or vial as described in Skills 29-2 and 29-3.	
10. **When all medications for one patient have been prepared, recheck the label with the MAR before taking them to the patient.**	This is a *third* check to ensure accuracy and to prevent errors. Some facilities require the third check to occur at the bedside, after identifying the patient and before administration.
11. Lock the medication cart before leaving it.	Locking the cart or drawer safeguards the patient's medication supply. Hospital accrediting organizations require medication carts to be locked when not in use.
12. Transport medications to the patient's bedside carefully, and keep the medications in sight at all times.	Careful handling and close observation prevent accidental or deliberate disarrangement of medications.
13. **Ensure that the patient receives the medications at the correct time.**	Check agency policy, which may allow for administration within a period of 30 minutes before or 30 minutes after the designated time.
14. Perform hand hygiene and put on PPE, if indicated.	Hand hygiene and PPE prevent the spread of microorganisms. PPE is required based on transmission precautions.
15. Identify the patient. Usually, the patient should be identified using two methods. Compare information with the CMAR or MAR.	Identifying the patient ensures the right patient receives the medications and helps prevent errors.
a. Check the name and identification number on the patient's identification band.	This is the most reliable method. Replace the identification band if it is missing or inaccurate in any way.
b. Ask the patient to state his or her name and birth date, based on facility policy.	This requires a response from the patient, but illness and strange surroundings often cause patients to be confused.
c. If the patient cannot identify him- or herself, verify the patient's identification with a staff member who knows the patient for the second source.	This is another way to double-check identity. Do not use the name on the door or over the bed because these may be inaccurate.
16. Close the door to the room or pull the bedside curtain.	This provides patient privacy.
17. Complete necessary assessments before administering medications. Check the patient's allergy bracelet or ask the patient about allergies. Explain the purpose and action of the medication to the patient.	Assessment is a prerequisite to administration of medications. Explanation provides rationale, increases knowledge, and reduces anxiety.
18. Scan the patient's bar code on the identification band, if required.	Scanning provides additional check to ensure that the medication is given to the right patient.
19. Put on clean gloves.	Gloves help prevent exposure to contaminants.
20. Select an appropriate administration site.	Appropriate site prevents injury and allows for accurate reading of the test site at the appropriate time.
21. Assist the patient to the appropriate position for the site chosen. Drape as needed to expose only area of site to be used.	Appropriate site prevents injury. Draping helps maintain the patient's privacy.
22. Identify the appropriate landmarks for the site chosen.	Good visualization is necessary to establish the correct location of the site and to avoid damage to tissues.

ACTION

RATIONALE

23. Cleanse the area around the injection site with an antimicrobial swab. Use a firm, circular motion while moving outward from the injection site (Figure 1). Allow area to dry.

Pathogens on the skin can be forced into the tissues by the needle. Moving from the center outward prevents contamination of the site. Allowing skin to dry prevents introducing alcohol into the tissue, which can be irritating and uncomfortable.

24. Remove the needle cap with the nondominant hand, pulling it straight off.

The cap protects the needle from contact with microorganisms. This technique lessens the risk of an accidental needlestick.

25. Grasp and bunch the area surrounding the injection site or spread the skin taut at the site (Figure 2).

Decision to create a skin fold is based on the nurse's assessment of the patient and needle length used. Pinching is advised for thinner patients and when a longer needle is used, to lift the adipose tissue away from underlying muscle and tissue. If pinching is used, once the needle is inserted, release the skin to avoid injecting into compressed tissue. If skin is pulled taut, it provides easy, less painful entry into the subcutaneous tissue.

FIGURE 1. Cleaning injection site.

FIGURE 2. Bunching tissue around injection site.

26. **Hold the syringe in the dominant hand between the thumb and forefinger. Inject the needle quickly at a 45- to 90-degree angle (Figure 3).**

Inserting the needle quickly causes less pain to the patient. Subcutaneous tissue is abundant in well-nourished, well-hydrated people and spare in emaciated, dehydrated, or very thin persons. For a person with little subcutaneous tissue, it is best to insert the needle at a 45-degree angle.

27. After the needle is in place, release the tissue. If you have a large skin fold pinched up, ensure that the needle stays in place as the skin is released. Immediately move your nondominant hand to steady the lower end of the syringe. Slide your dominant hand to the end of the plunger. Avoid moving the syringe.

Injecting the solution into compressed tissues results in pressure against nerve fibers and creates discomfort. If there is a large skin fold, the skin may retract away from the needle. The nondominant hand secures the syringe. Moving the syringe could cause damage to the tissues and inadvertent administration into incorrect area.

28. Inject the medication slowly (at a rate of 10 seconds per milliliter).

Rapid injection of the solution creates pressure in the tissues, resulting in discomfort.

29. Withdraw the needle quickly at the same angle at which it was inserted, while supporting the surrounding tissue with your nondominant hand.

Slow withdrawal of the needle pulls the tissues and causes discomfort. Applying counter traction around the injection site helps to prevent pulling on the tissue as the needle is withdrawn. Removing the needle at the same angle at which it was inserted minimizes tissue damage and discomfort for the patient.

30. Using a gauze square, apply gentle pressure to the site after the needle is withdrawn (Figure 4). Do not massage the site.

Massaging the site is not necessary and can damage underlying tissue and increase the absorption of the medication. Massaging after heparin administration can contribute to hematoma formation. Massaging after an insulin injection may contribute to unpredictable absorption of the medication.

(continued)

Skill · 29-6 Administering a Subcutaneous Injection *continued*

ACTION

FIGURE 3. Inserting needle.

RATIONALE

FIGURE 4. Applying pressure to the injection site.

31. Do not recap the used needle. Engage the safety shield or needle guard. Discard the needle and syringe in the appropriate receptacle.

Safety shield or needle guard prevents accidental needlestick. Proper disposal of the needle prevents injury.

32. Assist the patient to a position of comfort.

This provides for the well-being of the patient.

33. Remove gloves and additional PPE, if used. Perform hand hygiene.

Removing PPE properly reduces the risk for infection transmission and contamination of other items. Hand hygiene prevents the spread of microorganisms.

34. Document the administration of the medication immediately after administration. See Documentation section below.

Timely documentation helps to ensure patient safety.

35. Evaluate the response of the patient to the medication within an appropriate time frame for the particular medication.

The patient needs to be evaluated for therapeutic and adverse effects from the medication.

DOCUMENTATION

Record each medication given on the CMAR/MAR or record using the required format, including date, dose, time, and the site of administration, immediately after administration. If using a bar code system, medication administration is automatically recorded when scanned. PRN medications require documentation of the reason for administration. Prompt recording avoids the possibility of accidentally repeating the administration of the drug. If the drug was refused or omitted, record this in the appropriate area on the medication record and notify the primary care provider. This verifies the reason medication was omitted and ensures that the primary care provider is aware of the patient's condition.

UNEXPECTED SITUATIONS AND ASSOCIATED INTERVENTIONS

- *When skin fold is released, needle pulls out of skin:* Engage safety shield or needle guard. Appropriately discard needle. Attach new needle to syringe and administer injection.

- *Patient refuses to let nurse administer medication in a different location:* Explain the rationale behind rotating injection sites. Discuss other available injection sites with patient. If patient will still not allow injection in another area, administer medication to patient, document patient's refusal and discussion, and notify primary care provider.

- *Nurse sticks self with needle before injection:* Discard needle and syringe appropriately. Follow facility policy regarding needlestick injury. Prepare new syringe with medication and administer to patient. Complete appropriate paperwork and follow facility's policy regarding accidental needlestick injuries.

- *Nurse sticks self with needle after injection:* Discard needle and syringe appropriately. Complete appropriate paperwork and follow facility's policy regarding accidental needlestick injuries.

> • *During injection, patient pulls away from needle before medication is delivered fully:* Remove and appropriately discard needle. Attach a new needle to syringe and administer remaining medication at a different site. Document events and interventions according to facility policy.

SPECIAL CONSIDERATIONS

General Considerations

- Ongoing assessment is an important part of nursing care to evaluate patient response to administered medications and early detection of adverse effects. If an adverse effect is suspected, withhold further medication doses and notify the patient's primary healthcare provider. Additional intervention is based on type of reaction and patient assessment.

- Refer to the section on Drug-Specific Equipment and Techniques in this chapter for important guidelines for administering heparin and low-molecular-weight heparin preparations such as enoxaparin (Lovenox) subcutaneously (see Fig. 29-11).

Infant and Child Considerations

- Do not tell a child that an injection will not hurt. Describe the feel of the injection as a pinch or a sting. A child who believes you have been dishonest with him or her is less likely to cooperate with future procedures.

Older Adult Considerations

- Many elderly patients have less adipose tissue. Adjust the angle of the needle and angle of insertion accordingly. You do not want to inadvertently give a subcutaneous medication intramuscularly.

Home Care Considerations

- Reuse of syringes in the home setting is not recommended. Changes and improvements to insulin syringes to make injections painless have resulted in thinner, shorter, sharper, and better lubricated needles. As a result, after one injection, the tip of the fine needles can bend and form a hook that can tear tissue if reused. In addition, these fine needles can break and leave fragments in the skin and tissue if reused. Reuse results in more painful injections related to a reduction in needle lubricant and tip damage (Caffrey, 2003).

- Encourage patients to consult the policies of their local government regarding contaminated and sharps waste disposal. It is important to dispose of needles and syringes in a hard, plastic container. Liquid detergent or liquid fabric softener containers are good choices. Never use glass containers.

Skill • 29-7 Administering an Intramuscular Injection

EQUIPMENT

- Disposable gloves
- Additional PPE, as indicated
- Medication

- Sterile syringe and needle of appropriate size and gauge
- Antimicrobial swab

- Small gauze square
- Computer-generated Medication Administration Record (CMAR) or Medication Administration Record (MAR)

IMPLEMENTATION

ACTION	RATIONALE
1. Gather equipment. Check each medication order against the original order in the medical record according to facility policy. Clarify any inconsistencies. Check the patient's chart for allergies.	This comparison helps to identify errors that may have occurred when orders were transcribed. The primary care provider's order is the legal record of medication orders for each facility.
2. Know the actions, special nursing considerations, safe dose ranges, purpose of administration, and adverse effects of the medications to be administered. Consider the appropriateness of the medication for this patient.	This knowledge aids the nurse in evaluating the therapeutic effect of the medication in relation to the patient's disorder and can also be used to educate the patient about the medication.

(continued)

Skill · 29-7   Administering an Intramuscular Injection *continued*

ACTION	RATIONALE
3. Perform hand hygiene.	Hand hygiene prevents the spread of microorganisms.
4. Move the medication cart to the outside of the patient's room or prepare for administration in the medication area.	Organization facilitates error-free administration and saves time.
5. Unlock the medication cart or drawer. Enter pass code and scan employee identification, if required.	Locking of the cart or drawer safeguards each patient's medication supply. Hospital accrediting organizations require medication carts to be locked when not in use. Entering pass code and scanning ID allows only authorized users into the system and identifies user for documentation by the computer.
6. **Prepare medications for one patient at a time.**	This prevents errors in medication administration.
7. Read the CMAR/MAR and select the proper medication from the patient's medication drawer or unit stock.	This is the *first* check of the label.
8. Compare the label with the CMAR/MAR. Check expiration dates and perform calculations, if necessary. Scan the bar code on the package, if required.	This is the *second* check of the label. Verify calculations with another nurse to ensure safety, if necessary.
9. If necessary, withdraw medication from an ampule or vial, as described in Skills 29-2 and 29-3.	
10. **When all medications for one patient have been prepared, recheck the label with the MAR before taking them to the patient.**	This is a *third* check to ensure accuracy and to prevent errors. Some facilities require the third check to occur at the bedside, after identifying the patient and before administration.
11. Lock the medication cart before leaving it.	Locking the cart or drawer safeguards the patient's medication supply. Hospital accrediting organizations require medication carts to be locked when not in use.
12. Transport medications to the patient's bedside carefully, and keep the medications in sight at all times.	Careful handling and close observation prevent accidental or deliberate disarrangement of medications.
13. **Ensure that the patient receives the medications at the correct time.**	Check agency policy, which may allow for administration within a period of 30 minutes before or 30 minutes after designated time.
14. Perform hand hygiene and put on PPE, if indicated.	Hand hygiene and PPE prevent the spread of microorganisms. PPE is required based on transmission precautions.
15. Identify the patient. Usually, the patient should be identified using two methods. Compare information with the CMAR or MAR.	Identifying the patient ensures the right patient receives the medications and helps prevent errors.
a. Check the name and identification number on the patient's identification band.	This is the most reliable method. Replace the identification band if it is missing or inaccurate in any way.
b. Ask the patient to state his or her name and birth date, based on facility policy.	This requires a response from the patient, but illness and strange surroundings often cause patients to be confused.
c. If the patient cannot identify him- or herself, verify the patient's identification with a staff member who knows the patient for the second source.	This is another way to double-check identity. Do not use the name on the door or over the bed, because these may be inaccurate.
16. Close the door to the room or pull the bedside curtain.	This provides patient privacy.
17. Complete necessary assessments before administering medications. Check the patient's allergy bracelet or ask the patient about allergies. Explain the purpose and action of the medication to the patient.	Assessment is a prerequisite to administration of medications. Explanation provides rationale, increases knowledge, and reduces anxiety.
18. Scan the patient's bar code on the identification band, if required.	Provides additional check to ensure that the medication is given to the right patient.
19. Put on clean gloves.	Gloves help prevent exposure to contaminants.
20. Select an appropriate administration site.	Selecting the appropriate site prevents injury.
21. Assist the patient to the appropriate position for the site chosen. Drape as needed to expose only the area of site being used.	Appropriate positioning for the site chosen prevents injury. Draping helps maintain the patient's privacy.

ACTION

22. **Identify the appropriate landmarks for the site chosen.**

23. Cleanse the area around the injection site with an antimicrobial swab. Use a firm, circular motion while moving outward from the injection site. Allow area to dry.

24. Remove the needle cap by pulling it straight off. Hold the syringe in your dominant hand between the thumb and forefinger.

25. Displace the skin in a Z-track manner by pulling the skin down or to one side about 1″ (2.5 cm) with your nondominant hand and hold the skin and tissue in this position (Figure 1).

RATIONALE

Good visualization is necessary to establish the correct location of the site and to avoid damage to tissues.

Pathogens on the skin can be forced into the tissues by the needle. Moving from the center outward prevents contamination of the site. Allowing skin to dry prevents introducing alcohol into the tissue, which can be irritating and uncomfortable.

This technique lessens the risk of an accidental needlestick and also prevents inadvertently unscrewing the needle from the barrel of the syringe.

This ensures medication does not leak back along the needle track and into the subcutaneous tissue.

FIGURE 1. The Z-track or zigzag technique is recommended for intramuscular injections. (**A**) Normal skin and tissues. (**B**) Moving the skin to one side. (**C**) Needle is inserted at a 90-degree angle, and the nurse aspirates for blood. (**D**) Once the needle is withdrawn, displaced tissue is allowed to return to its normal position, preventing the solution from escaping from the muscle tissue.

26. Quickly dart the needle into the tissue so that the needle is perpendicular to the patient's body (Figure 2). This should ensure that it is given using an angle of injection between 72 and 90 degrees.

27. As soon as the needle is in place, use the thumb and forefinger of your nondominant hand to hold the lower end of the syringe. Slide your dominant hand to the end of the plunger. Inject the solution slowly (10 seconds per milliliter of medication).

28. Once the medication has been instilled, wait 10 seconds before withdrawing the needle.

29. Withdraw the needle smoothly and steadily at the same angle at which it was inserted, supporting tissue around the injection site with your nondominant hand.

30. **Apply gentle pressure at the site with a dry gauze (Figure 3).** Do not massage the site.

A quick injection is less painful. Inserting the needle at a 72- to 90-degree angle facilitates entry into muscle tissue.

Moving the syringe could cause damage to the tissues and inadvertent administration into incorrect area. Rapid injection of the solution creates pressure in the tissues, resulting in discomfort. An outdated practice is the inclusion of aspiration (process of pulling back on the plunger of the syringe before injection to ensure the medication is not injected into a blood vessel) has been part of this procedure in the past. According to the CDC (2009), this procedure is not required.

This allows medication to begin to diffuse into the surrounding muscle tissue (Nicoll & Hesby, 2002).

Slow withdrawal of the needle pulls the tissues and causes discomfort. Applying counter traction around the injection site helps to prevent pulling on the tissue as the needle is withdrawn. Removing the needle at the same angle at which it was inserted minimizes tissue damage and discomfort for the patient.

Light pressure causes less trauma and irritation to the tissues. Massaging can force medication into subcutaneous tissues.

(continued)

Skill · 29-7 **Administering an Intramuscular Injection** *continued*

ACTION

FIGURE 2. Darting the needle into the tissue.

31. Do not recap the used needle. Engage the safety shield or needle guard, if present. Discard the needle and syringe in the appropriate receptacle.

32. Assist the patient to a position of comfort.

33. Remove gloves and additional PPE, if used. Perform hand hygiene.

34. Document the administration of the medication immediately after administration. See Documentation section below.

35. Evaluate patient's response to medication within an appropriate time frame. Assess site, if possible, within 2 to 4 hours after administration.

RATIONALE

FIGURE 3. Applying pressure at the injection site.

Proper disposal of the needle prevents injury.

This provides for the well-being of the patient.

Removing PPE properly reduces the risk for infection transmission and contamination of other items. Hand hygiene prevents the spread of microorganisms.

Timely documentation helps to ensure patient safety.

The patient needs to be evaluated for therapeutic and adverse effects from the medication. Visualization of the site allows for assessment of any untoward effects.

DOCUMENTATION

Record each medication given on the CMAR/MAR or record using the required format, including date, time, and the site of administration, immediately after administration. If using a bar code system, medication administration is automatically recorded when scanned. PRN medications require documentation of the reason for administration. Prompt recording avoids the possibility of accidentally repeating the administration of the drug. If the drug was refused or omitted, record this in the appropriate area on the medication record and notify the primary care provider. This verifies the reason medication was omitted and ensures that the primary care provider is aware of the patient's condition.

UNEXPECTED SITUATIONS AND ASSOCIATED INTERVENTIONS

• *Nurse sticks self with needle before injection:* Discard needle and syringe appropriately. Follow agency policy regarding needlestick injury. Prepare new syringe with medication and administer to patient. Complete appropriate paperwork and follow facility's policy regarding accidental needlesticks.

• *Nurse sticks self with needle after injection:* Discard needle and syringe appropriately. Follow agency policy regarding needlestick injury. Complete appropriate paperwork and follow facility's policy regarding accidental needlesticks.

• *During injection, patient pulls away from needle before medication is delivered fully:* Remove and appropriately discard needle. Attach a new needle to syringe and administer remaining medication at a different site. Document events and interventions according to facility policy.

• *While injecting needle into patient, nurse hits patient's bone:* Withdraw and discard the needle. Apply new needle to syringe and administer in alternate site. Document incident in patient's medical record. Notify primary care provider. Complete appropriate paperwork related to special events according to facility policy.

SPECIAL CONSIDERATIONS

General Considerations

- Ongoing assessment is an important part of nursing care to evaluate patient response to administered medications and early detection of adverse effects. If an adverse effect is suspected, withhold further medication doses and notify the patient's primary healthcare provider. Additional intervention is based on the type of reaction and patient assessment.

Infant and Child Considerations

- The vastus lateralis is the preferred site for infants.

Older Adult Considerations

- Muscle mass atrophies as a person ages. Take care to evaluate the patient's muscle mass and body composition. Use appropriate needle length and gauge for patient's body composition. Choose appropriate site based on the patient's body composition.

Home Care Considerations

- Encourage patients to consult the policies of their local government regarding contaminated and sharps waste disposal. Explain that needles and syringes should be disposed of in a hard, plastic container. Liquid detergent or liquid fabric softener containers are good choices. Glass containers should not be used.

Skill · 29-8   Administering Medications by Intravenous Bolus or Push Through an Intravenous Infusion

EQUIPMENT

- Antimicrobial swab
- Watch with second hand, or stopwatch
- Clean gloves
- Additional PPE, as indicated
- Prescribed medication
- Syringe with a needleless device or 23- to 25-gauge, 1″ needle (follow facility policy)
- Syringe pump if necessary
- Computer-generated Medication Administration Record (CMAR) or Medication Administration Record (MAR)

IMPLEMENTATION

ACTION	RATIONALE
1. Gather equipment. Check medication order against the original order in the medical record, according to facility policy. Clarify any inconsistencies. Check the patient's chart for allergies. Verify the compatibility of the medication and IV fluid. Check a drug resource to clarify whether the medication needs to be diluted before administration. Check the infusion rate.	This comparison helps to identify errors that may have occurred when orders were transcribed. The primary care provider's order is the legal record of medication orders for each facility. Compatibility of medication and solution prevents complications. Delivers the correct dose of medication as prescribed.
2. Know the actions, special nursing considerations, safe dose ranges, purpose of administration, and adverse effects of the medications to be administered. Consider the appropriateness of the medication for this patient.	This knowledge aids the nurse in evaluating the therapeutic effect of the medication in relation to the patient's disorder and can also be used to educate the patient about the medication.
3. Perform hand hygiene.	Hand hygiene prevents the spread of microorganisms.
4. Move the medication cart to the outside of the patient's room or prepare for administration in the medication area.	Organization facilitates error-free administration and saves time.
5. Unlock the medication cart or drawer. Enter pass code and scan employee identification, if required.	Locking of the cart or drawer safeguards each patient's medication supply. Hospital accrediting organizations require medication carts to be locked when not in use. Entering pass code and scanning ID allows only authorized users into the system and identifies user for documentation by the computer.
6. **Prepare medication for one patient at a time.**	This prevents errors in medication administration.
7. Read the CMAR/MAR and select the proper medication from the patient's medication drawer or unit stock.	This is the *first* check of the label.

(continued)

Skill · 29-8 Administering Medications by Intravenous Bolus or Push Through an Intravenous Infusion *continued*

ACTION	RATIONALE
8. Compare the label with the CMAR/MAR. Check expiration dates and perform calculations, if necessary. Scan the bar code on the package, if required.	This is the *second* check of the label. Verify calculations with another nurse to ensure safety, if necessary.
9. If necessary, withdraw medication from an ampule or vial, as described in Skills 29-2 and 29-3.	
10. **Recheck the label with the MAR before taking it to the patient.**	This is a *third* check to ensure accuracy and to prevent errors. Some facilities require the third check to occur at the bedside, after identifying the patient and before administration.
11. Lock the medication cart before leaving it.	Locking the cart or drawer safeguards the patient's medication supply. Hospital accrediting organizations require medication carts to be locked when not in use.
12. Transport medications and equipment to the patient's bedside carefully, and keep the medications in sight at all times.	Careful handling and close observation prevent accidental or deliberate disarrangement of medications. Having equipment available saves time and facilitates performance of the task.
13. **Ensure that the patient receives the medications at the correct time.**	Check agency policy, which may allow for administration within a period of 30 minutes before or 30 minutes after designated time.
14. Perform hand hygiene and put on PPE, if indicated.	Hand hygiene and PPE prevent the spread of microorganisms. PPE is required based on transmission precautions.
15. Identify the patient. Usually, the patient should be identified using two methods. Compare information with the CMAR or MAR.	Identifying the patient ensures the right patient receives the medications and helps prevent errors.
a. Check the name and identification number on the patient's identification band.	This is the most reliable method. Replace the identification band if it is missing or inaccurate in any way.
b. Ask the patient to state his or her name and birth date, based on facility policy.	This requires a response from the patient, but illness and strange surroundings often cause patients to be confused.
c. If the patient cannot identify him- or herself, verify the patient's identification with a staff member who knows the patient for the second source.	This is another way to double-check identity. Do not use the name on the door or over the bed because these may be inaccurate.
16. Close the door to the room or pull the bedside curtain.	This provides patient privacy.
17. Complete necessary assessments before administering medications. Check the patient's allergy bracelet or ask the patient about allergies. Explain the purpose and action of the medication to the patient.	Assessment is a prerequisite to administration of medications. Explanation provides rationale, increases knowledge, and reduces anxiety.
18. Scan the patient's bar code on the identification band, if required.	Provides additional check to ensure that the medication is given to the right patient.
19. **Assess IV site for presence of inflammation or infiltration.**	IV medication must be given directly into a vein for safe administration.
20. If IV infusion is being administered via an infusion pump, pause the pump.	Pausing prevents infusion of fluid during bolus administration and activation of pump occlusion alarms.
21. Put on clean gloves.	Gloves prevent contact with blood and body fluids.
22. Select injection port on tubing that is closest to venipuncture site. Clean port with antimicrobial swab.	Using port closest to needle insertion site minimizes dilution of medication. Cleaning deters entry of microorganisms when port is punctured.
23. Uncap syringe. Steady port with your nondominant hand while inserting syringe into center of port.	This supports the injection port and lessens the risk for accidentally dislodging IV or entering the port incorrectly.
24. Move your nondominant hand to the section of IV tubing just above the injection port. Fold the tubing between your fingers.	This temporarily stops flow of gravity IV infusion and prevents medication from backing up tubing.
25. Pull back slightly on plunger just until blood appears in tubing.	This ensures injection of medication into the bloodstream.

ACTION

26. **Inject the medication at the recommended rate** (see Special Considerations below) (Figure 1).

27. Release the tubing. Remove the syringe. Do not recap the used needle, if used. Engage the safety shield or needle guard, if present. Release the tubing and allow the IV fluid to flow. Discard the needle and syringe in the appropriate receptacle.

28. Check IV fluid infusion rate. Restart infusion pump, if appropriate.

29. Remove gloves and additional PPE, if used. Perform hand hygiene.

30. Document the administration of the medication immediately after administration. See Documentation section below.

31. Evaluate patient's response to medication within appropriate time frame.

RATIONALE

This delivers correct amount of medication at proper interval according to manufacturer's directions.

FIGURE 1. Injecting medication while interrupting IV flow. *(Photo by B. Proud.)*

Proper disposal of the needle prevents injury.

Injection of bolus may alter rate of fluid infusion, if infusing by gravity.

Removing PPE properly reduces the risk for infection transmission and contamination of other items. Hand hygiene prevents the spread of microorganisms.

Timely documentation helps to ensure patient safety.

The patient needs to be evaluated for therapeutic and adverse effects from the medication.

DOCUMENTATION

Document the administration of the medication immediately after administration, including date, time, dose, route of administration, site of administration, and rate of administration on the CMAR/MAR or record using the required format. If using a bar code system, medication administration is automatically recorded when scanned. PRN medications require documentation of the reason for administration. Prompt recording avoids the possibility of accidentally repeating the administration of the drug. If the drug was refused or omitted, record this in the appropriate area on the medication record and notify the primary care provider. This verifies the reason medication was omitted and ensures that the primary care provider is aware of the patient's condition.

UNEXPECTED SITUATIONS AND ASSOCIATED INTERVENTIONS

• *Upon assessing IV site before administering medication, no blood return is aspirated:* If IV appears patent, without signs of infiltration, and IV fluid infuses without difficulty, proceed with administration. Observe closely for signs and symptoms of infiltration during and after administration.

• *Upon assessing patient's IV site before administering medication, nurse notes that IV has infiltrated:* Stop IV fluid and remove IV from extremity. Restart IV in a different location. Continue to monitor new IV site as medication is administered.

• *While administering medication, nurse notes a cloudy, white substance forming in IV tubing:* Stop IV from flowing and stop administering medication. Clamp IV at site nearest to patient. Change administration tubing and restart infusion. Check literature or consult pharmacist regarding compatibility of medication and IV fluid.

(continued)

Skill · 29-8   Administering Medications by Intravenous Bolus or Push Through an Intravenous Infusion *continued*

- *While nurse is administering medication, patient begins to complain of pain at IV site:* Stop medication. Assess IV site for any signs of infiltration or phlebitis. Flush the IV with normal saline to check for patency. If the IV site appears within normal limits, resume medication administration at a slower rate.

SPECIAL CONSIDERATIONS

- Facility policy may recommend the following variations when injecting a bolus IV medication:
  - Release folded tubing after each increment of the drug has been administered at prescribed rate to facilitate delivery of medication.
  - Use a syringe with 1 mL normal saline to flush tubing after an IV bolus is delivered to ensure that residual medication in tubing is not delivered too rapidly.
- Consider how fast IV fluid is flowing to determine whether a flush of normal saline is in order after administering medication. If IV fluid is flowing less than 50 mL per hour, it may take medication up to 30 minutes to reach patient. This depends on what type of tubing is being used in the agency.
- If the IV is a small gauge (22- to 24-gauge) placed in a small vein, a blood return may not occur even if IV is intact. Also, patient may complain of stinging and pain at site while medication is being administered due to irritation of vein. Placing a warm pack over the vein or slowing the rate may relieve discomfort.
- If the medication and IV solution are incompatible, a bolus may be given by flushing the tubing with normal saline before and after the medication bolus. Consult facility policy.
- Ongoing assessment is an important part of nursing care to evaluate patient response to administered medications and early detection of adverse effects. If an adverse effect is suspected, withhold further medication doses and notify the patient's primary healthcare provider. Additional intervention is based on type of reaction and patient assessment.

Skill · 29-9   Administering a Piggyback Intermittent Intravenous Infusion of Medication

EQUIPMENT

- Medication prepared in labeled small-volume bag
- Short secondary infusion tubing (micro-drip or macrodrip)
- IV pump
- Needleless connector, if required, based on facility system
- Antimicrobial swab
- Metal or plastic hook
- IV pole
- Date label for tubing
- Computer-generated Medication Administration Record (CMAR) or Medication Administration Record (MAR)
- PPE, as indicated

IMPLEMENTATION

ACTION	RATIONALE
1. Gather equipment. Check each medication order against the original order in the medical record, according to facility policy. Clarify any inconsistencies. Check the patient's chart for allergies.	This comparison helps to identify errors that may have occurred when orders were transcribed. The primary care provider's order is the legal record of medication orders for each facility.
2. Know the actions, special nursing considerations, safe dose ranges, purpose of administration, and adverse effects of the medications to be administered. Consider the appropriateness of the medication for this patient.	This knowledge aids the nurse in evaluating the therapeutic effect of the medication in relation to the patient's disorder and can also be used to educate the patient about the medication.
3. Perform hand hygiene.	Hand hygiene prevents the spread of microorganisms.
4. Move the medication cart to the outside of the patient's room or prepare for administration in the medication area.	Organization facilitates error-free administration and saves time.

ACTION	RATIONALE
5. Unlock the medication cart or drawer. Enter pass code and scan employee identification, if required.	Locking of the cart or drawer safeguards each patient's medication supply. Hospital accrediting organizations require medication carts to be locked when not in use. Entering pass code and scanning ID allows only authorized users into the system and identifies user for documentation by the computer.
6. **Prepare medications for one patient at a time.**	This prevents errors in medication administration.
7. Read the CMAR/MAR and select the proper medication from the patient's medication drawer or unit stock.	This is the *first* check of the label.
8. Compare the label with the CMAR/MAR. Check expiration dates. Confirm the prescribed or appropriate infusion rate. Calculate the drip rate if using gravity system. Scan the bar code on the package, if required.	This is the *second* check of the label. Verify calculations with another nurse to ensure safety, if necessary. Infusing medication at appropriate rate prevents injury.
9. **When all medications for one patient have been prepared, recheck the label with the MAR before taking them to the patient.**	This is a *third* check to ensure accuracy and to prevent errors. Some facilities require the third check to occur at the bedside, after identifying the patient and before administration.
10. Lock the medication cart before leaving it.	Locking the cart or drawer safeguards the patient's medication supply. Hospital accrediting organizations require medication carts to be locked when not in use.
11. Transport medications to the patient's bedside carefully, and keep the medications in sight at all times.	Careful handling and close observation prevent accidental or deliberate disarrangement of medications.
12. **Ensure that the patient receives the medications at the correct time.**	Check agency policy, which may allow for administration within a period of 30 minutes before or 30 minutes after designated time.
13. Perform hand hygiene and put on PPE, if indicated.	Hand hygiene and PPE prevent the spread of microorganisms. PPE is required based on transmission precautions.
14. Identify the patient. Usually, the patient should be identified using two methods. Compare information with the CMAR or MAR.	Identifying the patient ensures the right patient receives the medications and helps prevent errors.
a. Check the name and identification number on the patient's identification band.	This is the most reliable method. Replace the identification band if it is missing or inaccurate in any way.
b. Ask the patient to state his or her name and birth date, based on facility policy.	This requires a response from the patient, but illness and strange surroundings often cause patients to be confused.
c. If the patient cannot identify him- or herself, verify the patient's identification with a staff member who knows the patient for the second source.	This is another way to double-check identity. Do not use the name on the door or over the bed because these may be inaccurate.
15. Close the door to the room or pull the bedside curtain.	This provides patient privacy.
16. Complete necessary assessments before administering medications. Check the patient's allergy bracelet or ask the patient about allergies. Explain the purpose and action of the medication to the patient.	Assessment is a prerequisite to administration of medications. Explanation provides rationale, increases knowledge, and reduces anxiety.
17. Scan the patient's bar code on the identification band, if required.	Scanning provides an additional check to ensure that the medication is given to the right patient.
18. Assess the IV site for the presence of inflammation or infiltration.	IV medication must be given directly into a vein for safe administration.
19. Close the clamp on the short secondary infusion tubing. Using aseptic technique, remove the cap on the tubing spike and the cap on the port of the medication container, taking care to avoid contaminating either end.	Closing the clamp prevents fluid from entering system until the nurse is ready. Maintaining sterility of tubing and medication port prevents contamination.
20. Attach infusion tubing to the medication container by inserting the tubing spike into the port with a firm push and twisting motion, taking care to avoid contaminating either end.	Maintaining sterility of tubing and medication port prevents contamination.

(continued)

Skill · 29-9   Administering a Piggyback Intermittent Intravenous Infusion of Medication *continued*

ACTION	RATIONALE
21. Hang piggyback container on IV pole, positioning it higher than primary IV according to manufacturer's recommendations (Figure 1). Use metal or plastic hook to lower primary IV fluid container.	Position of containers influences the flow of IV fluid into primary setup.

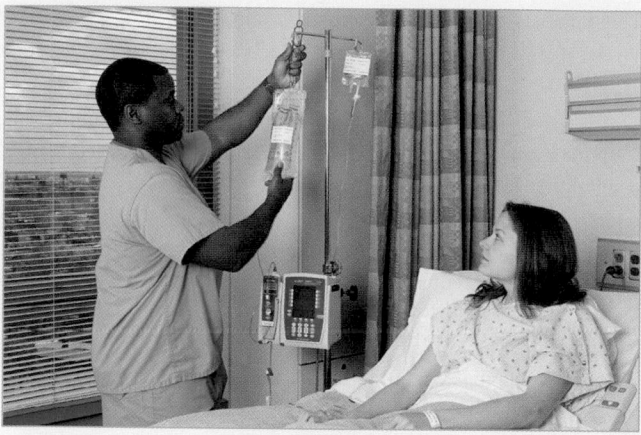

FIGURE 1. Positioning piggyback container on IV pole. *(Photo by B. Proud.)*

ACTION	RATIONALE
22. Place label on tubing with appropriate date.	Tubing for piggyback setup may be used for 48 to 96 hours, depending on agency policy. Label allows for tracking of the next date to change.
23. Squeeze drip chamber on tubing and release. Fill to the line or about half full. Open clamp and prime tubing. Close clamp. Place needleless connector on the end of the tubing, using sterile technique, if required.	This removes air from tubing and preserves sterility of setup.
24. Use an antimicrobial swab to clean the access port or stopcock above the roller clamp on the primary IV infusion tubing (Figure 2).	This deters entry of microorganisms when piggyback setup is connected to port. Backflow valve in primary line secondary port stops flow of primary infusion while piggyback solution is infusing. Once completed, backflow valves open and flow of primary solution resumes.
25. Connect piggyback setup to the access port or stopcock (Figure 3). If using, turn the stopcock to the open position.	Needleless systems and stopcock setup eliminate the need for a needle and are recommended by the Centers for Disease Control and Prevention.

FIGURE 2. Cleaning access port. *(Photo by B. Proud.)*

FIGURE 3. Connecting piggyback setup to access port. *(Photo by B. Proud.)*

ACTION

26. Open clamp on the secondary tubing. Set rate for secondary infusion on infusion pump and begin infusion (Figure 4). If using gravity infusion, use the roller clamp on the primary infusion tubing to regulate flow at prescribed delivery rate (Figure 5). Monitor medication infusion at periodic intervals.

RATIONALE

Backflow valve in primary line secondary port stops flow of primary infusion while piggyback solution is infusing. Once completed, backflow valves opens and flow of primary solution resumes. It is important to verify the safe administration rate for each drug to prevent effects.

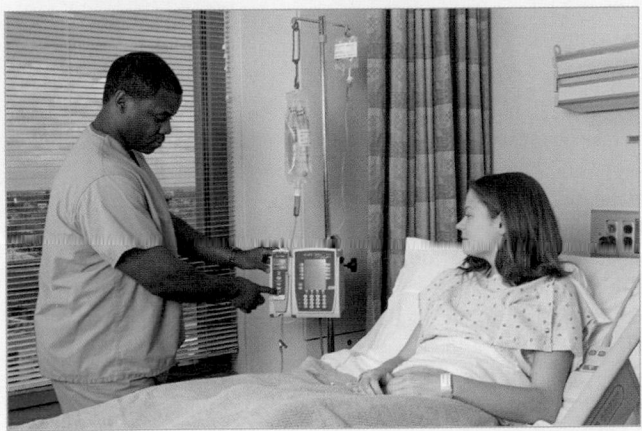

FIGURE 4. Setting rate on infusion pump. *(Photo by B. Proud.)*

FIGURE 5. Using roller clamp on primary infusion tubing to regulate gravity flow. *(Photo by B. Proud.)*

27. Clamp tubing on piggyback set when solution is infused. Follow facility policy regarding disposal of equipment.

28. Replace primary IV fluid container to original height. **Check primary infusion rate on infusion pump. If using gravity infusion, readjust flow rate of primary IV.**

29. Remove PPE, if used. Perform hand hygiene.

30. Document the administration of the medication immediately after administration. See Documentation section below.

31. Evaluate patient's response to medication within appropriate time frame. Monitor IV site at periodic intervals.

Most facilities allow the reuse of tubing for 48 to 96 hours. This reduces risk for contaminating primary IV setup.

Most infusion pumps automatically restart primary infusion at previous rate after secondary infusion is completed. If using gravity infusion, piggyback medication administration may interrupt normal flow rate of primary IV. Rate readjustment may be necessary.

Removing PPE properly reduces the risk for infection transmission and contamination of other items. Hand hygiene prevents the spread of microorganisms.

Timely documentation helps to ensure patient safety.

The patient needs to be evaluated for therapeutic and adverse effects from the medication.

DOCUMENTATION

Document the administration of the medication immediately after administration, including date, time, dose, route of administration, site of administration, and rate of administration on the CMAR/MAR or record using the required format. If using a bar code system, medication administration is automatically recorded when scanned. PRN medications require documentation of the reason for administration. Prompt recording avoids the possibility of accidentally repeating the administration of the drug. If the drug was refused or omitted, record this in the appropriate area on the medication record and notify the primary care provider. This verifies the reason medication was omitted and ensures that the primary care provider is aware of the patient's condition. Document the volume of fluid administered on the intake and output record, if necessary.

UNEXPECTED SITUATIONS AND ASSOCIATED INTERVENTIONS

• *Upon assessing the IV site before administering medication, the nurse notes that the IV has infiltrated:* Stop IV fluid and remove the IV from the extremity. Restart the IV in a different location. Continue to monitor the new IV site as medication is administered.

(continued)

Skill · 29-9   Administering a Piggyback Intermittent Intravenous Infusion of Medication *continued*

- *While administering medication, the nurse notes a cloudy, white substance forming in the IV tubing:* Stop the IV from flowing and stop administering the medication to prevent precipitate from entering the patient's circulation. Clamp the IV at the site nearest to the patient. Replace tubing on primary and secondary infusions. Check the literature regarding incompatibilities of medications before administering. Medication infusion may require second IV site or flushing of tubing before and after administration, using tandem system.

- *While nurse is administering medication, the patient begins to complain of pain at the IV site:* Stop the medication. Assess the IV site for any signs of infiltration or phlebitis. Flush the IV with normal saline to check for patency. If the IV site appears within normal limits, resume medication administration at a slower rate.

SPECIAL CONSIDERATIONS

General Considerations

- An alternate way to prime the secondary tubing, particularly if administration set is in place from previous infusion, is to "backfill" the secondary tubing. Attach the medication bag to the secondary infusion tubing. Lower the medication bag below the main IV solution container and open the clamp on the secondary infusion tubing. This allows the primary IV solution to flow up the secondary tubing to the drip chamber, "backfilling" the tubing. Allow the solution to enter the drip chamber until the drip chamber is half full. Close the clamp on the secondary tubing and hang the medication container on the IV pole. Proceed with administration by lowering the primary IV container, as described above. This "backfill" method keeps the infusion system intact, preventing introduction of microorganisms and prevents loss of medication when the tubing is primed. Check facility policy regarding the use of "backfilling."

- Ongoing assessment is an important part of nursing care to evaluate patient response to administered medications and early detection of adverse effects. If an adverse effect is suspected, withhold further medication doses and notify the patient's primary healthcare provider. Additional intervention is based on type of reaction and patient assessment.

Infant and Child Considerations

- Small infants and children with fluid restrictions may not tolerate the added IV fluid needed for administration with piggyback or volume-control systems. For these children, consider using the mini-infusion pump.

Skill · 29-10   Introducing Drugs Through a Medication or Drug-Infusion Lock (Intermittent Peripheral Venous Access Device) Using the Saline Flush

EQUIPMENT

- Medication
- Saline flushes (2), volume according to facility policy, usually 2 to 3 mL
- Antimicrobial swabs
- Watch with second hand or stopwatch feature
- Gloves
- Computer-generated Medication Administration Record (CMAR) or Medication Administration Record (MAR)

IMPLEMENTATION

ACTION

1. Gather equipment. Check the medication order against the original order in the medical record, according to agency policy. Clarify any inconsistencies. Check the patient's chart for allergies. Check a drug resource to clarify whether medication needs to be diluted before administration. Verify the recommended infusion rate.

RATIONALE

This comparison helps to identify errors that may have occurred when orders were transcribed. The physician's order is the legal record of medication orders for each agency. Compatibility of medication and solution prevents complications. Recommended infusion rate delivers the correct dose of medication as prescribed.

ACTION

2. Know the actions, special nursing considerations, safe dose ranges, purpose of administration, and adverse effects of the medications to be administered. Consider the appropriateness of the medication for this patient.

3. Perform hand hygiene.

4. Move the medication cart to the outside of the patient's room or prepare for administration in the medication area.

5. Unlock the medication cart or drawer. Enter pass code and scan employee identification, if required.

6. **Prepare medication for one patient at a time.**

7. Read the CMAR/MAR and select the proper medication from the patient's medication drawer or unit stock.

8. Compare the label with the CMAR/MAR. Check expiration dates and perform calculations, if necessary. Scan the bar code on the package, if required.

9. If necessary, withdraw medication from an ampule or vial, as described in Skills 29-2 and 29-3.

10. **When all medications for one patient have been prepared, recheck the label with the MAR before taking them to the patient.**

11. Lock the medication cart before leaving it.

12. Transport medications and equipment to the patient's bedside carefully, and keep the medications in sight at all times.

13. **Ensure that the patient receives the medications at the correct time.**

14. Perform hand hygiene and put on PPE, if indicated.

15. Identify the patient. Usually, the patient should be identified using two methods. Compare information with the MAR or CMAR.

   a. Check the name and identification number on the patient's identification band.

   b. Ask the patient to state his or her name and birth date, based on facility policy.

   c. If the patient cannot identify him- or herself, verify the patient's identification with a staff member who knows the patient for the second source.

16. Close the door to the room or pull the bedside curtain.

17. Complete necessary assessments before administering medications. Check the patient's allergy bracelet or ask the patient about allergies. Explain the purpose and action of the medication to the patient.

RATIONALE

This knowledge aids the nurse in evaluating the therapeutic effect of the medication in relation to the patient's disorder and can also be used to educate the patient about the medication.

Hand hygiene prevents the spread of microorganisms.

Organization facilitates error-free administration and saves time.

Locking of the cart or drawer safeguards each patient's medication supply. Hospital accrediting organizations require medication carts to be locked when not in use. Entering pass code and scanning ID allows only authorized users into the system and identifies user for documentation by the computer.

This prevents errors in medication administration.

This is the *first* check of the label.

This is the *second* check of the label. Verify calculations with another nurse to ensure safety, if necessary.

Allows administration of medication.

This is the *third* check to ensure accuracy and to prevent errors. Some facilities require the third check to occur at the bedside, after identifying the patient and before administration.

Locking the cart or drawer safeguards the patient's medication supply. Hospital accrediting organizations require medication carts to be locked when not in use.

Careful handling and close observation prevent accidental or deliberate disarrangement of medications. Having equipment available saves time and facilitates performance of the task.

Check facility policy, which may allow for administration within a period of 30 minutes before or 30 minutes after designated time.

Hand hygiene and PPE prevent the spread of microorganisms. PPE is required based on transmission precautions.

Identifying the patient ensures the right patient receives the medications and helps prevent errors.

This is the most reliable method. Replace the identification band if it is missing or inaccurate in any way.

This requires a response from the patient, but illness and strange surroundings often cause patients to be confused.

This is another way to double-check identity. Do not use the name on the door or over the bed because these may be inaccurate.

This provides patient privacy.

Assessment is a prerequisite to administration of medications. Explanation provides rationale, increases knowledge, and reduces anxiety.

(continued)

Skill · 29-10   Introducing Drugs Through a Medication or Drug-Infusion Lock (Intermittent Peripheral Venous Access Device) Using the Saline Flush *continued*

ACTION	RATIONALE
18. Scan the patient's bar code on the identification band, if required.	Scanning provides additional check to ensure that the medication is given to the right patient.
19. Assess IV site for presence of inflammation or infiltration.	IV medication must be given directly into a vein for safe administration.
20. Put on clean gloves.	Gloves protect the nurse's hands from contact with the patient's blood.
21. Clean the access port of the medication lock with antimicrobial swab (Figure 1).	Cleaning removes surface contaminants at the lock entry site.
22. Stabilize the port with your nondominant hand and insert the syringe, or needleless access device, of normal saline into the access port (Figure 2).	This allows for careful insertion into the center circle of the lock.
23. Release the clamp on the extension tubing of the medication lock. Aspirate gently and check for blood return (Figure 3).	This ensures the catheter of the medication lock is in a vein.

FIGURE 1. Cleaning access port. *(Photo by B. Proud.)*

FIGURE 2. Inserting syringe into access port. *(Photo by B. Proud.)*

FIGURE 3. Aspirating for blood return. *(Photo by B. Proud.)*

24. Gently flush with normal saline by pushing slowly on the syringe plunger. Observe the insertion site while inserting the saline. Remove syringe.	Saline flush ensures that the IV line is patent. Puffiness or swelling as the site is flushed could indicate infiltration of the catheter.

ACTION	RATIONALE
25. Insert syringe, or needleless access device, with medication into the port and gently inject medication, using a watch to verify correct administration rate. **Do not force the injection if resistance is felt.**	Easy installation of medication usually indicates that the lock is still patent and in the vein. If force is used against resistance, a clot may break away and cause a blockage elsewhere in the body.
26. Remove the medication syringe from the port. Stabilize the port with your nondominant hand and insert the syringe, or needleless access device, of normal saline into the port. Gently flush with normal saline by pushing slowly on the syringe plunger (Figure 4). **If medication lock is capped with positive pressure valve/device, remove syringe, and then clamp the IV tubing (Figure 5).** Alternately, to gain positive pressure if positive pressure valve/device is not present, clamp the IV tubing as you are still flushing the last of the saline into the medication lock. Remove syringe.	Positive pressure prevents blood from backing into catheter and causing the medication lock to clot off.

FIGURE 4. Flushing port with normal saline. *(Photo by B. Proud.)*

FIGURE 5. Clamping the access port. *(Photo by B. Proud.)*

27. Discard the syringe in the appropriate receptacle.	Proper disposal prevents injury.
28. Remove PPE, if used. Perform hand hygiene.	Removing PPE properly reduces the risk for infection transmission and contamination of other items. Hand hygiene prevents the spread of microorganisms.
29. Document the administration of the medication immediately after administration. See Documentation section below.	Timely documentation helps to ensure patient safety.
30. Evaluate the patient's response to medication within appropriate time frame.	The patient needs to be evaluated for therapeutic and adverse effects from the medication.
31. Check the medication lock site at least every 8 hours or according to facility policy.	This ensures patency of system.

DOCUMENTATION

Document the administration of the medication and/or saline flush, including date, time, dose, route of administration, site of administration, and rate of administration on the CMAR/MAR or record using the required format, immediately after administration. If using a bar code system, medication administration is automatically recorded when scanned. PRN medications require documentation of the reason for administration. Prompt recording avoids the possibility of accidentally repeating the administration of the drug. If the drug was refused or omitted, record this in the appropriate area on the medication record and notify the primary care provider. This verifies the reason medication was omitted and ensures that the primary care provider is aware of the patient's condition.

(continued)

Skill · 29-10 Introducing Drugs Through a Medication or Drug-Infusion Lock (Intermittent Peripheral Venous Access Device) Using the Saline Flush *continued*

UNEXPECTED SITUATIONS AND ASSOCIATED INTERVENTIONS

- *Upon assessing the medication lock site before administering medication, nurse notes that the medication lock has infiltrated:* Remove medication lock from extremity. Restart peripheral venous access in a different location. Continue to monitor new site as medication is administered.

- *While nurse is administering medication, patient begins to complain of pain at the site:* Stop the medication. Assess the medication lock site for signs of infiltration and phlebitis. Flush the medication lock with normal saline again to recheck patency. If the IV site appears within normal limits, resume medication administration at a slower rate. If pain persists, stop, remove medication lock and restart in a different location.

- *As nurse is attempting to access lock, tip of syringe touches patient's arm:* Discard syringe. Prepare a new dose for administration.

- *No blood return is noted upon aspiration:* If medication lock appears patent, without signs of infiltration, and normal saline fluid infuses without difficulty, proceed with administration. Observe closely for signs and symptoms of infiltration during and after administration.

SPECIAL CONSIDERATIONS

General Considerations

- If medication lock is not used, flush with saline every 8 to 12 hours to maintain patency, according to facility policy.

- Routinely change the medication lock site every 72 to 96 hours, according to facility policy. This reduces the risk of infection and emboli in the bloodstream.

- Intermittent infusions of small-volume IV medications can also be administered through the medication lock. Attach IV medication container to infusion tubing and prime. After flushing the medication lock with saline as outlined above, attach the infusion tubing to the medication lock. Adjust infusion rate with roller clamp on infusion tubing. After infusion is completed, remove tubing from lock and flush with saline as outlined above.

- Ongoing assessment is an important part of nursing care to evaluate patient response to administered medications and early detection of adverse effects. If an adverse effect is suspected, withhold further medication doses and notify the patient's primary healthcare provider. Additional intervention is based on type of reaction and patient assessment.

Infant and Child Considerations

- If the volume of medication being administered is small (<1.0 mL), always include the amount of flush solution as part of the total amount to be injected and take this into account when determining how fast to push a medication. For example, if the medication is to be injected at a rate of 1.0 mL per minute and the total amount of solution to be injected is 2.25 mL (0.25 mL medication volume plus 2.0 mL saline flush solution volume equals 2.25 mL), then the medication would be injected over a period of 2 minutes 15 seconds.

● Developing Critical Thinking Skills

1. You are scheduled to give an intramuscular injection in the ventrogluteal site and remember learning that it should be administered using the Z-track technique. When you mention this to the nurse in the hospital who has been taking care of your patient, she tells you to be sure to remember the air bubble. You remember your instructor telling you not to use an air bubble. What should you do?

2. You are caring for two patients and have just completed giving medications to the first when you realize that you gave her the medications ordered for your other patient. What should you do?

● Practicing for NCLEX

1. Which drug name is the name selected by the pharmaceutical company selling the drug and protected by trademark?
   a. Chemical name
   b. Generic name
   c. Official name
   d. Trade name

2. The process by which a drug is transferred from its site of entry into the body to the bloodstream is known as which of the following?
   a. Absorption
   b. Distribution
   c. Metabolism
   d. Excretion

3. A patient has an abnormal, unexpected response to a drug. This is defined as which of the following?
   a. Drug tolerance
   b. A cumulative effect
   c. An idiosyncratic effect
   d. An anaphylactic reaction

4. A medication order reads: "K-Dur, 20 mEq PO b.i.d." When does the nurse correctly give this drug?
   a. Daily before bedtime
   b. By mouth every other day
   c. Twice a day by the oral route
   d. Once a week after recording an apical rate

5. You are to administer a medication to Mr. Brown. In addition to checking his identification bracelet, you can correctly verify his identity by doing which of the following?
   a. Asking the patient his name
   b. Reading the patient's name on the sign over the bed
   c. Asking the patient's roommate to verify his name
   d. Asking, "Are you Mr. Brown?"

6. You are to administer a medication using a nasogastric tube. Before giving the medication, what should you do?
   a. Crush the enteric-coated pill for mixing in a liquid
   b. Flush open the tube with 60 mL of very warm water
   c. Check for proper placement of the nasogastric tube
   d. Take the patient's vital signs

7. The medication order reads: "Hydromorphone, 2 mg IV every 3 to 4 hours p.r.n. pain." The prefilled cartridge is available with a label reading "Hydromorphone 2 mg/ 1 mL." The cartridge contains 1.2 mL of hydromorphone. Which of the following actions is correct?
   a. Give all the medication in the cartridge because it expanded when it was mixed
   b. Call the pharmacy and request the proper dose
   c. Refuse to give the medication
   d. Dispose of 0.2 mL correctly before administering the drug

8. A patient requires 40 units of NPH insulin and 10 units of regular insulin daily subcutaneously. Which of the following gives the correct sequence when mixing insulins?
   a. Inject air into the regular insulin vial and withdraw 10 units; then, using the same syringe, inject air into the NPH vial and withdraw 40 units of NPH insulin.
   b. Inject air into the NPH insulin vial, being careful not to allow the solution to touch the needle; next, inject air into the regular insulin vial and withdraw 10 units; then, withdraw 40 units of NPH insulin.

c. Inject air into the regular insulin vial, being careful not to allow the solution to touch the needle; next, inject air into the NPH insulin vial and withdraw 40 units; then, withdraw 10 units of regular insulin.
   d. Inject air into the NPH insulin vial and withdraw 40 units; then, using the same syringe, inject air into the regular insulin vial and withdraw 10 units of regular insulin.

9. Ms. Hall has an order for hydromorphone, 2 mg, intravenously, q 4 hours p.r.n. pain. The nurse notes that according to Ms. Hall's chart, she is allergic to Dilaudid. The order for medication was signed by Dr. Long. Which of the following would be the correct procedure in this situation?
   a. Administer the medication; the doctor knows best.
   b. Call Dr. Long and ask that she change the medication.
   c. Ask the supervisor to administer the medication.
   d. Ask the pharmacist to provide a medication to take the place of Dilaudid.

10. The nurse manager on your unit prepared medications for Mr. Giles. She is called to the phone and asks you to give the patient his medications. Which is the best response to this request?
    a. Give Mr. Giles the medication and record it in his chart.
    b. Tell the nurse manager that you do not have time and ask her to get someone else.
    c. Tell the nurse manager that because you did not pour the medication, you cannot administer it.
    d. Give the medication to Mr. Giles but have the nurse manager chart it.

11. Why is the intravenous method of medication administration called the "most dangerous route of administration"?
    a. The vein can take only a small amount of fluid at a time.
    b. The vein may harden and become nonfunctional.
    c. Blood clots may become a serious problem.
    d. The drug is placed directly into the bloodstream, and its action is immediate.

12. Mr. King is receiving heparin subcutaneously. Which of the following demonstrates correct technique for this procedure?
    a. Aspirate before giving and gently massage after the injection.
    b. Do not aspirate; massage the site for 1 minute.
    c. Do not aspirate before or massage after the injection.
    d. Massage the site of the injection; aspiration is not necessary but will do no harm.

13. A patient refuses to take her noon medication, saying that she does not need it. Which of the following would be the best response?
    a. Tell her that she must take the medication because the doctor ordered it.
    b. Tell her that you went through a lot of preparation to get her medications ready, and it's the least she can do.

c. Tell her that you don't care whether she takes the medications or not.

d. Tell her that you will return the medications to the cart but would like to discuss her reasons for refusing to take the medications.

14. A nurse discovers that she has made a medication error. Which of the following should be her first response?

a. Record the error on the medication sheet.

b. Notify the physician regarding course of action.

c. Check the patient's condition to note any possible effect of the error.

d. Complete an incident report, explaining how the mistake was made.

15. The nurse takes an 8 a.m. medication to the patient and properly identifies her. The patient asks the nurse to leave the medication on the bedside table and states that she will take it with breakfast when it comes. What is the best response to this request?

a. Leave the medication and return later to make sure that it was taken.

b. Tell her that it is against the rules, and take the medication with you.

c. Tell her that you cannot leave the medication but will return with it when breakfast arrives.

d. Take the drug from the room and record it as refused.

● Answers With Rationale

1. *d.* The chemical name identifies the drug's chemical composition and molecular structure. The generic name is assigned by the manufacturer who develops the drug. The official name is the name that identifies the drug in the official publication.

2. *a.* Distribution, metabolism, and excretion occur after the drug has been absorbed.

3. *c.* Drug tolerance results when the body becomes accustomed to the drug over time. A cumulative effect occurs when the body cannot metabolize one dose of a drug before another one is given. An anaphylactic reaction is a life-threatening, immediate response to a drug.

4. *c.* The abbreviation "b.i.d." refers to twice-a-day administration.

5. *a.* A sign over the patient's bed may not always be current. The roommate is an unsafe source of information. The patient may not hear his name but may reply in the affirmative anyway (e.g., a person with a hearing deficit).

6. *c.* Tube placement should always be checked before administering any medication to prevent the possibility of aspiration if the tube is not in the stomach. Enteric-coated pills should never be crushed, and very warm water may injure stomach mucosa. Taking vital signs is not necessary unless a particular medication requires it before administration.

7. *d.* Many cartridges are overfilled, and some of the medication needs to be discarded. Always check the volume needed to provide the correct dose with the volume in the syringe. Giving the excess medication in the cartridge may result in adverse effects for the patient. For this dose, it is not necessary to call the pharmacy or refuse to give the medication, provided the order is written correctly.

8. *b.* Regular or short-acting insulin should never be contaminated with NPH or any insulin modified with added protein. Placing air in the NPH vial first without allowing the needle to contact the solution ensures that the regular insulin will not be contaminated.

9. *b.* The nurse is responsible for any medications he or she gives and must contact the doctor to inform her of the patient's allergy to the drug. The nurse should not give the medication and might speak with the supervisor only if he or she is uncomfortable with the physician's answer once she is notified. The nurse is legally unable to order a replacement medication, as is the pharmacist.

10. *c.* Nurses should never give medications prepared by someone else because they are responsible for what they administer.

11. *d.* The intravenous route is a direct access to the bloodstream, and medications act quickly when given intravenously. The condition of the veins is not as important as the rapid effect of the medication administered intravenously.

12. *c.* When giving heparin subcutaneously, do not aspirate or massage, so as not to cause trauma or bleeding in the tissues.

13. *d.* The patient has the right to refuse medications, but the nurse should assess the patient's reasons for refusal, document them, and report them to the physician.

14. *c.* The nurse's first responsibility is the patient, and careful observation is necessary to assess for any effect of the medication error. The other nursing actions are pertinent, but only after checking the patient's welfare.

15. *c.* Safe nursing practice requires that a medication never be left at the patient's bedside. It is not correct to say that the patient has refused medication in this situation.

● Medication Calculation Problems

1. Metoprolol (Lopressor), 25 mg PO, is ordered. Metoprolol is available as 50-mg tablets. How many tablets would the nurse administer?

2. Phenytoin (Dilantin), 100 mg PO, is ordered to be given through a nasogastric tube. Phenytoin is available as 30 mg/5 mL. How much would the nurse administer?

3. Captopril (Capoten), 12.5 mg PO, is ordered. Captopril is available as 25-mg tablets. How many tablets would the nurse administer?

4. Potassium chloride (K-Dur), 20 mEq, is ordered. Potassium chloride is available as 10 mEq per tablet. How many tablets would the nurse administer?

5. Digoxin (Lanoxin), 0.0625 mg PO, is ordered. Digoxin is available as 0.125-mg tablets. How many tablets would the nurse administer?

6. Propantheline bromide (Pro-Banthine), 15 mg, is ordered. Propantheline bromide is available as 7.5-mg tablets. How many tablets would the nurse administer?

7. Ciprofloxacin (Cipro), 500 mg PO, is ordered. Ciprofloxacin is available as 250-mg tablets. How many tablets would the nurse administer?

8. Furosemide (Lasix), 20 mg PO, is ordered. Furosemide is available as 40-mg tablets. How many tablets would the nurse administer?

9. Theophylline elixir, 100 mg PO, is ordered by way of a percutaneous endoscopic gastrostomy tube. Theophylline elixir is available as 80 mg/15 mL. How much would the nurse administer?

10. Clonidine (Catapres), 0.1 mg PO, is ordered. Clonidine is available as 0.2-mg tablets. How many tablets would the nurse administer?

11. Vitamin K, 10 mg given IM, is ordered. Vitamin K is available as 5 mg/mL. How much would the nurse administer?

12. Morphine Sulfate 10 mg IV is ordered. Morphine is available as 4 mg/mL. How much would the nurse administer?

13. Midazolam (Versed), 3 mg IM, is ordered. Midazolam is available as 5 mg/mL. How much would the nurse administer?

14. Ondansetron (Zofran) 0.15 mg/kg is ordered. Ondansetron is available 2 mg/mL. The patient weighs 30 kg. How much would the nurse administer?

15. Epoetin alfa (Epogen), 2,000 units SC, is ordered. Epoetin alfa is available as 4,000 units/mL. How much would the nurse administer?

16. Nalbuphine (Nubain), 1.5 mg IM, is ordered. Nalbuphine is available as 1 mg/mL. How much would the nurse administer?

17. Octreotide acetate (Sandostatin), 50 mcg SC, is ordered. Octreotide is available as 100 mcg/mL. How much would the nurse administer?

18. Lisinopril (Zestril) 40 mg once a day is ordered. Zestril is available as an oral solution 8 mg/mL. How much should the nurse administer via the enteral feeding tube?

19. Prochlorperazine (Compazine), 7.5 mg IM, is ordered. Prochlorperazine is available as 5 mg/mL. How much would the nurse administer?

20. Glycopyrrolate (Robinul), 0.4 mg IM, is ordered. Glycopyrrolate is available as 0.2 mg/mL. How much would the nurse administer?

● Answers to Medication Calculation Problems

1. $\dfrac{\text{dose on hand}}{\text{quantity on hand}} = \dfrac{\text{dose required}}{X \text{ (quantity desired)}}$

$$\frac{50 \text{ mg}}{1 \text{ tablet}} = \frac{25 \text{ mg}}{X}$$

cross-multiply:

$$50X = 25$$

$$X = 0.5 \text{ or } \tfrac{1}{2} \text{ tablet}$$

2. $\dfrac{\text{dose on hand}}{\text{quantity on hand}} = \dfrac{\text{dose desired}}{X \text{ (quantity desired)}}$

$$\frac{30 \text{ mg}}{5 \text{ mL}} = \frac{100 \text{ mg}}{X}$$

cross-multiply:

$$30X = 500$$

$$X = 16.66 \text{ or } 17 \text{ mL}$$

3. $\dfrac{\text{dose on hand}}{\text{quantity on hand}} = \dfrac{\text{dose desired}}{X \text{ (quantity desired)}}$

$$\frac{25 \text{ mg}}{1 \text{ tablet}} = \frac{12.5 \text{ mg}}{X}$$

cross-multiply:

$$25X = 12.5$$

$$X = 0.5 \text{ or } \tfrac{1}{2} \text{ tablet}$$

4. $\dfrac{\text{dose on hand}}{\text{quantity on hand}} = \dfrac{\text{dose desired}}{X \text{ (quantity desired)}}$

$$\frac{10 \text{ mEq}}{1 \text{ tablet}} = \frac{20 \text{ mEq}}{X}$$

cross-multiply:

$$10X = 20$$

$$X = 2 \text{ tablets}$$

5. $\dfrac{\text{dose on hand}}{\text{quantity on hand}} = \dfrac{\text{dose desired}}{X \text{ (quantity desired)}}$

$$\frac{0.125 \text{ mg}}{1 \text{ tablet}} = \frac{0.0625 \text{ mg}}{X}$$

cross-multiply:

$$0.125X = 0.0625$$

$$X = 0.5 \text{ or } \tfrac{1}{2} \text{ tablet}$$

6. $\dfrac{\text{dose desired}}{\text{quantity on hand}} \times \dfrac{\text{quantity}}{\text{on hand}} = X \text{ (desired quantity)}$

$\dfrac{15 \text{ mg}}{7.5 \text{ mg}} \times 1 \text{ tablet} = X$

$2 \times 1 = 2 \text{ tablets}$

7. $\dfrac{\text{dose desired}}{\text{dose on hand}} \times \dfrac{\text{quantity}}{\text{on hand}} = X \text{ (desired quantity)}$

$\dfrac{500 \text{ mg}}{250 \text{ mg}} \times 1 \text{ tablet} = X$

$2 \times 1 = 2 \text{ tablets}$

8. $\dfrac{\text{dose desired}}{\text{dose on hand}} \times \dfrac{\text{quantity}}{\text{on hand}} = X \text{ (desired quantity)}$

$\dfrac{20 \text{ mg}}{40 \text{ mg}} \times 1 \text{ tablet} = X$

$\frac{1}{2} \times 1 = X$

$X = \frac{1}{2} \text{ tablet}$

9. $\dfrac{\text{dose desired}}{\text{dose on hand}} \times \dfrac{\text{quantity}}{\text{on hand}} = X \text{ (desired quantity)}$

$\dfrac{100 \text{ mg}}{80 \text{ mg}} \times 15 \text{ mL} = X$

$\dfrac{1500}{80} = X$

$X = 18.75 = 19 \text{ mL}$

10. $\dfrac{\text{dose desired}}{\text{dose on hand}} \times \dfrac{\text{quantity}}{\text{on hand}} = X \text{ (desired quantity)}$

$\dfrac{0.1 \text{ mg}}{0.2 \text{ mg}} \times 1 \text{ tablet} = X$

$\frac{1}{2} \times 1 = X$

$X = \frac{1}{2} \text{ tablet}$

11. $\dfrac{\text{dose on hand}}{\text{quantity on hand}} = \dfrac{\text{dose desired}}{X \text{ (quantity desired)}}$

$\dfrac{5 \text{ mg}}{1 \text{ mL}} = \dfrac{10 \text{ mg}}{X}$

cross-multiply:

$5X = 10$

$X = 2 \text{ mL}$

12. $\dfrac{\text{dose on hand}}{\text{quantity on hand}} = \dfrac{\text{dose desired}}{\text{quantity desired}}$

$\dfrac{4 \text{ mg}}{1 \text{ mL}} = \dfrac{10 \text{ mg}}{X}$

cross-multiply:

$4X = 10$

$X = 2.5 \text{ mL}$

13. $\dfrac{\text{dose on hand}}{\text{quantity on hand}} = \dfrac{\text{dose desired}}{X \text{ (quantity desired)}}$

$\dfrac{5 \text{ mg}}{1 \text{ mL}} = \dfrac{3 \text{ mg}}{X}$

cross-multiply:

$5X = 3$

$X = 0.6 \text{ mL}$

14. $\dfrac{0.15 \text{ mg}}{1 \text{ kg}} = \dfrac{x}{30 \text{ kg}}$

$1x = 4.5 \text{ mg dose}$

$\dfrac{\text{dose on hand}}{\text{quantity on hand}} = \dfrac{\text{dose desired}}{\text{quantity desired}}$

$\dfrac{2 \text{ mg}}{1 \text{ mL}} = \dfrac{4.5 \text{ mg}}{X}$

cross-multiply:

$2X = 4.5$

$X = 2.25 \text{ mL}$

15. $\dfrac{\text{dose on hand}}{\text{quantity on hand}} = \dfrac{\text{dose desired}}{X \text{ (quantity desired)}}$

$\dfrac{4000 \text{ U}}{1 \text{ mL}} = \dfrac{2000 \text{ U}}{X}$

cross-multiply:

$4000X = 2000$

$X = \frac{1}{2} \text{ mL}$

16. $\dfrac{\text{dose desired}}{\text{dose on hand}} \times \dfrac{\text{quantity}}{\text{on hand}} = X \text{ (desired quantity)}$

$\dfrac{1.5 \text{ mg}}{1 \text{ mg}} \times 1 \text{ mL} = X$

$1.5 \times 1 = X$

$X = 1.5 \text{ mL}$

17. $\dfrac{\text{dose desired}}{\text{dose on hand}} \times \dfrac{\text{quantity}}{\text{on hand}} = X \text{ (desired quantity)}$

$\dfrac{50 \text{ mcg}}{100 \text{ mcg}} \times 1 \text{ mL} = X$

$\frac{1}{2} \times 1 = X$

$X = \frac{1}{2} \text{ mL}$

18. $\dfrac{\text{dose on hand}}{\text{quantity on hand}} = \dfrac{\text{dose desired}}{\text{quantity desired}}$

$\dfrac{8 \text{ mg}}{1 \text{ mL}} = \dfrac{40 \text{ mg}}{X}$

cross-multiply:

$8X = 40$

$X = 5 \text{ mL via enteral feeding tube}$

19. $\dfrac{\text{dose desired}}{\text{dose on hand}} \times \dfrac{\text{quantity}}{\text{on hand}} = X$ (desired quantity)

$$\dfrac{7.5 \text{ mg}}{5 \text{ mg}} \times 1 \text{ mL} = X$$

$$1.5 \times 1 = X$$

$$X = 1.5 \text{ mL}$$

20. $\dfrac{\text{dose desired}}{\text{dose on hand}} \times \dfrac{\text{quantity}}{\text{on hand}} = X$ (desired quantity)

$$\dfrac{0.4 \text{ mg}}{0.2 \text{ mg}} \times 1 \text{ mL} = X$$

$$2 \times 1 = X$$

$$X = 2 \text{ mL}$$

Taylor Suite Resources

The Taylor Suite offers these additional resources to enhance learning and facilitate understanding of this chapter:

- thePoint online resource, http://thepoint.lww.com/Taylor7E
- Student DVD-ROM included with the book
- Study Guide for Taylor's Fundamentals of Nursing
- Skill Checklists for Taylor's Fundamentals of Nursing
- Taylor's Clinical Nursing Skills: Chapter 5, *Medications*
- Taylor's Video Guide to Clinical Nursing Skills: *Oral and Topical Medications, Injectable Medications,* and *Intravenous Medications*

BIBLIOGRAPHY

Abrams, A., Lammon, C., Pennington, S., & Goldsmith, T. (2008). *Clinical drug therapy. Rationales for nursing practice* (9th ed.). Philadelphia: Wolters Kluwer Health/Lippincott Williams & Wilkins.

American Diabetes Association. (2004). Insulin administration: Position statement. *Diabetes Care, 27*(Supplement 1), S106–9.

American Society of Health-System Pharmacists (ASHP). (2009). ASHP statement on bar-code-enabled medication administration technology. *American Journal of Health-System Pharmacy, 66*(6), 588–590.

Annersten, M., & Willman, A. (2005). Performing subcutaneous injections: A literature review. *Worldviews on Evidence-Based Nursing, 2*(3), 122–130.

Aschenbrenner, D., & Venable, S. (2009). *Drug therapy in nursing* (3rd ed.). Philadelphia: Wolters Kluwer Health/Lippincott Williams & Wilkins.

Balas, M., Scott, L., & Rogers, A. (2004). The prevalence and nature of errors observed in 36 health care facilities. *Archives of Internal Medicine, 162*(16), 1897–1903.

Ball, A., & Smith, K. (2008). Optimizing transdermal drug therapy. *American Journal of Health-System Pharmacy, 65*(14), 1337–1346.

Barnsteiner, J. (2005). Medication reconciliation: Transfer of medication information across settings—keeping it free from error. *American Journal of Nursing, 105*(3 Suppl), 31–36.

Ben-Aharon, I., Gafter-Gvili, A., Paul, M., Leibovici, L., & Stemmer, S. M. (2008). Interventions for alleviating cancer-related dyspnea: A systematic review. *Journal of Clinical Oncology, 26*(14), 2396–2404.

Best practices for safe medication administration. (2006). *AORN Journal, 84*(Suppl. 1), S45–56, S58–60.

Bulechek, G., Butcher, H., & McCloskey Dochterman, J. (Eds.). (2008). *Nursing interventions classification (NIC)* (5th ed.). St. Louis: Mosby Elsevier.

Burke, K. (2005). Executive summary: The state of the science on safe medication administration symposium. *American Journal of Nursing, 105*(3 Suppl), 4–9.

Bushardt, R., & Jones, K. (2005). Nine key questions to address polypharmacy in the elderly. *Journal of the Academy of Physician Assistants, 18*(5), 32–40.

Caffrey, R. (2003). Diabetes under control: Are all syringes created equal? *American Journal of Nursing, 103*(6), 46–49.

Capriotti, T. (2004a). Any science behind the hype of "natural" dietary supplements? *MEDSURG Nursing, 13*(5), 339–344.

Capriotti, T. (2004b). Basic concepts to prevent medication calculation errors. *MEDSURG Nursing, 13*(1), 62–65.

Carpenito-Moyet, L. (2008). *Nursing diagnosis: Application to clinical practice* (12th ed.). Philadelphia: Wolters Kluwer Health/Lippincott Williams & Wilkins.

Carroll, P. (2003). Medication errors: The bigger picture. *RN, 66*(1), 52–58.

Carter-Templeton, H., & McCoy, T. (2008). Are we on the same page? A comparison of intramuscular injection explanations in nursing fundamental texts. *MEDSURG Nursing, 17*(4), 237–240.

Centers for Disease Control and Prevention (CDC). (2008a). Injection safety FAQs for providers. Available at www.cdc.gov/ncidod/dhqp/InjectionSafetyFAQs.html.

Centers for Disease Control and Prevention (CDC). (2008b). Injection safety information for providers. Available at www.cdc.gov/ncidod/dhqp/ps_providerInfo.html.

Centers for Disease Control and Prevention (CDC). (2009). *The pink book: Appendices. Epidemiology and prevention of vaccine preventable diseases* (11th ed.). Appendix D. Vaccine administration. Vaccine administration guidelines. Available at www.cdc.gov/vaccines/pubs/pinkbook/pink-appendx.htm#appd.

Cohen, M. (2007). *Medication errors* (2nd ed.). Washington, DC: American Pharmacists Association.

Craig, G. (2009). *Clinical calculations made easy* (4th ed.). Philadelphia: Wolters Kluwer Health/Lippincott Williams & Wilkins.

Cranwell-Bruce, L. (2009). Update in diabetes management. *MEDSURG Nursing, 18*(1), 51–54.

Elsner, F., Radbruch, L, Loick, G, Gärtner, J., Sabatowski, R. (2005). Intravenous versus subcutaneous morphine titration in patients with persisting exacerbation of cancer pain. *Journal of Palliative Medicine, 8*(4), 743–750.

Greenawalt, K. (2009). How are all those medications affecting your older patient? *Nursing, 39*(5), 56hn1–2.

Greenway, K. (2004). Using the vestrolgluteal site for intramuscular injection. *Nursing Standard, 18*(25), 39–42.

Grissinger, M., & Globus, N. J. (2004). How technology affects your risk of medication errors. *Nursing, 34*(1), 36–41.

Heyneman, C. (2003). Preoperative considerations: Which herbal products should be discontinued before surgery? *Critical Care Nurse, 23*(2), 116–123.

Hicks, R., Becker, C., & Jackson, D. (2008). Understanding medication errors: Discussion of a case involving a urinary catheter implicated in a wrong route error. *Urologic Nursing, 28*(6), 454–459.

Horner, S., & Fouladi, R. (2008). Improvement of rural children's asthma self-management by lay educators. *Journal of School Health, 78*(9), 506–513.

Hughes, R., & Ortiz, E. (2005). Medication errors. *American Journal of Nursing, 105*(3 Suppl), 14–24.

Hunter, J. (2008). Subcutaneous injection technique. *Nursing Standard, 22*(21), 41–44.

The Institute for Safe Medication Practices (ISMP). (2009). ISMP and FDA campaign to eliminate use of error-prone abbreviations. Available at www.ismp.org/tools/abbreviations/.

The Joint Commission (TJC). (2010). *National patient safety goals*. Available at http://www.jointcommission.org/PatientSafety/NationalPatientSafetyGoals/.

Kyle, T. (2008). *Essentials of pediatric nursing*. Philadelphia: Wolters Kluwer Health/Lippincott Williams & Wilkins.

Lannefors, L. (2006). Inhalation therapy: Practical considerations for nebulisation therapy. *Physical Therapy Reviews, 11*(1), 21–27.

Love, G. (2006). Administering an intradermal injection. *Nursing, 36*(6), 20.

McBride, D. (2009). Medication mistakes are important to identify in outpatient treatment. *ONS Connect, 24*(3), 21.

McIntyre, L., & Courey, T. (2007). Safe medication administration. *Journal of Nursing Care Quality, 22*(1), 40–42.

McRoberts, S. (2005). The use of bar code technology in medication administration. *Clinical Nurse Specialist, 19*(2), 55–56.

Moorhead, S., Johnson, M., Maas, M., Swanson, E. (Eds.). (2008). Nursing outcomes classification (NOC) (4th ed.). St. Louis: Mosby Elsevier.

Moshang, J. (2005). Making appoint about insulin pens. *Nursing, 35*(2), 46–47.

Mullan, J. (2005). Technology as an aid to the nurse–patient interaction at the bedside. *American Journal of Nursing, 105*(3 Suppl), 39.

Muñoz, C., & Hilgenberg, C. (2005). Ethnopharmacology. *American Journal of Nursing, 105*(8), 40–47.

NANDA International. (2009). *Nursing diagnoses: Definitions and classification 2009–2011*. Oxford, UK: Wiley-Blackwell.

Nicholas, P., & Agius, C. (2005). Toward safer IV medication administration. *American Journal of Nursing, 105*(3 Suppl), 25–30.

Nicoll, L., & Hesby, A. (2002). Intramuscular injection: An integrative research review and guideline for evidence-based practice. *Applied Nursing Research, 16*(2), 149–162.

Pape, T. (2003) Applying airline safety practices to medication administration. *Med Surg Nursing, 12*(2), 77–94.

Porth, C., & Matfin, G. (2009). *Pathophysiology: Concepts of altered health states* (8th ed.). Philadelphia: Wolters Kluwer Health/Lippincott Williams & Wilkins.

Purnell, L. (2009). *Guide to Culturally Competent Health Care*. (2nd ed.). Philadelphia: F. A. Davis.

Rosenkoetter, M., Bowcutt, M., Khasanshina, E., Chernecky, C., & Wall, J. (2008). Perceptions of the impact of "Smart Pumps" on nurses and nursing care provided. *Journal of the Association for Vascular Access, 13*(2), 60–69.

Rubin, B., & Durotoye, L. (2004). How do patients determine that their metered-dose inhaler is empty? *Chest, 126*(4), 1134–1137.

Rushing, J. (2004). How to administer a subcutaneous injection. *Nursing, 34*(6), 32.

Sander, N., Fusco-Walker, S. Harder, J., & Chipps, B. E. (2006). Dose counting and the use of pressurized metered-dose inhalers: running on empty. *Annals of Allergy, Asthma & Immunology, 97*(1), 34–38.

Sanofi Aventis. (2008). How to Self-inject Guide. Available at www.lovenox.com/consumer/prescribed-lovenox/self-inject/inject-lovenox.aspx. Accessed April 7, 2010.

Scarpaci, L., Tsoukleris, M., & McPherson, M. (2007). Assessment of hospice nurses' technique in the use of inhalers and nebulizers. *Journal of Palliative Medicine, 10*(3), 665–676.

Schaeffer, R. (2009). Closing the medication safety loop. *Health Management Technology, 30*(3), 30–32.

Scheiner, G., Sobel, R., Smith, D., Pick, A. Kruger, D., King, J., & Green, K. (2009). Insulin pump therapy: Guidelines for successful outcomes. *The Diabetes Educator, 35*(Supp. 2), 295–435.

Shane, R. (2009). Current status of administration of medications. *American Journal of Health-System Pharmacy, 66*(3 Suppl), S42–S47.

Simmons, D., Graves, K., & Flynn, E. (2009). Threading needles in the dark. The effect of the physical work environment on nursing practice. *Critical Care Nursing Quarterly, 32*(2), 70–74.

Small, S. (2004). Preventing sciatic nerve injury from intramuscular injections: Literature review. *Journal of Advanced Nursing, 47*(3), 287–296.

Smeltzer, S., Bare, B., Hinkle, J., Cheever, K. (2010). *Brunner & Suddarth's textbook of medical-surgical nursing* (12th ed.). Philadelphia: Wolters Kluwer Health/Lippincott Williams & Wilkins.

Stephens, M. (2003). Subcutaneous injections. *Nursing Times, 99*(26), 29.

Swanlund, S., Schcrck, K., Metcalfe, S., & Jesek-Hale, S. (2008). Keys to successful self-management of medications. *Nursing Science Quarterly, 21*(3), 238–246.

Tabloski, P. (2010). *Gerontological nursing: The essential guide to clinical practice* (2nd ed.). Upper Saddle River, NJ: Pearson Prentice Hall.

Thompson, R. (2008). Hold the insulin! Or maybe not. *Nursing, 38*(12), 28–31.

Toedter Williams, N. (2008). Medication administration through enteral feeding tubes. *American Journal of Health-System Pharmacy, 65*(24), 2347–2357.

U.S. Food and Drug Administration (FDA). (2009a). Information of Consumers (Drugs). Available at www.fda.gov/ResourcesForYou/Consumers/default.htm.

U.S. Food and Drug Administration (FDA). (2009b). Medication errors. Available at www.fda.gov/Drugs/DrugSafety/MedicationErrors/default.htm#abbreviations.

U.S. Food and Drug Administration (FDA). (2009c). MedWatch: The FDA safety, information, and adverse event reporting program. Available at www.fda.gov/Safety/MedWatch/default.htm.

U.S. Food and Drug Administration (FDA). (2009d). Dietary Supplements. Available at www.fda.gov/Food/DietarySupplements/default.htm.

Ward, H. (1988). *My friends' beliefs*. New York: Walker and Company.

Wright, K. (2009a). Administering medication to adult patients with dysphagia. *Nursing Standard, 23*(29), 61–68.

Wright, K. (2009b). Supporting the development of calculating skills in nurses. *British Journal of Nursing, 18*(7), 399–402.

Zaybak, A., Gunes, U., Tamsel, S., Khorshid, L., & Eser, I. (2007). Does obesity prevent the needle from reaching muscle in intramuscular injections? *Journal of Advanced Nursing, 58*(6), 552–556.

Perioperative Nursing

MOLLY GREENBAUM

Molly, a 38-year-old woman who is scheduled for a vaginal hysterectomy later in the day, arrives at the hospital at 6:30 a.m. With tears in her eyes and wringing her hands, she states, "I really didn't sleep very much last night. I kept thinking about the surgery."

MARCUS BENJAMIN

Marcus, a 73-year-old man, has just had a total hip replacement under general anesthesia and is transferred to the postanesthesia care unit (PACU). His vital signs are stable. He has an intravenous catheter in his right antecubital space, infusing at 125 mL/hr, and an indwelling urinary catheter in place, draining clear yellow urine. The dressing over the surgical site is clean and dry, without any drainage.

GABRIELLE McALLISTER

Gabrielle McAllister is a 5-year-old girl scheduled for a tonsillectomy and adenoidectomy at a hospital-based same-day surgery unit. She was born with a congenital cardiac defect and has had 6 prior surgeries. She is small for her age and is allergic to latex, but is an otherwise healthy kindergarten student.

After completing the chapter, you will be able to accomplish the following:

1. Describe the surgical experience, including perioperative phases, classifications of surgery, types of anesthesia, informed consent and advance directives, and outpatient/same-day surgery.

2. Conduct a preoperative nursing history and physical assessment to identify patient strengths as well as factors that increase risks for surgical and postoperative complications.

3. Prepare a patient physically and psychologically for surgery.

4. Identify assessments and interventions specific to the prevention of complications in the immediate and early postoperative phases.

5. Use the nursing process to develop an individualized plan of care for the surgical patient during each phase of the perioperative period.

KEY TERMS

anesthesia	moderate sedation/ analgesia
atelectasis	
deep vein thrombosis (DVT)	optional surgery
	perioperative nursing
elective surgery	perioperative period
embolus	pneumonia
emergency surgery	shock
hemorrhage	thrombophlebitis
hypothermia	urgent surgery

The treatment of many illnesses and injuries includes some type of surgical or procedural intervention. Surgery is an intervention in which the knowledge and skill of multiple care providers are combined for the welfare of the patient. Surgery may be done for a variety of reasons: to cure or minimize disease; to diagnose the specific presence of a disease or condition; to reconstruct or eliminate a defect; to enhance form and function; to prescribe appropriate postoperative treatment and prognosis; to palliate, or offer comfort, when cure is not possible; to follow up or monitor an incurable disease process; and to offer a preventative option when disease is inevitable, such as an elective, prophylactic mastectomy for a woman at high risk for breast cancer. Surgery may be planned or unplanned, elective/optional or necessary, major or minor, and may involve any body part or system. Surgery is a stressor that

requires physical and psychosocial adaptations for both the patient and the family. The patient's recovery from a surgical procedure requires skillful and knowledgeable nursing care, whether the surgery is done on an outpatient basis or in the hospital. (See the accompanying Reflective Practice box for an example of nursing care for a patient who has undergone surgery.)

Nursing care provided for the patient before, during, and after surgery is called **perioperative nursing.** The perioperative continuum encompasses the preoperative, intraoperative, and postoperative phases for the patient. This term is used by all members of the interdisciplinary team, including nursing. The nursing process is used to make assessments and provide interventions to promote the recovery of health, prevent further injury or illness, and facilitate coping with alterations in physical structure and function.

A conceptual model for perioperative nursing care is shown in Figure 30-1. In this model, the patient is at the center of all care activities. Surrounding the patient are four domains. Three of these domains, safety, physiologic responses, and the patient and family behavioral responses, are critical for patient care. The fourth domain, health system, represents the structure elements and other system activities that must be present to support safe, effective, high-quality patient care.

With this model, each domain has desired outcomes. These outcomes are identified first in the model because perioperative nursing is preventive in nature. This is in contrast to the usual progression of the nursing process, which begins with assessment. Thus, perioperative nurses base their plans of care on already known and recognized desired outcomes. The patient is assessed for the relevance of the outcome, nursing diagnoses are then identified, and interventions are planned.

The type of surgery scheduled influences the desired outcomes, nursing diagnoses, assessments, and interventions carried out by the nurse. For example, the nurse's role when caring for the patient having same-day surgery may involve providing patient care from admission through discharge. The nurse's role for hospital-based surgery is usually specific to one phase. The perioperative nursing goal is to promote and assist the patient and family to achieve a level of wellness equal to or greater than what they had prior to the procedure (Association of periOperative Registered Nurses [AORN], 2006c).

THE SURGICAL EXPERIENCE

Regardless of the surgical or interventional procedure required or the setting in which it is performed, all patients progress through specific phases, require some type of anesthesia and monitoring support, and must give their consent for surgery.

Phases of the Perioperative Period

The patient who is having surgery progresses through several distinct phases, called the **perioperative period.** The three phases of perioperative patient care are:

- The preoperative phase, beginning when the patient and surgeon mutually decide that surgery is necessary and

REFLECTIVE PRACTICE

Challenge to Intellectual Skills

During a recent clinical experience on a level II ICU, I worked with a Ron Johnson, a middle-aged male patient who had an extensive medical history that included gunshot wounds, bilateral leg amputations, paraplegia, and several surgeries. Because of this, he had lengthy hospital stays and was known by the staff as being a difficult and manipulative patient. During my encounter with him, he was first day postoperation from a urinary diversion surgery. The patient was ordered to be NPO for the first 2 to 3 days following the surgery. However, this patient claimed that his surgeon had told him that he would be able to eat the day after the surgery, and he was demanding that I give him food and fluids. "I want some food and I want it now!" I told the patient that I had to follow the orders in his chart and that it was unlikely that he would be able to have anything by mouth during my shift. He asked me to explain the reasons for being NPO after surgery, and I did my best under the time constraints by telling him that the bowel is affected by anesthesia and it is not ready to handle the intake of food and fluids. In all honesty, I did not know the major consequences of eating or drinking after surgery; however, I did not admit this to him. He was obviously not satisfied with my explanation because when I returned from my lunch break, he was sitting in front of a lunch tray with a large glass of fluids. He had talked some of the nursing assistants into getting him the items. He made the decision to act against my instructions and the instructions of his surgeon because I was not able to give him a clear, articulate explanation of his NPO status.

Thinking Outside the Box: Possible Courses of Action

- Tell the patient that I was unable to give him the best explanation of his NPO status, informing him that I would return in 5 to 10 minutes after consulting with a nurse and deciding the best way to articulate to him the consequences of ignoring the order.
- Avoid giving him any explanation at all, assuming that because of his extensive surgical history he knew the reasons why he must not eat or drink.

- Ask another nurse or even the dietitian to explain the NPO order.
- Alert the surgeon that this patient was at risk for being noncompliant and ask him to come to see the patient as soon as possible.

Evaluating a Good Outcome: How Do I Define Success?

- The patient verbalizes an understanding of my explanation and the consequences of his actions.
- The patient complies with the physician's orders and with my instructions.

- The patient remains free of injuries/complications.
- I feel competent in my explanations and actions.
- I am able to take responsibility for the patient's actions.

Personal Learning: Here's to the Future!

This patient taught me a great deal. He taught me that sometimes, rather than giving an inadequate explanation, it would be better to admit that you do not know or that your knowledge is not up to par in a particular area. I should have been honest with Mr. Johnson, admitting that I was unsure about why he wasn't allowed to eat or drink. It would have been more advantageous to consult with someone else before giving him a more thorough explanation. I also should have recognized that Mr. Johnson was exhibiting extreme frustration and depression, placing him at high risk for noncompliance. All he needed was someone to take the extra time with him, offering compassion and support. Unfortunately, the patient did not comply with the order and thus was at risk for developing serious complications, such as a bowel obstruction. I alerted the surgeon of the patient's actions, and luckily, the surgeon was understanding. In the future, I will make a major effort to gather the appropriate information to give patients a thorough, understandable explanation when they ask for specific information.

Colleen Kilcullen, Georgetown University

Reflection

How would you respond in a similar situation? Why? What does this tell you about yourself and about the adequacy of your skills for professional practice? What cognitive skills did the nursing student use? What cognitive skills were lacking or would have been helpful? How might the patient's past history have influenced the nursing student's actions? Explain. If you were this nursing student, would you have been influenced by his past history? Why or why not? Can you think of other ways to respond? What other skills (cognitive, interpersonal, technical, ethical/legal) would you need to respond well in this situation? Do you agree with the criteria to evaluate a successful outcome? Did this nursing student meet the criteria? Why or why not?

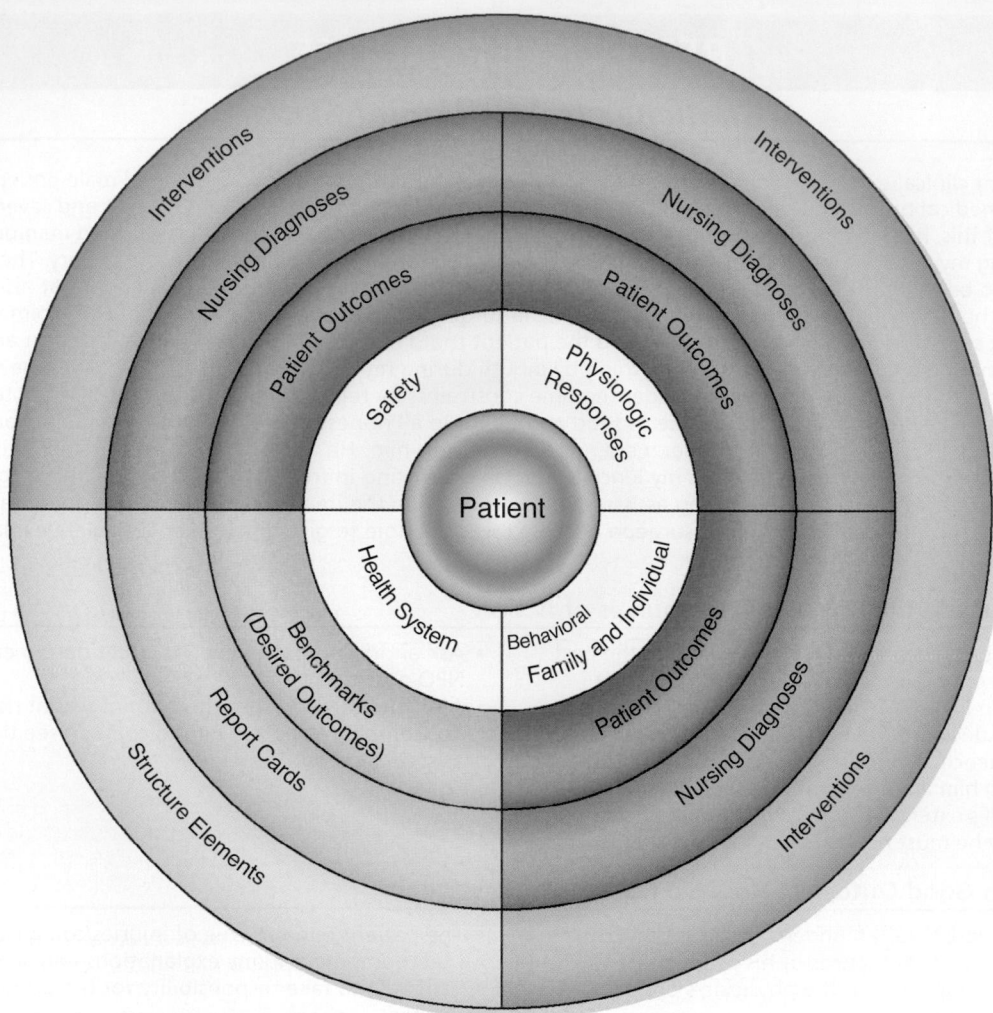

FIGURE 30-1. Association of periOperative Registered Nurses Perioperative Patient-Focused Model (Reproduced with permission, AORN Perioperative Patient-Focused Model. Copyright© AORN, Inc., 2170 S. Parker Road, Suite 300, Denver, CO 80231.)

will take place. It ends when the patient is transferred to the operating room (OR) or procedural bed.

• The intraoperative phase, beginning when the patient is transferred to the OR bed, also called a table, until transfer to the postoperative recovery area.

• The postoperative phase, lasting from admission to the recovery area to complete recovery from surgery and the last follow-up physician visit.

The postoperative phase can be further divided into phase I (providing patient care from a totally anesthetized state to one requiring less acute nursing interventions), phase II (preparing the patient for self or family care or for care in a phase III extended care environment), and phase III (providing ongoing care for patients requiring extended observation or intervention after transfer or discharge from phase I or II) (American Society of PeriAnesthesia Nurses (ASPAN), 2008).

With an increasing trend toward short-stay or same-day surgical treatment, the nursing interventions in each phase of perioperative nursing care may vary somewhat, but they

remain basically the same. The nursing process is used during each phase to meet physical and psychosocial needs and to facilitate the patient's return to health. Each of these phases, with related patient needs and nursing activities, is described in detail in this chapter.

Surgical Procedure Classification

Surgical procedures usually are classified according to urgency, risk, and purpose. Table 30-1 lists each classification, with purposes and examples for each. No matter what the defined degree of risk, any surgical procedure imposes physical and psychological stress and is seldom considered minor by the patient.

➤ *Recall Molly Greenbaum, the 38-year-old woman who is to undergo a vaginal hysterectomy. The nurse would incorporate knowledge about the various classifications of surgery to plan appropriate care before and after surgery.* ■

TABLE • 30-1 CLASSIFICATION OF SURGICAL PROCEDURES		
Classification	**Purpose**	**Examples**
Based on Urgency		
Elective: Delay of surgery has no ill effects; can be scheduled in advance based on patient's choice.	• To remove or repair a body part • To restore function • To improve health • To improve self-concept	Tonsillectomy, hernia repair, cataract extraction and lens implantation, hemorrhoidectomy, hip prosthesis, scar revision, facelift, mammoplasty
Urgent: Usually done within 24–48 hours	• To remove or repair a body part • To preserve or restore health • To prevent further tissue damage	Removal of gallbladder, coronary artery bypass, surgical removal of a malignant tumor, colon resection, amputation
Emergency: Done immediately	• To preserve life (plus purposes listed above)	Control of hemorrhage; repair of trauma, perforated ulcer, intestinal obstruction; tracheostomy
Based on Degree of Risk		
Major: May be elective, urgent, or emergency	• To preserve life • To remove or repair a body part • To restore function • To improve or maintain health	Carotid endarterectomy, cholecystectomy, nephrectomy, colostomy, hysterectomy, radical mastectomy, amputation, trauma repair
Minor: Primarily elective	• To remove skin lesions • To correct deformities	Teeth extraction, removal of warts, skin biopsy, dilation and curettage, laparoscopy, cataract extraction, arthroscopy
Based on Purpose		
Diagnostic	• To make or confirm a diagnosis	Breast biopsy, laparoscopy, bronchoscopy, exploratory laparotomy
Ablative	• To remove a diseased body part	Appendectomy, subtotal thyroidectomy, partial gastrectomy, colon resection, amputation
Palliative	• To relieve or reduce intensity of an illness; is not curative	Colostomy, nerve root resection, débridement of necrotic tissue, balloon angioplasties, arthroscopy
Reconstructive	• To restore function to traumatized or malfunctioning tissue • To improve self-concept	Scar revision, plastic surgery, skin graft, internal fixation of a fracture, breast reconstruction
Transplantation	• To replace organs or structures that are diseased or malfunctioning	Kidney, liver, cornea, heart, joints
Constructive	• To restore function in congenital anomalies	Cleft palate repair, closure of atrial–septal defect

Surgery Based on Urgency

Surgery is also categorized into broad categories that cross specialty areas:

• **elective surgery** is a procedure that is preplanned and based on the patient's choice and availability of scheduling for the patient, surgeon, and facility. This is a nonurgent procedure that does not have to be done immediately.
• **emergency surgery** must be done immediately to preserve life, a body part, or function.
• **urgent surgery** must be done within a reasonably short time frame to preserve health, but is not an emergency.
• **optional surgery** is not critical to survival or function.

Surgery Based on Degree of Risk

Surgery is classified as minor or major based on the degree of risk for the patient. Minor surgery is almost always per-

formed in settings such as a physician's office, an outpatient clinic, or a same-day, outpatient surgery setting. This classification means that the surgical procedure is usually brief, carries a low risk, and results in few complications. In contrast, major surgery may require hospitalization and specialized care, is usually prolonged, has a higher degree of risk, involves major body organs or life-threatening situations, and has a greater risk for postoperative complications. However, the major and minor nomenclature is not as descriptive of the actual procedures today because of the remarkable evolution of surgical science and technology. Advances in the use of laser techniques and minimally invasive approaches involving very small incisions have made major surgery less traumatic, requiring shortened hospital stays. Many surgical procedures, even though they are classified as major, may now be performed on an outpatient (same-day) basis or as a 23-hour hospital stay. Major procedures can be accomplished with minimal anesthesia in short time frames, permitting the patient to return home within the same day, with minimal pain and quick return to normal daily activities. New surgical approaches using minimally invasive techniques continue to evolve, which most likely continue to impact perioperative care.

Surgery Based on Purpose

Some terms used to classify surgical procedures based on purpose include diagnostic, curative, preventative, ablative, palliative, reconstructive, transplantation, and constructive (see Table 30-1).

Anesthesia

Anesthesia is a method and technique of making potentially uncomfortable interventions tolerable and safe. Anesthetic agents can be administered systemically, to the whole body, or regionally to block nerve conduction. General, or systemic, anesthesia is a balance of loss of consciousness, analgesia (pain relief), relaxation, and loss of reflexes (temporary paralysis). In contrast, regional anesthesia does not cause narcosis, or sleepiness, but results in analgesia and reflex loss. Anesthesiologists (medical doctors) or certified registered nurse anesthetists (CRNA) administer anesthetic agents while monitoring the patient's physiologic response and maintaining homeostasis throughout the procedure and recovery. Nurse anesthesia is an advanced nursing specialty. Both physicians and nurses who administer anesthesia perform preoperative physical assessments, conduct preoperative teaching, administer anesthesia during the surgical procedure, and oversee the patient's postoperative recovery from the anesthetic.

General Anesthesia

General anesthesia involves the administration of drugs by the inhalation or intravenous (IV) route to produce central nervous system depression. General anesthesia typically is a combination of both intravenous and inhalation anesthetics. The desired actions of general anesthesia are loss of consciousness, analgesia, relaxed skeletal muscles, and depressed reflexes. Choices of route and type of anesthesia are made primarily by the anesthesia provider after discussion with the patient. Many factors influence these choices, including the type and length of surgery and the physical and psychological status of the patient. Inhalation anesthesia is often used because it has the advantage of rapid induction, excretion, and reversal of effects.

The three phases of general anesthesia are induction, maintenance, and emergence. Induction begins with administration of the anesthetic agent and continues until the patient is ready for the incision. Maintenance continues from this point until near the completion of the procedure. Emergence starts as the patient begins to awaken from the altered state induced by the anesthesia and usually ends when the patient is ready to leave the operating room; the length of time depends on the depth

and length of anesthesia (Rothrock, 2007). New anesthetic agents enable patients to emerge from anesthesia and "wake up" in a fraction of the time required in the past. As these agents become more commonly used, patients will frequently bypass the PACU. This will enable more surgical procedures to be safely done in doctors' offices.

General anesthesia is advantageous because it can be used for patients of any age and for any surgical procedure, with the patient unaware of the physical trauma of the surgery. There are, however, major associated risks for circulatory and respiratory depression, postoperative nausea and vomiting, and alterations in thermoregulation.

> *Remember Marcus Benjamin, the 73-year-old man who had a total hip replacement. The nurse would need to incorporate knowledge about the risks associated with general anesthesia along with knowledge of the physiologic changes associated with aging when developing an appropriate plan of care for this patient. Key to this plan of care would be measures that prevent or minimize Mr. Benjamin's risk for complications.* ∎

Regional Anesthesia

Regional anesthesia occurs when an anesthetic agent is injected near a nerve or nerve pathway in or around the operative site, inhibiting the transmission of sensory stimuli to central nervous system receptors. The patient receiving regional anesthesia remains awake, but loses sensation in a specific area or region of the body. In some instances, reflexes may also be lost. Although regional anesthesia may be selected for numerous types of surgery and patients, it is especially useful in reducing postsurgical pain, bowel dysfunction, and length of hospital stay for older adult patients.

Regional anesthesia may be accomplished through major nerve blocks or through spinal (subarachnoid block), caudal, or epidural blocks.

- *Nerve blocks* are accomplished by injecting a local anesthetic around a nerve trunk supplying the area of surgery such as the jaw, face, and extremities. Onset and duration of the block depend on the anesthetic drug, its concentration, the amount injected, and the addition of epinephrine, which prolongs the block.
- *Spinal anesthesia* is achieved by injecting a local anesthetic into the subarachnoid space through a lumbar puncture, causing sensory, motor, and autonomic blockage. This type of anesthesia is used for surgery of the lower abdomen, perineum, and legs. Adverse effects of spinal anesthesia may include hypotension, headache, and urine retention.
- *Caudal anesthesia* is the injection of the local anesthetic into the epidural space through the caudal canal in the sacrum; it may be used for procedures on the lower extremities or perineum.

- *Epidural anesthesia* involves the injection of the anesthetic through the intervertebral spaces, usually in the lumbar region (although it may also be used in the thoracic or cervical regions). It is used for surgeries of the arms, shoulders, thorax, abdomen, pelvis, and legs.

Topical and Local Anesthesia

Topical anesthesia is used on mucous membranes, open skin surfaces, wounds, and burns. Cocaine in a 4% to 10% solution is the most commonly used agent; others are lidocaine and bupivicaine. Topical anesthetics may be sprayed, spread, or applied with a compress of drug-saturated gauze or cotton-tipped applicators.

Local anesthesia is the injection of an anesthetic agent such as lidocaine, bupivicaine, or tetracaine to a specific area of the body. It is administered by the surgeon in minor, short-term surgical or diagnostic procedures such as tissue biopsy. It bathes the tissue around a targeted nerve or infiltrates the underlying tissue in the operative area. Epinephrine may be mixed with the local anesthetic to minimize bleeding by causing local vasoconstriction. It also helps to prolong the length of analgesia by trapping the anesthetic in the tissue through slowed absorption that results from the vasoconstriction of the surrounding vessels. Local anesthesia may also be injected during general anesthetic procedures to prolong pain relief after the general anesthetic wears off.

Moderate Sedation/Analgesia

Moderate sedation/analgesia, also called conscious or procedural sedation, is used for short-term and minimally invasive procedures. The patient maintains cardiorespiratory function and can respond to verbal commands while the IV administration of sedatives and analgesics raises the pain threshold and produces an altered mood with some degree of amnesia (AORN, 2008c). The patient retains the ability to keep his/her airway open and can respond appropriately. This type of anesthesia is often administered by a perioperative, endoscopy, interventional radiology or interventional cardiology nurse with specialized training and competence in administering the medications and monitoring the patient's cardiac rate and rhythm, respiratory rate, oxygen saturation, level of consciousness, level of pain, blood pressure, and skin condition.

Informed Consent and Advance Directives

Informed consent is the patient's voluntary agreement to undergo a particular procedure or treatment (such as surgery) after having received the following information, which should be provided in understandable words (layman's terms) by the procedural physician:

- Description of the procedure or treatment along with potential alternative therapies

- The underlying disease process and its natural course
- Name and qualifications of the person performing the procedure or treatment
- Explanation of the risks involved, including risk for damage, disfigurement, or death, and how often they occur
- Explanation that the patient has the right to refuse treatment and that consent can be withdrawn
- Explanation of expected outcome, recovery, and rehabilitation plan and course

Informed consent protects the patient, the physician, and the healthcare institution. The signed form is a legal document as well as an ethical imperative. The responsibility for securing informed consent from the patient lies with the person who will perform the procedure. This is usually the physician. The nurse may sign as a witness, signifying that the patient signed the consent form without coercion and was alert and aware of the act. The patient always has the right to refuse treatment.

Consent forms are not legal if the patient is confused, unconscious, sedated, mentally incompetent, or a minor (as determined by state laws). Consent may be given in those instances by a parent, spouse, next of kin, or legal guardian. Most states have a list prioritizing authorized next of kin for signing operative consents. It is important to know who is authorized so that the proper person can be contacted in case a question arises. In emergency situations, the physician may obtain consent over the telephone or by court order. More detailed information about informed consent is included in Chapter 7.

Advance directives, also legal documents, allow the patient to specify instructions for healthcare treatment should he or she be unable to communicate these wishes postoperatively. This allows the patient to discuss his or her wishes with family members in advance of the surgery. Two common forms of advance directive include living wills and durable power of attorney for healthcare. If the patient should experience a serious, life-threatening complication, such as intraoperative cardiac arrest, the family has previous knowledge of the patient's wishes regarding cessation of treatment, resuscitative efforts, or end-of-life decisions. It is important to discuss and document the exact wishes of the patient and family members before surgery, especially related to resuscitation (do-not-resuscitate [DNR]).

Outpatient/Same-day Surgery

Surgical procedures performed in outpatient or same-day (also referred to as ambulatory) surgical settings have become common, as the healthcare system has reduced the length of hospital stays to lower healthcare costs. These surgical settings may be found as freestanding units, in hospitals, and in physicians' offices. Some freestanding surgery centers specialize in selected types of surgery, such as orthopedics or hernia repair. Others perform a wide variety of surgical interventions, including major surgical procedures that formerly required as much as a 3-week stay in a hospital.

Typically, patients are admitted to the healthcare setting the morning of surgery. Allowing the patient to spend the night before surgery at home and to return to his or her own home to recover, reduces much of the stress associated with surgery. Patients who are older or chronically ill or who do not have support systems or access to resources to provide the care needed after surgery may require additional teaching and referral for home care services.

THE NURSING PROCESS FOR PREOPERATIVE CARE

Patients who require surgical intervention and nursing care enter the healthcare setting in a wide variety of situations, ranging from essentially healthy people who have planned elective procedures to emergency admissions for treatment of trauma or serious illness (such as a cardiac arrest or stroke). Surgical patients may be of any age and at any point on the health–illness continuum. It is the nurse's responsibility to identify factors that affect the risk of a surgical procedure. This includes assessing the physical and psychosocial needs of the patient and family and establishing a plan of care based on appropriate nursing diagnoses. Interventions are designed to meet the patient's needs and facilitate recovery as the patient progresses through the perioperative period.

➤ *Consider Gabrielle McAllister, the 5-year-old girl scheduled for tonsillectomy and adenoidectomy (T & A). As a child with a history of cardiac defects, prior surgeries, and latex allergy, she is at risk for anesthesia complications related to her birth defects and allergic reaction if she is exposed to latex. The nurse would need to obtain a thorough history of the patient's previous surgeries, what happens when she is exposed to latex, and how she responded after the surgeries to identify the patient's risk for problems with the current surgical procedure and anesthesia.* ■

Some of the desired outcomes that frame the plan of care for the surgical patient, outlined by the AORN (2008d), state that the patient will meet the following goals:

- Be free from injury and adverse effects related to positioning, retained foreign objects, or chemical, physical, or electrical hazards
- Be free from infection
- Maintain fluid and electrolyte balance and skin integrity
- Maintain normal body temperature
- Be free from **deep vein thrombosis** (DVT, formation of a blood clot ["thrombus"] in a deep vein)
- Have their pain managed
- Demonstrate an understanding of the physiologic and psychological responses to the planned surgery
- Participate in a rehabilitation process following surgery

Assessing

The importance of preoperative assessment cannot be overemphasized. Surgery is a major trauma to the body, and preoperative assessments identify factors that may place the patient at greater risk for complications during and after surgery (see Examples of Nursing Interventions and Nursing Outcomes Classifications (NIC/NOC): Risk Identification).

Assessment of the surgical patient includes:

- Obtaining a health history and performing a physical assessment to establish a baseline data base
- Identifying risk factors and allergies that could pose surgical complications
- Identifying medications and treatments the patient is currently receiving
- Determining the teaching and psychosocial needs of the patient and family
- Determining postsurgical support and referral needs for recovery

---

Examples of Nursing Interventions and Nursing Outcomes Classifications (NIC/NOC)

Risk Identification

Nursing Interventions	Nursing Outcomes
• Review past medical history and documents for evidence of existing or previous medical and nursing diagnoses. • Identify patient(s) with continuing care needs. • Determine presence and quality of family support. • Determine presence/absence of basic living needs. • Set mutual goal setting, as appropriate.	• Risk Detection • Risk Control

Data from Bulechek, G., Butcher, H., & Dochterman, J. M. (Eds). (2008). *Nursing interventions classification (NIC)* (5th ed.). St. Louis: Mosby Elsevier, and Moorhead, S., Johnson, M., Maas, M., & Swanson, E. (Eds). (2008). *Nursing outcomes classification (NOC)* (4th ed.). St. Louis: Mosby Elsevier.

Box 30-1 PREOPERATIVE INFORMATION FOR OUTPATIENT/SAME-DAY SURGERY

Provide verbal and written instructions for patients having outpatient/same-day surgery as follows:

- List medications routinely taken, and ask the physician which should be taken or omitted the morning of surgery.
- Notify the surgeon's office if a cold or infection develops before surgery.
- List allergies, and be sure the operating staff is aware of these.
- Remove nail polish and do not wear makeup for the procedure.
- Leave all jewelry and valuables at home.
- Wear clothing that buttons in front; short-sleeved garments are better for surgery on the hands.
- Have someone available for transportation home after recovery from anesthesia.

Inform patient of:

- Limitations on eating or drinking before surgery, with a specific time to begin the limitations.
- When and where to arrive for the procedure, as well as the estimated time when the procedure will be performed.

The assessment is often conducted several days before surgery as part of preoperative laboratory screening and teaching; this is referred to as preadmission testing. It may be conducted in the hospital, a surgical clinic, an office, or even in the patient's home.

Preoperative nursing assessments and teaching are key care activities for patients who will be having outpatient or same-day surgery. Preoperative teaching can often be combined with preoperative screening tests, which are usually done up to 30 days before the scheduled surgery. Perioperative assessment and teaching for outpatient/same-day surgery includes instructions to the patient and family (Box 30-1).

Health History

The health history identifies risk factors and strengths in the patient's physical and psychosocial status and helps the nurse to individualize the preoperative assessment. Health history information significant to the surgical experience includes the patient's developmental level; medical history; medications; previous surgeries; perceptions and knowledge of the surgery to be done; nutrition; use of alcohol, illicit drugs, or nicotine; activities of daily living and occupation; coping patterns and support systems; and sociocultural needs.

DEVELOPMENTAL CONSIDERATIONS

Infants and older adults are at a greater risk from surgery than are children and young or middle-aged adults. The infant has a lower total blood volume, making even a small loss of blood a serious concern because of the risk for dehy-

dration and the inability to respond to the need for increased oxygen during surgery. In addition, the airway is small, soft, and pliable and infants and small children frequently have upper respiratory infections, such as colds, that can cause airway obstruction and hypoxia. This patient population can quickly develop bronchospasm, stridor, and respiratory arrest. If a child exhibits signs of even mild respiratory infections on the day of surgery, their procedure will be postponed until it resolves.

The infant also has difficulty maintaining stable body temperature during surgery because the shivering reflex is not well developed, making hypothermia or hyperthermia more likely. Their lower glomerular filtration rate and creatinine clearance can lead to a slower metabolism of drugs that require renal biotransformation. Because the liver is immature until after the first year of life, the effects of muscle relaxants and narcotics may be prolonged.

Physiologic changes associated with aging (described in Chapter 20) increase the surgical risk for older patients. These changes, summarized in the Focus on the Older Adult display, decrease older adults' ability to respond to the stress of surgery, alter the effects of preoperative and postoperative medications and anesthesia, and prolong or alter wound healing processes. With an increasing older adult population, assessing physiologic changes is crucial to providing knowledgeable, safe, holistic nursing care to older surgical patients. Chronic illnesses, more common in the older population, also increase surgical risk and may require alterations in usual perioperative procedures. For example, a patient with congestive failure may be more easily fatigued and thus unable to be up and about as rapidly after surgery.

> *Consider Marcus Benjamin, the 73-year-old man who had a total hip replacement. Due to his age, the nurse would need to be alert to potential complications specifically associated with age-related changes, reduced mobility, and use of general anesthesia, IV therapy, and urinary catheterization.* ∎

MEDICAL HISTORY

The medical history provides information about past and current illnesses. Pathologic changes associated with past and current illnesses increase surgical risk as well as the risk for postoperative complications. Preoperative assessments and documentation are necessary to provide a database for individualized assessments and interventions in the intraoperative and postoperative phases of care. Examples of diseases and associated risks may include:

- Cardiovascular diseases, such as thrombocytopenia, hemophilia, recent myocardial infarction or cardiac surgery, heart failure, and dysrhythmias, increase the risk for hemorrhage and hypovolemic shock, hypotension, venous stasis, thrombophlebitis, and overhydration with IV fluids.

FOCUS ON THE OLDER ADULT

NURSING INTERVENTIONS TO ADDRESS AGE-RELATED INCREASED SURGICAL RISK

Age Related Changes	Nursing Interventions
Cardiovascular Decreased cardiac output, stroke volume and cardiac reserve Decreased peripheral circulation Increased vascular rigidity	• Obtain and record baseline vital signs. • Assess peripheral pulses. • Teach leg exercises, turning, and ambulating. • Document normal activity levels and tolerance of fatigue. • Monitor fluid administration rate. • Allow sufficient time for effects of medications to occur.
Respiratory Reduced vital capacity Diminished cough reflex Decreased oxygenation of blood Decreased chest expansion and strength of intercostal muscles and diaphragm	• Obtain and record baseline respiratory depth and rate. • Teach coughing and deep-breathing exercises. • Teach use of incentive spirometer. • Assess color of skin. • Explain use of pulse oximeter for monitoring postoperative oxygenation.
Central Nervous System Decreased reaction time and coordination Reduced short-term memory Sensory deficits Decreased thermoregulation ability	• Orient to surroundings. • Institute safety measures, such as keeping environment clear of clutter and using a night light. • Allow additional time for teaching. • Use appropriate measures to conserve body heat.
Renal Decreased renal blood flow Reduced bladder capacity	• Monitor amount and times of voiding. • Monitor fluid and electrolyte status. • Maintain and record intake and output.
Gastrointestinal Increased gastric pH Prolonged gastric-emptying time Decreased hepatic blood flow, liver mass, and enzyme function	• Obtain baseline weight. • Monitor nutritional status (weight, laboratory data). • Observe for prolonged effects of medications.
Integumentary Decreased vascularity Decreased skin moisture and elasticity Decreased subcutaneous fat	• Assess skin status. • Monitor fluid status. • Pad and protect bony prominences. • Monitor skin for pressure areas. • Use minimal amounts of tape on dressings and intravenous sites.

• Respiratory disorders, such as pneumonia, bronchitis, asthma, emphysema, and chronic obstructive pulmonary diseases, increase the risk for respiratory depression from anesthesia as well as postoperative pneumonia, atelectasis, and alterations in acid–base balance.
• Kidney and liver diseases influence the patient's response to anesthesia, affect fluid and electrolyte as well as acid–base balance, alter the metabolism and excretion of drugs, and impair wound healing.
• Endocrine diseases, especially diabetes mellitus, increase the risk for hypoglycemia or acidosis, slow wound healing and present an increased risk for postoperative cardiovascular complications.

MEDICATIONS

The use of prescribed, over-the-counter, or herbal drugs can affect the patient's reaction to and increase the risk from the stress of surgery and the effects of the anesthetic agent. Some herbal products can increase bleeding while others may potentiate the actions of depressant anesthetic drugs. Surgical risk is increased by drugs in the following categories:

• Anticoagulants (may precipitate hemorrhage)
• Diuretics (may cause electrolyte imbalances, with resulting respiratory depression from anesthesia)
• Tranquilizers (may increase the hypotensive effect of anesthetic agents)

- Adrenal steroids (abrupt withdrawal may cause cardiovascular collapse in long-term users)
- Antibiotics in the mycin group (when combined with certain muscle relaxants used during surgery, may cause respiratory paralysis)
- Oral antidiabetic medications (such as metformin hydrochloride) may react with radiologic (x-ray) iodinized contrast dyes, and cause acute renal failure (Hodgson & Kizior, 2007).

Many medications are discontinued before the surgery, but the nurse should know the purposes and actions of the patient's drugs as well as the physician's orders. Specific medications may be given the morning of surgery with sips of water (e.g., patients with heart or cardiovascular problems or diabetes mellitus).

PREVIOUS SURGERY

Data about previous surgeries are important for meeting the patient's physical and psychological needs throughout the perioperative period. Physical implications of previous surgeries are important to the intraoperative and postoperative phases (e.g., previous heart or lung surgery may necessitate adaptations in anesthesia and in positioning during surgery). Complications during or after prior surgery, such as malignant hyperthermia, latex sensitivity, pneumonia, thrombophlebitis, or surgical site infection, may put the patient at risk during this surgery, necessitating individualized postoperative monitoring.

The patient's past experiences with surgery also affect the plan of care established in the preoperative phase, especially if a past experience was negative. When the interview elicits negative feelings about the surgical experience, pain management, or nursing interventions carried out to prevent complications during previous surgeries, teaching and mutual goal setting take on an even greater importance. For children, the most stressful events before surgery include the admission process, lab tests, injections, the timeframe before and during transport to the operating room, and the recovery period in PACU (Algren & Arnow, 2007).

In addition to experiences with past surgery, the patient's perceptions and knowledge of the surgical procedure to be performed should be assessed. The patient's questions or statements about the surgery are important for meeting psychological and family needs when preparing the patient for surgery and planning for patient and family teaching and preparation for discharge.

NUTRITIONAL STATUS

Both malnutrition and obesity increase surgical risk. Surgery increases the body's need for nutrients necessary for normal tissue healing and resistance to infection. A patient who is malnourished is at a higher risk for alterations in fluid and electrolyte balance, delay in wound healing, and wound infection. Obese patients are at increased risk for respiratory, cardiovascular, positional injury, deep vein thrombosis, and gastrointestinal problems. Overweight patients may have

obstructive sleep apnea, putting them at risk for reduced respiratory function. They may also have gastroesophageal reflux disease (GERD), putting them at risk for aspiration of stomach contents. Fatty tissue has a poor blood supply and, therefore, has less resistance to infection; as a result, postoperative complications of delayed wound healing, wound infection, and disruption in the integrity of the wound are more common.

USE OF ALCOHOL, ILLICIT DRUGS, OR NICOTINE

Patients with a large habitual intake of alcohol require larger doses of anesthetic agents and postoperative analgesics, increasing the risk for drug-related complications. Patients who use illicit drugs are at risk for interactions with anesthetic agents. These are specific to the illicit drug used and should be noted on the medical record for safe anesthetic management. IV drug use may render veins hardened, inflamed, and unusable for anesthesia drug administration.

Patients who smoke are at higher risk for respiratory complications after surgery. All patients retain pulmonary secretions during anesthesia, but smokers, who already have increased mucous secretions and decreased ciliary action in the tracheobronchial tree, have more difficulty clearing the respiratory passages after surgery. In addition, the tracheobronchial mucosa is chronically irritated in people who smoke; anesthesia increases this irritation. Patients who smoke are at risk for hypoxia and postoperative pneumonia. Smoking compromises wound healing by constricting blood vessels, impairing blood flow to healing tissues.

ACTIVITIES OF DAILY LIVING AND OCCUPATION

Exercise, rest, and sleep habits are important for preventing postoperative complications and facilitating recovery. A patient with a well-established exercise program has improved cardiovascular, respiratory, metabolic, and musculoskeletal function, thereby lowering the risks of surgery. Rest and sleep are essential to physical and emotional adaptation and recovery from the stress of surgery. Information from the health history allows the nurse to individualize interventions to promote rest and sleep.

Many surgical procedures require a delay in returning to a career or occupation or may affect how the patient earns a living. Knowledge of a patient's usual work and concerns about returning to work help the nurse plan necessary teaching and referrals.

COPING PATTERNS AND SUPPORT SYSTEMS

Assessing the patient's psychological, sociocultural, and spiritual dimensions is as important as the physical history and examination. Surgery is a major psychological stressor and affects coping patterns, support systems, and individual human needs. A surgical procedure, whether it is planned or unexpected, major or minor, causes anxiety and fear. While obtaining the health history, the nurse can use cues from the patient's and family's verbal and nonverbal communication to identify fears and concerns and to plan nursing interventions to provide the information and emotional support necessary to successful recovery from surgery.

Surgery is an unfamiliar experience over which a person has no control; the resulting anxiety and fear may be expressed in many ways such as anger, withdrawal, apathy, confrontation, or questioning. Patients often fear the unknown, pain or death, and changes in body image and self-concept. The patient typically has fears about the surgery itself—the anesthesia, the diagnosis, the future, financial and family responsibilities, response to pain, or possible disfigurement or disability. Common fears are that the anesthesia will not "put me to sleep," that death will occur during surgery, or that the patient will not be able to handle postoperative pain. Surgical procedures often leave the patient with permanent changes in body structure, function, or appearance from which patients commonly fear alterations in physical attractiveness, social relationships, lifestyle, and sexuality.

> *Remember Molly Greenbaum, the 38-year-old woman who is fearful of surgery. Her statements about the inability to sleep, in conjunction with the tears in her eyes and wringing of hands, would be cues that she is experiencing stress. Exploring Molly's fears, past coping mechanisms, and support systems would be valuable in developing the patient's plan of care, both before and after surgery. Doing so would help to promote a positive perioperative experience for her. In addition, the nurse would need to investigate what fears Molly may be experiencing related to a vaginal hysterectomy such as changes in physical attractiveness, marital relationship, and sexuality.* ∎

Therapeutic communication skills are essential for establishing the trusting nurse–patient relationship that is necessary to identify and resolve fear. Encourage the patient to identify and verbalize fears; often simply talking about fears helps to diminish their magnitude. At the same time, incorrect knowledge can be identified and corrected, strengths can be identified, and teaching can be done. The reduction of fear is of major importance in preoperative preparation; emotional stress added to the physical stress of surgery increases the surgical risk. The nursing history should elicit the ways in which a patient provides self-support to reduce stress. These are discussed in Chapter 42 and range from listening to music to practicing active relaxation techniques.

Coping with stress can be facilitated through the support systems identified in the assessment phase of preoperative nursing care. As much as possible, family members or significant others should be part of the initial interview and should be included in discussions of fears and concerns. Encourage family members to provide support before and after surgery. When permitted, encourage parents to accompany their child to the preoperative waiting area and bring them to the recovery area when the patient is awake.

Identifying the patient's spiritual beliefs aids in meeting the patient's spiritual needs. These needs can be met through acceptance, participation in prayer or other rituals, and/or referral to a spiritual leader. Faith in a higher being or source of personal strength provides support and helps to reduce fears in many people.

The need for other support systems can also be identified in the initial interview. For example, a patient having a colostomy, heart transplant, or mastectomy may have many questions answered and anxieties reduced by a preoperative visit from a person who has had the same operation and adapted successfully.

SOCIOCULTURAL NEEDS

A person's perceptions of and reactions to the surgical experience are influenced by individual factors, including family health beliefs and practices, economic factors, and cultural/ethnic background. A patient who requires surgery, but has grown up in a family that believes that surgical intervention is the last possible option for treating illness, may be hesitant about the surgery or may be convinced that death will result. The resulting anxiety may make this patient even more susceptible to surgical risk. Reactions to teaching, physical care, and pain are also influenced by family values and cultural/ethnic identity. For example, a male patient reared with the belief that it is unmanly to acknowledge pain may demonstrate a stoic acceptance of pain and refuse needed medications postoperatively.

Cultural and ethnic influences also affect the patient's responses to and perceptions of the surgical experience. The patient's cultural background may require that nursing interventions be individualized to meet needs in such areas as language, food preferences, family interactions and participation, personal space, and health beliefs and practices (see Chapter 2). For example, a patient from a culture that believes that bed rest is the most important treatment for illness or injury may have difficulty accepting the need for postoperative exercises and early ambulation.

Physical Assessment

Assessing the patient's current physical status provides data for interventions to decrease surgical risk and potential postoperative complications. Depending on the situation, the physical assessment is conducted as described in Chapter 25. See also Focused Assessment Guide 30-1 for key areas to assess.

Various presurgical screening tests provide objective data of normal body function. In cases of abnormalities, such tests provide data for medical interventions to improve the patient's physical status and thus decrease the risks for surgical complications. The nurse's role is to ensure that the tests are explained to the patient, appropriate specimens are collected, the results are documented in the patient's record before surgery, and abnormal findings are reported.

Usual presurgical screening tests include chest x-ray, electrocardiography, complete blood count, electrolyte levels, and urinalysis. Normal findings for laboratory tests are

FOCUSED ASSESSMENT GUIDE • 30-1

PREOPERATIVE PHYSICAL ASSESSMENT

Factors to Assess	Questions and Approaches
General survey	• Note general state of health. • Note body posture and stature. • Take and record vital signs.
Skin	• Inspect skin for color, characteristics, and location and appearance of lesions. • Assess skin over bony prominences. • Palpate skin turgor.
Chest and lungs	• Observe chest excursion and diameter and shape of thorax. • Auscultate breath sounds. • Palpate for any pain or tenderness.
Cardiovascular system	• Inspect for jugular vein distention. • Auscultate apical rate, rhythm, and character. • Auscultate heart sounds. • Assess for peripheral edema. • Palpate character of peripheral pulses.
Abdomen	• Ask time of last bowel movement. • Inspect abdominal contour. • Auscultate bowel sounds.
Neurologic system	• Note orientation, level of consciousness, awareness, and speech. • Assess reflexes. • Assess motor and sensory ability. • Assess visual and hearing ability.
Musculoskeletal system	• Inspect and note joint range of motion. • Palpate muscle strength. • Assess ability to ambulate.

found in Appendix B. Significant abnormal findings include an elevated white blood cell count (presence of infection), decreased hematocrit and hemoglobin level (presence of bleeding, anemia), hyperkalemia or hypokalemia (increased risk for cardiac problems), elevated blood urea nitrogen or creatinine levels (possible renal failure), and abnormal urine constituents (indicating infection or fluid imbalances).

Diagnosing

Nursing diagnoses for patients in the preoperative phase may be identified for various actual or potential problems for which a patient is at risk. These are derived from the analysis of subjective and objective data obtained from the health history and physical examination as well as information from other health team members and screening tests. Many diagnoses reflect assessment of risk and are made to guide interventions for patient needs in the intraoperative and postopera-

tive phases. Nursing care throughout the perioperative period must be consistent and documented; the preoperative nursing diagnoses provide the basis for consistent, holistic care from admission through recovery. See Examples of NANDA Nursing Diagnoses appropriate to the preoperative period.

Outcome Identification and Planning

Preoperative nursing care is affected by the length of the preoperative phase. There may not be enough time for comprehensive assessments and teaching for patients who enter the hospital through the emergency department needing immediate surgery and those who have outpatient/same-day surgery. In such cases, the nurse must use standardized preoperative plans and individualize the plans for the particular patient and family. Outcomes are standard for all patients having surgery, but nursing interventions are designed to meet the priority needs of individual patients and situations.

Examples of NANDA Nursing Diagnoses
The Preoperative Patient

Nursing Diagnoses	Related Factors	Sample Defining Characteristics
Grieving	Any condition that is perceived as a potential loss, such as physical ability and appearance following surgery	• Verbalizations of distress at the potential loss • Denial of the potential loss • Altered eating habits, sleep patterns, activity level, and/or libido
Anxiety	Any condition that is perceived as a threat or danger, such as effects of surgery on ability to carry out family roles and responsibilities. Any condition that is perceived as a danger, such as the possibility of dying while under anesthesia.	• Restlessness, poor eye contact, fidgeting, quivering voice, hand tremor • Increased pulse and respirations • Abdominal pain, sweating, dry mouth, fatigue, nausea, urinary frequency • Preoccupation, forgetfulness, decreased attention span • Verbalizations of distress, worry, being afraid
Risk for Infection	Any condition that interferes with normal inflammatory healing process	*Risk Factors* • Obesity • Aging • Immunosuppression • Malnutrition

Planning for the entire perioperative period is done in the preoperative phase and includes expected outcomes that are discussed and mutually agreed on by the nurse, the patient, and the family. Specific appropriate outcomes include that the patient:

• Is physically and emotionally prepared for surgery
• Demonstrates turning, coughing, and deep-breathing exercises
• Verbalizes understanding of postoperative pain management
• Maintains fluid intake and nutritional balance to meet needs

Implementing

Preoperative nursing interventions provide the patient with the necessary psychological and physical preparation for surgery and the postoperative phase. This section discusses implementing the plan of care to meet established patient goals. Skill 30-1, Providing Preoperative Patient Care: Hospitalized Patients, outlines the actions and rationale for preoperative patient care.

Preparing the Patient Psychologically Through Communicating

Surgery is almost always viewed as a life crisis and evokes anxiety and fear. Anxiety can be reduced and recovery facili-

tated by nursing actions that focus on therapeutic communication and patient and family teaching. Each patient is a unique individual and responds to the surgical experience in a unique way. One note of caution: Avoid false reassurance. In an attempt to allay anxiety and fear, the nurse may be tempted to reassure the patient that he or she will be fine. Such a response denies the patient's emotional needs, shuts off therapeutic communications and trust, and may not be true.

The nurse uses therapeutic communication skills and techniques, as described in Chapter 21, to establish a supportive and trusting nurse–patient relationship and to facilitate psychological safety and security. Nursing interventions to meet the psychological needs of the surgical patient through communication are outlined in Box 30-2.

Preparing the Patient Psychologically Through Teaching

Teaching about postoperative activities, a nursing responsibility, is implemented in the preoperative phase. Patients and families need to know about surgical events and sensations, how to manage pain, and how to perform the physical activities necessary to decrease the risk for postoperative complications and facilitate recovery. The teaching–learning process (see Chapter 22) is individualized to meet common and individual patient needs. The success of preoperative teaching varies with the timing of the teaching, the individual patient and his or her support systems, the type of surgery, and group

Box 30-2 NURSING INTERVENTIONS TO MEET PSYCHOLOGICAL NEEDS OF PATIENTS HAVING SURGERY

- Establish and maintain a therapeutic relationship, allowing the patient to verbalize fears and concerns.
- Use active listening skills to identify and validate verbal and nonverbal messages revealing anxiety and fear.
- Use touch, as appropriate, to demonstrate genuine empathy and caring.
- Be prepared to respond to common patient questions about surgery:
  Will I lose control of body functions while I'm having surgery?
  How long will I be in the operating room and PACU?
  Where will my family be?
  Will I have pain when I wake up?
  Will the anesthetic make me sick?
  Will I need a blood transfusion?
  How long will it be before I can eat?
  What kind of scar will I have?
  When will I be able to be sexually active?
  When can I go back to work?

versus individual sessions. Preoperative teaching has proven beneficial in decreasing postoperative complications and length of stay as well as positively influencing recovery. Patients who are well prepared with detailed preoperative instruction deal more effectively with their surgery and are better prepared to manage their pain and engage in appropriate self-care activities.

The timing of teaching is a significant consideration: Teaching too far in advance of surgery or when the patient is anxious is less effective. In today's healthcare system, patients often enter the hospital the day of surgery and teaching must be adapted to this schedule. Many institutions provide teaching sessions before admission to prepare the patient for surgery. Whether done before or after admission, a preoperative teaching checklist gives nurses organized and comprehensive guidelines for instruction. Box 30-3 provides a sample of preoperative teaching with associated surgical events.

TEACHING ABOUT SURGICAL EVENTS AND SENSATIONS

Patients and their families need to know when surgery is scheduled, about how long the surgery and postanesthesia

Box 30-3 SAMPLE PREOPERATIVE TEACHING: ACTIVITIES AND EVENTS FOR IN-HOSPITAL SURGERY

Preoperative Phase
- [ ] Exercises and physical activities
  - [ ] Deep-breathing exercises
  - [ ] Coughing
  - [ ] Incentive spirometry
  - [ ] Turning
  - [ ] Leg exercises
- [ ] Pain management
  - [ ] Meaning of PRN orders for medications
  - [ ] Timing for best effect of medications
  - [ ] Splinting incision
  - [ ] Nonpharmacologic pain management options
- [ ] Visit by anesthesiologist
- [ ] Physical preparation
  - [ ] NPO
  - [ ] Sleeping medication the night before
  - [ ] Preoperative checklist (review items)
- [ ] Visitors and waiting room
- [ ] Transported to operating room by stretcher

Intraoperative Phase
- [ ] Holding area
  - [ ] Skin preparation
  - [ ] Intravenous lines and fluids
  - [ ] Medications

- [ ] Operating room
  - [ ] Operating room bed
  - [ ] Lights and common equipment (e.g., cardiac monitor, pulse oximeter, warming device)
  - [ ] Safety belt
  - [ ] Sensations
  - [ ] Staff

Postoperative Phase
- [ ] Postanesthesia care unit
  - [ ] Frequent vital signs, assessments (e.g., orientation, movement of extremities, strength of grasp)
  - [ ] Dressings/drains/tubes/catheters
  - [ ] Intravenous lines
  - [ ] Pain medications/comfort measures
  - [ ] Family notification
  - [ ] Sensations
  - [ ] Airway/oxygen therapy/pulse oximetry
  - [ ] Staff
- [ ] Transfer to unit (on stretcher)
  - [ ] Frequent vital signs
  - [ ] Sensations
  - [ ] Pain medications/nonpharmacologic strategies
  - [ ] NPO, diet progression
  - [ ] Exercises
  - [ ] Early ambulation
  - [ ] Family visits

care will last, and what will be done before, during, and after surgery (e.g., procedures, medications, equipment). If the surgery is elective, a tour of the operating suite, or a video of the preoperative journey to the OR, may be helpful in reducing anxiety and fear of the unknown. A tour or video is especially helpful for children (Algren & Arnow, 2007). An explanation of surgical events includes a description of the various members of the healthcare team; where and when to report for admission; instructions for preoperative fasting and bowel prep, if ordered; instructions for taking special medications; and the importance of bringing a responsible adult to drive the patient home. Patients may not drive themselves home or take public transportation alone if they have had any anesthesia or sedation.

Patients also benefit from knowing sensory information they may experience during the perioperative period. Although the sensations differ depending on the type of surgery, teaching should include information about dry mouth and drowsiness from preoperative medications, a sore throat from the insertion of an endotracheal tube, a gradual return of feeling and movement after spinal anesthesia, and pain from the surgical incision. Patients should also be made aware of the coolness of the environment, firmness of the OR bed, the sounds and sights of multiple care providers wearing surgical masks, and the bright overhead lights. Assure the patient that he or she is the most important person in the room and will be well cared for and comforted.

TEACHING ABOUT PAIN MANAGEMENT

Pain is a normal part of the surgical experience and a major concern for the patient and family. Evidence-based guidelines for the management of acute surgical pain have been established by several professional agencies. The guidelines are based on these principles: (1) the pain reported by the patient is the determining factor of pain control, (2) pain must be assessed as often as every 2 hours after major surgery, and (3) the older patient is at risk for both undertreatment and overtreatment of pain. Continuing or unresolved pain can increase the patient's length of recovery and delay discharge. Unrelieved postoperative pain should be treated as a serious complication of surgery, not as a normal expectation. The nurse is responsible for assessment, implementation, evaluation of a pain management plan, and for teaching the patient preoperatively how to communicate and report pain (see Chapter 35) so it is manageable. Children can be introduced to an age-specific pain scale preoperatively (Jacob, 2007).

Teach the patient and family that medications to relieve pain will be ordered by the physician and administered by the nurse. The physician may order pain medications to be given on a regular basis or on an as-needed (p.r.n.) basis. If medication is ordered p.r.n., there is a time restriction between doses (e.g., every 2 or 4 hours). The patient needs to ask for the medication and should do so before the pain becomes severe. If the medication does not control the pain or if the patient has unpleasant side effects (such as nausea and vomiting), a different medication can be ordered. There is little danger of addiction to pain medications used in the postoperative management of pain. The use of relaxation techniques (e.g., deep breathing, music, and guided imagery) enhances the effects of pain medications (See the accompanying Research in Nursing box).

Alternative methods of pain control that may be used after surgery include transcutaneous electrical nerve stimulation (TENS), pressure-controlled pain pumps filled with local anesthetics with soaker drains placed inside the incision, patient-controlled analgesia (PCA), and patient-controlled epidural anesthesia. A discussion of TENS and information about nursing interventions when using PCA are in Chapter 35. The

---

RESEARCH IN NURSING
Bridging the Gap to Evidence-Based Practice

EFFECTS OF MUSIC INTERVENTION ON ANXIETY AND PAIN

The use of music in the healthcare environment has been credited with reducing patients' anxiety and fear, promoting comfort, distraction, and pleasure. Music has been used since ancient times to influence health. Florence Nightingale recognized the healing properties of soft continuous music on comfort.

Related Research

Nilsson, U. (2008). The anxiety- and pain-reducing effects of music interventions: A systematic review. *ADRN Journal, 87*(4), 780–807.

The nurse researcher reviewed 42 randomized controlled experimental research studies of the effect of music on patients in the perioperative setting having elective surgery. Music interventions, delivered by cassette player and headphones, had a positive influence on minimizing patient pain and anxiety in half of the studies.

Relevance to Nursing Practice

Recommendations from this review suggest that the best results can be achieved with slow and flowing music of 60 to 80 beats per minute, soft low volume, and nonlyrical. The patient should participate in choosing the music within appropriate selections, use suitable sound equipment, and listen for at least 30 minutes for the best effect. Music is an inexpensive intervention that may also reduce the use of analgesics and sedatives.

For additional research, visit thePoint.

patient should be taught how to use these methods of pain control before surgery and their effectiveness monitored after surgery.

TEACHING ABOUT PHYSICAL ACTIVITIES

The most common causes of postoperative complications are alterations in cardiovascular and respiratory function, including atelectasis, pneumonia, thrombophlebitis, and emboli. Physical activities to reduce the risk for these complications are deep breathing, coughing, incentive spirometry, leg exercises, and turning in bed. These activities are taught in the preoperative period. The patient should be able to state the purpose and demonstrate the activities before going to surgery. (This section gives the rationale for the activities; postoperative complications are discussed later in the chapter.)

Deep Breathing

During surgery, the cough reflex is suppressed, mucus accumulates in the tracheobronchial passageways, and the lungs do not ventilate fully. After surgery, respirations often are less effective as a result of the anesthesia, pain medications, and pain from the incision. Patients who have thoracic or high abdominal incisions are especially prone to shallow breathing because of incisional pain with deeper respirations. As a result, alveoli do not inflate and may collapse, and secretions are retained, increasing the risk for atelectasis and respiratory infection. Deep-breathing exercises hyperventilate the alveoli and prevent them from collapsing again, improve lung expansion and volume, help to expel anesthetic gases and mucus, and facilitate oxygenation of tissues. See Guidelines for Nursing Care 30-1 for how to teach the patient deep-breathing techniques.

Coughing

Coughing helps remove retained mucus from the respiratory tract and usually is taught in conjunction with deep breathing. Coughing is especially important in patients with an increased risk for respiratory complications. Because coughing is often painful, the patient should be taught how to splint the incision (i.e., support the incision with a pillow or folded bath blanket) and to use the period after pain medication has been administered to best advantage. See Guidelines for Nursing Care 30-2 on how to teach the patient how to cough effectively.

Incentive Spirometry

An incentive spirometer is often ordered for patients having surgery, and the proper technique for using it should be practiced preoperatively. This device helps to increase lung volume and inflation of alveoli and facilitates venous return. A gauge on the incentive spirometry device allows the patient to measure his or her progress and provides immediate positive reinforcement for the breathing efforts. See Chapter 39 for more information.

Leg Exercises

During surgery, venous blood return from the legs slows; in addition, some surgical positions, such as having the legs elevated in the lithotomy position (see illustration in Chapter 12) decrease venous return. With circulatory stasis in the legs, thrombophlebitis and resultant emboli are potential complications. Leg exercises increase venous return through flexion and contraction of the quadriceps and gastrocnemius muscles. Leg exercises must be individualized to patient needs, physical condition, physician preference, and agency protocol. Figure 30-2 highlights how to teach the patient to perform leg exercises.

Turning in Bed

Turning in bed improves venous return, respiratory function, and intestinal peristalsis and prevents the unrelieved skin pressure that would occur if the patient were to remain in only one position. Although turning in bed sounds like a simple procedure, incisional pain makes it difficult, underscoring the need for practicing it before surgery. To turn in bed, the patient should raise one knee, reach across to grasp the side rail on the side toward which he or she is turning,

Guidelines for Nursing Care • 30-1

TEACHING DEEP BREATHING TECHNIQUES

- Place the patient in semi-Fowler's position, with the neck and shoulders supported.
- Ask the patient to place the hands over the rib cage, so he or she can feel the chest rise as the lungs expand.
- Ask the patient to:
  - Exhale gently and completely.
  - Inhale through the nose gently and completely.
  - Hold his or her breath for 3 to 5 seconds and mentally count "one, one thousand, two, one thousand," and so forth.

- Exhale as completely as possible through the mouth with lips pursed (as if whistling).
- Repeat three times.
- This exercise should be done every 1 to 2 hours while the patient is awake for the first 24 hours after surgery and as necessary thereafter, depending on risk factors and pulmonary status.

Guidelines for Nursing Care • 30-2

EFFECTIVE COUGHING

- Place the patient in a semi-Fowler's position, leaning forward.
- Provide a pillow or folded bath blanket to use in splinting the incision.
- Ask the patient to:
  - Inhale and exhale deeply and slowly through the nose three times.
  - Take a deep breath and hold it for 3 seconds.
  - "Hack" out for three short breaths.
  - With mouth open, take a quick breath.
  - Cough deeply once or twice.
  - Take another deep breath.
- Repeat the exercise every 2 hours while awake.

Encouraging patient to "hack" out three short coughs after holding breath.

and roll over while pushing with the bent leg and pulling on the side rail. A small pillow is useful for splinting the incision while turning. The patient should turn and change positions in bed every 2 hours when awake.

Preparing the Patient Physically

The physical preparation of the patient for surgery varies, depending on the patient's physical status and special needs, type of surgery, and physician's orders. Certain nursing interventions are appropriate for all surgical patients in the areas of hygiene and skin preparation, elimination, nutrition and fluids, and rest and sleep. The nurse is also responsible for the preparation and safety of the patient on the day of surgery.

HYGIENE AND SKIN PREPARATION

Intact skin is the body's first line of defense against microorganisms, and the surgical incision provides a potential entry for infection. Therefore, the skin is prepared to minimize skin contamination and decrease the risk for postoperative surgical site infection.

The skin is cleaned at the operative site with an antibacterial soap or solution to remove bacteria. The patient can do this while taking a bath or shower. Ideally, a shower is taken the evening before and/or the morning of surgery. Children and adult inpatients may be bathed preoperatively with microfiber cloths impregnated with chlorhexidine gluconate antimicrobial skin antiseptic, which eliminates skin microorganisms and leaves an antimicrobial film on the skin to protect the surgical incision from infections (Edmiston, Krepel, Seabrook, Lewis, Brown, & Towne, 2008). Shampooing the hair and cleaning the fingernails also help to reduce the number of organisms present on the body.

Hair removal at the surgical site may be necessary before surgery. However, the need for hair removal depends on the amount of hair, the location of the incision, and the type of surgical procedure being performed. This may be done on the unit or in the surgical suite immediately before the operation, usually in the surgical holding area. If hair must be removed, AORN (AORN, 2008a) recommends using hair clippers, rather than shaving the area, as was done in the past (see the accompanying box, PICO in Practice: Asking Clinical Questions). If the surgeon requires that the patient be shaved, it should be done as close to the time of surgery as possible. The condition of the skin and method of hair removal and skin preparation must be documented on the patient record.

ELIMINATION

Emptying the bowel of feces is no longer a routine procedure before surgery, but the nurse should use preoperative assessments to determine the need for an order to facilitate bowel elimination. If the patient has not had a bowel movement for several days or has had preoperative barium diagnostic tests, an enema helps prevent postoperative constipation.

If the patient is scheduled for surgery of the gastrointestinal tract, a prescribed bowel prep and a cleansing enema are usually ordered. Peristalsis does not return for 24 to 48 hours after the bowel is handled, so preoperative cleansing helps to decrease postoperative constipation. An empty bowel also prevents contamination of the surgical area during surgery.

Insertion of an indwelling urinary catheter may be ordered before surgery, especially in patients having pelvic surgery, to prevent bladder distention or accidental injury. If an indwelling catheter is not in place, the patient should void immediately before receiving preoperative medications to ensure an empty bladder during surgery.

Lie in a semi-Fowler's position. Bend the knee, raise the foot, and keep it elevated for a few seconds.

Extend the lower leg

Lower the leg to the bed. Do this 5 times with one leg, then repeat with the other leg.

A — Point toes of both feet toward the foot of the bed. Relax both feet.

B — Pull toes toward the chin. Relax both feet.

C — Make circles with both ankles. First circle to the right, then to the feft. Repeat 3 times. Relax both feet.

FIGURE 30-2. Leg exercises to increase venous return.

NUTRITION AND FLUIDS

Patients need to be well nourished and hydrated before surgery to counterbalance fluid, blood, and electrolyte loss during surgery and to facilitate anesthesia delivery and tissue healing after surgery. Preoperative assessments provide a baseline for physical preparation for surgery, including the need for supplemental nutrition, fluids, or electrolytes. A patient who is undernourished may require parenteral nutrition (see Chapter 36) and IV electrolyte replacements. If the patient's screening tests show a hemoglobin level of less than 10 g/dL and a hematocrit of less than 33%, blood or

blood component therapy may be given preoperatively to maintain volume and increase the oxygenation of tissue during surgery.

Although maintaining a nothing by mouth (NPO) status for at least 8 hours prior to surgery was the standard for many years, the American Society of Anesthesiologists (1999) revised the practice guidelines for preoperative fasting. The diet order depends on the type of surgery and type of anesthesia to be used. Current practice is to allow patients to drink liquids or eat food up to 2 hours before surgery depending on the type of surgery and with the permission of the physician. If clear liquids are allowed, they should be carefully defined for the patient, and include water, fruit juices without pulp, carbonated beverages, clear tea, and

PICO IN PRACTICE
Asking Clinical Questions

Patient Scenario: You are a staff nurse who works in a same-day surgery center. You are asked to serve as a preceptor for a newly hired nurse, Terri, who has just finished a nurses' refresher course at the local community college. Terri worked as a perioperative nurse for over 12 years, but her practice was on hiatus while she stayed at home to raise two children for the past 15 years. One day, Terri asks you why it is no longer standard practice to shave patients' surgical sites to prepare them for surgery. She notes to you that this was standard protocol for patients 15 years ago and that it was thought to diminish the incidence of surgical site infections.

- POPULATION: Perioperative patients
- INTERVENTION: Surgical site shaving of hair
- COMPARISON: No surgical site shaving of hair
- OUTCOME: Lower rates of surgical site infections

PICO Question: Does preoperative shaving of the surgical site result in lower rates of surgical site infections?

Finding: From the Cochrane Collaboration: Tanner, J., Woodings, D., & Moncaster, K. (2006). Preoperative hair removal to reduce surgical site infections. *Cochrane Database of Systematic Reviews.* 3(CD004122).

Findings from this systematic review suggest that preoperative shaving of surgical sites is associated with higher rates of surgical site infections.

Level of Evidence: Level I—Systematic Review

Recommendation: You note to Terri that, although shaving surgical sites may have been standard practice 15 years ago, this practice actually results in higher rates of surgical site infections and is no longer advocated.

black coffee. Patients, especially children, may be less anxious, better hydrated, and experience fewer headaches and nausea after surgery if permitted selected fluids (including breast milk for infants) up to within 2 to 4 hours before surgery. Patients having a colonoscopy should be instructed to refrain from eating prepared foods that contain Olestra, a synthetic fat food additive used in potato chips. This chemical is not always totally eliminated from the bowel and causes yellow adhesive plaques to form on colonoscopes and surgical instruments. It also may cover mucosal tissue lesions.

The nurse explains the reason for being NPO to the patient and, at the appropriate time, removes all food and fluids from the bedside and places a sign over the bed so that all health team members and visitors know about the restriction. If the patient eats or drinks, the physician should be notified at once, as the procedure may have to be delayed or cancelled.

REST AND SLEEP

Rest and sleep are important in reducing the stress before surgery and for healing and recovery after surgery. The nurse can facilitate rest and sleep in the immediate preoperative period by meeting psychological needs, carrying out teaching, providing a quiet environment, encouraging relaxation or comfort measures that are personally effective for the individual patient, or administering the prescribed bedtime sedative medication for hospitalized surgical patients.

Preparing the Patient on the Day of Surgery

A preoperative checklist is often used to outline the nurse's responsibilities on the day of surgery; these activities must be completed and documented before the patient is transported to surgery. Some of these activities have already been described (e.g., NPO, preoperative teaching, informed consent, skin preparation, screening tests, bladder elimination).

Preoperative medications that might be prescribed are as follows:

- Sedatives, such as diazepam (Valium), midazolam (Versed), or lorazepam (Ativan) to alleviate anxiety and decrease recall of events related to surgery
- Anticholinergics, such as atropine and glycopyrrolate (Robinul), to decrease pulmonary and oral secretions and to prevent laryngospasm
- Narcotic analgesics, such as morphine and meperidine hydrochloride (Demerol), to facilitate patient sedation and relaxation and to decrease the amount of anesthetic agent needed
- Neuroleptanalgesic agents, such as fentanyl citrate-droperidol (Innovar), to cause a general state of calmness and sleepiness
- Histamine-2 receptor blockers, such as cimetidine (Tagamet) and ranitidine (Zantac), to decrease gastric acidity and volume

Guidelines for Nursing Care 30-3 provides further information about preoperative interventions the day of surgery for a hospitalized patient.

Evaluating

Evaluating the plan of care for the preoperative phase is based on the expected outcomes. The plan is effective if the patient is physically and emotionally prepared for surgery, verbalizes expected events and sensations of the perioperative period, and demonstrates postoperative exercises and activities.

THE NURSING PROCESS FOR INTRAOPERATIVE CARE

The intraoperative phase of surgery begins with admission of the patient to the surgical area and lasts until the patient is transferred to the PACU. Although the surgeon has a dominant role during this phase, the perioperative nurse has critical responsibilities and roles in collaboratively meeting patient needs. The nursing process uses the preoperative data and plan as a basis for the intraoperative plan of care.

Assessing

The first room the patient enters when transferred to the surgical area is the preoperative holding area. Nurses in surgical scrub attire identify the surgical patient, assess the patient's emotional and physical status, and verify the information on the preoperative checklist including assessment data, lab reports, and consents for surgery and blood transfusion. They may also carry out required immediate preoperative care, including performing skin preparation, starting IV fluids, placing sequential compression devices to prevent deep vein thrombosis (DVT), determining pain level, assuring patient and family, providing comfort, and giving preoperative medications. The patient's response to the procedures is assessed, and the events of surgery are explained.

The Joint Commission, an independent accrediting agency for healthcare organizations and agencies, has established a standard of universal protocol to ensure patient safety when having surgery by preventing wrong site, wrong procedure, and wrong person surgery. The universal protocol has three components: preoperative verification process, marking the operative site, and a final verification just prior to beginning a procedure (Joint Commission, 2010).

When the operating room is prepared, a perioperative nurse helps transport the patient to the operating room. In the operating room, the patient is positioned on the operating bed, identified again with the operative team using at least two identifiers (such as name, birth date, medical record number), and then anesthetized and draped. The perioperative nurse assesses the patient and reviews preoperative data, paying particular attention to factors that increase surgical risk. To maintain patient safety, the nurse also assesses the patient during positioning and monitors supplies used.

Diagnosing

Patient problems in the intraoperative period may occur as a result of the position of the patient during the procedure, the

Guidelines for Nursing Care • 30-3

PROVIDING PREOPERATIVE PATIENT CARE: HOSPITALIZED PATIENT (DAY OF SURGERY)

- Check that preoperative consent forms are signed, witnessed, and correct; that advance directives are in the medical record (as applicable); and that the patient's chart is in order.
- Gather the needed equipment and supplies.
- Perform hand hygiene.
- **Check vital signs.** Notify physician of any pertinent changes (i.e., rise or drop in blood pressure, elevated temperature, cough, symptoms of infection).
- Provide hygiene and oral care. Assess for loose teeth. **Remind patient of food and fluid restrictions before surgery.**
- Instruct the patient to remove all personal clothing including underwear and put on a hospital gown.
- Ask patient to remove cosmetics, jewelry including body piercing, nail polish, and prostheses (e.g., contact lenses, false eyelashes, dentures). Some facilities allow a wedding band to be left in place, depending on the type of surgery, provided it is secured to the finger with tape.
- If possible, give valuables to a family member or place valuables in an appropriate area, such as the hospital safe if this is not possible.
- **Have patient empty bladder before surgery.**

- Attend to any special preoperative orders, such as starting an IV line.
- Complete preoperative checklist and record of patient's preoperative preparation.
- **Administer preoperative medication as prescribed by physician/anesthesia provider.**
- Raise side rails of bed; place bed in lowest position. Instruct patient to remain in bed or on stretcher. If necessary, a safety belt may be used.
- Help move the patient from the bed to the transport stretcher if necessary. Reconfirm patient identification and ensure that all preoperative events and measures are documented.
- Tell the family of the patient where the patient will be taken after surgery and the location of the waiting area where the surgeon will come to explain the outcome of the surgery.
- After the patient leaves for the operating room, prepare the room and make a postoperative bed for the patient. Anticipate any necessary equipment based on the type of surgery and the patient's history.

effects of the anesthesia, equipment used and potential hazards, disruption of tissues during surgery, and the incision. See Examples of NANDA Nursing Diagnoses during the intraoperative period.

Outcome Identification and Planning

The planning phase of the nursing process focuses on identifying interventions most effective for preventing complications, resolving patient problems, and ensuring patient safety. Some expected outcomes are that the patient will:

- Remain free of neuromuscular injury
- Remain free from wrong site, wrong side, wrong procedure surgery
- Maintain fluid and electrolyte balance
- Maintain skin integrity (other than for the incision)
- Have symmetric breathing patterns

Examples of NANDA Nursing Diagnoses

The Intraoperative Patient

Nursing Diagnoses	Related Factors	Sample Defining Characteristics
Risk for Imbalanced Fluid Volume	Hemorrhage Failure of regulatory mechanisms	• Increased pulse rate with decreased volume • Decreased blood pressure
Risk for Perioperative Positioning Injury	Any lengthy surgical procedure requiring special intraoperative positioning	*Risk Factors* • Aging • Obesity • Anesthesia, with resulting sensory/perceptual alterations • Emaciation

- Be free of injury from burns, retained foreign objects (inaccurate count of supplies), and medication errors
- Remain free from surgical site infection
- Maintain normothermia

Implementing

During surgery, nurses function as scrub nurses and circulating nurses, in an expanded role as registered nurse first assistants (RNFAs), or in an advanced practice role as acute care nurse practitioners (Advanced Practice Nurses [APNs]).

The scrub nurse is a member of the sterile team who maintains surgical asepsis while draping and handling instruments and supplies. The circulating nurse identifies and assesses the patient on admission to the operating room, collaborates in safely positioning the patient on the operating bed, assists with monitoring the patient during surgery, provides additional supplies, maintains environmental safety, and counts the number of instruments, needles, and sponges used during the surgery to prevent the accidental loss of an item in the open incision. The RNFA actively assists the surgeon by providing exposure of the operative area, hemostasis (blood clotting), and wound closure. The APN coordinates care activities, collaborates with physicians and nurses in all phases of perioperative and postanesthesia care, and integrates case management, critical paths, and research into care of the surgical patient. Additional educational preparation is required for the roles of the RNFA and the APN (Rothrock, 2007).

Positioning

The patient is placed in a specific operative position after anesthesia has produced loss of consciousness and reflexes. Patient safety, comfort, and good body alignment in positioning must be ensured to prevent alterations in integumentary, respiratory, vascular, and neuromuscular function (Rothrock, 2007). The risk for skin injury is avoided by lifting, rather than rolling or pulling, the patient into the surgical position. Rolling or pulling can cause a shearing force, in which two or more tissue layers slide on each other, stretching subcutaneous blood vessels, obstructing blood flow, and contributing to pressure ulcers.

Although all of the operative positions are not described here, perioperative nurses need to know the position to be used and significant nursing considerations for that position. Two examples are the Trendelenburg position and the lithotomy position. The Trendelenburg position requires lowering the upper torso and raising the feet. It is commonly used in minimally invasive surgery of the lower abdomen or pelvis. The displacement of the abdominal viscera toward the head decreases diaphragmatic movement and respiratory exchange; blood pools in the upper torso, and blood pressure increases; hypotension can result with return to the supine position. Shearing with resultant tissue damage is also a significant risk in this position. The lithotomy position is used for gynecologic, rectal, and urologic procedures. The placement of legs in stirrups causes pooling of blood in the legs,

increasing the risk of thrombophlebitis. Pressure can also damage the peroneal nerve, with resultant foot drop.

Draping

Drapes are used to create and maintain a sterile field around the operative site, preventing the passage of microorganisms, particulate matter, and fluids between sterile and nonsterile areas. The only area left exposed is the incision site. In some cases, plastic adhesive drapes may be used to form a complete seal over the skin. With these drapes, skin color is visible, and the incision is made through the impermeable adhesive drape.

Documenting

Throughout surgery, the perioperative nurse documents ongoing patient assessment, item counts (sponges, sharps, instruments), monitoring data (e.g., vital signs, urine output, blood loss, pulse oximetry results), positioning, medications, dressings and drains, specimens, and responses to care on the intraoperative record. This documentation includes planning and implementation of perioperative nursing activities and evaluation of the achievement of patient outcomes.

Transferring to the Postanesthesia Care Unit

After the surgery, the patient is moved carefully from the operating bed to a stretcher or bed. This is a critical time: Sudden or rough handling can cause severe hypotension or potentially lethal cardiac or respiratory arrest. The patient is then transported to the PACU, and the OR nurse verbally communicates relevant preoperative and intraoperative assessments and interventions to the PACU nurses to ensure continuity of care. The primary objective of the hand-off report from OR nurse to PACU nurse is to provide accurate information about the patient's care, procedure, presenting condition, and any important events that occurred during the procedure. It allows for communication clarification and questions (Clancy, 2008; Odom-Forren, 2007).

Evaluating

Evaluation of the effectiveness of the plan of care for the intraoperative phase is based on the expected outcomes. If met, the plan was effective.

POSTOPERATIVE NURSING CARE

The postoperative phase can be divided into two stages—immediate care (usually provided in the PACU in both in-hospital and outpatient/same-day surgery centers) and ongoing postoperative care (lasting from return to the unit through convalescence). Nursing assessments and interventions are consistent with those in the preoperative and intraoperative phases and are carried out to maintain function, promote recovery, and facilitate coping with alterations in structure or function. (See the accompanying Through the Eyes of a Student.) Assessments and nursing interventions

Through the Eyes of a Student

The first time I took care of a patient with "multiple tubes," I was horrified at the thought of actually touching the patient. I hadn't really been exposed to that many critically ill patients until my last semester as a student nurse. I remember being assigned a patient in the cardiothoracic intensive care unit in the hospital where I trained. The patient was a "fresh heart"—a cardiopulmonary bypass graft patient who had just been operated on that morning.

I remember walking into the room and thinking, "What do I do with all of these tubes?" and then with horror thinking, "What if one of them falls out?" Needless to say, I was overwhelmed and frightened but at the same time excited at the challenge that faced me. I asked my preceptor what each tube was for and

where it was hooked up and whether it would fall out if I touched it. She answered all my questions with patience and understanding and asked me if I wanted to handle the lines. I looked at her as if she were insane, but went ahead and did it. Would you believe that nothing fell out! I must admit that the experience taught me a lot, but it also got me over the fear of tubes.

I now chuckle every time I see a nursing student's face with that same look of horror as I had, and I try to answer every question with the same degree of patience and understanding that my preceptor had for me.

—*Lynda L. Ullmer, RN*
Gaithersburg, MD

are combined in discussing immediate postoperative care; the phases of the nursing process are used to describe ongoing postoperative care.

Immediate Postoperative Assessment and Care

Care in the PACU involves assessing the postoperative patient, with emphasis on preventing complications from anesthesia or the surgery. Assessments are continuous, using preoperative and intraoperative data as bases for comparison. The assessments made in the PACU include respiratory status, cardiovascular status, central nervous system status, fluid status, wound status, and general condition. These assessments initially are made every 10 to 15 minutes. Children can quickly lose their airway and go into a crisis. Emergence delirium, where they wake up thrashing and disoriented, is common in children. They must be safeguarded from hurting themselves and often re-induced into general anesthesia to promote a smoother anesthesia emergence.

The average PACU stay is about 1 hour, but it will vary depending on the type of surgery, length of anesthesia, and patient response. Outpatient/same-day surgery patients return home after recovery in the PACU. The critical role functions of the PACU nurse include vigilant monitoring during emergence from anesthesia and the first hours after surgery, pain management, fluid and electrolyte balance, stabilization of physiologic parameters (such as heart and respiratory rate), and preparation for the next level of care (DeFazio-Quinn, 2009).

▶ *Mr. Benjamin, the older adult who has had a total hip replacement, will require frequent assessments during his stay in the PACU, specifically vital signs, cardiovascular status, respiratory status, IV therapy, wound status, and urinary elimination.* ■

Respiratory Status

Respiratory function is assessed by monitoring respiratory rate, rhythm, and depth; auscultating breath sounds; noting the oxygen saturation level; assessing skin color; and monitoring the cardiovascular and mental status. During a surgical procedure with general anesthesia, an endotracheal tube may be inserted to administer the anesthetic gases and maintain patent air passages. The airway is not removed until the laryngeal and pharyngeal reflexes return, allowing the patient to control the tongue, cough, and swallow. The airway is assessed for patency, humidified oxygen is administered, and pulse oximetry is initiated. Ineffective respiratory function is indicated by restlessness and anxiety; unequal chest expansion with use of accessory muscles; shallow, noisy respirations; cyanosis; and tachycardia.

Respiratory obstruction is the most common PACU emergency. It may occur as a result of secretion accumulation, obstruction by the tongue, laryngospasm (a sudden, violent contraction of the vocal cords), or laryngeal edema. Respiratory obstruction is indicated by assessments of ineffective respiratory function plus observing for wheezing or crowing sounds with respiratory effort. Positioning, administering humidified oxygen, encouraging the patient to take deep breaths, and suctioning may be used to maintain a patent airway and tissue oxygenation.

Cardiovascular Status

Cardiovascular function is assessed by taking vital signs, monitoring electrocardiogram rate and rhythm, and observing skin color and condition. Blood pressure findings are compared with baseline data from the preoperative period. Transient hypertension can occur as a result of anesthetic effects, respiratory insufficiency, the surgical procedure, or the excitement phase of recovery from anesthesia.

Hypotension may be the result of varied factors, including anesthetic agents, preoperative medications, position changes, blood loss, respiratory alterations, and peripheral blood pooling. Oxygen administration, deep breathing, leg exercises, verbal stimulation (to help expel anesthetic gases and facilitate increasing level of consciousness), and maintaining accurate IV flow rates can increase low blood pressure.

Patients are at risk for altered body temperature related to the surgical procedure, its length, anesthetic agents, a cool surgical environment, age, and use of cool irrigating or infusion fluids. Inadvertent **hypothermia** (temperature below 35.5°C [96°F]) can lead to complications of poor wound healing, hemodynamic stress, cardiac disturbances, coagulopathy, delayed emergence from anesthesia, and shivering and its associated discomfort (AORN, 2008b). Measure the patient's body temperature, usually by the temporal or tympanic route, and initiate interventions if the patient complains of being cold or is hypothermic. Warmed blankets placed on the patient's body and head and forced warm-air devices are used for rewarming.

All pulses are assessed for bilateral equality, rhythm, rate, and character. Of special significance are assessments of abnormal function—an irregular rhythm, absence of pulses, or tachycardia. Tachycardia, an early symptom of shock, must be carefully evaluated. Other related assessments for shock are a decreasing blood pressure, cyanosis, a cool skin temperature, and a decrease in urine output.

Central Nervous System Status

The return of central nervous system function is assessed through the patient's response to stimuli and orientation. Consciousness returns in reverse order, with the usual pattern being: (1) unconsciousness, (2) response to touch and sounds, (3) drowsiness, (4) awake but not oriented, and (5) awake and oriented. Nurses in the PACU verbally reorient the patient by gently touching and calling him or her by name.

Fluid Status

Fluid imbalance may result from factors such as preoperative fluid restriction, fluid loss during surgery, wound drainage, or the surgical stress response (with retention of sodium and water). Imbalanced fluid volume (deficit or excess) is a risk for all surgical patients but is an especially important consideration in children and older adults. Assessing fluid status includes skin turgor, vital signs, urine output, wound drainage, and IV fluid intake. IV fluid administration assessments include the type of fluid infused, the rate, location of lines, condition of the IV insertion site, and the security and patency of the tubing.

Wound Status

The nurse in the PACU assesses the dressing over the incision (the wound) for amount, consistency, and color of drainage as well as for any tubes or drains and the amount and type of drainage by that route. Large amounts of bright-red drainage, combined with other abnormal physical status assessments (restlessness, pallor, cold moist skin, decreasing blood pressure, increasing pulse and respiratory rates), may indicate hemorrhage and hypovolemic shock. Report these symptoms immediately.

Pain Management

Pain is both a subjective and an objective experience. Clinical practice guidelines developed by the Agency for Health Care Research and Quality recommend the assessment of pain using a rating scale. The scale may be verbal (ranging from no pain to worst possible pain), numeric (with 10 on a scale of 0 to 10 being the worst possible pain), or a "faces" rating scale, ranging from a smiley face indicating no pain to a face that has frowns and tears for worst possible pain (see Chapter 35). Early administration of analgesia, using nonsteroidal anti-inflammatory drugs and opiates, occurs in the PACU. Opiates may be delivered by PCA, allowing the patient to control the analgesic administration. Nonpharmacologic methods to decrease pain and improve comfort include positioning, verbal reassurance, and touch. Preoperative assessments of methods that are personally effective for the patient assist in effective implementation in the PACU. These should supplement, not substitute for, pharmacologic pain relief.

General Condition

Other assessments and interventions are made to ensure physical and emotional comfort and safety. Constant reorientation and reassurance that the surgery is completed provide psychological comfort. Careful assessments, proper positioning, and use of side rails maintain physical safety. The patient is discharged from the PACU when physical status and level of consciousness are considered stable. The family is notified that the patient is being transferred back to the room, and the PACU nurse gives a verbal report to the unit nurse about the assessments and interventions during the intraoperative and immediate postoperative phases.

Ongoing Postoperative Care

Ongoing postoperative care is planned to facilitate recovery from surgery and coping with alterations. The plan of care includes promoting physical and psychological health, preventing complications, and teaching self-care when the patient returns home. Skill 30-2, Providing Postoperative Care When Patient Returns to Room, outlines initial and ongoing postoperative patient care.

THE NURSING PROCESS FOR ONGOING POSTOPERATIVE CARE
Assessing

The nurse on the unit assists PACU personnel in transferring the patient to the bed in the unit and makes an initial assessment using data from the preoperative and intraoperative phases. A postoperative checklist or flow sheet may be used. The initial assessment is often combined with the implementation of postoperative physician's orders. See Table 30-2 for focused assessments and interventions.

After conducting the assessment, document the time of arrival and all assessment data. Agency protocol is followed

TABLE • 30-2	POSTOPERATIVE ASSESSMENTS AND INTERVENTIONS ON RETURN TO THE UNIT
Factors to Assess	**Assessments and Interventions**
Vital signs and oxygen saturation	• Temperature, blood pressure, pulse and respiratory rates; oxygen saturation • Note, report, and document deviations from preoperative and PACU data as well as symptoms of complications.
Color and temperature of skin	• Skin color (pallor, cyanosis), skin temperature, and diaphoresis
Level of consciousness	• Orientation to time, place, and person • Reaction to stimuli and ability to move extremities
Intravenous fluids	• Type and amount of solution, flow rate, security and patency of tubing • Infusion site
Surgical site	• Dressing and dependent areas for drainage (color, amount, consistency) • Drains and tubes; be sure they are intact, patent, and properly connected to drainage systems.
Other tubes	• Assess indwelling urinary catheter, gastrointestinal suction, and others for drainage, patency, and amount of output. • Be sure dependent drainage bags are hanging properly and suction drainage is attached and functioning. • If oxygen is ordered, ensure placement of ordered application and flow rate.
Comfort	• Assess pain (location, duration, intensity) and determine whether analgesics were given in the PACU. • Assess for nausea and vomiting. • Cover the patient with a blanket. • Reorient to the room as necessary. • Allow family members to remain with the patient after the initial assessment is completed.
Position and safety	• Place the patient in an ordered position, *or* • If the patient is not fully conscious, place in the side-lying position. • Elevate the side rails and place the bed in low position.

for assessment routines: Common time frames are every 15 minutes until stable, changing to every 1 to 2 hours for the first 24 hours, and every 4 hours thereafter. Although agency protocols are used for guidelines in the immediate postoperative period, the nurse is responsible for adjusting the frequency and priorities of assessment to the specific needs of each patient.

Diagnosing

Nursing diagnoses in the postoperative phase may represent actual problems or those for which the patient is at risk. When making nursing diagnoses, the nurse uses assessment data and plans of care established before and during surgery and includes the family. See Examples of NANDA Nursing Diagnoses appropriate to the postoperative period.

Outcome Identification and Planning

The plan of care in the postoperative phase begins in the preoperative phase, when nursing activities to reduce stress and teach postoperative activities are carried out. From admission, the patient and family are prepared for uneventful recovery and self-care after discharge. Specific expected

outcomes are individualized based on risk factors, the surgical procedure, and the patient's unique needs. Examples of desired postoperative outcomes for a patient after major surgery are as follows:

The patient will:

• Carry out leg exercises every 2 to 4 hours.
• Deep breathe and cough effectively every 2 hours.
• Verbalize decreasing levels of pain.
• Have a balanced intake and output.
• Regain normal bowel and bladder elimination.
• Exhibit a healing surgical incision.
• Remain free of infection.
• Verbalize any concerns about appearance of wound.
• Verbalize and demonstrate wound self-care.

Implementing

Many nursing interventions in the postoperative phase have already been discussed in this chapter or are fully discussed in other chapters; therefore, this section focuses on nursing interventions to meet the expected outcomes of the plan of care. Nursing care is discussed to prevent complications, promote a return to health, and facilitate coping with alterations.

Examples of NANDA Nursing Diagnoses

The Postoperative Patient

Nursing Diagnoses	Related Factors	Sample Defining Characteristics
Risk for Infection	Any condition that interferes with normal inflammatory healing process or provides an entry for infectious agents	*Risk Factors* • Obesity • Aging • Immunosuppression • Malnutrition • Presence of incision • Decreased ability to cough, deep breathe, use incentive spirometer • Presence of drains, tubes, and catheters • Insertion site for intravenous therapy
Disturbed Body Image	Any condition that causes confusion in the mental image of oneself, including surgical incision, removal of body part, and inability to use body as one did before surgery	• Verbalization of altered view of one's body in appearance, structure, or function • Refusal to look at incision or area of surgical treatment • Actual change in one's body from surgery or trauma • Actual missing body part • Verbalizations of negative feelings about body
Acute Pain	Any condition that causes actual tissue damage, such as the surgical incision	• Rating pain as severe on a scale of 1 to 10 (i.e., as a 9) • Positioning or guarding self to avoid pain • Inability to sleep • Loss of appetite • Diaphoresis, changes in vital signs, dilated pupils • Moaning, crying, sighing
Urinary Retention	Any condition that causes incomplete emptying of the bladder, such as neurologic effects of anesthesia	• Urine not eliminated for more than 8 hours • Distended, palpable bladder • Small, frequent voiding • Residual urine

A wide variety of factors increase the risk of postoperative complications, including age, health habits, physical condition, medical history, psychological status, and surgical intervention (e.g., anesthesia, positioning, wound). Ongoing postoperative assessments and interventions are implemented to decrease the risk for postoperative complications. If postoperative complications occur, the nurse provides physical assessments and care, provides emotional support to the patient and family, and carries out prescribed treatments. See Nursing Advocacy in Action for an example of a patient who may require an advocate.

Preventing Cardiovascular Complications

Nursing interventions to prevent or monitor for cardiovascular complications are listed in Box 30-4. Specific cardiovascular complications include hemorrhage, shock, thrombophlebitis, and pulmonary embolus.

HEMORRHAGE

Hemorrhage is an excessive internal or external blood loss, and may lead to hypovolemic shock. It may occur from a slipped suture, a dislodged clot in the wound, or stress on the surgical site; it may also be the result of pathophysiologic conditions or certain medications. Common manifestations of hemorrhage include restlessness, anxiety, and frank bleeding as well as hypotension; cold, clammy skin; a weak, thready, and rapid pulse; cool, mottled extremities; deep, rapid respirations; decreased urine output; thirst; and apprehension. The primary purposes of care for the patient experiencing a hemorrhage include stopping the bleeding and

NURSING ADVOCACY IN ACTION

Patient Scenario

Alex is a 28-year-old man admitted to the surgical intensive care unit after undergoing a partial gastric bypass surgical procedure. He originally weighed 700 lbs but lost 100 lbs prior to being approved for the surgery. Patients like Alex are usually admitted to the intensive care unit for airway management and to ensure strict adherence to fluid intake restrictions needed to maintain the integrity of the suture line. You are assigned to care for Alex. The nurse giving report says the following:

- "Alex is noncompliant with the fluid intake restrictions. He tries to sneak water. I don't know why we have to care for patients who are not willing to follow the medical treatment plan that they agreed to before surgery."
- "He should be repositioned hourly but since he's not motivated to participate with his ADLs, especially bathing and turning in bed, I wouldn't worry. Why should we take a risk of hurting ourselves when he obviously doesn't care?"
- "His mother told the charge nurse yesterday that caregivers were making comments related to his size and were not providing the same quality of care as they gave to other patients."

Implications for Nursing Advocacy

How will you respond if you are Alex's nurse? Talk with your classmates and experienced nurses about the questions that follow.

- If you elect to advocate for Alex, what practical steps can you take to ensure better health outcomes?
- What is reasonable to expect of a student nurse, a graduate nurse, and an experienced nurse in this situation?
- What advocacy skills are needed to effectively respond to this challenge?

replacing blood volume. If bleeding occurs, apply a pressure dressing to the bleeding site, notify the surgeon immediately, and be prepared to have the patient return to the operating room if bleeding cannot be stopped.

SHOCK

Shock is the body's reaction to acute circulatory failure as the result of an alteration in circulatory control or a loss of intravascular fluid. The type of shock most commonly seen in postoperative patients is hypovolemic shock, which occurs from a decrease in blood volume. Common manifestations of shock are the same as those for hemorrhage.

The primary purpose of care for a patient in shock is to improve and maintain tissue perfusion by eliminating the cause of the shock. Nursing interventions include notifying the surgeon immediately; establishing and maintaining the airway; placing the patient in a flat position with the legs elevated 30 to 45 degrees; administering oxygen; monitoring vital signs, hematocrit, and blood gas results; maintaining body warmth with covers; and administering medications. The nurse must also be prepared to assist with the insertion of IV lines and to administer fluids as well as whole blood or its components.

THROMBOPHLEBITIS

Thrombophlebitis is an inflammation of a vein associated with thrombus (blood clot) formation. Thrombophlebitis from venous stasis is most commonly seen in the legs of postoperative patients. Manifestations of thrombophlebitis are pain and cramping in the calf or thigh of the involved extremity, redness and swelling in the affected area, elevated temperature, and an increase in the diameter of the involved extremity.

Care for the patient with thrombophlebitis includes preventing a clot from breaking loose and becoming an embolus that travels to the lungs, heart, or brain and preventing further clot formation. Nursing interventions include administering medications (e.g., anti-inflammatory agents, anticoagulants, analgesics), maintaining the patient on bed rest, applying external heat, applying thigh-high antiembolic stockings or sequential pneumatic compression devices (Box 30-5), and measuring bilateral calf or thigh

---

Box 30-4 **NURSING INTERVENTIONS TO PREVENT OR MONITOR POSTOPERATIVE CARDIOVASCULAR COMPLICATIONS**

- Assess and document vital signs as ordered and as the patient's status dictates, using preoperative assessments as a baseline.
- Provide covers, forced warm air, or other warming device or techniques as necessary to prevent shivering and hypothermia.
- Maintain fluid balance.
- Maintain accurate intake and output.
- Monitor rate, type, and access site of intravenous fluids.
- Assess skin turgor and hydration of mucous membranes.
- Monitor amount, color, and consistency of wound drainage (dressings and drains or tubes).

- Implement leg exercises and turning in bed every 2 hours.
- Assist with ambulation. Ambulation usually begins the evening of surgery and increases as tolerated; blood pressure and pulse and respiratory rates are used to monitor tolerance.
- Apply and follow protocols for antiembolic stockings or compression devices, if ordered.
- Administer anticoagulant medications, if prescribed.
- Measure bilateral calf and thigh circumference daily.
- Avoid positioning that impedes venous return (e.g., do not mechanically raise the knee portion of the bed or place pillows under the knees).

Box 30-5   PNEUMATIC COMPRESSION DEVICES

Pneumatic compression devices are composed of an air pump, connecting tubes, and an extremity sleeve. The sleeve may cover the entire leg or may extend from the foot to the knee. A variety of types are available; the accompanying figure provides one example. The devices apply brief pressure to the legs to enhance blood flow and venous return, thereby decreasing the risk for thrombophlebitis after surgery. The devices may apply either intermittent or sequential pressure. Intermittent pneumatic compression devices fit over the entire leg, with inflation and deflation of the sleeve covering the leg alternating from one leg to the other by a preset timer. Sequential pneumatic compression devices are designed so that pressure moves up the leg in increments. They may inflate and deflate by alternating from one leg to the other, or they may do so for both legs at once.

Nursing Care

- Explain the purpose of the device to the patient.
- Apply the device so that two fingers fit between the leg and the sleeve.
- Position the tubing so the patient can move about without interrupting the air flow.
- Remove the sleeves at least once a day for skin care and assessment.

- Assess the extremities for peripheral pulses, edema, changes in sensation, and movement on a regular schedule.
- Ensure that all chambers are inflating in proper sequence once per shift.

Sleeve containing three chambers

Pump

First chamber inflated

---

circumference every shift. Teach the patient not to massage the legs.

Preventing Respiratory Complications

Nursing interventions to prevent or monitor for respiratory complications include monitoring vital signs; implementing deep breathing, coughing, and incentive spirometry; turning in bed every 2 hours; ambulating; maintaining hydration; avoiding positioning that decreases ventilation; and monitoring responses to narcotic analgesics. Specific respiratory complications include pulmonary embolus, pneumonia, and atelectasis.

PULMONARY EMBOLUS

An **embolus** is a blood clot or foreign substance that is dislodged and travels through the bloodstream until it lodges in a smaller vessel. In postoperative patients, the embolus is often part of a thrombus that breaks free from a vein wall. If the embolus lodges in the pulmonary vessels, it is called a pulmonary embolus. Manifestations of a pulmonary embolus include dyspnea, chest pain, cough, cyanosis, rapid respirations, tachycardia, and anxiety. This is a life-threatening condition and immediate treatment is necessary. The primary goals of care are to stabilize cardiovascular and respiratory function and to prevent further emboli. Nursing interventions include notifying the physician immediately, maintaining the patient on bed rest in the semi-Fowler's position, assessing vital signs frequently, administering oxygen, administering medications (e.g., anticoagulants, analgesics), and instructing the patient to avoid Valsalva's maneuver (forced exhalation against a closed glottis, such as straining to have a bowel

movement) to prevent increased intrathoracic pressure and, possibly, increased emboli.

PNEUMONIA

Pneumonia is an inflammation of the alveoli as the result of an infectious process or the presence of foreign material. Pneumonia may occur postoperatively as a result of aspiration, infection, depressed cough reflex, increased secretions from anesthesia, dehydration, and immobilization. Manifestations of pneumonia include fever, chills, a cough that produces rusty or purulent sputum, crackles and wheezes, dyspnea, and chest pain. The goals of care are to treat the underlying infection, maintain respiratory function, and prevent the spread of microorganisms. Nursing interventions include those used to prevent or monitor for respiratory complications and promoting full aeration of the lungs by positioning the patient in semi-Fowler's or Fowler's position, administering oxygen, administering medications (e.g., antibiotics, expectorants, analgesics), providing frequent oral hygiene, and ensuring rest and comfort.

ATELECTASIS

Atelectasis is the incomplete expansion or collapse of alveoli with retained mucus, involving a portion of lung and resulting in poor gas exchange. Manifestations of atelectasis include decreased lung sounds over the affected area, dyspnea, cyanosis, crackles, restlessness, and apprehension. The primary goals of care are to ensure oxygenation of tissues, prevent further atelectasis, and expand involved lung tissues. Nursing interventions include those used to prevent or monitor for respiratory complications, and positioning the patient in semi-Fowler's position, administering oxygen, and administering analgesics for pain.

Preventing Surgical Site Complications

The nurse assesses and cares for the surgical site to promote healing and prevent complications such as infection, dehiscence (wound closure separation), and evisceration (protrusion of intra-abdominal organs). Wound care is discussed in Chapter 32. Nursing interventions to prevent surgical site complications are assessing vital signs (especially for fever); maintaining hydration; maintaining nutritional status; encouraging a diet high in proteins, carbohydrates, calories, and vitamins; using proper hand hygiene; and following aseptic technique when changing dressings at the surgical site and exit sites for tubes and drains. Soiled gloves and dressings should be disposed of following standard precautions.

Promoting a Return to Health

Nurses provide interventions during postoperative recovery to promote physical and psychological functioning at as near a normal state as possible. The plan of care to achieve this goal includes activities to meet elimination, fluid and electrolyte, nutrition, and rest and comfort needs.

ELIMINATION NEEDS

Both urinary and bowel elimination can be altered by anesthesia, manipulation of organs during surgery, inactivity, and altered fluid and food intake during the perioperative period. Assessments and nursing interventions to promote the return of normal bowel and urinary elimination are outlined in Box 30-6.

FLUID AND NUTRITION NEEDS

Nursing assessments and interventions to meet fluid needs are met by monitoring patterns of intake and output, maintaining prescribed IV fluid infusion rates, and assessing skin turgor and mucous membranes for dehydration. Nutrition needs are met by monitoring weight, providing oral hygiene before meals and as needed, monitoring postoperative dietary progression (often from clear to full liquids, then from soft to regular diet), maintaining an environment conducive to appetite (clean, neat, free of odors), encouraging the patient to sit up in bed or a chair for meals, and encouraging family participation in meals.

COMFORT AND REST NEEDS

Comfort needs are a priority after surgery. Factors that interfere with comfort include nausea, vomiting, thirst, hiccups, and pain at the surgical site. Nursing interventions that promote rest and comfort by providing relief for these problems are listed in Guidelines for Nursing Care 30-4. Comfort and rest are also promoted by providing personal hygiene, keeping bed linens clean, providing quiet rest periods, and allowing family members to remain with the patient.

Helping the Patient Cope

Surgery may alter the patient's physical appearance as well as his or her physiologic function, leading to the risk for or actual alterations in self-concept and body image. Changes in a person's self-perception can influence all of the human dimensions and areas of human functioning, including self-esteem, relationships with others, sexual identity, spiritual beliefs, sociocultural values, and independent and fulfilling engagement in activities of daily living.

Many surgical patients have the same reaction to loss of a body part as to a death (see Chapter 43). The response and adaptation to the loss are influenced by multiple factors, including age, cultural values and beliefs, sociocultural background, significance of the body part, visibility of the body part, time to prepare for the change, and support people available. A surgical patient's grief is a normal, appropriate response. It is unique to the person experiencing it, and although there are stages and phases of grief, there is no timetable for it. The nurse must be aware of the patient's needs and provide interventions to meet those needs in coping with

---

Box 30-6   NURSING ASSESSMENTS AND INTERVENTIONS TO MEET POSTOPERATIVE ELIMINATION NEEDS

Bowel Elimination
- Assess for the return of peristalsis by auscultating bowel sounds every 4 hours when the patient is awake.
- Assess abdominal distention, especially if bowel sounds are not audible or are high pitched (indicative of possible paralytic ileus, which is an absence of intestinal peristalsis).
- Assess ability to pass flatus and stool.
- Assist with movement in bed and ambulation to relieve gas pains, a common postoperative discomfort.
- Encourage food and fluid intake when ordered, especially fruit juices and high-fiber foods.
- Maintain privacy when patient is using the bedpan, urinal, commode, or bathroom.
- Administer suppositories, enemas, or medications, such as stool softeners, as prescribed.

Urinary Elimination
- Monitor patterns of intake and output.
- Assist in assuming normal position to void by using an upright position when on a bedpan and using a bedside commode or bathroom when able, or by assisting the male patient to stand upright to void with a urinal.
- Assess for bladder distention by palpating above the symphysis pubis if the patient has not voided within 8 hours after surgery or if the patient has been voiding frequently in amounts of less than 50 mL; notify the physician of abnormal assessment results.
- Maintain prescribed intravenous fluid infusion rates.
- Encourage oral fluid intake when prescribed.
- Provide privacy when the patient is using bedpan, bedside commode, urinal, or bathroom.
- Initiate urinary catheterization, if prescribed.

Guidelines for Nursing Care • 30-4

PROMOTING POSTOPERATIVE REST AND COMFORT

Nausea and Vomiting

- Avoid giving the patient a large amount of fluids or food at one time, especially after being NPO.
- Administer prescribed medications.
- Provide oral hygiene, as needed.
- Maintain clean environment.
- Avoid use of a straw.
- Avoid strong-smelling food.
- Assess for possible allergy to medications, such as antibiotics or analgesics.
- Maintain bowel elimination.

Thirst

- Offer sips of water or ice chips when NPO (if permitted).
- Maintain oral hygiene.

Hiccups

- Have the patient do the following:
  - Take several swallows of water while holding the breath (if not NPO).
  - Rebreathe into a paper bag.
  - Eat a teaspoon of granulated sugar.

Surgical Pain

- Assess pain frequently; administer prescribed analgesics every 2 to 4 hours on a regular schedule during the first 24 to 36 hours after surgery.
- Reinforce preoperative teaching for pain management.
- Offer nonpharmacologic measures to supplement medications: massage, position changes, relaxation, guided imagery, meditation, music.

change. Nursing interventions to facilitate coping and adaptation are outlined in Box 30-7.

Providing Outpatient/Same-Day Surgery Postoperative Care

Evaluating the patient's postoperative status after outpatient/same-day surgery focuses on ensuring that the patient can be safely cared for at home. After surgery and recovery from the anesthetic, the patient is asked to sit up and drink liquids. A patient who is no longer drowsy or dizzy, has stable vital signs, and has voided is allowed to go home accompanied by a responsible adult. The patient is not allowed to drive a car or go home alone on public transportation. The usual length of time from completion of surgery to discharge is 1 to 3 hours, provided that established criteria have been met. Written and verbal instructions for home care are given to the patient and family.

Evaluating

The achievement of desired outcomes for postoperative recovery and rehabilitation may be evaluated in a number of ways. Because the final resolution of some desired outcomes may not be apparent or measurable at the time of discharge, many institutions use follow-up telephone calls or surveys that are mailed to patients. It may also be possible to collaborate with the physician's office to have a patient complete a survey on the first postoperative visit. Whatever mechanism is selected, important outcomes, such as the absence of surgical site infection, the patient's satisfaction with pain management measures, return to former levels of mobility and activity, and the absence of postoperative nausea and vomiting and other complications for which the patient was at risk, should be included as part of evaluative criteria.

See Nursing Care Plan 30-1 for examples of the nursing process related to perioperative care.

Box 30-7   NURSING INTERVENTIONS TO FACILITATE POSTOPERATIVE COPING AND ADAPTATION

- Accept each patient as a unique individual.
- Identify through verbal and nonverbal cues patients who are at risk for alteration in self-concept. The risk is increased if the patient has little support from others, a visible alteration, or an alteration that will seriously affect functional ability.
- Allow time for patients and families to verbalize their feelings about the alteration, and do not assume that all patients will have problems.

- Identify and support strengths and effective coping mechanisms.
- Encourage the patient and family to be part of goal setting and decision making throughout the surgical experience.
- Provide teaching and honest information to the patient and family about all aspects of care.
- Work collaboratively with other members of the health team to provide referrals and resources as necessary to meet physical, psychological, and spiritual needs.

NURSING PLAN OF CARE · 30-1

For Gabrielle McAllister

Remember Gabrielle McAllister, the 5-year-old admitted for removal of her tonsils and adenoids in same-day surgery? When she arrived, she was clinging to her mother and crying. Her mother said, "I don't think I can stand this again, but I know it has to be done." The admitting nurse made the following assessments:

- Five-year-old girl, small for age, with history of several previous surgeries for congenital cardiac defect.
- History of latex allergy.
- Crying, clinging to mother.
- Mother verbalizes fear of daughter having surgery again.

NURSING DIAGNOSIS Anxiety related to upcoming surgery manifested by child's crying and clinging to mother, mother's verbalization of fear.

EXPECTED OUTCOME 8/9/12—Prior to surgery, child (and mother, as appropriate) will:

- calmly sit on mother's lap
- verbalize decreased anxiety (mother)
- demonstrate knowledge of physiologic and psychological responses to surgery (mother)

Nursing Interventions	Rationale	Evaluative Statement
Assess patient and family knowledge base	Patient may be misinformed or unaware of her surgery or preop instructions. Prior surgery experience may have been different	8/9/12 Outcome met: Patient understands expectations for surgery, is calm and cuddled on her mother's lap, clutching her toy bunny named "Bunny."
Review preop teaching	Patient/family may need teaching or reinforcement	*C. Smith, RN*
Clarify understanding of questions and preop instructions and teaching	This ensures the patient and family understand and conveys caring and compassion from the nurse	
Provide appropriate emotional support and calm environment	Most patients respond positively to compassion and kindness	8/9/12 Outcome met: Patient is calm and quiet. States that she is ready to have her tonsils taken out so that she will not have any more sore throats. She knows that her parents will be waiting "just next door" until she is done. This is Bunny's 4th surgery.
Orient to OR environment with time and sensory information	Information and positive interpersonal communication may decrease anxiety	
Allow patient to take her stuffed toy bunny with her to the OR	Favorite toys will bring comfort and sense of not being alone	
Communicate unresolved issues to OR team	OR team will be able to continue support measures	*C. Smith, RN*

NURSING DIAGNOSIS Latex Allergy Response related to developed hypersensitivity to natural latex rubber from multiple exposures

EXPECTED OUTCOME 8/9/12—During the perioperative period, the child will:

- remain free of signs and symptoms of latex allergy

(continued)

NURSING PLAN OF CARE · 30-1

For Gabrielle McAllister (continued)

Nursing Interventions	Rationale	Evaluative Statement
Assess patient environment for latex-containing items	Patients with a latex allergy may have allergic response to any object containing latex.	8/9/12 Outcome met. Latex allergy bracelet applied to left wrist. No signs or symptoms of latex reaction on transfer to OR.
Provide latex-free or latex-safe substitutes	Safety for the patient with a latex allergy mandates the provision of latex-free objects and donning an allergy ID bracelet.	*C. Smith, RN*
Provide patient with allergy ID bracelet		
Notify OR team of patient's latex allergy	Anesthesia will have emergency drugs available if patient demonstrates intra-operative reaction. OR team will be able to continue to provide a latex-free intraoperative environment	

NURSING DIAGNOSIS   Acute pain (postoperative) related to effects of surgical removal of tonsils and adenoids

EXPECTED OUTCOME   8/9/12—Throughout the perioperative period, the child will:

- Verbalize decreased level of pain in her throat
- Demonstrate/report adequate pain control

Nursing Interventions	Rationale	Evaluative Statement
Assess for pain using age-appropriate pain scale and report to physician or anesthesiologist	Pain is subjective. Caregivers need to be aware of patient's perception. Pre-emptive (before the painful event) analgesia may protect the patient from awakening with severe postop pain, nausea, and vomiting.	8/9/12. Outcome met. CRNA gave 0.5 mg of midazolam IV before transfer to OR. Patient is sleeping quietly. *C. Smith, RN*
Implement pain control measures as needed	Pain control measures may be necessary to ensure patient's comfort.	8/10/12 Outcome met. Pain medication administered as requested by child's mother; child reports decreasing pain in her throat. *C. Smith, RN*

SAMPLE DOCUMENTATION   8/9/12

Patient and parent identified on admission to preop holding area. Patient expressed mild fear of procedure, and separation from parents. Patient made comfortable with warm blankets and sitting on mother's lap after donning OR pajamas. Assessed for knowledge of impending procedure. Preop teaching reinforced. Assurance given about pain and latex allergy management protocol. Concerns reported to anesthesia provider and OR team. CRNA gave 0.2 mg midazolam IV before transfer to OR. Patient calm and sleeping quietly on transfer. Patient accompanied by toy stuffed bunny named "Bunny." No signs or symptoms of latex reaction on transfer to OR.

C. Smith, RN

Skill · 30-1 Providing Preoperative Patient Care: Hospitalized Patient

EQUIPMENT (will vary depending on the type of surgery)

- Blood pressure cuffs
- Electronic blood pressure machine
- Pulse oximeter sensors
- IV pump
- Antiembolism stockings
- Pneumatic compression stockings
- Tubes, drains, vascular access tubing
- Incentive spirometer
- Small pillow
- Personal protective equipment (PPE), as indicated

IMPLEMENTATION

ACTION	RATIONALE
1. Check the patient's chart for the type of surgery and review the medical orders. Review the nursing database, history, and physical examination. Check that the baseline data are recorded; report those that are abnormal.	These checks ensure that the care will be provided for the right patient and any specific teaching based on the type of surgery will be addressed. Also, this review helps to identify patients who are at increased surgical risk.
2. **Check that diagnostic testing has been completed and results are available; identify and report abnormal results.**	This check may influence the type of surgery performed and anesthetic used, as well as the timing of surgery or the need for additional consultation.
3. Gather the necessary supplies and bring to the bedside stand or overbed table.	Preparation promotes efficient time management and organized approach to the task. Bringing everything to the bedside conserves time and energy. Arranging items nearby is convenient, saves time, and avoids unnecessary stretching and twisting of muscles on the part of the nurse.
4. Perform hand hygiene and put on PPE, if indicated.	Hand hygiene and PPE prevent the spread of microorganisms. PPE is required based on transmission precautions.
5. Identify the patient.	Identifying the patient ensures the right patient receives the intervention and helps prevent errors.
6. Close curtains around bed and close door to room if possible. Explain what you are going to do and why you are going to do it to the patient.	This ensures the patient's privacy. Explanation relieves anxiety and facilitates cooperation.
7. Explore the psychological needs of the patient related to the surgery as well as the family.	Meeting the psychological needs of the patient and family before surgery can have a beneficial effect on the postoperative course.
a. Establish the therapeutic relationship, encouraging the patient to verbalize concerns or fears.	
b. Use active learning skills, answering questions and clarifying any misinformation.	
c. Use touch, as appropriate, to convey genuine empathy.	
d. Offer to contact spiritual counselor (priest, minister, rabbi) to meet spiritual needs.	Spiritual beliefs for some patients and family can provide a source of support over the perioperative course.
8. **Identify learning needs of patient and family.** Ensure that the informed consent of the patient for the surgery has been signed, witnessed, and dated. Inquire if the patient has any questions regarding the surgical procedure (Figure 1). Check the patient's record to determine if an advance directive has been completed. If an advance directive has not been completed, discuss with the patient the possibility of completing as appropriate. If patient has had surgery before, ask about this experience.	This enhances surgical recovery and allays anxiety by preparing patient for postoperative convalescence, discharge plans, and self-care. The surgeon is responsible for explaining the details of the surgical procedure and potential risks and complications. The nurse is responsible for clarifying what the surgeon has explained to the patient and contacting the surgeon if the patient does not understand or has further questions. An advance directive provides written communication of the patient's wishes to the healthcare team related to the patient's desire for extraordinary life-sustaining treatments if the patient's condition is deemed unsalvageable. Previous surgical experience may impact preoperative care positively or negatively, depending on this past experience.

(continued)

Skill · 30-1   Providing Preoperative Patient Care: Hospitalized Patient   *continued*

ACTION	RATIONALE
9. Provide teaching about deep-breathing exercises. (See Guidelines for Nursing Care 30-1 for specific technique.)	Deep-breathing exercises improve lung expansion and volume, help expel anesthetic gases and mucus from the airway, and facilitate the oxygenation of body tissues.
10. Provide teaching regarding coughing and splinting (providing support to the incision). (See Guidelines for Nursing Care 30-2 for specific technique.)	Coughing helps remove retained mucus from the respiratory tract. Splinting minimizes pain while coughing or moving.
11. Provide teaching regarding incentive spirometer (Figure 2). (See Chapter 39, Guidelines for Nursing Care 39-1.)	Incentive spirometry improves lung expansion, helps expel anesthetic gases and mucus from the airway, and facilitates oxygenation of body tissues.

FIGURE 1. Identifying the needs of the patient and answering questions.

FIGURE 2. An incentive spirometer helps increase lung volume and promotes inflation of the alveoli.

12. Provide teaching regarding leg exercises (as appropriate).	Leg exercises assist in preventing muscle weakness, promote venous return, and decrease complications related to venous stasis. Leg exercises may be contraindicated for patients with certain conditions, such as lower extremity fractures.
13. Assist the patient in putting on antiembolism stockings and demonstrate how the pneumatic compression device operates. (Refer to Chapter 33 for specific information.)	Antiembolism stockings and pneumatic compression devices are used postoperatively for patients who are at risk for a deep-vein thrombosis (DVT) and pulmonary embolism.
14. Provide teaching regarding turning in the bed.	Turning and repositioning of the patient is important for prevention of postoperative complications and for minimizing pain.

a. Instruct the patient to use a pillow or bath blanket to splint where the incision will be. Ask the patient to raise his or her left knee and reach across to grasp the right side rail of the bed when he/she is turning toward his or her right side (Figure 3). If patient is turning to his or her left side, he or she will bend the right knee and grasp the left side rail.

b. When turning the patient onto his or her right side, ask the patient to push with bent left leg and pull on the right side rail (Figure 4). Explain to patient that the nurse will place a pillow behind his/her back to provide support, and that the call bell will be placed within easy reach (Figure 5).

c. Explain to the patient that position change is recommended every 2 hours.

ACTION

FIGURE 3. Instructing patient to raise the left knee and reach across to grasp the right side rail toward which she will be turning.

RATIONALE

FIGURE 4. Helping patient to roll over to her right side while she pushes with the left bent leg and pulls on the side rail.

FIGURE 5. After patient is turned, provide support with pillows behind the patient's back.

15. Provide teaching about pain management.

   a. Discuss past experiences with pain and interventions that the patient has used to reduce pain.

   b. Discuss the availability of analgesic medication postoperatively.

   c. Discuss the use of patient controlled analgesia (PCA), as appropriate. (Refer to Chapter 35.)

   d. Explore the use of other alternative and nonpharmacologic methods to reduce pain such as position change, massage, relaxation/diversion, guided imagery, and meditation.

Using ordered analgesics to minimize pain helps prevent postoperative complications.

Past experiences with pain can impact patient's ability to manage the pain of surgery. Pain is a subjective experience and individuals vary on what interventions are effective in reducing pain.

Depending on the physician's order, the patient may need to request analgesic medication as needed, or a PCA (patient-controlled analgesia) or epidural analgesia may be ordered, for which patient will need specific instruction on how to use. See Chapter 10 for more information.

Patient understanding of the use of PCA is crucial for effective, safe administration.

These measures may reduce anxiety and may decrease the amount of pain medication that is needed. Analgesic therapy should involve a multimodal approach influenced by age, weight, and comorbidities.

(continued)

Skill · 30-1   Providing Preoperative Patient Care: Hospitalized Patient *continued*

ACTION	RATIONALE
16. Review equipment that may be used.	
a. Show the patient various equipment such as IV pumps, electronic blood pressure cuff, tubes, and surgical drains.	Knowledge can reduce anxiety about equipment. The patient may need an indwelling urinary (Foley) catheter during and after surgery to keep the bladder empty and to monitor urinary output. Drains are frequently used to remove excess fluid around the surgical incision.
17. Provide skin preparation.	
a. **Ask the patient to bathe or shower with the antiseptic solution. Remind the patient to clean the surgical site.**	An antiseptic shower may be ordered 1 or 2 days before surgery and repeated the morning of surgery to begin the process of preparing the skin before surgery and to prevent infection. Recent research advises against hair removal of the surgical site due to increased potential for infection. The CDC recommends that if shaving is necessary, it should be performed immediately before the surgery, using disposable supplies and aseptic technique. Follow agency policy regarding skin preparation of the surgical patient. In addition, immediately before the surgical procedure, the skin of the patient's operative site will be cleansed with a product that is compatible with the antiseptic used for showering.
18. Provide teaching about following dietary/fluid restrictions.	
a. **Explain to the patient that both food and fluid will be restricted before surgery to ensure that the stomach contains a minimal amount of gastric secretions. This restriction is important to reduce the risk of aspiration. Emphasize to the patient the importance of avoiding food and fluids during the prescribed time period, since failure to adhere may necessitate cancellation of the surgery.**	Common practice in preparation for surgery has included having the patient fast after midnight, nothing by mouth (NPO) the night before surgery. At times, this restriction involved fasting up to 10 to 12 hours when surgery was performed in the later part of the next day. Recent research on both adults and children is challenging this NPO standard or fasting practice before surgery, claiming that a less restricted fluid intake of clear fluids could be safely taken up to 2 hours before surgery for individuals who are considered low risk for aspiration or regurgitation, depending on the type of surgery (America Society of Anesthesiologists, 1999). **Follow agency policy regarding the time period when this restriction will need to be followed.**
19. Provide intestinal preparation, as appropriate. In certain situations, the bowel will need to be prepared through the administering of enemas or laxatives to evacuate the bowel and to reduce the intestinal bacteria.	This preparation will be needed when major abdominal, perineal, perianal, or pelvic surgery is planned.
a. **As needed, provide explanation of the purpose of enemas or laxatives before surgery. If patient will be administering an enema, clarify the steps as needed.**	Enemas can be stressful, especially when repeated enemas are required to obtain a clear fluid return. Repeated enemas may cause fluid and electrolyte imbalance, orthostatic hypotension, and weakness. Follow safety precautions to guard against patient falls. Anesthetic agents and abdominal surgery can interfere with normal elimination function during the initial postoperative period. Refer to Chapter 13 to review skill for enema administration.
20. **Check administration of regularly scheduled medications.** Review with patient routine medications, over-the-counter medications, and herbal supplements that are taken regularly. Check the physician's orders and review with patient which meds he/she will be permitted to take the day of surgery.	Many patients take medications for a variety of chronic medical conditions. Adjustments in taking these medications may be needed before surgery. Certain medications such as aspirin are stopped days before surgery due to their anticoagulant effect. Certain cardiac and respiratory drugs may be taken the day of surgery per physician's order. If the patient is diabetic and takes insulin, the insulin dosage may be reduced.
21. Remove PPE, if used. Perform hand hygiene.	Removing PPE properly reduces the risk for infection transmission and contamination of other items. Hand hygiene prevents the spread of microorganisms.

DOCUMENTATION
Guidelines

Document that the patient's records were reviewed, including the history, physical assessment, and any laboratory values and diagnostic studies. Record that the surgeon was notified of any abnormal values. Document the components of perioperative teaching that were reviewed with the patient and family if present, such as use of the incentive spirometer, deep-breathing exercises, splinting, leg exercises, antiembolism (T.E.D.) stockings, and pneumatic compression devices. Record the patient's ability to demonstrate the skills and response to the teaching, and note if any follow-up instruction needs to be performed. Document other preoperative teaching, including pain management, intestinal preparation, medications, and preoperative skin preparation. Record any patient concerns about the surgery and whether the surgeon was contacted to provide any further explanations. Document the emotional support that was offered to the patient and if a spiritual counselor was notified per request of patient.

Sample Documentation

4/2/12 1030 Patient's records were reviewed and no abnormal results were identified. Perioperative teaching points reviewed with patient and her husband, including the rationale for each of these points. Patient demonstrated proper use of incentive spirometry, deep breathing, splinting while coughing, and leg exercises. Reviewed pain management, intestinal preparation, medications, and preoperative skin preparation. Patient stated that she was anxious about the surgery since this will be her first time to the operating room. Emotional support and reassurance were provided.

—J. Grabbs, RN

UNEXPECTED SITUATIONS AND ASSOCIATED INTERVENTIONS

- *A patient's laboratory results are noted to be abnormal:* Notify primary care provider. Some abnormalities, such as an elevated INR (indicating problems with the ability of the blood to clot) or abnormalities in the CBC may postpone the surgery.
- *A patient says to you, "I'm not sure I really want this surgery":* Discuss with the patient why he or she feels this way. Notify primary care provider. Patients should not undergo surgery until they are sure that surgery is what they want.

SPECIAL CONSIDERATIONS
General Considerations

- Obese patients are at greater risk of surgical complications and death compared to optimal-weight patients. In taking this patient's history, the nurse needs to be alert for other medical conditions such as diabetes, hypertension, and sleep apnea.

Infant and Child Considerations

- Children have special needs related to their overall health, age, and size. Easing preoperative anxiety of the child is crucial and includes using simple and concrete terms when providing information.
- The nurse needs to be sensitive to the anxiety level of the parent and provide support, explanations, and patient teaching as needed.
- Accurate weights are essential for correct medication dosages.
- Developmentally appropriate pain assessment and therapy needs to be followed to ensure adequate pain management.

Older Adult Considerations

- Age-related changes and preexisting chronic conditions can affect the postoperative course of the older adult patient.
- It is important to present preoperative teaching information slowly with reinforcement, since processing of information can be slower.
- Pain assessment and therapy may be suboptimal due to communication barriers and comorbidities present in many older adult patients. These patients may respond differently to pain medication, therefore, careful and individualized attention is required in this more vulnerable age group.

Skill · 30-2   Providing Postoperative Care When Patient Returns to Room

EQUIPMENT (will vary depending upon the surgery)

- Electronic blood pressure machine
- Blood pressure cuff
- Electronic thermometer
- Pulse oximeter

- Stethoscope
- IV pump, IV solutions
- Antiembolism stockings
- Pneumatic compression devices

- Tubes, drains, vascular access tubing
- Incentive spirometer
- PPE, as indicated
- Blankets, as needed

IMPLEMENTATION

ACTION

RATIONALE

Immediate Care

1. When patient returns from the PACU, obtain a report from the PACU nurse and review the operating room and PACU data.

Obtaining report ensures accurate communication and promotes continuity of care.

2. Perform hand hygiene and put on PPE, if indicated.

Hand hygiene and PPE prevent the spread of microorganisms. PPE is required based on transmission precautions.

3. Identify the patient.

Identifying the patient ensures the right patient receives the intervention and helps prevent errors.

4. Close curtains around bed and close door to room if possible. Explain what you are going to do and why you are going to do it to the patient.

This ensures the patient's privacy. Explanation relieves anxiety and facilitates cooperation.

5. **Place patient in safe position (semi- or high Fowler's or side-lying). Note level of consciousness.**

A sitting position facilitates deep breathing; the side-lying position with neck slightly extended prevents aspiration and airway obstruction. Alternate positions may be appropriate based on the type of surgery.

6. **Obtain vital signs. Monitor and record vital signs frequently.** Assessment order may vary, but usual frequency includes taking vital signs every 15 minutes the first hour, every 30 minutes the next 2 hours, every hour for 4 hours, and finally every 4 hours.

Comparison with baseline preoperative vital signs may indicate impending shock or hemorrhage. Some institutions use a paper or computer flow sheet to record initial postoperative data.

7. Assess the patient's respiratory status. (Refer to Chapter 25.) Measure the patient's oxygen saturation level (Figure 1).

Comparison with baseline preoperative respiratory assessment may indicate impending respiratory complications.

FIGURE 1. Obtaining postoperative oxygen saturation level.

8. Assess the patient's cardiovascular status. (Refer to Chapter 25.)

Comparison with baseline preoperative cardiovascular assessment may indicate impending cardiovascular complications.

9. Assess the patient's neurovascular status, based on the type of surgery performed. (Refer to Chapter 25.)

Comparison with baseline preoperative neurovascular assessment may indicate impending neurovascular complications.

ACTION

10. Provide for warmth, using heated or extra blankets as necessary (Figure 2). Assess skin color and condition.

11. Check dressings for color, odor, presence of drains, and amount of drainage (Figure 3). Mark the drainage on the dressing by circling the amount and include the time. Turn the patient to visually assess under the patient for bleeding from the surgical site.

RATIONALE

The operating room is a cold environment. Hypothermia is uncomfortable and may lead to cardiac arrhythmias and impaired wound healing.

Hemorrhage and shock are life-threatening complications of surgery and early recognition is essential.

FIGURE 2. Providing comfort and warmth to the patient.

FIGURE 3. Checking the dressings for color, odor, and amount of drainage.

12. Verify that all tubes and drains are patent and equipment is operative; note amount of drainage in collection device. If an indwelling urinary (Foley) catheter is in place, note urinary output.

13. Verify and maintain IV infusion at correct rate.

14. Assess for and relieve pain by administering medications ordered by physician. If patient has been instructed in use of PCA for pain management, review use. Check record to verify if analgesic medication was administered in the PACU.

15. Provide for a safe environment. Keep bed in low position with side rails up, based on facility policy. Have call bell within patient's reach.

16. Remove PPE, if used. Perform hand hygiene.

Ongoing Care

17. Promote optimal respiratory function.

    a. Assess respiratory rate, depth, quality, color, and capillary refill. Ask if the patient is experiencing any difficulty breathing.

This ensures maintenance of vital functions.

This replaces fluid loss and prevents dehydration and electrolyte imbalances.

Observe for nonverbal behavior that may indicate pain such as grimacing, crying, and restlessness. Analgesics and other nonpharmacologic pain strategies are used for relief of postoperative pain.

This prevents accidental injury. Easy access to call bell permits patient to call for nurse when necessary.

Removing PPE properly reduces the risk for infection transmission and contamination of other items. Hand hygiene prevents transmission of microorganisms.

Anesthetic agents may depress respiratory function. Patients who have existing respiratory or cardiovascular disease, have abdominal or chest incisions, who are obese, elderly, or in a poor state of nutrition are at greater risk for respiratory complications.

Postoperative analgesic medication can reduce the rate and quality of the respiratory effort.

(continued)

Skill · 30-2   Providing Postoperative Care When Patient Returns to Room   *continued*

ACTION

b. Assist with coughing and deep-breathing exercises (Refer to Guidelines for Nursing Care 30-1 and 30-2).

c. Assist with incentive spirometry.

d. Assist with early ambulation.

e. Provide frequent position change.

f. Administer oxygen, as ordered.

g. Monitor pulse oximetry.

18. Promote optimal cardiovascular function:

a. Assess apical rate, rhythm, and quality and compare to peripheral pulses, color, and blood pressure. Ask if the patient has any chest pains or shortness of breath.

b. Provide frequent position changes.

c. Assist with early ambulation.

d. Apply antiembolism stockings or pneumatic compression devices, if ordered and not in place. If in place, assess for integrity.

e. Provide leg and range-of-motion exercises if not contraindicated.

19. Promote optimal neurologic function:

a. Assess level of consciousness, motor, and sensation.

b. Determine the level of orientation to person, place, and time.

c. Test motor ability by asking the patient to move each extremity.

d. Evaluate sensation by asking the patient if he or she can feel your touch on an extremity.

20. Promote optimal renal and urinary function and fluid and electrolyte status. Assess intake and output, evaluate for urinary retention, and monitor serum electrolyte levels.

a. Promote voiding by offering bedpan at regular intervals, noting the frequency, amount, and if any burning or urgency symptoms.

b. Monitor urinary catheter drainage if present.

c. Measure intake and output.

21. Promote optimal gastrointestinal function and meet nutritional needs:

a. Assess abdomen for distention and firmness. Ask if patient feels nauseated, any vomiting, and if passing flatus.

b. Auscultate for bowel sounds.

c. Assist with diet progression, encourage fluid intake, and monitor intake.

d. Medicate for nausea and vomiting as ordered by physician.

RATIONALE

Preventive measures can improve venous return and circulatory status.

Anesthetic and pain management agents can alter neurological function.

Older patients may take longer to return to their level of orientation before surgery. Drug and anesthetics will delay this return.

Anesthesia alters motor and sensory function.

Anesthetic agents and surgical manipulation in the area may temporarily depress bladder tone and response causing urinary retention.

Frequency, burning, or urgency may indicate possible urinary tract abnormality.

The primary care provider needs to be notified if the urinary output is less than 30 mL/hr or 240 mL/8-hr period.

Intake and output are good indicators of fluid balance.

Anesthetic agents and narcotics depress peristalsis and normal functioning of gastrointestinal tract. Flatus indicates return of peristalsis.

Presence of bowel sounds indicates return of peristalsis.

Patients may experience nausea post surgery and are encouraged to resume diet slowly, starting with clear liquids and advancing as tolerated.

Antiemetics are frequently ordered to alleviate postoperative nausea.

ACTION

22. Promote optimal wound healing.

  a. Assess condition of wound for presence of drains and any drainage.

  b. Use surgical asepsis for dressing changes.

  c. Inspect all skin surfaces for beginning signs of pressure ulcer development and use pressure-relieving supports to minimize potential skin breakdown.

23. Promote optimal comfort and relief from pain.

  a. Assess for pain (location and intensity using scale).

  b. Provide for rest and comfort; provide extra blankets as needed for warmth.

  c. Administer pain medications, as needed, or other nonpharmacologic methods.

24. Promote optimal meeting of psychosocial needs:

  a. Provide emotional support to patient and family, as needed.

  b. Explain procedures and offer explanations regarding postoperative recovery as needed to both patient and family members.

RATIONALE

Alterations in nutritional, circulatory, and metabolic status may predispose patient to infection and delayed healing.

Surgical asepsis reduces the risk of infection.

Lying on the operating room table in the same position can predispose some patients to pressure ulcer formation, especially in patients who have undergone surgery lasting more than 4 hours.

This shortens recovery period and facilitates return to normal function.

Control of postoperative pain promotes patient comfort and recovery.

Patients may experience chilling in the postoperative period.

This facilitates individualized care, anxiety reduction, and patient's return to normal health.

DOCUMENTATION

Guidelines

Document the time that the patient returns from PACU to the surgical unit. Record the patient's level of consciousness, vital signs, all assessments, and condition of dressing. If patient has oxygen running, an IV, or any other equipment, record this information. Document the pain assessment and interventions that were instituted to alleviate this pain, as well as the patient's response to the interventions. Document any patient teaching that is reviewed with the patient, such as use of incentive spirometer.

Sample Documentation

4/10/12 1330 Patient returned to room at 1315, drowsy but easily answers to name. Patient's temperature 98.8°F, pulse 78, BP 122/84, O2 sat 96% on O2 2L/min. Right lower abdominal dressing dry and intact. Rates pain at a "4" on scale of 1–10, was medicated in PACU with 10-mg morphine sulfate IV at 10:30. Incentive spirometry completed × 10 cycles, 750 mL each. Patient deep breathing and coughing without production and turned to right side with HOB elevated. See flow sheet for additional system assessments.

—J. Grabbs, RN

UNEXPECTED SITUATIONS AND ASSOCIATED INTERVENTIONS

- *Vital signs are progressively increasing or decreasing from baseline:* Notify primary care provider. A continued decrease in blood pressure or an increase in heart rate could indicate internal bleeding.

- *Dressing was clean before but now has large amount of fresh blood:* Do not remove dressing. Reinforce dressing with more bandages. Removing the bandage could dislodge any clot that is forming and lead to further blood loss. Notify primary care provider.

- *Patient reports pain that is not relieved by ordered medication:* After fully assessing pain (location, description, alleviating factors, causal factors), notify primary care provider. Pain can be a clue to other problems, such as hemorrhage.

- *Patient is febrile within 12 hours of surgery:* Assist patient with coughing and deep breathing. If ordered, begin incentive spirometry. Continue to monitor vital signs and laboratory values, such as complete blood count (CBC).

(continued)

Skill · 30-2   Providing Postoperative Care When Patient Returns to Room   *continued*

- *Adult patient has a urine output of less than 30 mL per hour:* Unless this is expected, notify primary care provider. Urine output is a good indicator of tissue perfusion. Patient may need more fluid or may need medication to increase blood pressure if it is low.

SPECIAL CONSIDERATIONS

General Considerations

- Be aware of baseline sensory deficits. Ensure appropriate aids are in place, such as glasses or hearing aids. Lack of appropriate aids may impact postoperative assessments, such as level of consciousness.
- For patients undergoing throat surgery, such as a tonsillectomy, evaluate swallowing pattern. A patient who has had throat surgery and swallows frequently may be bleeding from the incision site.
- In the obese patient, medications may not perform as expected related to the lack of serum proteins that are needed to bind with drugs to support their effectiveness. Additionally, due to the larger kidney mass of the obese patient, renal elimination rates of certain drugs are increased, reducing the effectiveness of these drugs.
- Check to make sure that the mattress for the obese patient is of high quality, since this patient is at greater risk for skin breakdown due to the poor vascular supply of adipose tissue.
- Ensure that written postoperative instructions specific to the patient and follow-up appointments with the surgeon or other healthcare professionals are provided to each patient upon discharge from the hospital or outpatient center. Information such as signs and symptoms to report to the primary care provider as well as restrictions in activity and diet need to be addressed. In addition, patients discharged the same day as their surgery are required to have a responsible individual accompany them home, and a contact telephone number is to be provided in case of emergency. The patient should be alert and oriented, or mental status should be at the patient's baseline. The vital signs of the patient should be stable.

Infant and Child Considerations

- Postoperative complications are related to the respiratory system in this age group. After receiving general anesthesia, premature infants are at greater risk for apnea.
- Infants and children are at great risk for temperature-related complications since their body temperature can change rapidly. It is essential to have warmed blankets and other warming equipment available to avoid this complication.

Older Adult Considerations

- In the older adult patient, postoperative pneumonia can be a very serious complication resulting in death. Therefore, it is especially important to encourage and assist the patient in using the incentive spirometer and with deep-breathing exercises.
- Older patients may take longer to return to their level of orientation before surgery. Drugs and anesthetics will delay this return.

● Developing Critical Thinking Skills

1. You are providing the immediate preoperative care for a woman scheduled for surgery to remove a brain tumor. She tells you she does not want the surgery because she knows she is dying and just wants to go home to be with her husband and children. She also knows that her husband cannot accept the fact that she is dying and wants her to have the surgery. What do you do?

2. You are assigned to discharge a woman from your same-day surgery unit to her home. You strongly believe that she is not ready to go home, and there is no caregiver in her home. When you voice your concern to the surgeon, you are told that this is not your problem and that there is noth-ing anyone can do about the situation because her insurer will not approve hospitalization. How do you respond?

● Practicing for NCLEX

1. The nurse is preparing Mrs. Ogg for surgery for treatment of a ruptured spleen as the result of an automobile crash. The nurse knows that this type of surgery belongs in which of the following categories?
   a. Minor, diagnostic
   b. Minor, elective
   c. Major, emergency
   d. Major, palliative

2. A group of students are reviewing the purposes of general anesthesia in preparation for a test. The students demonstrate a need for additional study when they identify which of the following as a purpose?
   a. Loss of consciousness
   b. Relaxation of skeletal muscles
   c. Reduction of reflex action
   d. Localized loss of sensation

3. A nurse has been asked to witness a patient signature on an informed consent form for surgery. For which one of these patients would the document be valid?
   a. A 92-year-old patient who is severely confused
   b. A 45-year-old patient who is oriented and alert
   c. A 10-year-old patient who is oriented and alert
   d. A 36-year-old patient who has had a narcotic premedication

4. A 72-year-old woman is taking several medications on a regular basis. Which of the following categories of drugs would be most likely to increase her surgical risk?
   a. Anticoagulants
   b. Antacids
   c. Laxatives
   d. Sedatives

5. A nurse is caring for an obese patient who has surgery. The nurse monitors this patient for which of the following postoperative complications?
   a. Hunger
   b. Impaired wound healing
   c. Hemorrhage
   d. Gas pains

6. A nurse is teaching a man scheduled to have same-day surgery. Which teaching method would be most effective in preoperative teaching for ambulatory surgery?
   a. Lecture
   b. Discussion
   c. Audiovisuals
   d. Written instructions

7. Mr. Ying is scheduled for surgery. He says to the nurse, "I am so frightened—what if I don't wake up?" What would be the best response?
   a. "You have a wonderful doctor."
   b. "Let's talk about how you are feeling."
   c. "Everyone wakes up from surgery!"
   d. "Don't worry, you will be just fine."

8. A patient asks a nurse what a PCA pump does. The nurse explains that a PCA pump allows postoperative patients to:
   a. Be totally pain free
   b. Take unlimited amounts of medication
   c. Choose the type of pain medication
   d. Administer their own analgesics

9. Mr. Moreno has had a surgical procedure that necessitated a thoracic incision. The nurse anticipates that he will have a higher risk for postoperative complications involving which body system?
   a. Respiratory system
   b. Circulatory system
   c. Digestive system
   d. Nervous system

10. While assessing a patient in the PACU, the nurse notes increased wound drainage, restlessness, a decreasing blood pressure, and an increase in the pulse rate. The nurse interprets these findings as most likely indicating which of the following?
    a. Thrombophlebitis
    b. Atelectasis
    c. Infection
    d. Hemorrhage

11. A patient tells the nurse she is having pain in her right lower leg. How does the nurse assess for the presence of thrombophlebitis?
    a. By palpating the skin over the tibia and fibula
    b. By documenting daily calf circumference measurements
    c. By recording vital signs obtained four times a day
    d. By noting difficulty with ambulation

12. Gas pains are a common postoperative discomfort. Which of the following nursing actions implemented in the plan of care would be most likely to relieve gas pains?
    a. Cough and deep breathe every 2 hours.
    b. Maintain NPO status for 48 hours.
    c. Encourage frequent ambulation.
    d. Take vital signs every 4 hours.

13. Which of the following surgical patients is at a greater risk for alterations in body image?
    a. A 19-year-old woman who had a repair of large facial laceration
    b. A 42-year-old woman who has had gallbladder surgery
    c. A 14-year-old boy who underwent a repair of a fractured clavicle
    d. A 52-year-old man who has had an inguinal hernia repair

14. Older adults often have reduced vital capacity as a result of normal physiologic changes. Which nursing intervention would be most important for the postoperative care of an older surgical patient specific to this change?
    a. Take and record vital signs every shift.
    b. Turn, cough, and deep breathe every 4 hours.
    c. Encourage increased intake of oral fluids.
    d. Assess bowel sounds daily.

15. The nurse is explaining the rationale for performing leg exercises after surgery. Which reason would the nurse include in the explanation?
    a. Promote respiratory function
    b. Maintain functional abilities
    c. Provide diversional activities
    d. Increase venous return

● Answers With Rationale

1. *c.* This surgery would involve a major body organ, has the potential for postoperative complications, requires hospitalization, and must be done immediately to save the patient's life.

2. *d.* A localized loss of sensation occurs with a regional anesthetic.

3. *b.* A consent form is not legal if the patient signing the form is confused, sedated, or a minor.

4. *a.* Anticoagulant drug therapy would increase the risk for hemorrhage during surgery.

5. *b.* Fatty tissue is less vascular and, therefore, less resistant to infection and more prone to delayed wound healing.

6. *d.* Written instructions are most effective in providing information for same-day surgery.

7. *b.* This answer allows the patient to talk about his feelings and fears and is therapeutic.

8. *d.* A PCA pump allows the patient to administer his or her own analgesic.

9. *a.* A thoracic incision makes it more painful for the patient to take deep breaths or cough. Shallow respirations and ineffective coughing increase the risk for respiratory complications.

10. *d.* Increased wound drainage, restlessness, decreasing blood pressure, and increasing pulse rate are assessment findings that indicate hemorrhage.

11. *b.* Inflammation from thrombophlebitis increases the size of the affected extremity and can be assessed by measuring circumference on a regular basis.

12. *c.* Frequent ambulation stimulates peristalsis and relieves gas pains.

13. *a.* Large facial wounds increase the risk for an alteration in body image.

14. *b.* Reduced vital capacity in older adults increases the risk for respiratory complications, including pneumonia and atelectasis. Having the patient turn, cough, and deep breathe every 4 hours maintains respiratory function and helps to prevent complications.

15. *d.* Leg exercises in the postoperative period increase venous return. As a result, the patient has a decreased risk for thrombophlebitis and emboli.

Taylor Suite Resources

The Taylor Suite offers these additional resources to enhance learning and facilitate understanding of this chapter:

- thePoint online resource, http://thepoint.lww.com/Taylor7E
- Student DVD-ROM included with the book
- Study Guide for Taylor's Fundamentals of Nursing

- Skill Checklists for Taylor's Fundamentals of Nursing
- Taylor's Clinical Nursing Skills: *Chapter 6, Perioperative Nursing*
- Taylor's Video Guide to Clinical Nursing Skills: *Perioperative Nursing Care*

BIBLIOGRAPHY

Algren, C. L., & Arnow, D. (2007). Pediatric variations of nursing interventions. In M. J. Hockenberry & D. Wilson (Eds.), *Wong's nursing care of infants and children*, (8th ed.) (pp. 1083–1139). St. Louis: Saunders Elsevier.

American Society of Anesthesiologists, Inc. (1999). Practice guidelines for preoperative fasting and the use of pharmacologic agents to reduce the risk of pulmonary aspiration: Application to healthy patients undergoing elective procedures. *Anesthesiology, 90*, 896–905.

American Society of PeriAnesthesia Nurses (ASPAN). (2008). *Standards of perianesthesia nursing practice.* Thorofare, NJ: American Society of PeriAnesthesia Nurses.

Association of periOperative Registered Nurses (AORN). (2006a). Perioperative patient focused model. *Standards, recommended practices, and guidelines.* Denver: AORN, Inc.

Association of periOperative Registered Nurses (AORN). (2006b). *AORN's age-specific competency series.* Denver: AORN, Inc.

Association of periOperative Registered Nurses (AORN). (2006c). Perioperative patient focused model. In *Standards, recommended practices, and guidelines.* Denver, CO: Author.

Association of periOperative Registered Nurses (AORN). (2008a). *Perioperative standards and recommended practices.* Denver: AORN, Inc.

Association of periOperative Registered Nurses (AORN). (2008b). AORN guidance statement: Postoperative patient care in the ambulatory surgery setting. In *Perioperative standards and recommended practices* (pp. 219–226). Denver: AORN, Inc.

Association of periOperative Registered Nurses (AORN). (2008c). Recommended practices for managing the patient receiving moderate sedation/analgesia. In *Perioperative standards and recommended practices* (pp. 461–472). Denver: AORN, Inc.

Association of periOperative Registered Nurses (AORN). (2008d). Perioperative patient outcomes. In *Perioperative Standards and recommended practices* (pp. 37–46). Denver: AORN, Inc.

Barash, P. G., Cullen, B. F., & Stoelting, R. K. (2006). *Clinical anesthesia* (5th ed.). Philadelphia: Lippincott Williams & Wilkins.

Cantrel, S. W., Ward, K. S., & Van Wicklen, S. A. (2007). Translating research on venous thromboembolism into practice. *AORN Journal, 86*(4), 590–602.

Clancy, C. M. (2008). The importance of simulation: Preventing hand-off mistakes. *AORN Journal, 88*(4), 625–627.

Crenshaw, J., & Winslow, E. (2002). Preoperative fasting: Old habits die hard. *American Journal of Nursing, 102*(5), 36–45.

DeFazio-Quinn, D. M. (2009). Perianesthesia nursing as a specialty. In C. B. Drain & J. Odon-Forren (Eds.), *Perianesthesia nursing: A critical care approach* (5th ed.) (pp. 11–31). St. Louis: Saunders Elsevier.

DiPaola, C. A. (2008). Preventing deep vein thrombosis: A perioperative nursing imperative. *AORN Journal, 88*(2), 283–285.

Edmiston, C. E., Krepel, C. J., Seabrook, C. R., Lewis, B., Brown, K., & Towne, J. (2008). Preoperative shower revisited: Can high topical antiseptic levels be achieved on the skin surface before surgical admission? *Journal of the American College of Surgery, 207*(2), 233–239.

Hodgson, B. B., & Kizior, R. J. (2007). *Saunders nursing drug handbook.* St. Louis: Saunders Elsevier.

Jacob, E. (2007). Pain assessment and management in children. In Hockenberry, M.J, & Wilson, D. *Wong's nursing care of infants and children* (8th ed.) (pp. 205–642). St. Louis: Saunders Elsevier.

Joint Commission. (2010). *National patient safety goals.* Available at http://www.jointcommission.org.

Nilsson, U. (2008). The anxiety- and pain-reducing effects of music interventions: A systematic review. *AORN Journal,* *87*(4), 780–807.

Odom-Forren, J. (2007). Accurate patient handoffs: Imperative for patient safety. *Journal of Perianesthesia Nursing, 22*(4), 233–234.

Patel, N., Bagen, B., Vadera, S., Gil Maltenfort, M., Deutsch, H., Vaccaro, A. A., et al. (2007). Obesity and spine surgery: Rela-tion to perioperative complications. *Journal of Neurosurgery and Spine* 6(4), 291–297.

Pop, R. S., Manworren, R., Guzzetta, C., Hynan, L. (2007). Peri-anesthesia nurses' pain management after tonsillectomy and adenoidectomy: Pediatric patient outcomes. *Journal of Perianesthesia Nursing, 22*(2), 91–101.

Rothrock, J. (2007). *Alexander's care of the patient in surgery* (13th ed.). St. Louis: Mosby Elsevier.

Susleck, D., Willocks, A., Secrest, J., Norwood, B. K., Holweger, J., Davis, M., et al. (2007). The perianesthesia experience from the patient's perspective. *Journal of Perianesthesia Nursing, 22*(1), 10–20.

PROMOTING HEALTHY PHYSIOLOGIC RESPONSES

The art and science of caring are blended when nurses implement actions to meet basic human needs and to promote healthy physiologic responses. The chapters in Unit VII focus on information and guidelines essential to nursing practice in a wide variety of clinical settings and involving both healthy and ill patients of all ages. Included are nursing interventions to promote safety and comfort and to meet basic physiologic needs: hygiene, activity and rest, nutrition, elimination, oxygenation, and fluid–electrolyte balance.

Each basic physiologic need is discussed first with a review of concepts pertinent to the specific area of human function and response and then with an examination of factors that affect need satisfaction. The steps of the nursing process are used to provide guidelines and information necessary for making accurate assessments, establishing outcomes, and planning, implementing, and evaluating specific nursing interventions to meet needs and promote wellness.

The chapters in Unit VII enable the beginning nurse to integrate the knowledge and skills necessary to promote healthy physiologic responses in patients in any practice setting. Nursing process skills are further refined to ensure that care is holistic, comprehensive, and individualized.

> " . . . what nursing has to do is to put the patient in the best condition for nature to act upon him. "

FLORENCE NIGHTINGALE (1820–1910) • *a philosopher, theorist, statistician, humanitarian, and inspirational leader who founded modern nursing through a systematic method of training well-qualified nurses; she also initiated important reforms in military sanitation and hospital construction that greatly improved patient survival*

31 Hygiene

KYLIE SIMPSON

Kylie, age 20, is a student at a state university. She had been having vaginal itching and burning for 2 weeks and went to the campus health clinic. She was diagnosed with a vaginal infection. She asks the nurse at the campus health clinic, "This is terrible. It's the second infection in 7 months. Is there something wrong with me? Isn't there something I can do to keep this from happening again?"

SONYA DELAMORDO

Sonya is an older Hispanic woman who has had a stroke (brain attack) resulting in right-sided paralysis. She is being discharged from the hospital and will now live with her daughter, who will be her primary caregiver. Her daughter is eager to learn everything she can about caring for her mother and asks numerous questions, including the best way to keep her mother clean.

ANDREW CRAIG

Andrew, age 68, has multiple diagnoses and limited mobility. He lives in an extended-care facility. Andrew needs assistance with his morning care. He tells the nurse, "I've already had a complete bath."

LEARNING OBJECTIVES

After completing the chapter, you will be able to accomplish the following:

1. Identify factors affecting personal hygiene.

2. Assess the adequacy of hygiene practices and self-care behaviors using appropriate interview and physical assessment skills.

3. Assess the condition of the patient's skin, oral cavity, hair, and nails using appropriate interview and physical assessment skills.

4. Develop nursing diagnoses that identify hygiene problems amenable to nursing intervention.

5. Describe the priorities of scheduled hygiene care.

6. Demonstrate techniques for assisting patients with hygiene measures, including those used when administering various types of baths and those used in cleaning each part of the body.

7. Describe agents commonly used on the skin and scalp, including any precautions necessary for their use.

8. Plan, implement, and evaluate nursing care for common problems of the skin and mucous membranes.

KEY TERMS

alopecia	halitosis
caries	pediculosis
cerumen	periodontitis
cheilosis	plaque
gingivitis	stomatitis
glossitis	tartar

Measures for personal cleanliness and grooming, called personal hygiene, promote physical and psychological well-being. Personal hygiene practices vary widely among people. It is important that personal care be carried out conveniently and frequently enough to promote personal hygiene and wellness. Illness, hospitalization, and institutionalization generally require modifications in hygiene practices. In these situations, the nurse helps the patient to continue sound hygiene practices and can teach the patient and family members, when necessary, regarding hygiene. Nurses assisting patients with basic hygiene must respect individual patient preferences, providing only the care that patients cannot, or should not, provide for themselves. In addition, nurses

should value each patient as an individual and take into consideration his or her physical, mental, and emotional state of being while providing hygiene care (see the accompanying Reflective Practice box).

This chapter discusses multiple factors that affect personal hygiene and nursing measures that promote personal hygiene. A practical guide for assessing the adequacy of personal hygiene is presented. The data collected when assisting with hygiene may lead to the identification of multiple nursing diagnoses and collaborative problems. Examples of such diagnoses and problems are provided. Patient outcomes are presented, as are specific nursing strategies used when performing care of the skin, mouth, eyes, ears, nose, feet, perineal areas, and vaginal areas. The concluding nursing plan of care related to feminine hygiene illustrates how the nurse uses knowledge of personal hygiene practices and the integumentary system, along with specific nursing interventions, to resolve nursing diagnoses and to promote the patient's general sense of well-being.

HYGIENE PRACTICES

Hygienic practices include caring for the skin, hair, nails, mouth, teeth, and perineal area. There are strong links between good hygiene practices and the health of a person. Inadequate hygiene practices can contribute to alterations in the health of a person.

The skin, or integument, is the largest organ of the body and has multiple functions. The integumentary system is made up of the skin, the subcutaneous layer directly under the skin, and the appendages of the skin, including the hair and nails. Chapter 32 provides a description of the anatomy and physiology of the integumentary system and factors that affect skin integrity. Personal hygiene practices play an integral role in caring for the integumentary system.

Hair is an accessory structure of the skin. Good general health is essential for attractive hair and skin, and cleanliness is a positive influence. Illness affects the hair, especially when endocrine abnormalities, increased body temperature, poor nutrition, or anxiety and worry are present. Changes in the color or condition of the hair shaft are related to changes in hormonal activity or to changes in the blood supply to hair follicles.

The nails are an accessory structure of the skin composed of epithelial tissue. Healthy nailbeds are pink, convex, and evenly curved. With certain pathologic conditions, and to some extent with aging, the nails become ridged and areas become concave. Hygienic care includes keeping the nails trimmed and clean.

A person's general health influences the health of his or her mouth and teeth, and proper care of the mouth and teeth lends to overall health. For example, there is an established relationship between healthy teeth and a diet sufficient in calcium and phosphorus, along with vitamin D, which is necessary for the body to make use of these minerals. Maintaining good oral hygiene and dental care has several benefits. There is esthetic value in having a clean and healthy mouth. Having one's own teeth contributes to an intact body

REFLECTIVE PRACTICE

Challenge to Interpersonal Skills

It was our first day of clinical, sophomore year, and we were instructed to do complete a.m. care with our patients. My patient, Andrew Craig, was a 68-year-old man with multiple diagnoses and limited mobility. As I entered the room, he told me he had just had a bed bath a few hours earlier. I wasn't sure what to do, so I asked the tech if my patient had already had a complete bed bath. The tech pulled me into the patient's room and proceeded to scream at the patient, telling him not to lie to me and threatening to make him sit in the chair all day. This patient did not have a hip and had antibiotic beads in the area, so it was very painful for him to sit in a chair because the beads dug into his side. The tech then told me to do the bed bath and left the room. I was left in a very awkward position because the patient was mad at me and I was astounded by how the tech had treated this patient. I was extremely upset as a result of this confrontation.

The day was emotionally very difficult for me, and when I arrived home, I became even more upset. The manner in which the tech treated the patient, even though the patient had a tendency to be manipulative, was completely out of line.

Thinking Outside the Box: Possible Courses of Action

- Make the best of a bad situation, but do nothing to change the status quo: "Hey, I'm only a student, right?"
- Confront the tech and tell her about my outrage.
- Report the tech to her supervisor.
- Consult with my instructor about how a professional nurse should respond in a situation like this.
- Be prepared to "go to the top" if initial attempts to reform a bad system don't meet with success.

Evaluating a Good Outcome: How Do I Define Success?

- The patient's basic hygiene needs are met.
- The patient's humanity and integrity are respected.
- Healthcare professionals and technicians are held accountable for incompetent, unethical, and illegal behavior (the tech, nursing leadership, and administration in this nursing home).
- I learn how to be a successful patient advocate.

Personal Learning: Here's to the Future!

I proceeded to talk to my clinical instructor and the coordinator of the class about the incident. The coordinator contacted the nursing home and I had to give a formal statement about the incident. The nurse manager who took my statement was not very receptive and was actually very patronizing.

This entire experience helped me to recognize the type of nurse I want to be. First and foremost, I always want to ensure that I provide a high-quality patient care. At the time of my unfortunate experience, I did not respond immediately to the tech's inappropriate comments. But now that I have gained more experience and become more confident, I would definitely respond immediately if a similar situation ever arose again. I realize that I can't let fear stand in my way when the quality of patient care is suffering. I would encourage any nurse who sees a colleague or anyone treating a patient without the utmost respect and care to speak up and contact appropriate personnel to discuss the situation.

In addition to this one tech's inappropriate behavior, the overall conditions of this nursing home were appalling. I learned a lot this semester about the shortage of nurses (1 RN for 40 patients) and, consequently, how patient care is being jeopardized. During the unfortunate episode to which I was exposed, I was astonished and outraged, but I didn't take any steps to change the conditions except reporting this one incident. At the end of the semester, we reported the conditions to the class coordinator. Now I realize that as an individual, I could have done more to change the conditions in the nursing home. In retrospect, I should have taken a leadership role and notified the outside licensing agency about these conditions (the nursing home ended up losing its accreditation that summer). All nurses are responsible for ensuring the quality of care given to patients, and we must contact whomever necessary to ensure changes are made.

This experience was very difficult for me, but in the end, I think it opened my eyes to the importance of nurses acting as leaders.

Catherine Barrell, Georgetown University

Reflection

How do you think you would respond in a similar situation? Why? What does this tell you about yourself and about the adequacy of your skills for professional practice? Can you think of other ways to respond? What other skills (cognitive, interpersonal, technical, ethical/legal) would you need to respond well in this situation? What factors may have played a role in the tech's answer to the patient and nursing student? How did the nursing student's actions adhere to ethical and legal principles? Did the nursing student act as a patient advocate? Why or why not? Is it within the nursing student's scope of practice to individually contact a higher authority such as a licensing agency about the situation? Discuss your answer. Do you agree with the criteria to evaluate a successful outcome? Did the nursing student meet the criteria? Please explain your answer.

image. In addition, the beginning of the digestive process and gustatory pleasure are enhanced when the mouth and teeth are in good condition.

The perineal area is dark, warm, and often moist, providing conditions that favor bacterial growth. The patient who cannot clean the perineal area needs the nurse's assistance for this important part of personal hygiene. Neglecting perineal cleaning for the patient who cannot provide self-care often results in physical and psychological discomfort for the patient, skin breakdown, and offensive odors.

FACTORS AFFECTING PERSONAL HYGIENE

Hygiene practices vary widely among groups and individuals. Hygiene activities and practices can protect health and prevent disease. It is important to respect differences in patient hygiene practices and provide care and information in a nonjudgmental manner. The following factors may influence personal hygiene behaviors.

Culture

It is important to identify cultural variations that could affect a patient's personal hygiene preferences, such as typical bathing habits, and behaviors, such as use of various hygiene-related products. For example, people from some cultures place a high value on personal cleanliness and feel unclean unless they shower or bathe at least once daily. Many consider bathing incomplete without the use of products to reduce or mask normal body odors. Other people often find a weekly bath sufficient and may feel no need to mask normal body odors. Culture may also influence whether bathing is a private or communal activity.

> *Consider Sonya Delamordo, the Hispanic woman being discharged to her daughter's home after experiencing a stroke. Although the daughter is very eager to take care of her mother, the nurse would need to investigate the patient's culture to determine how the patient might feel about being cared for by her daughter. Typically, hygiene is a personal matter. The nurse needs to discuss this area with the patient and her daughter to ensure competent care.* ∎

Socioeconomic Class

A person's socioeconomic class and financial resources often define the hygiene options available to him or her. Access to assistive services, such as shelters, may be limited for some patients. For example, a person renting a room in a boarding house may have limited or no access to a tub or shower and may have limited finances to buy soap, shampoo, shaving cream, and deodorant. Homeless people, who often carry all their belongings in a car or shopping cart, may welcome the warm running water and soap available in roadside or public restrooms.

Spiritual Practices

Spiritual practices, including religious beliefs, may dictate ceremonial washings and purifications, sometimes as a prelude to prayer or eating. For example, in the Orthodox Jewish tradition, ritual baths are required for women after childbirth and menstruation. In some religions, contact with a deceased person or a deceased animal may make a person "unclean." Other religions dictate that no modern facilities be installed in homes. This would prohibit some people from having running water and toilets in their homes. As a result, they may bathe infrequently.

Developmental Level

Children learn hygiene practices while growing up. Family practices often dictate hygiene habits, such as morning or evening baths; the frequency of shampooing, tooth brushing, and clothing changes; feelings about nudity; and so on. As adolescents become more concerned about their personal appearance, they may adopt new hygiene measures, such as taking showers more frequently and wearing deodorant. Bathing frequency commonly decreases as a person ages, possibly due to limitations in mobility and the natural tendency toward drier skin with age. In addition, older people may avoid the use of deodorant soaps to prevent excessive drying of the skin.

Health State

Disease, surgery, or injury may reduce a person's ability to perform hygiene measures or motivation to follow usual hygiene habits. Weakness, dizziness, and fear of falling may prevent an individual from entering a tub or shower or from bending to wash the lower extremities. Illness may also create a demand for new or modified hygiene measures. For example, the peripheral vascular complications that often accompany diabetes mellitus require meticulous foot care. The presence of pain with an acute condition or chronic pain can affect a person's ability to perform and/or tolerate personal hygiene measures.

> *Remember Sonya Delamordo, who has right-sided paralysis as a result of a stroke. She will have to adapt to caring for herself, dealing with the mobility limitations of her right side, especially if she is right handed. Both she and her daughter will have to learn how to adapt personal hygiene practices, based on Sonya's abilities.* ∎

Personal Preferences

People have different preferences with regard to hygiene practices such as taking a shower versus a tub bath, using bar soap versus liquid soap, and washing to wake oneself or to relax before sleep. A person's self-concept and sexuality also influence personal hygiene practices. For example, in an effort to promote a positive self-image, older adults may use skin care products advertised to prevent wrinkles and diminish signs of aging. Women who are sexually active may use a variety of hygiene products following intercourse that promote cleanliness.

THE NURSING PROCESS FOR SKIN CARE AND PERSONAL HYGIENE

Nurses who role model good health behaviors are more effective teachers. Promoting Health 31-1 suggests general behaviors to maintain acceptable personal hygiene. Use this display for yourself before using it with others.

Assessing

The comprehensive nursing assessment uses interview and physical assessment skills to elicit data about the patient's hygiene status. When alterations in a patient's physical or mental health state result in impaired ability to maintain acceptable personal hygiene, additional specific assessment skills are needed to determine the patient's limitations.

Nursing History

Bathing practices and cleansing habits and rituals vary widely. A clear threat to health must exist before a nurse decides that an individual's hygiene practices are inadequate. The nurse assessing the adequacy of a patient's hygiene practices determines whether the patient has the knowledge, attitude, skills, and resources to care for the skin and mucous membranes. Refer to Focused Assessment Guide 31-1.

Hygiene practices include bathing and care of the skin and specific body areas, including the oral cavity, eyes, ears, nose, hair, nails, feet, and perineal and vaginal areas.

SKIN

Question the patient about any past or current problems (e.g., rashes, lumps, itching, dryness, lesions). When skin problems are present, ask the patient the following:

- How long have you had this problem?
- Does it bother you?
- How does it bother you? Does it itch?
- Have you found anything that helps relieve these symptoms?

When documenting the nursing history, be specific, clearly describing the patient's typical hygiene practices and any complaints. The following are two examples of documentation related to hygiene and skin care:

Hygiene: "Showers twice daily, once in the morning and after working out in the evening. Skin tends to be very dry, and moisturizing creams are used daily. Aveeno Oilated baths p.r.n. Allergic to deodorant soaps."

Integument: "History of athlete's foot since high school days with outbreaks every 2 to 3 months. Knowledgeable about appropriate foot care. Uses antifungal agent

---

PROMOTING HEALTH • 31-1

Hygiene

Patients view nurses as role models for achieving healthy lifestyles. Use the assessment checklist to determine how well you are meeting your hygiene needs. Then develop a prescription for self-care by choosing appropriate behaviors from the list of suggestions. Information to promote healthy hygiene practices, such as information about dental health, exercise and fitness, skin care, and hair loss is available online. Check out these sites: MedlinePlus at http://medlineplus.gov and the National Women's Health Resource Center at http://www.healthywomen.org.

Assessment Checklist

☐ almost always   ☐ sometimes   ☐ almost never

☐ ☐ ☐   1. I keep my hair clean and neatly styled.

☐ ☐ ☐   2. My skin is clean.

☐ ☐ ☐   3. The condition of my mouth indicates satisfactory oral hygiene.

☐ ☐ ☐   4. My nails are neatly manicured.

☐ ☐ ☐   5. My body is free of unpleasant odors.

Self-Care Behaviors

1. Ensure that diet and exercise are appropriate, since this contributes to clean and intact skin.
2. Brush and floss teeth regularly and visit the dentist at least annually.
3. Keep hair clean, combed, and brushed regularly.
4. Use certain hair care products (e.g., hair dyes) cautiously, since they may damage the hair.
5. Clean under nails and maintain nails at an appropriate length. Clip nails straight across and shape or smooth with an emery board or file, if necessary.
6. Bathe and cleanse skin regularly. Apply lotion or cream to dry skin, as necessary. Cleanse the axilla and perineal area thoroughly and apply deodorant or antiperspirant as needed.
7. Appreciate the relationship between hygiene and overall well-being.

FOCUSED ASSESSMENT GUIDE • 31-1

HYGIENE PRACTICES

Factors to Assess	Questions and Approaches
Daily and weekly bathing habits	Tell me about your daily and weekly bathing habits. Are there special bathing or hygiene products you routinely use or can't use? How can nurses best help you to meet your hygiene needs?
Factors interfering with hygiene practices (sensory, cognitive, endurance, mobility, or motivation)	What recently or in the past has interfered with your hygiene practices? Does anything interfere with your ability to be as clean as you would like?
Pain	Do you have pain? Describe characteristics, onset, location, duration, associated symptoms, and intensity. Does the pain interfere with your ability to perform personal hygiene tasks? Does caring for yourself cause pain or discomfort?
Exposure history	Do you sunbathe? How much sun or tanning-booth exposure do you get? Do you use sunscreen? Does your job or daily activities/hobbies expose you to chemicals, such as bleach, petroleum, paint, insecticides, or cleaning products?
History of skin or mucous membrane problems (nature, onset of problem and frequency, causes, severity, symptoms, interventions attempted, results)	Describe any skin problems with rashes, lumps, itching, dryness, lesions, ecchymosis, or masses. What have you used to relieve these symptoms?
Special hygiene practices	
• Mouth	How do you clean your teeth and gums? How often do you have a dental examination? Do you have any dental appliances? Are there any tender areas or lesions in your mouth?
• Eyes, ears, and nose	Do you wear glasses or contact lenses to improve your vision? Do you wear a hearing aid? Have you experienced any discharge or bleeding from or swelling of your eyes, ears, or nose?
• Hair	Have you noticed any unusual dryness of the scalp or changes in hair texture and amount?
• Feet and nails	Is the appearance of the nails normal? How do you normally care for and clean your nails? Is the skin intact on the feet? Have you noticed any swelling of one or both feet? Do you wear any special shoes?
• Perineum	Have you noticed any unusual discharge, swelling, itching, or inflammation? Are you able to complete your own perineal care? Do you follow any special hygiene practices during menstruation? What type of feminine hygiene products (e.g., pads, tampons, douches) do you use?
• Piercings	Do you have any body piercings on your face, neck, arms, legs, torso, navel, or genitals? Have you experienced any problems related to the procedure? How do you care for your piercing(s)?

such as terbinafine hydrochloride (Lamisil DermaGel) or tolnaftate (Tinactin cream), a topical fungicidal agent."

ORAL CAVITY

Assessment of the oral cavity involves obtaining a nursing history related to the oral cavity, including structures such as the teeth, tongue, and salivary glands. When obtaining the nursing history, identify the patient's normal oral hygiene practices and the variables influencing these practices. Note the history of any oral problems and related treatments.

Identify any variables known to cause oral problems, such as deficient self-care abilities, poor nutrition or excessive intake of refined sugars, family history of periodontal disease, or ingestion of chemotherapeutic agents that produce oral lesions. Patients at increased risk for oral problems include those who are seriously ill, comatose, dehydrated, confused, depressed, or paralyzed. Patients who are mouth breathers, those who can have no oral intake of nutrition or fluids, those with nasogastric tubes or oral airways in place, and those who have had oral surgery are also at increased risk.

EYES, EARS, AND NOSE

Ask the patient to identify any special eye, ear, or nose care that he or she performs. Also, address any specific care measures related to the use and care of visual aids or prosthetics (glasses, contact lenses, artificial eye) and hearing aids. Inquire about any history of eye, ear, and nose problems, and related treatments.

HAIR

Identify the patient's usual hair and scalp care practices, including styling preferences. Note any history of hair or scalp problems; possible causes of changes in the distribution, texture, or amount of hair; and related treatments. Be alert for any factors that are known to cause hair or scalp problems or that require special care such as deficient self-care abilities, immobility, malnutrition, and treatments known to result in hair loss (e.g., certain chemotherapeutic agents).

NAILS AND FEET

Gather information about the patient's normal nail and foot care practices. Include the type of footwear worn and any history of nail or foot problems and their treatments. Foot problems, particularly common in people with diabetes mellitus and peripheral vascular disease, often require hospitalization (Agency for Healthcare Research and Quality [AHRQ], 2005). A proactive educational approach can prevent many of the serious complications (e.g., ulcers, lower extremity amputations) associated with foot problems.

Identify any variables known to cause nail and foot problems, such as deficient self-care abilities, vascular disease, arthritis, diabetes mellitus, history of biting nails or trimming them improperly, frequent or prolonged exposure to chemicals or water, trauma, ill-fitting shoes, or obesity.

PERINEAL AND VAGINAL AREAS

Note any history of perineal or vaginal problems and related treatments. Identify any variables known to cause perineal or vaginal problems or to create a need for special care, such as urinary or fecal incontinence, an indwelling Foley catheter, childbirth, douching, rectal or genital surgery, and diseases such as urinary tract infection, diabetes mellitus, and certain sexually transmitted infections (STIs) (e.g., herpes).

Physical Assessment

An assessment of pertinent body systems can provide data about the patient's hygiene status and the patient's ability to maintain acceptable personal hygiene.

MUSCULOSKELETAL SYSTEM

Impairment of the musculoskeletal system can interfere with a patient's ability to perform tasks related to personal hygiene. The skills used to assess the musculoskeletal system are described in detail in Chapters 25 and 33. Many conditions produce muscle weakness, decreased range of motion, impaired balance, fatigue, and/or lack of coordination.

SKIN

The inspection and palpation skills used to assess the integumentary system are described in detail in Chapter 25. Assisting patients with basic hygiene measures provides an excellent opportunity for examining a patient's skin. Many individuals are unaware that they have skin lesions, such as precancerous moles, that if untreated could prove fatal. Early detection and treatment of skin problems are important nursing functions.

When examining the skin, pay careful attention to cleanliness, color, texture, temperature, turgor, moisture, sensation, vascularity, and any lesions. If a lesion is detected, document the type, color, size, distribution and grouping, location, and consistency. Terminology helpful in describing these findings is presented in Chapter 25. Follow these general guidelines for assessing the skin:

- Proceed systematically in a head-to-toe fashion.
- Use a good source of light, preferably daylight.
- Compare bilateral parts for symmetry.
- Use standard terminology to report and record findings.
- Allow data obtained in the nursing history to direct the skin assessment.
- Identify any variables known to cause skin problems, such as deficient self-care abilities, immobility, malnutrition, decreased hydration, decreased sensation, sun exposure, vascular problems (altered tissue perfusion or venous return), or the presence of irritants (body secretions or excretions on the skin, other chemicals, mechanical devices).

Because lifestyle factors, changes in health state, illness, and certain diagnostic and therapeutic measures may adversely affect the skin, be alert for patients who may be at high risk for skin problems, and perform the appropriate skin assessment. Assessment may reveal dry skin, acne, or skin rashes. Table 31-1 summarizes recommended treatments for these skin problems.

TABLE • 31-1   SKIN CARE PROBLEMS

Skin Problem	Definition	Treatment
Dry Skin	The skin loses moisture and may crack and peel, or become irritated and inflamed. Symptoms include scaling, flaking, itching, and cracks in the skin.	• Keep baths or showers short, and/or bathe less frequently. • Use warm, not hot water to bathe. • Use as little soap as possible. Try mild cleansers or soaps. • Dry skin thoroughly and gently. • Use moisturizers at least daily. • Drink plenty of water throughout the day. • Use a humidifier if the air is dry.
Acne	A skin condition that is characterized by plugged pores (blackheads and whiteheads) and inflamed pimples (pustules). Hormones stimulate the sebaceous glands of the skin to enlarge, produce oil, and plug the pores.	• Avoid squeezing or picking infected areas because this can spread the infection and cause scarring. • Gently wash the face twice a day with a mild cleanser and warm (not hot) water. • Oil-free, water-based moisturizers and make-up should be used. Look for products that are "noncomedogenic" or "nonacnegenic." Use cosmetics sparingly to avoid further blockage of the sebaceous ducts. • Keep hair off the face and wash hair daily. • Some acne treatments (both over-the-counter and prescription) can increase the skin's sensitivity to sunlight and ultraviolet light. Avoid sun/tanning booth exposure; use sunscreen.
Skin rashes	Eruptions or inflammations of the skin that may be found anywhere on the body. May be precipitated by skin contact with an allergen, overexposure to the sun, and/or systemic causes, like a reaction to a medication.	• Wash area thoroughly with mild cleansing agent and rinse well. • Use a moisturizing lotion on a dry rash to prevent itching and promote healing. • Use a drying agent on a wet rash. • Try tepid baths to help relieve inflammation and itching. • Use antiseptic sprays or lotions to help lessen itching, promote healing, and prevent skin breakdown. • Avoid exposure to causative agent, if known. • See a physician if symptoms do not respond to treatment or become worse.

When documenting a physical assessment of the skin, describe exactly what is observed or palpated, including appearance, texture, size, location or distribution, and characteristics of any findings. The following are two examples of documentation of the physical assessment of the skin:

"Skin is pink, warm, dry, and elastic; no petechiae, lesions, or excoriation; multiple moles of small size and regular border and surface."

"Red, macular rash generalized over trunk and thighs; semi confluent lesions measure 1 to 2 mm; abrupt onset."

ORAL CAVITY

A physical assessment of the oral cavity involves inspection of the oral cavity and surrounding structures, with particular attention to any unusual odors. When performing the physical assessment of the oral cavity, examine the following:

• Lips: color, moisture, lumps, ulcers, lesions, and edema
• Buccal mucosa: color, moisture, lesions, nodules, and bleeding
• Color of the gums and surface of the gums: lesions, bleeding, edema, and exudate
• Teeth: any loose, missing, or carious (decayed) teeth. Note the presence of dentures or other orthodontic devices.
• Tongue: color, symmetry, movement, texture, and lesions
• Hard and soft palates: intactness, color, patches, lesions, and petechiae
• Oropharynx: movement of the uvula and condition of tonsils, if present

Also, note unusual mouth odors and assess the adequacy of mastication and swallowing. Refer to Chapter 25 for further description of nursing assessment of the oral cavity.

When inspecting the oral cavity, observe for any oral problems. These problems may be benign or only mildly annoying to patients, but they may also be life threatening. Identifying the problem and its cause and initiating appropriate treatment are imperative. This may require consultation with a dentist or physician.

Dental Caries

The decay of teeth with the formation of cavities is called **caries.** Caries result from failure to remove **plaque,** an invisible, destructive, bacterial film that builds up on everyone's teeth and eventually leads to the destruction of tooth enamel. A successful plaque-fighting program includes limiting sweet snacks such as soft drinks, candy, gum, jams, and jellies between meals; thorough cleansing of the teeth; and regular dental checkups. The use of antiplaque fluoride toothpastes, mouth rinses, and flossing also help prevent dental caries.

Periodontal Disease

The major cause of tooth loss in adults older than 35 years of age is gum disease. **Gingivitis** is an inflammation of the gingiva, the tissue that surrounds the teeth. **Periodontitis,** or periodontal disease, is a marked inflammation of the gums that also involves degeneration of the dental periosteum (tissues) and bone. Symptoms include bleeding gums; swollen, red, painful gum tissues; receding gum lines with the formation of pockets between the teeth and gums; pus that appears when gums are pressed; and loose teeth. If unchecked, plaque builds up and, along with dead bacteria, forms hard deposits called **tartar** at the gum lines. The tartar attacks the fibers that fasten teeth to the gums and eventually attacks bone tissue also. The teeth then loosen and fall out. **Halitosis,** a strong mouth odor or a persistent bad taste in the mouth, may be the first indication of periodontal disease. Regular treatment by a dentist is imperative.

Other Oral Problems

Other oral problems that may be observed when inspecting the oral cavity include the following:

- **Stomatitis,** an inflammation of the oral mucosa, has numerous causes, such as bacteria, virus, mechanical trauma, irritants, nutritional deficiencies, and systemic infection. Symptoms may include heat, pain, increased flow of saliva, and halitosis.
- **Glossitis,** an inflammation of the tongue, can be caused by deficiencies of vitamin B_{12}, folic acid, and iron.
- **Cheilosis,** an ulceration of the lips (reddened fissures at the angles of the mouth), is most often caused by vitamin B complex deficiencies (especially riboflavin).
- Dry oral mucosa may simply be related to dehydration or may be caused by mouth breathing, an alteration in salivary functioning, or certain medications (e.g., anticholinergic drugs).
- Oral malignancies, appearing as lumps or ulcers, must be distinguished from benign mouth problems because early detection may lead to cure; later detection can lead to radical surgery or death. Teach patients to see their dentist immediately if they notice white or red patches, persistent sores, swelling, bleeding, numbness, or pain in the mouth.

EYES, EARS, AND NOSE

During the eye examination, note the position, alignment, and general appearance of the eye. Check that eyelashes are distributed equally and curl outward. Note the presence of lesions, nodules, redness, swelling, crusting, flaking, excessive tearing, or discharge of eyelids. Check the color of the conjunctivae and test the patient's blink reflex. Assess the patient's gross visual acuity by having the patient read newsprint.

When examining the ear, note its position, alignment, and general appearance. Pay particular attention to a build-up of wax in the canal, dryness, crusting, or the presence of any discharge or foreign body. Older adults can have a build-up of cerumen that can cause impaired hearing. This is a result of harder, drier cerumen and decreased motility of the cilia in the ear canal. Test the patient's gross hearing acuity.

While examining the nose, note its position and general appearance, patency of the nostrils, and presence of tenderness, dryness, edema, bleeding, discharge, or secretions.

Refer to Chapter 25 for additional information related to nursing assessment of the eyes, ears, and nose.

HAIR

Assess the condition of the hair. Inspect it for texture, cleanliness, and oiliness. Inspect the scalp for any scaling, lesions, inflammation, or infection. Note any abnormalities such as dandruff, hair loss, or infestations. Patients of African American descent may have very dry scalps and dry, fragile hair; patients of Asian descent tend to have straight hair that does not necessarily require special care. When in doubt, ask the patient, a family member, or significant other about the specific manner in which hair care is performed.

Dandruff

Dandruff is a condition characterized by itching and flaking of the scalp and may be complicated by the embarrassment it causes. Persistent, severe cases usually require medical attention, but daily brushing and shampooing with a medicated shampoo may be all that is needed to keep the scalp free of dandruff.

Hair Loss

Hair growth and hair loss are ongoing, daily processes; hair loss becomes a potential problem only when it exceeds hair growth. Absence or loss of hair is called **alopecia.** Alopecia on the head is also referred to as baldness. Alopecia can be a partial or complete, local or generalized, loss of hair. Patchy hair loss can result from infections of the scalp. Hair loss from plaiting, excessive backcombing and teasing, or the use of hair rollers is usually temporary, and hair returns when the tension on the hair shaft is halted.

Excessive generalized hair loss may occur with infection, especially with high fever, nutritional deficiencies, hormonal disorders, childbirth, general anesthesia, drug toxicity, chemotherapy, thyroid disease, liver disease, hepatic and renal failure, and radiation. Some believe that an excessive intake of vitamin A may play a role in hair loss. Alopecia can also occur as part of the aging process. Alopecia related to aging is more common in men than women. There is no known cure for baldness, although some medications are currently in use and others are being developed; their long-term efficacy is unknown. For example, minoxidil (Rogaine), a cardiovascular and antihypertensive drug, has reversed balding to some degree when applied to the scalp. Hairpieces, frequently worn by people who are bald, require the same care as normal hair but less frequent washing.

Hair transplantation is a surgical procedure for baldness. Hair is taken from donor sites, usually from the back or sides of the scalp, and transplanted to areas with no hair. The procedure is long and expensive but reportedly has decided benefits for people who find baldness psychologically unpleasant. Complications include serious scalp infections.

Pediculosis

Infestation with lice is called **pediculosis.** There are three common types of lice: pediculus humanus capitis, which infests the hair and scalp; pediculus humanus corporis, which infests the body; and Phthirus pubis, which infests the shorter hairs on the body, usually the pubic and axillary hair. Lice lay eggs, called nits, on the hair shafts. Nits are white or light gray and look like dandruff but cannot be brushed or shaken off the hair. Frequent scratching and scratch marks on the body and the scalp suggest the presence of pediculosis.

Pediculosis can be spread directly by contact with the hair of infested persons. It is less common for transmission to occur indirectly through contact with clothing, bed linen, brushes, and combs of infested persons. Teaching patients, especially children, not to share personal items is a good way to prevent transmission. The importance of environmental measures is controversial. When necessary, sealing clothing in a plastic bag for 10 to 14 days is effective to kill lice. Headgear, pillowcases, and towels should be washed in hot water and dried on the hot cycle of the dryer.

Several commercial preparations, called pediculicides, are available for the treatment of pediculosis. These drugs destroy the lice and their eggs or nits. However, two treatments are usually necessary before all the nits are destroyed. The procedures and the medications used for the treatment of pediculosis vary among health agencies. The infested hair may be shaved, especially when pubic and axillary hair is infested. In addition, the partners of patients with pubic infestation must be notified.

When educating the patient, stress the importance of finishing the treatment. Many times the patient will shampoo the hair once and not follow through with a second washing. Failure to complete the treatment has produced lice that are now resistant to many of the pediculicides on the market. See Teaching Tips 31-1: Dealing With Head Lice.

TEACHING TIPS • 31-1

DEALING WITH HEAD LICE

Health Topic	Teaching Tip	Why Is This Important?
Who is at risk for getting head lice?	Preschool- and elementary-aged children (age 3–10) and their families are most often infested; however, anyone coming in contact with someone who has lice can become infected.	Lice can infect any person, regardless of hygiene practices or social status.
How do you become infected with head lice?	By coming in close contact with anyone who has lice; sharing combs, hats, clothing, coats, and scarves with anyone who has lice; lying on a bed, couch, pillow, carpet, or stuffed animal that has recently been in contact with someone who has lice.	One way to prevent the spread of lice is to avoid sharing combs and clothing with people outside of the family.
What are the signs and symptoms of head lice infestation?	Tickling feeling on scalp; itching; sores on the head caused by scratching. The lice may also be seen, especially behind the ears and near the neckline at the back of the neck.	The faster the lice are noticed, the easier they are to eradicate.
How is head lice treated?	Apply a pediculicide* according to the manufacturer's directions. Machine wash all washable clothing and bed linens using a hot water cycle. Dry laundry using high heat for at least 20 minutes. Store all clothing, stuffed animals, comforters, and other material things that cannot be washed or dry cleaned in a plastic bag for 2 weeks. Soak all brushes for 1 hour in rubbing alcohol. *Note: Women who are pregnant or breastfeeding should not use pediculicides. Consult a healthcare provider before using pediculicides on a person who has allergies, asthma, or other medical conditions.	All head lice must be killed or removed or a reinfestation may occur.

Information obtained from Centers for Disease Control (CDC). *Lice.* Available at cdc.gov/lice/; and Directors of Health Promotion and Education (DHPE). *Infectious facts: Head lice.* Available at www.dhpe.org/infect/lice.html.

Ticks

Ticks are an important consideration because they can transmit serious diseases such as Lyme disease, Rocky Mountain spotted fever, and tularemia. Transmission of these diseases can be decreased if the tick is removed within 24 hours of becoming attached. To remove a tick, grasp it with tweezers close to the skin and then steadily pull the tick away (Stafford, 2007). Once the tick is removed, cleanse the area with soap and warm water.

NAILS AND FEET

Examine nails for intactness and cleanliness. Assess capillary refill and the contour of the nailbed. Observe the nail base for redness, swelling, bleeding, discharge, and tenderness. Patients with dark skin tones may have freckles or pigmented streaks in their nails and nails may be thicker. Examine the feet for cleanliness and intactness of skin, and note any swelling, inflammation, lesions, tenderness, or orthopedic problems. Examine carefully the skin between the toes. Refer to Chapter 25 for additional information on techniques for assessing the nails and feet.

PERINEAL AND VAGINAL AREAS

Examine the male genitalia for lesions, swelling, inflammation, excoriation, tenderness, and discharge (amount, color, odor, source). Examine the female genitalia for color, size, lesions, masses, swelling, inflammation, excoriation, tenderness, and discharge (amount, color, odor, source). Inspect the anal area for cracks, nodules, distended veins, masses, or polyps. Note any perineal odors. Refer to Chapter 25 for additional information about perineal assessment.

Diagnosing

A careful assessment of the adequacy of a patient's hygiene practices and the assessment of the skin, mucous membranes, and other body areas may lead to the identification of numerous patient problems that can be classified as nursing diagnoses. Each nursing diagnosis statement identifies a patient problem and suggests expected patient outcomes. The etiology of the problem directs nursing interventions. Problems concerning deficient hygiene are categorized as self-care deficits. Self-Care Deficit diagnoses address four specific activities necessary to meet daily needs: feeding, bathing and hygiene, dressing and grooming, and toileting. It is important to identify the cause of these problems correctly. If hygiene is deficient because of insufficient knowledge, health education may quickly remedy the problem. If, however, hygiene is viewed as a low priority by the individual or the person lacks the physical ability to perform hygiene measures, these problems must be addressed before health education can be effective. The following are examples of appropriate nursing diagnoses:

- Bathing Self-Care Deficit related to postoperative weakness
- Pain related to alteration in skin integrity
- Ineffective Coping related to chronic skin disease

- Ineffective Health Maintenance: dental caries related to deficient oral hygiene practices
- Impaired Oral Mucous Membrane related to malnutrition and dehydration
- Impaired Social Interaction related to negative body image: acne
- Imbalanced Nutrition: Less Than Body Requirements related to stomatitis

Examples of these diagnoses, etiologic factors, and defining characteristics appear in Examples of NANDA Nursing Diagnoses: Hygiene.

In certain situations, a wellness nursing diagnosis may be appropriate as the patient progresses toward an increased level of health awareness and wellness. An example of a wellness diagnosis may be Health-Seeking Behaviors related to oral hygiene practices.

Data collected during the nursing assessment may also lead to the identification of a collaborative problem. For example, a patient receiving intravenous chemotherapy is at risk for developing phlebitis, a complication requiring a collaborative approach. Therefore, when caring for a patient receiving intravenous chemotherapy, checking the infusion site every shift is a priority based on the nurse's knowledge that this complication can occur. In addition, careful preparation and administration of the drug according to the manufacturer's instructions, adherence to nursing protocols for the maintenance of intravenous infusions, and ongoing nursing assessment are key to helping reduce the risk for phlebitis. If redness, warmth, tenderness, or swelling is noted, immediate collaborative intervention is indicated.

Similarly, a nurse may notice a 1.5-cm mole with an irregular border on a patient's back during a bath. Prompt reporting of this finding to the physician may lead to the detection and early, successful treatment of the medical diagnosis of malignant melanoma.

Outcome Identification and Planning

The plan of nursing care identifies nursing measures to assist the patient to develop or maintain hygiene practices that contribute to a sense of well-being. Appropriate expected outcomes include the following: The patient will:

- Verbalize feeling comfortable and clean
- Participate fully in necessary hygiene measures according to cognitive, sensory, mobility, and endurance abilities
- Maintain intact skin and mucous membranes
- Demonstrate correct skin care measures (when indicated) such as oral care, care of eyes, ears, and nose, nail and foot care, and perineal and vaginal care
- Demonstrate signs of healing in existing lesions (oral, scalp, or perineal)
- Exhibit lips, oral mucosa, gums, and tongue that are intact, moist, and free of inflammation and lesions
- Verbalize importance of good teeth-brushing habits, fluoride use, and regular dental examinations
- Demonstrate healthy functioning of eyes, ears, and nose
- Exhibit eyes, ears, and nose that appear clean

Examples of NANDA Nursing Diagnoses

Hygiene

Nursing Diagnoses	Related Factors	Sample Defining Characteristics
Bathing Self-Care Deficit	Sensory, cognitive, endurance, mobility, or motivation deficits; low value attached to regular bathing, brushing, flossing, and dental examinations; pain	"I don't need a bath. I'm not dirty." Seventy-year-old man 5 days after a left thoracotomy. Transient confusion, generalized postoperative weakness. Unable to ambulate more than a few steps with assistance of two caregivers.
Impaired Oral Mucous Membrane	Ineffective oral hygiene, immunosuppression, malnutrition, NPO for more than 24 hours, dehydration	Fifty-year-old woman recently diagnosed with cancer, receiving chemotherapy. Resulting stomatitis. "My mouth is so painful! It's an 8 out of 10." Noted to have ulcers in mouth, inability to eat, oral liquid intake limited to tepid, non-acidic liquids. Leery of using soft toothette for oral care. Unable to verbalize importance of and technique for oral saline rinses.
Impaired Social Interaction	Negative body image, visual or auditory impairment	"I hate the way I look. Everyone stares at me. I don't even feel like going to school." Sixteen-year-old boy has come to the pediatrician's office for a physical for his driver's license permit. He has severe acne, involving his face, neck, and back.

- Demonstrate proper use and care of visual or auditory aids
- Exhibit clean hair
- Verbalize satisfaction with appearance
- Participate in hair and scalp care as able
- Exhibit intact, clean, and manicured nails
- Demonstrate intact, clean, and lesion-free foot skin
- Report reduced or absent nail and foot problems (specify: calluses, corns, plantar warts, ingrown nails, athlete's foot)

Implementing

When performing general hygiene measures, respect the patient's personal preferences, allow and encourage as much self-care as the patient can perform, meet the patient's need for privacy, and promote physiologic and psychological wellness. (Refer to the Nursing Advocacy in Action box.) The following sections discuss hygiene measures, including providing scheduled care; helping with bathing and skin care; massaging; providing routine head-to-toe hygiene care; providing environmental care, including making the bed; and teaching patients about skin care. Refer to the accompanying Focus on the Older Adult display for interventions related to hygiene for this age group.

Providing Scheduled Hygiene Care

When patients require nursing assistance with personal hygiene, provide this care at regular intervals. In most hospitals and long-term care settings, the following types of

hygiene care are provided. These are individualized according to the patient's personal and cultural preferences.

> Remember Andrew Craig, the older man in the extended-care facility who reported that he had already had a complete bath. The nurse would need to investigate this to determine if he had indeed received care. If he had not, then the nurse would need to seek additional information to explain his statement; perhaps the patient was too tired or did not like having to be helped with his care. This information is essential to plan the patient's care effectively.

EARLY MORNING CARE

Shortly after the patient awakens, assist him or her with toileting if necessary and then provide comfort measures to refresh the patient and prepare him or her for breakfast (or diagnostic tests). Nursing measures include washing the face and hands and providing mouth care. If needed, supplies necessary for morning care can be ordered at this time.

MORNING CARE (A.M. CARE)

After breakfast, complete morning care. Depending on the patient's self-care abilities, offer assistance with toileting, oral care, bathing, back massage, special skin care measures (e.g., pressure ulcer), hair care (includes shaving if indicated), cosmetics, dressing, and positioning for comfort. Cosmetics, if desired, can enhance morale in an ill patient.

NURSING ADVOCACY IN ACTION

Patient Scenario

Mr. John Doe has been in the emergency room all night. When you arrive for clinical the next morning, the charge nurse tells you to "clean up the frequent flyer in bed 10." She proceeds to tell you that he's a "homeless bum who appears every month or so to get a bath, shave, meal, and warm bed." She is clearly frustrated that the night shift "dumped him" on the day shift saying they wanted him to "sleep off his buzz."

When you walk to bed 10, you discover a foul-smelling, dirty, hairy man with vomit all over his shirt. He grabs your arm and demands something to eat and something for belly pain. When you walk out to check his orders, three older nurses tease you about your assignment and tell you to "not waste too much time on this creep." When you tell your nurse preceptor about his "belly pain," she tells you that he is just drug seeking and suggests you ignore him or try a placebo.

Implications for Nursing Advocacy

How will you respond if you are John Doe's nurse? Talk with your classmates and experienced nurses about the questions that follow.

- If you elect to advocate for Mr. John Doe, what practical steps can you take to ensure better health outcomes?
- What is reasonable to expect of a student nurse, a graduate nurse, and an experienced nurse in this situation?
- What advocacy skills are needed to effectively respond to this challenge?

Agency policies are followed for refreshing or changing bed linens, and the patient's bedside area is tidied. When morning care is completed, the patient should feel refreshed and should be in a comfortable and safe environment.

Morning care is often categorized as self-care, partial care, or complete care. Patients identified as self-care are capable of managing their personal hygiene independently once oriented to the bathroom. However, offer a back massage and spend time assessing the patient's day-to-day needs. Patients identified as partial care most often receive morning hygiene care at the bedside or seated near the sink in the bathroom. They usually require assistance with body areas that are difficult to reach. Patients identified as complete care require nursing assistance with all aspects of personal

FOCUS ON THE OLDER ADULT

NURSING STRATEGIES TO PROMOTE PERSONAL HYGIENE FOR AGE-RELATED CHANGES

Age-Related Changes	Nursing Strategies
Impaired Oral Mucous Membrane • Loss of elasticity, atrophy of epithelial cells, diminished blood supply to connective tissue • Decreased salivation • Use of medications for chronic conditions that may cause dry mouth	• Perform brushing, flossing, and rinsing after meals and before bedtime • Brush dentures daily and rinse with cool water • Avoid mouthwashes with alcohol content • Inspect mouth daily for lesions and inflammation • Use lubricant on lips • Suck on sugar-free candies, chew sugarless gum, use salivary substitutes • Continue with dental exams at the dentist every 6 months
Impaired Physical Mobility • Decreased range of motion • Presence of chronic conditions that compromise functional ability • Decreased muscle strength and agility	• Use adaptive devices for hygiene such as toothbrush with a large handle or extended handle, long-handled body sponge, shower chair, and grab bars • Provide for safety in the bathroom: use nonslip mats, grab bars
Risk for Impaired Skin Integrity • Diminished secretion of natural oils and perspiration • Loss of elasticity • Thinning of epidermis, loss of elastin and subcutaneous fat	• Use safe water temperatures to bathe • Shower instead of tub bath • Use moisturizers and lubricants at least daily • Bath less often (not every day)

hygiene. A complete bed bath is done, or the patient is taken to the shower.

AFTERNOON CARE (P.M. CARE)

Hospitalized patients frequently receive visitors in the afternoon or evening or use this time to rest when not scheduled for tests or therapies. Ensure the patient's comfort after lunch and offer assistance to nonambulatory patients with toileting, handwashing, and oral care. Straightening bed linens and helping patients with mobility problems to reposition themselves comfortably are other welcome nursing measures.

HOUR OF SLEEP CARE (H.S. CARE)

Shortly before the patient retires, again offer assistance with toileting, washing of the face and hands, and oral care. Because many patients find that a back massage helps them to relax and fall asleep, offer one routinely. Change any soiled bed linens or clothing, and position the patient comfortably. Ensure that the call light and any other objects the patient desires (e.g., urinal, radio, water glass) are within easy reach.

AS NEEDED CARE (P.R.N. CARE)

In addition to scheduled care, offer individual hygiene measures as needed. Some patients require oral care every 2 hours. Patients who are diaphoretic (sweating profusely) may need their clothing and bed linens changed several times a shift. At other times, a nurse may decide to forego hygiene measures because the patient's need for undisturbed rest may be a higher priority.

Helping With Bathing and Skin Care

Bathing serves a variety of purposes, including:

- Cleansing the skin
- Acting as a skin conditioner

- Helping to relax a restless person
- Promoting circulation by stimulating the skin's peripheral nerve endings and underlying tissues
- Serving as a musculoskeletal exercise through activity involved with bathing, thereby improving joint mobility and muscle tonus
- Stimulating the rate and depth of respirations
- Promoting comfort through muscle relaxation and skin stimulation
- Providing sensory input
- Helping to improve self-image
- Providing an excellent opportunity to strengthen the nurse–patient relationship, to thoroughly assess the patient's integumentary system, to observe the patient's physiologic and emotional status closely, to teach the patient as indicated, and to demonstrate care and interest in the patient's general welfare

The simple act of bathing a patient is a vital and caring intervention. The accompanying Examples of Nursing Interventions and Nursing Outcomes Classifications (NIC/NOC) box lists standardized nursing interventions and corresponding outcomes related to helping the patient promote cleaning of the body for relaxation, cleanliness, and healing. In recent years, this basic personal care measure has often been assigned to an unlicensed staff member rather than the professional nurse. It has become a task to be accomplished rather than an opportunity for therapeutic individualized intervention. Although unlicensed assistive personnel are increasingly performing hygiene measures, the nurse is responsible for ensuring that hygiene measures were performed satisfactorily. Refer to Chapter 15 for a discussion of the nurse's accountability when care is delegated. Nurses whose primary focus is the patient, however, can use the time spent on assisting with bathing to establish a rapport with the patient and to further assess the patient's integumentary system. See Through the Eyes of a Student.

Examples of Nursing Interventions and Nursing Outcomes Classifications (NIC/NOC)

Bathing

Nursing Interventions	Nursing Outcomes
- Monitor functional ability while bathing - Offer handwashing after toileting and before meals - Use fun bathing techniques with children, such as wash dolls or toys - Bathe in water of a comfortable temperature - Monitor skin condition while bathing - Apply lubricating ointment and cream to dry skin areas	- Self-care: Bathing - Patient Satisfaction: Functional assistance - Oral Hygiene - Motivation - Energy Conservation

From Bulechek, G., Butcher, H., & McCloskey Dochterman, J. (Eds.). (2008). *Nursing interventions classification (NIC)* (5th ed., p. 153). St. Louis, MO: Mosby Elsevier; and Moorhead, S., Johnson, M., Maas, M., Swanson, E. (Eds.). (2008). *Nursing outcomes classification (NOC)* (5th ed., p. 806). A full listing of nursing activities for each nursing intervention and outcomes can be found in these books.

Through the Eyes of a Student

I entered the room with a feeling of dread. How could I possibly bathe the sick, elderly, helpless woman lying in this hospital bed? I had never bathed anyone older than age 2 years, other than myself, of course. How would I be able to move her limp, seemingly lifeless old body? What would an 85-year-old body look like? I could not imagine. I've read all the manuals that describe this procedure, I know what to do, so why am I so nervous? I must be worried that I will hurt her in some way. Maybe she has not been cared for properly before and her hygiene is poor. Well, I might as well get this over with because I'll be doing it the rest of my life. I've got to learn sometime.

I've mustered up enough courage to enter my patient's room. Michelle, her primary nurse, offers to help me because the patient is so difficult to move. Boy, am I relieved! Right before Michelle and I are about to begin, my patient, Mrs. Ash, asks for her teeth. I assume this must mean her dentures and reassure her that I have not seen them but will be happy to look for them as soon as we have completed her bath. Michelle and I each take a side and begin to bathe her. It's truly amazing how those range-of-motion exercises come to mind so easily. I had thought they were long forgotten with the rest of the past semester. Wouldn't my instructors love to hear me now! Suddenly Mrs. Ash yells, "I need the bed pan!" "Oh no!" I thought, as I rushed to the bathroom with soapy gloved hands trying frantically to locate her bed pan before there could be an accident. Michelle, who remained calm during my frenzy, simply stated, "Don't worry,

she has an indwelling catheter. She says that every time I bathe her." I knew she had a catheter, how did I forget? Somewhat humbled, I returned to the procedure. I really wanted to put some lotion on her skin because it was so dry. When we were ready to do her back, we prepared to lift her. I pulled her toward me, and Michelle was to continue the bath. We were not prepared for what we saw underneath. Firmly cushioned in Mrs. Ash's lower left buttock were none other than her dentures! On removing them, Michelle and I had to smile at the periodontal grin implanted on Mrs. Ash's bottom. Michelle then asked her how her teeth had gotten to the location where we found them. All she seemed to know was that she needed those teeth back in her mouth NOW! She snatched the dentures from Michelle's hand and attempted to insert them. Michelle and I in unison blurted out, "No, Mrs. Ash, please wait until we clean your teeth before you put them back in your mouth!" Mrs. Ash, somewhat confused, begrudgingly handed over her teeth to be cleaned. Michelle had the honors while I finished the last touches of good hygiene for Mrs. Ash.

What a difference cleanliness can make, not only for the patient, but also for me, the student nurse. I felt better knowing that Mrs. Ash was clean and that this procedure was behind me. And to think that I was apprehensive! This was definitely an interesting learning experience.

—Marilyn Johnson
Holy Family College, Philadelphia

SHOWER AND TUB BATHS

A shower is the preferred method of bathing for hospitalized patients who are ambulatory and able to tolerate the activity. Tub baths may be an option, particularly in long-term care, depending on facility policy. For the most part, even though many patients can bathe on their own, the following responsibilities apply:

- Check to see that the bathroom is available, clean, and safe. Showers should have mats or nonskid strips to prevent patients from slipping and falling.
- Ensure that necessary articles, such as soap, a washcloth, a towel, and a gown, are available for the patient.
- Provide a place for a weak or physically disabled patient to sit in a shower. Most health agencies have a stool or chair that can be used in the shower and handheld showerheads may facilitate the process. Some nurses have reported that a commode chair with the pan removed serves effectively as a shower chair and offers the patient more support than a stool or chair.
- Assist the patient to the shower or bathroom, as indicated. Patients who are beginning ambulation often need assistance to help prevent falling or fainting.
- Check to see that the water temperature is safe and comfortable—110°F to 115°F (43°C–46°C). The lower

temperature is recommended for children and elderly patients.
- Ensure privacy for patients who can safely shower or bathe independently. See that a call device is handy, and make sure the patient knows what the button is for, so that the patient can obtain help if necessary.
- Help the patient get in and out of the bathtub, as indicated. Have the patient grasp the handrails at the side of the tub, or place a chair at the side of the tub. The patient sits on the chair and eases to the edge of the tub. After putting both feet into the tub, it is then relatively easy for the patient to reach the opposite side and ease down into the tub. The patient may kneel first in the tub and then sit in it; this process can be reversed when leaving the tub. Use a hydraulic lift, when available, to lower and lift patients who are unable to maneuver safely or completely bear their weight.
- Keep the bathroom door unlocked. Health personnel should be able to enter with ease if the patient needs help. A sign hung on the door ensures privacy. Never leave children or confused patients alone in the bathroom.
- Help to wash and dry areas of the body that the patient cannot reach, such as the back.
- Make any necessary adaptations. For example, if the patient is confused and becomes agitated as a result of

Box 31-1   MEETING THE BATHING NEEDS OF PATIENTS WITH DEMENTIA

- Shift the focus of the interaction from the "task of bathing" to the needs and abilities of the patient. Focus on comfort, safety, autonomy, and self-esteem, in addition to cleanliness.
- Individualize patient care. Consult the patient, the patient's record, family members, and other caregivers to determine patient preferences.
- Consider what can be learned from the behaviors associated with dementia about the needs and preferences of the patient. A patient's behavior may be an expression of unmet needs; unwillingness to participate may be a response to uncomfortable water temperatures or levels of sound or light in the room.
- Consider other methods for bathing. Showers and tub baths are not the only options in bathing. Towel baths, washing

under clothes, and bathing "body sections" one day at a time are other possible options.
- Maintain a relaxed demeanor. Use calming language. Try to determine phrases and terms the patient understands in relation to bathing and make use of them. Offer frequent reassurance.
- Explore the need for routine analgesia before bathing. Move limbs carefully and be aware of signs of discomfort during bathing.
- Wash the face and hair at the end of the bath or at a separate time. Water dripping in the face and having a wet head are often the most upsetting parts of the bathing process for people with dementia.

Adapted from Flori, L. (2007). Don't throw in the towel: Tips for bathing a patient who has dementia. *Nursing, 37*(7), 22–23; and Rader, J., Barrick, A., Hoeffer, B., Sloane, P. D., McKenzie, D., Talerico, K. A., et al. (2006). The bathing of older adults with dementia: Easing the unnecessarily unpleasant aspects of assisted bathing. *American Journal of Nursing, 106*(4), 40–49.

over stimulation when bathing, reduce the stimuli. Turn down the lights and play soft music and/or warm the room before taking the patient into it (Flori, 2007). Box 31-1 outlines possible measures to implement to meet the bathing needs of patients with dementia. Also, see the accompanying Research in Nursing box.

▶ *Recall Sonya Delamordo, the older Hispanic woman going to her daughter's home after a stroke. Although the responsibilities listed apply to a hospitalized patient, the nurse can incorporate these responsibilities into the teaching plan for Mrs. Delamordo's daughter to ensure the patient's safety with hygiene.* ∎

Figure 31-1 illustrates several features that add to the safety of a patient taking a shower. Ensure proper cleaning between patient uses to comply with infection control measures, according to facility policy.

BED BATHS

Some patients must remain in bed as a part of their therapeutic regimen but can still bathe themselves. Other patients are not on bed rest but require total or partial assistance with bathing in bed due to physical limitations, such as fatigue or limited range of motion. Implement the following nursing measures to help patients take a bath in bed:

- Provide the patient with articles for bathing and a basin of water that is a comfortable and safe temperature.

RESEARCH IN NURSING
Bridging the Gap to Evidence-Based Practice

ASSISTING COGNITIVELY IMPAIRED NURSING HOME RESIDENTS WITH BATHING

Persons with dementia experience altered abilities to think and function, and may experience changes in personality, mood, and behavior. These changes can present challenges for the patient and caregivers, making interaction during bathing and personal care activities potentially difficult and dangerous. Alternate techniques and interventions can reduce a patient's agitation and minimize potential problems.

Related Research

Hoeffer, B., Talerico, K., Rasin, J., Mitchell, C. M., Stewart, B. J., McKenzie, D., et al. (2006). Assisting cognitively impaired nursing home residents with bathing: Effects of two bathing interventions on caregiving. *The Gerontologist, 46*(4), 524–532.

This study addressed whether a person-centered approach with showering and the towel bath improved caregiving behaviors (gentleness and verbal support) and preparedness (confidence

and ease), and reduced distress (hassles) when assisting residents in a long-term care facility with bathing. Caregivers who received training in a person-centered approach significantly improved in the use of gentleness and verbal support and in the perception of ease of bathing.

Relevance to Nursing Practice

This study suggests that a person-centered approach with showering and with the towel bath improves how care is given to residents who become agitated and aggressive during bathing. In addition, caregivers experienced improvement in perception of their experience when bathing these residents. Facilities should consider individualizing the bathing experience to improve the quality of care and comfort of patients/residents and improve caregiver morale.

For additional research, visit the**Point**

FIGURE 31-1. Examples of features that add to the safety of a patient taking a shower or bath. (**A**) A call bell equipped with a pull cord. (**B**) A shower equipped with a safety seat and hand rail. *(Photo by B. Proud.)*

Place these items conveniently for the patient on a bedside stand or overbed table.

- Provide privacy for the patient. Make sure the call device is within reach.
- Remove the top linens from the patient's bed and replace them with a bath blanket.
- Place cosmetics in a convenient place for the patient. Provide a mirror, a good light, and hot water for patients who wish to shave with a razor.
- Assist patients who cannot bathe themselves completely. For example, some patients can wash only the upper parts of the body. Nursing personnel then complete the remainder of the bath.

Bathing procedures for patients who require total nursing assistance vary among health agencies. Skill 31-1 offers one example as a guide. It assumes that the patient can be raised or lowered in bed and that, although the patient may have limited movement, the nurse can manage the patient alone.

THE BAG BATH OR DISPOSABLE BATH

Some healthcare agencies recommend use of the "bag bath" as an alternative to the traditional bed bath. There are several variations of this bath. In one system, 8 to 10 washcloths are contained in a plastic bag and cleanser and warm water are added to prepare the bath. Another self-contained bathing system consists of a package containing 8 to 10 premoistened, disposable washcloths. The unopened package is warmed in the microwave or stored in a warmer until use. Each part of the patient's body is cleansed with a fresh cloth. No rinsing is required. The skin is allowed to air dry (for about 30 seconds) so that the emollient ingredient of the cleaner remains on the skin.

Feedback about this procedure has been overwhelmingly positive. Nursing staff value the time savings when compared with a traditional bed bath and find it effective and easy to perform. Most patients have commented favorably on the bag bath. Patients with mild to moderate skin impairments demonstrated an improved skin condition with consistent use of the bag bath.

PROMOTING SKIN HEALTH

An easy and effective way to promote the barrier function of the skin and keep the skin healthy is the daily use of soap substitutes, topical emollients, and barrier products (Watkins, 2008; Voegeli, 2008a). Soap cleans the skin, but at the same time it removes dirt from the surface, it affects the lipids that are present on the skin and the skin pH. This contributes to drier skin, damaging the barrier function of the skin. The substitution of a nonsoap emollient cleaning agent is an easy way to prevent drying and damage to the skin. The rinseless products mentioned in the description of a bag bath are examples of nonsoap emollient cleaning agents.

Topical emollient agents are also known as moisturizers and can be applied to the skin as a lotion, cream, gel, or ointment. They act to seal water into the skin and replace lipids in the skin, effectively hydrating the skin and recreating the waterproof barrier of the skin. Apply topical moisturizers after bathing. Ideally, they should be applied twice a day but may need more frequent application, depending on the skin condition and the product used.

Skin barrier products include creams, ointments, and films and are used to protect vulnerable skin. They are used to protect skin at risk for damage caused by excessive exposure to water and irritants, such as urine and feces. They are also used to prevent skin breakdown around stomas and wounds with excessive exudate. Application of one of these products forms a thin layer on the surface of the skin to repel potential irritants. Apply these products by following the manufacturer's recommendations and facility policy. Box 31-2 outlines general skin care principles.

MASSAGING THE BACK

A backrub generally follows the patient's bath. A backrub acts as a general body conditioner and can relieve muscle

---

Box 31-2 GENERAL SKIN CARE PRINCIPLES

- Assess the patient's skin daily
- Cleanse the skin when indicated, such as when soiled, using a no-rinse, pH balanced cleanser
- Avoid using soap and hot water; avoid excessive friction and scrubbing
- Minimize skin exposure to moisture (incontinence, wound leakage); use a skin barrier product as necessary
- Use emollients

Adapted from Voegeli, D. (2008). Care or harm: Exploring essential components in skin care regimens. *British Journal of Nursing, 17(1),* 24–30.; Registered Nurses' Association of Ontario Professional Association. (2005). Risk assessment & prevention of pressure ulcers. NGC: 004215. Available at http://www.guideline.gov/summary/summary.aspx?doc_id=7006&nbr=004215&string="wound&ostomy"+and+"continence+nurses+society."

tension and promote relaxation. Some nurses forego giving backrubs to patients due to time constraints. However, giving a backrub allows the nurse to observe the skin for signs of breakdown. A backrub improves circulation; can decrease pain, distress, and anxiety; can improve sleep quality; and provides a means of communication with the patient through the use of touch.

Because some patients may consider the backrub a luxury and be reluctant to accept it, be sure to communicate its importance and value to the patient. An effective backrub should take 4 to 6 minutes to complete. If a lotion is used, warm it before use.

Be aware of the patient's medical diagnosis when considering giving a backrub. A backrub is contraindicated, for example, if the patient has had back surgery or has fractured ribs. Position the patient on the abdomen or, if this is contraindicated, on the side. Recommended techniques for administering a backrub are outlined in Skill 35-1 in Chapter 35, Comfort.

Administering Oral Hygiene

The mouth requires care even during illness, but sometimes care must be modified to meet a patient's needs. Adequate oral hygiene care is imperative to promote the patient's sense of well being and prevent deterioration of the oral cavity. Poor oral hygiene is reported to lead to the colonization of the oropharyngeal secretions by respiratory pathogens. Diligent oral hygiene care can improve oral health and limit the growth of pathogens in the oropharyngeal secretions, decreasing the incidence of aspiration pneumonia and other systemic diseases (Yoon & Steele, 2007; AACN, 2006). Refer to the accompanying PICO in Practice box.

If the patient can assist with mouth care, provide the necessary materials (Skill 31-2). Physical limitations, such as those associated with aging, often lead to less than adequate oral hygiene. The dexterity required for adequate brushing and flossing may decrease with age or illness. Older patients may be dependent on caregivers for oral hygiene. Patients with cognitive impairment, such as dementia, are also at risk for inadequate oral hygiene (Bailey et al., 2005). If the patient is unable to perform oral hygiene, make certain that the mouth receives care as often as necessary to keep it clean and moist, as often as every 1 or 2 hours if necessary. This is especially important for patients who cannot drink or are not permitted fluids by mouth. Skill 31-3 gives techniques for administering oral hygiene to dependent patients. Moisten the mouth with water, if allowed, and lubricate the lips often enough to keep the membranes well moistened. Following the steps for

---

PICO IN PRACTICE
Asking Clinical Questions

Scenario: You are the nurse educator for three adult critical care units at a health science center university hospital. While attending the monthly multidisciplinary Critical Care Quality Improvement Committee meeting, you note with concern that the rates of pneumonia among patients receiving mechanical ventilation (i.e., ventilator-associated pneumonia [VAP]) this past quarter was higher than expected, according to national standards. You have read several articles in the literature that suggest that assuring good oral hygiene in patients receiving mechanical ventilation is associated with lower rates of VAP. Your three units meet the hospital's policy that patients receiving mechanical ventilation receive oral care every four hours. However, you know that there is no standard policy for how oral care is provided to patients receiving mechanical ventilation, and you know that different nurses on each unit deliver oral care using different methods and oral care products. You decide to investigate whether the evidence-based literature supports use of a standard oral care protocol for patients receiving mechanical ventilation.

- POPULATION: Critically ill adult patients receiving mechanical ventilation
- INTERVENTION: Standard oral care protocol
- COMPARISON: None
- OUTCOME: Decreased rates of VAP

PICO Question: Does implementation of a standard oral care protocol for adult patients receiving mechanical ventilation reduce rates of VAP?

Finding: From a CINAHL database search: Weitzel, T., Robinson, S. B., & Holmes, J. (2006). Preventing nosocomial pneumonia: Routine oral care reduced the risk of infection at one facility. *American Journal of Nursing, 106*(9), 72A–72B, 72E–72G.

These researchers implemented a standard oral care protocol for mechanically ventilated patients and then tracked rates of VAP utilizing a retrospective chart review. They found that the rates of VAP significantly dropped after the protocol was implemented.

Level of Evidence: Level IV

Recommendation: You present these research findings to your colleagues on the Critical Care Quality Improvement Committee and recommend that the protocol outlined in this study be replicated on your three critical care units. You offer to provide the education necessary to the staff nurses who work on these units so that they may provide standardized oral care to their mechanically ventilated patients. After oral care for mechanically ventilated patients is standardized on these units, you intend to closely scrutinize the rates of VAP to assure that they are lower. If they do not improve, then the protocol may need to be revised and other methods targeted at decreasing the rates of VAP may need to be considered.

cleaning the mouth thoroughly is more important than the agent used. This supports the personal experience of many people that no mouthwash, breath freshener, ointment, or paste replaces a thorough mechanical cleaning of the oral cavity.

TOOTH BRUSHING AND FLOSSING

A soft bristled toothbrush should be small enough to reach all teeth. Clean and dry all brushes between uses. Most damage is done by bacteria directly after eating, so make sure the patient brushes the teeth immediately after eating or drinking. The tongue should also be cleaned with the brush. Use a toothbrush even when the patient has no or few teeth. It is the only effective way to remove plaque and debris (Holman, Roberts, & Nicol, 2005).

Automatic toothbrushes, electric or battery operated, are simple to use and are as good as manual brushes for removing debris and plaque. Pressurized water spray units are available to assist with oral hygiene. However, if too much water pressure is used, particles of debris may be forced into tissue pockets, leading to gum damage. Therefore, discuss their use with a dentist.

The toothbrush cannot reach areas between the teeth where food lodges, so flossing once a day is recommended. Flossing removes the debris that the brush cannot and helps to break up colonies of bacteria.

Toothpastes and powders aid the brushing process and usually have a pleasant taste that encourages brushing, especially by children. Most dentifrices are safe to use, but those containing harsh abrasives may scratch the enamel of the teeth and, therefore, are not recommended. Salt and sodium bicarbonate are far less expensive than proprietary products on the market and just as effective for short-term use. However, these products lack fluoride and should not be used exclusively. Dentifrices containing stannous fluoride and antitartar, and antiplaque rinses decrease dental caries and thus are recommended by many dentists.

MOUTHWASHES

An offensive breath odor (halitosis) is often systemic in nature. For example, the odor of onions and garlic on the breath comes from the lungs, where the oils are being removed from the bloodstream and eliminated with respiration. A mouthwash cannot remove halitosis when odors are being eliminated by respiration.

If the cause of halitosis is poor oral hygiene, cleaning reduces the odor. Commercial mouthwashes may also be helpful. Therapeutic mouth rinses that reduce bacteria can help reduce plaque, gingivitis, and bad breath. Anticavity rinses with fluoride help protect tooth enamel and are often used with children (American Dental Association (ADA), 2008; Mayo Foundation for Medical Education and Research (MFMER), 2007d). If concentrated mouthwashes are used frequently in debilitated patients, however, they may injure oral tissue.

DENTURE CARE

Failing to wear dentures for a long period allows the gum line to change, thus affecting the fit of the dentures. If the patient has been instructed to remove dentures while sleep-

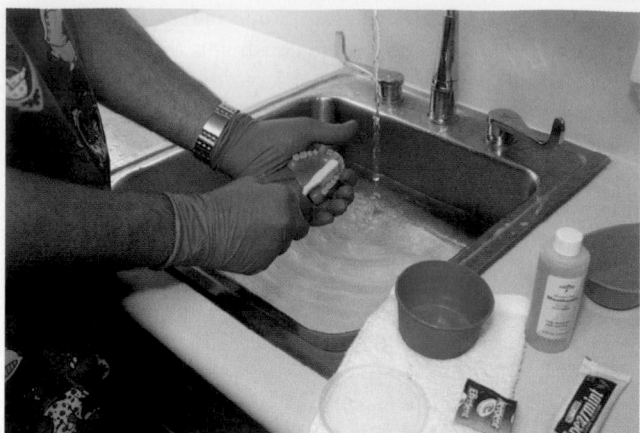

FIGURE 31-2. Proper method of cleaning dentures.

ing, a disposable denture cup is convenient and easy to use. Advise the patient not to wrap dentures in toilet tissue or disposable wipes because these are likely to be thrown away.

Patients with dentures are more likely to keep them in the mouth if they are kept clean. If the patient cannot care for them, the nurse must ensure that the dentures are clean. Use care when handling a patient's dentures because they represent a considerable financial investment, and replacement for damage or loss is expensive.

When cleaning dentures, put on gloves and hold them over a basin of water or a sink lined with a washcloth or soft towel (Fig. 31-2) so that if they slip from your grasp, they will not fall onto a hard surface and break. If necessary, grasp the dentures with a 4″ × 4″ piece of gauze to help prevent them from slipping out of your gloved hands. Use cool or lukewarm water to cleanse them. Hot water may warp the plastic material of which most dentures are made. Use a soft toothbrush and toothpaste. Dentures may be soaked in commercial preparations to help remove stains and hardened particles and then rinsed well after cleaning. Give the patient the opportunity to brush the gums and tongue and rinse his or her mouth before the dentures are replaced. Assist the patient with care as necessary. Store dentures in cold water when not in the patient's mouth. Leaving dentures to dry can cause warping, leading to discomfort when worn (Holman, Roberts, & Nicol, 2005).

The following is an example of documentation for oral care:

10/20/12—Patient generally breathes with mouth open. Mucous membranes and lips appear dry. Teeth brushed with morning care; toothettes moistened with water used for mouth moisturizing every 4 hours. Lubricating ointment applied to lips.

—D. Sadowski, RN

Providing Eye Care

Normally, the eyes are kept clean with lacrimal secretions. During illness, the eyes may produce more secretions than normal and may appear glasslike. Use the following techniques when secretions adhere to the eyelashes and become dry and crusty or when discharge is present:

• Wear gloves during the cleaning procedure.

- Use water or normal saline and cotton balls or a clean washcloth or compress to clean the eyes. Never use soap to clean the eyes because soap is irritating to eye tissues.
- Position the patient on the same side as the eye to be cleaned so that solution and debris do not run across the bridge of the nose and contaminate the other eye.
- Dampen a washcloth or cotton ball with the solution of choice and wipe once while moving the cotton ball from the inner canthus to the outer canthus of the eye. This technique minimizes the risk for forcing debris into the area drained by the nasolacrimal duct. Turn the washcloth and use a different section for each stroke. Alternately, discard the used cotton ball.
- Continue this technique, using a different section of the washcloth or one cotton ball for each stroke, until the eye is clean.
- Turn the patient to the opposite side and clean the other eye in the same manner.
- Wipe the lashes dry with a paper tissue or a clean washcloth, exposing a clean area of the tissue or cloth with each stroke.
- If the eyelashes are matted with secretions or debris that cannot be removed by wiping, apply a warm wet compress to the closed eye for 3 to 5 minutes to loosen the secretions so that they may be removed in a painless manner.

CARE OF THE UNCONSCIOUS PATIENT'S EYES

Patients with diminished or absent blink (corneal) reflexes and patients whose eyelids remain open require frequent eye care, at least every 4 hours. If the eye is not kept moist, corneal ulceration may result from excessive drying of the eye. Nursing measures include using saline or artificial tears, based on the medical orders, to lubricate the eye and a protective eye shield to keep the eye closed.

EYEGLASS CARE

Eyeglasses are essential for many people and represent a considerable financial investment. Take special precautions to prevent them from being broken or lost. Encourage patients who need glasses to wear them to avoid eyestrain.

Many eyeglasses have plastic lenses, which are considerably lighter in weight than glass lenses but correct vision just as well. Plastic lenses scratch easily. Whenever setting down glasses, make sure they are placed with the lenses up.

Clean eyeglasses over a terry towel, so that if they slip they will not become scratched or broken. Use warm water and soap or a special cleansing preparation. Hot water may warp plastic lenses and frames. Rinse the glasses well after cleaning them with soap and water and dry with a clean, soft cotton cloth, such as a cotton handkerchief or a special eyeglass cleaning cloth. Paper products that are made of wood pulp increase the risk of scratching the lenses, so do not use a dry paper tissue to clean eyeglasses. Do not use silicone tissues to clean plastic lenses.

CONTACT LENS CARE

A contact lens is a small disc worn directly on the eyeball. It stays in place by surface tension of the eye's tears. Contact lenses are either hard or soft. The older hard lenses are not gas permeable; newer ones are gas permeable and are more comfortable because they allow oxygen to pass directly through the lens to the cornea. Soft lenses are made of a plastic material that absorbs water to become soft and pliable. They are brittle when dehydrated and absorb water when placed in a solution, usually normal saline, or when in contact with tears. Soft lenses may be used for daily wear or extended wear. Disposable soft lenses are also available.

People who wear contact lenses, and the nurses caring for them, need to take special precautions to keep the lenses free of microorganisms that may lead to eye infections and to avoid injuring or scratching the surface of the eye. When providing contact lens care, always perform meticulous hand hygiene and put on gloves before touching eye surfaces and lenses. Caution lens wearers about eye irritation in the presence of noxious vapors or smoke. Also, remind lens wearers that lenses should not come into contact with cosmetics, soaps, or hair sprays because eye irritation may result. Urge the patient to report immediately to the prescribing physician any adverse reaction related to contact lens use.

The cornea, which consists of dense connective tissue, does not have its own blood supply. It is nourished primarily by oxygen from the atmosphere and from tears. In a patient who wears contact lenses, the cornea requires more than its normal supply of oxygen because its metabolic rate increases. To allow the cornea to receive a maximal supply of oxygen, hard lenses should not be worn for more than 12 to 16 hours and should be removed before sleeping. Extended-wear soft lenses can be left in place for 1 to 30 days, depending on the manufacturer. Individuals wearing extended-wear lenses should clean them at least once a week. The time that disposable soft lenses should be worn also varies according to the type and the manufacturer. A new type of disposable lens is replaced daily, whereas other options include lenses that can be worn day and night for 7 days or during waking hours only for 14 days. Excessive tearing, pain, and redness signal the need to remove lenses.

If a patient wears contact lenses but cannot remove them, the nurse is responsible for removing them. This may occur, for example, when the nurse is caring for an unconscious patient. Whenever an unconscious patient is admitted without any family present, always assess the patient to determine whether he or she wears contact lenses. Leaving contact lenses in place for long periods could result in permanent eye damage.

Before removing hard or gas-permeable lenses, use gentle pressure to center the lens on the cornea. A small suction device can also be used in an emergency situation to remove gas-permeable or hard lenses. Figure 31-3 demonstrates removal of hard and soft lenses. Once the lens is removed, identify it as being for the right or left eye, because the two lenses are not necessarily identical. If an eye injury is present, do not try to remove lenses because of the danger of causing an additional injury.

ARTIFICIAL EYE CARE

Most patients who wear an artificial eye prefer to care for it themselves. Encourage them to do so when possible. The necessary equipment includes a small basin, soap and water for

Removing Hard Contact Lenses

If the lens is not centered over the cornea, apply gentle pressure on the lower eyelid to center the lens.

Gently pull the outer corner of the eye toward the ear.

Position the other hand below the lens to receive it and ask the patient to blink.

Or

Gently spread the eyelids beyond the top and bottom edges of the lens.

Gently press lower eyelid up against the bottom of the lens.

After the lens is tipped slightly, move eyelids towards one another to cause the lens to slide out between the eyelids.

Removing Soft Contact Lenses

Storing Lenses

Have the patient look forward. Retract the lower lid with one hand. Using the pad of the index finger on the other hand, move the lens down the sclera.

Using the pads of the thumb and index finger, grasp the lens with a gentle pinching motion and remove.

Because lenses may be different for each eye, storage cases are marked L and R, designating left and right lenses. It is important to place the first lens in its designated cup in the storage case before removing the second lens to avoid mixing them up.

FIGURE 31-3. Removing contact lenses.

washing, and solution for rinsing the prosthesis. Normal saline or tap water can be used for rinsing. Most people have their own method for cleaning the eye socket and the area around it. Ask the patient how he or she does this, and enable the patient to continue with the usual practice. When the nurse is performing the care, the patient should be lying down so that the prosthesis does not accidentally fall to the floor. Flush the socket with normal saline before replacing the prosthesis.

Providing Ear Care

Other than cleaning the outer ears, little intervention is needed for routine hygiene of the ear. After the ears are washed, dry them carefully with a soft towel so that water and **cerumen** (wax) are removed by capillary action. Forcing the towel into the ear for drying or using a cotton-tipped applicator may aid in the formation of wax plugs. Using bobby pins, hairpins, paper clips, or fingernails to remove wax from the ear is extremely dangerous because these may injure or puncture the eardrum.

If the patient uses a hearing aid, check the batteries routinely and clean the earpieces or ear mold daily with mild soap and water. A whistling sound that is audible when the hearing aid is held in the hand with the power on and the volume high indicates that the battery is functioning properly. Refer to Chapter 21 for strategies nurses can use to promote communication with a hearing-impaired patient. If hearing loss is mild and the patient is not using a hearing aid, the following suggestions may help to improve hearing and should be included in any patient teaching:

- Avoid noisy places for conversation.
- Choose well-lit places where it is easier to look at the speaker's face, lips, and hands for cues to the conversation.
- Cup your hand behind your ear.
- Ask people to face you when they are speaking to you.
- Ask people to repeat what they said, if it was not clear to you, and to speak slowly.
- Consider buying amplitude devices so that you can hear your television and radio without turning up the sound.

Figure 31-4 illustrates three types of hearing aids.

Providing Nose Care

The best way to clean the nose is to blow it gently. Both nostrils should be open while doing this. Closing one nostril adds to the danger of forcing debris into the eustachian tubes. Irrigations are usually contraindicated because of the danger of forcing material into the sinuses.

If the external nares are crusted, applying a warm, moist compress helps to soften and remove the crusts. Disposable paper tissues are recommended for nasal secretions. A cotton-tipped applicator may be used to clean the nares, but with great care to avoid injury. Never introduce the applicator into the nares.

Providing Hair Care

Daily brushing of the hair helps keep it clean and distributes oil along the shaft of each hair. Brushing also stimulates blood circulation in the scalp. Hair that becomes entangled is difficult to comb. Combing tiny sections of hair at a time may be necessary if a patient's hair has not been combed for even 1 day. The best way to protect long hair from matting and tangling is to ask the patient for permission to braid it. Patients usually consent to the procedure if it increases their comfort. Parting the hair in the middle on the back of the head and making two braids, one on either side, prevents the discomfort of lying on one heavy braid on the back of the head. When braiding a patient's hair, ensure that the hair is not pulled too tightly.

Occasionally, a patient's hair is almost hopelessly matted, and cutting the hair may be necessary. Before a patient's hair is cut, usually the patient signs a written consent. Also, as appropriate, discuss with a member of the patient's immediate family the necessity of cutting the hair.

Tightly curled (kinky) hair usually requires special attention. It is normally dry and curly and becomes matted and tangled easily. Use a comb with wide-spaced teeth and work the hair through from the neckline upward toward the forehead.

Some people have their hair straightened, but even after this process, it may be difficult to untangle the hair when the person is confined to bed. Some African Americans style their hair in small braids. The braids are not undone for shampooing and may need to have a lubricant or oil applied daily to prevent hair strands from breaking. Demonstrate cultural consideration by grooming the patient's hair in the style preferred by the patient.

Behind the ear (moderate to severe loss)   **In the ear** (mild to severe loss)   **In the canal** (mild to moderate loss)

FIGURE 31-4. Several types of hearing aids.

SHAMPOOING THE HAIR

The hair, which is exposed to the same dirt and oil as the skin, requires washing as often as necessary to keep it clean. Wash the comb and brush each time the hair is washed and as frequently as necessary between shampoos. Many health agencies have beauticians and barbers to assist with hair care, including shampooing, but this does not relieve the nurse of the responsibility.

Before shampooing the hair, brush or have the patient brush and comb the hair well to stimulate the scalp and undo tangled hair. The patient may then shampoo the hair while showering, if able. In some hospitals, a physician's order is required for shampooing a patient's hair.

If the patient is on bed rest, whether at home or in the hospital, and unable to shampoo his or her own hair, use the following as a guide:

* Prepare several pitchers of water of a suitably warm temperature for a thorough washing and rinsing, shampoo, one or two towels for drying, and a receptacle to receive wash and rinse water.
* Place a protective pad and a plastic hair-washing tray if one is available (Fig. 31-5) under the head.
* Place the patient in a position over the pad so that water drainage is directed into the receptacle.
* Wet the hair, apply shampoo, and massage the scalp well while washing the hair.
* Rinse the hair and reapply shampoo for a second washing, if indicated.
* Rinse the hair thoroughly.
* Apply conditioner if requested or if the scalp appears dry.
* Dry the hair as quickly as possible to prevent the patient from becoming chilled, and arrange the hair according to the patient's preference.

If regular shampooing is inappropriate or is contraindicated by the patient's condition, other products for use at the bedside are available. Products for use at the bedside do not require rinsing and are available as foams, concentrates, and dry powders. After application of a foam or concentrate cleaner, lather the product and then towel-dry the hair. Comb and style the hair as per the patient's preference. Keep the head covered with

FIGURE 31-5. The nurse uses a protective pad and plastic tray to prepare for shampooing a patient's hair.

FIGURE 31-6. Using a shampoo cap to clean a patient's hair.

a towel until the hair dries to help minimize chilling of the patient. Alternately, shampoo caps are available, and are being used with increasing frequency (Figure 31-6). These commercially prepared, disposable caps contain a rinseless shampoo product. Warm the cap in the microwave or store it in a warmer until use. Place the cap on the patient's head and massage the hair and scalp through the cap, to lather the shampoo. After shampooing for the manufacturer's suggested length of time, remove and discard the cap. Finally, towel dry the patient's hair and style it according to the patient's preference.

SHAVING

Grooming of body hair other than hair on the head can be an important part of a patient's self-esteem and well-being. Patients with beards or mustaches may require nursing assistance to keep the beard and mustache clean. Never trim or shave a patient's beard or mustache without the patient's consent. Female patients may require assistance with shaving underarm and leg hair, depending on the patient's personal preference and abilities. Blade razors tend to give a closer shave than do electric razors, but many patients find electric razors more convenient and practical. Electric shavers are usually recommended when the patient is receiving anticoagulant therapy or has a bleeding disorder and are especially convenient for ill and bedridden patients. Shaving after a warm bath or shower softens the hair, making the process easier (MFMER, 2007c). The technique for shaving patients who cannot shave themselves is described in Guidelines for Nursing Care 31-1.

Providing Fingernail Care

The following are recommended techniques for the care of fingernails:

* File the nails to form an oval at the ends. Do not trim so far down on the sides that the skin and cuticle are injured.
* Remove hangnails, which are broken pieces of cuticle, by cutting them off. Avoid injury to tissue with the cuticle scissors.
* Gently push cuticles back off the nail when soft and pliable after a soaking in warm water.
* Push back cuticles with a blunt instrument or a terry cloth.

Guidelines for Nursing Care • 31-1

SHAVING

- Perform hand hygiene and put on disposable gloves (contact with blood is possible if any skin nicks occur).
- Cover patient's chest with a towel or waterproof pad. Fill bath basin with warm (43° to 46°C [110° to 115°F]) water. Press a warm washcloth on the patient's facial skin to soften the hair.
- Dispense shaving cream into palm of hand. Rub hands together, then apply to area to be shaved in a layer approximately 0.5″ thick.
- With one hand, pull the skin taut at the area to be shaved. Using a smooth stroke, begin shaving. *If shaving the face,* shave with the direction of hair growth in downward, short strokes. *If shaving a leg,* shave against the hair in upward, short strokes.
- Wash off residual shaving cream.
- If patient requests, apply aftershave or lotion to area shaved.
- Remove and discard gloves and perform hand hygiene.

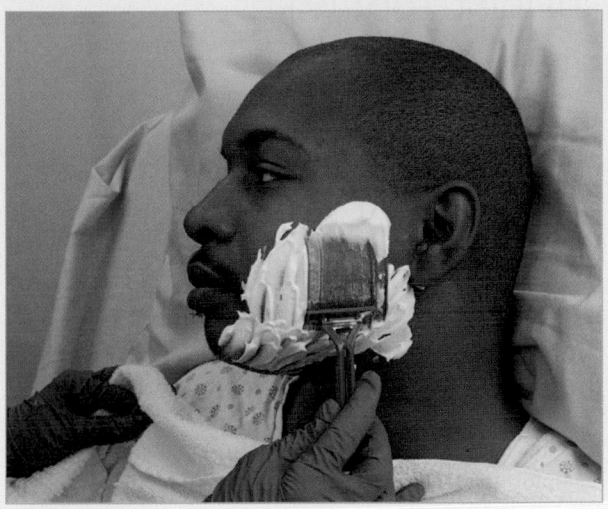

Shaving the face.

- Apply an emollient to the cuticle to help prevent hangnails.
- Clean under the nails with a blunt instrument, being careful not to injure the area where the nail is attached to the underlying tissue.

Splitting and peeling of the nails are usually caused by dryness. Teach the patient to avoid contact with soap and water as much as possible, use a good hand cream frequently, and avoid using polish remover with acetone, which tends to dry the nails (MFMER, 2007b).

Providing Foot Care

Proper foot care is important at any age. It becomes even more so with aging and when conditions such as circulatory disturbances or diabetes mellitus are present. Guidelines for Nursing Care 31-2 highlights the appropriate techniques related to foot care.

The following is an example of documentation of foot care:

10/20/12—Patient states, "I guess I cut that nail too short. It's been hurting for 2 months now." Great toe on right foot is swollen, red, and painful. Skin at base of nail is white. Limps when walking. After bath, patient soaked right foot and dried it carefully.

—*A. Jones, RN*

Providing Perineal Care

Perineal cleaning is performed in a matter-of-fact and dignified manner. If this approach is followed, patients generally do not find care by a person of the opposite gender to be offensive or embarrassing.

> *Remember Sonya Delamordo, who is going home after a stroke to her daughter's home. The patient may be embar-*

rassed to have her daughter help with perineal care. The nurse would encourage the patient to do as much as she is able, using her left side. By doing so, the patient maintains some control over the situation, thereby promoting her self-esteem and fostering personal hygiene and independence. ∎

In some cases, a sitz bath may be used to clean and irrigate the perineal and anal areas. The portable type is especially handy in situations where moving a patient to a stationary sitz tub would be cumbersome. The skills associated with administering a sitz bath are discussed in Chapter 32.

Perineal care may be carried out while the patient remains in bed. When performing perineal care, follow these guidelines:

- Assemble supplies, and provide for privacy.
- Explain the procedure to the patient, perform hand hygiene, and put on disposable gloves.
- Wash and rinse the groin area (both male and female patients). Use a small amount of mild, unscented soap and water.
- For a female patient, spread the labia and move the washcloth from the pubic area toward the anal area to prevent carrying organisms from the anal area back over the genital area (Fig. 31-7). Always proceed from the least contaminated area to the most contaminated area. Use a clean portion of the washcloth for each stroke. Rinse the washed areas well with plain water.
- For a male patient, clean the tip of the penis first, moving the washcloth in a circular motion from the meatus outward. Wash the shaft of the penis using downward strokes toward the pubic area (Fig. 31-7). Always proceed from the least contaminated area to the most contaminated area. Rinse the washed areas well with plain water. In an *uncircumcised male patient* (teenage or older), retract the

Guidelines for Nursing Care • 31-2

PROVIDING FOOT CARE

- Bathe the feet thoroughly in a mild soap and tepid water solution. Avoid soaking the feet. Be sure to clean the interdigital area.
- Rinse the feet to remove soap residue that can dry and irritate the skin.
- Dry feet thoroughly, including the area between the toes.
- Apply a moisturizer to feet if they are dry. Include the area between the toes. Patients with diabetes should apply moisturizer on the tops and bottoms of the feet to keep the skin soft. These patients should sprinkle talcum powder or cornstarch between the toes to keep the skin dry (MFMER, 2007a).
- Use an antifungal foot powder if necessary to prevent fungal infections, such as athlete's foot.
- Patients with diabetes should file the nails; avoid using scissors or nail clippers, which may slip and injure tissues. Nondiabetic patients should avoid digging into or cutting the toenails at the lateral corners when trimming the nails.
- Do not cut off corns or calluses. Commercial removers should be avoided because they may contain ingredients that can lead to development of infection and ulcers. Con-

sult a *podiatrist*, a physician who treats foot disorders, when corns or calluses are present.
- Explain the dangers of going barefoot. Skin on the feet may be injured, or athlete's foot may be acquired in public showers.
- Advise to wear appropriate footwear. Break in new shoes gradually. Improperly fitting shoes can lead to corns, calluses, bunions, and blisters. The soles should be flexible and non-slippery and the heel heights should be safe and offer appropriate support. Shoes with rough ridges, wrinkles, or tears in the linings should be discarded or repaired.
- Advise to wear cotton socks, which provide warmth and absorb perspiration.
- Teach to avoid wearing knee-high stockings, and do not sit with the knees crossed because this can obstruct the circulation to the lower extremities and feet.
- Prop the feet up above the level of the hips a few minutes several times a day if the feet swell.
- Avoid using heating pads and hot-water bottles because of the danger of blistering and burning the feet.
- Report any signs of foot problems to your physician. This is especially important for patients with diabetes.

foreskin (prepuce) while washing the penis. Pull the *uncircumcised male patient's* foreskin back into place over the glans penis to prevent constriction of the penis, which may result in edema and tissue injury. It is not recommended to retract the foreskin for cleaning during infancy and childhood, as injury and scarring could occur (MedlinePlus, 2007b). Wash and rinse the male patient's scrotum. Handle the scrotum, which houses the testicles, with care because the area is sensitive.
- Dry the cleaned areas and apply an emollient as indicated. Avoid the use of powder. Powder may become a medium for the growth of bacteria.

- Turn the patient on his or her side and continue with cleansing the anal area. Continue in the direction of least contaminated to most contaminated area. In the female, cleanse from the vagina toward the anus. In both female and male patients, change the washcloth with each stroke until the area is clean. Rinse and dry the area.
- Remove gloves and perform hand hygiene. Continue with additional care as necessary.

If the patient has an indwelling catheter and the agency recommends daily care for the catheter, this is usually done after perineal care. Care of an indwelling catheter is discussed in Chapter 37.

FIGURE 31-7. Performing normal perineal care.

Incontinent patients require special attention to perineal care. Patients with urinary or fecal incontinence are at risk for perineal skin damage. This damage is related to moisture, changes in the pH of the skin, overgrowth of bacteria and infection of the skin, and erosion of perineal skin from friction on moist skin. Skin care for these patients should include measures to reduce overhydration (excess exposure to moisture), contact with ammonia and bacteria, and friction. Remove soil and irritants from the skin during routine hygiene, and clean the area when the skin becomes exposed to irritants. Avoid using soap and excessive force for cleaning. The use of perineal skin cleansers, moisturizers, and barriers is recommended for skin care for the incontinent patient. These products help promote healing and prevent further skin damage. Incontinence, and nursing care of the patient with incontinence, is discussed further in Chapters 32, 37, and 38.

Providing Vaginal Care

Vaginal mucous secretions are odor free until they combine with air and perspiration. Thus, for vaginal care, using plain soap and water is the most effective means to control odor. In normal, healthy women, daily douching is believed to be unnecessary and unwise because it tends to remove normal bacterial flora from the vagina, and an acidic solution may irritate or injure normal cells. Douching has also been linked to vaginal irritation, bacterial vaginosis, pelvic inflammatory disease, and sexually transmitted infections (STIs) (National Women's Health Information Center, 2005). Although douching is occasionally ordered to treat a vaginal infection, it is not recommended as a routine hygiene measure.

Deodorants to control odor around the vaginal orifice are unnecessary. No therapeutic benefit from their use has been proven to date. Use of these special deodorants is not a substitute for keeping the area clean, and female patients often require teaching on this subject.

If patients insist on using them, explain that, although these deodorants do not contain aluminum salts, which are irritating to the mucous membrane, they are intended for external use only. They should not be placed on sanitary napkins or tampons. Some sprays have been reported as possibly harmful when sprayed into the vagina. Repeated use is not generally recommended because of reported irritation and rashes. In addition, the sprays should not be used on broken skin areas.

Providing Care for Body Piercing

Body piercing has increased in popularity and acceptance over recent years, regardless of socioeconomic and cultural background. Piercings can be found on the face (tongue, lips, nose, eyebrows), ears, neck, arms, legs, torso, navel, and genitals of patients. Nurses and other healthcare providers need to provide safe and effective care for patients with body piercings, including accurate assessment and site care. Basic wound care used for body piercings are usually called "aftercare." Aftercare techniques are used for the new piercing and whenever the piercing fistula has become disrupted through injury or exhibits signs of infection or inflammation (MFMER, 2008; Halliday, 2005). Guidelines for Nursing Care 31-3 provides appropriate techniques related to piercing site care.

Providing Environmental Care

The environment can improve or detract from the patient's sense of well-being. The patient's environment consists of the bedside unit and the furnishings and equipment in the space around the bed. Ensure that this area is clean and clutter-free, safe, and pleasant.

Basic furniture includes the bed, overbed table, bedside stand, and chairs. Standard equipment in the healthcare environment includes the call light, oxygen, suction, and electrical outlets; light fixtures; bath basin; emesis basin; bedpan or urinal; water pitcher and glass; and bed linens. One nursing responsibility is ensuring that necessary equipment and items are in their proper place and functioning properly.

Patients usually store personal items in the bedside stand. Always request permission from alert patients before opening the stand to obtain the bath basin, lotion, or other items. When assisting with hygiene, respecting the patient's right to privacy and ownership of personal goods decreases the patient's sense of powerlessness.

Before leaving the bedside, get into the habit of saying to the patient, "Is there anything else I can do to make you more comfortable?" Checking with the patient communicates genuine caring and can correct for any oversights. In

Guidelines for Nursing Care • 31-3

PROVIDING BODY PIERCING CARE

- Perform hand hygiene before providing care. Put on gloves.
- Jewelry and the piercing site should be cleansed of all crust and debris. Rinse the site with warm water and use a cotton swab to gently remove any crusting.
- Apply a dab of liquid medicated cleanser to the area. Turn the jewelry back and forth to work the cleanser around the opening. Rinse well.
- Advise patients to avoid the use of alcohol, peroxide, and ointments at the site.
- Oral piercing aftercare includes rinsing with an antibacterial, alcohol-free mouthwash for 30 to 60 seconds after meals and at bedtime. The patient should brush the teeth with a new, soft-bristled toothbrush.
- Advise patients to avoid oral tobacco use.
- Most piercings take 6 to 8 weeks to heal, but some may take several months or a year to heal.

the case of manipulative patients, set limits regarding what comfort and hygiene measures can be performed.

Good ventilation in patient rooms is imperative to limit pathogens and unpleasant odors associated with body secretions and excretions, for example, urine, stool, vomitus, draining wounds, or body odors. Decrease odors by emptying bedpans, urinals, and emesis basins promptly. When the waste receptacle in the patient's room is used to dispose of soiled dressings or anything with a strong odor, be sure to remove the trash before leaving the room. Dispose of the trash according to facility policy. Room deodorizers may need to be used.

Patient preferences for room temperature often vary widely. Whenever possible, respect the patient's preference when determining the room temperature. In general, the room temperature should be between 20°C and 23°C (68°F–74°F).

Many patients find it difficult to sleep in a healthcare facility. Patients are often disturbed frequently for assessment or treatment purposes. Care should be taken to reduce harsh lighting and noises whenever possible, although adequate lighting is necessary for all nursing procedures. Whenever possible, avoid carrying on conversations immediately outside the patient's room. Many patients find this stressful because the noise disturbs them and because they believe whatever is being said involves them.

BED SAFETY AND COMFORT

Many people who are ill and hospitalized or are being cared for at home spend a large portion of the day—if not the entire day—in bed, so the bed is an important part of the patient's environment. Nursing responsibilities include ensuring a safe and comfortable bed.

The typical hospital bed has a motorized metal frame in three sections, which allows the height of the bed to be raised or lowered and the head and foot to be adjusted. Know how to operate the bed and be ready to explain it to the patient. Bed positions are described in Chapter 33.

Hospital beds can also be ordered for use in the home. Because certain positions may be harmful to some patients, instruct the patient and family about advisable bed positions and the use of the bed controls. Historically, hospital beds have been generally 26 inches (66 cm) from the floor. This is higher than most beds at home, thus enabling the nurse or caregiver to reach the patient without undue musculoskeletal strain. However, many manufacturers are making low-height beds available to healthcare facilities. These beds have a minimum height of 7 to 15 inches from the floor.

Side rails are used to provide assistance with moving in bed, and access to bed controls is often on the side rails. See Chapter 26 for additional discussion about the use of side rails. Use side rails when indicated and according to facility policy. Also, lock the wheels or casters on the hospital bed whenever the bed is stationary to prevent the bed from moving when the patient is moving from the bed to an upright position or being transferred. The headboard of most hospital beds is removable to allow close patient contact in an emergency situation.

Nurses are responsible for ensuring the safety and comfort of the patient at the bedside. To promote bed safety while maintaining patient comfort, ensure the following before leaving the patient's bedside:

- The bed is in its lowest position.
- The bed position is safe for the patient.
- The bed controls are functioning (bed is electrically safe).
- Call light functioning and always within reach
- Side rails are raised if indicated.
- The wheels or casters are locked.

The hospital mattress is firm and generally covered with a water-repellent material that can be easily wiped with a bactericidal solution between patients. A variety of therapeutic beds and mattresses are available to reduce or relieve the effects of pressure on the skin (Fig. 31-8). These are discussed in more detail in Chapter 32.

Agency policies usually dictate the availability and use of bed linens. Bed linens include mattress covers, sheets, incontinence pads, pillowcases, blankets, bedspreads, and bath blankets. Changing the bed linen is often not the nurse's responsibility and is delegated. The nurse is responsible for coordinating with assistive personnel to ensure patient comfort. To promote bed comfort, ensure the following before leaving a patient:

- Linens are clean and free of crumbs and wrinkles.
- The patient feels comfortably warm.
- Pressure areas are protected from rough sheets, hem edges, and water-repellent material. This is especially important for patients with a nursing diagnosis of Risk for Impaired Skin Integrity.

MAKING A BED

A comfortable bed and appropriate bedding contribute to a patient's sense of well-being. Usually bed linens are changed after the bath, but some agencies change linens only

FIGURE 31-8. This special bed is an air-flotation, low-air-loss support surface that provides pressure relief. In this KinAir III, there is a microprocessor computer control panel that controls air flow and temperature precisely. A built-in digital scale and heater are included. The bed also has a quick-release level for CPR. *(Photo courtesy of KCI Therapeutic Services, San Antonio, TX.)*

Through the Eyes of a Student

One of my first patients was a man in his late 60s who had suffered a stroke. I was assigned to care for him, and his care included a bed bath and complete linen change—with him in the bed. I was determined to complete this task totally on my own, without asking anyone for help. This was my first mistake.

The patient yelled out a lot and had very rough mannerisms. I kept thinking to myself, "I must treat him with gentle care and not show any fear." Inside I was shaking furiously.

I managed to complete his bath and then began to change the sheets. I helped the patient to turn to one side, tucking the dirty linens close to him. I applied the fitted sheets to the upper portion of the bed . . . so far, so good. Immediately going to the foot

of the bed, I applied the bottom portion. The top portion popped off—I ran to the top of the bed, reapplied the top portion—the bottom portion popped off—I reapplied it. . . . I must have spent 15 minutes running back and forth trying to get both ends to stay on. By this time, sweat was pouring off my face.

When I finally cried "Uncle," I discovered that certain fitted sheets just didn't fit all the mattresses. The usual routine in this case is to walk to the linen closet and get another fitted sheet. That probably takes about 15 seconds!

—*Linda A. Keough*
Delaware County Community College, Media Pennsylvania

when soiled. The bed is made for the ambulatory patient, as described in Skill 31-4. If the patient is bedridden, the occupied bed is made, as described in Skill 31-5.

Although there are variations in the procedure for making an occupied bed, these minor differences have no real effect on the patient's comfort. In some instances, creativity and flexibility are necessary when changing linens because of the patient's condition, orthopedic appliances on the bed, or treatments that may be in progress. Refer to Through the Eyes of a Student.

Teaching Patients About Skin Care

Teaching about skin care can occur at different times. For example, teaching can be done informally during assessment and care procedures. Here, the nurse shares information about general skin care measures, including ways to prevent or reduce a patient's risk for skin problems. Teaching addressing a specific topic, such as dry skin, diabetic foot care, or acne, may be addressed as part of the nursing care plan. The following section describes common topics related to skin care and skin problems.

SOAPS AND DETERGENTS

A wide variety of soaps and detergents are available. Soaps are often made from vegetable and animal fats, whereas most detergents are made from petroleum derivatives. Studies have shown that expensive cleansing agents are no more effective than their less expensive counterparts. Patients who experience dry skin or other alterations in skin health may benefit from using nonsoap cleaning agents. See discussion in "Promoting Skin Health."

DEODORANTS AND ANTIPERSPIRANTS

Perspiration is essentially odorless, although it contains some waste products, such as uric acid and ammonia. The odor of perspiration results when bacteria, normally present on everyone's skin, act on the skin's normal secretions.

Inform patients that keeping the body and clothing clean is the best way to prevent body odors. Recommend the use of deodorants and antiperspirants after the skin is clean.

Deodorants mask odor, and antiperspirants are intended to reduce the amount of perspiration. They act as astringents and tend to close the exits of the sweat glands. Advise patients to use antiperspirants and deodorants with care and according to directions to prevent skin irritation. Keep in mind that these products are contraindicated in some situations, such as before mammography and during the postoperative period for a patient who has had a mastectomy.

COSMETICS

Cosmetics frequently enhance the appearance of clean and healthy skin. Cosmetics can be used judiciously to help disguise blemishes, improve skin coloring, and make wrinkles appear less obvious. However, certain cultural and religious groups discourage their use.

Periodically, cosmetics containing harmful ingredients have appeared on the market. Be alert to such agents and help consumers avoid their use. The U.S. Department of Health and Human Services Food and Drug Administration (FDA) enforces federal laws on the purity of foods, drugs, and cosmetics and on the advertising claims of their manufacturers. The FDA is a good source of information.

Remind patients that cosmetics often become contaminated with bacteria and fungi. Teach patients not to share cosmetics and advise them to discard cosmetics after they are 2 to 4 months old, especially those applied near the eyes (U.S. Department of Health and Human Services Food and Drug Administration [FDA], 2008). Encourage patients to keep makeup applicators and puffs immaculately clean.

Evaluating

Performing or assisting with the performance of hygiene measures provides a means of at least daily contact with the patient to determine whether the patient is achieving outcomes related to hygiene and skin care. Indicators that can be used to determine outcome achievement include the following:

- Level of patient's participation in hygiene program
- Elimination of, reduction in, or compensation for factors interfering with the patient's independent execution of

hygiene measures, for example, weakness, decreased motivation, and lack of knowledge

- Changes related to specific skin problems, for example, healing of skin lesions, elimination or reduction in causative factors, and independent patient management of the prescribed treatment program

The following are examples of evaluation related to hygiene:

10/26/12—Outcome partially met. Patient's oral mucosa is intact, but thick, dry secretions continue to build up on oral mucosa and gums despite every-4-hour care.
Revision: Increase frequency of oral hygiene to every 2 hours. Instruct family.

—N. Glynn, RN

10/24/12—Outcome met. Patient demonstrated correct care (cleaning) of artificial eye for the past two mornings. States, "I guess I should be happy to be alive and still able to see."

—N. Glynn, RN

10/27/12—Outcome partially met. Patient reports that she is uncomfortable wearing a wig but feels better since its purchase.

Revision: Patient still has many questions about effects of chemotherapy; continue teaching and use opportunities to build self-esteem.

—A. Jones, RN

10/27/12—Expected outcome met. Patient correctly verbalized rationale for diabetic foot care program and expressed interest in attending the diabetic classes.

—A. Diaz, RN

11/20/12—Outcome partially met. Child returned to clinic with clean perineal area and relief of painful urination. Mother reports child spends half the time with her and half with father (parents separated) and that father is not committed to hygiene practices.

Revision: Stress again to child importance of retracting foreskin during perineal care.

—C. Moser, RN

Ongoing evaluation helps adjust the nursing plan of care. For examples of the nursing process for hygiene, see the accompanying Nursing Plan of Care 31-1 for Kylie Simpson.

NURSING PLAN OF CARE • 31-1

For Kylie Simpson and Female University Students

Glenda Davis is a nurse practitioner who works in a campus health clinic at a state university. Kylie Simpson met with Glenda Davis at the clinic. Kylie had been having vaginal itching and burning for 2 weeks. She was diagnosed with a vaginal infection. She asks Glenda, "This is terrible. It's the second infection in 7 months. Is there something wrong with me? Isn't there something I can do to keep this from happening again?"

Frequently, women ask Glenda questions about feminine hygiene. Realizing that each woman who presents with a question probably represents many other women with similar unvoiced questions, Glenda talks with Kylie, including patient teaching regarding feminine hygiene in their discussion. Glenda decides to develop an insert entitled *Self-Care: Feminine Hygiene* for the campus newspaper. The information she plans to include and the population she will address in her checklist are based on the following assessment data:

- Heterogeneous female population is of various ages, cultures, religions, sexual orientation, and family and lifestyle backgrounds.

- Knowledge about feminine hygiene varies widely from almost no knowledge to students who are well read or members of women's health professions.
- Students who present with questions are mostly concerned about the risk of acquiring an STI or the dangers of certain products (e.g., tampons and toxic shock syndrome) or have questions related to intercourse and contraception.
- Numerous students report to the clinic with vaginal infections and urinary tract infections.
- Interest is high; ability to comprehend written materials is high.

NURSING DIAGNOSIS   Self-Care Deficit: Feminine Hygiene related to knowledge deficit as manifested by female students presenting to the campus clinic with questions about feminine hygiene; high incidence of vaginal and urinary tract infections; negative attitudes about feminine body frequently expressed.

EXPECTED OUTCOME   Students will:

Express positive body image, valuing their uniqueness

(continued)

NURSING PLAN OF CARE · 31-1

For Kylie Simpson and Female University Students (continued)

Nursing Interventions	Rationale	Evaluative Statement
With each student who presents at the clinic for help with a gynecologic concern or problem, take the time to assess her knowledge of the female body and her acceptance of her body and comfort with it.	The women's health movement has encouraged women to feel ownership of their bodies, to appreciate their uniqueness as women, and to increase their awareness of their physical bodies and the feelings associated with them. Many women still feel that the genital area and cyclic phenomena such as the menstrual cycle and the female sexual response cycle are "dirty," and symptoms in this area may evoke fear, guilt, anxiety, and shame.	*Six-month evaluation:* 6/30/12 Outcome partially met: Students are beginning to discuss gynecologic concerns more freely, yet great hesitance persists. *Revision:* Continue to help women to know, understand, and accept their bodies and to talk about their bodies. Make this a priority of the nursing staff at the clinic. *G. Davis, RN*
Counsel appropriately.	It is important for nurses to provide women with information about their bodies.	

EXPECTED OUTCOME Students will:

- Correctly describe feminine hygiene self-care behaviors they are willing to incorporate into their daily lifestyles

Nursing Interventions	Rationale	Evaluative Statement
Assess with each patient her knowledge of feminine hygiene practices (correct any misconceptions) and motivation to use them consistently.	Many women have never been instructed about feminine hygiene, and harmful practices may be "picked up" from the media and other sources (e.g., the use of frequent douching and deodorants to eliminate normal body odors).	6/30/12 Outcome met. Following publication of the *Self-Care: Feminine Hygiene* feature and one-on-one counseling using this printed handout, patients are knowledgeable about preventive hygiene measures. *G. Davis, RN*
Address specific concerns related to menstruation, intercourse, other maturational events.	Maturational events, such as menstruation, becoming sexually active, and pregnancy, may result in a need for new or modified hygiene practices.	
Teach the importance of using preventive hygiene measures to reduce the likelihood of acquiring a urinary tract or vaginal infection. Distribute the *Self-Care: Feminine Hygiene* handout and discuss this with the patient.	It is better to prevent a genitourinary infection than to treat it.	

EXPECTED OUTCOME Campus health clinic records will:

- Demonstrate a reduction in both new and recurrent genitourinary infections

(continued)

NURSING PLAN OF CARE · 31-1

For Kylie Simpson and Female University Students *(continued)*

Nursing Interventions	Rationale	Evaluative Statement
Educate women regarding preventive hygiene measures (refer to the *Self-Care* handout).	It is better to prevent a genitourinary infection than to treat it.	6/30/12 Outcome met. Six months after publication and use of the *Self-Care: Feminine Hygiene* handout, the incidence of genitourinary infections is reduced 10%. Will continue to keep education in this regard a priority.
Educate women to distinguish normal from abnormal findings (vaginal discharge, pain, bleeding, problems with urination) and to seek help when appropriate. Nursing measures include teaching preventive measures, instructing in recognition of symptoms, and assisting with self-care activities to prevent and treat infections, including the securing of assistance when indicated.	Early treatment of genitourinary infections reduces the likelihood of residual problems.	*G. Davis, RN*
Document new and recurrent genitourinary infections; identify predisposing factors.	Documentation facilitates on-going management of a recurring problem.	

SAMPLE DOCUMENTATION

6/15/12
Nursing Student visited clinic and expressed need for information about feminine hygiene practices in general as well as those specific hygiene measures for use after intercourse. Also related concern about contracting an STI from partners. Reported that she became sexually active this year and has sexual intercourse once or twice weekly. Stated that "many of my friends use douches" and questioned whether any particular douche products are recommended. We discussed the *Self-Care: Feminine Hygiene* handout and reviewed various healthcare practices. Clarified for student her misconception regarding the advisability of douching. Also counseled her about her right to talk with a sexual partner about STIs and previous contacts with infected individuals. Advised that she refrain from contact or use a condom when she has intercourse. Student reported feeling more "in charge" of body and better able to care for it. Discussed all topics on plan of care and encouraged her to revisit clinic in 6 months for further clarification and evaluation.

G. Davis, RN

Skill · 31-1   Giving a Bed Bath

EQUIPMENT

- Washbasin and warm water
- Personal hygiene supplies (deodorant, lotion, others)
- Skin-cleaning agent

- Emollient and skin barrier, as indicated
- Towels (2)
- Washcloths (2)
- Bath blanket

- Gown or pajamas
- Bedpan or urinal
- Laundry bag
- Nonsterile gloves; other PPE as indicated

IMPLEMENTATION

ACTION	RATIONALE
1. Review chart for any limitations in physical activity.	Identifying limitations prevents patient discomfort and injury.
2. Bring necessary equipment to the bedside stand or overbed table.	Bringing everything to the bedside conserves time and energy. Arranging items nearby is convenient, saves time, and avoids unnecessary stretching and twisting of muscles on the part of the nurse.
3. Perform hand hygiene and put on gloves and/or other PPE, if indicated.	Hand hygiene and PPE prevent the spread of microorganisms. PPE is required based on transmission precautions.
4. Identify the patient. Discuss procedure with patient and assess patient's ability to assist in the bathing process, as well as personal hygiene preferences.	Identifying the patient ensures the right patient receives the intervention and helps prevent errors. Discussion promotes reassurance and provides knowledge about the procedure. Dialogue encourages patient participation and allows for individualized nursing care.
5. Close curtains around bed and close door to room if possible. Adjust the room temperature if necessary.	This ensures the patient's privacy and lessens the risk for loss of body heat during the bath.
6. Remove sequential compression devices and antiembolism stockings from lower extremities according to agency protocol.	Most manufacturers and agencies recommend removal of these devices before the bath to allow for assessment.
7. Offer patient bedpan or urinal.	Voiding or defecating before the bath lessens the likelihood that the bath will be interrupted, because warm bath water may stimulate the urge to void.
8. Remove gloves and perform hand hygiene.	Hand hygiene deters the spread of microorganisms.
9. Adjust the bed to a comfortable working height; usually elbow height of the caregiver (VISN 8, 2009).	Having the bed at the proper height prevents back and muscle strain.
10. Put on gloves. Lower side rail nearer to you and assist patient to side of bed where you will work. Have patient lie on his or her back.	Gloves prevent transmission of microorganisms. Having the patient positioned near the nurse and lowering the side rail prevent unnecessary stretching and twisting of muscles on the part of the nurse.
11. Loosen top covers and remove all except the top sheet. Place bath blanket over patient and then remove top sheet while patient holds bath blanket in place. If linen is to be reused, fold it over a chair. Place soiled linen in laundry bag. Take care to prevent linen from coming in contact with your clothing.	The patient is not exposed unnecessarily, and warmth is maintained. If a bath blanket is unavailable, the top sheet may be used in place of the bath blanket.
12. Remove patient's gown and keep bath blanket in place. If patient has an IV line and is not wearing a gown with snap sleeves, remove gown from other arm first. **Lower the IV container and pass gown over the tubing and the container. Rehang the container and check the drip rate.**	This provides uncluttered access during the bath and maintains warmth of the patient. IV fluids must be maintained at the prescribed rate.
13. **Raise side rails.** Fill basin with a sufficient amount of comfortably warm water (110°–115°F). Add the skin cleanser, if appropriate, according to manufacturer's directions. Change as necessary throughout the bath. Lower side rail closer to you when you return to the bedside to begin the bath.	Side rails maintain patient safety. Warm water is comfortable and relaxing for the patient. It also stimulates circulation and provides for more effective cleansing.
14. Put on gloves, if necessary. Fold the washcloth like a mitt on your hand so that there are no loose ends (Figures 1–3).	Gloves are necessary if there is potential contact with blood or body fluids. Having loose ends of cloth drag across the patient's skin is uncomfortable. Loose ends cool quickly and feel cold to the patient.

(continued)

Skill · 31-1 Giving a Bed Bath *continued*

ACTION	RATIONALE
15. Lay a towel across patient's chest and on top of bath blanket.	This prevents chilling and keeps bath blanket dry.
16. **With no cleanser on the washcloth, wipe one eye from the inner part of the eye, near the nose, to the outer part (Figure 4). Rinse or turn the cloth before washing the other eye.**	Soap is irritating to the eyes. Moving from the inner to the outer aspect of the eye prevents carrying debris toward the nasolacrimal duct. Rinsing or turning the washcloth prevents spreading organisms from one eye to the other.

FIGURE 1. Folding washcloth in thirds around hand to make a bath mitt.

FIGURE 2. Straightening washcloth before folding into mitt.

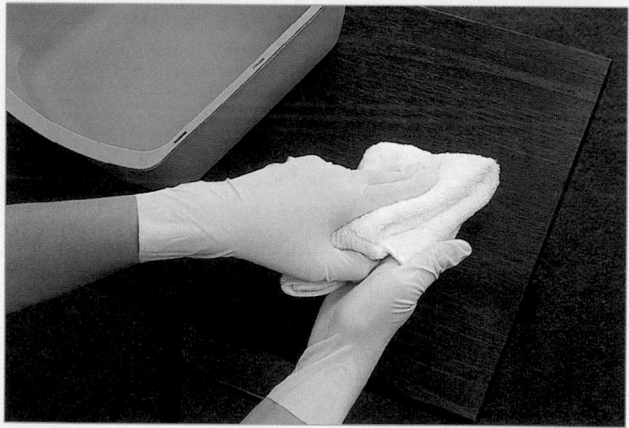

FIGURE 3. Folding ends over and tucking ends under folded washcloth over palm.

FIGURE 4. Washing from the inner corner of the eye outward.

17. Bathe patient's face, neck, and ears. Apply appropriate emollient.	Use of emollients is recommended to restore and maintain skin integrity (Voegeli, 2008a; Watkins, 2008; Brown & Butcher, 2005).
18. Expose patient's far arm and place towel lengthwise under it. Using firm strokes, wash hand, arm, and axilla, lifting the arm as necessary to access axillary region (Figure 5). Rinse, if necessary, and dry. Apply appropriate emollient.	The towel helps to keep the bed dry. Washing the far side first eliminates contaminating a clean area once it is washed. Gentle friction stimulates circulation and muscles and helps remove dirt, oil, and organisms. Long, firm strokes are relaxing and more comfortable than short, uneven strokes. Rinsing is necessary when using some cleansing products. Use of emollients is recommended to restore and maintain skin integrity (Voegeli, 2008a; Watkins, 2008; Brown & Butcher, 2005).

ACTION

19. Place a folded towel on the bed next to the patient's hand and put basin on it. Soak the patient's hand in basin (Figure 6). Wash, rinse if necessary, and dry hand. Apply appropriate emollient.

RATIONALE

Placing the hand in the basin of water is an additional comfort measure for the patient. It facilitates thorough washing of the hands and between the fingers and aids in removing debris from under the skin. Use of emollients is recommended to restore and maintain skin integrity (Voegeli, 2008a; Watkins, 2008; Brown & Butcher, 2005).

FIGURE 5. Exposing the far arm and washing it.

FIGURE 6. Soaking hand in basin.

20. Repeat Actions 15 and 16 for the arm nearer you. An option for the shorter nurse or one prone to back strain might be to bathe one side of the patient and move to the other side of the bed to complete the bath.

21. Spread a towel across patient's chest. Lower bath blanket to patient's umbilical area. Wash, rinse, if necessary, and dry chest. Keep chest covered with towel between the wash and rinse. Pay special attention to the folds of skin under the breasts.

22. Lower bath blanket to the perineal area. Place a towel over patient's chest.

23. Wash; rinse, if necessary; and dry abdomen (Figure 7). Carefully inspect and clean umbilical area and any abdominal folds or creases.

24. Return bath blanket to original position and expose far leg. Place towel under far leg. Using firm strokes, wash; rinse, if necessary; and dry leg from ankle to knee and knee to groin (Figure 8). Apply appropriate emollient.

25. Wash, rinse if necessary, and dry the foot. Pay particular attention to the areas between toes. Apply appropriate emollient.

26. Repeat Actions 24 and 25 for the other leg and foot.

27. Make sure patient is covered with bath blanket. Change water and washcloth at this point or earlier if necessary.

28. Assist patient to prone or side-lying position. Put on gloves, if not applied earlier. Position bath blanket and towel to expose only the back and buttocks.

Exposing, washing, rinsing, and drying one part of the body at a time avoids unnecessary exposure and chilling. Areas of folds of skin may be sources of odor and skin breakdown if not cleaned and dried properly.

Keeping the bath blanket and towel in place avoids exposure and chilling.

Skin-fold areas may be sources of odor and skin breakdown if not cleaned and dried properly.

The towel protects linens and prevents the patient from feeling uncomfortable from a damp or wet bed. Washing from ankle to groin with firm strokes promotes venous return. Use of emollients is recommended to restore and maintain skin integrity (Voegeli, 2008a; Watkins, 2008; Brown & Butcher, 2005).

Drying of the feet is important to prevent irritation, possible skin breakdown, and infections (NIA, 2009). Use of emollients is recommended to restore and maintain skin integrity (Voegeli, 2008a; Watkins, 2008; Brown & Butcher, 2005).

The bath blanket maintains warmth and privacy. Clean, warm water prevents chilling and maintains patient comfort.

Positioning the towel and bath blanket protects the patient's privacy and provides warmth. Gloves prevent contact with body fluids.

(continued)

Skill · 31-1   Giving a Bed Bath   *continued*

FIGURE 7. Washing the abdomen, with perineal and chest areas covered.

FIGURE 8. Washing and drying far leg, keeping the other leg covered.

29. Wash; rinse, if necessary; and dry back and buttocks area (Figure 9). **Pay particular attention to cleansing between gluteal folds, and observe for any redness or skin breakdown in the sacral area.**

Fecal material near the anus may be a source of microorganisms. Prolonged pressure on the sacral area or other bony prominences may compromise circulation and lead to development of decubitus ulcer.

FIGURE 9. Washing the upper back.

30. If not contraindicated, give patient a backrub, as described in Chapter 10. Back massage may be given also after perineal care. Apply appropriate emollient and/or skin barrier product.

A backrub improves circulation to the tissues and is an aid to relaxation. A backrub may be contraindicated in patients with cardiovascular disease or musculoskeletal injuries. Use of emollients is recommended to restore and maintain skin integrity (Voegeli, 2008a; Watkins, 2008; Brown & Butcher, 2005). Skin barriers protect the skin from damage caused by excessive exposure to water and irritants, such as urine and feces (Voegeli, 2008a).

31. Raise the side rail. Refill basin with clean water. Discard washcloth and towel. Remove gloves and put on clean gloves.

The washcloth, towel, and water are contaminated after washing the patient's gluteal area. Changing to clean supplies decreases the spread of organisms from the anal area to the genitals.

32. Clean perineal area or set up patient so that he or she can complete perineal self-care. If the patient is unable, lower the side rail and complete perineal care, following guidelines in the chapter text. Apply skin barrier, as indicated. Raise side rail, remove gloves, and perform hand hygiene.

Providing perineal self-care may decrease embarrassment for the patient. Effective perineal care reduces odor and decreases the risk for infection through contamination. Skin barriers protect the skin from damage caused by excessive exposure to water and irritants, such as urine and feces (Voegeli, 2008a).

ACTION

33. Help patient put on a clean gown and assist with the use of other personal toiletries, such as deodorant or cosmetics.

34. Protect pillow with towel and groom patient's hair.

35. **When finished, make sure the patient is comfortable, with the side rails up and the bed in the lowest position.**

36. Change bed linens, as described in Skills 31-4 and 31-5. Dispose of soiled linens according to agency policy. Remove gloves and any other PPE, if used. Perform hand hygiene.

RATIONALE

This provides for the patient's warmth and comfort.

Proper positioning with raised side rails and proper bed height provides for patient comfort and safety.

Removing PPE properly reduces the risk for infection transmission and contamination of other items. Hand hygiene prevents the spread of microorganisms.

DOCUMENTATION

Guidelines

Record any significant observations and communication on chart. Document the condition of the patient's skin. Record the procedure, amount of assistance given, and patient participation. Document the application of skin care products, such as a skin barrier.

Sample Documentation

7/14/12 2130 Bath provided with complete assistance; reddened area (3 cm × 3 cm) noted on patient's sacral area; skin-care team consultation made.

—C. Stone, RN

UNEXPECTED SITUATIONS AND ASSOCIATED INTERVENTIONS

- *Patient becomes chilled during bath:* If the room temperature is adjustable, increase it. Another bath blanket may be needed.

- *The patient becomes unstable during the bath:* Critically ill patients often need to be bathed in stages. For instance, the right arm is bathed, and then the patient is allowed to rest for a short period before the left arm is bathed. The amount of rest time needed depends on how unstable the patient is and which parameter is being monitored. If the blood pressure drops when the patient is stimulated, the nurse may watch the blood pressure while bathing the patient and stop when it begins to decrease. Once the blood pressure returns to the previous level, the nurse can begin to bathe the patient again.

SPECIAL CONSIDERATIONS

General Considerations

- To remove the gown from a patient with an IV line, take the gown off the uninvolved arm first and then thread the IV tubing and bottle or bag through the arm of the gown. To replace the gown, place the clean gown on the unaffected arm first and thread the IV tubing and bottle or bag from inside the arm of the gown on the involved side. Never disconnect IV tubing to change a gown because this causes a break in a sterile system and could introduce infection.

- Lying flat in bed during the bed bath may be contraindicated for certain patients. The position may have to be modified to accommodate their needs.

- Incontinent patients require special attention to perineal care. Patients with urinary or fecal incontinence are at risk for perineal skin damage. This damage is related to moisture, changes in the pH of the skin, overgrowth of bacteria and infection of the skin, and erosion of perineal skin from friction on moist skin. Skin care for these patients should include measures to reduce overhydration (excess exposure to moisture), reduce contact with ammonia and bacteria, and reduce friction. Remove soil and irritants from the skin during routine hygiene, as well as cleansing when the skin becomes exposed to irritants. Avoid using soap and excessive force for cleaning. The use of perineal skin cleansers, moisturizers, and moisture barriers are recommended for skin care for the incontinent patient. These products help promote healing and prevent further skin damage.

- If the patient has an indwelling catheter and the agency recommends daily care for the catheter, this is usually done after perineal care. Agency policy may recommend use of an antiseptic cleaning agent or plain soap and water on a clean washcloth. Put on clean gloves before cleaning the catheter. Clean 6″ to 8″ of the catheter, moving from the meatus downward. Be careful not to pull or tug on the catheter during the cleaning motion. Also, inspect the meatus for drainage and note the characteristics of the urine.

(continued)

Skill · 31-1   Giving a Bed Bath   *continued*

Infant and Child Considerations	• When bathing an infant or young child, have supplies within easy reach and support or hold the child securely at all times to ensure safety.
	• Never leave the child alone.
Older Adult Considerations	• Check the temperature of the water carefully before bathing an older patient because sensitivity to temperature may be impaired in older persons.
	• An older, continent patient may not require a full bed bath with soap and water every day. If dry skin is a problem, water and skin lotion or bath oil may be used on alternate days. If applying lotion, place the lotion dispenser in warm bath water while bathing the patient. This will warm the lotion before it is applied to the patient.
	• Refer to Box 31-1 for guidelines to assist in meeting hygiene needs for patients with dementia.
Home Care Considerations	• Evaluate the safety of the bathing area in the home. Tub mats, adhesive strips, grab bars, and shower stools can help prevent falls.
	• Use plastic trash bags or a plastic shower-curtain liner to protect the mattress when bathing or shampooing a patient in bed. Disposable washcloths may also be an option to consider. A large plastic container or baby bathtub can effectively serve as a shampoo basin.
	• If linens are soiled with blood or body fluids, instruct family members to wear gloves when handling them. They should be rinsed first in cold water and then washed separately from other household wash, using hot water, laundry detergent, and bleach.
	• Teach a family member or caregiver how to perform comfort measures, such as a backrub.
	• Instruct patients at home with an indwelling catheter, or their caregivers, to wash the urinary meatus and perineal area twice daily with soap and water. The anal area should also be cleaned after each bowel movement. Careful hand washing is imperative.

Skill · 31-2   Assisting the Patient With Oral Care

EQUIPMENT

- Toothbrush
- Toothpaste
- Emesis basin
- Glass with cool water

- Disposable gloves
- Additional PPE, as indicated
- Towel
- Mouthwash (optional)

- Washcloth or paper towel
- Lip lubricant (optional)
- Dental floss

IMPLEMENTATION

ACTION	RATIONALE
1. Perform hand hygiene and put on gloves if assisting with oral care, and/or other PPE, if indicated.	Hand hygiene and PPE prevent the spread of microorganisms. PPE is required based on transmission precautions.
2. Identify the patient. Explain procedure to patient.	Identifying the patient ensures the right patient receives the intervention and helps prevent errors. Explanation facilitates cooperation.
3. Assemble equipment on overbed table within patient's reach.	Organization facilitates performance of task.
4. Close the room door or curtains. Place the bed at an appropriate and comfortable working height, usually elbow height of the caregiver (VISN 8, 2009).	Closing the door or curtains provides privacy. Proper bed height helps reduce back strain while performing the procedure.
5. Lower side rail and assist patient to sitting position if permitted, or turn patient onto side. Place towel across patient's chest. Raise bed to a comfortable working position.	The sitting or side-lying position prevents aspiration of fluids into the lungs. The towel protects the patient from dampness.

<table>
<tr><td>

ACTION

6. Encourage patient to brush own teeth, or assist if necessary.

  a. Moisten toothbrush and apply toothpaste to bristles.

  b. Place brush at a 45-degree angle to gum line (Figure 1) and brush from gum line to crown of each tooth (Figure 2). Brush outer and inner surfaces. Brush back and forth across biting surface of each tooth.

  c. Brush tongue gently with toothbrush (Figure 3).

  d. Have patient rinse vigorously with water and spit into emesis basin (Figure 4). Repeat until clear. Suction may be used as an alternative for removal of fluid and secretions from mouth.

</td><td>

RATIONALE

Water softens the bristles.

Facilitates removal of plaque and tartar. The 45-degree angle of brushing permits cleansing of all surface areas of the tooth.

Removes coating on the tongue. Gentle motion does not stimulate gag reflex.

The vigorous swishing motion helps to remove debris. Suction is appropriate if patient is unable to expectorate well.

</td></tr>
</table>

FIGURE 1. Placing brush at a 45-degree angle to the gum line.

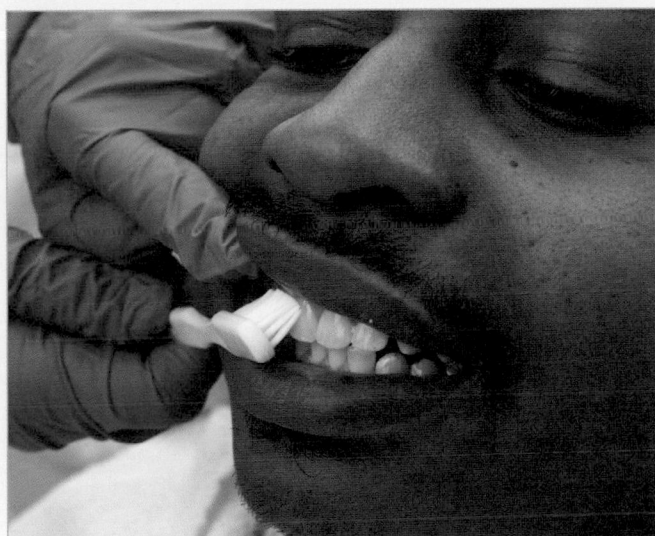

FIGURE 2. Brushing from the gum line to the crown of each tooth.

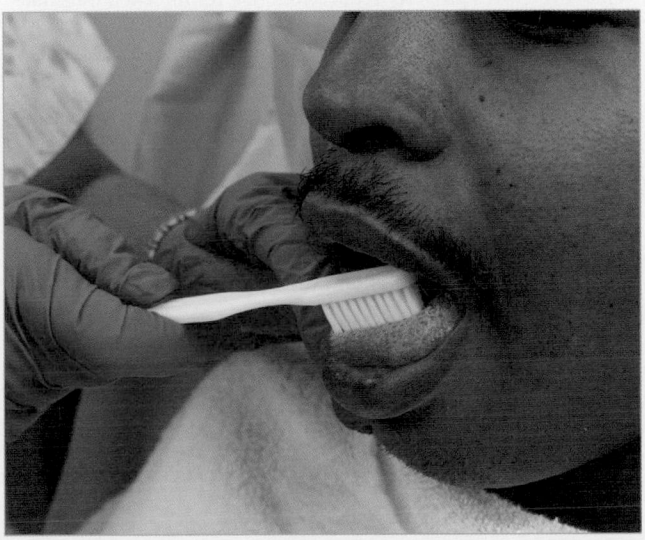

FIGURE 3. Brushing the tongue.

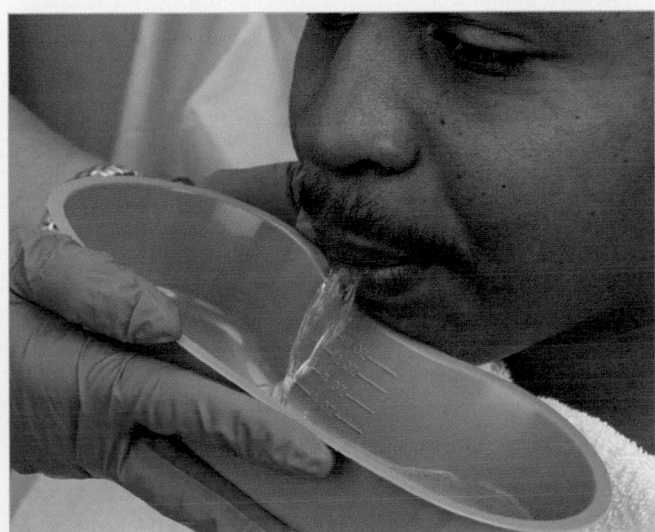

FIGURE 4. Holding emesis basin for patient to rinse and spit.

(continued)

Skill · 31-2   Assisting the Patient With Oral Care   *continued*

ACTION

7. Assist patient to floss teeth, if appropriate:

    a. Remove approximately 6″ of dental floss from container or use a plastic floss holder. Wrap the floss around the index fingers, keeping about 1″ to 1.5″ of floss taut between the fingers.

    b. Insert floss gently between teeth, moving it back and forth downward to the gums.

    c. Move the floss up and down, first on one side of a tooth and then on the side of the other tooth, until the surfaces are clean (Figure 5). Repeat in the spaces between all teeth.

    d. Instruct patient to rinse mouth well with water after flossing.

RATIONALE

Flossing aids in removal of plaque and promotes healthy gum tissue.

The floss must be held taut to get between the teeth.

Trauma to the gums can occur if floss is forced between teeth.

This ensures that the sides of both teeth are cleaned.

Vigorous rinsing helps to remove food particles and plaque that have been loosened by flossing.

FIGURE 5. Flossing the teeth.

8. Offer mouthwash if patient prefers.

9. Offer lip balm or petroleum jelly.

10. Remove equipment. Remove gloves and discard. Raise side rail and lower bed. Assist patient to a position of comfort.

11. Remove any other PPE, if used. Perform hand hygiene.

Mouthwash leaves a pleasant taste in the mouth.

Lip balm lubricates lips and prevents drying.

Removing gloves properly reduces the risk for infection transmission and contamination of other items. These actions promote patient comfort and safety.

Removing PPE properly reduces the risk for infection transmission and contamination of other items. Hand hygiene prevents the spread of microorganisms.

DOCUMENTATION

Guidelines

Record oral assessment, significant observations, and unusual findings, such as bleeding or inflammation. Document any teaching done. Document procedure and patient response.

Sample Documentation

10/20/12 0930 Patient performed oral care with minimal assistance. Oral-cavity mucosa pink and moist. No evidence of bleeding or ulceration. Lips slightly dry; lip moisturizer applied. Reinforcement provided related to importance of flossing teeth every day. Patient demonstrates appropriate flossing technique.

—*L. Schneider, RN*

UNEXPECTED SITUATIONS AND ASSOCIATED INTERVENTIONS

- *While cleaning the teeth, you notice a large amount of bleeding from the gum line:* Stop brushing. Allow patient to gently rinse mouth with water and spit into emesis basin. Before brushing again, check most recent platelet level. Consider the use of a toothette to provide oral hygiene.
- *Patient has braces on teeth:* Brush extra thoroughly. Braces collect food particles.

SPECIAL CONSIDERATIONS
General Considerations

- Use a soft bristled toothbrush with a small head even when the patient has no or few teeth. It is the only effective way to remove plaque and debris from the teeth, gums, and tongue (Holman, Roberts, & Nicol, 2005).
- A patient receiving chemotherapy medication may have bleeding gums and extremely sensitive mucous membranes. Use a soft sponge toothette for cleaning, and a saltwater rinse (half teaspoon salt in 1 cup of warm water) (Polovich et al., 2009).

Infant and Child Considerations

- When assisting small children with oral care, do not use toothpaste that contains fluoride if the child cannot spit out excess. Excessive amounts of ingested fluoride can lead to a discoloration of the teeth.
- Oral hygiene should begin as soon as an infant's teeth erupt. Clean teeth and gums by wiping with a damp cloth. As the infant gets more teeth, introduce a small toothbrush. Use water to clean an infant's teeth, not toothpaste.

Skill · 31-3   Providing Oral Care for the Dependent Patient

EQUIPMENT

- Toothbrush
- Toothpaste
- Emesis basin
- Glass with cool water
- Disposable gloves
- Additional PPE, as indicated
- Towel
- Mouthwash (optional)
- Dental floss (optional)
- Denture-cleaning equipment (if necessary)
- Denture cup
- Denture cleaner
- 4 × 4 gauze
- Washcloth or paper towel
- Lip lubricant (optional)
- Sponge toothette
- Irrigating syringe with rubber tip (optional)
- Suction catheter with suction apparatus (optional)

IMPLEMENTATION

ACTION	RATIONALE
1. Perform hand hygiene and put on PPE, if indicated.	Hand hygiene and PPE prevent the spread of microorganisms. PPE is required based on transmission precautions.
2. Identify the patient. Explain procedure to patient.	Identifying the patient ensures the right patient receives the intervention and helps prevent errors. Explanation facilitates cooperation.
3. Assemble equipment on overbed table within reach.	Organization facilitates performance of task.
4. Close the room door or curtains. Place the bed at an appropriate and comfortable working height, usually elbow height of the caregiver (VISN 8, 2009). Lower one side rail and position patient on the side, with head tilted forward. Place towel across patient's chest and emesis basin in position under chin. Put on gloves.	Cleaning another person's mouth is invasive and may be embarrassing (Holman, Roberts, & Nicol, 2005). Closing the door or curtains provides privacy. Proper bed height helps reduce back strain while performing the procedure. The side-lying position with head forward prevents aspiration of fluid into lungs. Towel and emesis basin protects patient from dampness. Gloves prevent the spread of microorganisms.

(continued)

Skill · 31-3 **Providing Oral Care for the Dependent Patient** *continued*

ACTION	RATIONALE
5. Gently open the patient's mouth by applying pressure to lower jaw at the front of the mouth. Remove dentures, if present. Brush the teeth and gums carefully with toothbrush and paste (Figure 1). Lightly brush the tongue.	Toothbrush provides friction necessary to clean areas where plaque and tartar accumulate.
6. Use toothette dipped in water to rinse the oral cavity. If desired, insert the rubber tip of the irrigating syringe into patient's mouth and rinse gently with a small amount of water (Figure 2). **Position patient's head to allow for return of water or use suction apparatus to remove the water from oral cavity (Figure 3).**	Rinsing helps clean debris from the mouth. Forceful irrigation may cause aspiration.

FIGURE 1. Carefully brushing patient's teeth.

FIGURE 2. Using irrigating syringe and a small amount of water to rinse mouth.

FIGURE 3. Using suction to remove excess fluid.

ACTION	RATIONALE
7. Clean the dentures before replacing.	Cleaning maintains dentures and oral hygiene. Plaque can accumulate on dentures and can promote oropharyngeal colonization of pathogens (Yoon & Steele, 2007).
8. Apply lubricant to patient's lips.	This prevents drying and cracking of lips.
9. Remove equipment and return patient to a position of comfort. Remove your gloves. Raise side rail and lower bed.	Promotes patient comfort and safety. Removing gloves properly reduces the risk for infection transmission and contamination of other items.
10. Remove additional PPE, if used. Perform hand hygiene.	Removing PPE properly reduces the risk for infection transmission and contamination of other items. Hand hygiene prevents the spread of microorganisms.

DOCUMENTATION

Guidelines

Record oral assessment, significant observations, and unusual findings, such as bleeding or inflammation. Document any teaching done. Document procedure and patient response.

Sample Documentation

7/10/12 0945 Oral care performed. Oral cavity mucosa pink and moist. Small amount of bleeding noted from gums after using soft-bristled toothbrush. Resolved spontaneously when brushing completed. No evidence of ulceration. Lips slightly dry; lip moisturizer applied.

—C. Stone, RN

UNEXPECTED SITUATIONS AND ASSOCIATED INTERVENTIONS

- *Patient begins to bite the toothbrush:* Do not jerk the toothbrush out. Wait for patient to relax mouth before removing the toothbrush and continuing with care.
- *Mouth is extremely dry with crusts that remain after oral care provided:* Increase frequency of oral hygiene. Apply mouth moisturizer to oral mucosa.

SPECIAL CONSIDERATIONS

General Considerations

- Suction toothbrushes may be used with patients with dysphagia, including those on enteral feedings (Yoon & Steele, 2007).
- A patient receiving chemotherapy medication may have bleeding gums and extremely sensitive mucous membranes. Use a soft sponge toothette for cleaning, and a saltwater rinse (half teaspoon salt in 1 cup of warm water) (Polovich et al., 2009).
- Use a soft bristled toothbrush with a small head even when the patient has no or few teeth. It is the only effective way to remove plaque and debris from the teeth, gums, and tongue (Holman, Roberts, & Nicol, 2005).

Skill · 31-4   Making an Unoccupied Bed

EQUIPMENT

- One large flat sheet
- One fitted sheet
- Drawsheet (optional)
- Blankets
- Bedspread
- Pillowcases
- Linen hamper or bag
- Bedside chair
- Waterproof protective pad (optional)
- Disposable gloves
- Additional PPE, as indicated

IMPLEMENTATION

ACTION	RATIONALE
1. Assemble equipment and arrange on a bedside chair in the order in which items will be used.	Organization facilitates performance of task.
2. Perform hand hygiene. Put on PPE, as indicated.	Hand hygiene and PPE prevent the spread of microorganisms. PPE is required based on transmission precautions.
3. Adjust the bed to a comfortable working height, usually elbow height of the caregiver (VISN 8, 2009). Drop the side rails.	Having the bed at the proper height prevents back and muscle strain. Having the side rails down reduces strain on the nurse while working.
4. Disconnect call bell or any tubes from bed linens.	Disconnecting devices prevents damage to the devices.
5. Put on gloves. Loosen all linen as you move around the bed, from the head of the bed on the far side to the head of the bed on the near side.	Gloves prevent the spread of microorganisms. Loosening the linen helps prevent tugging and tearing on linen. Loosening the linen and moving around the bed systematically reduce strain caused by reaching across the bed.

(continued)

Skill · 31-4   Making an Unoccupied Bed   *continued*

ACTION	RATIONALE
6. Fold reusable linens, such as sheets, blankets, or spread, in place on the bed in fourths and hang them over a clean chair.	Folding saves time and energy when reusable linen is replaced on the bed. Folding linens while they are on the bed reduces strain on the nurse's arms. Some agencies change linens only when soiled.
7. Snugly roll all the soiled linen inside the bottom sheet and place directly into the laundry hamper (Figure 1). **Do not place on floor or furniture. Do not hold soiled linens against your uniform.**	Rolling soiled linens snugly and placing them directly into the hamper helps prevent the spread of microorganisms. The floor is heavily contaminated; soiled linen will further contaminate furniture. Soiled linen contaminates the nurse's uniform, and this may spread organisms to another patient.
8. If possible, shift mattress up to head of bed. If mattress is soiled, clean and dry according to facility policy before applying new sheets.	This allows more foot room for the patient.
9. Remove your gloves, unless indicated for transmission precautions. Place the bottom sheet with its center fold in the center of the bed. Open the sheet and fan-fold to the center (Figure 2).	Gloves are not necessary to handle clean linen. Removing gloves properly reduces the risk for infection transmission and contamination of other items. Opening linens on the bed reduces strain on the nurse's arms and diminishes the spread of microorganisms. Centering the sheet ensures sufficient coverage for both sides of the mattress.

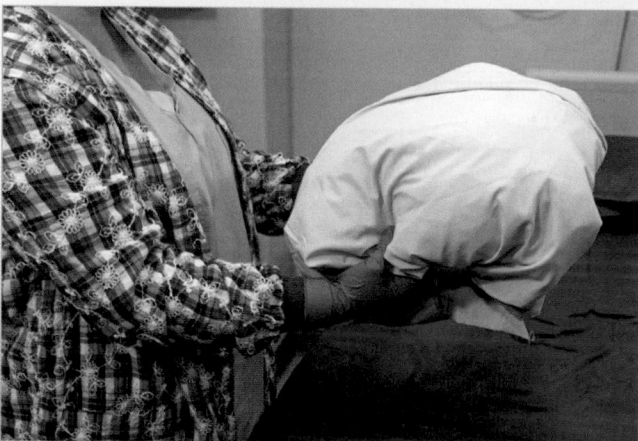

FIGURE 1. Bundling soiled linens in bottom sheet and holding them away from body.

FIGURE 2. Opening bottom sheet and fan-folding to center of bed.

10. If using, place the drawsheet with its center fold in the center of the bed and positioned so it will be located under the patient's midsection. Open the drawsheet and fan-fold to the center of the mattress (Figure 3). If a protective pad is used, place it over the drawsheet in the proper area and open to the center fold. Not all agencies use drawsheets routinely. The nurse may decide to use one. In some institutions, the protective pad doubles as a drawsheet.	If the patient soils the bed, drawsheet and pad can be changed without the bottom and top linens on the bed. Having all bottom linens in place before tucking them under the mattress avoids unnecessary moving about the bed. A drawsheet can aid moving the patient in bed.
11. Pull the bottom sheet over the corners at the head and foot of the mattress. Tuck the drawsheet securely under the mattress.	Making the bed on one side and then completing the bed on the other side saves time. Having bottom linens free of wrinkles reduces patient discomfort.
12. Move to the other side of the bed to secure bottom linens. Pull the bottom sheet tightly and secure over the corners at the head and foot of the mattress. Pull the drawsheet tightly and tuck it securely under the mattress.	This removes wrinkles from the bottom linens, which can cause patient discomfort and promote skin breakdown.

ACTION

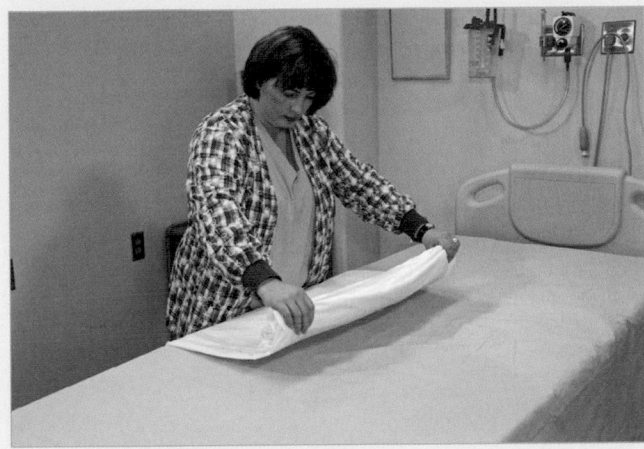

FIGURE 3. Placing drawsheet on bed.

RATIONALE

13. Place the top sheet on the bed with its center fold in the center of the bed and with the hem even with the head of the mattress. Unfold the top sheet. Follow same procedure with top blanket or spread, placing the upper edge about 6″ below the top of the sheet.

14. Tuck the top sheet and blanket under the foot of the bed on the near side. Miter the corners (Figure 4).

15. Fold the upper 6″ of the top sheet down over the spread and make a cuff.

16. Move to the other side of the bed and follow the same procedure for securing top sheets under the foot of the bed and making a cuff (Figure 5).

Opening linens by shaking them spreads organisms into the air. Holding linens overhead to open them causes strain on the nurse's arms.

This saves time and energy and keeps the top linen in place.

This makes it easier for the patient to get into bed and pull the covers up.

Working on one side of the bed at a time saves energy and is more efficient.

FIGURE 4. Mitering corner of top sheet and spread.

FIGURE 5. Cuffing top linens.

(continued)

Skill · 31-4 **Making an Unoccupied Bed** *continued*

ACTION	RATIONALE
17. Place the pillows on the bed. Open each pillowcase in the same manner as you opened other linens. Gather the pillowcase over one hand toward the closed end. Grasp the pillow with the hand inside the pillowcase. Keep a firm hold on the top of the pillow and pull the cover onto the pillow. Place the pillow at the head of the bed (Figure 6).	Opening linens by shaking them causes organisms to be carried on air currents. Covering the pillow while it rests on the bed reduces strain on the nurse's arms and back.
18. Fan-fold or pie-fold the top linens.	Having linens opened makes it more convenient for the patient to get into bed.
19. Secure the signal device on the bed according to agency policy (Figure 7).	The patient will be able to call for assistance as necessary. Promotes patient comfort and safety.

FIGURE 6. Placing pillow on bed.

FIGURE 7. Securing signal device to bed.

20. Raise side rail and lower bed.	Promotes patient comfort and safety.
21. Dispose of soiled linen according to agency policy.	Deters the spread of microorganisms.
22. Remove any other PPE, if used. Perform hand hygiene.	Removing PPE properly reduces the risk for infection transmission and contamination of other items. Hand hygiene prevents the spread of microorganisms.

DOCUMENTATION	Changing of bed linens does not need to be documented. The use of a specialty bed, or bed equipment, such as Balkan frame or foot cradle, should be documented.
UNEXPECTED SITUATIONS AND ASSOCIATED INTERVENTIONS	• *Drawsheet is not available:* A flat sheet can be folded in half to substitute for a drawsheet, but extra care must be taken to avoid wrinkles in the bed. • *Patient is frequently incontinent of stool or urine:* More than one protective pad can be placed under the patient to protect the bed, but care must be taken to ensure that the patient is not lying on wrinkles from linens.

Skill · 31-5 Making an Occupied Bed

EQUIPMENT

- One large flat sheet
- One fitted sheet
- Drawsheet (optional)
- Blankets

- Bedspread
- Pillowcases
- Linen hamper or bag
- Bedside chair

- Protective pad (optional)
- Disposable gloves
- Additional PPE, as indicated

IMPLEMENTATION

ACTION	RATIONALE
1. Check chart for limitations on patient's physical activity.	This facilitates patient cooperation, determines level of activity, and promotes patient safety.
2. Assemble equipment and arrange on bedside chair in the order the items will be used.	Organization facilitates performance of task.
3. Perform hand hygiene. Put on PPE, as indicated.	Hand hygiene and PPE prevent the spread of microorganisms. PPE is required based on transmission precautions.
4. Identify the patient. Explain what you are going to do.	Patient identification validates the correct patient and correct procedure. Discussion and explanation allay anxiety and prepare the patient for what to expect.
5. Close curtains around bed and close door to room if possible.	This ensures the patient's privacy.
6. Adjust the bed to a comfortable working height, usually elbow height of the caregiver (VISN 8, 2006).	Having the bed at the proper height prevents back and muscle strain.
7. Lower side rail nearest you, leaving the opposite side rail up. Place bed in flat position unless contraindicated.	Having the mattress flat makes it easier to prepare a wrinkle-free bed.
8. Put on gloves. Check bed linens for patient's personal items. **Disconnect the call bell or any tubes/drains from bed linens.**	Gloves prevent the spread of microorganisms. It is costly and inconvenient when personal items are lost. Disconnecting tubes from linens prevents discomfort and accidental dislodging of the tubes.
9. Place a bath blanket over patient. Have patient hold on to bath blanket while you reach under it and remove top linens (Figure 1). Leave top sheet in place if a bath blanket is not used. Fold linen that is to be reused over the back of a chair. Discard soiled linen in laundry bag or hamper. **Do not place on floor or furniture. Do not hold soiled linens against your uniform.**	The blanket provides warmth and privacy. Placing linens directly into the hamper helps prevent the spread of microorganisms. The floor is heavily contaminated; soiled linen will further contaminate furniture. Soiled linen contaminates the nurse's uniform, and this may spread organisms to another patient.
10. If possible and another person is available to assist, grasp mattress securely and shift it up to head of bed.	This allows more foot room for the patient.

FIGURE 1. Removing top linens from under bath blanket.

(continued)

Skill · 31-5   Making an Occupied Bed   *continued*

ACTION	RATIONALE
11. Assist patient to turn toward opposite side of the bed, and reposition pillow under patient's head.	This allows the bed to be made on the vacant side.
12. Loosen all bottom linens from head, foot, and side of bed.	This facilitates removal of linens.
13. Fan-fold soiled linens as close to patient as possible (Figure 2).	This makes it easier to remove linens when the patient turns to the other side.
14. Use clean linen and make the near side of the bed. Place the bottom sheet with its center fold in the center of the bed (Figure 3). Open the sheet and fan-fold to the center, positioning it under the old linens (Figure 4). Pull the bottom sheet over the corners at the head and foot of the mattress.	Opening linens on the bed reduces strain on the nurse's arms and diminishes the spread of microorganisms. Centering the sheet ensures sufficient coverage for both sides of the mattress. Positioning under the old linens makes it easier to remove linens.
15. If using, place the drawsheet with its center fold in the center of the bed and positioned so it will be located under the patient's midsection. Open the drawsheet and fan-fold to the center of the mattress. Tuck the drawsheet securely under the mattress (Figure 5). If a protective pad is used, place it over the drawsheet in the proper area and open to the center fold. Not all agencies use drawsheets routinely. The nurse may decide to use one.	If the patient soils the bed, drawsheet and pad can be changed without the bottom and top linens on the bed. A drawsheet can aid moving the patient in bed.

FIGURE 2. Moving soiled linen as close to patient as possible.

FIGURE 3. Placing bottom sheet with center fold in center of bed.

FIGURE 4. Fan-folding bottom sheet to the center, positioning it under the old linens.

FIGURE 5. Tucking drawsheet tightly.

ACTION

16. Raise side rail. Assist patient to roll over the folded linen in the middle of the bed toward you. Reposition pillow and bath blanket or top sheet. Move to other side of the bed and lower side rail.

17. Loosen and remove all bottom linen (Figure 6). Discard soiled linen in laundry bag or hamper. **Do not place on floor or furniture. Do not hold soiled linens against your uniform.**

18. Ease clean linen from under the patient. Pull the bottom sheet taut and secure at the corners at the head and foot of the mattress. Pull the drawsheet tight and smooth. Tuck the drawsheet securely under the mattress.

19. Assist patient to turn back to the center of bed. Remove pillow and change pillowcase. Open each pillowcase in the same manner as you opened other linens. Gather the pillowcase over one hand toward the closed end. Grasp the pillow with the hand inside the pillowcase. Keep a firm hold on the top of the pillow and pull the cover onto the pillow. Place the pillow under the patient's head.

20. Apply top linen, sheet, and blanket if desired, so that it is centered. Fold the top linens over at the patient's shoulders to make a cuff. Have patient hold on to top linen and remove the bath blanket from underneath (Figure 7).

21. Secure top linens under foot of mattress and miter corners. Loosen top linens over patient's feet by grasping them in the area of the feet and pulling gently toward foot of bed.

22. Return patient to a position of comfort. Remove your gloves. Raise side rail and lower bed. Reattach call bell.

RATIONALE

This ensures patient safety. The movement allows the bed to be made on the other side. The bath blanket provides warmth and privacy.

Placing linens directly into the hamper helps prevent the spread of microorganisms. The floor is heavily contaminated; soiled linen will further contaminate furniture. Soiled linen contaminates the nurse's uniform, and this may spread organisms to another patient.

This removes wrinkles and creases in the linens, which are uncomfortable to lie on.

Opening linens by shaking them causes organisms to be carried on air currents.

This allows bottom hems to be tucked securely under the mattress and provides for privacy.

This provides for a neat appearance. Loosening linens over the patient's feet gives more room for movement.

Promotes patient comfort and safety. Removing gloves properly reduces the risk for infection transmission and contamination of other items.

FIGURE 6. Removing soiled bottom linens from other side of bed.

FIGURE 7. Removing bath blanket from under top linens.

(continued)

Skill · 31-5 Making an Occupied Bed *continued*

ACTION	RATIONALE
23. Dispose of soiled linens according to agency policy.	Deters the spread of microorganisms.
24. Remove any other PPE, if used. Perform hand hygiene.	Removing PPE properly reduces the risk for infection transmission and contamination of other items. Hand hygiene prevents the spread of microorganisms.

DOCUMENTATION

Changing of bed linens does not need to be documented. The use of a specialty bed, or bed equipment, such as Balkan frame or foot cradle, should be documented. Document any significant observations and communication.

UNEXPECTED SITUATIONS AND ASSOCIATED INTERVENTIONS

• *Dirty linens are grossly contaminated with urinary or fecal drainage:* Obtain an extra towel or protective pad. Place the pad under and over the soiled linens so that new linens will not be in contact with soiled linens. Clean and dry the mattress according to facility policy before applying new sheets.

SPECIAL CONSIDERATIONS
Older Adult Consideration

• Using a soft bath blanket, or a flannelette blanket as a bottom sheet may solve the problem of "coldness" for elderly patients with vascular problems or arthritis.

● Developing Critical Thinking Skills

1. Practice the art of back massage with a willing partner until you feel comfortable and confident including this nursing measure in your routine care. Discuss with other students the therapeutic benefits of massage, and identify nursing situations for which it may be the primary therapy.

2. Interview people of different ages and cultural backgrounds about their hygiene practices. Ask specific questions about the type of nursing assistance they would require if hospitalized and unable to meet their hygiene needs independently. Are there special products or equipment they would need? To what extent are nurses obliged to respect the hygiene preferences of patients?

● Practicing for the NCLEX

1. When planning for completion of a patient's personal hygiene, it is most important to consider which of the following?
   a. When the patient had his or her most recent bath
   b. The patient's usual hygiene practices and preferences
   c. Where the bathing fits in the nurse's schedule
   d. The time that is convenient for the patient care assistant

2. Why is adequate oral hygiene an essential part of nursing care? Select all that apply.
   a. It promotes the patient's sense of well-being.
   b. It prevents deterioration of the oral cavity.
   c. It contributes to decreased incidence of aspiration pneumonia.
   d. It eliminates the need for flossing.
   e. It decreases oropharyngeal secretions.

3. During a bath, the nurse observes that a patient has dry skin. Which action would be best?
   a. Bathe the patient more frequently.
   b. Use an emollient on the dry skin.
   c. Massage the skin with alcohol.
   d. Discourage fluid intake.

4. Which recommendation by the nurse to an adolescent patient with acne would be most appropriate?
   a. Wash the skin twice a day.
   b. Use cosmetics liberally to cover blackheads.
   c. Use emollients on the area.
   d. Squeeze blackheads as they appear.

5. The nurse observes a marked inflammation of the gums, and recession and bleeding of the gums and documents this observation using which term?
   a. Glossitis
   b. Caries
   c. Cheilosis
   d. Periodontitis

6. Which action would be the priority when administering oral care to a dependent patient?
   a. Assisting the patient to the dorsal recumbent position
   b. Wearing disposable gloves
   c. Using a firm toothbrush to cleanse teeth and gums
   d. Irrigating forcefully with hydrogen peroxide

7. Mr. James has an eye infection with a moderate amount of discharge. Which action would be most appropriate for the nurse to use when cleaning his eyes?
   a. Using hydrogen peroxide
   b. Wiping from the outer canthus to the inner canthus
   c. Positioning him on the same side as the eye to be cleansed
   d. Using only one cotton ball per eye

8. Which of the following interventions would the nurse include in the plan of care when providing foot care to an older patient?
   a. Using scissors to correct an ingrown toenail
   b. Trimming toenails as short as possible
   c. Using an alcohol rub if the feet are dry
   d. Bathing the feet at least daily

9. Providing perineal care to a patient requires which of the following?
   a. Using a clean portion of the washcloth for each stroke
   b. Moving from most contaminated to least contaminated area
   c. Using sterile gloves
   d. Leaving the foreskin undisturbed in an uncircumcised adult male

10. A nurse is caring for an 80-year-old patient who has become weak and fatigues easily. He is unable to wash his body and always asks the nurse to brush his teeth. Based on this information, which of the following is an appropriate nursing diagnosis for this patient?
    a. Risk for Impaired Skin Integrity related to immobility
    b. Bathing/Hygiene Self-Care Deficit related to decreased strength and endurance
    c. Social Isolation related to lack of visitors
    d. Impaired Oral Mucous Membrane related to inability to brush his teeth

11. An older patient with an unsteady gait requests a tub bath. Which of the following actions would be most appropriate?
    a. Add Alpha-Keri oil to the water to prevent dry skin.
    b. Allow the patient to lock the door to guarantee privacy.
    c. Assist the patient in and out of the tub to prevent falling.
    d. Keep the water temperature very warm because the patient chills easily.

12. During morning care, the patient asks the nurse to shave him with a disposable razor. Before shaving him, what should the nurse do?
    a. Have him sign a permission form.
    b. Check to see if the patient is taking anticoagulants.
    c. Tell him that only a family member may shave a patient.
    d. Position him flat in bed.

13. An unresponsive patient is wearing gas-permeable contact lenses. How would the nurse remove these lenses?

a. Gently irrigate the eye with an irrigating solution from the inner canthus outward.
b. Grasp the lens with a gentle pinching motion.
c. Don sterile gloves before attempting the removal procedure.
d. Ensure that the lens is centered on the cornea before gently manipulating the lids to release it.

14. The nurse is about to bathe a female patient who has an intravenous access in place in her forearm. The patient's gown, which does not have snaps on the sleeves, needs to be removed prior to bathing. What should the nurse do?
    a. Temporarily disconnect the IV tubing at a point close to the patient and thread it through the gown sleeve.
    b. Cut the gown with scissors to allow arm movement.
    c. Thread the bag and tubing through the gown sleeve, keeping the line intact.
    d. Temporarily disconnect the tubing from the IV container, threading it through the gown.

15. When making an occupied bed, which of the following is most important for the nurse to do?
    a. Keep the bed in the low position
    b. Use a bath blanket or top sheet for warmth and privacy
    c. Constantly keep the side rails raised on both sides
    d. Move back and forth from one side to the other when adjusting the linens

● Answers With Rationale

1. *b.* Bathing practices and cleansing habits and rituals vary widely. The patient's preferences should always be taken into consideration, unless there is a clear threat to health. The patient and nurse should work together to come to a mutually agreeable time and method to accomplish the patient's personal hygiene. The availability of staff to assist may be important, but the patient's preferences are a higher priority.

2. *a, b, c.* Adequate oral hygiene is essential for promoting the patient's sense of well-being and preventing deterioration of the oral cavity. Diligent oral hygiene care can also improve oral health and limit the growth of pathogens in the oropharyngeal secretions, decreasing the incidence of aspiration pneumonia and other systemic diseases (Yoon & Steele, 2007; AACN, 2006). Oral care does not eliminate the need for flossing (*d*) or decrease oropharyngeal secretions (*e*).

3. *b.* An emollient soothes dry skin, whereas frequent bathing increases dryness, as does alcohol. Discouraging fluid intake leads to dehydration and, subsequently, dry skin.

4. *a.* Washing the skin removes oil and debris, whereas liberal use of cosmetics and emollients can clog the pores. Squeezing blackheads is always discouraged because it may lead to infection.

5. *d.* Periodontitis is a marked inflammation of the gums, whereas caries refers to the presence of tooth decay.

Cheilosis is ulceration of the lips, and glossitis is an inflammation of the tongue.

6. **b.** Disposable gloves provide a barrier to protect the nurse and patient. The dorsal recumbent position is unsafe because the patient may easily aspirate any secretions or fluids. A soft toothbrush is recommended to avoid causing irritation and bleeding, and forceful irrigation is never safe. Water would be the choice for any gentle irrigation.

7. **c.** Positioning the patient on the same side as the involved eye discourages contamination of the other eye. Always cleanse from the inner canthus to the outer canthus to avoid forcing debris into the nasolacrimal duct. Water or normal saline should be used for cleansing the eye of any discharge, and one cotton ball should be used for each stroke.

8. **d.** An older patient should have foot care once daily. Correcting an ingrown toenail should be done by a podiatrist, and trimming the toenails may require a physician's order. Cutting the toenails as short as possible exposes tender areas to friction and may lead to the skin being cut during trimming. Alcohol is drying and should not be used when dry skin is usually already a problem.

9. **a.** A clean portion of the washcloth should be used for each stroke to prevent contamination of other areas. Cleansing should always proceed from the least contaminated to the most contaminated area. Clean gloves, not sterile gloves, are used to provide perineal care. The foreskin in an uncircumcised male should be pulled back to allow cleansing underneath and then gently returned to its former position.

10. **b.** Risk for Impaired Skin Integrity, Social Isolation, and Impaired Oral Mucous Membrane may be appropriate nursing diagnoses for this patient. However, not enough is known, based on the information given, to formulate these diagnoses. The priority at this time, based on the given information, is Bathing/Hygiene Self-Care Deficit.

11. **c.** Safe nursing practice requires that the nurse assist a patient with an unsteady gait in and out of the tub. Adding Alpha-Keri oil to the bath water is dangerous for this patient because it makes the tub slippery. Although privacy is important, if the patient locks the door, the nurse cannot help if there is an emergency. The water should be comfortably warm at 43° to 46°C. Older patients have an increased susceptibility to burns due to diminished sensitivity.

12. **b.** A patient who is taking anticoagulants should be shaved with an electric razor rather than a blade razor. Shaving a patient does not require a permission form be signed and can be completed by either the caregiver or a family member. A shave is best completed with the patient in a Fowler's or semi-Fowler's position to prevent soap and water from running behind the patient's head.

13. **d.** The lens must be situated on the cornea, not the sclera, before removal. To remove hard contact lenses, the upper and lower eyelids are gently maneuvered to

help loosen the lens and slide it out of the eye. An attempt to grasp a hard lens might result in a scratch on the cornea. Clean, not sterile, gloves are used.

14. **c.** Threading the bag and tubing through the gown sleeve keeps the system intact. Opening an IV line, even temporarily, causes a break in a sterile system and introduces the potential for infection. Cutting a gown is not an alternative except in an emergency.

15. **b.** Using the bath blanket or top sheet keeps the patient warm and provides privacy. Keeping the bed in the low position and working over raised side rails may strain the nurse's back. Continually moving back and forth to tuck and arrange linen is time consuming and disorganized.

Taylor Suite Resources

The Taylor Suite offers these additional resources to enhance learning and facilitate understanding of this chapter:

- thePoint online resource, http://thepoint.lww.com/Taylor7E
- Student DVD-ROM included with the book
- Study Guide for Taylor's Fundamentals of Nursing
- Skill Checklists for Taylor's Fundamentals of Nursing
- Taylor's Clinical Nursing Skills: *Chapter 7, Hygiene*
- Taylor's Video Guide to Clinical Nursing Skills: *Hygiene*

BIBLIOGRAPHY

Agency for Healthcare Research and Quality (AHRQ). (2005). *Economic and health costs of diabetes*. HCUP highlight 1. AHRQ publication no. 05-0034. Rockville, MD: Author. Available at http://ahrq.gov/data/hcup/highlight/high1.html.

American Academy of Dermatology. (2008). *Acne*. Available at www.aad.org/public/publications/pamphlets/common_acne.html. Accessed August 2, 2008.

American Academy of Dermatology. (2010). *12 ways to get better results from acne treatment*. Available at www.skincarephysicians.com/acnenet/twelve_results. html. Accessed April 21, 2010.

American Association of Critical-Care Nurses (AACN). (2006). *Practice Alert: Oral care in the critically ill*. Available at www.aacn.org/WD/Practice/Content/practicealerts.pcms?pid= 1&&menu. Accessed July 31, 2008.

American Association of Critical-Care Nurses (AACN). (2005). *Practice Alert. Deep vein thrombosis prevention*. Available at www.aacn.org/WD/Practice/Content/practicealerts.pcms?pid= 1&&menu=practice. Accessed July 31, 2008.

American Dental Association (ADA). (2008). ADA seal of acceptance program. Mouthrinses. Available http://www.ada.org/ada/seal/mouthrinses.asp. Accessed November 13, 2008.

Andrews, M., & Boyle, J. (2008). *Transcultural Concepts in Nursing Care* (5th ed.). Philadelphia: Lippincott Williams & Wilkins.

Bailey, R., Gueldner, S., Ledikwe, J., et al. (2005). The oral care of older adults. *Journal of Gerontological Nursing, 31*(7), 11–17.

Bloomfield, J., Pegram, A., & Jones, A. (2008). Recommended procedure for bedmaking in hospital. *Nursing Standard, 22*(23), 41–44.

Brown, A., & Butcher, M. (2005). A guide to emollient therapy. *Nursing Standard, 19*(24), 68–75.

Bulechek, G., Butcher, H., & McCloskey Dochterman, J. (Eds.). (2008). *Nursing interventions classification (NIC)* (5th ed.). St. Louis, MO: Mosby Elsevier.

Burr, S., & Penzer, R. (2005). Promoting skin health. *Nursing Standard, 19*(36), 57–65.

Carpenito-Moyet, L. (2008). *Nursing diagnosis: Application to clinical practice.* (12th ed.). Philadelphia: Wolters Kluwer Health/Lippincott Williams & Wilkins.

Centers for Disease Control (CDC). *Lice.* Available at cdc.gov/lice/. Accessed July 29, 2008.

Ciancio, S. (2008). Mouth rinses and their impact on oral hygiene. *Access, 22*(5), 24–29.

Cleveland Clinic. (2008). *Contact lens care.* Available at http://my.clevelandclinic.org/devices/vision_correction/Contact_Lenses/hic_Contact_Lens_Care.aspx. Accessed August 9, 2008.

Cohen, B., & Taylor, J. (2005). *Memmler's structure and function of the human body* (8th ed.) Philadelphia: Lippincott Williams & Wilkins.

Costello, T., & Coyne, I. (2008). Nurses' knowledge of mouth care practices. *British Journal of Nursing, 17*(4), 264–268.

DeBoer, S., Amundson, T., & Angel, E. (2006). Managing body jewelry in emergency situations: Misconceptions, patient care, and removal techniques. *Journal of Emergency Nursing, 32*(2), 159–164.

Directors of Health Promotion and Education (DHPE). *Infectious Facts: Head Lice.* Available at www.dhpe.org/infect/lice.html. Accessed July 29, 2008.

Downey, L. (2008). Bed bathing patients in hospital. *Nursing Standard, 22*(34), 35–40.

Flori, L. (2007). Don't throw in the towel: Tips for bathing a patient who has dementia. *Nursing, 37*(7), 22–23.

Halliday, K. (2005). Body piercing: Issues and challenges for nurses. *Journal of Forensic Nursing, 1*(2), 47–56.

Hess, C. (2008). *Skin & wound care.* (6th ed.). Philadelphia: Lippincott Williams & Wilkins.

Hoeffer, B., Talerico, K., Rasin, J., et al. (2006). Assisting cognitively impaired nursing home residents with bathing: Effects of two bathing interventions on caregiving. *The Gerontologist, 46*(4), 524–532.

Holman, C., Roberts, S., & Nicol, M. (2005). Practice update: Clinical skills with older people. Promoting oral hygiene. *Nursing Older People, 16*(10), 37–38.

Jarvis, C. (2008). *Physical Examination & Health Assessment.* (5th ed.). St. Louis: Saunders/Elsevier.

Kyle, T. (2008). *Essentials of Pediatric Nursing.* Philadelphia: Lippincott Williams & Wilkins.

Mayo Foundation for Medical Education and Research (MFMER). (2008). *Piercings: Proper care can help prevent complications.* Available at www.mayoclinic.com/print/piercings/SN00049/METHOD=print. Accessed July 30, 2008.

Mayo Foundation for Medical Education and Research (MFMER). (2007a). *Amputation and diabetes: How to protect your feet.* Available at www.mayoclinic.com/health/amputation-and-diabetes/DA00140. Accessed July 31, 2008.

Mayo Foundation for Medical Education and Research (MFMER). (2007b). *Nails: How to keep your fingernails health and strong.* Available at www.mayoclinic.com/health/nails/WO00020. Accessed July 31, 2008.

Mayo Foundation for Medical Education and Research (MFMER). (2007c). *Skin care: Top 5 habits for health skin.* Available at www.mayoclinic.com/health/skin-care/SN00003.

Mayo Foundation for Medical Education and Research (MFMER). (2007d). *Oral health: Tips for proper dental care.* Available at www.mayoclinic.com/health/dental/DE00003.

MedlinePlus. (2007a). *Dry skin.* Available at www.hlm.nih.gov/medlineplus/ency/article/003250.htm. Accessed August 2, 2008.

MedlinePlus. (2007b). *Penis care (uncircumcised).* Available at www.nlm.nih.gov/medlineplus/ency/article/001917.htm. Accessed July 31, 2008.

MedlinePlus. (2007c). *Rashes.* Available at www.nlm.nih.gov/medlineplus/ency/article/003220.htm#Home%20Care. Accessed August 2, 2008.

Meltzer, D. (2005). Complications of body piercing. *American Family Physician, 72*(10), 2029–2034.

Miller, C. (2008). Communication difficulties in hospitalized older adults with dementia: Try these techniques to make communicating with patients easier and more effective. *American Journal of Nursing, 108*(3), 58–66.

Moorhead, S., Johnson, M., Maas, M., et al. (Eds). (2008). Nursing Outcomes Classification (NOC). (4th ed.). St. Louis, MO: Mosby Elsevier.

The National Women's Health Information Center. U.S. Department of Health and Human Services. (2005). *Douching.* Available at www.4woman.gov/faq/douching.htm.

NANDA International. (2009). *Nursing diagnoses: Definitions and classification 2009–2011.* West Sussex, UK: Wiley-Blackwell.

National Institute on Aging (NIA). (2009). Age page. Foot Care. Available at www.nia.nih.gov/HealthInformation/Publications/footcare.htm. Accessed April 21, 2010.

Pegram, A., Bloomfield, J., & Jones, A. (2007). Clinical skills: Bed bathing and personal hygiene needs of patients. *British Journal of Nursing, 16*(6), 356–358.

Pellatt, G. (2007). Clinical skills: Bed making and patient positioning. *British Journal of Nursing, 16*(5), 302–305.

Polovich, M., White, J., & Kelleher, L. (2009). *Chemotherapy and biotherapy guidelines and recommendations for practice.* (3rd ed.). Oncology Nursery Society.

Purnell, L., & Paulanka, B. (2005). *Guide to culturally competent health care.* Philadelphia: F. A. Davis Company.

Rader, J., Barrick, A., Hoeffer, B., et al. (2006). The bathing of older adults with dementia: Easing the unnecessarily unpleasant aspects of assisted bathing. *American Journal of Nursing, 106*(4), 40–49.

Registered Nurses' Association of Ontario Professional Association. (2005). *Risk assessment & prevention of pressure ulcers. NGC: 004215.* Available at http://www.guideline.gov/summary/summary.aspx?doc_id=7006&nbr=004215&string="wound &ostomy"+and+"continence+nurses+society."

Smeltzer, S., Bare, B., Hinkle, J., et al. (2010). *Brunner & Suddarth's Textbook of Medical-Surgical Nursing.* (12th ed.). Philadelphia: Lippincott Williams & Wilkins.

Stafford, K.C. [2007]. *Tick management handbook.* New Haven, CT: Connecticut Agricultural Experiment Station. Available at www.cdc.gov/ncidod/dvbid/Lyme/resources/handbook.pdf. Accessed July 29, 2008.

National Women's Health Information Center. (2004). *Cosmetics and your health.* Available at http://womenshealth.gov/faq/cosmetics.pdf. Accessed July 31, 2008.

U.S. Food and Drug Administration. (2008). *A guide to bed safety. Bed rails in hospitals, nursing homes and home health care: The facts.* Available at http://www.fda.gov/cdrh/beds/bed_brochure.html. Accessed July 29, 2008.

U.S. Food and Drug Administration (FDA). (2008). *Use eye cosmetics safely.* Available at www.fda.gov/consumer/updates/eyecosmetics041708.html. Accessed July 31, 2008.

VISN8 Patient Safety Center. (2009). Safe patient handling and movement algorithms. Tampa, FL: Author. Available at www.visn8.va.gov/patientsafetycenter/safePthandling/default.asp.

Voegeli, D. (2008a). Care or harm: Exploring essential components in skin care regimens. *British Journal of Nursing, 17*(1), 24–30.

Voegeli, D. (2008b). The effect of washing and drying practices on skin barrier function. *Journal of Wound, Ostomy & Continence Nursing, 35*(1), 84–90.

Voegeli, D. (2007). The role of emollients in the care of patients with dry skin. *Nursing Standard, 22*(7), 62, 64–8.

Watkins, P. (2008). Using emollients to restore and maintain skin integrity. *Nursing Standard, 22*(41), 51–58, 60.

Weber, J., & Kelley, J. (2007). *Health assessment in nursing* (3rd ed.). Philadelphia: Lippincott Williams & Wilkins.

Yoon, M., & Steele, C. (2007). The oral care imperative: The link between oral hygiene and aspiration pneumonia. *Topics in Geriatric Rehabilitation, 23*(3), 280–288.

32 Skin Integrity and Wound Care

MARY BIESICKER

Mary, who is 84 years of age, has been cared for at home by her daughter since being hospitalized last year for a cerebrovascular accident (stroke). She has been unable to take care of herself, finds it harder and harder to get out of bed, and is having increasingly frequent episodes of incontinence. According to her daughter, Mary has developed a "blister" on her back. She is being assessed by the home health nurse at the request of her daughter, who is finding it increasingly difficult to care for her mother alone.

LUCIUS EVERLY

Lucius, who has a history of diabetes and circulatory problems, underwent abdominal surgery several days ago and is in the critical care unit. He is slouched down in bed; his abdominal dressing is moist, and only part of the tape securing the dressing is adhering to the skin. His level of consciousness is decreased, and he responds only to moderate touch and pain. Further assessment reveals the beginning of a pressure ulcer on his heel.

SAM BENTZ

Sam, a 56-year-old man, has been admitted to the hospital for aggressive treatment of a bone infection that has not responded to usual methods.
Mr. Bentz is 5 feet 4 inches tall and weighs more than 300 pounds. He tells you, "Last time I was here, my skin got really irritated and I developed several skin wounds."

LEARNING OBJECTIVES

After completing the chapter, you will be able to accomplish the following:

1. Discuss the processes involved in wound healing.

2. Identify factors that affect wound healing.

3. Identify patients at risk for pressure ulcer development.

4. Describe the method of staging of pressure ulcers.

5. Accurately assess and document the condition of wounds.

6. Provide nursing interventions to prevent pressure ulcers.

7. Implement appropriate dressing changes for different kinds of wounds.

8. Provide information to patients and caregivers for self-care of wounds at home.

9. Apply hot and cold therapy effectively and safely.

KEY TERMS

bandage	maceration
débridement	necrosis
dehiscence	negative-pressure wound therapy (NPWT)
dermis	
desiccation	pressure ulcer
dressing	purulent drainage
epidermis	sanguineous drainage
eschar	scar
evisceration	serosanguineous drainage
exudate	
fistula	serous drainage
friction	shear
granulation tissue	subcutaneous tissue
ischemia	wound

The skin is the body's first line of defense, protecting the underlying structures from invasion by organisms. Maintaining an intact skin surface is important because a break or disruption in this integrity is potentially dangerous and possibly life threatening. The nurse plays a major role in maintaining the patient's skin integrity, in identifying risk factors that predispose a patient to a break in integrity, in intervening to prevent or reduce a patient's risk for impaired skin integrity, and in providing specific wound care when breaks in

integrity arise. Additional information related to general skin care is discussed in Chapter 31.

Knowledgeable and skilled wound care is an essential component of nursing care. Using the nursing process, an individualized plan of care is developed to assess the patient and the wound, identify and prevent complications, implement and evaluate skills essential to wound care, and provide physical and emotional support to facilitate healing, adaptation, and self-care. Wound care may be required in any healthcare setting, and increasingly complex wounds are being cared for at home.

This chapter provides information about disruptions in skin and tissue integrity, including wounds and pressure ulcers. Because applications of heat and cold are used to treat altered skin integrity, the discussion of those treatment modalities is also included. Refer to the Reflective Practice display for an illustration of nursing care issues related to skin integrity.

ANATOMY AND PHYSIOLOGY OF THE INTEGUMENTARY SYSTEM

Structures of the Skin

The skin, or integument, is the largest organ of the body and has multiple functions. The integumentary system is made up of the skin, the subcutaneous layer directly under the skin, and the appendages of the skin, including glands in the skin, hair, and nails. The integumentary system also includes the blood vessels, nerves, and sensory organs of the skin. The skin is essential for maintaining life.

The skin has two layers. An underlying layer, the subcutaneous layer, is sometimes included in descriptions as the third layer of the skin (Burr & Penzer, 2005; Hess, 2008; Jarvis, 2008; Porth & Matfin, 2009). The top layer, or outermost portion, is the **epidermis.** The epidermis is composed of layers of stratified epithelial cells. These cells fuse to form a protective, waterproof layer of keratin material. Epithelial cells have no blood vessels of their own and depend on underlying tissues for nourishment and waste removal. When well nourished, epithelium regenerates relatively easily and quickly.

The second layer of skin, the **dermis,** consists of a framework of elastic connective tissue. Nerves, hair follicles, glands, and blood vessels are located in this layer. Each hair consists of the shaft, which projects through the dermis beyond the surface of the skin, and the hair follicle, which lies in the dermis.

The dermis rests on the **subcutaneous tissue,** the underlying layer that anchors the skin layers to the underlying tissues of the body. The subcutaneous tissue consists of adipose tissue, made up of lobules of fat cells, and connective tissue. This layer stores fat for energy, serves as a heat insulator for the body, and provides a cushioning effect for protection. This fatty tissue layer contains blood and lymph vessels, nerves, and fat cells.

The skin covers the entire body and is continuous with mucous membranes at normal body orifices. A cross-section of normal skin is illustrated in Figure 32-1.

REFLECTIVE PRACTICE

Challenge to Ethical and Legal Skills

I had a tough clinical 2 weeks ago while caring for Lucius Everly, a critical care postop patient with a history of diabetes and circulation problems. The nurse I was working with had floated to the unit on this day, but I didn't know that at the time. Mr. Everly appeared to be neglected by other caregivers, and because he was not communicating and had a decreased level of consciousness, he could not express his needs. I saw that he needed bathing, wound care, repositioning in bed, and some additional attention. While in the room, the nurse spoke about Mr. Everly as though he was deaf. In my opinion, the nurse did not respect his inability to communicate. I became frustrated because she did not share my sense of concern for him. I became irritated when I asked what we could do to care for the poor circulation to his feet. My irritation increased when I realized that he was developing a pressure sore on his heel.

Thinking Outside the Box: Possible Courses of Action

- Tell my clinical instructor of my frustrations earlier in the day so my patient's care could have been addressed earlier and my frustrations wouldn't have built up.
- Go to my nurse and tell her that I disagreed with the care she was providing, insisting that more needed to be done for this patient.
- Ask the charge nurse to assess the quality of care that my patient was getting compared to what he needed to be receiving.

Evaluating a Good Outcome: How Do I Define Success?

- Patient receives a higher quality of care.
- The nurse is not insulted by hearing feedback about the care she is providing.
- By addressing the problem earlier in the process, my frustrations do not interfere with the rest of my day.
- The patient is not discriminated against and neglected based on his inability to communicate and his decreased level of consciousness.

Personal Learning: Here's to the Future!

Happy and sad outcome. Although this patient was not verbally communicating, I held his hand, talked to him, and felt that he was able to recognize my caring presence. After our lunch break, I verbalized my frustration about the lack of care to my clinical instructor and I asked if she would come meet him and help me provide the care I saw was due. My clinical instructor agreed that this patient was in need of more care. She, unlike my nurse, did not speak about his condition in front of him as though he could not hear. My instructor also made sure we did everything possible so that this patient was as comfortable as possible. She talked to him as though he was able to hear. In addition, my instructor called in the charge nurse to point out the lack of care this patient had been receiving, wanting to ensure that his future level of care improved. My instructor and the charge nurse, in a professional, nondegrading way, expressed to the assigned nurse that this patient needed a higher quality of care due to his critical condition. Having my teacher agree with my concerns for this patient and address the nurse and charge nurse made me feel much better about the care my patient would then receive. I later told my teacher that I was frustrated because I felt all the nurse was concerned about was "giving all the medications, and signing off on the right pages," when in fact talking to this patient, holding his hand, and making him more comfortable was definitely more important. Two days later the patient died. I was sad but so honored to have been able to care for him and hold his hand in his last days.

Although I think I should have gone to my clinical instructor earlier in the day to explain the problem I was having, telling her was the right decision. My instructor took my concerns seriously and first helped me care for the patient, then went straight to the charge nurse to ensure proper skin and wound care for the patient. Lastly, she was able to address the nurse without insulting her to make sure we were all on the same page about the care this patient needed but had not been getting. By speaking up, I was able to leave my clinical assignment feeling positive about my actions and advocating for this patient. I still felt frustrated with how he had been cared for and realized that all too often as care providers we get too involved in the routine of charting, distributing medications, and so on and can forget how important some simple measures are such as offering a gentle touch, positioning, providing hygiene and wound care, and just spending time with the patient.

Carrie Staines, Georgetown University

Reflection

How do you think you would respond in a similar situation? Why? What does this tell you about yourself and about the adequacy of your skills for professional practice? What factors might have affected the assigned nurse's response to the patient? Would the student have been affected by any of these same factors? Explain. What evidence from the scenario would lead you to suspect that the patient is at risk for impaired skin integrity? What preventive measures might be appropriate? Can you think of other ways to respond? What other skills (cognitive, interpersonal, technical, ethical/legal) would you need to respond well in this situation? What, if any, ethical and legal principles were demonstrated by the nursing student's actions? Do you agree with the criteria to evaluate a successful outcome? Did the nursing student validate the rationale for the outcome? Would other criteria be appropriate to include? If so, explain.

FIGURE 32-1. A cross-section of normal skin.

Functions of the Skin and Mucous Membranes

The skin provides multiple functions: protection, temperature regulation, psychosocial, sensation, vitamin D production, immunological, absorption, and elimination. See Table 32-1 for details of each of these functions.

Mucous membranes line body cavities that open to the outside of the body, joining with the skin. They can also be found in the digestive tract, the respiratory passages, and

TABLE • 32-1	FUNCTIONS OF THE SKIN
Function	**Mechanisms**
Protection	• Acts as a barrier to water, microorganisms, and damaging ultraviolet rays of the sun. • Protection against infection. • Injury to underlying tissues and organs is decreased by intact skin. • Prevents loss of moisture from the surface and underlying structures.
Temperature Regulation	• The evaporation of perspiration draws heat from the skin. • Blood vessels in the skin dilate to dissipate heat. • In cold conditions, blood vessels in the skin constrict to diminish heat loss. • In cold conditions, contraction of pilomotor muscles cause the hair to stand on end, forming a layer of air on the body for insulation (gooseflesh or goose bumps).
Psychosocial	• External appearance is a major contributor to self-esteem. • Important role in identification and communication.
Sensation	• Millions of nerve endings in the skin provide the sense of touch, pain, pressure, and temperature. • Sensory impulses from the skin allow the body to adjust to the environment, in conjunction with the brain and spinal cord.
Vitamin D Production	• A precursor for vitamin D is present in the skin, which, in conjunction with ultraviolet rays from the sun, produces vitamin D.
Immunological	• A breach in the surface of the skin triggers immunological responses in the skin.
Absorption	• Substances, such as medications, can be absorbed through the skin for local and systemic effect.
Elimination	• Water, electrolytes, and nitrogenous wastes are excreted in small amounts in sweat.

TABLE • 32-2 FACTORS PLACING AN INDIVIDUAL AT RISK FOR SKIN ALTERATIONS

Factor	Nursing Implications
Lifestyle Variables	
Homosexuality, history of multiple sexual partners; intravenous drug users; hemophiliacs; bisexual male; partners of the above	• These patients are at high risk for infection with human immunodeficiency virus (HIV) and acquired immunodeficiency syndrome (AIDS). • Assessment needs to include careful examination of the skin for purple blotches that may be indicative of Kaposi's sarcoma.
Occupation or other activity that gives an individual prolonged exposure to the sun	• Places individual at high risk for developing skin cancer, which has an excellent prognosis if detected and treated in its early stages but which may be fatal if treatment is delayed. • Assessment needs to include careful examination for a sore that does not heal or a change in size or color of a wart or mole.
Body piercing	• Potential interference with airway management. Potential risk for bacterial and viral infections, scarring, nerve damage, tissue trauma, and deformity. • Assess patient's knowledge of symptoms of infection at the site and when to seek medical care. • Assess piercing site(s) for redness, swelling, discharge, or excessive pain at the site.
Changes in Health State	
Dehydration or malnutrition	• If fluid, protein, and vitamin C intake is deficient, skin loses elasticity and becomes prone to breakdown. • Nursing care is directed toward preventing skin breakdown: frequent changes of patient's position with skin assessment at each change, special mattresses and protection of bony prominences, use of lotions, and attention to fluid and nutritional status.
Reduced sensation (paralysis, local nerve damage, circulatory insufficiency)	• Patient's inability to sense temperature extremes, pressure, friction, and other such factors can easily result in injury. • Nursing care incorporates special attention to safety.
Illness	
Diabetes mellitus	• Numerous factors combine to cause skin problems in diabetic patients: cuts and sores that do not heal, lesions on the lower extremities that ulcerate and become necrotic, and recurrent bacterial and fungal infections. • The diabetic patient must be taught special hygiene measures to prevent trauma to the skin and learn to assess the skin carefully to detect any alteration.
Diagnostic Measures	
Gastrointestinal (GI) series	• The GI cleansing preparations administered to patients having GI studies done may result in diarrhea, which irritates the sensitive skin in the perianal area—especially if the patient had bouts of diarrhea before the studies; anticipating the problem, noting redness and inflammation, and beginning warm baths and ointments are welcome nursing measures that patients may be too embarrassed to seek.
Therapeutic Measures	
Bed rest	• Bed rest predisposes patients to skin breakdown; the harsh detergents used on hospital laundry compound this problem. • Pressure points need to be examined frequently and protected.
Casts	• Casts easily irritate the skin; careful assessment, covering the rough edges of the cast, and skin care are indicated.
Aquathermia unit	• Wet heat has therapeutic benefit but, if applied to the skin for too long, may macerate the skin; follow protocol in length of application, examine skin carefully between treatments, and allow to dry.
Medications	• Medications may cause allergic skin reactions, such as rashes. • When evaluating the patient's response to a new drug, examine the skin for redness and itching.
Radiation Therapy	• Radiation therapy exposes normal skin cells as well as cancer cells in treatment field to effects of radiation, with the potential for erythema and moist desquamation (loss of skin integrity).

the urinary and reproductive tracts. Epithelium covers the mucous membrane surfaces and contains cells that secrete mucus. Mucous membranes have receptors that offer the body protection; for example, an irritating substance in the upper respiratory tract causes a person to sneeze, and food caught in the larynx or trachea causes a person to cough. Sneezing and coughing are protective mechanisms that help rid the body of foreign materials. Mucous membranes are insensitive to temperature, except in the mouth and rectum, but are sensitive to pressure. Mucous membranes also function to absorb substances from their surface; for example, digested food is absorbed through the mucous membrane in the small intestine.

Factors Affecting Skin Integrity

Basic principles related to integrity of the skin and mucous membranes include the following:

- Unbroken and healthy skin and mucous membranes serve as the first lines of defense against harmful agents.
- Resistance to injury of the skin and mucous membranes varies among people. Factors influencing resistance include the person's age, the amount of underlying tissues, and illness conditions.
- Adequately nourished and hydrated body cells are resistant to injury. The better nourished the cell is, the better able it is to resist injury and disease.
- Adequate circulation is necessary to maintain cell life. When circulation is impaired for any reason, cells receive inadequate nourishment and cannot remove wastes efficiently.

Table 32-2 identifies some factors that place a patient at risk for skin alterations.

Developmental Considerations

Specific characteristics of the skin are associated with different developmental stages. Hygiene practices at every age have a direct influence on the status and appearance of the skin.

- In children younger than 2 years, the skin is thinner and weaker than it is in adults.
- An infant's skin and mucous membranes are injured easily and are subject to infection. Careful handling of infants is required to prevent injury to and infection of the skin and mucous membranes.
- A child's skin becomes increasingly resistant to injury and infection.
- The structure of the skin changes as a person ages. The maturation of epidermal cells is prolonged, leading to thin, easily damaged skin. Circulation and collagen formation are impaired, leading to decreased elasticity and increased risk for tissue damage from pressure. Changes that occur in the skin with aging are discussed in Focus on the Older Adult.

State of Health

The state of a person's health and therapeutic treatments have a direct effect on the condition of the skin. Proper nutrition, adequate circulation, and good overall health are important for healthy skin.

- Very thin and very obese people tend to be more susceptible to skin irritation and injury.

FOCUS ON THE OLDER ADULT

NURSING STRATEGIES TO ADDRESS AGE-RELATED SKIN ALTERATIONS

Age-Related Changes	Nursing Strategies
Subcutaneous and dermal tissue become thin: • Skin is more easily injured. • Skin has less capacity to insulate. • Skin wrinkles more easily. • Sensation of pressure and pain is reduced.	• Do not apply tape to skin unless necessary. • Check skin frequently to observe for any signs of a pressure ulcer. • Pad bony prominences if necessary. • Assess pressure tolerance by checking pressure points for redness after 30 minutes.
Activity of the sebaceous and sweat gland decreases: • Skin becomes dryer. • Pruritus (itching) may occur.	• Clean perineal area daily but do not bathe full body on a daily basis. • Apply lotions as needed. • Encourage adequate hydration.
Cell renewal is shorter: • Healing time is delayed.	• Perform careful skin assessments, looking for signs of skin breakdown.
Melanocytes (cells that make the pigment that colors hair and skin) decline in number: • Hair becomes gray-white. • Skin may be unevenly pigmented.	• Assist patient with skin checks, observing for any signs of melanoma or other skin abnormalities.
Collagen fiber is less organized: • Skin loses elasticity.	• Check skin frequently for tears, irritation, or breakdown.

TABLE • 32-3   TYPES OF WOUNDS

Type	Cause
Incision	Cutting or sharp instrument; wound edges in close approximation and aligned
Contusion	Blunt instrument, overlying skin remains intact, with injury to underlying soft tissue; possible resultant bruising and/or hematoma
Abrasion	Friction; rubbing or scraping epidermal layers of skin; top layer of skin abraded
Laceration	Tearing of skin and tissue with blunt or irregular instrument; tissue not aligned, often with loose flaps of skin and tissue
Puncture	Blunt or sharp instrument puncturing the skin; intentional (such as venipuncture) or accidental
Penetrating	Foreign object entering the skin or mucous membrane and lodging in underlying tissue; fragments possibly scattering throughout tissues
Avulsion	Tearing a structure from normal anatomic position; possible damage to blood vessels, nerves, and other structures
Microbial	Secretion of exotoxins or release of endotoxins by living organisms
Chemical	Toxic agents such as drugs, acids, alcohols, metals, and substances released from cellular necrosis
Thermal	High or low temperatures; cellular necrosis as a possible result
Irradiation	Ultraviolet light or radiation exposure
Pressure ulcers	Compromised circulation secondary to pressure or pressure combined with friction
Venous ulcers	Injury and poor venous return, resulting from underlying conditions, such as incompetent valves or obstruction
Arterial ulcers	Injury and underlying ischemia, resulting from underlying conditions, such as atherosclerosis or thrombosis
Diabetic ulcers	Injury and underlying diabetic neuropathy, peripheral arterial disease, diabetic foot structure

Adapted from: Harvey, C. (2005). Wound healing. *Orthopaedic Nursing, 24*(2), 143–157; Hess, C. (2008). *Skin & wound care* (6th ed.). Philadelphia, Wolters Kluwer Health/Lippincott Williams & Wilkins; Porth, C., & Matfin, G. (2009). *Pathophysiology: Concepts of altered health states* (8th ed.). Philadelphia: Wolters Kluwer Health/Lippincott Williams & Wilkins; Smeltzer, S., Bare, B., Hinkle, J. H. & Cheever, K. H. (2010). *Brunner & Suddarth's textbook of medical-surgical nursing* (12th ed., p. 2528 [Chart 71-6]). Philadelphia: Lippincott Williams & Wilkins.; and Snyder, L., & Moore, D. (2008). Wound basics: Types, treatment, and care. *RN, 71*(8), 32–37.

- Fluid loss through fever, vomiting, or diarrhea reduces the fluid volume of the body. This is termed "dehydration" and makes the skin appear loose and flabby.
- Excessive perspiration, often associated with being ill, predisposes the skin to breakdown, especially in skin folds.
- Jaundice, a condition caused by excessive bile pigments in the skin, results in a yellowish skin color. The skin is often itchy and dry, and patients with jaundice are more likely to scratch their skin and cause an open lesion with the potential for infection.
- Diseases of the skin such as eczema and psoriasis may have a genetic predisposition and often cause lesions that require special care.

WOUNDS

A **wound** is a break or disruption in the normal integrity of the skin and tissues. That disruption may range from a small cut on a finger to a third-degree burn covering almost all of the body. Wounds may result from mechanical forces (such as surgical incisions) or physical injury (such as a burn). Examples of types of wounds and their causes are highlighted in Table 32-3.

Wound Classification

Wounds are classified in many different ways, including intentional or unintentional (based on how they were acquired), open or closed, and acute or chronic (based on the length of time the patient has had the wound). Wounds may also be classified as partial-thickness (all or a portion of the dermis is intact), full-thickness (the entire dermis and sweat glands and hair follicles are severed), or complex (the dermis and underlying subcutaneous fat tissue are damaged or destroyed).

Intentional Wounds and Unintentional Wounds

An intentional wound is the result of planned invasive therapy or treatment. These wounds are purposefully created for therapeutic purposes. Examples of intentional wounds include those that result from surgery, intravenous therapy, and lumbar puncture. The wound edges are clean, and bleeding is usually controlled. Because the wound was made under sterile conditions with sterile supplies and skin preparation, the risk for infection is decreased, and healing is facilitated.

> *Think back to Lucius Everly, the patient who had abdominal surgery and is in the critical care unit. His postoperative treatments would necessitate the placement of one or more intravenous accesses. His venous access and surgical wound would be considered intentional wounds. The nurse would incorporate an understanding of the principles of surgical asepsis when caring for these wound sites to prevent infection.* ■

Unintentional wounds are accidental. These wounds occur from unexpected trauma, such as from accidents, forcible injury (such as a stabbing or a gunshot), and burns. Because the wounds occur in an unsterile environment, contamination is likely. Wound edges are usually jagged, multiple traumas are common, and bleeding is uncontrolled. These factors create a high risk for infection and a longer healing time.

Open and Closed Wounds

An open wound occurs from intentional or unintentional trauma. The skin surface is broken, providing a portal of entry for microorganisms. Bleeding, tissue damage, and increased risk for infection and delayed healing may accompany open wounds. Examples include incisions and abrasions.

A closed wound results from a blow, force, or strain caused by trauma such as a fall, an assault, or a motor vehicle crash. The skin surface is not broken, but soft tissue is damaged, and internal injury and hemorrhage may occur. Examples include ecchymosis and hematomas.

Acute and Chronic Wounds

Acute wounds, such as surgical incisions, usually heal within days to weeks. The wound edges are well approximated (edges meet to close skin surface) and the risk of infection is lessened. Acute wounds usually move through the healing process without difficulty. Chronic wounds, in contrast, do not progress through the normal sequence of repair. The healing process is impeded. The wound edges are often not approximated, the risk of infection is increased, and the normal healing time is delayed. Chronic wounds remain in the inflammatory phase of healing. The inflammatory phase is discussed below. Chronic wounds include any wound that does not heal along the expected continuum, such as wounds related to arterial or venous insufficiency, and pressure ulcers.

Wound Healing

Wound healing is a process of tissue response to injury. Injured tissues are repaired by physiologic mechanisms that regenerate functioning cells and replace connective tissue cells with scar tissue. The healing process fills the gap caused by tissue destruction, restoring the structural integrity of the damaged tissue through the orderly release of growth factors and chemical mediators (Porth & Matfin, 2009). These substances help to increase the blood supply to the damaged area, wall off and remove cellular and foreign debris, and initiate cellular development.

Normally, the healing process occurs without assistance. However, interventions can help to support the process. For example, tissue healing is promoted by keeping the injured area free of debris through proper cleaning. Positioning the wounded area to promote circulation to that part helps to promote tissue healing. These interventions are based on the principles of wound healing outlined in Box 32-1.

Wound repair occurs by primary intention, secondary intention, or tertiary intention (Hess, 2008). Wounds healed by primary intention are well approximated (skin edges tightly together). Intentional wounds with minimal tissue loss, such as those made by a surgical incision with sutured approximated edges, usually heal by primary intention. Wounds healed by secondary intention have edges that are not well approximated. Large, open wounds, such as from burns or major trauma, which require more tissue replacement and are often contaminated, commonly heal by secondary intention. If a wound that is healing by primary intention becomes infected, it will heal by secondary intention. Wounds that heal by secondary intention take longer to heal and form more scar tissue (Porth & Matfin, 2009). Connective tissue healing and repair follow the same phases in healing, although differences occur in the length of time required for each phase and in the extent of granulation tissue formed. Wounds healed by tertiary, or delayed primary, intention are those wounds left open for several days to allow edema or infection to resolve or exudate to drain, and then are closed (Hess, 2008).

Phases of Wound Healing

The wound healing process can be divided into phases; depending on the reference, healing occurs in three or four phases. These four phases systematically lead to repair of the injury: hemostasis, inflammation, proliferation, and maturation (Hess, 2008). If three stages are identified, hemostasis is included as part of the inflammatory stage.

HEMOSTASIS

Hemostasis occurs immediately after the initial injury. Involved blood vessels constrict and blood clotting begins through platelet activation and clustering. After only a brief period of constriction, these same blood vessels dilate and capillary permeability increases, allowing plasma and blood components to leak out into the area that is injured, forming a liquid called **exudate.** The accumulation of exudate causes swelling and pain. Increased perfusion results in heat and redness. If the wound is small, the clot loses fluid and a hard scab is formed to protect the injury. The platelets are also responsible for releasing substances that stimulate other

Box 32-1   PRINCIPLES OF WOUND HEALING

- Intact skin is the first line of defense against microorganisms. A break in the integrity of the skin increases the risk for infection. Careful hand hygiene before caring for a wound is probably the single most effective method for preventing wound infections.
- The body responds systemically to trauma in any of its parts. For example, a surgical incision can cause a variety of systemic reactions, including increased body temperature, increased heart and respiratory rates, anorexia or nausea and vomiting, musculoskeletal tension, and hormonal changes.
- An adequate blood supply is essential for the body's normal response to any injury. The blood transports increased numbers of leukocytes, erythrocytes, and platelets to the site of injury. Antibodies are carried by the plasma. Increased circulation to the injured part removes toxins and debris and provides nutrients and oxygen. Areas of the body with a good blood supply, such as the head and the neck, heal faster than areas in which the blood supply is not as great, such as the distal part of an extremity.
- Normal healing is promoted when the wound is free of foreign material, such as excessive exudate, dead or damaged tissue cells, pathogenic organisms, or embedded fragments of bone, metal, glass, or other substances. In some situations, a collection of pus or foreign body is walled off and healing occurs around it to form an abscess.

- The ability to handle altered skin integrity depends on the extent of the damage and the person's general state of health. The capacity to deal adequately with a wound is limited when a healthy person sustains a massive injury, when the patient has a chronic illness or a depressed immune system, or when the patient is very young or very old.
- The body's response to a wound is more effective if proper nutrition has been maintained.
  - Undernourished patients are at greater risk for developing a wound infection because they have difficulty mounting their cell-mediated defense system associated with T-lymphocyte activity, and some leukocytic functions are diminished in the presence of protein deficiency.
  - Although the role of fatty acids in wound healing is not well understood, certain quantities of glucose are necessary to meet the energy requirements for wound healing.
  - Various vitamins, minerals, and trace elements are also needed for efficient wound healing. Vitamin A is necessary for collagen synthesis and epithelialization. Vitamin B complex serves as a cofactor of enzyme reactions needed for wound healing. Vitamin C is needed for collagen synthesis, capillary formation, and resistance to infection. Vitamin K is needed for the synthesis of prothrombin. Zinc, copper, and iron assist in collagen synthesis. Manganese serves as an enzyme activator.

cells to migrate to the injury to participate in the other phases of healing.

INFLAMMATORY PHASE

The inflammatory phase follows hemostasis and lasts about 4 to 6 days. White blood cells, predominantly leukocytes and macrophages, move to the wound. Leukocytes arrive first to ingest bacteria and cellular debris. About 24 hours after the injury, macrophages (a larger phagocytic cell) enter the wound area and remain for an extended period. Macrophages are essential to the healing process. They not only ingest debris, but also release growth factors that are necessary for the growth of epithelial cells and new blood vessels. These growth factors also attract fibroblasts that help to fill in the wound, which is necessary for the next stage of healing. Acute inflammation is characterized by pain, heat, redness, and swelling at the site of the injury. During the inflammatory phase, the patient has a generalized body response, including a mildly elevated temperature, leukocytosis (increased number of white blood cells in the blood), and generalized malaise.

PROLIFERATION PHASE

The proliferation phase is also known as the fibroblastic, regenerative, or connective tissue phase. The proliferation phase lasts for several weeks. New tissue is built to fill the wound space, primarily through the action of fibroblasts. Fibroblasts are connective tissue cells that synthesize and secrete collagen and produce specialized growth factors responsible for inducing blood vessel formation as well as increasing the number and movement of endothelial cells.

Capillaries grow across the wound, bringing oxygen and nutrients required for continued healing. Fibroblasts form fibrin that stretches through the clot. A thin layer of epithelial cells forms across the wound, and blood flow across the wound is reinstituted. The new tissue, called **granulation tissue,** forms the foundation for scar tissue development. It is highly vascular, red, and bleeds easily. In wounds that heal by first intention, epidermal cells seal the wound within 24 to 48 hours, so the granulation tissue is not visible.

Collagen synthesis and accumulation continue, peaking in 5 to 7 days. Depending on the size of the wound, collagen deposit continues for several weeks or even years. By the end of the second week following the injury, the majority of white blood cells have left the wound area, and the wound is lighter in color. The systemic symptoms now typically disappear. During this phase, adequate nutrition and oxygenation, as well as prevention of strain on the suture line, are important patient care considerations.

Wounds that heal by secondary intention eventually follow the same process but take longer to heal and form more scar tissue (Porth & Matfin, 2009). Granulation tissue fills the wound and is then covered by skin cells that grow over the granulation tissue. Connective tissue healing and repair follow the same phases in healing, although differences occur in the length of time required for each phase and in the extent of granulation tissue formed.

MATURATION PHASE

The final stage of healing begins about 3 weeks after the injury, possibly continuing for months or years. Collagen that was haphazardly deposited in the wound is remodeled, making the healed wound stronger and more like adjacent tissue. New collagen continues to be deposited, which compresses the blood vessels in the healing wound, so that the **scar,** an avascular collagen tissue that does not sweat, grow hair, or tan in sunlight, eventually becomes a flat, thin line. Scar tissue is strong but less elastic than uninjured tissue. Wounds that heal by secondary intention take longer to remodel and form a scar smaller than the original wound; if the scar is over a joint or other body structure, it may limit movement and cause disability.

> ➤ *Recall Sam Bentz, the 56-year-old man admitted for treatment of a bone infection. The nurse would apply the knowledge about the phases of wound healing when reviewing this patient's past history (the wounds he developed on his last admission). In addition, this knowledge would help form the basis for the patient's plan of care should another wound occur during this hospitalization.* ■

Factors Affecting Wound Healing

Wound healing is affected by a variety of factors. Local factors, those occurring directly in the wound, include pressure, **desiccation** (dehydration), **maceration** (overhydration), trauma, edema, infection, and **necrosis** (death of tissue). Systemic factors, those occurring throughout the body, include age, circulation to and oxygenation of tissues, nutritional status, wound condition, health status, immunosuppression, and medication use (Harvey, 2005; Hess, 2008; Porth & Matfin, 2009).

LOCAL FACTORS

Wound healing can be prolonged by factors occurring local to the wound itself. These factors are discussed in the following sections.

Pressure

Pressure disrupts the blood supply to the wound area. Persistent or excessive pressure interferes with blood flow to the tissue and delays healing.

Desiccation

Desiccation is the process of drying up. Cells dehydrate and die in a dry environment. This cell death causes a crust to form over the wound site and delays healing. Wounds that are kept moist (not wet) and hydrated experience enhanced epidermal cell migration, which supports epithelialization (epithelial cell migration to the wound bed) (Hess, 2008).

Maceration

Overhydration of cells related to urinary and fecal incontinence can lead to impaired skin integrity. This damage is related to moisture, changes in the pH of the skin, overgrowth of bacteria and infection of the skin, and erosion of skin from friction on moist skin. Refer to Chapter 31 for further discussion of maceration.

Trauma

Repeated trauma to a wound area results in delayed healing or the inability to heal.

Edema

Edema at a wound site interferes with the blood supply to the area, resulting in an inadequate supply of oxygen and nutrients to the tissue.

Infection

Bacteria in a wound increase stress on the body, requiring increased energy to deal with the invaders. Infection requires large amounts of energy be spent by the immune system to fight the microorganisms, leaving little or no reserves to attend to the job of repair and healing. In addition, toxins produced by bacteria and released when bacteria die interfere with wound healing and cause cell death.

Necrosis

Dead tissue present in the wound delays healing. Dead tissue appears as slough, moist, yellow stringy tissue, and eschar appears as dry, black, leathery tissue. Healing of the wound will not take place with necrotic tissue in the wound. Removal of the dead tissue must occur for healing to begin (Hess, 2008; Snyder & Moore, 2008).

SYSTEMIC FACTORS

Wound healing also can be prolonged by factors not related to the wound location itself. These factors are discussed in the following sections.

Age

The major skin layers arise from different embryologic origins, resulting in poor adherence between the epidermis and the dermis. This loose binding between the layers causes the layers to separate easily during an inflammatory process, placing infants and small children at risk for impaired skin integrity. Epidermal stripping, the unintentional removal of the epidermis with tape removal, is one type of such injury. Care should be taken to minimize tension, traction, and wrinkles on the skin when using tape on these patients.

Children and healthy adults, however, heal more rapidly than do older adults, in whom physiologic changes caused by aging result in diminished fibroblastic activity and circulation. Older adults are more likely to have one or more chronic illnesses, with pathologic changes that impede the healing process. See the accompanying Focus on the Older Adult display for other age-related factors affecting wound healing.

Circulation and Oxygenation

Adequate blood flow to deliver nutrients and oxygen and to remove local toxins, bacteria, and other debris is essential for wound healing. Certain physical conditions, because of their effect on circulation and oxygenation, can affect wound healing.

FOCUS ON THE OLDER ADULT

AGE-RELATED FACTORS AFFECTING WOUND HEALING

Age-Related Changes	Nursing Interventions
Skin loses turgor and is more fragile.	• Maintain hydration with intravenous fluids as prescribed. • Maintain record of intake and output. • Use caution when removing tape.
Decreased secretion of enzymes and absorption of nutrients and minerals may increase risk for delayed wound healing.	• Maintain intake of adequate kilocalories with oral, enteral, or parenteral feedings. • Ensure diet is high in protein, vitamin A, vitamin C, and trace elements (zinc and copper). • Monitor lab results such as serum albumin, total protein.
Risk of infection increases from: • Slower inflammatory response • Reduced antibody production and endocrine system function • Increased incidence of chronic illnesses, such as diabetes mellitus and cardiovascular disease, that compromise circulation and tissue oxygenation	• Maintain careful hand hygiene and surgical asepsis with dressing changes and care of tubes or drains. • Take and record vital signs, noting and reporting increased temperature. • Monitor wound for manifestations of infection. • Administer medications as prescribed. • Administer supplemental oxygen as prescribed.

➤ *Recall Lucius Everly, the patient described in the Reflective Practice display. The nurse's ability to integrate knowledge of the effects of diabetes on circulation would be important in planning measures to ensure adequate circulation to his extremities as a means to prevent skin breakdown.* ▪

Large amounts of subcutaneous and tissue fat (which has fewer blood vessels) in people who are obese may slow wound healing because fatty tissue is more difficult to suture, is more prone to infection, and takes longer to heal.

➤ *Remember Sam Bentz, the middle-aged patient with a bone infection described at the beginning of the chapter. The nurse would incorporate an understanding of this patient's past history and large size to develop an appropriate plan of care to prevent future occurrences of skin breakdown.* ▪

Circulation may be impaired in older adults and in people with peripheral vascular disorders, cardiovascular disorders, hypertension, or diabetes mellitus. Oxygenation of tissues is decreased in people with anemia or chronic respiratory disorders and in those who smoke.

Nutritional Status

Wound healing requires adequate proteins, carbohydrates, fats, vitamins, and minerals. Calories and protein are necessary to rebuild cells and tissues. Vitamins A and C are essential for epithelialization and collagen synthesis. Zinc plays a role in proliferation of cells. Fluids are necessary for optimal function of cells. All phases of the wound healing process are slowed or inadequate in the patient with poor nutritional status and fluid balance. Nutrition is further discussed in Chapter 36.

Wound Condition

The condition of the wound also affects how quickly and effectively it heals. For example, large, contaminated, infected wounds or wounds that retain foreign bodies heal slowly. Sutures are needed to close surgical wounds. However, sutures also act as foreign bodies, so they are removed as soon as possible.

Medications and Health Status

Patients who are taking corticosteroid drugs or require postoperative radiation therapy are at high risk for delayed healing and wound complications. Corticosteroids decrease the inflammatory process, which may delay healing. Radiation depresses bone marrow function, resulting in decreased leukocytes and an increased risk of infection. The presence of a chronic illness (such as cardiovascular disease or diabetes mellitus) or impaired immune function can impair wound healing. Chemotherapeutic agents impair or stop proliferation of all rapidly growing cells, including cells involved in wound healing (Scott, 2008). Prolonged antibiotic therapy increases a patient's risk for secondary infection and superinfection (Harvey, 2005).

Immunosuppression

Suppression of the immune system as a result of disease (e.g., AIDS, lupus), medication (e.g., chemotherapy), or age (e.g., changes associated with advancing age) can delay wound healing.

Wound Complications

Wound complications include infection, hemorrhage, dehiscence, evisceration, and fistula. These complications increase the risk for generalized illness and death, lengthen the patient's need for healthcare interventions, and add to healthcare costs.

INFECTION

Bacteria can invade a wound at the time of trauma, during surgery, or at any time after the initial wound occurs. A contaminated wound is more likely to become infected than one that is not contaminated. Additionally, the risk of infection is increased in a surgical wound created during a procedure involving the intestines because the risk for contamination with fecal material is high. Wound infections also occur as a result of hospital-acquired infections (HAIs). Symptoms of wound infection usually become apparent within 2 to 7 days after the injury or surgery; often, the patient is at home. Symptoms of infection include purulent drainage; increased drainage, pain, redness, and swelling in and around the wound; increased body temperature; and increased white blood cell count. Wound infections can lead to other complications, including osteomyelitis (bone infection) and sepsis (presence of pathogenic organisms in the blood or tissues).

HEMORRHAGE

Hemorrhage may occur from a slipped suture, a dislodged clot at the wound site, infection, or the erosion of a blood vessel by a foreign body, such as a drain. Check the dressing and the wound under the dressing, if possible, frequently during the first 48 hours after the injury, and no less than every 8 hours thereafter. If excessive bleeding does occur, additional pressure dressings or packing may be necessary, fluid replacement is probably necessary, and surgical intervention may be required. Internal hemorrhage causes the formation of a hematoma. If the bleeding leads to a large accumulation of blood, it can put pressure on surrounding blood vessels and cause tissue ischemia (deficiency of blood to an area). See Chapter 30 for more information about hemorrhage.

DEHISCENCE AND EVISCERATION

Dehiscence and evisceration (Fig. 32-2) are the most serious postoperative wound complications. **Dehiscence** is the partial or total separation of wound layers as a result of excessive stress on wounds that are not healed. **Evisceration** is the most serious complication of dehiscence (Harvey, 2005; Smeltzer et al., 2010). The wound completely separates, with protrusion of viscera through the incisional area. Patients at greater risk for these complications include those who are obese or malnourished, smoke tobacco, use anticoagulants, have infected wounds, or experience excessive coughing, vomiting, or straining (Harvey, 2005; Smeltzer et al., 2010). An increase in the flow of fluid from the wound between postoperative days 4 and 5 may be a sign of an impending dehiscence. The patient may say that "something has suddenly given way." If dehiscence occurs, cover the wound area with sterile towels moistened with sterile 0.9% sodium chloride solution and notify the physician. Once dehiscence occurs, the wound is managed like any open wound. Dehiscence and evisceration of an abdominal incision is a medical emergency. Place the patient in the low Fowler's position and cover the exposed abdominal contents, as discussed previously. Do not leave the patient alone. Notify the primary care

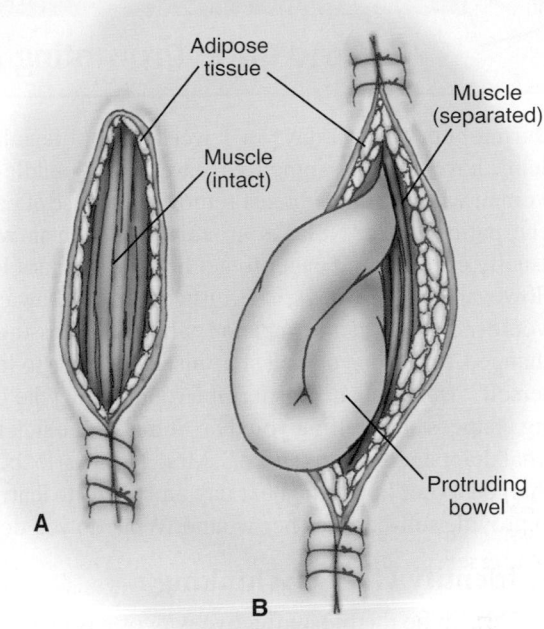

FIGURE 32-2. Wound complications. (**A**) Dehiscence. (**B**) Evisceration.

provider immediately. This situation is an emergency that requires prompt surgical repair (Harvey, 2005).

FISTULA FORMATION

A **fistula** is an abnormal passage from an internal organ to the outside of the body or from one internal organ to another. Fistulas may be created purposefully; for example, an arteriovenous fistula is created surgically to provide circulatory access for kidney dialysis. However, fistula formation is often the result of infection that has developed into an abscess, which is a collection of infected fluid that has not drained. Accumulated fluid applies pressure to surrounding tissues, leading to the formation of the unnatural passage. The presence of a fistula increases the risk for delayed healing, additional infection, fluid and electrolyte imbalances, and skin breakdown.

Psychological Effects of Wounds

Because the skin is a sensory organ and plays a major role in communication with others and self-image, wounds require emotional as well as physical adaptation. Although stress and adaptation vary greatly among individuals, actual and potential emotional stressors are common in all patients with wounds. These stressors include pain, anxiety, fear, and changes in body image.

Pain

Pain is part of almost any trauma, from a small cut on the finger to a large incision made during abdominal surgery. Although pain can be considered a physical complication, it

FOCUSED CRITICAL THINKING GUIDE • 32-1

Wound Care: Promoting Acceptance of Changes in Body Image

During both clinical days in 1 week, you (a female student) have been assigned to care for a middle-aged woman who has had a breast removed because of cancer. The patient, Mrs. Nola, is an attractive woman who is usually cheerful and eager to get better and return home. However, on both days, she turned her head away and would not look at the incision when her dressing was changed. She tells you that she "just can't stand to look at herself." Her husband has left the room during the dressing changes after telling you that "it makes me sick to see what happened to my wife." Mrs. Nola is to be discharged to her home the next day and needs to learn how to provide self-care for her wound. What do you do?

1. Identify Goal of Thinking

Determine the most effective way of ensuring wound care and at the same time assisting Mrs. Nola in accepting her altered self-image.

2. Assess Adequacy of Knowledge

Pertinent circumstances: The diagnosis of cancer was made only 1 day before the surgical removal of the breast. The patient is to be discharged to her home the next day. The wound from her mastectomy has not completely healed and will require dressing changes for another 3 or 4 days. Mrs. Nola has had a disfiguring surgery and is coping with not only a change in body image, but also the diagnosis of cancer. She has never before been seriously ill nor had surgery. She has a strong, loving relationship with her husband, but he is unable to deal with the physical disfigurement at this time.

Prerequisite knowledge: Before you decide what to do in this situation, you need to know at what level Mrs. Nola is in coping with the diagnosis of cancer. If she is still in denial about the disease, it is likely that she is also denying the surgical procedure and the changes in her body. You will need to review responses to the diagnosis of cancer as well as the stages of grief and loss. You will have to learn what her sources of support are and how she can best access and use them. You will need to assess how best to help her achieve wound care in the face of her continued refusal even to look at the wound.

Room for error: If she is forced to look at the wound or made to feel inadequate because of her inability to do so, she will feel threatened and most likely will become angry in response to the perceived threat.

Time constraints: Some decision about wound care must be made before her discharge the next day.

3. Address Potential Problems

There are several potential obstacles to critical thinking in this situation. As a student, you want to exhibit safe, knowledgeable care, and the importance of teaching for home care has been an emphasis in this course. As a woman, you have a sense of what the loss of a breast must mean. Having had a family member die of cancer, you find yourself wanting to do everything for Mrs. Nola. As a novice in nursing, you find it difficult to handle these emotional components of patient care and find yourself wanting to scold both the patient and her husband for being so silly about something as simple as a dressing.

4. Consult Helpful Resources

You must first understand the loss and grief Mrs. Nola is experiencing, and you must then relate that to her response to self-care of the wound. Your best source of information about her coping methods and sources of personal strength is Mrs. Nola herself. You also discuss the most effective way of providing wound care at home with your instructor and the case manager for Mrs. Nola.

5. Critique Judgment/Decision

After talking to Mrs. Nola, your instructor, and the case manager, you mutually agree that Mrs. Nola cannot be hurried into acceptance of her medical diagnosis or her body changes. The case manager consults with Mrs. Nola's physician, who writes an order for a home health nurse to visit for the next 4 days and complete the dressing change. After talking with Mrs. Nola, you identify that she is still very much in denial. You discuss with her the possibility of having a visitor from "Reach to Recovery," a support group for women with breast cancer who have had a mastectomy. Mrs. Nola tells you that she thinks she would like to talk to someone with the same problem, and you call a referral for her. When you tell Mrs. Nola that a home health nurse will be visiting her for the first few days at home to change her dressing, tears come into her eyes. She says "I am so scared, I just don't know what to do." You realize that insisting that Mrs. Nola do her own dressing would have been extremely stressful for her and that you would have considered the wound as more important than the patient. When you share the situation in postconference, your clinical group supports your decision.

also has a large psychological component. Pain from wounds is often increased by activities such as ambulating, coughing, moving in bed, and dressing changes. The actual pain might be worsened by the patient's apprehension about such activities. Nursing interventions to reduce pain can greatly reduce emotional stress. See Chapter 35 for a more in-depth discussion of pain.

Anxiety and Fear

Anxiety and fear are common responses to a wound. Patients are apprehensive about the possibility of the wound opening, how much privacy will be lost as the wound is being cared for, and how they and others will react to the appearance and smell of the wound. When caring for patients with wounds, demonstrating acceptance and empathy, encouraging the expression of feelings, answering questions accurately and honestly, and avoiding excessive exposure of body parts when giving wound care are essential.

Changes in Body Image

Body image reflects a person's view of himself or herself as a whole entity. When the skin and tissues are traumatized, that image is changed, requiring the person to adapt and reformulate the concept of self. Wounds and scars that are visible to others, especially on the face, can result in feelings of conspicuousness, ugliness, and diminished self-worth. Large scars, such as from removal of a breast or from creation of a colostomy opening, can seriously affect the person's sexuality, social relationships, and self-concept. Referral to support groups or counselors may be necessary to facilitate coping and acceptance of changes in body structure or function. See the Focused Critical Thinking Guide 32-1: Wound Care: Promoting Acceptance of Changes in Body Image. In addition, Chapter 41 contains more information about self-concept.

PRESSURE ULCERS

A **pressure ulcer** is a wound with a localized area of tissue necrosis. Depending on the depth of the ulcer, a pressure ulcer may be an acute wound or a chronic wound. The underlying cause is pressure. Most pressure ulcers develop when soft tissue is compressed between a bony prominence and an external surface for a prolonged period of time, or when soft tissue undergoes pressure in combination with shear and/or friction (Hess, 2008; National Pressure Ulcer Advisory Panel [NPUAP], 2007c). The terms "decubitus ulcer," "pressure sore," and "bedsore" are also used to refer to this type of wound. The term "pressure ulcer" is considered the most appropriate term because pressure is the most prominent underlying cause.

Pressure ulcers are costly in terms of patient discomfort, disfigurement, decreased quality of life, and healthcare expenditures (Brillhart, 2006; Elliott, McKinley, & Fox, 2008). Most pressure ulcers occur in older adults as a result of a combination of factors, including aging skin, chronic illnesses, immobility, malnutrition, fecal and urinary incontinence, and altered level of consciousness. Other significant at-risk populations include individuals with spinal cord injuries, traumatic brain injuries, or neuromuscular disorders. When pressure ulcers occur, aggressive intervention and treatment can spare the patient unnecessary pain and discomfort, prevent further tissue deterioration, hasten wound healing, and save millions of healthcare dollars. See the accompanying Research in Nursing box, which highlights the importance of the nurse's role in providing pressure ulcer prevention and treatment.

Factors in Pressure Ulcer Development

Pathologic changes at a pressure ulcer site result from blood vessel collapse caused by pressure, usually from body weight. Necrosis eventually occurs, leading to the characteristic ulcer. Two mechanisms contribute to pressure ulcer development: (1) external pressure that compresses blood vessels and (2) friction and shearing forces that tear and injure blood vessels and abrade the top layer of skin.

External Pressure

Pressure ulcers usually occur over bony prominences where body weight is distributed over a small area without much subcutaneous tissue to cushion damage to the skin. Common sites for pressure ulcers are illustrated in Figure 32-3. Of the susceptible areas, most pressure ulcers occur over the sacrum and coccyx, followed by the trochanter and the calcaneus (heel).

The major predisposing factor for a pressure ulcer is external pressure applied over an area, which results in occluded blood capillaries and poor circulation to tissues. Insufficient circulation deprives tissues of oxygen and nutrients, which leads to **ischemia** (deficiency of blood in a particular area), hypoxia (inadequate amount of oxygen available to cells), edema, inflammation, and, ultimately, necrosis and ulcer formation. A pressure ulcer may form in as little as 1 to 2 hours if the patient has not moved or been repositioned to allow circulation to flow to dependent areas. Patients with casts, orthopedic devices, or support stockings require routine assessment of areas where inadequate circulation may be a contributing factor to the development of a pressure ulcer.

> *Consider Mr. Everly, the postoperative patient in the critical care unit described in the Reflective Practice display. The nurse would integrate knowledge of the patient's condition, including his decreased level of consciousness and confinement in bed, to plan measures such as a turning schedule, proper positioning, and activities to promote movement in bed, thereby preventing body parts from exposure to prolonged pressure. ∎*

Friction and Shear

Friction occurs when two surfaces rub against each other. The injury, which resembles an abrasion, also can damage

RESEARCH IN NURSING
Bridging the Gap to Evidence-Based Practice

PRESSURE ULCERS IN INTENSIVE CARE

Critically ill patients are at increased risk for pressure ulcers, which negatively affect a patient's quality of life and patient outcomes. Factors contributing to this increased risk include a greater severity of illness, increased length of stay, poor tissue perfusion due to hemodynamic instability, sensory impairment, and poor nutritional status. Facilities usually have policies and protocols in place, as well as products and procedures, addressing pressure ulcer prevention and treatment. These policies and procedures are not always implemented for each and every patient. Prevention of pressure ulcers is a fundamental aspect of intensive care nursing and nursing initiatives to provide care in a cost-effective manner are of utmost importance.

Related Research

Franz, R., Gardner, S., Specht, J., McIntire, G. (2002). Integration of pressure ulcer treatment protocols into practice: Clinical outcomes and care environment attributes. *Outcomes Management for Nursing Practice, 5*(3), 112–120.

The purpose of this quality improvement project was to improve patient outcomes by reducing the prevalence of pressure ulcers, identify areas for improvement in prevention of pressure ulcers, and increase the adoption of preventive strategies in an intensive care unit (ICU). Surveys of patient's skin

For additional research, visit the Point.

were performed and one-on-one clinical instruction was provided to bedside nurses caring for these patients over a 26-month period of time. Pressure ulcer data was displayed in the clinical area and updated regularly. The frequency of pressure ulcers of all stages showed an overall downward trend, and the prevalence decreased from 50% to 8%. The appropriate allocation of pressure-relieving devices increased from 75% up to 95% to 100%. The origin of the ulcer (community or hospital acquired) and the anatomical site of the pressure ulcers did not change during the study period. The authors concluded that the program was successful in reducing the prevalence of pressure ulcers among intensive care patients. They also concluded that quality improvement interventions are a highly effective formula for improving patient outcomes and are easily implemented using clinical expertise and existing resources.

Relevance to Nursing Practice

Nurses must be able to provide care based on knowledge and skill, but they must also be managers of resources and costs of services provided in any setting. It is vital that nurses be familiar with and implement facility policies to prevent pressure ulcers. This study demonstrates that a relatively simple protocol was successful in ensuring implementation for each and every patient.

---

superficial blood vessels directly under the skin. A patient who lies on wrinkled sheets is likely to sustain tissue damage as a result of friction. The skin over the elbows and heels often is injured due to friction when patients lift and help move themselves up in bed with the use of their arms and feet. Friction burns can also occur on the back when patients

are pulled or slid over sheets while being moved up in bed or transferred onto a stretcher.

Shear results when one layer of tissue slides over another layer. Shear separates the skin from underlying tissues. The small blood vessels and capillaries in the area are stretched and possibly tear, resulting in decreased circulation to the

FIGURE 32-3. Common sites for development of pressure ulcers.

FIGURE 32-4. Shearing forces can occur when a patient is moved carelessly or slides down in bed.

tissue cells under the skin. Figure 32-4 illustrates how shearing forces occur. Patients who are pulled, rather than lifted, when being moved up in bed or from bed to chair or stretcher are at risk for injury from shearing forces. A patient who is partially sitting up in bed is susceptible to shearing force when the skin sticks to the sheet and underlying tissues move downward with the body toward the foot of the bed. This may also occur in a patient who sits in a chair but slides down.

Risks for Pressure Ulcer Development

In addition to pressure, friction, and shear, a combination of causes contributes to ulcer development. These include immobility, nutrition and hydration, skin moisture, mental status, and age; these factors are addressed here. Additional risk factors are outlined in Box 32-2.

Immobility

Patients who spend long periods of time in bed or seated without shifting their body weight properly are at great risk for development of a pressure ulcer (Hess, 2008). Individuals who are ambulatory usually do not develop this type of injury because no part of the body experiences prolonged pressure. In addition, when asleep, healthy people tend to move about in bed freely. Patients who are unconscious and paralyzed, those with cognitive impairments, or have other physical limitations, such as a fracture, are subject to pressure ulcers if they are allowed to remain in any one position for an extended period. Persons who are emotionally depressed ordinarily do not move around a great deal, placing them at risk for pressure ulcer formation. Additional

factors that cause immobility and may result in this serious problem include surgery and the use of tranquilizers or sedatives.

Nutrition and Hydration

Protein–calorie malnutrition predisposes a person to pressure ulcer formation because poorly nourished cells are damaged easily. Protein deficiency leading to a negative nitrogen balance, electrolyte imbalances, and insufficient caloric intake also predisposes the skin to injury. Other deficiencies can increase risk. For example, vitamin C deficiency causes capillaries to become fragile, with resultant poor circulation to the area. The condition of the teeth or fit of dentures may also exacerbate the problem of inadequate dietary intake. Dehydration as well as edema can interfere with circulation and subsequent cell nourishment.

Moisture

Primary sources of skin moisture include perspiration, urine, feces, and drainage from wounds (Butler, 2006). Prolonged moisture on the skin reduces the skin's resistance to trauma, particularly damage from friction and shear. When skin is damp, less friction is required to blister and abrade skin. Additionally, the moisture associated with urinary and fecal incontinence is believed to increase the risk for skin damage due to the chemical irritation from the ammonia in the urine. Ammonia also raises the alkalinity of the skin pH, altering the function of the normally acidic skin. A more alkaline pH promotes premature shedding of skin cells and decreases the skin's defense against bacteria, which results in enhanced growth of pathogens, such as yeast and staphylococci.

Box 32-2 RISK FACTORS FOR PRESSURE ULCER DEVELOPMENT

Immobility, nutrition and hydration, skin moisture, mental status, and age are factors in the development of pressure ulcers. In addition, patients compromised by the following conditions are at risk for pressure ulcer development:

- Dehydration
- Incontinence
- Skin hygiene
- Diabetes mellitus
- Diminished pain awareness
- Fractures
- History of corticosteroid therapy
- Immunosuppression
- Multisystem trauma
- Poor circulation
- Previous pressure ulcers
- Significant obesity or thinness

Adapted from Benbow, M. (2008). Pressure ulcer prevention and pressure–relieving surfaces. *British Journal of Nursing, 17*(13), 830–835; and Hess, C. (2008). *Wound care* (6th ed.). Philadelphia: Wolters Kluwer Health/Lippincott Williams & Wilkins; National Pressure Ulcer Advisory Panel (NPUAP). (2001a) Pressure ulcer prevention: a competency-based curriculum. Available at www.npuap.org/PDF/prevcurr.pdf.

Mental Status

The more alert an individual is, the more likely he or she is to protect skin integrity by relieving pressure periodically and maintaining adequate skin hygiene. Apathy, confusion, or a comatose state can diminish these self-care abilities and increase the likelihood of skin breakdown.

Age

Older adults are at a greater risk for pressure ulcer formation because the aging skin is more susceptible to injury. Chronic and debilitating diseases, more common in this age group, may adversely affect circulation and oxygenation of dermal structures. Other problems, such as malnutrition and immobility, compound the risk of pressure ulcer development in older adults.

Pressure Ulcer Staging

The first indication that a pressure ulcer may be developing is blanching (becoming pale and white) of the skin over the area under pressure. This ischemia makes the skin appear paler than in areas where circulation is adequate. When pressure is relieved, ischemia is rapidly followed by hyperemia. Reactive hyperemia is a blanchable reddening of the skin that occurs when pressure is removed. The body literally floods the area with blood to nourish and remove wastes from the cells. The area appears red and feels warm, but blanches when slight pressure is applied. Reactive hyperemia is not a pressure ulcer. After a patient who has been lying supine for 2 hours is repositioned onto the side, any reddened area due to reactive hyperemia should fade within 60 to 90 minutes. In patients with darkly pigmented skin, it may be best to assess for hyperemia by touch; the skin feels warm. Also, assess for some change in color relative to the surrounding skin.

If the pressure continues after ischemia occurs, circulation is further impaired and a pressure ulcer develops. Appropriate intervention depends on early recognition of the stage of development of the pressure ulcer. Pressure ulcers are commonly classified according to six stages (four numbered and two unnumbered)—suspected deep-tissue injury, stage I, stage II, stage III, stage IV, and unstageable.

Suspected deep-tissue injury presents as purple or maroon localized area of discolored intact skin or blood-filled blister due to damage of underlying soft tissue from pressure and/or shear. It may initially present as a painful, firm, mushy, boggy, warmer, or cooler area as compared to adjacent tissue (NPUAP, 2007c).

A stage I pressure ulcer is a defined area of intact skin with nonblanchable redness of a localized area usually over a bony prominence. Darkly pigmented skin may not have visible blanching; its color may differ from the surrounding skin. The area may be painful, firm, soft, warmer, or cooler as compared to adjacent tissue (NPUAP, 2007c). A stage II pressure ulcer involves partial thickness loss of dermis and presents as a (NPUAP, 2007c). A stage III ulcer presents with full thickness tissue loss. Subcutaneous fat may be visible but bone, tendon, or muscle is not exposed. Slough that may be present does not

obscure the depth of tissue loss. May include undermining and tunneling (NPUAP, 2007c). Stage IV ulcers involve full thickness tissue loss with exposed bone, tendon, or muscle. Slough or eschar may be present on some part of the wound bed and often include undermining and tunneling.

Pressure ulcers are classified as unstageable when the base of the ulcer is covered by slough (yellow, tan, gray, green, or brown) and/or eschar (tan, brown, or black) in the wound bed. **Eschar** is a thick, leathery scab or dry crust that is necrotic (dead tissue) and must be removed before the stage can be determined accurately. However, stable (dry, adherent, intact, without erythema or fluctuance) eschar on the heels serves as "the body's natural (biological) cover" and should not be removed (NPUAP, 2007c).

Detailed descriptions of these stages and a visual representation are presented in Box 32-3.

THE NURSING PROCESS FOR WOUNDS
Assessing
Nursing History

When obtaining the nursing history, include questions about the appearance of the skin and patient activities that may contribute to the development of a pressure ulcer. Often a combination of factors places the patient at greatest risk for a pressure ulcer.

Question the patient and family about recent changes in the appearance or condition of the skin and any skin care regimens. Also, assess activity status, nutritional state, elimination patterns, and cognitive state.

Evaluate the patient's general condition and laboratory test results. Be alert for signs and symptoms of infection, which may cause generalized malaise, increased pain, anorexia, and an elevated body temperature and pulse rate. Laboratory data indicating an infection include an elevated white blood cell count and, if a wound culture has been done, a causative organism.

The accompanying Focused Assessment Guide 32-1 provides additional suggestions for gathering a nursing history.

Skin Assessment

Skin assessment should be an integral part of every patient's care. It is important to provide patients with a proactive strategy for skin care. Many conditions and wounds, particularly pressure ulcers, can be prevented or minimized with early interventions. Skin assessment provides needed information for developing an appropriate plan of care. The inspection and palpation skills used to assess the integumentary system are described in detail in Chapter 25. Be sure to inspect the skin systematically in a head-to-toe fashion, including bony prominences, on admission and then at regular intervals for all at-risk patients. Reassessment is recommended (National Pressure Ulcer Advisory Panel [NPUAP], 2007a), as follows:

- Acute care setting: On admission, then reassessed at least every 48 hours or if the patient's condition changes. Reassess stable patients in intensive care units daily; reassess unstable patients every shift.

| Box 32-3 | COMPARISON OF STAGES OF PRESSURE ULCERS |

Suspected Deep Tissue Injury

Purple or maroon localized area of discolored intact skin or blood-filled blister due to damage of underlying soft tissue from pressure and/or shear. Deep tissue injury may be difficult to detect in individuals with dark skin tones. The area may be preceded by tissue that is painful, firm, boggy, warmer, or cooler as compared to adjacent tissue. Evolution may include a thin blister over a dark wound bed. The wound may further evolve and become covered by a thin eschar. Evolution may be rapid, exposing additional layers of tissue even with optimal treatment.

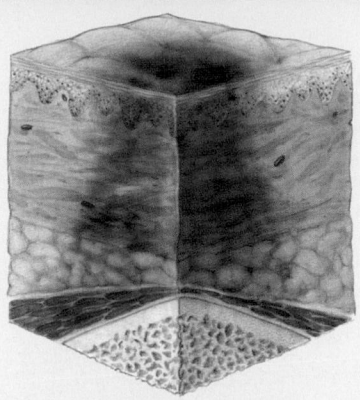

Stage I

Intact skin with nonblanchable redness of a localized area usually over a bony prominence. Darkly pigmented skin may not have visible blanching; its color may differ from the surrounding area. The area may be painful, firm, soft, warmer, or cooler as compared to adjacent tissue. Stage I may be difficult to detect in individuals with dark skin tones. Stage I may indicate "at risk" persons.

Stage II

Partial thickness loss of dermis presenting as a shallow open ulcer with a red pink wound bed, without slough. Presents as a shiny or dry shallow ulcer without slough or bruising (which indicates suspected deep tissue injury). May also present as an intact or open/rupture serum-filled blister. This stage should not be used to describe skin tears, tape burns, perineal dermatitis, maceration, or excoriation.

(continued)

Box 32-3   COMPARISON OF STAGES OF PRESSURE ULCERS   *(continued)*

Stage III

Full thickness tissue loss. Subcutaneous fat may be visible, but bone, tendon, or muscle are not exposed. Bone/tendon is not visible or directly palpable. Slough may be present but does not obscure the depth of tissue loss. May include undermining and tunneling. The depth of a stage III pressure ulcer varies by anatomical location. The bridge of the nose, ear, occiput, and malleolus do not have subcutaneous tissue, and stage II ulcers at these locations can be shallow. In contrast, areas with significant adipose tissue can develop extremely deep Stage III pressure ulcers.

Stage IV

Full thickness tissue loss with exposed bone, tendon, or muscle. Exposed bone/tendon is visible or directly palpable. Slough or eschar may be present on some parts of the wound bed. Often include undermining and tunneling. The depth of a stage IV pressure ulcer varies by anatomical location. The bridge of the nose, ear, occiput, and malleolus do not have subcutaneous tissue and these ulcers can be shallow at these locations. Stage IV ulcers can extend into muscle and/or supporting structures (e.g., fascia, tendon, or joint capsule), making osteomyelitis possible.

Unstageable

Full thickness tissue loss in which the base of the ulcer is covered by slough (yellow, tan, gray, green, or brown) and/or eschar (tan, brown, or black) in the wound bed. Until enough slough and/or eschar is removed to expose the base of the wound, the true depth, and therefore stage, cannot be determined. Stable (dry, adherent, intact, without erythema, or fluctuance) eschar on the heels serves as "the body's natural (biological) cover" and should not be removed.

From National Pressure Ulcer Advisory Panel (NPUAP). (2007c). Updated staging system. Pressure ulcer stages revised by NPUAP. Available at www.npuap.org/pr2.htm.; and Porth, C., & Matfin, G. (2009). *Pathophysiology: Concepts of altered health states* (8th ed.). Philadelphia: Lippincott Williams & Wilkins.

Illustrations from National Pressure Ulcer Advisory Panel (NPUAP). (2007b). Resources. Staging illustrations. Available at www.npuap.org/resources.htm.

FOCUSED ASSESSMENT GUIDE • 32-1

SKIN INTEGRITY

Factors to Assess	Questions and Approaches
Appearance of skin	• Do you have any skin areas that are discolored? • Do some areas of skin on your body feel warmer or colder than others? • Describe the moisture in your skin: is it damp, dry, oily? • Have you noticed that your skin seems to be thinner? Where? • Have you noticed any swelling in your feet, ankles, or fingers? • Tell me about how you take care of your skin. For example, do you take a tub bath or shower? How often? Do you use oils or lotions?
Recent changes in skin	• Do you have any sores on your body? If so, how many, and where are they? Have they changed in size? Do you have any drainage from them? • Have you noticed that the skin over your hips or backbone gets red if you sit or lie in one position for a long time? Does this disappear in a short time when you are up?
Activity/mobility	• Do you need assistance to walk or move? If so, how much? • Are you confined to your bed or a chair when up? • Can you change your position when you want to?
Nutrition	• Have you gained or lost weight recently? • Describe your usual meals each day. • How many glasses or cups of liquid do you drink each day? • Do you take any food supplements or vitamins? • Do you prepare your own meals? • Do you wear dentures? How do they fit? • Do you have any difficulty swallowing? • Has a doctor ever told you that you are anemic?
Pain	• If you have a sore, is it painful? • Do you take anything for pain? If so, what do you take, and how often? Does it help?
Elimination	• Have you noticed any problems with your bowels or urination? If so, describe. • Have you ever used pads or special pants because you can't control your urine or stools?

• Long-term care setting: On admission, then reassess every 48 hours for the first week, weekly for the first month, followed by monthly to quarterly assessments; more frequently if the patient's condition changes.

• Home healthcare: On admission, then reassess at every visit.

Early detection and treatment of skin problems are important nursing functions. Interventions to promote skin health are discussed in Chapter 31. Physical assessment of the skin is included as part of the initial database collection.

Pressure Ulcer Assessment

Many pressure ulcers can be prevented. It is a nursing priority to perform a comprehensive assessment in all settings and identify patients at risk for pressure ulcers, predisposing factors, or evidence of actual pressure ulcers.

RISK ASSESSMENT

An aggressive approach to prevent a pressure ulcer or manage the care of a patient who already has impaired skin integrity begins with a risk assessment form, which should be simple to use, reliable, and cost-effective. Several different scales are available to assess risk, such as the Norton scale (physical condition, mental condition, activity, mobility, incontinence) and the Braden scale (mental status, continence, mobility, activity, nutrition; Fig. 32-5). With these tools, a numeric score is assigned to each assessment area. The degree of risk is based on the patient's total score. Using the Braden scale, a score of 19 to 23 indicates no risk; 15 to 18, mild risk; 13 to 14, moderate risk; 10 to 12, high risk; and 9 or lower, very high risk (Braden & Maklebust, 2005).

Once a patient's risk has been identified, agencies use different approaches. Appropriate interventions are initiated based on the patient's identified risk. Many healthcare facilities

Braden Scale for Predicting Pressure Sore Risk

Sensory Perception: Ability to respond meaningfully to pressure-related discomfort
1. **Completely Limited:** Unresponsive (does not moan, flinch, or grasp) to painful stimuli, due to diminished level of consciousness or sedation, OR limited ability to feel pain over most of body surface.
2. **Very Limited:** Responds only to painful stimuli. Cannot communicate discomfort except by moaning or restlessness, OR has a sensory impairment which limits the ability to feel pain or discomfort over half of body.
3. **Slightly Limited:** Responds to verbal commands but cannot always communicate discomfort or need to be turned, OR has some sensory impairment which limits ability to feel pain or discomfort in 1 or 2 extremities.
4. **No Impairment:** Responds to verbal commands. Has no sensory deficit which would limit ability to feel or voice pain or discomfort.

SCORE

Moisture: Degree to which skin is exposed to moisture
1. **Constantly Moist:** Skin is kept moist almost constantly by perspiration, urine, etc. Dampness is detected every time patient is moved or turned.
2. **Very Moist:** Skin is often but not always moist. Linen must be changed at least once a shift.
3. **Occasionally Moist:** Skin is occasionally moist, requiring an extra linen change approximately once a day.
4. **Rarely Moist:** Skin is usually dry: linen requires changing only at routine intervals.

SCORE

Activity: Degree of physical activity
1. **Bedfast:** Confined to bed.
2. **Chairfast:** Ability to walk severely limited or non-existent. Cannot bear own weight and/or must be assisted into chair or wheelchair.
3. **Walks Occasionally:** Walks occasionally during the day, but for very short distances, with or without assistance. Spends majority of each shift in bed or chair.
4. **Walks Frequently:** Walks outside the room at least twice and inside room at least once every 2 hours during waking hours.

SCORE

Mobility: Ability to change and control body position
1. **Completely immobile:** Does not make even slight changes in body or extremity position without assistance.
2. **Very Limited:** Makes occasional slight changes in body or extremity position but unable to make frequent or significant changes independently.
3. **Slightly Limited:** Makes frequent though slight changes in body or extremity position independently.
4. **No Limitation:** Makes major and frequent changes in position without assistance.

SCORE

Nutrition: Usual food intake pattern
1. **Very Poor:** Never eats a complete meal. Rarely eats more than 1/3 of food offered. Eats 2 servings or less of protein (meat or dairy products) per day. Takes fluids poorly. Does not take a liquid dietary supplement, OR is NPO and/or maintained on clear liquids or IV for more than five days.
2. **Probably Inadequate:** Rarely eats a complete meal and generally eats only about half of any food offered. Protein intake includes only 3 servings of meat or dairy products per day. Occasionally will take a dietary supplement, OR receives less than optimum amount of liquid diet or tube feeding.
3. **Adequate:** Eats over half of most meals. Eats a total of 4 servings of protein (meat, dairy products) each day. Occasionally will refuse a meal, but will usually take a supplement if offered, OR is on a tube feeding or TPN regimen, which probably meets most of nutritional needs.
4. **Excellent:** Eats most of every meal. Never refuses a meal. Usually eats a total of 4 or more servings of meat and dairy products. Occasionally eats between meals. Does not require supplementation.

SCORE

Friction and Shear
1. **Problem:** Requires moderate to maximum assistance in moving. Complete lifting without sliding against sheets is impossible. Frequently slides down in bed or chair, requiring frequent repositioning with maximum assistance. Spasticity, contractures, or agitation leads to almost constant friction.
2. **Potential Problem:** Moves feebly or requires minimum assistance. During a move skin probably slides to some extent against sheets, chair, restraints, or other devices. Maintains relatively good position in chair or bed most of the time but occasionally slides down.
3. **No Apparent Problem:** Moves in bed and in chair independently and has sufficient muscle strength to lift up completely

SCORE

	Risk Level	
3 or 4 = Moderate to Low Impairment	19-23 Not at risk	NPO: Nothing by Mouth
Total Points Possible: 23	15-18 low risk	IV: Intravenously
Risk Predicting Score: 16 or Less	13-14 moderate risk	TPN: Total parenteral nutrition
	10-12 high risk	
	≤ 9 very high risk	

Total Score:

FIGURE 32-5. Braden scale for predicting pressure ulcer risk. *(Copyright 1988 by Barbara Braden and Nancy Bergstrom. Reprinted with permission. All rights reserved.)*

use a special pressure ulcer assessment form. Documenting assessments is essential to ensure continuity of care, providing the foundation on which to develop the skin plan of care. All caregivers in the home or healthcare agency need to be aware of specific assessments, *including mobility, nutritional status, and moisture and incontinence.*

MOBILITY

Assessing a patient's mobility status includes evaluating the patient's ability to move, turn, and reposition the body. A patient who is confined to bed or a chair or has limited range of motion is at increased risk for a pressure ulcer. This assessment of activity status is done upon admission to the healthcare facility or during the initial home care interview. The use of any assistive devices to maintain mobility and activity is noted. Additional suggestions for gathering information about mobility are described in Chapter 33.

NUTRITIONAL STATUS

The importance of sound nutrition in the prevention and treatment of a pressure ulcer is well established. Older adults, in particular, need adequate nutrition for optimal health and wound healing. Nutritional assessment is described in Chapter 36. The following laboratory criteria indicate that a patient is nutritionally at risk for development of a pressure ulcer:

- Albumin level <3.2 mg/dL (normal, 3.5–5 mg/dL).
- Prealbumin <19 mg/dL (normal 16–40 mg/dL)
- Body weight decrease of >15%

Additional laboratory tests to consider in patients at risk for or presenting with pressure ulcers include:

- Total lymphocyte count <1,800/mm^3 (normal, 1,000–4,000/mm^3)
- Hemoglobin A1C >8% (normal <6%)
- Glucose >120 mg/dL (normal 70–120 mg/dL)

MOISTURE AND INCONTINENCE

Many studies have documented that moisture makes the skin more susceptible to injury. Whether the moisture is from perspiration, wound drainage, urine, or stool, the skin is compromised. Moisture can create an environment in which microorganisms can multiply and the skin is more likely to blister, suffer abrasions, and become macerated (softening or disintegration of the skin in response to moisture). Chapters 37 and 38 have additional assessment information related to incontinence.

EVALUATION OF EXISTING PRESSURE ULCER

Skin assessment for a pressure ulcer specifically includes inspection of the following (Agency for Health care Research and Quality, NPUAP, 2001b; Hess, 2008):

- Location of any lesion or ulcer
- Identification of the stage (see Box 32-3)
- Size of the ulcer: length, width, depth (see Guidelines for Nursing Care 32-1); presence of undermining, a hollow

between the skin surface and the wound bed, resulting from death of the underlying tissue

- Color and type of wound tissue
- Presence of any abnormal pathways in the wound, such as a sinus tract (a cavity or channel underneath the wound that has the potential for infection) or tunneling (a passageway or opening that may be visible at skin level, but with most of the tunnel under the surface of the skin). See Guidelines for Nursing Care 32-1.
- Visible necrotic tissue; necrotic tissue that is in the process of separating from viable portions of the body is referred to as slough.
- Presence of an exudate or drainage (amount and type)
- Presence of odor
- Presence or absence of granulation tissue
- Visible evidence of epithelialization
- Periwound skin condition

The RYB Wound Classification (see Box 32-4) can also be used to aid in assessment and description of the pressure ulcer appearance.

Wound Assessment

Wound assessment involves inspection (sight and smell) and palpation for appearance, drainage, odor, and pain. Wound assessment determines the status of the wound, identifies barriers to the healing process, and signs of complications. Accurate assessment provides essential baseline data and information to judge the effectiveness of treatment and wound healing progression. Skin integrity and wound assessment are performed at regular intervals, based on the nature of the wound and facility policy.

APPEARANCE OF THE WOUND

Note the location of the wound. Location is described in relation to the nearest anatomic landmark, such as bony prominences. Document the size of the wound. Measurements are taken in millimeters or centimeters, measuring length, width, and depth. Refer to Guidelines for Nursing Care 32-1 for details on measuring a wound.

Assess wounds for the approximation of the wound edges (edges meet) and signs of dehiscence or evisceration. Assess the color of the wound and surrounding area. Note the presence of drains, tubes, staples, and sutures. The edges of a healthy healing surgical wound appear clean and well approximated, with a crust along the wound edges. Initially, the edges are reddened and slightly swollen. After approximately 1 week, the skin is closer to normal in appearance, with wound edges healing together. The skin surrounding the wound may at first be bruised, but this too returns to normal as blood is reabsorbed.

When infection is present, the wound is swollen and deep red. It feels hot on palpation, and drainage is increased and possibly purulent. If dehiscence is impending or present, the wound edges are separated. If the wound edges have separated and the wound is open, describe the type of tissue in the wound: granulation, slough, or eschar (see Box 32-4).

Guidelines for Nursing Care • 32-1

MEASURING WOUNDS AND PRESSURE ULCERS

Size of the Wound

- Draw the shape and describe it.
- Measure the length, width, and diameter (if circular).

Depth of the Wound

- Use Standard Precautions; use appropriate Transmission-Based Precautions when indicated.
- Perform hand hygiene. Put on gloves.
- Moisten a sterile, flexible applicator with saline and insert it gently into the wound at a 90-degree angle with the tip down (Figure A).
- Mark the point on the swab that is even with the surrounding skin surface, or grasp the applicator with the thumb and forefinger at the point corresponding to the wound's margin (Figure B).
- Remove the swab and measure the depth with a ruler (Figure C).

Wound Tunneling

- Use Standard Precautions; use appropriate Transmission-Based Precautions when indicated.
- Perform hand hygiene. Put on gloves.
- Determine direction: Gently insert a sterile applicator into the site where tunneling occurs. View the direction of the applicator as if it were the hand of a clock (Figure D). The direction of the patient's head represents 12 o'clock. Moving in a clockwise direction, document the deepest sites where the wound tunnels.
- Determine the depth: While the applicator is inserted into the tunneling, mark the point on the swab that is even with the wound's edge, or grasp the applicator with the thumb and forefinger at the point corresponding to the wound's margin. Remove the swab and measure the depth with a ruler (see Figure C).
- Document both the direction and depth of tunneling.

FIGURE A

FIGURE B

FIGURE C

FIGURE D

Adapted from Hess, C. (2008). *Skin & wound care* (6th ed.). Philadelphia: Wolters Kluwer Health/Lippincott Williams & Wilkins.

Assess for the presence of odor, but only after the wound has been cleaned. The presence of odor can be indicative of certain types of bacteria.

DRAINAGE

The inflammatory response results in the formation of exudate, which then drains from the wound. The exudate is composed of fluid and cells that escape from blood vessels and are deposited in or on tissue surfaces. This exudate is called wound drainage and is described as serous, sanguineous, serosanguineous, or, if infected, purulent.

- **Serous drainage** is composed primarily of the clear, serous portion of the blood and from serous membranes. Serous drainage is clear and watery.
- **Sanguineous drainage** consists of large numbers of red blood cells and looks like blood. Bright-red sanguineous drainage is indicative of fresh bleeding, whereas darker drainage indicates older bleeding.
- **Serosanguineous drainage** is a mixture of serum and red blood cells. It is light pink to blood tinged.
- **Purulent drainage** is made up of white blood cells, liquefied dead tissue debris, and both dead and live

Box 32-4 RYB WOUND CLASSIFICATION

A color classification system termed "R(red) Y(yellow) B(black)" can be used for wound assessment and to help direct treatment for open wounds (healing by secondary intention) (Hess, 2008; Krasner, 1995; Stotts, 1990). This classification, with related interventions, is based on the assessment of wound color. However, many wounds have red, yellow, and black components and are categorized as mixed wounds (see Figure). When all colors are present, the wound is treated first for the most serious color: black, followed by yellow, and finally red.

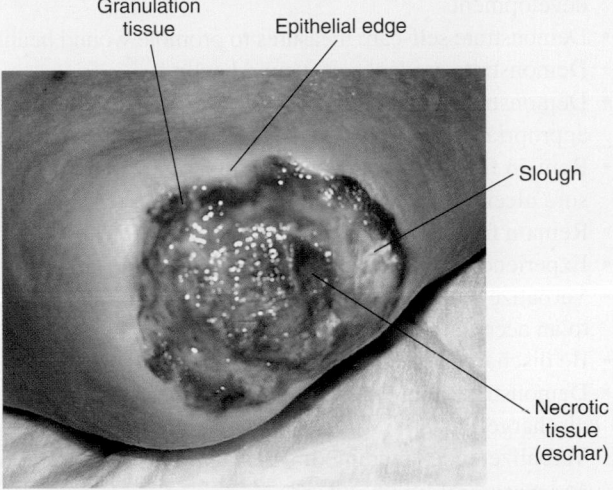

Granulation tissue — Epithelial edge — Slough — Necrotic tissue (eschar)

R = Red = Protect
Red wounds are in the proliferative stage of healing and reflect the color of normal granulation tissue. Wounds in this stage need protection with nursing interventions that include gentle cleansing, use of moist dressings, and changing of the dressing only when necessary, and/or based on product manufacturer's recommendations.

Y = Yellow = Cleanse
Yellow color in the wound may indicate the presence of exudate (drainage) or slough and requires wound cleaning. These wounds are characterized by oozing from the tissue covering the wound, often accompanied by purulent drainage. Drainage can be whitish yellow, creamy yellow, yellowish green, or beige. To cleanse these wounds, nursing interventions include the use of wound cleansers and irrigating the wound.

B = Black = Débride
Black in the wound may indicate the presence of an eschar (necrotic tissue), which is usually black but may also be brown, gray, or tan. The eschar requires débridement (removal) before the wound can heal. These wounds are often cared for by advanced practice nurses who are educated in the care of more complex wounds. After débridement, the wound is treated as a yellow wound and then, as healing progresses, a red wound.

---

bacteria. Purulent drainage is thick, often has a musty or foul odor, and varies in color (such as dark yellow or green), depending on the causative organism.

Drains may be inserted in or near a wound to promote drainage, thereby reducing the risk of abscess formation and promoting wound healing. Various types of drains are described in Table 32-4 and discussed later in this chapter.

Assess the amount, color, odor, and consistency of wound drainage. The amount and color depend on the wound location and size. Typically, larger wounds have more drainage than do smaller wounds. Assess wound drainage on the wound, on the dressings, in drainage bottles or reservoirs, or, depending on the location of the wound and the amount of drainage, under the patient.

SUTURES AND STAPLES
Skin sutures are used to hold tissue and skin together. Sutures may be black silk, synthetic material, or fine wire. Sutures are removed when enough tensile strength has developed to hold the wound edges together during healing. The time frame varies depending on the patient's age, nutritional status, and wound location. Frequently, after skin sutures are removed, small wound-closure strips of adhesive are applied across the wound to give additional support as it continues to heal. Figure 32-6 shows an example of an incision with sutures. Retention sutures are used to provide extra support for patients who are obese and for wounds with an increased risk for dehiscence.

Pain Assessment

Nurses have long recognized that patients with alterations in skin integrity, including surgical wounds, traumatic wounds, and pressure ulcer wounds, experience pain. Focus assessment on whether dressing changes, positioning in bed or in a

TABLE • 32-4 COMMON TYPES OF DRAINS

Type	Purpose	Example
Penrose	Provides sinus tract	After incision and drainage of abscess, in abdominal surgery
T-tube	For bile drainage	After gallbladder surgery
Jackson-Pratt	Decrease dead space by collecting drainage	After breast removal, abdominal surgery
Hemovac	Decrease dead space by collecting drainage	After abdominal, orthopedic surgery
Gauze, iodoform gauze, NuGauze	Allow healing from base of wound	Infected wounds, after removal of hemorrhoids

FIGURE 32-6. Incision with sutures.

chair, or movement elicits any expressions of pain. Perform a pain assessment at each dressing change; measure and document the level of pain before, during, and after a procedure (Lloyd Jones, 2008). Even if pain is never verbalized or expressed, always assume that pain is a definite possibility, and focus on comfort needs. Ask the patient about pain from the wound. If the patient experiences increased or constant pain from the wound, further assessments are necessary. Pain, especially when accompanied by an increased or purulent flow of drainage, may indicate delayed healing or an infection. Surgical incisional pain is usually most severe for the first 2 to 3 days and then progressively diminishes. Detailed assessment of pain is discussed in Chapter 35.

Diagnosing

Data that the nurse collects may lead to the development of several nursing diagnoses related to skin integrity and wound care. Each nursing diagnosis statement identifies a patient problem and suggests expected patient outcomes. The etiology of the problem directs nursing interventions. The following are examples of appropriate nursing diagnoses:

- Disturbed Body Image
- Deficient Knowledge related to wound care
- Acute Pain
- Chronic Pain
- Impaired Tissue Integrity
- Readiness for Enhanced Knowledge: Wound Care may be appropriate for patients who request information about wound care at home
- Impaired Skin Integrity
- Activity Intolerance
- Self-care Deficit
- Risk for Impaired Skin Integrity
- Risk for Trauma

Examples of diagnoses, etiologic factors, and defining characteristics appear in Examples of NANDA Nursing Diagnoses: Patient with a Wound or Pressure Ulcer.

Outcome Identification and Planning

When nurses care for patients who have or are at risk for impaired skin and tissue integrity, nursing interventions are planned toward facilitating the patient's return to health by providing interventions that facilitate wound healing, reducing the risk for complications, and promoting psychosocial adaptation. The following are examples of appropriate outcomes. The patient will:

- Maintain skin integrity
- Demonstrate self-care measures to prevent pressure ulcer development
- Demonstrate self-care measures to promote wound healing
- Demonstrate evidence of wound healing
- Demonstrate increase in body weight and muscle size, if appropriate
- Remain free of infection at the site of the wound or pressure ulcer
- Remain free of signs and symptoms of infection
- Experience no new areas of skin breakdown
- Verbalize that the pain management regimen relieves pain to an acceptable level
- Be discharged to home within established parameters
- Demonstrate appropriate wound care measures before discharge
- Verbalize understanding of signs and symptoms to report and necessary follow-up care

Implementing

Provide preventative measures for patients at risk. Teach patients about their health conditions and provide information and support to improve health literacy by their patients. Refer to the accompanying Promoting Health Literacy display.

When caring for the patient with a wound or pressure ulcer, nursing interventions focus on preventing infection, promoting wound healing, preventing further injury or alteration in skin integrity, promoting physical and emotional comfort, and facilitating coping. The accompanying Nursing Interventions and Nursing Outcomes Classifications (NIC/NOC) box offers suggested nursing interventions and outcomes related to Risk for Impaired Skin Integrity. It is often appropriate and necessary to consult with the wound care specialist, often a wound certified nurse specialist, to plan and coordinate the most effective care for the patient.

Preventing Pressure Ulcers

Tissue load management refers to therapeutic means to manage pressure, friction, and shear on tissues (Hess, 2008). Interventions to prevent injury to the skin and promote optimal health are outlined in Guidelines for Nursing Care 32-2. Additional interventions related to personal hygiene and maintaining skin health are discussed in Chapter 31. Implement interventions related to tissue load management as part of the nursing plan of care for patients at risk for developing pressure ulcers or who have a pressure ulcer. This includes interventions that can be implemented while the patient is in bed and sitting in chairs or wheelchairs.

Examples of NANDA Nursing Diagnoses

Patient With a Wound or Pressure Ulcer

Nursing Diagnoses	Related Factors	Sample Defining Characteristics
Impaired Skin Integrity	Any condition that alters the dermis and/or epidermis, such as a surgical incision or traumatic wound; moisture, physical immobilization	• Presence of intentional or unintentional wound • Presence of a pressure ulcer
Risk for Infection	Any condition that interferes with normal inflammatory healing process or provides an entry for infectious agents	Risk factors: • Disruption in skin integrity • Contaminated wounds • Chronic wounds • Extremes of age • Obesity or malnutrition • Presence of drains, tubes, or catheters • Immunosuppression
Acute Pain	Any condition that causes actual tissue damage, including intentional and unintentional wounds	• Presence of wound • "On a 1-to-10 scale, my pain is 9." • Positioning or guarding self or body part to avoid pain • "I hurt so much that I can't sleep or eat." • Diaphoresis, changes in vital signs, dilated pupils • Moaning, sighing, crying
Disturbed Body Image	Any condition that causes confusion in the mental image of oneself, such as a surgical or traumatic wound	• "I just don't feel like I'm the same person I used to be." • "I'll never be able to do my job if this arm doesn't work." • Refusal to look at incision or area of surgical treatment • Actual change in one's body from surgery or trauma • Actual missing body part
Impaired Tissue Integrity	Any condition that causes damage to dermal, epidermal, and subcutaneous tissues, such as pressure, friction, shear, or altered circulation	• Presence of suspected deep tissue injury or pressure ulcer
Chronic Pain	Any condition that causes potential or actual damage to tissues with pain that is constant or recurring without a predictable end and lasts longer than 6 months, such as from a chronic wound or pressure ulcer	• "I've had this bad pain for over a year now." • "I am so tired because this constant pain won't let me sleep." • "I can't do the things I used to do because it just hurts too much." • Presence of pressure ulcer for extended period of time

Promoting Health Literacy

IN PATIENTS WITH BREAST CANCER

Patient Scenario

Tashana Douglas, 42, has been diagnosed with breast cancer. She had a modified mastectomy 3 weeks ago and has returned to the clinic to discuss the rest of her treatment. She is going to have several weeks of outpatient radiation therapy. She states, "I feel pretty good, and the surgeon said my cancer is gone. Why do I need more treatment? My neighbor told me her sister had radiation and had terrible side effects." Ms. Douglas appears anxious as she relates that the neighbor's sister was extremely tired and had a "terrible rash or burn with her treatment. It took a long time to get better and really hurt." She states, "I don't know if I want to risk having that happen to me!" Ms. Douglas verbalizes concern that she will "give the radiation to others in her home and make them sick." She asks, "Do you think I should have this radiation stuff?"

Nursing Considerations: *Tips for Improving Health Literacy*

Review with Ms. Douglas the appropriate interventions she should be using to ensure her surgical site heals, including skin care. Provide Ms. Douglas with easy to read information about radiation therapy and potential side effects, as well as interventions she can implement to prevent and/or minimize the side effects of radiation therapy, particularly side effects related to skin integrity. Encourage her to ask her primary care provider, as well as the radiologist, as many questions as needed to understand her condition and the planned radiation treatment. Encourage Ms. Douglas to ask her primary care provider the following three questions:

- What is my main problem?
- What do I need to do?
- Why is it important for me to do this?

What additional measures can you take to help increase health literacy in this patient? What other measures would be helpful if Ms. Douglas does not speak English, cannot read, or has other learning deficits?

To protect patients at risk from the adverse effects of pressure, implement turning and positioning schedules, as well as the use of appropriate support surfaces (tissue load management surfaces). Reposition patients at least every 2 hours (Hess, 2008). Older adult patients tend to have less tissue tolerance, necessitating more frequent repositioning if redness on bony prominences is noted. The oblique position, an alternative to the side-lying position, results in significantly less pressure on the trochanter area.

Positioning devices such as pillows, foam wedges, or pressure-reducing boots can prove helpful to keep body weight off bony prominences. For example, a standard pillow placed under the calves raises the heels off the bed and alleviates pressure. Never use ring cushions, or "donuts," because they increase venous pressure. Minimize the effects of shearing force by limiting the amount of time the head of the bed is elevated, when possible.

Support surfaces are an important part of managing pressure, friction, and shear on tissues (Hess, 2008). A support surface is a specialized device for pressure redistribution designed for management of tissue loads (Benbow, 2008b; Hess, 2008). Support surfaces are available in sizes and shapes to be used on beds, chairs, examination tables, and operating room tables. Support surfaces are pressure-reducing or pressure-relieving

Examples of Nursing Interventions and Nursing Outcomes Classifications (NIC/NOC)

Risk for Impaired Skin Integrity

Nursing Interventions	Nursing Outcomes
• Bedrest Care • Incision Site Care • Wound Care • Pressure Management • Pressure Ulcer Prevention • Skin Surveillance	• Wound Healing: Primary Intention • Immobility Consequences: Physiological • Tissue Integrity: Skin and Mucous Membranes

From Bulechek, G., Butcher, H., & McCloskey Dochterman, J. (Eds.) (2008). *Nursing interventions classification (NIC)* (5th ed., p. 336). St. Louis, MO: Mosby Elsevier; and Moorhead, S., Johnson, M., Maas, M., Swanson, E. (Eds.). (2008). *Nursing outcomes classification (NOC)* (5th ed., p. 746). A full listing of nursing activities for each nursing intervention and outcomes can be found in these books.

Guidelines for Nursing Care • 32-2

PREVENTING PRESSURE ULCERS

- Assess the skin of patients at risk on a daily basis. Pay particular attention to bony prominences.
- Cleanse the skin routinely and whenever any soiling occurs. Use a mild cleansing agent, minimal friction, and avoid hot water.
- Maintain higher humidity in the environment and use skin moisturizers for dry skin.
- Avoid massage over bony prominences.
- Protect the skin from moisture associated with episodes of incontinence or exposure to wound drainage.
- Minimize skin injury from friction and shearing forces by using proper positioning, turning, and transferring

techniques. Use lubricants, protective films, dressings, and padding to diminish the effects of friction on the skin.
- Investigate reasons for inadequate dietary intake of protein and calories. Administer nutritional supplements or more aggressive nutritional intervention as needed.
- Continue efforts to improve mobility and activity. If this is unrealistic, attempt to maintain current level of activity, mobility, and range of motion.
- Document measures used to prevent pressure ulcers and the results of these interventions.

devices. The most common support surfaces are seating devices (air, fluid foam, or gel cushions), air-, gel-, or water-filled mattress overlays; static flotation mattresses; alternating air mattresses; low-air-loss beds; and air-fluidized beds (Hess, 2008). It is important to individualize the type of support surface based on the patient's needs. Because none of these devices totally relieves pressure, continue to perform position changes at regular intervals.

The use of appropriate devices to ensure safe patient handling and movement is an important part of tissue load management. Use devices, such as friction reducing sheets and lifting devices, with patients who cannot assist during transfers and position changes. These interventions and devices are discussed at length in Chapter 33.

Wound Care/Wound Management

The goal of wound care is to promote tissue repair and regeneration so that skin integrity is restored. Wounds can be treated by leaving them open to air; no **dressing** (protective covering placed over a wound) is applied. Wounds left open to the air heal more slowly because wound drying produces a dried eschar or scab. If the scab is removed accidentally before healing is complete, reinjury occurs, and the new delicate cells are exposed. Wounds left open are exposed to more environmental factors and potential injury.

Closed wound care uses dressings to keep the wound moist, promoting healing. A moist environment is best for wound healing. When a dressing is placed over a wound, the wound fluid keeps the surface of the wound moist. As a result, epidermal cells migrate more rapidly, maximizing healing. In addition, covered wounds can help patients cope with alterations in body image.

Many different types of dressings are available, but all have essentially the same purposes:

- Provide physical, psychological, and aesthetic comfort
- Prevent, eliminate, or control infection
- Absorb drainage
- Maintain a moist wound environment
- Protect the wound from further injury

- Protect the skin surrounding the wound
- Remove necrotic tissue, if appropriate

There is no standard frequency for how often dressings should be changed. It depends on the amount of drainage, the primary practitioner's preference, the nature of the wound, and the particular wound care product being used. It is customary for the surgeon or other advanced practice professional to perform the first dressing change on a surgical wound, usually within 24 to 48 hours after surgery.

> *Consider the care needed by Lucius Everly, the patient in the critical care unit. Although he has multiple needs, performing incisional wound care cannot be overlooked; otherwise, his risk of infection may increase.* ■

Wound contamination occurs through a moist medium. Microorganisms can move from the external surface through the dressing to the wound if a dressing remains in place until it is saturated. Microorganisms can also move from the wound to the outer surface of a saturated dressing. For these reasons, always replace dressings with fresh dressings or reinforce the dressing with additional dressings before drainage causes saturation.

Dressing changes provide an excellent opportunity for teaching, especially important when the patient will be changing dressings at home. Encourage the patient to help as much as possible, if appropriate.

The sight of the wound may disturb a patient. Listen carefully to what the patient is saying and observe nonverbal communication as well. In some instances, the patient may not want to look at the wound, particularly with a wound that involves a change in normal body functions or appearance, such as a wound resulting from the removal of a breast, the amputation of an extremity, or the placement of a tube in a draining wound. With patience and emotional support, patients can learn to cope with and adapt to their wound.

TYPES OF WOUND DRESSINGS

The items needed for a dressing change may be gathered individually or may be packaged in a sterile dressing tray, depending on the healthcare setting. Wound care in the home may depend on the supplies provided by the patient or family.

The number and type of dressings used depend on the location and size of the wound, type and depth of wound, the presence of infection, the need for **débridement** (removal of devitalized tissue and foreign material), and the amount and type of drainage.

Dry gauze dressings can be used to cover wounds, commonly closed surgical wounds. These dressings come in various sizes (2×2 inches, 4×4 inches, 4×8 inches) and are commercially packaged as single units or in packs. Gauze dressings often consist of three layers. The first layer of dressing material applied directly to a draining wound is often nonabsorbent but hydrophilic (i.e., capable of carrying moisture). This type of material allows drainage from the wound to move into overlying absorbent layers of dressing, helping to prevent maceration and reinfection. Moreover, this type of dressing is less likely to stick to the wound, making dressing changes more comfortable for the patient.

Material to absorb and collect drainage is then placed over the first layer of nonabsorbent material. This material acts as a wick, pulling drainage out by capillary action. Absorbent cotton has far greater capillarity than untreated cotton. Therefore, cotton-lined gauze sponges soak up more liquid than do unlined sponges. The number of gauze sponges used in the dressing depends on the amount of drainage. Loosely packed gauze, the threads of which act as numerous wicks, enhances capillarity and directs drainage upward and away from the wound. Fluffed and loosely packed dressings are more absorbent than tightly packed dressings. The top of the dressing may be further protected by surgical or abdominal pads, which are thick, absorbent pads that help to absorb profuse drainage.

Nonadherent gauzes include sterile petrolatum gauze and Telfa gauze. Telfa's shiny outer surface is applied to the wound. These dressings allow drainage to pass through and be absorbed by the outer absorbent layer but prevent outer dressings from adhering to the wound and causing further injury when removed.

Special gauze dressings (e.g., Sof-Wick) are precut halfway to fit around drains or tubes. Larger dressings (8×10 bandages, abdominal pads [ABDs], Surgi-Pads) are placed over the smaller gauze dressings and absorb drainage and protect the wound from contamination or injury.

Transparent films (e.g., OpSite) are semipermeable membrane dressings that are adhesive and waterproof. These dressings are occlusive, decreasing the possibility of contamination, while allowing visualization of the wound. This type of dressing is often used over peripheral intravenous sites, central venous access device insertion sites, and noninfected healing wounds.

> *Think back to Lucius Everly, the patient in the critical care unit. The nurse most likely would use a transparent dressing on his venous access sites, thereby allowing frequent assessment of the sites.* ∎

When caring for open wounds and pressure ulcers, it is necessary to keep the wound tissue moist and the surrounding skin dry (Hess, 2008; Snyder, 2008). Therefore, use dressings that continuously keep the wound moist, placing the moist dressing only on the wound surface and keeping the intact, healthy skin surrounding the ulcer dry because it is susceptible to damage. Select a dressing that absorbs exudate, if present, but still maintains a moist environment for healing. Use a skin sealant or moisture-barrier ointment on the surrounding skin and secure the dressing with the least amount of tape or other material to secure that is necessary.

The presence of foreign matter and/or devitalized, injured, infected tissue in a wound may indicate the need for débridement to promote wound healing (Hess, 2008; Snyder, 2008; Stephen-Haynes & Thompson, 2007). Débridement can be accomplished through several different methods. Autolytic débridement uses occlusive dressings, such as hydrocolloids or transparent films, and uses the body's own enzymes and defense mechanisms to loosen and liquefy necrotic tissue. This type of débridement can be used on any type of wound (Snyder, 2008). Biosurgical débridement involves the use of sterile fly larvae. The larvae secrete an enzyme that liquefies dead tissue, which is ingested by the larvae, clearing the wound of bacteria and infection (Stephen-Haynes & Thompson, 2007). Enzymatic débridement involves the application of commercially prepared enzymes to speed up the body's autolytic process. Mechanical débridement uses external physical force to dislodge and remove debris and necrotic tissue. This could be achieved by wound irrigation with pulsed pressure lavage (washing), whirlpool therapy, ultrasound or laser treatment, or with surgical débridement (Hess, 2008; Snyder, 2008; Stephen-Haynes & Thompson, 2007). In the past, wet-to-dry gauze dressings have been used to débride wounds; this is no longer considered good practice. This type of dressing damages healthy wound bed tissue and can be painful (Snyder, 2008; Stephen-Haynes & Thompson, 2007). Concern exists that complete drying of the gauze disrupts angiogenesis. However, despite concerns by wound care experts, these dressings are often still prescribed by physicians for wound débridement (Armstrong & Price, 2004).

There are many other wound care products/dressings available, each with distinctive actions, as well as indications, contraindications, advantages, and disadvantages. It is very important for the nurse to be aware of the products available in a particular facility and be familiar with the indications for, and correct use of, each type of dressing and wound care product. Generally, a wound with heavy exudate will need a more absorptive dressing and a dry wound will require rehydration with a dressing that keeps the wound moist (Benbow, 2008a; Hess, 2008; Snyder, 2008). Table 32-5 outlines the purposes and uses for several wound dressing/product categories.

CHANGING THE DRESSING

Prepare the patient for the dressing change before starting the procedure by explaining what will be done. If wound

TABLE • 32-5 EXAMPLES OF WOUND DRESSINGS/PRODUCTS

Type	Purposes	Use
Transparent films, such as: Bioclusive DermaView Mefilm Polyskin Uniflex OpSite Tegaderm	• Allow exchange of oxygen between wound and environment • Are self-adhesive • Protect against contamination; waterproof • Prevent loss of wound fluid • Maintain a moist wound environment • Facilitate autolytic debridement • No absorption of drainage • Allow visualization of wound • May remain in place for 24 to 72 hours, resulting in less interference with healing	• Wounds with minimal drainage • Wounds that are small; partial-thickness • Stage I pressure ulcers • Cover dressings for gels, foams, and gauze • Secure intravenous catheters, nasal cannulas, chest tube dressing, central venous access devices
Hydrocolloid dressings, such as: DuoDerm Comfeel PrimaCol Ultec Exuderm	• Are occlusive or semi-occlusive, limiting exchange of oxygen between wound and environment • Minimal to moderate absorption of drainage • Maintain a moist wound environment • Are self-adhesive • Provide cushioning • Facilitate autolytic débridement • Protect against contamination • May be left in place for 3 to 7 days, resulting in less interference with healing	• Partial- and full-thickness wounds • Wounds with light to moderate drainage • Wounds with necrosis or slough • Not for use with wounds that are infected
Hydrogels, such as: IntraSite Gel Aquasorb ClearSite Hypergel ActiFormCool	• Maintain a moist wound environment • Minimal absorption of drainage • Facilitate autolytic débridement • Do not adhere to wound • Reduce pain • Most require a secondary dressing to secure	• Partial- and full-thickness wounds • Necrotic wounds • Burns • Dry wounds • Wounds with minimal exudate • Infected wounds
Alginates, such as: Sorbsan AlgiCell Curasorb AQUACEL KALGINATE Melgisorb	• Absorb exudate • Maintain a moist wound environment • Facilitate autolytic débridement • Requires secondary dressing • Can be left in place for 1 to 3 days	• Infected and noninfected wounds • Wounds with moderate to heavy exudate • Partial- and full-thickness wounds • Tunneling wounds • Moist red and yellow wounds • Not for use with wounds with minimal drainage or dry eschar
Foams, such as: LYOfoam Allevyn Biatain Mepilex Optifoam	• Maintain a moist wound environment • Do not adhere to wound • Insulate wound • Highly absorbent • Can be left in place up to 7 days • Some products need a secondary dressing to secure	• Absorb light to heavy amounts of drainage • Use around tubes and drains • Not for use with wounds with dry eschar
Antimicrobials, such as: SilvaSorb Acticoat Excilon Silverlon	• Antimicrobial or antibacterial action • Reduce infection • Prevent infection	• Draining, exuding, and nonhealing wounds to protect from bacterial contamination and reduce bacterial contamination • Acute and chronic wounds
Collagens, such as: BGC Matrix Stimulin PROMOGRAN Matrix	• Absorbent • Maintain a moist wound environment • Do not adhere to wound • Compatible with topical agents • Nonadherent • Conform well to the wound surface • Require secondary dressing to secure	• Partial- or full-thickness wounds • Infected and noninfected • Skin grafts • Donor sites • Tunneling wounds • Moist red and yellow wounds • Wounds with minimal to heavy exudate

(continued)

TABLE • 32-5   EXAMPLES OF WOUND DRESSINGS/PRODUCTS *(continued)*

Type	Purposes	Use

Composites, such as:
    Alldress
    Covaderm
    StrataSorb
	• Combine two or more physically distinct products in a single dressing with several functions
	• Allow exchange of oxygen between wound and environment
	• May facilitate autolytic débridement
	• Provide physical bacterial barrier and absorptive layer
	• Semiadherent or nonadherent
	• Primary or secondary dressing
		• Partial- and full-thickness wounds
		• Wounds with minimal to heavy exudate
		• Necrotic tissue
		• Mixed (granulation and necrotic tissue) wounds
		• Infected wounds

Adapted from Benbow, M. (2008a). Exploring the concept of moist wound healing and its application in practice. *British Journal of Nursing (Tissue viability supplement, 17*(15), S4–S16; Bookout, K. (2008). Wound care product primer for the nurse practitioner: Part I. *Journal of Pediatric Health Care, 22*(1), 60–63; Hess, C. (2008). *Skin & wound care* (6th ed.). Philadelphia: Wolters Kluwer Health/Lippincott Williams & Wilkins; and Snyder, L. (2008). Wound basics: Types, treatment, and care. *RN, 71*(8), 32–37.

care is uncomfortable, administer a prescribed analgesic 30 to 45 minutes before changing the dressing. Also, plan to change the dressing midway between meals so that the patient's appetite and mealtimes are not disturbed.

Provide privacy by properly screening the patient; close the room door and curtain. Then help the patient into a position that is comfortable and also convenient for changing the dressing. Expose only the area necessary to perform the wound care while maintaining proper draping.

Using appropriate aseptic techniques when changing the dressing is crucial. Be especially vigilant in performing hand hygiene thoroughly before and after changing dressings and in adhering to Standard Precautions and Transmission-Based Precautions, when necessary. Among the most common causes of hospital-acquired infections is carelessness in practicing asepsis during dressing changes. Surgical wounds that have dehisced require the use of sterile technique. Pressure ulcers are nonsterile wounds. There is no need to use sterile dressings on these wounds, and non-sterile gloves can be used for wound care (NPUAP, 2007d).

Removing a Dressing

Remove any dressing currently in place (Hess, 2008).

• Use Standard Precautions; use appropriate Transmission-Based Precautions when indicated.
• Perform hand hygiene and put on clean (nonsterile) gloves.
• Remove tapes and dressings in the direction of hair growth to minimize trauma to the skin. Use a push–pull method; lift a corner of the dressing away from the skin, then gently push the skin away from the dressing.
• Carefully lift the adhesive barrier from the surrounding skin. If there is resistance, use a silicone-based adhesive remover, as this allows for the easy, rapid, and painless removal without the associated problems of skin stripping (Rudoni, 2008; Stephen-Haynes, 2008).
• Slowly remove the dressing, noting the amount, type, color, and odor of the drainage.

• Discard the dressing according to facility policy.
• Remove gloves and perform hand hygiene.

Cleaning the Wound

Perform wound cleaning to remove microorganisms and debris with as little chemical and mechanical force as possible and protect healthy granulation tissue. Normal saline solution (0.9% sodium chloride) is usually the agent of choice, particularly when cleaning pressure ulcer wounds. There are also commercially prepared cleansing sprays available for use.

Wounds are cleaned initially and before applying any new dressing. Guidelines for Nursing Care 32-3 outlines the techniques for cleaning a wound with approximated edges, such as a surgical incision, and for cleaning a wound with unapproximated edges, to remove cellular debris and drainage. It is also used to apply local heat or an antiseptic to an area. Wound irrigation is a directed flow of solution over tissues. Sterile equipment and solutions are required for irrigating an open wound, even in the presence of an existing infection. Sterile 0.9% sodium chloride or sterile water, an antiseptic, or an antibiotic solution may be used, depending on the condition of the wound and the primary practitioner's order. A sterile, large-volume syringe is used to direct the flow of the solution. After irrigation, open wounds may be packed with appropriate dressing materials to absorb additional drainage and allow healing by secondary intention to take place (Hess, 2008). Nonsterile solutions are generally used to clean the skin surface if the wound edges are approximated.

Applying a New Dressing

Apply a skin protectant or barrier to the healthy skin around the wound. This is particularly important if there is drainage from the wound. The skin protectant prevents skin irritation and excoriation from tape, adhesives, and wound drainage.

The nurse should be familiar with and follow the manufacturer's guidelines for the specific dressing in use.

Guidelines for Nursing Care • 32-3

CLEANING WOUNDS

Cleaning Wounds with Approximated Edges

- Use Standard Precautions; use appropriate Transmission-Based Precautions when indicated.
- Moisten a sterile gauze pad or swab with the prescribed cleansing agent.
- Use a new swab or gauze for each downward stroke.
- Clean from top to bottom.
- Work outward from the incision in lines parallel to it (Figure A).
- Wipe from the clean area toward the less clean area.

Cleaning Wounds with Unapproximated Edges

- Use Standard Precautions; use appropriate Transmission-Based Precautions when indicated.
- Moisten a sterile gauze pad or swab with the prescribed cleansing agent and squeeze out excess solution.
- Use a new swab or gauze for each circle.
- Clean the wound in full or half circles, beginning in the center and working toward the outside (Figure B).
- Clean to at least 1 inch beyond the end of the new dressing.
- If a dressing is not being applied, clean to at least 2 inches beyond the wound margins.

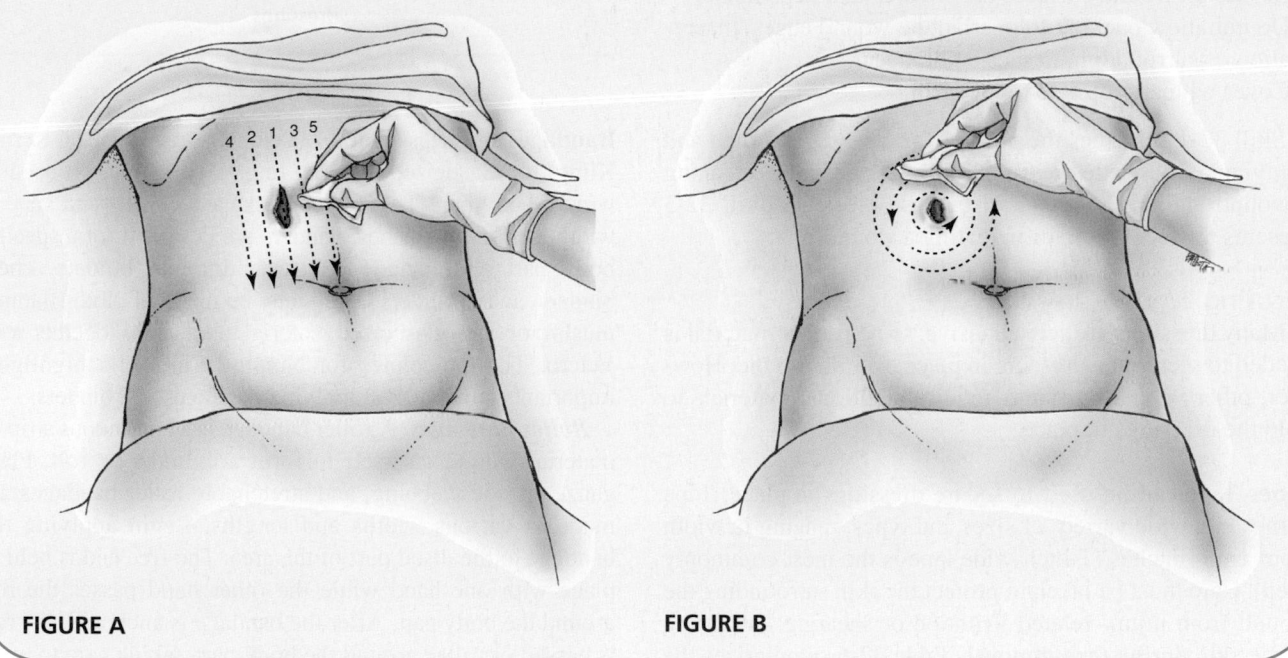

FIGURE A   **FIGURE B**

From Hess, C. (2008). *Wound care* (6th ed.). Philadelphia: Wolters Kluwer Health/Lippincott Williams & Wilkins.

General guidelines for applying a new dressing include (Hess, 2008):

- Check the wound care order or nursing care plan.
- Perform hand hygiene
- Use Standard Precautions; use appropriate Transmission-Based Precautions when indicated.
- Check the patient's identification.
- Explain what you are going to do to the patient.
- Provide privacy by closing the door to the room and pulling the bedside curtain.
- Put on gloves.
- Cleanse the wound, and periwound skin, as prescribed.
- Apply a skin barrier, such as Skin Prep®, to the areas of skin where the dressing adhesive or tape will be placed; to areas around wound where drainage may come in contact with skin.

- Gently place the dressing at the wound center and extend it at least 1 inch beyond the wound in each direction. Alternately, follow the manufacturer's directions for application.
- Remove gloves when the dressing is in place, before handling tape, if used.
- Do not apply tape under tension to prevent blisters and skin shearing.
- Perform hand hygiene.

Some wounds require packing with dressing material as part of treatment. It is important to be familiar with and follow the manufacturer's guidelines for the specific product in use. To pack a wound:

- Check the wound care order or nursing care plan.
- Perform hand hygiene

- Use Standard Precautions; use appropriate Transmission-Based Precautions when indicated.
- Check the patient's identification.
- Explain what you are going to do to the patient.
- Provide privacy by closing the door to the room and pulling the bedside curtain.
- Cleanse the wound and periwound skin, as prescribed.
- Apply a skin barrier, such as Skin Prep, to the areas of skin where the dressing adhesive or tape will be placed; to areas around wound where drainage may come in contact with skin.
- Moisten packing material, as necessary and as indicated by the manufacturer's directions or medical orders.
- Loosely pack the wound cavity just until the wound surfaces and edges are covered. If tunneling is present, pack the tunneling area first, then the base of the wound. Alternately, follow the manufacturer's directions for application.
- Ensure all wound surfaces are covered and kept moist.
- Do not allow packing to overlap the wound edges; maceration of surrounding tissues could occur.
- Cover with appropriate top dressing.

Skill 32-1 describes the process for cleaning a wound and applying a dry sterile dressing. Skill 32-2 describes cleaning a wound and applying a moist sterile dressing. Skill 32-3 presents the technique for irrigating a wound.

Securing Wound Dressings

Many dressings are self-adhesive, so no further material is needed to secure the dressing in place over the wound. However, other wound dressings require additional materials to hold the dressings in place.

Tape. Tape can be used to secure dressings in place. Tape comes in a wide variety of sizes and types, ranging in width from 1 to 4 inches (1-inch-wide tape is the most commonly used). Care must be taken to protect the skin surrounding the wound from injury-related irritation or shearing, or tearing of the skin during tape removal. Table 32-6 summarizes the types and purposes of different tapes.

Bandages and Binders. Bandages and binders are used to secure dressings, apply pressure, and support the wound.

TABLE • 32-6	TYPES OF TAPE
Type	**Purpose**
Adhesive (can cause occlusion, allergy, skin maceration, shearing)	Used for strength, support, and economy • To secure dressings and splints • To strap joints to prevent athletic injuries • To immobilize or stabilize body parts • To provide pressure • To approximate wound edges
Paper, plastic, acetate	Increased comfort, decreased allergic and skin problems • To close small wounds • To secure dressings
Microfoam	Used for compression or pressure dressings

Bandages are strips of cloth, gauze (e.g., roller gauze, Kerlix, Kling), or elasticized material (e.g., Ace bandages) used to wrap a body part. They come packaged in rolls and vary in width from 1 to 6 inches. Binders are designed for a specific body part and include slings, abdominal binders, chest binders, and T-binders. They may be made of cloth (flannel, muslin) or of an elasticized material that fastens together with Velcro. The Guidelines for Nursing Care 32-4 highlights important principles for applying bandages and binders.

Roller Bandages. A roller bandage is a continuous strip of material wound on itself to form a cylinder or roll. Plain gauze, elastic webbing, and stretchable roller bandages are made in various widths and lengths. Begin applying the bandage to the distal part of the area. The free end is held in place with one hand while the other hand passes the roll around the body part. After the bandage is anchored, the roll is passed or rolled around the body part, taking care to exert equal tension in all turns and rolling toward the heart, to avoid causing venous stasis and resulting edema. The bandage can be applied using a circular turn, spiral turn, or figure-of-eight turn (Fig. 32-7). For each technique, keep tension

Guidelines for Nursing Care • 32-4

APPLYING BANDAGES AND BINDERS

- Clean the area to be covered and dry it thoroughly before applying a bandage or binder, because prolonged heat and moisture on the skin may cause skin breakdown.
- Bandage the body part in the normal functioning position to prevent deformities and discomfort.
- Apply the bandage or binder with sufficient pressure to provide the amount of immobilization or support desired, to

remain in place, and to secure a dressing when present. Do not apply pressure to such a degree that circulation to the body part involved is impeded.

- Maintain equal tension with all bandage turns; avoid unnecessary and uneven overlapping of turns.
- After application, assess circulation and comfort at regular intervals.

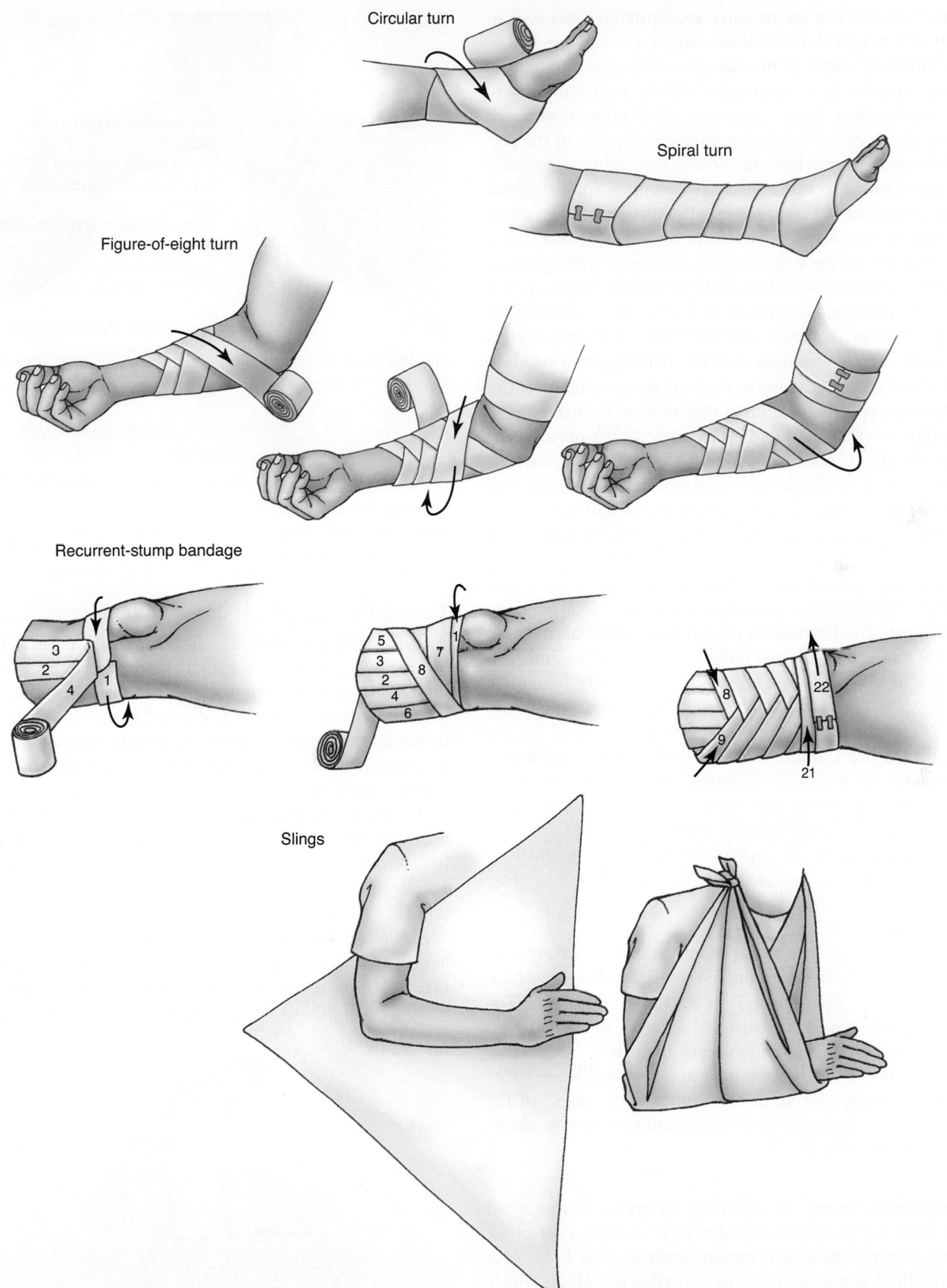

Circular turn

Spiral turn

Figure-of-eight turn

Recurrent-stump bandage

Slings

FIGURE 32-7. Techniques for applying various bandages.

equal by unwinding the bandage gradually and only with as much of a length as is required. Evenly overlap one-half to two-thirds the width of the bandage with each turn, except for the circular turn. A circular turn is used primarily to anchor a bandage. In a circular turn, the bandage is wrapped around the body part with complete overlapping of the previous bandage turn. Once the circular turn anchors the bandage, application continues, ascending in a spiral manner using a spiral turn. Each turn overlaps the preceding one by one-half or two-thirds the width of the bandage. The spiral turn is useful for the wrist, fingers, and trunk. The figure-of-eight turn consists of making oblique overlapping turns that ascend and descend alternately. It is effective for use around joints, such as the knee, elbow, ankle, and wrist. When removing a roller bandage, cut the bandage with bandage scissors to prevent excessive manipulation of the part. Cut on the side opposite the injury or the wound, from one end to the other, so that the bandage can be folded open for its entire length. If the bandage is to be reused, it may be unwound by keeping the loose end together and passing it as a ball from one hand to the other while unwinding it.

Recurrent Stump Bandage. When applying a recurrent stump bandage, a few circular turns are made to anchor the bandage, and the initial end of the bandage is placed in the center of the body part being bandaged, well back from the tip to be covered. The bandage is passed back and forth over the tip, first on the one side and then on the other side of the centerpiece of the bandage. Figure 32-7 shows how to apply a recurrent bandage to a stump, using the figure-of-eight turn to finish the bandage. Recurrent bandages are used for fingers, for the head, and for the stump of an amputated limb.

Binders. Of the many different kinds of binders, those used most commonly include straight binders, T-binders, and slings. A straight binder is a straight piece of material, usually about 15 to 20 cm (6 to 8 inches) wide and long enough to more than circle the torso. It is used for the chest and the abdomen. Straight binders may be pinned or, more commonly, fastened with Velcro.

A T-binder might be used to secure dressings on the rectum and perineum and in the groin. The single T-binder is used for female patients, the double T-binder for male patients. The belt is passed around the waist and secured, and the tails are passed between the legs and fastened to the belt.

A sling is used to support an arm. Most healthcare agencies use commercial strap slings or sleeve slings. In the home, a large piece of cloth folded into a triangle can be used as a sling (see Fig. 32-7).

Montgomery Straps. Montgomery straps use ties attached to an adhesive backing to hold dressings in place. Protect the patient's skin with a skin barrier, such as Skin Prep, or a hydrocolloid dressing, prior to applying the Montgomery straps. The adhesive backing is applied to the skin adjacent to the wound, with the ties extending over the wound area. When the dressing is changed, the strips are untied and turned back to allow for wound care. After applying the new dressing, the straps are tied over the dressing to hold it in

FIGURE 32-8. Montgomery straps make it possible to care for a wound without removing adhesive strips with each dressing change.

place (Fig. 32-8). Montgomery straps can be useful in preventing skin irritation and damage due to constant retaping with dressing changes. Montgomery straps should be changed when they become moist or soiled.

Caring for Patients with Wound Drains

A variety of drains, catheters, or tubes may be inserted into or near a wound when it is anticipated that a collection of fluid in a closed area would delay healing. After a surgical procedure, the surgeon places one end of the tube or drain in or near the area to be drained and passes the other end through the skin, either directly through the incision or through a separate opening called a stab wound. Wound drains are either open systems that drain into dressings or closed systems that drain into a suction device. Drains and tubes may or may not be sutured in place.

OPEN DRAINAGE SYSTEMS

A Penrose drain is soft and flexible. This drain does not have a collection device. It empties into absorptive dressing material. It promotes drainage passively, with the drainage

FIGURE 32-9. Penrose drain.

FIGURE 32-10. Jackson-Pratt drain.

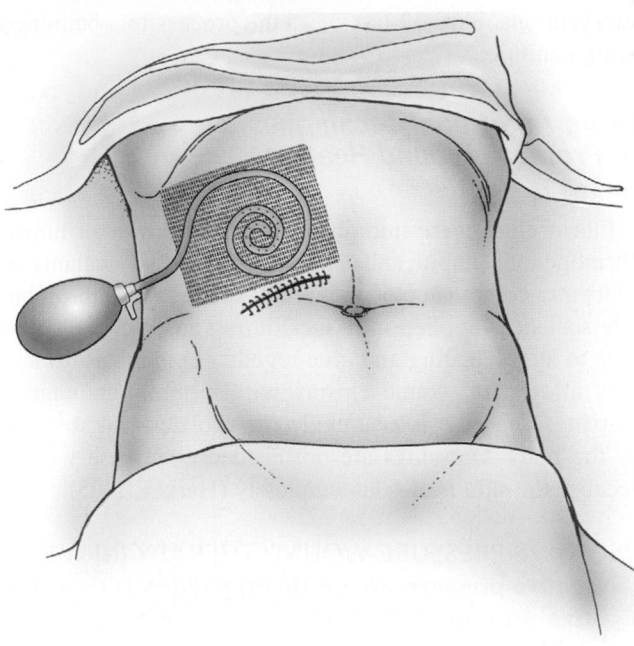

moving from the area of greater pressure, in the wound or surgical site, to the area of less pressure, the dressing. They are not sutured in place. A sterile, large safety pin is often attached to the outer portion to prevent the drain from slipping back into the incised area (Fig. 32-9). Care is necessary to ensure that these drains are not dislodged during dressing changes. Sometimes the physician orders a Penrose drain that is to be shortened each day. To do so, grasp the end of the drain with sterile forceps, pull it out a short distance while using a twisting motion, and cut off the end of the drain with sterile scissors. Place a new sterile pin at the base of the drain, as close to the skin as possible.

CLOSED DRAINAGE SYSTEMS

Closed drainage systems consist of a drainage tube that may be connected to an electrical suction device or have a portable built-in reservoir to maintain constant low suction. Examples include Jackson-Pratt drainage tubes (Fig. 32-10) and Hemovacs (Fig. 32-11). These tubes are usually sutured

to the skin. The closed drainage system prevents microorganisms from entering the wound from saturated dressings. Closed drainage systems also allow accurate measurement of drainage. Be sure to know which type of drain or tube was inserted during surgery to ensure accurate assessments and interventions. These systems must be emptied and the suction reestablished according to the directions for each device. This usually involves compressing the container while the port is open, then closing the port after the device is compressed. Skills 32-4 and 32-5 outline the procedures for caring for Jackson-Pratt and Hemovac drains. Wear gloves when emptying the drainage and do not touch the open port to avoid contaminating the port.

Collecting a Wound Culture

If assessment of the wound indicates a possible infection, it is important to culture the wound. Culturing the wound allows identification of the infecting organism(s) and appropriate

FIGURE 32-11. Hemovac drain.

interventions. Skill 32-6 reviews the process for obtaining a wound culture.

Using Additional Techniques to Promote Wound Healing

FIBRIN SEALANTS

Fibrin glues were initially mixtures of bovine or human fibrinogen, thrombin, and calcium. Newer fibrin sealants are concentrated human clottable proteins and human thrombin. The sealant is applied to tissues during an operative procedure to stop bleeding and glue together epidermal surfaces. This allows for wound closure with minimal drainage or scarring. The glue is eventually metabolized and absorbed by the body. Dressings are not needed over these wounds because the skin is closed completely (Harvey, 2005).

NEGATIVE-PRESSURE WOUND THERAPY (NPWT)

Negative-pressure wound therapy (NPWT) (or topical negative pressure [TNP]) promotes wound healing and wound closure through the application of uniform negative pressure on the wound bed, reduction in bacteria in the wound, and the removal of excess wound fluid, while providing a moist wound healing environment. The negative pressure results in mechanical tension on the wound tissues, stimulating cell proliferation, blood flow to wounds, and the growth of new blood vessels. It is used to treat a variety of acute or chronic wounds, wounds with heavy drainage, wounds failing to heal, or wounds healing slowly. Examples of such wounds include pressure ulcers; arterial, venous, and diabetic ulcers; dehisced surgical wounds; infected wounds; skin graft sites; and burns. NPWT is not considered for use in the presence of active bleeding; wounds with exposed blood vessels, organs, or nerves; malignancy in wound tissue; presence of dry/necrotic tissue; or with fistulas of unknown origin (Hess, 2008; Preston, 2008; Thompson, 2008). Cautious use is indicated in the presence of unrelieved pressure, anticoagulant therapy, poor nutritional status, and immunosuppressant therapy (Preston, 2008). Assess candidates for pre-existing bleeding disorders or the use of anticoagulants and other medications or supplements that prolong bleeding times, such as aspirin or ginkgo biloba (Malli, 2005; Preston, 2008). Skill 32-7 outlines the procedure for applying NPWT.

GROWTH FACTORS

Growth factors are naturally occurring proteins. They are applied to the wound bed, where they bind to cells to promote granulation, cell proliferation, and cell migration. They are used during the proliferative phase of wound healing in patients with chronic nonhealing wounds.

OXYGEN THERAPY

Oxygen therapy is sometimes used to facilitate repair of slowly healing wounds. It involves placing patients in a hyperbaric, pressurized chamber, where they breathe 100% oxygen. The tissues are exposed to the high-concentration oxygen environment, which promotes cell proliferation,

blood flow to wounds, and the growth of new blood vessels. The action of white blood cells is also enhanced.

HEAT AND COLD THERAPY

The application of heat or cold is sometimes used as part of the treatment of wounds. The application of heat accelerates the inflammatory response to promote healing. The local application of cold constricts peripheral blood vessels, reduces muscle spasms, and promotes comfort. The use of these therapies is discussed later in the chapter.

OTHER TREATMENT OPTIONS FOR PRESSURE ULCERS

When other treatment options have failed, surgery may be considered. Surgical procedures may include direct closure of the wound, skin grafting, or various skin flap procedures. The decision is based on the patient's condition and the severity of the ulcer. After surgery, vigilantly protect the surgical site from pressure and contamination.

Several other treatment modalities are being investigated. They include electrical stimulation, laser irradiation, ultrasound, and miscellaneous topical agents and systemic drugs.

Removing Sutures or Staples

Sutures are removed when the wound has developed enough tensile strength to hold the wound edges together during healing. This stage varies from patient to patient, depending on age, nutritional status, and wound location. Silk sutures typically are removed within 6 to 8 days to prevent suture marks, even though collagen formation and remodeling take a total of at least 21 days. This means the scar may still stretch and widen after the silk sutures have been removed. Special subcutaneous techniques have been developed to minimize this problem.

Sutures are removed with a suture removal set; staples are removed with a special staple remover. The steps in removing sutures and staples are summarized in the accompanying Guidelines for Nursing Care 32-5. After the removal of skin sutures small adhesive wound-closure strips, that look something like tape, are sometimes applied across the healing wound to help hold it together and give additional support as it continues to heal (Fig. 32-12). Unless otherwise directed, these adhesive strips are not removed during wound care.

Teaching Wound Care at Home

GENERAL GUIDELINES

With the increase in ambulatory surgery and earlier discharge of patients from inpatient settings to home care, teaching patients and their families about wound care is important. Although a nurse may be needed to change dressings and provide wound care in complex situations, family members often are taught how to perform the procedure. To provide the continuity of care that is necessary to prevent infection and promote healing, be sure to include teaching about wound care as part of discharge planning and in interactions with home care patients and families. A summary of

Guidelines for Nursing Care • 32-5

REMOVING STAPLES AND SUTURES

The removal of staples or sutures may be done by the physician or by the nurse with a physician's order. Always follow agency protocol; keep in mind these general guidelines:

- Use sterile techniques, following recommended CDC guidelines for care of wounds.

- Perform hand hygiene before and after the procedure.

- Explain the procedure to the patient. Describe the sensation that will be experienced as a pulling or slightly uncomfortable experience.

- Use proper technique to remove and dispose of old dressings.

- Clean the incision from the center of the wound outward, according to agency policy and procedure for type of agent.

- Remove every other suture or staple to be sure wound edges are healed; if they are, remove remaining sutures or staples as ordered.

- Remove or reapply dressing, depending on physician preference and agency policy.

- Remember that some physicians order Steri-Strip application to the healed wound after removal of staples or sutures to give additional support to the wound as it continues to heal. Follow agency protocol and physician preference for placement of these tapes.

Specifics for Suture Removal

1. Use a sterile suture removal kit.

2. Using the sterile forceps, grasp the knot of the first suture and gently lift the knot.

3. Using the sterile scissors, cut one side of the suture below the knot close to the skin (Figure A).

4. Grasp the knot with the forceps and pull the cut suture through the skin (be sure to pull through the healed wound only the portion of the suture that has been inside the tissue).

Specifics for Staple Removal

1. As directed on the package, gently position the sterile staple remover under the staple to be removed.

2. Firmly close the staple remover to straighten the staple ends (do not lift upward while disengaging staple ends) (Figure B).

3. Carefully lift upward with the closed staple remover to remove the staple from the incision line. It may be necessary to remove one end of the staple and then the other if it does not easily lift out.

FIGURE A. Removing sutures.

FIGURE B. Removing staples.

teaching content is outlined in Teaching Tips 32-1: Wound Care and Healing.

PRESSURE ULCER PREVENTION AND CARE

Teaching patients and caregivers how to prevent pressure ulcers requires a comprehensive, organized educational effort. Initially, the healthcare provider presents basic information that explains the terminology, identifies risk factors, explains where and how pressure ulcers develop, and describes various prevention strategies and options. Illustrated instructions written at the level of the learner are a valuable resource. The protocols listed in the Guidelines for Nursing Care boxes serve as a model for development of a teaching plan that incorporates basic principles and targets individuals at risk. As new information becomes available, education for prevention of pressure ulcers requires updating.

FIGURE 32-12. Applying Steri-Strips on an incision.

Involve the patient and caregivers in the plan of care and provide them with a good understanding about causative factors for the pressure ulcer. Instruct them in proper hand hygiene techniques and how to identify the signs and symptoms of infection. Provide the patient and caregivers with simple, easy-to-read instructions. Encourage frequent consultation with the primary healthcare provider about the progress of wound healing and products used. In addition, ensure that the patient, family, or caregivers understand the need for adequate nutrition to aid in wound healing. Assess the patient's nutritional status and suggest consultation with a dietitian for dietary deficiencies, if necessary.

If dressing changes or wound care is painful, teach the patient to use pain medication as prescribed 30 to 60 minutes before the procedure. Reinforce the importance of hand hygiene before and after the dressing change.

Documenting Wound Care

Documentation related to wound care is an important nursing responsibility. Clear and accurate documentation is essential for communication of wound status and tracking of the progression of healing (Hess, 2008). Precise documentation contributes to continuity of care, accurate evaluation of care, and appropriate changes in wound care, if necessary. Use a skin and wound assessment tool to accurately record assessment findings and treatment interventions. Figure 32-13 shows an example of a paper skin and wound assessment/documentation tool and Figure 32-14 shows an example of a computer documentation tool.

Evaluating

Evaluation of wound and pressure ulcer care involves reassessment at regular intervals to monitor response to the treatment, determine the effectiveness of the treatment, and allow for necessary changes in the plan of care. The plan of care for the patient with a wound is evaluated based on the expected outcomes. Evaluation is ongoing throughout the care of the patient, with the plan being effective if no complications have occurred during wound healing, wound is progressing through the healing stages, and the patient or family has the knowledge and skill necessary for wound care at home, if appropriate.

Tips

TEACHING TIPS · 32-1

WOUND CARE AND HEALING

Health Topic	Suggested Content
Supplies	• Methods for obtaining dressing supplies such as purchasing from pharmacies, drug stores, discount stores, and medical supply stores • Considerations for costs and ease of use • Investigation about reimbursement by insurance company or other source of healthcare financing for supplies
Infection prevention	• Signs and symptoms of infection to be immediately reported to the healthcare provider • Need to watch for increased body temperature, red or separated wound edges, increased pain in the wound, and increased drainage that is thick and has a foul odor • Wearing of disposable gloves when changing the dressing • Hand hygiene before putting on and after removing the gloves • Proper methods for disposal of old dressing, such as wrapping old dressing in several layers of newspaper or putting it in a plastic bag before disposal in a trash container
Wound healing	• Importance of eating well-balanced meals that are high in protein and vitamins • Need to drink 6 to 8 glasses of fluids each day • Rest periods during the day • Modifications in activities of daily living and exercise until healing is complete and approval is given by healthcare provider

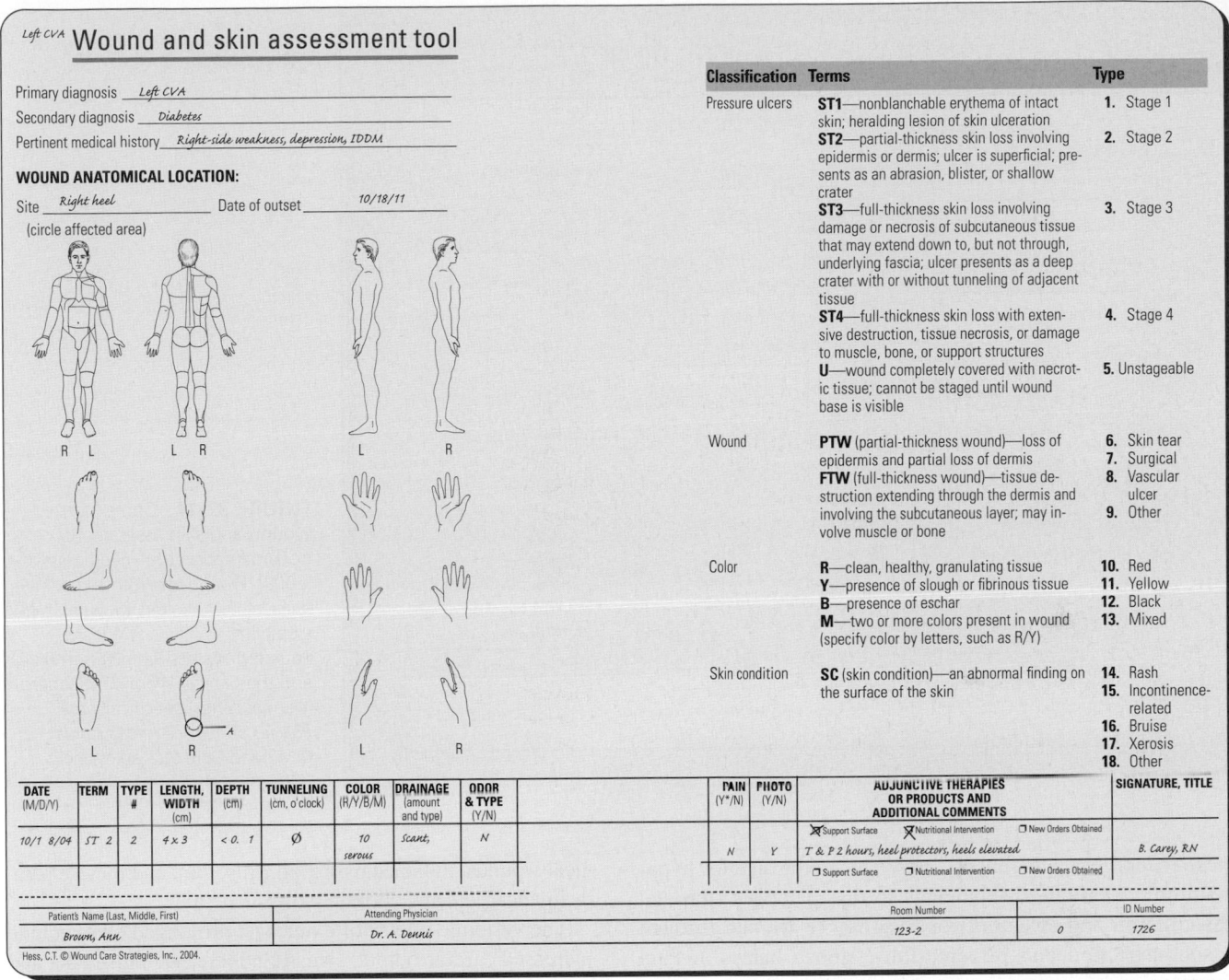

FIGURE 32-13. Wound and skin assessment/documentation tool. (From Hess, C. [2008]. *Wound care* [6th ed.; pp. 110–111]. Philadelphia: Wolters Kluwer Health/Lippincott Williams & Wilkins.)

When evaluating the effectiveness of a plan of care designed to prevent the development of pressure ulcers or treat pressure ulcers or other wounds already present, the nurse uses each nurse–patient interaction to determine if the patient has met the individualized expected outcomes in the plan of care. Nursing care is considered effective if the patient, family member, or caregiver expresses satisfaction with prevention and treatment measures and is able to accomplish the following:

- Participate effectively in preventive and treatment regimens
- Prevent development of any additional areas of skin breakdown
- Demonstrate progressive healing of pressure ulcer or other wound
- Improve overall physical condition (including nutritional state and mobility status)
- Remain free of infection at any pressure ulcer or other wound site
- Communicate the need for additional support (environmental, physical, psychosocial)

Evaluation is a continuous process that involves ongoing assessment and revised plans and implementations. Color photographs are an excellent method of evaluating the progression of wound healing, allowing visual comparison of the wound at the initial assessment and throughout the plan of care through the recovery stages.

HEAT AND COLD THERAPY

Heat and cold are applied to a specific part or all of a patient's body to bring about a local or systemic change in body temperature for various therapeutic purposes. Physiologic responses to heat and cold are modified by the method and duration of application, the degree of heat and cold applied, the patient's age and physical condition, and the amount of body surface covered by the application. Nurses use heat and cold as nursing interventions in both hospital- and community-based settings.

Body temperature is regulated by cells in the hypothalamus in response to signals from thermal (heat and cold) receptors located close to the skin's surface. Stimulation of

FIGURE 32-14. Computerized wound and skin assessment/documentation tool. (From Hess, C. [2008]. *Wound care* [6th ed.; p. 109]. Philadelphia: Wolters Kluwer Health/Lippincott Williams & Wilkins. Source: TriAssess Premier Software and the *Clinical Wound Manager Manual Series,* specifically the *Policies and Procedures Manual.* © Wound Care Strategies, Inc., 2003.)

these receptors sends sensory messages to the anterior hypothalamus to initiate mechanisms to dissipate heat (through vasodilation and sweating) or to preserve warmth through vasoconstriction and piloerection ("goose bumps"). Pain receptors, also located near the skin's surface, are also affected by heat and cold as painful stimuli, with excessive heat perceived as burning and excessive cold experienced as numbness followed by pain.

Effects of Applying Heat

The application of local heat dilates peripheral blood vessels, increases tissue metabolism, reduces blood viscosity and increases capillary permeability, reduces muscle tension, and helps relieve pain. Vasodilation increases local blood flow. In turn, the supply of oxygen and nutrients to the area is increased, and venous congestion is decreased. As local blood flow increases, the viscosity of blood is reduced and increased capillary permeability improves the delivery of leukocytes and nutrients while also facilitating the removal of wastes and prolonging clotting time. These actions, combined with increased tissue metabolism, accelerate the inflammatory response to promote healing.

Heat reduces muscle tension to promote relaxation and helps to relieve muscle spasms and joint stiffness. Heat also helps relieve pain by stimulating specific nerve fibers, closing the gate that allows the transmission of pain stimuli to centers in the brain. Because of these local physiologic effects, heat in various forms is used to treat infections, sur-

gical wounds, inflamed tissue, arthritis, joint and muscle pain, dysmenorrhea, and chronic pain.

The systemic effects of extensive, prolonged heat include increased cardiac output, sweating, increased pulse rate, and decreased blood pressure. This response occurs when heat is applied to a large body area, increasing the blood flow to that area while decreasing it to another part of the body, in effect, causing hypovolemic shock.

Effects of Applying Cold

The local application of cold constricts peripheral blood vessels, reduces muscle spasms, and promotes comfort. Cold reduces blood flow to tissues and decreases the local release of pain-producing substances such as histamine, serotonin, and bradykinin. This action in turn reduces the formation of edema and inflammation. Decreased metabolic needs and capillary permeability, combined with increased coagulation of blood at the wound site, facilitate the control of bleeding and reduce edema formation.

Cold also reduces muscle spasm, alters tissue sensitivity (producing numbness), and promotes comfort by slowing the transmission of pain stimuli. Cold, for these effects, is used after direct trauma, for dental pain, for muscle spasms, after sprains, and to treat some chronic pain syndromes.

Exposure to prolonged or extensive environmental cold produces systemic effects of increased blood pressure, shivering, and goose bumps. Although shivering is a normal body response to cold, prolonged cold may cause tissue injury.

Physiologic Considerations

The rebound phenomenon is important to the therapeutic value of heat and cold and to the safety of patients receiving such therapy. Heat produces maximum vasodilation in 20 to 30 minutes; if heat is continued beyond that time, tissue congestion and vasoconstriction occurs (for unknown reasons). With cold, maximum vasoconstriction occurs when the skin reaches 15°C (60°F); then vasodilation begins.

The ability of the body to adapt to heat and cold is an important consideration when applying heat or cold and when teaching patients and caregivers about heat and cold therapy. Initially, heat and cold skin receptors are stimulated strongly by sudden changes in temperature. For the first few seconds after being stimulated, the response decreases rapidly; it then decreases more slowly for the next 30 minutes, as the receptors adapt to the temperature. A hot application, even if the temperature remains constant, does not feel as warm after adaptation has taken place. Be sure to inform patients that increasing the temperature or lengthening the time of application can seriously damage tissues.

THE NURSING PROCESS FOR HEAT AND COLD THERAPY
Assessing

Before initiating heat or cold therapy, assess the patient's physical and mental status, the condition of the body area to be treated with heat or cold, and the condition of the equipment to be used. Carefully evaluate factors influencing the patient's ability to tolerate heat and cold applications. These factors are the basis for the following considerations:

- How long will the heat or cold be applied? Prolonged exposure increases tolerance, and rebound effects are undesirable.
- What body part is involved? Some body areas, such as the neck, perineum, and inner aspects of the wrist and forearm, are more sensitive to thermal changes.
- Is the skin intact? Open tissue or abraded skin is more sensitive to thermal changes.
- How large is the area? Applications of heat or cold to large areas of the body cause systemic responses and lower tolerance of temperature change.
- What is the patient's age? Infants, children, and older adults do not tolerate temperature changes as well as adults.
- What is the patient's physical condition? Patients with certain alterations in health, such as those with cardiovascular or peripheral vascular diseases, might have reduced response to or tolerance of thermal changes.

Assessing Overall Status

Assessing the patient's overall status includes obtaining a health history and completing a physical examination. A history of cardiovascular or peripheral vascular impairment, sensory impairment, and alterations in mental status, such as confusion or decreased level of consciousness, indicates the

need for caution when using heat or cold because of the danger of tissue damage. Assessments include response to stimuli (sharp and dull), color and appearance of body tissues, circulation (pulses, blanching sign, temperature, color), level of consciousness, and orientation.

> ➤ *Consider Mr. Everly, the postoperative patient in the critical care unit. Imagine that the physician had ordered heat or cold applications for this patient. The nurse would need to obtain a thorough assessment of his physical status when planning this care because his history of diabetes and circulation problems, in conjunction with his decreased level of consciousness, would place him at high risk for injury and tissue damage. In addition, the nurse would need to assess him frequently during the application of heat or cold to ensure his safety.* ∎

Do not apply heat to an open wound immediately after the trauma; during hemorrhage; over noninflammatory edema; to an acutely inflamed area, a localized malignant tumor, the testes, or the abdomen of a pregnant woman; or over metallic implants. Conversely, do not use cold for open wounds or for patients with impaired peripheral circulation or allergy to cold.

Assessing the Area of Application

Perform baseline assessments to ensure safety and to evaluate the outcomes of therapy. The risk for damage to tissues is increased if the area is traumatized or has altered integrity. Assess for open lesions, blisters, wounds, edema, bleeding, or drainage or evidence of altered circulation such as changes in color, temperature, pulses, and sensation. As with any assessment, compare body parts bilaterally for changes. Tissues with decreased or absent pulses, those that appear pale or cyanotic, and those that feel cold to the touch indicate a decrease in circulation. Subsequently, the risk for injury from heat and cold applications increases.

When the heat or cold is applied, make ongoing assessments to ensure patient safety and comfort. When heat is applied, assess the patient for undesired responses, including localized redness, blistering, and pain (symptoms of burning), along with possible systemic responses, such as hypotension and changes in consciousness. When cold is applied, assess for localized responses, including pallor, cyanosis, numbness, and pain.

Assessing the Condition of Equipment

The nurse is responsible for checking the equipment used and for maintaining patient safety. Included in this responsibility is checking the condition of cords, plugs, and heating or cooling elements. In addition, inspect the equipment for fluid leaks. Also, check to ensure that the equipment distributes and maintains the constant temperature. Do not use faulty equipment; if faulty equipment is found, it should be returned for repair.

Diagnosing

The patient's need for and response to the heat or cold suggest possible nursing diagnoses, including the following:

- Ineffective Thermoregulation
- Ineffective Tissue Perfusion
- Acute Pain
- Chronic Pain
- Risk for Injury
- Risk for Trauma

Outcome Identification and Planning

Heat and cold are used for a variety of therapeutic purposes that are an essential part of planning individualized care and forming the basis for patient outcomes. When applications of heat or cold are part of a plan of care, the following outcomes are appropriate; specific outcomes should be chosen based on the purpose of the application. The patient will:

- Verbalize increased comfort
- Demonstrate evidence of wound healing, decreased muscle spasms, decreased edema, and increased comfort
- Verbalize and demonstrate safe hot or cold application

Implementing

Heat and cold applications may be moist or dry, using many forms and methods. The prescription for the heat and cold application should include the type of application, the body area to be treated, and the frequency and length of time for the applications.

Explain to the patient the purpose and steps of the application and the sensations that will be experienced. In the hospital, provide a timer or clock and have the call bell within reach. In the home, teach the patient or family member to check the equipment each time to ensure that it is in good working order, avoid lying or leaning on the equipment, cover the heating device with a protective cloth, apply heat only for the prescribed time period, and report any changes in sensation or discomfort to the healthcare provider.

Applying Heat

Heat is applied by both dry and moist methods. Hot water bags, electric heating pads, aquathermia pads, or chemical heat packs provide local dry heat by conduction. Hot compresses or packs, sitz baths, or soaks provide moist heat by conduction.

DRY HEAT
Hot Water Bags

Hot water bags are a method of dry heat application. Although relatively easy and inexpensive to use, they have disadvantages. They may leak, and often the weight of the bag or bottle on the patient's body part can be uncomfortable. Moreover, there is a danger of burns from improper use.

Electric Heating Pads

An electric heating pad can be used to apply dry heat locally. It is easy to apply, is relatively safe to use, and provides constant and even heat. Improper use can, however,

result in injury. When applying a heating pad, follow these recommendations:

- Avoid using pins to secure a heating pad. There is a danger of electric shock if a pin touches a wire.
- Place a covering over the pad, preferably one that is moisture proof. Also, prevent wet and moist conditions around the pad. Short-circuiting the heating element may cause an electric shock. Do not cover the heating pad with anything that might be heavy; heat may accumulate and burn the patient when it cannot dissipate normally from the pad.
- Place a heating pad anteriorly or laterally to, not under, the body part. If the heating pad is between the patient and the mattress, heat dissipation may be inadequate, leading to burning of the patient or the bed linens.
- Use a heating pad with a selector switch that cannot be turned up beyond a safe temperature. After heat has been applied and a certain amount of adaptation of heat receptors takes place, the patient often increases the heat when the switch is not permanently preset because the pad does not seem sufficiently warm. Many people have been burned by turning up the heat in an electric pad because they thought the pad was too cool.
- Assess the skin at regular intervals for the effects of excessive exposure to heat such as increased skin redness, changes in sensation, or discomfort.
- Check agency protocol for the use of heating pads; a release form may need to be signed.

Aquathermia Pads

Aquathermia (Aqua-K) pads are commonly used in healthcare agencies and homes for various health problems, including back pain, muscle spasms, thrombophlebitis, and mild inflammation. These devices are safer to use than a heating pad, but they too must be checked carefully. Guidelines for using an aquathermia pad are given in Skill 32-8.

Hot Packs

Commercial hot packs provide a specified amount of dry heat for a specific period. Instructions on the package describe how to activate the pack, either by striking it on a firm surface or by squeezing or kneading it. Follow the same precautions as for other types of dry heat applications.

MOIST HEAT
Warm Moist Compresses

Warm moist compresses are used to promote circulation and healing and to reduce edema. Because moist heat evaporates and cools rapidly, change these compresses frequently and cover them with a heating agent (hot water bottle, heating pad, Aqua-K pad). Skill 32-9 describes the application of warm compresses.

Sitz Baths

Sitz baths are a method of applying tepid or warm water to the pelvic or rectal area by sitting in a tub, special chair, or basin filled with sufficient water to reach the umbilicus.

Guidelines for Nursing Care • 32-6

ASSISTING WITH A SITZ BATH

- Test the water in a sitz bath with a thermometer before the patient enters the water.
- If the purpose of the sitz bath is to apply heat, use water at a temperature of 34° to 37°C (93° to 99°F) for 15 minutes to produce relaxation of the parts involved after a short initial period of contraction. Do not use warm water if considerable congestion is already present.
- If the purpose of the sitz bath is to produce relaxation or to promote healing in a wound by cleansing it of discharge and debris, use water at a temperature of 34° to 37°C (93° to 99°F). Check agency protocols for the correct temperature.
- Assist the patient into the tub or onto the sitz bath and position properly. The patient should be able to sit in the basin or tub with the feet flat on the floor without any pressure on the sacrum or thighs.

- Wrap a blanket around the shoulders to protect from chilling and exposure.
- Monitor the patient closely for signs of weakness and fatigue, and discontinue the bath if faintness, pallor, a rapid pulse rate, or nausea is noted.
- Test the water in the tub several times, and keep it at the desired temperature. Additional hot water may be added by pouring it slowly from a pitcher or by opening the hot water faucet slightly. Agitate the water by stirring it as the hot water is added to prevent burning the patient.
- Do not leave the patient alone if there are any questions about safety.
- Help the patient out of the tub when the bath is completed. A sitz bath should take 15 to 20 minutes. Help the patient dry, and cover him or her adequately.

Special basins that fit onto the toilet seat are available. They are designed so that the patient's buttocks fit into a rather deep seat that is filled with water of the desired temperature; the legs and feet remain out of the water. The basins are disposable and economical for home or healthcare agency use. A regular bathtub is not as satisfactory for a sitz bath because the heat causes generalized vasodilation, altering the effect desired. Techniques for administering a sitz bath are given in Guidelines for Nursing Care 32-6.

Warm Soaks

The immersion of a body area into warm water or a medicated solution is called a soak. The purposes of soaks vary: to increase blood supply to a locally infected area; to aid in cleaning large, sloughing wounds, such as burns; to improve circulation; and to apply medication to a locally infected area. A soak has the added advantage of making manipulation of a painful area much easier because the body part is buoyed by the weight of water it displaces. If a warm soak is ordered, follow these general guidelines:

- If a soak is prescribed for a large wound (e.g., an entire arm or lower leg or even an area of the torso), expect to adapt sterile technique. For example, sterilize the container into which the body area is placed before use if possible; if not, clean the container scrupulously. Tap water may be used for soaks because it is accepted as being free from pathogens.
- Unless the temperature of the soak is prescribed otherwise, set the temperature of the water within a range of 105°F to 109°F (40.5°C to 43°C), which is considered to be physiologically effective and comfortable for the patient.
- Position the container holding the fluid so that the part to be immersed is comfortable and the patient is in good body alignment.

- During the treatment, which usually takes 15 to 20 minutes per soak, maintain the temperature of the soak as constant as possible. This may be done by discarding some of the fluid every 5 minutes and replacing it or by adding solutions at a higher temperature while agitating the water. When replacing or adding fluids, have the patient remove the extremity from the soak.

Applying Cold

Cold is applied by both dry and moist methods. Dry cold is provided with ice bags, cold packs, or a hypothermia blanket (or pad). Cold compresses are a method of applying moist cold.

DRY COLD
Ice Bags

Ice bags, like their counterpart hot water bottles or bags, are relatively easy and inexpensive methods for applying cold to an area. They have essentially the same disadvantages as hot water bags. When using an ice bag, follow these recommendations:

- Fill the bag with small pieces of ice to about two-thirds full. This makes the bag light in weight. Using ice chips, rather than cubes, makes it easier to mold the bag to the body part.
- Remove air from the ice bag in the same manner as removing air from a hot water bag.
- After securing the cap, test the ice bag for leaks and wipe off excess moisture.
- Place a cover on the ice bag to provide comfort and to absorb moisture that may accumulate on the outside of the bag.

- Apply an ice bag for 30 minutes and then remove it for about an hour before reapplying it. This technique prevents the effects of prolonged exposure to cold.
- In the home setting, a bag of frozen vegetables (such as peas) makes a good substitute for an ice bag.

Cold Packs

Commercially prepared ice packs are available in many healthcare agencies and may be purchased commercially. These bags are sealed containers filled with a chemical or a nontoxic substance. Depending on the type, the bags are frozen in the freezer or (if not frozen) are squeezed to activate the chemical that produces the cold. These packs are advantageous because the frozen solution remains pliable and can be easily molded to fit the body part. They are covered with a ribbed cotton sleeve so that the bag can be slipped onto an extremity, or the bag can simply be placed on a body part, such as the head. Assess the skin beneath the pack periodically for symptoms of numbness and pain.

MOIST COLD

Moist, cold local applications are called cold compresses. They might be used for an injured eye, a headache, a tooth extraction, and sometimes for hemorrhoids. The texture and thickness of the material used depend on the area to which it is applied. For example, eye compresses could be prepared from surgical gauze compresses, which have a small amount of cotton filling. A washcloth makes an excellent compress for the head or face.

Immerse the material used for the application in a clean basin that contains pieces of ice and a small amount of water. Wring the compress thoroughly before applying it to avoid dripping. Dripping is uncomfortable for the patient and may result in wetting the patient's clothing or bed linens. Change the compress frequently, continuing the application for 20 minutes. Repeat the application every 2 to 3 hours as ordered. Ice bags or commercial devices are available for keeping the compresses cold, helping to decrease the frequency with which they must be changed.

Evaluating

The expected outcomes for applying heat and cold when included as part of a plan of care are used to evaluate the effectiveness of the planned interventions. Although the specific outcomes depend on the purpose of the application, nursing care is considered effective if the patient is able to:

- Verbalize increased comfort
- Verbalize increased ability to rest and sleep
- Demonstrate evidence of wound healing
- Demonstrate a decrease in symptoms of muscle spasms, inflammation, and edema
- Verbalize and demonstrate safe hot and cold applications

Ongoing evaluation of skin integrity is needed to determine needs and the effectiveness of any interventions, including heat and cold therapy. (See the accompanying concept map for Lucius Everly and the Nursing Plan of Care 32-1 for Mary Biesicker.)

NURSING PLAN OF CARE · 32-1

for Mary Biesicker

Mary Biesicker, who is 84 years of age, has been cared for at home by her daughter since being hospitalized last year for a stroke. During the past several months, Mary has been confined to her bed, has had minimal appetite, and has occasionally been confused and disoriented. During the past week, she has had several episodes of bowel and bladder incontinence. Her daughter also reports that Mary has developed a "blister on her lower back at the end of her backbone." She is scheduled for an assessment visit by the nurse from a local home care agency because her daughter is finding it increasingly difficult to care for her mother alone.

The nurse's initial assessment of Mary, relative to skin integrity, revealed the following:

Skin status: Presence of a nickel-sized open area on the sacrum (stage II pressure ulcer), 2 cm in diameter and 1 cm in depth. No abnormal pathways noted. Reddened area (0.5 cm) surrounding lesion. No drainage noted. Reddened area (2.5 cm) also noted on right elbow. Skin dry over all body surfaces.

Nutritional status: Daughter states, "usual weight is 115 to 120 lb, and she has definitely lost some weight." Poor skin turgor.

Elimination status: Wearing "adult diaper," diaper damp with urine and small amount of light brown liquid stool.

Activity status: Lying quietly in bed, moans when area around lesion is palpated.

NURSING DIAGNOSIS	Impaired Skin Integrity related to mechanical factors, inactivity, altered nutritional intake, and incontinence as manifested by stage II pressure ulcer on sacral area and reddened area on right elbow
EXPECTED OUTCOME	6/6/12—at weekly visit, the patient will:

- Experience reduction of pressure on bony prominences (absence of any additional reddened areas)

(continued)

NURSING PLAN OF CARE · 32-1

for Mary Biesicker (continued)

Nursing Interventions	Rationale	Evaluative Statement
Assess skin for development of any pressure areas (use agency tool).	Pressure results in poor circulation that causes skin breakdown.	6/13/12 Outcome met. Patient has been turned from side to side every 2 hours. Reddened area on right elbow measures 1.25 cm in diameter. No new reddened areas observed. *Recommendation:* Arrange for delivery of hospital bed with overbed trapeze setup. Secure a home health aide for limited period of time to assist with repositioning during the night and allow daughter time to rest.
Avoid sitting or lying on a pressure ulcer.	This facilitates pressure relief in the area and allows blood to reenter capillaries and provide oxygen to the area.	
Reposition from side to side at least every 2 hours.	The duration of pressure is more devastating to skin than the amount of pressure.	
Use pillows to maintain side-lying or oblique position in bed and support right elbow off bed surface.	Pillows relieve pressure on lesion and areas at risk and promote improved circulation to those areas.	*M. Lieb, RN*
Place foam overlay mattress on bed.	Static device provides support and relieves pressure on skin surface.	

EXPECTED OUTCOME   6/6/12—at weekly visit, the patient will:

- Demonstrate a reduction in the size of the stage II pressure ulcer on sacrum

Nursing Interventions	Rationale	Evaluative Statement
Assess condition of pressure ulcer at time of dressing change (refer to previous assessments).	Signs of infection and deterioration can be recognized and treatment plan revised.	6/13/12 Outcome met. Pressure ulcer has decreased slightly in size— 1.7 cm in diameter, depth remains the same. No apparent infection noted. Will continue with present treatment regimen.
Irrigate wound with normal saline using a 60-mL piston syringe with a catheter tip.	Normal saline cleanses the wound without harming tissues.	
Dry skin thoroughly surrounding the ulcer.	Moisture makes intact skin more susceptible to injury.	*M. Lieb, RN*
Apply moisture-retentive dressing (Tegasorb).	Moisture-retentive dressings create a healing environment by allowing epithelial cells to bridge the wound gap and close it.	
Use clean technique for the dressing change.	In the home, the risk is minimal for cross-contamination of microorganisms.	

(continued)

NURSING PLAN OF CARE • 32-1

for Mary Biesicker (continued)

EXPECTED OUTCOME 6/6/12—at weekly visit, the patient/caregiver will:

• Demonstrate skills required to promote skin integrity and care for a pressure ulcer

Nursing Interventions	Rationale	Evaluative Statement
Assess caregiver's (daughter) motivation and ability to manage treatment regimen.	Motivation influences readiness to learn and contributes to positive learning outcomes.	6/13/12 Outcome partially met. Daughter able to recognize appearance of pressure areas on skin. Stated she would like to review treatment routine again. Daughter performed assessment and dressing change satisfactorily with nurse in attendance. Clarified and reviewed written instructions again. Daughter states, "I feel much more confident now." *M. Lieb, RN*
Instruct daughter about causes, skin assessment techniques, and individualized treatment regimen. Provide written instructions and illustrations when possible.	A clear concise teaching guide provides consistent education and is available for reinforcement.	
Provide information about community resources available for assistance with care of mother.	Resources provide opportunity for support and problem solving.	

SAMPLE DOCUMENTATION

6/20/12 Home care visit (nursing)
Mrs. Biesicker was revisited in her home for continued assessment and treatment of pressure ulcer. Nursing diagnosis: Impaired Skin Integrity related to pressure, inactivity, inadequate nutritional intake, and incontinence. According to daughter, patient was turned and repositioned every 2 hours. Foam mattress and pillow supports used for support and pressure reduction. Dressing on pressure ulcer changed. Wound cleansed with normal saline, intact skin surrounding wound, and Tegasorb dressing applied. Granulation tissue noted in wound bed, no evidence of drainage or reddened area around wound. Ulcer has decreased to 1½ cm in size. Reddened area not apparent on right elbow. Reviewed written instructions with daughter for 6/23/12 to discuss healthcare options. Will continue current plan of care and visits every other day.

M. Lieb, RN

Lucius Everly, who has a history of diabetes and circulatory problems, underwent abdominal surgery several days ago and is now in the critical care unit. When you enter, he is slouched down in bed. Assessment reveals that his abdominal dressing is moist, and only part of the tape securing the dressing is adhering to the skin. His level of consciousness is decreased, and he responds only to moderate touch and pain. With repositioning, he moans. Further assessment reveals the beginning of a pressure ulcer on his heel. He is NPO and has a central intravenous catheter in place for administration of total parenteral nutrition (TPN). An indwelling catheter is in place to accurately measure intake and output. He is currently afebrile but has been prescribed antibiotics prophylactically.

Priority 1

Risk for Infection related to surgical incision and invasive therapy
Supporting Data:
• Abdominal surgical incision with moist dressing
• Pressure ulcer on heel
• Weakened defenses from chronic illness, such as diabetes and circulatory problems
• Central venous catheter
• Indwelling urinary catheter
• Afebrile
• IV antibiotics prescribed

Outcome:
Patient will remain afebrile with absence of redness or purulent drainage at surgical site. Urine will remain clear.

Nursing Interventions:
• Maintain aseptic technique with dressing change, parenteral therapy, and indwelling urinary catheter
• Use proper handwashing technique
• Dispose of soiled dressings appropriately
• Change dressing as needed
• Note appearance of pressure ulcer, incision, and IV insertion sites
• Monitor characteristics of urine
• Monitor temperature every 4 hours

Evaluation: Lucius is afebrile. His urine is clear. No drainage is noted from pressure ulcer. His surgical incision is draining serosanguineous material. Continue interventions.

Priority 2

Impaired Skin Integrity related to surgical incision and parenteral therapy
Supporting Data:
• Abdominal surgical incision
• Moist dressings, loosely secured
• History of factors impeding healing (diabetes and circulatory problems)
• Central venous catheter
• NPO receiving TPN

Outcome: Patient will demonstrate signs of a healing incision, absence of skin irritation, absence of IV infiltration, and will maintain optimal nutrition

Nursing Interventions:
• Change abdominal dressing daily and as needed to prevent saturated dressings
• Inspect surgical incision for signs of healing
• Cleanse surgical incision
• Use Montgomery straps to secure dressing and prevent skin irritation from tape
• Use transparent dressing to cover central venous catheter insertion site to allow inspection of insertion site
• Inspect insertion site frequently and administer TPN as prescribed to meet nutritional needs and promote healing

Evaluation: Surgical dressings have been changed as needed to minimize moisture against skin. Pink granulation tissue is noted at the surgical incision. Nutrition has been maintained as noted by stable weight and a prealbumen level within normal limits. Parenteral therapy maintained without signs of infiltration.

Priority 3

Impaired Tissue Integrity related to altered mobility and chronic illness
Supporting Data:
• Decreased level of consciousness
• Unable to turn independently
• Pressure ulcer on heel
• History of circulatory problems and diabetes

Outcome:
Patient will demonstrate signs of healing in pressure ulcer on heel; no further skin breakdown will occur.

Nursing Interventions:
• Inspect skin, noting areas that are reddened
• Use Braden scale to assess risk for pressure ulcer
• Turn and reposition patient at least every 2 hours, using padded devices
• Use linen to assist in position change to decrease shearing force
• Apply heel protectors
• Avoid pressure on heels by placing pillow under calves when patient is supine position
• Cover pressure ulcer on heel with appropriate protective dressing
• Consider consult with wound care specialist

Evaluation: Lucius has been consistently turned every 2 hours; healthy granulation tissue is noted in wound bed.

- - - - - **Relationship**   ▉ **Assessment**   ▉ **Nursing Diagnosis**   ▉ **Outcome Identification**   ▉ **Interventions**   ▉ **Evaluation**

Concept map displaying the nursing process for Lucius Everly.

Skill · 32-1 Cleaning a Wound and Applying a Dry, Sterile Dressing

EQUIPMENT

- Sterile gloves
- Clean disposable gloves
- Additional PPE, as indicated
- Gauze dressings
- Surgical or abdominal pads
- Sterile dressing set or suture set (for the sterile scissors and forceps)

- Sterile cleaning solution as ordered (commonly 0.9% normal saline solution, or a commercially prepared wound cleanser)
- Sterile basin (may be optional)
- Sterile drape (may be optional)
- Plastic bag or other appropriate waste container for soiled dressings

- Waterproof pad and bath blanket
- Tape or ties
- Bath blanket or other linens for draping patient
- Additional dressings and supplies needed or required by the physician's order

IMPLEMENTATION

ACTION	RATIONALE
1. Review the medical orders for wound care or the nursing plan of care related to wound care.	Reviewing the order and plan of care validates the correct patient and correct procedure.
2. Gather the necessary supplies and bring to the bedside stand or overbed table.	Preparation promotes efficient time management and organized approach to the task. Bringing everything to the bedside conserves time and energy. Arranging items nearby is convenient, saves time, and avoids unnecessary stretching and twisting of muscles on the part of the nurse.
3. Perform hand hygiene and put on PPE, if indicated.	Hand hygiene and PPE prevent the spread of microorganisms. PPE is required based on transmission precautions.
4. Identify the patient.	Identifying the patient ensures the right patient receives the intervention and helps prevent errors.
5. Close curtains around bed and close door to room if possible. Explain what you are going to do and why you are going to do it to the patient.	This ensures the patient's privacy. Explanation relieves anxiety and facilitates cooperation.
6. Assess the patient for possible need for nonpharmacologic pain-reducing interventions or analgesic medication before wound care dressing change. Administer appropriate prescribed analgesic. Allow enough time for analgesic to achieve its effectiveness.	Pain is a subjective experience influenced by past experience. Wound care and dressing changes may cause pain for some patients.
7. Place a waste receptacle or bag at a convenient location for use during the procedure.	Having a waste container handy means the soiled dressing may be discarded easily, without the spread of microorganisms.
8. Adjust bed to comfortable working height, usually elbow height of the caregiver (VISN 8, 2009).	Having the bed at the proper height prevents back and muscle strain.
9. Assist the patient to a comfortable position that provides easy access to the wound area. Use the bath blanket to cover any exposed area other than the wound. Place a waterproof pad under the wound site.	Patient positioning and use of a bath blanket provide for comfort and warmth. Waterproof pad protects underlying surfaces.
10. Check the position of drains, tubes, or other adjuncts before removing the dressing. Put on clean, disposable gloves and loosen tape on the old dressings (Figure 1). If necessary, use an adhesive remover to help get the tape off.	Checking ensures that a drain is not removed accidentally if one is present. Gloves protect the nurse from contaminated dressings and prevent the spread of microorganisms. Adhesive-tape remover helps reduce patient discomfort during removal of dressing.
11. Carefully remove the soiled dressings (Figure 2). If there is resistance, use a silicone-based adhesive remover to help remove the tape. If any part of the dressing sticks to the underlying skin, use small amounts of sterile saline to help loosen and remove (Figure 3).	Cautious removal of the dressing is more comfortable for the patient and ensures that any drain present is not removed. A silicone-based adhesive remover allows for the easy, rapid, and painless removal without the associated problems of skin stripping (Rudoni, 2008; Stephen-Haynes, 2008). Sterile saline moistens the dressing for easier removal and minimizes damage and pain.
12. After removing the dressing, note the presence, amount, type, color, and odor of any drainage on the dressings (Figure 4). Place soiled dressings in the appropriate waste receptacle. Remove your gloves and dispose of them in an appropriate waste receptacle (Figure 5).	The presence of drainage should be documented. Proper disposal of soiled dressings and used gloves prevents spread of microorganisms.

FIGURE 1. Loosening dressing tape.

FIGURE 2. Removing dressing.

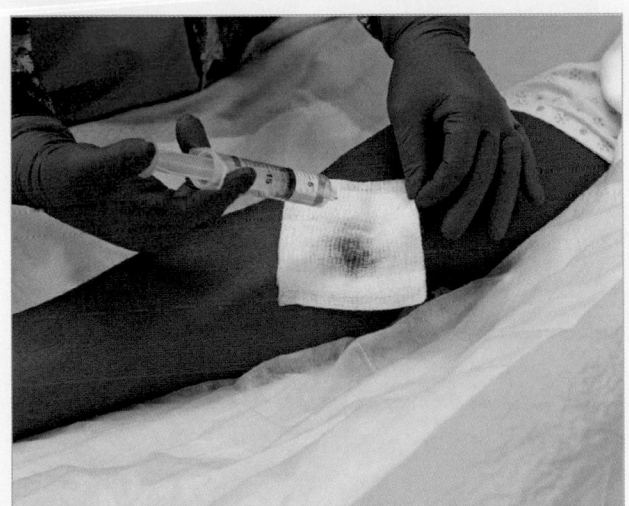

FIGURE 3. Using saline to aid in removing dressing.

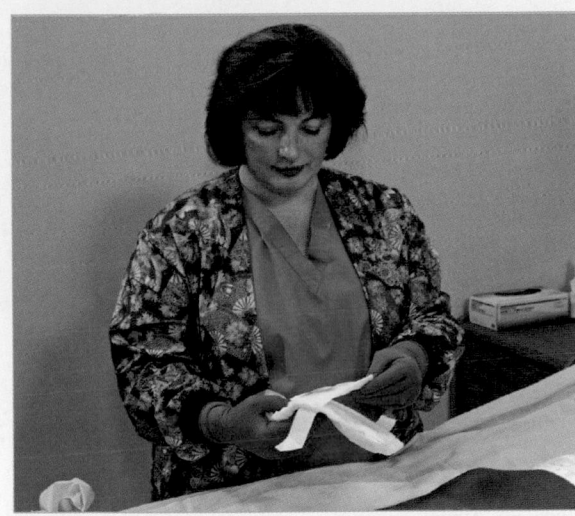

FIGURE 4. Assessing dressing that has been removed.

FIGURE 5. Removing gloves.

(continued)

Skill · 32-1   **Cleaning a Wound and Applying a Dry, Sterile Dressing**   *continued*

ACTION

13. Inspect the wound site for size, appearance, and drainage. Assess if any pain is present. Check the status of sutures, adhesive closure strips, staples, and drains or tubes, if present. Note any problems to include in your documentation.

14. **Using sterile technique, prepare a sterile work area and open the needed supplies (Figure 6).**

15. Open the sterile cleaning solution. Depending on the amount of cleaning needed, the solution might be poured directly over gauze sponges over a container for small cleaning jobs, or into a basin for more complex or larger cleaning.

16. Put on sterile gloves (Figure 7).

RATIONALE

Wound healing or the presence of irritation or infection should be documented.

Supplies are within easy reach and sterility is maintained.

Sterility of dressings and solution is maintained.

Use of sterile gloves maintains surgical asepsis and sterile technique and reduces the risk for spreading microorganisms.

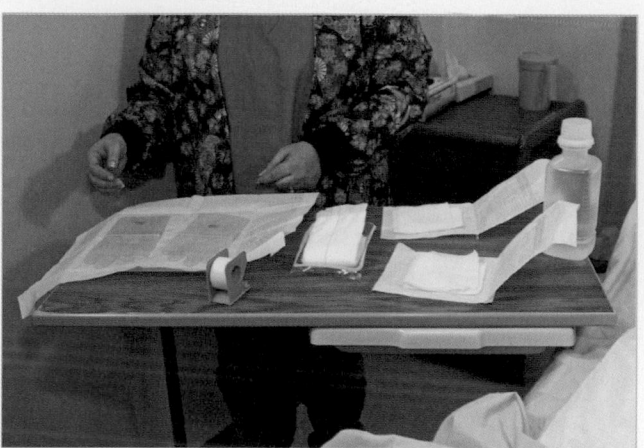

FIGURE 6. Setting up sterile field.

FIGURE 7. Putting on sterile gloves.

17. Clean the wound. **Clean the wound from top to bottom and from the center to the outside (Figure 8). Following this pattern, use new gauze for each wipe, placing the used gauze in the waste receptacle. Alternately, spray the wound from top to bottom with a commercially prepared wound cleanser.**

Cleaning from top to bottom and center to outside ensures that cleaning occurs from the least to most contaminated area and a previously cleaned area is not contaminated again. Using a single gauze for each wipe ensures that the previously cleaned area is not contaminated again.

FIGURE 8. Cleaning wound with dampened gauze.

ACTION

18. Once the wound is cleaned, dry the area using a gauze sponge in the same manner. Apply ointment or perform other treatments, as ordered (Figure 9).

19. If a drain is in use at the wound location, clean around the drain.

20. Apply a layer of dry, sterile dressing over the wound (Figure 10). Forceps may be used to apply the dressing.

21. Place a second layer of gauze over the wound site.

22. Apply a surgical or abdominal pad (ABD) over the gauze at the site as the outermost layer of the dressing (Figure 11).

RATIONALE

Moisture provides a medium for growth of microorganisms. The growth of microorganisms may be inhibited and the healing process improved with the use of ordered ointments or other applications.

Cleaning the insertion site helps prevent infection.

Primary dressing serves as a wick for drainage. Use of forceps helps ensure that sterile technique is maintained.

A second layer provides for increased absorption of drainage.

The dressing acts as additional protection for the wound against microorganisms in the environment.

FIGURE 9. Applying antimicrobial ointment to wound with cotton applicator.

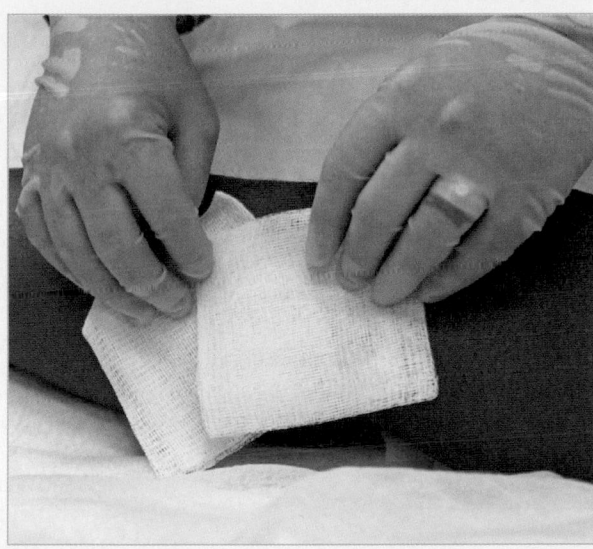

FIGURE 10. Applying dry dressing to site.

FIGURE 11. Applying a surgical pad over dressing and securing with tape.

(continued)

Skill · 32-1 Cleaning a Wound and Applying a Dry, Sterile Dressing *continued*

ACTION	RATIONALE
23. Remove and discard gloves. Apply tape, Montgomery straps, or roller gauze to secure the dressings. Alternately, many commercial wound products are self-adhesive and do not require additional tape.	Proper disposal of gloves prevents the spread of microorganisms. Tape or other securing products are easier to apply after gloves have been removed.
24. After securing the dressing, label dressing with date and time. Remove all remaining equipment; place the patient in a comfortable position, with side rails up and bed in the lowest position.	Recording date and time provides communication and demonstrates adherence to the plan of care. Proper patient and bed positioning promotes safety and comfort.
25. Remove PPE, if used. Perform hand hygiene.	Removing PPE properly reduces the risk for infection transmission and contamination of other items. Hand hygiene prevents the spread of microorganisms.
26. Check all wound dressings every shift. More frequent checks may be needed if the wound is more complex or dressings become saturated quickly.	Checking dressings ensures the assessment of changes in patient condition and timely intervention to prevent complications.

DOCUMENTATION

Guidelines

Document the location of the wound and that the dressing was removed. Record your assessment of the wound including approximation of wound edges, presence of sutures, staples or adhesive closure strips, and the condition of the surrounding skin. Note if redness, edema, or drainage is observed. Document cleansing of the incision with normal saline and any application of antibiotic ointment as ordered. Record the type of dressing that was reapplied. Note pertinent patient and family education and any patient reaction to this procedure, including patient's pain level and effectiveness of nonpharmacologic interventions or analgesia if administered.

Sample Documentation

9/8/12 0600 Dressing removed from left lateral calf incision. Scant purulent secretions noted on dressing. Incision edges approximately 1 mm apart, red, with ecchymosis and edema present. Small amount of purulent drainage from wound noted. Area cleansed with normal saline, dried, antibiotic ointment applied per order. Surrounding tissue red and ecchymotic. Redressed with nonadhering dressing, gauze, and wrapped with stretch gauze. Patient reports adequate pain control after preprocedure analgesic; states pain is dull ache, 1/10 on pain scale.

—N. Joiner, RN

UNEXPECTED SITUATIONS AND ASSOCIATED INTERVENTIONS

- *The previous wound assessment states that the incision was clean and dry and the wound edges were approximated, with the staples and surgical drain intact. The surrounding tissue was without inflammation, edema, or erythema. After the dressing is removed, the nurse notes the incision edges are not approximated at the distal end, multiple staples are evident in the old dressing, the surrounding skin tissue is red and swollen, and purulent drainage is on the dressing and leaking from the wound:* Assess the patient for any other signs and symptoms such as pain, malaise, fever, and paresthesias. Place a dry sterile dressing over the wound site. Report the findings to the physician and document the event in the patient's record. Be prepared to obtain a wound culture and implement any changes in wound care as ordered.

- *After the nurse has put on sterile gloves, the patient moves too close to the edge of the bed and the nurse must support her with his hands to prevent the patient from falling:* If nothing else in the sterile field was touched, remove the contaminated gloves and put on new sterile gloves. If you did not bring a second pair, use the call bell to summon a coworker to provide a new pair of gloves.

- *The nurse has set up dressing supplies, removed the old dressing, and put on sterile gloves to clean the wound. The nurse then realizes that a necessary piece of dressing material has been forgotten:* Ask the patient to press the call bell to summon a coworker to provide the missing supplies.

SPECIAL CONSIDERATIONS

General Considerations

- Instruct the patient, if appropriate, and ancillary staff members to observe for excessive drainage that may overwhelm the dressing. They should also report when dressings become soiled or loosened from the skin.

Older Adult Considerations

- The skin of older adults is less elastic and more sensitive; use paper tape, Montgomery straps, or roller gauze (on extremities) to prevent tearing of the skin.

Skill · 32-2 Applying a Saline-Moistened Dressing

EQUIPMENT

- Clean disposable gloves
- Sterile gloves, if indicated
- Additional PPE, as indicated
- Sterile dressing set or suture set (for the sterile scissors and forceps)
- Sterile thin-mesh gauze dressing for packing, if ordered
- Sterile gauze dressings

- Surgical or abdominal pads
- Skin-protectant wipes
- Sterile basin
- Sterile cleaning solution as ordered (commonly 0.9% normal saline solution)
- Sterile saline
- Tape or ties

- Plastic bag or other appropriate waste container for soiled dressings
- Sterile cotton-tipped applicators
- Supplies for wound cleansing or irrigation, as necessary
- Waterproof pad and bath blanket

IMPLEMENTATION

ACTION	RATIONALE
1. Review the medical orders for wound care or the nursing plan of care related to wound care.	Reviewing the order and plan of care validates the correct patient and correct procedure.
2. Gather the necessary supplies and bring to the bedside stand or overbed table.	Preparation promotes efficient time management and organized approach to the task. Bringing everything to the bedside conserves time and energy. Arranging items nearby is convenient, saves time, and avoids unnecessary stretching and twisting of muscles on the part of the nurse.
3. Perform hand hygiene and put on PPE, if indicated.	Hand hygiene and PPE prevent the spread of microorganisms. PPE is required based on transmission precautions.
4. Identify the patient.	Identifying the patient ensures the right patient receives the intervention and helps prevent errors.
5. Close curtains around bed and close door to room if possible. Explain what you are going to do and why you are going to do it to the patient.	This ensures the patient's privacy. Explanation relieves anxiety and facilitates cooperation.
6. Assess the patient for possible need for nonpharmacologic pain-reducing interventions or analgesic medication before wound care dressing change. Administer appropriate prescribed analgesic. Allow enough time for analgesic to achieve its effectiveness.	Pain is a subjective experience influenced by past experience. Wound care and dressing changes may cause pain for some patients.
7. Place a waste receptacle or bag at a convenient location for use during the procedure.	Having a waste container handy means the soiled dressing may be discarded easily, without the spread of microorganisms.
8. Adjust bed to comfortable working height, usually elbow height of the caregiver (VISN 8, 2009).	Having the bed at the proper height prevents back and muscle strain.

(continued)

Skill · 32-2 **Applying a Saline-Moistened Dressing** *continued*

ACTION	RATIONALE
9. Assist the patient to a comfortable position that provides easy access to the wound area. Position the patient so the wound cleanser or irrigation solution will flow from the clean end of the wound toward the dirtier end, if being used (see Skill 32-3 for irrigation techniques). Use the bath blanket to cover any exposed area other than the wound. Place a waterproof pad under the wound site.	Patient positioning and use of a bath blanket provide for comfort and warmth. Gravity directs the flow of liquid from the least contaminated to the most contaminated area. Waterproof pad protects underlying surfaces.
10. Put on clean gloves. Carefully and gently remove the soiled dressings. If there is resistance, use a silicone-based adhesive remover to help remove the tape. If any part of the dressing sticks to the underlying skin, use small amounts of sterile saline to help loosen and remove.	Gloves protect the nurse from handling contaminated dressings. Cautious removal of the dressing is more comfortable for the patient and ensures that any drain present is not removed. A silicone-based adhesive remover allows for the easy, rapid, and painless removal without the associated problems of skin stripping (Rudoni, 2008; Stephen-Haynes, 2008). Sterile saline moistens the dressing for easier removal and minimizes damage and pain.
11. After removing the dressing, note the presence, amount, type, color, and odor of any drainage on the dressings. Place soiled dressings in the appropriate waste receptacle.	The presence of drainage should be documented. Discarding dressings appropriately prevents the spread of microorganisms.
12. Assess the wound for appearance, stage, the presence of eschar, granulation tissue, epithelialization, undermining, tunneling, necrosis, sinus tract, and drainage. Assess the appearance of the surrounding tissue. Measure the wound.	This information provides evidence about the wound healing process and/or the presence of infection.
13. Remove your gloves and put them in the receptacle.	Discarding gloves prevents the spread of microorganisms.
14. Using sterile technique, open the supplies and dressings. Place the fine-mesh gauze into the basin and pour the ordered solution over the mesh to saturate it.	Gauze touching the wound surface must be moistened to increase the absorptive ability and promote healing.
15. Put on the sterile gloves. Alternately, clean gloves (clean technique) may be used to clean a chronic wound.	Sterile gloves maintain surgical asepsis. Clean technique is appropriate when cleaning chronic wounds.
16. Clean the wound. Refer to Skill 32-1. Alternately, irrigate the wound, as ordered or required (see Skill 32-3).	Cleaning the wound removes previous drainage and wound debris.
17. Dry the surrounding skin with sterile gauze dressings.	Moisture provides a medium for growth of microorganisms.
18. Apply a skin protectant to the surrounding skin, if needed.	A skin protectant prevents skin irritation and breakdown.
19. If not already on, put on sterile gloves. Squeeze excess fluid from the gauze dressing. Unfold and fluff the dressing.	Sterile gloves prevent contamination of the dressing material. The gauze provides a thin, moist layer to contact all the wound surfaces.
20. Gently press to loosely pack the moistened gauze into the wound (Figure 1). If necessary, use the forceps or cotton-tipped applicators to press the gauze into all wound surfaces (Figure 2).	The dressing provides a moist environment for all wound surfaces. Avoid overpacking the gauze; loosely pack to prevent too much pressure in the wound bed, which could impede wound healing.

FIGURE 1. Gently pressing gauze into wound.

FIGURE 2. Using a cotton-tipped applicator to press gauze into all wound surfaces.

ACTION	**RATIONALE**
21. Apply several dry, sterile gauze pads over the wet gauze.	Dry gauze absorbs excess moisture and drainage.
22. Place the ABD pad over the gauze.	The ABD pad prevents contamination.
23. Remove and discard gloves. Apply tape, Montgomery straps, or roller gauze to secure the dressings. Alternately, many commercial wound products are self-adhesive and do not require additional tape.	Proper disposal of gloves prevents the spread of microorganisms. Tape or other securing products are easier to apply after gloves have been removed.
24. After securing the dressing, label dressing with date and time. Remove all remaining equipment; place the patient in a comfortable position, with side rails up and bed in the lowest position.	Recording date and time provides communication and demonstrates adherence to plan of care. Proper patient and bed positioning promotes safety and comfort.
25. Remove PPE, if used. Perform hand hygiene.	Removing PPE properly reduces the risk for infection transmission and contamination of other items. Hand hygiene prevents the spread of microorganisms.
26. Check all wound dressings every shift. More frequent checks may be needed if the wound is more complex or dressings become saturated quickly.	Checking dressings ensures the assessment of changes in patient condition and timely intervention to prevent complications.

DOCUMENTATION

Guidelines

Document the location of the wound and that the dressing was removed. Record your assessment of the wound, including evidence of granulation tissue, presence of necrotic tissue, stage (if appropriate) and characteristics of drainage. Include the appearance of the surrounding skin. Document the cleansing or irrigation of the wound and solution used. Record the type of dressing that was reapplied. Note pertinent patient and family education and any patient reaction to this procedure, including patient's pain level and effectiveness of nonpharmacologic interventions or analgesia if administered.

Sample Documentation

> <u>11/20/11</u> 1645 Healing abdominal incision with granulating tissue noted. Open area 2 cm × 4 cm × 0.5 cm depth in center of incision. No evidence of necrosis or tunneling. Scant amount of serous drainage. Saline-moistened dressing applied to open wound; covered loosely with ABD dressing. Patient denies pain from incision. Instructed patient that moist saline gauze will facilitate the healing process and to notify nurse for any discomfort related to incision.
>
> —R. Dobbins, RN

UNEXPECTED SITUATIONS AND RELATED INTERVENTIONS

- *When removing a patient's dressing, the assessment reveals eschar in the wound:* Notify the primary care provider or wound care specialist, as a different treatment modality and/or débridement may be necessary. The presence of eschar in a wound precludes the staging of the wound. The eschar must be removed for adequate pressure ulcer staging to be done. Stable (dry, adherent, intact, without erythema or fluctuance) eschar on the heels serves as "the body's natural (biological) cover" and should not be removed (NPUAP, 2007c).

- *The wound assessment reveals several depressions or craterlike areas on inspection of a wound:* Notify the primary care provider or wound care specialist, who may order the wound to be packed. Pack wound cavities loosely with dressing material. Overpacking may increase pressure and interfere with tissue healing.

- *The nurse notes that the wound dressing is dry upon removal:* Reduce the time interval between changes to prevent drying of the materials, which may disrupt healing tissue.

(continued)

Skill · 32-2   Applying a Saline-Moistened Dressing *continued*

SPECIAL CONSIDERATIONS

- Make sure ancillary staff understand the importance of reporting excessive drainage from the dressing, and any soiled or loose dressings.
- Guidelines from the Wound, Ostomy, Continence Nurses Society (WOCN) and National Pressure Ulcer Advisory Panel (NPUAP) recommend that clean gloves may be used to treat chronic wounds and pressure ulcers as long as the infection-control procedures are followed. The *no-touch technique* may be used within these guidelines. Clean gloves are used to handle dressing material. Irrigants and dressings are sterile. The wound is redressed by picking up dressing materials by the corner and placing the untouched side over the wound (NPUAP, 2007d; Wooten & Hawkins, 2005).
- Many products are available to treat chronic wounds and pressure ulcers. Treatment varies based on facility policy, nursing protocol, clinical specialist referrals, primary care provider orders, and product in use.

Skill · 32-3   Performing Irrigation of a Wound

EQUIPMENT

- A sterile irrigation set, including a basin, irrigant container, and irrigation syringe
- Sterile irrigation solution as ordered by the physician, warmed to body temperature, commonly 0.9% normal saline solution
- Plastic bag or other waste container to dispose of soiled dressings
- Sterile gloves
- Sterile drape (may be optional)
- Clean disposable gloves
- Moisture-proof gown, mask, and eye protection
- Additional PPE, as indicated
- Sterile dressing set or suture set (for the sterile scissors and forceps)
- Waterproof pad and bath blanket, as needed
- Sterile gauze dressings
- Sterile packing gauze, as needed
- Tape or ties
- Skin-protectant wipes

IMPLEMENTATION

ACTION	RATIONALE
1. Review the medical orders for wound care or the nursing plan of care related to wound care.	Reviewing the order and plan of care validates the correct patient and correct procedure.
2. Gather the necessary supplies and bring to the bedside stand or overbed table.	Preparation promotes efficient time management and organized approach to the task. Bringing everything to the bedside conserves time and energy. Arranging items nearby is convenient, saves time, and avoids unnecessary stretching and twisting of muscles on the part of the nurse.
3. Perform hand hygiene and put on PPE, if indicated.	Hand hygiene and PPE prevent the spread of microorganisms. PPE is required based on transmission precautions.
4. Identify the patient.	Identifying the patient ensures the right patient receives the intervention and helps prevent errors.
5. Close curtains around bed and close door to room if possible. Explain what you are going to do and why you are going to do it to the patient.	This ensures the patient's privacy. Explanation relieves anxiety and facilitates cooperation.
6. Assess the patient for possible need for nonpharmacologic pain-reducing interventions or analgesic medication before wound care and/or dressing change. Administer appropriate prescribed analgesic. Allow enough time for analgesic to achieve its effectiveness before beginning procedure.	Pain is a subjective experience influenced by past experience. Wound care and dressing changes may cause pain for some patients.
7. Place a waste receptacle or bag at a convenient location for use during the procedure.	Having a waste container handy means the soiled dressing may be discarded easily, without the spread of microorganisms.

ACTION

8. Adjust bed to comfortable working height, usually elbow height of the caregiver (VISN 8, 2009).

9. Assist the patient to a comfortable position that provides easy access to the wound area. Position the patient so the irrigation solution will flow from the clean end of the wound toward the dirtier end. Use the bath blanket to cover any exposed area other than the wound. Place a waterproof pad under the wound site.

10. Put on a gown, mask, and eye protection.

11. Put on clean gloves. Carefully and gently remove the soiled dressings. If there is resistance, use a silicone-based adhesive remover to help remove the tape. If any part of the dressing sticks to the underlying skin, use small amounts of sterile saline to help loosen and remove.

12. After removing the dressing, note the presence, amount, type, color, and odor of any drainage on the dressings. Place soiled dressings in the appropriate waste receptacle.

13. Assess the wound for appearance, stage, the presence of eschar, granulation tissue, epithelialization, undermining, tunneling, necrosis, sinus tract, and drainage. Assess the appearance of the surrounding tissue. Measure the wound.

14. Remove your gloves and put them in the receptacle.

15. Set up a sterile field, if indicated, and wound cleaning supplies. Pour warmed sterile irrigating solution into the sterile container. Put on the sterile gloves. Alternately, clean gloves (clean technique) may be used when irrigating a chronic wound.

16. Position the sterile basin below the wound to collect the irrigation fluid.

17. Fill the irrigation syringe with solution (Figure 1). **Using your nondominant hand, gently apply pressure to the basin against the skin below the wound to form a seal with the skin (Figure 2).**

18. **Gently direct a stream of solution into the wound (Figure 3). Keep the tip of the syringe at least 1 inch above the upper tip of the wound. When using a catheter tip, insert it gently into the wound until it meets resistance. Gently flush all wound areas.**

19. Watch for the solution to flow smoothly and evenly. When the solution from the wound flows out clear, discontinue irrigation.

20. Dry the surrounding skin with gauze dressings (Figure 4).

21. Apply a skin protectant to the surrounding skin.

RATIONALE

Having the bed at the proper height prevents back and muscle strain.

Patient positioning and use of a bath blanket provide for comfort and warmth. Gravity directs the flow of liquid from the least contaminated to the most contaminated area. Waterproof pad protects underlying surfaces.

Using personal protective equipment, such as gowns, masks, and eye protection, is part of Standard Precautions. A gown protects clothes from contamination should splashing occur. Goggles protect mucous membranes of eyes from contact with irrigant fluid or wound drainage.

Gloves protect the nurse from handling contaminated dressings. Cautious removal of the dressing is more comfortable for the patient and ensures that any drain present is not removed. A silicone-based adhesive remover allows for the easy, rapid, and painless removal without the associated problems of skin stripping (Rudoni, 2008; Stephen-Haynes, 2008). Sterile saline moistens the dressing for easier removal and minimizes damage and pain.

The presence of drainage should be documented. Discarding dressings appropriately prevents the spread of microorganisms.

This information provides evidence about the wound healing process and/or the presence of infection.

Discarding gloves prevents the spread of microorganisms.

Using warmed solution prevents chilling of the patient and may minimize patient discomfort. Sterile technique and gloves maintain surgical asepsis. Clean technique is appropriate for irrigating chronic wounds.

Patient and bed linens are protected from contaminated fluid.

The solution will collect in the basin and prevent the irrigant from running down the skin. Patient and bed linens are protected from contaminated fluid.

Debris and contaminated solution flow from the least contaminated to most contaminated area. High-pressure irrigation flow may cause patient discomfort as well as damage granulation tissue. A catheter tip allows the introduction of irrigant into a wound with a small opening or one that is deep.

Irrigation removes exudate and debris.

Moisture provides a medium for growth of microorganisms. Excess moisture can contribute to skin irritation and breakdown.

A skin protectant prevents skin irritation and breakdown.

(continued)

Skill · 32-3   Performing Irrigation of a Wound   *continued*

ACTION

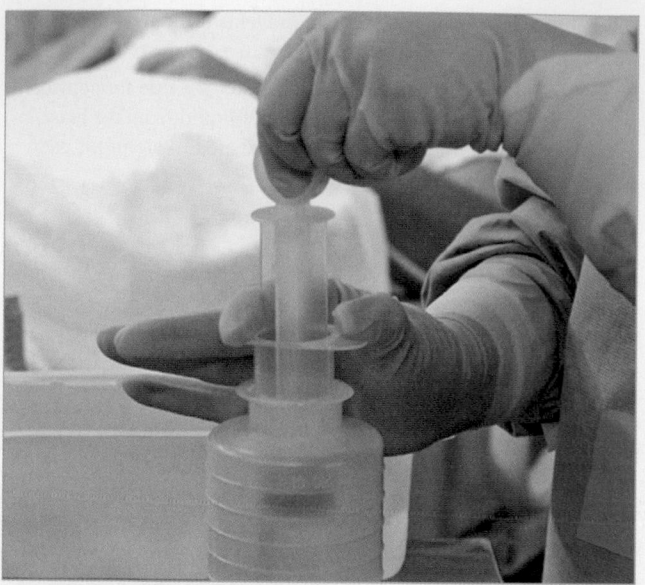

FIGURE 1. Drawing up sterile solution from sterile container into irrigation syringe.

FIGURE 3. Irrigating wound with a gentle stream of solution. Solution drains into collection container.

22. Apply a new dressing to the wound (see Skill 32-1) (Figure 5).

23. Remove and discard gloves. Apply tape, Montgomery straps, or roller gauze to secure the dressings. Alternately, many commercial wound products are self-adhesive and do not require additional tape.

24. After securing the dressing, label dressing with date and time. Remove all remaining equipment; place the patient in a comfortable position, with side rails up and bed in the lowest position.

RATIONALE

FIGURE 2. Patient lying on side with wound exposed, sterile collection container placed against skin, bed protected with waterproof pad.

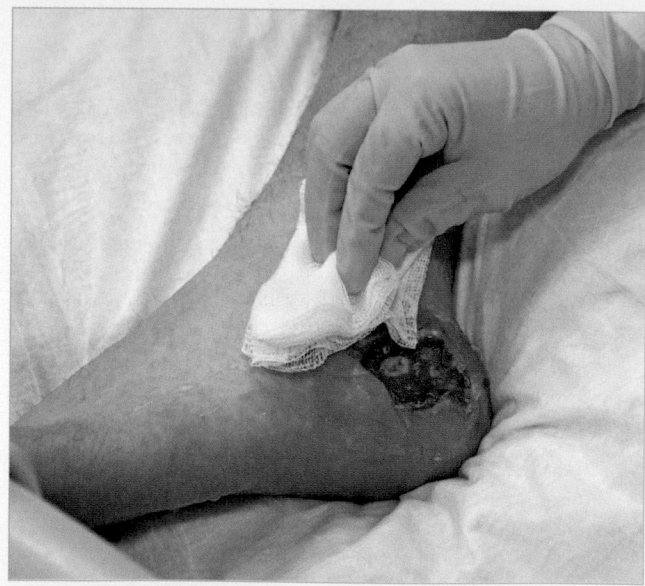

FIGURE 4. Drying around wound, not in wound, with sterile gauze pad.

Dressings absorb drainage, protect the wound, and promote healing.

Tape or other securing products are easier to apply after gloves have been removed. Proper disposal of gloves prevents the spread of microorganisms.

Recording date and time provides communication and demonstrates adherence to plan of care. Proper patient and bed positioning promotes safety and comfort.

ACTION   **RATIONALE**

FIGURE 5. Applying a new dressing.

25. Remove remaining PPE. Perform hand hygiene.

Removing PPE properly reduces the risk for infection transmission and contamination of other items. Hand hygiene prevents the spread of microorganisms.

26. Check all wound dressings every shift. More frequent checks may be needed if the wound is more complex or dressings become saturated quickly.

Checking dressings ensures the assessment of changes in patient condition and timely intervention to prevent complications.

DOCUMENTATION

Guidelines

Document the location of the wound and that the dressing was removed. Record your assessment of the wound, including evidence of granulation tissue, presence of necrotic tissue, stage (if appropriate), and characteristics of drainage. Include the appearance of the surrounding skin. Document the irrigation of the wound and solution used. Record the type of dressing that was applied. Note pertinent patient and family education and any patient reaction to this procedure, including patient's pain level and effectiveness of nonpharmacologic interventions or analgesia if administered.

Sample Documentation

3/5/12 1700 Dressing removed from left outer heel area. Minimal serosanguineous drainage noted on dressings. Wound 4 × 5 × 2 cm, pink, with granulation tissue evident. Surrounding skin tone consistent with patient's skin, no edema or redness noted. Irrigated with normal saline and hydrogel dressing applied.

—J. Lark, RN

UNEXPECTED SITUATIONS AND ASSOCIATED INTERVENTIONS

• *The patient experiences pain when the wound irrigation is begun:* Stop the procedure and administer an analgesic as ordered. Obtain new sterile supplies and begin the procedure after an appropriate amount of time has elapsed to allow the analgesic to begin working. Note the patient's pain on the nursing plan of care so that pain medication can be given before future wound treatments.

• *During the wound irrigation, the nurse notes bleeding from the wound. This has not been documented as happening with previous irrigations:* Stop the procedure. Assess the patient for other symptoms. Obtain vital signs. Report the findings to the primary care provider and document the event in the patient's record.

Skill · 32-4   Caring for a Jackson-Pratt Drain

EQUIPMENT

- Graduated container for measuring drainage
- Clean disposable gloves
- Additional PPE, as indicated
- Cleansing solution, usually sterile normal saline
- Sterile gauze pads
- Skin-protectant wipes
- Dressing materials for site dressing, if used

IMPLEMENTATION

ACTION	RATIONALE
1. Review the medical orders for wound care or the nursing plan of care related to wound/drain care.	Reviewing the order and plan of care validates the correct patient and correct procedure.
2. Gather the necessary supplies and bring to the bedside stand or overbed table.	Preparation promotes efficient time management and organized approach to the task. Bringing everything to the bedside conserves time and energy. Arranging items nearby is convenient, saves time, and avoids unnecessary stretching and twisting of muscles on the part of the nurse.
3. Perform hand hygiene and put on PPE, if indicated.	Hand hygiene and PPE prevent the spread of microorganisms. PPE is required based on transmission precautions.
4. Identify the patient.	Identifying the patient ensures the right patient receives the intervention and helps prevent errors.
5. Close curtains around bed and close door to room if possible. Explain what you are going to do and why you are going to do it to the patient.	This ensures the patient's privacy. Explanation relieves anxiety and facilitates cooperation.
6. Assess the patient for possible need for nonpharmacologic pain-reducing interventions or analgesic medication before wound care dressing change. Administer appropriate prescribed analgesic. Allow enough time for analgesic to achieve its effectiveness before beginning procedure.	Pain is a subjective experience influenced by past experience. Wound care and dressing changes may cause pain for some patients.
7. Place a waste receptacle at a convenient location for use during the procedure.	Having a waste container handy means that the soiled dressing may be discarded easily, without the spread of microorganisms.
8. Adjust bed to comfortable working height, usually elbow height of the caregiver (VISN 8, 2009).	Having the bed at the proper height prevents back and muscle strain.
9. Assist the patient to a comfortable position that provides easy access to the drain and/or wound area. Use a bath blanket to cover any exposed area other than the wound. Place a waterproof pad under the wound site.	Patient positioning and use of a bath blanket provide for comfort and warmth. Waterproof pad protects underlying surfaces.
10. Put on clean gloves; put on mask or face shield if indicated.	Gloves prevent the spread of microorganisms; mask reduces the risk of transmission should splashing occur.
11. Place the graduated collection container under the outlet of the drain. Without contaminating the outlet valve, pull the cap off. The chamber will expand completely as it draws in air. **Empty the chamber's contents completely into the container (Figure 1). Use the gauze pad to clean the outlet. Fully compress the chamber with one hand and replace the cap with your other hand (Figure 2).**	Emptying the drainage allows for accurate measurement. Cleaning the outlet reduces the risk of contamination and helps prevent the spread of microorganisms. Compressing the chamber reestablishes the suction.
12. Check the patency of the equipment. Make sure the tubing is free from twists and kinks.	Patent, untwisted, or unkinked tubing promotes appropriate drainage from wound.
13. Secure the Jackson-Pratt drain to the patient's gown below the wound with a safety pin, making sure that there is no tension on the tubing.	Securing the drain prevents injury to the patient and accidental removal of the drain.
14. Carefully measure and record the character, color, and amount of the drainage. Discard the drainage according to facility policy. Remove gloves.	Documentation promotes continuity of care and communication. Appropriate disposal of biohazard material reduces the risk for microorganism transmission. Proper disposal of gloves deters transmission of microorganisms.

ACTION

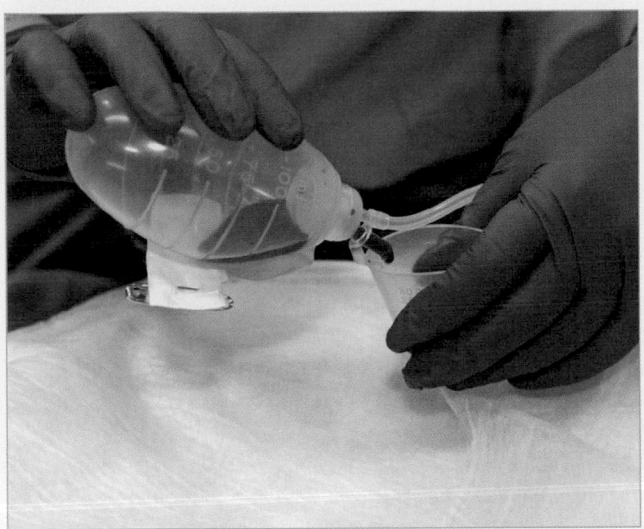

FIGURE 1. Emptying contents of Jackson-Pratt drain into collection device.

RATIONALE

FIGURE 2. Compressing Jackson-Pratt drain and replacing cap.

15. Put on clean gloves. If the drain site has a dressing, redress the site. Include cleaning of the sutures with the gauze pad moistened with normal saline. Dry sutures with gauze before applying new dressing.

16. If the drain site is open to air, observe the sutures that secure the drain to the skin. Look for signs of pulling, tearing, swelling, or infection of the surrounding skin. Gently clean the sutures with the gauze pad moistened with normal saline. Dry with a new gauze pad. Apply skin protectant to the surrounding skin if needed.

17. Remove and discard gloves. Remove all remaining equipment; place the patient in a comfortable position, with side rails up and bed in the lowest position.

18. Remove additional PPE, if used. Perform hand hygiene.

19. Check drain status at least every 4 hours. Check all wound dressings every shift. More frequent checks may be needed if the wound is more complex or dressings become saturated quickly.

Dressing protects the site. Cleaning and drying sutures deters growth of microorganisms.

Early detection of problems leads to prompt intervention and prevents complications. Gentle cleaning and drying prevent the growth of microorganisms. Skin protectant prevents skin irritation and breakdown.

Proper removal and disposal of gloves prevents spread of microorganisms. Proper patient and bed positioning promotes safety and comfort.

Removing PPE properly reduces the risk for infection transmission and contamination of other items. Hand hygiene prevents the spread of microorganisms.

Checking drain ensures proper functioning and early detection of problems. Checking dressings ensures the assessment of changes in patient condition and timely intervention to prevent complications.

DOCUMENTATION
Guidelines

Document the location of the wound and drain, the assessment of the wound and drain site, and patency of the drain. Note if sutures are intact. Document the presence of drainage and characteristics on the old dressing upon removal. Include the appearance of the surrounding skin. Document cleansing of the drain site. Record any skin care and the dressing applied. Note that the drain was emptied and recompressed. Note pertinent patient and family education and any patient reaction to this procedure, including patient's pain level and effectiveness of nonpharmacologic interventions or analgesia if administered. Document the amount and characteristics of drainage obtained on the appropriate intake and output record.

(continued)

Skill · 32-4 Caring for a Jackson-Pratt Drain *continued*

Sample Documentation

2/7/12 2400 Right chest incision and drain open to air. Wound edges approximated, slight ecchymosis, no edema, redness, or drainage. Steri-Strips intact. J-P drain patent and secured with suture. Exit site without edema, drainage, or redness. Drain emptied and recompressed. 40 mL sanguineous drainage recorded.

—Carol White, RN

UNEXPECTED SITUATIONS AND ASSOCIATED INTERVENTIONS

• *A patient has a Jackson-Pratt drain in the right lower quadrant following abdominal surgery. The record indicates it has been draining serosanguineous fluid, 40 to 50 mL every shift. While performing your initial assessment, you note that the dressing around the drain site is saturated with serosanguineous secretions and there is minimal drainage in the collection chamber:* Inspect the tubing for kinks or obstruction. Assess the patient for changes in condition. Remove the dressing and assess the site. Often, if the tubing becomes blocked with a blood clot or drainage particles, the wound drainage will leak around the exit site of the drain. Cleanse the area and redress the site. Notify the primary care provider of the findings and document the event in the patient's record.

• *Your patient calls you to the room and says, "I found this in the bed when I went to get up." He has his Jackson-Pratt drain in his hand. It is completely removed from the patient:* Assess the patient for any new and abnormal signs or symptoms, and assess the surgical site and drain site. Apply a sterile dressing with gauze and tape to the drain site. Notify the primary care provider of the findings and document the event in the patient's record.

SPECIAL CONSIDERATIONS

• Often patients have more than one Jackson-Pratt drain. Number or letter the drains for easy identification. Record the drainage from each drain separately, identified by the number or letter, on the intake and output record.

• When the patient with a drain is ready to ambulate, empty and compress the drain before activity. Secure the drain to the patient's gown below the wound, making sure there is no tension on the drainage tubing. This removes excess drainage, maintains maximum suction, and avoids strain on the drain's suture line.

Skill · 32-5 Caring for a Hemovac Drain

EQUIPMENT

• Graduated container for measuring drainage
• Clean disposable gloves
• Additional PPE, as indicated

• Cleansing solution, usually sterile normal saline
• Sterile gauze pads

• Skin-protectant wipes
• Dressing materials for site dressing, if used

IMPLEMENTATION

ACTION	RATIONALE
1. Review the medical orders for wound care or the nursing plan of care related to wound/drain care.	Reviewing the order and plan of care validates the correct patient and correct procedure.
2. Gather the necessary supplies and bring to the bedside stand or overbed table.	Preparation promotes efficient time management and organized approach to the task. Bringing everything to the bedside conserves time and energy. Arranging items nearby is convenient, saves time, and avoids unnecessary stretching and twisting of muscles on the part of the nurse.
3. Perform hand hygiene and put on PPE, if indicated.	Hand hygiene and PPE prevent the spread of microorganisms. PPE is required based on transmission precautions.

ACTION

4. Identify the patient.

5. Close curtains around bed and close door to room if possible. Explain what you are going to do and why you are going to do it to the patient.

6. Assess the patient for possible need for nonpharmacologic pain-reducing interventions or analgesic medication before wound care dressing change. Administer appropriate prescribed analgesic. Allow enough time for analgesic to achieve its effectiveness before beginning procedure.

7. Place a waste receptacle at a convenient location for use during the procedure.

8. Adjust bed to comfortable working height, usually elbow height of the caregiver (VISN 8, 2009).

9. Assist the patient to a comfortable position that provides easy access to the drain and/or wound area. Use a bath blanket to cover any exposed area other than the wound. Place a waterproof pad under the wound site.

10. Put on clean gloves; put on mask or face shield if indicated.

11. Place the graduated collection container under the outlet of the drain. Without contaminating the outlet, pull the cap off. The chamber will expand completely as it draws in air. **Empty the chamber's contents completely into the container (Figure 1). Use the gauze pad to clean the outlet. Fully compress the chamber by pushing the top and bottom together with your hands. Keep the device tightly compressed while you apply the cap (Figure 2).**

RATIONALE

Identifying the patient ensures the right patient receives the intervention and helps prevent errors.

This ensures the patient's privacy. Explanation relieves anxiety and facilitates cooperation.

Pain is a subjective experience influenced by past experience. Wound care and dressing changes may cause pain for some patients.

Having a waste container handy means that the soiled dressing may be discarded easily, without the spread of microorganisms.

Having the bed at the proper height prevents back and muscle strain.

Patient positioning and use of a bath blanket provide for comfort and warmth. Waterproof pad protects underlying surfaces.

Gloves prevent the spread of microorganisms; mask reduces the risk of transmission should splashing occur.

Emptying the drainage allows for accurate measurement. Cleaning the outlet reduces the risk of contamination and helps prevent the spread of microorganisms. Compressing the chamber reestablishes the suction.

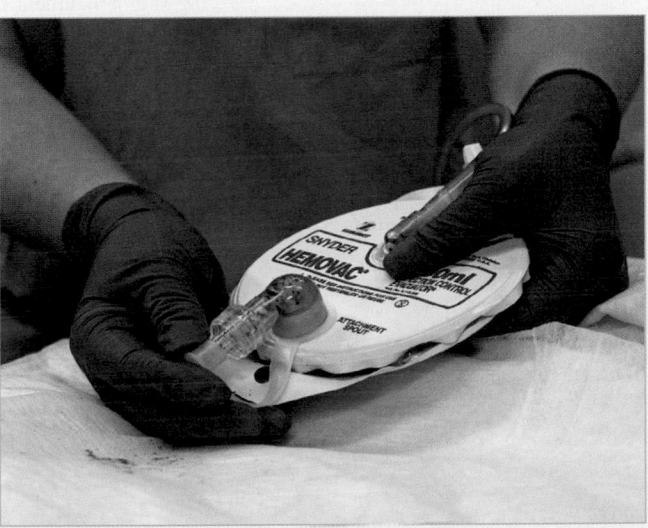

FIGURE 1. Emptying Hemovac drain into collection device.

FIGURE 2. Compressing the Hemovac and securing the cap.

(continued)

Skill · 32-5 **Caring for a Hemovac Drain** *continued*

ACTION	RATIONALE
12. Check the patency of the equipment. Make sure the tubing is free from twists and kinks.	Patent, untwisted, or unkinked tubing promotes appropriate drainage from wound.
13. Secure the Hemovac drain to the patient's gown below the wound with a safety pin, making sure that there is no tension on the tubing.	Securing the drain prevents injury to the patient and accidental removal of the drain.
14. Carefully measure and record the character, color, and amount of the drainage. Discard the drainage according to facility policy.	Documentation promotes continuity of care and communication. Appropriate disposal of biohazard material reduces the risk for microorganism transmission.
15. Put on clean gloves. If the drain site has a dressing, redress the site. Include cleaning of the sutures with the gauze pad moistened with normal saline. Dry sutures with gauze before applying new dressing.	Dressing protects the site. Cleaning and drying sutures deters growth of microorganisms.
16. If the drain site is open to air, observe the sutures that secure the drain to the skin. Look for signs of pulling, tearing, swelling, or infection of the surrounding skin. Gently clean the sutures with the gauze pad moistened with normal saline. Dry with a new gauze pad. Apply skin protectant to the surrounding skin if needed.	Early detection of problems leads to prompt intervention and prevents complications. Gentle cleaning and drying prevent the growth of microorganisms. Skin protectant prevents skin irritation and breakdown.
17. Remove and discard gloves. Remove all remaining equipment; place the patient in a comfortable position, with side rails up and bed in the lowest position.	Proper removal of gloves prevents spread of microorganisms. Proper patient and bed positioning promotes safety and comfort.
18. Remove additional PPE, if used. Perform hand hygiene.	Removing PPE properly reduces the risk for infection transmission and contamination of other items. Hand hygiene prevents the spread of microorganisms.
19. Check drain status at least every 4 hours. Check all wound dressings every shift. More frequent checks may be needed if the wound is more complex or dressings become saturated quickly.	Checking drain ensures proper functioning and early detection of problems. Checking dressings ensures the assessment of changes in patient condition and timely intervention to prevent complications.

DOCUMENTATION

Guidelines

Document the location of the wound and drain, the assessment of the wound and drain site, and patency of the drain. Note if sutures are intact. Document the presence of drainage and characteristics on the old dressing upon removal. Include the appearance of the surrounding skin. Document cleansing of the drain site. Record any skin care and any dressing applied. Note that the drain was emptied and recompressed. Note pertinent patient and family education and any patient reaction to this procedure, including patient's pain level and effectiveness of nonpharmacologic interventions or analgesia if administered. Document the amount and characteristics of drainage obtained on the appropriate intake and output record.

Sample Documentation

1/18/12 1000 Hemovac drain in place in left lower extremity, site open to air. Suture intact; exit site slightly pink, without redness, edema, or drainage. Surrounding skin without edema, ecchymosis, or redness. Exit site and suture cleansed with normal saline. Hemovac emptied of 9 mL sanguineous secretions and recompressed.

—A. Smith, RN

UNEXPECTED SITUATIONS AND ASSOCIATED INTERVENTIONS	• *A patient has a Hemovac drain placed in the left knee following surgery. The record indicates it has been draining serosanguineous secretions, 40 to 50 mL every shift. While performing your initial assessment, you note that the collection chamber is completely expanded. The nurse empties the device and compresses to resume suction. A short time later, the nurse observes that the chamber is completely expanded again:* Inspect the tubing for kinks or obstruction. Inspect the device, looking for breaks in the integrity of the chamber. Make sure the cap is in place and closed. Assess the patient for changes in condition. Remove the dressing and assess the site. Make sure the drainage tubing has not advanced out of the wound, exposing any of the perforations in the tubing. If you are not successful in maintaining the suction, notify the primary care provider of the findings and interventions and document the event in the patient's record.
SPECIAL CONSIDERATIONS	• When the patient with a drain is ready to ambulate, empty and compress the drain before activity. Secure the drain to the patient's gown below the wound, making sure there is no tension on the drainage tubing. This removes excess drainage, maintains maximum suction, and avoids strain on the drain's suture line.

Skill · 32-6   Collecting a Wound Culture

EQUIPMENT

- A sterile Culturette kit (aerobic or anaerobic) with swab, or a culture tube with individual sterile swabs
- Sterile gloves
- Clean disposable gloves
- Additional PPE, as indicated

- Plastic bag or appropriate waste receptacle
- Patient label for the sample tube
- Biohazard specimen bag
- Bath blanket (if necessary to drape the patient)

- Supplies to clean the wound and reapply a sterile dressing after obtaining the culture.

IMPLEMENTATION

ACTION	RATIONALE
1. Review the medical orders for obtaining a wound culture.	Reviewing the order and plan of care validates the correct patient and correct procedure.
2. Gather the necessary supplies and bring to the bedside stand or overbed table.	Preparation promotes efficient time management and organized approach to the task. Bringing everything to the bedside conserves time and energy. Arranging items nearby is convenient, saves time, and avoids unnecessary stretching and twisting of muscles on the part of the nurse.
3. Perform hand hygiene and put on PPE, if indicated.	Hand hygiene and PPE prevent the spread of microorganisms. PPE is required based on transmission precautions.
4. Identify the patient.	Identifying the patient ensures the right patient receives the intervention and helps prevent errors.
5. Close curtains around bed and close door to room if possible. Explain what you are going to do and why you are going to do it to the patient.	This ensures the patient's privacy. Explanation relieves anxiety and facilitates cooperation.
6. Assess the patient for possible need for nonpharmacologic pain-reducing interventions or analgesic medication before obtaining the wound culture. Administer appropriate prescribed analgesic. Allow enough time for analgesic to achieve its effectiveness before beginning procedure.	Pain is a subjective experience influenced by past experience. Wound care and dressing changes may cause pain for some patients.
7. Place an appropriate waste receptacle within easy reach for use during the procedure.	Having the waste container handy means that soiled materials may be discarded easily, without the spread of microorganisms.

(continued)

Skill · 32-6 **Collecting a Wound Culture** *continued*

ACTION

RATIONALE

8. Adjust bed to comfortable working height, usually elbow height of the caregiver (VISN 8, 2009).

Having the bed at the proper height prevents back and muscle strain.

9. Assist the patient to a comfortable position that provides easy access to the wound. If necessary, drape the patient with the bath blanket to expose only the wound area. Place a waterproof pad under the wound site. Check the culture label against the patient's identification bracelet (Figure 1).

Patient positioning and use of a bath blanket provide for comfort and warmth. Checking the culture label with the patient's identification ensures the correct patient and the correct procedure.

FIGURE 1. Checking culture label with the patient's identification band.

10. If there is a dressing in place on the wound, put on clean gloves. Carefully and gently remove the soiled dressings. If there is resistance, use a silicone-based adhesive remover to help remove the tape. If any part of the dressing sticks to the underlying skin, use small amounts of sterile saline to help loosen and remove.

Gloves protect the nurse from handling contaminated dressings. Cautious removal of the dressing is more comfortable for the patient and ensures that any drain present is not removed. A silicone-based adhesive remover allows for the easy, rapid, and painless removal without the associated problems of skin stripping (Rudoni, 2008; Stephen-Haynes, 2008). Sterile saline moistens the dressing for easier removal and minimizes damage and pain.

11. After removing the dressing, note the presence, amount, type, color, and odor of any drainage on the dressings. Place soiled dressings in the appropriate waste receptacle.

The presence of drainage should be documented. Discarding dressings appropriately prevents the spread of microorganisms.

12. Assess the wound for appearance, stage, the presence of eschar, granulation tissue, epithelialization, undermining, tunneling, necrosis, sinus tract, and drainage. Assess the appearance of the surrounding tissue. Measure the wound.

This information provides evidence about the wound healing process and/or the presence of infection.

13. Remove your gloves and put them in the receptacle.

Discarding gloves prevents the spread of microorganisms.

14. Set up a sterile field, if indicated, and wound cleaning supplies. Put on the sterile gloves. Alternately, clean gloves (clean technique) may be used when cleaning a chronic wound.

Sterile gloves maintain surgical asepsis. Clean technique is appropriate when cleaning chronic wounds.

15. Clean the wound. Refer to Skill 32-1. Alternately, irrigate the wound, as ordered or required (see Skill 32-3).

Cleaning the wound removes previous drainage and wound debris, which could introduce extraneous organisms into the collected specimen, resulting in inaccurate results.

16. Dry the surrounding skin with gauze dressings. Put on clean gloves.

Moisture provides a medium for growth of microorganisms. Excess moisture can contribute to skin irritation and breakdown. The use of a culture swab does not require immediate contact with the skin or wound, so clean gloves are appropriate to protect the nurse from contact with blood and/or body fluids.

ACTION

17. Twist the cap to loosen the swab on the Culturette tube, or open the separate swab and remove the cap from the culture tube. **Keep the swab and inside of the culture tube sterile (Figure 2).**

18. If contact with the wound is necessary to separate wound margins to permit insertion of the swab deep into the wound, put a sterile glove on one hand to manipulate the wound margins. Clean gloves may be appropriate for contact with pressure ulcers and chronic wounds.

19. **Carefully insert the swab into the wound. Press and rotate the swab several times over the wound surfaces. Avoid touching the swab to intact skin at the wound edges (Figure 3). Use another swab if collecting a specimen from another site.**

RATIONALE

Supplies are ready to use and within easy reach, and aseptic technique is maintained.

If contact with the wound is necessary to collect the specimen, a sterile glove is necessary to prevent contamination of the wound.

Cotton tip absorbs wound drainage. Contact with skin could introduce extraneous organisms into the collected specimen, resulting in inaccurate results. Using another swab at a different site prevents cross-contamination of the wound.

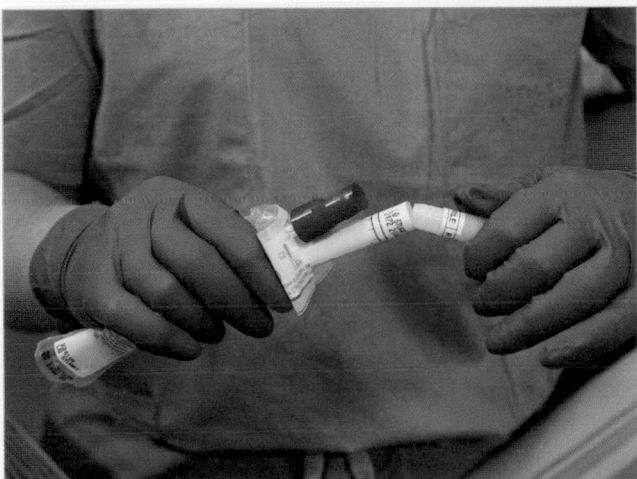

FIGURE 2. Removing cap from culture tube.

FIGURE 3. Swabbing the wound.

20. Place the swab back in the culture tube (Figure 4). **Do not touch the outside of the tube with the swab.** Secure the cap. Some swab containers have an ampule of medium at the bottom of the tube. It might be necessary to crush this ampule to activate. Follow the manufacturer's instructions for use.

21. Remove gloves and discard them accordingly.

22. Put on gloves. Place a dressing on the wound, as appropriate, based on medical orders and/or the nursing plan of care. Remove gloves.

23. After securing the dressing, label dressing with date and time. Remove all remaining equipment; place the patient in a comfortable position, with side rails up and bed in the lowest position.

24. Label the specimen according to your institution's guidelines and send it to the laboratory in a biohazard bag (Figure 5).

25. Remove PPE, if used. Perform hand hygiene.

The outside of the container is protected from contamination with microorganisms, and the sample is not contaminated with organisms not in the wound. Surrounding the swab with culture medium is necessary for accurate culture results.

Removing gloves properly reduces the risk for infection transmission and contamination of other items.

Wound dressings protect, absorb drainage, provide a moist environment, and promote wound healing. Removing gloves properly reduces the risk for infection transmission and contamination of other items.

Recording date and time provides communication and demonstrates adherence to plan of care. Proper patient and bed positioning promotes safety and comfort.

Proper labeling ensures proper identification of the specimen.

Removing PPE properly reduces the risk for infection transmission and contamination of other items. Hand hygiene prevents the spread of microorganisms.

(continued)

Skill · 32-6   **Collecting a Wound Culture**   *continued*

FIGURE 4. Placing applicator swab in the culture tube.

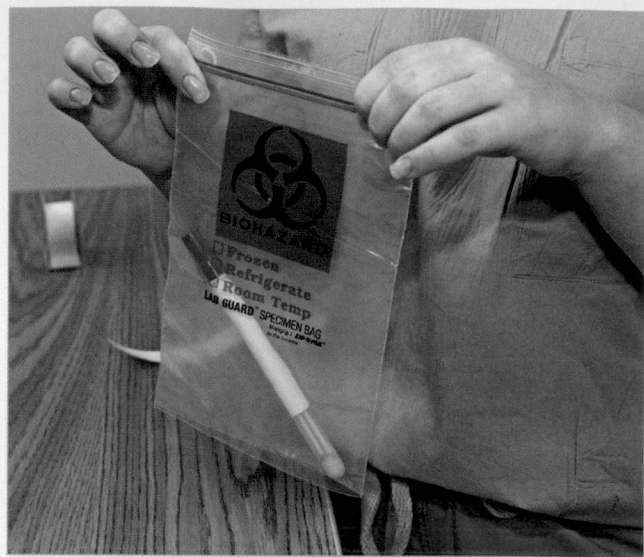

FIGURE 5. Culture container in biohazard bag.

DOCUMENTATION

Guidelines

Document the location and the assessment of the wound, including type of tissue present, presence of necrotic tissue, stage (if appropriate), and characteristics of drainage. Include the appearance of the surrounding skin. Document cleansing of the wound and the obtaining of the culture. Record any skin care and/or dressing applied. Note pertinent patient and family education and any patient reaction to this procedure, including patient's pain level and effectiveness of nonpharmacologic interventions or analgesia if administered.

Sample Documentation

6/22/12 2100 Wound noted on patient's hand 2 cm × 3 cm × 1 cm, red, tender, with purulent drainage present. Edges macerated, without erythema and tenderness. Wound cleaned with normal saline, culture obtained. Skin barrier applied to surrounding area, wound packed with moist saline gauze, dressed with dry gauze and Kling, hand elevated. Culture labeled and sent to lab.

—*J. Wentz, RN*

UNEXPECTED SITUATIONS AND ASSOCIATED INTERVENTIONS

- *The nurse has inserted the culture swab into the patient's wound to obtain the specimen and realizes that the wound was not cleaned:* Discard this swab. Obtain the additional supplies needed to clean the wound according to facility policy and a new culture swab. Cleaning the wound prior to obtaining a specimen for culture removes previous drainage, wound debris, and skin flora, which could introduce extraneous organisms into the specimen, resulting in inaccurate results. Clean the wound and then proceed to obtain the culture specimen.

- *As the nurse prepares to insert the culture swab into the wound, the nurse inadvertently touches the swab to the patient's bedclothes:* Discard this swab, obtain a new culture swab, and collect the specimen.

Skill · 32-7 Applying Negative-Pressure Wound Therapy

EQUIPMENT

- Negative-pressure unit (V.A.C. ATS unit)
- Evacuation/collection canister
- V.A.C. Foam dressing
- V.A.C. Drape
- T.R.A.C. Pad
- Skin-protectant wipes
- Sterile gauze sponge

- A sterile irrigation set, including a basin, irrigant container, and irrigation syringe
- Sterile irrigation solution as ordered by the physician, warmed to body temperature
- Waste receptacle to dispose of contaminated materials
- Sterile gloves (2 pairs)

- Sterile scissors
- Clean disposable gloves
- Gown, mask, eye protection
- Additional PPE, as indicated
- Sterile scissors
- Waterproof pad and bath blanket

IMPLEMENTATION

ACTION	RATIONALE
1. Review the medical order for the application of NPWT therapy, including the ordered pressure setting for the device.	Reviewing the order validates the correct patient and correct procedure.
2. Gather the necessary supplies and bring to the bedside stand or overbed table.	Preparation promotes efficient time management and organized approach to the task. Bringing everything to the bedside conserves time and energy. Arranging items nearby is convenient, saves time, and avoids unnecessary stretching and twisting of muscles on the part of the nurse.
3. Perform hand hygiene and put on PPE, if indicated.	Hand hygiene and PPE prevent the spread of microorganisms. PPE is required based on transmission precautions.
4. Identify the patient.	Identifying the patient ensures the right patient receives the intervention and helps prevent errors.
5. Close curtains around bed and close door to room if possible. Explain what you are going to do and why you are going to do it to the patient.	This ensures the patient's privacy. Explanation relieves anxiety and facilitates cooperation.
6. Assess the patient for possible need for nonpharmacologic pain-reducing interventions or analgesic medication before wound care dressing change. Administer appropriate prescribed analgesic. Allow enough time for analgesic to achieve its effectiveness before beginning procedure.	Pain is a subjective experience influenced by past experience. Wound care and dressing changes may cause pain for some patients.
7. Adjust bed to comfortable working height, usually elbow height of the caregiver (VISN 8, 2009).	Having the bed at the proper height prevents back and muscle strain.
8. Assist the patient to a comfortable position that provides easy access to the wound area. Position the patient so the irrigation solution will flow from the clean end of the wound toward the dirty end. Expose the area and drape the patient with a bath blanket if needed. Put a waterproof pad under the wound area.	Patient positioning and draping provide for comfort and warmth. Gravity directs the flow of liquid from the least contaminated to the most contaminated area. Waterproof pad protects the patient and the bed linens.
9. Have the disposal bag or waste receptacle within easy reach for use during the procedure.	Having the waste container handy means that soiled dressings and supplies may be discarded easily, without the spread of microorganisms.
10. Using sterile technique, prepare a sterile field and add all the sterile supplies needed for the procedure to the field. Pour warmed, sterile irrigating solution into the sterile container.	Proper preparation ensures that supplies are within easy reach and sterility is maintained. Warmed solution may result in less discomfort.
11. Put on a gown, mask, and eye protection.	Use of personal protective equipment is part of Standard Precautions. A gown protects your clothes from contamination if splashing should occur. Goggles protect mucous membranes of your eyes from contact with irrigant fluid.

(continued)

Skill · 32-7   Applying Negative-Pressure Wound Therapy   *continued*

ACTION	RATIONALE
12. Put on clean gloves. Carefully and gently remove the dressing. If there is resistance, use a silicone-based adhesive remover to help remove the drape. **Note the number of pieces of foam removed from the wound. Compare with the documented number from the previous dressing change.**	Gloves protect the nurse from handling contaminated dressings. A silicone-based adhesive remover allows for the easy, rapid, and painless removal without the associated problems of skin stripping (Rudoni, 2008; Stephen-Haynes, 2008). Counting the number of pieces of foam assures the removal of all foam that was placed during the previous dressing change.
13. Discard the dressings in the receptacle. Remove your gloves and put them in the receptacle.	Proper disposal of dressings and used gloves prevents the spread of microorganisms.
14. Put on sterile gloves. Using sterile technique, irrigate the wound (see Skill 32-3).	Irrigation removes exudate and debris.
15. Clean the area around the skin with normal saline. Dry the surrounding skin with a sterile gauze sponge.	Moisture provides a medium for growth of microorganisms.
16. Assess the wound for appearance, stage, the presence of eschar, granulation tissue, epithelialization, undermining, tunneling, necrosis, sinus tract, and drainage. Assess the appearance of the surrounding tissue. Measure the wound.	This information provides evidence about the wound healing process and/or the presence of infection.
17. **Wipe intact skin around the wound with a skin-protectant wipe and allow it to dry well.**	Skin protectant provides a barrier against irritation and breakdown.
18. Remove gloves if they become contaminated and discard them into the receptacle.	Proper disposal of gloves prevents spread of microorganisms.
19. Put on a new pair of sterile gloves, if necessary. **Using sterile scissors, cut the foam to the shape and measurement of the wound. Do not cut foam over the wound.** More than one piece of foam may be necessary if the first piece is cut too small. Carefully place the foam in the wound. **Ensure foam-to-foam contact if more than one piece is required. Note the number of pieces of foam placed in the wound.**	Aseptic technique maintains sterility of items to come in contact with wound. Foam should fill the wound but not cover intact surrounding skin. Foam fragments may fall into wound if cutting is performed over the wound. Foam-to-foam contact allows for even distribution of negative pressure. Recording the number of pieces of foam aides in assuring the removal of all foam with next dressing change.
20. Trim and place the V.A.C. Drape to cover the foam dressing and an additional 3 to 5 cm border of intact periwound tissue. V.A.C. Drape may be cut into multiple pieces for easier handling.	The occlusive air-permeable V.A.C. Drape provides a seal, allowing the application of the negative pressure.
21. Choose an appropriate site to apply the T.R.A.C. Pad.	T.R.A.C. Pad should be placed in the area where the greatest fluid flow and optimal drainage is anticipated. Avoid placing over bony prominences or within creases in the tissue.
22. Pinch the Drape and cut a 2 cm hole through the Drape. Apply the T.R.A.C. Pad (Figure 1). Remove V.A.C. Canister from package and insert into the V.A.C. Therapy Unit until it locks into place. Connect T.R.A.C. Pad tubing to canister tubing (Figure 2) and check that the clamps on each tube are open. Turn on the power to the V.A.C. Therapy Unit and select the prescribed therapy setting.	A hole in the drape allows for removal of fluid and/or exudate. The canister provides a collection chamber for drainage.
23. Assess the dressing to ensure seal integrity. The dressing should be collapsed, shrinking to the foam and skin.	Shrinkage confirms good seal, allowing for accurate application of pressure and treatment.
24. Remove and discard gloves. Apply tape, Montgomery straps, or roller gauze to secure the dressings. Alternately, many commercial wound products are self-adhesive and do not require additional tape.	Tape or other securing products are easier to apply after gloves have been removed. Proper disposal of gloves prevents the spread of microorganisms.
25. Label dressing with date and time. Remove all remaining equipment; place the patient in a comfortable position, with side rails up and bed in the lowest position.	Recording date and time provides communication and demonstrates adherence to plan of care. Proper patient and bed positioning promotes safety and comfort.
26. Remove PPE, if used. Perform hand hygiene.	Removing PPE properly reduces the risk for infection transmission and contamination of other items. Hand hygiene prevents the spread of microorganisms.

ACTION

FIGURE 1. Applying T.R.A.C. pad.

RATIONALE

FIGURE 2. Connecting T.R.A.C. tubing to collection canister tubing.

27. Check all wound dressings every shift. More frequent checks may be needed if the wound is more complex or dressings become saturated quickly.

Checking dressings ensures the assessment of changes in patient condition and timely intervention to prevent complications.

DOCUMENTATION
Guidelines

Record your assessment of the wound, including evidence of granulation tissue, presence of necrotic tissue, and stage (if appropriate) and characteristics of drainage. Include the appearance of the surrounding skin. Document the cleansing or irrigation of the wound and solution used. Document the application of the NPWT, noting the pressure setting, patency, and seal of the dressing. Describe the color and characteristics of the drainage in the collection chamber. Record pertinent patient and family education and any patient reaction from this procedure, including the presence of pain and effectiveness or ineffectiveness of pain interventions.

Sample Documentation

4/5/12 0800 NPWT dressing intact with good seal maintained, V.A.C. system patent, pressure setting 50 mm Hg. Purulent, sanguineous drainage noted in collection chamber and tubing. Surrounding tissue without edema, redness, ecchymosis, or signs of irritation. Patient verbalizes an understanding of movement limitations related to the system.

—B. Clark, RN

UNEXPECTED SITUATIONS AND ASSOCIATED INTERVENTIONS

- *While assessing the patient, the nurse notes that the seal between the transparent dressing and the foam and skin is not tight:* Check the dressing seals, tubing connections, and canister insertion, and ensure the clamps are open. If a leak in the transparent dressing is identified, the appropriate pressure is not being applied to the wound. Apply additional transparent dressing to reseal. If this application does not correct the break, change the dressing.

- *The patient complains of acute pain while NPWT is operating:* Assess the patient for other symptoms, obtain vital signs, assess the wound, and assess the vacuum device for proper functioning. Report your findings to the primary care provider and document the event in the patient's record. Administer analgesics, as ordered. Continue or change the wound therapy, as ordered.

(continued)

Skill · 32-7   Applying Negative-Pressure Wound Therapy   *continued*

SPECIAL CONSIDERATIONS

- Change the wound dressing every 48 hours for noninfected wounds, or every 12 to 24 hours for infected wounds. Time dressing changes to allow for wound assessment by the other members of the healthcare team.
- Measure and record the amount of drainage each shift as part of the intake and output record.
- Be alert for audible and visual alarms on the vacuum device to alert you to problems such as tipping of the device greater than 45 degrees, a full collection canister, an air leak in the dressing, or dislodgment of the canister.
- NPWT should operate for 24 hours. It should not be shut off for more than 2 hours in a 24-hour period. When NPWT is restarted, irrigate the wound per medical order or facility policy, and apply a new NPWT dressing.
- When maceration of the surrounding skin beneath the occlusive dressing occurs, this may be treated by placing a barrier/wafer dressing beneath the transparent dressing to protect the skin. Verify with facility policy as needed.

Skill · 32-8   Applying an External Heating Pad

Heat applications accelerate the inflammatory response, promoting healing. Heat is also used to reduce muscle tension, relieve muscle spasm, and relieve joint stiffness. Heat also helps relieve pain. It is used to treat infections, surgical wounds, inflammation, arthritis, joint pain, muscle pain, and chronic pain.

Heat is applied by moist and dry methods. The medical order should include the type of application, the body area to be treated, the frequency of application, and the length of time for the applications. Water used for heat applications needs to be at the appropriate temperature to avoid skin damage: 115° to 125°F for older children and adults and 105° to 110°F for infants, young children, older adults, and patients with diabetes or those who are unconscious.

Common types of external heating devices include Aquathermia pads (one brand) and crushable, microwaveable hot packs. Aquathermia pads are used in healthcare agencies and are safer to use than heating pads. The temperature setting for an Aquathermia pad should not exceed 105° to 109.4°F, depending on facility policy. Microwaveable packs are easy and inexpensive to use but have several disadvantages. They may leak and pose a danger from burns related to improper use. They are used most often in the home setting.

EQUIPMENT

- Aquathermia heating pad (or other brand) with electronic unit
- Distilled water
- Cover for the pad, if not part of pad
- Gauze bandage or tape to secure the pad
- Bath blanket
- PPE, as indicated

IMPLEMENTATION

ACTION	RATIONALE
1. Review the medical order for the application of heat therapy, including frequency, type of therapy, body area to be treated, and length of time for the application.	Reviewing the order and plan of care validates the correct patient and correct procedure.
2. Gather the necessary supplies and bring to the bedside stand or overbed table.	Preparation promotes efficient time management and organized approach to the task. Bringing everything to the bedside conserves time and energy. Arranging items nearby is convenient, saves time, and avoids unnecessary stretching and twisting of muscles on the part of the nurse.
3. Perform hand hygiene and put on PPE, if indicated.	Hand hygiene and PPE prevent the spread of microorganisms. PPE is required based on transmission precautions.
4. Identify the patient.	Identifying the patient ensures the right patient receives the intervention and helps prevent errors.

ACTION

5. Close curtains around bed and close door to room if possible. Explain what you are going to do and why you are going to do it to the patient.

6. Adjust bed to comfortable working height, usually elbow height of the caregiver (VISN 8, 2009).

7. Assist the patient to a comfortable position that provides easy access to the area where the heat will be applied; use a bath blanket to cover any other exposed area.

8. Assess the condition of the skin where the heat is to be applied.

9. Check that the water in the electronic unit (Figure 1) is at the appropriate level. Fill the unit two-thirds full or to the fill mark, with distilled water, if necessary. Check the temperature setting on the unit to ensure it is within the safe range.

10. Attach pad tubing to electronic unit tubing (Figure 2).

RATIONALE

This ensures the patient's privacy. Explanation relieves anxiety and facilitates cooperation.

Having the bed at the proper height prevents back and muscle strain.

Patient positioning and use of a bath blanket provide for comfort and warmth.

Assessment supplies baseline data for post-treatment comparison and identifies conditions that may contraindicate the application.

Sufficient water in the unit is necessary to ensure proper function of the unit. Tap water leaves mineral deposits in the unit. Checking the temperature setting helps to prevent skin or tissue damage.

Allows flow of warmed water through heating pad.

FIGURE 1. External heating pad electronic unit.

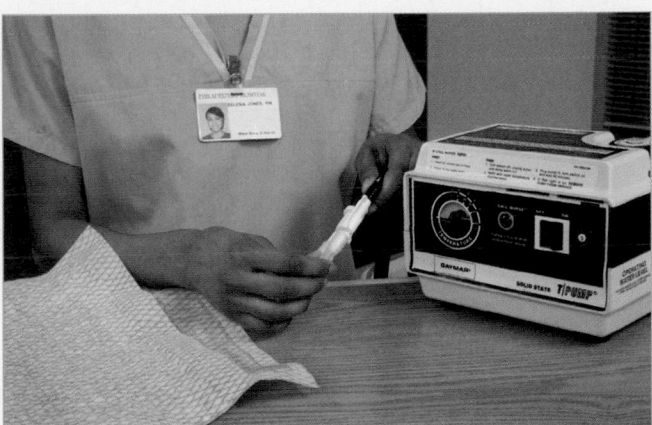

FIGURE 2. Attaching pad tubing to electronic unit tubing.

11. Plug in the unit and warm the pad before use. Apply the heating pad to the prescribed area (Figure 3). Secure with gauze bandage or tape.

12. **Assess the condition of the skin and the patient's response to the heat at frequent intervals, according to facility policy. Do not exceed the prescribed length of time for the application of heat.**

13. Remove gloves and discard. Remove all remaining equipment; place the patient in a comfortable position, with side rails up and bed in the lowest position.

Plugging in the pad readies it for use. Heat travels by conduction from one object to another. Gauze bandage or tape holds the pad in position; **do not use pins, as they may puncture and damage the pad.**

Maximum vasodilation and therapeutic effects from the application of heat occur within 20 to 30 minutes. Using heat for more than 45 minutes results in tissue congestion and vasoconstriction, known as the rebound phenomenon. Also, prolonged heat application may result in an increased risk of burns.

Proper removal of gloves prevents spread of microorganisms. Proper patient and bed positioning promotes safety and comfort.

(continued)

Skill · 32-8 Applying an External Heating Pad *continued*

ACTION

FIGURE 3. Applying the heating pad.

RATIONALE

14. Remove additional PPE, if used. Perform hand hygiene.

Removing PPE properly reduces the risk for infection transmission and contamination of other items. Hand hygiene prevents the spread of microorganisms.

15. Remove after the prescribed amount of time. Reassess the patient and area of application, noting the effect and presence of adverse effects.

Removal reduces risk of injury due to prolonged heat application. Heat applications are used to promote healing, reduce muscle tension, relieve muscle spasm, relieve joint stiffness, relieve pain, and treat infections, surgical wounds, inflammation, arthritis, joint pain, muscle pain, and chronic pain. Assessment provides input as to the effectiveness of the treatment.

DOCUMENTATION

Guidelines

Document the rationale for application of heat therapy. If patient is receiving heat therapy for pain, document the assessment of pain pre- and postintervention. Specify the type of heat therapy and location where it is applied, as well as length of time. Record the condition of the skin, noting any redness or irritation before the heat application and after the application. Document the patient's reaction to the heat therapy. Record any appropriate patient or family education.

Sample Documentation

> 9/13/12 2300 Patient complaining of pain, rating it 5 out of 10. Aquathermia pad applied to patient's lower back for 30 minutes; now rating pain as 2 out of 10. Skin without signs of redness or irritation before and after application.
>
> —M. Martinez, RN

UNEXPECTED SITUATIONS AND ASSOCIATED INTERVENTIONS

- *When performing a periodic assessment of the site during the application of heat, the nurse notes excessive swelling and redness at the site and the patient complains of pain that was not present prior to the application of heat:* Remove the heat source. Assess the patient for other symptoms and obtain vital signs. Report your findings to the primary care provider and document the interventions in the patient's record.

SPECIAL CONSIDERATIONS

General Considerations

- Direct heat treatment is contraindicated for patients at risk for bleeding, patients with a sprained limb in the acute stage, or patients with a condition associated with acute inflammation. Use cautiously with children and older adults. Patients with diabetes, stroke, spinal cord injury, and peripheral neuropathy are at risk for thermal injury, as are patients with very thin or damaged skin. Be extremely careful when applying to heat-sensitive areas, such as scar tissue and stomas.

- Instruct the patient not to lean or lie directly on the heating device, as this reduces air space and increases the risk of burns.
- Check the water level in the Aquathermia unit periodically. Evaporation may occur. If the unit runs dry, it could become damaged. Refill with distilled water periodically.

Home Care Considerations

- A hot water bag or commercially prepared hot pack may be used in the home to apply heat. If using a hot water bag, fill with hot tap water to warm the bag, then empty it to detect any leaks. Check the temperature of the water with the bath thermometer or test on your inner wrist, adjusting the temperature as ordered (usually 115° to 125°F for adults). Checking the temperature ensures that the heat applied is within the acceptable range of temperatures. Fill the bag one-half to two-thirds full. Partial filling keeps the bag lightweight and flexible so that it can be molded to the treatment area. Squeeze the bag until the water reaches the neck; this expels air, which would make the bag inflexible and would reduce heat conduction. Fasten the top and cover the bag with an absorbent cloth. The covering protects the skin from direct contact with the bag. If using a commercially prepared hot pack, follow manufacturer's directions and carefully assess skin before and after heat application.

Skill · 32-9 Applying a Warm Compress

EQUIPMENT

- Prescribed solution to moisten the compress material, warmed to 105° to 110°F
- Container for solution
- Gauze dressings or compresses
- Alternately, obtain the appropriate number of commercially packaged prewarmed dressings from the warming device
- Clean disposable gloves
- Additional PPE, as indicated
- Waterproof pad and bath blanket
- Dry bath towel
- Tape or ties
- Aquathermia or other external heating device, if ordered or required to maintain the temperature of the compress

IMPLEMENTATION

ACTION	RATIONALE
1. Review the medical order for the application of a moist warm compress, including frequency, and length of time for the application.	Reviewing the order and plan of care validates the correct patient and correct procedure.
2. Gather the necessary supplies and bring to the bedside stand or overbed table.	Preparation promotes efficient time management and organized approach to the task. Bringing everything to the bedside conserves time and energy. Arranging items nearby is convenient, saves time, and avoids unnecessary stretching and twisting of muscles on the part of the nurse.
3. Perform hand hygiene and put on PPE, if indicated.	Hand hygiene and PPE prevent the spread of microorganisms. PPE is required based on transmission precautions.
4. Identify the patient.	Identifying the patient ensures the right patient receives the intervention and helps prevent errors.
5. Assess the patient for possible need for nonpharmacologic pain-reducing interventions or analgesic medication before beginning the procedure. Administer appropriate analgesic, consulting physician's orders, and allow enough time for analgesic to achieve its effectiveness before beginning procedure.	Pain is a subjective experience influenced by past experience. Depending on the site of application, manipulation of the area may cause pain for some patients.
6. Close curtains around bed and close door to room if possible. Explain what you are going to do and why you are going to do it to the patient.	This ensures the patient's privacy. Explanation relieves anxiety and facilitates cooperation.

(continued)

Skill · 32-9   Applying a Warm Compress   *continued*

ACTION

7. If using an electronic heating device, check that the water in the unit is at the appropriate level. Fill the unit two-thirds full with distilled water, or to the fill mark, if necessary. Check the temperature setting on the unit to ensure it is within the safe range. (Refer to Skill 32-8.)

8. Assist the patient to a comfortable position that provides easy access to the area. Use a bath blanket to cover any exposed area other than the intended site. Place a waterproof pad under the site.

9. Place a waste receptacle at a convenient location for use during the procedure.

10. Pour the warmed solution into the container and drop the gauze for the compress into the solution. Alternately, if commercially packaged prewarmed gauze is used, open packaging.

11. Put on clean gloves. Assess the application site for inflammation, skin color, and ecchymosis.

12. **Retrieve the compress from the warmed solution, squeezing out any excess moisture (Figure 1). Alternately, remove prewarmed gauze from open package. Apply the compress by gently and carefully molding it to the intended area. Ask patient if the application feels too hot.**

13. Cover the site with a single layer of gauze (Figure 2) and with a clean dry bath towel (Figure 3); secure in place if necessary.

RATIONALE

Sufficient water in the unit is necessary to ensure proper function of the unit. Tap water leaves mineral deposits in the unit. Checking the temperature setting helps to prevent skin or tissue damage.

Patient positioning and use of a bath blanket provide for comfort and warmth. Waterproof pad protects underlying surfaces.

Having a waste container handy means that the used materials may be discarded easily, without the spread of microorganisms.

Prepares compress for application.

Gloves protect the nurse from potential contact with microorganisms. Assessment provides information about the area, the healing process and about the presence of infection and allows for documentation of the condition of the area before the compress is applied.

Excess moisture may contaminate the surrounding area and is uncomfortable for the patient. Molding the compress to the skin promotes retention of warmth around the site.

Towel provides extra insulation.

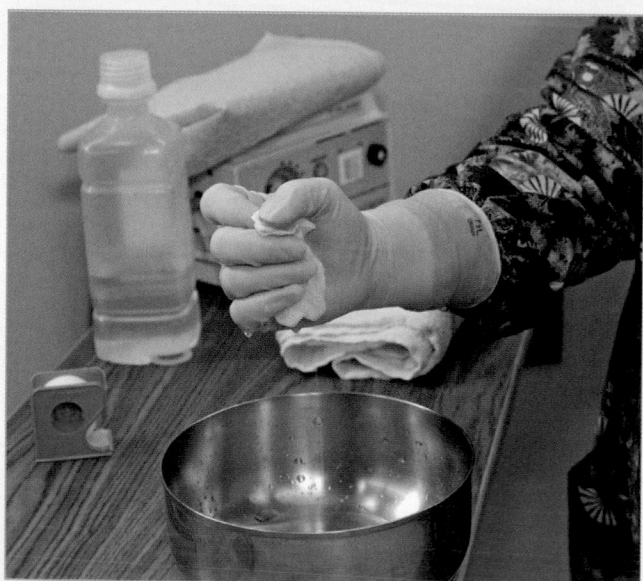

FIGURE 1. Squeezing excess solution out of a dressing.

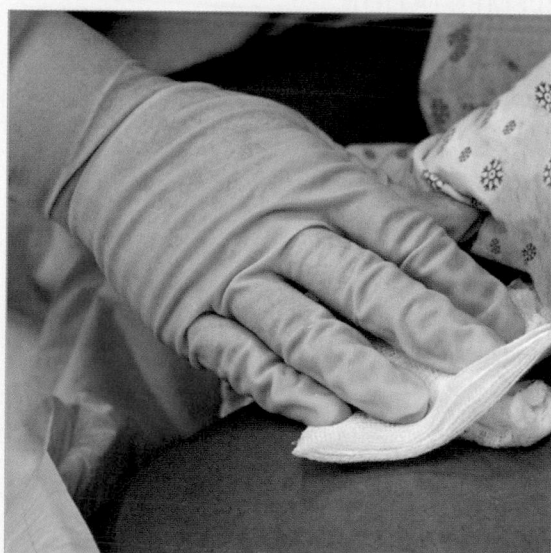

FIGURE 2. Applying single layer of gauze.

FIGURE 3. Applying clean bath towel.

14. Place the Aquathermia or heating device, if used, over the towel.

Use of heating device maintains the temperature of the compress and extends the therapeutic effect.

15. Remove gloves and discard them appropriately. Perform hand hygiene, and remove additional PPE, if used.

Hand hygiene prevents the spread of microorganisms, removing PPE properly reduces the risk for infection transmission and contamination of other items.

16. **Monitor the time the compress is in place to prevent burns and skin/tissue damage. Monitor the condition of the patient's skin and the patient's response at frequent intervals.**

Extended use of heat results in an increased risk for burns from the heat. Impaired circulation may affect the patient's sensitivity to heat.

17. After the prescribed time for the treatment (up to 30 minutes), remove the external heating device (if used) and put on gloves.

Gloves protect the nurse from potential contact with microorganisms.

18. Carefully remove the compress while assessing the skin condition around the site and observing the patient's response to the heat application. Note any changes in the application area.

Assessment provides information about the healing process; the presence of irritation or infection should be documented.

19. Remove gloves. Place the patient in a comfortable position. Lower the bed. Dispose of any other supplies appropriately.

Repositioning promotes patient comfort and safety.

20. Remove additional PPE, if used. Perform hand hygiene.

Removing PPE properly reduces the risk for infection transmission and contamination of other items. Hand hygiene prevents the spread of microorganisms.

DOCUMENTATION

Guidelines

Document the procedure, the length of time the compress was applied, including use of an Aquathermia pad. Record the temperature of the Aquathermia pad and length of application time. Include a description of the application area, noting any edema, redness, or ecchymosis. Document the patient's reaction to the procedure including pain assessment. Record any patient and family education that was provided.

(continued)

Skill · 32-9   Applying a Warm Compress   *continued*

Sample Documentation

7/6/12 0900 Left forearm with positive radial pulse, sensation and movement within normal limits, skin pale with brisk capillary refill. Left medial forearm (IV access infiltration site) positive for redness, edema; no evidence of maceration or drainage. Moist saline compress applied with Aquathermia pad set at 100°F for 30 min. Site assessed every 10 min; no evidence of injury noted. Left arm elevated on pillows.

—S. Tran, RN

UNEXPECTED SITUATIONS AND ASSOCIATED INTERVENTIONS

• *The nurse is monitoring a patient with a warm compress. Procedure requires that the nurse check the area of application every 5 minutes for tissue tolerance. The nurse notes excessive redness and slight maceration of the surrounding skin, and the patient verbalizes increased discomfort:* Stop the heat application. Remove the compress. Assess the patient for other symptoms. Obtain vital signs. Report the findings to the primary care provider and document the event in the patient's record.

SPECIAL CONSIDERATIONS

General Considerations

• Patients with diabetes, stroke, spinal cord injury, and peripheral neuropathy are at risk for thermal injury, as are patients with very thin or damaged skin.

• Be extremely careful when applying to heat-sensitive areas, such as scar tissue and stomas.

● Developing Critical Thinking Skills

1. How would you individualize your teaching about needed supplies, wound care, and resources for the following patients?
   • A homeless man admitted to the hospital for gangrene of the big toe. The toe has been amputated.
   • A teenage gang member treated in the emergency department for a superficial (but long) knife wound
   • An infant who has had abdominal surgery and is now having diarrhea
   • A frail, 80-year-old man who needs daily dressing changes on a draining wound and lives with his blind wife

2. Describe the nursing interventions you would include in a plan of care to prevent pressure ulcers in the following patients:
   • A middle-aged woman, 70 pounds over normal body weight, who has a fractured femur and is recovering at home (she lives alone)
   • A 90-year-old man with cognitive impairment who is confined to bed
   • A 17-year-old girl who is paralyzed from the waist down after a diving accident and is wheelchair dependent

● Practicing for NCLEX

1. Thirty-six hours after having surgery, a patient has a slightly elevated body temperature and generalized malaise, as well as pain and redness at the surgical site. Which intervention is most important to include in this patient's nursing care plan?
   a. Document the findings and continue to monitor the patient.
   b. Administer antipyretics, as ordered.
   c. Increase the frequency of assessment to every hour and notify the patient's physician.
   d. Increase the frequency of wound care and contact the physician for an antibiotic order.

2. Which term would the nurse use to document wound drainage that is thick, odorous, and green?
   a. Serous
   b. Sanguineous
   c. Serosanguineous
   d. Purulent

3. A patient who has a large abdominal wound suddenly calls out for help because she feels as though something is falling out of her incision. Inspection reveals a gaping open wound with tissue bulging outward. In which order should the nurse perform the following interventions? (Arrange from first to last.)
   a. Notify the physician immediately of the situation.
   b. Cover the exposed tissue with sterile towels moistened with sterile NSS
   c. Place the patient in the low Fowler's position

4. A patient, age 16, was in an automobile accident and received a wound across her nose and cheek. After

CHAPTER 32 Skin Integrity and Wound Care

surgery to repair the wound, the patient says, "I am so ugly now." Based on this statement, what nursing diagnosis would be most appropriate?

a. Pain
b. Impaired Skin Integrity
c. Disturbed Body Image
d. Disturbed Thought Processes

5. A patient is admitted with a nonhealing surgical wound. Which nursing action is most effective in preventing a wound infection?

a. Using sterile dressing supplies
b. Suggesting dietary supplements
c. Applying antibiotic ointment
d. Performing careful hand hygiene

6. During a dressing change, inspection of the wound reveals what appears to be reddish-pink tissue in the wound. The nurse interprets this as most likely indicating:

a. A sign of infection
b. Eschar
c. Exudate
d. Granulation tissue

7. The nurse is performing a sterile irrigation of an open abdominal wound. Which intervention should be done first?

a. Direct a stream of solution into the wound.
b. Position the patient so the irrigation solution will flow from clean to dirty.
c. Assess the wound and surrounding tissue.
d. Put on sterile gloves.

8. The nurse is developing a plan of care for an 86-year-old woman who has been admitted for right hip arthroplasty (hip replacement). Which assessment finding(s) indicate a high risk for pressure ulcer development for this patient? Select all that apply.

a. The patient takes time to think about her responses to questions.
b. The patient's age of 86 years.
c. Patient reports inability to control urine.
d. A scheduled hip arthroplasty
e. Lab findings include BUN 12 (elderly normal 8-23 mg/dL) and creatinine 0.9 (adult female normal 0.61.1 mg/dL).
f. Patient reports increased pain in right hip when repositioning in bed or chair.

9. The nurse is explaining to a patient the anticipated effect of the application of cold to an injured area. What response indicates the patient understands the explanation?

a. "I can expect to have more discomfort in the area where the cold is applied."
b. "I should expect more drainage from the incision after the ice has been in place."
c. "I should see less swelling and redness with the cold treatment."

d. "My incision may bleed more when the ice is first applied."

10. The nurse is providing patient teaching regarding the use of negative pressure wound therapy. Which explanation provides the most accurate information to the patient?

a. The therapy is used to collect excess blood loss and prevent the formation of a scab.
b. The therapy will prevent infection, ensuring the wound heals with less scar tissue.
c. The therapy provides a moist environment and stimulates blood flow to the wound.
d. The therapy irrigates the wound to keep it free from debris and excess wound fluid.

11. After an initial assessment, the nurse documents the presence of a reddened area that has blistered. According to recognized staging systems, as what stage would this ulcer be classified?

a. Stage I
b. Stage II
c. Stage III
d. Stage IV

12. An older confused patient sits and slumps in her chair most of the day. She is most likely to develop a pressure ulcer because of what factor?

a. Malnutrition
b. Shearing forces
c. Edema
d. A chronic disease

13. The nurse assesses a stage III pressure ulcer manifested as:

a. Redness that persists when pressure is relieved
b. An open lesion with full thickness tissue loss and visible subcutaneous fat
c. A necrotic area extending through the fascia to bone
d. A reddened area with an abrasion and pain

14. Which action would be a priority in preventing a patient from developing a pressure ulcer?

a. Using waterproof material on the bed
b. Massaging any reddened area frequently
c. Using an air-inflated ring to relieve pressure on areas
d. Using a mild cleansing agent when cleansing the skin

15. In which sequence should the nurse implement the interventions to clean a surgical wound with dehisced edges?

a. Clean the wound in full or half circles, beginning in the center and working toward the outside
b. Moisten sterile gauze or swab with prescribed cleansing agent
c. Clean to at least 1 inch beyond the end of the new dressing
d. Explain the procedure to the patient

● Answers With Rationale

1. ***a.*** The assessment findings are normal for this stage of healing following surgery. The patient is in the inflammatory phase of the healing process, which involves a response by the immune system. This acute inflammation is characterized by pain, heat, redness, and swelling at the site of the injury (surgery, in this case). The patient also has a generalized body response, including a mildly elevated temperature, leukocytosis, and generalized malaise.

2. ***d.*** Purulent drainage is the result of an infection and is thick, odorous, and colored.

3. ***c, b, a.*** Dehiscence and evisceration is a postoperative emergency that requires prompt surgical repair. The correct order of implementation by the nurse is to place the patient in the low Fowler's position, cover the exposed tissue with sterile towels moistened with sterile NSS, and notify the physician immediately of the situation.

4. ***c.*** Wounds cause emotional as well as physical stress.

5. ***d.*** Although all of the answers may help in preventing wound infections, careful handwashing (medical asepsis) is the most important.

6. ***d.*** Granulation tissue is new tissue composed of many small blood vessels, is pinkish red, and fills an open wound when it starts to heal.

7. ***b.*** Positioning the patient in a comfortable position that provides easy access to the wound area and allows gravity to direct the flow of liquid from the least contaminated to the most contaminated area. Positioning should occur before beginning the actual procedure to limit the amount of time the wound is exposed. Nonsterile gloves, as well as gown, mask, and eye protection need to be put on before beginning the actual procedure, after the patient is properly positioned. Then, the old dressing can be removed, the irrigation prepared, and sterile gloves applied to perform the irrigation, with the stream of liquid flowing from the least contaminated to the most contaminated area.

8. ***b, c, d, f.*** Pressure, friction and shear, as well as other factors usually combine to contribute to pressure ulcer development. The skin of older adults is more susceptible to injury; incontinence contributes to prolonged moisture on the skin, as well as negative effects related to urine in contact with skin; hip surgery involves decreased mobility during the postoperative period, as well as pain with movement, contributing to immobility; and increased pain in hip may contribute to increased immobility; all these factors are related to an increased risk for pressure ulcer development. Apathy, confusion, and/or altered mental status are risk factors for pressure ulcer development. Dehydration (indicated by an elevated BUN and creatinine) is a risk for pressure ulcer development.

9. ***c.*** The local application of cold constricts peripheral blood vessels, reduces muscle spasms, and promotes comfort. Cold reduces blood flow to tissues, decreases the local release of pain-producing substances, decreases metabolic needs, and capillary permeability. The resulting effects include decreased edema, coagulation of blood at the wound site, promotion of comfort, decreased drainage from wound, and decreased bleeding.

10. ***c.*** Negative-pressure wound therapy (or topical negative pressure [TNP]) promotes wound healing and wound closure through the application of uniform negative pressure on the wound bed, reduction in bacteria in the wound, and the removal of excess wound fluid, while providing a moist wound healing environment. The negative pressure results in mechanical tension on the wound tissues, stimulating cell proliferation, blood flow to wounds, and the growth of new blood vessels. It is used to treat a variety of acute or chronic wounds, wounds with heavy drainage, wounds failing to heal, or healing slowly.

11. ***b.*** A stage II pressure ulcer involves partial thickness loss of dermis and presents as a shallow open ulcer with a red pink wound bed, without slough. It may also present as an intact or open/ruptured serum-filled blister.

12. ***b.*** Sitting slumped in a chair for an extended period can easily result in shearing force, causing a pressure ulcer. Malnutrition, edema, and the presence of chronic disease may certainly be risk factors for the development of a pressure ulcer, but the most likely cause in this situation is shearing force.

13. ***b.*** A stage III pressure ulcer presents as full thickness tissue loss; subcutaneous fat may be visible but bone, tendon, or muscle are not exposed. Slough may be present but does not obscure the depth of tissue loss. May include undermining and tunneling.

14. ***d.*** A mild cleaning agent is less irritating. The skin should be rinsed, if necessary for the product used, and dried thoroughly.

15. ***d, b, a.*** Cleaning a wound removed microorganisms and debris without introducing microorganisms to the wound or damaging healthy granulation tissue.

Taylor Suite Resources

The Taylor Suite offers these additional resources to enhance learning and facilitate understanding of this chapter:

- thePoint online resource, http://thepoint.lww.com/Taylor7E
- Student DVD-ROM included with the book
- Study Guide for Taylor's Fundamentals of Nursing
- Skill Checklists for Taylor's Fundamentals of Nursing
- Taylor's Clinical Nursing Skills: *Chapter 8, Skin Integrity and Wound Care*
- Taylor's Video Guide to Clinical Nursing Skills: *Skin Integrity and Wound Care*

BIBLIOGRAPHY

Andrews, M., & Boyle, J. (2008). *Transcultural concepts in nursing care* (5th ed.). Philadelphia: Wolters Kluwer Health/Lippincott Williams & Wilkins.

Armstrong, M., & Price, P. (2004). Wet-to-dry gauze dressing: fact and fiction. *Wounds, 16*(2), 56–62.

Association for Professionals in Infection Control and Epidemiology (APEC). Guideline for prevention of surgical site infection. Source: Center for Disease Control and Prevention (CDC). Hospital Infection Control Practices Advisory Committee. Mangram, A., Horan, T., & Jarvise, W. (1999). *American Journal of Infection Control, 27*(2), 97–132. Available at www.apic.org/AM/Template.cfm?Section=Guidelines-_and_Standards&template=/CM/ContentDisplay.cfm&section=Topics1&ContentID=1148.

Benbow, M. (2008a). Exploring the concept of moist wound healing and its application in practice. *British Journal of Nursing (Tissue viability supplement), 17*(15), S4–S16.

Benbow, M. (2008b). Pressure ulcer prevention and pressure–relieving surfaces. *British Journal of Nursing, 17*(13), 830–835.

Bergstrom, N., Braden, B., Laguzza, A., & Holman, V. (1987). The Braden scale for predicting pressure sore risk. *Nursing Research, 36*(4), 205–210.

Bookout, K. (2008). Wound care product primer for the nurse practitioner: Part I. *Journal of Pediatric Health Care, 22*(1), 60–63.

Braden, B., & Maklebust, J. (2005). Preventing pressure ulcers with the Braden scale. *American Journal of Nursing, 105*(6), 70–72.

Brillhart, B. (2006). Preventive skin care for older adults. *Geriatrics & Aging, 9*(5), 334–339.

Bulechek, G., Butcher, H., & McCloskey Dochterman, J. (Eds.). (2008). *Nursing interventions classification (NIC)* (5th ed.). St. Louis: Mosby Elsevier.

Burr, S., & Penzer, R. (2005). Promoting skin health. *Nursing Standard, 19*(36), 57–65.

Butler, C. (2006). Pediatric skin care: Guidelines for assessment, prevention, and treatment. *Pediatric Nursing, 32*(5), 443–450.

Carpenito-Moyet, L. (2008). *Nursing diagnosis: Application to clinical practice* (12th ed.). Philadelphia: Wolters Kluwer Health/Lippincott Williams & Wilkins.

Edmonds, J. U. (2007). Nutrition and wound healing: Putting theory into practice. *Wound Care, 12*(12), S31–S34.

Elliott, R., McKinley, S., & Fox, V. (2008). Quality improvement program to reduce the prevalence of pressure ulcers in an intensive care unit. *American Journal of Critical Care, 17*(4), 328–335.

Fischbach, F., & Dinning M. (2009). *A manual of laboratory and diagnostic tests* (8th ed.). Philadelphia: Wolters Kluwer Health/Lippincott Williams & Wilkins.

Flores, A. (2008). Sterile versus non-sterile glove use and aseptic technique. *Nursing Standard, 23*(6), 35–39.

Gray, M. (2007). Incontinence-related skin damage: Essential knowledge. *Ostomy Wound Management, 53*(12), 28–32.

Halliday, K. (2005). Body piercing: Issues and challenges for nurses. *Journal of Forensic Nursing, 1*(2), 47–56.

Harvey, C. (2005). Wound healing. *Orthopaedic Nursing, 24*(2), 143–157.

Hess, C. (2008). *Skin & wound care* (6th ed.). Philadelphia: Wolters Kluwer Health/Lippincott Williams & Wilkins.

Hockenberry, M. (2005). *Wong's essentials of pediatric nursing* (7th ed.). St. Louis: Elsevier Mosby.

Jarvis, C. (2008). *Physical examination & health assessment* (5th ed.). St. Louis: Saunders/Elsevier.

Krasner, D. (1995). Wound care: How to use the red-yellow-black system. *American Journal of Nursing, 5*(95), 44–47.

Kyle, T. (2008). *Essentials of Pediatric Nursing.* Philadelphia: Wolters Kluwer/Lippincott Williams & Wilkins.

Lindgren, M., Unosson, M., Krantz, A., & Ek, A. C. (2005). Pressure ulcer risk factors in patients undergoing surgery. *Journal of Advanced Nursing, 50*(6), 605–612.

Lloyd Jones, M. (2008). Assessing and managing wound pain during dressing changes. *Nursing & Residential Care, 10*(7), 325–330.

Malli, S. (2005). Device safety. Keep a close eye on vacuum-assisted wound closure. *Nursing, 35*(7), 25.

Meltzer, D. (2005). Complications of body piercing. *American Family Physician, 72*(10), 2029–2034.

Mendez-Eastman, S. (2005). Using negative-pressure for positive results. *Nursing, 35*(5), 48–50.

Moorhead, S., Johnson, M., Maas, M., Swanson, E. (Eds). (2008). *Nursing outcomes classification (NOC)* (4th ed.). St. Louis: Mosby Elsevier.

National Pressure Ulcer Advisory Panel (NPUAP). (2001a). Pressure ulcer prevention: A competency-based curriculum. Available at www.npuap.org/PDF/prevcurr.pdf.

National Pressure Ulcer Advisory Panel (NPUAP). (2001b). Pressure ulcer treatment: A competency-based curriculum. Available at www.npuap.org/PDF/treatment_curriculum.pdf.

National Pressure Ulcer Advisory Panel (NPUAP). (2007a). Pressure ulcer prevention points. Available at www.npuap.org/PU_Prev_Points.pdf.

National Pressure Ulcer Advisory Panel (NPUAP). (2007b). Resources. Staging illustrations. Available www.npuap.org/resources.htm.

National Pressure Ulcer Advisory Panel (NPUAP). (2007c). Updated staging system. Pressure ulcer stages revised by NPUAP. Available www.npuap.org/pr2.htm.

National Pressure Ulcer Advisory Panel (NPUAP). (2007d). Updated staging system. Wound infection and infection control. Available www.npuap.org/pr2.htm.

Negative Pressure. (2008). *British Journal of Nursing, 2008–2009: Wound care handbook.* Author. P. 164–8. CINAHL AN: 2010031958.

NANDA International. (2009). *Nursing diagnoses: Definitions and classification 2009–2011.* West Sussex, UK: Wiley-Blackwell.

Porth, C., & Matfin, G. (2009). *Pathophysiology: Concepts of altered health states* (8th ed.). Philadelphia: Wolters Kluwer Health/Lippincott Williams & Wilkins.

Preston, G. (2008). An overview of topical negative pressure therapy in wound care. *Nursing Standard, 23*(7), 62–8.

Preston, R. (2005). Aseptic technique: Evidence-based approach for patient safety. *British Journal of Nursing, 14*(10), 540–542, 544–546.

Reddy, M., Gill, S., & Rochon, P. (2006). Preventing pressure ulcers: A systematic review. *Journal of the American Medical Association (JAMA), 296*(8), 974–984, 1020.

Rudoni, C. (2008). A service evaluation of the use of silicone-based adhesive remover. *British Journal of Nursing, Stoma Care Supplement, 17*(2), S4, S6, S8–9.

Saver, C. (2008). Cool kids: Children's Hospital of Philadelphia uses therapeutic hypothermia in pediatric cases. *Nursing Spectrum, 17*(22), 14–15.

Scardillo, J. (2005). Postoperative care of patients with surgical drains. *Perspectives in Nursing, 4*(4), 1, 4–6.

Scott, A. (2008). Wound care & cancer. *Advance for Nurses, 10*(19), 29–30.

Smeltzer, S., Bare, B., Hinkle, J. H., & Cheever, K. H. (2010). *Brunner & Suddarth's textbook of medical-surgical nursing* (12th ed.). Philadelphia: Wolters Kluwer Health/Lippincott Williams & Wilkins.

Snyder, L., & Moore, K. (2008). Wound basics: Types, treatment, and care. *RN, 71*(8), 32–37.

Stephen-Haynes, J. (2008). Skin integrity and silicone: APPEEL 'no-sting' medical adhesive remover. *British Journal of Nursing, 17*(12), 792–795.

Stephen-Haynes, J., & Thompson, G. (2007). The different methods of wound debridement. *British Journal of Community Nursing, 12*(6), Wound Care: S6, S8–10, S12–4.

Stotts, N. (1990). Seeing red, yellow and black: The three-color concept of wound care. *Nursing, 20*(2), 59–61.

Thompson, G. (2008). An overview of negative pressure wound therapy (NPWT). *Wound Care,* 13(6), Wound Care: S23–4, S26, S28–30.

Vanderwee, K., Grypdonck, M., De Bacquer, D., Defloor, T. (2007). Effectiveness of turning with unequal time intervals on the incidence of pressure ulcer lesions. *Journal of Advanced Nursing, 57*(1), 59–68.

VISN 8 Patient Safety Center. (2009). Safe patient handling and movement algorithms. Tampa, FL: Author. Available at www.VISN8.va.gov/patientsafetycenter/safePtHandling. Accessed April 23, 2010.

Voegeli, D. (2008). Care or harm: Exploring essential components in skin care regimens. *British Journal of Nursing, 17*(1), 24–29.

Walker, J. (2007). Patient preparation for safe removal of surgical drains. *Nursing Standard, 21*(49), 39–41.

Weber, J., & Kelley, J. (2007). *Health assessment in nursing* (3rd ed.). Philadelphia: Lippincott Williams & Wilkins.

Wooten, M., & Hawkins, K. (2005). WOCN position statement. Clean versus sterile: Management of chronic wounds. Available at www.wocn.org/pdfs/WOCN_Library/Position_Statements/c/vst.pdf. Accessed May 15, 2010.

Worley, C. (2005a). So, what do I put on this wound? The wound dressing puzzle: Part I. *Dermatology Nursing, 17*(2), 143–144.

Worley, C. (2005b). So, what do I put on this wound? The wound dressing puzzle: Part II. *Dermatology Nursing, 17*(3), 204–205.

Worley, C. (2005c). So, what do I put on this wound? The wound dressing puzzle: Part III. *Dermatology Nursing, 17*(4), 299–300.

Activity | 33

QUAN HONG NGUYEN

Mr. Nguyen is a 75-year-old man who had an ischemic stroke (cerebrovascular accident or "brain attack") secondary to thrombosis (formation of a blood clot). His neurological deficits have remained unchanged for the 2 days he has been in the hospital. He is alert, but has hemiplegia on his left side. His wife states, "It will be quite a bit of work to care for Quan at home. My bones and joints hurt all the time. He needs a lot of help turning, moving, and getting out of bed. How will I manage?"

KELSI LESTER

Kelsi is a 10-year-old girl in the pediatric unit as a result of a skiing accident. Unconscious at present, she may or may not regain consciousness. She is on complete bed rest and requires both frequent positioning to maintain correct body alignment and attention to her range of motion.

MAGGIE WYATT

Maggie, a woman in her 30s with a fractured right tibia, is being treated with an external fixation device that has caused an infection. Following therapy for the infection, the patient is being discharged and requires transfer from the wheelchair to her mother's car.

This chapter describes the physiology of movement and factors affecting body alignment and mobility. A comprehensive section on exercise differentiates the types of exercise, explores the role of exercise in disease prevention and health promotion, notes risks related to exercise, and assists in the design of individualized exercise programs. The effects of immobility on body systems are discussed along with related nursing interventions. A practical guide for assessing body alignment and mobility states is included, with pertinent interview questions and physical assessment techniques. Analysis of patient mobility data may lead to the nursing diagnoses of Impaired Physical Mobility or Activity Intolerance or to diagnoses identifying effects of mobility problems on other areas of human functioning. Examples of nursing diagnoses are included. Expected outcomes are identified, and specific nursing strategies are presented. The concluding Nursing Plan of Care illustrates how the nurse uses knowledge of mobility and knowledge of safe patient-handling techniques along with specific nursing interventions to promote fitness and to resolve mobility problems. The Reflective Practice box highlights important considerations to keep in mind when caring for patients with activity deficits.

PHYSIOLOGY OF MOVEMENT AND ALIGNMENT

Purposeful, coordinated movement of the body and maintenance of alignment require the integrated functioning of the musculoskeletal and nervous systems. The following sections review concepts related to movement and alignment.

Skeletal System

The framework of bones, the joints between them, and cartilage that protects our organs and allows us to move is called the skeletal system. Functions of this system include the following:

- Supporting the soft tissues of the body (maintains body form and posture)
- Protecting crucial components of the body (brain, lung, heart, spinal cord)
- Furnishing surfaces for the attachments of muscles, tendons, and ligaments, which, in turn, pull on the individual bones and produce movement
- Providing storage areas for minerals (such as calcium) and fat
- Producing blood cells (hematopoiesis)

The 206 bones in the human body are classified by their shape. Long bones, found in the upper and lower extremities (e.g., humerus and femur), contribute to height and length. Short bones, located in the wrist and ankle, contribute to movement. Flat bones are relatively thin (e.g., ribs and several of the skull bones) and contribute to shape (structural contour). Irregular bones are all those bones not included in the preceding classifications (e.g., bones of the spinal column and jaw).

REFLECTIVE PRACTICE
Challenge to Technical Skills

Last year during my medical–surgical clinical experience, I was taking care of Maggie Wyatt, a female patient in her 30s, with an external fixation device on her right leg. The patient had broken her tibia, and this was the third surgery to try to correct the fracture. The external device had caused an infection for which Maggie was being treated. I was assigned to care for her on the day that she was being discharged. Throughout the day, I formed a close bond with her, and the nurse asked me to bring Maggie to her car when she was ready to leave. I was a little apprehensive about being able to help her into the car with the external fixator in place because she could not bend her leg at all. I had a couple of choices—I could take her down to the car myself and hope that there wouldn't be any problem helping her get into the car, or I could tell the nurse I didn't feel comfortable bringing the patient to the car because I didn't have any experience transferring patients with a device such as this one. However, I really wanted to bring this patient down and see her through the final stage of discharge.

Thinking Outside the Box: Possible Courses of Action

- Take the patient down to the car by myself and do the best I can to help transfer her to the car.
- Explain to the nurse that I don't feel that I have the skills to bring this patient down on my own and ask her to do it.
- Explain to the nurse that I would really like to bring the patient down to the car but that I do not feel that I have the experience to do it on my own; ask her to assist me.
- Ask the nurse, before bringing the patient down, what is the best way to transfer the patient to the car.

Evaluating a Good Outcome: How Do I Define Success?

- Patient receives the highest quality of care and has the least amount of pain possible during the transfer.
- I learn from the experience and gain skills and knowledge for the future.
- Patient is at least not harmed and is possibly benefited by my action.

Personal Learning: Here's to the Future!

Unfortunately, in this case I did not make the right decision. I convinced myself that it could not be that difficult to transfer this very cooperative patient to her car with her mother's assistance. However, I was very wrong. I definitely should have asked for assistance. The car was extremely small, and it was hard to get her to sit across the back seat while keeping her leg completely straight. The patient was experiencing a fair amount of pain from the device. So, every time we tried to get her into the car, she experienced more pain. Fortunately, a physical therapist came outside to help another patient and then also helped us. I realized that not only did I not have the skills to transfer her myself, but also that this was really a two-person job. The physical therapist taught me the best way to transfer this patient, and I learned a great deal from the experience. I was very lucky that my patient was very understanding and accommodating in this situation. I learned how to transfer a patient properly, but most importantly, I realized how important it is to trust your instincts and ask for help when you think you may need it—it's always better to be over prepared than under prepared.

Catherine Barrell, Georgetown University

Reflection

How do you think you would respond in a similar situation? Why? What does this tell you about yourself and about the adequacy of your skills for professional practice? Can you think of other ways to respond? What other skills (cognitive, interpersonal, technical, ethical/legal) would you need to respond well in this situation? What factors do you think might have influenced the nursing student's actions? Suppose that the patient was using crutches or a walker instead of having the fixation device in place. How might the nursing student's actions been different? Imagine that the physical therapist did not arrive on the scene. What would have been the nursing student's next best action? Do you agree with the criteria to evaluate a successful outcome? Did the nursing student meet the criteria? Please explain your response.

Bones are too rigid to bend without damage. Therefore, all movements that change the positions of the bony parts of the body occur at joints. The terms articulation and joint refer to the area where a bone meets another bone. Joints are classified according to the amount of movement they permit and on the basis of the material between the adjoining bones. Types of joints are outlined in Table 33-1. Diarthroses or synovial joints, joints in which there is a potential space between the articulating bones, are freely moving joints. Freely movable joints are discussed here in relation to the topic of activity.

Several types of freely movable joints are found in the body. These include the following:

- *Ball-and-socket joint:* The rounded head of one bone fits into a cuplike cavity in the other; flexion–extension,

TABLE • 33-1   **JOINTS**

Type	Movement	Material Between the Bones	Examples
Fibrous	Immovable (synarthrosis)	No joint cavity; fibrous connective tissue between bones	Sutures between bones of skull
Cartilaginous	Slightly movable (amphiarthrosis)	No joint cavity; cartilage between bones	Pubic symphysis; joints between bodies of vertebrae
Synovial	Freely movable (diarthrosis)	Joint cavity containing synovial fluid	Gliding, hinge, pivot, condyloid, saddle, ball-and-socket joints

From Cohen, B. J., & Taylor, J. (2005). *Memmler's structure and function of the human body* (8th ed.). Philadelphia: Lippincott Williams & Wilkins.

abduction–adduction, and rotation can occur (e.g., shoulder and hip joints).
- *Condyloid joint:* The oval head of one bone fits into a shallow cavity of another bone; flexion–extension and abduction–adduction can occur (e.g., wrist joint).
- *Gliding joint:* Articular surfaces are flat; flexion–extension and abduction–adduction can occur (e.g., carpal bones of wrist and tarsal bones of feet).
- *Hinge joint:* A spool-like surface of one bone fits into a concave surface of another bone; only flexion–extension can occur (e.g., elbow, knee, ankle joints).
- *Pivot joint:* A ringlike structure that turns on a pivot; movement is limited to rotation, for example, turning a

doorknob (e.g., joints between the atlas and axis and between the proximal ends of the radius and the ulna).
- *Saddle joint:* Bone surfaces are convex on one side and concave on the other; movements are side to side and back and forth (e.g., joint between the trapezium and metacarpal of the thumb).

Movements possible at diarthrodial joints include abduction, adduction, flexion, extension, and rotation. Special movements of the forearm, ankle, and clavicle include supination, pronation, inversion, and eversion. These movements are defined in Table 33-2 and illustrated in Skill 33-6, Providing Range-of-Motion Exercises, later in the chapter.

TABLE • 33-2	TERMS COMMONLY USED TO DESCRIBE BODY POSITIONS AND MOVEMENTS
Term	**Definition and Example**
Abduction	Lateral movement of a body part away from the midline of the body. *Example:* A person's arm is abducted when it is moved away from the body.
Adduction	Lateral movement of a body part toward the midline of the body. *Example:* A person's arm is adducted when it is moved from an outstretched position to a position alongside the body.
Circumduction	Movement of the distal part of the limb to trace a complete circle while the proximal end of the bone remains fixed. *Example:* The leg is outstretched and moved in a circle.
Flexion	The state of being bent. *Example:* A person's cervical spine is flexed when the head is bent forward chin to chest.
Extension	The state of being in a straight line. *Example:* A person's cervical spine is extended when the head is held straight on the spinal column.
Hyperextension	The state of exaggerated extension. It often results in an angle greater than 180 degrees. *Example:* A person's cervical spine is hyperextended when looking overhead, toward the ceiling.
Dorsiflexion	Backward bending of the hand or foot. *Example:* A person's foot is in dorsiflexion when the toes are brought up as though to point them at the knee.
Plantar flexion	Flexion of the foot. *Example:* A person's foot is in plantar flexion in the footdrop position.
Rotation	Turning on an axis; the turning of a body part on the axis provided by its joint. *Example:* A thumb is rotated when it is moved to make a circle.
Internal rotation	A body part turning on its axis toward the midline of the body. *Example:* A leg is rotated internally when it turns inward at the hip and the toes point toward the midline of the body.
External rotation	A body part turning on its axis away from the midline of the body. *Example:* A leg is rotated externally when it turns outward at the hip and the toes point away from the midline of the body.
Special Movements	
Pronation	The assumption of the prone position. *Example:* A person is in the prone position when lying on the abdomen; a person's palm is prone when the forearm is turned so that the palm faces downward.
Supination	The assumption of the supine position. *Example:* A person is in the supine position when lying on the back; a person's palm is supine when the forearm is turned so that the palm faces upward.
Inversion	Movement of the sole of the foot inward (occurs at the ankle)
Eversion	Movement of the sole of the foot outward (occurs at the ankle)

The strength and flexibility of the skeletal system also depend on ligaments, tendons, and cartilage. **Ligaments** are tough fibrous bands of connective tissue that bind joints together and connect bones and cartilage. **Tendons** are strong, flexible, inelastic fibrous bands and flattened sheets of connective tissue that attach muscle to bone. **Cartilage** is hard nonvascular connective tissue found in the joints as well as in the nose, ear, thorax, trachea, and larynx. Cartilage in joints functions as a shock absorber and as a bearing surface that reduces friction between the moving parts of the joint. Fat may also provide padding at joints.

Muscular System

The muscular system is composed of three types of muscles: (1) skeletal, (2) cardiac, and (3) smooth or visceral muscles. Muscle tissue produces movement by contraction of its cells. Skeletal muscle works with tendons and bones to move the body. Cardiac muscle forms the bulk of the heart and produces the regular contractions that create the heartbeat. Smooth muscle forms the walls of the hollow organs (such as the stomach and intestines), and is in the walls of blood vessels and other hollow tubes (such as ureters) that connect internal organs. Skeletal muscle is discussed here in relation to the topic of activity.

The skeletal muscle system includes the skeletal muscle tissue and connective tissue that comprise individual muscle organs, such as the biceps. Bones and joints provide form to the body and serve as the levers and fulcrums that make body movement possible. Movement results from a skeletal muscle contracting and exerting force on a tendon, which, in turn, pulls on a bone. Muscles have two differing points of attachment: (1) the attachment of a muscle to the more stationary bone is called the point of origin, and (2) the attachment to the more movable bone is the point of insertion. Between these two points is the fleshy "belly" of the muscle. The excitability, contractility, extensibility, and elasticity of muscles enable them to perform three important functions for the body through contraction:

- Motion
- Maintenance of posture (skeletal muscle contractions hold the body in stationary positions)
- Heat production (skeletal muscle contractions produce heat and help maintain body temperature)

Figure 33-1 illustrates the relationship of skeletal muscles to bones and the use of bones as levers and of joints as fulcrums to produce body movement.

Nervous System

The skeletal and muscular systems cannot produce purposeful movement without a functioning nervous system.

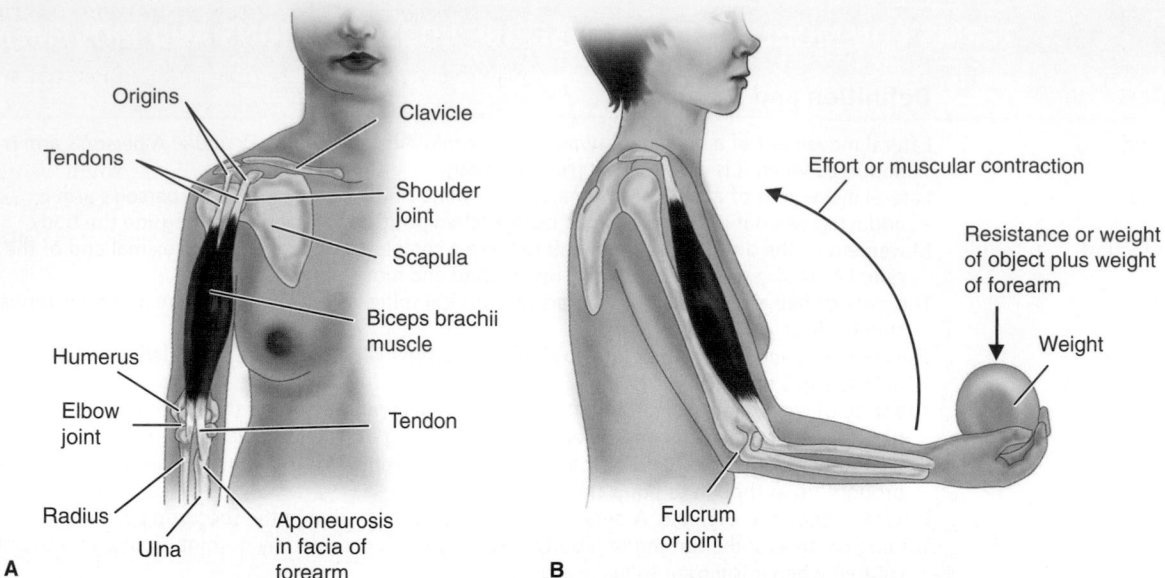

FIGURE 33-1. Relationship of skeletal muscles to bones. (**A**) Skeletal muscles produce movements by pulling on bones. (**B**) Bones serve as levers, and joints act as fulcrums for the levers. The lever and fulcrum principle is illustrated by the movement of the forearm lifting a weight.

Nerve impulses stimulate muscles to contract. More specifically:

- Nerve cells called **neurons** conduct impulses from one part of the body to another.
- The afferent nervous system conveys information from receptors in the periphery of the body to the central nervous system (CNS) (e.g., light pressure on nose).
- This information is processed by the CNS, leading to a response (e.g., "There is a fly on my nose. I want to brush it off.").
- The efferent system conveys the response from the CNS to skeletal muscles by way of the somatic nervous system (e.g., muscles in the arm, wrist, and hand contract, and the fingers brush the fly from the face).

Normal Movement and Alignment

The following concepts are an important part of normal movement and musculoskeletal functioning, and contribute to a person's overall well-being.

Body Alignment or Posture

Good posture, or good body alignment, is the alignment of body parts that permits optimal musculoskeletal balance and operation and promotes healthy physiologic functioning. A person in correct alignment is experiencing no undue strain on the joints, muscles, tendons, or ligaments while balance is maintained.

> Consider Maggie Wyatt, the woman being discharged with an external fixation device in place. Although the device is heavy and awkward and requires her to keep her right leg extended, body alignment is crucial for Maggie to prevent undue strain on other parts of her body. ∎

The criteria for correct alignment in the standing, sitting, and reclining positions are described in the Assessing section later in this chapter.

Balance

A body in correct alignment is balanced. An object is balanced when its center of gravity is close to its base of support, the line of gravity goes through the base of support, and the object has a wide base of support. The center of gravity of an object is the point at which its mass is centered. In humans, the center of gravity when standing is located in the center of the pelvis about midway between the umbilicus and the symphysis pubis. The line of gravity is a vertical line that passes through the center of gravity. The base of support is the foundation that provides for an object's stability. The wider the base of support and the lower the center of gravity, the greater the stability of the object will be. Figure 33-2 illustrates body balance.

Body balance increases when individuals spread the feet farther apart, thereby broadening the base of support, and flex the hips and knees, thus lowering the center of gravity. These two simple maneuvers are important interventions that can decrease the musculoskeletal strain that occurs with excessive stretching or overexertion of a muscle or muscle–tendon unit. Musculoskeletal strain most commonly affects the lower back and cervical spine region. Trauma to the musculoskeletal system is discussed later in the chapter.

Coordinated Body Movement

Using major muscle groups, rather than weaker ones, and taking advantage of the body's natural levers and fulcrums

FIGURE 33-2. The effect of the base of support and gravity on balance is shown. (**A**) The line of gravity passes through the wide base of support. This person is the most stable of the three. (**B**) The line of gravity also passes through the base of support, although the base is narrower. This person is less stable than the person in **A**. (**C**) The line of gravity does not pass through the base of support. This person is unstable.

facilitates the actions of lifting, carrying, pushing, pulling, and moving objects. Major muscle groups include the flexors, extensors, and abductors of the thighs; flexors and extensors of the knees; and flexors and extensors of the upper and lower arms. Use of the arm bones as levers and the elbows as fulcrums facilitates lifting a weight against resistance, the force of gravity—the lever and fulcrum principle (see Fig. 33-1).

Postural Reflexes

Integrated functioning of the musculoskeletal and nervous systems is essential for body alignment and balance. Postural tonus, the sustained contraction of select skeletal muscles that keeps the human body in an upright position against the force of gravity, depends on the functioning of several postural reflexes:

- *Labyrinthine sense:* This sense of position and movement is provided by the sensory organs in the inner ear, which are stimulated by body movement (changes in head position) and transmit these impulses to the cerebellum.
- *Proprioceptor or kinesthetic sense:* This informs the brain of the location of a limb or body part as a result of joint movements stimulating special nerve endings in muscles, tendons, and fascia.

- *Visual or optic reflexes:* Visual impressions contribute to posture by alerting the person to spatial relationships with the environment (nearness of ceilings, walls, furniture, condition of floor, etc.).
- *Extensor or stretch reflexes:* When extensor muscles are stretched beyond a certain point (e.g., when knees buckle under), their stimulation causes a reflex contraction that aids a person to reestablish erect posture (e.g., straighten the knee).

Body Mechanics

Body mechanics is the application of mechanical laws to the human body, specifically in regard to structure, function, and position of the body (VISN 8 Patient Safety Center, 2005). It includes proper body movement in daily activities, the prevention and correction of problems associated with posture, and the enhancement of coordination and endurance. It is important to use the principles of body mechanics during activity and during rest periods, to prevent injury and to prevent sore muscles and joints. The principles of body mechanics are also used to assess and maintain the alignment of patients. The correct use of body mechanics is a part of illness prevention and health promotion. Many activities in which the nurse engages, from as simple an activity as moving a chair, repositioning the medication cart, or reaching to silence a monitor alarm, require understanding and using these principles. Nurses who consciously develop good habits can demonstrate to others proper ways of using the musculoskeletal system. The application of body mechanics is discussed in the Implementing section of the Nursing Process, later in the chapter.

Patient Care Ergonomics

Patient-handling tasks are the primary cause of musculoskeletal disorders among nurses (American Nurses Association [ANA], 2004). Nurses who retire from or leave nursing often cite back, shoulder, and neck injuries as an influencing factor. Forty-seven percent (47%) of nurses in the United States have reported injuries to their back (Nelson, Fragala, & Menzel, 2003). Many nurses say they have had episodes of occupation-related back problems and accept back pain as a routine consequence of the job—which it need not be. Variables that can lead to back injuries or back pain for healthcare workers include:

- Uncoordinated lifts
- Manual lifting and transferring of patients without assistive devices
- Lifting when fatigued
- Lifting after recent recovery from a back injury
- Repetitive movements such as lifting, transferring, and repositioning patients
- Standing for long periods of time
- Transferring patients from beds to stretchers and chairs, wheelchairs, or operating tables; repositioning patients in bed

- Repetitive tasks
- Transferring/repositioning uncooperative or confused patients (ANA, 2004; Occupational Safety & Health Administration [OSHA], 2003)

Patient care ergonomics is the practice of designing equipment and work tasks to conform to the capability of the worker in relation to patient care. It is very important to incorporate patient care ergonomics into nursing practice and patient care. Frequently, it is necessary to move a patient who is weak or unable to move on his or her own. However, as discussed, manual lifting, transferring, and repositioning of patients that involves lifting most or all of a patient's weight are high-risk activities for nurses and patients. A more effective approach to safe patient transfers is thought to include patient assessment criteria; algorithms for patient handling and movement decisions; specialized patient handling equipment, used properly and operated using good body mechanics; and the use of lift teams. The use of mechanical lifts and other patient handling devices reduces the effect of cumulative trauma and injuries in nursing that occur slowly over time because of repeated musculoskeletal stress and decreases healthcare worker fatigue (VISN 8 Patient Safety Center, 2007; Nelson & Baptiste, 2006; Nelson, Fragala, et al., 2003). In addition, the use of assistive patient handling equipment contributes to patient comfort and protects patient dignity, while increasing safety. Patients are less subjected to awkward or forceful handling that can be experienced when lifting, transferring, or repositioning is done manually (VISN 8 Patient Safety Center, 2007; ANA, 2008b).

Research conducted at the VISN 8 Patient Safety Center of Inquiry at the James A. Haley Veterans Hospital Veterans Administration Medical Center, and other institutions, supports the consistent use of standardized protocols and mechanical lifting devices as a more effective approach to decrease the risk of injury for healthcare workers, rather than just using proper body mechanics (Nelson & Baptiste, 2006; Nelson, Fragala, et al., 2003; Nelson, Owen, et al., 2003). The Occupational Safety & Health Administration (OSHA, 2003) recommends minimizing manual lifting of patients/residents in all cases and eliminating lifting when possible. Even routine repetitive care activities such as changing bed linens and bathing patients have the potential to cause back injury. Preventive measures should focus on careful assessment of the patient care environment so that patients can be moved safely and effectively. The use of a back belt does not prevent back injury. In some institutions, specially trained staff members who function as "back injury resource nurses" are responsible for assisting nurses to assess patients. Other institutions have created "lift teams" or "patient lift teams" as part of their institution's safe patient handling policy. Lift teams are groups of specially trained staff that provide safe patient transfers (VISN 8 Patient Safety Center, 2005). The application of patient care ergonomics, specifically safe patient handling and movement, is discussed in detail later in this chapter, in the Implementation section of the Nursing Process.

Orthopedics

Orthopedics refers to the correction or prevention of disorders of body structures used in locomotion. Nurses have long recognized that basic orthopedic principles apply in all areas of nursing, not just to patients with bone fractures or other pathologic skeletal changes. For example, a person who has a sedentary occupation and engages in little physical activity may have poorly developed muscles. A patient who is on complete bed rest is in danger of losing muscle tonus. **Tonus** is the term used to describe the state of slight contraction—the usual state of skeletal muscles. If bed rest is prolonged, there is danger of developing **contractures** (permanent contraction of a muscle) if the patient does not have exercise and joint motion and if good posture is not maintained. The functioning of various internal body processes is also influenced by position and movement or by their absence.

FACTORS AFFECTING MOVEMENT AND ALIGNMENT

Numerous factors, including growth and development, physical health, mental health, lifestyle variables, attitude and values, fatigue and stress, and external factors such as weather, influence an individual's posture, movement, and daily activity level.

Developmental Considerations

A person's age and degree of neuromuscular development markedly influence body proportions, posture, body mass, movements, and reflexes. To promote neuromuscular development in patients of all ages and to facilitate each patient's use of the body to perform self-care actions, nurses need to be familiar with developmental variations in body proportions and neuromuscular development. These variations are presented in Table 33-3 with related nursing assessment priorities and nursing interventions.

> Recall Kelsi Lester, the 10-year-old girl in a coma. Typically, children of this age are highly active and mobile. However, Kelsi is confined to bed due to her accident. The nurse would obtain a history of Kelsi's activity level before the accident to determine her neuromuscular development. The nurse would then use this information to develop an age-appropriate plan of care to maximize Kelsi's level of function. ∎

Physical Health

Problems in the musculoskeletal or nervous systems can have a negative influence on body alignment and movement. Similarly, illness or trauma involving other body systems may interfere with movement because of either the underlying pathology or the treatment regimen. Be sensitive to how both acute and chronic health problems affect a patient's general appearance (posture, body proportions, movements)

TABLE • 33-3	ACTIVITY VARIATIONS BASED ON DEVELOPMENTAL LEVEL: ASSESSMENT PRIORITIES AND NURSING INTERVENTIONS	
Developmental Level	**Assessment Priorities**	**Nursing Interventions**
Infant • Periods of activity and alertness alternate with quiet periods and sleep. • At 3 months: may raise chest and head when prone • By 5 months: head control usually achieved	Assess the following key developmental milestones at these ages: **3 to 6 mo** • Ability to sit • Head control **6 to 9 mo** • Sits steadily • Rolls over • Creeps on all fours • Pulls to a standing position • Has improved hand–eye coordination **9 to 12 mo** • Progresses toward unassisted walking • Is able to pick up small objects	• Encourage parents to examine their baby (e.g., count fingers and toes). • Respond to concerns that parents have about minor variations in newborn's appearance or behavior. • Emphasize that individual variation in activity patterns and neuromuscular development should be expected. • Account for any prematurity when discussing normal developmental progression of preterm infants.
Toddler • Gross and fine motor development continue rapidly. • By 15 months: most can walk unassisted • At 18 months: most can run • At 2 years: can jump • At 3 years: most can stack blocks, string large beads, work simple puzzles, and dress themselves	• Assess progress in walking, running, and jumping. • Assess small muscle coordination (e.g., ability to dress themselves, wash hands, brush teeth). • Distinguish slow developers who fall within normal range from those with developmental lags.	• Help parents to learn and accept their child's uniqueness. • Teach parents the importance of providing a safe environment. • Enthusiastically reinforce and praise toddler's mastery of new skills. • Set limits so that toddler does not overextend himself or herself in drive for mastery of skills.
Child • Muscles, bones, and nervous system develop, allowing greater gross and fine motor control • By age 4: negotiate stairs, walk backward, and hop on one foot • By age 5: skip, jump rope, and jump off heights of several steps • Able to manipulate writing materials • Has acquired all basic mechanisms for physical locomotion	• Use developmental charts to assess gross and fine motor development. • Determine activity level and types of play that involve physical exertion.	• Teach parents that attitudes about the body and exercise are developed during this period. • Counsel as appropriate.
Adolescent • Size increases: growth spurt • Secondary sex characteristics appear • If physically fit: can be a time of boundless energy and great athletic performance • If inactive: may begin a lifelong pattern of unhealthy behavior	• Determine activity level and type of regular exercise. • Evaluate safety of recreational choices. • Screen for scoliosis (lateral curvature of the spine). • Examine muscle mass, tone, and strength and joint mobility.	• Encourage physical activity and limitation of sedentary hobbies. • Lifestyle counseling regarding the importance of exercise and fitness is critical. • Encourage to exercise regularly if necessary. • Caution about gauging physical limits and not "pushing too hard."
Adult • Stands and sits erect and is capable of balanced and coordinated, purposeful movement • During pregnancy: center of gravity shifts because of developing fetus • Activity levels vary greatly	• Assess balance between activity and rest in person's lifestyle. • Note any lifestyle factors or illnesses that interfere with mobility or ability to carry out activities of daily living.	• Fitness counseling is important. • Clarify misconceptions about exercise. • Design and monitor safe exercise programs. • Those with mobility alterations may require special care.

(continued)

TABLE • 33-3	ACTIVITY VARIATIONS BASED ON DEVELOPMENTAL LEVEL: ASSESSMENT PRIORITIES AND NURSING INTERVENTIONS *(continued)*		
Developmental Level	**Assessment Priorities**	**Nursing Interventions**	
Older Adult • Increased convexity in the thoracic spine (kyphosis) from disk shrinkage and decreased height • Flexed posture • Loss of muscle tone • Subcutaneous fat loss • Arthritic joint changes may be present	• Assess general ease of movement and gait. • Assess alignment. • Check joints and their function. • Assess muscle mass, tone, and strength.	Teach and counsel about: • Importance of regular exercise • Need to maintain proper weight • Need for high protein, calcium, and vitamin D–enriched diet • Pacing activities • Using assistive devices safely when needed • Safety-proof homes to reduce falls	

and ability to move purposefully to perform activities of daily living (ADLs). When assessing a patient's response to a mobility deficit, work to:

• Reinforce behaviors that promote healthy functioning (e.g., congratulate a patient who manages transfers well despite left-sided weakness or paralysis)
• Correct behaviors that compound the mobility deficit over time (e.g., a patient with arthritis who severely restricts movement because of joint stiffness and tenderness learns successful adaptive strategies that can be shared with other patients and families; or energy-conservation measures are used by patients with emphysema who have greatly decreased activity tolerance)

Muscular, Skeletal, or Nervous System Problems

Problems with the musculoskeletal or nervous systems may involve one or more of the following health issues.

CONGENITAL OR ACQUIRED POSTURAL ABNORMALITIES

A newborn with developmental hip dysplasia or a clubfoot, a teenager with scoliosis (lateral curvature of the spine), and an older person with kyphosis (increased convexity in the curvature of the thoracic spine) are all experiencing postural abnormalities that affect their appearance and mobility. Nursing responsibilities may include the following:

• Early detection of and referral for these problems
• Exploration and selection of patient education, counseling, and support as treatment options
• Careful attention to positioning, transfers, and exercise
• Education of the patient and family regarding safe self-care activities

PROBLEMS WITH BONE FORMATION OR MUSCLE DEVELOPMENT

Problems with bone formation may include any of the following:

• Congenital problems, such as achondroplasia, in which premature bone ossification leads to dwarfism, or osteo-

genesis imperfecta, which is characterized by excessively brittle bones and multiple fractures both at birth and later in life
• Nutrition-related problems, such as vitamin D deficiency, which results in deformities of the growing skeleton (rickets)
• Disease-related problems, such as Paget's disease, in which excessive bone destruction and abnormal regeneration result in skeletal pain, deformities, and pathologic fractures
• Age-related problems, such as osteoporosis, in which bone destruction exceeds bone formation and in which the resultant thin, porous bones fracture easily

The muscular dystrophies are a group of genetically transmitted disorders that share a common progressive degeneration and weakness of skeletal muscles. They vary in terms of the muscle groups involved and their clinical course. Myasthenia gravis is a weakness of the skeletal muscles caused by an abnormality at the neuromuscular junction that prevents muscle fibers from contracting.

Nursing responsibilities for patients with problems of bone formation and muscle development and functioning include the following:

• Careful collaboration with the physician and healthcare team to determine the motor capacities of the individual
• Patient and family education aimed at developing optional mobility
• Having a solid knowledge base about the underlying disease process
• The ability to position, transfer, and exercise the patient safely, with attention to patient comfort

PROBLEMS AFFECTING JOINT MOBILITY

Inflammation, degeneration, and trauma can all interfere with joint mobility. The term arthritis describes more than 100 different diseases that affect areas in or around joints, characterized by inflammation, pain, damage to joint cartilage, and/or stiffness (Arthritis Foundation, 2007b). Osteoarthritis, also termed degenerative joint disease, is a noninflammatory, progressive disorder of movable joints, particularly weight-bearing joints, characterized by the deterioration of articular cartilage and pain with motion. Once the articular cartilage is damaged, bony deposits (bone spurs) may form in the joints, causing more pain with movement of the joint.

> *Remember Mrs. Nguyen, the older woman concerned about caring for her husband at home. The nurse would need to consider the impact of possible age-related problems as contributing to Mrs. Nguyen's current problems with bone and joint pain. Due to her older adult status, the likelihood of osteoporosis and degenerative joint disease is high. Therefore, teaching to minimize stress on the joints when assisting with her husband's care would be important in preventing possible bone and joint injuries and reducing pain.* ■

Trauma to a joint may result in a sprain, in which the wrenching or twisting of a joint results in a partial tear or rupture to its attachments, or a dislocation, the displacement of a bone from a joint with tearing of ligaments, tendons, and capsules. Any condition restricting joint mobility has potentially crippling effects.

Nurses caring for patients with joint problems work collaboratively with physicians, physical therapists, and other healthcare professionals to maintain joint mobility. Patient education is directed to the patient's mastery of an exercise and care program, which fosters tissue repair and maximal independence in ADLs.

> *Think back to Maggie Wyatt, the woman being discharged after treatment for a fractured tibia. The nurse would need to work closely with other members of Maggie's healthcare team to ensure that joint mobility is maintained, even with the device in place. The discharge teaching plan would include measures to maintain function of the right leg while the external fixation device immobilizes the fractured area.* ■

TRAUMA TO THE MUSCULOSKELETAL SYSTEM

Injury to the musculoskeletal system can result in fractures and soft tissue injuries. A fracture, a break in the continuity of a bone or cartilage, may result from a traumatic injury or some underlying disease process. Healing requires realignment of the bone fragment, immobilization, and restoration of the bone's function. Soft tissue injuries include sprains, strains, and dislocations (dislocations and sprains are discussed in Problems Affecting Joint Mobility). A strain, the least serious of these injuries, is a stretching of a muscle. Nurses need to be knowledgeable in first-aid measures for musculoskeletal trauma as well as in acute and rehabilitative care.

PROBLEMS AFFECTING THE CENTRAL NERVOUS SYSTEM

A problem in any of the principal parts of the brain or spinal cord involved with skeletal muscle control can affect mobility. The cerebral motor cortex assumes the major role of controlling precise, discrete movements. A cerebrovascular accident (stroke) or head trauma may damage the motor cortex and produce temporary or permanent voluntary motor impairment. Basal ganglia integrate semivoluntary movements such as walking, swimming, and laughing. In Parkinson's disease, there is progressive degeneration of the basal ganglia of the cerebrum. Unnecessary skeletal movements result in tremors and muscle rigidity, which interfere with voluntary movement. The cerebellum assists the motor cortex and basal ganglia by making body movements smooth and coordinated. In multiple sclerosis, the myelin sheaths of neurons in the CNS deteriorate to hardened scars or plaques. Plaque formation in the cerebellum may produce lack of coordination of one hand.

The pyramidal pathways convey voluntary motor impulses from the brain through the spinal cord by way of two major pathways: (1) the pyramidal pathway and (2) the extrapyramidal pathway. With trauma to the spinal cord, transection of these motor pathways results in complete bilateral loss of voluntary movement below the level of the trauma.

Patients with injury to the CNS often verbalize that no one talks with them (or with their families) about how the disease may progress and affect their functioning. Nurses caring for these patients need to be knowledgeable about the pathology and clinical course of these diseases to provide appropriate patient education and counseling.

> *Recall Kelsi Lester, the 10-year-old in a coma after a skiing accident. Although Kelsi is unconscious, the nurse must communicate with her, making sure to explain all that is happening to her and all that is being done. In addition, the nurse would need to communicate with Kelsi's family to ensure that they understand what is happening. For example, the nurse needs to explain the reasons for frequent turning, position changes, and exercises while Kelsi is unconscious.* ■

Problems Involving Other Body Systems

The pathology of numerous other acute and chronic illnesses may also affect mobility. Chronic obstructive lung disease and conditions such as ascites may alter posture. Any illnesses that interfere with oxygenation at the cellular level decrease the amount of oxygen available to the muscles for work and thus decrease activity tolerance. These illnesses include anemia, angina, cardiac arrhythmias, heart failure, and chronic obstructive pulmonary disease. Diseases characterized by a larger breakdown of protein than that which is manufactured leads to a **negative nitrogen balance** (e.g., anorexia nervosa and certain cancers) that results in muscle wasting and decreased physical energy for movement and work. Symptoms accompanying many illnesses, such as fatigue, muscle aches, and pain, may also lead to immobility. Bed rest is an important component of treatment for many diseases or trauma states, such as myocardial infarction,

TABLE • 33-4	COMPARISON OF EFFECTS OF EXERCISE AND IMMOBILITY ON BODY SYSTEMS	
Body System	**Effects of Exercise**	**Effects of Immobility**
Cardiovascular System	↑Efficiency of heart ↓Resting heart rate and blood pressure ↑Blood flow and oxygenation of all body parts	↑Cardiac workload ↑Risk for orthostatic hypotension ↑Risk for venous thrombosis
Respiratory System	↑Depth of respiration ↑Respiratory rate ↑Gas exchange at alveolar level ↑Rate of carbon dioxide excretion	↓Depth of respiration ↓Rate of respiration Pooling of secretions Impaired gas exchange
Gastrointestinal System	↑Appetite ↑Intestinal tone	Disturbance in appetite Altered protein metabolism Altered digestion and utilization of nutrients
Urinary System	↑Blood flow to kidneys ↑Efficiency in maintaining fluid and acid–base balance ↑Efficiency in excreting body wastes	↑Urinary stasis ↑Risk for renal calculi ↓Bladder muscle tone
Musculoskeletal System	↑Muscle efficiency ↑Coordination ↑Efficiency of nerve impulse transmission	↓Muscle size, tone, and strength ↓Joint mobility, flexibility Bone demineralization ↓Endurance, stability ↑Risk for contracture formation
Metabolic System	↑Efficiency of metabolic system ↑Efficiency of body temperature regulation	↑Risk for electrolyte imbalance Altered exchange of nutrients and gases
Integument	Improved tone, color, and turgor, resulting from improved circulation	↑Risk for skin breakdown and formation of pressure ulcers
Psychological Well-Being	Energy, vitality, general well-being Improved sleep Improved appearance Improved self-concept Positive health behaviors	↑Sense of powerlessness ↓Self-concept ↓Social interaction ↓Sensory stimulation Altered sleep–wake pattern ↑Risk for depression

surgery, and fractures. Although rest is essential for the healing process, immobility associated with bed rest may cause its own problems. Table 33-4 outlines a comparison of the effects of immobility and exercise on body systems. Nurses need to be vigilant in determining the effects of any injury or illness on mobility and in providing care to facilitate optimal mobility.

Mental Health

Just as an individual's physical health influences body appearance and movement, so also does the person's mental health. Body processes tend to slow down in depression, and there is a lack of visible energy and enthusiasm. Body posture also may be affected. For example, the person with depression often sits with head bowed and shoulders slumped and may lack the energy to eat or even to use the toilet. Even facial movement may be decreased to the point at which the individual's face registers no emotion (termed a flat affect). On the other hand, individuals who are not depressed are more likely to have erect posture and animated facial features.

Lifestyle

An individual's lifestyle, whether active or sedentary, is influenced by many variables, including the individual's occupation, leisure activity preferences, and cultural influences. Activities in many occupations are sedentary. Therefore, individuals wishing to exercise regularly need to plan ahead for these leisure activities by preparing to exercise before or after work hours or during a lunch break. Patients may also participate in leisure activities that are sedentary in nature such as reading, debating, crafts, and watching television. In addition, a person's diet and smoking history are other lifestyle variables that influence mobility. Culture and gender may also play a role, encouraging or discouraging exercise.

Nurses, particularly those involved in community health activities, need to consider appropriate forms of exercise and geographic location before making recommendations to patients from diverse cultures. For example, walking is a commonly prescribed exercise. However, walking may pose a threat to the individual in unsafe environments, such as high-crime areas. Identifying culturally acceptable physical activities is an important step in planning a program of physical activity. Physical activities that are congruent with overall lifestyle and cultural context will be easier to incorporate into daily living (Andrews & Boyle, 2008). An exercise prescription for a Native American might include suggestions for exploring nearby mountain areas, hunting, or even participating in Native American dances as more acceptable methods for increasing activity level.

Attitude and Values

In some families, such as those who hike, swim, or play ball together, children learn early to value regular exercise. As these children mature, they often continue to value exercise and find new ways to incorporate regular exercise into their daily routine. On the other hand, children may be raised in families who are sedentary and where watching sports is the closest anyone comes to exercise. Attitudes and values learned early may be internalized for a lifetime. Individual values also influence the exercise options people make. Individuals who place a high value on physical attractiveness may be highly committed to regular exercise because it helps produce the body they want. Another individual may exercise because of the desire for physical strength, relating strength with power. However, someone more disposed to intellectual pursuits may perceive body development as simply wasting time that could be better used to develop the mind. Sometimes, exercise is viewed as too much of a chore. As a result, individuals avoid exercise. Offer suggestions for

how to incorporate exercise into the person's daily routine, thus making exercise less of a chore.

Fatigue and Stress

Chronic stress may deplete body energy to the point that fatigue makes even the thought of exercise overwhelming. Ironically, regular exercise is energizing and can better equip a person to deal with daily stresses. Refer to the accompanying Research in Nursing display regarding exercise and fatigue in patients with multiple sclerosis. Excessive exercise, however, may stress the body and lead to injury as well as to fatigue.

External Factors

Many external factors can influence activity and mobility. Among these, weather probably exerts the greatest influence over outside exercise. A brisk, clear day is invigorating and invites increased activity. High humidity, very hot and very cold temperatures, rain, and snow, on the other hand, discourage outdoor exercise. Sufficient financial resources for gym memberships, access to exercise equipment, safe outdoor parks and sports areas, the availability of malls for early-morning walkers, support people, and occupational or insurance rewards for exercise can all encourage regular exercise. Discouraging factors include lack of free time, insufficient financial resources for equipment purchase or gym membership, air pollution, unsafe neighborhoods, and lack of support and reinforcement.

EXERCISE

Active exertion of muscles involving the contraction and relaxation of muscle groups is termed **exercise.** Each of the

---

RESEARCH IN NURSING
Bridging the Gap to Evidence-Based Practice

EXERCISE AND FATIGUE

Physical deconditioning contributes to fatigue and impaired health in persons with multiple sclerosis, as well as the general population. Long-term deconditioning contributes to a higher risk of chronic illnesses, such as diabetes and cardiovascular disease. Exercise improves physical fitness, and has the potential to improve other factors, such as quality of life and fatigue. Nurses are in ideal positions to offer guidance, teaching, and support to assist patients in dealing with the often-overwhelming effects of multiple sclerosis, as well as other diseases.

Related Research

McCullagh, R., Fitzgerald, A., Murphy, R., Cooke, G. (2008). Long-term benefits of exercising on quality of life and fatigue in multiple sclerosis patients with mild disability: A pilot study. *Clinical Rehabilitation, 22*(3), 206–214.

Aerobic exercise has been shown to improve fitness in patients with multiple sclerosis. This randomized controlled trial set

out to determine the longer-term benefits of exercise on patients with multiple sclerosis, particularly to look at the effect of exercise on quality of life and fatigue. Participants attended twice-weekly exercise classes and exercised independently once a week for 3 months. The exercised group had significantly greater improvements in quality of life and level of fatigue at the end of the trial, and these benefits continued at 6 months.

Relevance for Nursing Practice

Exercise appears to be a safe, feasible intervention that can have a positive effect in improving the quality of life and reducing fatigue for patients with multiple sclerosis. Discussions about methods to assist patients in maintaining or increasing physical activity should be a part of routine nursing care.

For additional research, visit thePoint.

many different types of exercise can produce different physiologic and psychological benefits.

Types of Exercise

Exercise can be divided into two major types. One is based on the type of muscle contraction occurring during the exercise. The second is based on the type of body movement occurring and the health benefits achieved.

Muscle Contraction

Exercise may be categorized according to the type of muscle contraction involved as being isotonic, isometric, or isokinetic (Fig. 33-3).

Isotonic exercise involves muscle shortening and active movement. Examples include carrying out ADLs, independently performing range-of-motion exercises, and swimming, walking, jogging, and bicycling. Potential benefits include increased muscle mass, tone, and strength; improved joint mobility; increased cardiac and respiratory function; increased circulation; and increased osteoblastic or bone-building activity. When the nurse or family member performs passive range-of-motion exercises for a patient, the patient's muscles do not exert effort. Therefore, although still beneficial, the overall potential benefits are reduced.

Isometric exercise involves muscle contraction without shortening (i.e., there is no movement or only a minimum shortening of muscle fibers). Examples include contractions of the quadriceps and gluteal muscles. Potential benefits are increased muscle mass, tone, and strength; increased circulation to the exercised body part; and increased osteoblastic activity. Nurses encourage both isotonic and isometric exercises for hospitalized patients with limited mobility.

Isokinetic exercise involves muscle contractions with resistance. The resistance is provided at a constant rate by an external device, which has a capacity for variable resistance. Examples include rehabilitative exercises for knee and elbow injuries and lifting weights. Using the device, the person takes the muscles and joint through a complete range of motion without stopping, meeting resistance at every point.

> *Consider Maggie Wyatt, the woman being discharged with an external fixation device in place. A specific exercise routine that includes isotonic and isometric exercises would most likely be prescribed for Maggie. Later in the course of Maggie's treatment after her fracture has healed, isokinetic exercises may be included to strengthen her right leg.* ∎

Body Movement

Exercise activities may also be categorized according to the type of body movement involved and the health benefits they produce. Types of exercise involving body movement include aerobic exercises, stretching exercises, strength and endurance exercises, and movement and ADLs.

FIGURE 33-3. Three types of exercise. *Isotonic exercise* involves muscle shortening and active movement. *Isometric exercise* involves muscle contraction without shortening. *Isokinetic exercise* involves muscle contraction with resistance.

Aerobic exercise refers to sustained (often rhythmic) muscle movements that increase blood flow, heart rate, and metabolic demand for oxygen over time, promoting cardiovascular conditioning. Examples of aerobic activities include swimming, walking, jogging, cross-country skiing, aerobic dancing, bicycling, jumping rope, and racquetball. Aerobic exercise may be further distinguished as having high or low impact. The number of injuries, such as shin splints, related to high-impact aerobic workouts led to the development of low-impact workouts that place less stress on the musculoskeletal system.

Stretching exercises involve movements that allow muscles and joints to be stretched gently through their full range of motion, increasing flexibility. Specific warm-up and cooldown exercises, Hatha yoga, and some forms of dance are examples. Benefits include increased range-of-joint movements, improved circulation and posture, and relaxation.

Strength and endurance exercises are components of a variety of muscle-building programs. Weight training, calisthenics, and specific isometric exercises can build both strength and endurance, increasing the power of the musculoskeletal system and generally improving the whole body. They may or may not have aerobic benefit.

Movement and ADLs include housecleaning, running after playful toddlers, climbing stairs instead of riding in elevators, and so on. Household activities can also contribute to an active lifestyle.

Effects of Exercise on Major Body Systems

The human body was designed for motion, and regular exercise is necessary for its healthy functioning. Individuals who choose inactive lifestyles or who are forced into inactivity by illness or injury place themselves at high risk for serious health problems. The effects of regular exercise on major body systems are explored in the following sections and outlined previously in Table 33-4. Individuals differ in the benefits they receive from exercise based on the patient's age and overall health status.

Cardiovascular System

To meet the demand for oxygen created by the rhythmic contraction and relaxation of skeletal muscle groups, the supply of oxygenated blood to skeletal muscle needs to be increased. The cardiovascular system meets this challenge by increasing the heart rate, increasing the contractile strength of the myocardium, and increasing stroke volume (volume of blood ejected), thus increasing cardiac output. Arterial (systolic) blood pressure is increased, and blood is shunted from the nonexercising tissues to the heart and muscles. Exercise also improves venous return because the contracting muscles compress superficial veins and push blood back to the heart against gravity. Over time, with cardiovascular conditioning, regular exercise produces the following benefits:

- Increased efficiency of the heart
- Decreased heart rate and blood pressure
- Increased blood flow to all body parts
- Increased circulating fibrinolysin (substance that breaks up small clots)

Respiratory System

The respiratory and cardiovascular systems work together to make increased oxygen available to the muscles. During exercise, the depth of respiration, respiratory rate, gas exchange at the alveolar level, and rate of carbon dioxide excretion are increased. Over time, regular exercise leads to improved pulmonary functioning.

Musculoskeletal System

The rhythmic contraction and relaxation of muscle groups during exercise result in increased muscle mass, tone, strength, and increased joint mobility. The more a person exercises, the more strength he or she has to exercise or work in the future. Regular exercise produces the following benefits:

- Increased muscle efficiency (strength) and flexibility
- Increased coordination
- Increased efficiency of nerve impulse transmission

Regular exercise is also believed to slow the effects of aging. For example, exercise has been shown to help prevent **osteoporosis** (the process of bone demineralization) associated with aging. Exercise has also been associated with minimizing bone loss during chemotherapy. Refer to the accompanying Research in Nursing display regarding exercise and bone mineral density.

Metabolic Processes

The metabolic rate increases during exercise so that sufficient glucose and fatty acids can be converted to provide the energy needed for increased muscle function. During strenuous exercise, the metabolic rate can increase to up to 20 times normal. Increased body heat and waste products are also produced. With regular exercise, the efficiency of metabolism and body temperature regulation is increased.

Gastrointestinal System

During exercise, blood is shunted away from the stomach and intestines to the exercising muscles. With regular exercise:

- Appetite is increased.
- Intestinal tone is increased, which improves digestion and elimination.
- Weight may be controlled.

Urinary System

Regular exercise increases blood circulation, including improved blood flow to the kidneys. This allows the kidneys to maintain the body's fluid balance and acid–base balance more efficiently and to excrete body wastes.

Skin

Increased circulation resulting from regular exercise nourishes the skin. Thus, regular exercise aids in promoting the overall general health of the skin.

Psychosocial Outlook

Some of the most important benefits of regular exercise are psychological. These benefits include:

- Increased energy, vitality, and general well-being
- Improved sleep
- Improved appearance (body image)

RESEARCH IN NURSING
Bridging the Gap to Evidence-Based Practice

EXERCISE, BONE MINERAL DENSITY, AND CHEMOTHERAPY

Significant bone loss is an adverse effect of breast cancer treatment that often goes undetected and untreated in pre- and postmenopausal women. Osteoporosis is becoming a long-term complication of breast cancer treatment. Breast cancer survivors are almost five times as likely to experience a vertebral fracture in the year following treatment than healthy women. Nurses are in ideal positions to offer guidance, teaching, and support to assist cancer patients in dealing with the potential for this devastating adverse effect of the disease and treatment.

Related Research

Schwartz, A., Winters-Stone, K., Ballucci, B. (2007). Exercise effects on bone mineral density in women with breast cancer receiving adjuvant chemotherapy. *Oncology Nursing Forum, 34*(3), 627–633.

In this randomized clinical trial, the effects of aerobic and resistance exercise on changes in bone mineral density was examined. Participants were randomized to aerobic or resistance exercise and usual care. Patients completed exercise testing and bone mineral density assessment at the beginning

For additional research, visit thePoint.

of their chemotherapy treatment and at 6 months. Aerobic exercise preserved bone mineral density significantly better compared to usual care. Resistance exercise also reduced treatment-related bone loss to a lesser degree. In addition, participants in the aerobic and resistance exercise groups experienced improved aerobic capacity and muscle strength.

Implications for Nurses

This study suggests that weight bearing aerobic exercise reduces declines in bone mineral density experienced by women receiving chemotherapy. It also suggests that moderate intensity exercise maintains, and may improve, aerobic capacity and muscle strength in women undergoing chemotherapy. Encouraging women receiving chemotherapy to exercise may prevent or at least minimize bone loss as a result of chemotherapy and may prevent or delay the long-term effects of osteoporosis and improve overall physical well-being. Discussions about methods to assist patients in maintaining or increasing physical activity during or following cancer treatment should be a part of routine nursing care.

- Improved self-concept
- Increased positive health behaviors

Risks Related to Exercise

A common reason many people offer for not exercising is fear of experiencing personal harm. Personal harm can include cardiovascular events, muscle injuries, or falling. Be responsive to these fears with realistic knowledge of the risks associated with exercise and specific prevention strategies.

Precipitation of a Cardiac Event

Although the risk of exercise precipitating a major cardiac event in a healthy individual is minimal, the risk is much higher for individuals with known or suspected cardiovascular disease. Thus, a pre-exercise medical examination, medical supervision during exercise, and an individually designed exercise plan are recommended for sedentary people older than 35 years of age and for any person with a past or current cardiovascular condition, diabetes, osteoporosis, asthma, or obesity (NIH, 2005).

Orthopedic Discomfort and Disability

Orthopedic problems caused by irritation of bones, tendons, ligaments, and sometimes muscles are the most common injuries associated with exercise. This irritation may result from added weight-bearing stress or from collision with the ground, an object, or another person. Teach patients to follow the guideline of rest, ice, compression, and elevation (RICE) if injury occurs. While the injured area is rested, recommend

the application of ice to minimize pain and edema, an elastic bandage for compression, and elevation of the injured area to help reduce edema. Advise the patient to contact a physician immediately to diagnose the extent of the injury. Instruct the patient to discontinue exercise until the injury is healed.

Other Health Problems

Other types of health problems may be associated with different types of exercise, depending to a large extent on external factors (temperature on a given day, humidity, pollution index, safety of the neighborhood) as well as internal factors (age, history of previous injury, overuse, obesity, health history). Examples of other health problems related to exercise include heat exhaustion or heat stroke, exercise-induced asthma, and chest pain related to overexertion.

Effects of Immobility on the Body

Lack of exercise, inactivity, or immobility related to illness or injury place a person at high risk for serious health problems. Immobility can affect the major body systems and has been linked to a predisposition to many chronic health problems (Peterson, 2007). Like the benefits a person receives from exercise, complications resulting from immobility differ in their occurrence and severity based on the patient's age and overall health status.

Cardiovascular System

The primary and serious effects of immobility on the cardiovascular system include increased cardiac workload, orthostatic hypotension, and venous stasis, with resulting venous thrombosis. Immobility results in an increased workload for the heart. With immobility, the skeletal muscles that normally compress valves in the leg veins and help to pump the blood back to the right side of the heart do not adequately contract. There is less resistance offered by the blood vessels and blood pools in the veins, thus increasing the venous blood pressure and changing the distribution of blood in the immobile person. As a result, the heart rate, cardiac output, and stroke volume increase.

Immobility predisposes the patient to thrombi formation because of venous stasis, especially in the legs, where normal muscular activity helps move blood toward the central circulatory system. During periods of immobility, calcium leaves the bones and enters the blood, where it influences blood coagulation, leading to an increased risk of thrombus formation.

A person who is immobile is more susceptible to developing orthostatic hypotension. The normal neurovascular adjustments that occur to maintain systemic blood pressure with position changes are not used during periods of inactivity and become inoperative. A drop in blood pressure may occur as a result of a lack of vasoconstriction when changing from a supine to an upright position. The person tends to feel weak and faint when this condition occurs. See Chapter 24 for additional discussion of orthostatic hypotension.

Respiratory System

The effects of immobility on the respiratory system are related to decreased ventilatory effort and increased respiratory secretions. Immobility causes a decrease in the depth and rate of respirations, in part because of a reduced need for oxygen by body cells. When areas of lung tissues are not used over time, atelectasis (incomplete expansion or collapse of lung tissue) may occur. Immobility results in a poor exchange of carbon dioxide and oxygen, upsets their balance in the body, and eventually causes an acid–base imbalance.

When a person is immobile, the movement of secretions in the respiratory tract is decreased, causing secretions to pool and leading to respiratory congestion. These conditions predispose the person to respiratory tract infections. Hypostatic pneumonia is a type of pneumonia that results from inactivity and immobility. The situation worsens when the person is dehydrated or using pharmacologic agents that increase the tenacity of secretions, depress the coughing mechanism, and/or depress respirations.

Decreased movement in the thoracic cage during respirations also occurs with immobility. This decrease may be due to loss of tonus in muscles involved with respirations, pressure on the chest wall because of the patient's position in bed, or depression of the respiratory system by various pharmaceutical agents.

Musculoskeletal System

Effects of immobility on the musculoskeletal system are rapidly seen in patients confined to bed. People attempting to walk after several days of bed rest are often surprised to find how weak their legs have become. Immobility (musculoskeletal disuse) leads to decreased muscle size (**atrophy**), tone, and strength; decreased joint mobility and flexibility; bone demineralization; and limited endurance, resulting in problems with ADLs.

Immobility is often the cause of contractures and **ankylosis,** a consolidation and immobilization of a joint. Contractures result from atrophy of muscles, with subsequent inability to function, and from a decrease in the muscle's strength, coordination, and endurance. A joint can be permanently fixed when ankylosed.

The process of bone demineralization (osteoporosis) is also increased in immobile patients. Normally, the stress and strain of weight-bearing activity stimulate bone formation and balance it with the natural destruction of bone. With immobility, however, bone formation slows while breakdown increases, resulting in a net loss of bone calcium, phosphorus, and bone matrix. This condition, disuse osteoporosis, is characterized by bones that may be either spongy or brittle. Bone demineralization may result in pathologic fractures related to the bone's brittleness, bone deformities related to the bone's sponginess, arthropathy (joint disease) related to calcium depletion in the joints, or renal calculi (stones) related to the excessive excretion of calcium through the kidneys and urinary tract.

Metabolic Processes

Because the resting body requires less energy, the cellular demand for oxygen is decreased, leading to a decreased metabolic rate. In many immobilized patients, however, factors such as fever, trauma, chronic illness, or poor nutrition can actually increase the body's metabolic demands and increase catabolism (the breakdown of the body's protein stores to provide energy to meet the body's energy requirements). If unchecked, this process results in muscle wasting and a negative nitrogen balance. Anorexia, or decreased appetite, often accompanies and compounds this problem. Negative nitrogen balance and poor nutrition thus worsen the muscle atrophy and weakness already resulting from immobility. Numerous fluid and electrolyte imbalances, alterations in the exchange of nutrients and gases at the cellular level, and gastrointestinal (GI) problems can all result from metabolic disturbances.

Gastrointestinal System

Immobility leads to disturbances in appetite, decreased food intake, altered protein metabolism, and poor digestion and utilization of food. If individuals increase food intake while decreasing energy expenditure, weight gain will result. Normal muscular activity in the GI tract also slows down in an immobile person, which often results in constipation, poor defecation reflexes, and an inability to expel feces and gas adequately.

Urinary System

In a nonerect patient, the kidneys and ureters are level, and urine remains in the renal pelvis for a longer period of time

FOCUSED ASSESSMENT GUIDE • 33-1

MOBILITY AND EXERCISE

Factors to Assess	Questions and Approaches
Daily activity level	Describe the activities you normally carry out during a routine day. What type of physical exercise is a part of your daily lifestyle? • Activities of daily living • Type, frequency, duration of physical exercise • Past history of activity and exercise; recent changes
Endurance	Describe how much and what type of activity makes you tired. • History of dizziness, dyspnea, frequent pauses in activity to rest, or marked increase in respiratory rate after moderate activity
Exercise/fitness goals	What exercise or fitness goals are you currently working on? • Attitudes about exercise and physical fitness • Knowledge of the benefits of exercise • Motivation to exercise • Current exercise and fitness goals
Mobility problems	Do you experience any problems with movement or with more vigorous activity or exercise? If yes, please describe these problems. • Nature of the problem • Onset of disturbance and frequency • Known causes • Severity • Symptoms • Effect of problem on everyday functioning • Interventions attempted and results
Physical or mental health alterations	Are there any physical or mental health problems that may be affecting your mobility? Tell me about them. • Decrease of strength or endurance (e.g., myocardial infarction, congestive heart failure, cardiomyopathy, chronic obstructive pulmonary disease, cancer, gastrointestinal disorders) • Neuromuscular impairment (multiple sclerosis, Parkinson's disease, spinal injuries) • Musculoskeletal impairment (arthritis, fractures, muscular dystrophy) • Perceptual or cognitive impairment (cerebrovascular accident, brain tumor or trauma, vision disorders) • Pain or discomfort (burns, rheumatoid arthritis, chronic pain syndrome, postoperative pain) • Depression or severe anxiety (neurosis, schizophrenia)
External factors affecting mobility	Is there anything else you can think of that limits your ability to get around? • Environmental factors (stairs, lack of railings or other assistive devices, unsafe neighborhood) • Financial resources

before gravity causes it to move into the ureters and bladder. Urinary stasis favors the growth of bacteria that, when present in sufficient quantities, may cause urinary tract infections. Poor perineal hygiene, incontinence, decreased fluid intake, or an indwelling urinary catheter can increase the risk for urinary tract infection in an immobile patient.

Immobility also predisposes the patient to renal calculi, or kidney stones, which are a consequence of high levels of urinary calcium; urinary retention and incontinence resulting from decreased bladder muscle tone; the formation of alkaline urine, which facilitates growth of urinary bacteria; and decreased urine volume.

Skin

In patients who are immobile, especially those who are older or debilitated, the impaired circulation that accompanies immobility may result in serious skin breakdown. Prolonged pressure over bony prominences produces areas of breakdown, leading to pressure ulcers. Pressure ulcers can progress from stage 1, redness, to stage 4, destruction of subcutaneous tissue and muscle. Pressure ulcers are described in detail in Chapter 32.

Psychosocial Outlook

When a person can no longer move the body purposefully and needs to depend on someone else for assistance with simple self-care activities, the person's sense of self is often threatened. Skeletal deformities can influence body image, an inability to meet role expectations can decrease self-concept, and a prolonged period of lying dependent in bed can lead to feelings of worthlessness and diminished self-esteem.

Immobility can produce exaggerated emotional responses to the stresses of everyday living. Patients can become apathetic, possibly because of decreased sensory stimulation, and develop altered thought processes. Lack of mobility can also diminish an individual's opportunities to interact socially and deprive that person of normal support systems. Coping difficulties are common for both immobilized patients and their families. Furthermore, the amount of time immobilized patients spend resting often disrupts their usual sleep–wake patterns and may interfere with both the quantity and quality of their sleep.

> *Remember Kelsi Lester, the 10-year-old girl who is unconscious. Due to her current state, Kelsi is at high risk for developing any or all of the possible complications associated with immobility, including thrombi, pneumonia, constipation, urinary tract infection, and skin breakdown. Although she is unconscious, the effects of immobility ultimately can affect her psychosocial outlook. The nurse would integrate knowledge of the effects of immobility when developing Kelsi's plan of care that would include close frequent assessment, early detection, and prompt intervention to prevent any possible complications. Vigilant nursing care is essential.* ∎

THE NURSING PROCESS
Assessing

The comprehensive nursing assessment uses both interview and physical assessment skills to elicit data about the patient's mobility status. When alterations in a patient's physical or mental health state result in impaired mobility, additional specific assessment skills are needed to determine the patient's physical limitations.

Nursing History

During the nursing history, interview patients regarding their daily activity level, endurance, exercise and fitness goals, mobility problems, physical or mental health alterations that affect mobility, and external factors affecting mobility. Questioning patients about their fitness goals is important to provide an indication of the patient's view of health. This interviewing strategy communicates to patients that you expect them to be exercising and is itself a powerful teaching tool.

The accompanying Focused Assessment Guide illustrates elements common to obtaining a mobility status history. When a problem exists, assess the nature of the problem, its onset and frequency, known causes, severity and symptoms, effects on everyday functioning, the interventions attempted by the patient, and the results.

Physical Assessment

Physical assessment of mobility status includes an assessment of general ease of movement and gait; alignment, joint structure, and function; muscle mass, tone, and strength; and endurance. Table 33-5 provides normal findings and significant alterations. During this assessment, direct attention to both structure and function. The patient's ability to stand, walk, sit up, and grasp are important because these enable the patient to wash, dress, and feed himself or herself and perform other basic ADLs.

Older adults make up an increasingly larger part of the general, as well as hospital, population. Functional decline (inability to care for oneself by bathing, dressing, toileting, eating, transferring, and/or maintaining continence) in hospitalized patients can have severe consequences. Changes in mobility status contribute to this functional decline. Assessment of an older patient's ability to care for her- or himself is an important part of a mobility assessment; this assessment can provide clues to changes in health and prevent, or prevent further, functional decline. See the accompanying Focus on the Older Adult for an example of a tool to use to measure older adults' capacity to care for themselves and assist nurses to detect subtle changes in health and prevent functional decline.

GENERAL EASE OF MOVEMENT AND GAIT

Begin the physical assessment of an ambulatory patient the moment the patient walks into the room. Voluntarily controlled, fluid, and coordinated body movements are keys to the integrated functioning of the skeletal, muscle, and nervous systems. Note whether the patient's body movements are quick and sure or slow and deliberate. These observations communicate both a sense of the person's emotional status and self-care abilities. Common involuntary movements that may be observed include tremors (continuous quivering of whole muscles or major portions of a muscle) and tics (irregularly occurring spasmodic movements such as winking, grimacing, or shoulder shrugging).

Note the gait of the patient who is ambulatory. The patient's movements while walking should be coordinated

TABLE • 33-5 OVERVIEW OF THE PHYSICAL ASSESSMENT OF MOBILITY STATUS

Component	Normal Finding	Significant Alterations
General ease of movement	Body movements are: • Voluntarily controlled (purposeful) • Fluid • Coordinated	Involuntary movements: • Tremors • Tics • Chorea • Athetosis • Dystonia • Fasciculations • Myoclonus • Oral–facial dyskinesias
Gait and posture	Head erect, vertebrae are straight Knees and feet point forward Arms at side with elbows flexed Arms swing freely in alternation with leg swings While one leg is in the stance phase, the other is in the swing phase	Abnormalities of gait and posture: • Spastic hemiparesis • Scissors gait • Steppage gait • Sensory ataxia • Cerebellar ataxia • Parkinsonian gait • Gait of old age • Use of assistive devices for ambulation
Alignment	Independent maintenance of correct alignment: • In the standing and sitting position, a straight line can be drawn from the ear through the shoulder and hip • In bed, the head, shoulders, and hips are aligned	Abnormal spinal curvatures Inability to maintain correct alignment independently
Joint structure and function	Absence of joint deformities Full range of motion	Limitation in the normal range of motion Increased joint mobility Swelling or tenderness in or around the joint Heat or redness Crepitation Deformities Muscle atrophy, nodules, skin changes Asymmetry of involvement
Muscle mass, tone, and strength	Adequate muscle mass, tone, and strength to accomplish movement and work	Atrophy, hypertrophy Hypotonicity (flaccidity), spasticity Paresis or paralysis
Endurance	Ability to turn in bed, maintain correct alignment when sitting and standing, ambulate, and perform self-care activities	Physiologic or psychological inability to tolerate an increase in activity: • Significantly increased pulse, respiration, blood pressure after rest • Shortness of breath, dyspnea • Weakness • Pallor • Confusion • Vertigo • Pain

and the posture well balanced. The arms should swing freely in a rhythm alternating with the legs. Figure 33-4 illustrates stance and swing, the two phases of the normal gait. The heel of the right foot strikes the ground (stance), while the toe of the left foot pushes off and leaves the ground, moving the leg from behind to in front of the body (swing). While one leg is in the stance phase, the other is in the swing phase. Detection of gait abnormalities is impor-

tant because they may place the individual at risk for injury and also because they may indicate intoxication or a neuromuscular disorder.

Note whether the patient uses any assistive devices such as wheelchair, brace, cane, walker, or crutches to aid in ambulation. Also, determine whether this aid is meeting the patient's needs, if the aid is required for mobility, and if the aid is being used safely.

FOCUS ON THE OLDER ADULT

KATZ INDEX OF INDEPENDENCE IN ACTIVITIES OF DAILY LIVING

ACTIVITIES POINTS (1 OR 0)	INDEPENDENCE: (1 POINT) **NO** supervision, direction, or personal assistance	DEPENDENCE: (0 POINTS) **WITH** supervision, direction, personal assistance, or total care
BATHING POINTS:_____	**(1 POINT)** Bathes self completely or needs help in bathing only a single part of the body such as the back, genital area, or disabled extremity.	**(0 POINTS)** Needs help with bathing more than one part of the body, getting in or out of the tub or shower. Requires total bathing.
DRESSING POINTS:_____	**(1 POINT)** Gets clothes from closets and drawers and puts on clothes and outer garments complete with fasteners. May have help tying shoes.	**(0 POINTS)** Needs help with dressing self or needs to be completely dressed.
TOILETING POINTS:_____	**(1 POINT)** Goes to toilet, gets on and off, arranges clothes, cleans genital area without help.	**(0 POINTS)** Needs help transferring to the toilet, cleaning self, or uses bedpan or commode.
TRANSFERRING POINTS:_____	**(1 POINT)** Moves in and out of bed or chair unassisted. Mechanical transferring aides are acceptable.	**(0 POINTS)** Needs help in moving from bed to chair or requires a complete transfer.
CONTINENCE POINTS:_____	**(1 POINT)** Exercises complete self-control over urination and defecation.	**(0 POINTS)** Is partially or totally incontinent of bowel or bladder.
FEEDING POINTS:_____	**(1 POINT)** Gets food from plate into mouth without help. Preparation of food may be done by another person.	**(0 POINTS)** Needs partial or total help with feeding or requires parenteral feeding.

TOTAL POINTS = _____   6 = High (patient independent) 0 = Low (patient very dependent)

Slightly adapted from Katz, S., Down, T.D., Cash, H.R., & Grotz, R.C. (1970). Progress in the development of the index of ADL. *The Gerontologist*, 10(1), 20-30. Copyright © The Gerontological Society of America. Reproduced [Adapted] by permission of the publisher.

ALIGNMENT

Correct body alignment permits optimal musculoskeletal balance and operation and promotes good physiologic functioning. Deviations in body alignment may result from chronic poor posture, trauma, muscle damage, or nerve dysfunction. Fatigue and a person's mental and emotional status may also influence alignment.

Observe alignment when a patient is standing, sitting, or lying (Fig. 33-5). Note whether the patient is able to maintain correct alignment independently.

A patient's body is in correct body alignment when standing when:

- The head is held erect.
- The face is in the forward position, in the same direction as the feet.
- The chest is held upward and forward.
- The spinal column is upright, and the curves of the spine are within normal limits.
- The abdominal muscles are held upward and the buttocks downward.

Swing phase
begins

Stance
phase

Swing phase
completed

Normal gait

FIGURE 33-4. The stance and swing phases of normal gait.

FIGURE 33-5. Adequate posture. In the sitting and standing positions, a straight line can be drawn from the ear through the shoulder and hip. In bed, the head, shoulders, and hips are aligned.

- The knees are extended—not bent or hyperextended in the knee-locked position.
- The feet are at right angles to the lower legs.
- The line of gravity goes through the center of the knees and in front of the ankle joints.
- The base of support is on the soles of the feet, and weight is distributed through the soles and heels.

Correct body alignment when sitting is similar to correct alignment when standing except that the hips are flexed, the knees are flexed and not crossed, and the base of support is on the buttocks and upper thighs. The popliteal area should be free of the edge of the chair to prevent circulatory stasis and possible nerve injury.

JOINT STRUCTURE AND FUNCTION

Use inspection and palpation to examine joints, their range of motion, and the surrounding tissue. **Range of motion** is the complete extent of movement of which a joint is normally capable. (Skill 33-6 later in this chapter illustrates the range of motion of selected joints.) When assessing joint mobility, note the following:

- Size, shape, color, and symmetry of joints. Note any masses, deformities, or muscle atrophy.
- Range of motion of each joint.
- Any limitation in the normal range of motion or any unusual increase in the mobility of a joint (instability). Range of motion varies among individuals and decreases with aging.

- Muscle strength when performing range-of-motion exercises against resistance.
- Any swelling, heat, tenderness, pain, nodules, or crepitation (palpable or audible crunching or grating sensation produced by motion of the joint).
- Compare findings in one joint with those of the opposite joint.

MUSCLE MASS, TONE, AND STRENGTH

Adequate skeletal muscle mass, tone, and strength are prerequisites to body movement and work performance. Mass refers to muscle size. Assess muscle mass throughout the body and compare one muscle group to another using tape measurements. Atrophy describes muscle mass that is decreased through disuse or neurologic impairment. Hypertrophy refers to increased muscle mass resulting from exercise or training. Patients experiencing muscle wasting as a result of a chronic disease process such as cancer may report visible changes in muscle mass.

The slight residual tension that remains in a resting normal muscle with an intact nerve supply is termed muscle tone. Assess muscle tone by flexing and extending the elbow or knee and noting the degree of resistance to these movements. Decreased tone, hypotonicity, or **flaccidity** results from disuse or neurologic impairments. **Spasticity,** increased tone that interferes with movement, is also caused by neurologic impairments.

> *The nurse would need to assess closely the muscle tone of Kelsi Lester, the 10-year-old girl who is unconscious.*

Due to her current neurologic status of being unconscious, this assessment information would provide a means to evaluate her nervous system function. In addition, the nurse would be alert for evidence of flaccidity, which could result from lack of use or possibly impairment of her nervous system due to the accident. ■

Muscle strength varies greatly from one individual to another and within the same individual and is affected by muscle use. Test muscle strength by asking the patient to move actively against resistance. For example, instruct the patient to push the examiner's palms apart or to push the foot against the examiner's palm. When comparing muscle groups, remember that a person's dominant side tends to be stronger.

Impaired muscle strength or weakness is termed **paresis.** The absence of strength secondary to nervous impairment is called **paralysis.** Hemiparesis refers to weakness of one half of the body, and hemiplegia is paralysis of one half of the body. Paraplegia is paralysis of the legs, and quadriplegia is paralysis of the arms and legs.

The patient's muscle strength should be adequate for the performance of tasks the patient deems necessary. For example, a patient whose primary means of ambulation is a wheelchair requires upper body strength.

ENDURANCE

When assessing endurance, evaluate the patient's ability to turn in bed, maintain correct alignment when sitting or standing, ambulate, and perform self-care activities. When a physical or psychological factor is believed to be affecting endurance, accomplish the following:

- Obtain vital signs while the patient is at rest.
- Instruct the patient to perform the activity (e.g., ambulation).
- Observe the patient's response during and after the activity.
- Take the vital signs immediately after the activity.
- Reassess the vital signs after the patient has rested for 3 minutes.

Significant findings indicating that a person's exercise tolerance has been reached include noticeably increased pulse, respirations, and blood pressure; shortness of breath; dyspnea; weakness; pallor; confusion; and vertigo.

Diagnosing

Recognizing cues that indicate both potential and actual problems is essential when analyzing data about a patient's mobility status. Because the problems associated with immobility can seriously undermine the patient's well-being and often require complex and costly treatment, prepare to direct interventions aimed at preventing these problems whenever possible. The plan of care for the patient with an alteration in mobility should include nursing diagnoses that identify the complications of immobility for which the patient is at greatest risk.

Nursing diagnoses specifically addressing problems of mobility include:

- Activity Intolerance
- Impaired Physical Mobility

Examples of related factors and defining characteristics are listed in the accompanying Examples of NANDA Nursing Diagnoses box.

A patient's mobility status also may affect other areas of human functioning. Examples of nursing diagnoses related to problems of mobility may include:

- Chronic Pain related to inability to change body position independently, limited range of motion, and muscle atrophy
- Impaired Walking related to development of footdrop
- Impaired Transfer Ability related to generalized weakness
- Ineffective Health Maintenance related to lack of mobility to procure needed services—no support persons
- Impaired Home Maintenance related to immobility
- Noncompliance With Exercise Prescription related to decreased endurance, decreased motivation
- Bathing, Feeding, Dressing, Toileting Self-Care Deficit related to physical weakness (decreased muscle mass and strength), altered mobility (upper or lower extremities)
- Sexual Dysfunction related to neuromuscular impairment

Outcome Identification and Planning

If the patient is not experiencing any mobility problems, expected patient outcomes are directed toward the promotion of physical fitness. For example, the patient will:

- Follow a program of regular physical exercise that improves cardiovascular function, endurance, flexibility, and strength

To achieve this long-term expected outcome, numerous short-term expected outcomes may be needed. An example follows.

By the next visit, 8/20/12, the patient will:

- Identify four personal benefits of regular exercise
- Describe an exercise program (activities, frequency, duration) the patient is willing to follow
- Identify his target heart range
- Obtain medical clearance for the exercise program if at high risk for complications
- List support systems that will reinforce exercise efforts

Patients at high risk for specific mobility problems require different expected outcomes. For example, the patient will:

- Demonstrate correct body alignment whenever observed (alignment)
- Adhere to an every-2-hour positioning schedule (alignment)
- Demonstrate full range of joint motion (joint mobility)
- Demonstrate adequate muscle mass, tone, and strength to perform functional ADLs (muscle mass, tone, strength)

Examples of NANDA Nursing Diagnoses
Mobility

Nursing Diagnoses	Related Factors	Sample Defining Characteristics

Activity Intolerance	• Any condition that interferes with the transport of oxygenated blood to tissue (e.g., cardiac problems such as congestive heart failure and arrhythmias; respiratory problems, especially chronic obstructive pulmonary disease; circulatory problems; diabetes mellitus)
	• Any condition that causes fatigue (depression, pain, sleep disturbances, prolonged bed rest, sedentary lifestyle)
		• Decreased ability to perform basic self-care activities: turning in bed, changing position, ambulating, washing, dressing, eating, and so on
		• Altered response to activity:
		  • Dyspnea, shortness of breath, excessive increase in respiratory rate
		  • Weak pulse, excessive increase in pulse rate, change in rhythm
		  • Blood pressure that fails to increase with activity or that decreases
		  • Weakness, pallor, confusion, vertigo

Impaired Physical Mobility	• Neuromuscular impairment (stroke, Parkinson's disease) • Musculoskeletal impairment (fracture, arthritis) • Decreased strength and endurance • Pain or discomfort • Depression	• Physical inability to move purposefully or a reluctance to move • Limited range of motion • Decreased muscle mass, tone, or strength • Therapy-related restrictions on movement (e.g., an order for bed rest, traction, cast, or splints)

Patients who are immobile require outcomes directed toward preventing complications related to inactivity and its effects on the body systems. For example, the patient will:

• Be free from signs of skin breakdown.
• Change from a lying to a standing position safely, without injury
• Show signs of adequate venous return
• Be free of contractures

Outcomes need to be individualized for more specific problems (e.g., for the patient learning to walk with crutches or needing to master transfer techniques with only upper body mobility).

> *Consider Maggie Wyatt, the woman being discharged after treatment for a fracture. An appropriate outcome for Ms. Wyatt would be that she demonstrates ability to transfer herself from the bed to the chair and then to the car, with the assistance of a support person.* ■

Implementing

The use of body mechanics to reduce the risk of injury when providing patient care and safe patient handling and movement strategies are discussed in the following sections. Nursing strategies designed to promote correct body alignment, mobility, and fitness are described, as well as interventions to prevent complications from immobility. Techniques for positioning patients, performing range-of-motion exercises, moving, lifting, and ambulating patients, and designing exercise programs are included.

Application of Body Mechanics

Providing patient care places demands on the nurse's musculoskeletal system. These demands are a result of movement and use of equipment necessary to providing care and the handling of patients. Nurses lift, carry, push, pull, and move objects and people in the course of their work. Performing these actions correctly is necessary to avoid musculoskeletal strain and injury. Body mechanics include proper body movement in daily activities, the prevention and correction of problems associated with posture, and the enhancement of coordination and endurance. The guidelines listed below for body mechanics are important to anyone, including nurses, who are engaged in physical activity both at home and at work. Overexertion injuries to workers' necks, shoulders, and backs are the most costly work-related injury for healthcare facilities (UCLA, 2008b; Waters, Collins, Galinsky, & Caruso, 2006; ANA, 2004; Converso & Murphy, 2004).

Techniques to prevent back stress that should be included routinely in injury-prevention programs include the following:

• Develop a habit of erect posture (correct alignment). Slouching can strain neck and back muscles. When sitting, use the chair back to support the whole spine, keeping shoulders back but relaxed. Balance the head over the shoulders, avoid leaning forward, and hold in the stomach muscles.

- Use the longest and the strongest muscles of the arms and the legs to help provide the power needed in strenuous activities. The muscles of the back are less strong and more easily injured when used improperly.
- Use the internal girdle and a long midriff to stabilize the pelvis and to protect the abdominal viscera when stooping, reaching, lifting, or pulling. The internal girdle is made by contracting the gluteal muscles in the buttocks downward and the abdominal muscles upward. It is helped further by making a long midriff by stretching the muscles in the waist. Figure 33-6 illustrates the internal girdle.
- Work as closely as possible to an object that is to be lifted or moved. This brings the body's center of gravity close to that of the object being moved, thereby permitting most of the burden to be borne by the leg and arm

FIGURE 33-7. (*Left*) A good position for lifting is illustrated. This person is using the long and strong muscles of the arms and legs and holding the object so that the line of gravity falls within the base of support. (*Right*) This is an incorrect position for lifting because pull is exerted on the back muscles and leaning causes the line of gravity to fall outside the base.

muscles, rather than the back. Figure 33-7 illustrates a proper and an improper way to pick up an object.

- Face the direction of your movement. Avoid twisting your body.
- Use the weight of the body as a force for pulling or pushing, by rocking on the feet or leaning forward or backward. This reduces the amount of strain placed on the arms and the back.
- Slide, roll, push, or pull an object, rather than lift it, to reduce the energy needed to lift the weight against the pull of gravity.
- Use the weight of the body to push an object by falling or rocking forward and to pull an object by falling or rocking backward.
- Push rather than pull equipment when possible. Keep arms close to your body and push with your whole body, not just your arms.
- Begin activities by broadening the base of support. Spread the feet to shoulder width.
- Make sure that the surface is dry and smooth when moving an object to decrease the effects of friction. Rough, wet, or soiled surfaces can contribute to increased friction, increasing the amount of effort required to move an object.
- Flex the knees, put on the internal girdle, and come down close to an object that is to be lifted.
- Break up heavy loads into smaller loads. The National Institute for Occupational Safety and Health (NIOSH) recommends manual load lifting limits of 51 pounds (Converso & Murphy, 2004). Take breaks from lifting or moving to relax and recover.

Ensuring Safe Patient Handling and Movement

Safe patient handling and transfers involve the use of patient assessment criteria, algorithms for patient handling decisions, and proper use of patient handling equipment. Keep the patient in good alignment and protect him or her from injury while being moved.

FIGURE 33-6. (*Left*) Internal girdle "on." Abdominal muscles contracted, giving a feeling of upward pull, and gluteal muscles contracted, giving a downward pull. (*Right*) Slouch position, showing abdominal muscles relaxed and body out of good alignment.

SAFE PATIENT TRANSFER

Follow these recommended guidelines when moving and lifting patients:

- Assess the patient. Know the patient's medical diagnosis, capabilities, and any movement not allowed. Put in place braces or any device the patient wears before helping from bed.
- Assess the patient's ability to assist with the planned movement. Patients should be encouraged to assist in their own transfers. Encouraging the patient to perform tasks that are within his capabilities promotes independence. Eliminating or reducing unnecessary tasks by the nurse reduces the risk of injury.
- Assess the patient's ability to understand instructions and cooperate with the staff to achieve the movement. Box 33-1 outlines general guidelines to consider related to mobility and safe handling of people with dementia.
- Use an assessment tool to aid in patient assessment and decision making regarding safe patient handling and movement. An example of a tool can be found in Figure 33-8.
- During any patient transferring task, if any caregiver is required to lift more than 35 pounds of a patient's weight, then the patient should be considered to be fully dependent and assistive devices should be used for the transfer.
- Ensure enough staff is available and present to safely move the patient. See the Reflective Practice box at the beginning of the chapter.
- Assess the area for clutter, accessibility to the patient, and availability of devices. Remove any obstacles that may make moving and lifting inconvenient.
- Decide which equipment to use. Step-by-step protocols or algorithms are available to aid decision making to prevent injury to staff and patients (Fig. 33-9). Use handling

aids, transfer equipment, and assistive devices (discussed below), whenever possible to help reduce risk of injury to yourself and the patient.

- Plan carefully what you will do before moving or lifting a patient. Assess the mobility of attached equipment. You may injure the patient or yourself if you have not planned well. If necessary, enlist the support of another nurse. This reduces the strain on everyone involved. Communicate the plan with staff and the patient to ensure coordinated movement.
- Explain to the patient what you plan to do. Then use what abilities the patient has to assist you. This technique often decreases the effort required and the possibility of injury to you.
- If the patient is in pain, administer the prescribed analgesic sufficiently in advance of the transfer to allow the patient to participate in the move comfortably.
- Elevate the bed as necessary so that you are working at a height that is comfortable and safe for you.
- Lock the wheels of the bed, wheelchair, or stretcher so that they do not slide while you are moving the patient.
- Be sure the patient is in good body alignment while being moved and lifted to protect the patient from strain and muscle injury.
- Support the patient's body well. Avoid grabbing and holding an extremity by its muscles.
- Avoid friction on the patient's skin during moving.
- Use friction-reducing devices whenever possible, especially during lateral transfers.
- Move your body and the patient in a smooth, rhythmic motion. Jerky movements tend to put extra strain on muscles and joints and are uncomfortable for the patient.
- Use mechanical devices such as lifts, slides, transfer chairs, or gait belts for moving patients. Be sure that you understand how the device operates and that the patient is properly secured and informed of what will

Box 33-1 SAFE HANDLING OF PATIENTS WITH DEMENTIA

- Be aware that communication problems and weakness can make the handling of patients with dementia challenging.
- Keep in mind that instructions to patients experiencing dementia can be misconstrued due to slow mental processing.
- Determine if the patient experiencing dementia has receptive aphasia. This inability to understand what is being said results in noncompliance with verbal instructions.
- Phrase instructions positively. For example, remind the patient to "Stand up" until the chair is correctly positioned, instead of saying "Don't sit down." The patient may not register the "Don't" and will try to sit too early. Positive instructions are more likely to result in successful maneuvers.
- Get the patient's attention, make eye contact, and speak directly to the patient. Give instructions that are clear and short.

- Ask one question at a time, allow the patient to answer, and repeat the question if necessary.
- Allow the patient to focus on the task; avoid correcting the process of the action unless it would be dangerous to the patient not to do so.
- Identify the patient's established patterns of behavior, customs, traits, and everyday habits and try to incorporate these habits into desired activities. For instance, a patient with dementia may resist or become frightened when a morning shower is attempted if the patient was accustomed to evening baths. Another individual may have difficulty getting out of bed in the morning for the simple reason that he is being asked to get out on what he considers the wrong side of the bed.

(Adapted from Miller, C. [2008]. Communication difficulties in hospitalized older adults with dementia: Try these techniques to make communicating with patients easier and more effective. American Journal of Nursing, 108[3], 58–66; Smith, M. & Buckwalter, K. [2005]. Behaviors associated with dementia: Whether resisting care or exhibiting apathy, an older adult with dementia is attempting communication. Nurses and other caregivers must learn to "hear" this language. American Journal of Nursing, 105[7], 40–52; and Wright, K. [2005]. Mobility and safe handling of people with dementia. Nursing Times, 101[17], 38–40.)

Assessment Criteria and Care Plan for Safe Patient Handling and Movement

I. Patient's Level of Assistance:

_____ Independent—Patient performs task safely, with or without staff assistance, with or without assistive devices.

_____ Partial Assist—Patient requires no more help than standby, cueing, or coaxing, or caregiver is required to lift no more than 35 lbs of a patient's weight.

_____ Dependent—Patient requires nurse to lift more than 35 lbs of the patient's weight, or patient is unpredictable in the amount of assistance offered. In this case assistive devices should be used.

An assessment should be made prior to each task if the patient has varying level of ability to assist due to medical reasons, fatigue, medications, etc. When in doubt, assume the patient cannot assist with the transfer/repositioning.

II. Weight-Bearing Capability

_____ Full

_____ Partial

_____ None

III. Bilateral Upper-Extremity Strength

_____ Yes

_____ No

IV. Patient's level of cooperation and comprehension:

_____ Cooperative—may need prompting; able to follow simple commands.

_____ Unpredictable or varies (patient whose behavior changes frequently should be considered as unpredictable), not cooperative, or unable to follow simple commands.

V. Weight: _____   Height: _____

Body Mass Index (BMI) [needed if patient's weight is over 300 lbs][1]: _____

If BMI exceeds 50, institute Bariatric Algorithms

The presence of the following conditions are likely to affect the transfer/repositioning process and should be considered when identifying equipment and technique needed to move the patient.

VI. Check applicable conditions likely to affect transfer/repositioning techniques.

_____ Hip/Knee/Shoulder Replacements	_____ Respiratory/Cardiac Compromise	_____ Fractures
_____ History of Falls	_____ Wounds Affecting Transfer/Positioning	_____ Splints/Traction
_____ Paralysis/Paresis	_____ Amputation	_____ Severe Osteoporosis
_____ Unstable Spine	_____ Urinary/Fecal Stoma	_____ Severe Pain/Discomfort
_____ Severe Edema	_____ Contractures/Spasms	_____ Postural Hypotension
_____ Very Fragile Skin	_____ Tubes (IV, Chest, etc.)	

Comments:_____

_____

_____

VII. Appropriate Lift/Transfer Devices Needed:

Vertical Lift: _____

_____

Horizontal Lift: _____

_____

Other Patient Handling Devices Needed: _____

_____

Sling Type: Seated _____   Seated (Amputee) _____   Standing _____   Supine _____   Ambulation _____   Limb Support _____

Sling Size: _____

Signature: _____   **Date:** _____

[1]If patient's weight is over 300 lbs, the BMI is needed. For Online BMI table and calculator see: http://www.nhlbi.nih.gov/guidelines/obesity/bmi_tbl.htm

FIGURE 33-8. Sample assessment tool for safe patient handling and movement. (VISN 8 Patient Safety Center. [2009]. *Safe patient handling and movement algorithms.* Tampa, FL: Author. Available at www.visn8.med.gov/patientsafetycenter/safePtHandling.)

Algorithm 4: Reposition in Bed: From Side to Side or Up

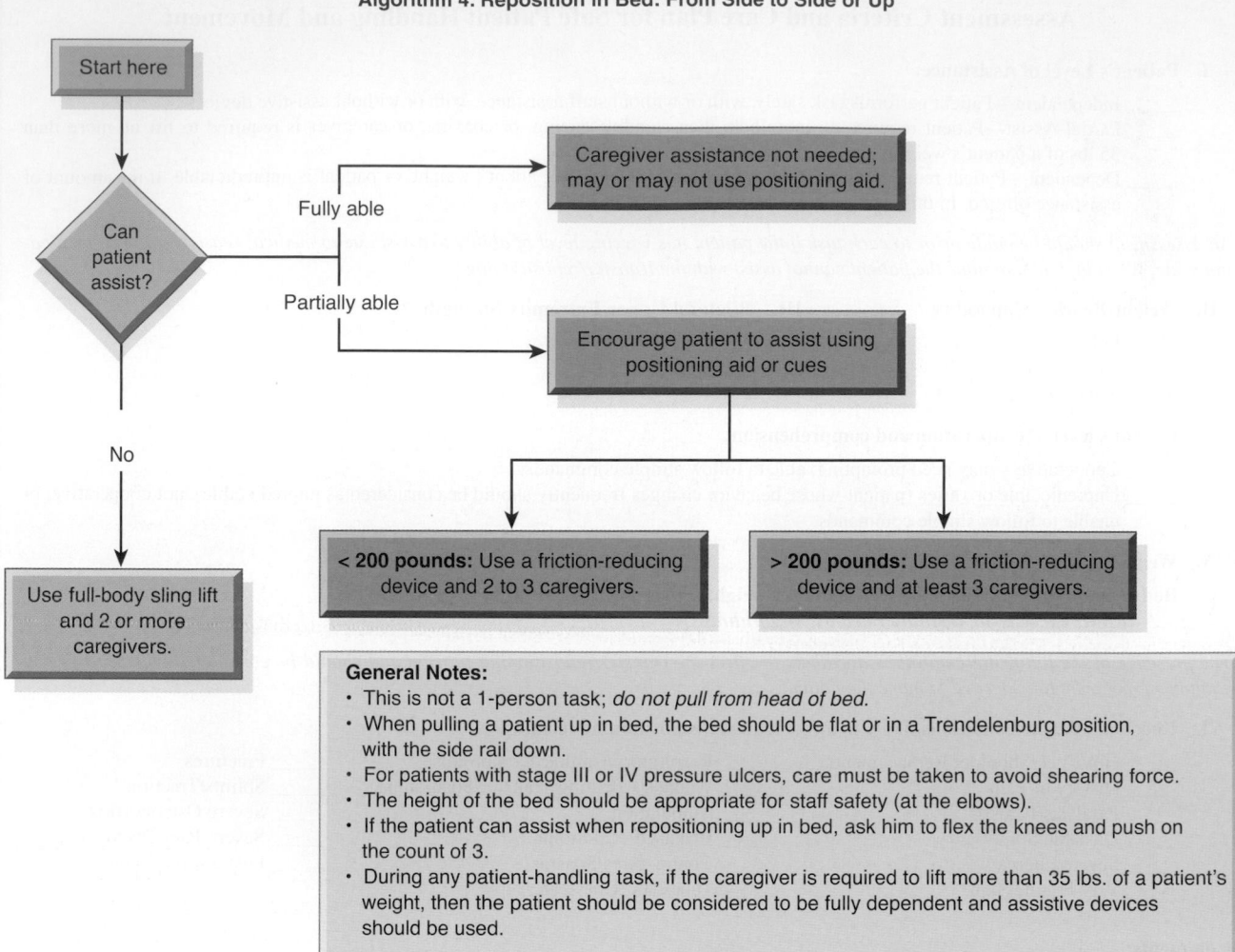

FIGURE 33-9. Step-by-step procedure or algorithm used to outline safe technique for repositioning a patient in bed. (VISN 8 Patient Safety Center. [2009]. *Safe patient handling and movement algorithms.* Tampa, FL: Author. Available at http://www.visn8.med.gov/patientsafetycenter/safePtHandling.)

occur. Patients who do not understand or are afraid may be unable to cooperate and may suffer injury as a result.

• Assure that the equipment used meets weight requirements. Bariatric patients (BMI greater than 50) require bariatric transfer aids and equipment. Bariatric transfer aids and equipment are designed to be used with persons who are obese.

➤ *Consider Mrs. Nguyen, the woman caring for her husband at home. The nurse would evaluate the need for assistive devices and secure the identified items for patient care. The nurse would incorporate safe patient handling and moving guidelines when role modeling the proper techniques for moving and lifting Mr. Nguyen. In addition, the nurse would use these guidelines to develop a teaching plan for Mrs. Nguyen to ensure safety for all involved when moving and lifting Mr. Nguyen.* ∎

EQUIPMENT AND ASSISTIVE DEVICES

Many devices and equipment are available to aid in transferring, repositioning, and lifting patients. It is important to use the right equipment and appropriate device based on patient assessment and desired movement.

Gait Belts

A gait belt is a device used for transferring patients and assisting with ambulation (Fig. 33-10). The belt, which often has handles, is placed around the patient's waist and secured by Velcro fasteners. The handles can be placed in a variety of configurations so the caregiver can have better access to, improved grasp, and control of the patient (VISN 8, 2005; Nelson, Fragala, et al., 2003). Some belts are hand-held slings that go around the patient, providing a firm grasp for the caregiver and facilitating the transfer (Nelson, Owen, et al., 2003). The gait belt is used to help the patent stand and provides stabilization during pivoting. Gait belts also allow the nurse to assist in ambulating patients who have leg strength, can cooperate, and require minimal assistance.

FIGURE 33-10. Gait belts.

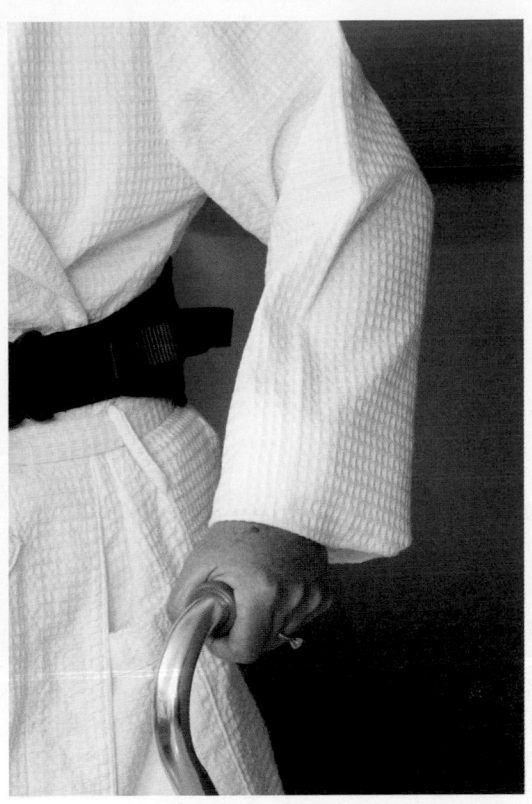

Gait belts should not be used on patients with abdominal or thoracic incisions (Blocks, 2005).

Stand-Assist and Repositioning Aids

Some patients need minimal assistance to stand up. With an appropriate support to grasp, they can lift themselves. Many types of devices can help a patient to stand. These devices can be freestanding or attached to the bed or wheelchair. Other aids have a pull bar to assist the patient to stand, and then a seat unfolds under the patient. After the patient sits on the seat, the device can be wheeled to the toilet, chair, shower, or bed.

Lateral-Assist Devices

Lateral-assist devices reduce patient-surface friction during side-to-side transfers. Roller boards, slide boards, transfer boards, inflatable mattresses, and friction-reducing lateral-assist devices are examples of these devices that make transfers safer and more comfortable for the patient. For example, an inflatable lateral-assist device is a flexible mattress that is placed under the patient. An attached, portable air supply then inflates the mattress, which provides a layer of air under the patient. This air cushion allows nursing staff to perform the move with much less effort (Baptiste, Boda, Nelson, Lloyd, & Lee, 2006; Nelson, Owen, et al., 2003). Another example is a transfer board, usually made of smooth, rigid, low-friction material (such as coated wood or plastic). The board, which is placed under the patient, provides a slick surface for the patient during transfers, thereby reducing

friction and the force required to move the patient. A third type of lateral sliding aid is made of a special fabric that reduces friction. Some devices have long handles that reduce reaching by staff to improve safety and make the transfer easier (Fig. 33-11).

Friction-Reducing Sheets

Friction-reducing sheets can be used under patients to prevent skin shearing when moving patients in bed and when assisting with lateral transfers. Their use reduces friction and the force required to move patients.

FIGURE 33-11. Lateral-assist device with long handles to reduce reaching by staff.

FIGURE 33-12. Mechanical lateral-assist device.

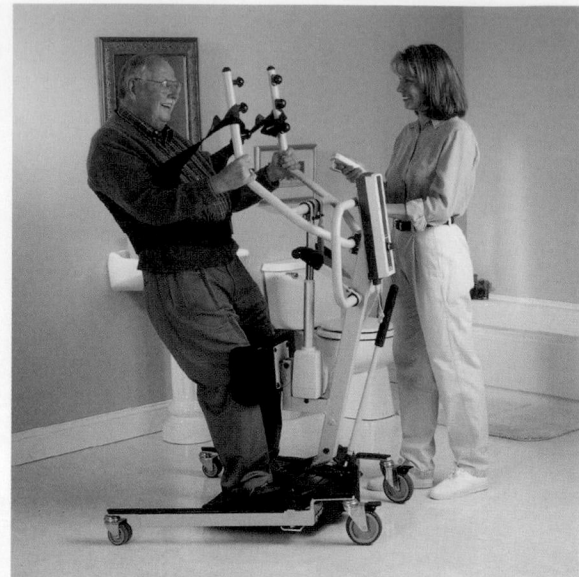

FIGURE 33-13. Stand-assist aid.

Mechanical Lateral-Assist Devices

Mechanical lateral-assist devices include specialized stretchers and eliminate the need to slide the patient manually. Some devices are motorized, whereas others use a hand crank. A portion of the device moves from the stretcher to the bed, sliding under the patient, bridging the bed and stretcher (Fig. 33-12). The device is then returned to the stretcher, effectively moving the patient without any pulling by staff members.

Transfer Chairs

Chairs that can convert into stretchers are available. These are useful with patients who have no weight-bearing capacity, cannot follow directions, and/or cannot cooperate. The back of the chair bends back and the leg supports elevate to form a stretcher configuration, eliminating the need for lifting the patient. Some of these chairs have built-in mechanical aids to perform the patient transfer, as detailed above.

Powered Stand-Assist and Repositioning Lifts

These devices can be used with patients who can bear weight on at least one leg, can follow directions, and are cooperative. A simple sling is placed around the patient's back and under the arms. The patient rests his feet on the device's footrest and places his hands on the handle. The device mechanically assists the patient to stand, without any assistance from the nurse (Fig. 33-13). Once the patient is standing, the device can be wheeled to a chair, the toilet, or bed. Some devices have removable footrests and can be used as a walker. Some have scales incorporated into the device that can be used to weigh the patient.

Powered Full-Body Lifts

These devices are used with patients who cannot bear any weight to move them out of bed, into and out of a chair, and to a commode or stretcher. A full-body sling is placed under the patient's body, including head and torso, then the sling is

attached to the lift (Fig. 33-14). The device slowly lifts the patient. Some devices can be lowered to the floor to pick up a patient who has fallen. These devices are available on portable bases and ceiling-mounted tracks.

Positioning Patients

Positioning that maintains correct body alignment and facilitates physiologic functioning contributes to the patient's psychological and physical well-being. The force of gravity pulls parts of the body out of alignment unless adequate support is provided. Various positions are, therefore, protective in nature only when the patient is positioned properly.

COMMON DEVICES TO PROMOTE CORRECT ALIGNMENT

Many devices can help maintain good body alignment and muscle tonus while the patient is in bed and can alleviate discomfort or pressure on various parts of the body.

FIGURE 33-14. Powered full-body lift.

Pillows

Pillows are used primarily to provide support or to elevate a body part. Pillows of different sizes are useful for different parts. Those intended for the head are usually full-sized or large-sized pillows. Small pillows are ideal for support or elevation of the extremities, shoulders, or incisional wounds. Specially designed heavy pillows are useful to elevate the upper part of the body when an adjustable bed is unavailable, such as at home.

Mattresses

For a mattress to be comfortable and supportive, it must be firm but have sufficient "give" to permit good body alignment. A patient who must remain in a bed with a nonsupportive mattress may complain of backache and other discomforts.

Special mattresses, pads, and types of beds used to help prevent pressure ulcers are discussed in Chapter 32.

Adjustable Beds

The head of an adjustable bed can be elevated to the desired degree. This positioning is discussed later in the chapter. The foot of an adjustable bed can also be elevated as desired. Some adjustable beds allow the bed to be "broken," or gatched, so that the mattress is flexed at the level of the knees. This position is rarely recommended because it can cause pressure on the popliteal space behind the knee, resulting in impaired circulation to the lower extremity and an increased risk for clot formation.

The adjustable bed can also be changed so that the distance from the bed to the floor can be altered. Position the bed at the height that will let the patient stand with the least amount of effort. Healthcare workers use the higher positions so that they do not strain their backs while providing bed care. General guidelines for safe use of beds are discussed in Chapter 31.

Many beds being used in patient care environments have improvements to support transfer and repositioning of the patient. Some beds easily convert to a chair, bypassing the need for bed-to-chair transfers. Other beds are designed to align the patient's hip with the pivot point in the bed, minimizing slippage toward the foot of the bed when the head of the bed is raised, reducing the need to reposition the patient. Many new mattress surfaces are designed to eliminate the need for frequent repositioning by the nurse; some provide a cushion of air under the patient during movement, reducing friction; and others have surfaces that can rotate to move the patient as needed for care.

> *Consider Mrs. Nguyen, the older woman caring for her husband after his stroke. If necessary and not already in the home, an adjustable bed could be recommended to help her provide care to her husband. This would be beneficial to both Mrs. Nguyen and her husband.* ■

Trapeze Bar

A trapeze bar (Fig. 33-15) is a handgrip suspended from a frame near the head of the bed. The patient can grasp the bar

FIGURE 33-15. A trapeze device makes it possible for the patient to lift part of the body from the bed, thus facilitating turning and moving up in bed.

with one or both hands and then raise the trunk from the bed. The trapeze makes moving and turning considerably easier for many patients and facilitates transfers into and out of bed. It can also be used when a patient needs to perform exercises that strengthen some muscles of the upper extremities (e.g., biceps).

Additional Equipment

The greatest danger to the feet occurs when they are unsupported in the dorsiflexion position. The toes drop downward, and the feet are in plantar flexion. Because of the pull of gravity, this position of the feet occurs naturally when the body is at rest. If maintained for extended periods, plantar flexion can cause an alteration in the length of muscles, and the patient may develop a complication called **foot drop.** In this position, the foot is unable to maintain itself in the perpendicular position, heel–toe gait is impossible, and the patient experiences extreme difficulty in walking. The use of a foot support, such as a foot boot or high-top sneakers, helps avoid this complication. Figure 33-16 demonstrates a foot in plantar flexion versus the dorsiflexion position maintained by wearing a high-top canvas sneaker.

If top bedding must be kept off the patient's lower extremities, a device called a cradle is used. A cradle is usually a metal frame that supports the bed linens away from the patient while providing privacy and warmth. There are a number of sizes and shapes of cradles. If used, the cradle should be fastened securely to the bed so that it does not slide or fall on the patient.

Sandbags, available in various sizes, can be used to immobilize an extremity and support body alignment. When properly filled, they should be pliable enough to be shaped to body contours to provide support. Avoid hard or firmly packed sandbags. Position a sandbag to avoid creating pressure on a bony prominence.

Trochanter rolls are used to support the hips and legs so that the femurs do not rotate outward. Figure 33-17 illustrates and describes how to use trochanter rolls. Properly placed pillows can also be used to help prevent the thighs

A

B

FIGURE 33-16. (**A**) Plantar flexion occurs when the foot is not supported. (**B**) When high-top sneakers support the feet, the dorsiflexion position is maintained.

from turning outward, but they tend to slip out of place and require frequent adjustment to be effective.

If a patient is paralyzed or unconscious, hand–wrist splints or hand rolls may be necessary to provide a means for keeping the thumb in the correct position, that is, slightly adducted and in apposition to the fingers. A hand roll can be created by folding a washcloth, rolling it, and securing it in place with tape. Once placed against the palm of the hand, it can effectively keep the hand in a functional position (Fig. 33-18). A commercial plastic or aluminum splint also may be used to hold the thumb in place regardless of the hand position. Encourage patients who are not moving their fingers to do finger exercises, with special attention to having the thumb touch the tip of each finger.

Side rails can assist the patient in rolling from one side to the other or to sitting up without calling for assistance. Using the side rails can help the patient retain or regain muscle effi-

ciency. When using side rails, be sure to explain their use to patients and their families and follow the protocol of the healthcare agency. If a patient requests that side rails be raised for additional security, the patient must have the ability to raise and lower the side rails independently. Safe use of side rails is discussed in Chapter 26.

PROTECTIVE POSITIONING

Patients accustomed to an active lifestyle who generally use a bed only for sleep are often unaware of the importance of correct body alignment and regular position changes when on prescribed bed rest. Whenever possible, teach both the patient and family the following:

- Correct positioning techniques
- The need to change positions frequently, at least every 2 hours
- The importance of using the time allotted to position changes to exercise the extremities and to assess and massage pressure areas (reddened areas should not be massaged)

When the patient is unable to change position independently, use a turn schedule, posted at the bedside to assist with and document the rotation of positions. Table 33-6 describes common bed positions and nursing measures to prevent complications associated with these positions.

FIGURE 33-17. Trochanter rolls prevent the external rotation of the hips of a bedridden patient. The patient is placed on a folded sheet so that the top edge is at the hips and the lower edge is about one third of the way down the thighs. Towels or bath blankets are rolled under each side until the roll is snugly against the patient's hips and thighs. The support cannot unroll, and the weight of the patient keeps it secure.

FIGURE 33-18. A hand roll holds the hand in functional position.

TABLE • 33-6   **COMMON BED POSITIONS AND PROTECTIVE NURSING ACTIONS**

Position	Complication to Be Prevented	Suggested Preventive Actions
Fowler's Position	Flexion contracture of the neck	Allow the head to rest against the mattress or be supported by a small pillow only.
	Exaggerated curvature of the spine	Use a firm support for the back; position the patient so that the angle of elevation starts at the hips.
	Dislocation of the shoulder	Support the forearms on pillows to elevate them sufficiently so that no pull is exerted on the shoulders.
	Flexion contracture of the wrist	Support the hand on pillows so that it is in natural alignment with the forearm.
	Edema of the hand	Support the hand so that it is slightly elevated in relation to the elbow.
	Flexion contractures of the fingers and abduction of the thumbs	Provide hand–wrist splints if necessary.
	Impaired lower extremity circulation and knee contracture, pressure on heels	Elevate the knees for only brief periods; place one or two pillows under the lower legs from below the knees to the ankles; avoid pressure on the popliteal vessels; avoid using the knee gatch.
	External rotation of the hips	Use trochanter roll.
	Footdrop	Support the feet in dorsal flexion. Use footboard; high-top sneakers can also be used.
Protective Supine Position	Exaggerated curvature of the spine and flexion of the hips	Provide a firm supportive mattress; use a bed board if necessary.
	Flexion contracture of the neck	Place pillows under the upper shoulders, the neck, and the head so that the head and the neck are held in the correct position.
	Internal rotation of the shoulders and extension of the elbows (hunch shoulders)	Place pillows or arm supports under the forearms so that the upper arms are alongside the body and the forearms are pronated slightly.
	Flexion of the lumbar curvature	Place rolled towel or small pillow under lumbar curvature if needed.
	Extension of the fingers and abduction of the thumbs (clawhand deformities)	Use hand–wrist splints if appropriate.
	External rotation of the femurs	Place sandbags or a trochanter roll alongside the hips and the upper half of the thighs.
	Hyperextension of the knees	Place a pillow under the lower legs from below the knees to the ankles.
	Footdrop	Use a footboard or make an improvised firm foot support to hold the feet in dorsal flexion; high-top sneakers may also be recommended.
Protective Side-Lying or Lateral Position	Lateral flexion of the neck	Place a pillow under the head and the neck.
	Inward rotation of the arm and interference with respiration	Place a pillow under the upper arm; lower arm should be flexed and positioned comfortably.
	Extension of the finger and abduction of the thumbs	Provide hand–wrist splint if necessary.
	Internal rotation and adduction of the femur	Use one or two pillows as needed to support the leg from the groin to the foot.
	Twisting of the spine	Ensure that the two shoulders are aligned with the two hips.

(continued)

TABLE • 33-6   COMMON BED POSITIONS AND PROTECTIVE NURSING ACTIONS *(continued)*

Position	Complication to Be Prevented	Suggested Preventive Actions
Protective Sims' Position	Lateral flexion of the neck	Place a small pillow under the head unless the drainage of oral secretions is desired.
	Damage to nerves and blood vessels in the axillae of the lower arm	Carefully position lower arm behind and away from the patient's back.
	Internal shoulder rotation and adduction	Abduct the upper shoulder slightly so that shoulder and elbow are flexed; place a pillow between the chest and upper arm.
	Internal rotation and adduction of the hip; lumbar lordosis	Place a pillow under the upper flexed leg from the groin to the foot.
	Twisting of the spine	Ensure that the two shoulders are aligned with the two hips.
	Footdrop	Support the lower foot in dorsal flexion with a sandbag.
Protective Prone Position	Flexion on the cervical spine	Place a small pillow under the head.
	Hyperextension of the spine; impaired respirations	Place some suitable support under the patient between the end of the rib cage and the upper abdomen if this facilitates breathing and if there is space there.
	Footdrop	Move the patient down in bed so that the feet are over the mattress, or support the lower legs on a pillow just high enough to keep the toes from touching the bed.

Fowler's Position

The semi sitting position, or Fowler's position, calls for the head of the bed to be elevated 45 to 60 degrees. This position is often used to promote cardiac and respiratory functioning because abdominal organs drop in this position, thereby providing maximal space in the thoracic cavity. This is also the position of choice for eating, conversation, vision, and urinary and intestinal elimination.

Variations of Fowler's position include high Fowler's and low Fowler's or semi-Fowler's position. In the high Fowler's position, the head of the bed is elevated 90 degrees. When a bedside table with a pillow on top of it is placed in front of the patient in high Fowler's position, the patient can lean forward and rest the arms on the pillow, assuming a posture that allows for maximal lung expansion. In low Fowler's or semi-Fowler's position, the head of the bed is elevated only 30 degrees.

In Fowler's position, the buttocks bear the main weight of the body. In this position, the heels, sacrum, and scapulae are at risk for skin breakdown and require frequent assessment. See Table 33-6 for information about correct positioning and nursing actions to prevent complications associated with this position.

Supine or Dorsal Recumbent Position

In the supine position, the patient lies flat on the back with the head and shoulders slightly elevated with a pillow unless contraindicated, such as spinal anesthesia or surgery on the spinal vertebrae. Correct alignment in the supine position is illustrated in Table 33-6.

Side-lying or Lateral Position

In the side-lying position, the patient lies on the side and the main weight of the body is borne by the lateral aspect of the lower scapula and the lateral aspect of the lower ilium. Because many people routinely fall asleep in the side-lying position, this is a comfortable alternative to the supine position for the patient on bed rest. Although it relieves pressure on the scapulae, sacrum, and heels and allows the legs and feet to be comfortably flexed, support pillows are needed for correct positioning (see Table 33-6).

The oblique position, a variation of the side-lying position, is recommended as an alternative to the side-lying position because it places significantly less pressure on the trochanter region. The patient turns toward the side with the hip of the top leg flexed at a 30-degree angle and the knee flexed at 35 degrees. The calf of the upper leg is positioned slightly behind the body's midline. Pillows support the patient's back and calf of the top leg (Fig. 33-19).

Another variation of the lateral position is Sims' position. In this position, the patient again lies on the side, but the lower arm is behind the patient and the upper arm is flexed at both the shoulder and the elbow. In this position, the main body weight is borne by the anterior aspects of the humerus, clavicle, and ilium. Thus, the major pressure points differ from those in the lateral and other bed-lying positions (see Table 33-6).

Prone Position

In the prone position, the person lies on the abdomen with the head turned to the side. The body is straight in the prone

FIGURE 33-19. Modified lateral position (oblique position) is an alternative to the side-lying position and results in significantly less pressure on the trochanter area.

position because the shoulders, head, and neck are in an erect position, the arms are easily placed in correct alignment with the shoulder girdle, the hips are extended, and the knees can be prevented from flexing or hyperextending. When patients on bed rest use this position periodically, it helps to prevent flexion contractures of the hips and knees. However, the pull of gravity on the trunk when the patient lies prone produces a marked lordosis or forward curvature of the lumbar spine. The position is thus contraindicated for people with spinal problems. The pull of gravity on the feet may result in plantar flexion unless the legs and feet are positioned carefully (see Table 33-6).

Antiembolism Stockings and Pneumatic Compression Devices

Venous stasis and the development of venous thrombosis are potential complications of immobility. Antiembolism stockings and pneumatic compression devices are passive interventions prescribed to aid in the prevention of venous stasis and the development of venous thrombosis.

ANTIEMBOLISM STOCKINGS

Antiembolism stockings are often used for patients at risk for deep vein thrombosis, pulmonary embolism, and to help prevent phlebitis (described in Chapter 30). Manufactured by several companies, they are made of elastic material and are available in either knee-high or thigh-high length. By applying pressure, antiembolism stockings increase the velocity of blood flow in the superficial and deep veins and improve venous valve function in the legs, promoting venous return to the heart. A physician's order is required for their use. When assisting with antiembolism stockings, follow these general nursing guidelines:

- Measure the patient's legs to determine the proper size of stocking. Each leg should have a correct fitting stocking; if measurements are different, then two different sizes of stocking need to be ordered to ensure correct fitting on each leg (Walker & Lamont, 2008). The manufacturer whose stockings are being used gives directions for measuring. Some stockings fit either leg; others are designated right or left. An improperly fitting stocking is uncomfortable and ineffective and possibly even harmful (Walker & Lamont, 2007).
- Assess the skin condition and neurovascular status of the legs. Report abnormalities before continuing with the application of the stockings.

- Be prepared to apply the stockings in the morning before the patient is out of bed and while the patient is supine. If the patient is sitting or has been up and about, have the patient lie down with legs and feet elevated for at least 15 minutes before applying the stockings. Otherwise, the leg vessels are congested with blood, reducing the effectiveness of the stockings.
- Do not massage the legs. If a clot is present, it may break away from the vessel wall and circulate in the bloodstream.
- Check the legs regularly for redness, blistering, swelling, and pain. Some recommend checking the legs at least once every 8 hours; others recommend twice a day. Remove the stockings completely once a day to bathe the legs and feet.
- Launder the stockings as necessary, but at least every 3 days. Soiled stockings irritate the skin. Dry the stockings on a flat surface to prevent them from stretching. The patient may need two pairs of stockings so that he or she can wear one pair while the second pair is being cleaned.

Always remove antiembolism stockings during morning care and inspect the legs. Then reapply the stockings before the patient is out of bed, as shown in Skill 33-1.

PNEUMATIC COMPRESSION DEVICES

Intermittent pneumatic compression devices may be used in conjunction with antiembolism stockings. They are composed of an air pump, connecting tubes, and extremity sleeves. They require a physician's order and are often prescribed for high-risk surgical patients, patients with decreased mobility, patients with chronic venous disease, and patients at risk for deep-vein disorders. Pneumatic compression devices apply intermittent or sequential pressure to the leg to enhance blood flow and venous return, simulating the normal muscle-pumping action in the legs.

Turning the Patient in Bed

Frequently, a patient cannot turn in bed without assistance. Nurses need to use their knowledge of correct alignment to turn the patient from the back onto the side, from the back onto the abdomen, and from the abdomen onto the back. A suggested decision-making strategy is outlined in Figure 33-9, Algorithm 4: Reposition in Bed: From Side to Side or Up (VISN 8, 2009). If the patient is unable to assist with movement, a full-body sling and two or more caregivers are required. When turning the patient, the bed should be at the height of the caregivers' elbows, to ensure a comfortable working height. The technique for turning a patient in bed is described and illustrated in Skill 33-2. Mastering this turning technique helps nurses adhere to an every-2-hour turn schedule for an immobile patient.

> *Consider Genevieve Augustus, the older woman caring for her husband at home and Kelsi Lester, the 10-year-old girl who is unconscious. Teaching Mrs. Augustus how to properly turn her husband in bed and assist him in doing so would be crucial to minimize stress and strain on Mrs. Augustus' back and legs. Turning Kelsi every 2 hours would be essential to prevent skin breakdown.* ∎

Moving a Patient Up in Bed

A suggested decision-making strategy is outlined in Figure 33-9, Algorithm 4: Reposition in Bed: From Side to Side or Up (VISN 8, 2009). The first decision point is whether or not the patient can assist. If they are fully able, caregiver assistance is not needed and the patient may or may not use a positioning aid. If the patient is fully able to assist in moving up in the bed, allow the patient to complete the movement independently, with safe supervision. The patient assists movement either by pushing with the feet flat against the bed or by using an overbed trapeze. If they are only par-

tially able, encourage the patient to assist using a positioning aid or cues. If the patient is less than 200 pounds, use a friction-reducing device and two to three caregivers. If the patient is over 200 pounds, use a friction-reducing device and at least three caregivers. If the patient is not able to assist, use a fully-body sling lift and two or more caregivers. Friction-reducing sheets or other devices should be used to minimize shearing forces and work effort. A technique used to move a patient up in bed when the patient is partially able to assist and two caregivers are available is described and illustrated in Skill 33-3.

Moving a Patient From Bed to Stretcher

Considerable care must be taken when moving a patient from a bed to a stretcher, or vice versa, to prevent injury to the patient and the caregivers. A suggested decision-making strategy is outlined in Figure 33-20, Algorithm 2: Lateral Transfer to and From: Bed to Stretcher, Trolley (VISN 8, 2009). If the patient is fully able to assist in the transfer, allow the patient to complete the movement independently, with supervision for safety. If the patient is partially able or not able to assist at all, and the patient weighs less than 200 pounds, use a friction-reducing device. If the patient weighs more than 200 pounds, a friction-reducing device and three caregivers are required. If the patient is unconscious or weakened, additional nurses are needed to support the extremities and the head. These actions

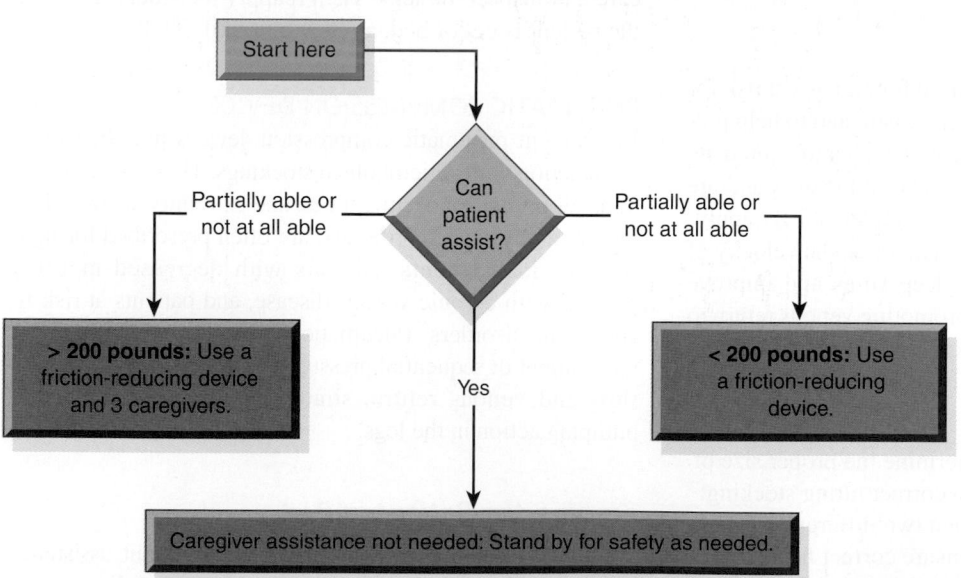

Algorithm 2: Lateral Transfer to and From: Bed to Stretcher, Trolley

FIGURE 33-20. Step-by-step procedure used to make decisions for safely transferring a patient from bed to stretcher. (VISN 8 Patient Safety Center. [2009]. *Safe patient handling and movement algorithms.* Tampa, FL: Author. Available at http://www.visn8.med.gov/patientsafetycenter/safePtHandling.)

Comments:
- Surfaces should be even for all lateral patient moves.
- For patients with stage III or IV pressure ulcers, care must be taken to avoid shearing force.
- During any patient transferring task, if any caregiver is required to lift more than 35 lbs. of a patient's weight, then the patient should be considered to be fully dependent and assistive devices should be used for the transfer.

are described in Skill 33-4. When returning the patient to the bed from the stretcher, the same techniques are used.

Moving a Patient From Bed to Chair

Safety and comfort are key concerns when assisting the patient out of bed. Preliminary assessment of vital signs provides baseline data, and subsequent recordings determine the effect of this activity on the patient. The position of the nurse as he or she prepares to move the patient and placement of the chair are critical elements in the transfer. The patient's apparel should be sufficient to prevent embarrassment and provide warmth yet not impede movement.

Assess the patient's ability to bear weight when deciding the appropriate method for transfer and transfer aid. Patients who are unable to bear partial weight or full weight or who are uncooperative should be transferred using a full-body sling lift with two caregivers. The technique for assisting a patient to transfer from bed to chair is described in Skill 33-5.

> *Recall Maggie Wyatt, the woman being discharged with an external fixation device in place. In assessing the situation, the nurse would need to determine how much Maggie can help with the transfer. From there, the nurse would then determine if another person is needed to help transfer Maggie. Realizing that the device is heavy and cumbersome, the nurse would determine that most likely two persons are needed.* ■

FIGURE 33-21. Logrolling by two or three nurses aids in turning a patient with a spinal injury. One nurse stands on the side, holding the drawsheet taut. The patient is moved toward the other two nurses on a predetermined signal.

Logrolling a Patient

When a patient has a spinal injury or is recovering from neck, back, or spinal surgery, it is often necessary to keep the body in straight alignment when turning the patient. Two or three nurses can accomplish this safely by logrolling a patient (Fig. 33-21). Do not try to logroll the patient without enough help. Do not twist the patient's head, spine, shoulders, knees, or hips while logrolling. Refer to the accompanying Guidelines for Nursing Care 33-1: Logrolling a Patient.

Assisting With Range-of-Motion Exercises

Range of motion is the complete extent of movement of which a joint is normally capable. Engaging in routine tasks, such as bathing, eating, dressing, and writing, helps use muscle groups that keep many joints in effective range of motion. When all or some of normal ADLs are impossible, attention should be given to the joints not being used at all or to those that are limited in their use.

Unless contraindicated, active, active-assistive, or passive range-of-motion exercises should be encouraged regularly and included in the patient's plan of care. In **active exercise,** the patient independently moves joints through their full range of motion (isotonic exercise). In active-assistive exercise, the nurse may provide minimal support, whereas in **passive exercise,** the patient is unable to move independently, and the nurse moves each joint through its range of motion. Both active and passive exercises improve joint mobility and increase circulation to the affected part, but only active exercise increases muscle mass, tone, and strength and improves cardiac and respiratory functioning. Thus, exercises should be as active as the patient's physical condition permits. It is also helpful to teach isometric exercises to patients to increase muscle mass, tone, and strength.

Include directives in the nursing plan of care for range-of-motion exercises, specifying what, how, and when, so that all who care for the patient observe the same routine. In some institutions, nurses work closely with physiotherapists in designing and implementing exercise programs. Refer to Table 33-2 for an explanation of terms related to movement. The following are basic guidelines when helping to put the patient's joints through range of motion:

- Teach the patient what exercise is being undertaken, why, and how it will be done. A show-and-tell technique is often helpful.
- Avoid overexertion and using exercises to the point that the patient develops fatigue. The exercises are not to

Guidelines for Nursing Care • 33-1

LOGROLLING A PATIENT

- Use a friction-reducing sheet, or if not available, a drawsheet, to facilitate smooth movement. Ensure the sheet extends from above the patient's shoulders to below the hips.
- Perform hand hygiene.
- Provide privacy by closing the door and/or pulling the bedside curtain.
- Explain what you are going to do to the patient.
- Perform a baseline assessment of the patient's neurologic status.
- Raise the bed to a comfortable working height and lower the side rails, if in raised position.
- Have the patient cross his or her arms on the chest.
- Place a pillow between the knees.
- Have two nurses stand on one side of the bed opposite the direction the patient will be turned. The third helper stands on the other side.

- Fanfold or roll the drawsheet tightly against the patient and carefully slide him or her to the side of the bed toward the two nurses.
- Have one helper then move to the other side of the bed, so two nurses are on the side to which the patient is turning.
- Face the patient. Everyone moves on a predetermined signal. Holding the rolled drawsheet taut to support the body, turn the patient as a unit toward the two nurses. The patient's head, shoulders, spine, hips, and knees should turn simultaneously.
- Use pillows to support the patient's back, buttocks, and legs in straight alignment in a side-lying position.
- Raise the side rails, lower the bed, and place the call bell within the patient's reach.
- Reassess the patient's neurological status and comfort level.
- Document the procedure and the patient's response.

exhaust or tax the patient. Certain exercises may need to be delayed until the patient's condition allows.
- Avoid neck hyperextension and attempts to achieve full range of motion in all joints with older patients. These movements may prove painful. Encourage adequate range of motion in those joints necessary to perform ADLs.
- Start gradually and work slowly. All movements should be smooth and rhythmic. Irregular and jerky movements are uncomfortable for patients.
- Move each joint until there is resistance but not pain. Uncomfortable reactions should be reported and exercises halted until further instructions are obtained.
- While exercising joints, use a variety of support measures to prevent muscle strain or injury to the patient, as demonstrated in Figure 33-22:
  - *Cupping*—placing a cupped hand under the joint to support it (e.g., under the elbow)
  - *Cradling*—supporting the joint with one hand while cradling the distal portion of the extremity with the remaining arm (e.g., the calf or forearm might be cradled while the knee or elbow is supported)
  - *Supporting* the joint by holding the adjacent distal and proximal muscular areas (indicated when a joint is painful); grasping muscle groups or major tendons is likely to cause injury to the tissues
- Return the joint to a neutral position, that is, its normal position of alignment, when finishing each exercise.
- Keep friction at a minimum when moving extremities to avoid injuring the skin.
- Use range-of-motion exercises twice a day, and do the exercises regularly to build up muscle and joint capabilities.

Each exercise is carried out two to five times. Many of the exercises can be carried out when the patient is being bathed and become part of that procedure. Encourage routine tasks such as eating, dressing, self-bathing, and writing to help to put certain joints through range of motion.
- Expect the patient's respiratory and heart rate to increase during exercising, which is good. These rates should return to usual resting levels within 3 minutes. If they do not, the exercises are probably too strenuous for the patient.
- Use passive exercises as necessary, but encourage active exercises of the same kind when the patient is able to do so independently. Exercises should continue at home after a period of hospitalization, as necessary.

▶ *Think back to Maggie Wyatt, the woman being discharged after treatment for a fracture. Range-of-motion exercises are essential for Maggie to maintain function. Although physical therapy would probably develop the exercise regimen, the nurse would need to reinforce these instructions with Maggie before discharge. In addition, the nurse would observe Maggie performing the active range-of-motion exercises and would assist with the passive exercises until she goes home.* ∎

The goal of range-of-motion exercises is to keep the patient in the best possible physical state when bed rest is necessary. When range of motion exercises are not considered as routine measures, consult the patient's physician.

FIGURE 33 22. Support measures used to prevent muscle strain or injury to the patient during range-of-motion exercises. (**A**) Using a cupped hand to support a joint. (**B**) Supporting the joint by holding the distal and proximal areas adjacent to the joint. (**C**) Cradling the distal portion of a lower extremity.

Skill 33-6 illustrates the normal movements incorporated in passive range-of-motion exercises.

Helping Patients Ambulate

Fortunately, for most patients, prolonged periods of bed rest are no longer considered necessary during most illnesses. Activity, even as mild as a short walk around the room, down the hall, from the bedroom to the living room, or out into the yard, is a protective measure for the body.

PHYSICAL CONDITIONING

Patients who are not confined to bed for long periods, who sleep well, and who experience possibly short periods of rest during the day may not require special considerations for increased physical activity in preparation for ambulation. However, others have to be prepared for the day when ambulation is resumed. Certain exercises that strengthen the overall efficiency of the musculoskeletal system can be done in bed. Check for physical activity restrictions or other contraindications before beginning any exercises.

Quadriceps and Gluteal Setting Drills (Sets)

Quadriceps drills are an isometric exercise—an exercise in which muscle tension occurs without a significant change in the length of the muscle. One of the most important mus-

cle groups used in walking is the quadriceps femoris. This muscle group helps extend the leg and flex the thigh. To help reduce weakness and make first attempts at walking easier, encourage bedridden patients to contract this muscle group frequently. Following are techniques for quadriceps drills:

* Have the patient contract or tighten the muscles on the front of the thighs. The patient has the feeling of pushing the knees downward into the mattress and pulling the feet upward.
* Have the patient hold the position just described while counting slowly to four, and then relax the muscles for an equal count. Emphasize that relaxation is important to prevent muscle fatigue.
* Caution the patient not to hold his or her breath during these exercises to avoid straining the heart.
* Teach the patient to do quadriceps drills two or three times each hour, four to six times a day.
* Instruct the patient to stop the exercise short of muscle fatigue.

The muscles in the buttocks can be exercised in the same way by pinching the buttocks together and then relaxing them. This is called gluteal setting. Tightening and holding the abdominal muscles for 6 seconds and then relaxing them also strengthens this muscle group to facilitate walking.

Pushups

The muscles of the arms and shoulders may also need strengthening before the patient is ready to be out of bed. Exercises should improve the strength needed to hold onto or get into a chair and to move about with greater ease. They are part of the preparation for patients who must learn to walk on crutches.

A trapeze attached to the bed of a patient who has limited use of the lower part of the body helps the patient to move about in bed and strengthens muscles in the upper part of the body. However, this does not strengthen the triceps, which is the muscle group necessary for crutch walking or for moving from a bed to a chair. More suitable exercises are pushups, which are done as follows:

- While sitting up in bed without support, the patient can do pushup exercises to strengthen the triceps. Instruct the patient to lift the hips off the bed by pushing down with the hands on the mattress. If the mattress is too soft, a block of books can be placed on the bed under the patient's hands.
- Pushups may also be done with the patient lying in bed on the abdomen. Instruct the patient to place the hands near the outstretched body at about shoulder level, with palms down on the mattress and elbows bent sharply. Then have the patient straighten the elbows to lift the head and shoulders off the bed.
- Pushups may also be done when the patient sits in an armchair or wheelchair. The patient places the hands on the arms of the chair and then raises the body out of the seat.
- Pushups should be done three or four times a day at first, with the number increased as upper body strength is increased.

> *Remember Maggie Wyatt, the woman with a fracture being discharged? Due to bed rest, her physical conditioning may be less than what it was before the fracture. Therefore, exercises, such as quadriceps and gluteal setting exercises and pushups in bed could help to improve Maggie's conditioning, allowing her to participate more fully in her care, including when she transfers from the bed to the chair or from the chair to the car.* ■

Dangling

Dangling refers to the position in which the person sits on the edge of the bed with legs and feet over the side of the bed. This exercise helps prepare patients for being out of bed. It is carried out as follows:

- Place the patient in the sitting position in bed for a few minutes. This will accustom the patient to this position and help prevent feelings of faintness.
- Place the bed in the low position or have a footstool handy on which the patient can rest the feet while dangling.

- Move the patient toward the side of the bed near you so that you do not stretch and strain while turning the patient.
- Pivot the patient a quarter of a turn by supporting the shoulders and legs. Swing the patient's legs over the side of the bed. The patient may place his or her hands on your shoulders.
- Rest the patient's feet on the floor or on a footstool. This gives a sense of security, and lessens the likelihood that the patient will slide off the bed.
- Have the patient move the feet using an up-and-down, marching motion. This promotes circulation in the legs.
- Remain with the patient and be ready to place the patient back to a lying position if he or she feels faint, to prevent falling out of bed.

Daily Activities for Purposeful Exercise

Many activities can be carried out in ways that encourage patients to move and thereby gain the benefit of exercise, improving physical conditioning. When patients understand the purpose, they often adopt other exercises for themselves. For example, position the bedside stand so that the patient must use shoulder and arm muscles to reach it, instead of placing it so that little effort is required to take things from it. Place the signal cord so that the patient must move either the arm or shoulder to reach it, as long as it is definitely within reach. Encourage patients to sit up and reach for the overbed table, to pull it close, and then to push it back in place. In addition, encourage patients to try to wash their back independently or put on socks while still in bed.

In a hospital setting, ADLs may be one of the few independent activities that a patient can perform. Allowing the patient to do as much as he or she can accomplish independently is vital. Be sure to offer encouragement and praise. "Learned dependency," which often occurs with the older adult population, can lead to a decrease in self-esteem and depression. Collaborate with the occupational therapist when necessary to determine types of adaptive equipment that would help the patient achieve maximal functional independence. Box 33-2 provides examples of available adaptive equipment. Providing the

---

Box 33-2   ADAPTIVE EQUIPMENT TO ASSIST WITH ACTIVITIES OF DAILY LIVING

- Long-handled bath sponges
- Reachers
- Long-handled shoe horns and sock aids
- Elastic shoelaces
- Utensils that are enlarged, specially angulated, or have special grips
- Velcro devices
- Feeding devices such as plates or bowls with suction-cup bottoms
- Splints and positioning equipment
- Environmental adaptations

A **B**

FIGURE 33-23. (**A**) One nurse guiding a patient to the floor. (**B**) Two nurses lowering a patient to the floor.

necessary adaptive tools, coupled with encouraging independence, will create the optimal outcome.

ASSISTANCE WITH WALKING

Many patients who have been confined to bed for an extended period find that they must almost learn to walk all over again. Often, nurses play a major role in the patient's recovery, mental outlook, hope, and faith, especially when the patient must adhere to a rigid and often difficult schedule of reeducating muscle groups. A patient who is able to raise the leg only 2.5 cm (1 inch) from the bed possesses sufficient power to begin walking.

Because muscle reeducation is a major task, the patient needs the assistance of experts in physical medicine. However, nurses can assist patients out of bed and help them walk when a physical therapist is not present. Plan to walk with a patient who is walking for the first few times after a period of bed rest.

Before getting the patient out of bed, do the following:

- Assess the patient's ability to walk and the need for assistance (one nurse, two nurses, walker, cane, walking belt, or crutches).
- Explain to the patient exactly what is to be done: transfer technique from bed to erect position, projected distance to be ambulated, assistance available, and the correct manner of using it. Instruct the patient to alert the nurse immediately if feeling dizzy or weak.
- Ensure that the patient has a clear path for ambulation.

Assist the patient to an erect position for ambulation, pausing after the patient is seated at the edge of the bed and again after the patient first stands, to ensure that the patient feels steady. Use a gait belt, if necessary, to prevent injury to the nurse and patient. Reinforce the need to stand erect and to hold the head high to achieve the full benefits of walking.

Patients who are fearful of walking often tend to look at their feet. Remind the patient to take deep breaths to aerate the lungs while walking. Because patients who are walking for the first time after prolonged bed rest often feel faint or weak, plan ambulation for a short distance, gradually increasing the distance as tolerated. As this distance is increased, have chairs readily available should the patient need to rest. Should a patient faint or begin to fall while walking, stand with feet apart to create a wide base of support and rock the pelvis out on the side facing the patient. With arms under the patient's axillae and encircling the patient, slide the patient down one's body to the floor, carefully protecting the patient's head (Fig. 33-23A). If the patient is wearing a gait belt, use the belt to ease the patient backward against one's own body and gently ease the patient to the floor while protecting the patient's head. When two nurses are assisting a patient who starts to fall or faint, they both should use one hand to grasp the gait belt to support the patient and grasp the patient's hand or wrist with their other hand. After they have steadied the patient, they can slowly lower him or her to a chair or the floor (Fig. 33-23B). Practice these maneuvers before they are needed in an emergency situation.

One-Nurse Assist

Patients who require minimal nursing assistance may walk well with the nurse walking alongside. Provide support by standing at the patient's side and placing both hands at the patient's waist. Supporting the patient at the waist helps the patient to maintain an erect posture and prevents unintentionally pulling the patient to one side. Use of a gait belt snugly secured around the patient's waist also provides this type of support. Grasp the belt securely in the back and walk behind and slightly to the side of the patient (Fig. 33-24).

Frequently, it is necessary to assist the patient with intravenous (IV) therapy equipment to walk. Secure a portable IV pole that moves easily. The patient walks with

FIGURE 33-24. Assistance with ambulation. The nurse stands on the patient's weaker side and grasps the gait belt.

the assistance of the nurse and the portable IV pole. Ensure that all the equipment is secure before walking and be alert for any tension or sudden action that might dislodge or interfere with the infusion. Also, consider reviewing this technique with family members who are assisting with ambulation and are unfamiliar with how to steady the patient, maneuver equipment, and navigate through crowded or narrow areas.

When a patient has weakness or paralysis on one side, stand on the weaker or affected side and stabilize the patient by grasping the gait belt. Support the patient's weak arm by using one hand to support the patient's forearm and hand.

Two-Nurse Assist

A two-nurse assist is the safer method to use when there is uncertainty about the patient's ability to walk. Use of a gait belt snugly secured around the patient's waist provides a safe place for the nurses to support the patient. Each nurse should grasp the belt securely with the hand nearest the patient at the handle on each side of the patient. Support the patient's near arm by holding the patient's lower arm or hand. Walk slightly behind and to the side of the patient.

MECHANICAL AIDS FOR WALKING

Various devices can assist a patient with walking. These devices enhance the patient's balance and ability to bear weight. The most common are walkers, canes, braces, and crutches. Typically, a patient is fitted for a device and instructed in its use in the department of physical medicine or physical therapy. In this instance, the nurse's concern is chiefly to reinforce the teaching the patient has received and

to ensure that the patient continues to use the device properly to assist in safe ambulation. In some healthcare settings, however, nurses may be responsible for fitting patients with the device. Whenever you assess a patient who has been using a walker, cane, brace, or crutches for a period of time, determine whether the device is still needed, whether it continues to meet the patient's needs, and whether the patient continues to use it properly.

Some older patients consider the use of a mobility aid a visible symbol of weakness or an indication of decline in capabilities and loss of independence. Many patients refuse to use them and keep them out of sight. If the mobility aid is intended for short-term use (e.g., after hip replacement surgery), the response is usually more positive. Be sensitive to a patient's perspective regarding these devices and focus on the meaning the aid has for the patient, rather than simply emphasizing how to use it. Allow patients some control over their mobility decisions while still ensuring a safe environment. General guidelines for helping patients who need the assistance of a walker, cane, brace, or crutches include the following:

- Whenever possible, instruct the patient and family members in the correct use of the device before it is needed (e.g., before surgery). If family members are knowledgeable, they can reinforce the teaching as needed.
- When ready to begin walking with the new device, make sure the patient is wearing rubber-soled, well-fitting shoes and that there is a clear path for ambulation (clean, flat, dry, well lit). Use a gait belt, especially if the patient is at high risk for falls.
- Before moving, make sure the patient is steady on the feet when standing; instruct the patient to stand erect, looking straight ahead. The nurse should walk behind and slightly to one side of the patient (in cases of hemiparesis or hemiparalysis, walk on the patient's affected side). Should the patient lose balance, be prepared to grasp the patient's shoulder and the gait belt to steady the patient.

Walker

A walker is a lightweight metal frame (usually aluminum) with four legs (Fig. 33-25A). Walkers improve balance by increasing the patient's base of support, enhancing lateral stability, and supporting the patient's weight. The walker provides a sense of security and support. There are several types of walkers, specified according to the arm strength and balance of the patient. Most walkers have four legs with rubber tips. Some walkers have wheels on the front legs. These walkers are best for patients with a gait that is too fast for a walker without wheels and for patients who have difficulty lifting a walker. Because lifting repeatedly is not required, energy expenditure and stress to the back and upper extremities is lower than with a standard walker (Mincer, 2007). Walkers also are available with wheels on all four legs. These can be used by patients who require a larger base of support and do not rely on the walker to bear weight. If full

FIGURE 33-25. Mechanical aids to walking. (**A**) A walker is a lightweight metal frame with a broad, four-point base of support. The walker should be adjusted to the height of the patient's hip joint so that the patient's elbows are flexed about 30 degrees. (**B**) Three types of canes. Single-ended canes with half-circle handles are recommended for patients requiring minimal support. Single-ended canes with straight handles are recommended for patients with hand weakness. Three- or four-prong canes are recommended for patients with poor balance

body weight is applied to this type of walker, it could roll away, resulting in a fall. Wheeled walkers are best for patients who need minimal weight bearing from the walker. Walkers often prove to be difficult to maneuver through doorways and congested areas. They should not be used on stairs (Mincer, 2007).

When the patient stands between the back legs of the walker with arms relaxed at the side, the top of the walker should line up with the crease on the inside of the patient's wrist. When the patient's hands are placed on the grips, elbows should be flexed about 30 degrees (Mayo, 2007). The walker's rubber tips should be intact to prevent slipping. Generally, the patient lifts the walker without wheels ahead of himself or herself and steps into it. Instruct a patient using a walker to do the following:

- Wear nonskid shoes or slippers.
- When rising from a seated position, use the chair arms for support. Once standing, place one hand at a time on the walker and move forward into it.
- Begin by pushing the walker forward, keeping the back upright. Place one leg inside the walker, keeping the walker in place. Then, step forward with the remaining leg into the walker, keeping the walker still. Repeat the process by moving the walker forward again.
- Caution the patient to avoid pushing the walker out too far in front and leaning over the walker. The

patient should always step into the walker, rather than walking behind it, staying upright as they move (Mayo, 2007).
- Never attempt to use a walker on stairs.

Canes

Canes widen a person's base of support, providing increased balance (Mincer, 2007). Canes come in three variations (see Fig. 33-25B): single-ended canes with half-circle handles (recommended for patients requiring minimal support and those who will be using stairs frequently), single-ended canes with straight handles (recommended for patients with hand weakness because the handgrip is easier to hold but not recommended for patients with poor balance), canes with three (tripod) or four prongs (quad cane) or legs to provide a wide base of support (recommended for patients with poor balance).

Many canes are adjustable; fit them so that when the patient stands with the cane's tip 4 inches (10 cm) to the side of the foot, the cane extends from the floor to the patient's hip joint. The elbow should be flexed 30 degrees when holding the cane. Rubber tips on the cane prevent slipping and accidents. Inspect these regularly to ensure they are intact. Teach patients to stand erect when walking with a cane and not to lean out over the cane.

When walking with a cane, instruct patients to hold the cane in the opposite hand from the leg with the most severe deficit (Mincer, 2007). Ambulation proceeds in the following fashion:

1. The patient stands with weight evenly distributed between the feet and the cane.
2. The cane is held on the patient's stronger side and is advanced 4 to 12 inches (10 to 30 cm).
3. Supporting weight on the stronger leg and the cane, the patient advances the weaker foot forward, parallel with the cane.
4. Supporting weight on the weaker leg and the cane, the patient next advances the stronger leg forward ahead of the cane (heel slightly beyond the tip of the cane).
5. The weaker leg is moved forward until even with the stronger leg, and the cane is once again advanced as in step 2.

When less support is required from the cane, the patient can advance the cane and weaker leg forward while the stronger leg supports the patient's weight. Teach patients to position their canes within easy reach when they sit down so that they can rise easily.

Braces

Braces that support weakened leg muscles are available in many variations. Nursing responsibilities include knowing when the brace is to be worn and the correct technique for applying the brace, monitoring to ensure correct use of the brace by the patient, and observing for any untoward problems the brace might cause (e.g., skin irritation). Muscle changes such as those occurring with growth and development or brought about by illness (atrophy) may require the brace to be refitted to maintain its effectiveness.

Crutches

Sometimes it is necessary for patients to use crutches for a time to avoid using one leg or to help strengthen one or both legs. The two types of crutches most commonly used are axillary crutches and the forearm crutches (Fig. 33-26).

Forearm crutches are used for patients requiring long-term support for ambulation (Mincer, 2007). A supportive frame extends beyond the handgrip for the lower arm to help guide the crutch. These crutches are more likely to be used by patients who have permanent limitations and will always need crutch assistance for ambulation.

Axillary crutches are used to provide support for patients who have temporary restrictions on ambulation. These crutches require significant strength to use. Patients must

FIGURE 33-26. Axillary (*left*) and forearm (*right*) support crutches.

have adequate upper body and upper arm strength to use this type of crutch.

The procedure for crutch walking is usually taught by a physical therapist, but it is important for the nurse to be knowledgeable about the patient's progress and the gait being taught. Be prepared to guide the patient at home or in the hospital after the initial teaching is completed. Remind the patient that the support of body weight should come primarily on the hands and arms while using the crutches, not in the axillary areas, where pressure may damage nerves and cut off circulation. Also, the crutches should not be forced into the axillae each time the body moves forward. Teaching Tips 33-1 summarizes the important content to reinforce regarding crutch walking.

Promoting Exercise

PREVENTING ILLNESS AND PROMOTING WELLNESS THROUGH EXERCISE

According to Healthy People 2010, regular physical activity helps prevent certain chronic diseases such as hypertension, type 2 diabetes, cardiovascular disease, obesity, and osteoporosis (U.S. Department of Health and Human Services, 2000). Vigorous physical activity is not always needed to achieve positive results. Studies have shown that moderate physical activity can be beneficial when incorporated into daily routines (National Institutes of Health [NIH], 2005).

Nurses who role model healthy behaviors are more effective teachers. Use the Promoting Health Display 33-1: Activity for yourself before using it with others. This display reflects on self-care behaviors vital for maintaining a healthy level of activity. Promoting exercise and emphasizing wellness behaviors are challenging opportunities for nurses. It is important to be committed to assisting and supporting patients to make lifestyle changes that improve the patients' health and well-being.

Advanced age has traditionally been associated with a decline in muscle strength and reluctance to exercise. Maintaining balance during exercise is frequently a concern of patients and caregivers. The accompanying Examples of Nursing Interventions and Nursing Outcomes Classifications (NIC/NOC) box lists standardized nursing interventions and corresponding outcomes related to helping the patient with impaired physical mobility. As researchers focus on the potential of regular exercise activities to slow the aging process, nurses intervene to prevent the deleterious effects associated with decreased physical activity. See the accompanying Focus on the Older Adult display for a summary of the benefits of exercise and specific precautions related to exercise for this age group.

An ongoing program of exercise for older patients also promotes confidence, improves outlook, offers opportunities for socialization, and fosters continued independence, while lessening the potential for falls and other injuries (Haines, 2007; Tseng, Chen, Wu, & Lin, 2007). Older people who integrate a

CRUTCH WALKING

Health Topic	Teaching Tip	Why Is This Important?
Correct positioning for use of crutches	Prevent pressure on the axillae. Keep elbows close to sides. Prevent crutches from getting closer than 12 inches to feet.	Pressure placed on the axillae can cause damage to nerves and circulation. This helps stabilize the crutches to prevent the patient from falling. This prevents the patient from tripping over the crutches.
Functioning at home	*To rise from a chair:* Slide forward to the edge of the chair. Extend the injured leg to prevent any weight bearing. Place crutches on unaffected side, lean forward, and push off using the crutches. *To climb stairs:* Advance unaffected leg past crutches, then place weight on unaffected leg. Advance affected leg and then crutches to the step. Continue with this order until top of stairs is reached. *To descend stairs:* Move crutches and affected leg first, followed by the unaffected leg.	Patient needs to learn that everyday occurrences may be challenging and, if not done correctly, may end up with injury to affected leg.

planned exercise regimen into their daily routine benefit physiologically and report improved self-esteem.

DESIGNING EXERCISE PROGRAMS

The benefits of exercise for each of the major body systems are so significant that designing individualized exercise programs for patients is an important nursing responsibility, often in conjunction with the physical therapist. Such a program should incorporate ADLs and planned exercise sessions. Depending on the patient's physical condition, exercise is designed to promote optimal fitness.

The individual's commitment to a program of regular exercise depends on the following:

- Knowledge of the benefits of exercise and the problems related to immobility
- Appreciation of the fact that in society, sedentary lifestyles are common and most people must consciously choose to exercise
- Belief that each person is responsible for his or her own health and that exercise is essential to one's well-being

Foster a commitment to regular exercise by teaching and counseling patients about exercise. To do this, be knowledgeable about the types and benefits of exercise as well as the risks associated with exercise.

When working with a patient to develop an individualized exercise prescription, use the following guidelines:

- Explore the patient's fitness goals, interests, skills, exercise opportunities, and exercise capacity.

- Assist the patient in obtaining medical clearance for exercise.
- Explore feasible exercise activities with the patient, considering the health benefits sought, the time involved, cost, any need for special equipment, precautions, and risks.
- Develop an exercise program that specifies warm-up and cool-down activities (walking, stretching) and three or four major exercise activities from which the patient can choose.
- Specify the frequency, duration, and intensity of the exercise activity. The recommended frequency for most types of exercise is at least 30 minutes a day of at least moderate-intensity physical activity on most, and preferably all, days of the week (Marcus et al., 2006). Moderate-intensity physical activity produces a noticeable increase in heart rate and breathing, working hard enough to raise heart rate and breathing, yet able to carry on a conversation. Aerobic activities of daily living that would meet this intensity level include washing windows and sweeping floors (Aquaro Sebastian, 2007).
- Encourage the patient to complement the exercise program with everyday activities that require exercise.
- Try to identify with the patient any potential threats to the exercise program's successful implementation. Plan support strategies.
- Use ongoing evaluation to determine whether the exercise prescription is meeting the patient's needs and whether the patient is adhering to the prescription.

PROMOTING HEALTH • 33-1

Activity

Patients view nurses as role models for achieving healthy lifestyles. Use the following assessment checklist to determine how well you are meeting your need for exercise. Then develop a prescription for self-care by choosing appropriate behaviors from the list of suggestions.

Assessment Checklist

☐ almost always   ☐ sometimes   ☐ almost never

☐ ☐ ☐ 1. My lifestyle demonstrates that I place a high value on exercise as a component of wellness (e.g., I use stairs instead of elevators).

☐ ☐ ☐ 2. I exercise for 30 to 45 minutes three or four times per week.

☐ ☐ ☐ 3. I have sufficient energy for each day's tasks.

☐ ☐ ☐ 4. I maintain my target weight/BMI.

Self-Care Behaviors

1. Decide to make the most of everyday opportunities for exercise: use stairs instead of elevators, walk instead of ride, park the car farther from your destination than usual and walk the distance briskly, and so forth.
2. Choose exercise activities you enjoy and plan three or four 30- to 45-minute exercise sessions weekly.

3. Obtain medical clearance for exercise if you fall in a high-risk group. Learn and observe the appropriate exercise safeguards (e.g., wear running shoes with the proper support).
4. Alternate types of exercise to avoid boredom.
5. Use part of your lunchtime for brisk walking or other exercise.
6. Invite a friend to exercise with you so you have the added support of a buddy or join a spa, health club, or exercise group.
7. Consistently use principles of body mechanics in both leisure and work activities.
8. Build up exercise sessions gradually to avoid overexertion and injury to muscles.
9. Evaluate your lifestyle to see what prevents you from exercising regularly and address these factors (low value attached to health or exercise, low motivation, lack of time, lack of rest, or faulty nutrition).

Information to promote activity and exercise is available online. Check out these sites: NHLBI Aim for a Healthy Weight at www.nhlbi.nih.gov/health/public/heart/obesity/lose_wt; President's Council on Physical Fitness and Sports at www.fitness.gov; and the American Dietetic Association at www.eatright.org.

Examples of Nursing Interventions and Nursing Outcomes Classifications (NIC/NOC)

Exercise Therapy: Balance

Nursing Interventions

- Determine patient's ability to participate in activities requiring balance.
- Evaluate sensory functions (e.g., vision, hearing, proprioception).
- Provide safe environment for practice of exercises.
- Encourage patient to maintain wide base of support, if needed.
- Assist to stand (or sit) and rock body from side to side to stimulate balance mechanisms.
- Assist patient to practice standing with eyes closed for short periods at regular intervals to stimulate proprioception.
- Monitor patient's response to balance exercises.

Nursing Outcomes

- Activity tolerance
- Coordinated movement
- Endurance
- Patient satisfaction: Functional assistance
- Vital signs

From Bulechek, G., Butcher, H., & McCloskey Dochterman, J. (Eds.). (2008). *Nursing interventions classification (NIC)* (5th ed., p. 336). St. Louis, MO: Mosby Elsevier; and Moorhead, S., Johnson, M., Maas, M., Swanson, E. (Eds.). (2008). *Nursing outcomes classification (NOC)* (5th ed., p. 746). A full listing of nursing activities for each nursing intervention and outcomes can be found in these books.

FOCUS ON THE OLDER ADULT

NURSING STRATEGIES TO PROMOTE EXERCISE AND ACTIVITY FOR AGE-RELATED CHANGES

Age-Related Changes	Nursing Strategies
Activity Intolerance	
• Decreased respiratory vital capacity	• Encourage patient to gradually increase physical activity and to listen to cues from his or her own body.
• Decreased transport of oxygenated blood to tissue (as in chronic obstructive pulmonary disease or decreased cardiac output)	• Instruct patient to avoid sudden position changes that may cause dizziness.
	• Instruct patient to avoid extreme temperatures if exercising.
	• Provide for sufficient hydration.
	• Encourage patient to avoid exercise if weak or ill.
	• Instruct patient to stop exercising if chest pain occurs, and consult with physician before resuming activity.
	• Instruct patient to respect fatigue. Do not push to the point of exhaustion.
Impaired Physical Mobility	
• Decreased range of motion	• Encourage patient to warm up before beginning exercises and to cool down after exercising.
• Decreased stability of gait	• Encourage patient to modify exercises versus forcing joints beyond the natural range of motion.
	• Discuss safety precautions that patient may take when exercising, such as walk in a gym or mall versus on an uneven sidewalk.
	• Recommend that patient wear proper footwear when exercising.

Box 33-3 identifies characteristics of a successful exercise program and prevention strategies to avoid the risks associated with exercise.

Evaluating

When evaluating the effectiveness of a plan of care designed to help patients enhance, maintain, or regain mobility and fitness goals, use each nurse–patient interaction to evaluate the patient in the following respects:

• General ease of movement and gait
• Body alignment
• Joint structure and function
• Muscle mass, tone, and strength
• Endurance

An excellent time to assess these essential ingredients of well-being is when the patient is performing simple everyday tasks such as walking, undertaking hygiene measures, dressing, and eating. Because illness and enforced inactivity can affect these tasks negatively, ongoing evaluation is necessary if serious problems are to be avoided. For examples of the nursing process for activity, see the accompanying concept map for Kelsi Lester and Nursing Plan of Care 33-1 for Quan Hong Nguyen.

Box 33-3 CHARACTERISTICS OF A SUCCESSFUL EXERCISE PROGRAM

• The program is individually designed (considers the individual's fitness goals, interests, skills, exercise opportunities, and exercise capacity).
• The program specifies warm-up and cool-down activities and a variety of major exercise activities—variety is preferable to a single-exercise activity.
• The program specifies frequency, intensity, and duration of exercise.
• The program is convenient to perform, compatible with the individual's lifestyle, and fun!
• The individual in such a program should understand the program and feel confident that exercise will result in definite health benefits.

Prevention Strategies to Avoid Risks Associated With Exercise
People beginning exercise programs should be familiar with the following guidelines:

• Obtain a pre-exercise medical examination and medical supervision during exercise if older than age 35 years and sedentary or if there is any past or current cardiovascular condition.
• Begin a new exercise program slowly and allow your body's support structure time to accommodate to the new stress.
• Know your body and respect its limitations. Never force a joint beyond its natural range of motion.
• Respect fatigue. Whenever you feel tingling, pain, or burning in a muscle, stop and rest the muscle for 15 minutes before continuing to exercise.
• Follow the safety guidelines for specific exercises; for example, joggers are advised to run on soft surfaces as opposed to cement or asphalt, to wear well-constructed shoes with thick soles and arch supports, and to run in a safe environment with a low pollution index.

Kelsi Lester is a 10-year-old girl in the pediatric unit as a result of a skiing accident. She is unconscious and may or may not regain consciousness. She is on complete bed rest. She requires frequent positioning to maintain correct body alignment and attention to her ROM. She responds to painful stimuli with slight nonpurposeful withdrawal. No spontaneous movements are noted. Ultrasound of lower extremities was negative for deep vein thrombosis (DVT). Subcutaneous heparin administration has been prescribed to prevent thrombus formation. Continuous tube feedings and intravenous therapy are prescribed to meet Kelsi's fluid and nutritional needs. Kelsi has been incontinent of stool and has an indwelling urinary catheter. Her heels are reddened, but otherwise her skin is intact. Kelsi's mother is at the bedside; she states, "I feel so helpless."

Priority 1	Priority 2	Priority 3
Nursing Diagnosis: Ineffective Tissue Perfusion: Potential for Thrombus Formation related to altered mobility. **Supporting Data:** • Unconscious • No spontaneous movements • No swelling or redness areas noted in calf • Ultrasound of lower extremities was negative for DVT	**Nursing Diagnosis: Impaired Physical Mobility** related to altered neurological functioning. **Supporting Data:** • Unconscious • No spontaneous movements noted • Responds to painful stimuli with nonpurposeful withdrawal • Complete bed rest	**Nursing Diagnosis: Impaired Skin Integrity** related to altered mobility from skiing accident. **Supporting Data:** • No spontaneous movements • Heels reddened • Incontinent of stool • Continuous tube feedings • Foley catheter and IV in place • Complete bed rest
Outcome: Patient will remain free of DVT.	**Outcome:** Patient will maintain neurological function and be free from muscular contractures.	**Outcome:** Patient will maintain intact skin integrity.
Nursing Interventions: • Maintain anti-embolism stockings and sequential pneumatic compression devices • Turn and reposition at least every 2 hours • Perform passive ROM exercises 3 times a day • Maintain adequate hydration with parenteral therapy and tube feedings as prescribed • Monitor for side effects of anticoagulant therapy	**Nursing Interventions:** • Assess motor function • Turn and reposition at least every 2 hours • Support proper body alignment using positioning devices • Use foot boot to prevent foot drop • Use wrist splints and hand rolls to maintain functional position • Perform passive ROM 3 times a day; teach parents to assist with exercises • Consult physical therapy and occupational therapy • Explain procedures to Kelsi prior to performing activity	**Nursing Interventions:** • Assess skin every 8 hours • Use Braden scale to assess risk for pressure ulcer • Maintain nutrition by monitoring tube feedings as prescribed • Use alternating pressure mattress • Turn and reposition every 2 hours • Remove protective devices and splints periodically to assess for skin irritation • Assess IV insertion site for any redness or swelling • Document any areas of skin breakdown • Check for incontinence frequently and cleanse perirectal area; apply barrier cream • Use bed linens to reposition to avoid shearing pressure force
Evaluation: Kelsi has no occurrences of DVT. Anti-embolism stockings, sequential pneumatic compression devices, and activity have been maintained.	**Evaluation:** Kelsi is being turned every 2 hours. Positioning devices are being used. No contractures or foot drop is noted. Parents are assisting in turning and ROM exercises.	**Evaluation:** Kelsi's heels are no longer reddened. She shows no signs of skin breakdown.

- - - - - Relationship   Assessment   Nursing Diagnosis   Outcome Identification   Interventions   Evaluation

Concept map displaying the nursing process for Kelsi Lester.

NURSING PLAN OF CARE · 33-1
For Quan Hong Nguyen

Quan Hong Nguyen is an alert, 57-year-old married man who was admitted to the hospital with a diagnosis of an ischemic stroke (cerebrovascular accident or 'brain attack' [Smeltzer, Bare, Hinkle, & Cheever, 2010]) secondary to thrombosis (formation of a blood clot). He has a history of hypertension. This is his second hospital day, and the attending physicians have termed the stroke a *completed stroke*; that is, Mr. Nguyen's neurologic deficits have been unchanged for 2 days, and he is believed to be ready for more aggressive rehabilitative treatment. On hospital day 2, an assessment of Mr. Nguyen's mobility status and ability to participate in activities of daily living revealed the following data:

- *Mental status*—basically alert and able to follow simple commands; expresses his needs verbally when encouraged, but speech is slow; seems forgetful of usual routine for basic self-care activities
- *Neuromuscular status*—hemiplegia; severe motor and sensory deficits of the left side of the face and the left arm and leg

- *Muscle mass, tone, and strength*—well-developed muscles in all extremities; history of a lifetime of sports, most recently played tennis two to four times weekly; decreased muscle tone (hypotonicity, flaccidity) in left arm and leg motor function is absent in left arm and very weak in left leg; strong motor function on right extremities; incapable of weight-bearing on left side; incapable of independent turning, sitting, standing, transferring, or ambulation
- *Joint mobility*—decreased on left side; otherwise full range of motion; no contractures
- *Endurance*—fatigues quickly (e.g., during complete bath)
- Some deficit in spatial–perceptual orientation (e.g., ignores objects on his left side), but it is difficult to assess this completely yet

NURSING DIAGNOSIS Impaired Physical Mobility (turning in bed, sitting, standing, transferring, ambulating) related to left hemiplegia and weakness as manifested by: motor function absent in left arm and weak in left leg, decreased joint mobility in left extremities, fatigue

EXPECTED OUTCOME 1/25/12 Whenever observed, the patient will:

- Be in correct body alignment with (1) each joint on the left side higher than the joint proximal to it and (2) supportive devices in place (bed board, footboard, trochanter roll, hand–wrist splint, shoulder sling, pillows)

Nursing Interventions

At each position change (as dictated by every-2-hour turn schedule posted at the bedside), make sure that the patient is in correct alignment. Follow agency positioning guidelines for the supine, side-lying (lies on unaffected side), and prone positions.

Rationale

Correct positioning prevents contractures, relieves pressures, and maintains alignment.
- Positioning each joint higher than the preceding one prevents edema and its resulting fibrosis.
- Placing the patient in the prone position for 30 minutes two or three times daily helps prevent knee and hip flexion contractures.

Evaluative Statement

1/27/12 Outcome being met. Every-2-hour positioning schedule being followed with patient in correct body alignment to prevent contractures.

S. Beecher, RN

(continued)

NURSING PLAN OF CARE · 33-1

For Quan Hong Nguyen (continued)

Nursing Interventions	Rationale	Evaluative Statement
Use the following supportive devices: firm mattress, footboard, trochanter roll, shoulder sling when patient is in upright position, volar resting splint, and pillows.	Support devices aid in maintaining the patient in correct positioning. • Firm mattress provides skeletal support. • Footboard during flaccid period prevents footdrop, heel cord shortening, and plantar flexion. • Trochanter roll prevents external rotation of hip when patient is in dorsal position. • Shoulder sling during flaccid period prevents shoulder subluxation and shoulder–hand syndrome. • Volar resting splint supports the wrist and hand in a functional position. • A pillow in the axilla of the left side prevents adduction of the affected side.	
Teach both the patient and family the importance of correct positioning.	Teaching promotes self-care and lays the foundation for successful rehabilitation.	
Allow the family to participate in helping the patient to get comfortable in the different positions.	Involving the family in the patient's care facilitates the coping process.	

EXPECTED OUTCOME   By hospital day 7, 1/30/12, the patient will:

• Replace the passive range-of-motion exercises the nurse is now performing four times daily to all joints with (1) the patient's active exercise of the left arm and left leg and (2) the patient's active range-of-motion exercises for all other joints

Nursing Interventions	Rationale	Evaluative Statement
Assess the patient's knowledge of the importance of exercise and ability and motivation to exercise.	Unless the patient understands the reason for exercise and is physically, mentally, and attitudinally capable of exercise, he will not follow through.	1/30/12 Outcome partially met. Patient has successfully demonstrated complete set of range-of-motion exercises (to both left and right sides); however, he tires during the exercises and stops unless verbally encouraged.
Teach the patient how to exercise his left arm and leg by using his unaffected (right) extremities.	Active exercise maintains joint mobility, prevents contracture development in the paralyzed extremity, prevents further deterioration of the neuromuscular system, helps to regain motor control, and increases circulation.	*Revision:* Monitor patient's exercise four times daily; continue to enlist family's support. *S. Beecher, RN*
Demonstrate a complete set of range-of-motion exercises to the patient and family and have the patient return the demonstrations.	Involving the family helps ensure the success of the exercise program because it requires a big time and effort commitment.	

NURSING PLAN OF CARE · 33-1

For Quan Hong Nguyen (continued)

EXPECTED OUTCOME   By hospital day 7, 1/30/12, the patient will:

- Perform quadriceps, gluteal, and abdominal settings five times daily

Nursing Interventions	Rationale	Evaluative Statement
Teach the patient and family how to tighten the quadriceps, gluteal, and abdominal muscles and hold them for 6 seconds (slow count to 4) before relaxing. A 2-minute rest should be allowed between contractions and the patient cautioned not to hold his breath during these exercises because this places strain on the heart. The exercises should be stopped short of muscle fatigue.	These exercises will maintain muscle mass, tone, and strength (while the patient is on bed rest); and prevent atrophy. They also increase circulation to the exercised body parts.	1/30/12 Outcome partially met. Patient has demonstrated exercises correctly; however, he needs to be reminded to perform them. Family is effective in this regard. *Revision:* Compliment family on excellent job they are doing and reinforce importance of exercise to maximize rehabilitative potential. *S. Beecher, RN*

EXPECTED OUTCOME   By hospital day 7, 1/30/12, the patient will:

- Participate in the every-2-hour positioning schedule by assisting with turning to the degree he is able

Nursing Interventions	Rationale	Evaluative Statement
Teach the patient how he can help to reposition himself by grabbing onto the side rail with his right hand and also by placing his unaffected leg under the left one to move himself.	The more the patient can do independently, the more in control he will feel. These activities will pave the way to increasing independence in self-care activities.	1/27/12 Outcome met. Patient consistently assists in repositioning. Seems pleased to be able to help the nurses in this way. *S. Beecher, RN*

EXPECTED OUTCOME   By hospital day 7, 1/30/12, the patient will:

- Demonstrate a safe pivot transfer from bed to chair and chair to bed

Nursing Interventions	Rationale	Evaluative Statement
Assess the stage of recovery of muscle function.	Most patients will begin to show signs of spasticity with exaggerated reflexes within 48 hours—this denotes progress. If muscles are still flaccid after several weeks, prognosis for regaining function is poor.	1/30/12 Outcome met. Patient can safely transfer from bed to chair and chair to bed but requires nursing assistance. *S. Beecher, RN*

(continued)

NURSING PLAN OF CARE • 33-1

For Quan Hong Nguyen (continued)

EXPECTED OUTCOME By hospital day 7, 1/30/12, the patient will:

- Demonstrate standing balance

Nursing Interventions	Rationale	Evaluative Statement
Assess activity tolerance by taking vital signs before attempting balance training and transfers.	Vital signs and the patient's physical condition should be assessed before a new activity, during the activity, and shortly afterward to assess activity tolerance.	1/30/12 Outcome not met. Patient has not demonstrated standing balance; falls to left side without nursing support. *Revision:* Allow more time for goal achievement.
Precede transfers with balance training. Assist the patient to a sitting position at the edge of the bed and observe for steadiness and the ability to maintain an erect posture.	The patient needs sitting and standing balance before progressing to harder tasks. Dizziness or syncope may signal vasomotor instability.	*S. Beecher, RN*
Place the chair by the bed on the patient's unaffected side and assist the patient to dress. Initially, the nurse helps the patient to stand by placing his or her right knee against the patient's strong knee, grasping the patient around the waist with both arms, and pulling the patient forward while rocking back on the left leg (nurse's knees are slightly flexed).	This prevents the patient's knees from buckling and the pressure of the nurse's knee forces the patient to straighten the strong knee and bear weight on it. In this position, the patient's feet cannot slip forward. In this position, the nurse is using good principles of body mechanics.	
Once the patient is standing, assess standing balance and observe for signs of activity intolerance (pallor, shortness of breath, excessive increase in pulse rate, perspiration). Direct the patient to (1) grab the far arm of the chair with his strong arm, (2) turn on his strong foot, and (3) sit down. The nurse's right leg and the patient's strong leg are used as a pivot.	Using the unaffected extremity facilitates movement and provides stability.	
Pivot patient out of bed to chair three times a day (may pivot out of bed to bedside commode). Gradually increase time in chair based on patient's tolerance. Correctly align patient in chair using supportive devices as necessary.	Increasing exercise to the patient's tolerance level promotes improved muscle strength and maintenance of range of motion.	

(continued)

NURSING PLAN OF CARE · 33-1

For Quan Hong Nguyen (continued)

EXPECTED OUTCOME   On discharge to rehabilitation center, the patient will:

- Be free of contractures

Nursing Interventions	Rationale	Evaluative Statement
Implement previously stated nursing actions.	These actions promote independence and return to activities of daily living.	1/30/12 Outcome met. Patient has no contractures. *S. Beecher, RN*

NURSING DIAGNOSIS   Self-Care Deficit (all basic self-care activities) related to decreased alertness and left-sided motor and sensory deficits as manifested by: inability to use left arm (is right-handed), inability to ambulate, forgetfulness, fatigue.

EXPECTED OUTCOME   By hospital day 7, 1/30/12, the patient will:

- Demonstrate beginning ability to resume self-care activities despite motor and sensory deficits of left side; use right arm to (1) assist in morning hygiene; (2) feed himself (finger foods, beverages); and (3) exercise

Nursing Interventions	Rationale	Evaluative Statement
Continue to assess extent of patient's motor and sensory deficits and ability to perform self-care activities.	This facilitates recognition of any recovery of function and allows setting of appropriate goals.	1/29/12 Outcome met. For the past 2 days, patient has washed his left arm, abdomen, and legs; combed his hair; fed himself; and performed range-of-motion exercises. *S. Beecher, RN*
Set realistic short-term goals for each session with patient and reward progress: "This morning we'll see how much of your bath you are able to manage yourself!" "It must feel good to be able to do this for yourself again."	Adding *realistic* new tasks for each day gives the patient a goal to work toward; a pattern of *noticed* success encourages continued efforts.	
Approach patient from his unaffected side, and place call bell, bedside table, phone, and so on, on this side.	This helps the patient to compensate for alterations in sensory perception.	
Teach patient how to transfer all self-care activities to the unaffected side and how to use one-handed techniques and adaptive equipment.	There is never only one way to do anything.	
Encourage patient to brush his teeth, comb his hair, bathe and feed himself, and to assist in toileting. Explain to the family why it is critical to allow him to do these things himself, even if movements are tiring, clumsy, and initially frustrating.	This improves the patient's sense of control of his own activities of daily living and improves morale.	

(continued)

NURSING PLAN OF CARE · 33-1

For Quan Hong Nguyen (continued)

Nursing Interventions	Rationale	Evaluative Statement
Continually reevaluate the patient's need for gentle care versus firm, directive encouragement. Involve the family in this process.	Emotional lability is common after stroke. Patients fluctuate between heroic efforts toward independent self-care and whining demands to be totally cared for. The appropriate nursing response varies from moment to moment and runs the range of tender care to unrelenting firm direction. All nursing responses need to communicate the nurse's sincere care for the patient and commitment to developing his best potential.	

EXPECTED OUTCOME   On discharge to rehabilitation center, the patient will:

- Show signs of physical and mental readiness to acquire increasing independence in self-care

Nursing Interventions	Rationale	Evaluative Statement
Implement previously stated nursing actions.	These actions help the patient toward regaining control of his daily living and improve morale.	1/31/12 Outcome met. Patient's muscle strength and joint mobility maintained during hospitalization. Patient is now participating in self-care activities and is eager to learn skills to become more independent. *S. Beecher, RN*

SAMPLE DOCUMENTATION

1/25/12 3 p.m., Nursing

Dr. Steel examined the patient at 1 p.m. and noted he is now in "completed stroke stage and ready for more aggressive rehabilitative treatment." This was explained to patient, his wife, and son. The patient smiled and seemed to understand that he is out of immediate danger. Initial instructions given to the patient on how he can assist with position changes and actively exercise his left arm and leg. Correctly demonstrated these maneuvers with verbal cuing. Motor function still absent in left arm and weak in left leg. Plan of care revised to incorporate new exercise goals.

S. Beecher, RN

Skill · 33-1 — Applying and Removing Antiembolism Stockings

EQUIPMENT

- Elastic antiembolism stockings in ordered length in correct size. See Assessment for appropriate measurement procedure.
- Measuring tape
- Talcum powder (optional)
- Skin cleanser, basin, towel
- Nonsterile gloves
- Additional PPE as indicated

IMPLEMENTATION

ACTION	RATIONALE
1. Review the medical record and medical orders to determine the need for antiembolism stockings.	Reviewing the medical record and order validates the correct patient and correct procedure.
2. Perform hand hygiene. Put on PPE, as indicated.	Hand hygiene and PPE prevent the spread of microorganisms. PPE is required based on transmission precautions.
3. Identify the patient. Explain what you are going to do and the rationale for use of elastic stockings.	Patient identification validates the correct patient and correct procedure. Discussion and explanation allay anxiety and prepare the patient for what to expect.
4. Close curtains around bed and close door to room if possible.	This ensures the patient's privacy.
5. Adjust the bed to a comfortable working height, usually elbow height of the caregiver (VISN 8, 2009).	Having the bed at the proper height prevents back and muscle strain.
6. Assist patient to supine position. If patient has been sitting or walking, have him or her lie down with legs and feet well elevated for at least 15 minutes before applying stockings.	Dependent position of legs encourages blood to pool in the veins, reducing the effectiveness of the stockings if they are applied to congested blood vessels.
7. Expose legs one at a time. Wash and dry legs, if necessary. Powder the leg lightly unless patient has a breathing problem, dry skin, or sensitivity to the powder. If the skin is dry, a lotion may be used. Powders and lotions are not recommended by some manufacturers; check the package material for manufacturer specifications.	Helps maintain patient's privacy. Powder and lotion reduce friction and make application of stockings easier.
8. Stand at the foot of the bed. Place hand inside stocking and grasp heel area securely. Turn stocking inside out to the heel area, leaving the foot inside the stocking leg (Figure 1).	Inside-out technique provides for easier application; bunched elastic material can compromise extremity circulation.
9. With the heel pocket down, ease the foot of stocking over foot and heel (Figure 2). Check that patient's heel is centered in heel pocket of stocking (Figure 3).	Wrinkles and improper fit interfere with circulation.
10. Using your fingers and thumbs, carefully grasp edge of stocking and pull it up smoothly over ankle and calf, toward the knee (Figure 4). Make sure it is distributed evenly.	Easing the stocking carefully into position ensures proper fit of the stocking to the contour of the leg. Even distribution prevents interference with circulation.

FIGURE 1. Pulling antiembolism stocking inside out.

FIGURE 2. Putting foot of stocking onto patient.

(continued)

Skill · 33-1 Applying and Removing Antiembolism Stockings *continued*

ACTION

FIGURE 3. Ensuring heel is centered after stocking is on.

RATIONALE

FIGURE 4. Pulling the stocking up the leg.

ACTION	RATIONALE
11. Pull forward slightly on toe section. If the stocking has a toe window, make sure it is properly positioned. Adjust if necessary to ensure material is smooth.	Ensures toe comfort and prevents interference with circulation.
12. If the stockings are knee-length, make sure each stocking top is 1 to 2 inches below the patella. Make sure the stocking does not roll down.	Prevents pressure and interference with circulation. Rolling stockings may have a constricting effect on veins.
13. If applying thigh-length stocking, continue the application. Flex the patient's leg. Stretch the stocking over the knee.	This ensures even distribution.
14. Pull the stocking over the thigh until the top is 1 to 3 inches below the gluteal fold (Figure 5). Adjust the stocking as necessary to distribute the fabric evenly. Make sure the stocking does not roll down.	Prevents excessive pressure and interference with circulation. Rolling stockings may have a constricting effect on veins.

FIGURE 5. Pulling the stocking up over the thigh.

15. Remove equipment and return patient to a position of comfort. Remove your gloves. Raise side rail and lower bed.	Promotes patient comfort and safety. Removing gloves properly reduces the risk for infection transmission and contamination of other items.
16. Remove any other PPE, if used. Perform hand hygiene.	Removing PPE properly reduces the risk for infection transmission and contamination of other items. Hand hygiene prevents the spread of microorganisms.

Removing Stockings

17. To remove stocking, grasp top of stocking with your thumb and fingers and smoothly pull stocking off inside out to heel. Support foot and ease stocking over it.	This preserves the elasticity and contour of the stocking. It allows assessment of circulatory status and condition of skin on lower extremity and for skin care.

DOCUMENTATION

Guidelines

Document the patient's leg measurements as a baseline. Document the application of the stockings, size stocking applied, skin and leg assessment, and neurovascular assessment.

Sample Documentation

> <u>7/22/12</u> 0945 Leg measurements: calf 14$\frac{1}{2}$", length heel to knee 16". Measurements equal bilaterally. Knee-high antiembolism stockings (medium/regular) applied bilaterally. Posterior tibial and dorsalis pedal pulses +2 bilaterally; capillary refill <2 seconds and skin on toes consistent with rest of skin and warm. Skin on lower extremities is intact bilaterally.
>
> —*C. Stone, RN*

UNEXPECTED SITUATIONS AND ASSOCIATED INTERVENTIONS

- *Patient's leg measurements are outside the guidelines for the available sizes:* Notify prescriber. Patient may require custom-fitted stockings.
- *Patient has large amount of pain with application of stockings:* If pain is expected (e.g., if the patient has a leg incision), the patient may be premedicated and the stockings applied once the medication has had time to take effect. If the pain is unexpected, a physician may need to be notified because the patient may be developing a deep-vein thrombosis.
- *Patient has an incision on the leg:* When applying and removing stockings, be careful not to hit the incision. If the incision is draining, apply a small bandage to the incision so that it does not drain onto the stockings. If the stockings become soiled by drainage, wash and dry according to instructions.
- *Patient is to ambulate with stockings:* Place skid-resistant socks or slippers on before patient attempts to ambulate.

SPECIAL CONSIDERATIONS

General Considerations

- Remove stockings once every shift for 20 to 30 minutes. Wash and air-dry as necessary, according to manufacturer's directions.
- Assess at least every shift for skin color, temperature, sensation, swelling, and the ability to move. If complications are evident, remove the stockings and notify the physician or primary care provider.
- Evaluate stockings to ensure the top or toe opening does not roll with movement. Rolled stocking edges can cause excessive pressure and interfere with circulation.
- Despite the use of elastic stockings, a patient may develop deep-vein thrombosis or phlebitis. A unilateral swelling, redness, tenderness, pain, and warmth are possible indicators of these complications. Notify the primary care provider of the presence of any symptoms.

Home Care Considerations

- Make sure that the patient has an extra pair of stockings ordered during hospitalization before discharge (for payment and convenience purposes).
- Stockings may be laundered with other "white" clothing. Avoid excessive bleach. Remove from dryer as soon as "low heat" cycle is complete to avoid shrinkage. Stockings may also be air-dried. Check manufacturer's directions.

Skill · 33-2   Assisting a Patient With Turning in Bed

EQUIPMENT

- Friction-reducing sheet or draw sheet
- Bed surface that inflates to aid in turning
- Pillows or other supports to help the patient maintain the desired position
- after turning and to maintain correct body alignment for the patient
- Additional caregivers to assist, based on assessment
- Nonsterile gloves, if indicated; other PPE as indicated

IMPLEMENTATION

ACTION	RATIONALE
1. Review the physician's orders and nursing plan of care for patient activity. Identify any movement limitations and the ability of the patient to assist with turning. Consult patient-handling algorithm, if available, to plan appropriate approach to moving the patient.	Checking the physician's order and plan of care validates the correct patient and correct procedure. Identification of limitations and ability and use of an algorithm helps to prevent injury and aids in determining best plan for patient movement.
2. Gather any positioning aids or supports, if necessary.	Having aids readily available promotes efficient time management.
3. Perform hand hygiene. Put on PPE, as indicated.	Hand hygiene and PPE prevent the spread of microorganisms. PPE is required based on transmission precautions.
4. Identify the patient. Explain the procedure to the patient.	Patient identification validates the correct patient and correct procedure. Discussion and explanation help allay anxiety and prepare the patient for what to expect.
5. Close the room door or curtains. Position at least one nurse on either side of the bed. Place pillows, wedges, or any other support to be used for positioning within easy reach. Place the bed at an appropriate and comfortable working height, usually elbow height of the caregiver (VISN 8, 2009). Lower both side rails.	Closing the door or curtain provides privacy. Proper bed height helps reduce back strain while performing the procedure. Proper positioning and lowering the side rails facilitate moving the patient and minimize strain on the nurses.
6. If not already in place, position a friction-reducing sheet under the patient.	Sheets aid in preventing shearing and reducing friction and the force required to move the patient.
7. Using the friction-reducing sheet, move the patient to the edge of the bed, opposite the side to which he or she will be turned. Raise the side rails.	With this placement, the patient will be on the center of the bed after turning is accomplished. Raising side rails ensures patient safety.
8. If the patient is able, have the patient grasp the side rail on the side of the bed toward which they are turning (Figure 1). Alternately, place the patient's arms across his or her chest and cross his or her far leg over the leg nearest you.	Encourages the patient to assist as much as possible with the movement. This facilitates the turning motion and protects the patient's arms during the turn.

FIGURE 1. Having the patient grasp the side rail on the side of the bed toward which they are turning. *(Note: Patient's covers have been pulled back in this series of photos to show skill action. Covers should be folded back just enough to work, not expose patients unnecessarily.)* (Photo by B. Proud.)

ACTION

9. If available, activate the bed mechanism to inflate the side of the bed behind the patient's back.

10. **The nurse on the side of the bed toward which the patient is turning should stand opposite the patient's center with his or her feet spread about shoulder width and with one foot ahead of the other (Figure 2). Tighten your gluteal and abdominal muscles and flex your knees. Use your leg muscles to do the pulling. The other nurse should position his or her hands on the patient's shoulder and hip, assisting to roll the patient to the side. Instruct the patient to pull on the bed rail at the same time. Use the friction-reducing sheet to gently pull the patient over on his or her side (Figure 3).**

RATIONALE

Activating the turn mechanism inflates the side of the bed for approximately 10 seconds, aiding in propelling the patient to turn, and reducing the work required by the nurse. This helps avoid straining the nurse's lower back.

The nurse is in a stable position with good body alignment and prepared to use large muscle masses to turn the patient. These maneuvers support the patient's body and make use of the nurse's weight to assist with turning.

FIGURE 2. Standing opposite the patient's center with feet spread about shoulder width and with one foot ahead of the other. *(Photo by B. Proud.)*

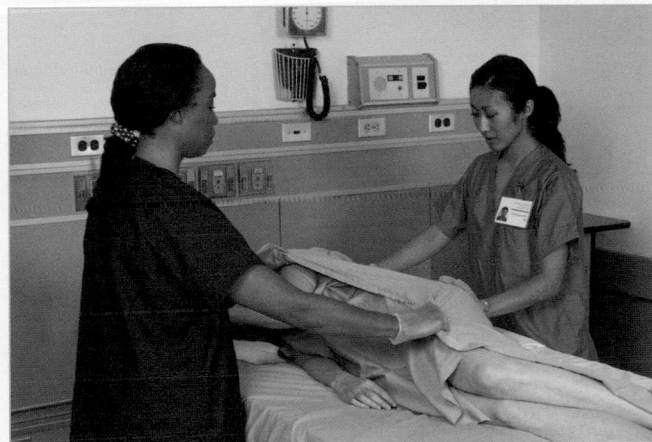

FIGURE 3. Working together to position patient over on her side. *(Photo by B. Proud.)*

11. Use a pillow or other support behind the patient's back. Pull the shoulder blade forward and out from under the patient.

12. Make the patient comfortable and position in proper alignment, using pillows or other supports under the leg and arm as needed. Readjust the pillow under the patient's head. Elevate the head of the bed as needed for comfort.

13. **Place the bed in the lowest position, with the side rails up. Make sure the call bell and other necessary items are within easy reach.**

14. Clean transfer aids per facility policy, if not indicated for single patient use. Remove gloves and other PPE, if used. Perform hand hygiene.

Pillow will provide support and help the patient maintain the desired position. Positioning the shoulder blade removes pressure from the bony prominence.

Positioning in proper alignment with supports ensures that the patient will be able to maintain the desired position and will be comfortable.

Adjusting the bed height ensures patient safety.

Proper cleaning of equipment between patient use prevents the spread of microorganisms. Removing PPE properly reduces the risk for infection transmission and contamination of other items. Hand hygiene prevents the spread of microorganisms.

DOCUMENTATION

Guidelines

Many facilities provide areas on the bedside flow sheet to document repositioning. Be sure to document the time of the patient's change of position, use of supports, and any pertinent observations, including skin assessment. Document the patient's tolerance of the position change. Document aids used to facilitate movement.

(continued)

Skill · 33-2   Assisting a Patient With Turning in Bed   *continued*

Sample Documentation

> <u>11/10/12</u> 1130 Patient repositioned from right side to left side; alignment maintained with wedge support behind back and pillow between legs. Skin on pressure points on right side without signs of irritation, edema, or redness. Patient reports no pain with movement. Friction-reducing sheet used to facilitate transfer and left in place under patient. Three caregivers required for repositioning.
>
> —*B. Clapp, RN*

UNEXPECTED SITUATIONS AND ASSOCIATED INTERVENTIONS

- *You are turning a patient by yourself, but you realize that the patient cannot help as much as you thought and is heavier than you anticipated:* Use the call bell to summon assistance from a coworker. Alternatively, cover the patient, make sure all rails are up, lower the bed to the lowest position, and get someone to assist you. Consider using a friction-reducing sheet and two to three additional caregivers.

Skill · 33-3   Moving a Patient Up in Bed With the Assistance of Another Nurse

EQUIPMENT

- Friction-reducing sheet or other friction-reducing device
- Nonsterile gloves, if indicated
- Additional caregivers to assist, based on assessment
- Full-body sling lift and cover sheet, if necessary, based on assessment and availability

IMPLEMENTATION

ACTION	RATIONALE
1. Review the medical record and nursing plan of care for conditions that may influence the patient's ability to move or to be positioned. Assess for tubes, intravenous lines, incisions, or equipment that may alter the positioning procedure. Identify any movement limitations. Consult patient handling algorithm, if available, to plan appropriate approach to moving the patient.	Reviewing the order and plan of care validates the correct patient and correct procedure. Identification of limitations and ability and use of an algorithm helps to prevent injury and aids in determining best plan for patient movement.
2. Perform hand hygiene and put on PPE, if indicated.	Hand hygiene and PPE prevent the spread of microorganisms. PPE is required based on transmission precautions.
3. Identify the patient. Explain the procedure to the patient.	Patient identification validates the correct patient and correct procedure. Discussion and explanation help allay anxiety and prepare the patient for what to expect.
4. Close the room door or curtains. Place the bed at an appropriate and comfortable working height, usually elbow height of the caregiver (VISN 8, 2009). Adjust the head of the bed to a flat position or as low as the patient can tolerate. Placing the bed in slight Trendelenburg position aids movement, if the patient is able to tolerate it.	Closing the door or curtain provides for privacy. Proper bed height helps reduce back strain while you are performing the procedure. Flat positioning helps to decrease the gravitational pull of the upper body.
5. Remove all pillows from under the patient. Leave one at the head of the bed, leaning upright against the headboard.	Removing pillows from under the patient facilitates movement; placing a pillow at the head of the bed prevents accidental head injury against the top of the bed.
6. Position at least one nurse on either side of the bed, and lower both side rails.	Proper positioning and lowering the side rails facilitate moving the patient and minimize strain on the nurses.
7. If a friction-reducing sheet (or device) is not in place under the patient, place one under the patient's midsection.	A friction-reducing device supports the patient's weight and reduces friction during the repositioning.

ACTION	RATIONALE
8. Ask the patient (if able) to bend his or her legs and put his or her feet flat on the bed to assist with the movement.	Patient can use major muscle groups to push. Even if the patient is too weak to push on the bed, placing the legs in this fashion will assist with movement and prevent shearing of the skin on the heels.
9. Have the patient fold the arms across the chest. Have the patient (if able) lift the head with chin on chest.	Positioning in this manner provides assistance, reduces friction, and prevents hyperextension of the neck.
10. One nurse should be positioned on each side of the bed, at the patient's midsection with feet spread shoulder width apart and one foot slightly in front of the other.	Doing so positions each nurse opposite the center of the body mass, lowers the center of gravity, and reduces the risk for injury.
11. If available on bed, engage mechanism to make the bed surface firmer for repositioning.	Decreases friction and effort needed to move the patient.
12. Grasp the friction-reducing sheet securely, close to the patient's body.	Having the sheet close to the body brings the patient's center of gravity closer to each nurse and provides for a secure hold.
13. Flex your knees and hips. Tighten your abdominal and gluteal muscles and keep your back straight.	Using the legs' large muscle groups and tightening muscles during transfer to prevent back injury.
14. Shift your weight back and forth from your back leg to your front leg and count to three (Figure 1). On the count of three, move the patient up in bed. If possible, the patient can assist with the move by pushing with the legs (Figure 2). Repeat the process if necessary to get the patient to the right position.	The rocking motion uses the nurses' weight to counteract the patient's weight. Rocking develops momentum, which provides a smooth lift with minimal exertion by the nurses. If the patient assists, less effort is required by the nurses.

FIGURE 1. Nurses positioned at the patient's midsection, shifting weight from back leg to front leg in preparation for move. *(Note: Patient's covers have been pulled back in this series of photos to show skill action. Covers should be folded back just enough to work, not expose patients unnecessarily.)*

FIGURE 2. Patient moved up in bed.

15. **Assist the patient to a comfortable position and readjust the pillows and supports as needed. Return bed surface to normal setting, if necessary. Raise the side rails. Place the bed in the lowest position (Figure 3).**	Readjusting the bed with supports and side rails ensures patient safety and comfort.

(continued)

Skill · 33-6   **Providing Range-of-Motion Exercises**   *continued*

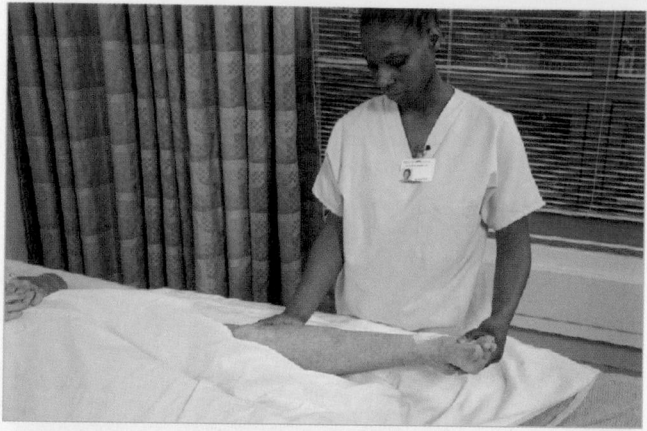

FIGURE 21. Turning the patient's foot and leg toward the opposite leg to rotate it internally.

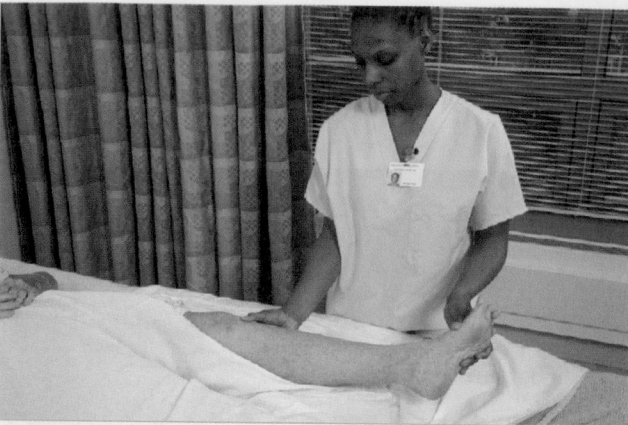

FIGURE 22. Turning the patient's foot and leg outward away from the opposite leg to rotate it externally.

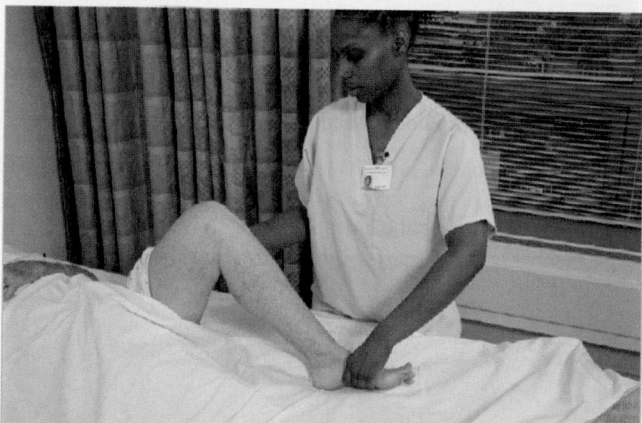

FIGURE 23. Bending the patient's leg and bringing the heel toward the back of the leg.

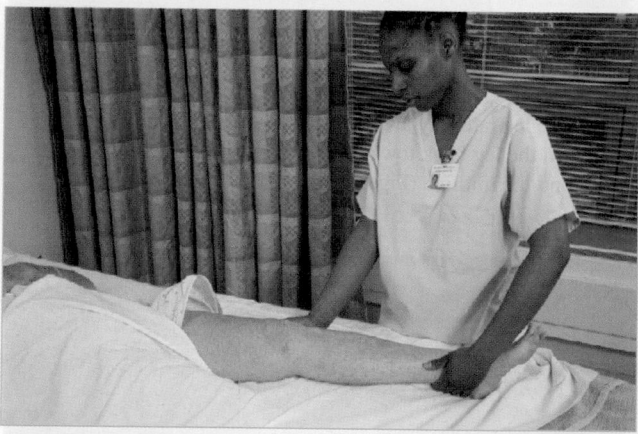

FIGURE 24. Returning the leg to a straight position.

FIGURE 25. At the ankle, moving the patient's foot up and back until the toes are upright.

FIGURE 26. Moving the patient's foot with the toes pointing down.

ACTION

FIGURE 27. Turning the sole toward the midline.

RATIONALE

FIGURE 28. Turning the sole outward.

23. Curl the toes downward (Figure 29), and then straighten them out (Figure 30). Spread the toes apart (Figure 31) and bring them together (Figure 32).

These movements provide for flexion, extension, abduction, and adduction of the toes.

FIGURE 29. Curling the patient's toes down.

FIGURE 30. Straightening the patient's toes.

FIGURE 31. Spreading the patient's toes apart.

FIGURE 32. Bringing the patient's toes together.

(continued)

Skill · 33-6 Providing Range-of-Motion Exercises *continued*

ACTION	RATIONALE
24. Repeat these exercises on the other side of the body. Encourage the patient to do as many of these exercises by himself or herself as possible.	Repeating motions on the other side provides exercise for the entire body.
25. When finished, make sure the patient is comfortable, with the side rails up and the bed in the lowest position.	Proper positioning with raised side rails and proper bed height provides for patient comfort and safety.
26. Remove gloves and any other PPE, if used. Perform hand hygiene.	Removing PPE properly reduces the risk for infection transmission and contamination of other items. Hand hygiene prevents the spread of microorganisms.

DOCUMENTATION

Guidelines

Document the exercises performed, any significant observations, and the patient's reaction to the activities.

Sample Documentation

5/1/12 0945 Range-of-motion exercises performed to all joints. Patient able to perform active range of motion of head, neck, shoulders, and arms. Required moderate assistance with ROM to lower extremities. Denied any complaints of pain during exercises. Patient tolerated exercise session well. Sitting in semi-Fowler's position with side rails up, watching television.

—J. Chrisp, RN

UNEXPECTED SITUATIONS AND ASSOCIATED INTERVENTIONS

- *While you are performing range-of-motion exercises, the patient complains of feeling tired:* Stop the activity for that time. Reevaluate the nursing plan of care. Space the exercises out at different times of the day. Schedule exercise times for the parts of the day the patient is typically feeling more rested.

- *While exercising your patient's leg, he complains of sudden, sharp pain:* Stop the exercises. Assess the patient for other symptoms. Notify the physician of the event and your findings. Joints should be moved until there is resistance but not pain. Uncomfortable reactions should be reported and exercises halted. The activity plan may have to be revised.

SPECIAL CONSIDERATIONS

General Considerations

- Many of these exercises can be incorporated into daily activities, such as during bathing.

- A physician's order and specific instructions should be obtained to perform range-of-motion exercises for patients with acute arthritis, fractures, torn ligaments, joint dislocation, acute myocardial infarction, and bone tumors or metastases.

Older Adult Considerations

- Avoid neck hyperextension and attempts to achieve full range of motion in all joints with older patients.

● Developing Critical Thinking Skills

1. Pretend that you have a mobility impairment (i.e., you have to use crutches or a walker, cane, or wheelchair), and attempt to perform your usual daily activities, ideally including visiting a public place, such as a school or mall. How did you feel about the restriction of your movement? How can nurses best assist patients who are coping with these restrictions? How did the public respond to your impairment, and what effects might such responses have on individuals with mobility impairments? Are public spaces adequately adapted to meet the needs of those with mobility impairments? What measures are needed to address any deficiencies? Did you identify any safety needs?

2. Suppose a friend is confined to bed for several months after a motorcycle accident that resulted in severe orthopedic and internal injuries. What nursing measures would you recommend to avoid the hazards of immobility?

● Practicing for NCLEX

1. What term would the nurse use to identify the strong, flexible, inelastic fibrous bands and flattened sheets of connective tissue that attach muscle to bone?
   a. Tendons
   b. Ligaments
   c. Cartilage
   d. Joints

2. Why are mechanical aids necessary for patient handling and movement?
   a. Nurses do not have sufficient training using proper body mechanics to be safe.
   b. Manual lifting techniques are not sufficient to protect nurses from injury.
   c. They reduce the time and number of staff needed to move the patient.
   d. Nurses are not as physically fit as they should be.

3. A patient performs rehabilitative exercises with resistance after a knee injury. The nurse interprets this type of exercise as which of the following?
   a. Isotonic
   b. Isokinetic
   c. Isometric
   d. Aerobic

4. Which of the following would the nurse expect to assess when a patient experiences a greater breakdown of protein than that which is manufactured?
   a. Fluid volume excess
   b. A contracture
   c. Osteoporosis
   d. Negative nitrogen balance

5. When explaining the cause of frequent urinary tract infections related to immobility, the nurse understands that immobility may result in which of the following?
   a. Improved renal blood supply to the kidneys
   b. Urinary stasis
   c. Decreased urinary calcium
   d. Acidic urine formation

6. Mr. Brown is experiencing some difficulty breathing. The nurse most appropriately assists him into which position?
   a. Dorsal recumbent position
   b. Lateral position
   c. Fowler's position
   d. Sims' position

7. While doing range-of-motion exercises with a patient who is bedridden, the nurse is aware of which of the following considerations?
   a. Neck hyperextension should be encouraged, particularly in older people.
   b. Exercises should be continued until the patient is fatigued.
   c. Exercises should be done frequently to lessen pain for the patient.

   d. Each joint is exercised to the point of resistance but not pain.

8. The nurse is assisting a patient with conditioning exercises to prepare for ambulation. The nurse correctly instructs the patient to do what?
   a. Do full-body pushups in bed six to eight times daily
   b. Breathe in and out smoothly during quadriceps drills
   c. Dangle on the side of the bed for 30 to 60 minutes
   d. Allow the nurse to bathe the patient completely to prevent fatigue

9. In many situations, a patient has sufficient strength to walk if he or she can do which of the following?
   a. Lie prone for 1 hour
   b. Bathe him- or herself
   c. Raise the foot off the bed 1 inch
   d. Sit up in bed for 1 hour

10. Mrs. Eden tells the nurse she feels faint while walking in the corridor with the nurse. What should the nurse do?
    a. Instruct the patient to quicken her pace so they can return to her room
    b. Leave her momentarily to find another nurse to help
    c. Advise her to look down at her feet to help maintain her balance
    d. Guide her to a nearby chair, easing her onto it to rest

11. When a patient is using a cane for maximal support, the nurse is aware that the patient should do which of the following?
    a. Hold the cane on the weaker side
    b. Distribute weight evenly between the feet and the cane
    c. Keep the elbow that is holding the cane straight and stiff
    d. Advance the weaker foot ahead of the cane

12. The use of patient care ergonomics is associated with which of the following patient outcomes?
    a. Increased patient comfort, security, and dignity during lifts and transfers
    b. Increased patient falls, skin tears, and abrasions
    c. Decreased patient movement and independence
    d. Increased friction and shearing

13. Which of the following should the nurse do when assisting the patient to ambulate?
    a. Place a hand under the axilla to provide support
    b. Ensure the patient walks as far as possible for as long as possible
    c. Use a gait belt to provide support
    d. Encourage the patient to watch their feet to ensure a steady gait

14. When working with an older patient to develop an exercise program, the nurse would recommend which of the following?
    a. A frequency of six times a week
    b. Exercising to the point of breathlessness when trying to speak

c. Maintaining a target heart rate of 220 plus age

d. Obtaining medical clearance before beginning the program

15. A bedridden patient who is blind is admitted to a healthcare facility from his or her home with pressure ulcers on the sacral area. Which nursing diagnosis would be a priority?

a. Risk for Imbalanced Body Temperature related to stage 2 pressure ulcer

b. Impaired Skin Integrity related to immobility

c. Feeding Self-Care Deficit related to blindness

d. Activity Intolerance related to prolonged bed rest

● Answers With Rationale

1. *a.* Tendons are the strong fibrous bands and flattened sheets of connective tissue that attach muscle to bone. Ligaments (*b*) bind joints together and connect bones and cartilage, whereas cartilage (*c*) is nonvascular connective tissue found in the joints as well as in the nose, ear, thorax, trachea, and larynx. Joints (*d*) are areas in which one bone comes into close contact with another bone.

2. *b.* The use of assistive equipment as part of a safe patient handling and movement program can significantly reduce the risk of musculoskeletal disorders and contributes to patient comfort. The use of "body mechanics" (*a*) has been shown to be unsafe in relation to the transfer and movement of patients. The time and number of staff (*c, d*) needed for transfer may or may not be affected by the use of mechanical aids.

3. *b.* Isokinetic exercise involves muscle contraction with resistance, whereas isotonic exercise (*a*) involves muscle shortening and active movement. Isometric exercise (*c*) involves muscle contraction without shortening, and aerobic exercise (*d*) is sustained muscle movements that increase blood flow, heart rate, and metabolic demand for oxygen over time, promoting cardiovascular conditioning.

4. *d.* Negative nitrogen balance results when the body excretes more nitrogen than it takes in. Contractures (*b*) are permanent contraction states of muscles, and osteoporosis (*c*) involves bone demineralization. Fluid volume excess (*a*) is indirectly related to protein manufacture or breakdown.

5. *b.* In a nonerect patient, the kidneys and ureters are level, and urine remains in the renal pelvis for a longer period of time before gravity causes it to move into the ureters and bladder, resulting in urinary stasis. Urinary stasis favors the growth of bacteria that may cause urinary tract infections. Regular exercise, not immobility, improves blood flow to the kidneys (*a*). Immobility predisposes the patient to *increased* levels of urinary calcium and alkaline urine (*c* and *d*), contributing to renal calculi and urinary tract infection, respectively.

6. *c.* Fowler's position promotes maximal breathing space in the thoracic cavity and is the position of choice when someone is having difficulty breathing. Lying flat on the back or side (*a, b*) or Sims' position (*d*) would not facilitate respiration and would be difficult for the patient to maintain.

7. *d.* Joints should be exercised slowly, smoothly, and rhythmically to the point of resistance but not pain. Joints should never be exercised to the point of pain or fatigue (*b*). Neck hyperextension (*a*) should be avoided in older patients and may prove painful.

8. *b.* Breathing in and out smoothly during quadriceps drills maximizes lung inflation. The patient should never hold his or her breath during exercise drills because this places a strain on the heart. Pushups are usually done three or four times a day and involve only the upper body (*a*). Dangling for 30 to 60 minutes is unsafe (*c*). The nurse encourages the patient to be as independent as possible to prepare for return to normal ambulation and ADLs.

9. *c.* Being able to raise the foot 1 inch off the bed frequently indicates sufficient strength for walking. Lying prone (*a*), bathing himself or herself (*b*), or sitting up in bed (*d*) do not necessarily indicate the muscle coordination and strength necessary in the lower limbs for walking.

10. *d.* Guiding the patient to a chair in the hall and easing her into it is the safest action. Asking her to walk faster (*a*) and leaving her alone (*b*) are definitely unsafe actions. If the patient looks down at her feet, she may become dizzy and unbalanced (*c*).

11. *b.* The patient's weight should be evenly distributed between his or her feet and the cane. Holding the cane on the weaker side (*a*) is difficult and unsafe. The elbow should be flexed at a 30-degree angle when holding the cane. The cane is advanced first, then the weaker foot.

12. The correct response is *a.* The use of patient care ergonomics is associated with increased patient safety and comfort, as well as *decreased* patient falls, skin tears and abrasions (*b*), *increased* patient movement and independence (*c*), and *decreased* friction and shearing (*d*).

13. *c.* A gait belt is a device used for transferring patients and assisting with ambulation, giving the caregiver better access to, improved grasp, and control of the patient. Pulling on patient's axilla (*a*) could result in injury to the patient and should not be attempted. Ambulation should begin with a short distance, gradually increasing the distance as tolerated (*b*). The patient should stand erect and hold the head high to achieve the full benefits of walking (*d*).

14. *d.* Patients older than 35 years should always get medical clearance before initiating an exercise program. Frequency is initially three times a week, and exercise should be maintained so that the patient is able to talk

without becoming breathless. The target heart rate is calculated as 60% to 90% of the maximal heart rate (220 – age).

15. **b.** The priority nursing diagnosis for this patient at this moment is Impaired Skin Integrity related to immobility. An end result of the immobility is the development of a pressure ulcer. The other nursing diagnoses may be appropriate but are not the priority on admission to the healthcare facility.

Taylor Suite Resources

The Taylor Suite offers these additional resources to enhance learning and facilitate understanding of this chapter:

- thePoint online resource, http://thepoint.lww.com/Taylor7E
- Student DVD-ROM included with the book
- Study Guide for Taylor's Fundamentals of Nursing
- Skill Checklists for Taylor's Fundamentals of Nursing
- Taylor's Clinical Nursing Skills: *Chapter 9, Activity*
- Taylor's Video Guide to Clinical Nursing Skills: *Activity*

BIBLIOGRAPHY

American Association of Critical-Care Nurses (AACN). (2005). *Practice alert. Deep vein thrombosis prevention.* Available at www.aacn.org/WD/Practice/Content/practicealerts.pcms?pid=1&&menu=practice.

American Nurses Association (ANA). (2004). *Position statement on elimination of manual patient handling to prevent work-related musculoskeletal disorders.* Silver Spring, MD: Author.

American Nurses Association (ANA). (2008a). Ergonomics/Handle with Care. Silver Spring, MD: Author. Available at: http://nursingworld.org/MainMenuCategories/Occupationaland Environmental/occupationalhealth/handlewithcare.aspx.

American Nurses Association (ANA). (2008b). *Handle with care.* Fact sheet. Silver Spring, MD: Author. Available at: http://nursingworld.org/MainMenuCategories/OccupationalandEnvironmental/occupationalhealth/handlewithcare/Resources/FactSheet.aspx.

Andrews, M., & Boyle, J. (2008). *Transcultural concepts in nursing care* (5th ed.). Philadelphia: Wolters Kluwer Health/Lippincott Williams & Wilkins.

Aquaro Sebastian, L. (2007). Exercise recommendations. *Advance for Nurses, 9*(27), 33–35.

Arthritis Foundation. (2007a). Osteoarthritis. Available at: http://www.arthritis.org/disease-center.php?disease_id=32.

Arthritis Foundation. (2007b). What is arthritis? Available at: http://www.arthritis.org/what-is-arthritis.php.

Baptiste, A., Boda, S., Nelson, A., Lloyd, J., & Lee, W. (2006). Friction-reducing devices for lateral patient transfers: A clinical evaluation. *AAOHN Journal, 54*(4), 173–180.

Blocks, M. (2005). Practical solutions for safe patient handling. *Nursing, 35*(10), 44–45.

Brace, T. (2005). The dynamics of pushing and pulling in the workplace. Assessing and treating the problem. *AAOHN Journal, 53*(5), 224–229.

Bulechek, G., Butcher, H., & McCloskey Dochterman, J. (Eds.). (2008). *Nursing interventions classification (NIC)* (5th ed.). St. Louis: Mosby Elsevier.

Carpenito-Moyet, L. (2008). *Nursing diagnosis: Application to clinical practice* (12th ed.). Philadelphia: Wolters Kluwer Health/Lippincott Williams & Wilkins.

Chavez, C. (2005). Lifting safety and ergonomics. *Radiologic Technology, 76*(6), 469–472.

Cohen, B. J., & Taylor, J. (2005). *Memmler's structure and function of the human body* (8th ed.). Philadelphia: Lippincott Williams & Wilkins.

Collins, J., Wolf, L., Bell, J., & Evanoff, B. (2004). An evaluation of a "best practices" musculoskeletal injury prevention program in nursing homes. *Injury Prevention, 10*(4), 206–211.

Converso, A., & Murphy, C. (2004). Winning the battle against back injuries. *RN, 67*(2), 52–57.

Fernandes, T. (2006a). Moving and handling: Hoists and slings. *Nursing and Residential Care, 8*(12), 548–551.

Fernandes, T. (2006b). Suitable moving and handling equipment: A guide. *International Journal of Therapy and Rehabilitation, 13*(10), 477–481.

Fletcher, K. (2005). Immobility: Geriatric self-learning module. *Medsurg Nursing, 14*(1), 35–37.

Fralick-Ball, S. (2008). Ergonomics in healthcare. *Advance for Nurses, 10*(10), 39–41.

Geraghty, M. (2005). Nursing the unconscious patient. *Nursing Standard, 20*(1), 54–64.

Gillis, A., & MacDonald, B. (2005). Prevention: Deconditioning in the hospitalized elderly. *Canadian Nurse, 101*(6), 16–20.

Griffiths, H., & Gallimore, D. (2005). Positioning critically ill patients in hospital. *Nursing Standard, 19*(42), 56–64.

Haines, T. (2007). Additional exercise for older subacute hospital inpatients to prevent falls: Benefits and barriers to implementation and evaluation. *Clinical Rehabilitation, 21*(8), 742–753.

Hobbs, T., Wolverton, C., & Clevenger, K. (2007). Lift team technologies elevate positive outcomes. *Nursing Management, 38*(7), 50–52.

Jarvis, C. (2008). *Physical examination & health assessment* (5th ed.). St. Louis: Saunders/Elsevier.

Kato, M., Izumi, K., Hiramatsu, T., & Shogenji, M. (2006). Development of an exercise program for fall prevention for elderly persons in a long-term care facility. *Japan Journal of Nursing Science, 3*(2), 107–117.

Kyle, T. (2008). *Essentials of pediatric nursing.* Philadelphia: Wolters Kluwer Health/Lippincott Williams & Wilkins.

Kirshbaum, M. (2006). A review of the benefits of whole body exercise during and after treatment for breast cancer. *Journal of Clinical Nursing, 16*(1), 104–121.

Marcus, B., Williams, D., Dubbert, P., Sallis, J., King, A., Yancey, A., et al. (2006). Physical activity intervention studies: What we know and what we need to know: A scientific statement from the American Heart Association Council on nutrition, physical activity, and metabolism. *Circulation, 114*(24), 2739–2752.

Mayo Clinic. (2007). *How to choose and use a walker.* Available at www.mayoclinic.com/health/walker/HA00060.

McCoskey, K. (2007). Ergonomics and patient handling. *AAOHN Journal, 55*(11), 454–461.

McCullagh, R., Fitzgerald, A., Murphy, R., & Mater, C. (2008). Long-term benefits of exercising on quality of life and fatigue in multiple sclerosis patients with mild disability: A pilot study. *Clinical Rehabilitation, 22*(3), 206–214.

Miller, C. (2008). Communication difficulties in hospitalized older adults with dementia: Try these techniques to make communicating with patients easier and more effective. *American Journal of Nursing, 108*(3), 58–66.

Mincer, A. (2007). Assistive devices for the adult patient with orthopaedic dysfunction: Why physical therapists choose what they do. *Orthopaedic Nursing, 26*(4), 226–233.

Moorhead, S., Johnson, M., Maas, M., Swanson, E. (Eds.). (2008). *Nursing outcomes Classification (NOC)* (4th ed.). St. Louis: Mosby Elsevier.

NANDA International. (2009). *Nursing diagnoses: Definitions and classification 2009–2011.* West Sussex, UK: Wiley-Blackwell.

National Institutes of Health (NIH), & National Heart, Lung and Blood Institute. (2005). *Aim for a healthy weight.* NIH Publication No. 05-5213. Bethesda, MD: Author.

National Osteoporosis Foundation. (2008). *Fast facts on osteoporosis.* Available at http://www.nof.org/osteoporosis/diseasefacts.htm.

Nelson, A., & Baptiste, A. (2004). Evidence-based practices for safe patient handling and movement. *Online Journal of Issues in Nursing, 9*(3), Manuscript 3.

Nelson, A., & Baptiste, A. (2006). Update on evidence-based practices for safe patient handling and movement. *Orthopaedic Nursing, 25*(6), 367–368.

Nelson, A., Collins, J., Knibbe, H, Cookson, K., de Castro, A. B., & Whipple, K. L. (2007). Safer patient handling. *Nursing Management, 38*(3), 26–33.

Nelson, A., Fragala, G., & Menzel, N. (2003). Myths and facts about back injuries in nursing. *American Journal of Nursing, 103*(2), 32–40.

Nelson, A., Matz, M., Chen, F., Siddharthan, K., Lloyd, J., & Fragala, G. (2006). Development and evaluation of a multifaceted ergonomics program to prevent injuries associated with patient handling tasks. *International Journal of Nursing Studies, 43*(6), 717–733.

Nelson, A., Owen, B., Lloyd, J., Fragala, G., Matz, M., Amato, M., et al. (2003). Safe patient handling & movement: Preventing back injury among nurses requires careful selection of the safest equipment and techniques. *American Journal of Nursing, 103*(3), 32–43.

NIOSH sets 35-lb limit as the max for safe lifts. (2007). *Hospital employee health, 26*(12), 136–137.

Occupational Safety & Health Administration (OSHA), U.S. Department of Labor. (2003). *HealthCare wide hazards module-ergonomics.* Washington, DC: Author. Available at www.osha.gov/SLTC/etools/hospital/hazards/ergo/ergo.html.

Pellatt, G. (2005). Safe handling. The safety and dignity of patients and nurses during patient handling. *British Journal of Nursing, 14*(21), 1150–1156.

Pellat, G. (2007). Clinical skills: Bed making and patient positioning. *British Journal of Nursing, 16*(5), 302–305.

Peterson, J. (2007). Get moving! Physical activity counseling in primary care. *Journal of the American Academy of Nurse Practitioners, 19*(7), 349–357.

Porth, C. & Matfin, G. (2009). *Pathophysiology: Concepts of altered health states* (8th ed.). Philadelphia: Wolters Kluwer Health/Lippincott Williams & Wilkins.

Rinds, G. (2007). Moving and handling: Part one. *Nursing & Residential Care, 9*(6), 260–262.

Rinds, G. (2007). Moving and handling, Part two: Risk management. *Nursing & Residential Care, 9*(7), 306–309.

Schwartz, A., Winters-Stone, K., & Gallucci, B. (2007). Exercise effects on bone mineral density in women with breast cancer receiving adjuvant chemotherapy. *Oncology Nursing Forum, 34*(3), 627–633.

Smeltzer, S., Bare, B., Hinkle, J., & Cheever, K. H. (2010). *Brunner & Suddarth's textbook of medical-surgical nursing* (12th ed.). Philadelphia: Wolters Kluwer Health/Lippincott Williams & Wilkins.

Smith, M., & Buckwalter, K. (2005). Behaviors associated with dementia: Whether resisting care or exhibiting apathy, an older adult with dementia is attempting communication. Nurses and other caregivers must learn to 'hear' this language. *American Journal of Nursing, 105*(7), 40–52.

Stenger, K. (2007). Ergonomics and economics of safe patient lifting. *Healthcare Purchasing News, 31*(3), 68–69.

Swann, J. (2006). Keeping mobile: Part one. *Nursing & Residential Care, 8*(12), 566–568.

Tseng, C.N., Chen, C.C.H., Wu, S.C., & Lin, L.C. (2007). Effects of a range-of-motion exercise programme. *Journal of Advanced Nursing, 57*(2), 181–191.

UCLA Office of Environment, Health, and Safety. (2008a). UCLA Ergonomics. *Back Safety.* Available at http://ergonomics.ucla.edu/back.html.

UCLA Office of Environment, Health, and Safety. (2008b). UCLA Ergonomics. *Injury Prevention.* Available at: http://ergonomics.ucla.edu/back.html.

University of Iowa Hospitals and Clinics. (2006). *Using crutches safely.* Iowa City, Iowa: Author. Available at www.uihealthcare.com/topics/bonesjointsmuscles/bone3458.html.

U.S. Department of Health and Human Services. (2000). *Healthy People 2010, conference edition.* Washington, DC: Author. Available at http://www.health.gov/healthypeople/Document/HTML/Volume2/22Physical.htm.

VISN 8 Patient Safety Center. (2005). Patient care ergonomics resource guide: Safe patient handling and movement. Tampa, FL: Available at http://www.visn8.med.va.gov/patientsafetycenter/safePtHandling/default.as.

VISN 8 Patient Safety Center. (2007). *Safe patient handling nursing school curriculum module.* Tampa, FL: Author. Available at http://www.visn8.med.va.gov/PatientSafetyCenter/safePtHandling/SPHMToolkit_Final.DOC.

VISN 8 Patient Safety Center. (2009). *Safe patient handling and movement algorithms.* Tampa, FL: Author. Available at http://www.visn8.med.gov/patientsafetycenter/safePtHandling.

Walker, L., & Lamont, S. (2007). The use of antiembolic stockings. Part 1: A literature review. *British Journal of Nursing, 16*(22), 1408–1412.

Walker, L., & Lamont, S. (2008). Graduated compression stockings to prevent deep vein thrombosis. *Nursing Standard, 22*(40), 35–38.

Wallace, M., & Shelkey, M. (2008). Monitoring functional status in hospitalized older adults. *American Journal of Nursing, 108*(4), 64–71.

Waters, T., Collins, J., Galinsky, T., & Caruso, C. (2006). NIOSH research efforts to prevent musculoskeletal disorders in the healthcare industry. *Orthopaedic Nursing, 25*(6), 380–389.

Weber, J., & Kelley, J. (2007). *Health assessment in nursing* (3rd ed.). Philadelphia: Wolters Kluwer/Lippincott Williams & Wilkins.

White, K., & Jacques, P. (2007). Combined diet and exercise intervention in the workplace: Effect on cardiovascular disease risk factors. *AAOHN Journal, 55*(3), 109–114.

Wright, K. (2005). Mobility and safe handling of people with dementia. *Nursing Times, 101*(17), 38–40.

Rest and Sleep | 34

JEANETTE AND ABBY CLARK

Jeanette accompanies her 15-year-old daughter, Abby, to the clinic. While the daughter is having some routine laboratory testing done in another department, Mrs. Clark says, "She always seems to be tired. When she was small, I could never get her to sleep. Now all she wants to do is sleep. It's all I can do to get her up for school each morning."

THE OMEARA FAMILY

Lydia Omeara asks whether she should let her infant twins sleep in bed with her and her husband. "They have their own beds, of course, but at night, when they get up, they like to be in bed with us. Plus, I still breastfeed my babies, so having them nearby would really make it easier for me."

CHARLIE BITNER

Charlie is an 86-year-old man who has recently been admitted to a long-term care facility. He tells his daughter that "even though I go to bed around 9 p.m., I don't fall asleep until after midnight and then I'm up twice to go to the bathroom and have a lot of trouble falling back to sleep." His daughter has mentioned to the nurse that her father spends a lot of time napping during the day.

LEARNING OBJECTIVES

After completing the chapter, you will be able to accomplish the following:

1. Describe the functions and physiology of sleep.

2. Identify variables that influence rest and sleep.

3. Describe nursing implications that address age-related differences in the sleep cycle.

4. Perform a comprehensive sleep assessment using appropriate interview questions, a sleep diary when indicated, and physical assessment skills.

5. Describe common sleep disorders, noting key assessment criteria.

6. Develop nursing diagnoses that correctly identify sleep problems that may be treated through independent nursing interventions.

7. Describe nursing strategies to promote rest and sleep based on scientific rationale.

8. Plan, implement, and evaluate nursing care related to selected nursing diagnoses involving sleep problems.

KEY TERMS

circadian rhythm	parasomnias
delta sleep	rapid eye movement (REM) sleep
dyssomnias	
enuresis	rest
hypersomnia	restless leg syndrome (RLS)
insomnia	
melatonin	sleep
narcolepsy	sleep apnea
nocturnal myoclonus	sleep cycle
non–rapid eye movement (NREM) sleep	sleep deprivation
	sleep hygiene
	somnambulism

In this chapter, **rest** connotes a condition in which the body is in a decreased state of activity, with the consequent feeling of being refreshed. Many factors affect a person's ability to rest. Adults juggling the demands of their job and family responsibilities often find little opportunity for rest and relaxation during the course of a day. Children involved in numerous extracurricular activities, as well as trying to excel academically, also do not have the opportunity to rest and relax during the day. Even when rest is possible, one's environment is not always conducive to physical and mental relaxation. Suggestions for preparing a restful environment and promoting relaxation are discussed later in the chapter.

Sleep is a state of rest accompanied by altered consciousness and relative inactivity. It is a complex rhythmic state involving a progression of repeated cycles, each representing different phases of body and brain activity. Although sensitivity to external stimuli is diminished during sleep, this sensitivity can be readily reversed.

Most people can fall asleep easily and remain asleep until the desired waking time. Conversely, others rarely fall asleep without a struggle, and then when they do, sleep is fragmented. Many people have sleep disturbances that go undetected for years, progressively undermining their energy and destroying their sense of self. Sleep loss that results in fatigue and decreased competence increases the risk of a sleep-related motor vehicle accident. The National Sleep Foundation's 2005 Sleep in America poll reported that 32% of Americans admitted driving while feeling drowsy at least once per month during the past year. More than one-third (36%) admitted they have fallen asleep while driving (National Sleep Foundation [NSF], 2008a). Driver fatigue, according to conservative estimates by the National Highway Traffic Safety Administration, is responsible for 100,000 police-reported accidents, 1,550 fatalities, and 76,000 injuries each year (Goldsmith, 2007). In addition, studies of physicians' and nurses' work habits have concluded that sleep deprivation from extended work schedules may be a causative factor in a substantial number of adverse medical events and errors (Trinkoff, Geiger-Brown, Brady, Lipscomb, & Muntaner, 2006).

The discomfort produced by illness and the need for hospitalization and treatment may interfere dramatically with a patient's ability to sleep. Consequently, nurses need to be vigilant in detecting and treating sleep disturbances (see the accompanying Reflective Practice display for an example).

This chapter provides the nurse with knowledge of the functions and physiology of sleep and factors affecting sleep. Practical suggestions for performing a comprehensive sleep assessment are included. Sample interview questions for a general sleep history are presented, along with information on sleep diaries and pertinent physical assessment data. The importance of analyzing these data is explained, and numerous examples of nursing diagnoses are given. Expected patient outcomes and specific nursing strategies for promoting rest and sleep are described. The concluding nursing plan of care illustrates how the nurse's knowledge of rest and sleep, combined with skilled nursing interventions and caring, can resolve sleep problems.

PHYSIOLOGY OF SLEEP

Two systems in the brainstem, the reticular activating system (RAS) and the bulbar synchronizing region, are believed to work together to control the cyclic nature of sleep. The RAS extends upward through the medulla, the pons, the midbrain, and into the hypothalamus. It facilitates reflex and voluntary movements as well as cortical activities related to a state of alertness. The RAS comprises many nerve cells and fibers.

REFLECTIVE PRACTICE

Challenge to Intellectual Skills

I was working in our well-baby clinic today when a mother, Lydia Omeara, asked my advice about letting her infant twins sleep in bed with her and her husband: "They have their own beds, of course, but at night, when they get up, they seem to like to be in bed with us. Plus, I still breastfeed my babies, so having them nearby would really make it easier for me." She mentioned reading an article recently about this, noting that while this custom is usual in other countries, it had been discouraged until recently in the United States. According to the article, she said that it seems that more and more U.S. parents are doing this now. She asked for my advice, and I had no idea how to respond. Clearly, anything that resulted in better rest for the parents—who are up many times each night if the babies aren't sleeping well—would seem to be a good idea. However, I vaguely remembered learning that small children are at increased risk for sudden infant death syndrome in an adult bed. I needed to find the best way to respond to Mrs. Omeara.

Thinking Outside the Box: Possible Courses of Action

- Make up an answer: "Yes, it's OK" or "No way! What are you, crazy?"
- Refer her to a nurse with more experience.

- Tell her that I honestly don't know the answer but I will find out more about this and then get back to her.

Evaluating a Good Outcome: How Do I Define Success?

- A decision is made about where the children sleep that protects them and promotes rest, health, and well-being for each member of the family.
- I learn more about what science dictates is the best recommendation.

- I am faithful to my professional obligations to be knowledgeable about matters like this.

Personal Learning: Here's to the Future!

Since I don't have children myself and couldn't ever remember spending the night in my parents' bed or having a conversation with them about this, I certainly couldn't draw on personal experience in responding to this mother. In addition, we had never studied anything about this topic. I did remember a recent article in "Newsweek" magazine raising the issue, but I didn't remember this article proposing a scientifically grounded recommendation. As a result, I did some research on this issue and learned that there is a wide range of opinion on this matter. I did

my best to summarize the arguments, pro and con, and then I shared these with Mrs. Omeara so that she and her husband could make an informed decision.

This little experience has taught me a lot about the power of my profession to influence—literally—how people are born, live, and die. I want to have enough knowledge to help people make the best possible life choices, never leading them astray by virtue of my ignorance!

Amy Norris, Georgetown University

Reflection

How do you think you would respond in a similar situation? Why? What does this tell you about yourself and about the adequacy of your skills for professional practice? Can you think of other ways to respond? Research the Internet for the "Newsweek" article referred to by the nursing student. What information does this article provide? Would this article be a reliable research article? Please explain why or why not. What other skills (cognitive, interpersonal, technical, ethical/legal) would you need to respond well in this situation? What information would be necessary for the nursing student to obtain from the patient to provide an overall picture of the family situation? Create a sleep history tool that the nursing student could use to assess the patient's sleep. Do you agree with the criteria to evaluate a successful outcome? Did the nursing student meet the criteria? Please explain your answer.

The fibers have connections that relay impulses into the cerebral cortex and spinal cord.

During sleep, the RAS experiences few stimuli from the cerebral cortex and the periphery of the body. Wakefulness occurs when this system is activated with stimuli from the cerebral cortex and from periphery sensory organs and cells (see Chap. 44, Fig. 44-1). For example, an alarm clock awakens us from sleep to a state of consciousness, in which we realize that we must prepare for the day. Sensations such as pain, pressure, and noise produce wakefulness by means of peripheral organs and cells.

The hypothalamus has control centers for several involuntary activities of the body, one of which concerns sleeping and waking. Injury to the hypothalamus may cause a person to sleep for abnormally long periods.

Various neurotransmitters are involved with the sleeping process. Norepinephrine and acetylcholine, in addition to dopamine, serotonin, and histamine, are involved with excitation. Gamma-aminobutyric acid (GABA) appears to be necessary for inhibition. However, research has yet to prove exactly how biochemical changes and hormones function in sleep.

Circadian Rhythms

Rhythmic biologic clocks are known to exist in plants, animals, and humans. Influenced by both internal and external factors, they regulate certain biologic and behavioral functions in humans. Some cycles are monthly, such as a woman's menstrual cycle. **Circadian rhythms** complete a full cycle every 24 hours. "Circa" in Latin means "approximately" and "diem" is the Latin word for "day"; circadian represents approximately 1 day (Porth, 2007). Fluctuations in a person's heart rate, blood pressure, body temperature, hormone secretions, metabolism, and performance and mood depend in part on circadian rhythms.

Sleep is one of the body's most complex biologic rhythms. Circadian synchronization exists when an individual's sleep–wake patterns follow the inner biologic clock. When physiologic and psychological rhythms are high or most active, the person is awake; when these rhythms are low, the person is asleep. Although light and dark appear to be powerful regulators of the sleep–wake circadian rhythm, they do not exert primary control. The regulating mechanism is the person's individual biologic clock, which is subject to numerous influences, such as occupational demands and social pressures. For example, nurses who work the night shift may routinely sleep from 2 p.m. to 8 p.m., and peak physiologic activity may occur between 10 p.m. and 6 a.m. during work. Problems of desynchronization occur when sleep–wake patterns are frequently altered and the person attempts to sleep during high-activity rhythms or to work when the body is physiologically prepared to rest.

> ▶ *Think back to Charlie Bitner, the older man living in a long-term care facility. The nurse would need to assess Mr. Bitner, gathering data about his circadian rhythm. This knowledge would be important in developing an individualized plan of care for the patient to promote adequate sleep.* ∎

Stages of Sleep

Research reveals that there are two major stages of sleep: **non–rapid eye movement (NREM) sleep** and **rapid eye movement (REM) sleep.** These stages have been studied and analyzed with the help of the electroencephalograph (EEG), which receives and records electrical currents from the brain; the electrooculogram (EOG), which records eye movements; and the electromyograph (EMG), which records muscle tone (Fig. 34-1).

NREM Sleep

NREM sleep (comprising about 75% of total sleep) consists of four stages. Stages I and II, consuming about 5% and 50% of a person's sleep time, respectively, are light sleep. During these stages, the person can be aroused with relative ease. Stages III and IV, each representing about 10% of total sleep time, are deep-sleep states, termed **delta sleep** or slow-wave sleep. The arousal threshold (intensity of stimulus required to awaken) is

FIGURE 34-1. Sleep is determined in the laboratory by measuring the electrical activity of the brain and muscles and the movement of the eyes, using techniques of electrooculography, electromyography, and electroencephalography.

usually greatest in stage IV NREM. Throughout the stages of NREM sleep, the parasympathetic nervous system dominates, and decreases in pulse, respiratory rate, blood pressure, metabolic rate, and body temperature are observed. Characteristics of the four stages of NREM sleep are summarized in Box 34-1.

REM Sleep

It is more difficult to arouse a person during REM sleep than during NREM sleep. In normal adults, the REM state consumes 20% to 25% of a person's nightly sleep time. People who are awakened during the REM state almost always report that they have been dreaming. They can usually vividly recall their dreams even if they were absurd or have no sensible meaning for them. Everyone dreams.

During REM sleep, the pulse, respiratory rate, blood pressure, metabolic rate, and body temperature increase, whereas general skeletal muscle tone and deep tendon reflexes are depressed. REM sleep is believed to be essential to mental and emotional equilibrium and to play a role in learning, memory, and adaptation.

A person who is deprived of REM sleep for several nights generally then spends more time in REM sleep on successive nights. This phenomenon, termed REM rebound, allows the total amount of REM sleep to remain fairly constant over time. See Box 34-1 for characteristics of REM sleep.

Sleep Cycle

Normally during a **sleep cycle,** a person passes consecutively through the four stages of NREM sleep. This pattern is then

Box 34-1   CHARACTERISTICS OF NREM AND REM SLEEP

NREM Sleep

Stage I
- The person is in a transitional stage between wakefulness and sleep.
- The person is in a relaxed state but still somewhat aware of the surroundings.
- Involuntary muscle jerking may occur and waken the person.
- The stage normally lasts only minutes.
- The person can be aroused easily.
- This stage constitutes only about 5% of total sleep.

Stage II
- The person falls into a stage of sleep.
- The person can be aroused with relative ease.
- This stage constitutes 50% to 55% of sleep.

Stage III
- The depth of sleep increases, and arousal becomes increasingly difficult.
- This stage composes about 10% of sleep.

Stage IV
- The person reaches the greatest depth of sleep, which is called *delta sleep.*

- Arousal from sleep is difficult.
- Physiologic changes in the body include the following:
  - Slow brain waves are recorded on an EEG.
  - Pulse and respiratory rates decrease.
  - Blood pressure decreases.
  - Muscles are relaxed.
  Metabolism slows and the body temperature is low.
  This constitutes about 10% of sleep.

REM Sleep
- Eyes dart back and forth quickly.
- Small muscle twitching, such as on the face
- Large muscle immobility, resembling paralysis
- Respirations irregular; sometimes interspersed with apnea
- Rapid or irregular pulse
- Blood pressure increases or fluctuates
- Increase in gastric secretions
- Metabolism increases; body temperature increases
- Encephalogram tracings active
- REM sleep enters from stage II of NREM sleep and reenters NREM sleep at stage II: arousal from sleep difficult
- Constitutes about 20% to 25% of sleep

---

reversed, and the person returns from stage IV to stage III to stage II. Instead of reentering stage I and awakening, the person enters into the REM stage of sleep, after which he or she reenters NREM sleep at stage II and returns to stages III and IV. If a person is awakened from sleep at any time, he or she returns to sleep again by starting at stage I of NREM sleep.

> ▶ *Consider Charlie Bitner, the long-term care resident described at the beginning of the chapter. When evaluating Mr. Bitner's sleep cycle, the nurse would need to keep in mind that each time Mr. Bitner awakes, his sleep cycle is starting all over again. Subsequently, he is experiencing light sleep, characteristic of sleep stages I and II.* ■

Most people go through four or five cycles of sleep each night. On average, each cycle lasts about 90 to 100 minutes. The term "sleep architecture" is used to describe this alternating between REM and NREM sleep during these cycles (Cole & Richards, 2007). The cycles tend to become longer as morning approaches. Ordinarily, more deep sleep occurs in the delta stage in the first half of the night, especially if one is tired or has lost sleep.

Figure 34-2 illustrates the normal sleep pattern of young adults. Variations in the sleep cycle occur according to age, as Figure 34-3 illustrates.

Sleep Requirements and Patterns

For no known reason, 8 hours of sleep a night has been the accepted standard for adults, despite obvious variations seen in the general population. No rigid formula exists for the regular intervals and duration of sleep. It is important, however, that each person follows a pattern of rest that maintains well-being.

Despite individual variations, some generalities can be stated. On the average, infants require 14 to 20 hours each day. Growing children require from 10 to 14 hours of sleep.

FIGURE 34-2. A single normal sleep cycle. In the normal nocturnal pattern, the shaded cycle is repeated four or five times. Periods of REM sleep generally increase in duration, and periods of deep sleep (stage IV) progressively decrease as morning approaches.

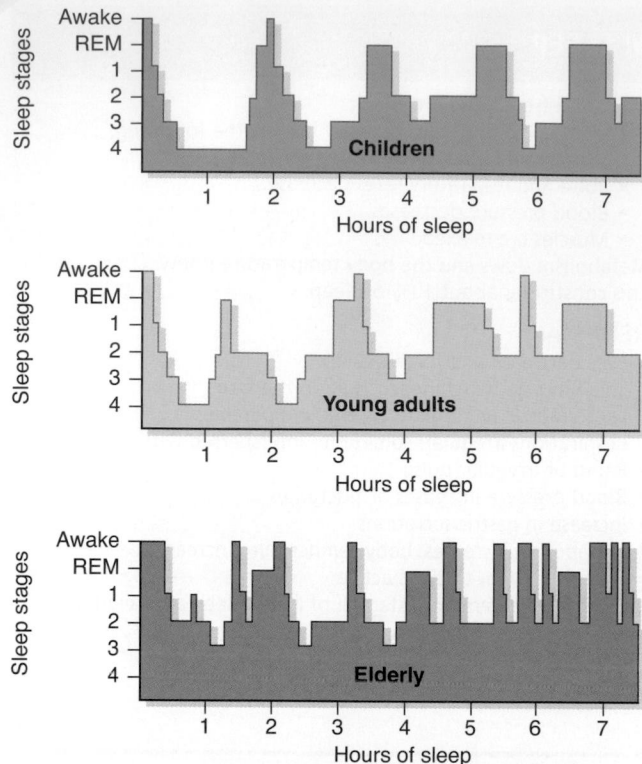

FIGURE 34-3. A comparison of developmental differences in NREM and REM cycles during nocturnal sleep for children, young adults, and older people.

> *Recall Jeanette Clark, the mother of an adolescent girl who seems to want to sleep all the time. When discussing this issue with Mrs. Clark, the nurse would need to integrate information about the adolescent's developmental stage—that is, that adolescence is a period of tremendous growth.* ■

The recommended amount of sleep for adults is 7 to 9 hours. Those who are able to relax and rest easily, even while awake, often find that less sleep is needed, whereas others may find that more sleep is required to overcome fatigue. Fatigue can be considered a normal, protective body mechanism and nature's warning that sleep is necessary. Chronic fatigue, however, is abnormal and is often a symptom of illness.

Sleep patterns of older adults vary, but 23% to 40% report recurring insomnia at least a few nights a month (Cole & Richards, 2007). Older people often need more time to fall asleep, wake earlier and more frequently during the night, and are less able to cope with changes in their usual sleep patterns than are younger people. Many older individuals nap during the day, which often results in sleeping fewer hours at night. Illnesses in older adults may also affect their sleep patterns. For instance, many older men have enlargement of the prostate gland, which may cause them to awaken throughout the night to use the bathroom.

Patterns of sleep periodicity appear to be learned. For example, most people learn to sleep at night and to be awake and work during the day. However, many night workers learn to sleep equally well during the day.

FACTORS AFFECTING SLEEP

A variety of factors influence both the quality and quantity of sleep.

Developmental Considerations

Variations in sleep patterns are related to age. Box 34-2 highlights these variations and associated nursing implications. For example, children at 3 years of age who sleep less than 12 hours nightly are more likely to be overweight (Traveras et al., 2008). Insufficient sleep may also affect normal growth and development and be a contributing factor in performance deficits and behavioral problems. Routine assessment of sleepiness or short sleep patterns in children is a first step in identifying the existence of a sleep problem and factors interfering with a child's sleep. Parents also reported that physicians do not routinely query them during childhood health examinations about their child's sleep patterns and habits.

Motivation

A desire to be wakeful and alert helps overcome sleepiness and sleep. For example, a tired person may be wakeful and alert when at a party or when attending an interesting play or concert. The opposite is also true: When there is minimal motivation to be awake, sleep generally follows. For example, a student who is bored and disinterested in a lecture or class may doze during the lecture.

Culture

An individual's cultural beliefs and practices can influence rest and sleep. Although developmental stages are similar, children's bedtime rituals, sleeping position and place, and pattern of sleep may vary based on culture. Methods to enhance or foster sleep may also be culturally influenced. For example, an older Asian patient may choose herbal tea rather than a sleeping medication to promote relaxation and sleep. A cultural orientation toward privacy and quiet makes sleep difficult in a busy special care unit where male and female patients sleep in close proximity. Sensitivity to a patient's culture must be included in the plan of care for preparing the patient for an evening's sleep.

> *Think back to Mrs. Omeara, the mother of infant twins, who is wondering whether she should let her twins sleep in her and her husband's bed. The nurse would need to investigate the family's cultural background to determine any influences it may have on the patient's question. The nurse would then use this information to develop an individualized, culturally appropriate plan of care for dealing with this question.* ■

Box 34-2 DEVELOPMENTAL PATTERNS OF SLEEP

Newborns and Infants

Sleep Pattern

- *Newborn:* Sleeps an average of 16 hours/24 hours; averages about 4 hours at a time.
- Each infant's sleep pattern is unique. On average, infants sleep 10 to 12 hours at night with possibly several naps during the day.
- Usually by 8 to 16 weeks of age, an infant sleeps through the night.
- REM sleep constitutes much of the sleep cycle of a young infant.

Nursing Implications

- Teach parents to position infant on the back. Sleeping in the prone position increases the risk for sudden infant death syndrome (SIDS).
- Advise parents that eye movements, groaning, grimacing, and moving are normal activities at this age.
- Encourage parents to have infant sleep in a separate area rather than their bed.
- Caution parents about placing pillows, crib bumpers, quilts, stuffed animals, and so on in the crib because this may pose a suffocation risk.

Toddlers

Sleep Pattern

- Need for sleep declines as this stage progresses. May initially sleep 12 hours at night with two naps during the day and end this stage sleeping 8 to 10 hours a night and napping once during the day.
- Toddlers may begin to resist naps and going to bed at night.
- They may move from crib to youth bed or regular bed around 2 years.

Nursing Implications

- Establish a regular bedtime routine (e.g., reading a story, singing a lullaby, saying prayers).
- Advise parents of the value of a routine sleeping pattern with minimal variation.
- Encourage attention to safety once child moves from crib to bed. If child attempts to wander out of room, a folding gate may be necessary across the door of the room.

Preschoolers

Sleep Pattern

- Children in this stage generally sleep 9 to 16 hours at night, with 12 hours being the average.
- The REM sleep pattern is similar to that of an adult.
- Daytime napping decreases during this period, and by the age of 5 years, most children no longer nap.
- This age group may continue to resist going to bed at night.

Nursing Implications

- Encourage parents to continue bedtime routines.
- Advise parents that waking from nightmares or night terrors (awakening screaming about 20 minutes after falling asleep) are common during this stage. Waking the child and comforting him or her generally helps. Sometimes use of a night light is soothing.

School-Aged Children

Sleep Pattern

- Younger school-aged children may require 10 to 12 hours nightly, whereas older children in this stage may average 8 to 10 hours
- Sleep needs usually increase when physical growth peaks.

Nursing Implications

- Discuss the fact that the stress of beginning school may interrupt normal sleep patterns.
- Advise that a relaxed bedtime routine is most helpful at this stage.
- Inform parents about child's awareness of the concept of death possibly occurring at this stage. Encourage parental presence and support to help alleviate some of the child's concerns.

Adolescents

Sleep Pattern

- Sleep needs of teenagers vary widely. The growth spurt that normally occurs at this stage may necessitate the need for more sleep; however, the stresses of school, activities, and part-time employment may cause adolescents to have a restless sleep.
- Many adolescents do not get enough sleep.

Nursing Implications

- Advise parents that complaints of fatigue or inability to do well in school may be related to not enough sleep. *Excessive daytime sleepiness (EDS)* may also make the teenager more vulnerable to accidents and behavioral problems.

Young Adults

Sleep Pattern

- The average amount of sleep required is 8 hours, but in fact, many young adults require less sleep.
- Sleep is affected by many factors: physical health, type of occupation, exercise. Lifestyle demands may interfere with sleep patterns.
- REM sleep averages about 20% of sleep.

Nursing Implications

- Reinforce that developing good sleep habits has a positive effect on health, particularly as an individual ages.
- If loss of sleep is a problem, explore lifestyle demands and stress as possible causes.
- Suggest use of relaxation techniques and stress-reduction exercises rather than resorting to medication to induce sleep. Sleep medications decrease REM sleep, may be habit forming, and frequently lose their effectiveness over time.

Middle-Aged Adults

Sleep Pattern

- Total sleep time decreases during these years with a decrease in stage IV sleep.
- The percentage of time spent awake in bed begins to increase.
- Individuals become more aware of sleep disturbances during this period.

Nursing Implications

- Encourage adults to investigate consistent sleep difficulties to exclude pathology or anxiety and depression as causes.
- Encourage adults to avoid use of sleep-inducing medication on a regular basis.

Older Adults

Sleep Pattern

- An average of 5 to 7 hours of sleep is usually adequate for this age group.
- Sleep is less sound, and stage IV sleep is absent or considerably decreased. Periods of REM sleep shorten.
- Elderly people frequently have great difficulty falling asleep and have more complaints of problems sleeping.

(continued)

Box 34-2   **DEVELOPMENTAL PATTERNS OF SLEEP** *(continued)*

- Decline in physical health, psychological factors, effects of drug therapy (e.g., nocturia), or environmental factors may be implicated as causes of inability to sleep.

Nursing Implications
- A comprehensive nursing assessment and individualized interventions may be effective in the long-term care of this age group.

- Emphasize concern for a safe environment because it is not uncommon for older people to be temporarily confused and disoriented when they first awake.
- Use sedatives with extreme caution because of declining physiologic function and concerns about polypharmacy.
- Encourage people to discuss sleep concerns with their physicians.

Lifestyle and Habits

Various lifestyle factors can affect a person's ability to sleep well. People working a shift other than the day shift must reorganize their priorities, or sleep difficulties may occur. Based on the circadian cycle, the body prepares for sleep at night by decreasing the body temperature and releasing **melatonin** (a natural chemical produced at night that decreases wakefulness and promotes sleep). Working the night shift disrupts this natural process and can result in loss of sleep and other adverse effects, such as anxiety, personal conflicts, loneliness, depression, gastrointestinal symptoms, and substance abuse (Guterl, 2008; Leap, 2008; Mason, 2008).

Developing a sleep pattern is especially difficult if the shift changes periodically. Nurses who work long hours and varying shifts have difficulty finding time to exercise and this can promote weight gain. The longer work hours have also been identified as a factor in an increase in the number of errors while at work (Guterl, 2008). The following Web site offers tips to help an individual on night shift adjust to a reversal of circadian rhythms: www.cdc.gov/niosh/topics/workschedules.

Sleep can be affected by watching some types of television shows, participating in stimulating outside activities, and taking part in activity or exercise. One's abilities to relax from work-related pressures and to put aside home stresses are also important factors in the ability to fall asleep (Promoting Health 34-1: Rest and Sleep).

Physical Activity and Exercise

Activity and exercise increase fatigue and, in many instances, promote relaxation that is followed by sleep. It appears that physical activity increases both REM and NREM sleep.

Moderate exercise is a healthy way to promote sleep, but exercise that occurs within a 2-hour interval before normal bedtime can hinder sleep. The fatigue that results from normal work activities or exercise is believed to contribute to a

---

PROMOTING HEALTH • 34-1

Rest and Sleep

Use the assessment checklist to determine how well you are meeting needs for rest and sleep. Then develop a prescription for self-care by choosing appropriate behaviors from the list of suggestions.

Assessment Checklist

| ❑ almost always | ❑ sometimes | ❑ almost never |

❑ ❑ ❑ 1. I feel rested and refreshed when I get up in the morning.

❑ ❑ ❑ 2. I have energy to carry out normal activities of daily living.

❑ ❑ ❑ 3. I understand the normal changes in sleep and rest requirements and patterns that occur with aging.

❑ ❑ ❑ 4. I set aside time for quiet recreation and restful activities each day.

Self-Care Behaviors

1. Follow a regular routine for bedtime and morning awakening.
2. Accept individual differences in need for sleep.
3. Use relaxation exercises to relax before bedtime, especially if feeling stressed.
4. Avoid caffeine, smoking, and alcohol before bedtime.
5. Adjust bedcoverings, room temperature, and lighting to your preferences.
6. Eat a small carbohydrate snack before going to bed.
7. Be aware of the potential dangers of sleeping pills.
8. Use some part of each day for quiet, enjoyable activities such as crafts, hobbies, reading, watching television, listening to music, and visiting with friends.
9. Incorporate three or four periods of regular exercise into each week.

restful sleep, whereas excessive exercise or exhaustion can decrease the quality of sleep.

> *Remember Jeanette Clark, the mother of the adolescent girl who seems to be sleeping all the time. As part of the health promotion teaching plan, the nurse would need to explain to Mrs. Clark about the changes occurring during adolescence. In addition to this stage being a period of rapid growth, it is also a time of increased activity—physically, emotionally, and socially. All of these may be affecting her daughter's sleep patterns.* ∎

Dietary Habits

It has long been believed that the dietary amino acid L-tryptophan acts to promote sleep. A small protein-containing snack before bedtime used to be recommended for patients with insomnia. However, as nutritionists have studied the effects of various foods on mood, new information has emerged. Protein may actually increase alertness and concentration, whereas carbohydrates appear to affect brain serotonin levels and promote calmness and relaxation. Therefore, a small protein- and carbohydrate-containing snack may be effective.

ALCOHOL INTAKE

Alcoholic beverages, when used in moderation, appear to induce sleep in some people. However, large quantities have been found to limit REM and delta sleep (Goldsmith, 2007). This effect may partially explain the phenomenon of a hangover after excessive alcohol consumption. Most recommendations to promote effective sleep recommend that alcohol and products containing alcohol should not be used within 6 hours of sleep (Gevirtz, 2007).

CAFFEINE-CONTAINING BEVERAGES

Caffeine is a central nervous system stimulant. For many people, beverages containing caffeine interfere with the ability to fall asleep. Examples of beverages containing caffeine include coffee, tea, and most cola drinks. Chocolate also contains caffeine.

SMOKING

Nicotine has a stimulating effect, and smokers usually have a more difficult time falling asleep. They are more easily aroused once asleep and may describe themselves as light sleepers. Eliminating cigarette smoking after the evening meal appears to improve the smoker's ability to fall asleep. People usually report improved sleep patterns after discontinuing nicotine use.

Total withdrawal from smoking may be associated with temporary sleep disturbances. Patients who stop smoking often have more daytime sleepiness and report significantly more restlessness at night. Whether this is a short-term effect or is related to nicotine's effect on the central nervous system is uncertain.

Environmental Factors

Most people sleep best in their usual home environments. Sleeping in a strange or new environment tends to influence both REM and NREM sleep. People accustomed to sleeping in a noisy environment, such as a busy large city, actually have a hard time falling asleep in an area that is extremely quiet. By turning on a radio or other noise, the person may actually be able to rest in the new environment. Likewise, if a patient is accustomed to sleeping in a quiet environment, a room next to a high-traffic area, such as the nurse's desk, may not be the best place for this patient to rest.

Psychological Stress

Psychological stress such as from illness and various life situations tend to disturb sleep. Generally, psychological stress affects sleep in two ways: (1) the person experiencing stress may find it difficult to obtain the amount of sleep he or she needs, and (2) REM sleep decreases in amount, which tends to add to anxiety and stress.

> *Consider Mrs. Omeara, the mother described in the beginning of the chapter and in the Reflective Practice display. The nurse would need to gather additional information about Mrs. Omeara's current situation to determine if any stressors might be affecting her ability to obtain adequate rest and sleep. Areas to address may include her typical daily activities, amount of time spent caring for each child, employment, and amount of assistance and support from others. In addition, the nurse would need to investigate the reasons underlying Mrs. Omeara's question about the babies sleeping in the parents' bed.* ∎

Illness

Illness, a physiologic as well as a psychological stressor, influences sleep. Certain illnesses are more closely related to sleep disturbances than others. For example:

- Gastric secretions increase during REM sleep. Many people with peptic ulcers awaken at night with pain. They find that eating a snack or using antacids to neutralize stomach acidity often relieves discomfort and promotes sleep.
- The pain associated with coronary artery disease and myocardial infarction is more likely with REM sleep.
- Epilepsy seizures are most likely to occur during NREM sleep and appear to be depressed by REM sleep.
- Liver failure and encephalitis tend to cause a reversal in day–night sleeping habits.
- Hypothyroidism tends to decrease the amount of NREM sleep, especially stages II and IV, while hyperthyroidism may result in difficulty falling asleep.
- End stage renal disease (ESRD) disrupts nocturnal sleep and leads to excessive daytime sleepiness. Patients with ESRD who receive dialysis also have a higher incidence of

restless leg syndrome (discussed later in the chapter), which possibly is related to the iron deficiency common in ESRD.

Chronotherapeutics is a growing field of study that involves the strategic use of time in the administration of medicine. Researchers have determined that certain treatments for disease are more effective when body rhythms are taken into account. For example, a larger midafternoon dose of asthma medication may be more effective in preventing attacks that commonly occur at night during sleep. The timing of antihypertensive medication administration may need to be adjusted to provide peak protection during early-morning hours, when heart attacks are more common. Cancer chemotherapy appears to be less toxic when administered at certain times of the day. Paying attention to biologic rhythms may influence drug tolerance and medication effectiveness.

Medications

Sleep quality is also influenced by certain drugs. Drugs that decrease REM sleep include barbiturates, amphetamines, and antidepressants. Diuretics, antiparkinsonian drugs, some antidepressants and antihypertensives, steroids, decongestants, caffeine, and asthma medications are seen as additional common causes of sleep problems. For short-term use, zaleplon (Sonata) and zolpidem tartrate (Ambien) are often prescribed to promote sleep in older adults because there is less residual sleepiness (Lilley, Harrington, & Snyder, 2007). Eszopiclone (Lunesta) is prescribed for longer-term treatment of chronic insomnia.

COMMON SLEEP DISORDERS

A nurse who interviews a patient to obtain a sleep history needs to understand common sleep disturbances to recognize significant data. The most recent classification of sleep disorders categorized by the International Classification of Sleep Disorders includes four major categories of disturbances:

- Dyssomnias
- Parasomnias
- Sleep disorders associated with medical or psychiatric disorders
- Other proposed disorders

The more common sleep disorders are the dyssomnias and parasomnias. **Dyssomnias** are sleep disorders characterized by insomnia or excessive sleepiness. **Parasomnias** are patterns of waking behavior that appear during sleep. A brief description of these disturbances follows.

Dyssomnias
Insomnia

Insomnia is characterized by difficulty falling asleep, intermittent sleep, or early awakening from sleep. It is the most common of all sleep disorders. People older than 60 years of age, women (especially after menopause), and persons with a history of depression are more likely to experience insomnia. This sleep disorder can also occur during periods of stress, in

situations involving some change in the normal environment, after traveling across time zones (jet lag), and as a result of the side effects of medications.

Usually, people reporting insomnia have been observed to fall asleep more quickly and sleep more than they report they do. However, the condition can lead to such distress that further wakefulness results. A person with insomnia often reports feeling tired, lethargic, and irritable during the day. Difficulty concentrating is also a common manifestation.

Treatment of insomnia is usually unnecessary because most episodes last for only a short period. Insomnia that lasts less than 4 weeks is termed acute while chronic insomnia persists for 5 weeks to 6 months. Chronic insomnia is frequently listed as the motivating factor for a visit to a sleep disorder clinic. Insomnia that lasts more than 6 months may be termed persistent and may even continue throughout life (Goldsmith, 2007).

According to the Centers for Disease Control and Prevention (CDC) (2008), nearly 10% of the U.S. population suffers from chronic insomnia. Certain health conditions have been associated with chronic insomnia. They include obesity; type 2 diabetes; psychiatric disorders, such as depression; and cardiovascular disorders such as heart failure, stroke, hypertension, and myocardial infarction (heart attack). The misuse of alcohol or caffeine can have an adverse effect on insomnia and stopping these behaviors may reduce or eliminate the insomnia (Goldsmith, 2007; O'Brien, 2007).

Nonpharmacological approaches should be attempted initially to resolve the insomnia. Cognitive Behavioral Therapy (CBT) is a safe, effective means of managing chronic insomnia and may include sleep hygiene measures, stimulus control, and sleep restriction therapy (NSF, 2008b). CBT involves meeting with a therapist and working through maladaptive sleep beliefs. It may also include biofeedback and relaxation techniques. When used in conjunction with these other complementary therapies, CBT is very successful. If, however, these measures prove ineffective, pharmacologic treatment may be necessary. Pharmacologic options include the use of sedatives and hypnotics. However, only short-term use, at the lowest dose, is recommended.

Sleep hygiene refers to nonpharmacologic recommendations that help an individual get a better night's sleep. These entail reviewing and changing lifestyles and environment. Sleep hygiene suggestions include the following:

- Restricting the intake of caffeine, nicotine, and alcohol, especially later in the day.
- Avoiding activities after 5 p.m. that are stimulating.
- Avoiding naps.
- Eating a light meal before bedtime.
- Sleeping in a cool, dark room.
- Eliminating use of a bedroom clock.
- Taking a warm bath before bedtime.
- Trying to keep the sleep environment as quiet as possible (Gevirtz, 2007).

Stimulus control involves using the bedroom for sex and sleep only. People with insomnia who have problems initiating sleep should stay in the bedroom for only 15 to 20 minutes. If after this time they cannot fall asleep, they should leave the room and return only when they feel sleepy. Getting up at the same time every day, no matter what time the person fell asleep, and refraining from napping during the day are recommended.

Sleep restriction is based on the theory of limiting the time in bed to actual sleep time. It is thought that excessive time in bed may result in fragmented sleep, which may exacerbate the insomnia. A sleep diary helps to determine sleep patterns. The focus of sleep restriction is to avoid naps and early bedtimes and, actually, change the way an individual sleeps.

Relaxation therapy involves any type of relaxation, such as progressive muscle relaxation, imagery training, or meditation. Not all relaxation methods are beneficial for all patients. Relaxation therapy and biofeedback are discussed in detail in Chapter 42.

Hypersomnia

Hypersomnia is a condition characterized by excessive sleep, particularly during the day. A person may fall asleep for intervals during work, while eating, or even during conversations. These naps do not usually relieve their symptoms. When they awake, they are often disoriented, irritated, restless, and have slower speech and thinking processes.

Causes of hypersomnia are varied. They may include:

- Another sleep disorder, such as sleep apnea
- Drug or alcohol abuse
- Head trauma or other injury to the central nervous system
- Effect of certain medications
- Depression
- Obesity
- Other medical conditions (multiple sclerosis, epilepsy).

Some individuals may have a genetic predisposition to hypersomnia. It appears most often in adolescents and young adults.

Treatment of hypersomnia is symptomatic in nature. Stimulant drugs may prove effective, or in some cases, antidepressants may be prescribed. Attention to diet (avoidance of alcohol and caffeine) and behavioral changes (avoidance of night work and social activities later in the evening) may offer some relief from such episodes. Although not usually life threatening, hypersomnia can have some serious consequences, such as motor vehicle accidents that occur because of drowsiness or falling asleep while driving. These attacks may occur indefinitely (National Institute of Neurological Disorders and Stroke, 2006).

Narcolepsy

Narcolepsy is a condition characterized by an uncontrollable desire to sleep. A person with narcolepsy can literally fall asleep standing up, while driving a car, in the middle of a conversation, or while swimming. Individuals with narcolepsy tend to fall asleep quickly, find it difficult to wake up, sleep fewer hours than others, and sleep restlessly.

Narcolepsy is considered a neurologic disorder. The condition usually begins in susceptible people during adolescence or early adulthood and continues through life. Between 50,000 and 2.4 million people in the United States have this disorder (National Heart Lung and Blood Institute, 2008).

Sleepiness during the day is often the first symptom of narcolepsy, which usually occurs several years before experiencing any difficulty with nighttime sleep. Common features of narcolepsy include the following:

- Sleep attacks: irresistible urge to sleep, regardless of the type of activity in which the patient is engaged
- Cataplexy: sudden loss of motor tone that may cause the person to fall asleep; usually experienced during a period of strong emotion
- Hypnagogic hallucinations: nightmares or vivid hallucinations
- Sleep-onset REM periods: during a sleep attack, the person moves directly into REM sleep
- Sleep paralysis: skeletal paralysis that occurs during the transition from wakefulness to sleep

The presence of any two symptoms helps to confirm the diagnosis. Undiagnosed, a person with narcolepsy is potentially dangerous to himself or herself and others. In some countries, a person with a diagnosis of narcolepsy is not permitted to drive a motor vehicle. A central nervous system stimulant (e.g., methylphenidate [Ritalin]) that causes wakefulness may be used to control narcolepsy. Additional medications such as modafinil (Provigil), a wakefulness-promoting compound, and sodium oxybate (Xyrem), a sedative used for treating disturbed nocturnal sleep, have proved effective in treating narcoleptic symptoms (Lilley et al., 2007). People using such drugs should take them faithfully because with discontinuation of use, the uncontrollable desire to sleep returns.

Sleep Apnea

Sleep apnea is a condition in which a person experiences the absence of breathing (apnea) or diminished breathing efforts (hypopnea) during sleep between snoring intervals. Breathing may cease for 10 to 20 seconds, possibly as long as 2 minutes. During long periods of apnea, the oxygen level in the blood drops, the pulse usually becomes irregular, and the blood pressure often increases. Many people experience sleep apnea without symptoms, but excessive daytime sleepiness is commonly reported. Although it occurs most commonly in middle-aged men who are obese and have short thick necks, women and people of other ages may also experience it.

Obstructive sleep apnea (OSA) can result when the airway is occluded because of the collapse of the hypopharynx (Fig. 34-4) or from other structural abnormalities such as enlarged tonsils and adenoids, a deviated nasal septum, and thyroid enlargement. Narrowing of nasal passageways caused by allergic rhinitis or nasal polyps is another factor contributing to OSA (Goldberg, 2007). Sleep apnea affects more than 18 million American adults but most of these people are never diagnosed and treated. Approximately 2% to 3% of children may also have OSA (NSF, 2009).

Normal unoccluded airway

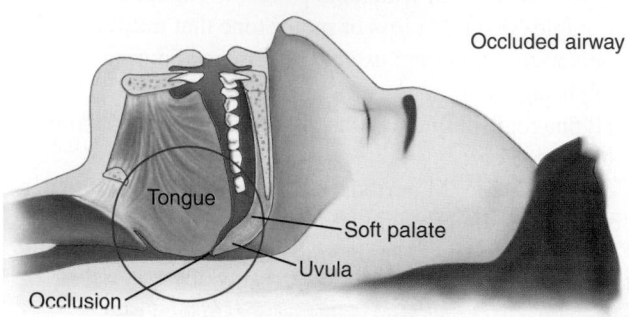

Occluded airway

Tongue

Soft palate

Uvula

Occlusion

FIGURE 34-4. Obstructive sleep apnea occurs when the airway is occluded due to collapse of the hypopharynx. Normally the airway remains open during sleep (see inset).

Some investigators have theorized that sleep apnea may explain certain cases of death that occur during sleep. According to recent research, individuals with OSA had "more than twice the number of cardiac deaths during sleeping hours compared to the general population" (O'Brien, 2007). In healthy people, OSA may impair cardiac function over time and lead to the development of heart failure. If heart failure has already been diagnosed, OSA may result in progression of this condition. Sleep apnea and heart failure are a dangerous combination, making it even more important to recognize and treat OSA.

Clinical information and polysomnography can confirm the diagnosis of sleep apnea. This overnight sleep study consists of an EEG recording of the stages of sleep and any episodes of apnea, an electrooculogram that detects eye movements, and an electromyographic recording of muscle movement (Shields, 2008). Cardiopulmonary monitoring of the arterial oxygen saturation and an electrocardiogram (ECG) to detect any cardiac arrhythmias can also assist in the diagnosis of obstructive sleep apnea.

People with obstructive sleep apnea may become irritable during the day, fall asleep during monotonous activities, have difficulty concentrating, and exhibit slower reaction times. They are also more likely to be involved in motor vehicle accidents. Alcohol, tobacco, and sleeping pills increase the breathing disruption that occurs in sleep apnea and should be avoided.

Treatment of moderate obstructive sleep apnea may consist of removing the tonsils or using an oral appliance when sleeping. If this is ineffective, continuous positive airway pressure (CPAP) may be recommended. CPAP is noninvasive

and consists of a mask connected to an air pump that is worn during sleep. This device delivers positive air pressure that holds the airway open. Many patients discontinue use of CPAP because of a sensation of claustrophobia, discomfort exhaling against air inflow, or dryness and skin irritation. If conservative treatment methods fail, surgery to remove soft tissue at the back of the mouth may be an option. This surgery is not without risks and poses significant postoperative issues for the patient. Individuals who opt for the procedure need continued support and comprehensive teaching, including coping strategies, for the immediate postoperative period (Caballer, 2007).

Restless Leg Syndrome

People with **restless leg syndrome (RLS)** cannot lie still and report unpleasant creeping, crawling, or tingling sensations in the legs. Usually, these sensations are in the calf, but they may occur anywhere from the ankle to the thigh. Patients describe an irresistible urge to move the legs when these sensations occur, usually during the evening and night. In some cases, symptoms may affect both sides of the body. Almost one-fourth of the individuals diagnosed with RLS have an iron deficiency but the reason for this association is unclear. RLS is also seen in patients with end-stage renal disease (ESRD) and in pregnant women. Over the counter medications such as antihistamines can exacerbate the symptoms of RLS. This disorder has no cure.

Although restless leg syndrome is a common sleep disorder that affects up to 15% of the population, many healthcare workers are unaware of its existence. The acronym URGE summarizes the symptoms and criteria for diagnosis of RLS:

U – urge to move the legs

R – rest-induced

G – gets better with activity

E – evening symptoms more severe (Taverno & Pavlovich-Danis, 2008).

Massaging the legs, walking, doing knee bends, and moving the legs sometimes bring relief. Research continues into additional treatment options, but the following may prove effective:

- Eliminating use of caffeine, tobacco, and alcohol.
- Taking a mild analgesic at bedtime (provided it is compatible with the current medical regimen).
- Applying heat or cold to the extremity.
- Using relaxation techniques. Biofeedback and transcutaneous electrical nerve stimulation (TENS) may also relieve symptoms (see the accompanying Promoting Health Literacy display).

Ropinirole (Requip), a drug used to treat symptoms of Parkinson's disease, has been approved by the FDA to treat restless leg syndrome. A newer drug in the same category, pramipexole dihydrochloride (Mirapex), has also proved effective for relief of the symptoms of RLS.

The Restless Legs Syndrome Foundation (http://www.rls.org) is a support group available for the millions of people with this disorder who experience chronic sleep loss.

Promoting Health Literacy
IN PATIENTS WITH RESTLESS LEG SYNDROME

Patient Scenario

Mary Weymouth is a 40-year-old woman who has an appointment to see her primary physician because of a "strange sensation in her legs that is keeping her awake at night." When asked by the nurse to further describe her symptoms, Mary explains that she has this feeling that "something is crawling up her lower leg." She keeps moving her leg from side to side until she finally just gets out of bed and walks around for a while. She states that movement seems to "make it better" but this does not work all the time. Sometimes, she also gets "pretty severe cramping pain" that can last several hours. Mary relates that this has been happening 2 or 3 nights a week for at least 1 month and she finds that she is "very sleepy" the following day. At times when she is at work, she said that she finds herself starting to "nod off" and is afraid that someone might notice and she could lose her job. She's tried drinking a few glasses of wine at night to relax her and has also occasionally taken some Tylenol PM to see if that will help her sleep through the night. Nothing seems to help. After the physician examined her, he asked if anyone in her family had similar symptoms. Mary remembered that her mother used to tell her that she sometimes had "nervous legs" at night. The physician reviews her history and tells Mary that her symptoms indicate that she has Restless Leg Syndrome. At this time, he prefers not to prescribe medication for her but wants her to try some nonpharmacologic measures to see if they ease her symptoms. As Mary is making another appointment, she tells the nurse that "she doesn't know how much longer she can manage without a good night's sleep most nights. I may just have to give Tylenol PM another try."

Nursing Considerations: *Tips for Improving Health Literacy*

Provide Mary with some specific information about measures that may ease her symptoms of RLS and allow her to get a restful sleep. Recommend that she avoid alcohol, caffeine, and any over-the-counter sleeping medications because they contain antihistamines that may aggravate the symptoms of RLS. Encourage her to participate in and incorporate into her daily life any regular, moderate physical activity to promote a better sleep at night. Suggest using a heating pad or warm bath or an ice pack to possibly help with these sensations. Explain to Mary that there is no specific diagnostic test for RLS, but if her symptoms are not relieved by these other measures, there is a medication that the physician might prescribe. Also, give her information about the Web site that is specifically for patients with RLS. When Mary returns for her follow-up appointment, she needs to be prepared to ask her physician the following questions:

- What is my main problem? Can anything else be associated with this Restless Leg Syndrome?
- What else do I need to do?
- Why is it important for me to do this?
- What can you do if you prescribe a medication and it does not help with my symptoms?

What additional measures can you take to help increase health literacy in this patient? What other measures would be helpful if Mary did not speak English, could not read, or had other learning deficits?

Sleep Deprivation

Sleep deprivation refers to a decrease in the amount, consistency, or quality of sleep. It may result from decreased REM sleep or NREM sleep. Total sleep deprivation is rarely seen, other than in experimental settings. There are many causes, and the manifestations progress from irritability and impaired mental abilities to a total disintegration of personality. In general, the effects of sleep deprivation become increasingly apparent after 30 hours of continual wakefulness.

Partial sleep deprivation may result in loss of concentration, inattention, and impaired information processing and poses serious safety risks. Excessive daytime sleepiness, a form of partial sleep deprivation, impairs performance at times when individuals need to be alert. The strange environment of the hospital, physical discomfort and pain, the effects of medications, and the need for 24-hour nursing care may also contribute to sleep deprivation in hospitalized patients.

It is unclear whether irreversible damage to body tissue results from prolonged or chronic sleep deprivation. However, sleep deprivation clearly produces changes in physical and mental functioning, supporting the belief that sleep is essential for well-being. Even mild OSA with its accompanying decreased quality of sleep and constant fatigue is thought to "put stress on the body equivalent to five years of aging" (Schaller, 2008). Sleep deprivation may be caused by shorter periods of sleep, which over time can cause impairment. Whether it occurs as a result of a disorder or it is voluntary sleep curtailment, sleep deprivation has wide-ranging negative consequences for human health and well-being.

> *Recall Charlie Bitner, the long-term care facility resident complaining of sleep problems. From the patient's statements, the nurse would identify that Mr. Bitner is at*

risk for developing sleep deprivation. Therefore, the nurse would work with Mr. Bitner to establish measures that would promote effective sleep patterns. ■

Parasomnias

Parasomnias are patterns of waking behavior that appear during REM or NREM stages of sleep. Common examples are **somnambulism** (sleepwalking), sleeptalking, night terrors (screaming upon awakening due to a perceived threat), bruxism (grinding of teeth during sleep), and **enuresis** (urinating during sleep). They are more commonly seen in children. Although parasomnias are commonly outgrown before adulthood, safety and prevention of injury are paramount concerns.

A type of parasomnia that is gaining more attention is sleep-related eating disorder, which is when the patient eats but does not remember eating in the morning. People with sleep-related eating disorder can gain weight and experience injury either from cooking in their sleep or eating potentially dangerous raw food. They also may experience sleep disruption.

THE NURSING PROCESS FOR REST AND SLEEP
Assessing
Sleep History

Interview questions help identify the patient's sleep–wakefulness patterns, the effect of these patterns on everyday functioning, the patient's use of sleep aids, and the presence of sleep disturbances and contributing factors. If the patient's sleep is adequate and poses no problems, the sleep history may be brief (four questions), or it may be more detailed. When the patient's response to any of the interview questions indicates a potential problem, open-ended questions may be used to gather more data (Focused Assessment Guide 34-1).

If the patient is being admitted to a care facility, assess his or her usual times for retiring and waking, bedtime rituals, and preferences regarding sleep environment so that these can be incorporated into the plan of care, if possible. Patients in hospitals often receive fragmented sleep. Their sleep may be disrupted by routine care measures, noise in the environment, and lighting (see the accompanying Nursing Advocacy in Action display). One study involving patients in an ICU discovered that more interruptions in sleep were due to patient care than environmental noises (Cole & Richards, 2007). Paying attention to small matters can make the difference between a patient's having a good night of sleep or no sleep.

When a sleep disturbance is noted, ask about the following when obtaining the history:

- The nature of the problem
- Its cause
- The related signs and symptoms
- When it began and how often it occurs
- How it affects everyday living
- The severity of the problem and whether it can be treated independently by nurses or needs to be referred to another professional
- How the patient is coping with the problem and the success of any treatments attempted

NURSING ADVOCACY IN ACTION

Patient Scenario

Maria was born premature. After surgery on her bowel, she was placed on the transplantation list for a new liver and small bowel and started on total parenteral nutrition. She is now 9 months old but has spent the last 4 weeks in the hospital with fungemia, a fungus infection spread throughout the bloodstream. Her single mother, Ms. Gomez, practically lives at the hospital and in recent days has annoyed the nurses with her complaints about the nursing care. Her English is limited, but she is able to express her annoyance at the many times Maria is awakened during the night for treatment and care. "Why can't the nurses do several things at once so Maria can at least get a few hours of uninterrupted sleep?!" Recently the nurses complained to the medical director and he informed Ms. Gomez that if she doesn't stop interfering with Maria's care, the doctors will take Maria off the transplantation list. The nurse giving you report repeats this story and tells you "not to take any complaints or grief from the mom." When you meet Ms. Gomez and listen to her story, you admire her love for Maria and willingness to advocate for her. You also sense the mother's frustration with the system. She asks you tearfully, "They can't take Maria off the list, can they? I am only trying to be a good mother." Ms. Gomez appears to have no family or other support network.

Implications for Nursing Advocacy

How will you respond if you were the nurse assigned Maria as a patient? Talk with your classmates and experienced nurses about the questions that follow.

- Is it fair to say that Ms. Gomez is being threatened for trying to advocate for her baby? If you elect to advocate for Maria and her mother, what practical steps can you take to remedy this situation?
- What is it reasonable to expect of a student nurse, graduate nurse, and an experienced nurse in this situation?
- What advocacy skills are needed to effectively respond to this challenge?

FOCUSED ASSESSMENT GUIDE • 34-1

REST AND SLEEP

Factors to Assess	Questions and Approaches
Usual sleep–wakefulness pattern: Recent changes Usual sleeping and waking times	Do you set an alarm and hit "snooze" before getting up? How many hours of sleep do you usually get in a day? Do you wake up earlier in the morning than you would like and find it difficult to fall back asleep? Have there been any recent changes in your usual sleep–wake patterns? If yes, describe them and tell me if they are causing any problems for you. Do you usually go to bed and wake up about the same time each day?
Number of hours of undisturbed sleep	How have you been sleeping? Do you have any difficulty falling asleep? Do you wake up frequently during the night? Do you dream at night? Are your dreams frightening?
Quality of sleep Number and duration of naps	How much sleep do you think you need to feel rested? Do you take naps throughout the day?
Effect of sleep pattern on everyday functioning Energy level (ability to perform activities of daily living)	In what way does the sleep you get each day affect your everyday living? Has this sleep disturbance caused any change in your sex life? Do you feel rested and ready to start the day when you wake up? Are there times during the day or certain activities when you feel especially tired? What happens when you don't get enough sleep? Are you having difficulty concentrating?
Sleep aids Means of relaxing before bedtime	What do you do to relax before you get ready for bed?
Bedtime rituals Sleep environment	Describe what you usually do to help yourself fall asleep. Tell me how you like your room (lights, noises, ventilation, position of door, temperature) and bed (mattress, pillows, blankets) when you are sleeping.
Pharmacologic aids	Do you take any medications to help you sleep? Are you taking any medicine at all?
Sleep disturbances and contributing factors Nature of the sleep disturbance	Tell me about your sleep problem.
Onset of disturbance Causes (physical, psychosocial, medicine related)	How often does it occur? Are you doing anything differently now that might be causing the problem?
Severity Symptoms	Do you wake up gasping for air? Do you snore? Do you recall changing your position frequently during the night?
Interventions attempted and results	What have you been doing to deal with the problem? How effective were these measures?

> *Think back to Lydia Omeara, the mother of two infants who was asking about allowing the infants to sleep in their parents' bed. The nurse would need to obtain a sleep history from Mrs. Omeara to ascertain her sleep pattern. This information would be helpful in determining the reasons for allowing the children to sleep in their parents' bed.* ∎

Assistance from the patient's bed partner may be needed to aid in data collection and provide more accurate information regarding his or her sleep patterns. The patient's record may also contain pertinent information (e.g., a history of illnesses that influence sleep).

Sample records of a sleep history in a comprehensive nursing assessment are as follows:

Reports needs 8 to 9 hours of sleep to feel his best and usually gets this without problem.

RESEARCH IN NURSING
Bridging the Gap to Evidence-Based Practice

INCLUDING SLEEP ISSUES IN HEALTHCARE SCREENING

There is increased recognition that more than one-third of the U.S. population suffer from insomnia and daytime sleepiness. Research has also documented that insufficient sleep and sleep disorders significantly impact quality of life in multiple ways. Although family practice physicians and nurse practitioners consistently query patients about their diet, pattern of exercise, weight management, and mental health/stress management strategies, there is minimal, if any, mention of sleep issues at these office appointments. Unhealthy sleep patterns and the resulting negative consequences are rarely topics of discussion in health history databases at family medicine clinics. Considering that sleep occupies approximately one-third of our life, it is disconcerting that alterations in sleep are not more commonly addressed.

Related Research

Sorscher, A. (2008). How is your sleep: A neglected topic for health care screening. *The Journal of the American Board of Family Medicine, 21*(2), 141–148.

This study examined the general topics for healthcare screening, focusing on the frequency of questions relating to sleep and/or sleeping patterns. The health history databases at 121 primary care clinics in the Twin Cities metropolitan area were surveyed. This analysis involved the practices of 75% of the Family Practice physicians at this location. Results of this research indicated that the majority (57%) of the health assessments had no

For additional research, visit the **Point**

content on sleep issues while 43% of the surveys included 1 or 2 sleep-related questions. The United States Preventative Services Task Force oversees the routine preventative practices recommended for primary care physicians. Their latest guideline makes no mention of healthy sleep issues. Additionally, two major insurance providers for health maintenance organizations, Aetna and Kaiser-Permanente, do not ask questions about sleep practices in their standard health habits questionnaire. As evidence-based information accumulates about the vital role sleep plays in a healthy lifestyle, sleep disorder medicine will soon become more of a focus for primary care physicians. In the future, it may well be standard to have a section on sleep patterns and issues in all screening forms.

Relevance to Nursing Practice

Nurses in all settings need an awareness of the extent of sleep problems in all populations. If even the slightest suspicion of a sleep problem arises, nurses should question patients about sleeping patterns and normal sleep hygiene issues. As this research confirmed, inadequate sleep and its consequences are infrequently documented in health histories. Once healthcare providers recognize that a patient has difficulty sleeping, a more thorough assessment should be made to explore sleep hygiene practices and other factors that may affect sleep quality. Nursing care that is holistic and individualized must address rest and sleep issues.

Generally retires at 11:30 p.m. and rises at 7:30 a.m. No special sleep rituals.

Mother reports toddler has erratic sleep patterns. May nap at any time in the afternoon or evening and sleep from 1 to 3 hours. Depending on nap, goes to bed anywhere from 7 to 11 p.m. and sleeps about 11 to 13 hours. Resists falling asleep and wants "water, story, snack, kisses, etc." Parents' lifestyle is constantly changing—little consistency for the child regarding sleep expectations.

In outpatient settings and physician's offices, the issue of healthy sleep practices and the presence of sleep disorders are not routinely assessed. Given that the need for adequate sleep has become a national health problem, it can be expected that this will become a focus in future patient interactions (see the accompanying Research in Nursing display).

Sleep Diary

A sleep diary or log provides more specific data on the patient's sleep–wakefulness patterns over a long period. It summarizes information about these patterns, possibly indicating activities and behaviors that affect the quality and quantity of sleep. Generally, the diary is kept for 14 days and typically includes a graph of the total number of hours of sleep per day. Depending on the nature of the problem,

graphs may be made of the number of undisturbed hours of sleep, number of awakenings, and so forth. In addition, a daily record is completed addressing the following:

- Time patient retires
- Time patient tries to fall asleep
- Approximate time patient falls asleep
- Time of any awakenings during the night and when sleep was resumed
- Time of awakening in the morning
- Presence of any stressors patient believes are affecting his or her sleep
- A record of any food, drink, or medication patient believes has positively or negatively influenced his or her sleep (include time of ingestion)
- Record of physical activities—type, duration, and time
- Record of mental activities—type, duration, and time
- Record of activities performed 2 to 3 hours before bedtime, bedtime rituals, changes in sleep environment
- Presence of any worries or anxieties patient believes are affecting his or her sleep

> *Remember Jeanette Clark, the mother of the adolescent girl who seems to be sleeping all the time. Having Mrs. Clark's daughter complete a sleep diary might be helpful in*

obtaining a better picture of what is happening and helping rule out other causes for the daughter's increased fatigue and sleeping. These underlying causes could be wide ranging, including such conditions as depression, physical illness, or increased activity or schoolwork. ■

It is helpful if the patient has a bed partner who can assist with the diary. The patient needs to understand that the diary is simply a diagnostic tool. If keeping the diary causes too much stress for the patient and further interferes with his or her ability to sleep restfully, it should be discontinued.

Physical Assessment

The findings in the physical assessment may either confirm that the patient is getting sufficient rest to provide energy for the day's activities or validate the existence of a sleep disturbance that is decreasing the quantity or quality of sleep. Key findings include energy level (presence of physical weakness, fatigue, lethargy, or decreased energy), facial characteristics (narrowing or glazing of eyes, swelling of eyelids, decreased animation), or behavioral characteristics (yawning, rubbing eyes, slow speech, slumped posture). Physical data suggestive of potential sleep problems (e.g., obesity, enlarged neck, deviated nasal septum) may also be noted.

If the nurse or a bed partner can observe the patient sleeping, other sleep characteristics to assess include restlessness, sleep postures, and sleep activities such as snoring or leg jerking (nocturnal myoclonus).

SNORING

Snoring is caused by an obstruction to airflow through the nose and mouth. Other than disturbing others in the same bedroom, snoring is not ordinarily a sleeping disorder. However, snoring accompanied by apnea can present a problem. When snoring changes from the characteristic sawing-wood sound to a more irregular silence followed by a snort, this indicates obstructive apnea.

NOCTURNAL MYOCLONUS

Observed in 10% to 20% of chronic insomniacs, **nocturnal myoclonus** involves marked muscle contractions that result in the jerking of one or both legs during sleep. The jerking lasts about 28 seconds, on average; may arouse the sleeper; and contributes to insomnia.

Diagnosing

Disturbed Sleep Pattern as the Problem

When assessment data point to a sleep problem that is amenable to nursing therapy, it receives the label Disturbed Sleep Pattern if the problem is time limited or Sleep Deprivation if the problem is prolonged. Common etiologies for these nursing diagnoses may include the following:

- Physical discomfort or pain
- Emotional discomfort or pain caused by anxiety and stress

- Changes in bedtime rituals or sleep environment
- Disruption of circadian rhythm
- Exercise just before sleep
- Caffeine, nicotine, or alcohol intake after dinner
- Drug dependency and withdrawal
- Symptoms of physical illness

Examples of nursing diagnoses in which the disturbed sleep pattern is the primary problem are presented in the accompanying NANDA box.

Disturbed Sleep Pattern as the Etiology

The disturbed sleep pattern may affect many other areas of human functioning. In the nursing diagnoses that follow, the disturbed sleep pattern is the cause of another problem:

- Anxiety related to inability to fall asleep, inability to control behavior while asleep, and sleep apnea (threat of death)
- Activity Intolerance related to sleep deprivation
- Fatigue related to prolonged excessive role demands
- Ineffective Coping related to insomnia: insufficient quantity and quality of sleep
- Fear related to narcoleptic patient's potential to harm self or others
- Impaired Gas Exchange related to sleep apnea (oxygen saturation of the blood)
- Risk for Injury related to somnambulism, narcolepsy, sleep apnea
- Risk for Acute Confusion related to fluctuation in sleep–wake cycle, use of diphenhydramine (Benadryl) to aid sleep
- Deficient Knowledge (e.g., nonpharmacologic remedies for insomnia) related to misinformation, lack of interest in learning, cognitive limitation
- Risk for situational low self-esteem related to effects of sleep deprivation (e.g., sleep apnea syndrome)
- Anxiety related to nocturnal enuresis
- Impaired Social Interaction related to excessive daytime sleeping, sleep deprivation
- Disturbed Thought Processes related to chronic insomnia, sleep deprivation

Important Distinctions

Because the problem statement of the nursing diagnosis identifies what is wrong with the patient and suggests the expected outcomes and the etiology of the problem directs nursing interventions, analysis of the assessment data is essential when deciding whether the sleep data indicate the problem, contribute to a different problem, or are signs or symptoms of the problem. Sleep data potentially fit in all three categories. For example, when a disturbed sleep pattern involving altered sleep–wake patterns is assessed in a graduate nurse who is getting adjusted to a new full-time job, shift work, and increased independence, three different diagnoses might be written:

Disturbed Sleep Pattern associated with altered sleep–wake patterns related to shift work and stress of new

Examples of NANDA Nursing Diagnoses

Sleep

Nursing Diagnoses	Related Factors	Sample Defining Characteristics
Disturbed Sleep Pattern: Difficulty Falling Asleep	Worries about family and lack of destressing rituals	• "At least 4 or 5 nights a week, I lay in bed awake for 3 or 4 hours before I finally fall asleep. Sometimes it is 2 or 3 in the morning and I'm still awake worrying about the kids. I've tried getting up and reading or paying my bills, but even that doesn't make me sleepy." • Reports problem falling asleep for past 6 months; is widowed and very concerned about two teenage sons. Never sleeps until both sons are home. States she does nothing special to relax. Feels her worries are "her business"—no support person with whom she shares these.
Disturbed Sleep Pattern: Difficulty Remaining Asleep	Noise of hospital environment and need for periodic treatments	• Admitted to hospital 3/6/11; cholecystectomy 3/7/11 • "I don't think I've had one decent night's sleep since my surgery. I've been falling asleep about 9 p.m. and then someone wakes me up for my medicine. I just about get back to sleep and someone's putting the light on to poke at my dressing or to check this tube. I know I'm getting grouchy." • Orders include every-4-hour vital signs; nursing assessment of the incision, nasogastric tube, intravenous therapy; and medication for pain and for sleep.
Disturbed Sleep Pattern: Premature Awakening	Barbiturate dependency and lack of knowledge of nonpharmacologic aids for insomnia	• Patient has history of mild to moderate depression, related to loss of job and perceived role inadequacy, for the past 3 years; has been taking secobarbital (Seconal), a barbiturate hypnotic, 100 mg by mouth nightly for the past year and a half. • "I seem to be waking up earlier and earlier, can't fall back asleep, and I start each day feeling like I have a hangover." • "I'd like to get off these drugs, but I'm terrified that without them I won't sleep at all."
Disturbed Sleep Pattern: Excessive Daytime Sleeping	Effects of biologic aging (moderate increase in stage I and II sleep; slow-wave sleep, stages III and IV, decreases by 50% or more)	• Male patient, aged 74, complains during his annual physical that he seems to be napping more during the day, yet when he tries to fall asleep at night he often cannot. • "I'm spending more time in bed, but I'm less rested. Worst of all is not knowing whether or not I'll be awake enough to drive my car or enjoy a good card game."
Disturbed Sleep Pattern: Altered Sleep–Wake Patterns	Frequent rotations of shift and overtime	• Graduate nurse, 24 years old, who has been working on a busy medical floor for 6 months; rotates 11–7 and 7–3 shifts; recently a problem with staffing has necessitated frequent rotations. Patient often volunteers (two or three times a week) for overtime. • "I don't know what is wrong with me. I'm so tired anymore and don't feel at all like myself. All I want to do when I'm off is to sleep—but often I can't fall asleep when I lay down. Please help!"

job as manifested by complaints of always feeling tired and not getting enough sleep: The disturbed sleep pattern involving the altered sleep–wake pattern is the problem statement; priority nursing energies are directed toward changing this pattern and helping the patient achieve both the necessary quantity and quality of sleep.

Ineffective Coping related to multiple stresses of new job and altered sleep–wake pattern (sleep deprivation) as manifested by statements such as, "I don't know how much longer I can do this," "I'm always tired, and all I want to do is sleep," "I'm so grouchy—people must hate me!" Here, the altered sleep–wake pattern is just one of the factors contributing to the patient's problem of ineffective coping; priority nursing energies are directed toward improving the patient's coping skills by teaching the patient how to increase the quantity and quality of sleep.

Ineffective Coping related to multiple stressors and lack of stress-relieving rituals as manifested by inability to fall asleep, excessive fatigue, and feelings that personality is changing: In this instance, the altered sleep–wake pattern is merely a symptom of the patient's actual problem—ineffective coping. The expectation is that when the coping problem is resolved, the symptom will disappear.

None of the preceding diagnoses is more correct than the others. With each patient, the nurse must review each cluster of significant data and identify the key problem, contributing factors, and related signs and symptoms. The exact nature of the nursing diagnosis directs the nursing interventions.

Outcome Identification and Planning

Rest and sleep are essential components of well-being. Planning for patient care, especially in a healthcare facility, involves planning with the patient suitable measures to promote rest and sleep. Whenever nurses care for a patient, nursing measures support the following expected patient outcomes: The patient will:

- Maintain a sleep–wake pattern that provides sufficient energy for the day's tasks
- Demonstrate self-care behaviors that provide a healthy balance between rest and activity
- Identify stress-relieving rituals that enable the patient to fall asleep more easily
- Demonstrate decreased signs of sleep deprivation
- Verbalize feeling less fatigued and more in control of life activities

Implementing

In most cases, sleep problems are not the primary reason for a patient's interaction with the healthcare system. Communicating with the patient while displaying a nonjudgmental, caring attitude often is the key to detecting a patient's sleep problem. Patients who believe the nurse is generally concerned about their well-being are not reluctant to discuss their insomnia or their concern about a child who is a bed wetter. In order to correct a sleep problem, the patient needs to believe that the nurse cares and will provide extra help to promote rest and sleep. The accompanying box lists Examples of Nursing Interventions and Nursing Outcomes Classifications (NIC/NOC) that aid in sleep promotion.

Preparing a Restful Environment

A comfortable bed helps promote rest and sleep. The bottom linen should be tight and clean. The upper linen, while secure, should allow freedom of movement and should not exert pressure, especially over the legs and feet. Good body alignment is conducive to relaxation. For patients who must assume unusual positions because of their illness, ingenuity and skill are necessary to minimize muscle strain and discomfort. For example, patients who must remain in the orthopneic position to aid breathing should be well supported in a manner that relieves muscle strain.

A quiet and darkened room with privacy is relaxing for nearly everyone. In a strange environment, unfamiliar noises, such as people walking by or entering and leaving the room and the sounds of elevator doors, bring complaints from most hospitalized patients. Although some of these sounds are difficult to control, make every effort to reduce disturbances and to promote relaxation and sleep. Many healthcare facilities have made attempts to transform their patient care areas into quieter settings that facilitate rest and sleep. Attention to design features with a focus on eliminating environmental noise, providing patients with private rooms, and formal quiet times on units all are aimed at creating a more supportive environment that is conducive to good sleep.

The temperature of the room, the amount of ventilation, and the amount of bed covering are matters of individual choice. Meet the patient's wishes when at all possible. Many older patients cannot sleep if they feel cold. Thermal blankets or comforters, insulated bed socks, cotton flannel sheets, leg warmers, long underwear, and a stockinette cap help patients stay warm and promote comfort and sleep. See Focus on the Older Adult for additional suggestions.

> *Recall Charlie Bitner, the older man living in a long-term care facility. The nurse would work with Mr. Bitner to ensure that his sleeping area is as comfortable and restful as possible. Making sure that he is warm enough, dimming the lights, closing the door (as much as allowed), and minimizing disturbances outside his room would be key.* ■

Promoting Bedtime Rituals

Most people have bedtime rituals to help them relax and promote sleep. Reading, listening to the radio, watching television, talking to a family member, and praying are common before-sleep activities. Children may take a favorite doll, stuffed toy, or blanket to bed; listen to a bedtime story; kiss everyone good night; and say prayers before bed (Fig. 34-5).

> ## Examples of Nursing Interventions and Nursing Outcomes Classifications (NIC/NOC)
> ### *Sleep Enhancement*
>
> **Nursing Interventions**
>
> - Approximate patient's regular sleep–wake cycle in planning care.
> - Determine the effects of the patient's medications on sleep pattern.
> - Adjust environment (e.g., light, noise, temperature, mattress, bed) to promote sleep.
> - Encourage patient to establish a bedtime routine to facilitate transition from wakefulness to sleep.
> - Facilitate maintenance of patient's usual bedtime routines, presleep cues/props, and familiar objects (e.g., for children, a favorite blanket/toy, rocking, pacifier, or story; for adults, a book to read, etc.) as appropriate.
> - Instruct patient to avoid bedtime foods and beverages that interfere with sleep.
> - Instruct patient how to perform autogenic muscle relaxation or other nonpharmacologic forms of sleep inducement.
> - Initiate/implement comfort measures of massage, positioning, and affective touch.
> - Discuss with patient and family sleep-enhancing techniques.
>
> **Nursing Outcomes**
>
> - Motivation
> - Rest
> - Sleep
> - Comfort Status: Environment
> - Personal Well-Being
> - Stress Level

Bulechek, G., Butcher, H., & Dochterman, J. (2008). *Nursing interventions classification (NIC)* (5th ed., p. 665). St. Louis: C. V. Mosby Inc. A full listing of nursing activities for each nursing intervention can be found in this book.
Moorhead, S., Johnson, M., Maas, M., & Swanson, E. (2008). *Nursing outcomes classification (NOC)* (p. 815). St. Louis: C.V. Mosby. A full listing of nursing outcomes for each nursing diagnosis can be found in this book.

FIGURE 34-5. A bedtime routine helps promote sleep in children.

FOCUS ON THE OLDER ADULT

AGE-RELATED CHANGES AND NURSING STRATEGIES FOR REST AND SLEEP

Age-Related Changes	Nursing Strategies
Disturbed Sleep Pattern: Initiation of Sleep • Decreased physical activities • Tired and fatigued throughout day • Depression • Polypharmacy	• Encourage patient to engage in some type of physical activity, such as walking or water aerobics. • Discourage napping throughout day. • Arrange for assessment for depression and treatment. • Review medications that patient is taking and assess for any side effects of sleep pattern disturbances.
Disturbed Sleep Pattern: Maintaining Sleep • Nocturia • Sleep-related movement disturbances (e.g., restless leg syndrome)	• Decrease fluids during the evening. • Take diuretics in the morning or early evening. • Discuss problems with healthcare provider.

Readiness for sleep follows a personal hygiene routine for many people, such as brushing teeth, washing hands and face, voiding, or taking a bath or shower. Snacks are important elements in the bedtime rituals of many children and adults. Although eating the wrong foods may produce a bad night's sleep, going to bed hungry may also interfere with sleep.

> Teaching Mrs. Omeara about the importance of bedtime rituals for her two infants may promote the children's sleep. In addition, the nurse would need to reinforce the need for her own bedtime rituals to ensure that the sleep she obtains is restful. ∎

To promote relaxation and sleep, be alert to the patient's bedtime rituals and observe them as much as possible. Include these rituals in the patient's plan of care so that all health personnel can observe them.

Offering Appropriate Bedtime Snacks and Beverages

Because carbohydrates seem to promote sleep, there appears to be justification for offering a snack or beverage high in carbohydrates before bedtime, such as toast, a small bagel, crackers, or a glass of fruit juice, if this is allowed in the patient's regimen. An alcoholic beverage helps to promote sleep for some people. However, alcohol after dinner generally should be avoided because it may interrupt the normal sleep cycle and interfere with deep sleep. For most patients, beverages containing caffeine should be avoided for at least 4 to 5 hours before bedtime. Recommend that the patient take fluids during the day but avoid excessive fluid intake before bedtime so that he or she will not have to use the bathroom during the night.

Promoting Relaxation

One can relax without sleeping, but sleep rarely occurs until one is relaxed. Stress and anxiety interfere with a person's ability to relax, rest, and sleep. Means for dealing with worries include dealing with problems as they arise, conditioning yourself to consider stressful issues only at certain times, teaching yourself that worrying never solves problems and is counterproductive, and giving the worries over to another (e.g., a trusted family member, friend, caregiver, or God). The distraction and relaxation techniques described in Chapters 35 and 42 may be beneficial for a patient whose worries are contributing to a sleep disturbance. A backrub, a warm bath, and washing the face if the patient is bedridden are typical nursing measures to help patients relax. The technique for back massage is described in Skill 35-1 in Chapter 35.

Promoting Comfort

One of the greatest deterrents to rest and sleep is pain, and pain commonly occurs in illness. Depending on the cause and severity of the discomfort or pain, appropriate nursing measures include remaining with a lonely and frightened child or adult, using the simple strategy of caring presence and touch, offering a back massage, obtaining an extra blanket, or administering an analgesic. These and other nursing techniques to promote comfort are described in Chapter 35. Be sensitive to the patient's discomfort to recognize and relieve it.

Respecting Normal Sleep–Wake Patterns

Make every effort to allow the patient to experience his or her normal period of sleep. In many instances, insisting that all patients retire and awaken at specific times is not necessary. For example, is there a good reason to wake a patient at 7 a.m. if the patient ordinarily sleeps until 9 a.m.? The patient's normal napping habits should also be followed when possible. REM sleep is more common during morning naps, whereas NREM sleep is more common during naps later in the day. With this knowledge, help the patient plan napping periods that best fit his or her needs and least interfere with nighttime sleeping.

Scheduling Nursing Care to Avoid Unnecessary Disturbances

Many patients complain that they are awakened to take sleeping pills and are aroused in the early morning to prepare for breakfast long before it is served. Consider these common complaints when developing the patient's plan of care to promote rest and sleep.

Whenever possible, provide care during periods when the patient is normally awake. When this is not feasible, avoid awakening the patient during REM sleep, when the rapid eye movements can be observed. Because a patient's need for sleep is important, examine priorities for nursing care. For example, consider whether checking a vital sign or carrying out a particular nursing measure is more important than the patient's sleep (see Focused Critical Thinking Guide 34-1).

Using Medications to Produce Sleep

Medications for sleep are often ordered for patients. Sedative-hypnotics induce sleep; antianxiety drugs reduce anxiety and tension. However, the sleep produced by sedative-hypnotics is an unnatural sleep. All these drugs disturb either REM or NREM sleep to some degree. Although most sedative-hypnotics provide several nights of excellent sleep, the medication often loses its effect after 1 or 2 weeks. At this point, many people increase the dosage of the medication or complement the drug with alcohol. Vigorous nursing intervention is needed to prevent a patient from developing a pattern of drug dependency and alcohol abuse.

The most commonly prescribed sleep aids belong to the sedative-hypnotic class of benzodiazepines. These drugs include flurazepam (Dalmane) and temazepam (Restoril). When used to induce sleep, both these drugs have the potential to produce daytime drowsiness, a morning hangover effect, and physical and psychological dependence. Drugs in a newer class of nonbenzodiazepines are less likely to cause adverse effects and have a lower risk of abuse. These more commonly prescribed drugs include eszopiclone (Lunesta) and zolpidem (Ambien). The most recently approved sleep medication is ramelteon (Rozerem). This drug is classified as a melatonin receptor agonist and it normalizes sleep cycles by enabling the body's supply of melatonin to naturally promote sleep (Goldsmith, 2007).

Sleep medications are often ordered on a p.r.n. (as needed) basis. Administer these medications only when indicated and always with the full knowledge of their limitations. Provide thorough patient education about these medications. In addition, help patients develop other self-care strategies, including developing healthy sleep and lifestyle behaviors. Use alternative nonpharmacologic measures to promote sleep when appropriate. Over-the-counter (OTC) sleep medications most often contain antihistamines and should only be used on a short-term basis because of the potential for adverse effects and their lack of effectiveness over a lengthy time period (Wooten, 2007).

> ➤ *Remember Charlie Bitner, the older man living in the long-term care facility. Nonpharmacologic measures would be helpful to promote sleep. Having Mr. Bitner consume a warm beverage before bedtime, listen to soft music, or receive a backrub may promote relaxation, thereby enhancing the effectiveness of the prescribed sleep medication.* ∎

Teaching About Rest and Sleep

A well-informed person is better able to cope with distressing situations. Teach patients and their families about the nature of rest and sleep and their importance to well-being. For example, the fact that children and adults are getting less sleep has been implicated as a contributing factor to the obesity epidemic in the United States (CDC, 2008; Goldsmith, 2007). Various studies confirm that adults and children who slept less than their recommended hours per night were more likely to be overweight. This sleep–weight link is possibly related to two hormones: leptin and ghrelin. Leptin signals the brain to stop eating, whereas ghrelin promotes continued eating. Research suggests that sleep deprivation lowers leptin levels and elevates ghrelin levels, thus increasing one's appetite. To compound the problem, a drop in leptin also can be interpreted by the brain as a sign of starvation. Unfortunately, the brain then signals the body to eat more while it simultaneously lowers the body's metabolic rate. When this happens, people are more likely to gain weight, even if food intake is decreased. This information appears to verify that lack of sleep affects not just the brain, but also the entire body (Schardt, 2005).

Also teach patients about normal variations in sleep patterns and common measures to promote relaxation and sleep (Teaching Tips 34-1). Discuss the plan of care with the patient and make sure it is acceptable to him or her. If a sleep disorder becomes a problem and common nursing measures are inadequate, the nurse may need to refer the patient to a health practitioner prepared to deal with it.

Evaluating

The nurse evaluates the effectiveness of the plan of care to promote rest and sleep by checking whether the patient has met the individualized expected outcomes specified in the plan. See Nursing Plan of Care 34-1 for Mr. Bitner.

Nursing care is considered effective if the patient is able to:

- Verbalize feeling rested or having had a restful night's sleep
- Identify factors that interfere with or disrupt the normal sleep pattern
- Use techniques that promote sleep and provide a restful environment
- Concentrate and function effectively during waking hours
- Eliminate behaviors related to sleep deprivation

FOCUSED CRITICAL THINKING GUIDE • 34-1

Sleep

You have just arrived on the unit and checked your clinical assignment. You have two patients today and about 30 minutes before preconference. Your routine is to review their charts for pertinent information, go and introduce yourself to them, and take their morning vital signs before preconference. With 10 minutes to spare, you visit your second patient and find that he is sound asleep. Remembering that he had a fractured hip repaired 2 days ago and that the night nurse had stated in his note that the patient was restless and awake until 4:00 a.m., you are reluctant to awaken him. On the other hand, at your midterm conference your instructor commented that you need to improve your organizational skills. If you don't have your vital signs recorded until after preconference, then breakfast arrives, doctors make rounds, and you're that much further behind in your morning care and documentation. When you look at the flow sheet at the foot of the bed, you note that the last set of vitals were taken at midnight and were within normal limits. You're attempting to reconcile several things—the importance of these morning vital signs, the patient's need for sleep, and your need to accomplish your tasks on time and receive a good evaluation. What should you do?

1. Identify Goal of Thinking

Determine whether it is more important to awaken your patient for morning vital signs or let him sleep at least until after your preconference.

2. Assess Adequacy of Knowledge

Pertinent circumstances: Your patient had major surgery 2 days ago, did not have a restful night, but is sleeping peacefully now. You realize that his vital signs can be an important indicator of a complication. You also need to accomplish your tasks in a timely and organized manner.

Prerequisite knowledge: To make your decision, you need knowledge about his postoperative condition and assessment data that indicate he is recovering or developing a complication. You are aware that sleep is vital to promote tissue repair, physical recovery, and mental well-being. You also need to review the tasks that you need to accomplish this morning and decide how and if priorities could be shifted.

Room for error/time constraints: Will a delay in taking vital signs cause injury to this patient? You are not planning to omit this task but just questioning whether to postpone it and allow the patient to have some additional sleep.

3. Address Potential Problems

Waking your patient for vital signs may be disturbing for him and interfere with his need for rest. A decision to postpone morning vital signs might also cause several problems. If the patient has developed a complication, such as an infection, his elevated temperature may go undetected for at least another hour. By the time you come out of preconference, the patient may be eating his breakfast, which further delays recording of vital signs. You perceive that you are already falling behind on your schedule and are really intent on completing your responsibilities on time today.

4. Consult Helpful Resources

Before you make your decision, you should check the patient's flow sheet and note whether the previous set of vital signs were within normal limits. The primary nurse and your instructor may also help you sort through your priorities in this situation.

5. Critique Judgment/Decision

You have two choices here. If you wake your patient up and take his vital signs, you are disturbing him when he is sleeping soundly, risking the fact that he may be angry with you but are on schedule for the day's activities. By postponing his vital signs at least until after postconference, you provide additional rest for the patient but know that you are already behind schedule and worry that your instructor will view you as disorganized. After reviewing your options and checking his chart again, you decide to allow him to sleep and plan to take them as soon as possible after your preconference. During preconference, when your instructor reviews your priorities for the day, she comments positively that you have individualized care based on your particular patient's needs at the moment. In your mind, you determine that the vital signs are your next priority and will take minimal time, and you should still be able to complete care and documentation in a competent manner and on time.

TEACHING TIPS • 34-1

REST AND SLEEP

Health Topic	Suggested Content	Why Is This Important?
Activity	• Find an activity that can be done daily and involves physical exertion, such as walking. • Do not participate in any physical activities right before bedtime.	• Sleep is easier to obtain if some physical activity has been completed. • Many people find it hard to rest and sleep right after a physical activity.
Diet	• Avoid food, beverages, or OTC medications that contain caffeine in the evening. • Eat a light dinner. • Eat a light carbohydrate-containing snack at bedtime if hungry.	• Caffeine is a stimulant and may prolong the time it takes to fall asleep. • Eating a large meal before bedtime may produce heartburn, delaying sleep. • Carbohydrates may affect the serotonin levels in the brain and thus promote sleep.
Sleep Patterns	• Keep to usual waking time every day, even if previous night's bedtime was later than usual or sleep was restless. • Get out of bed if unable to fall asleep within 30 minutes, and go into another room.	• Keeping the same pattern helps the body's circadian rhythms. • By using the bedroom for only sleep and sexual activity, the mind begins to associate this room with sleep.

NURSING PLAN OF CARE • 34-1

For Mr. Bitner

Mr. Bitner is an alert, widowed, 86-year-old man who was admitted to a nursing home 2 months ago. He is ambulatory and performs most of his self-care. His admitting medical diagnoses include diabetes mellitus and hypertension. He adds to this list "a touch of arthritis." His daughter complains to the charge nurse that her father seems to be spending more and more time during the day napping and that he says he does not sleep well at night. A comprehensive sleep assessment of Mr. Bitner after his daughter's expression of concern reveals the following data.

SLEEP–WAKEFULNESS PATTERN

• Patient goes to bed between 8 and 9 p.m. and gets out of bed between 7 and 8 a.m. because the staff are getting his roommate out of bed at this time. He states he never falls asleep before midnight because he always watched the late news at home. He usually wakes twice during the night to void and often cannot go back to sleep.
• During the day, patient is frequently observed dozing in his chair. If not discouraged, he returns to his room midmorning and afternoon for a 1-hour nap.

EFFECT OF SLEEP PATTERN ON EVERYDAY LIVING

• Patient states: "I'm always tired. I don't seem to have much energy anymore."

• Patient has not socialized yet with other residents and, without strong encouragement, does not participate in group activities.
• From his point of view, life holds little reason for him to be awake. "I worked for the railroad for almost 50 years and I never overslept once."

SLEEP AIDS

• Patient denies ever using medication to fall asleep. States he often relaxed at home in the evening with a couple of beers.
• Patient likes a dim light on during the night so that he can find the bathroom easily and likes his bedroom door ajar.
• Patient sleeps with two blankets and is often still cold.

SLEEP DISTURBANCES AND CONTRIBUTING FACTORS

• Patient states: "Ever since my wife died, I'm just not getting enough sleep, and since I came here it's worse. I don't know why I don't fall asleep when I go to bed or why I wake up so much. It sure makes the nights long."
• Patient has no regular periods of exercise and drinks black coffee with every meal and one or two diet colas in the evening.

(continued)

NURSING PLAN OF CARE · 34-1

For Mr. Bitner (continued)

NURSING DIAGNOSIS — Disturbed Sleep Pattern: involving difficulty falling asleep and remaining asleep related to new sleep environment and schedule, evening caffeine intake, and insufficient meaningful daytime activity

EXPECTED OUTCOME — By the next monthly assessment, 1/20/11, the patient will:

- Retire after viewing the 11 p.m. news in the TV room with Mr. Sparter

Nursing Interventions	Rationale	Evaluative Statement
Assess advisability of reestablishing Mr. Bitner's usual retiring pattern of going to bed after the 11 p.m. news. Assess how patient spends the time from the evening meal to 11 p.m.—explore relaxing alternatives with him. Investigate possibility that he and Mr. Sparter might become social partners.	Strengthens the natural rhythm of his sleep–wake cycle. Elimination of evening naps will facilitate his falling asleep more easily.	1/18/11 Outcome met. Patient does not go to bed until after the news and has been observed talking with Mr. Sparter. *Recommendation:* Continue to develop evening activities with him—he finds that the time after supper "drags." *M. LeBon, RN*

EXPECTED OUTCOME — By the next monthly assessment, 1/20/11, the patient will:

- Report that he falls asleep within 1 hour of getting into bed

Nursing Interventions	Rationale	Evaluative Statement
Continue to assess how long it takes patient to fall asleep after getting into bed.	In elderly patients, stage I time is increased.	1/18/11 Outcome partially met. Three or four nights a week, he falls asleep within 30 minutes of going to bed. States he really misses comfort of his wife.
Explore with patient means to relax before falling asleep—deep breathing, imagery, prayer.	Activities that calm and relax the person prepare the body for sleep.	*Revision:* Investigate patient's sense of loss and need for touch. May be a good candidate for pet therapy program.
Teach the importance of using the bed only as a place to sleep. Advise patient when he cannot sleep to get out of bed and to go to another room where he can perform some monotonous activity (watching television, listening to radio).	This maintains the bed as a powerful stimulus for sleep and helps to prevent "conditioned" insomnia ("Well, here I am in bed now and I know sleep won't come").	*M. LeBon, RN*

EXPECTED OUTCOME — By the next monthly assessment, 1/20/11, the patient will:

- Decrease nighttime awakenings to one, after which he returns to a sound sleep

(continued)

NURSING PLAN OF CARE · 34-1

For Mr. Bitner (continued)

Nursing Interventions	Rationale	Evaluative Statement
Assess and manipulate factors that contribute to nighttime awakenings: • Need to void (time of day diuretic is taken, amounts of fluid intake in the evening) • Roommate's wakefulness, snoring, or need for care • Uncomfortableness in strange environment • Comfort (e.g., temperature)	Individualizing the patient's bedtime environment and meeting comfort needs (warmth, soft light, and so forth) promote sleep onset and maintenance.	1/18/11 Outcome partially met. Nighttime awakenings vary from none to three nightly. See previous revision. *M. LeBon, RN*
Teach patient how, on awakening, to concentrate on breathing until he falls back to sleep.	This uses the power of positive thinking to facilitate return to sleep.	

EXPECTED OUTCOME   By the next monthly assessment, 1/20/11, the patient will:

• Attend the center's exercise sessions Monday through Friday at 10 a.m.

Nursing Interventions	Rationale	Evaluative Statement
Assess whether patient understands the relation between daily exercise and his ability to sleep.	Regular exercise throughout the day is known to increase physical fatigue and to promote sleep. Exercise or stimulating activities immediately before retiring interfere with sleep's onset.	1/20/11 Outcome met. Patient has become an enthusiastic participant in exercise sessions—attends daily. *M. LeBon, RN*
Determine how his exercise needs can best be met (i.e., through a group program or an individualized program of walking, or other program).	Exercise program must be individualized based on physical state and interests of patient.	
Use positive verbal reinforcement to communicate to patient that someone cares that he is using positive means to remedy his sleep disturbance and increase his well-being.	Activity provides the opportunity for socialization and improvement of a self-image. Positive reinforcement promotes continued participation.	
Encourage patient's daughter to go for walks with him when she visits and to question him about his exercise program.	Communications and interaction with family members helps the elderly patient to maintain self-esteem and to feel valuable and loved.	

(continued)

NURSING PLAN OF CARE · 34-1

For Mr. Bitner (continued)

EXPECTED OUTCOME By the next monthly assessment, 1/20/11, the patient will:

- Substitute caffeine-free beverages for coffee and cola at supper and evening snack

Nursing Interventions	Rationale	Evaluative Statement
Assess patient's willingness to substitute caffeine-free beverages for coffee and cola.	Caffeine is a stimulant that can cause difficulty sleeping.	1/20/11 Outcome met. Patient now drinks decaffeinated coffee with meals and milk in the evening. Dislikes caffeine-free sodas.
Consult with dietary department and his daughter about options. Experiment with options until his preferences are determined.	Caffeine-free versions of beverages are often available and can be used based on patient acceptance.	*M. LeBon, RN*
Gradually reduce his caffeine intake, especially from evening meal onward. Offer a carbohydrate evening snack.	Carbohydrate snack appears to promote sleep.	

SAMPLE DOCUMENTATION

12/20/11 Nursing
Family conference to discuss Mr. Bitner's sleep disturbance initiated by daughter's concern. Present were Mr. Bitner and his daughter (A. Jelner), K. Behner (social worker), W. Quing (activity director), and M. LeBon (primary nurse). Primary nurse presented findings from comprehensive sleep assessment: Nursing diagnosis: Disturbed Sleep Pattern: difficulty falling asleep and remaining asleep related to new sleep environment and schedule, evening caffeine intake, and insufficient meaningful daytime activity. Discussion centered on strategies to help Mr. Bitner develop interests in the center, including possibilities for increased physical exercise, decrease his evening caffeine intake (daughter to bring noncaffeinated colas), and reestablish usual retiring and waking times. See plan of care. Patient's progress will be evaluated at next monthly assessment, 1/20/11.

M. LeBon, RN

● Developing Critical Thinking Skills

1. Interview three adults of varying ages (young, middle, elderly) about their sleep and rest patterns, using the Focused Assessment Guide in this chapter. Explore the special problems experienced by each of the adults, the efficacy of the self-help measures they use to cope, and helpful nursing interventions.

2. Interview three practicing nurses who are recent graduates. Using the Focused Assessment Guide in the text, ask them: if they are getting adequate rest, what factors are compromising their rest (e.g., working double or rotating shifts), how any lack of rest is affecting their practice, and what self-help measures have they used or would be appropriate. Discuss with your classmates the situation of practicing nurses with sleep alterations, the factors that place nurses at risk for sleep alterations, and what students can learn to lower their risk.

● Preparing for NCLEX

1. Assessment of a patient's body temperature in the late afternoon is 37.2°C (99°F). The nurse assesses this as most likely due to what?
   a. A sign of an infection
   b. Result of a normal circadian rhythm
   c. Hyperpyrexia
   d. Due to a warm environment

2. Which of the following records muscle tone?
   a. Electroencephalograph (EEG)
   b. Electrocardiograph (ECG)
   c. Electrooculograph (EOG)
   d. Electromyograph (EMG)

3. The nurse observes some involuntary muscle jerking in a sleeping patient. The nurse determines that the patient is most likely in which stage of sleep?
   a. Stage I NREM sleep
   b. Stage II NREM sleep
   c. Stage IV NREM sleep
   d. REM sleep

4. The nurse observes a slight increase in a patient's vital signs while he is sleeping during the night. According to the patient's stage of sleep, the nurse expects which of the following to be true?
   a. He is aware of his surroundings at this point.
   b. He is in delta sleep at this time.
   c. It would be most difficult to awaken him at this time.
   d. This is most likely an NREM stage.

5. How many cycles of sleep does a person typically go through each night?
   a. 2 or 3
   b. 4 or 5
   c. 10 to 12
   d. 20 to 25

6. The nurse is discussing with an older woman the factors that induce sleep. Which of the following does the nurse teach her?
   a. A cup of regular tea may induce sleep.
   b. Large quantities of alcohol promote a deep sleep.
   c. The amount of REM sleep decreases with age.
   d. Physical activity decreases REM and NREM sleep.

7. A patient falls asleep in the middle of a conversation. The nurse would suspect which disorder?
   a. Hypersomnia
   b. Narcolepsy
   c. Somnambulism
   d. Sleep apnea

8. Which of the following descriptions is true of the diagnostic tool called a sleep diary?
   a. It is generally kept for 1 week
   b. It includes a record of daily physical activity
   c. It includes a record of body temperature taken each evening
   d. It reports primarily subjective data about sleep activities

9. To help a patient get to sleep, the nurse suggests that he do which of the following?
   a. Follow his usual bedtime routine if possible
   b. Drink two or three glasses of water at bedtime
   c. Have a large snack at bedtime
   d. Take a sedative-hypnotic every night at bedtime

10. Which of the following is the most common complaint of patients visiting sleep disorder clinics?
    a. Hypersomnia
    b. Narcolepsy
    c. Chronic insomnia
    d. Enuresis

11. A prolonged pattern of REM deprivation may result in which of the following?
    a. Symptoms of psychosis
    b. Increased episodes of dreaming
    c. Decreased sensitivity to pain
    d. Increased mental alertness

12. Active dreaming occurs during what stage of sleep?
    a. Stage II NREM sleep
    b. Stage III NREM sleep
    c. Stage IV NREM sleep
    d. REM sleep

13. When describing illness as a stressor that can influence sleep during various stages, which example would be most appropriate for the nurse to use?
    a. Hypothyroidism can result in a decrease in the amount of certain stages of NREM sleep.
    b. A person with heart disease is more likely to have chest pain during NREM sleep.
    c. A patient with epilepsy is more likely to have seizures during REM sleep.
    d. An increase in gastric secretions in a person with an ulcer will most likely occur during NREM sleep.

14. Caffeine is a known stimulant, and its intake should be:
    a. Avoided at least 30 minutes before bedtime
    b. Combined with milk to counteract its effect
    c. Avoided at least 4 to 5 hours before bedtime
    d. Encouraged during waking hours to counteract the effects of sleeplessness

15. Medications that induce sleep (sedative-hypnotics) may disturb REM or NREM sleep. The nurse should be aware of which of the following considerations?
    a. They should be taken with alcohol for increased effect.
    b. They usually become ineffective after several weeks.
    c. They can usually be given at intervals during the night.
    d. They should be combined with daytime amphetamines to counteract hangover effect.

● Answers With Rationale

1. *b.* A slight increase in body temperature in the late afternoon is the result of a normal circadian rhythm. This slight variation from normal does not necessarily mean an infection is present, nor is it hyperpyrexia (high fever). A warm environment might cause an elevation in body temperature, but the most likely cause is normal circadian rhythm.

2. *d.* An EMG measures muscle tone, an EEG records electrical currents from the brain, an EOG records eye movements, and an ECG records cardiac activity.

3. *a.* Involuntary muscle jerking occurs in stage I NREM sleep. In the other stages, the muscles proceed from a relaxed state to large muscle immobility.

4. *c.* During REM sleep, it is difficult to arouse a person, and the vital signs increase. Delta sleep is NREM stages III and IV sleep.

5. *b.* A person goes through probably four or five cycles of sleep each night, with each cycle lasting 90 to 100 minutes.

6. *c.* The nurse would teach the older woman that the amount of REM sleep decreases with age. Regular tea contains caffeine and increases alertness. Large quantities of alcohol limit REM and delta sleep. Physical activity increases both REM and NREM sleep.

7. *b.* Narcolepsy is an uncontrollable desire to sleep. Hypersomnia refers to excessive sleep, somnambulism is sleepwalking, and sleep apnea is a condition in which breathing ceases for a period of time between snoring.

8. *b.* A sleep diary includes activities during the day because they have an effect on sleep, is usually kept for at least 14 days, and is more helpful if objective comments from a bed partner are included. A record of body temperature is insignificant.

9. *a.* Drinking two or three glasses of water at bedtime will probably cause the patient to awaken during the night to void. A large snack may be uncomfortable right before bedtime. Taking a sedative-hypnotic every night disturbs REM and NREM sleep, and sedatives also lose their effectiveness quickly.

10. *c.* Chronic insomnia is the most common reason people visit a sleep disorder clinic.

11. *a.* Prolonged episodes of REM deprivation may cause symptoms of psychosis. With REM deprivation, dreaming is absent, sensitivity to pain increases, and mental alertness decreases.

12. *d.* Active dreaming occurs during REM sleep.

13. *a.* Hypothyroidism can interfere with stages II and IV of NREM sleep. Chest pain occurs more frequently during REM sleep. Epileptic seizures occur more frequently during NREM sleep. Gastric secretions increase during REM sleep.

14. *c.* Caffeine should be avoided at least 4 to 5 hours before bedtime. Milk does not counteract its effect, and caffeine use is never recommended, even during waking hours.

15. *b.* Sedative-hypnotics should never be taken with alcohol because alcohol potentiates their effect. They are usually ordered only at bedtime and may have one repeat order if the patient cannot fall asleep, but they are not given at intervals during the night. Amphetamine use is never recommended.

Taylor Suite Resources

The Taylor Suite offers these additional resources to enhance learning and facilitate understanding of this chapter:

- thePoint online resource, http://thepoint.lww.com/Taylor7E
- Student DVD-ROM included with the book
- Study Guide for Taylor's Fundamentals of Nursing

BIBLIOGRAPHY

Arora, V., Georgitis, E., Siddique, J. Vekhter, B., Woodruff, J., Humphrey, H., et al. (2008). Association of workload of on call medical interns with on-call sleep duration, shift duration, and participation in educational activities. *JAMA, 300*(10), 1146–1153.

Barton-Burke, M. (2006). Cancer-related fatigue and sleep disturbances. *American Journal of Nursing, 106*(3), 72–77.

Bulechek, G., Butcher, H., & Dochterman, J. (2008). *Nursing interventions classification (NIC)* (5th ed., p. 665). St. Louis: C.V. Mosby.

Caballer, L. (2007). Sound advice about surgery for sleep apnea. *Nursing, 37*(11), 56hn5–56hn6.

Centers for Disease Control and Prevention (CDC). (2008). *Sleep and sleep disorders: A public health challenge.* Available at: http://www.cdc.gov/sleep/

Cole, C., & Richards, K. (2007). Sleep disruption in older adults. *American Journal of Nursing, 107*(5), 40–50.

Gevirtz, C. (2007). Treating sleep disturbances in patients with chronic pain. *Nursing, 37*(4), 26–27.

Goldberg, R. (2007). Obstructive sleep apnea. *Advance for Nurses: Pennsylvania, New Jersey, Delaware, 9*(14), 25–27.

Goldsmith, C. (2007). Insomnia: Sleepless in America. *Nursing Spectrum, 16*(5), 16–19.

Guterl, G. (2008). Your internal clock. *Advance for Nurses: Pennsylvania, New Jersey, Delaware, 10*(1), 15–16.

Hartner, K. (2008). Top priority: Good sleep is important to keep your body and mind rested and healthy. *Advance for Nurses: Pennsylvania, New Jersey, Delaware, 10*(6), 44.

Keefe, S. (2007). ZZZs & healing. *Advance for Nurses: Pennsylvania, New Jersey, Delaware, 9*(11), 33–34.

Leap, E. (2008). These shifts are killing me. *American Journal of Nursing, 108*(3), 13.

Lilley, L., Harrington, S., & Snyder, J. (2007). *Pharmacology & the nursing process* (5th ed.). St. Louis: Mosby.

Mason, D. (2008). Sleep on it. *American Journal of Nursing, 108*(3), 11.

McMillan, S., Tofthagen, C., & Morgan, M. (2008). Relationships among pain, sleep disturbances, and depressive symptoms in outpatients from a comprehensive cancer center. *Oncology Nursing Forum, 35*(4), 603–611.

Moorhead, S., Johnson, M., Maas, M., & Swanson, E. (2008). *Nursing outcomes classification (NOC)* (p. 815). St. Louis: C.V. Mosby.

National Heart Lung and Blood Institute. (2008). *What is narcolepsy?* Available at http://www.nhlbi.nih.gov/health/dci/Diseases/nar/nar_what.html.

National Institute of Neurological Disorders and Stroke. (2006). NINDS hypersomnia information page. Available at http://www.ninds.nih.gov/disorders/hypersomnia/hypersomnia.htm.

National Sleep Foundation (NSF). (2008a). *2008 sleep in America poll.* Available at www.sleepfoundation.org/sites/default/files/2008%20POLL%20SOF.PDF

National Sleep Foundation (NSF). (2008b). *Cognitive behavioral therapy for insomnia.* Available at http://www.sleepfoundation.org/article/hot-topics/cognitive-behavioral-therapy-insomia_Therapy_for_Insomnia

National Sleep Foundation (NSF). (2008c). *Longer work days leave Americans nodding off on the job.* Available at http://www.sleepfoundation.org/article/press-release/long-work-days-leave-americans-nodding-the-job.

National Sleep Foundation (NSF). (2009). *Sleep apnea and sleep.* Available at http://www.sleepfoundation.org/article/sleep-related-problems/obstructive-sleep-apnea-and-sleep.

O'Brien, M. (2007). ZZZs & your heart. *Advance for Nurses: Pennsylvania, New Jersey, Delaware, 9*(19), 22–24.

Porth, C. (2007). *Essentials of pathophysiology: Concepts of altered health states* (2nd ed.). Philadelphia: Lippincott Williams & Wilkins.

Proctor, S. (2008). Long-term effects of a good night's sleep. *Advance for Nursing: Pennsylvania, New Jersey, Delaware, 10*(8), 13.

Schaller, J. (2008). Myths & facts . . . About obstructive sleep apnea. *Nursing, 38*(1), 27.

Schardt, D. (2005). How sleep affects your weight. *Nutrition Action Newsletter, 32*(6), 10–11.

Shields, J. (2008). Sleep apnea: Diagnosis and treatment improve quality of life. *Nursing Spectrum, 17*(6), 36–37.

Smyth, C. (2008). Evaluating sleep quality in older adults. *American Journal of Nursing, 108*(5), 42–51.

Sorscher, A. (2008). How is your sleep: A neglected topic for health care screening. *The Journal of the American Board of Family Medicine, 21*(2), 141–148.

Taverno, T., & Pavlovich-Danis, S. (2008). Strange sensations invade the extremities in restless legs syndrome. *Nursing Spectrum, 17*(20), 22–27.

Taveras, E., Rifas-Shiman, S. Oken, E., Gunderson, E., & Gillman, M. (2008). Short sleep duration in infancy and risk of childhood overweight. *Archives of Pediatrics & Adolescent Medicine, 162*(4), 305–311.

Trinkoff, A., Geiger-Brown, J., Brady, B. Lipscomb, J., & Muntaner, C. (2006). How long and how much are nurses now working? *American Journal of Nursing, 106*(4), 60–71.

Wooten, J. (2007). Managing OTC insomnia remedies. *RN, 70*(11), 23.

Comfort | 35

CARLA POTTER

Carla is a 26-year-old white woman. She experiences "bad cramps" and periodic fatigue, anxiety, irritability, and mood swings approximately 1 week before the start of her menses. She told the nurse practitioner that her job as a computer programmer is stressful and these monthly symptoms are affecting her job performance and relationships.

SHEREE LINCOLN

Sheree, who has just undergone abdominal surgery, returns to the medical–surgical unit. Patient-controlled analgesia (PCA) is prescribed. Approximately 2 hours after returning from surgery, the patient is complaining of pain. Assessment reveals that she has not been using the PCA device.

XAVIER MALTON

Xavier, a 5-year-old boy diagnosed with ulcerative colitis, is in the bathroom with his mother. He suddenly grabs his belly while on the toilet and starts to scream, "Something hurts really bad!" His mother pulls the emergency call bell. He is doubled over in pain and can't get off the toilet. After being assisted back to his bed and receiving the smallest dose of pain medication possible as per the physician's order, Xavier continues to scream for half an hour more as he curls up in a fetal position on his bed. "The pain is so bad, it will never go away!"

After completing the chapter, you will be able to accomplish the following:

1. Describe specific elements in the pain experience.

2. Compare and contrast acute and chronic pain.

3. Identify factors that may affect an individual's pain experience.

4. Obtain a complete pain assessment using appropriate interviewing and physical assessment skills.

5. Develop nursing diagnoses that correctly identify pain problems and demonstrate the relationship between pain and other areas of human functioning.

6. Demonstrate the correct use of nonpharmacologic pain relief measures.

7. Administer analgesic agents safely to produce the desired level of analgesia without causing undesirable side effects.

8. Collaborate with the members of other health disciplines, using different treatment modalities to promote pain relief.

9. Use teaching and counseling skills to empower patients to direct their own pain management programs.

KEY TERMS

acute pain	nociceptors
addiction	opioid
adjuvant	pain threshold
analgesic	pain tolerance
breakthrough pain	perception
chronic pain	phantom pain
cutaneous pain	physical dependence
dynorphin	placebo
endorphins	psychogenic pain
enkephalins	referred pain
exacerbation	remission
gate control theory	somatic pain
intractable	tolerance
modulation	transduction
neuromodulators	transmission
neuropathic pain	visceral pain
neurotransmitters	

A person in pain often experiences it as an all-consuming reality and wants only one intervention—pain relief. If pain relief were as simple as rubbing a back or administering a prescribed analgesic, nursing's task would be easy. However, no two people experience pain exactly the same way. Differences in individual pain perception and response to pain, as well as the multiple and diverse causes of pain, require the use of highly specialized abilities to promote comfort and to relieve pain. The most essential of these are the nurse's belief that the patient's pain is real, the willingness to become involved in the patient's pain experience, and a competence in developing effective pain management regimens. (See the accompanying Reflective Practice box for an example.)

Although pain is often an all-consuming priority for patients, it can be easily missed because it is intangible. As a result, it becomes easier to overlook a patient's poorly communicated pain than it is to ignore a dressing that needs to be changed, or the need for assistance with walking, or the administration of a prescribed medication. Nurses who somehow manage to practice nursing while remaining insensitive to the comfort needs of their patients do a grave disservice to these patients and to the nursing profession itself.

Nurses are not alone in undervaluing the need for pain management. Although pain is a common reason for seeing a physician and for taking medication, medical science still is ill equipped to deal with its widespread occurrence. Research indicates that 30% of hospitalized patients do not receive adequate treatment for pain and that outmoded regimens to treat pain, such as intramuscular injections and the use of meperidine (Demerol) for postoperative pain are still being prescribed (D'Arcy, 2007c). Pain also affects the body in many ways, including hyperglycemia, immune system dysfunction, altered coagulation, gastrointestinal (GI) ileus, urinary retention, decreased lung volume, sympathetic nervous system stimulation, and psychological distress (Smeltzer, Bare, Hinkle, & Cheever, 2010). Scientists and clinicians have united in their efforts to ensure that pain management is a high priority in our healthcare system. New advances in understanding and treating pain have focused on the real possibility of controlling most human pain. The Joint Commission (TJC) supports the patient's right to pain management and published standards for assessment and management of pain in hospitals, ambulatory care settings, and home care settings (TJC, 2008a). The Joint Commission recommendations include teaching all patients to use a pain rating scale and determining a pain rating goal with each patient. In 2006, according to data collected by The Joint Commission (2007), 85% of accredited hospitals were compliant with assessment and treatment of pain once it was identified.

This chapter discusses the pain experience and factors that influence it. A detailed guide to assessing pain is presented, along with numerous examples of nursing diagnoses and specific nursing strategies for promoting comfort and assisting patients to achieve pain management goals. The concluding nursing plan of care illustrates how to use specific nursing interventions based on knowledge of and

REFLECTIVE PRACTICE

Challenge to Interpersonal and Ethical Skills

While working as a childcare technician one summer, I took my job quite seriously. As a nurse-in-training, I saw this job as an extension of my nursing education. I believed that the standards of care to which I held myself in my clinical rotations, and to which my professors held me, applied just as diligently in this job. I quickly found that I was the only childcare technician on the floor who held myself, let alone everyone else, to such high standards. In addition, I was quite dismayed to find that my standards for quality were actually higher than those of most of the registered nurses (RNs) employed on that unit. Nonetheless, I did not let that dissuade me. I sought out the few RNs whose standards were on par with mine, and I tried to work with them as often as possible.

One particular evening, about 15 minutes before our 12 1/2-hour shift was finally over, I was very grateful to be working with one such nurse. The quality of care that one of my patients was receiving from the physicians during an episode of acute pain was what I could only kindly call substandard.

I was caring for Xavier Malton, a 5-year-old boy diagnosed with ulcerative colitis, a form of inflammatory bowel disease (IBD). Suddenly, at the end of this relatively quiet shift, the emergency call bell alarm sounded. Frantically searching the switchboard for the source of the alarm, I realized that it was coming from Xavier's bathroom. As I ran the 10 feet to his room, thoughts of him bleeding internally or perforating his bowel ran through my head. I got there at the same time his nurse did, only to discover that his mother had pulled the alarm because her son had suddenly grabbed his belly while on the toilet and had started screaming that something was hurting very much. He was so doubled over in pain that he could not even get off the toilet. Having Crohn's disease myself, another form of IBD, I knew that the pain this boy was experiencing was excruciating and not imagined.

Over the course of the next half hour, his physicians reluctantly allowed us to drag them into his room, but they would only examine him after we insisted it was necessary because they could be dealing with an obstruction or a perforated bowel that might need surgery. Their attitude was that since he had IBD, abdominal pain was part of that, and that we should just "Let it pass" uneventfully, giving him the smallest dose of pain medication possible—which we did.

However, Xavier continued to scream, literally, for half an hour more, as he lay curled up in a fetal position on his bed. From across the hallway, I could hear him screaming that the pain was "so bad" and that it would never go away.

Thinking Outside the Box: Possible Courses of Action

- I can "give up" and try not to care since this system clearly is not committed to meeting comfort needs. But this means abandoning my patients.
- I could be persistent about advocating for this patient until his pain is relieved—trying to get as many healthcare professionals on my side as possible.
- I can consult with a colleague whom I respect about the best way to accomplish the above, since I don't want to alienate caregivers with whom I will need to continue to work.

Evaluating a Good Outcome: How Do I Define Success?

- Patient's pain is relieved and patient reports feeling comfortable.
- Colleagues are newly committed to the responsibility of EVERYONE to adequately manage pain.
- My working relationships with other professional caregivers are not compromised by my fierce advocacy for this patient.
- My personal and professional integrity remains intact.

Personal Learning: Here's to the Future!

Forty-five minutes after our shift had ended, Xavier's nurse and I were still following the physicians around, demanding that they reassess the patient and prescribe additional pain medication for him. Finally, we simply refused to leave the hospital until Xavier's pain was properly treated. We threatened to report them to the Joint Commission for substandard care, for allowing a 5-year-old child to scream and writhe in pain when all they needed to do was write a p.r.n. order for additional pain medication.

Finally, they wrote the order. Unfortunately, the narcotic they ordered was in short supply in the hospital, and we had none on the floor. The pharmacy had none to give. We spent the next 15 minutes tracking some down. Finally, we did give Xavier additional pain medication— and ultimately, it did relieve his pain and he was able to fall asleep. However, we left the hospital almost an hour and a half after our shift had ended, time that was lost to Xavier and time for which we would not receive compensation.

Transforming the culture of healthcare is a daunting task. Challenging the traditionally all-powerful physician takes courage and commitment. Demanding an unacceptable situation be remedied requires an absolute belief in the rights of the patient. The situation was indeed unacceptable—even when everyone else thinks it is acceptable. Any RN facing a situation that has the potential to transform the culture of healthcare for the better has the responsibility to take advantage of that situation, no matter what the professional risk. I would recommend that any RN in a similar situation take the same steps that Xavier's nurse and I did. Fight for what you believe is right. Do not be afraid to challenge others whom you think are wrong, even physicians. Be confident in your opinions. Refuse to back down. Remember that if you do not ensure that your patient's needs are met, maybe no one else will either. Advocate at all times for high-quality care, never settling for less.

Tracey Sara Miller, Georgetown University

(continued)

REFLECTIVE PRACTICE

Challenge to Interpersonal and Ethical Skills (continued)

Reflection

How do you think you would respond in a similar situation? Why? What does this tell you about yourself and about the adequacy of your skills for professional practice? What responses to pain did Xavier exhibit that would indicate to the nurse and nursing student that Xavier was in pain? What factors and misconceptions may have played a role in this situation? Propose possible strategies that might be appropriate to remedy these factors or correct these misconceptions. Can you think of other ways to respond? What other skills (cognitive, interpersonal, technical, ethical/legal) would you need to respond well in this situation? Explain how the nurse and nursing student advocated for Xavier. Would you use the same methods to advocate for Xavier? If so, why? If not, please explain why not. Do you agree with the criteria to evaluate a successful outcome? Did the nursing student meet the criteria? Please explain.

sensitivity to the patient's pain experience to resolve pain problems successfully.

THE PAIN EXPERIENCE

Pain is an elusive and complex phenomenon, and despite its universality, its exact nature remains a mystery. It is one of the human body's defense mechanisms that indicates the person is experiencing a problem. Margo McCaffery (1979, p. 11) offers the definition of pain that is probably of greatest benefit to nurses and their patients: "Pain is whatever the experiencing person says it is, existing whenever he (or she) says it does." This definition rests on the belief that the only one who can be a real authority on whether, and how, an individual is experiencing pain is that individual.

Pain is present whenever a person says it is, even when no specific cause of the pain can be found. Health practitioners must rely on the patient's description of the pain because it is a subjective symptom that only the patient can identify and describe.

> ➤ *Consider Xavier Malton, the 5-year-old boy with ulcerative colitis who suddenly develops acute pain. The nurse demonstrates understanding that Xavier is indeed experiencing pain because of his screaming that something hurts. Furthermore, his screaming is validated by his body posture and inability to get off the toilet.* ■

Types of Pain

Pain may be classified according to its duration, its location or source, its mode of transmission, or its etiology.

Duration of Pain

Perhaps the most common distinction involves the duration of pain. **Acute pain** is generally rapid in onset, varies in intensity from mild to severe. It is protective in nature; that is, it warns the individual of tissue damage or organic disease. After its underlying cause is resolved, acute pain disappears. It should end once healing occurs. Causes of acute pain include a pricked finger, sore throat, or surgery.

Chronic pain is pain that may be limited, intermittent, or persistent but that lasts beyond the normal healing period. The most recent definition of chronic pain no longer mentions the previous guideline of 3 to 6 months duration for pain to be considered chronic. Commonly, people with chronic pain experience periods of **remission** (when the disease is present but the person does not experience symptoms) or **exacerbation** (the symptoms reappear). Pain associated with cancer or other progressive disorders is termed chronic malignant pain. Pain in people whose tissue injury is nonprogressive or healed is termed chronic nonmalignant pain.

Patients have difficulty describing chronic pain because it may be poorly localized. Moreover, healthcare personnel have difficulty assessing it accurately because of the unique responses of individual patients to persistent pain. Unlike acute pain, chronic pain is often perceived as meaningless and may lead to withdrawal, depression, anger, frustration, and dependency. In addition, the misconceptions and personal biases of caregivers can adversely affect the management of patients with chronic pain. Individuals with chronic pain may be viewed, in general, by healthcare personnel as hysterical personalities, malingerers, or hypochondriacs. On the other hand, nurses who have experienced chronic pain or struggled through the experience with a loved one have a special awareness of its debilitating, destructive nature. Nurses need an awareness of their own personal feelings toward pain and the factors that affect pain if they are to assess and manage their patient's pain creatively and effectively. See Promoting Health 35-1 for a checklist of behaviors to foster one's self-awareness of comfort needs and pain.

Source of Pain

Pain can also be categorized according to its location. **Cutaneous pain** (superficial pain) usually involves the skin or subcutaneous tissue. A paper cut that produces sharp pain with a burning sensation is an example of cutaneous pain. Deep **somatic pain** is diffuse or scattered and originates in tendons, ligaments, bones, blood vessels, and nerves. Strong pressure on a bone or damage to tissue that occurs with a sprain causes deep somatic pain. **Visceral pain** is poorly localized and originates in body organs in the thorax, cranium, and abdomen. This pain occurs as organs stretch abnormally

---

PROMOTING HEALTH • 35-1

Comfort

Use the assessment checklist to determine how well you are meeting comfort needs. Then, develop a prescription for self-care by choosing appropriate behaviors from the list of suggestions.

Assessment Checklist

☐ almost always   ☐ sometimes   ☐ almost never

☐ ☐ ☐ 1. Obtain a medical evaluation when acute or chronic pain is present.

☐ ☐ ☐ 2. Respect pain as the body's means of signaling that all is not well.

☐ ☐ ☐ 3. Control stress in the environment.

☐ ☐ ☐ 4. Avoid excessive fatigue.

☐ ☐ ☐ 5. Practice stress reduction or diversionary behaviors when pain is present.

☐ ☐ ☐ 6. Become aware of personal preconceived notions that affect your perception of pain in others.

Self-Care Behaviors

1. I seek medical attention when pain persists.
2. I am aware of my usual behavioral responses to pain.
3. I use stress reduction techniques regularly.
4. I am able to have a restful sleep at night.
5. I have a positive outlook about my present situation.
6. I am aware of how to use distraction strategies to deal with pain.

---

and become distended, ischemic, or inflamed. A reflex contraction or spasm of the abdominal wall, called guarding, may occur as a protective mechanism to prevent additional trauma to underlying structures. An individual automatically tenses their abdomen when an acute abdominal pain condition is present. This prevents underlying tissues and organs from being palpated or touched.

> *Think back to Sheree Lincoln, the woman who has had abdominal surgery. Based on the nurse's understanding of the sources of pain, the nurse would identify that Sheree is most likely experiencing visceral pain, secondary to the effects of surgery on the abdominal organs.* ■

Mode of Transmission

Pain also can be classified based on its mode of transmission. Pain can originate in one part of the body but be perceived in an area distant from its point of origin. This is known as **referred pain.** Pain associated with a myocardial infarction, or heart attack, is frequently referred to the neck, shoulder, or arms (often the left arm). Referred pain is transmitted to a cutaneous (skin) site different from where it originated. This is possible because the pain can travel to other areas of the body innervated by the affected nerve root. Figure 35-1 illustrates cutaneous areas to which pain from various organs is usually referred.

Etiology

Pain also is classified by its cause, which can be highly varied. **Neuropathic pain** results from an injury to or abnormal

functioning of peripheral nerves or the central nervous system (CNS). The exact cause of neuropathic pain is unknown, and it can occur in many forms. Neuropathic pain can be of short duration or lingering and is often described as burning or stabbing. Allodynia, a characteristic feature of neuropathic pain, is pain that occurs after a normally weak or nonpainful stimuli, such as a light touch or a cold drink. Numerous pain syndromes have been identified that produce neuropathic pain. Several common examples are included in Table 35-1. All of these pain syndromes are capable of causing severe pain. Appropriate treatment of these syndromes is often delayed as a result of misdiagnosis; nursing can play an important role in their early detection.

When pain is resistant to therapy and persists despite a variety of interventions, it is referred to as **intractable.** Nurses and physicians together need to determine the appropriate pain treatment for each case of intractable pain so that an individual can regain a healthy quality of life.

The pain that is often referred to an amputated leg where receptors and nerves are clearly absent is a real experience for the patient. This type of pain is called **phantom pain** or phantom limb pain and is without demonstrated physiologic or pathologic substance. One theory suggests that sensory misrepresentations from the missing limb may still remain in the brain thereby causing phantom pain.

Pain may originate from physical causes; that is, a physical cause for the pain can be identified. Pain may also have a psychogenic origin (**psychogenic pain**), meaning that a physical cause for the pain cannot be identified. However, it has been observed that a pure origin is probably rare, and pain usually has both physical and psychogenic components. Furthermore, pain that results from a mental event can be just as intense as pain that results from a physical event.

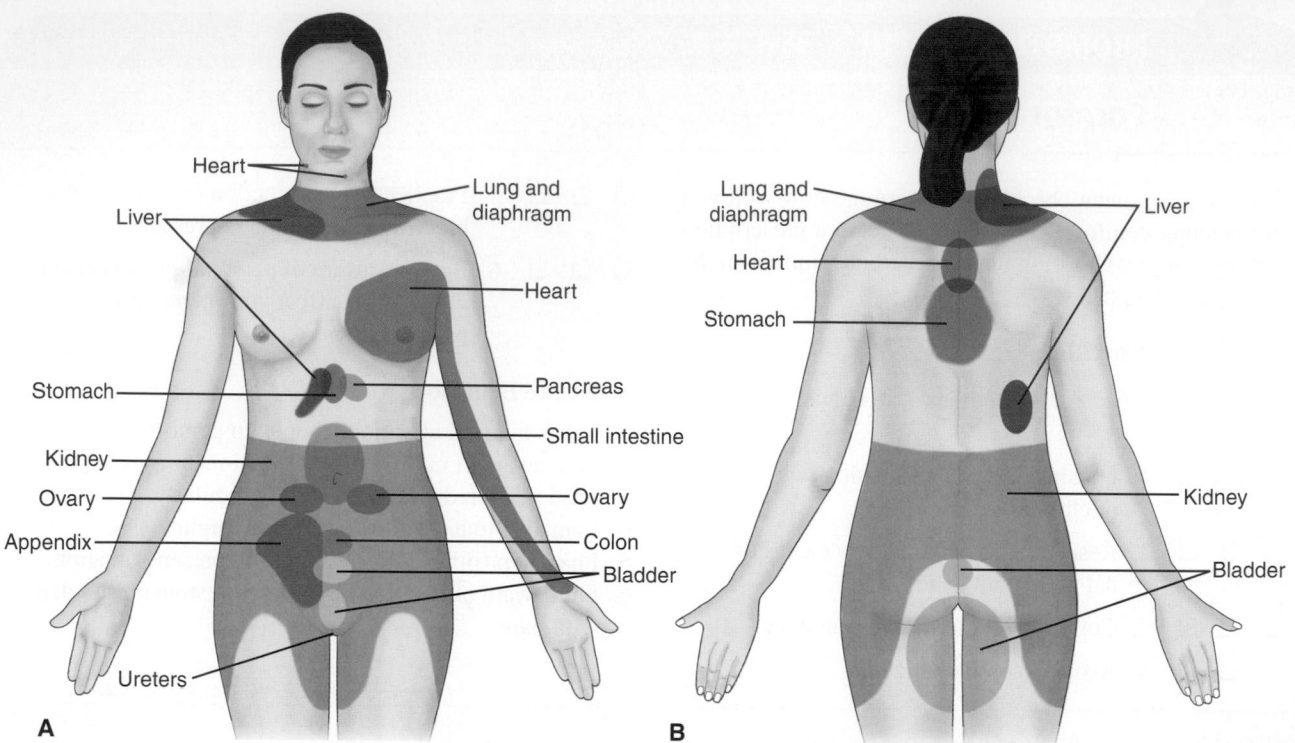

FIGURE 35-1. These drawings representing the anterior (**A**) and posterior (**B**) views of the body illustrate areas to which various organs refer pain.

Responses to Pain

The three types of responses to pain are physiologic, behavioral, and affective. Examples of these responses are listed in Box 35-1, Common Responses to Pain. The severity of pain and its duration affect responses to pain. Research has indicated that increases in vital signs may occur briefly in acute pain and may be absent in chronic pain states (D'Arcy, 2008c).

▶ *Recall Xavier Malton, the child with ulcerative colitis experiencing an acute episode of pain. The nurse assesses*

TABLE • 35-1	COMMON PAIN SYNDROMES
Pain Syndrome	**Description**
Complex regional pain syndrome (causalgia)	Pain occurs in the area of a partially injured peripheral nerve (the most common lesions are of the brachial plexus or median or sciatic nerve). The pain is described as burning, severe, diffuse, and persistent and is elicited by minimal movement or touch of the affected area. It increases with repeated stimulation and continues even after stimulation ceases.
Postherpetic neuralgia	Pain syndrome follows an acute central nervous system infection, such as herpes zoster (shingles). The herpes syndrome is characterized by a vesicular eruption and neuralgic pain, which is usually unilateral and encircles the body in band-like clusters. The severity of the pain may be mild to severe. Intractable pain may persist for months to years.
Phantom limb pain	Pain that may occur in any person who has had a body part amputated either surgically or traumatically. Pain varies and may be a severe, burning, fiery sensation; crushing; cramping; a sense that the limb is edematous; or a sensation that the limb is being twisted and distorted. It may be triggered by the sensation of touching the stump, the occurrence of another illness, fatigue, atmospheric changes, and emotional stress.
Trigeminal neuralgia	Paroxysms of lightning-like stabs of intense pain in the distribution of one or more divisions of the trigeminal nerve, the fifth cranial nerve. Pain is usually experienced in the mouth, gums, lips, nose, cheek, chin, and surface of the head and may be triggered by everyday activities like talking, eating, shaving, or brushing one's teeth.
Diabetic neuropathy	A common complication of long-term diabetes mellitus. Metabolic and vascular changes result in damage to peripheral and autonomic nerves. Sensory loss can result when peripheral nerves are involved and eventually lead to injury progressing to infection and gangrene. Symptoms include sensations of numbness, prickling, or tingling (paresthesias).

COMMON RESPONSES TO PAIN

Behavioral (Voluntary) Responses
Moving away from painful stimuli
Grimacing, moaning, and crying
Restlessness
Protecting the painful area and refusing to move

Physiologic (Involuntary) Responses
Typical Sympathetic Responses When Pain Is Moderate and Superficial
Increased blood pressure*
Increased pulse and respiratory rates*
Pupil dilation
Muscle tension and rigidity
Pallor (peripheral vasoconstriction)
Increased adrenalin output
Increased blood glucose

Typical Parasympathetic Responses When Pain Is Severe and Deep
Nausea and vomiting
Fainting or unconsciousness
Decreased blood pressure
Decreased pulse rate
Prostration
Rapid and irregular breathing

Affective (Psychological) Responses
Exaggerated weeping and restlessness
Withdrawal
Stoicism
Anxiety
Depression
Fear
Anger
Anorexia
Fatigue
Hopelessness
Powerlessness

*An increase in vital signs may occur briefly in acute pain but may not occur when chronic pain is present.

that Xavier is in pain first by his screams. Additionally, the nurse interprets his behavioral and affective responses, such as his body posture, inability to get off of the toilet, and later his fetal position in bed. Moreover, the nurse would validate these findings with physiologic responses such as skin color, and muscle tension and possibly vital signs. ∎

Mild pain experienced briefly may produce little or no behavioral response, whereas intense pain experienced briefly usually results in reflex action to escape the cause. Pain that continues for a relatively short time, such as for a few days or a week, is often accepted by the patient without it being all-consuming. The patient expects relief and believes the cause is self-limiting. However, anxiety is ordinarily present. On the other hand, chronic pain tends to consume the entire person. It demands total attention so that the patient has limited resources to take care of other matters of daily living. It is physically and emotionally exhausting and tends to result

in depression and irritability. Chronic fatigue usually accompanies chronic pain.

Lack of an obvious response to pain does not mean the patient is without pain. Careful assessment is especially important to understand what the patient is experiencing.

The Pain Process

The mechanism or process of pain is believed to involve four stages: transduction, transmission, perception, and modulation of pain (Lewis, Heitkemper, O'Brien, & Bucher, 2007).

Transduction

The activation of pain receptors is referred to as **transduction.** It involves conversion of painful stimuli into electrical impulses that travel from the periphery to the spinal cord at the dorsal horn. The peripheral nerve fibers that transmit pain are called **nociceptors.** Additionally, when the threshold of perception for pain has been reached and when there is injured tissue, it is believed that the injured tissue releases chemicals that excite or activate nerve endings. For example, a damaged cell releases histamine, which excites nerve endings. Lactic acid accumulates in tissues injured by lack of blood supply and is believed to excite nerve endings and cause pain or to lower the threshold of nerve endings to other stimuli (e.g., heat or pressure). The prolonged effect of pain stimuli acting on the central nervous system can lead to sensitization, meaning that the threshold for activation of pain is lowered. At that point, even harmless stimuli can trigger pain; pain signals are faster and feel more intense (D'Arcy, 2006c).

Other substances are also released that stimulate nociceptors or pain receptors. These include bradykinin, prostaglandins, and substance P:

- Bradykinin, a powerful vasodilator that increases capillary permeability and constricts smooth muscle, plays an important role in the chemistry of pain at the site of an injury even before the pain message gets to the brain. It also triggers the release of histamine and, in combination with it, produces the redness, swelling, and pain typically observed when an inflammation is present.
- Prostaglandins are hormone-like substances that send additional pain stimuli to the CNS.
- Substance P sensitizes receptors on nerves to feel pain and also increases the rate of firing of nerves.

Prostaglandins, substance P, and serotonin (a hormone that can act to stimulate smooth muscles, inhibit gastric secretion, and produce vasoconstriction) are **neurotransmitters** or substances that either excite or inhibit target nerve cells.

Receptors in the skin and superficial organs, although incapable of responding selectively, may also be stimulated by mechanical, thermal, chemical, and electrical agents. Friction from bed linens and pressure from a cast are mechanical stimulants. Sunburn and cold water on a tooth with caries are thermal stimulants. An acid burn is the result of a chemical stimulant. The jolt of a static charge is an electrical stimulant.

Transmission of Pain Stimuli

Pain sensations from the site of an injury or inflammation are conducted along pathways to the spinal cord and then on to higher centers. These pathways are rather clearly defined in certain areas, but are still somewhat unclear in other areas. The overall process is known as **transmission.** No specific pain organs or cells exist in the body. Rather, an interlacing network of undifferentiated free nerve endings receives painful stimuli. Free nerve ending pain receptors include the afferent (those fibers carrying impulses from the pain receptors toward the brain) fast-conducting A-delta-fibers and the slow-conducting C-fibers. The larger A-delta-fibers transmit acute, well-localized pain, whereas the smaller C-fibers convey diffuse, visceral pain that is often described as burning and aching. It is estimated that there are several million of these nerve endings in the body, numerous in the layers of the skin and in some internal tissues, such as the joint surfaces. In the deeper tissues of the body, the pain receptors are diffusely but unevenly spread.

A protective pain reflex is responsible for withdrawal of an endangered tissue from a damaging stimulus. Sensory impulses travel over A-fibers through the dorsal root ganglion to the dorsal horn of the spinal cord. At this point, the sensory nerve impulse synapses with a motor neuron, and the impulse is carried along efferent nerve pathways back to the site of the painful stimulus in a reflex arc. This results in an immediate muscle contraction that removes the injured part from the source of the pain. Figure 35-2 illustrates the transmission of the pain sensation, the initiation of the protective reflex response, and conscious awareness of the location, intensity, and quality of the pain after the impulse reaches the cortex.

Perception of Pain

The **perception** of pain involves the sensory process that occurs when a stimulus for pain is present. It includes the person's interpretation of the pain. The threshold of perception, the **pain threshold,** is the lowest intensity of a stimulus that causes the subject to recognize pain. This threshold is remarkably similar for everyone, but some studies have reached the conclusion that women have lower thresholds than men (Smeltzer et al., 2010). The possibility that men and women have different expectations relative to pain perception may be a contributing factor to pain threshold. Still, it is theorized by at least some authorities that the phenomenon of adaptation does occur, that is, the pain threshold can be changed within a certain range. This phenomenon has been studied, for example, when prisoners of war reported that the pain of repeated torture was not as acute as it would have been under different circumstances. Many factors might well have played a role, but at least some adaptation appears likely.

Adaptation may also be demonstrated when a person's hand is immersed in warm water. A sensation of pain eventually occurs as the water is heated. However, the person can tolerate a higher temperature as water is gradually heated to

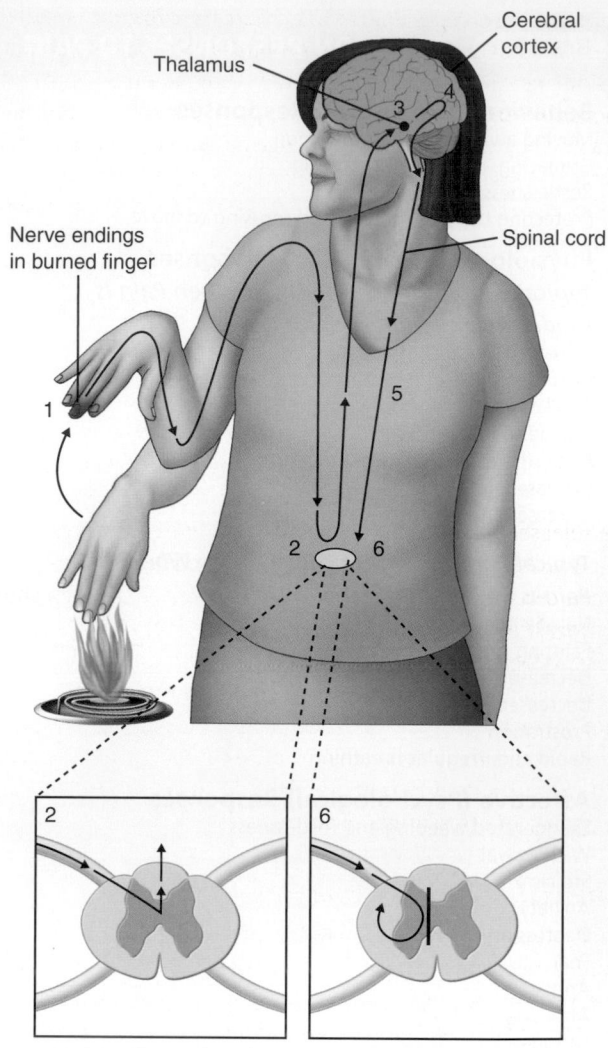

FIGURE 35-2. Pain sensation and relief. (1) Pain's path begins as a message and is received by nerve endings in a burned finger. Potent chemicals (substance P, bradykinin, prostaglandins) are released, sensitizing the nerve endings, helping to transmit the pain message from the injured finger toward the brain, and setting the stage for healing (inflammatory response). (2) The pain signal from the burned finger travels as an electrochemical impulse along the length of the nerve to the dorsal horn on the spinal cord, a region that runs the length of the spine and receives signals from all over the body. (3) The message is relayed to the thalamus, a sensory center in the brain where sensations such as heat, cold, pain, and touch first become conscious. (4) It then travels on to the cortex, where the intensity and location of pain are perceived. Little is known about factors that influence the individual's perception of pain at this point, the meaning attributed to the pain, and the voluntary responses elicited. (5) Pain relief begins as a signal from the brain and descends by way of the spinal cord. (6) In the dorsal horn, chemicals such as endorphins are released to diminish the pain message from the injured finger.

the pain level than if the hand had been plunged into hot water without any preparation.

Modulation of Pain

The process by which the sensation of pain is inhibited or modified is referred to as **modulation.** The sensation of pain appears to be regulated or modified by substances called neuromodulators. These **neuromodulators** are endogenous opioid compounds, meaning they are naturally present, morphine-like chemical regulators in the spinal cord and brain. They appear to have analgesic activity and alter the perception of pain. These endogenous opioid compounds are believed to produce their analgesic effects by binding to specific opioid receptor sites throughout the CNS, blocking the release or production of pain-transmitting substances. Both pain and stress appear capable of activating the endogenous opiate system.

Endorphins and enkephalins are opioid neuromodulators. **Endorphins** are produced at neural synapses at various points along the CNS pathway. They are powerful pain-blocking chemicals that have prolonged analgesic effects and produce euphoria. It is suggested that endorphins may be released when certain measures are used to relieve pain, such as skin stimulation and relaxation techniques, and when certain pain-relieving drugs are used. The endorphin, **dynorphin,** has the most potent analgesic effect. However, many questions remain about endorphins.

Enkephalins, which are widespread throughout the brain and dorsal horn of the spinal cord, are considered less potent than endorphins. Enkephalins are thought to reduce pain sensation by inhibiting the release of substance P from the terminals of afferent neurons.

The Gate Control Theory of Pain

Many theories have attempted to explain the mechanism of pain. However, the **gate control theory** provides the most practical model regarding the concept of pain. It describes the transmission of painful stimuli and recognizes a relation between pain and emotions. The theory states that certain nerve fibers, those of small diameter, conduct excitatory pain stimuli toward the brain, but nerve fibers of a large diameter appear to inhibit the transmission of pain impulses from the spinal cord to the brain. There is a gating mechanism that is believed by some to be located in substantia gelatinosa cells in the dorsal horn of the spinal cord. The exciting and inhibiting signals at the gate in the spinal cord determine the impulses that eventually reach the brain. Thus, only a limited amount of sensory information can be processed by the nervous system at any given moment. When too much information is sent through, certain cells in the spinal column interrupt the signal as if closing a gate.

The brain can also influence the gating mechanism. Past experiences and learned behaviors, which are interpreted by the brain, regulate or adjust the eventual behavioral responses to pain. Thus, the gating mechanism appears to be influenced by the amount of activity in large and small afferent fibers in addition to nerve impulses that descend from the brain. This helps explain why similar painful stimuli are interpreted differently by different people. Although not everyone accepts the gate control theory, it appears to explain why mechanical and electrical interventions or heat and pressure may provide effective pain relief. Nursing measures, such as massage or a warm compress to a painful lower back area, stimulate large nerve

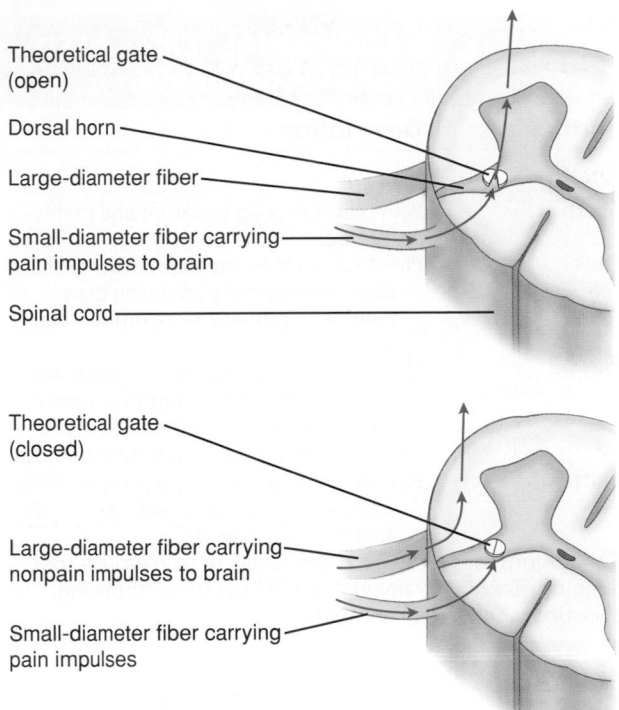

FIGURE 35-3. An illustration of the gate control theory of pain.

fibers to close the gate, thus blocking pain impulses from that area. Figure 35-3 illustrates the gate control theory of pain.

FACTORS AFFECTING THE PAIN EXPERIENCE

Pain is a highly personal experience. Many factors influence the comfort status of a person at any given moment. When an individual experiences pain, almost anything can influence how the painful stimulus is transmitted to the brain, how it is perceived, and the response that is made to it.

A person learns to know what causes unpleasantness and what to interpret as pain. Each person's interpretation is influenced by background, such as how he or she has experienced and dealt with pain in the past, and what culture has taught the person about pain. Through past experiences, each person also learns to differentiate among the various types of pain and to associate pain with certain descriptive words. Table 35-2 lists common definitions for additional terms used by patients to describe pain.

Culture

Cultural norms dictate much of our daily behavior, attitudes, and values. Therefore, it is natural that culture influences the individual's response to pain. Nurses need to understand that there are ways other than their own of responding to pain. Nurses, as a subculture, value self-control and the ability to function under stress. As a result, nurses may expect patients in pain to display a similarly calm, objective, uncomplaining approach to pain. It is particularly important to avoid stereotyping responses to pain because the nurse frequently

Table • 35-2	ADDITIONAL TERMS USED TO DESCRIBE PAIN
Term	**Description**
Quality	
Sharp	Pain that is sticking in nature and that is intense.
Dull	Pain that is not as intense or acute as sharp pain, possibly more annoying than painful. It is usually more diffuse than sharp pain.
Diffuse	Pain that covers a large area. Usually, the patient is unable to point to a specific area without moving the hand over a large surface, such as the entire abdomen.
Shifting	Pain that moves from one area to another, such as from the lower abdomen to the area over the stomach.
Other terms used to describe the quality of pain include sore, stinging, pinching, cramping, gnawing, cutting, throbbing, shooting, and vise-like pressure.	
Severity	
Severe or excruciating Moderate Slight or mild	These terms depend on the patient's interpretation of pain. Behavioral and physiologic signs help assess the severity of pain. On a scale of 1 to 10, slight pain could be described as being between about 1 and 3; moderate pain, between about 4 and 7; and severe pain, between about 8 and 10.
Periodicity	
Continuous	Pain that does not stop.
Intermittent	Pain that stops and starts again.
Brief or transient	Pain that passes quickly.

encounters patients who are in pain or anticipating that it will develop. A form of pain expression that is frowned on in one culture may be desirable in another cultural group. Be knowledgeable about cultural variations and develop an understanding of cultural influences on pain tolerance, expressions of pain, and alternative practices used to manage pain.

Ethnic Variables

Much research has been done on ethnic and cultural influences on pain. The classic study on behavioral responses to pain in people of similar ethnic origin was done by Zborowski (1969). He studied men in the 1950s and 1960s in four cultural groups—"Old American" (American-born, white, Protestant, and without identification with any foreign group), Jewish, Italian, and Irish. According to Zborowski, Old American and Irish men typically minimized and controlled their expression of pain, whereas Jewish and Italian men tended to be more vocal and outwardly emotional with their expressions of pain. Today, the ethnic heritage of many people is mixed, thereby making it more difficult to anticipate individual responses to pain. Healthcare providers increase their respect and sensitivity for diversity if they

understand the effects of culture and ethnicity on the pain experience. Table 35-3 describes typical pain responses in selected ethnocultural groups. The nurse working with other ethnic groups can find pertinent studies in the literature and on various web sites (Narayan, 2010). Additional information on cultural influences on pain is presented in Chapter 2.

Family, Gender, and Age Variables

Other culturally related variables are family, gender, and age. An individual's response to pain or symptoms may be affected or influenced by the response of family members. Spouses also may reinforce pain behavior in their partners. Children growing up in different families may learn to "be brave" and ignore pain or to use the pain experience to secure attention and service from family members. Family size and birth order do not appear to be significant in distinguishing chronic pain sufferers.

Similarly, children may learn that there are gender differences in pain expression—it may be acceptable for a little girl to run home crying with a scraped knee, but a little boy may be told that he should be brave and not cry. Adult men and women may hold on to gender expectations regarding pain communication and incorrectly interpret the presence or absence of pain expressions in others. Women are more comfortable communicating the discomfort associated with pain, but this ability to verbalize may cause some to view the pain as emotionally or psychologically based. Several studies report that pain in women needs to be addressed more aggressively because their pain management is consistently reported as inadequate.

In addition, different age groups have different beliefs and norms regarding pain sensation and response. At one time, the infant's inability to communicate pain led healthcare practitioners to the erroneous assumption that pain sensation was diminished or absent. More recently, it has been demonstrated that infants and small children are sensitive to and experience pain. Among older people, pain has often been viewed as a natural component of the aging process, being ignored or undertreated by healthcare providers. On the other hand, conditions normally painful in young adults (e.g., myocardial infarction) may result in minimal pain complaints in older people. That an older person does not complain of pain may indicate that he or she fears the treatment for the pain or just refuses to give in to the pain. For many older adults, pain has become accepted as a daily occurrence and is regarded as part of the normal aging process. These variables, which influence pain sensation, perception, and response, make pain assessment a complex task for the nurse.

Religious Beliefs

Religious beliefs can be a powerful influence on the individual's experience of pain. In some religions, individuals view pain and suffering as a "lack of goodness" in themselves. Thus, pain and suffering are viewed as a means of purification or of making up for individual and community sin. This meaning helps the individual to cope with pain, thus becoming a

TABLE • 35-3	PAIN EXPRESSION IN SELECTED ETHNOCULTURAL GROUPS
Ethnic Group	**Response to Pain**
African Americans	Often viewed as a sign of illness or disease. Some believe that suffering and pain are inevitable. Spiritual and religious beliefs may contribute to high tolerance for pain. Some believe that praying and laying on of hands may aid in deliverance from pain and suffering.
Arab Americans	Often view pain as unpleasant and something that should be controlled. Tend to express pain openly with family members but may act in a more restrained manner in the presence of health professionals. Usually expect positive response from Western medical interventions to control pain.
Chinese Americans	Expressions of pain are usually similar to those of Americans. Often believe pain is related to the influence of imbalances in the yin and yang. Usually cope with pain by using externally applied oils and massage as well as warmth, sleeping on the area of pain, relaxation, and aspirin.
Greek Americans	Ponos (pain) is viewed by most as an evil that needs to be eradicated. Physical and emotional pain are usually shared with the family. Family is considered a resource for pain relief because they act as advocates and provide emotional support.
Mexican Americans	Most delay seeking medical help for pain and hope, instead, that it will go away; consider it a necessary part of life. Seem to experience more pain than other ethnic groups but report it less frequently. Often see a direct relationship between pain and suffering and immoral behavior.
Navajo Indians	Do not usually openly express their pain or request pain medication. Adequate pain control is often difficult because they may mask the actual intensity of their pain. May prefer herbal medicines and use them without the knowledge of the healthcare provider.

Adapted from Purnell, L., & Paulanka, B. (2003). *Transcultural health care: A culturally competent approach* (2nd ed.). Philadelphia: F. A. Davis.

source of strength. Patients with this belief may refuse analgesics and other pain relief measures, feeling that this lessens their suffering. On the other hand, illness and pain may also be viewed as punishment from a vengeful God. Individuals may find their faith shaken and question the existence of a loving God. How can belief in a loving God be compatible with their present experience of pain? Anger, resentment, and depression may compound the pain experience. Patients may find it helpful to confer with a spiritual adviser about their pain experience.

Environment and Support People

An individual's environment and the presence or absence of caring support people may also influence the experience of pain. Many people find that the strangeness of the healthcare environment, especially the lights, noise, lack of sleep, and constant activity of a critical care unit, compounds the experience of pain. The sense of powerlessness that accompanies admission to an institution may decrease the individual's ability to cope with pain.

➤ *Recall Sheree Lincoln, the postoperative patient in pain described at the beginning of the chapter. In addition to the pain related to surgery, the nurse would need to assess the effect of the environment on Sheree's pain. For example,*

she may be frightened by equipment being used postoperatively. Additionally, she may feel alone and powerless due to her current condition. Assessment also would need to include information about past experiences with pain, support persons available, and teaching she received preoperatively. ■

Depersonalization or separation from a favorite pillow, pet, or source of music may further decrease the person's sense of comfort. For some, the presence of a loved family member or friend is essential to their sense of well-being. Others prefer to be alone when in pain and may become agitated in the presence of a family member.

Some patients may use their pain to acquire secondary gains, such as special attention and services from their families. If unchecked, this tendency usually leads to resentment and anger in family members and their eventual avoidance of the patient. Intervening and attempting an honest discussion of this problem is important.

Anxiety and Other Stressors

Anxiety, which is almost always present when pain is anticipated or being experienced, tends to increase the perceived intensity of pain. The threat of the unknown is ordinarily more devastating and anxiety producing than a threat for which one has been prepared. Studies have indicated that patients who were taught preoperatively about what to expect postoperatively did not require as much medication for pain as those who had similar operative procedures but did not receive this teaching (Van Steenacker, 2007). See Chapter 30 for additional discussion of pain management during the perioperative experience.

Although a cause-and-effect relationship has not clearly been verified, pain may be aggravated with anxiety, muscular tension, and fatigue. The rested and relaxed person can often cope with more discomfort than someone who is suffering from a lack of sleep.

> *Think back to Carla Potter, the young woman experiencing "bad cramps" prior to her menses. She also reports anxiety, fatigue, and mood swings in addition to other symptoms. In order to individualize her plan of care, the nurse needs to gather additional data and investigate the possibility of specific relaxation measures that may effectively help Carla Potter to reduce some of the anxiety that she reports.* ■

An individual who is greatly fatigued and who has no competing demands requiring attention may experience pain more acutely. For example, many people have discovered that the pain of a foot ache or an ingrown toenail that was only mildly annoying during the day's work becomes unbearable at night when there is nothing else to distract the mind from the pain.

Past Pain Experience

An individual's experience of pain in the past and the qualities of that experience profoundly affect new pain experiences:

• Some patients have never known severe pain and have no fear of pain, not realizing how intense the sensation can be.
• Some patients have experienced severe acute or chronic pain in the past but received immediate and adequate pain relief. These patients are generally unafraid of pain and initiate appropriate requests for assistance.
• Some patients have known severe pain in the past and were unable to secure relief. Even the suggestion of new pain can lead to acute feelings of fear, despair, and hopelessness.
• An individual whose past pain experience led to correction of unhealthy behavior and produced a greater sense of health and well-being may respect and value pain and consider the meaning and significance of a new pain carefully.
• In general, people who have experienced more pain than usual in their lifetimes tend to anticipate more pain and to exhibit increased sensitivity to pain.
• Some pain memories are virtually unerasable; new contact with conditions similar to those that caused the earlier pain can provoke a violent response.

THE NURSING PROCESS FOR COMFORT
Assessing

Because the pain experience is unique to each individual, the nurse who wants to help the patient achieve comfort and pain control needs sophisticated pain assessment skills. Assessing all factors that affect the pain experience—psychological, emotional, and sociocultural, as well as physiologic—is essential. Pain is complex and difficult to interpret and requires a reliable assessment tool.

Pain as the Fifth Vital Sign

In an effort to improve patients' quality of life and make pain management a priority, the American Pain Society, in 1995, encouraged caregivers to include assessment for pain as the fifth vital sign. Routine measurement of vital signs accompanied by a pain assessment raises awareness of the existence of pain, places additional emphasis on optimizing pain relief, and moves patients more quickly toward comfort and recovery.

The Joint Commission (TJC), in an effort to improve pain management, also developed accreditation standards that included emphasis on the patient's right to effective assessment and treatment of pain. These standards include the following (Burney, 2001).

• Patients have the right to appropriate assessment and management of their pain.
• Ongoing assessment of the existence of pain should also include the nature and intensity of the pain in all patients.
• Assessment results should be recorded in a manner that promotes regular reassessment and follow-up.
• Staff, including new clinical staff, must be oriented and competent in assessment and management of pain.
• Policies and procedures that support prescription or ordering of pain medications must be in place.
• Pain must be managed so it does not interfere with a patient's participation in rehabilitation.
• Patients and families require education about effective pain management.
• Discharge planning should address the patient's needs for management of pain symptoms.
• Data must be collected to monitor the appropriateness and effectiveness of the facility's pain management plan.

Common Misconceptions

Many patient misconceptions interfere with the patient's ability to communicate pain. Examples of common patient beliefs related to pain and communicating it include the following:

• The doctor has ordered pain-relieving medication for me, which I will be given routinely.
• If I ask for something for my pain, I may become addicted to the medication.
• Sometimes it is better to put up with the pain than to deal with the side effects of the pain medication.

- I should somehow be able to control my pain. It is immature to talk about pain.
- It is better to wait until the pain gets really bad before asking for help. If I take the medication now for moderate pain, it won't relieve severe pain later on.
- I don't want to bother anyone—I know how busy they are.
- It's natural for me to have pain after surgery. After a few days, I should notice it lessening.

> *Recall Sheree Lincoln, the woman who has undergone abdominal surgery. It would be important for the nurse to investigate Sheree's understanding of her postoperative pain and what her expectations are. Doing so would provide clues for the nurse indicating possible patient misconceptions about pain and pain relief, thereby providing a basis for teaching and correcting these misconceptions.* ■

Additional misconceptions and prejudices about pain and pain relief that hamper the nurse's assessment and treatment of the patient with pain have been summarized by McCaffery and Pasero (1999) and are presented in Table 35-4.

Components of a Pain Assessment

Various forms used to help guide the assessment of pain have been described in the nursing literature. The primary purposes of using a guide to assess pain are to eliminate guesswork and biases when dealing with the patient's pain, to understand what the person is experiencing, to analyze findings that will help prepare an appropriate nursing response to the patient's pain, and to facilitate improved outcomes, such as fewer complications, shorter hospital stays, and improved quality of life.

Characteristics of pain generally assessed include the following:

- Patient's verbalization and description of the pain
- Duration of the pain
- Location of the pain
- Quantity and intensity of the pain
- Quality of the pain
- Chronology of the pain
- Aggravating factors
- Alleviating factors
- Physiologic indicators of pain
- Behavioral responses
- Effect of the pain experience on activities and lifestyle

A comprehensive pain assessment must also include discussion of the patient's expectations for pain relief. The patient and healthcare team need to select a realistic goal or a number on the pain scale that is acceptable and satisfactory and that facilitates recovery. This helps the patient recognize and report pain that is unacceptable and also allows caregivers to evaluate more readily the effectiveness of their pain management techniques. The Focused Assessment Guide 35-1 suggests questions or approaches helpful in assessing the various pain factors.

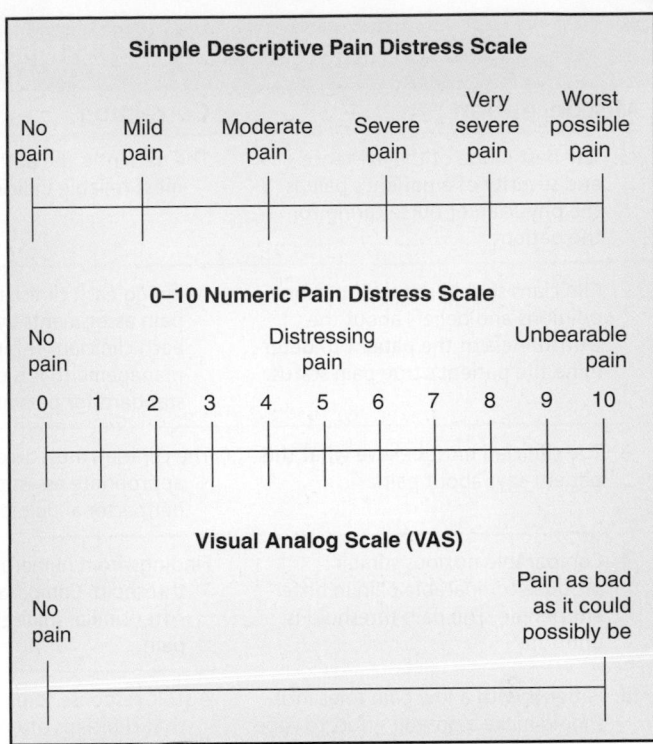

FIGURE 35-4. Pain distress scales. (From AHCPR, Acute Pain Management Guide Panel, 1992.)

For continued assessment of pain and evaluation of pain control measures, a pain scale allows the patient to rate effectively the pain he or she is experiencing on a continual basis. Figure 35-4 shows examples of several pain-intensity rating scales that can be used by verbally communicative patients, including the numerical pain scale that is currently the national standard. It is best to use the same scale to rate a patient's pain throughout a hospital stay.

When assessing an individual's pain, McCaffery and Pasero (1999) list these basic methods:

- Patient's self-report
- Report of family member, other person close to the patient, or caregiver who is familiar with the patient
- Nonverbal behaviors (restlessness, grimacing, crying, clenching fists, protecting the painful area)
- Physiologic measures (increased blood pressure and pulse) although most research verifies that reliance on vital signs to indicate the presence of pain should be minimized. The absence of an increase in vital signs does not mean that pain is not present.

Pain must not be overlooked in patients who have difficulty with communication. Their pain requires adequate treatment. Examples of pain rating scales that can be used with patients who are nonverbal or have difficulty communicating verbally include the Payen behavioral pain scale for use with critically ill patients who are intubated and the Face Legs Activity Cry and Consolability (FLACC) pain scale for use with infants and young children (from ages 2 months to 7 years) and with older adults who can't speak (Herr et al., 2006).

TABLE • 35-4   BARRIERS TO THE ASSESSMENT AND TREATMENT OF PAIN

Misconception	Correction
1. The best judge of the existence and severity of a patient's pain is the physician or nurse caring for the patient.	The patient is the authority about his or her pain. The patient's self-report is the most reliable indicator of the existence and intensity of pain.
2. Clinicians should use their personal opinions and beliefs about the truthfulness of the patient to determine the patient's true pain status.	Allowing each clinician to act on personal beliefs presents the potential for different pain assessments by different clinicians, leading to different interventions from each clinician. This results in inconsistent and often inadequate pain management. It is essential to establish the patient's self-report of pain as the standard for pain assessment.
3. The clinician must believe what the patient says about pain.	The clinician must accept and respect the patient's report of pain and proceed with appropriate assessment and treatment. The clinician is always entitled to his or her personal opinion, but this cannot be allowed to guide professional practice.
4. Comparable noxious stimuli produce comparable pain in different people. The pain threshold is uniform.	Findings from numerous studies have failed to support the notion of a uniform pain threshold. Comparable stimuli do not result in the same pain in different people. After similar injuries, one person may suffer moderate pain and the other severe pain.
5. Patients with a low pain tolerance should make a greater effort to cope with pain and should not receive as much analgesia as they desire.	A stoic response to pain is valued in this society and many others. Research shows that clinicians often do not like patients with a low pain tolerance. However, imposing these values on the patient and withholding analgesics is inappropriate.
6. There is no reason for patients to hurt when no physical cause for pain can be found.	Pain is a new science, and it would be foolish of us to think that we will be able to determine the cause of all the pains that patients report.
7. Patients should not receive analgesics until the cause of pain is diagnosed.	Pain is no longer the clinician's primary diagnostic tool. Symptomatic relief of pain should be provided while the investigation of cause proceeds. Early use of analgesics is now advocated for patients with acute abdominal pain.
8. Visible signs, either physiologic or behavioral, accompany pain and can be used to verify its existence and severity.	Even with severe pain, periods of physiologic and behavioral adaptation occur, leading to periods of minimal or no signs of pain. Lack of pain expression does not necessarily mean lack of pain.
9. Anxiety makes pain worse.	Anxiety is often associated with pain, but the cause-and-effect relationship has not been established. Pain often causes anxiety, but it is not clear that anxiety necessarily makes pain more intense.
10. Patients who are knowledgeable about opioid analgesics and who make regular efforts to obtain them are "drug seeking" (addicted).	Patients with pain should be knowledgeable about their medications, and regular use of opioids for pain relief is not addiction. When a patient is accused of "drug seeking," it may be helpful to ask, "What else could this behavior mean? Might this patient be in pain?"
11. When the patient reports pain relief after a placebo, this means that the patient is a malingerer or that the pain is psychogenic.	About one third of patients who have obvious physical stimuli for pain (e.g., surgery) report pain relief after a placebo injection. Therefore, placebos cannot be used to diagnose malingering, psychogenic pain, or any psychological problem. Sometimes, placebos relieve pain, but why this happens remains unknown.
12. The pain rating scale preferred for use in daily clinical practice is the Visual Analogue Scale (VAS).	For patients who are verbal and can count from 0 to 10, the Numerical Rating Scale (NRS) pain rating scale is preferred. It is easy to explain, measure, and record, and it provides numbers for setting pain management goals.
13. Cognitively impaired elderly patients are unable to use pain rating scales.	When an appropriate pain rating scale (e.g., 0–5) is used and the patient is given sufficient time to process information and respond, many cognitively impaired elderly patients can use a pain rating scale.

FOCUSED ASSESSMENT GUIDE • 35-1

THE PAIN EXPERIENCE

Factors to Assess	Questions and Approaches
Characteristics of the pain Location	*"Where is your pain? Is it external or internal?"* (Asking the patient with acute pain to point to the painful area with one finger may help to localize the pain. Patients with chronic pain may have difficulty trying to localize their pain, however.)
Duration	*"How long have you been experiencing pain? How long does a pain episode last? How often does a pain episode occur?"*

Quantity	Ask the patient to indicate the degree (amount) of pain currently experienced on the scale below:
	
	0 1 2 3 4 5 6 7 8 9 10
	No Mild Moderate Severe Pain as
	pain bad as
	                                                    it can
	                                                  be
	
	It is also helpful to ask how much pain the patient has (on the same scale) when the pain is at its least and at its worst:
	
	Least _____ Worst _____

Quality	*"What words would you use to describe your pain?"*
Chronology	*"How does the pain develop and progress?"* (If pattern can be identified, interventions early in a pain sequence will often be far more effective than those used after the pain is well established.) *"Has the pain changed since it first began? If so, how?"*
Aggravating factors	*"What makes the pain occur or increase in intensity?"*
Alleviating factors	*"What makes the pain go away or lessen? What methods of relief have you tried in the past? How long were they used? How effective were they?"* (Methods of relief currently in effect for hospitalized patients should be apparent from the chart. It is important to verify the use of current orders and their effectiveness with the patient. Outpatients may need to be asked to record a medication profile, a thorough and accurate account of all medications they are taking.)
Associated phenomena	*"Are there any other factors that seem to relate consistently to your pain? Any other symptoms that occur just before, during, or after your pain?"*
Physiologic responses Vital signs (blood pressure, pulse, respirations) Skin color Perspiration Pupil size Nausea	Signs of sympathetic stimulation may occur with acute pain but need not be present to verify the presence of pain. Signs of parasympathetic stimulation (decreased blood pressure and pulse, rapid and irregular respirations, pupil constriction, nausea and vomiting, and warm, dry skin) may occur, especially in prolonged, severe pain, visceral, or deep pain.
Muscle tension	Observe. Ask the patient whether he or she is aware of any tight, tense muscles.
Anxiety	Are signs of anxiety evident? (May include decreased attention span or ability to follow directions, frequent asking of questions, shifting of topics of conversation, avoidance of discussion of feelings, acting out, somatizing.)
Behavioral responses Posture, gross motor activities	Does patient rub or support a particular area? Make frequent position changes? Walk, pace, kneel, or assume a rolled-up position? Does patient rest a particular body part? Protect an area from stimulation? Lie quietly? (In acute pain, postural and gross motor activities are often altered; in chronic pain, the only signs of change may be postures characteristic of withdrawal.)
Facial features	Does the patient have a pinched look? Are there facial grimaces? Knotted brow? Overall taut, anxious appearance? (A look of fatigue is more characteristic of chronic pain.)
Verbal expressions	Does the patient sigh, moan, scream, cry, repetitively use the same words?

(continued)

FOCUSED ASSESSMENT GUIDE • 35-1

THE PAIN EXPERIENCE *(continued)*

Factors to Assess	Questions and Approaches
Affective responses	
Anxiety	*"Do you feel anxious? Are you afraid? If so, how bad are these feelings?"*
Depression	*"Do you feel depressed, down, or low? If so, how bad are these feelings? Are your feelings about yourself mostly good or bad? Do you have feelings of failure? Do you see yourself or your illness as a burden to those you care about?"*
Interactions with others	How does the patient act when he or she is in pain in the presence of others? How does the patient respond to others when he or she is not in pain? How do significant others and caregivers respond to the patient when the patient is in pain? When the patient is not in pain?
Degree to which pain interferes with patient's life (use past performance as baseline)	*"Does the pain interfere with sleep? If so, to what extent? Is fatigue a major factor in the pain experience? Is the conduct of intimate or peer relationships affected by the pain? Is work function affected? Participation in recreational–diversional activities?"* (An activity diary is often helpful—sometimes crucial. One to several weeks of hourly activity recorded by the patient may be necessary. Levels of pain, intake of food, and sleep–rest periods are noted along with activities performed. Separate diaries for inpatient and outpatient episodes may be necessary because hospitalization markedly affects the nature and type of activities performed.)
Perception of pain and meaning to patient	*"Are you worried about your illness? Do you see any connection between your pain and the nature or course of illness? If so, how do you see them as related? Do you find any meaning in your pain? If so, is this beneficial or detrimental to you? Are you struggling to find some meaning for your pain?"*
Adaptive mechanisms used to cope with pain	*"What do you usually do to relieve stress? How well do these things work? What techniques do you use at home to help cope with the pain? How well have they worked? Do you use these in the hospital? If not, why not?"*
Outcomes	*"What would you like to be doing right now, this week, this month, if the pain were better controlled? How much would the pain have to decrease (on the 0–10 scale) for you to begin to accomplish these goals?"*

Assessment of Special Populations

Pain rating scales attempt to confirm and, if possible, quantify the presence of pain in a variety of populations and situations. Alternative approaches to pain assessment ensure that unacceptable levels of pain are addressed and treated.

CHILDREN

In recent years, healthcare personnel have become much more concerned about addressing pain relief in infants and children. Previously, it was believed that young children lacked the neurologic development to sense pain the way adults do. Thus, pain relief was not a priority when children were hospitalized. Young children frequently received no treatment for pain during their entire hospital stay. Infants, particularly premature infants, are as sensitive to painful stimuli as older children and adults. Current thinking is that inadequately controlled pain during infancy and childhood may alter a person's response to pain in adulthood. Pain is frustrating for children because they are unable to understand the concept and cause of pain and may have difficulty describing it. Depending on age, the child may see the pain as a form of punishment for something that he or she has done. It is thought that children are able to indicate that pain is present at approximately 2 years of age (Herr et al., 2006).

Current methods of assessing and measuring children's pain frequently involve use of more than one technique for assessment. A pain history provides information about the language the child uses to indicate pain, how and to whom this pain is usually reported, and indications of previous pain experiences and coping strategies. Self-report is usually the most reliable account of pain. Communication with parents, guardians, or other important family members is vital for accurate pediatric pain assessment and management. In addition, the following observations may provide an indication of the presence and severity of pain in a child:

- Irritability and restlessness
- Crying, screaming, or other verbal expression of pain
- Grimacing, grinding of teeth, or clenching fists
- Touching or grabbing of painful body part
- Kicking, thrashing, or attempting to move away from a painful stimulus

Numerous scales and tools can be used to assess a child's pain (Table 35-5). One commonly used pain assessment scale, the Wong-Baker FACES pain rating scale (Fig. 35-5), asks children to compare their pain to a series of faces ranging from a broad smile to a tearful grimace. The Oucher pain

Table • 35-5	PAIN ASSESSMENT SCALES	
Resource	**Website**	**Indications**
COMFORT Scale	http://painconsortium.nih.gov/pain_scales/index.html	Infants, children, adults who are unable to use NRS or Wong–Baker FACES Pain Rating Scale
CRIES Pain Scale	http://painconsortium.nih.gov/pain_scales/index.html	Neonates (ages 0–6 months)
FLACC Scale	http://painconsortium.nih.gov/pain_scales/index.html	Infants and children (2 months–7 years) who are unable to validate the presence of or quantify the severity of pain
Wong–Baker Faces Pain Rating Scale	http://painconsortium.nih.gov/pain_scales/index.html	Adults and children (>3 years old) in all patient care settings
0–10 Numeric Rating Scale	http://painconsortium.nih.gov/pain_scales/index.html	Adults and children (>9 years old) in all patient care settings who are able to use numbers to rate the intensity of their pain
Checklist of Non-Verbal Indicators	http://painconsortium.nih.gov/pain_scales/index.html	Adults who are unable to validate the presence of or quantify the severity of pain using either the Numeric Rating Scale or Wong–Baker FACES Pain Rating Scale
Oucher Pain Scale	http://www.oucher.org/history.html	Young children who can point to a face to indicate their level of pain
PAINAD Scale	http://links.lww.com/A251	Patients whose dementia is so advanced that they can't verbally communicate
FPS-R (FACES Pain Scale – Revised)	www.painsourcebook.ca	Young children in parallel with numerical self-rating scales (0–10). Patients choose the depiction of a facial expression that best corresponds with their pain.
Payen Behavioral Pain Scale	http://www.nursingcenter.com/prodev/ce_article.asp?tid=574382	Useful with intubated, critically ill patients; measurement of bodily indicators of pain; and tolerance of intubation.

scale, developed by Beyer and others (1992) for use in young patients, combines a 0-to-100 scale with six photographic images of children in pain. This scale is helpful for use with older children. Adaptations of the Oucher pain scale are also available for various ethnic groups.

The CRIES Pain Scale is a tool intended for use with neonates and infants from 0 to 6 months. The COMFORT Scale used to assess pain and distress in critically ill pediatric patients relies on six behavioral and two physiologic factors that determine the level of analgesia needed to adequately

1. Explain to the child that each face is for a person who feels happy because he or she has no pain (hurt, or whatever word the child uses) or feels sad because he or she has some or a lot of pain.
2. Point to the appropriate face and state, "This face . . .":
   0—"is very happy because he [or she] doesn't hurt at all."
   1—"hurts just a little bit."
   2—"hurts a little more."
   3—"hurts even more."
   4—"hurts a whole lot."
   5—"hurts as much as you can imagine, although you don't have to be crying to feel this bad."
3. Ask the child to choose the face that best describes how he or she feels. Be specific about which pain (eg, "shot" or incision) and what time (eg, Now? Earlier before lunch?)

FIGURE 35-5. Wong-Baker FACES Pain Rating Scale for use with children. (From Hockenberry, M. J. [2005]. *Wong's essentials of pediatric nursing* [7th ed.]. St. Louis: Mosby. Used with permission.)

relieve pain in these children (van Dijket et al., 2005). The FLACC scale (F – Faces, L – Legs, A – Activity, C – Cry, C – Consolability) designed for infants and children from age 2 months to 7 years who are unable to validate the presence or severity of pain rates each of the five categories on a 0-to-2 scale. Additionally, children may be asked to record their pain experiences in a daily diary. Detecting and accurately assessing pediatric pain have resulted in new and innovative approaches toward pain control in children.

A recent study documented efforts to identify the presence of pain in preterm neonates who were on a ventilator. Facial expressions, high activity level, and poor response to handling were viewed as indicators of the presence of pain in this population (Boyle et al., 2006).

> *Think back to Xavier Malton, the 5-year-old with acute pain. Incorporating the use of an age-appropriate pain assessment tool would be crucial in assessing Xavier's pain. Because Xavier is 5 years old, he may have difficulty describing his pain and its severity. For example, according to Xavier, "Something was hurting very much." Using the FACES scale or the Oucher scale would help the nurse to quantify the severity of Xavier's pain, providing objective evidence from which to intervene appropriately. The tool also would be extremely useful in determining the effectiveness of pain relief interventions, providing objective evidence denoting any changes in the pain's severity. This evaluation would serve as a basis for continuing pain management.* ∎

COGNITIVELY IMPAIRED PATIENTS

Assessment of pain in people who are cognitively impaired presents special challenges to nurses. It is generally recognized that cognitively impaired individuals are frequently undertreated because they may be unable to report pain verbally or describe the dimensions of their pain. Horgas and Miller (2008) estimate that 43% to 71% of cognitively impaired older adults may be experiencing some degree of pain. Pain has been demonstrated as a possible cause of aggressive behavior in cognitively impaired older adults.

To manage pain effectively, nurses must rely on their own careful assessments, their empathic qualities, and the expectation that a cognitively impaired patient will experience pain if a verbal patient usually reports this event as painful. The combination of a history of pain, observations of a patient's pain by families and caregivers, and the presence of medical diagnoses associated with pain also facilitates pain assessment in this population. Moreover, special efforts are needed to identify accurate methods for assessing their pain. The Pain Assessment in Advanced Dementia (PAINAD) scale has been developed to assess pain in this population. It relies on observation of five specific items: breathing, vocalization, facial expression, body language, and consolability (Horgas & Miller, 2008). Refer to Table 35-5 for additional information regarding the PAINAD scale.

OLDER ADULTS

Assessing pain in the older adult can be challenging. Adults over the age of 65 years experience pain more frequently than do younger adults and endure moderate to severe pain for twice as long as younger adults (Eliopoulos, 2005). The Centers for Disease Control and Prevention (CDC) reported that one fifth of adults age 65 and older experienced pain persisting for more than 24 hours in the past month and three-fifths of these adults stated that the pain had lasted for 1 year or more (National Center for Health Statistics, 2006). As mentioned, many see pain in the elderly as part of the normal aging process. Because many older people have chronic disease, pain is a common occurrence.

Assessment of pain in the older adult can be problematic. Visual or hearing impairments may influence the assessment format. Multiple-drug regimens that are common in older people can also affect reliable reporting of pain. One myth held by many is that older patients have a decreased sensitivity to pain and, therefore, a heightened pain tolerance. Pain is seen by many elderly patients as a forecast of serious illness or death. Boredom, loneliness, and depression may affect an older person's perception and report of pain.

Experts agree that pain can be adequately assessed in most older adults using common rating scales. The Wong-Baker FACES Pain Rating Scale (see Fig. 35-5), recommended for pain assessment in children, may also be effective for this age group because a 0-to-5 scale is easier to use. The Numeric Rating Scale, the verbal descriptor scale, and the Faces Pain Scale-Revised (FPS-R; see Table 35-5) are additional pain rating scales that are also widely used for assessing pain in older adults (Flaherty, 2008). Special attention and consideration of an older patient's and the younger patient's pain can positively affect the nurse's ability to assess pain accurately.

Diagnosing

Pain is such a complex phenomenon that its analysis often requires multidisciplinary collaboration. Although nursing has much to offer individuals experiencing both acute and chronic pain, the data collected by the nurse during the comprehensive pain assessment benefit the patient most when shared with physicians and other members of the healthcare team.

Attempting to intervene before an accurate assessment has been completed may mask the real cause of the patient's pain and lead to false assumptions and even further progression of symptoms and the disease process. The nurse who notes a pattern of headaches in a patient and relates this to the patient's description of recent stress (divorce, relocation, new job) may erroneously assume that the headaches are merely stress related and devise and implement a plan of relaxation exercises. A more careful analysis of patient data, however, may reveal that the headaches are of vascular origin, are migraine in nature, and that medical intervention is indicated. The headaches may also be symptomatic of intracranial disease such as a brain tumor, in which case delay in diagnosis could decrease the possibility of treatment and cure.

When a nursing diagnosis of acute or chronic pain is developed, the diagnostic statement and plan of care should identify the following:

- Type of pain
- Etiologic factors, to the extent that they are known and understood
- Patient's behavioral, physiologic, and affective responses
- Other factors affecting pain stimulus, transmission, perception, and response

Pain or Chronic Pain as the Problem

Many diagnoses can be developed for pain problems. The importance of identifying these problems and including them as priorities in the plan of care cannot be overstated. See the accompanying box for examples of NANDA nursing diagnoses.

Pain or Chronic Pain as the Etiology

Because the experience of pain affects so many other aspects of human functioning, pain may be the etiology of numerous other nursing diagnosis statements, including but not limited to:

- Ineffective Airway Clearance related to postoperative incisional pain
- Anxiety related to pain anticipation and inadequate pain management in the past
- Constipation related to chronic use of narcotic analgesics
- Compromised Family Coping related to father's inability to allow family to share his pain experience
- Ineffective Coping related to failure of chronic pain management strategies to date
- Ineffective Health Maintenance related to loss of will to live secondary to prolonged chronic pain
- Hopelessness related to belief that present pain means imminent death
- Risk for Injury related to decreased pain sensation
- Deficient Knowledge: Angina Pain Management related to belief that nothing will help the pain
- Fatigue related to lack of relief from chronic pain
- Fear related to possible significance of pain
- Impaired Physical Mobility related to arthritic pain
- Imbalanced Nutrition: Less Than Body Requirements related to gastrointestinal distress
- Dressing Self-Care Deficit related to painful movement of joints
- Ineffective Sexuality Patterns related to painful intercourse
- Disturbed Sleep Pattern from inability to fall asleep related to pain's worsening at night
- Risk for Spiritual Distress related to belief that God is unfairly causing this pain as some sort of undeserved punishment
- Disturbed Thought Processes related to effects of chronic pain and overmedication
- Risk for Self-Directed Violence related to loss of will to live with unrelieved chronic pain

Outcome Identification and Planning

After the diagnosis of a pain problem is made, developing a plan of care that, when implemented, demonstrates nursing's commitment to assist the patient to develop effective pain management strategies is crucial.

Nursing measures are directed toward the achievement of the following patient outcomes for individuals whose pain is acute in nature (i.e., it is expected that with healing the pain will subside and eventually disappear). The patient will:

- Describe a gradual reduction of pain, using a scale ranging from 0 (no pain) to 10 (pain as bad as it can be)
- Demonstrate competent execution of successful pain management program (specify)

When pain or chronic pain is the etiology in nursing diagnosis statements, outcomes will be specific to the underlying interference with health that is associated with the pain.

For patients whose pain is chronic in nature, an expected outcome may be contacting a hospice or a pain clinic. Hospice care (also mentioned in Chapters 8 and 10) addresses the physical, spiritual, social, and economic needs of terminally ill patients and their families in either the home or a hospice center. Pain relief is a priority in this setting. Numerous outpatient centers are also available to support patients with chronic pain and to improve their pain management through a variety of approaches. The physician, nurse, and other members of the healthcare team collaborate to develop the optimal pain-treatment plan for each patient with chronic pain.

Implementing

After the plan of care is developed, the nurse implements the nursing strategies that are most likely to assist the patient to achieve pain relief outcomes, whether at home or in a healthcare facility. Nursing interventions described in this chapter include establishing a trusting nurse–patient relationship, manipulating factors that affect the pain experience, initiating nonpharmacologic pain relief measures, managing pharmacologic interventions, reviewing additional pain control measures, ensuring ethical and legal responsibility to relieve pain, and teaching the patient about pain See the accompanying box for Examples of Nursing Intervention and Nursing Outcome Classifications (NIC/NOC) for management of pain.

Establishing a Trusting Nurse–Patient Relationship

Most patients with pain feel better, suffer less, and experience less anxiety when they believe that a competent nurse cares about their experience of pain and is available for help and support. Without the confidence developed in a good nurse–patient relationship, nothing seems to work. With it, amazing results have been obtained by using measures that ordinarily are only modestly effective. Measures that help strengthen the nurse–patient relationship and promote pain relief include discussing pain with the patient, allowing the

Examples of NANDA Nursing Diagnoses

Pain

Nursing Diagnoses	Related Factors	Sample Defining Characteristics
Pain: Acute Postoperative	Fear of taking prescribed analgesics	• Recent cholecystectomy • Face is pale and drawn; vital signs elevated from baseline • States, "I don't like to ask for anything for pain because I know people often get addicted."
Pain: Left Leg	Fractured femur and multiple lacerations; unsuccessful attempts to determine effective analgesic	• Recent motor vehicle accident • Grimaces whenever left leg is moved • Directs abusive language to anyone who touches left leg • Refuses to have dressing changed on left leg • Reports analgesic "only takes the edge off" the pain
Pain	Prolonged labor (dystocia) and commitment to natural childbirth	• Admitted to labor unit 18 hours ago with moderate contractions 2 minutes apart • Strength of contractions weakening; progress of dilation and effacement slow; failure to progress • "I'll feel like a failure if I take anything for pain. I want to 'go natural.' I know I can do it. Besides, the drugs would only hurt my baby."
Pain: Heightened Anticipation	Child's history of undergoing frequent painful procedures	• Child diagnosed at age 3 years with acute nonlymphoid leukemia • History of bone marrow aspirations, spinal taps, platelet transfusions, chemotherapy, and other such procedures • Child "freezes" when unfamiliar healthcare worker enters room
Pain: Chest	Decreased blood supply to myocardium (angina) and fear	• "I never know when it will grab me next. I get this crushing pain in my chest and can't do anything. Usually one or two of those nitro tablets bring me relief. I'm always scared, though, that the pain won't go away."
Chronic Pain: Headaches	Inadequate pain management secondary to belief that somehow patient "deserves this pain"	• Reports history of migraine headaches for past 5 years • Never sought treatment • "My mother told me that we all get the pain in life that we deserve—goodness, I've been no saint."
Chronic Pain	Inadequate pain management of metastatic cancer involving bone	• "I can't help feeling, though, that no one is meant to live like this." • Diagnosed with cancer of bladder 2 years ago; presently metastatic spread to spine • Rates pain 10 on a scale of 1 (minimal) to 10 (greatest) • "I haven't been taking as much of this pain medicine as the doctor said I could because if I get used to it now nothing will work when the pain gets even worse later." • "When I told the nurse in the hospital about my pain she said I'd have to get used to it." • "I don't want to burden my wife and kids with my pain."
Chronic Pain	Rheumatoid arthritis and inappropriate activity during exacerbations	• Stiffness of joints, limitation of motion, heat, swelling, and tenderness • States pain is often intense after activity • "I can't accept not being able to do all I want to do for my husband and children."

Examples of Nursing Intervention and Nursing Outcome Classifications (NIC/NOC)

Pain Management

Nursing Interventions	Nursing Outcomes
• Perform a comprehensive assessment of pain to include location, characteristics, onset/duration, frequency, quality, intensity, and precipitating factors. • Consider cultural influences on pain response. • Explore with patient factors to relieve/worsen pain. • Ensure that patient receives attentive analgesic care.	• Comfort level • Symptom level • Pain level • Pain control • Patient satisfaction: symptom control

Bulechek, G., Butcher, H., & Dochterman, J. (2008). *Nursing Interventions Classification (NIC)* (5th ed., p. 532–533). St. Louis: C.V. Mosby. A full listing of nursing activities for each nursing intervention can be found in this book.
Moorhead, S., Johnson, M., Maas, M., & Swanson, E. (2008). *Nursing Outcomes Classification (NOC)* (p. 793). St. Louis: C.V. Mosby. A full listing of nursing outcomes for each nursing diagnosis can be found in this book.

patient to help choose a method of pain relief, and visiting and remaining with the patient in pain. These measures promote a collaborative relationship in which the patient's pain is treated with respect (see the accompanying box, Through the Eyes of a Patient).

Manipulating Factors Affecting the Pain Experience

There are many ways to manage pain. In addition to pharmacologic and nonpharmacologic measures, simple nursing interventions can positively alter patients' pain experience and speed their recovery.

REMOVING OR ALTERING THE CAUSE OF PAIN

Removing or altering the cause of the pain is ideal and sometimes possible. Possible measures that promote comfort and help in pain relief include removing or loosening a tight binder, if permissible; seeing to it that a distended bladder is emptied; taking steps to relieve constipation and flatus; changing body positions and ensuring correct body alignment; and changing soiled linens and dressings that may be irritating the skin. A hungry or thirsty patient may need a snack or a drink to feel more comfortable.

Certain drugs are useful for removing or altering the intensity of painful stimuli. For example, drugs that decrease smooth muscle spasms in the GI tract and those that decrease contractions of skeletal muscles reduce discomfort.

ALTERING FACTORS AFFECTING PAIN TOLERANCE

As a result of the pain assessment and the trusting relationship he or she has established, the nurse is better able to identify those factors that are increasing the patient's pain experience and decreasing his or her pain tolerance. **Pain tolerance** is the point beyond which a person is no longer willing to endure pain. These factors should be alleviated whenever possible. For example, patients whose families

Through the Eyes of a Patient

I've always thought of myself as a "take charge" kind of person. It's important for me in my business to be calm and always in control of my emotions. The "big C" changed everything for me. A recent hospitalization made me take time to think about what's happening to me.

Even in the hospital, I had a steady stream of visitors—some friends and some business associates. Even the mayor stopped by to see me! For all of them, I was my usual self—smiling, joking, and acting as if everything was normal. I made sure I took my pain medicine before they came. I kept all my fears about cancer and dying hidden behind my smiling face. I never broke down—not even in front of my wife! Men aren't supposed to cry, you know!

One nurse's simple gesture changed all that. One evening after all my visitors, my wife, and my son had left, she must have sensed something. She came over, stood next to me, put her arm around my shoulders and quietly said, "You know, Bob, it's alright to cry." It was like the dam opened up. I looked at her, my face cracked, and all of a sudden I couldn't stop sobbing. She must have known that I needed to talk about what was happening to me. I needed to say those words out loud to someone—"I'm afraid the pain will get too bad! I'm afraid of dying. I can't let my family see me this way!" She just let me cry, kept holding my hands, and just by being there and listening, helped me at that particular moment in ways that you will never know.

have never acknowledged their pain and who have repeatedly been told that their pain is all in their head may experience a greater ability to deal with their pain when someone finally takes the pain seriously. Nursing measures include communication to the patient that responses to pain are acceptable and education of the patient's family.

Fatigue tends to increase pain; therefore, promoting rest is helpful. The patient in pain usually feels more comfortable when the environment is quiet and restful. Although sensory restrictions, such as eliminating unnecessary noise and bright lights, are usually indicated, it is rarely helpful to leave the patient alone in an environment with little sensory input. The patient is then more likely to focus on self and the discomfort.

Lack of knowledge, finding no meaning in the pain, being pessimistic about its relief, and fear may also interfere with the patient's ability to deal with pain. Common fears include a loss of control and embarrassment by being unable to deal with the pain maturely. Another fear may be a fear of taking pain relief medication. The patient may view the need for medication as a sign of weakness or may fear addiction or loss of the effectiveness at a later date. Older patients, in particular, are frequently frustrated by similar concerns about pain management.

Initiating Nonpharmacologic (Complementary and Alternative) Relief Measures

Although analgesics are usually the primary treatment measure for pain, a growing trend is seen involving integration of complementary, nonpharmacologic measures with conventional medical treatment. These interventions are varied and can be practiced in all healthcare settings by most members of the healthcare team. Refer to Chapter 28 for additional discussion of complementary and alternative relief measures.

USING DISTRACTION

Conscious attention often appears to be necessary to experience pain, whereas preoccupation with other things has been observed to distract the patient from pain. Distraction requires the patient to focus attention on something other than the pain. It is not entirely clear whether distraction raises the threshold of pain or increases pain tolerance. Many patients whose pain is relieved by distraction report being able to place pain in the periphery of awareness. This is compatible with the theory that if the reticular formation in the brainstem receives sufficient sensory input, it can ignore or block out select sensations such as pain. The Lamaze method of childbirth is one common example involving the use of distraction.

Distraction alone may relieve mild pain. However, it is most effective when used before pain begins or soon thereafter. It has also been proven effective when used with analgesics for treatment of a brief episode of severe pain (e.g., pain that accompanies a diagnostic procedure). Distraction may also be used successfully with children.

Recall Xavier Mullon, the child with ulcerative colitis in severe pain. The nurse could incorporate the use of

nonpharmacologic measures for pain relief, such as distraction, to enhance the effectiveness of analgesics. ■

Techniques that distract attention include the following:

- Visual distractions: counting objects, reading, or watching TV
- Auditory distractions: listening to music
- Tactile kinesthetic distractions: holding or stroking a loved person, pet, or toy; rocking; slow rhythmic breathing
- Project distractions: playing a challenging game, performing meaningful play or work

EMPLOYING HUMOR

Humor can be an effective distraction, can help an individual cope with pain, and may even have a positive effect on the immune system. It has been proven particularly effective before painful procedures, and many pain, cancer, and ambulatory care centers encourage patients to view humorous videos before a painful, tedious procedure (Christie & Moore, 2005). Facente (2006) discussed the potential effects of laughter on a patient's ability to cope with pain and discomfort. These are highlighted in Box 35-2.

Remember to use humor only with patients who are responsive to its use and wish to use it. Humor should not be used in patients with moderate to severe pain, nor should it be a replacement for pharmacologic analgesia. In addition, humor must be patient specific. Thus, the nurse will need to determine what makes a patient laugh, how the patient has used humor or play in the past, and how it helped. Let the patient select the humorous materials, and when possible, incorporate strategies that include the patient's family and friends.

LISTENING TO MUSIC

Listening to music can relax, soothe, decrease pain, and provide distraction. By stimulating the release of endorphins, music enhances one's sense of well-being and decreases the need for pain medication. Patients can select the music they

Box 35-2 THERAPEUTIC EFFECTS OF LAUGHTER

Laughter causes the following physiological and psychological effects:
- Decreases levels of epinephrine (the stress hormone)
- Activates the immune system
- Elevates the threshold for pain and can minimize the pain sensation
- Promotes spiritual and psychological coping
- Helps one to face difficult or unpleasant procedures
- Creates a more positive atmosphere
- Increases heart rate and stimulates circulation
- Deepens respirations
- Causes muscles to contract

Adapted from Facente, A. (2006). Humor in health care: Irreverent or invaluable? Nursing, 36(4), 64hn6–7.

prefer to be used for relaxation before, during, and after surgical experiences, or to help focus on breathing techniques during labor. Some evidence has indicated that music may be effective for soothing agitated newborns and comatose patients (Cepeda, Carr, & Alvarez, 2006).

USING IMAGERY

Patients who use imagery (an example of mind–body interaction) to decrease pain sensation imagine something that involves one or all of the senses, concentrate on that image, and gradually become less aware of the pain. Imagery may be as simple as a child thinking of "happy things" (a beloved pet, lollipops, Christmas morning, Grandmom's lap), or as involved as an adult recreating a favorite place and then experiencing the healing presence or touch of a loved person or the healing energies of nature in that setting. The imagery technique has also been used to create an image in which the cause of the pain is visualized and then overcome or counteracted by some more powerful image.

Imagery has been found to be more effective for patients with chronic pain than for patients with acute, severe pain. General techniques for successfully guiding a patient to use imagery include the following:

- Help the patient to identify the problem or goal.
- Suggest that the patient begin the imagery with several minutes of focused breathing, relaxation, or meditation.
- Help the patient to develop images of the problem, as well as personal internal resources (e.g., coping strategies) and external healing therapies (e.g., medications, treatments).
- Encourage images of the desired state of well-being at the end of the session.

If the patient becomes restless or upset, the imagery experience is terminated and attempted later when the patient seems better disposed. Guided imagery is also discussed in Chapter 42.

EMPLOYING RELAXATION

Relaxation techniques reduce skeletal muscle tension and lessen anxiety. By assisting the patient with relaxation techniques, the nurse acknowledges the patient's pain and expresses a willingness to help the patient relieve the distress caused by his or her pain. The positive effects of relaxation for the person with pain include the following (LeMone & Burke, 2008):

- Improved quality of sleep
- Distraction from the pain
- Decreased fatigue
- Increased confidence and sense of self-control in coping with pain
- Lessening of the detrimental physiologic effects of continued or repeated stress from pain
- Increased effectiveness of other pain relief measures
- Improved ability to tolerate pain
- Decreased distress or fear during anticipation of pain
- Reassurance that the nurse is aware of his or her problem and wants to help

Relaxation is most effective as a pain relief measure when combined with slow, deep, easy breathing from the abdomen or diaphragm, with the patient's eyelids closed or with the individual focusing on a real or imagined fixed spot. Researchers who studied the effect of relaxation measures for pain relief have reported that progressive muscle relaxation seems to have a positive effect on arthritis pain. Support was also found for the use of jaw relaxation and systematic relaxation techniques for relieving postoperative pain (Kwekkeboom & Gretarsdottir, 2006). Relaxation techniques are also discussed in Chapters 28 and 42.

> *Consider Carla Potter, the young woman with apparent symptoms of PMS. Relaxation techniques may help her to better manage her periods of anxiety. The first step is to assess her familiarity with relaxation techniques and discuss which of these measures are adaptable to her work environment and acceptable to her.* ■

USING CUTANEOUS STIMULATION

The success of cutaneous stimulation (techniques that stimulate the skin's surface) in relieving pain is often explained using the gate control theory. The gate control theory of pain postulates that cutaneous nerve fibers are large-diameter fibers carrying impulses to the CNS. When the skin is stimulated, pain is believed to be controlled by closing the gating mechanism in the spinal cord. This decreases the number of pain impulses that reach the brain for perception. These techniques can be used in all healthcare settings to supplement a pain-control regimen. Some forms of cutaneous stimulation include the following:

- Massage (with or without analgesic ointments or liniments containing menthol); see Skill 35-1: Giving a Back Massage.
- Application of heat or cold, or both intermittently (see detailed discussion in Chapter 32)
- Acupressure
- Transcutaneous electrical nerve stimulation (TENS)

Acupressure, a modern-day Western descendant of acupuncture, involves the use of the fingertips to create gentle but firm pressure to usual acupuncture sites. This technique of holding and releasing various pressure points has a calming effect, most likely related to the body's release of endorphins and enkephalins. Acupressure is easily taught to patients and families. Because patients can perform acupressure on themselves, it gives them a feeling of control in their care.

TENS is a noninvasive alternative technique that involves electrical stimulation of large-diameter fibers to inhibit transmission of painful impulses carried over small-diameter fibers. The TENS unit consists of a battery-powered portable unit, lead wires, and cutaneous electrode pads that are applied to the painful area (Fig. 35-6). The use of TENS requires a physician's order.

TENS therapy has reportedly been effective in reducing postoperative pain and improving mobility after surgery.

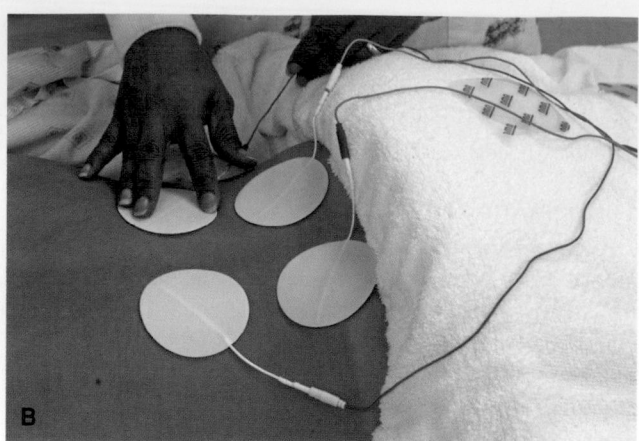

FIGURE 35-6. (**A**) TENS unit. (**B**) Applying TENS electrodes.

Positive results have also been noted when it is used as an adjunct with physical therapy and for patients with low back pain. The TENS unit may be applied intermittently throughout the day or worn for extended periods of time, depending on the physician's order.

Use of cutaneous stimulation is limited because the pain must be localized. Otherwise, it is most likely too diffuse to be effective. In addition, most individuals cannot tolerate stimulation of the painful area; they may, however, be helped by stimulation of the surrounding or contralateral area.

USING ACUPUNCTURE

Acupuncture is a technique that uses needles of various lengths inserted into specific parts of the body to produce insensitivity to pain. The technique was developed in China and has been used for centuries in many Asian countries. It has gained acceptance in the Western world as an alternative intervention to help control discomfort from disorders such as headaches, menstrual cramps, postoperative dental pain, low back pain, and carpal tunnel syndrome. The relief of pain by acupuncture is generally explained on the basis of the gate control theory. Self-hypnosis may also account for some of acupuncture's success. Repeated treatments are often needed.

Percutaneous electrical nerve stimulation (PENS) is a complementary therapy used particularly for the management of acute and chronic pain syndromes. This form of acupuncture combines the advantages of both electroacupuncture and TENS and consists of needle probes being placed into soft tissue to stimulate peripheral sensory nerves that relate to the area of injury or pain. The electrical stimulus that is delivered bypasses the skin barrier and goes directly to the involved nerve. PENS has been shown to be effective when dealing with chronic low back pain as well as diabetic neuropathy pain.

USING HYPNOSIS

Hypnosis, a technique that produces a subconscious state accomplished by suggestions made by a hypnotist, has been used successfully in many instances to control pain. The person's state of consciousness is altered by suggestions so that pain is not perceived as it normally would be. According to

many hypnotists, it also alters the physical signs of pain. Many people can be taught autohypnosis, that is, self-induced hypnosis, for the control of pain. It is generally believed that a successful response to hypnosis is related to the individual's openness to suggestion, belief that hypnosis will work, and emotional readiness.

EMPLOYING BIOFEEDBACK

Biofeedback is a technique that uses a machine to monitor physiologic responses through electrode sensors on the patient's skin. The feedback signal or unit transforms the physiologic data into a visual display. Upon seeing pain-related responses, such as increased muscle tension or elevated blood pressure, the patient is taught to regulate this physiologic response and control pain by practicing techniques such as deep-breathing exercises, progressive relaxation exercises, or visual imagery. Biofeedback decreases the individual's pain by reducing the anxiety associated with lack of control over bodily functions, distracts the person's attention from the pain to concentration on the person's inner state and the feedback signal, and reduces the cause of the pain. Eventually, the desired effect is for an individual to produce the expected effect without the use of the biofeedback machinery. Limitations of this method include the high degree of motivation needed and difficulty of maintaining control after the training program.

PROVIDING THERAPEUTIC TOUCH

Therapeutic Touch is an alternative therapy that involves using one's hands to direct an energy exchange consciously from the practitioner to the patient to facilitate healing or pain relief. It is viewed by many as a powerful adjunct to pain relief therapy. Patients who have received therapeutic touch state that it helps with feelings of comfort, calmness, and well-being. It is derived from the ancient practice of laying on of hands, but nurses skilled in Therapeutic Touch never actually touch their patients when using this technique. Therapeutic Touch was developed by nurses, does not require a physician's order, and can be used in any setting. Nurses caring for patients with terminal diseases relate that

RESEARCH IN NURSING
Bridging the Gap to Evidence-Based Practice

USING THERAPEUTIC TOUCH TO EASE A PATIENT'S PAIN

There are more than 10 million people with cancer in the United States. In addition to the pain that can accompany this diagnosis, a sense of anxiety and fear is not uncommon at varying points from diagnosis through treatment. Nurses are familiar with the traditional approaches to pain relief but complementary therapies offer nurses an additional method to ease a patient's pain and relieve the anxiety and fear that are often also present. Therapeutic Touch is a complementary nonpharmacological approach to pain relief for cancer patients.

Related Research

Jackson, E., Kelley, M., McNeil, P., Meyer, E., Schlegel, L., & Eaton, M. (2008). Does therapeutic touch help reduce pain and anxiety in patients with cancer? *Clinical Journal of Oncology Nursing, 12*(1), 113–120.

Therapeutic Touch was introduced in the early 1970s and involves the use of the hands to balance the body's energy flow, thus promoting healing. The authors used 12 research studies to review and analyze evidence regarding the effectiveness of Therapeutic Touch to relieve pain and anxiety in cancer patients. Research in this field is limited but the authors included only higher-level evidence-based research in their review. One group of researchers concluded that Therapeutic Touch was a "promising therapy" to relieve cancer pain but that evidence, at this point, is not conclusive enough to recommend it as an effective therapy for this disease. Four studies confirmed that Therapeutic Touch did improve physical and psychological symptoms as evidenced by increased sense of

well-being, improvements in pain and anxiety, and reductions in heart rate, respiratory rate, and blood pressure. In these research studies, experimental groups where patients received Therapeutic Touch therapy demonstrated improvements in anxiety, mood, fatigue, and pain versus the results seen in the control groups. One study concluded that experienced practitioners achieved better results and were more effective using Therapeutic Touch to relieve pain and anxiety. The authors of this article concluded after their review that Therapeutic Touch is effective as a treatment modality to relieve cancer pain and anxiety. More research is needed, especially since this is a nontraditional approach to pain relief.

Relevance to Nursing Practice

As nurse researchers gather data and information related to Therapeutic Touch, it is also important to educate patients about nonpharmacologic therapies that complement traditional approaches. Patients, obviously, have to be open to the use of Therapeutic Touch. Not all healthcare practitioners are aware of the potential benefits of Therapeutic Touch and other complementary therapies. Continuing education programs should consider this topic for programs for registered nurses. Since research continues to confirm that Therapeutic Touch is an effective pain relief measure and the role of nursing is holistic, undergraduate nursing programs should also consider curricular content on Therapeutic Touch and complementary measures to relieve pain.

For additional research, visit thePoint.

therapeutic touch complements their efforts to alleviate suffering and can be used to promote comfort during the final stages of life. Refer to the accompanying Nursing Research box for a discussion of the effectiveness of Therapeutic Touch in easing cancer patients' pain.

Managing Pharmacologic Relief Measures

Whether pain is acute or chronic, measures exist to control most pain experiences. However, many misconceptions still exist about pain relief, and because of this, many people still receive inadequate pain treatment and suffer needlessly. To make informed decisions and individualize care, nurses need updated information and ongoing education about drug therapy, the cornerstone of many pain-treatment regimens.

ADMINISTERING ANALGESICS

An **analgesic** is a pharmaceutical agent that relieves pain. Analgesics function to reduce the person's perception of pain and to alter the person's responses to discomfort. There are three general classes of drugs used for pain relief:

- Nonopioid analgesics (acetaminophen and nonsteroidal anti-inflammatory drugs [NSAIDs])

- **Opioid** analgesics (all controlled substances; e.g., morphine, codeine, meperidine, hydromorphone, methadone)
- Adjuvant drugs (anticonvulsants, antidepressants, multipurpose drugs)

The nurse administering analgesics needs to combine a healthy respect for the drug being administered with a thorough knowledge of its mechanism of action, side effects, and administration guidelines. This combination of knowledge of and respect for the drug should result in analgesics being used wisely to produce their desired effect.

Knowledge of common analgesics enables the nurse to tailor the patient's regimen and communicate professionally with physicians about a patient who is being undermedicated or who needs a different drug or route of administration. Nurses should not refrain from using analgesics or reduce their doses because of an unrealistic fear of their potency and side effects.

Repeated studies have confirmed improvement in pain assessment and documentation but not in pain relief. Pain is still undertreated and frequently unrelieved. Physician, nurse, and patient variables all contribute to this situation. Physicians often prescribe insufficient analgesic doses because of a tendency to overestimate the efficacy and duration of analgesics, underestimate the pain experience, and worry excessively about the possibility of respiratory problems and addiction. Nurses, who ideally spend the most time with the patient and who are supposed experts in human responses (e.g., the response to pain), often compound this problem by further reducing the insufficient analgesic dose or by not administering the medication at all. Nurse variables include the low priority given to pain management, arbitrary pain assessments and erroneous judgments about a patient's pain and need for analgesia, and fear of being the person who administers the drug that causes respiratory depression or another serious side effect. According to Pasero, Manworren, and McCaffery (2007), healthcare providers need to be held accountable for their failure to provide optimum pain relief for all individuals. The inability of many patients to discuss their pain and to request pain assistance perpetuates this problem.

Opioid Analgesics

Opioids, formerly called narcotic analgesics, are generally considered the major class of analgesics used in the management of moderate to severe pain because of their effectiveness. In sufficient dosage, they are considered capable of relieving pain of virtually every nature. Opioids produce analgesia by attaching to opioid receptors in the brain. New research on pain management has indicated that a person's response to opioids may be affected by individual differences in opioid binding sites. Enzymes that promote binding at a site may be missing meaning that less of the particular opioid will bind to the site and be activated. This is referred to as opioid polymorphism and may explain why responses vary to specific opioid medication (D'Arcy, 2008c).

Morphine, the prototype opioid, is available in multiple dosage forms, has a fairly predictable action, and is relatively inexpensive. The most common side effects associated with opioid use are sedation, nausea, and constipation. Most side effects disappear with prolonged use, but if constipation persists, it usually responds to treatment with increased fluids and fiber and use of a mild laxative or stool softener.

Respiratory depression is a commonly feared side effect of opioid use. In reality, it is an uncommon occurrence in long-term therapy because patients have usually developed a tolerance to the drug and its respiratory depressant effects. If respiratory depression is suspected, it is usually preceded by sedation. Nursing assessment using the numeric sedation scale can determine those patients at risk for respiratory depression (McCaffery & Pasero, 1999). The numeric sedation scale is as follows:

- 1 = awake and alert; no action necessary
- 2 = occasionally drowsy but easy to arouse; requires no action
- 3 = frequently drowsy and drifts off to sleep during conversation; decrease the opioid dose
- 4 = somnolent with minimal or no response to stimuli; discontinue the opioid and consider use of naloxone

If respiratory depression is suspected and the opioid dose is withheld, the patient may be physically stimulated by shaking or using a loud sound, along with reminders every few minutes to breathe deeply. If this is ineffective, naloxone (Narcan), an opioid antagonist that reverses the respiratory-depressant effect of an opioid, can be used. Naloxone is administered intravenously at a very slow rate. Within 1 to 2 minutes, the patient usually opens his or her eyes and is able to respond to the nurse. When the patient is alert again and the respiratory rate is greater than 9 breaths/min, the opioid may be resumed.

Many myths and irrational fears persist concerning the use of opioid analgesics. Patients and caregivers cite fear of addiction as a reason for ineffective treatment of pain. Because of this, nurses are concerned about administering prescribed doses of opioids, physicians underprescribe pain medication, and patients refuse or take less than prescribed doses of the drugs. Physical dependence and tolerance are frequently confused with addiction. **Physical dependence** is a phenomenon in which the body physiologically becomes accustomed to the opioid and suffers withdrawal symptoms if the opioid is suddenly removed or the dose is rapidly decreased. **Tolerance** occurs when the body becomes accustomed to the opioid and needs a larger dose each time for pain relief. **Addiction** is a pattern of compulsive opioid use for means other than pain control. According to D'Arcy (2007c), the four characteristics that define addiction are a craving for the substance, compulsive use, lack of control over the drug, and continued use despite harm. Less than 1% of patients with pain become addicted to opioids, yet many nurses surveyed seriously overestimated the likelihood of addiction when opioids are used for pain relief. In reality, physical dependence and tolerance are expected responses; patients treated with opioids for pain rarely develop addiction (D'Arcy, 2007c). The tolerance and physical dependence that can occur after 4 weeks of regular opioid use and result in a decrease in analgesic effect can be treated by increasing the dose until pain control is again apparent.

When individuals report that pain is present, research confirms that each patient's expression and self-report of pain are unique even if they have the same degree of pain. McCaffery, Pasero, and Ferrell (2007) list important factors to consider when administering an opioid analgesic. These include:

- the patient's pain rating
- the sedation level
- the patient's comfort-function goal (the pain rating that allows a patient to perform necessary or desired activities)

Continuous intravenous infusion of opioids has proved effective for the relief of acute postoperative pain. In 2004, the American Society for Pain Management recommended the development of guidelines for the practice of using range orders to administer IV opioids to patients in acute pain. Pasero, Manworren, and McCaffery (2007) define a range order as "a medication order in which the dosage or time period or both are specified according to a range . . . depending on the patient's pain level and condition." An example of a range order is: Morphine 2 to 8 mg IV every 2 hours as needed for pain.

Controversy and confusion exist regarding the use of these range orders for the delivery of IV opioids. The Joint Commission now includes an accreditation criterion stating that hospitals must have a clear policy regarding range orders but hospitals are struggling with establishing the protocols and defining exactly how nurses should interpret these orders. However, if hospitals have a clear protocol regarding range orders, nurses have the opportunity to address each patient's individual pain experience while protecting against adverse effects. Although there are many parameters to consider, ultimately, a nurse requires excellent assessment skills and good clinical judgment to use range orders safely and effectively.

Nonopioid Analgesics

Nonopioid analgesics, such as acetaminophen and nonsteroidal anti-inflammatory drugs (NSAIDs), are usually the drugs of choice for mild to moderate pain. The simplest dosage schedules and least invasive pain management modalities should be used first. Many times, these drugs alone can provide adequate pain relief. Many of these medications are over-the-counter (OTC) products, whereas some are available by prescription only. Some can cause gastric side effects, but these symptoms may be preventable if the drug is taken with food or antacids.

NSAIDs also have an anti-inflammatory effect. Individual responses to the NSAIDs vary, but these agents are contraindicated in patients with bleeding disorders (their action may interfere with platelet function) or probable infections (NSAIDs can mask the signs of an infection). An FDA advisory committee has recommended that the labels on all NSAIDs warn the consumer about the potential for gastric bleeding if certain risk factors are present and the caution that NSAIDs should be taken for the shortest times needed. The combination of nonopioid analgesics and opioids provides more analgesia than either drug taken alone.

The COX-2 inhibitors, a class of NSAIDs, have a lower risk of gastrointestinal bleeding but are thought to significantly increase cardiovascular risks. Two of the COX-2 inhibitors, rofecoxib (Vioxx) and valdecoxib (Bextra), have been withdrawn from the market because of increased evidence of adverse cardiac events. Celecoxib (Celebrex), another COX-2 inhibitor, is available in the United States and used for treatment of osteoarthritis and rheumatoid arthritis (Flasar & Wentz, 2006). The recommendation is that NSAIDs appear to be safe in low doses for short periods of time.

Adjuvant Drugs

Adjuvant drugs are typically used for other purposes but are also used to enhance the effect of opioids by providing additional pain relief. They may also reduce side effects from prescribed opioids or lessen anxiety about the pain experi-

ence. Research has indicated that antidepressants and anticonvulsants are also effective for neuropathic pain (Keller, 2006).

APPLYING GENERAL PRINCIPLES FOR ANALGESIC ADMINISTRATION

When using medications for pain relief, the nurse must first assess the patient's pain and understand the patient's goals for pain relief. In the home as well as in acute care settings, nurses provide quality nursing care when they empower patients to take charge of their own pain relief measures. The following guidelines are recommended for effective, individualized pain management in any setting:

- Review the pain scale of choice thoroughly.
- Discuss the benefits of using a pain scale.
- Try various pain control measures.
- Use pain control measures before pain increases in severity.
- Ask the patient what has proved effective for pain relief in the past.
- Select and modify pain control measures based on the patient's response.
- Encourage the patient to try the pain treatment several times before labeling it ineffective.
- Be open-minded about alternative pain relief strategies.
- Be persistent.
- Be a safe practitioner.

Various organizations and groups have made recommendations for pain control in a variety of settings. These include the American Pain Society, the American Society for Pain Management Nursing, the National Institutes of Health Pain Consortium, and the American Nurses Association. The revised Joint Commission standards ensure that pain management is a quality-assurance issue in healthcare agencies (TJC, 2008b).

In the home, oral morphine is still the drug of choice to control chronic pain and to control moderate severe acute pain. This method is less expensive and easy to administer, but requires that the patient is able to swallow and retain food and fluids.

Accurate documentation is imperative to determine effectiveness of the current regimen or the need to change pain control measures if relief is not obtained. Pain diaries provide a method for individuals to document their particular pain experience, list medication or alternative therapies that were used to treat the pain, and record their effectiveness (Aguirre, Nevidjon, & Clemens, 2008). Attempts to recall particular aspects of a painful experience are not always accurate. Pain diaries can be used in a variety of settings and help improve the overall management of pain. Effective patient and family teaching is the cornerstone of pain relief therapy in the home.

Ongoing Assessment

Just as the pain experience of each patient is unique, so too is the response of each patient to a prescribed analgesic.

The nurse continually needs to evaluate whether the medication is producing the desired analgesic effect; identify changes in the patient's condition (correction or worsening of pathology, increased drug tolerance) that necessitate changes in the analgesic agent, dose, or route of administration; and identify the development of side effects of the analgesic that may warrant its discontinuance. As long as the patient's pain exists, ongoing assessment and documentation of pain control is imperative. Fundamental to this assessment is the knowledge of the basic action, doses, and routes of administration; side effects; and administration guidelines of the analgesic being administered.

Timing is an important consideration when administering analgesics. To time analgesics appropriately, know the average duration of action for the drug and time administration so that the peak analgesic effect occurs when the pain is expected to be most intense. For example, an analgesic would be offered before ambulating a patient postoperatively.

A p.r.n. (as needed) drug regimen has not been proven effective for people experiencing acute pain. In the early postoperative period, when pain is expected, this protocol may result in an intense pain experience for the patient. Later, however, in the postoperative course, a p.r.n. schedule may be acceptable to relieve occasional pain episodes. Continuous intravenous infusion has proved effective for the relief of acute postoperative pain. Patient-controlled analgesia and epidural analgesia are discussed later in the chapter.

The p.r.n. protocol is totally inadequate for patients experiencing chronic pain. Regular administration of analgesics, or around-the-clock (ATC) administration (at regularly scheduled intervals), has been shown to offer superior pain management for chronic cancer pain. Long-acting controlled-release oral morphine or oxycodone or use of a fentanyl patch have been proven effective for this type of pain. The FDA issued its second warning regarding safe use of the fentanyl patch. It is intended for use in patients who are opioid-tolerant and have chronic pain; it should not be used to treat acute pain. Patients need instruction to apply the patch according to the time interval prescribed, avoid the application of heat in areas where the patch is in place, and dispose of used patches appropriately (U.S. Food and Drug Administration, 2010).

Management of Breakthrough Pain

Breakthrough pain (BTP) is a temporary flare-up of moderate to severe pain that occurs even when the patient is taking ATC medication for persistent pain. This pain is often not diagnosed correctly and is frequently undertreated. Breakthrough pain can be classified as incident pain (e.g., pain caused by movement), idiopathic (spontaneous pain due to an unknown cause), or end-of-dose pain, where the pain occurs before the next dose of analgesic is due. Although it usually occurs in patients with chronic pain, it can occur in acute situations, such as a patient with postoperative pain. Incident BTP is treated more effectively with supplemental doses of a short-acting opioid

taken on a p.r.n. or "as needed" basis, rather than with an increase in the dose of the ATC medication or shortening of the interval between doses, which typically is more effective with end-of-dose pain. However, the treatment for idiopathic BTP is more difficult and usually requires adjustment of the dose and dosing interval to relieve this pain. Effective management of BTP requires a medication with rapid onset and short duration of effect (Prommer, 2009).

USING ACUTE PAIN MANAGEMENT TREATMENT REGIMENS

As a patient's advocate, ensure that a strong emphasis is placed on the need for aggressive, individualized strategies that can minimize or eliminate acute pain and promote positive patient outcomes. Preventing pain is easier than treating it once it has occurred. Discuss pain control options with patients before surgery, and address the patient's responsibility regarding reporting pain. Additional nursing interventions that can eliminate acute postoperative pain include maintaining a steady serum level of the analgesic (PCA or epidural analgesia can help here), treating side effects quickly and aggressively, encouraging use of nonpharmacologic complementary therapies as adjuncts to the medical regimen, and expecting incident pain and dealing with it.

Undertreatment of pain that accompanies procedures, whether performed in a hospital, home, or outpatient clinic, is a common occurrence. If there is any doubt about the likelihood of pain resulting from a procedure, analgesia should be provided. In situations where the patient is unable to report the presence of pain (e.g., an unconscious patient), the nurse needs to consider pain relief if a procedure is planned that normally elicits a complaint of pain. This could include turning a patient or a dressing change. In this case, the acronym APP (assume pain present) should be documented (Pasero, 2007). In some instances, for example, if the patient is unable to communicate verbally but capable of some response, it may be necessary to provide a method for the patient to indicate that pain is occurring during a procedure. The simple raising of a finger or hand or squeeze of a squeak toy can alert the caregiver that analgesia is needed.

Multiple studies have reported that racial differences exist when opioids are prescribed for pain control. Black and Hispanic patients were 8% less likely than white patients to receive opioids for treatment of acute pain (McCarberg, 2008; Mennick, 2008). Gender can also be a factor. For example, a study reported that a group of physicians in one study were more likely to prescribe optimal pain medication for men versus woman following surgery (McCarberg, 2008).

EMPLOYING CANCER OR CHRONIC PAIN MANAGEMENT TREATMENT REGIMENS

Individuals with cancer sometimes suffer needlessly from pain. This pain, surprisingly, remains undertreated in both children and adults, and nurses need to act as advocates for pain relief for these patients. The major principles that guide treatment for cancer or chronic pain include:

- Giving medications orally, if possible.
- Administering medication ATC rather than on a p.r.n. basis.
- Adjusting the dose to achieve maximum benefits with minimal side effects.
- Allowing patients as much control as possible over their medication regimen.

Recently, opioid contracts are being used in settings where patients with chronic pain are treated. These written agreements document the person's informed consent, define treatment goals, and outline the risks and goals associated with opioid therapy (D'Arcy, 2008c). They are not legally binding but encourage patients to follow prescribed protocols.

In an effort to alleviate unnecessary pain and suffering, the World Health Organization (WHO) devised a three-step analgesic ladder (Fig. 35-7) that recommends the appropriate progression of drugs and dosages that should be used to manage chronic pain effectively. Emphasis is on individualizing treatment and using the analgesic ladder to provide attentive, aggressive pain relief. The effectiveness of the WHO analgesic ladder is widely acknowledged, and this regimen provides relief to 70% to 90% of patients with cancer pain. Some clinicians have suggested that the WHO three-step analgesic ladder may require some adjustment based on the clinical experience that has occurred in the 20 years since the ladder was proposed. The 10% to 30% of patients with severe pain who do not obtain satisfactory pain relief using this guideline may require alternative routes of drug administration, nerve blocks, or other invasive procedures to relieve their pain. Study continues in an effort to

provide the data needed to effect a change or adjustment if one is justified in the WHO analgesic ladder (Time to modify the WHO analgesic ladder?, 2005).

PROVIDING PAIN TREATMENT IN SPECIAL POPULATIONS

Children and older adults need accurate assessment and treatment of pain. Their behavioral indicators of pain are unique and this necessitates special approaches to determine the presence and level of pain as well as individualized techniques to relieve the pain.

Children

Effective pain management in children requires careful assessment; good communication among patient, family, and caregivers; and a thorough understanding of the actions and side effects of drugs used to relieve pain. The child is still the best source of information about the pain, and various assessment tools mentioned previously help to measure the intensity of the pain.

> ➤ *Remember Xavier Malton, the child with ulcerative colitis in acute pain? The nurse needs to assess Xavier continually for effectiveness of the prescribed analgesic and request changes in any orders if the analgesic is not effective. Considering Xavier's current state, suggesting that the physician change the analgesic administration from p.r.n. dosing to around-the-clock dosing may be appropriate for a short period of time.* ■

In postoperative situations, children need analgesics ATC or by continuous infusion. Opioids are the drug of choice for moderate to severe pain. Pain management for cancer pain or chronic pain in children follows the prescription outlined in the WHO analgesic ladder. Withholding opioid drugs from children with cancer because of fear of addiction is unjustified because current knowledge does not indicate they are vulnerable to this problem.

Children also require pain management to minimize or alleviate the pain and distress associated with some procedures. The misconception persists that children experience pain differently; if a procedure is painful for an adult, then it is also painful for a child (Puchalski, 2008). Adequate education before the procedure and using drug and nondrug therapies to complement each other can take the pain and fear out of the experience. This is especially important for children with a chronic disease who must undergo multiple procedures as part of the treatment regimen.

Older Adults

Little research exists about pain management in older adults. Persistent or chronic pain is a common occurrence in older adults living in the community as well as residents of long-term care facilities. Many healthcare providers, and older individuals as well, expect that pain is a natural outcome

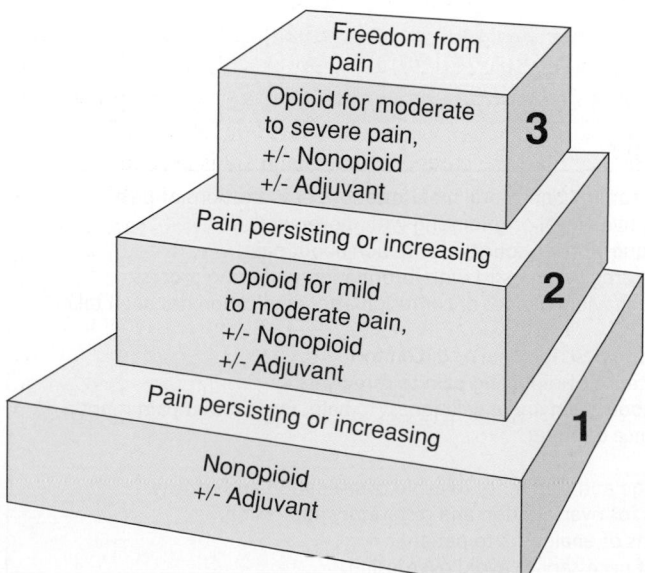

FIGURE 35-7. The WHO three-step pain relief ladder. (© World Health Organization. Redrawn with permission.)

of the aging process. As stated previously, pain is routinely undertreated in this population. Recommendations for analgesic administration for older adults include the following:

- Acetaminophen may be used cautiously for mild to moderate pain. NSAIDs have the potential for renal and gastric complications and a proton pump inhibitor should also be prescribed (D'Arcy, 2009).
- Administer medications, if possible, via the oral route.
- Use IM and IV analgesics cautiously because decreased circulation poses a risk for reduced absorption of opioids (Lilley, Harrington, & Snyder, 2007).

Opioid drugs can be used safely for older adult patients as long as appropriate precautions are taken, pain is conscientiously assessed, and potential side effects are monitored. Dosage and dosing intervals should be adjusted for the older adult based on therapeutic response to the drug and the presence of adverse effects. The accompanying Focus on the Older Adult box describes additional strategies pertinent to this age group.

ADMINISTERING ANALGESICS BY OTHER METHODS

In addition to the variety of drugs used to treat pain, multiple options exist for drug delivery systems. Patient-controlled analgesia, epidural analgesia, and other advanced interventions have improved pain management and the quality of life for many individuals.

Patient-Controlled Analgesia

Patient-controlled analgesia (PCA) provides effective individualized analgesia and comfort (Figure 35-8). This

FIGURE 35-8. A patient-controlled analgesia unit allows the patient to regulate the intravenous infusion of small amounts of analgesic as needed.

method of analgesia therapy may be used to manage acute and chronic pain in a healthcare facility or the home. PCA effectively relieves pain associated with operative procedures, labor and delivery, trauma situations, and cancer. This device is most commonly used to deliver analgesics intravenously or via the epidural route. The most frequently prescribed drugs for PCA administration are morphine, fentanyl, and hydromorphone.

The PCA system consists of a computerized portable infusion pump containing a chamber for a bag or syringe that is prefilled with the prescribed opioid analgesic. Both the Joint Commission (JC) and the Institute for Safe Medication Practices (ISMP) recommend standard doses and concentrations

FOCUS ON THE OLDER ADULT

NURSING STRATEGIES TO ADDRESS PHYSIOLOGIC CHANGES AFFECTING COMFORT

Age-Related Changes	Nursing Strategies
Communication Difficulties	• Observe carefully for any behavioral manifestations or indications of pain (e.g., change in activity level or grimacing with movement). • Use open-ended questions to solicit information about pain. • Rely on family or caregiver to assist with information-gathering process. • Monitor for any behavior changes or confusion after medication has been taken.
Denial of Pain	• Clarify terms used to describe pain or discomfort. • Emphasize importance of reporting pain to caregivers. • Express concern about pain and a willingness to help. Explain that pain is not a normal consequence of aging.
Altered Physiologic Response to Analgesics	• Be aware of dosage and frequency to avoid oversedation and toxicity. • Monitor carefully for oversedation and respiratory depression. • Explain side effects of analgesics to patient. • Use memory aid if necessary to avoid overdosing. • Discourage self-medication. • Caution about use of alcohol with analgesics. • Caution about driving or operating machinery when taking analgesics.

prepared in prefilled syringes and bags (D'Arcy, 2008b). Initially, a loading dose is administered to raise blood levels to a therapeutic level and control the pain. When the sensation of pain reoccurs, the patient pushes a button that activates the PCA device to deliver a small preset bolus dose of the analgesic. A dose interval that is programmed into the PCA unit (usually, 6–8 minutes) prevents reactivation of the pump and administration of another dose during that period of time. The pump mechanism can also be programmed to deliver only a specified amount of analgesic within a given time interval (the lock-out interval). This is most commonly every hour or, occasionally, every 4 hours. The 4-hour lock-out is not viewed as favorably now because the shorter interval allows for closer monitoring of pain relief (D'Arcy, 2008b). These safeguards limit the possibility of possible overmedication. In addition, time is provided for the patient to evaluate the effect of the previous dose. PCA pumps also have a locked safety system that prohibits any tampering with the device.

The proper selection of patients for PCA analgesia is vital for a positive experience. Suitable candidates for this type of delivery system include individuals who are alert and capable of controlling the unit. The Joint Commission and ISMP both identify individuals who are not recommended for this type of pain relief. These include confused elderly patients, infants and very young children, any cognitively impaired patient, those with conditions where oversedation poses a significant risk (e.g., asthma and sleep apnea), and patients who are taking other medications that potentiate opioids (D'Arcy, 2007b).

PCA has many advantages:

- Consistent analgesic blood level is maintained rather than the inconsistent analgesia obtained with periodic intramuscular injections, which results in sharp rises and falls of serum opioid levels.
- The analgesic is delivered intravenously or epidurally so that absorption is faster and more predictable than with the intramuscular route.
- The patient is in charge of the pain management program.
- The patient tends to use less medication because it is self-administered before the pain becomes too severe.
- The patient is able to ambulate earlier, which promotes less pulmonary complications.
- The patient is more satisfied and has improved pain relief.

PCA by proxy, which means that someone other than the patient activates the pump, continues to be a controversial issue. Unauthorized family members or caregivers (instead of the patient) who administer PCA by pushing the dosage button can cause serious analgesic overdoses resulting in oversedation, respiratory depression, and death. Some clinicians argue that in a pediatric setting, Nurse-Controlled Analgesia or Caregiver Controlled Analgesia is appropriate (Wuhrman et al., 2006). For this to be safe, rigid agency protocols need to be in place. The Joint Commission has issued a Sentinel Event Alert on patient-controlled analgesia and does not recommend PCA by proxy (D'Arcy, 2007b). It also

recommends that warning labels stating, "Only the patient should press this button" be attached to PCA pumps (Pasero & McCaffery, 2005). Refer to Chapter 26 for a discussion of Sentinel Event Alerts. The Joint Commission also advises that caregivers need to carefully monitor patients for respiratory depression using pulse oximetry and capnography (measurement of carbon dioxide concentrations) as appropriate. The carbon dioxide level in a patient's expirations can be measured by a sensor contained in a mask or nasal cannula that the patient is wearing. This provides a more reliable measure of impending respiratory depression (D'Arcy, 2007b).

Setting up the PCA system and ensuring that it is functioning properly are nursing responsibilities. Improper programming of the pump is the most common human error associated with this therapy. Both the Joint Commission and the ISMP recommend that another nurse checks the patient ID, drug dose and concentrations, PCA pump settings, and the infusion tubing and site prior to the initiation of PCA (D'Arcy, 2008b).

> *Recall Sheree Lincoln, the postoperative woman who is to use PCA system for pain control. Two hours after surgery, the patient is complaining of pain but has not used the PCA system. The nurse would need to determine the underlying reasons for not using the device. This assessment would include investigation of Sheree's knowledge base and what, if any, teaching she received preoperatively. For example, Sheree may have received teaching on how to use PCA but not have understood when or why to use it. Possibly she may be wanting to avoid use of any medication. The nurse would use this opportunity to reinforce instructions for using PCA and also for other nonpharmacologic measures for pain relief such as distraction, relaxation, massage, or imagery.* ■

Newer patient-controlled analgesia devices include a transdermal system that allows patients to self-administer doses of fentanyl over 24 hours for moderate to severe postoperative pain, the On-Q C-bloc system, and a Medication on Demand oral PCA device. The fentanyl iontophoretic transdermal system (ITS) is the size of a credit card, has adhesive backing, and is attached to the patient's upper arm or chest. The patient presses a button and the medication is delivered through the skin via a low-intensity direct current. Studies have indicated that pain control with this device is good to excellent (D'Arcy, 2007d). The On-Q C-bloc system delivers a local anesthetic through a small ball connected to a catheter that is placed near an incision or nerve close to a surgical site. Patients can press a button to deliver additional doses of the local anesthetic while the catheter delivers a continuous dose that helps to prevent breakthrough pain (Gevirtz, 2010). The Medication on Demand (MOD) device is an oral PCA device attached to an IV pole and requires that the patient wear a "radio frequency identification" wristband that allows access to the MOD. In order to receive a dose of medication, the patient records his level of pain, swipes his wristband over the device, and removes a single dose once the drawer is opened. The interval between medication doses is programmed into the MOD as per the physician's order. When this lock-out interval has passed, a green "ready light" appears on the device. Increased patient satisfaction is an expected outcome with MOD (Stett, 2010).

Epidural Analgesia

Epidural analgesia can be used to provide pain relief during the immediate postoperative phase (particularly after thoracic, abdominal, orthopedic, and vascular surgery) and for chronic pain situations. Epidural pain management is also being used for children with terminal cancer and for children undergoing hip, spinal, or lower extremity surgery. It is contraindicated if the patient is unable to give an informed consent, takes systemic anticoagulants, or has a history of long-term use of aspirin products or NSAIDs (Schwartz, 2006). The anesthesiologist usually inserts the catheter in the midlumbar region into the epidural space between the walls of the vertebral canal and the dura mater or outermost connective tissue membrane surrounding the spinal cord. For temporary therapy, the catheter exits directly over the spine, and the tubing is positioned over the patient's shoulder, with the end of the catheter taped to the person's chest. For long-term therapy, the catheter is usually tunneled subcutaneously and exits on the side of the body or on the abdomen (Fig. 35-9).

The narcotic or opioid acts directly on the opiate receptors in the spinal cord, and pain relief is achieved with smaller doses and less severe side effects. The epidural analgesia can be administered as a bolus dose (either one time or intermittent) via a continuous infusion pump, or by means of a patient-controlled epidural analgesia (PCEA) pump (Schwartz, 2006). The drug of choice is usually preservative-free morphine or fentanyl. Because the epidural space contains blood vessels, nerves, and fat, lipid-soluble fentanyl is readily dissolved and has a rapid onset of action (5 minutes) but a short duration of action (approximately 2 hours). Morphine is a hydrophilic opioid, meaning that this drug has a high affinity for water. It has a slower onset of action but may exert its analgesic effect for as long as 24 hours because it remains longer in the cerebrospinal fluid (CSF) and spinal tissue (Pasero, 2003). Epidural catheters used for the management of acute pain are typically removed between 36 and 72 hours after surgery, when oral medication can be substituted for relief of pain.

Nursing responsibilities vary among institutions but must include careful monitoring of the patient's response to therapy, with particular attention to the respiratory rate and pattern (Guidelines for Nursing Care 35-1). Too much narcotic or a displaced catheter may allow the medication to have a depressant effect on the brainstem center, causing life-threatening respiratory depression. Other potential side

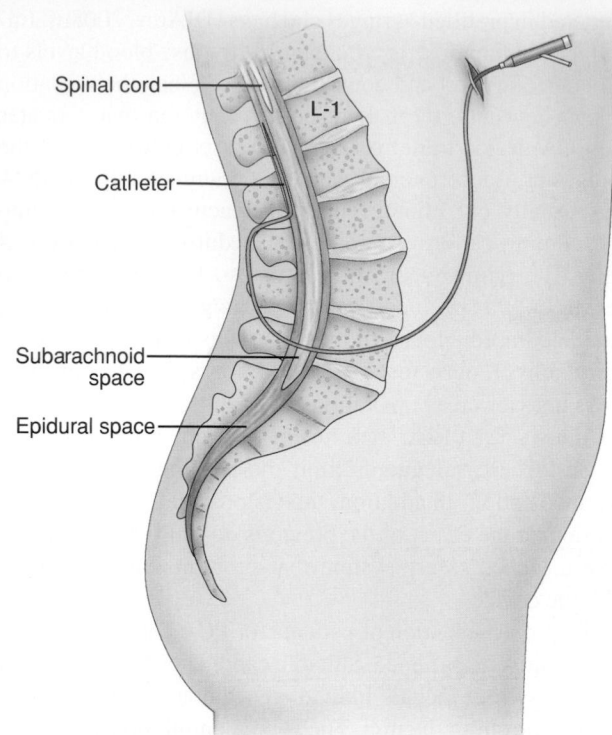

FIGURE 35-9. Placement of an epidural catheter for long-term use.

effects include hypotension, pruritus, urinary retention, nausea and vomiting, and infection or contamination.

Local Anesthesia

Anesthetic agents may be applied topically to the skin or mucous membranes or injected into the body to produce a temporary loss of sensation and motor and autonomic function in a localized area. The agents work by chemically blocking the nerve pathways involved in pain sensation and response and are sometimes called nerve blocks. Many people have experienced nerve blocks during dental work, when having a wound sutured, during delivery of a newborn, or for some minor surgical procedures. Nursing measures include noting any allergic responses the patient has had in the past to anesthetic agents, alerting the patient to the pain associated with the initial injection of the anesthetic if the physician does not numb the area first, offering emotional support to the patient during the procedure, observing for any untoward effects, and protecting the patient from injury until sensory and motor functions return. Two topical anesthetic creams (EMLA, which contains 2.5% lidocaine and 2.5% prilocaine, and ELA-Max, a 4%-lidocaine cream) provide safe, effective analgesia for children before painful procedures such as phlebotomy, lumbar puncture, or bone marrow aspiration. EMLA cream is prescribed by the physician and must be covered by an occlusive dressing for at least 1 hour before the procedure to provide local pain relief. After the time period, the cream is removed. ELA-MAX is an OTC preparation that takes effect in 30 minutes or less (Pillitteri, 2007).

Guidelines for Nursing Care • 35-1

CARING FOR PATIENTS RECEIVING EPIDURAL OPIOIDS

Nursing Action	Rationale
Verify the physician's order for analgesia, drug preparation, and rate of infusion with another RN.	Verification provides for safe administration of the correct dose at the correct rate.
Keep an ampule of 0.4 mg of naloxone (Narcan) and a syringe at the bedside.	Naloxone reverses the respiratory depressant effect of opioids.
Label tubing and pump apparatus "For Epidural Infusion Only."	Labeling prevents inadvertent administration of other intravenous medications through this setup.
Assess and record sedation level (using a sedation scale) and respiratory status, including pulse oximetry, q1h for the first 24 hours followed by q4h intervals (or according to agency policy). Notify MD for the following: sedation rating of 3, ↓ in depth and respiratory rate below 8 breaths/min.	Opioids can depress respiratory center in the medulla. Change in level of consciousness is usually the first sign of altered respiratory function.
Keep head of bed elevated 30 degrees unless this is contraindicated.	Elevation of the patient's head minimizes upward migration of opioid in the spinal cord, thus decreasing risk for respiratory depression.
Record level of pain and effectiveness of pain relief.	Referencing helps in determining need for subsequent "breakthrough" pain medication.
Monitor urinary output and assess for bladder distention.	Opioids can cause urinary retention.
Assess motor strength q4h.	Catheter may migrate into the intrathecal space and allow opioids to block transmission of nerve impulses completely through the spinal cord to the brain.
Monitor for side effects (pruritus, nausea, vomiting).	Opioids may spread into the trigeminal nerve causing itching or result in nausea and vomiting due to slowed gastrointestinal function or stimulation of a chemoreceptor trigger zone in the brain. Medications are available to treat these side effects.
Assess for signs of infection at the insertion site.	Inflammation or local infection may develop at the catheter insertion site. Strict aseptic technique and sterile dressing and tubing changes according to agency policy can prevent this complication.
Do not administer any other narcotics or adjuvant drugs without approval of clinician responsible for epidural injection.	Additional medication may potentiate the action of the opioid, thus increasing the risk for respiratory depression.

Teaching the Patient and Family About Pain

Often, a well-informed person can cope better with the distress of pain and tends to experience less anxiety about pain. See the Promoting Health Literacy box for suggestions regarding communicating with your healthcare practitioner to ensure improved outcomes related to pain management.

Teaching about pain should include family members so that they understand the concept of pain and are able to help the person in pain. The patient and family need information about the nature and causes of pain, explanation about a pain scale that can be used easily, practice with this assessment tool, and assistance to set goals for comfort and either optimal function or recovery. Teaching Tips 35-1 includes specific suggestions related to safety concerns about pain control in the home setting. In addition, provide the patient and family with information about available resources including reputable online sources for pain control and treatment and encourage them to use them. Table 35-6 provides information about online resources related to control and treatment of pain.

Play may be used effectively to discover a child's experience of pain and to teach the child how to cope with pain. Children are usually receptive to using dolls to act out pain experiences.

Ensuring the Ethical and Legal Responsibility to Relieve Pain

Quality pain management results when patients have access to safe, effective pain relief measures. Healthcare providers, in addition to monitoring, delivering, and documenting administration of analgesics, also have responsibility to inform patients that effective pain relief is vital to their treatment. Patients also have the right to expect that their statements of pain will be heeded quickly. Institutions must

Promoting Health Literacy
IN PATIENTS WITH PAIN

Patient Scenario

Jennifer Tyler, 44, has had several visits to her primary physician about her pain. She told the office nurse that she "doesn't know how much more of this I can take." Her history reveals that she has had an "aching pain, literally all over my body" for the last 3 months. Jennifer states that "It's taking over my life now. Everything I do hurts, and to make it worse, I don't sleep well at night and I can't even think straight." Additional symptoms she reported include fatigue, occasional muscle spasms in her legs, headaches that are occurring on a more frequent basis, and general anxiety about her health. Jennifer reports that initially she tried Advil off and on with some mild relief and even admits taking some "old muscle relaxants" that her husband had from a back injury. Despite the antidepressants and sleeping pills that were prescribed for her, she has not been able to get much in the way of pain relief. After his initial examination, her physician has ordered a variety of laboratory studies to try and determine exactly what is causing Ms. Tyler's pain. At this visit, he told Ms. Tyler that he suspects fibromyalgia may be the cause of her pain and other symptoms. He prescribes pregabalin (Lyrica) and wants to see her again in 3 weeks to see how this medication is working for her. As she is making the next appointment, Jennifer tells the nurse, "I sure hope this new medicine works. I'm running out of hope here. What kind of a life is this?"

Nursing Considerations: *Tips for Improving Health Literacy*

Provide Ms. Tyler with printed literature about fibromyalgia. Explain that this disease is difficult to diagnose and that this medication has recently been approved by the Food and Drug Administration (FDA) to treat fibromyalgia. Tell Ms. Tyler that the doctor may adjust her dose depending on how she tolerates the medicine and what kind of results she is getting from the drug. Caution her that dizziness and blurred vision may occur as side effects. Tell her if she has any signs of an allergic reaction, she should immediately stop taking the medication and report this to the physician. Inform her that she should avoid alcohol consumption while taking Lyrica and not to drive if she experiences any dizziness and blurred vision. Explain to her that the doctor may prescribe additional therapies to help her deal with rehabilitation as she recovers from this disease. Encourage Ms. Tyler when she returns for her next visit to be prepared to ask her physician the following questions:

- What is my main problem?
- What do I need to do?
- Why is it important for me to do this?
- What can you do if this new medication is not working?
- What else can you or I do to treat my pain?

What additional measures can you take to help maintain health literacy in this patient? What other measures would be helpful if Ms. Tyler did not speak English, could not read, or had other learning deficits?

TEACHING TIPS • 35-1

COMFORT

Health Topic	Teaching Tip	Why Is This Important?
Safety	Do not drive vehicle or operate heavy machinery after taking pain medication. Avoid alcohol and other CNS depressants while taking pain medication. Do not smoke without someone else present while taking pain medication. Do not walk without assistance while taking pain medication. Keep record or pain diary of level of pain, medication taken, and effect of medication.	Reflexes may be slowed and cognitive thinking decreased due to pain medications. Alcohol may interact with the pain medication and further depress the CNS, leading to respiratory failure. The patient may become tired due to the medication, fall asleep while smoking, and start a house fire. Some pain medications can cause drowsiness, dizziness, and blurred vision. Provides more accurate documentation of pain experience and prevents overdoses.
Diet	Do not take pain medication on an empty stomach.	Many patients become nauseated if pain medication is taken on an empty stomach.
Miscellaneous	Do not breastfeed without checking with your physician while taking pain medication.	Many pain medications can be found in breast milk and may harm the baby.

TABLE • 35-6   ONLINE RESOURCES FOR PAIN MANAGEMENT

Resource	Website	Information Provided
American Pain Foundation	http://www.painfoundation.org	Raises awareness about pain for people with pain and healthcare professionals
American Pain Society	http://ampainsoc.org	Provides current information about pain, including position statements and patient guides
American Society for Pain Management Nursing (ASPMN)	http://www.aspmn.org/index.htm	Promotes education, research, advocacy, and development of pain management standards
The City of Hope Pain/Palliative Care Resource Center	http://www.cityofhope.org/prc	Discusses pain assessment tools, pain management, and end-of-life care; has free publications and patient education materials
The National Foundation for the Treatment of Pain	http://www.paincare.org/	Support for patients with intractable pain and their caregivers
NIH Pain Consortium	http://painconsortium.nih.gov	Extensive review of research and current pain study findings
American Chronic Pain Association	http://www.theacpa.org/	Information about support groups for people with pain

assign and educate clinicians to address these issues in a timely, knowledgeable manner. The rights of patients with pain highlighted in Box 35-3 recognize the multidimensional aspects of the pain experience and an individual's right to have pain controlled as soon as possible. Also, as mentioned previously in this chapter, a patient's right to effective pain control is a focus of the Joint Commission.

In 2008, the American Pain Foundation proposed the National Pain Care Policy Act in an effort to improve pain care in the United States. This landmark policy was passed by both the U.S. House of Representative and U.S. Senate. In addition to expanding pain research, this act also provided grants for healthcare providers to improve their understanding and ability to treat pain and initiated a national outreach campaign that identified pain as a public health problem. Some of the provisions from this act are included in the new health reform bill passed in 2010 (American Pain Society, 2010).

> *Consider Xavier Malton, the child with acute pain. The nurses in the scenario advocated for Xavier, reinforcing his rights to have pain controlled as soon as possible.* ∎

Understanding the Placebo Controversy

The term **placebo** comes from the Latin word meaning "I shall please." According to McCaffery and Pasero (1999), a placebo is defined as "any medication or procedure, including surgery, that may produce an effect because of its implicit or explicit intent and not because of its specific physical or chemical properties." The person, unaware of the placebo's properties, may find it to be effective for the relief of pain because of the perception that it will provide comfort and because of belief in the person administering it. It is an injustice to judge a person experiencing relief from pain after the use of a placebo as a malingerer or as mentally ill. Various researchers have reported that a positive placebo effect may be related to a physiologic response (release of endorphins) or the patient's cultural expectations, attitudes, health beliefs, or anticipation of a positive response.

The use of placebos, however, raises serious ethical questions. Is lying to a patient justifiable? A nurse who administers a placebo must be willing to risk the possible consequence of the patient becoming aware of the duplicity and then refusing to trust the nurse or any other healthcare professional again. Patients who feel themselves to be in pain are vulnerable. If such a patient discovers a seeming plot to trick him or her into feeling better, it is unlikely that the patient will respect or appreciate the intentions of the physicians and

Box 35-3   A BILL OF RIGHTS FOR PEOPLE WITH PAIN

1. I have the right to have my reports of pain accepted and acted on by healthcare professionals.
2. I have the right to have my pain controlled, no matter what its cause or how severe it may be.
3. I have the right to be treated with respect at all times. When I need medication for pain, I should not be treated like a drug abuser.

May be duplicated for use in clinical practice. From McCaffery, M., & Pasero, C. (1999). *Pain: Clinical manual* (p. 13). Copyright © 1999, Mosby, Inc. St. Louis.

nurses involved. The long-term effects of this practice far outweigh any of its benefits. The Oncology Nursing Society and the American Nurses Association in addition to other professional organizations oppose placebo use. The American Society for Pain Management Nursing (ASPMN) agrees that placebo use is fraudulent and deceptive when used to assess and treat pain but supports placebo use in clinical trials in which the patient has signed an informed consent and the institutional review board has approved the research (McCaffery & Arnstein, 2006). The nurse has firm legal and ethical grounds for refusing to administer a placebo.

Evaluating

As soon as a pain problem is identified and a treatment plan developed and implemented, evaluation becomes ongoing. Evaluation is directed toward the changing nature of the pain experience, the treatment modalities (pain management program), and the patient's and family's response to the plan of care, all of which overlap.

The Pain Experience

The pain the patient is experiencing may change in many ways, and the nurse must be careful not to make a judgment about this too quickly. For example, if the pain lessens in intensity or disappears, it may mean that the underlying cause of the pain is diminished or absent and that treatment should be stopped, or it may mean that the pain management program is effective and should be continued. When pain intensity increases, it may simply indicate the need for more aggressive therapy, or it may be a warning that the underlying pathology has changed or worsened and that new medical intervention is required. Often, a new problem amenable

to treatment is masked by "old pain," and its detection may be delayed to the point that treatment is useless.

Management Regimens

The use of both noninvasive and invasive therapies must be continually evaluated to determine whether they are the best possible means the patient could use to obtain pain relief and whether they are effective with only minimal risk to the patient. Too often, a patient stays with the first analgesic prescribed without questioning whether it is the most effective drug for the particular pain, whether the dosage and timing guidelines are correct for the patient, and whether the analgesic is perhaps producing annoying or even harmful side effects that another drug would not produce.

Similarly, one patient may take to progressive relaxation exercises and find them helpful, whereas another patient may obtain similar benefits from a daily walking program. Nursing time spent evaluating the effectiveness of each pain relief therapy is well spent and results in a pain management program that is truly individualized to the patient.

Patient and Family Response

Ultimately, the plan of care is unsuccessful unless the patient and family are satisfied with the results. A successful plan of care results in the achievement of specified patient outcomes valued by the patient. Whenever possible, nursing care should terminate when the patient and family can independently direct the pain management program with the assistance of appropriate resources.

Refer to Table 35-6 for a listing of online sites for healthcare professionals, patients, and families related to management of pain. Nursing Plan of Care 35-1 highlights the nursing process related to pain for Carla Potter.

NURSING PLAN OF CARE · 35-1

For Carla Potter

Carla Potter is a 26-year-old white woman. She is unmarried and has no children. She is employed at a large company as a computer programmer. During the past 7 months, she has been experiencing periodic fatigue, anxiety, irritability, depression, and mood swings. Her general health is excellent. The nurse practitioner at the gynecologist's office believes Ms. Potter may be suffering from premenstrual syndrome. The nurse practitioner who interviewed Ms. Potter noted the following data:

• Patient has generalized discomfort—fatigue, anxiety, irritability, depression, and mood swings—about

1 week before her menses; discomfort subsides after onset of menses.
• Discomforts are believed to be heightened by stress at work but do not depend on this. Patient denies any new or unusual stress in life but believes symptoms are affecting her job performance and relationships.
• Patient relates history of "bad cramps" ever since periods started. Patient lacks knowledge of appropriate dietary and stress management techniques.
• Patient relates she has occasionally taken some of her friend's "tranquilizers" to ease her through a bad day—but she prefers not to take medication.

(continued)

NURSING PLAN OF CARE · 35-1

For Carla Potter *(continued)*

NURSING DIAGNOSIS   Ineffective Coping related to discomforts of premenstrual symptoms as manifested by reports of fatigue, anxiety, irritability, depression, and mood swings

EXPECTED OUTCOME   By the next monthly assessment, 10/30/11, patient will:

- Use relaxation techniques during periods of anxiety

Nursing Interventions	Rationale	Evaluative Statement
Assess patient's knowledge of relaxation techniques and motivation to use them.	Effective use of relaxation techniques requires a motivated patient.	10/30/11 Outcome partially met, patient used relaxation techniques during two periods of anxiety. Was driving on expressway during another period of anxiety, which made relaxation difficult.
Instruct patient regarding the use of progressive relaxation exercises and controlled breathing during periods of anxiety. For example, "Find a quiet, comfortable place and sit down. Consciously contract and relax the muscles of the whole body starting at the head and neck and working down to the feet until completely relaxed. At the same time, take slow, rhythmic breaths. Continue until anxiety passes."	Relaxation and controlled breathing are used to decrease anxiety and increase coping mechanisms.	*R. Gordon, RNC*

EXPECTED OUTCOME   By the next monthly assessment, 10/30/11, the patient will:

- Use a meal plan that includes three balanced meals per day and excludes caffeine, sugar, and sodium

Nursing Interventions	Rationale	Evaluative Statement
Assess patient's nutritional intake. Have patient identify current food preferences high in caffeine, sugar, and sodium and discuss substitutes. Teach patient rationale for decreasing intake of caffeine, sugar, and sodium.	Refined sugar and caffeine contribute to feelings of tension and irritability. Sodium contributes to water retention in the body.	10/30/11 Outcome met. Patient used meal plan for three balanced meals per day and eliminated all sugar, caffeine, and sodium from diet.
Instruct patient in developing a meal plan that includes three balanced meals per day.	Balanced meals provide optimal nutrition.	*R. Gordon, RNC*

EXPECTED OUTCOME   By the next monthly assessment, 10/30/11, the patient will:

- Incorporate exercise into routine

(continued)

NURSING PLAN OF CARE · 35-1

For Carla Potter (continued)

Nursing Interventions	Rationale	Evaluative Statement
Assess value patient attaches to physical fitness and regular periods of aerobic exercise; explore preferences.	Exercise can alleviate symptoms of depression, tension, anxiety, fatigue, and irritability. Exercise also serves as a distraction from discomforts.	10/30/11 Outcome met. Patient includes daily brisk walk around her neighborhood in her routine. *R. Gordon, RNC*
Instruct patient in use of regular daily exercise; design exercise prescription.	The fitness produced by regular exercise contributes to self-esteem.	

EXPECTED OUTCOME By the next monthly assessment, 10/30/11, the patient will:

- Supplement her diet with 50 mg of vitamin B_6 daily

Nursing Interventions	Rationale	Evaluative Statement
Instruct patient on daily use of vitamin B_6.	Vitamin B_6 may be effective in relieving symptoms of irritability, fatigue, and depression.	10/30/11 Outcome met. Patient supplements her diet daily with 50 mg of vitamin B_6. *R. Gordon, RNC*

EXPECTED OUTCOME By the next monthly assessment, 10/30/11, the patient will:

- Continue use of daily record of premenstrual syndrome (PMS) symptoms

Nursing Interventions	Rationale	Evaluative Statement
Instruct patient to continue use of daily record of PMS symptoms throughout the menstrual cycle.	Record keeping allows evaluation of the effectiveness of care plan.	10/30/11 Outcome met. Patient continued daily record, which illustrated drastic reduction in occurrence of PMS symptoms. Patient expressed delight in greater feeling of control she now has over how she feels. "I never realized that so many things affect my comfort level and health." *R. Gordon, RNC*

SAMPLE DOCUMENTATION

8/13/11 Nursing

Consultation with patient regarding apparent symptoms of PMS. She stated she experiences fatigue, anxiety, irritability, depression, and mood swings about 1 week before her menses. She states these symptoms interfere with her job performance and relationships. She also states that these symptoms seem to subside after onset of her menses. Patient admits to use of tranquilizers but prefers not to use medication. Advised patient to keep daily record of symptoms for one complete menstrual cycle. Patient indicated understanding of all instructions. She will return to office after completion of daily record for its analysis and to begin treatment, if indicated.

R. Gordon, RNC

Courtesy of Ruth E. Gordon, RNC, CRNP, DEd, Assistant Professor, Department of Nursing, Millersville University, Millersville, PA.

Skill · 35-1   Giving a Back Massage

EQUIPMENT

- Massage lubricant or lotion, warmed
- Pain assessment tool and/or scale
- Powder, if not contraindicated
- Bath blanket
- Towel
- Nonsterile gloves, if indicated
- Additional PPE, as indicated

IMPLEMENTATION

ACTION	RATIONALE
1. Perform hand hygiene and put on PPE, if indicated.	Hand hygiene and PPE prevent the spread of microorganisms. PPE is required based on transmission precautions.
2. Identify the patient.	Identifying the patient ensures the right patient receives the intervention and helps prevent errors.
3. Offer a back massage to the patient and explain the procedure.	Explanation encourages patient understanding and cooperation and reduces apprehension.
4. Put on gloves, if indicated.	Gloves are not usually necessary. Gloves prevent contact with blood and body fluid.
5. Close room door and/or curtain.	Closing the door or curtain provides privacy, promotes relaxation, and reduces noise and stimuli that may aggravate pain and reduce comfort.
6. Assess the patient's pain, using an appropriate assessment tool and measurement scale.	Accurate assessment is necessary to guide treatment/relief interventions and to evaluate the effectiveness of pain control measures.
7. Raise bed to a comfortable working position, usually elbow height of the caregiver (VISN 8, 2009), and lower the side rail.	Having the bed at the proper height prevents back and muscle strain.
8. Assist the patient to a comfortable position, preferably the prone or side-lying position. Remove the covers and move the patient's gown just enough to expose the patient's back from the shoulders to sacral area. Drape the patient as needed with the bath blanket.	This position exposes an adequate area for massage. Draping the patient provides privacy and warmth.
9. Warm the lubricant or lotion in the palm of your hand, or place the container in small basin of warm water. **During massage, observe the patient's skin for reddened or open areas. Pay particular attention to the skin over bony prominences.**	Cold lotion causes chilling and discomfort. Pressure may interfere with circulation and lead to pressure ulcers.
10. Using light gliding strokes (*effleurage*), apply lotion to patient's shoulders, back, and sacral area (Figure 1).	Effleurage relaxes the patient and lessens tension.

FIGURE 1. Using effleurage on a patient's back.

(continued)

Skill · 35-1   Giving a Back Massage   *continued*

ACTION

11. Place your hands beside each other at the base of the patient's spine and stroke upward to the shoulders and back downward to the buttocks in slow, continuous strokes (Figure 2). Continue for several minutes.

FIGURE 2. Stroking upward to the shoulders.

12. Massage the patient's shoulder, entire back, areas over iliac crests, and sacrum with circular stroking motions. **Keep your hands in contact with the patient's skin.** Continue for several minutes, applying additional lotion as necessary.

13. Knead the patient's skin by gently alternating grasping and compression motions (*pétrissage*) (Figure 3).

14. Complete the massage with additional long stroking movements that eventually become lighter in pressure (Figure 4).

RATIONALE

Continuous contact is soothing and stimulates circulation and muscle relaxation.

A firm stroke with continuous contact promotes relaxation.

Kneading increases blood circulation.

Long stroking motions are soothing and promote relaxation; continued stroking with gradual lightening of pressure helps extend the feeling of relaxation.

FIGURE 3. Using pétrissage.

FIGURE 4. Using light strokes with lessening pressure.

ACTION	RATIONALE
15. Use the towel to pat the patient dry and to remove excess lotion.	Drying provides comfort and reduces the feeling of moisture on the back.
16. Remove gloves, if worn. Reposition patient gown and covers. Raise side rail and lower bed. Assist patient to a position of comfort.	Repositioning bedclothes, linens, and the patient helps to promote patient comfort and safety.
17. Remove additional PPE, if used. Perform hand hygiene.	Removing PPE properly reduces the risk for infection transmission and contamination of other items. Hand hygiene prevents transmission of microorganisms.
18. Evaluate the patient's response to interventions. Reassess level of discomfort or pain using original assessment tools. Reassess and alter plan of care as appropriate.	Reassessment allows for individualization of plan of care and promotes optimal patient comfort.

DOCUMENTATION

Guidelines

Document pain assessment and other significant assessments. Document the use of and length of time of massage and patient response. Record alternative treatments to consider, if appropriate.

Sample Documentation

12/6/12 2330 Patient reports inability to sleep and increased pain at surgical site, rated 3/10. Medicated with propoxyphene 100 mg and acetaminophen 650 mg as ordered. Back massage administered × 10 minutes. Skin intact without redness. Patient reports increased comfort and relaxation; "I feel like I could sleep now."

—*B. Black, RN*

12/6/12 2400 Patient reports pain level 0/10.

—*B. Black, RN*

UNEXPECTED SITUATIONS AND ASSOCIATED INTERVENTIONS

- *Your patient cannot lie prone, so you are giving him a back massage while he is lying on his side. However, as you begin to massage the back, the patient cannot maintain the side-lying position:* If possible, have the patient hold on to the side rail on the side to which he is facing. If this is not possible or the patient cannot assist, use pillows and bath blankets to prevent the patient from rolling. If necessary, enlist the help of another person to maintain the patient's position. If possible, experiment with other positions based on the patient's condition and comfort, such as leaning forward against a pillow on the bedside table while sitting in a chair.

- *While massaging the patient's back, you notice a 2″ reddened area on the patient's sacrum:* Note this observation in the patient's medical record and report it to the physician. Do not massage the area. When the back massage is completed, position the patient off the sacral area, using pillows to maintain the patient's position, and institute a turning schedule.

SPECIAL CONSIDERATIONS

General Considerations

- Before giving a back massage, assess the patient's body structure and skin condition, and tailor the duration and intensity of the massage accordingly. If you are giving a back massage at bedtime, have the patient ready for bed beforehand so the massage can help him or her fall asleep.

- If the patient has oily skin, substitute a talcum powder or lotion of the patient's choice. However, to avoid aspiration, do not use powder if the patient has an endotracheal or tracheal tube in place. Avoid using powder and lotion together because this may lead to skin maceration.

- When massaging the patient's back, stand with one foot slightly forward and your knees slightly bent to allow effective use of your arm and shoulder muscles.

Infant and Child Considerations

- Hold infants and small children in a comfortable, well-supported position, such as against the chest or across the lap.

Older Adult Considerations

- Be gentle with massage. The skin on the elderly is often fragile and dry.

● Developing Critical Thinking Skills

1. Interview a nurse who specializes in pain management. Ask the nurse to describe the various physiologic and emotional responses to pain that she has observed in patients with acute and chronic pain. Question her about the different nursing interventions most likely to be effective for patients, in general, experiencing either acute or chronic pain. Inquire about specific pain management information and guidelines that she usually includes in discharge planning and teaching.

2. Consider what you personally believe about pain: what it is, what causes it, what is most likely to relieve it. Determine how pain is currently being managed within the tradition of Western medicine and what role nursing plays in keeping patients pain free. Visit nontraditional health centers where practitioners use a variety of noninvasive pain relief modalities, such as acupressure, relaxation techniques, imagery, and massage. In what ways, if any, has this new learning experience modified your beliefs about pain? Will it change your ability to design effective pain management regimens for your patients?

● Preparing for NCLEX

1. A patient complains of abdominal pain that is difficult to localize. The nurse categorically interprets this as which type of pain?
   a. Causalgia
   b. Visceral
   c. Superficial
   d. Psychogenic

2. A patient complains of pain in a site that is different from where it originates. The nurse documents this as what type of pain?
   a. Transient pain
   b. Superficial pain
   c. Phantom pain
   d. Referred pain

3. A patient who has fallen and injured his wrist carefully cradles it with the other hand. The patient is demonstrating which of the following responses to pain?
   a. Behavioral
   b. Affective
   c. Physiologic
   d. Involuntary

4. To help relieve her pain, Ann concentrates on a favorite vacation setting. The nurse interprets this technique as which of the following?
   a. Distraction
   b. Relaxation
   c. Recall
   d. Imagery

5. Which of the following descriptions does the nurse use to best describe intractable pain?
   a. Intermittent in nature
   b. Resistant to treatment
   c. Excruciating
   d. Widespread

6. Applying the gate control theory of pain, which of the following would be an effective nursing intervention for a patient with lower back pain?
   a. Encouraging regular use of analgesics
   b. Applying a moist heating pad to the area at prescribed intervals
   c. Reviewing the pain experience with the patient
   d. Ambulating the patient after administering medication

7. Which of the following would the nurse expect to assess as a physiologic response to moderate pain?
   a. Pupil dilation
   b. Restlessness
   c. Decreased pulse rate
   d. Protection of the painful area

8. Mrs. Young is receiving ATC medication for treatment of terminal cancer. She has recently reported several episodes of breakthrough pain. What treatment is most effective to manage these sudden flare-ups of pain?
   a. Increasing the dose of her ATC medication
   b. Restricting her physical activity
   c. Doing nothing more since her cancer is terminal
   d. Supplementing with doses of a short-acting opioid

9. When assessing pain in a child, the nurse needs to be aware of which of the following considerations?
   a. Immature neurologic development results in reduced sensation of pain.
   b. Inadequate or inconsistent relief of pain is widespread.
   c. Reliable assessment tools are currently unavailable.
   d. Narcotic analgesic use should be avoided.

10. Mr. Wright is recovering from abdominal surgery. When the nurse assists him to walk, she observes that he grimaces, moves stiffly, and becomes pale. She is aware that he has consistently refused his pain medication. Which of the following would be a priority nursing diagnosis?
    a. Acute Pain related to fear of taking prescribed postoperative medications
    b. Impaired Physical Mobility related to surgical procedure
    c. Anxiety related to outcome of surgery
    d. Risk for Infection related to surgical incision

11. When planning strategies for pain control in older patients, the nurse should be aware of which of the following?
    a. Pain is a natural outcome of the aging process.
    b. Sensitivity to pain increases with age.
    c. Narcotic use should be avoided.
    d. Denial of pain may occur.

12. When developing the plan of care for a patient with chronic pain, the nurse plans interventions based on the knowledge that chronic pain is most effectively relieved when analgesics are administered in what matter?
    a. On a p.r.n. (as needed) basis
    b. Conservatively
    c. Around the clock (ATC)
    d. Intramuscularly

13. Which of the following descriptions is true of using a placebo for pain control without the patient's consent?
    a. Widespread practice
    b. Consistently effective
    c. Deceptive
    d. Justified to determine whether the pain is real

14. The nurse provides vigilant monitoring of a patient receiving epidural analgesia to prevent the occurrence of which of the following?
    a. Pruritus
    b. Urinary retention
    c. Vomiting
    d. Respiratory depression

15. When assessing a patient receiving a continuous opioid infusion, the nurse immediately notifies the physician when the patient has which of the following findings?
    a. A respiratory rate of 10/min with normal depth
    b. A sedation level of 4
    c. Mild confusion
    d. Reported constipation

● Answers With Rationale

1. **b.** The patient's pain would be categorized as visceral pain, which is poorly localized and can originate in body organs in the abdomen. It is not complex regional pain syndrome (causalgia), which is pain that occurs in the area of injured peripheral nerves; cutaneous pain, which is superficial and usually involves the skin or subcutaneous tissue; or psychogenic pain, in which a physical cause for the pain cannot be identified.

2. **d.** Referred pain is perceived in an area distant from its point of origin, whereas transient pain is brief and passes quickly. Superficial pain originates in the skin or subcutaneous tissue. Phantom pain may occur in a person who has had a body part amputated, either surgically or traumatically.

3. **a.** Protecting or guarding a painful area is a behavioral response. Affective responses are psychological ones, and examples of a physiologic or involuntary response would be increased blood pressure or dilation of the pupils.

4. **d.** Imagery is a mind–body interaction that decreases pain sensation by focusing on pleasurable images. Distraction involves preoccupation with other things to relieve pain, and relaxation is a technique that reduces skeletal muscle tension and lessens anxiety. Recall is not a noninvasive relief measure.

5. **b.** Intractable pain is severe pain that is resistant to relief measures. The other terms do not describe this resistance to treatment.

6. **b.** Nursing measures such as applying warmth to the lower back stimulate the large nerve fibers to close the gate and block the pain. The other choices do not involve attempts to stimulate large nerve fibers that interfere with pain transmission as explained by the gate control theory.

7. **a.** Dilation of pupils is a physiologic or involuntary response to moderate pain, whereas decreased pulse rate, also a physiologic or involuntary response, occurs when pain is severe and deep. Restlessness and protection of the painful area are behavioral responses.

8. **d.** Breakthrough pain is best addressed by administering a short-acting opioid similar to her ATC medication. Increasing the dose of her ATC medication also increases her risk for developing side effects. All pain can be treated effectively, and limiting physical activity will not affect her breakthrough pain but may negatively affect her current lifestyle and self-esteem.

9. **b.** Healthcare personnel are only now becoming aware of pain relief as a priority for children in pain. The evidence supports the fact that children do indeed feel pain and reliable assessment tools are available specifically for use with children. Opioid analgesics may be safely used with children as long as they are carefully monitored.

10. **a.** Mr. Wright's immediate problem is his pain that is unrelieved because he refuses to take his pain medication for an unknown reason. The other nursing diagnoses are plausible, but not a priority in this situation.

11. **d.** Older people frequently deny pain because they view it as an ominous sign that may interfere with their independence. Pain sensitivity may decrease with age, but even this assumption is unsafe. Pain is not a natural outcome of the aging process. Opioid medications can be used if the older patient's response is carefully monitored and evaluated.

12. **c.** The p.r.n. protocol is totally inadequate for patients experiencing chronic pain. ATC doses of analgesics are more effective, whereas conservative pain management for whatever reason may also prove ineffective. Intramuscular administration is not practical on a long-range basis for a patient with chronic pain.

13. **c.** Using a placebo to control pain creates distrust in the nurse–patient relationship and is considered unethical behavior. It is not a widespread practice, is ineffective, and is never used to determine whether pain is real. Pain exists when the patient says it does.

14. **d.** Too much of an opioid drug given by way of an epidural catheter or a displaced catheter may result in the occurrence of respiratory depression. Pruritus, urinary retention, and vomiting may occur but are not life threatening.

15. **b.** Sedation level is more indicative of respiratory depression because it usually precedes it. A sedation level of 4 calls for immediate action because the patient has minimal or no response to stimuli. A respiratory level of 10 with normal depth of breathing is usually not a cause for alarm. Mild confusion may be evident with the initial dose and then disappear; additional observation is necessary. Constipation should be reported to the physician, but is not the priority in this situation.

Taylor Suite Resources

The Taylor Suite offers these additional resources to enhance learning and facilitate understanding of this chapter:

- thePoint online resource, http://thepoint.lww.com/Taylor7E
- Student DVD-ROM included with the book
- Study Guide for Taylor's Fundamentals of Nursing
- Skill Checklists for Taylor's Fundamentals of Nursing
- Taylor's Clinical Nursing Skills: *Chapter 10, Comfort*

BIBLIOGRAPHY

Aguirre, L., Nevidjon, B., & Clemens, A. (2008). Pain diaries. *American Journal of Nursing, 108*(6), 36–39.

American Pain Society. (2003). *Principles of analgesic use in the treatment of acute pain and cancer pain* (5th ed.). Glenview, IL: American Pain Society.

American Pain Society. (2005). *Guideline for the management of cancer pain in adults and children.* Glenview, IL: American Pain Society.

American Pain Society. (2008). *Advocacy.* Available at http://www.ampainsoc.org/advocacy/legislative.htm

American Pain Society. (2010). *Pain care provisions included in the new health reform bill.* Available at http://www.ampainsoc.org:8000/advocacy/legislative.htm

American Society for Pain Management. (2004). *The use of "as needed" range orders for opioid analgesics in the management of acute pain: A consensus statement of the American society for pain management nursing and the American pain society.* Lenexa, KS: The Society.

American Society for Pain Management & American Nurses Association. (2005). *Pain management nursing: Scope & Standards of practice.* Silver Spring, MD: Author.

Beyer, J., Denyes, M. J., & Villarruel, A. M. (1992). The creation, validation, and continuing development of the Oucher: A measure of pain intensity in children. *Journal of Pediatric Nursing, 7*(5), 335–346.

Boyle, E., Freer, Y., Wong, C. McIntosh, N., & Anand, K. J. (2006). Assessment of persistent pain or distress and adequacy of analgesia in preterm ventilated infants. *Pain, 124*(1–2), 87–91.

Bulechek, G., Butcher, H., & Dochterman, J. (2008). *Nursing interventions classification (NIC)* (5th ed., p. 532–533). St. Louis: C.V. Mosby.

Burney, R. (2001). Taking a look at pain in your organization. *Joint Commission Perspectives, 21*(2), 8–10.

Cepeda, M., Carr, D., & Alvarez, H. (2006). Music for pain relief. *The Cochrane Database of Systematic Reviews,* Issue 2. Chichester, UK: John Wiley and Sons, Ltd.

Christie, W., & Moore, C. (2005). The impact of humor on patients with cancer. *Clinical Journal of Oncology Nursing, 9*(2), 211–218.

Damsky, D. (2007). Getting the point about fibromyalgia. *Nursing, 37*(2), 61–64.

D'Arcy, Y. (2005). Conquering pain: Have you tried these new techniques? *Nursing, 35*(3), 36–41.

D'Arcy, Y. (2006a). Hot topics in pain management: Using NSAIDs safely. *Nursing, 36*(2), 22–23.

D'Arcy, Y. (2006b). Treating pain after a total joint replacement. *Nursing, 36*(5), 26–28.

D'Arcy, Y. (2006c). Which analgesic is right for my patient? *Nursing, 36*(7), 50–55.

D'Arcy, Y. (2007a). Eyeing capnography to improve PCA safety. *Nursing, 37*(9), 18–19.

D'Arcy, Y. (2007b). Knocking out pain safely with PCA. *Nursing Spectrum, 16*(15), 16–18.

D'Arcy, Y. (2007c). Managing pain in a patient who's drug-dependent. *Nursing, 37*(3), 36–40.

D'Arcy, Y. (2007d). New pain management options: Delivery systems and techniques. *Nursing, 37*(2), 26–27.

D'Arcy, Y. (2007e). Pain management by the numbers: Using rating scales effectively. *Nursing, 37*(11), 14–15.

D'Arcy, Y. (2008a). Does preemptive analgesia work? *Nursing, 37*(4), 52–55.

D'Arcy, Y. (2008b). Keep your patient safe during PCA. *Nursing, 38*(1), 50–55.

D'Arcy, Y. (2008c). Pain management survey report. *Nursing, 38*(6), 42–50.

D'Arcy, Y. (2009). Are opioids safe for your patient? *Nursing, 39*(4), 40–44.

Eliopoulos, C. (2005). *Gerontological nursing* (6th ed.). Philadelphia: Lippincott Williams & Wilkins.

Ezenwa, M., Ameringer, S., Ward, S., & Serlin, R. C. (2006). Racial and ethnic disparities in pain management in the United States. *Journal of Nursing Scholarship, 38*(30), 225–233.

Facente, A. (2006). Humor in health care: Irreverent or invaluable? *Nursing, 36*(4), 64hn6–7.

Flaherty, E. (2008). Using pain-rating scales with older adults. *American Journal of Nursing, 108*(6), 40–47.

Flasar, C., & Wentz, J. (2006). Are NSAIDs safe for arthritis pain? *Nursing, 36*(12), 24.

Gevirtz, C. (2010). Getting current with iontophoretic fentanyl. *Nursing, 40*(2), 65.

Herr, K., Coyne, P., Key, T., Manworren, R., McCaffery, M., Merkel, S., et al. (2006). Pain management in the non-verbal patient. *American Society for Pain Management Nursing, 7*(2), 44–52.

Horgas, A., & Miller, L. (2008). Pain assessment in people with dementia. *American Journal of Nursing, 108*(7), 62–70.

Hughes, D., Ladas, E., Rooney, D., & Kelly, K. (2008). Massage therapy as a supportive intervention for children with cancer. *Oncology Nursing Forum, 35*(3), 431–442.

Jackson, E., McNeil, P., & Schlegel, L. (2008). Does therapeutic touch help reduce pain and anxiety in patients with cancer? *Clinical Journal of Oncology Nursing, 12*(1), 113–120.

The Joint Commission. (2004). *Sentinel event alert: Patient controlled analgesia by proxy.* Available at http://www.jointcommission.org/SentinelEvents/SentinelEventAlert/sea_33.htm

The Joint Commission. (2007). Improving America's Hospitals: A Report on Quality & Safety. Available at http://www.jointcommission.org/NR/rdonlyres/505C10E1-6190-441F-B553-B59F4C30F963/0/2006_Annual_Report.pdf

The Joint Commission. (2008a). *News room: Health care issues.* Available at http://www.jointcommission.org/Newsroom/health_care_issues.htm#9

The Joint Commission. (2008b). Nutritional, functional, and pain assessments and screens. Available at http://www.jointcommission.org/AccreditationPrograms/Hospitals/Standards/09_FAQs/PC/Nutritional_+Functional_Pain_+Assessments.htm

Kapustin, J. (2008). Pain, pain, go away: A new medication for fibromyalgia sufferers. *Advance for Nurses: Pennsylvania, New Jersey, Delaware, 10*(6), 41.

Kean, M. (2007). Assessing complex pain behaviors. *Nursing, 37*(12), 18–19.

Keller, D. (2006). Pain relievers. *RN, 69*(4), 22–27.

Kwekkeboom, K., & Gretarsdottir, E. (2006). Systematic review of relaxation interventions for pain. *Journal of Nursing Scholarship, 38*(3), 269–277.

LeMone, P., & Burke, K. (2008). *Medical–surgical nursing: Critical thinking in client care* (4th ed.). Upper Saddle River, NJ: Pearson/Prentice Hall.

Lewis, S., Heitkemper, M., Dirksen, S., O'Brien, P., & Bucher, L. (2007). *Medical–surgical nursing: Assessment and management of clinical problems* (7th ed.). St. Louis: Mosby.

Lilley, L., Harrington, S., & Snyder, J. (2007). *Pharmacology and the Nursing Process* (5th ed.). St. Louis: Mosby, Inc.

Managing opioid-induced constipation. (2008). *Nursing, 38*(7), 55.

McCaffery, M. (1979). *Nursing management of the patient with pain* (2nd ed.). Philadelphia: J. B. Lippincott.

McCaffery, M., & Arnstein, P. (2006). The debate over placebos in pain management. *American Journal of Nursing, 106*(2), 62–66.

McCaffery, M., & Beebe, A. (1989). *Pain: Clinical manual for nursing practice.* St. Louis: C. V. Mosby.

McCaffery, M., & Pasero, C. (1999). *Pain: Clinical manual* (2nd ed.). St. Louis: C. V. Mosby.

McCaffery, M., Pasero, C., & Ferrell, B. (2007). Nurses' decisions about opioid dose. *American Journal of Nursing, 107*(12), 35–39.

McCarberg, B. (2008). What are we afraid of? Barriers to providing adequate pain relief. *Medscape.* Available at http://www.medscape.com/viewarticle/571671

Melzak, R., & Wall, P. (1968). Gate control theory of pain. In A. Soulairac, J. Cahn, & J. Carpentier (Eds.), *Pain: Proceedings of the international association on pain.* Baltimore: Williams & Wilkins.

Mennick, F. (2008). Racial disparities in ED pain treatment. *American Journal of Nursing, 108*(4), 18.

National Center for Health Statistics. (2006). *Health, United States, 2006. With chartbook on trends in the health of Americans. Special feature: Pain.* Hyattsville, MD: Centers for Disease Control and Prevention. Available at http://www.cdc.gov/nchs/data/hus/hus06.pdf#chartbookontrends.

NANDA International. (2009). *NANDA nursing diagnosis: Definitions & classification: 2009–2011.* West Sussex, UK: Wiley-Blackwell.

Narayan, M.C. (2010). Culture's effects on pain assessment and management. *American Journal of Nursing, 110*(4), 38–49.

Pasero, C. (2003). Epidural analgesia for postoperative pain: Excellent analgesia and improved patient outcomes after major surgery. *American Journal of Nursing, 103*(10), 62–64.

Pasero, C. (2007). Pain assessment in preterm neonates. *American Journal of Nursing, 107*(4), 30–31.

Pasero, C., & McCaffery, M. (2005). Authorized and unauthorized use of PCA pumps. *American Journal of Nursing, 105*(7), 30–32.

Pasero, C., Manworren, R. & McCaffery, M. (2007). IV opioid range orders for acute pain management. *American Journal of Nursing, 107*(2), 52–59.

Pillitteri, A. (2007). *Maternal and child health nursing: Care of the childbearing & childrearing family* (5th ed.). Philadelphia: Lippincott Williams & Wilkins.

Plaisance, L., & Logan, C. (2006). Nursing students' knowledge and attitudes regarding pain. *Pain Management Nursing, 7*(4), 167–175.

Puchalski, M. (2008). How should I manage postoperative pain in children? *Medscape.* Available at http://www.medscape.com/viewarticle/570716

Schwartz, A. (2006). Learning the essentials of epidural anesthesia. *Nursing, 36*(1), 44–49.

Slatkin, N., & Rhiner, M. (2008). Breakthrough pain: Improving recognition and management to enhance quality of life. *Medscape.* Available at http://www.medscape.com/viewprogram/9080

Smeltzer, S., Bare, B., Hinkle, J., & Cheever, K. (2010). *Textbook of medical-surgical nursing* (12th ed.). Philadelphia: Lippincott Williams & Wilkins.

Stett, G. (2010). Meet MOD – medication on demand. Available at http://www.avancen.com/about_the_mod.php

Swanson, B. (2008a). Managing older adults' pain: Part I- Overview and pharmacologic strategies. *Advance for Nurses: Pennsylvania, New Jersey, Delaware, 10*(20), 33–37.

Swanson, B. (2008b). Managing older adults' pain: Part II- Complementary and alternative therapies. *Advance for Nurses: Pennsylvania, New Jersey, Delaware, 10*(21), 25–28.

Time to modify the WHO analgesic ladder? (2005). *Pain Clinical Updates, 13*(5), 1–4.

U.S. Food and Drug Administration (FDA). (2010). *Second safety warning on fentanyl skin patch.* Available at http://www.fda.gov/ForConsumers/ConsumerUpdates/ucm100223.htm

Using pain relievers safely. (2008). *Nursing, 38*(8), 41.

van Dijk, M., Peters, W., van Deventer, P., & Tibboel, D. (2005). The COMFORT behavior scale. *American Journal of Nursing, 105*(1), 33–36.

Van Steenacker, D. (2007). Let patients control their pain. *Nursing Spectrum, 16*(21), 12.

VISN 8 Patient Safety Center. (2009). *Safe patient handling and movement algorithms.* Tampa, FL: Author. Available at http://www.visn8.va.gov/patientsafetycenter/safePtHandling. Accessed April 23, 2010.

World Health Organization (WHO). (1990). *Cancer pain relief and palliative care: Report of a WHO expert committee.* WHO Technical Report Series, No. 804. Geneva: Author.

Wuhrman, E., Cooney, M., Dunwoody, C., Eksterowicz, N., Merkel, S., & Oakes, L. (2006). Patient controlled analgesia (PCA). *Pain Management Nursing, 7*(4), 134–147.

Zborowski, M. (1969). *People in pain.* San Francisco: Jossey-Bass.

36 Nutrition

SUSAN OAKLAND

Susan Oakland, a 21-year-old student, is pregnant with her first child. Susan is in the ninth week of her pregnancy. She is experiencing persistent nausea, vomiting, and fatigue. She has had difficulty eating, with a resulting weight loss of 3 pounds since her first prenatal visit at 5 weeks gestation.

WILLIAM JOHNSTON

William, a 42-year-old executive, is newly diagnosed with high blood pressure and high cholesterol. He confides that his health has been the last thing on his mind and that his health habits are less than admirable. "I usually eat on the run, often fast food, or big dinners with lots of alcohol. I can't remember the last time I worked out or did any exercise, unless running from my car to the train counts! I guess it's no wonder I've gained a few pounds over the years!"

CHARLES GALLAGHER

Charles is the husband of a 67-year-old woman in the end stages of advanced dementia. She had a percutaneous endoscopic gastrostomy (PEG) inserted during her last hospitalization 6 weeks ago due to recurrent episodes of aspiration pneumonia from an inability to swallow. He states, "I was talking to the chaplain at the nursing home, and he questioned the wisdom of this tube. I respect him but we really don't have an option here, do we? I mean, if they take the tube out she'll starve to death—right?"

LEARNING OBJECTIVES

After completing the chapter, you will be able to accomplish the following:

1. List the six classes of nutrients, explaining the significance of each.

2. Identify risk factors for poor nutritional status.

3. Describe how nutrition influences growth and development throughout the life cycle.

4. Discuss the components of a nutritional assessment.

5. Evaluate a diet using the MyPyramid Food Guide.

6. Develop nursing diagnoses that correctly identify nutritional problems that may be treated by independent nursing interventions.

7. Describe nursing interventions to help patients achieve their nutritional goals.

8. Plan, implement, and evaluate nursing care related to select nursing diagnoses that involve nutritional problems.

9. Identify nursing interventions to safely deliver enteral nutrition.

10. Identify nursing interventions to safely deliver parenteral nutrition.

KEY TERMS

absorption	lipid
anorexia	minerals
anorexia nervosa	nasogastric (NG) tube
anthropometric	nasointestinal (NI) tube
aspiration	
basal metabolism	NPO
body mass index (BMI)	nutrient
bulimia	nutrition
calorie	obesity
carbohydrate	parenteral nutrition
cholesterol	percutaneous endoscopic gastrostomy tube (PEG)
clear liquid diet	
digestion	peripheral parenteral nutrition (PPN)
dysphagia	
enteral nutrition	protein
full liquid diet	recommended dietary allowance (RDA)
gastrostomy	
ketosis	residual

soft diet	trans fat
total parenteral nutrition (TPN)	triglycerides
	vitamins

This chapter provides information about basic nutrition theory, focusing on the six classes of nutrients, energy balance, choices for an adequate diet, food patterns and habits, and factors affecting nutrition. Components of simple screening and in-depth nutritional assessments are outlined. Two sets of nursing diagnoses are provided, and patient outcomes for healthy nutrition are discussed. The accompanying plan of care illustrates the significance of nutrition in nursing care. Nutrition is vital for life and health, and poor nutrition can seriously decrease one's level of wellness, which makes it a vital component of nursing. See the accompanying Reflective Practice display for an example.

PRINCIPLES OF NUTRITION

The science of **nutrition** is the study of how food nourishes the body. It encompasses the study of nutrients and how they are handled by the body as well as the impact of human behavior and environment on the process of nourishment. As such, this discipline involves physiology, psychology, and socioeconomics.

Nutrients are specific biochemical substances used by the body for growth, development, activity, reproduction, lactation, health maintenance, and recovery from illness or injury. The metabolic processes involved in these functions are complex. Subsequently, most nutrients work better together than they do alone. Also, nutrient needs change throughout the life cycle in response to changes in body size, activity, growth, development, and state of health.

Some nutrients are considered *essential* because either they are not synthesized in the body or are made in insufficient amounts. Essential nutrients must be provided in the diet or through supplements. Essential nutrients that supply energy and build tissue (such as carbohydrates, fats, protein) are referred to as *macronutrients. Micronutrients,* such as vitamins and minerals, are required in much smaller amounts to regulate and control body processes.

Nonessential nutrients do not have to be supplied through dietary sources because they either are not required for body functioning or are synthesized in the body in adequate amounts. Some nutrients can be converted to others in the body. For instance, the body converts excess carbohydrates and protein into fat and stores them as triglycerides.

Of the six classes of nutrients, three supply energy (carbohydrates, protein, lipids [fats]) and three are needed to regulate body processes (vitamins, minerals, water).

Energy Balance

The body needs energy to function. Energy is derived or obtained from foods consumed. Energy in the diet is measured

REFLECTIVE PRACTICE
Challenge to Legal and Ethical Skills

Mrs. Constance Gallagher is only 67 years old, but she is in the end stages of advanced dementia. She can no longer swallow and has had several hospitalizations in the past year for aspiration pneumonia. She lives in a nursing home (where I am doing a clinical rotation for my gerontologic nursing experience) and has a devoted family, husband, son, and daughter, who all visit regularly. For the last 6 weeks, she has received enteral feedings from a percutaneous endoscopic gastrostomy (PEG) tube that was placed during her last hospitalization. Mrs. Gallagher's husband confided to me that the chaplain at the nursing home, whom he respects and likes, questioned the wisdom of the feeding tube. He then asked me, "But we really don't have an option here, do we? I mean, if they take the tube out, she'll starve to death, no?" I had no idea how to respond.

Thinking Outside the Box: Possible Courses of Action

- Simply refer Mr. Gallagher to someone more experienced about these things (since I am clearly over my head).
- Find out more about this myself and then get back to him.

- Request an ethics consult to explore how we can best respond to the husband's questions about what is in his wife's best interests, especially given the role the home's chaplain is playing.

Evaluating a Good Outcome: How Do I Define Success?

- The patient's medical goals are met, including, if the family wishes, a dignified death.
- The Gallagher family feels at peace with their decisions and the results of these decisions.
- An ethically justified decision is made about continuing or withdrawing artificial nutrition and hydration that is

respectful of Mrs. Gallagher's wishes (to the extent that these are known) and compatible with her beliefs and interests.
- I develop skill in assisting with tough end-of-life decisions and learn more about how an ethics consult functions.

Personal Learning: Here's to the Future!

When I reported my exchange with Mr. Gallagher to the charge nurse, she said we might want to call an ethics consult because there were actually a few similar situations pending and not everyone on the unit seemed comfortable with the lead role the chaplain was taking in recommending the withdrawal of nutritional support. The consult was a great experience. All of the patient's family members attended, plus the medical director of the home, the nurses on the patient's unit, as well as the chaplain, the social worker, the home's ethicist, and myself. After the medical director described the natural progression of advanced dementia, the ethicist noted that there is a difference between dying of starvation (which only happens if food is withdrawn but fluids continue to hydrate) and dying of dehydration (which will happen if we pull the PEG tube and discontinue all

enteral feedings, and which is not believed to be painful). The ethicist then asked the family if they knew what the patient would want done if she could be asked if the benefits of continuing nutritional support outweighed the accompanying burdens of having her wrists restrained so she wouldn't pull out the tube, skin problems, etc. After some discussion, they were in agreement that she would not want to live this way. Since the Gallaghers were Catholic, the Catholic chaplain was invited to describe what the Roman Catholic Church teaches about this. After a rather lengthy discussion, a decision was made to withdraw enteral feedings. The family seemed at peace with their decision.

Through this experience, I learned how an ethics consult works and can see the advantages of tapping this resource in the future.

Reflection

How do you think you would respond in a similar situation? Why? What does this tell you about yourself and about the adequacy of your skills for professional practice? How did the ethics consult facilitate decision making? What ethical and legal principles were maintained? Investigate your agency for this service. What other services or resources might be available to aid in this type of decision-making process? Can you think of other ways to respond? What other skills (cognitive, interpersonal, technical, ethical/legal) would you need to respond well in this situation? How did the nursing student act as a patient advocate? Was the human dignity of the patient and the patient's family maintained? Why or why not? Do you agree with the criteria to evaluate a successful outcome? Did the nursing student meet these criteria?

in the form of kilocalories, commonly abbreviated as **calories,** or cal. Only carbohydrates, protein, and fat provide energy. Vitamins and minerals, needed for the metabolism of energy, do not provide calories.

Total energy intake for a meal, a day, or longer, can be calculated by using food composition tables: The values given

for total calories for each food eaten can simply be added, or the grams of carbohydrate, protein, and fat for each food eaten can be added and multiplied by the appropriate calorie level (4, 4, and 9 cal, respectively).

Energy in the body is used to carry on any kind of activity, whether voluntary or involuntary. A person's total daily energy expenditure is the sum of all the calories used to perform physical activity, maintain basal metabolism, and digest, absorb, and metabolize food.

If a person's daily energy intake is equal to total daily energy expenditure, the person's weight will remain stable. However, if the energy intake is less than the energy expended, the person's weight will decrease. If the energy intake exceeds energy expenditure, weight will increase.

Metabolic Requirements

Basal metabolism is the energy required to carry on the involuntary activities of the body at rest—the energy needed to sustain the metabolic activities of cells and tissues (Porth & Matfin, 2009). These activities include actions such as maintaining body temperature and muscle tone, producing and releasing secretions, propelling food through the gastrointestinal (GI) tract, inflating the lungs, and contracting the heart muscle. As the amount of energy used on physical activity declines, the proportion of calories used for basal metabolism increases; it accounts for more than half of most people's total energy requirements. Because of their larger muscle mass, men have a higher basal metabolic rate (BMR) than women. BMR is about 1 cal/kg of body weight per hour for men and 0.9 cal/kg per hour for women.

> ▶ *Think back to William Johnston, the middle-aged man with hypertension and high cholesterol. Based on the patient's gender, the nurse would expect his BMR to be greater than that for a woman. The nurse would need to consider this fact when planning the patient's care.* ■

Other factors that increase BMR include growth, infections, fever, emotional tension, extreme environmental temperatures, and elevated levels of certain hormones, especially epinephrine and thyroid hormones. Aging, prolonged fasting, and sleep all decrease BMR. Most nutritionists agree that fasting or following a very–low-calorie diet defeats a weight-loss plan because the body interprets this eating pattern as starvation and compensates by slowing down the resting metabolic rate, making it even more difficult to lose weight.

Body Weight Standards

As previously discussed, if a person's energy intake does not equal energy expenditure, weight will fluctuate. Ideal body weight (IBW) or healthy body weight is an estimate of optimal weight for optimal health. A general guideline, often called the rule-of-thumb method, determines ideal weight based on height. This formula is as follows:

For adult females:

> 100 lb. (for height of 5 ft) + 5 lb. for each
> additional inch over 5 ft

For adult males:

> 106 lb. (for height of 5 ft) + 6 lb. for each
> additional inch over 5 ft

(Add or deduct 10% from this figure based on body frame size.) Using this method can result in unrealistically low figures for adults who are very short or very tall. (Height and weight tables are commonly used for infants and children.)

The more preferred methods to establish ideal body weight include **body mass index (BMI)** (adults and children) and measurement of waist circumference (adults) (National Institutes of Health [NIH], 2008). The BMI, or Quetelet Index (W/H^2), is a ratio of weight (in kilograms) to height (in meters). The BMI is a reliable indicator of total body fat stores in the general population. Health practitioners use this more accurate weight calculation as an initial assessment of nutritional status. The BMI does not differentiate according to gender and is calculated in the following manner:

Using kilograms and meters:

$$BMI = \frac{\text{weight in kilograms}}{(\text{height in meters}) \times (\text{height in meters})}$$

Using pounds and inches:

$$BMI = \frac{\text{weight in pounds}}{(\text{height in inches}) \times (\text{height in inches})} \times 703$$

BMI also provides an estimation of relative risk for diseases such as heart disease, diabetes, and hypertension. However, it is important to note the BMI may not be accurate for people such as athletes, with a large muscle mass, or people with edema or dehydration, and older persons and others who have lost muscle mass (NIH, 2008; Dudek, 2006).

According to the most recent BMI guidelines published by the National Heart, Lung, and Blood Institute, a person with a BMI below 18.5 is underweight, a BMI of 25 to 29.9 indicates an overweight individual, a BMI of 30 or greater indicates obesity, and a BMI of 40 or greater indicates extreme obesity (NIH, 2008).

A significant intentional or unintentional change in the patient's weight can also indicate poor nutritional status and/or health problems. Significant weight change is determined by how much weight is lost per unit of time. To calculate the percent of weight change, use the following formula.

usual weight − present weight ÷ usual weight × 100

Weight loss is considered significant if it falls into the following guidelines (Dudek, 2006):

- 1% to 2% in 1 week
- 5% in 1 month
- 7.5% in 3 months
- 10% in 6 months

Waist circumference is measured by placing a measuring tape snugly around the patient's waist at the level of the umbilicus (Fig. 36-1). This measurement is a good indicator of abdominal fat. Where excess body fat is deposited is thought to be an important and reliable indicator of risk for disease, such as type 2 diabetes, dyslipidemia, hypertension, and cardiovascular disease (Dudek, 2006). This risk increases with a waist measurement of over 40 inches in men and

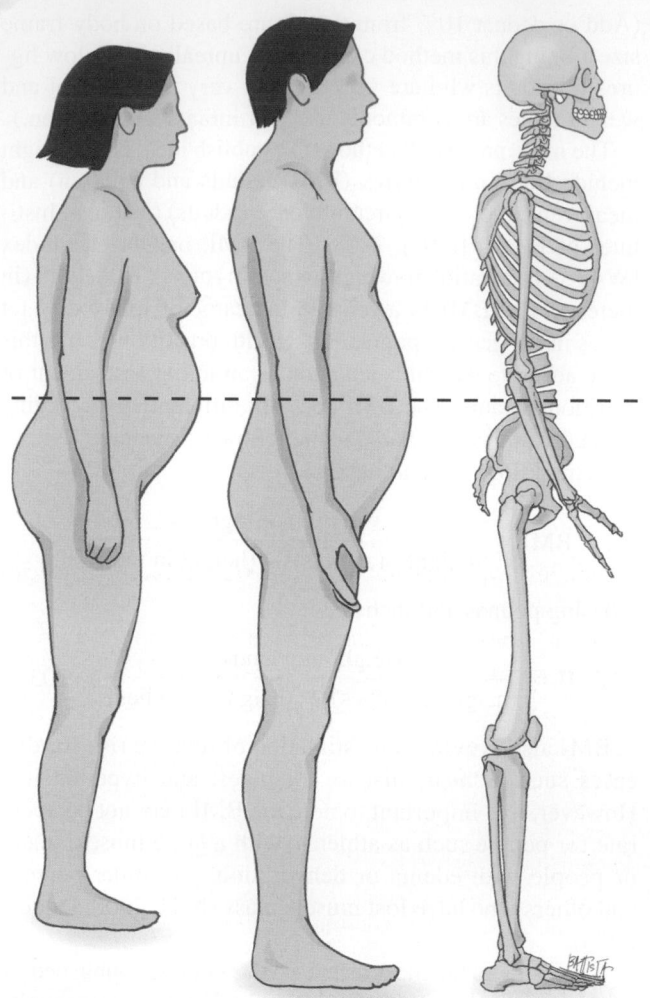

FIGURE 36-1. Positioning of measuring tape at the level of the umbilicus for waist circumference.

35 inches in women (NIH, 2000b). Table 36-1 displays the relationship of the risks of obesity-associated diseases and conditions by BMI and waist circumference.

Caloric Requirements

Just as healthy body weight or IBW can be determined in a variety of ways, so can a person's calorie requirements. Box 36-1 illustrates one method to determine calorie requirements. After calorie requirements have been determined, adjustments can be made for weight gain or loss, as needed. For instance, 1 lb (0.45 kg) of body fat equals about 3,500 cal. Therefore, to gain or lose 1 lb (0.45 kg) in a week, daily calorie intake should be increased or decreased, respectively, by 500 cal (3,500 cal divided by 7 days = 500 cal/d). Similarly, a weight gain or loss of 2 lb (0.9 kg) per week would require an adjustment of 1,000 cal/d. Because it becomes increasingly difficult to plan an adequate diet as the calorie level drops, diets that result in more than a 2-lb (0.9-kg) weight loss per week are not recommended.

➤ *Consider William Johnston, the man with poor health habits. The nurse would work with Mr. Johnston to develop an appropriate weight-loss plan that would contain adequate calories yet still foster a weight loss of 1 to 2 lb/week. Doing so would promote weight loss while still allowing for adequate nutritional intake.* ■

Energy Nutrients

Carbohydrates, protein, and fats are potential sources of energy for the body.

TABLE • 36-1	RISK OF OBESITY-ASSOCIATED DISEASES AND CONDITIONS BY BMI AND WAIST CIRCUMFERENCE RELATIVE TO NORMAL WEIGHT AND WAIST CIRCUMFERENCE (DISEASE RISK FOR TYPE 2 DIABETES, HYPERTENSION, AND CARDIOVASCULAR DISEASE)	
		Waist Circumference
	BMI (kg/m^2)	**Men ≤40 Inches (102 cm)** **Women ≤35 Inches (88 cm)**	**Men >40 Inches (102 cm)** **Women >35 Inches (88 cm)**
Underweight	<18.5	NA	NA
Normal	18.5–24.9	NA	NA
Overweight	25.0–29.9	Increased	High
Obesity, Class I	30.0–34.9	High	Very high
Obesity, Class II	35.0–39.9	Very high	Very high
Extreme Obesity	40.0 +	Extremely high	Extremely high

*Increased waist circumference can also be a marker for increased risk even in persons of normal weight.
(National Institutes of Health, National Heart, Lung and Blood Institute. [2000b]. NHLBI Obesity Education Initiative. *The practical guide: Identification, evaluation, and treatment of overweight and obesity in adults.* NIH publication no. 00-4084. October 2000. Available at www.nhlbi.nih.gov/guidelines/obesity/prctgd_c.pdf.)

(Adapted from Dudek, S. G. [2006]. *Nutrition essentials for nursing practice* [5th ed.]. Philadelphia: Lippincott Williams & Wilkins.)

Box 36-1   METHOD OF CALCULATING CALORIC REQUIREMENTS

- Estimate the basal metabolic rate (BMR) or the amount of calories necessary to maintain the body at rest. Because men usually have a greater muscle mass than women, their caloric requirements are slightly higher. A rule-of-thumb guideline for calculating BMR is to multiply healthy weight (in pounds) by 10 for women and 11 for men. For a person who is overweight, multiply by the average weight within the healthy weight range. For example:

  Male: 130 lb × 11 cal/lb = 1,430 cal/day

  Female: 130 lb × 10 cal/lb = 1,300 cal/day

- Estimate the total calories according to usual activity level. Choose the category that describes usual activities.

- 1.2   Sedentary: mostly sitting, driving, sleeping, standing, reading, typing, other low-intensity activities
- 1.3   Light activity: light exercise, such as walking not more than 2 hours per day
- 1.4   Moderate activity: moderate exercise such as heavy housework, gardening, and very little sitting
- 1.5   High activity: active in physical sports or a labor-intensive occupation, such as construction work

- Multiply the BMR by the number associated with the activity level. For example, the above female's BMR = 1,300 calories per day. She engages in light activity.

  1,300 × 1.3 = 1,690 total daily calories

Carbohydrates

Carbohydrates, commonly known as sugars and starches, are organic compounds composed of carbon, hydrogen, and oxygen. They serve as the structural framework of plants. The only animal source of carbohydrate in the diet is lactose, or "milk sugar."

The significance of carbohydrates cannot be overstated. They are relatively easy to produce and store, making them the most abundant and least expensive source of calories in the diet worldwide. In countries where grains are the dietary staple, carbohydrates may contribute as much as 90% of total calories. Table 36-2 summarizes the sources, functions, and significance of dietary carbohydrates. Carbohydrate intake is often correlated to income. As income increases, carbohydrate intake decreases and protein intake, a more expensive form of energy, increases.

CLASSIFICATION AND METABOLISM

The number of molecules within the structure determines the classification of carbohydrates. They are classified as simple (monosaccharide and disaccharide) or complex (polysaccharide) sugars.

Carbohydrates are more easily and quickly digested than protein and fat. Ninety percent of carbohydrate intake is digested. This percentage decreases as fiber intake increases. All carbohydrates are converted to glucose for transport through the blood or for use as energy. Glucose is an efficient fuel that certain tissues, particularly the central nervous system, rely on almost exclusively for energy. Glucose is transported from the GI tract, through the portal vein, to the liver. The liver stores glucose and regulates its entry into the blood. Hormones, especially insulin and glucagon, are responsible for keeping serum glucose levels fairly constant during both feasting and fasting.

Through a series of steps, cells oxidize (burn) glucose to provide energy, carbon dioxide, and water. Depending on a person's state of energy balance, the period between when carbohydrate is consumed and when it is used for energy may vary from minutes to months or longer. Unlike protein and fat, glucose is burned efficiently and completely and does not leave a toxic product for the kidneys to excrete.

When the supply of glucose exceeds what is needed for energy and for maintaining serum levels, it is stored. If muscle or liver glycogen stores are deficient, glucose is converted to glycogen and stored (glycogenesis). Conversely, glycogen is broken down in time of need to supply a ready source of glucose (glycogenolysis). When glycogen stores are adequate, the body converts excess glucose to fat and stores it as triglycerides in adipose tissue.

FUNCTIONS AND RECOMMENDED DIETARY ALLOWANCE

The primary function of carbohydrates is to supply energy. Except for indigestible fiber, all carbohydrates provide 4 calories per gram, regardless of the source.

The **recommended dietary allowance (RDA)** of essential nutrients refers to recommendations for average daily amounts that healthy population groups should consume over time. Although an exact requirement for carbohydrates has not been established, at least 50 to 100 g are needed daily to prevent **ketosis** (an abnormal accumulation of ketone bodies that is frequently associated with acidosis). The *Dietary Guidelines for Americans 2005* (United States Department of Agriculture [USDA] & Department of Health and Human Services [DHHS], 2005) recommends that carbohydrates provide 45% to 65% of total calories, mostly in the form of complex carbohydrates. Sugars added to foods supply calories but few or no nutrients. Refer to Table 36-2 for more information regarding the sources, functions, and significance of carbohydrates.

Protein

Protein is a vital component of every living cell. Within the human body, more than 1,000 different proteins are made by combining various amounts and proportions of the 22 basic building blocks known as amino acids. Although amino acids, like carbohydrates, contain carbon, hydrogen, and oxygen, they differ in that amino acids also contain nitrogen. Nine amino acids are classified as essential because they cannot be

TABLE • 36-2	SOURCES, FUNCTIONS, AND SIGNIFICANCE OF CARBOHYDRATES, PROTEIN, AND FAT		
Nutrient	**Sources**	**Functions**	**Significance**
Carbohydrates			
Simple sugars and starch	Fruits Vegetables Grains: rice, pasta, breads, cereals Dried peas and beans Milk (lactose) Sugars: white and brown sugar, honey, molasses, syrup	Provide energy Spare protein so it can be used for other functions Prevent ketosis from inefficient fat metabolism	Provide about 46% of the calories in the typical American diet; many believe carbohydrate intake should be increased to 50%–60% of total calories. Low carbohydrate intake can cause ketosis; high simple sugar intake increases the risk for dental caries.
Cellulose and other water-insoluble fibers	Whole wheat flour and wheat bran Vegetables: cabbage, peas, green beans, wax beans, broccoli, brussel sprouts, cucumber skins, peppers, carrots Apples	Absorb water to increase fecal bulk Decrease intestinal transit time	Are nondigestible; therefore, are excreted Help relieve constipation North Americans are urged to eat more of all types of fiber. Excess intake can cause gas, distention, and diarrhea.
Water-soluble fibers	Oat bran and oatmeal Dried peas and beans Vegetables Prunes, pears, apples, bananas, oranges	Slow gastric emptying Lower serum cholesterol level Delay glucose absorption	Help improve glucose tolerance in diabetics
Protein	Milk and milk products Meat, poultry, fish Eggs Dried peas and beans Nuts	Tissue growth and repair Component of body framework: bones, muscles, tendons, blood vessels, skin, hair, nails Component of body fluids: hormones, enzymes, plasma proteins, neurotransmitters, mucus Helps regulate fluid balance through oncotic pressure Helps regulate acid–base balance Detoxifies harmful substances Forms antibodies Transports fat and other substances through the blood Provides energy when carbohydrate intake is inadequate	Most North Americans consume twice the RDA (RNI) for protein. Experts recommend that we eat less animal protein and more vegetable protein. Protein deficiency is characterized by edema, retarded growth and maturation, muscle wasting, changes in the hair and skin, permanent damage to physical and mental development (in children), diarrhea, malabsorption, numerous secondary nutrient deficiencies, fatty infiltration of the liver, increased risk for infections, and high mortality. Except for elderly people, fad dieters, hospitalized patients, and people of low income, protein deficiency is rare in the United States and Canada.
Fat	Butter, oils, margarine, lard, salt pork, salad dressings, mayonnaise, bacon Whole milk and whole milk products High-fat meats Nuts	Provides energy Provides structure Insulates the body Cushions internal organs Necessary for the absorption of fat-soluble vitamins	Fat supplies about 37% of total calories in the typical North American diet; experts suggest a reduction to 30% or less of total calories. High-fat diets increase the risk for heart disease and obesity and are correlated with an increased risk for colon and breast cancers.

(Dudek, S. G. [2006]. *Nutrition essentials for nursing practice* [5th ed.]. Philadelphia: Lippincott Williams & Wilkins.)

synthesized in the body; they must be obtained from the diet. The remaining 13 amino acids are no less important, but because the body can make them as long as a supply of nitrogen is available, they are termed nonessential. Proteins are required for the formation of all body structures, including genes, enzymes, muscle, bone matrix, skin, and blood.

CLASSIFICATION AND METABOLISM

Dietary proteins may be labeled complete (high quality) or incomplete (low quality), based on their amino acid composition. Complete proteins contain sufficient amounts and proportions of all the essential amino acids to support growth, whereas incomplete proteins are deficient in one or more essential amino acids. Generally, animal proteins (eggs, dairy products, meats) are complete, and plant proteins (grains, legumes, vegetables) are incomplete. The only exception is soy, a plant protein that is considered a complete protein. Because different sources of plant proteins lack different amino acids, a plant protein can be complemented by combining it with a different plant protein or by adding a small amount of an animal protein to supply a complete protein. Examples of complementary vegetable proteins include corn tortilla and refried beans and lentil rice soup. Complementary proteins that use a small amount of animal protein include cereal with milk, rice pudding, and a cheese sandwich.

Dietary protein is broken down into amino acid particles by pancreatic enzymes in the small intestine. These are absorbed through the intestinal mucosa to be transported to the liver. In the liver, amino acids are recombined into new proteins or are released into the bloodstream for use in protein synthesis by tissues and cells. Excess amino acids are converted to fatty acids, ketone bodies, or glucose and are stored or used as metabolic fuel.

The body's protein tissues are in a constant state of flux. Tissues are continuously being broken down (catabolism) and replaced (anabolism). Nitrogen balance, a comparison between catabolism and anabolism, can be measured by comparing nitrogen intake (protein intake) and nitrogen excretion (nitrogen lost in urine, urea, feces, hair, nails, skin). When catabolism and anabolism are occurring at the same rate, as in healthy adults, the body is in a state of neutral nitrogen balance (i.e., nitrogen intake equals nitrogen excretion). A positive nitrogen balance occurs when nitrogen intake is greater than excretion—for example, during periods of growth, pregnancy, lactation, and recovery from illness. A negative nitrogen balance occurs when more nitrogen is excreted than is ingested. This undesirable state occurs in situations such as starvation and the catabolism that immediately follows surgery, illness, trauma, and stress.

FUNCTIONS AND RECOMMENDED DIETARY ALLOWANCE

The major function of protein is to maintain body tissues that break down from normal wear and tear and to support the growth of new tissue. Protein can be oxidized to provide 4 calories per gram. Using protein for energy is more expensive both financially and physiologically than using carbohydrates.

The nitrogen remaining after protein is metabolized burdens the kidneys. In addition, energy must be used to excrete the nitrogen. Like carbohydrates, protein consumed in excess of need can be converted to and stored as fat.

The recommended daily intake for protein for adults is 0.8 g/kg of desirable body weight, or about 56 g for the average woman and 63 g for the average man. Protein intake should contribute 10% to 20% of total caloric intake (Dudek, 2006). Refer to Table 36-2 for more information about the sources, functions, and significance of protein.

Fats

Fats in the diet, or **lipids,** are insoluble in water and, therefore, insoluble in blood. Like carbohydrates, they are composed of carbon, hydrogen, and oxygen. Ninety-five percent of the lipids in the diet are in the form of **triglycerides,** the predominant form of fat in food and the major storage form of fat in the body. Compound lipids (such as phospholipids, in which a lipid is combined with another substance) and derived lipids (such as cholesterol) constitute the remainder of the lipids ingested.

CLASSIFICATION AND METABOLISM

Food fats contain mixtures of saturated and unsaturated fatty acids. The difference in degree of saturation depends on the amount of hydrogen in fat molecules. Saturated fats contain more hydrogen than unsaturated fats. Most animal fats are considered saturated and have a solid consistency at room temperature. Conversely, most vegetable fats are considered unsaturated, remain liquid at room temperature, and are referred to as oils. Saturated fats tend to raise serum cholesterol levels, whereas unsaturated fats lower serum cholesterol levels. When manufacturers partially hydrogenate liquid oils, they become more solid and more stable. This substance is referred to as **trans fat.** Trans fat raises serum cholesterol. Therefore, it is to be counted in with the total number of saturated fats in a day. The U.S. Food and Drug Administration (FDA) requires that food nutrition labels must list trans fat so that consumers may make healthy choices in their diet.

Cholesterol is a fatlike substance found only in animal products. It is not an essential nutrient; the body makes sufficient amounts (Dudek, 2006; Sizer & Whitney, 2006). Cholesterol is an important component of cell membranes and is especially abundant in brain and nerve cells. It also is used to synthesize bile acids and is a precursor of the steroid hormones and vitamin D. Although cholesterol serves many important functions in the body, high serum levels are clearly associated with an increased risk for atherosclerosis. To help lower serum cholesterol levels, researchers recommend limiting cholesterol intake, eating less total fat—especially saturated and trans fat—eating more unsaturated fat, and increasing fiber intake, which increases fecal excretion of cholesterol.

▶ *Remember William Johnston, the middle-aged executive with hypertension and high cholesterol? Due to*

Mr. Johnston's "on-the-run" lifestyle, developing an individualized nutritional plan might be somewhat challenging. Based on an assessment of Mr. Johnston's eating habits, likes, and dislikes, the nurse would work with him to develop a plan that promotes weight loss and includes limiting cholesterol and total fat intake and consuming more foods containing unsaturated fats and fiber. Adapting the plan will help to promote adherence to it, thereby increasing the chances for success. ∎

Fat digestion occurs largely in the small intestine. Bile, secreted by the gallbladder, emulsifies fat to increase the surface area so that pancreatic lipase can break down fat more effectively. Through a complex series of events, most fats are absorbed into the lymphatic circulation with the help of a protein carrier and are transported to the liver. Of 100 grams eaten, only about 3 grams are excreted in the feces.

FUNCTIONS AND RECOMMENDED DIETARY ALLOWANCE

Fats are the most concentrated source of energy in the diet, providing 9 calories for every gram. Fat increases the palatability of the diet (e.g., to most people, filet mignon tastes better than flank steak) and has a high satiety value because it delays gastric emptying time. In the body, fat aids in the absorption of the fat-soluble vitamins and provides insulation, structure, and temperature control. Refer to Table 36-2 for more information about the sources, functions, and significance of fat.

The *Dietary Guidelines for Americans 2005* recommends that fat intake be no more than between 20% and 35% of total caloric intake, with less than 10% of fat calories from saturated fats and less than 300 mg/day of cholesterol (USDA & DHHS, 2005).

Regulatory Nutrients

Vitamins, minerals, and water are regulatory nutrients because they are needed by the body for the metabolism of energy nutrients.

Vitamins

Vitamins are organic compounds needed by the body in small amounts. Most vitamins are active in the form of coenzymes, which, together with enzymes, facilitate thousands of chemical reactions in the body. Although vitamins do not provide energy (calories), they are needed for the metabolism of carbohydrates, protein, and fat. Vitamins are essential in the diet because most are not synthesized in the body or are made in insufficient quantities. The absence or insufficient use of vitamins in the body causes specific deficiency syndromes.

Vitamins are present in foods in only small amounts. Fresh foods are higher in vitamins than processed foods because vitamins may be destroyed by light, heat, air, and during preparation. The exception is when vitamins not naturally occurring in a food are added, such as vitamin D-fortified milk. This process is called fortification.

In the United States, severe vitamin deficiencies are uncommon. Mild or subclinical deficiencies of vitamin A, vitamin C, folate, and vitamin B_6, however, may affect a significant proportion of the population, especially those who (1) are members of certain age groups or patient groups (infants, adolescents, pregnant and lactating women, older people); (2) smoke, abuse alcohol, or use medications on a long-term basis; (3) are chronically ill, either physically or psychologically; or (4) are poor or finicky eaters, such as chronic dieters, strict vegetarians, and food faddists.

Vitamins are classified as either water soluble or fat soluble. Water-soluble vitamins include vitamin C and the B-complex vitamins (ascorbic acid, thiamin, riboflavin, niacin, pyridoxine, biotin pantothenic acid, folate, cobalamin). They are absorbed through the intestinal wall directly into the bloodstream. Although some tissues are able to hold limited amounts of water-soluble vitamins, they usually are not stored in the body. Deficiency symptoms are apt to develop quickly when intake is inadequate; therefore, a daily intake is recommended. However, because water-soluble vitamins are not stored, amounts consumed in excess of need are excreted in the urine. Toxicities are not likely, although megadoses of certain water-soluble vitamins can be harmful.

Vitamins A, D, E, and K, the fat-soluble vitamins, are absorbed with fat into the lymphatic circulation. Like fat, they must be attached to a protein to be transported through the blood. Secondary deficiencies of the fat-soluble vitamins can occur anytime fat digestion or absorption is altered, such as during malabsorption syndromes and pancreatic and biliary diseases. The body stores excesses of the fat-soluble vitamins mostly in the liver and adipose tissue. Because they are stored, a daily intake is not imperative and deficiency symptoms may take weeks, months, or years to develop. Excessive intake, particularly of vitamins A and D, is toxic.

Many studies have attempted to evaluate the relationship of vitamin intake to diseases ranging from cardiovascular disease, osteoporosis, and neural tube defects to some types of cancers (NIH, 2007). Although scrutiny and research continue about vitamin supplements and their long-term effects, most nutritionists agree that vitamins will never be a substitute for good nutrition and healthy lifestyle practices (NIH, 2007: Dudek, 2006; Lichtenstein & Russell, 2005; USDA & DHHS, 2005). The *Dietary Guidelines for Americans 2005* (USDA & DHHS, 2005) recommends the nutrient needs should be met primarily through consuming foods. Supplements may be useful when they fill a specific identified nutrient gap that cannot or is not otherwise being met by the individuals' intake of food (NIH, 2007; USDA & DHHS, 2005). Supplementation can ensure adequate intakes of specific nutrients because of physiologic limitations or changes (Lichtenstein & Russell, 2005). For example, folate supplementation during pregnancy has significantly decreased the risk of children born with neural tube defects (Lichtenstein & Russell, 2005). Table 36-3 summarizes water- and fat-soluble vitamins.

TABLE • 36-3	**SUMMARY OF VITAMINS**			
Nutrient and Adult RDA	**Sources**	**Functions**	**Signs and Symptoms of Deficiency**	**Signs and Symptoms of Excess**
Water-Soluble Vitamins				
Vitamin C (ascorbic acid) 75–90 mg (additional 35 mg/day for smokers)	Citrus fruits, broccoli, green pepper, strawberries, greens	Collagen formation, antioxidant, enhances iron absorption	Scurvy, hemorrhaging, delayed wound healing	Hot flashes, headache, nausea, diarrhea
Vitamin B complex				
Thiamin 1.1–1.2 mg	Pork, liver, whole and enriched grains, legumes	Coenzyme in key reactions that produce energy from glucose	Beriberi, mental confusion, fatigue	None known
Riboflavin 1.1–1.3 mg	Milk, organ meats, enriched grains, greens	Carbohydrate, protein, and fat metabolism	Dermatitis, glossitis, photophobia	None known
Niacin 14–16 mg	Kidney, grains, lean meat, nuts	Carbohydrate, protein, and fat metabolism	Pellagra, dermatitis	Flushing and itching, nausea, vomiting, liver damage
B_6 (pyridoxine) 1.3–1.7 mg	Yeast, banana, cantaloupe, broccoli, spinach	Coenzyme in protein, fat, carbohydrate metabolism	Microcytic anemia, CNS problems	Difficulty walking, numbness of feet and hands
Folate 400 mcg	Green leafy vegetables, liver	RNA and DNA synthesis, formation and maturation of RBC	Macrocytic anemia: fatigue, weakness, pallor	None known
B_{12} (cyanocobalamin) 2.4 mcg	Animal products: organ meats, seafood	Coenzyme in protein metabolism and formation of heme portion of hemoglobin	Pernicious anemia (B_{12} deficiency related to impaired absorption due to lack of intrinsic factor)	None known
Pantothenic acid 5 mg	Widespread in foods; meat, poultry, fish, whole grain cereals	Carbohydrate, protein, and fat metabolism	None known	None known
Biotin 30 mcg	Liver, egg yolk	Carbohydrate, protein, and fat metabolism	Rare; dry skin, anorexia, fatigue	None known
Fat-Soluble Vitamins				
Vitamin A (retinol, retinal, retinoic acid) 700–900 mcg	Liver, carrots, egg yolk, fortified milk	Visual acuity in dim light, formation and maintenance of skin and mucous membranes; immune function	Night blindness, rough skin, bone growth ceases	Anorexia, loss of hair, dry skin, bone pain, vomiting, birth defects during pregnancy
Vitamin D (cholecalciferol, ergosterol) 5 mcg	Sunlight, fortified milk, fish liver oils	Calcium and phosphorus metabolism, stimulates calcium absorption	Retarded bone growth, bone malformation	Excessive calcification of bones, renal calculi, nausea, headache
Vitamin E (tocopherol) 15 mcg	Vegetable oils, wheat germ, whole grain products	Antioxidant, protects vitamin A, heme synthesis	Increased RBC hemolysis and macrocytic anemia in premature infants	Relatively nontoxic, although large doses can cause fatigue, diarrhea, and enhance action of anticoagulant medications
Vitamin K 90–125 mcg	Dark, green leafy vegetables; synthesized in intestines from gut bacteria	Synthesis of certain proteins necessary for blood clotting	Hemorrhagic disease of newborn, delayed blood clotting	Hemolytic anemia and liver damage with synthetic vitamin K

(Dudek, S. G. [2006]. *Nutrition essentials for nursing practice* [5th ed.]. Philadelphia: Lippincott Williams & Wilkins; and Sizer, F., & Whitney, E. [2006]. *Nutrition. Concepts and controversies* (10th ed.). Belmont, CA: Thomson Wadsworth.)

> *Think back to Susan Oakland, the young woman who is pregnant. She will be advised to take a daily multivitamin supplement as part of her prenatal care. Supplements are used in conjunction with an optimal diet, to meet the increased nutrient requirements of pregnancy.* ■

Minerals

Minerals are inorganic elements found in all body fluids and tissues in the form of salts (e.g., sodium chloride) or combined with organic compounds (e.g., iron in hemoglobin). Some minerals function to provide structure within the body, whereas others help to regulate body processes. Minerals, which are elements, are not broken down or rearranged in the body but, rather, are contained in the ash that remains after digestion. Excessive soaking and cooking in water can cause loss of minerals from food. However, minerals are commonly not destroyed by food processing.

Macrominerals (bulk minerals), minerals needed by the body in amounts greater than 100 mg/day, include calcium, phosphorus (phosphates), sulfur (sulfate), sodium, chloride, potassium, and magnesium. Microminerals, or trace elements, are minerals needed by the body in amounts less than 100 mg/day. Microminerals that have recommended dietary intake established include iron, zinc, manganese, chromium, copper, molybdenum, selenium, fluoride, and iodine. Additional trace elements included arsenic, boron, nickel, silicon, cobalt, and vanadium. Dietary guidelines for these elements have not been established. Ultratrace elements are elements that are consumed in microgram quantities each day. They occur in very low quantities in human tissues and their essentiality is uncertain. These elements include aluminum, lithium, nickel, silicon, tin, and vanadium. Macrominerals and microminerals that have recommended intake guidelines are summarized in Table 36-4.

Water

As the major body constituent present in every body cell, water accounts for between 50% and 60% of the adult's total weight. Infants have proportionately more water accounting for body weight. About two thirds of the body's water is contained within the cells (intracellular fluid [ICF]); the remainder is called extracellular fluid (ECF), which includes all other body fluids, such as plasma and interstitial fluid. Total body water and ECF decrease with age; ICF increases with an increase in body mass. Refer to Chapter 40 for more information on water in the body.

Water is more vital to life than food because it provides the fluid medium necessary for all chemical reactions, it participates in many reactions, and it is not stored in the body. Water acts as a solvent that dissolves many solutes, thereby aiding digestion, absorption, circulation, and excretion. Through evaporation from the skin, water helps to regulate body temperature. As a lubricant, water is needed both for mucous secretions and for movement between joints.

> *Think back to Charles Gallagher, husband of the woman with advanced dementia receiving enteral nutrition. During the group meeting about continuing or withdrawing the enteral nutrition, Mr. Gallagher learns that withdrawal of the feedings would also involve limited water intake. This information is important in helping Mr. Gallagher and his family arrive at an informed decision about whether or not to continue the enteral feedings.* ■

Sources of water in the diet include not only beverages but also solid foods, which contain from 10% to 98% water. Water is also produced through the metabolism of carbohydrates, protein, and fat. It leaves the body through urine, feces, expired air, and perspiration. Water intake (an average of 2,000 to 3,000 mL/day for adults [Sizer & Whitney, 2006]) usually equals water output. Water balance may be seriously affected when intake (such as in individuals who are elderly or in comatose states) or output (such as in patients with altered renal function, profuse perspiration, diarrhea, vomiting, fistulas, drainage tubes, hemorrhage, severe burns) is altered.

ANATOMY AND PHYSIOLOGY OF THE DIGESTIVE SYSTEM

The food consumed by a person supplies the essential nutrients needed for cells to perform their necessary functions, but the cells cannot use food in its consumed form. The gastrointestinal system breaks down the food into particles small enough to pass into the cells and be used by the cells. This breakdown process is called **digestion.** Digestion begins in the mouth where food is taken in, mixes with saliva, is pushed into the pharynx by the tongue, and then continues into the esophagus. Peristalsis moves the food through the esophagus and into the stomach. The stomach churns the ingested food, mixing it with substances to break down the food and convert it to a semiliquid mixture. The food leaves the stomach and enters the small intestine. The small intestine secrets enzymes that digest the food, along with secretions from the liver and pancreas. The digested nutrients are then transferred into the person's circulation (**absorption**), to be transported throughout the body. Most absorption of digested food and minerals, and some absorption of water, occurs through the walls of the small intestine. Undigested waste materials continue through the gastrointestinal tract and are eliminated. Elimination of these waste products is discussed in Chapter 38. Figure 38-1 in Chapter 38 illustrates the organs of the gastrointestinal tract.

ADEQUATE DIET SELECTION

An adequate diet provides a balanced intake of all essential nutrients in appropriate amounts. However, what constitutes an adequate diet is less obvious. Tools for planning or evaluating a diet for adequacy include the "MyPyramid" food guidance system, the RDA (Recommended Dietary Allowance),

TABLE • 36-4	SUMMARY OF MACROMINERALS AND MICROMINERALS			
Nutrient and Adult RDA	Sources	Functions	Signs and Symptoms of Deficiency	Signs and Symptoms of Excess
Macrominerals				
Calcium 1,000 mg	Milk and dairy products, canned fish with bones, greens	Bone and tooth formation, blood clotting, nerve transmission, muscle contraction	Tetany, osteoporosis	Renal calculi in susceptible people
Phosphorus 700 mg	Milk and milk products, soft drinks, processed foods	Bone and tooth formation, acid–base balance, energy metabolism	Hypophosphatemia: anorexia, muscle weakness	Hyperphosphatemia: symptoms of hypocalcemic tetany
Magnesium 310–420 mg	Green leafy vegetables, nuts, beans, grains	Bone and tooth formation, protein synthesis, carbohydrate metabolism	Hypomagnesemia: weakness, muscle pain, poor heart function	Hypermagnesemia: CNS depression, coma, hypotension
Sulfur (provided by adequate amounts of protein)	Meat, eggs, milk, dried peas and beans, nuts	Promotes certain enzyme reactions and detoxification reactions	None known	None known
Sodium 1,500 mg	Salt, processed foods	Major ion of extracellular fluid, fluid balance, acid–base balance	Hyponatremia: muscle cramps, cold and clammy skin	Edema, weight gain, high blood pressure if susceptible
Potassium 4,700 mg	Whole grains, fruits, leafy vegetables	Major ion of intracellular fluid, fluid balance, acid–base balance	Hypokalemia: muscle cramps and weakness, irregular heartbeat	Hyperkalemia: irritability, anxiety, cardiac arrhythmia, heart block
Chloride 2,300 mg	Salt	Component of HCl in stomach, fluid balance, acid–base balance	Hypochloremia: muscle spasms, alkalosis, depressed respirations	Hyperchloremia: acidosis
Microminerals				
Iron 8–18 mg	Liver, lean meats, enriched and whole grain breads and cereals	Oxygen transport by way of hemoglobin, constituent of enzyme systems	Microcytic anemia, pallor, decreased work capacity, fatigue, weakness	Hemosiderosis; acute iron poisoning from accidental overdose leads to GI symptoms and possible shock
Iodine 150 mg	Iodized salt, seafood, food additives	Component of thyroid hormones	Goiter	Acne-like lesions
Zinc 8–11 mg	Oysters, liver, meats, dried peas and beans, nuts	Tissue growth, sexual maturation, immune response	Impaired growth, sexual maturation, immune system functioning	Anorexia, nausea, vomiting, diarrhea, muscle pain, lethargy
Copper 900 mcg	Liver, shellfish, grains, dried peas and beans	Aids in iron metabolism and activity of some enzymes	Anemia, altered bone formation, hypercholesterolemia	Nervous system disturbances, vomiting
Manganese 1.8–2.3 mg	Whole grains, nuts, dried peas and beans, fruit	Part of enzymes needed for protein and energy metabolism	Poor reproductive performance, growth retardation	None known
Fluoride 3–4 mg (estimated safe, adequate intake)	Fluoridated water, fish, tea	Tooth formation and integrity, bone formation and integrity	Tooth decay; may increase risk for osteoporosis	Mottling and discoloration of tooth enamel
Chromium 25–35 mcg	Whole grains, meats	Cofactor for insulin, proper glucose metabolism	Impaired glucose tolerance, insulin resistance	None known
Selenium 55 mcg	Wheat (if grown in high-selenium soil), organ meats	Antioxidant	None known	Loss of hair, brittle fingernails, fatigue
Molybdenum 45 mg (estimated safe, adequate intake)	Liver, whole grains, dried peas and beans, organ meats	Oxidizes sulfur and products of sulfur metabolism	None known	Interferes with copper metabolism
Cobalt Unknown–apparently minute	Organ meats	Essential component of vitamin B_{12}	None known	None known

(Dudek, S. G. [2006]. *Nutrition essentials for nursing practice* [5th ed.]. Philadelphia: Lippincott Williams & Wilkins; and Sizer, F., & Whitney, E. [2006]. *Nutrition. Concepts and controversies* (10th ed.). Belmont, CA: Thomson Wadsworth.)

and dietary recommendations and guidelines issued from health and U.S. governmental agencies. The task of promoting health through proper nutrition has been made easier by labeling regulations that provide specific information about food contents and their comparison to recommended daily intakes.

Dietary Recommendations

The *Dietary Guidelines for Americans* are science-based strategies compiled by The Public Health Service of the Department of Health and Human Services and the U.S. Department of Agriculture. These guidelines provide advice to promote health and to reduce risk for major chronic diseases through diet and physical activity. Although these diet recommendations are not guaranteed to prevent diseases, many experts believe that most Americans can reduce their risk for chronic diet-related diseases, such as diabetes, certain types of cancer, and heart disease, by modifying the typical diet. The Public Health Service of the Department of Health and Human Services and the U.S. Department of Agriculture together update the *Dietary Guidelines for Americans* every 5 years. A summary of the Dietary Guidelines 2005 appears in Box 36-2. The complete guidelines are available at www.healthierus.gov/dietaryguidelines (USDA & DHHS, 2005).

Recommended Dietary Allowance

The recommended dietary allowances (RDA) are the recommended average daily dietary intake levels to meet the nutri-ent requirements for healthy individuals by life stage and gender (Dudek, 2006). Unlike a requirement, which is the amount of a nutrient needed to prevent a deficiency, an allowance has a safety factor built in to account for individual variations. Because the RDA is intended for populations and not individuals, some people may not be able to meet their individual requirements, despite consuming the RDA. Likewise, it is possible for some people to eat less than the RDA and still avoid deficiencies. Although the RDA is defined for age and gender and is revised about every 5 years as new information becomes available, it has not been established for all nutrients. Variety is recommended.

MyPyramid Food Guide

In April 2005, the U.S. Department of Agriculture (USDA) released the "MyPyramid: Steps to a Healthier You" food guidance system graphic (Fig. 36-2) to help consumers implement the 2005 dietary guidelines and RDA recommendations. It provides specific recommendations for making food choices to improve the American diet. The goals of the recommendations are to increase the intake of vitamins, minerals, and dietary fiber; lower the intake of saturated fats, trans fats, and cholesterol; increase the intake of fruits, vegetables, and whole grains; and support a calorie intake balanced with energy needs to promote a healthy weight. MyPyramid encourages eating a variety of foods from all food groups and being physically active every day. Each color band represents one of the five food groups and oils,

---

Box 36-2 **SUMMARY OF DIETARY GUIDELINES FOR AMERICANS 2005**

To achieve adequate nutrients within energy needs:
- Consume a variety of nutrient-dense foods and beverages within and among the basic food groups. Limit the intake of saturated and trans fats, cholesterol, added sugars, salt, and alcohol.
- Meet recommended intakes within energy needs by adopting a balanced eating pattern.

For weight management:
- Balance calories from foods and beverages with calories expended to maintain body weight in a healthy range.
- Make small decreases in food and beverage calories and increase physical activity to prevent gradual weight gain over time.

Guidelines for physical activity include:
- Engage in regular physical activity and reduce sedentary activities to promote health, psychological well-being, and a healthy body weight.
- Achieve physical fitness by including cardiovascular conditioning, stretching exercises for flexibility, and resistance exercises or calisthenics for muscle strength and endurance.

Food groups to encourage include:
- Consume a sufficient amount of fruits and vegetables, milk and milk products, and whole grains, while staying within energy needs.

- Choose a variety of fruits and vegetables each day from all vegetable subgroups.
- Choose at least half the grain selections from whole grains.

Guidelines for fats include:
- Keep total fat intake between 20% and 35% of calories, with most fats coming from sources of polyunsaturated and monounsaturated fats such as fish, nuts, and vegetable oils.
- Choose lean, low-fat, or fat-free meats, poultry, dry beans, and milk or milk products.

Guidelines for carbohydrates include:
- Choose fiber-rich fruits, vegetables, and whole grains often.
- Choose and prepare foods with little added sugars or caloric sweeteners.

Guidelines for sodium and potassium include:
- Consume less than 2,300 mg (approximately 1 teaspoon of salt) of sodium per day.
- Choose and prepare foods with little salt.
- Consume potassium-rich foods, such as fruits and vegetables.

Guidelines for alcoholic beverages include:
- Consume alcoholic beverages sensibly and in moderation. Consume up to one drink per day for women and up to two drinks per day for men.

(United States Department of Agriculture [USDA] and U.S. Department of Health and Human Services [DHHS]. [2005]. *Dietary guidelines for Americans 2005*. Available at www.health.gov/dietaryguidelines/dga2005/document/.)

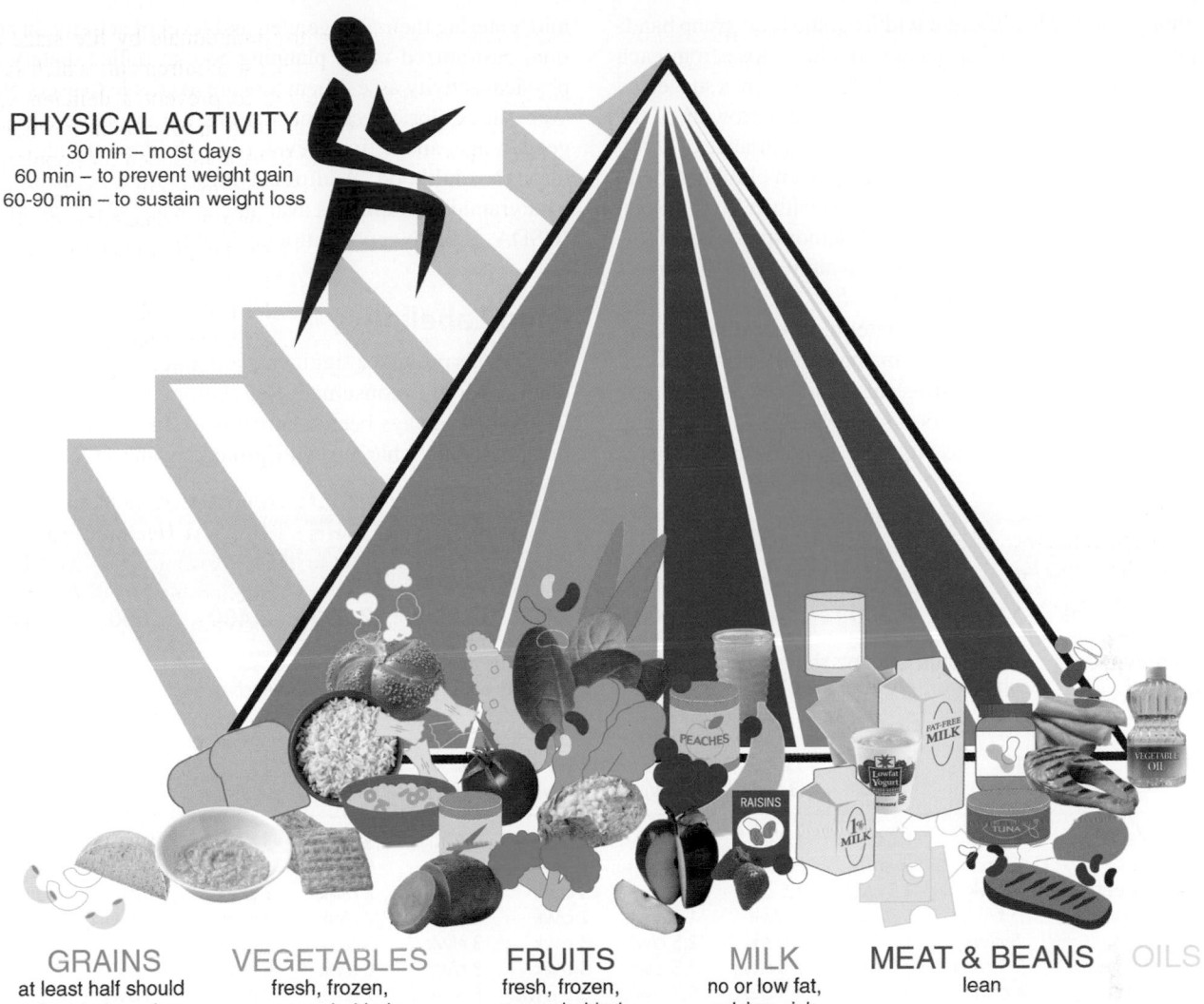

PHYSICAL ACTIVITY
30 min – most days
60 min – to prevent weight gain
60-90 min – to sustain weight loss

GRAINS	VEGETABLES	FRUITS	MILK	MEAT & BEANS	OILS
at least half should be whole grain	fresh, frozen, canned, dried	fresh, frozen, canned, dried	no or low fat, calcium rich	lean	

GRAINS	VEGETABLES	FRUITS	MILK	MEAT & BEANS
Make half your grains whole	Vary your veggies	Focus on fruits	Get your calcium-rich foods	Go lean with protein
Eat at least 3 oz. of whole-grain cereals, breads, crackers, rice, or pasta every day 1 oz. is about 1 slice of bread, about 1 cup of breakfast cereal, or ½ cup of cooked rice, cereal, or pasta	Eat more dark-green veggies like broccoli, spinach, and other dark leafy greens Eat more orange vegetables like carrots and sweetpotatoes Eat more dry beans and peas like pinto beans, kidney beans, and lentils	Eat a variety of fruit Choose fresh, frozen, canned, or dried fruit Go easy on fruit juices	Go low-fat or fat-free when you choose milk, yogurt, and other milk products If you don't or can't consume milk, choose lactose-free products or other calcium sources such as fortified foods and beverages	Choose low-fat or lean meats and poultry Bake it, broil it, or grill it Vary your protein routine – choose more fish, beans, peas, nuts, and seeds

For a 2,000-calorie diet, you need the amounts below from each food group. To find the amounts that are right for you, go to MyPyramid.gov.

Eat 6 oz. every day	Eat 2½ cups every day	Eat 2 cups every day	Get 3 cups every day; for kids aged 2 to 8, it's 2	Eat 5½ oz. every day

Find your balance between food and physical activity
- Be sure to stay within your daily calorie needs.
- Be physically active for at least 30 minutes most days of the week.
- About 60 minutes a day of physical activity may be needed to prevent weight gain.
- For sustaining weight loss, at least 60 to 90 minutes a day of physical activity may be required.
- Children and teenagers should be physically active for 60 minutes every day, or most days.

Know the limits on fats, sugars, and salt (sodium)
- Make most of your fat sources from fish, nuts, and vegetable oils.
- Limit solid fats like butter, margarine, shortening, and lard, as well as foods that contain these.
- Check the Nutrition Facts label to keep saturated fats, *trans* fats, and sodium low.
- Choose food and beverages low in added sugars. Added sugars contribute calories with few, if any, nutrients.

FIGURE 36-2. The MyPyramid.gov Food Guide. (Source: U.S. Department of Agriculture. [2008]. Available at www.mypyramid.gov.)

showing variety. The different widths of the food group bands suggest how much food a person should choose from each group; notice the proportion of each. Moderation is suggested by the narrowing of each food group by the narrowing of the color bars at the top of the pyramid. The importance of activity is represented by the steps and the person climbing them. The MyPyramid.gov URL, "Steps to a Healthier You" slogan, and person climbing the pyramid all demonstrate the importance of personalization. "Steps to a Healthier You" illustrates the theme of gradual improvement.

Information and educational materials are available on an interactive food guidance system that offers a customized food intake pattern for 12 different caloric levels, outlining suggested daily amounts of food from each basic food group (Table 36-5). Visitors to the Web site can customize a pyramid, entering their age, gender, and level of activity. In addition, customized menu planning and an online dietary and physical activity assessment tool are available to users of the Web site. Caloric recommendations are available based on gender, age, and activity level, from children of toddler age through adulthood. Additional information regarding the MyPyramid guidelines is available at www.MyPyramid.gov (USDA, 2008; Nappo-Dattoma, 2005).

Food Labeling

Food labels provide a significant amount of nutritional information for the consumer. Regulations that control food labels have always been controversial. In 1975, the FDA, a federal agency charged with protecting the U.S. food and

TABLE • 36-5 DAILY AMOUNT OF FOOD FROM EACH GROUP (VEGETABLE SUBGROUP AMOUNTS ARE PER WEEK)

Calorie Level	1,000	1,200	1,400	1,600	1,800	2,000	2,200	2,400	2,600	2,800
Food group	Food group amounts shown in cup (c) or ounce-equivalents (oz-eq), with number of servings (srv) in parentheses when it differs from the other units. See note for quantity equivalents for foods in each group. Oils are shown in grams (g).									
Fruits	1 c (2 srv)	1 c (2 srv)	1.5 c (3 srv)	1.5 c (3 srv)	1.5 c (3 srv)	2 c (4 srv)	2 c (4 srv)	2 c (4 srv)	2 c (4 srv)	2.5 c (5 srv)
Vegetables	1 c (2 srv)	1.5 c (3 srv)	1.5 c (3 srv)	2 c (4 srv)	2.5 c (5 srv)	2.5 c (5 srv)	3 c (6 srv)	3 c (6 srv)	3.5 c (7 srv)	3.5 c (7 srv)
Dark green veg.	1 c/wk	1.5 c/wk	1.5 c/wk	2 c/wk	3 c/wk	3 c/wk	3 c/wk	3 c/wk	3 c/wk	3 c/wk
Orange veg.	.5 c/wk	1 c/wk	1 c/wk	1.5 c/wk	2 c/wk	2 c/wk	2 c/wk	2 c/wk	2.5 c/wk	2.5 c/wk
Legumes	.5 c/wk	1 c/wk	1 c/wk	2.5 c/wk	3 c/wk	3 c/wk	3 c/wk	3 c/wk	3.5 c/wk	3.5 c/wk
Starchy veg.	1.5 c/wk	2.5 c/wk	2.5 c/wk	2.5 c/wk	3 c/wk	3 c/wk	6 c/wk	6 c/wk	7 c/wk	7 c/wk
Other veg.	4 c/wk	4.5 c/wk	4.5 c/wk	5.5 c/wk	6.5 c/wk	6.5 c/wk	7 c/wk	7 c/wk	8.5 c/wk	8.5 c/wk
Grains	3 oz-eq	4 oz-eq	5 oz-eq	5 oz-eq	6 oz-eq	6 oz-eq	7 oz-eq	8 oz-eq	9 oz-eq	10 oz-eq
Whole grains	1.5	2	2.5	3	3	3	3.5	4	4.5	5
Other grains	1.5	2	2.5	2	3	3	3.5	4	4.5	5
Lean meat and beans	2 oz-eq	3 oz-eq	4 oz-eq	5 oz-eq	5 oz-eq	5.5 oz-eq	6 oz-eq	6.5 oz-eq	6.5 oz-eq	7 oz-eq
Milk	2 c	2 c	2 c	3 c	3 c	3 c	3 c	3 c	3 c	3 c
Oils	15 g	17 g	17 g	22 g	24 g	27 g	29 g	31 g	34 g	36 g
Discretionary calorie allowance	165	171	171	132	195	267	290	362	410	426

Quantity equivalents for each food group:
  Grains—The following each count as 1 ounce-equivalent (1 serving) of grains: 1 cup cooked rice, pasta, or cooked cereal; 1 ounce dry pasta or rice; 1 slice bread; 1 small muffin (1 oz); 1 cup ready-to-eat cereal flakes.
  Fruits and vegetables—The following each count as 1 cup (2 servings) of fruits or vegetables: 1 cup cut up raw or cooked fruit or vegetable, 1 cup fruit or vegetable juice, 2 cups leafy salad greens.
  Meat and beans—The following each count as 1 ounce-equivalent: 1 ounce lean meat, poultry, or fish; 1 egg; ¼ cup cooked dry beans or tofu; 1 tablespoon peanut butter; 1 ounce nuts or seeds.
  Milk—The following each count as 1 cup (1 serving) of milk: 1 cup milk or yogurt, 1fi ounces natural cheese such as cheddar cheese or 2 ounces processed cheese. Discretionary calories must be counted for all choices, except fat-free milk.
Discretionary calorie allowance is: the remaining number of calories that can be from added sugars and fat in food preparation, sugars added to beverages, canned fruit; higher fat products.
For more information, refer to the Dietary Guidelines for Americans 2005 at www.healthierus.gov.
Source: National Institutes of Health, National Heart, Lung, and Blood Institute. (2005) *Aim for a healthy weight* (p. 8). NIH publication no. 05-5213.

drug supply, enacted legislation for a standardized label format that was considered a positive step toward educating the consumer about nutrition. Confusion and misinformation resulted as food manufacturers oversimplified or exaggerated health claims for their products. In 1990, Congress passed the Nutritional Labeling and Education Act, which required all foods, including fruits and vegetables, to be clearly labeled. Four broad categories are addressed in this legislation. They include nutrition labeling, serving sizes, descriptors, and health claims. Starting January 1, 2006, labels were required to include information related to the amount of trans fat (trans fatty acids) on nutrition fact labels. Consumers should be easily able to identify the amount of saturated fat, trans fat, cholesterol, and dietary fiber included in a product, and the number of calories from fat, in addition to viewing a listing of other nutritional information. Figure 36-3 illustrates a sample label with explanation of terms. The food label is a tool to educate the public about nutrition and aid in choosing foods wisely.

FACTORS AFFECTING NUTRITION

A person's food patterns and habits have a great impact on overall food intake. Food habits are a product of many evolving variables, such as physiologic and physical factors that influence nutrient requirements (e.g., stage of development, state of health, medications) and physical, sociocultural, and psychosocial factors that influence food choices (e.g., economics, culture, religion, tradition, education, politics, social status, food ideology [the meaning of food for an individual], learned aversions). These variables alone or in combination also can affect food intake and overall nutrition.

Physiologic and Physical Factors That Influence Nutrient Requirements

There are various reasons a person's nutrient requirements may differ. Some are permanent, such as gender, whereas others are temporary, such as pregnancy.

Developmental Considerations

Throughout the life cycle, nutrient needs change in relation to growth, development, activity, and age-related changes in metabolism and body composition. Periods of intense growth and development, such as during infancy, adolescence, pregnancy, and lactation, cause an increase in nutrient needs. Nutrient needs stabilize during adulthood, although older people may need more or less of some nutrients. Age influences not only nutrient requirements, but also food intake. The consistency of food consumed, eating patterns, and the significance of food change with physical and psychosocial development.

> ➤ *Remember Susan Oakland, the student who is pregnant, and William Johnston, the executive with hypertension and high cholesterol, described at the beginning of the chapter? The nurse would need to incorporate knowledge of each patient's developmental level when planning care.* ■

INFANTS

The period from birth to 1 year of age is the most rapid period of growth. Birth weight doubles in 4 to 6 months and triples by 1 year of age. Length increases 50% in the first year. Muscle control and the development of hand–eye coordination allow the infant to progress to sitting upright and self-feeding. The iron stores present at birth start to become depleted between 3 and 4 months of age. The immune system matures between 4 and 6 months of age.

Nutritional needs per unit of body weight are greater than at any other time in the life cycle. Breastfeeding is recommended as the major source of nutrition for the first 6 to 12 months of life. If the infant is not breastfed, the infant should receive one of the commercially prepared iron-fortified infant formulas. Cow's milk is not recommended for infants under the age of 1 year. Supplemental vitamins may be prescribed. Generally, solid foods are not introduced before the infant is developmentally ready, usually between 4 and 6 months of age. At this age, the infant gains control of the head, neck, jaw, and tongue; develops hand–eye coordination; and the ability to sit, chew, and drink. New foods should be introduced one at a time for a period of 5 to 7 days so that any allergic reaction can be easily identified (Dudek, 2006). By 1 year of age, the infant typically is eating table food. Iron-fortified foods are recommended.

TODDLERS AND PRESCHOOLERS

During this stage, the growth rate slows (Kyle, 2008). Mobility, autonomy, and coordination increase, as do muscle mass and bone density. Language skills improve, and the 3- to 5-year-old child also develops attitudes toward food.

Nutritionally, toddlers and preschoolers can feed themselves, verbalize food likes and dislikes, and occasionally use food to manipulate their parents. Appetite dramatically decreases and becomes erratic. Inappropriate use of food (i.e., to punish, reward, bribe, convey love) may lead to inappropriate food attitudes. Children in this age group often experience an inadequate intake of fruits and vegetables and/or excessive intake of sweetened fruit drinks.

SCHOOL-AGED CHILDREN

The 6- to 12-year-old child has an uneven, individualized, sometimes erratic growth pattern. Permanent teeth erupt as the digestive system matures. Socialization and independence increase. At this stage, the body accumulates reserves in preparation for the upcoming adolescent growth spurt.

Nutritional implications for the school-aged child focus on health promotion. Increasing energy requirements need to be balanced with foods of high nutritional value. The appetite improves but still may be irregular. The parents' role as the primary regulator of food intake diminishes, and advertising has more of an impact on the child's food choices.

ADOLESCENTS

Adolescence is a period of rapid physical, emotional, social, and sexual maturation. The growth spurt begins at different ages among individuals. Girls begin menstruation

Total Fat

Aim low: Most people need to cut back on fat! Too much fat may contribute to heart disease and cancer. Try to limit your calories from fat. For a healthy heart, choose foods with a big difference between the total number of calories and the number of calories from fat.

Saturated Fat

A new kind of fat? No — saturated fat is part of the total fat in food. It is listed separately because it's the key player in raising blood cholesterol and your risk of heart disease. Eat less!

Trans Fat

Trans fat contributes to higher cholesterol. Eat less!

Cholesterol

Too much cholesterol — a second cousin to fat — can lead to heart disease. Challenge yourself to eat less than 300 mg each day.

Sodium

You call it "salt," the label calls it "sodium." Either way, it may add up to high blood pressure in some people. So, keep your sodium intake low — 2,400 to 3,000 mg or less each day.*

* The AHA recommends no more than 3,000 mg sodium per day for healthy adults.

Daily Value

Feel like you're drowning in numbers? Let the Daily Value be your guide. Daily Values are listed for people who eat 2,000 or 2,500 calories each day. If you eat more, your personal daily value may be higher than what's listed on the label. If you eat less, your personal daily value may be lower.

For fat, saturated fat, cholesterol and sodium, choose foods with a low **% Daily Value**. For total carbohydrate, dietary fiber, vitamins and minerals, your daily value goal is to reach 100% of each.

g = grams (About 28 g = 1 ounce)
mg = milligrams (1,000 mg = 1 g)

Nutrition Facts

Serving Size 1/2 cup (114g)
Servings Per Container 4

Amount Per Serving

Calories 90   Calories from Fat 30

	% Daily Value*
Total Fat 3g	5%
Saturated Fat 0g	0%
Trans Fat 1g	
Cholesterol 0mg	0%
Sodium 300mg	13%
Total Carbohydrate 13g	4%
Dietary Fiber 3g	12%
Sugars 3g	
Protein 3g	

Vitamin A 80%	•	Vitamin C 60%
Calcium 4%	•	Iron 4%

* Percent Daily Values are based on a 2,000 calorie diet. Your daily values may be higher or lower depending on your caloric needs:

	Calories	2,000	2,500
Total Fat	Less than	65g	80g
Sat Fat	Less than	20g	25g
Cholesterol	Less than	300mg	300mg
Sodium	Less than	2,400mg	2,400mg
Total Carbohydrate		300g	375g
Fiber		25g	30g

Calories per gram:
Fat 9 • Carbohydrate 4 • Protein 4

More nutrients may be listed on some labels.

Serving Size

Is your serving the same size as the one on the label? If you eat double the serving size listed, you need to double the nutrient and caloric values. If you eat one-half the serving size shown here, cut the nutrient and caloric values in half.

Calories

Are you overweight? Cut back a little on calories! Look here to see how a serving of the food adds to your daily total. A 5'4", 138-lb. active woman needs about 2,200 calories each day. A 5'10", 174-lb. active man needs about 2,900. How about you?

Total Carbohydrate

When you cut down on fat, you can eat more carbohydrates. Carbohydrates are in foods like bread, potatoes, fruits and vegetables. Choose these often! They give you nutrients and energy.

Dietary Fiber

Grandmother called it "roughage," but her advice to eat more is still up-to-date! That goes for both soluble and insoluble kinds of dietary fiber. Fruits, vegetables, whole-grain foods, beans and peas are all good sources and can help reduce the risk of heart disease and cancer.

Protein

Most Americans get more protein than they need. Where there is animal protein, there is also fat and cholesterol. Eat small servings of lean meat, fish and poultry. Use skim or low-fat milk, yogurt, and cheese. Try vegetable proteins like beans, grains and cereals.

Vitamins & Minerals

Your goal here is 100% of each for the day. Don't count on one food to do it all. Let a combination of foods add up to a winning score.

FIGURE 36-3. Sample nutritional label with explanation of terms. (Source: U.S. Food and Drug Administration (US FDA). (2006). *How to understand and use the nutrition facts label*. Available at www.cfsan.fda.gov/~acrobat/nutfacts.pdf.)

and experience fat deposition, whereas males experience an increase in muscle mass, lean body tissue, and bones. Adolescence is also marked by intense psychosocial growth, family conflict, and social and peer pressure. Childhood nutrition problems often worsen during adolescence. Adolescents tend to skip breakfast, contributing to a lower-quality diet and decreased performance in school. Children in this age group tend to consume inadequate amounts of fruits, vegetables, and dairy products (Dudek, 2006).

Nutrient needs, especially for calories, protein, calcium, and iron, increase to support growth. Weight consciousness becomes compulsive in 1 of 100 teenaged girls and results in **anorexia nervosa,** an eating disorder characterized by extreme weight loss, muscle wasting, arrested sexual development, refusal to eat, and bizarre eating habits. **Bulimia,** another eating disorder characterized by gorging followed by purging with self-induced vomiting, diuretics, and laxatives, also becomes more common in this age group. Although contrasts exist, there is also some overlap between these diseases. Both conditions are serious health and nutritional problems, and individuals with these disorders require professional medical help and counseling. Other unhealthy diet practices include fasting, the use of diet pills, and laxative abuse.

Adolescents often eat their food rapidly, leading to overconsumption before satiety is experienced. Food is often eaten away from home, consisting of products from fast food restaurants, convenience stores, and vending machines—foods high in fat, sugar, and salt (Jenkins & Horner, 2005). These factors need to be considered when planning dietary interventions for adolescents.

If a teenage pregnancy occurs, both mother and child are at increased nutritional risk due to competition for the nutrients between the adolescent mother's body and that of the fetus. Nutritional needs may be harder to meet because fewer meals are eaten at home, and peer influence and busy schedules have an impact. Proper nutrition may help to reduce the incidence of preterm births, pregnancy-induced hypertension, and anemia, which are common in adolescent pregnancies (Dudek, 2006).

ADULTS

With adulthood, growth ceases. This age is also marked by a decline in the BMR with each decade. Adults may become more aware of the preventive role of exercise, or pressures of work and family may lead to a decline in physical activity and exercise.

Nutritional needs level off in adulthood, and fewer calories are required because of the decrease in BMR. Weight gain results if adjustments in caloric intake are not made.

PREGNANT AND LACTATING WOMEN

During pregnancy, the fetus, maternal tissues, and placenta grow dramatically. Weight gain occurs, and GI changes as a result of the pregnancy may result in nausea, vomiting, heartburn, or constipation. The quantity of breast milk produced depends on an adequate supply of nutrients.

Nutrient needs during pregnancy increase to support growth and maintain maternal homeostasis, particularly during the second and third trimesters. During the last two trimesters, normal-weight women need approximately 300 extra calories per day (Dudek, 2006). Key nutrient needs include protein, calories, iron, folic acid, calcium, and iodine. Caloric needs are higher for lactation than pregnancy, and the nutritional quality of breast milk is maintained at the expense of maternal nutrition if dietary intake is inadequate.

OLDER ADULTS

Because of the decreases in BMR and physical activity and loss of lean body mass, energy expenditure decreases. Loss of teeth and periodontal disease may make chewing more difficult. A decrease in peristalsis can result in constipation. Loss of taste between sweet and salty begins between 55 and 59 years of age, but discrimination between bitter and sour remains intact. The sensation of thirst also decreases. Degenerative diseases and the use of medications are more common with aging. It is not uncommon for social isolation, poor self-esteem, or loss of independence to affect nutritional intake negatively.

Because of the changes related to aging, the caloric needs of the body decrease. The need for nutrients, however, stays the same or increases (Dudek, 2006). Foods that are difficult to chew may need to be eliminated, whereas an increase in fiber and fluid intake can relieve constipation. Elderly people are also prone to dehydration, and lack of interest in eating is common. Nutrient intake, digestion, absorption, metabolism, or excretion may be altered because of the physiologic changes common to this age. Dietary restrictions related to chronic illness, limited income, isolation, and age-related physiologic changes place persons in this age group at risk for malnutrition (DiMaria-Ghalili & Amella, 2005).

Gender

Men differ from women in their nutrient requirements due to differences in body composition and reproductive function. Their larger muscle mass translates into higher caloric and protein requirements (therefore, slightly higher needs for B vitamins that metabolize calories and protein) because muscle is more metabolically active than adipose tissue (women have proportionately more adipose tissue). Women of childbearing age have higher iron requirements related to menstruation.

State of Health

The alteration in nutrient requirements that results from illness and trauma varies with the intensity and duration of the stress. For instance, fevers increase the need for calories and water. Unlike fevers related to septicemia, however, fevers caused by a mild case of the flu require few dietary adjustments.

Trauma, like major surgery, burns, and crush injuries, is followed by hormonal changes that profoundly affect the body's use of nutrients. To preserve or replenish body nutrient stores and to promote healing and recovery, nutrient requirements increase dramatically in the adaptive phase after stress. In some cases of severe trauma, such as major burns, the rehabilitative phase of recovery, characterized by the gradual normalization of nutrient needs, may last for years.

Chronic disorders, like diabetes mellitus, renal disease, hypertension, heart disease, GI disorders, and cancer, can alter nutrient requirements by influencing nutrient intake, digestion, absorption, metabolism, utilization, or excretion.

Mental health problems, such as depression and confusion, can cause a patient to forget to eat or lack the motivation to eat, leading to malnutrition.

Alcohol Abuse

Alcohol can alter the body's use of nutrients, and thereby its nutrient requirements, by numerous mechanisms. The toxic effect of alcohol on the intestinal mucosa interferes with normal nutrient absorption; thus, requirements increase as the efficiency of absorption decreases. Need for B vitamins increases because they are used to metabolize alcohol. Alcohol can also influence nutrient metabolism by impairing nutrient storage, increasing nutrient catabolism, and increasing nutrient excretion. Alcohol abuse that results in liver damage has profound effects on the body's nutrient metabolism and requirements.

Medication

Many drugs have the potential to influence nutrient requirements. Nutrient absorption may be altered by drugs that (1) change the pH of the GI tract, (2) increase GI motility, (3) damage the intestinal mucosa, or (4) bind with nutrients, rendering them unavailable to the body. Nutrient metabolism can be altered by drugs that (1) act as nutrient antagonists, (2) alter the enzyme systems that metabolize nutrients, or (3) alter nutrient degradation. Some drugs alter the renal reabsorption of nutrients and, therefore, may increase or decrease nutrient excretion.

Megadoses of Nutrient Supplements

Because some nutrients compete against each other for absorption, an excess of one nutrient can lead to a deficiency (or increase the requirement) of another, especially if one is absorbed preferentially. For instance, a delicate balance exists between zinc and copper. People who take therapeutic levels of zinc run the risk of developing a copper deficiency—which is otherwise rare—unless they also increase their intake of copper.

Dietary supplements can have drug-like effects and may interact with food and medication (Yen, 2005). Accurate information regarding the patient's use of dietary supplements is imperative to provide safe and appropriate care. The use of herbs, vitamins, minerals and other supplements can impact a patient's plan of care and must be considered by all members of the healthcare team. For example, a patient taking ginkgo biloba (an herbal), aspirin, and vitamin E (dietary supplement) may have to have surgery postponed due to an

---

| Box 36-3 | **RESOURCES FOR INFORMATION ABOUT HERBS, VITAMINS, MINERALS, AND OTHER DIETARY SUPPLEMENTS** |

- MedlinePlus: Herbs and Supplements, http://www.nlm.nih.gov/medlineplus/druginfo/herb_All.html
- National Center for Complementary and Alternative Medicine: Dietary and Herbal Supplements, http://nccam.nih.gov/health/supplements
- National Institutes of Health: Office of Dietary Supplements, http://dietary-supplements.info.nih.gov/

---

increased risk for excessive bleeding, because each of these substances have blood-thinning properties (Yen, 2005). Box 36-3 lists accurate reliable sources for the latest information about specific herbs and supplements based on scientific evidence.

Physical, Sociocultural, and Psychosocial Factors That Influence Food Choices

Dietary choices or restrictions also are influenced by economics, culture, religion, and personal feelings and meanings associated with food. The financial income of the patient or the patient's household can directly impact the ability to purchase sufficient food and/or food of high nutritional value. Diverse lifestyles and eating habits directly impact a person's nutritional health and well-being. Religious restrictions and beliefs or cultural practices may affect the patient's acceptance of, response to, and compliance with dietary therapies. Healthcare providers need an understanding of a patient's cultural values, beliefs, and practices to provide culturally acceptable care (Andrews & Boyle, 2008; Purnell & Paulanka, 2005).

Economic Factors

The adequacy of a person's food budget affects dietary choices and patterns. The increasing cost of food, coupled with limited purchasing power, may result in a decrease in the nutritional quality of the diet. Many variables influence the types of foods purchased. Creative use of the food dollar means using unit pricing to determine cost per serving (e.g., comparing the unit price of 39¢ per serving with a similar product's 45¢ per serving), selecting foods that contain adequate nutrients, and buying seasonal foods that are more economical and can be prepared easily at home. Avoiding convenience foods and meals purchased away from home can save food dollars.

Religion

Dietary restrictions associated with religions might affect a patient's nutritional requirements. Many religions eschew certain types of food products. For example, Mormons do not use coffee, tea, or alcohol, and are encouraged to limit meat consumption. Hindus do not eat beef because cows are considered sacred, and many are vegetarian, adhering to the concept of nonviolence as applied to foods (Dudek, 2006). Alternative food choices or meal patterns may be necessary. Kosher dietary laws require special food preparation techniques and prohibit intake of pork and shellfish. Thus, a patient's religious affiliation may affect his or her nutritional regimen. Patients should be asked regarding any preferences or restrictions. Kosher diets and other special diets are available in hospitals, nursing homes, retirement homes, and programs, such as Meals on Wheels.

Meaning of Food

Food means different things to different people, with food playing multiple roles in the lives of most individuals. In addition to satisfying hunger and providing nutrition, food may signify a celebration, a social gathering, or a reward. Some people use various foods to indicate caring or to give comfort and reassurance during times of stress or unhappiness. Mealtime may evoke memories of family discussions, laughter, and enjoyable times. Some may remember conflicts associated with eating or avoid eating because it reminds them of their loneliness and isolation. Others, because of society's emphasis on being thin, may resort to fad or crash-reducing diets to resolve eating conflicts and lose weight rapidly. This initial weight reduction seldom is sustained for an extended period, and a cycle of yo-yo dieting frequently results. Drastic weight loss is followed by an eating binge that causes the dieter to regain all the lost weight and, possibly, some additional weight each time the sequence occurs. Nutritional deficiencies may occur and place the person at risk for other diseases. Losing weight and keeping it off require a change in eating habits as part of the overall commitment to health.

Culture

Nutritional diversity is common among cultural or ethnic groups. The variety and selections are unique to each group and represent their personal beliefs and customs. Culture influences what is eaten or considered edible, how it is prepared, and what combinations of food are permitted. Herbal treatments that are popular in some cultures may interfere with or counteract the action of prescribed medication. The variations in food choices within a culture also depend on income levels and availability of foods. General and specific cultural knowledge allows the healthcare provider to ask the right questions when interacting with patients of varying backgrounds. Nurses who are aware of the specific needs and beliefs of culturally diverse patient populations are better able to communicate effectively and provide optimal care. Box 36-4 suggests guidelines for effective communication about nutrition with culturally diverse patients.

If a patient of a different culture is to be placed on a specific diet, discussing food choice options is necessary to customize the diet to meet the person's cultural demands. Discussing ways to integrate cultural food preferences into current nutrition guidelines is an important part of nursing care.

Additional Sociocultural Factors Affecting Nutritional Intake

In addition to the previously mentioned factors, the following issues need to be considered to determine their impact on a patient's nutritional status (Dudek, 2006):

- Illiteracy
- Language barriers
- Knowledge of nutrition
- Lack of caregiver or social support
- Social isolation
- Limited ability to obtain or purchase food

Box 36-4 **COMMUNICATING EFFECTIVELY ABOUT NUTRITION WITH CULTURALLY DIVERSE PATIENTS**

- Acquire basic information about health beliefs and practices of various cultural groups in your healthcare setting. This provides a basis for assessing patient's beliefs and practices. Recognize, however, that within all cultures and ethnic groups, there are members that do not hold all the values of the group.
- Ask specifically about the use of folk or home remedies prescribed by a nontraditional healer.
- Determine the patient's language preferences for spoken and written communication.
- Utilize printed or audiovisual information that is in the language spoken by your patients.
- Promote healthy food choices by identifying healthy traditional food practices and encourage their use.

- Support healthy new food practices.
- Discourage the adoption of less healthy American dietary practices.
- Encourage cultural sensitivity in healthcare workers in your particular setting.
- Recognize that diversity exists within cultural groups. For example, the Hispanic population includes Mexicans, Cubans, Puerto Ricans, and other Latino groups.
- Emphasize threads or messages in health teaching that are common to all cultures (e.g., concern about family, faith, home).
- Help culturally diverse patients to value and understand the importance of communicating concerns and asking questions about prescribed dietary practices.

(Adapted from Andrews, M., & Boyle, J. (2008). *Transcultural concepts in nursing care* (5th ed.). Philadelphia: Wolters Kluwer Health/Lippincott Williams & Wilkins; Dudek, S. [2006]. *Nutrition essentials for nursing practice* [5th ed.]. Philadelphia: Lippincott Williams & Wilkins; and Purnell, L., & Paulanka, B. [2005]. *Guide to culturally competent health care*. Philadelphia: F. A. Davis.)

• Lack of or inadequate cooking and/or food preparation arrangements

Food Intake

At times, a combination of physiologic and physical factors that influence nutrient requirements and, or in combination with, sociocultural and psychosocial factors can affect an individual's nutritional intake. Subsequently, these factors can result in a decrease or increase in food intake.

Decreased Food Intake

Food intake may decrease for various reasons. Patients with a BMI of less than 18.5 are considered underweight. **Anorexia,** or the lack of appetite, may be related to systemic and local diseases; numerous psychosocial causes, such as fear, anxiety, depression, pain; and impaired ability to smell and taste—or it may occur secondary to drug therapy or medical treatments. Others who may have limited food intake include those who have difficulty chewing and swallowing, those who experience chronic GI problems or undergo certain surgical procedures, those with certain chronic illnesses (such as cancer), and those with inadequate food budgets.

> *Consider Charles Gallagher, whose wife is receiving enteral feedings. The underlying reason for insertion of the PEG tube was her inability to swallow and subsequent development of aspiration pneumonia that required numerous hospitalizations. The nurse would need to communicate this information to Mr. Gallagher to ensure that he understands the rationale for the feeding. This understanding is important for decision making.* ∎

Increased Food Intake

Increased food intake may lead to obesity. Obesity presents a serious health problem physically, socially, and emotionally. **Obesity** is defined as body weight 20% or more above ideal weight or having a BMI of 30 or more. A positive caloric balance, resulting from an excess caloric intake or a decrease in energy expenditure, leads to the gradual accumulation of weight. This excess weight increases the risk for numerous medical problems; increases the risks associated with surgery; increases the risk for complications during pregnancy, labor, and delivery; and increases morbidity and mortality. People who are obese are often discriminated against in social, educational, and employment settings. In a society that values thinness, obesity can cause one to feel desperate, frustrated, depressed, and rejected, and to perceive oneself as a failure. About two thirds of adults in the United States are overweight and nearly one-third are considered obese (have a BMI ≥30) (Weight-control Information Network [WIN], 2007). In addition, approximately 17.5% of school-aged children and 17% of adolescents are overweight today (WIN).

Numerous theories about the cause of obesity have been proposed. According to genetic theories, a low resting metabolic rate or an inherited family tendency contribute to obesity. Physiologic factors that have been implicated include an increased number of fat cells, a lowered basal metabolic rate set point, a decreased amount of brown fat that burns kilocalories, insulin resistance, and hormone imbalance. A food and family environment that encourages overeating, a lifestyle in which exercise is minimal, and the availability of foods in a multitude of settings at all times are environmental factors that contribute to obesity (WIN, 2008). Additionally, many identify psychological reasons for obesity, including compulsiveness, using food to satisfy emotional needs, relying on food for compensation for lack of affection and companionship, and overeating as a release mechanism for boredom, anxiety, and feelings of inadequacy. Obesity is resistant to treatment, and weight loss is temporary at best unless behavior modification and exercise are incorporated into the dietary plan.

THE NURSING PROCESS
Assessing

Nutritional status has a significant impact on both health and disease. For well patients, good nutritional status can help to maintain health, promote normal growth and development, and protect against disease. During illness, good nutritional status can reduce the risk for complications and speed recovery time. Conversely, poor nutritional status can increase the risk for illness or death.

Like other aspects of nursing care, nutritional assessment is a systematic approach used to identify the patient's actual or potential needs, formulate a plan to meet those needs, initiate the plan or assign others to implement it, and evaluate

---

Box 36-5 **NUTRITIONAL ASSESSMENT CONSIDERATIONS FOR OLDER ADULTS***

Biochemical Data
• Low serum albumin level (below 3.5 mg/dL) may be a reflection of the aging process rather than a nutritional risk factor. Albumin synthesis declines with age.
• Hemoglobin levels that are lower than normal may only reflect anemia observed in elderly people as part of the aging process.

Anthropometric Data
• Because of age-related changes in body composition, skin-fold measurements, if used, should be taken from several body sites.

Dietary Data
• Dietary recall may be inaccurate because of vision and memory problems.
• Question use of vitamin and mineral supplements.
• Gather information concerning medication regimen (prescribed and over-the-counter) to assess for food–drug interactions and adverse effects of medications.

*Specific clinical data for older adults may be found in the Focus on the Older Adult display.

the effectiveness of the plan. The level of assessment may range from simple screening to a comprehensive, in-depth assessment, depending on individual circumstances. Regardless of the level of assessment, nutritional assessment is appropriate for all patients. Nurses can collect assessment data through history taking (dietary, medical, socioeconomic data), physical assessments (anthropometric and clinical data), and laboratory data. When performing a nutritional assessment, nurses need to be aware of the specific changes in older people that may reflect on the accuracy of the assessment process (Box 36-5).

Nurses, by nature of their caring role and personal encounters, serve as nutritional role models and are ideally situated to identify nutritional needs and assess and monitor for nutritional risks. Nurses who role model good health behaviors are more effective teachers. Use the Promoting Health Display 36-1: Nutrition for yourself before using it with others.

Dietary Data

Dietary data may be collected from the patient or family and can be evaluated according to the *Dietary Guidelines,* RDA,

or the MyPyramid Food Guide, depending on the purpose of the assessment.

NUTRITIONAL SCREENING

Nutritional screening is an important part of the nursing assessment. The acronym DETERMINE can be used to screen for warning signs of poor nutritional health (American Society on Aging, 2006).

- **D**isease: Any disease, illness, or chronic condition that causes a change in the way a person eats or makes it hard to eat
- **E**ating poorly: Eating too little or too much; skipping meals; eating the same foods all the time
- **T**ooth loss/mouth pain: Missing, loose, or rotten teeth or dentures that don't fit well or cause mouth sores make it hard to eat
- **E**conomic hardship: Having less or choosing to spend less on food makes it difficult to eat the foods needed to stay healthy
- **R**educed social contact: Being with people has a positive effect on eating and well-being

PROMOTING HEALTH • 36-1

Nutrition

Patients view nurses as role models for achieving healthy lifestyles. Use the assessment checklist to determine how well you are meeting your nutritional needs. Then develop a prescription for self-care by choosing appropriate behaviors from the list of suggestions.

Assessment Checklist

❑ almost always   ❑ sometimes   ❑ almost never

❑ ❑ ❑   1. I know and use the recommended dietary guidelines and servings.

❑ ❑ ❑   2. My weight is within 10% of the ideal for my height and body frame.

❑ ❑ ❑   3. I maintain an appropriate balance between exercise and food intake.

❑ ❑ ❑   4. I limit my fat, sugar, salt, and red meat intake.

❑ ❑ ❑   5. I limit my caffeine intake.

❑ ❑ ❑   6. I use alcoholic beverages in moderation.

❑ ❑ ❑   7. I make an effort to eat high-fiber foods.

Self-Care Behaviors

1. Maintain desirable weight, eating a variety of foods in adequate amounts from each of the food groups.

2. Eat slowly, take smaller portions, and avoid second helpings if trying to control overeating.
3. Eat a variety of foods low in calories and high in nutrients to lose weight.
4. Obtain medical clearance before starting a weight-loss program.
5. Avoid too many foods high in cholesterol (milk, egg yolk, organ meats, fats, oils); instead choose lean meat, fish, poultry, and beans.
6. Eat foods high in fiber: whole-grain breads and cereals, fruits, vegetables, dry beans.
7. Avoid excess use of salt and sugar.
8. Begin an exercise program and maintain it.
9. Learn healthy eating habits; read labels, become familiar with healthy fast-food and restaurant menus; and drink alcohol moderately (if at all).
10. Substitute healthy rewards for yourself that do not include high-calorie, low-nutrition snacks and beverages.

Information to promote effective nutrition, dietary supplement use, and safety; nutrient recommendations; and database resources are available online. Check out these sites: Office of Dietary Supplements at http://dietary-supplements.info.nih.gov/Health_ Information/Health_Information.aspx; Healthier US.gov at http://www.healthierus.gov/index.html.

- **M**ultiple medicines: The more medicines taken, the greater the risk for side effects, such as increased/decreased appetite, change in taste, constipation, weakness, drowsiness, diarrhea, and nausea. Vitamins or minerals taken in large doses act like drugs and can cause harm.
- **I**nvoluntary weight loss/gain: A large weight loss or gain can be a sign of serious health problems.
- **N**eeds assistance in self-care: Difficulty walking, shopping, purchasing, and cooking food interferes with the ability to meet nutrition needs.
- **E**lder years above age 80: As age increases, risk of frailty and health problems increase

The Mini Nutritional Assessment tool (MNA) is used to detect elderly persons at risk for malnutrition before changes in albumin level and the BMI. The MNA is a combination of screening questions followed by anthropometric measurements, including BMI, midarm and calf circumference, and weight loss. The MNA is fast and easy, and recommended for use with all elderly patients, whether they are community dwelling, hospitalized, or in long-term care settings (DiMaria-Ghalili & Guenter, 2008).

After a screening tool identifies a patient at risk, such as in a group of older adults, it is imperative that a nutritional assessment be completed as a follow-up. When this is combined with other methods of assessing nutritional status, the nurse is better prepared to coordinate a focused strategy to combat malnutrition.

ASSESSING DIETARY INTAKE

Many different methods can be used to assess actual dietary intake.

24-Hour Recall Method

The easiest way to collect dietary data is to obtain a 24-hour recall of all food and beverages the patient normally consumes during an average day. Ask the patient to recall details related to nutritional intake from the prior 24 hours. This method includes the patient's portion sizes, meal and snack patterns, meal timing, and location where food is eaten. Because this method relies on memory and accurate interpretation of portion sizes, the information may not be reliable.

Food Diaries/Calorie Counts

Food diaries and calorie counts require documentation of actual intake for a specified period of time. In an outpatient setting, ask the patient to record everything he has had to eat or drink, including portion size, over a set period of time. In the hospital setting, documentation is usually completed by the nursing staff. These tools may provide a better overall picture of nutrient intake because all food and beverages consumed in a specified period, usually 3 to 7 days, are recorded.

Food Frequency Record

Food frequency records give a general picture of nutritional consumption. Ask patients questions to elicit an average number of times certain foods or food groups are con-

sumed in a given period of time: per day, per week, or per month. For example, ask, "How many times in the last week have you eaten fresh fruit or fish?" or "How many times in the last week have you had a glass of milk?"

Diet History

A more comprehensive approach to diet assessment is a full diet history. In addition to a 24-hour food recall, calorie counts/food diaries, and food-frequency record, interview questions are geared to provide information on past and present food intake and habits. Sample questions are included in the accompanying Focused Assessment Guide 36-1.

> *Consider William Johnston, the man who has less-than-healthful dietary and health habits. The nurse could use a diet history to obtain specific information about Mr. Johnston's actual intake. Analysis of this information would reveal his actual dietary intake and identify potential and actual nutritional problems.* ■

Medical and Socioeconomic Data

Medical, social, and economic factors, as well as cultural and psychological influences, require evaluation for their impact on nutritional requirements and food choices. A nutritional assessment should include the following medical, social, and economic information (DiMaria-Ghalili & Amella, 2005; Dudek, 2006). Medical data include:

- Current illness as well as medical and surgical history
- Past and current drug history
- History of drug dependence or abuse
- Ability to chew and swallow, including condition of mouth, missing teeth, or dentures
- Appetite, food intolerance and allergies, and bowel habits

Social data include:

- Age, gender, family history, lifestyle (e.g., those at extremes in age are most at risk)
- Educational background
- Information about occupation, exercise, and sleep patterns
- Religious affiliation, cultural and ethnic background
- Use of alcohol and tobacco

Economic Data include:

- Source of income
- Food budget

Anthropometric Data

Anthropometric measurements are used to determine body dimensions. In children, anthropometric measurements are used to assess growth rate; in adults, they can give indirect measurements of body protein and fat stores. For the data to be accurate and reliable, standardized equipment and procedures must be used, and the data must be compared with the appropriate reference standards for the patient's age and sex.

FOCUSED ASSESSMENT GUIDE • 36-1

NUTRITION

Factors to Assess	Questions and Approaches
Usual dietary intake	Does your current intake differ from your usual intake?
	If so, is the reason a loss of appetite, changes in smell or taste, difficulty chewing and swallowing, hospitalization, a modified diet?
	With whom do you usually eat meals?
Food allergies or intolerances	Do you have any food allergies or intolerances?
Food preparation and storage	Who does the food shopping?
	Who prepares the meals?
	How is the food normally prepared? For instance, is food usually fried, baked, or broiled?
	Do you have adequate food storage space and preparation equipment?
Type of diet Dietary practices	Do you now or have you in the past followed a modified diet prescribed by a physician?
	Do you now or have you in the past used a fad diet, health foods, or self-prescribed supplements?
Eating disorder patterns	Do you view yourself as overweight?
	Do you weigh yourself frequently during one day?
	How is your appetite?
	Do you binge on large amounts of food in a short period?
	Have you ever caused yourself to vomit after eating a meal?
	Have you used laxatives, diuretics, herbal supplements, or over-the-counter weight-loss pills to lose weight?

Height and weight, the most common anthropometric measurements, are obtained when the patient is admitted to the healthcare facility and periodically thereafter or assessed in a home care environment. Weigh a patient on the same scale each time and at the same time of day, preferably before breakfast. Height and weight are used to calculate the patient's BMI. Because actual weight may be increased if the patient has edema, consider hydration status. Although self-reported weight may be recorded when actual weight is unobtainable, it is highly inaccurate and must be noted. Record an actual weight as soon as feasibly possible. Self-reported height in the elderly can be inaccurate related to shortening of the spine (DiMaria-Ghalili & Amella, 2005). Record an actual height as soon as possible.

Additional anthropometric measurements include triceps skin-fold measurements, a measure of subcutaneous fat stores; midarm circumference, a measure of skeletal muscle mass; and midarm muscle circumference, a measure of both skeletal muscle mass and fat stores.

Body Mass Index and Waist Circumference

Calculate the patient's body mass index (BMI) and measure their waist circumference, as discussed earlier in the chapter. Compare results with the established guidelines to deter-

mine patient's ideal body weight and identify potential health risks. Refer to Table 36-1.

Clinical Data

Although signs and symptoms of altered nutrition may be observed during a physical assessment (Table 36-6), they usually do not appear until the condition is advanced. In addition, further investigation is necessary to determine whether abnormal findings are actually caused by a nutritional deficiency, are possibly related to a nutritional deficiency, or are unrelated to nutritional status.

Assess for barriers to eating. **Dysphagia** (difficulty swallowing or the inability to swallow) can be the result of poor dental health, cancer, or a neurologic disease, such as stroke, Parkinson's disease, or dementia, and may reduce the patient's nutritional intake (Coxall et al., 2008; Metheny, 2007). Dysphagia also is associated with an increased risk for **aspiration**, the misdirection of oropharyngeal secretions or gastric contents into the larynx and lower respiratory tract (Metheny, 2007). Dental problems are associated with impaired chewing and avoidance of foods that may be difficult to chew, such as meat, fruit, and vegetables. Patients who experience weakness and fatigue may find eating to be a chore to avoid. Diminished sensor abilities, such as sight,

TABLE • 36-6   CLINICAL OBSERVATIONS FOR NUTRITIONAL ASSESSMENT

Body Area	Signs of Good Nutritional Status	Signs of Poor Nutritional Status
General appearance	Alert, responsive	Listless, apathetic, and cachetic
General vitality	Endurance, energetic, sleeps well, vigorous	Easily fatigued, no energy, falls asleep easily, looks tired, apathetic, depressed mood
Weight	Normal for height, age, body build	Overweight or underweight
Hair	Shiny, lustrous, firm, not easily plucked, healthy scalp	Dull and dry, brittle, loss of color, easily plucked, thin and sparse
Face	Uniform skin color; healthy appearance, not swollen	Dark skin over cheeks and under eyes, flaky skin, facial edema (moon face), pale skin color
Eyes	Bright, clear, moist, no sores at corners of eyelids, membranes moist and healthy pink color, no prominent blood vessels	Pale eye membranes, dry eyes (xerophthalmia); Bitot's spots, increased vascularity, cornea soft (keratomalacia), small yellowish lumps around eyes (xanthelasma), dull or scarred cornea
Lips	Good pink color, smooth, moist, not chapped or swollen	Swollen and puffy (cheilosis), angular lesion at corners of mouth or fissures or scars (stomatitis)
Tongue	Deep red, surface papillae present	Smooth appearance, beefy red or magenta colored, swollen, hypertrophy or atrophy
Teeth	Straight, no crowding, no cavities, no pain, bright, no discoloration, well-shaped jaw	Cavities, mottled appearance (Fluorosis), malpositioned, missing teeth
Gums	Firm, good pink color, no swelling or bleeding	Spongy, bleed easily, marginal redness, recessed, swollen and inflamed
Glands	No enlargement of the thyroid, face not swollen	Enlargement of the thyroid (goiter), enlargement of the parotid (swollen cheeks)
Skin	Smooth, good color, slightly moist, no signs of rashes, swelling, or color irregularities	Rough, dry, flaky, swollen, pale, pigmented, lack of fat under the skin, fat deposits around the joints (xanthomas), bruises, petechiae
Nails	Firm, pink	Spoon shaped (koilonychia), brittle, pale, ridged
Skeleton	Good posture, no malformations	Poor posture, beading of the ribs, bowed legs or knock-knees, prominent scapulas, chest deformity at diaphragm
Muscles	Well developed, firm, good tone, some fat under the skin	Flaccid, poor tone, wasted, underdeveloped, difficulty walking
Extremities	No tenderness	Weak and tender, edema of lower extremities
Abdomen	Flat	Swollen
Nervous system	Normal reflexes, psychological stability	Decrease in or loss of ankle and knee reflexes, psychomotor changes, mental confusion, depression, sensory loss, motor weakness, loss of sense of position, loss of vibration, burning and tingling of the hands and feet (paresthesia)
Cardiovascular system	Normal heart rate and rhythm, no murmurs, normal blood pressure for age	Cardiac enlargement, tachycardia, abnormal blood pressure
GI system	No palpable organs or masses (liver edge may be palpable in children)	Enlarged liver or spleen

(Adapted from Dudek, S. G. [2006]. *Nutrition essentials for nursing practice* [5th ed.]. Philadelphia: Lippincott Williams & Wilkins; and Mahan, L., & Jarvis, C. [2008]. *Physical examination & health assessment* [5th ed.]. St. Louis: Saunders Elsevier.)

taste, smell, and hearing, may also impact a patient's nutritional intake (Holmes, 2006).

Biochemical Data

Laboratory tests, which measure blood and urine levels of nutrients or biochemical functions that depend on an adequate supply of nutrients, can objectively detect nutritional problems in their early stages. Most routine biochemical tests measure protein status; measures of body vitamin, mineral, and trace element status are also available.

Hemoglobin, the oxygen-carrying protein of the red blood cells, and hematocrit, the volume of red blood cells packed by centrifugation in a given volume of blood, are measures of plasma protein that also reflect a person's iron status. Protein status can also be determined by measuring serum albumin and transferrin levels and by a total lymphocyte count. Serum albumin levels are a good indicator of a patient's nutritional status a few weeks prior to when the blood is drawn and can help identify chronic nutrition problems. The albumin level does not change with increasing age, but malnutrition and various disease states cause its level to decrease. Serum albumin levels can also be affected by the patient's hydration status; overhydration can cause a low albumin level and dehydration may cause a very high level (Fischbach & Dunning, 2009). Prealbumin levels indicate short-term nutritional status and can be used to detect daily changes in a patient's protein status (Fischbach & Dunning, 2006). Transferrin acts as an iron-transporting protein but because it is related to iron levels, may not always be an accurate indicator of nutritional status. The total lymphocyte count reflects immune status and is directly affected by impaired nutritional states.

Blood glucose, blood cholesterol, and blood triglycerides are additional laboratory tests relative to nutritional status. Twenty-four-hour urine tests used to measure protein metabolism include urine creatinine excretion and urine urea nitrogen. Urea, a breakdown product of amino acids, can be measured in the urine and blood. It reflects protein intake and the body's ability to detoxify and excrete this metabolic byproduct. Creatinine levels are directly proportional to the body's muscle mass, and a reduction in this value reflects severe malnutrition. These biochemical indicators with nutritional implications are summarized in Box 36-6.

Diagnosing

Assessment data may reveal actual or potential nutritional problems. As soon as problems are identified, refer the patient to appropriate services, including a dietitian.

Imbalanced Nutrition as the Problem

Data that the nurse collects may lead to the development of several nursing diagnoses related to nutrition. The following nursing diagnoses may be made when imbalanced nutrition is the cause of the patient's disorder:

- Imbalanced Nutrition: Less Than Body Requirements related to nothing by mouth (NPO), inadequate tube

Box 36-6 BIOCHEMICAL DATA WITH NUTRITIONAL IMPLICATIONS

- Hemoglobin (normal = 12–18 g/dL) decreased → anemia
- Hematocrit (normal = 40%–50%) decreased → anemia increased → dehydration
- Serum albumin (normal = 3.5–5.5 g/dL) decreased → malnutrition (prolonged protein depletion), malabsorption
- Prealbumin (normal = 23–43 mg/dL) decreased → protein depletion, malnutrition
- Transferrin (normal = 240–480 mg/dL) decreased → anemia, protein deficiency
- Blood urea nitrogen (normal = 17–18 mg/dL) increased → starvation, high protein intake, severe dehydration decreased → malnutrition, overhydration
- Creatinine (normal = 0.4–1.5 mg/dL) increased → dehydration decreased → reduction in total muscle mass, severe malnutrition

(Dudek, S. (2006). *Nutrition essentials for nursing practice* [5th ed.]. Philadelphia: Lippincott Williams & Wilkins; and Fischbach, F., & Dunning, M. [2006]. *Common laboratory & diagnostic tests* [4th ed.]. Philadelphia: Lippincott Williams & Wilkins.)

feeding, prolonged use of a clear liquid diet, numerous food intolerance or allergies, excessive dieting, anorexia, chewing or swallowing difficulties, nausea, vomiting, chronic diarrhea, malabsorption, psychological eating disorders (anorexia nervosa, bulimia), alcoholism, metabolic and endocrine disorders, inappropriate use of supplements
- Imbalanced Nutrition: More Than Body Requirements related to overeating, inactivity, metabolic and endocrine disorders, inappropriate use of supplements
- Risk for Imbalanced Nutrition: More Than Body Requirements related to inappropriate eating, closely spaced pregnancies, metabolic and endocrine disorders, inappropriate use of supplements

See specific examples in the accompanying NANDA Nursing Diagnoses box.

Imbalanced Nutrition as the Etiology

Data that the nurse collects may lead to the development of several nursing diagnoses related to nutrition. Nutritional problems may affect other areas of human functioning. In the following nursing diagnoses, the nutritional problem is the cause of another problem.

- Activity Intolerance related to inadequate caloric intake, obesity, iron-deficiency anemia
- Impaired Dentition related to nutritional deficits
- Ineffective Health Maintenance related to lack of knowledge about adequate nutrition
- Anxiety related to obesity

Examples of NANDA Nursing Diagnoses

Nutrition

Nursing Diagnoses	Related Factors	Sample Defining Characteristics
Imbalanced Nutrition: Less Than Body Requirements	Malabsorption	• "I seem to eat all day long and yet I keep losing weight." • Reports losing 15 lb within the past 3 weeks. Has 8 to 10 bowel movements daily of frothy, odorous stools that float. Fecal fat excretion test indicates steatorrhea. Patient appears fatigued and undernourished; muscle wasting is evident. Laboratory data reveal low serum albumin level (protein deficiency) and iron-deficiency anemia.
Imbalanced Nutrition: More Than Body Requirements	Decreased thyroid function leading to a decrease in metabolism	• "I don't eat enough to keep a bird alive, but I just keep getting fatter and fatter. I don't know what else to do unless I stop eating altogether." • Patient reports a 10-lb weight gain within the past month despite following a 1,200-calorie diet. Other symptoms noted include fatigue, amenorrhea, and dry skin. Laboratory data indicate low serum thyroxine (T_4) level, protein-bound iodine, and elevated serum thyroid-stimulating hormone and cholesterol levels. Radioactive iodine uptake was low.
Risk for Imbalanced Nutrition: More Than Body Requirements	Inappropriate use of supplements	• "I sent a sample of my hair away for a nutritional analysis, and the report came back saying that I should take supplements of zinc, iron, potassium, and magnesium." • For the past week, patient has been taking supplements of 500% of the RDA for zinc and magnesium. She takes twice as much iron as recommended, and large doses of potassium ad lib.

• Constipation related to inadequate fluid or fiber intake
• Diarrhea related to overeating, excessive fiber intake, excessive sorbitol intake (sugar alcohol)
• Deficient Fluid Volume related to inadequate fluid intake
• Risk for Infection related to inadequate calorie intake, inadequate protein intake
• Impaired Home Maintenance Management related to inability to purchase, store, or prepare food for family
• Impaired Skin Integrity related to protein malnutrition, vitamin A deficiency
• Deficient Knowledge related to new medical diet, nutrition misinformation, lack of interest in nutrition, intellectual deficit
• Noncompliance to a particular diet order related to lack of motivation, misinformation
• Chronic Low Self-Esteem related to obesity
• Disturbed Sleep Pattern related to excessive caffeine intake
• Social Isolation related to obesity

Wellness Diagnosis

Data that the nurse collects may lead to the development of several nursing diagnoses related to nutrition. For patients who are incorporating sound nutritional practices in their daily routine, the following wellness diagnosis may be appropriate: Readiness for Enhanced Nutrition associated with food safety.

Outcome Identification and Planning

Expected outcomes are derived from the actual or potential nutritional problems diagnosed. The goal is to maintain or restore optimal nutritional status using foods the patients like and tolerate as appropriate for their situation. Goals should also include those to alleviate symptoms or side effects of disease or treatment and to prevent complications or diet-related chronic diseases. General patient outcomes are listed here. Actual patient outcomes should list specific behaviors and criteria individualized for the patient situation. The patient will:

- Attain and maintain ideal body weight, as indicated by BMI and waist circumference.
- Eat a diet adequate but not excessive, in all nutrients, based on the MyPyramid Food Guideline system, the RDA, and dietary recommendations and guidelines issued from health and U.S. governmental agencies.
- Eat a variety of food in each of three or more meals.
- Follow the appropriate modified diet, when necessary, to restore health, avoid disease recurrences, and prevent or delay potential complications.

> *Remember Charles Gallagher, the husband of the woman receiving enteral nutrition. Initially, outcomes would focus on maintaining his wife's nutritional status. However, the informed decision made to withdraw the nutritional support would lead the nurse to revise the outcomes. Therefore, the outcomes then would focus on emotional comfort for the Gallagher family and a peaceful, dignified death for Mrs. Gallagher.* ∎

Implementing

Providing proper and adequate nourishment to the patient is a team effort implemented in a variety of settings. Diet orders are written by the physician in the inpatient setting, confirmed by the dietitian, and frequently explained to the patient by the nurse. The nurse may also be responsible for screening patients at home who are at nutritional risk, observing intake and appetite, evaluating the patient's tolerance, assisting the patient with eating, administering enteral and parenteral feedings, consulting with the dietitian and physician when dietary problems arise, addressing the potential for drug–nutrient reactions, obtaining more food or snacks for the patient when appropriate, monitoring food brought by visitors, and participating in nutrition education efforts. The accompanying Examples of Nursing Intervention and Nursing Outcome Classifications (NIC/NOC) box

lists standardized nursing interventions and corresponding outcomes related to nutrition.

Teaching Nutritional Information

For the greatest chance of success, tailor diet instructions individually to the patient's lifestyle, culture, intellectual ability, and level of motivation. Although strict guidelines and printed handouts may seem ideal, in practice, simplicity and compromise are often the keys to patient compliance.

> *Recall William Johnston, the patient with hypertension and high cholesterol. The nurse would need to consider Mr. Johnston's lifestyle when developing a teaching plan for him. As a result of his "on-the-run" lifestyle, the nurse would need to adapt the teaching plan, making sure that it is realistic for his needs. For example, the nurse might teach Mr. Johnston about reading food labels to ensure that his selections, when he is "on the run" are low in fat and cholesterol. In addition, the nurse would also provide Mr. Johnston with appropriate suggestions for choices when dining out. Doing so will help communicate to him that the plan is workable, enhancing the chances of Mr. Johnston complying with the plan, thereby achieving success.* ∎

Include information about food safety issues in patient teaching. This includes safe handling of foods, food storage, and preventing food-borne illness. Encourage patients to wash hands and clean food contact surfaces frequently when handling and preparing foods. Wash fruits and vegetables before eating or preparation. This helps prevent contamination of food with bacteria and viruses. Teach patients to cook foods to a safe temperature, 135° Fahrenheit or higher, to kill microorganisms. Also, explain that raw, cooked, and ready-to-eat foods should be separated during shopping and preparation and should

---

Examples of Nursing Intervention and Nursing Outcome Classifications (NIC/NOC)

Nutrition

Nursing Interventions	Nursing Outcomes
- Nutrition Management	- Nutritional Status
- Nutrition Therapy	- Appetite
- Nutritional Counseling	- Weight: Body Mass
- Nutritional Monitoring	- Knowledge: Diet
- Exercise Promotion	- Self Care: Eating
- Weight Management	

From Bulechek, G., Butcher, H., & McCloskey Dochterman, J. (Eds.). (2008). *Nursing interventions classification (NIC)* (5th ed., p. 336). St. Louis: Mosby Elsevier; and Moorhead, S., Johnson, M., Maas, M., Swanson, E. (Eds.). (2008). *Nursing outcomes classification (NOC)* (5th ed., p. 746). A full listing of nursing activities for each nursing intervention and outcome can be found in these books.

FOCUS ON THE OLDER ADULT

NURSING STRATEGIES TO ADDRESS AGE-RELATED CHANGES AFFECTING NUTRITION

Age-Related Changes	Nursing Strategies
Altered ability to chew related to loss of teeth, ill-fitting dentures, and gingivitis	• Encourage and instruct patient to care for and retain own teeth and dentures. • Encourage proper toothbrushing and use of special toothpaste if gums and teeth are sensitive. • Chop, shred, or puree foods that are difficult to chew. • Select ground meat, fish, or poultry as protein sources more easily chewed.
Loss of senses of smell and taste	• Serve food that is attractive and at proper temperature. • Serve one food at a time rather than mixing foods. • Serve foods with different textures and aromas.
Decreased peristalsis in the esophagus	• Avoid cold liquids. • Avoid emotional upsets and stress-producing situations. • Take anticholinergic drugs as ordered by physician.
Gastroesophageal reflux	• Avoid overeating. • Avoid juices, chocolate, and fat. • Avoid alcohol and smoking. • Elevate the head of the bed 30 to 40 degrees when sleeping. • Lose weight if necessary. • Avoid bending over. • Take antacids or other medications as ordered by physician. • Avoid eating right before bedtime.
Decreased gastric secretions	• Chew food thoroughly. • Eat meals on a regular schedule. • Use antacids or other medications as prescribed by physician. • Be alert for symptoms of deficiency of nutrients, particularly iron, calcium, fat, protein, and vitamin B_{12}.
Slowed intestinal peristalsis	• Eat a high-fiber diet. • Remain as active as possible. • Increase fluid intake. • Avoid laxative use. • Eat meals at a regular time. • Drink prune juice or eat prunes every morning.
Lowered glucose tolerance	• Eat more complex carbohydrates. • Avoid sugar-rich foods.
Reduction in appetite and thirst sensation	• Offer fluids at regular intervals and at preferred temperature. • Be alert for symptoms of dehydration and electrolyte imbalance. • Offer small meals at frequent intervals.
Nutritional deficiencies related to alcohol intake	• Encourage diet high in protein and carbohydrates. • Offer small, frequent meals to maintain caloric intake. • Restrict sodium and fluids if edema is present. • Take multivitamin supplements, as ordered by physician.
Loss of appetite associated with depression and loneliness	• Promote mealtime as a social event. • Set an attractive table in a pleasant setting. • Eat outdoors whenever possible. • Invite guests as often as possible. • Participate in special programs for senior citizens.
Physical handicaps	• Open cartons and assist with setup of meal. • Arrange for home-delivered meals. • Conserve energy when preparing meals (sit on a stool, etc.). • Provide transportation and assistance to obtain food.

(continued)

FOCUS ON THE OLDER ADULT

NURSING STRATEGIES TO ADDRESS AGE-RELATED CHANGES AFFECTING NUTRITION *(continued)*

Age-Related Changes	Nursing Strategies
Low income	• Buy specials when available at food store. • Use generic brands. • Use coupons. • Cook larger quantities than necessary and freeze the leftovers for future use. • Substitute eggs, skim milk powder, and beans for meat. • Check for any community resources available to elderly.
Malnutrition	• Eat essential foods first. • Select nutrient-dense foods. • Monitor for signs of nutritional deficiencies. • Encourage eating by planning special events.
Increased risk for drug–nutrient interactions	• Avoid unnecessary drugs; monitor for polypharmacy. • Be aware of drug actions and interactions. • Check with pharmacist to determine if medication may or may not be taken with food. • Assess for confusion and inability to manage medication regimen.

be stored separately. This prevents cross-contamination with microorganisms. Chill (refrigerate) perishable food promptly and keep cold foods at 41°F or lower to prevent the growth of pathogens. Advise patients to avoid raw (unpasteurized) milk and products made from unpasteurized milk and raw eggs. Teach patients to avoid undercooked meat and poultry, unpasteurized juices, and raw sprouts (USDA & DHHS, 2005; Yen, 2005).

Monitoring Nutritional Status

Nurses are aware that malnourished patients are more likely to have slower wound healing and to develop complications. Prevention of malnutrition can have a positive effect on patient outcomes. In the hospital, shortened stays limit the time available for nutritional screening and intervention. Patients are often acutely ill and uninterested or unable to absorb and retain any nutritional instruction. It may also be difficult to include a family member or caregiver responsible for food preparation in scheduled teaching sessions. In many situations, the home healthcare nurse has the opportunity to have a significant impact on nutritional health. Instruction can be provided in a relaxed setting that allows insight into a patient's cultural orientation and family patterns and traditions. This environment also encourages modification and adjustments in the nurse's approach to nutritional instruction. Investigate the variety of community services and programs that are available to provide nutritional support to patients at home. The accompanying box, Focus on the Older Adult, includes teaching content and strategies for the specific nutritional challenges facing the older adult.

Stimulating Appetite

Pain, illness, anxiety, and medications can contribute to anorexia and poor intake when in a healthcare facility or in the home. To the hospitalized patient, food and eating may take on much greater meaning. Loss of control over food choices, the way food is prepared, when and how food is served, and eating alone may do little to encourage normal eating. Make every effort to ensure that the proper food is not only served, but also eaten. The additional time and attention spent when encouraging a person to eat may have a positive effect on dietary intake. The following measures may help to stimulate appetite in any setting:

- Serve small, frequent meals to avoid overwhelming the individual with large amounts of food.
- Solicit food preferences and encourage favorite foods from home or prepared when at home, if possible.
- Provide encouragement and a pleasant eating environment.
- Be sure that any prepared food looks attractive.
- Schedule procedures and medications at times when they are least likely to interfere with appetite.
- Control pain, nausea, or depression with medications.
- Offer alternatives for items that a person cannot or will not eat.
- Encourage or provide good oral hygiene. Ensure that the patient's dentures are well-fitting and in place, if applicable.
- Remove clutter from the eating area.
- Keep eating area free from irritating odors.
- Arrange food tray so that an individual can easily reach food.

Box 36-7 SPECIAL CONSIDERATIONS AND INTERVENTIONS FOR FEEDING PATIENTS WITH DEMENTIA OR OTHER ALTERATIONS IN COGNITION

- Change the environment in which meals occur.
- Assess the area where meals are served. Create a home-like environment by preparing food close to the place where it will be served to stimulate senses.
- Observe as many former rituals as possible, such as handwashing and saying a blessing.
- Avoid clutter and distractions.
- Maintain a pleasant, well-lighted room.
- Keep food as close to its original form as possible.
- Serve meals in the same place at the same time.
- Closely supervise mealtime.
- Check food temperatures to prevent accidental mouth burns.
- Assist as needed. Be alert for cues from the patient. Turning away may signal the patient has had enough to eat or that he needs to slow down. Leaning forward with
an open mouth usually means the patient is ready for more food.
- Stroking the underside of the chin may help promote swallowing.
- Provide one food at a time; a whole tray of food may be overwhelming.
- Ensure the patient's glasses and hearing aid are working properly.
- Demonstrate what you want the patient to do. State the goal clearly, and then mimic the action with exaggerated motions.
- Provide between-meal snacks that are easy to consume using the hands.
- Use adaptive feeding equipment as needed such as weighted utensils, large-handled cups, and larger or smaller silverware than standard.

(Adapted from Dudek, S. [2006]. *Nutrition essentials for nursing practice* [5th ed.]. Philadelphia: Lippincott Williams & Wilkins; DiMaria-Ghalili, R., & Amella, E. [2005] Nutrition in older adults. *American Journal of Nursing, 105*(3), 40–51; and Hallpike, B. (2008). Promoting good nutrition in patients with dementia. *Nursing Standard, 22*(29), 37–43.

- Provide a comfortable position.
- Ask about any rituals during mealtimes at home and include them if possible.
- If patients are absent from their rooms during mealtime, order a late food tray or keep food warm until they return.
- Mealtime should be undisturbed; don't interrupt patients for nonurgent procedures during mealtime.

Assisting with Eating

The loss of independence that comes with the inability to self-feed can be a severe blow to a person's self-esteem. The following measures may help a person maintain dignity while being fed:

- Involve the person as much as possible. Solicit his or her preferences regarding the order of items eaten and the eating pace.
- Provide appropriate drinks.
- Sit at the patient's eye level and make eye contact to create a more relaxed atmosphere.
- Engage the individual in pleasant conversation to ease tension.
- Place a napkin, not a bib, over the person's clothes for protection.
- Use straws or special eating utensils whenever possible.
- Ensure that if a person wears dentures, hearing aids, or glasses, they are in place before mealtime.
- Open containers, cut meat, or apply condiments to the prepared food only if the person wishes.
- When assisting visually impaired patients:
  - Explain placement of foods on plates and food tray. Relating items on plate to the location on a clock face may be helpful.
  - Provide special plate guards, utensils, double handles, and compartmentalized plates.

- Place foods and dishes in similar locations at each meal.
- Use straws for beverages, if not contraindicated by the presence of dysphagia.
- Provide supervision as needed.

Box 36-7 outlines special considerations and interventions for feeding patients with dementia or other alterations in cognition. Box 36-8 highlights nursing considerations for feeding patients with dysphagia.

Box 36-8 SPECIAL CONSIDERATIONS AND INTERVENTIONS FOR FEEDING PATIENTS WITH DYSPHAGIA

- Provide at least a 30-minute rest period prior to mealtime. A rested person will likely have less difficulty swallowing (Metheny, 2007).
- Sit the patient upright, preferably in a chair. If bedrest is mandatory, elevate the head of the bed to a 90-degree angle.
- Avoid rushed or forced feeding. Adjust the rate of feeding and size of bites to the patient's tolerance.
- Initiate a nutrition consult for appropriate diet modification such as chopping, mincing, or pureeing of foods and liquid consistency.
- Alternate solids and liquids.
- Assess for signs of aspiration during eating: sudden appearance of severe coughing; choking; cyanosis; voice change, hoarseness, and/or gurgling after swallowing; frequent throat clearing after meals; or regurgitation through the nose or mouth.

(Holmes, S. [2008]. Nutrition and eating difficulties in hospitalized older adults. *Nursing Standard, 22*(26), 47–57; Metheny, N. [2007]. Try this: Best practices in nursing care to older adults. The Hartford Institute for Geriatric Nursing. Preventing aspiration in older adults with dysphagia. Issue Number 20. Available http://consultgerirn.org/uploads/File/trythis/issue_20.pdf.)

Providing Nutrition in Special Situations

A variety of normal and modified diets are available in healthcare settings and may be prescribed for use at home. Normal, regular, or house diets are designed to maintain optimal nutritional status by providing adequate amounts of all nutrients. The diet's actual composition varies with the quantity and types of food selected; the average calorie content ranges from 1,400 to 2,500 calories.

LIQUID DIETS

Liquid diets are used most often as transitional diets when eating resumes after acute illness, surgery, or parenteral nutrition. The decision to advance a patient's diet is based on the return of gastrointestinal function, the absence of symptoms related to a particular disease process, or the resolution of whatever prompted the dietary restriction. Often, medical orders are written to begin the patient on a clear liquid diet and advance to another diet as tolerated. This allows the nurse to assess the patient's tolerance of the beginning diet and change, or advance, the diet based on the assessments. The diet would progress from clear liquids to full liquids to a soft diet, then to a normal or modified diet, based on their condition and tolerance. Tolerance of diet can be assessed by the following: absence of nausea, vomiting, and diarrhea; absence of feelings of fullness; absence of abdominal pain and distention; feelings of hunger; and the ability to consume at least 50% to 75% of the food on the meal tray. For example, a postoperative patient may have an order to begin a clear liquid at breakfast and advance to a house diet as tolerated. The patient would receive a clear liquid diet for breakfast. The nurse would assess the patient's ability to ingest the clear liquids and then make a decision regarding progression of the diet.

Clear liquid diets contain only foods that are clear liquids at room or body temperature—gelatin, fat-free broth, bouillon, ice pops, clear juices, carbonated beverages, regular and decaffeinated coffee, and tea. Because clear liquid diets are inadequate in calories, protein, and most nutrients, progression to more nutritious alternatives is recommended as soon as possible. **Full liquid diets** contain all the items on a clear liquid diet. Additional items allowed include milk and milk drinks, puddings, custards, plain frozen desserts, pasteurized eggs, cereal gruels, vegetable juices, and milk and egg substitutes in addition to clear liquids. A full liquid diet contains liquids that can be poured at room temperature. High-calorie, high-protein supplements are recommended if a full liquid diet is used for more than 3 days.

SOFT DIETS

Soft diets are usually regular diets that have been modified to eliminate foods that are hard to digest and to chew, including those that are high in fiber, high in fat, and highly seasoned. Soft diets may also be called bland or low-fiber diets. Soft diets are adequate in calories and nutrients and may be used on a long-term basis.

Many other types of diets are used in the inpatient setting to aid in the treatment of disease or illness; many are prescribed

to be continued by the patient after discharge. Table 36-7 outlines information about the soft diet and other diets that may be prescribed for patients.

VEGETARIAN DIETS

Some patients may prefer a vegetarian diet for a variety of reasons, such as religious preference, ethical belief that killing animals for food is unjust, fear of contamination with pesticides, or health concerns about the cholesterol and saturated fats found in meats. There are many different forms of vegetarianism, ranging from avoidance of red meat to complete elimination of all animal products. Meats are usually replaced with legumes, grains, and vegetables, and, if well planned, this type of diet can satisfy all nutritional requirements. Because fewer or no animal products are consumed, vegetarians consume less saturated fat, cholesterol, and animal protein and greater amounts of carbohydrates, fiber, and other important nutrients. Vitamin B_{12}, vitamin A, and iron are nutrients that may require supplementation in some vegetarian diets, but most vegetarian diets are not deficient in any nutrients. Support patients who follow a vegetarian diet by assisting them or their caregiver to select nutritious food items from the large variety of foods available within their dietary framework.

NOTHING BY MOUTH

In some cases, such as before surgery to prevent aspiration related to anesthesia and after surgery until bowel sounds return, patients may be ordered nothing by mouth **(NPO).** NPO may also be necessary for patients undergoing certain medical tests; for patients experiencing severe nausea and vomiting, an inability to chew or swallow, or various acute or chronic GI abnormalities; for those who are comatose; and for women during labor and delivery.

The following measures may provide comfort to patients who are ordered NPO:

- Encourage or provide good oral hygiene.
- Provide the patient with ice chips or sips of water as allowed.
- Urge the patient to avoid watching others eat. Suggest alternate activities at mealtimes.

Well-nourished patients can easily withstand the stress of NPO for a short period, but being NPO for an extended period of time poses a nutritional challenge for many individuals. Patients with increased nutritional requirements and those who will be NPO for more than 2 days may require nutritional support from **enteral nutrition,** administering nutrients directly into the stomach, or **parenteral nutrition,** providing nutrition via IV therapy.

Providing Enteral Nutrition

Oral feeding is the preferred and most effective method of feeding patients. However, at times, a patient will be unable to meet nutritional needs through oral intake of an adequate diet. When this circumstance is present, an alternate feeding method may be necessary. Selection of a feeding tube may

TABLE • 36-7   SELECTED DIETS AND EXAMPLES OF INCLUDED/EXCLUDED FOODS

Diet and Description	Foods Allowed	Foods Excluded
Soft Diet: An adequate diet that is moderately low in fiber and lightly seasoned. Often used for patients after surgery or those with mild gastrointestinal distress. May also be used as a transition between liquids and a regular diet.	• All items on the full liquid diet • Cooked vegetables • Cooked or canned fruit • Banana • Avocado • Lettuce in small amounts • Melon • Potatoes, rice, barley, pasta • Lean, tender meats; fish; poultry • Eggs, mild cheese, smooth peanut butter • Soybeans • Yogurt and mild salad dressings	• Raw fruits and vegetables • Coarse breads and cereals • Potentially gas-forming foods, such as cabbage and broccoli
Fat-Restricted Diet: Low-fat diets are intended to lower the patient's total intake of fat. This diet may be used, for example, with patients experiencing chronic cholecystitis (inflammation of the gallbladder) to decrease gallbladder stimulation and as part of dietary interventions for patients with cardiovascular disease, to help prevent atherosclerosis. Total amount of servings would be individually prescribed for each patient.	• Skim milk; coffee, tea, fruit juice • Plain, nonfat cereals, spaghetti, noodles, rice, plain whole-grain or enriched breads • Cottage cheese, low-fat cheeses (containing less than 5% butterfat) • Nonfat frozen yogurt and nondairy desserts, fruit ice, sorbet gelatin, puddings made with skim milk, angel food cake, vanilla wafers • Egg whites as desired, 3 whole eggs per week, low-fat egg substitutes • 1 serving of fat (1 tsp butter, 1 tsp oil or shortening, 1 tsp mayonnaise, 6 small nuts, 5 small olives, 2 tsp Italian dressing, 2 tbsp light cream, ⅛ avocado) • Fruit as desired • Poultry without skin, fish, veal, liver, beef, pork, lamb, ¼ cup water packed tuna, 3 oz tofu • Bouillon, clear broth, cream soup made with skim milk • Jelly, jam, honey, molasses, sugar, gumdrops, jelly beans • All plainly prepared vegetables	• Whole milk, chocolate milk • Biscuits, pancakes, doughnuts, fritters, muffins • Whole-milk cheeses • Cake, pastry, pie, ice cream, chocolate • More than 1 egg/day, unless substituted for part of the meat allowed • Fat in excess of allowed amount • Avocado in excess of allowed amount • Fried meats, sausage, scrapple, hot dogs, spareribs, duck, peanut butter, salt pork, goose • All other soups • Any candy made with chocolate, nuts, butter, cream, or fat • Potato chips, fried potatoes, buttered, au gratin, or creamed vegetables
Pureed Diet: Also known as a blenderized liquid diet because the diet is made up of liquids and foods blenderized to liquid form. Used after oral or facial surgery and for patients with chewing and swallowing difficulties.	• All foods, unless otherwise contraindicated. Consistency is changed to liquid. • Broth, gravy, cream soups, cheese, tomato sauce, milk, and fruit juice are often used because of their higher calorie and nutritional value.	Thickness and viscosity is based on patient tolerance.
Mechanical Soft Diet: Regular diet with modifications for texture. Used for patients with limited chewing ability or who have had surgery to the head, neck, or mouth	• Chopped, ground, mashed, pureed foods • Mashed, soft ripened fruit, such as bananas, peaches, pears • Cooked, mashed soft vegetables, such as peas, carrots, yams	• Most raw fruits and vegetables • Foods containing seeds, nuts, dried fruit

be appropriate, because the next best method of feeding is via the enteral route. Enteral nutrition involves passing a tube into the GI tract to administer a formula containing adequate nutrients. Gastric feedings have the advantage of allowing the stomach to be used as a natural reservoir, regulating the amount of foods and liquids released into the small intestine. This alternate feeding method may deliver total or supplemental nutrition over a short-term period or for longer intervals. Consider factors related to selection of a feeding tube, including aspiration risk, the anticipated duration of the feeding tube, the function of the gastrointestinal (GI) tract, and the patient's overall condition and prognosis. Also, it is important to consider the ethical implications surrounding initiation of tube feedings, which entail knowledge of the patient's wishes concerning this intervention.

The decision to place, maintain, and/or discontinue feeding tubes can be a source of much turmoil in the lives of patients and their families. There are many emotional, physical, psychological, and cultural aspects to the institution, maintenance, and withdrawal of nutrition. Nurses can be a source of great support and information to aid patients and their families in making nutrition-related healthcare decisions.

SHORT-TERM NUTRITIONAL SUPPORT

For short-term use (less than 4 weeks), a nasogastric or nasointestinal route is usually selected. A **nasogastric (NG) tube** is inserted through the nose and into the stomach. However, the patient is at risk for aspirating the tube feeding solution into the lungs, a disadvantage for using this route. Patients with a dysfunctional gag reflex, high risk of aspiration, gastric stasis, gastroesophageal reflux, nasal injuries, and those who are unable to have the head of the bed elevated during feedings are not candidates for nasogastric feeding (Best, 2005).

Traditional nasogastric tubes are firm and large in diameter. One example is a Levin tube. A Levin tube is a flexible rubber or plastic single-lumen tube with holes at the stomach end and a connector at the opposing end. The connector allows for attachment to a feeding apparatus and medication administration (Fig. 36-4). Occasionally, a smaller, softer, more pliable polyurethane tube may be inserted via the nose into the stomach or small intestine. This type of tube is advantageous, providing greater patient comfort and less trauma to the nares. A Dobbhoff tube is an example of this type of tube (Fig. 36-5). However, the smaller tube diameter makes checking tube placement and medication administration more difficult than with the larger-diameter tubes. The method of inserting a nasogastric tube is described in Skill 36-1. Insertion, which requires skill and accuracy, is frequently done by the nurse.

A **nasointestinal (NI) tube** is passed through the nose and into the upper portion of the small intestine. It may be indicated for a patient with increased risk for aspiration due to a diminished gag reflex or slow gastric motility. Administration of the feeding solution into the small intestine also avoids the potential for gastric reflex. Some medical conditions (delayed gastric emptying, gastric tumor) also necessitate the use of a nasointestinal tube. However, when

FIGURE 36-5. Dobbhoff tube.

formula is delivered directly into the intestine, a type of dumping syndrome may develop because the pyloric valve in the stomach, which normally slows transit of food into the intestine, is bypassed. Rapid administration of hypertonic feeding solution into the proximal small intestine causes the movement of extracellular fluid from the vascular system into the small intestine. Distention of the small intestine occurs, with accompanying gas, bloating, nausea, diarrhea, cramping, and lightheadedness.

CONFIRMATION OF NG FEEDING TUBE PLACEMENT

Verify correct placement of the nasogastric tube after the initial insertion, before beginning a feeding or instilling liquids, and at regular intervals during continuous feedings. This ensures that the tip of the tube is situated in the stomach or intestine, preventing inadvertent administration of substances into the wrong place. A misplaced feeding tube in the lungs or pulmonary tissue places the patient at risk for aspiration. Radiographic examination, measurement of Aspirate pH, visual assessment of aspirate, measurement of tube length and measurement of tube marking, and monitoring of carbon dioxide are used to confirm feeding tube placement. With the exception of radiographic examination, the use of several of these techniques in conjunction with each other increases the likelihood of correct tube placement. An old technique of auscultation of air injected into a feeding tube has proved unreliable and may result in tragic consequences if used as an indicator of tube placement (AACN, 2005; Best, 2005; Khair, 2005; Sanko, 2004; Sweeney, 2005). Therefore, do not use it to confirm feeding tube placement.

Radiographic Examination

This is the standard procedure to verify initial placement of a feeding tube (AACN, 2005; Best, 2005; Ellet, 2004; Khair, 2005; Metheny et al., 2004). However, radiographs expose the patient to radiation, must be interpreted by a physician, are costly if done on a routine basis, and may be inaccessible. A radiograph only confirms the position of the tube at the time it was taken. The tube may have moved at any point thereafter. Also, as previously stated, placement must be checked frequently while the tube is in place.

FIGURE 36-4. Levin tube.

Measurement of Aspirate pH and Visual Assessment of Aspirate

The recommended method for checking placement, other than radiograph, is measuring the pH of the aspirate (AACN, 2005; Best, 2005; Earley, 2005; Ellet, 2004; Khair, 2005; May, 2007; Smeltzer et al., 2010). However, when continuous feedings are in use, pH becomes less helpful, because the nutritional formula buffers the pH of gastrointestinal secretions (Metheny et al., 2005). Visual assessment of aspirated gastric contents is also suggested as a tool to check placement (Padula et al., 2004; Smeltzer et al., 2010). Refer to Guidelines for Nursing Care 36-1: Visual Assessment and pH Measurement of Gastric Contents.

Aspiration of fluid through the feeding tubes is sometimes difficult, especially if a smaller diameter tube is used. Because they are less rigid, they may be more likely to collapse when negative pressure is applied during aspiration. More than likely, the difficulty is a result of a blocked tube. Additionally, the ports on the tip of the tube may not be positioned in fluid. Research by clinicians has demonstrated that aspiration is easier in small-bore tubes if there are multiple ports rather than a single port. Several attempts may be necessary to aspirate gastric contents. If repeated instillations of 30 mL of air and repositioning prove ineffective, tube placement should be checked by radiograph after obtaining a physician's order.

Measurement of Tube Length and Measurement of Tube Marking

Another way to verify tube placement is to measure the length of the exposed tube after insertion and document this measurement. Then, before each feeding, check tube length and compare findings with the initial measurement, in conjunction with pH measurement and visual assessment of aspirate. Any increase in the length of the exposed tube may indicate dislodgement (Bourgault et al., 2007; Smeltzer et al., 2010). Marking the tube with an indelible marker at the nostril and then assessing this marking each time the tube is used ensures that the tube has not become displaced.

Carbon Dioxide Monitoring

Monitoring for carbon dioxide to determine nasogastric tube position and/or dislodgement has been evaluated (May, 2007; Munera-Seeley et al., 2008). This involves the use of a capnograph or a colorimetric end-tidal CO_2 detector to detect the presence of carbon dioxide, which would indicate

---

Guidelines for Nursing Care • 36-1

VISUAL ASSESSMENT AND pH MEASUREMENT OF GASTRIC CONTENTS

Allow 1-hour interval after patient has received medication or completed an intermittent feeding before testing pH of gastric fluid. If feeding is continuous, plan pH testing at a time when feeding can be withheld.

- Insert 30 mL of air into tube before aspirating GI contents to flush out contents of tube.
- Withdraw small amount (5–10 mL) of gastric secretions.
- If unable to obtain specimen, reposition the patient and flush tube again with 30 mL of air. It may be necessary to retry several times.
- Place drop of gastric secretions onto pH paper or place small amount in plastic cup and dip the pH paper into it. Within 30 seconds, compare the color on the paper with the chart supplied by the manufacturer. (A pH meter and color chart is also an option.)
- Document results on the patient's flow sheet. The following are indications of placement:

pH
- Stomach: pH less than 5.5 (If the patient is taking an acid-inhibiting agent, the range may be 4.0–6.0)

- Intestines: pH 7.0 or higher
- Respiratory tract: pH 6.0 or higher

Color of Aspirate
- Stomach: grassy green, tan, off-white, bloody, or brown
- Intestines: medium to deep golden-yellow (may be greenish-brown if stained with bile)
- Respiratory tract: off-white and tinged with mucus

(American Association of Critical-Care Nurses (AACN). (2005). *Practice Alert: Verification of feeding tube placement.* Available at www.aacn.org/WD/Practice/Content/practicealerts.pcms?pid=1&&menu=.; Best, C. [2005]. Caring for the patient with a nasogastric tube. *Nursing Standard, 20*(3), 59–65; Khair, J. [2005]. Guidelines for testing the placing of nasogastric tubes. *Nursing Times, 101*(20), 26–27; May, S. (2007). Testing nasogastric tube positioning in the critically ill: Exploring the evidence. *British Journal of Nursing, 16*(1), 414–410; and Murray, J. [2005]. Clinical queries: How do I verify NG tube placement? *Nursing, 35*(8), 25.)

RESEARCH IN NURSING
Bridging the Gap to Evidence-Based Practice

CONFIRMATION OF NASOGASTRIC TUBE PLACEMENT

Inadvertent placement of nasogastric feeding tubes into the tracheopulmonary system during insertion and displacement at a time following initial insertion are potential life-threatening problems. The only absolutely reliable method to determine accurate placement is radiography. However, repeated radiographic testing is not practical or safe. Several methods of bedside testing, including evaluation of tube aspirate, measurement of aspirate pH, and measurement of exposed tube length, are in use; there is a continued need to strive for more conclusive methods to determine tube placement.

Related Research

Munera-Seeley, V., Ochoa, J., Brown, N., et al. (2008). Use of a colorimetric carbon dioxide sensor for nasoenteric feeding tube placement in critical care patients compared with clinical methods and radiography. *Nutrition in Clinical Practice, 23*(3), 318–321.

This study evaluated the use of a new commercial CO_2 sensor that was developed to assist in evaluating the placement of nasogastric feeding tubes. Nurses who performed placement of

For additional research, visit the **Point**.

nasogastric feeding tubes completed questionnaires following each procedure. The nurses recorded the clinical methods used to determine proper insertion and, based on them, where the tube was located. The nurses then evaluated nasogastric feeding tube insertion with the CO_2 sensor. From the readings, they recorded where the tube was located. Confirmation of tube placement was performed radiographically. The authors of the study evaluated 424 nasogastric feeding tube insertions. Of these, 15 (3.5%) were incorrectly placed into the airway and 409 were correctly placed into the stomach via the esophagus. The CO_2 sensor correctly assessed tube placement in 421 (99%) of the 424 cases. The authors of the study found the device to have a sensitivity of 86.7% and a specificity of 99.8%.

Relevance to Nursing Practice

The CO_2 sensor is a helpful bedside tool to use in conjunction with clinical methods during nasogastric feeding tube insertions. Nurses should consider investigating the use of these devices for use in their individual clinical facilities.

tube positioning in the patient's airway instead of the stomach. See the accompanying Research in Nursing display regarding the use of one of these tools.

Confirming Nasointestinal Tube Placement

After an initial x-ray for placement, the nurse can validate that the tube is still in the small intestine by checking the pH of the aspirate (pH >7 and bile-stained, ranging in color from light to golden yellow or brownish-green) (AACN, 2005).

LONG-TERM NUTRITIONAL SUPPORT

When enteral feeding is required for a long-term period, an enterostomal tube may be placed through an opening created into the stomach (gastrostomy) or into the jejunum (jejunostomy) (Smeltzer et al., 2010). Placement of a tube into the stomach can be accomplished by a surgeon or gastroenterologist via a **percutaneous endoscopic gastrostomy (PEG)** or a surgically (open or laparoscopically) placed **gastrostomy** tube. PEG tube insertion is often used because, unlike a traditional, surgically placed gastrostomy tube, it usually does not require general anesthesia. Use of a PEG tube or other type of gastrostomy tube requires an intact, functional GI tract. Insertion of a PEG tube involves local anesthesia, passage of an endoscope into the stomach, a small incision or stab wound through the skin of the abdomen, pushing a cannula through the small incision, insertion of a guide wire or suture material through the cannula, and introduction and placement of the PEG tube through one of several methods (Fig. 36-6 illustrates a PEG tube in place in the stomach).

In long-term feeding situations in which gastric problems exist, the jejunostomy is an alternate method through which

nutrition can be delivered. These tubes may be inserted surgically or with endoscopic or laparoscopic guidance (Fig. 36-7 illustrates a PEG/J tube in the jejunum). Gastrostomy or jejunostomy tubes are not easily dislodged.

For patients who are active yet require long-term continuous or intermittent feedings, a low-profile gastrostomy device (LPGD) may be an option (Fig. 36-8). Children are also excellent candidates for LPGDs. The external apparatus is minimal and consists of a button or skin disk that is stable, less irritating to the skin, and has no external tubing so it is easier to

FIGURE 36-6. Percutaneous endoscopic gastrostomy tube in place in the stomach. (Smeltzer, S. C., Bare, B. G., Hinkle, J. H., & Cheever, K. H., [2010]. *Brunner and Suddarth's textbook of medical surgical nursing* [12th ed., p. 1032.]. Philadelphia: Lippincott Williams & Wilkins.)

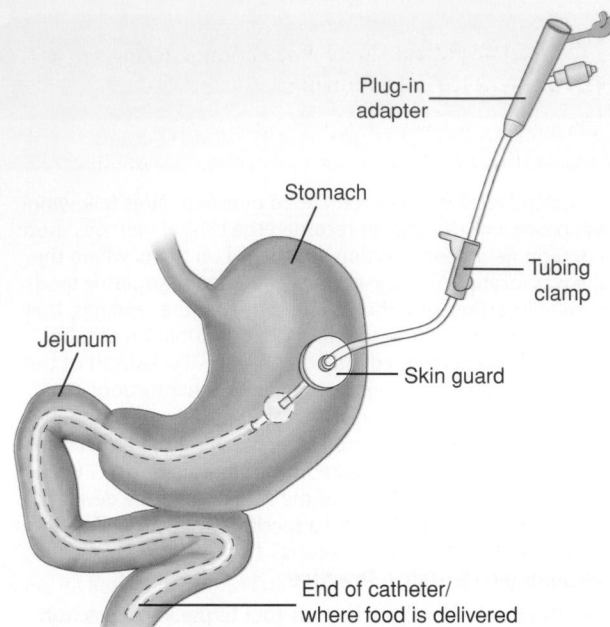

FIGURE 36-7. PEG/J tube inserted in the jejunum.

conceal with clothing. Additional advantages include the fact that it can be immersed in water, is less noticeable, and is less likely to migrate or become dislodged. The device has a cap, which is opened to access the feeding tube and connect with the administration set.

Checking placement of a gastrostomy or jejunostomy tube requires regular comparisons (according to agency policy) of the tube length to the measurement (inches or centimeters) that was documented after insertion. An indelible marker can be used to identify the exit point of the tube from the abdominal wall.

TUBE FEEDING ADMINISTRATION
Feeding Schedule
Based on the patient's physical, medical, and nutritional condition, the nutritionist usually makes recommendations concerning the feeding pattern or schedule.

FIGURE 36-8. Low-profile gastrostomy device (LPGD).

Continuous feedings allow gradual introduction of the formula into the GI tract, promoting maximal absorption. They require use of an enteral feeding pump, which limits the patient's mobility and increases cost. Continuous feeding into the stomach, however, is controversial because of the risk for reflux and aspiration.

Feedings into the intestine are always continuous to avoid triggering dumping syndrome, as the natural reservoir of the stomach is bypassed. Dumping syndrome is caused by overdistention of the small intestine. The use of intermittent or bolus feedings would provide larger than normal amounts of food and liquid in the proximal small intestine, causing overdistention, leading to nausea, diarrhea, cramping, and lightheadedness (Dudek, 2006).

Intermittent feedings are the preferred method for gastric feeding. Intermittent feedings are delivered at regular intervals in equal portions, introducing the formula gradually over a set period of time via gravity or a feeding pump. Alternately, bolus intermittent feedings, where a syringe is used to deliver the formula quickly into the stomach, may place the patient at risk for aspiration or cause distention. They are usually not recommended but may be used in long-term situations if tolerated by the patient. Intermittent feedings resemble a more normal pattern of intake and allow the patient freedom of movement between feedings (Dudek, 2006).

Another option is cyclic feeding. This involves administering continuous feeding for a portion of the 24-hour period. The usual routine is to feed the patient for 12 to 16 hours, most often overnight. Cyclic feeding allows the patient to attempt eating regular meals during the day, if this is possible, making ambulation and activity easier. Skill 36-2 describes administering a tube feeding.

Enteral Feeding Formulas
Many enteral feeding formulas are available. The nutritional composition of tube feedings depends on the feeding route, the patient's ability to digest and absorb nutrients, and his or her nutrient and fluid requirements. Other considerations include the availability and cost of the formula, medical conditions that require diet modifications, food intolerance, and allergies. Standard formulas contain intact molecules of protein, carbohydrates, and fats and require the patient to have normal digestion and absorption. Hydrolyzed formulas contain proteins and other nutrients in simple forms that require little or no digestion. These formulas are used with patients with impaired digestion or absorption. In addition to being nutritionally balanced, formulas may be high in calories, contain fiber, contain additional protein, or be especially formulated for patients with respiratory, renal, or other health problems. Detailed information about their composition and caloric value (most formulas contain 1 cal/mL, although 2 cal/mL concentrations are available) can be obtained from the product label.

Feedings are initiated at full strength. The rate of infusion begins at 10 to 40 mL per hour, depending on facility policy. The rate is then advanced by 10 to 20 mL per hour every 8 to 12 hours until the desired rate is achieved. Rate advancement is based on patient tolerance. Starting the feeding at a slower rate and progressing slowly improves tolerance. The previous practice of diluting feedings has not been shown to improve feeding tolerance and prolongs the period of inadequate nutrition support (Dudek, 2006). Criteria to consider when evaluating patient feeding tolerance includes:

- Absence of nausea, vomiting
- Minimal or no gastric residual
- Absence of diarrhea and constipation
- Absence of abdominal pain and distention
- Presence of bowel sounds within normal limits

Enteral Feeding Pumps

An enteral feeding pump regulates the amount of feeding solution that is delivered to the patient. The newer pumps are user friendly, have built-in safeguards that protect the patient from complications, and can be used in both institutions and the home. Safety features include automatic tube flush, cassettes that prevent free flow of formula, safety tips that prevent accidental attachment to an IV setup, and various audible and visible alarms. Most pumps can operate for up to 8 hours on battery. However, manufacturers recommend using the pump plugged into an electrical outlet for recharging whenever the patient is seated or resting for a period of time.

NURSING CONSIDERATIONS WITH TUBE FEEDING

Agency protocols may differ and should be followed, but nursing actions that contribute to successful tube feedings focus on patient safety, monitoring for complications, comfort, and education.

Promoting Patient Safety

To promote patient safety when administering a tube feeding, be sure to do the following:

- Check tube placement before administering any fluids, medications, or feeding using multiple techniques: x-ray, pH testing, aspirate characteristics, external length marking, and carbon dioxide monitoring. (Refer to Guidelines for Nursing Care 36-1.)
- Check **residual** (feeding remaining in the stomach) before each feeding or every 4 to 6 hours during a continuous feeding (according to institution policy). High gastric residual volumes (200 to 250 mL or greater) can be associated with high risk for aspiration and aspiration-related pneumonia (Bourgault, Ipe, Weaver, Swartz, & O'Dea, 2007; Metheny, 2008). Record residuals on flow sheet or in progress notes. Follow the clinician's order or facility policy for withholding feedings based on the residual. A residual of more than 10% to 20% above the hourly rate for the feeding may indicate that the feeding should be interrupted or delayed. Some experts now recommend that the patient's pattern of residual is more important than the amount (Bourgault et al.; Metheny). It is important to note that it is important to flush the feeding tube with water after checking gastric residual, to help prevent tube occlusions (Bourgault et al.; Metheny). Refer to the accompanying Through the Eyes of a Student display for a student nurse's experience with residual and a tube feeding.
- Assess the abdomen for abnormalities. Assess for bowel sounds at least once per shift to check for the presence

---

Through the Eyes of a Student

She looked lost in that big hospital bed, so thin and frail. Her hair was as white as her pillowcase and blankets, and her skin looked almost transparent. And then, I saw it. Snaking under her blankets into her belly was the feeding tube surrounded by thick, green, smelly discharge.

During preconference, my instructor had told me that I needed to check residual every 2 hours to monitor her absorption rate. The first time, with my instructor standing beside me like my guardian angel (or my patient's guardian angel, I'm not sure which), the procedure naturally went off without a hitch. I could do this, I thought, feeling more confident.

Because my patient had chronic diarrhea as well as skin breakdown at her sacrum, the next 2 hours flew by in a whirlwind of bathing. But now, the time had come. This is it, I thought. I'm on my own for the second residual check. And, again, I breathed a sigh of relief when the procedure was completed with no problems.

As the day progressed, I got myself a little behind schedule because I was determined to remove the hardened crusts from underneath her nails. Before I knew it, I got the message from another student that it was postconference time. Oh no! I didn't do my last residual check yet. Quickly, I emptied the basin I was

using on her fingernails and grabbed the plunger. I reached into my pocket for my hemostat to clamp off the line and the next thing I saw was Jevity squirting all over the bed, my patient, the clean Chux and me! I had cut the line instead of clamping it!

I quickly pinched both ends to stop the Jevity from squirting and frantically called for help. While waiting for rescue, I checked on my patient's response, not knowing how she was going to react. Thankfully, she was sound asleep, soothed by her recent nail massage. It seemed like forever before my instructor rushed in. With my eyes filling up, I attempted to explain that I had grabbed the scissors from my pocket instead of the hemostat. Guardian angel that she was (I think she was both of ours), my instructor calmly and efficiently proceeded to attach both ends of the tube together with the use of an adapter. Then we let the patient's physician know what happened.

Many lessons were learned that day, such as don't attempt a procedure in haste, and have all your supplies readily at hand. But the one thing I'll never, ever forget is that the scissors are the crooked ones!

—Eileen Cooper
Delaware County Community College, Media, PA

of peristalsis and a functional intestinal tract. Experts, however, have recently concluded that it is common for acutely ill patients to have delayed gastric emptying; therefore, delaying enteral feedings based on hypoactive bowel sounds may place a patient at risk for malnutrition. Gastric distention, nausea, vomiting, bloating, or pain may be a better indicator of how well a patient is tolerating a tube feeding (Palmer & Metheny, 2008; Sweeney, 2005).

- Make sure the patient is as upright as possible during feeding. If the patient is in bed during feedings, elevate the head of the bed at least 30 degrees during feeding and for 1 hour afterward to prevent reflux and aspiration. Pause the feeding if the patient has to be repositioned or temporarily laid flat. Resume the feeding only after the patient's head is returned to at least a 30-degree elevation.
- Prevent contamination during enteral feedings by maintaining the integrity of the feeding system and using proper technique. Closed systems, consisting of a sterile, prefilled, ready-to-hang container, reduce the opportunity for bacterial contamination of the feeding formula. An open system exists when formula from a can or bottle is added to a feeding setup. Always check the expiration date of formula. Perform hand hygiene and put on nonsterile gloves before preparing, assembling, and handling any part of the feeding system. Disinfect the opening and rim of any cans to be opened before opening. Label all equipment with the patient's name, date, and time the feeding was hung, and cap or cover any disconnected tubing. Clean a reusable feeding system with soap and hot water every 24 hours; replace a disposable feeding apparatus for open systems every 24 hours. Closed systems can be used up to 48 hours; check manufacturer's guidelines and facility policy.
- Medications may be administered through a feeding tube, but never give them while a feeding is being infused. Administer liquid forms of medications whenever possible. Never add medications directly to the formula; some drugs become ineffective when mixed with feeding formulas; medications mixed in feeding formulas may cause clogging of the feeding tube. It is very important to flush the tube with water before, between, and after the administration of medications. Administering medications through an enteral feeding tube is discussed in depth in Chapter 29.

Monitoring for Complications

Patients receiving tube feedings are at risk for several complications. Table 36-8 summarizes nursing measures to prevent selected complications. In addition, prevent the tube from becoming clogged or obstructed. Common causes of clogged enteral tubes include aspirated stomach contents, residue from medications, feeding flow rate of less than 50 mL/h, infrequent or inadequate addition of water to the system, and using a tube with a small lumen (Bourgault et al., 2007; Dudek, 2006). After checking placement, flush tube with 30 to 50 mL of water before and after each feeding or introduction of medications, at least every 4 hours during a continuous feeding, and after aspirating a tube for gastric contents

(Sudakin, 2006). After flushing the tube, be sure to document the amount on the intake and output record. Use of a feeding pump helps to prevent clogging. If an occlusion occurs, use a 60-mL syringe containing 30 to 60 mL of warm water to attempt to unclog the tube.

Providing Comfort Measures

Patients with nasogastric tubes often experience discomfort related to irritation to nasal and throat mucosa and drying of the oral mucous membranes. Implement several nursing interventions to ensure the patient's comfort and prevent alterations in the integrity of these tissues.

- Administer oral hygiene frequently (every 2 to 4 hours) to prevent drying of tissues and to relieve thirst. Offer the patient the opportunity to rinse the mouth with warm water and mouthwash solution frequently. Lubricate the lips generously.
- Keep the nares clean, especially around the tube, where secretions tend to accumulate. Using a lubricant after cleaning the nares is recommended.
- Help control local irritation from the tube in the throat. Analgesic throat lozenges or anesthetic sprays may be effective.
- Encourage the patient, if able, to verbalize concerns about tube feeding and presence of tube. A visit from another person who has learned to cope with this alternate feeding method may prove helpful.
- Ensure the tube is secured to the patient's nose and gown to prevent tension and tugging on the tube, causing trauma to the nares, and potential displacement.
- Be aware that some studies indicate that patients report being able to taste the feedings even though they are being fed through a gastric tube. If available and not contraindicated, offer the patient a choice of flavors.

> *Recall Charles Gallagher, the husband of the woman with advanced dementia receiving enteral nutrition. The nurse could teach Mr. Gallagher how to provide oral hygiene for his wife, including lubricating her lips. Doing so would allow Mr. Gallagher to feel some control over the situation. In addition, he would be helping to meet his wife's comfort needs and his own needs.* ∎

Providing Instruction

Often patients will continue to receive enteral feedings at home. Teaching Tips 36-1 outlines important points to review with patients and families in the home setting. Provide the patient and family with individualized instructions in written form as a reference for the patient and caregivers. Be sure to include the following in the teaching plan:

- Information about the administration of feedings, operation of the pump, formula, instructions regarding rate and how to check for tube placement, as well as what to do if the tube becomes dislodged

TABLE · 36-8 PREVENTING COMPLICATIONS OF ENTERAL FEEDING

Potential Complication	Preventive Interventions
Aspiration	• Use appropriate measures to check tube placement. • Elevate head of bed at least 30 degrees during feeding and for 1 hour afterward. • Give small, frequent feedings. • Avoid oversedation of patient. • Check residual volume per policy.
Clogged tube	• Flush tube before and after feeding, every 4 hours during continuous feeding, and after withdrawing aspirate. • Instill 30 mL of warm water with 50-mL or 60-mL syringe to attempt to unclog tube.
Nasal erosion with nasogastric or nasointestinal tubes	• Check nostrils every shift for signs of pressure. • Clean and moisten nares every 4 to 8 hours. • Start feeding at slow rate.

Diarrhea	• Prevent contamination in both open and closed systems:
	  • Change delivery set every 12 to 24 hours according to agency policy.
	  • Refrigerate opened cans of formula and discard after 24 hours.
	  • Limit hang time to 8 hours when using open system.
	• Use aseptic technique for patients who are immunosuppressed or acutely ill.
	• Assess for fecal impaction.

Other GI symptoms (nausea, vomiting, distention)	• Check residual prior to intermittent feedings and every 4 hours during continuous feedings. • Avoid oversedating client (delays gastric emptying). • Administer GI motility medications (Metoclopramide), as ordered.
Unplanned extubation	• Anchor tube adequately with tape. • Check on patient frequently. • Measure external length of tubing at regular intervals. • Restrain patient only if necessary, with physician's order.
Stoma infection	• Clean skin every shift with soap and warm water. Dry thoroughly. • Use topical antibiotics, as ordered. • Assess for signs of infection. • Request consult with wound care specialist, as needed.

• Care of the tube insertion site and possible complications that need to be reported
• Proper preparation, cleaning, and disposal of equipment
• Emergency telephone numbers, including the number for the home healthcare agency and the physician
• Arrangements for follow-up from the home health nurse as soon as possible after discharge

REMOVAL OF NASOGASTRIC TUBE
Removing the nasogastric tube as carefully as it is inserted is important to avoid causing the patient undue discomfort. After the tube is removed, provide for oral hygiene to remove disagreeable tastes and odors. Thorough oral hygiene is crucial when the tube has been in the intestinal tract and in contact with intestinal contents. Directions for removing the nasogastric tube are given in Skill 36-3.

NASOENTERIC TUBES FOR DECOMPRESSION
In addition to providing enteral feedings, nasogastric tubes can be used for other purposes. They may be inserted to decompress or drain the stomach of fluid, unwanted stomach contents, such as poison or medication and air, allowing it to rest, or before or after surgery, to promote healing. Nasogastric tubes may also be used to monitor GI bleeding and prevent intestinal obstruction. Tubes used for these purposes and associated nursing care are discussed in detail in Chapter 38.

Providing Parenteral Nutrition
Parenteral nutrition is the administration of nutritional support via the intravenous route. Patients who can't meet their nutritional needs by the oral or enteral routes may require intravenous nutritional supplementation. Intravenous supplementation may be prescribed for patients who have nonfunctional gastrointestinal (GI) tracts, who are comatose, or those who have high caloric and nutritional needs due to illness or injury; patients undergoing aggressive cancer therapy and those recovering from extensive burns, surgery, sepsis, or multiple fractures, for instance. Parenteral nutrition can be administered centrally, through a central venous access device (TPN), or peripherally (PPN), through a short-term intravenous access in

Tips

TEACHING TIPS • 36-1

HOME ENTERAL FEEDINGS

Health Topic	Teaching Tip	Why Is This Important?
Cleaning around a gastric tube insertion site	Use of soap and water, making sure that area is adequately rinsed Rotation of the guard after cleaning around it	If soap is left under the gastric tube guard, it can lead to skin irritation. The guard can put pressure on the skin, leading to skin breakdown.
Checking residuals	Method and reason for checking residual contents, as well as what to do with residual contents	Residual contents should not be routinely discarded to prevent an acid–base imbalance; however, the patient or caregiver should know when discarding is appropriate to prevent aspiration of stomach contents.
Delivering tube feedings	Head elevation while delivering a gastric feeding and for approximately an hour after the feeding Method of administration such as delivering the feedings via continuous or bolus method, and steps for carrying out the feeding	Keeping the head elevated helps to prevent aspiration of gastric tube feedings. Some patients do not tolerate the bolus method without vomiting. The patient or caregiver should know how to operate the machinery if it is to be delivered via continuous method or how to set up for a bolus feeding.
Leaking of gastric contents	Method of checking for problems (is guard too loose or balloon not filled adequately) if gastric tube is leaking stomach contents around insertion site	If gastric tube is leaking acidic stomach contents, the area around the insertion site can quickly break down.
Placement check	Methods to check placement to ensure tube has not migrated inward or outward	Gastrostomy tubes can be marked with an indelible marker. The mark should be checked to make sure it is at the level of the abdominal wall. If the marking is not visible, the tube may have migrated inward. If the mark is away from the abdominal wall, the tube may no longer be in the stomach. Patients may also measure the length of the tube from the skin and record the measurement. This measurement should be confirmed to ensure the tube has not migrated. (Tracey & Patterson, 2006)

a peripheral vein. The basic difference between the two types is the concentration of the solutions infused.

Total parenteral nutrition (TPN) is a highly concentrated, hypertonic nutrient solution. TPN provides calories, restores nitrogen balance, and replaces essential fluids, vitamins, electrolytes, minerals, and trace elements. TPN can also promote tissue and wound healing and normal metabolic function. It provides the bowel a chance to heal and reduces activity in the gallbladder, pancreas, and small intestine. TPN may be used to improve a patient's response to surgery (Fluids & electrolytes, 2006). TPN meets the patient's nutritional needs by way of nutrient-filled solutions administered intravenously through a central venous access device, such as a multilumen, nontunneled catheter into the subclavian vein, or a peripherally inserted central catheter (PICC). Hyperalimentation is another term sometimes used synonymously with parenteral nutrition.

Assessment criteria used to determine the need for TPN include an inability to absorb nutrients from the GI tract for more than 10 days; the presence of a debilitating illness lasting more than 2 weeks; loss of 10% or more of preillness weight; serum albumin level less than 3.5 g/dL; excessive nitrogen loss from wound infection, fistula, or abscess; renal or hepatic failure; and nonfunction of the GI tract for 5 to 7 days (Fluids & electrolytes, 2006).

Peripheral parenteral nutrition (PPN) is a less concentrated nutrient solution sometimes prescribed for patients who have a malfunctioning gastrointestinal tract and need short-term nutrition lasting less than 2 weeks (Fluids & electrolytes made incredibly easy, 2008). PPN is administered through a peripheral vein. Peripheral veins cannot tolerate highly concentrated solutions, so the solution is not as nutrient dense as TPN.

PARENTERAL NUTRITION SOLUTIONS AND ADMINISTRATION

TPN solutions are hypertonic. TPN contains the three primary components necessary to maintain nutrition: proteins,

TABLE • 36-9	COMMON COMPONENTS OF TPN
Additive	**Purpose**
Dextrose	Calories for metabolism
Amino acids	Protein for tissue repair
Lipids	Essential fatty acids and calories for metabolism, wound healing, red blood cell production
Acetate	Prevents metabolic acidosis
Calcium	Development of bones and teeth; aids in blood clotting
Chloride	Regulates acid–base balance; maintains osmotic pressure
Folic acid	DNA formation; promotes growth and development
Magnesium	Carbohydrate and protein absorption
Phosphorus	Cell energy and calcium balance
Potassium	Cellular activity and cardiac function
Sodium	Control water distribution; maintain normal fluid balance
Vitamin B complex	Carbohydrate absorption
Vitamin C	Wound healing
Vitamin D	Bone metabolism; maintain serum calcium levels
Vitamin K	Prevent bleeding disorders
Micronutrients, such as zinc, cobalt, and manganese	Wound healing; red blood cell synthesis

(Source: *Fluids & electrolytes made incredibly easy.* [2008]. [4th ed.]. Philadelphia: Wolters Kluwer Health/Lippincott Williams & Wilkins; and *Fluids & electrolytes. A 2-in-1 reference for nurses.* [2006]. Philadelphia: Lippincott Williams & Wilkins.)

carbohydrates, and fats. Additional components of parenteral nutrition include electrolytes, vitamins, and trace elements. The TPN formula is tailored to the individual patient's specific needs. Common components of TPN are listed in Table 36-9. Fat or lipid emulsions and dextrose add caloric value that the body needs to meet energy requirements. Because of the high glucose concentration, usually about 25% (thus, a hypertonic solution), it is important to monitor blood glucose levels (Skill 36-4).

PPN solutions are isotonic. PPN solutions contain components similar to those of TPN but in lesser concentrations and amounts. They contain low concentrations of dextrose and amino acids. PPN solutions provide fewer calories and supplement a patient's inadequate oral intake. This solution usually contains 10% glucose, which is suitable for administration into a peripheral vessel.

Physical incompatibility between the intravenous nutrition formula and other intravenous solutions, especially medications, is a potential problem and must be addressed. If the patient has a multilumen catheter in place, dedicate one lumen for the administration of the parenteral nutrition. Do not use that lumen or administration set for any other purpose. Not only does this prevent incompatibility problems, but it also reduces the risk for infection (Hadaway, 2005). If the patient's intravenous catheter has only one lumen, attempt to obtain a peripheral intravenous access for the administration of additional solutions. Consider discussing the potential for a midline or peripherally inserted central catheter with the patient's healthcare team. If an additional access is not available, research the compatibility of the solutions to be administered. Little research exists on the stability and compatibility of parenteral nutrition solutions and most medications. If compatible medications or other solutions must be given through the same lumen as parenteral nutrition, attach the administration set as close to the catheter hub as possible to limit the amount of contact between the drug (or solution) and the parenteral nutrition solution.

Pharmacists can add certain medications, such as regular insulin, heparin, cimetidine, ranitidine, famotidine or metoclopramide, into the parenteral nutrition solution, but medication should never be added to parenteral nutrition solutions after they are dispensed from the pharmacy (Hadaway, 2005).

PREVENTING COMPLICATIONS

TPN therapy is costly, requires constant monitoring, and has the potential for causing infections and metabolic and mechanical complications. It should be used only when enteral intake is inadequate or contraindicated and should be gradually discontinued as soon as possible. Prevention of potential complications associated with TPN requires vigilance and careful monitoring by the nurse. Potential complications include the following (Fluids & electrolytes, 2008; Fluids & electrolytes, 2006; Smeltzer et al., 2010):

- Complications related to the use of central venous access devices, such as pneumothorax and thromboembolism (inflammation of a blood vessel and formation of a thrombus [blood clot])
- Infection and sepsis
- Metabolic alterations, such as hyperglycemia or hypoglycemia
- Fluid, electrolyte, and acid–basc imbalances
- Phlebitis
- Hyperlipidemia
- Liver and gallbladder disease

Guidelines for Nursing Care 36-2 lists nursing guidelines for monitoring administration of parenteral nutrition.

PARENTERAL NUTRITION IN THE HOME SETTING

Many patients require long-term parenteral nutrition and continue such therapy in the home. Individuals with acquired immunodeficiency syndrome (AIDS), advanced cancer, difficulty swallowing, or chronic bowel problems are candidates for this type of nutritional support. Nurses are involved in educating the patient and caregiver about the techniques and responsibilities associated with parenteral nutrition, providing technical and psychological support, and documenting the assessments that allow parenteral nutrition to be continued in the home. Patient education should specifically include:

- Basic information about what TPN is and what it is used for
- Adverse reactions or catheter complications
- Circumstances that require contacting the physician
- Basic care of the venous access device used to administer
- Maintenance of equipment
- Frequency for measuring the patient's weight, intake and output, and monitoring glucose levels.

Evaluating

The effectiveness of the plan of care is evaluated as the last step in the nursing process. On an ongoing basis, the nurse accomplishes the following:

- Evaluates the patient's progress toward meeting nutritional outcomes
- Evaluates the patient's tolerance and adherence to the diet, when appropriate
- Assesses the patient's level of understanding of the diet and the need for further diet instruction or reinforcement
- Communicates findings to other members of the health-care team
- Revises the plan of care, as needed, or terminates nursing care

For samples of the nursing process for nutrition, see the accompanying concept map for William Johnston and the Nursing Plan of Care 36-1 for Susan Oakland.

Guidelines for Nursing Care • 36-2

MONITORING ADMINISTRATION OF PARENTERAL NUTRITION

- Use the same catheter lumen for administration of parenteral nutrition each time the tubing is changed.
- Use a pump to administer infusion of parenteral nutrition.
- If administration of parenteral nutrition is interrupted, administer a 5% to 10% dextrose solution to prevent hypoglycemia, based on facility policy.
- Discard unused parenteral nutrition solution within 24 hours of starting its administration.
- Check vital signs every 4 hours to monitor for development of infection or sepsis.
- Monitor blood glucose levels every 6 hours.
- Use aseptic technique when changing solution, tubing, filter, or dressings according to agency policy. Most infection-control practitioners recommend changing infusion administration sets every 24 hours.

- Change dressings at least three times per week, according to agency protocol. Some transparent semipermeable dressings are changed once per week. Change dressings if they become wet, soiled, or nonocclusive.
- Check that all connections are securely taped, catheter is clamped before opening the system, and insertion site is covered with sterile dressing.
- Compare the patient's daily weight to fluid intake and output. Total weight gain should not be greater than 3 lb per week. Weight gain greater than 1 lb per day indicates fluid retention.
- Assess serum protein and electrolyte levels for signs of imbalance.
- Because of the high glucose concentration, use tubing with an in-line filter.

William Johnston, a 42-year-old executive, is newly diagnosed with high blood pressure and high cholesterol. He confides that his health habits are less than admirable. "I usually eat on the run, often fast food, or big dinners with lots of alcohol. I can't remember the last time I worked out or did any exercise, unless running from my car to the train counts! I guess it's no wonder I've gained a few pounds over the years." He reports that he is 6 feet tall and currently weighs 213 lbs. His body mass index (BMI) is 29. During this office visit, the physician prescribes an antihypertensive medication and an antihyperlipidemic medication for his hypertension (HTN) and high cholesterol.

Priority 1

Nursing Diagnosis: Imbalanced Nutrition: More Than Body Requirements related to overeating and lack of exercise.
Supporting Data:
• Weight, 213 lbs; Height, 6 feet
• BMI is 29
• Diet consists of fast foods & big dinners
• Does not exercise
• Heavy alcohol use

Outcome:
Patient will identify ideal body weight and safely reduce weight towards this goal.

Nursing Interventions:
• Identify desired caloric intake
• Teach patient to weigh self weekly
• Assess typical dietary choices by having patient keep a food diary for 3 days
• Review dietary intake with the patient and compare to ideal meal plan using food pyramid guidelines
• Encourage gradual weight loss of 1–2 lbs/week
• Encourage/assist in plan of exercise (30–45 minutes, 5 days per week)
• Discuss ways of reducing stress

Evaluation: William stated he is committed to losing weight. He is walking briskly for 30 minutes at lunch time, 5 days a week. He has lost 2 lbs the first week.

Priority 2

Nursing Diagnosis: Ineffective Health Maintenance related to lack of knowledge about dietary restrictions to modify heart risk.
Supporting Data:
• Newly diagnosed HTN and high cholesterol
• Eating fast foods
• Heavy alcohol use
• Eats out frequently

Outcome:
Patient will demonstrate appropriate food choices within dietary restrictions.

Nursing Interventions:
• Assess willingness and motivation to learn
• Note patient's support systems
• Provide information regarding a diet low in sodium, cholesterol, and saturated fat
• Discuss strategies to maintain dietary restrictions when eating out
• Limit alcohol intake to decrease triglycerides
• Identify high nutritional value snacks that are portable when on the run
• Consult dietitian
• Provide printed instructions for ongoing reference

Evaluation: William developed a sample meal plan for a busy day, picking appropriate food choices, but states he might be too busy to think about this every day. Encourage consultation with dietitian.

Priority 3

Nursing Diagnosis: Deficient Knowledge related to newly diagnosed hypertension and hypercholesterolemia.
Supporting Data:
• Hypertension
• Hypercholesterolemia
• Poor health habits
• Hectic lifestyle
• Antihypertensive and antihyperlipidemic medications

Outcome:
Patient will verbalize understanding of management of HTN and hypercholesterolemia and will demonstrate behaviors to maintain health.

Nursing Interventions:
• Assess level of current knowledge
• Assess preferences for method of learning
• Provide printed material for future reference
• Teach the names, dose, times, actions, and side effects of medications he is taking
• Teach patient to take pulse and blood pressure every day and report significant changes to healthcare provider
• Teach patient the impact of hypertension and high cholesterol on the development of heart disease

Evaluation: William states his father died from heart disease; he doesn't want of follow in his footsteps. During a 2-week follow-up visit, you note he recorded his daily BP and pulse. His BP today is 123/82 mm Hg.

- - - - - **Relationship** **Assessment** **Nursing Diagnosis** **Outcome Identification** **Interventions** **Evaluation**

Concept map displaying the nursing process for William Johnston.

NURSING PLAN OF CARE • 36-1

For Susan Oakland

Susan Oakland, a 21-year-old student, was seen at the prenatal clinic for her first pregnancy at 5 weeks' gestation. On her next visit, 4 weeks later, she complained of nausea and vomiting and had lost 3 lb (1.4 kg).

ASSESSMENT FINDINGS

A comprehensive nutritional assessment revealed the following data:

Anthropometric Data

Usual body weight: 112 lb (50.8 kg)
Weight at 9-weeks' gestation: 109 lb (49.4 kg)
Height: 5 feet 5 inches (165.1 cm)
Ideal body weight: 125 lb (56.7 kg; range is 113 to 137 lb [51.3 to 62.1 kg])
Expected weight gain for 9-weeks' gestation: 1 to 2 lb (0.45 to 0.9 kg)

Biochemical Data

Laboratory data revealed low hemoglobin level and hematocrit.

Medical and Socioeconomic Data

- Patient complains of nausea and vomiting, which begin in the morning and continue until midafternoon. Her appetite is poor. She also states, "I'm always tired."
- Patient and her husband are first-semester graduate students; their source of income is graduate assistantships, and their food budget is limited.
- Patient states that she did not intend to become pregnant, but both she and her husband are excited about becoming parents. She plans to take a leave of absence from school for one semester when the baby is born; she wants to breastfeed.

Clinical Data

Patient appears pale. No other abnormal physical findings were noted.

Dietary Data

- Patient's 24-hour recall revealed an inadequate intake from the milk group and a marginal intake from the grain and meat groups. She skips breakfast because of a hurried schedule, which is now complicated by nausea; lunch comprises soup, salad, and fruit; dinner usually comprises chicken; cooked vegetables; pasta, rice, or potatoes; and fruit. Patient dislikes red meat and eats it only once or twice a month. She also dislikes milk and substitutes sugar-free soft drinks and water. Before becoming pregnant, she drank five or six cups of black coffee a day, but now she avoids it. Her snacks usually consist of fresh fruit and vegetables.
- Patient is very weight conscious; she periodically crash diets to maintain her weight at 112 lb (50.8 kg).
- Patient does not take vitamins, medications, or drugs; she drinks socially, one or two times per month.
- Nutritional problems and contributing factors include the following:
  - Inadequate intake of milk and calories contributed to by nausea and vomiting, dislike for milk, limited food budget, weight consciousness
  - Poor iron intake contributed to by lack of good sources of iron in her diet, no supplemental iron intake
  - Meal-skipping contributed to by nausea and vomiting, hurried schedule
  - Underweight or weight loss contributed to by weight consciousness, nausea, and vomiting

NURSING DIAGNOSIS *Imbalanced Nutrition:* Less Than Body Requirements related to increased requirements imposed by pregnancy, nausea and vomiting, weight consciousness, hurried schedule, food dislikes as manifested by: reports of anorexia, fatigue, 3-lb weight loss in 4-weeks' time, pale color, and low hemoglobin and hematocrit values.

EXPECTED OUTCOME By the next monthly assessment, 6/26/12, the patient will:

- Eat three or more small meals a day

(continued)

NURSING PLAN OF CARE · 36-1

For Susan Oakland (continued)

Nursing Interventions	Rationale	Evaluative Statement
Determine how the patient's schedule may be altered to allow time for meals. Encourage the patient to have easy-to-eat foods available for quick snacks, like cartons of yogurt; cheese and crackers; muffins; and fresh fruit.	Patient complained that her current schedule prevents regular meals. Easy-to-eat foods may be more acceptable and can be nutritionally comparable to traditional meals.	6/26/12 Outcome met. Patient eats three meals daily. Tries snacking on easy-to-eat foods when possible.
Advise the patient that nausea may be lessened by avoiding periods of hunger, and that later in the pregnancy, avoiding hunger will help ensure a steady supply of nutrients to the fetus.	Low blood glucose may contribute to nausea early in pregnancy; later in pregnancy, low blood glucose and resultant ketosis may be harmful to the fetus.	*Recommendation:* Encourage more snacking to increase overall food intake. *L. Swift, RN*

EXPECTED OUTCOME   By the next monthly assessment, 6/26/12, the patient will:

- Eat dry crackers, bread sticks, or dry cereal 30 minutes before rising.

Nursing Interventions	Rationale	Evaluative Statement
Advise the patient to eat a source of dry carbohydrates before getting up in the morning.	Eating dry carbohydrates 30 minutes before rising helps avoid nausea.	6/26/12 Outcome met. Patient eats dry crackers every morning 30 minutes before getting out of bed. Reports that it prevents morning nausea. *L. Swift, RN*

EXPECTED OUTCOME   By the next monthly assessment, 6/26/12, the patient will:

- Eat 6 small meals per day.

Nursing Interventions	Rationale	Evaluative Statement
Advise the patient to eat 6 small meals per day.	Small meals are easier to digest. Low glucose may contribute to nausea.	6/26/12 Outcome met. Patient eats at least 6 small meals per day. Nausea is occurring less frequently throughout the day.

EXPECTED OUTCOME   By the next monthly assessment, 6/26/12, the patient will:

- Avoid diet soft drinks

(continued)

NURSING PLAN OF CARE · 36-1

For Susan Oakland (continued)

Nursing Interventions

Advise the patient to avoid diet soft drinks. Recommend acceptable nutritional alternatives to the patient.

Rationale

Saccharin and aspartame have not been proved safe for the fetus. The diet sodas are filling but offer no calories for fetus.

Evaluative Statement

6/26/12 Outcome partially met. Patient reports that she drinks two or three cans of diet soft drinks a week at school to relieve thirst because nothing else is available.

Recommendation: Encourage the patient to bring something to drink during the day from home, such as frozen drink boxes of 100% fruit juice, which will thaw at room temperature, or an insulated container of ice water or milk flavored with vanilla (dislikes plain milk).

L. Swift, RN

EXPECTED OUTCOME By the next monthly assessment, 6/26/12, the patient will:

• Eat the recommended number of servings from each food group as suggested by the daily food guide for pregnancy.

Nursing Interventions

Provide the patient with a daily food guide for pregnancy, and explain the rationale for the increased recommendations. Investigate acceptable alternatives for red meat and milk, which the patient normally does not consume.

Rationale

Because this is the patient's first pregnancy, she is not aware of the recommendations for eating during pregnancy. Although no one particular food is essential during pregnancy, red meat is essential during pregnancy and an excellent source of iron, and milk is an excellent source of calcium, two minerals important for the developing fetus. If the patient is not provided with nutritionally equivalent alternatives, her diet may not be optimal, even if she consumes the recommended number of servings from the meat and milk groups (i.e., patient may not be getting as much iron as she can from her diet if she relies on fish, cheese, and white-meat poultry to satisfy the meat group recommendations).

Evaluative Statement

6/26/12 Outcome partially met. Patient's intake is improved: Intake from the grain and meat groups is adequate instead of marginal. However, the patient still has difficulty consuming enough items from the milk group.

Recommendation: Continue encouraging the patient to consume more items from the milk group such as cheese, yogurt, and pudding. Will advise the patient to add skim milk powder whenever possible to fortify home-cooked and home-baked products. Will recommend that the patient increase her intake of nondairy sources of calcium, such as broccoli, spinach, and greens or breakfast cereal, fruit juice, and soy beverages with added calcium. Iron may also be consumed through turkey dark meat, shellfish, or spinach.

L. Swift, RN

(continued)

NURSING PLAN OF CARE · 36-1

For Susan Oakland (continued)

EXPECTED OUTCOME   By the next monthly assessment, 6/26/12, the patient will:

- Gain 1 to 2 lb

Nursing Interventions	Rationale	Evaluative Statement
Advise the patient on the recommended rate and amount of weight gain. Stress the importance of quality weight gain.	Patient needs to understand that a 25- to 35-lb gradual weight gain is considered optimal for fetal development, and results in little gain in maternal fat tissue. However, because the fetus and maternal tissues require nutrients along with calories, it is essential that the weight gain comes from eating nutrient-dense calories instead of empty calories.	6/26/12 Outcome met. Noting a relief from nausea and an increase in the number of daily meals, the patient gained 2 lb. *L. Swift, RN*

EXPECTED OUTCOME   By the next monthly assessment, the patient will:

- Take prenatal vitamins as prescribed by the physician.

Nursing Interventions	Rationale	Evaluative Statement
Advise the patient to take the supplement as prescribed and that the supplements are not a substitute for an adequate diet.	Supplements are intended to be used in conjunction with an optimal diet, not in place of one, because they do not provide optimal amounts of all required nutrients. Because the requirements for folic acid and iron during pregnancy are usually not met through diet alone, supplements of these two nutrients in particular are necessary.	6/26/12 Outcome met. Patient reports taking supplement as prescribed. No adverse effects noted. *Recommendation:* Will continue to monitor patient's tolerance of supplement.
Advise the patient that the iron content in the supplements may cause constipation and the stools to become black.	Common adverse effects of large iron doses are constipation and black stools.	Will continue to implement plan and reassess at next monthly appointment, 7/28/12. *L. Swift, RN*

SAMPLE DOCUMENTATION

5/22/12 Nursing

Mrs. Oakland was seen for routine prenatal checkup at 9-weeks' gestation. Assessment findings reveal that the patient is underweight, has lost 3 lb (1.4 kg) in the past 4 weeks, is experiencing nausea and vomiting, has a deficient hemoglobin and hematocrit, and is fatigued. Other contributing factors include weight consciousness, hurried schedule, and food dislikes. Discussion centered on maintaining good dietary habits, improving overall intake and meal patterns to meet the demands of pregnancy and subsequent lactation, initiating dietary changes aimed at avoiding nausea and vomiting, and increasing iron intake. See plan of care. Patient's progress will be evaluated at the next monthly visit, 6/26/12.

L. Swift, RN

Skill · 36-1 Inserting a Nasogastric (NG) Tube

The nasogastric (NG) tube is passed through the nose and into the stomach. This type of tube permits the patient to receive nutrition through a tube feeding using the stomach as a natural reservoir for food. Another purpose of an NG tube may be to decompress or to drain unwanted fluid and air from the stomach. This application would be used, for example, to allow the intestinal tract to rest and promote healing after bowel surgery. The NG tube can also be used to monitor bleeding in the gastrointestinal (GI) tract, to remove undesirable substances (lavage) such as poisons, or to help treat an intestinal obstruction. Refer to Chapter 38.

EQUIPMENT

- Nasogastric tube of appropriate size (8–18 French)
- Stethoscope
- Water-soluble lubricant
- Normal saline solution or sterile water, for irrigation, depending on facility policy
- Tongue blade

- Irrigations set, including a Toomey (20–50 mL)
- Flashlight
- Nonallergenic tape (1″ wide)
- Tissues
- Glass of water with straw
- Topical anesthetic (lidocaine spray or gel) (optional)
- Clamp

- Suction apparatus (if ordered)
- Bath towel or disposable pad
- Emesis basin
- Safety pin and rubber band
- Nonsterile disposable gloves
- Additional PPE, as indicated
- Tape measure, or other measuring device
- Skin barrier
- pH paper

IMPLEMENTATION

ACTION	RATIONALE
1. Verify the medical order for insertion of an NG tube.	Ensures the patient receives the correct treatment.
2. Perform hand hygiene and put on PPE, if indicated.	Hand hygiene and PPE prevent the spread of microorganisms. PPE is required based on transmission precautions.
3. Identify the patient.	Identifying the patient ensures the right patient receives the intervention and helps prevent errors.
4. Explain the procedure to the patient and provide the rationale as to why the tube is needed. Discuss the associated discomforts that may be experienced and possible interventions that may allay this discomfort. Answer any questions, as needed.	Explanation facilitates patient cooperation. Some patient surveys report that of all routine procedures, the insertion of an NG tube is considered the most painful. Lidocaine gel or sprays are possible options to decrease discomfort during NG tube insertion.
5. Gather equipment, including selection of the appropriate NG tube.	This provides for an organized approach to task. NG tubes should be radioopaque, contain clearly visible markings for measurement, and may have multiple ports for aspiration.
6. Close the patient's bedside curtain or door. Raise bed to a comfortable working position, usually elbow height of the caregiver (VISN 8, 2009). Assist the patient to high Fowler's position or elevate the head of the bed 45 degrees if the patient is unable to maintain upright position. Drape chest with bath towel or disposable pad. Have emesis basin and tissues handy.	Closing curtains or door provides for patient privacy. Having the bed at the proper height prevents back and muscle strain. Upright position is more natural for swallowing and protects against bronchial intubation aspiration, if the patient should vomit. Passage of tube may stimulate gagging and tearing of eyes.
7. **Measure the distance to insert tube by placing tip of tube at patient's nostril and extending to tip of earlobe and then to tip of xiphoid process (Figures 1 and 2).** Mark tube with an indelible marker.	Measurement ensures that tube will be long enough to enter patient's stomach.
8. Put on gloves. Lubricate tip of tube (at least 2″–4″) with water-soluble lubricant. Apply topical anesthetic to nostril and oropharynx, as appropriate.	Lubrication reduces friction and facilitates passage of the tube into stomach. Water-soluble lubricant will not cause pneumonia if tube accidentally enters the lungs. Topical anesthetics act as local anesthetics, reducing discomfort. Consult the physician for an order for a topical anesthetic such as lidocaine gel or spray if needed.
9. After selecting the appropriate nostril, ask patient to slightly flex head back against the pillow. Gently insert the tube into the nostril while directing the tube upward and backward along the floor of the nose (Figure 3). Patient may gag when tube reaches pharynx. Provide tissues for tearing or watering of eyes. Offer comfort and reassurance to the patient.	Following the normal contour of the nasal passage while inserting the tube reduces irritation and the likelihood of mucosal injury. The tube stimulates the gag reflex readily. Tears are a natural response as the tube passes into the nasopharynx. Many patients report that gagging and throat discomfort can be more painful than passing through the nostrils.

ACTION

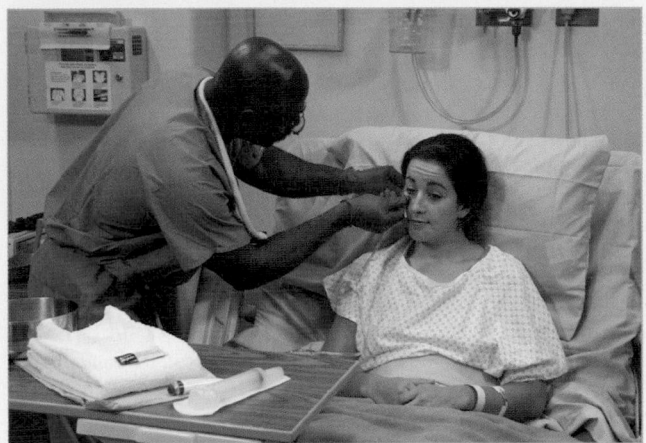

FIGURE 1. Measuring NG tube from nostril to tip of earlobe.

RATIONALE

FIGURE 2. Measuring NG tube from tip of earlobe to xiphoid process.

10. When pharynx is reached, instruct patient to touch chin to chest. Encourage patient to sip water through a straw or swallow even if no fluids are permitted. Advance tube in downward and backward direction when patient swallows (Figure 4). Stop when patient breathes. **If gagging and coughing persist, stop advancing the tube and check placement of tube with tongue blade and flashlight.** If tube is curled, straighten the tube and attempt to advance again. Keep advancing tube until pen marking is reached. **Do not use force. Rotate tube if it meets resistance.**

Bringing the head forward helps close the trachea and open the esophagus. Swallowing helps advance the tube, causes the epiglottis to cover the opening of the trachea, and helps to eliminate gagging and coughing. Excessive coughing and gagging may occur if the tube has curled in the back of throat. Forcing the tube may injure mucous membranes.

FIGURE 3. Beginning insertion with patient positioned with head up.

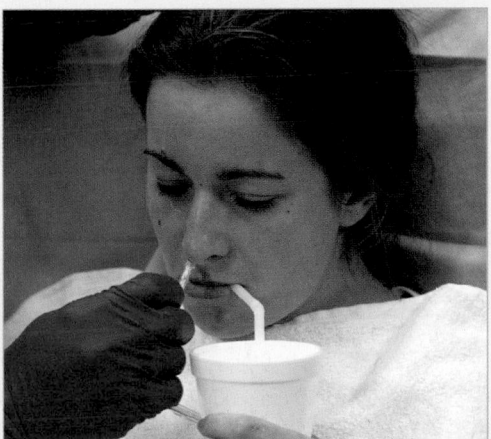

FIGURE 4. Advancing tube while patient drops chin to chest and swallows.

11. **Discontinue procedure and remove tube if there are signs of distress such as gasping, coughing, cyanosis, and inability to speak or hum.**

The tube is in the airway if the patient shows signs of distress and cannot speak or hum. If after three attempts, nasogastric insertion is unsuccessful, another nurse may try or the patient should be referred to another healthcare professional.

(continued)

Skill · 36-1   Inserting a Nasogastric (NG) Tube   *continued*

ACTION

12. Secure the tube loosely to the nose or cheek until it is determined that the tube is in the patient's stomach:

   a. Attach syringe to end of tube and aspirate a small amount of stomach contents.

   b. Measure the pH of aspirated fluid using pH paper or a meter. Place a drop of gastric secretions onto pH paper or place small amount in plastic cup and dip the pH paper into it. Within 30 seconds, compare the color on the paper with the chart supplied by the manufacturer (Figure 5).

   c. Visualize aspirated contents, checking for color and consistency.

   d. Obtain radiograph (x-ray) of placement of tube, based on facility policy (and ordered by physician).

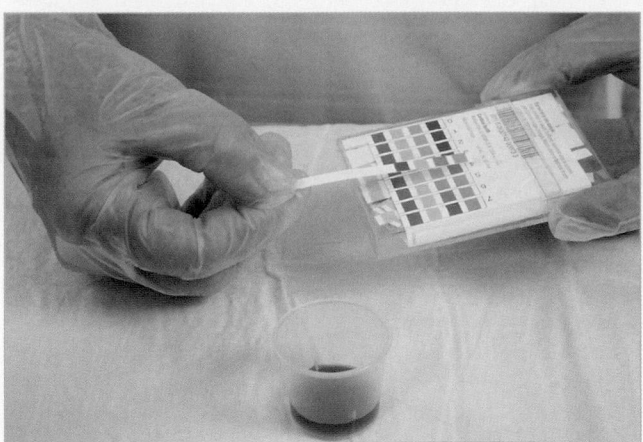

RATIONALE

Securing with tape stabilizes the tube while position is being determined.

The tube is in the stomach if its contents can be aspirated: pH of aspirate can then be tested to determine gastric placement. If unable to obtain specimen, reposition the patient and flush the tube with 30 mL of air. This action may be necessary several times. Current literature recommends that the nurse ensures proper placement of the NG tube by relying on multiple methods and not on one method alone.

Current research demonstrates that the use of pH is predictive of correct placement. The pH of gastric contents is acidic (less than 5.5). If patient is taking an acid-inhibiting agent, the range may be 4.0 to 6.0. The pH of intestinal fluid is 7.0 or higher. The pH of respiratory fluid is 6.0 or higher. This method will not effectively differentiate between intestinal fluid and pleural fluid.

Gastric fluid can be green with particles, off-white, or brown if old blood is present. Intestinal aspirate tends to look clear or straw-colored to a deep golden-yellow color. Also, intestinal aspirate may be greenish-brown if stained with bile. Respiratory or tracheobronchial fluid is usually off-white to tan and may be tinged with mucus. A small amount of blood-tinged fluid may be seen immediately after NG insertion.

The x-ray is considered the most reliable method for identifying the position of the NG tube.

FIGURE 5. Checking pH of gastric fluid.

13. Apply skin barrier to tip and end of nose and allow to dry. Remove gloves and secure tube with a commercially prepared device (follow manufacturer's directions) or tape to patient's nose. To secure with tape:

   a. Cut a 4″ piece of tape and split bottom 2″ or use packaged nose tape for NG tubes (Figure 6).

   b. Place unsplit end over bridge of patient's nose (Figure 7).

   c. Wrap split ends under tubing and up and over onto nose (Figure 8). **Be careful not to pull tube too tightly against nose.**

14. Put on gloves. Clamp tube and remove the syringe. Cap the tube or attach tube to suction according to the medical orders.

Skin barrier improves adhesion and protects skin. Constant pressure of the tube against the skin and mucous membranes may cause tissue injury. Securing tube prevents migration of the tube inward and outward.

Suction provides for decompression of stomach and drainage of gastric contents.

FIGURE 6. Making a 2″ cut into a 4″ strip of tape.

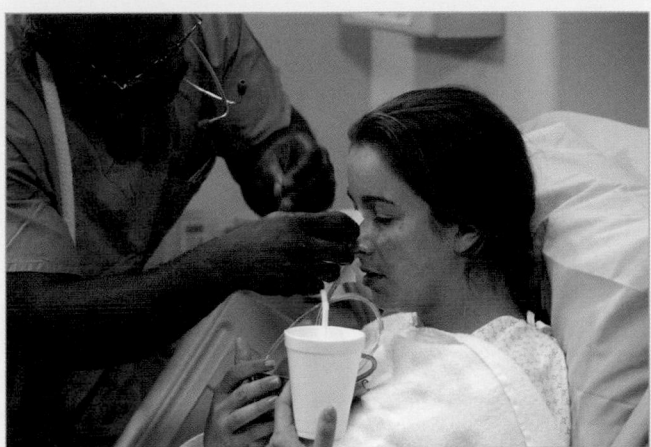

FIGURE 7. Applying tape to patient's nose.

FIGURE 8. Wrapping split ends around NG tube.

15. Measure length of exposed tube. Reinforce marking on tube at nostril with indelible ink. Ask the patient to turn their head to the side opposite the nostril the tube is inserted. Secure tube to patient's gown by using rubber band or tape and safety pin. For additional support, tube can be taped onto patient's cheek using a piece of tape. **If a double-lumen tube (e.g., Salem sump) is used, secure vent above stomach level.** Attach at shoulder level (Figure 9).

Tube length should be checked and compared with this initial measurement, in conjunction with pH measurement and visual assessment of aspirate. An increase in the length of the exposed tube may indicate dislodgement (Bourgault et al., 2007; Smeltzer et al., 2010). The tube should be marked with an indelible marker at the nostril. This marking should be assessed each time the tube is used to ensure the tube has not become displaced. Securing prevents tension and tugging on the tube. Turning the head ensures adequate slack in the tubing to prevent tension when the patient turns their head. Securing the double-lumen tube above stomach level prevents seepage of gastric contents and keeps the lumen clear for venting air.

16. Assist with or provide oral hygiene at 2- to 4-hour intervals. Lubricate the lips generously, clean nares, and lubricate, as needed. Offer analgesic throat lozenges or anesthetic spray for throat irritation if needed.

Oral hygiene keeps mouth clean and moist, promotes comfort, and reduces thirst.

17. Remove equipment and return patient to a position of comfort. Remove gloves. Raise side rail and lower bed.

Promotes patient comfort and safety. Removing gloves properly reduces the risk for infection transmission and contamination of other items.

(continued)

Skill · 36-1   Inserting a Nasogastric (NG) Tube   *continued*

ACTION	RATIONALE

FIGURE 9. Patient with Salem sump tube (NG) secured. Note blue vent at patient's shoulder.

18. Remove additional PPE, if used. Perform hand hygiene.	Removing PPE properly reduces the risk for infection transmission and contamination of other items. Hand hygiene prevents transmission of microorganisms.

DOCUMENTATION

Guidelines

Document the size and type of NG tube that was inserted and the measurement from tip of the nose to the end of the exposed tube. Also, document the results of the x-ray that was taken to confirm the position of the tube, if applicable. Record a description of the gastric contents, including the pH of the contents. Document the naris where the tube is placed and the patient's response to the procedure. Include assessment data, both subjective and objective, related to the abdomen. Record the patient teaching that was discussed.

Sample Documentation

> 10/4/12 0945 Abdomen slightly distended and taut; hypoactive bowel sounds. Patient reports transient nausea. 14-Fr Levin tube inserted via R naris, 20 cm of tube from naris to end of tube; gastric contents aspirated, pH 4, contents light green; patient tolerated without incident.
>
> —S. Essner, RN

UNEXPECTED SITUATIONS AND ASSOCIATED INTERVENTIONS

- *As a tube is passing through the pharynx, patient begins to retch and gag:* This is common during placement of an NG tube. Ask the patient if he/she wants the nurse to stop the procedure, allowing the patient to gain composure from the gagging episode. Continue to advance tube if the patient relates that he/she agrees. Have the emesis basin nearby in case patient begins to vomit.

- *The nurse is unable to pass the tube after trying a second time down the one nostril:* If the patient's condition permits, inspect the other nostril and attempt to pass the nasogastric tube down this nostril. If unable to pass down this nostril, consult another health professional.

- *As tube is passing through pharynx, patient begins to cough and shows signs of respiratory distress:* **Stop advancing the tube!** The tube is most likely entering the trachea. Pull tube back into nasal area. Support patient as he/she regains normal breathing ability and composure. If patient feels that he/she can tolerate another attempt, ask patient to keep chin on chest and swallow as tube is advanced to help prevent the tube from entering the trachea. Begin to advance tube, watching for any signs of respiratory distress.

- *No gastric contents can be aspirated:* If patient is comatose, check oral cavity. If tube is in gastric area, small air boluses may need to be given until gastric contents can be aspirated.

SPECIAL CONSIDERATIONS

General Considerations

To promote patient safety when administering a tube feeding, be sure to do the following:

- To promote patient safety, check tube placement before administering any fluids, medications, or feedings. Use multiple techniques: x-ray, external length marking/measurement, pH testing, and aspirate characteristics.
- Some patients require a nasointestinal tube. To insert a nasointestinal tube:
  - Measure tube from tip of nose to ear lobe and from ear lobe to xiphoid process. Add 8″ to 10″ for intestinal placement. Mark tubing at desired point.
  - Place patient on his or her right side. Nasointestinal tube is usually placed in the stomach and allowed to advance through peristalsis through the pyloric sphincter (may take up to 24 hours).
  - Administer medications to enhance GI motility, such as metoclopramide (Reglan), if ordered.
  - Test pH of aspirate when tube has advanced to marked point to confirm placement in intestine. Confirm position by radiograph. Secure with tape once placement is confirmed.
- Monitoring for carbon dioxide to determine nasogastric tube position and/or dislodgement has been investigated (May, 2007; Munera-Seeley et al., 2008). This involves the use of a capnograph or a colorimetric end-tidal CO_2 detector to detect the presence of carbon dioxide, which would indicate tube positioning in the patient's airway instead of the stomach.

Infant and Child Considerations

- Infants are obligate nose breathers; insertion of the tube via the mouth may be appropriate (orogastric tube) (Kyle, 2008).
- Age-specific equations are available to predict insertion distance and are the best method to determine insertion distance based on age and height for infants and children, 2 weeks to 19 years of age. Where age-specific prediction methods cannot be used, the next best choice is the nose or mouth to ear-mid-xiphoid-umbilicus span (Beckstrand, Cirgin Ellet, & McDaniel, 2007).

Skill · 36-2   Administering a Tube Feeding

EQUIPMENT

- Prescribed tube feeding formula at room temperature
- Feeding bag or prefilled tube feeding set
- Stethoscope
- Nonsterile gloves
- Additional PPE, as indicated
- Alcohol preps
- Disposable pad or towel
- Asepto or Toomey syringe
- Enteral feeding pump (if ordered)
- Rubber band
- Clamp (Hoffman or butterfly)
- IV pole
- Water for irrigation and hydration as needed
- pH paper
- Tape measure, or other measuring device

IMPLEMENTATION

ACTION	RATIONALE
1. Assemble equipment. Check amount, concentration, type, and frequency of tube feeding on patient's chart. Check expiration date of formula.	This provides for organized approach to task. Checking ensures that correct feeding will be administered. Outdated formula may be contaminated.
2. Perform hand hygiene and put on PPE, if indicated.	Hand hygiene and PPE prevent the spread of microorganisms. PPE is required based on transmission precautions.
3. Identify the patient.	Identifying the patient ensures the right patient receives the intervention and helps prevent errors.
4. Explain the procedure to the patient and why this intervention is needed. Answer any questions as needed.	Explanation facilitates patient cooperation.
5. Assemble equipment on overbed table within reach.	Organization facilitates performance of task.

(continued)

Skill · 36-4   **Obtaining a Capillary Blood Sample for Glucose Testing**   *continued*

ACTION	RATIONALE
8. Put on nonsterile gloves.	Gloves protect nurse from exposure to blood or body fluids.
9. Prepare lancet using aseptic technique.	Aseptic technique maintains sterility.
10. Remove test strip from the vial. **Recap container immediately.** Test strips also come individually wrapped. **Check that code number for the strip matches code number on monitor screen.**	Immediate recapping protects strips from exposure to humidity, light, and discoloration. Matching code numbers on the strip and glucose monitor ensures that the machine is calibrated correctly.
11. Insert strip into the meter according to directions for that specific device.	Correctly inserted strip allows meter to read blood glucose level accurately.
12. For adult, massage side of finger toward puncture site.	Massage encourages blood to flow to the area.
13. **Have patient wash hands with soap and warm water and dry thoroughly. Alternately, cleanse the skin with an alcohol swab. Allow skin to dry completely.**	Washing with soap and water or alcohol cleanses the puncture site. Warm water also helps to cause vasodilation. Alcohol can interfere with accuracy of results if not completely dried.
14. Hold lancet perpendicular to skin and pierce site with lancet (Figure 1).	Holding lancet in proper position facilitates proper skin penetration.
15. Wipe away first drop of blood with gauze square or cotton ball, if recommended by manufacturer of monitor.	Manufacturers recommend discarding the first drop of blood, which may be contaminated by serum or cleansing product, producing an inaccurate reading.
16. Encourage bleeding by lowering hand, making use of gravity. Lightly stroke the finger, if necessary, until sufficient amount of blood has formed to cover the sample area on the strip, based on monitor requirements (check instructions for monitor). Take care not to squeeze the finger, not to squeeze at puncture site, or not to touch puncture site or blood.	An appropriate-sized droplet facilitates accurate test results. Squeezing can cause injury to the patient and alter the test result (Ferguson, 2005).
17. Gently touch a drop of blood to pad to the test strip without smearing it (Figure 2).	Smearing blood on strip may result in inaccurate test results.

FIGURE 1. Piercing patient's finger with lancet.

FIGURE 2. Applying blood to test strip.

18. Press time button if directed by manufacturer.	Correct timing produces accurate results.
19. Apply pressure to puncture site with a cotton ball or dry gauze. **Do not use alcohol wipe.**	Pressure causes hemostasis. Alcohol stings and may prolong bleeding.
20. Read blood glucose results and document appropriately at bedside. Inform patient of test result.	Timing depends on type of meter.
21. Turn meter off, remove test strip and dispose of supplies appropriately. Place lancet in sharps container.	Proper disposal prevents exposure to blood and accidental needlestick.
22. Remove gloves and any other PPE, if used. Perform hand hygiene.	Removing PPE properly reduces the risk for infection transmission and contamination of other items. Hand hygiene reduces the transmission of microorganisms.

DOCUMENTATION

Guidelines

Document blood glucose level on a flow sheet in the medical record, according to facility policy. Document pertinent patient assessments, any intervention related to glucose level, and any patient teaching. Report abnormal results and/or significant assessments to primary healthcare provider.

Sample Documentation

> 11/1/12 0800 Patient performed own fingerstick blood glucose test with minimal guidance. Verbalized rationale for fasting measurement and able to state symptoms of hypoglycemia. Patient's fingerstick blood glucose level 168. 4 units regular Humulin insulin given per sliding scale, in addition to 10 units NPH Humulin insulin scheduled for 0800. Patient encouraged to review written guidelines for subcutaneous insulin administration; will review procedure and plan to have patient administer insulin at dinnertime. Patient verbalized an understanding.
>
> —B. Clapp, RN

UNEXPECTED SITUATIONS AND ASSOCIATED INTERVENTIONS

- *Extremity is pale and cool to the touch:* Begin by warming the extremity. Have adult patients warm their hands by rubbing them together. Warm moist compresses also may be used.

- *Blood glucose level results are above or below normal parameters:* Assess the patient for signs of hyperglycemia or hypoglycemia, respectively. Check medical record for ordered interventions, such as insulin dosage or carbohydrate administration. Notify healthcare provider of results and assessment.

SPECIAL CONSIDERATIONS

General Considerations

- Sampling of blood from an alternative site other than fingertips may have limitations. Blood in the fingertips show changes in glucose levels more quickly than blood in other parts of the body. This means that alternative site test results may be different from fingertip test results when glucose levels are changing rapidly (e.g., after a meal, taking insulin or during or after exercise) because the actual glucose concentration is different. Patients should be cautioned to use a fingertip sample if it is less than 2 hours after eating; less than 2 hours after injecting rapid-acting insulin; during exercise or within 2 hours of exercise; when sick or under stress; when having symptoms of hypoglycemia; if patient is unable to recognized symptoms of hypoglycemia; or if site results do not agree with the way the patient feels (Dale, 2006).

- Meters require calibration at least monthly or according to the manufacturer's recommendation, and when a new bottle of test strips is opened. Manufacturer's directions for calibration should be followed. After calibration, the meter is checked for accuracy by testing a control solution containing a known amount of glucose.

- Inadequate sampling can cause errors in the results. It is very important to be aware of requirements for specific monitor used.

- Monitors that measure glucose collected from the skin have recently become available. One of these devices use electrical stimulation to draw interstitial fluid through intact skin into a transdermal pad worn like a watch and provides a reading every 20 minutes. Another device is a monitor worn on a belt that uses a fine needle worn in the subcutaneous tissue to measure interstitial fluid glucose levels and transmit the results to a computer (Brown, 2008).

Infant and Child Considerations

- In infants and young children, use the heel to obtain the blood specimen. In an infant, use the outer aspect of the heel.
- If the heel is cool, place a warm compress on the foot.

Older Adult Considerations

- Meters are available with large digital readouts or audio components for patients with visual impairments.

Home Care Considerations

- Patients monitor blood glucose levels routinely at home.
- There are many different types of monitors available. Assist patients to identify desirable features for individual use.

● Developing Critical Thinking Skills

1. Prepare a diet for an economically disadvantaged family consisting of a single working mother and her three children, ages 3 to 14 years, taking into consideration the family's culture (specify a minority culture in your locale) and yearly income (below poverty level).

2. Prepare a 1-day menu that meets the recommended daily allowance of essential nutrients for the following patients:
   - An obese teenager
   - A child vegetarian
   - An executive with high blood pressure who dines out frequently with clients
   - A woman running a minimum of 12 miles daily as she trains for a marathon

● Practicing for NCLEX

1. When reviewing a patient's dietary intake, the nurse would identify which nutrient as providing the most concentrated source of energy in the body?
   a. Protein
   b. Carbohydrates
   c. Fat
   d. Macrominerals

2. Which of the following would the nurse need to keep in mind when teaching a patient about the current MyPyramid Food Guide?
   a. Meat and dairy products are located at the peak.
   b. All food groups are equally emphasized.
   c. Consumption of nutrient dense foods is promoted.
   d. The Pyramid focuses on deficiencies in our diet.

3. Which laboratory test result would the nurse interpret as indicating that a patient is at risk for poor nutritional status?
   a. Decreased serum albumin level
   b. Increased lymphocyte count
   c. Decreased blood urea nitrogen level
   d. Increased platelet count

4. Mr. Yow is refusing to eat. Which intervention would be most helpful in stimulating his appetite?
   a. Administering pain medication after meals
   b. Encouraging food from home when possible
   c. Scheduling his respiratory therapy before each meal
   d. Reinforcing the importance of his eating exactly what is delivered to him

5. Mrs. James has progressed to a full liquid diet. Which items would the nurse expect to see on the patient's meal tray?
   a. Apple juice and bouillon
   b. Water ice and ginger ale
   c. Puréed beef and cream of broccoli soup
   d. Custard and a glass of milk

6. When explaining parenteral nutrition, the nurse would describe this method as providing nutrients to the patient by way of which of the following?
   a. Gastrostomy tube
   b. Intravenous access
   c. Nasogastric tube
   d. Jejunostomy tube

7. The nurse completing anthropometric measurements for a patient collects which of the following information?
   a. Height and weight
   b. Serum hemoglobin and hematocrit levels
   c. Diet history
   d. Intake and output

8. When discussing a weight-reduction plan with Mrs. Young, the nurse would explain that 1 lb of body fat is equal to about how many calories?
   a. 1,500 cal
   b. 2,400 cal
   c. 3,500 cal
   d. 5,000 cal

9. Mr. White has been admitted to the alcoholic referral unit in the local hospital. Based on an understanding of the effects of alcohol on the GI tract, which of the following would the nurse be most alert for nutritionally?
   a. Vitamin B malnutrition
   b. Obesity
   c. Dehydration
   d. Vitamin C deficiency

10. A patient has a nasogastric tube inserted for feeding purposes. Using the stomach as a reservoir for food is advantageous in preventing what complication?
    a. Dumping syndrome
    b. Duodenal ulcers
    c. Hyperglycemia
    d. Gastric ulcers

11. Mrs. Lonte is ordered a clear liquid diet for breakfast, to advance to a house diet as tolerated. Which of the following assessments would indicate her diet should not be advanced?
    a. Mrs. Lonte consumed 75% of the liquids on her breakfast.
    b. Mrs. Lonte tells you she is hungry.
    c. Mrs. Lonte's abdomen is soft, nondistended, with bowel sounds.
    d. Mrs. Lonte reports fullness and diarrhea after breakfast.

12. Mr. Lang is receiving continuous tube feedings through a small-bore nasogastric tube. Which method is the most accurate in verifying correct tube placement?
    a. Auscultatory method
    b. Measurement of the gastric aspirate pH
    c. Measurement of the amount of residual
    d. Radiographic examination

13. Which of the following nursing diagnoses would probably be appropriate for a patient with a body mass index (BMI) of 39?
    a. Risk for Imbalanced Nutrition: More Than Body Requirements
    b. Imbalanced Nutrition: More Than Body Requirements
    c. Readiness for Enhanced Nutrition
    d. Imbalanced Nutrition: Less Than Body Requirements

14. A patient's history reveals gorging followed by purging with self-induced vomiting. The nurse interprets this as suggesting which disorder?
    a. Anorexia
    b. Morbid obesity
    c. Bulimia
    d. Cachexia

15. Which plant protein contains all the essential amino acids necessary to support growth?
    a. Grains
    b. Soy
    c. Vegetables
    d. Legumes

Answers With Rationale

1. *c.* Fat provides 9 cal for every gram compared with 4 cal/g each for protein (*a*) and carbohydrates (*b*). Macrominerals (*d*) are regulatory nutrients, not energy nutrients.

2. *c.* The broad bases at the bottom of the pyramid represent nutrient-dense foods that should make up the bulk of the diet. The focus of the MyPyramid Food Guide (*d*) is on wellness and prevention of nutritionally related diseases. Meats and dairy products are represented by the purple and blue bands (*a*), whereas the different band widths suggest the proportional contribution of each food group to a healthy diet (*b*).

3. *a.* A decreased serum albumin level may indicate protein malnutrition. The other test results do not represent a nutritional risk.

4. *b.* Food from home that the patient enjoys may stimulate him to eat. Pain medication (*a*) should be given before meals, respiratory therapy (*c*) should be scheduled after meals, and telling the patient what he must eat (*d*) is no guarantee that he will comply.

5. *d.* Custard and milk are items found in a full liquid diet. Apple juice and bouillon (*a*) and water ice and ginger ale (*b*) are clear liquids, and puréed beef and cream of broccoli soup (*c*) are more likely to be found in a soft diet.

6. *b.* Parenteral nutrition is given intravenously. Gastrostomy tube (*a*), nasointestinal route (*c*), and jejunostomy tube (*d*) are routes for enteral feedings.

7. *a.* Height and weight are the most common anthropometric measurements obtained. Intake and output measurements (*d*) indicate fluid balance, hemoglobin and hematocrit (*b*) are biochemical data, and a diet history (*c*) is used to complete dietary data.

8. *c.* One pound of body fat is equal to about 3,500 cal.

9. *a.* The need for B vitamins is increased in alcoholics because these nutrients are used to metabolize alcohol, thus depleting their supply. Alcohol abuse specifically affects the B vitamins. Obesity (*b*), dehydration (*c*), and vitamin C deficiency (*d*) may be present, but these are not directly related to the effect of alcohol on the GI tract.

10. *a.* When the stomach is used as a reservoir, the formula is released at a controlled rate, preventing the occurrence of the dumping syndrome. Duodenal (*b*) or gastric (*d*) ulcers are not commonly associated with enteral nutrition. Feeding solutions would not precipitate hyperglycemia (*c*) because they contain balanced amounts of nutrients.

11. *d.* Tolerance of diet can be assessed by the following: absence of nausea, vomiting, and diarrhea; absence of feelings of fullness; absence of abdominal pain and distention (*c*); feelings of hunger (*b*); and the ability to consume at least ½ to ¾ of the food on the meal tray (*a*).

12. *d.* Although a radiographic examination exposes the patient to radiation and is costly, it is still the most accurate method to check correct tube placement. Other methods that can be used are aspiration of gastric contents and measurement of the pH of the aspirate (*b*). The recommended method for checking placement, other than radiograph, is measuring the pH of the aspirate. Visual assessment of aspirated gastric contents is also suggested as a tool to check placement. In addition, the length of the exposed tube is measured after insertion and documented. Tube length should be checked and compared with this initial measurement, in conjunction with the previous two methods for checking tube placement. The auscultatory method (*a*) is considered inaccurate and unreliable. Measurement of residual amount (*c*) does not confirm placement.

13. *b.* A patient with a body mass index (BMI) of 39 is considered obese. She is not at risk for imbalanced nutrition (*a*) because it is already a problem and certainly is not experiencing nutrition that is less than body requirements (*d*). Readiness for Enhanced Nutrition (*c*) is appropriate when there is a healthy pattern of nutrient intake that is sufficient for meeting metabolic needs and can be strengthened and enhanced.

14. *c.* Bulimia is the only eating disorder mentioned that involves the cycle of gorging and purging. Anorexia (*a*) refers to a lack of appetite, whereas cachexia (*c*) reflects a state of malnutrition and wasting. Morbid obesity (*b*) indicates extreme obesity that interferes with normal activities.

15. **b.** Soy is considered a complete plant protein that contains all of the essential amino acids. Grains (*a*), vegetables (*c*), and legumes (*d*) are incomplete proteins.

Taylor Suite Resources

The Taylor Suite offers these additional resources to enhance learning and facilitate understanding of this chapter:

- thePoint online resource, http://thepoint.lww.com/Taylor7E
- Student DVD-ROM included with the book
- Study Guide for Taylor's Fundamentals of Nursing
- Skill Checklists for Taylor's Fundamentals of Nursing
- Taylor's Clinical Nursing Skills: *Chapter 11, Nutrition*
- Taylor's Video Guide to Clinical Nursing Skills: *Nutrition*

BIBLIOGRAPHY

American Association of Critical-Care Nurses (AACN). (2005). *Practice alert: Verification of feeding tube placement.* Available at www.aacn.org/WD/Practice/Content/practicealerts.pcms?menu=Practice.

American Dietetic Association. (2008). Position of the American Dietetic Association: Ethical and legal issues in nutrition, hydration, and feeding. *Journal of the American Dietetic Association, 108*(5), 873–882.

American Society on Aging. (2006). *Screening Tools and Surveys. Nutrition Screening Initiative.* Available www.asaging.org/cedc/module8/phase5/phase5_2a3.cfm. Accessed July 2, 2010.

Andrews, M., & Boyle, J. (2008). *Transcultural concepts in nursing care* (5th ed.). Philadelphia: Wolters Kluwer Health/Lippincott Williams & Wilkins.

Beckstrand, J., Cirgin Ellet, M., & McDaniel, A. (2007). Predicting internal distance to the stomach for positioning nasogastric and orogastric feeding tubes in children. *Journal of Advanced Nursing, 59*(3), 274–289.

Best, C. (2005). Caring for the patient with a nasogastric tube. *Nursing Standard, 20*(3), 59–65.

Best, C. (2007). Nasogastric tube insertion in adults who require enteral feeding. *Nursing Standard, 21*(40), 39–43.

Best, C. (2008). Enteral tube feeding and infection control: How safe is our practice? *British Journal of Nursing, 17*(16), 1036–1041.

Bourgault, A., Ipe, L., Weaver, J., Swartz, S., & O'Dea, P. J. (2007). Development of evidence-based guidelines and critical care nurses' knowledge of enteral feeding. *Critical Care Nurse, 27*(4), 17–29.

Brown, A.W. (2008). Clinician's guide to diabetes gadgets and gizmos. *Clinical Diabetes, 26*(2), 66–71.

Btaiche, I., & Khalidi, N. (2004a). Metabolic complications of parenteral nutrition in adults, part 1. *American Journal of Health-System Pharmacists, 61*(18), 1938–1949.

Btaiche, I., & Khalidi, N. (2004b). Metabolic complications of parenteral nutrition in adults, part 2. *American Journal of Health-System Pharmacists, 61*(19), 2050–2059.

Bulechek, G., Butcher, H., & McCloskey Dochterman, J. (Eds.). (2008). *Nursing interventions classification (NIC)* (5th ed.). St. Louis: Mosby Elsevier.

Carpenito-Moyet, L. (2008). *Nursing diagnosis: Application to clinical practice* (12th ed.). Philadelphia: Wolters Kluwer Health/Lippincott Williams & Wilkins.

Coxall, K., Dawes, E., Forsyth, E., et al. (2008). Applying the key principles of nutrition to nursing practice. *Nursing Standard, 22*(36), 44–48.

Dale, L. (2006). Make a point about alternate site blood glucose sampling. *Nursing, 36*(2), 52–53.

DiMaria-Ghalili, R., & Amella, E. (2005). Nutrition in older adults. *American Journal of Nursing, 105*(3), 40–51.

DiMaria-Ghalili, R., & Guenter, P. (2008). The mini nutritional assessment. *American Journal of Nursing, 108*(2), 50–59.

Dudek, S. (2006). *Nutrition essentials for nursing practice* (5th ed.). Philadelphia: Lippincott Williams & Wilkins.

Earley, T. (2005). Using pH testing to confirm nasogastric tube position. *Nursing Times, 101*(38), 26–28.

Edwards, S., & Metheny, N. (2000). Measurement of gastric residual volume: State of the science. *Medsurg Nursing, 9*(3), 125–128.

Ellet, M. (2004). What is known about methods of correctly placing gastric tubes in adults and children. *Gastroenterology Nursing, 27*(6), 253–261.

Fellows, L., Miller, E., Frederickson, M., Bly, B., & Felt, P. (2000). Evidence-based practice for enteral feedings: Aspiration prevention strategies, bedside detection, and practice change. *Medsurg Nursing, 9*(1), 27–31.

Ferguson, A. (2005). Blood glucose monitoring. *Nursing Times, 101*(38), 28–29.

Fischbach, F., & Dunning, M. (2006). *Common laboratory & diagnostic tests* (4th ed.). Philadelphia: Lippincott Williams & Wilkins.

Fischbach, F., & Dunning, M. (2009). *A manual of laboratory and diagnostic tests* (8th ed.). Philadelphia: Wolters Kluwer Health/Lippincott Williams & Wilkins.

Fluids & electrolytes. A 2-in-1 reference for nurses. (2006). Philadelphia: Lippincott Williams & Wilkins.

Fluids & electrolytes made incredibly easy. (2008). (4th ed.). Philadelphia: Wolters Kluwer Health/Lippincott Williams & Wilkins.

Guigoz, Y., Lauque, S., & Vellas, B. (2002). Identifying the elderly at risk for malnutrition: The mini nutritional assessment. *Clinics in Geriatric Medicine, 18*(4), 735–757.

Hadaway, L. (2005). Administering parenteral nutrition with other I.V. drugs. *Nursing, 35*(2), 26.

Hallpike, B. (2008). Promoting good nutrition in patients with dementia. *Nursing Standard, 22*(29), 37–43.

Hockenberry, M. (2005). *Wong's essentials of pediatric nursing* (7th ed.). St. Louis: Elsevier Mosby.

Holman, D., Roberts, S., & Nicol, M. (2005). Promoting adequate nutrition. *Nursing Older People, 17*(6), 31–32.

Holmes, S. (2006) Barriers to effective nutritional care for older adults. *Nursing Standard, 21*(3), 50–54.

Holmes, S. (2008). Nutrition and eating difficulties in hospitalised older adults. *Nursing Standard, 22*(26), 47–57.

Jarvis, C. (2008). *Physical examination & health assessment* (5th ed.). St. Louis: Saunders/Elsevier.

Jenkins, S., & Horner, S. (2005). Barriers that influence eating behaviors in adolescents, *Journal of Pediatric Nursing, 20*(4), 258–267.

Keithley, J.K., & Swanson, B. (2004). Clinical know-how: Nutrition Central Nutrition: An update on practice recommendations. *MEDSURG Nursing, 13*(2), 131–134.

Khair, J. (2005). Guidelines for testing the placing of nasogastric tubes. *Nursing Times, 101*(20), 26–27.

Kyle, T. (2008). *Essentials of Pediatric Nursing.* Philadelphia: Wolters Kluwer/Lippincott Williams & Wilkins.

Lichtenstein, A., & Russell, R. (2005). Essential nutrients: Food or supplements? Where should the emphasis be? *JAMA: Journal of the American Medical Association, 294*(3), 351–358.

May, S. (2007). Testing nasogastric tube positioning in the critically ill: Exploring the evidence. *British Journal of Nursing, 16*(7), 414–418.

McClave, S., Lukan, J., Stefater, J., Lowen, C. C., Looney, S. W., Matheson, P. J., et al. (2005). Poor validity of residual volumes as a marker for risk of aspiration in critically ill patients. *Critical Care Medicine, 33*(2), 324–330.

Metheny, N. (2002). Inadvertent intracranial nasogastric tube placement. *American Journal of Nursing, 102*(8), 25–27.

Metheny, N. (2007). Try this: Best practices in nursing care to older adults. The Hartford Institute for Geriatric Nursing. Preventing aspiration in older adults with dysphagia. Issue Number 20. Available at http://consultgerirn.org/uploads/File/trythis/issue_20.pdf.

Metheny, N. (2008). Residual volume measurement should be retained in enteral feeding protocols. *American Journal of Critical Care, 17*(1), 62–64.

Metheny, N., & Meert, K. (2004). Monitoring feeding tube placement. *Nutrition in Clinical Practice, 19*(5), 487–542.

Metheny, N., Schnelker, R., McGinnis, J., et al. (2005). Indicators of tubesite during feedings. *Journal of Neuroscience Nursing, 37*(6), 320–325.

Metheny, N., & Stewart, B. (2002). Testing feeding tube placement during continuous tube feedings. *Applied Nursing Research, 15*(4), 254–258.

Metheny, N., & Titler, M. (2001). Assessing placement of feeding tubes. *American Journal of Nursing, 101*(5), 36–45.

Miller, C. (2008). Communication difficulties in hospitalized older adults with dementia: Try these techniques to make communicating with patients easier and more effective. *American Journal of Nursing, 108(3),* 58–66.

Molle, E. (2005). Caring for older adults. Keep the upper GI tract from going downhill. *Nursing, 35*(10), 28–29.

Moorhead, S., Johnson, M., Maas, M., Swanson, E. (Eds). (2008). Nursing outcomes classification (NOC) (4th ed.). St. Louis: Mosby Elsevier.

Munera-Seeley, V., Ochoa, J., Brown, N., Bayless, A., Correia, M., Bryk, J., et al. (2008). Use of a colorimetric carbon dioxide sensor for nasoenteric feeding tube placement in critical care patients compared with clinical methods and radiography. *Nutrition in Clinical Practice, 23*(3), 318–321.

NANDA-I. (2009). *Nursing diagnoses: Definitions and classification 2009–2011.* West Sussex, UK: Wiley-Blackwell.

Nappo-Dattoma, L. (2005). 2005 USDA nutrition guidelines. *Access, 19*(8), 29–35.

National Institutes of Health (NIH). National Heart, Lung and Blood Institute. (2000a). NHLBI Obesity Education Initiative. *Aim for a healthy weight: Information for patients and the public.* Available at www.nhlbi.nih.gov/health/public/heart/obesity/lose_wt/patmats.htm. Accessed June 1, 2010.

National Institutes of Health (NIH). National Heart, Lung and Blood Institute. (2000b). NHLBI Obesity Education Initiative. *The practical guide: Identification, evaluation, and treatment of overweight and obesity in adults.* NIH publication no. 00-4084. October 2000. Available at www.nhlbi.nih.gov/guidelines/obesity/prctgd_c.pdf.

National Institutes of Health (NIH). National Heart, Lung and Blood Institute. (2005). *Aim for a healthy weight.* NIH publication no. 05-5213. Bethesda, MD: Author. Available www.nhlbi.nih.gov/health/public/heart/obesity/aim_hwt.htm.

National Institutes of Health (NIH). National Heart, Lung and Blood Institute. (2008). Diseases and conditions index: Overweight and obesity. Available at nhlbi.nih.gov/health/dci/Diseases/obe/obe_whatare.html.

National Institutes of Health. NIH State-of-the-Science Panel. NIH State-of-the-Science Conference Statement: Multivitamin/mineral supplements and chronic disease prevention. (2007). *Journal of Clinical Nutrition, 85*(1), Supplement: 257S–64S.

Padula, C. Kenny, A., Olandion, C., et al. (2004). External feedings: What the evidence says: Avoid contamination of feedings and its sequelae with this research-based protocol. *American Journal of Nursing, 104*(7), 62–28.

Palmer, J., & Metheny, N. (2008). Preventing aspiration during nasogastric, nasointestinal, or gastrostomy tube feedings. *American Journal of Nursing, 108*(2), 40–4, 47–9.

Phillips, M., & Nay, R. (2007). Nursing administration of medication via enteral tubes in adults: A systematic review. *International Journal of Evidence Based Healthcare, 5*(3), 324–353.

Porth, C., & Matfin, G. (2009). *Pathophysiology: Concepts of altered health states* (8th ed.). Philadelphia: Wolters Kluwer Health/Lippincott Williams & Wilkins.

Purnell, L., & Paulanka, B. (2005). *Guide to culturally competent health care.* Philadelphia: F. A. Davis Company.

Roberts, E. (2007). Nutritional support via enteral tube feeding in hospital patients. *British Journal of Nursing, 16*(17), 1058–1062.

Sanko, J. (2004). Aspiration assessment and prevention in critically ill enterally fed patients: Evidence-based recommendations for practice. *Gastroenterology Nursing, 27*(6), 279–285.

Sizer, F., & Whitney, E. (2006). *Nutrition: Concepts and controversies* (10th ed.). Belmont, CA: Thomson Wadsworth.

Smeltzer, S., Bare, D., Hinkle, J., & Cheever, K. (2010). *Brunner & Suddarth's textbook of medical-surgical nursing* (12th ed.). Philadelphia: Wolters Kluwer Health/Lippincott Williams & Wilkins.

Sudakin, T. (2006). Supporting nutrition with T.E.N. or T.P.N. *Nursing, 36*(32), 52–55.

Sweeney, J. (2005). Clinical queries: How do I verify NG tube placement? *Nursing, 35*(8), 25.

Tracey, D., & Patterson, G. (2006). Care of the gastrostomy tube in the home. *Home Healthcare Nurse, 24*(6), 381–386.

United States Department of Agriculture (USDA). (2008). MyPyramid.gov. Steps to a healthier you. Available at www.mypyramid.gov.

United States Department of Agriculture (USDA) & Department of Health and Human Services (DHHS). (2005). *Dietary guidelines for Americans 2005.* Available at www.health.gov/dietaryguidelines/dga2005/document/.

U.S. Food and Drug Administration (US FDA). (2006). *How to understand and use the nutrition facts label.* Available at www.cfsan.fda.gov/~acrobat/nutfacts.pdf.

VISN 8 Patient Safety Center. (2009). Safe patient handling and movement algorithms. Tampa, FL: Author. Available at http://www.visn8.va.gov/patientsafetycenter/safePtHandling. Accessed April 23, 2010.

Weight-control Information Network (WIN): National Institute of Diabetes and Digestive and Kidney Diseases (NDDK). (2007). Prevalence statistics related to overweight and obesity. Available at www.win.niddk.nih.gov/statistics/index.htm#preval.

Weight-control Information Network (WIN): National Institute of Diabetes and Digestive and Kidney Diseases (NDDK). (2008). Better health and you: Tips for adults. Why do people become overweight? Available at www.win.niddk.nih.gov/publications/better_health.htm.

Why assess for aspiration in patients with dysphagia? (2008). *American Journal of Nursing, 108*(2), 42–44.

Yen, P. (2005). Nutrition and well-being: Food and supplement safety. *Geriatric Nursing, 26*(5), 279–280.

37 Urinary Elimination

ELANA JASPERS

Elana Jaspers, age 83, has experienced decreased ability to perform ADLs related to arthritis, necessitating a move to an extended care facility. A short time after her arrival in her new home, Mrs. Jaspers began having difficulty with urinary incontinence.

ANNA GALINSKI

Anna, age 85, is frail and has numerous medical problems. She lives in a nursing home and like many of the residents was on a toileting regimen. Not long after a new charge nurse arrived, Anna and the other residents who used to be on toileting regimens had indwelling catheters inserted.

MIDORI MORITA

Midori, age 69, is taking care of her 70-year-old husband at home. She asks, "Should I talk with my husband's doctor about getting him a urinary catheter? Ever since he came back from the hospital this last time, he seems unable to use the urinal. He dribbles constantly and I can't keep up with the laundry. He had a catheter in the hospital."

LEARNING OBJECTIVES

After completing the chapter, you will be able to accomplish the following:

1. Describe the physiology of the urinary system.

2. Identify variables that influence urination.

3. Assess urinary elimination, using appropriate interview questions and physical assessment skills.

4. Perform the following assessment techniques: measure urine output, collect urine specimens, determine the presence of select abnormal urine constituents, determine urine specific gravity, and assist with diagnostic tests and procedures.

5. Develop nursing diagnoses that correctly identify urinary problems amenable to nursing therapy.

6. Demonstrate how to promote normal urination; facilitate use of the toilet, bedpan, urinal, and commode; perform catheterizations; and assist with urinary diversions.

7. Describe nursing interventions that can be used to manage urinary incontinence effectively.

8. Describe nursing interventions that can prevent the development of urinary tract infections.

9. Plan, implement, and evaluate nursing care related to selected nursing diagnoses associated with urinary problems.

KEY TERMS

autonomic bladder
bacteriuria
enuresis
external condom catheter
functional incontinence
hematuria
ileal conduit
indwelling urethral catheter
intermittent urethral catheter
Kegel exercises
micturition
mixed incontinence
nephrotoxic

nocturia
overflow incontinence
postvoid residual (PVR)
reflex incontinence
specific gravity
stress incontinence
suprapubic catheter
total incontinence
transient incontinence
urge incontinence
urinary diversion
urinary incontinence
urinary retention
urination
voiding

Elimination from the urinary tract helps to rid the body of waste products and materials that exceed bodily needs. This chapter describes the anatomy and physiology of the urinary system and factors that affect urination. A practical guide for assessing urinary elimination is included, along with detailed information on specific assessment measures, such as monitoring fluid intake, collecting urine specimens, testing urine, and assisting with other diagnostic procedures. Analysis of urinary assessment data may lead to the identification of one or more nursing diagnoses or to the early detection of a medical problem. When planning care, expected patient outcomes are established for which specific nursing strategies are presented. The concluding patient care study illustrates how the nurse's knowledge of the urinary system and urinary pathology forms the foundation for specific nursing interventions to resolve urinary problems.

Problems involving urinary elimination can be so embarrassing to patients that they may no longer participate in activities outside the home. Nurses assisting patients with urinary elimination problems or intervening to resolve health problems related to urination utilize many specialized skills. Refer to the Reflective Practice box.

ANATOMY AND PHYSIOLOGY
Kidneys and Ureters

The kidneys are located on either side of the vertebral column behind the peritoneum, in the upper abdominal cavity. One of the more significant functions of the kidneys is to help maintain the composition and volume of body fluids. About once every 30 minutes, the body's total blood volume passes through the kidneys for waste removal. The kidneys filter and excrete blood constituents that are not needed and retain those that are. Despite varying kinds and amounts of food and fluids ingested, body fluids remain relatively stable if the kidneys are functioning properly. Urine, the waste product excreted by the kidneys, contains organic, inorganic, and liquid wastes.

The nephron is the basic structural and functional unit of the kidneys. There are about 1 million nephrons in each kidney. Each nephron consists of a complicated system of arterioles, capillaries, and tubules. Nephrons remove the end products of metabolism, such as urea, creatinine, and uric acid from the blood plasma and form urine. The nephrons maintain and regulate fluid balance through the mechanisms of selective reabsorption and secretion of water, electrolytes, and other substances.

Once formed, urine from the nephrons empties into the pelvis of each kidney. From each kidney, urine is transported by rhythmic peristalsis through the ureters to the urinary bladder. The ureters enter the bladder obliquely. A fold of membrane in the bladder closes the entrance to the ureters so that urine is not forced up the ureters to the kidneys when pressure exists in the bladder. Figure 37-1 shows the male and female urinary systems and the position of the kidneys and ureters in the abdomen.

REFLECTIVE PRACTICE

Challenge to Ethical Skills

We had a strange experience during our rotation in a community nursing home. I was assigned to care for Anna Galinski, an 85-year-old frail woman with numerous medical problems. She, like many of the residents, was on a toileting regimen. In the middle of our 7-week experience, a new charge nurse started working on our unit. All of a sudden, Anna and the other residents who used to be on toileting regimens were given indwelling catheters. Knowing the greatly increased risk of infections with indwelling catheters, we suspected that the decision to rely on indwelling catheters was more a matter of convenience for the staff than what was in the best interests of the residents. The problem, how do you challenge a charge nurse?

Thinking Outside the Box: Possible Courses of Action

- Don't rock the boat! In 3 weeks, we'd be out of there. Keep our mouths shut and don't challenge authority.
- Ask for a meeting with the new charge nurse to explain our concerns, bringing our instructor for support. Be willing to go higher if the charge nurse cannot justify her decision and refuses to respond to our concerns.
- Work around the problem and try to get the residents' families to raise the issue.

Evaluating a Good Outcome: How Do I Define Success?

- Decisions are made about indwelling catheters that benefit and do not harm residents.
- I am faithful to my advocacy responsibilities within the current scope of my practice as a third-year student.
- I learn how to make the healthcare system work for patients/residents.
- I learn how to constructively challenge a physician or colleague.

Personal Learning: Here's to the Future!

This turned into a painful experience that made me realize just how difficult it can be to be an effective advocate for patients and residents. I am also newly aware of just how vulnerable nursing home residents are. A group of four students and myself asked to meet with the charge nurse. When we told her our concerns, she tried to justify her decision, but we still couldn't see any proof that the decision was made to benefit residents. Regrettably, she didn't respond to our concerns about infections at all. Because she was adamant about keeping the catheters, we told her that we would take the matter higher. Ulti- mately, we had to go all the way to the medical director, after thoroughly researching our concerns and getting lots of support for the argument we were making. In the process, the charge nurse made horrible accusations about us, threatening to ensure that students from our school would never work in this home again. Eventually, all was well that ended well. The charge nurse was "relieved of her administrative responsibilities" and our good names were restored. However, the process that we went through was difficult.

Reflection

How do you think you would respond in a similar situation? Why? What does this tell you about yourself and about the adequacy of your skills for professional practice? Can you think of other ways to respond? Did the nursing students act appropriately? Legally? Ethically? Why or why not? What issues or factors might have played a role in the charge nurse's response? The students' responses? Do you think that the charge nurse would have responded differently if the students had included their instructor in the meeting? What other skills (cognitive, interpersonal, technical, ethical/legal) would you need to respond well in this situation? Do you agree with the criteria to evaluate a successful outcome? Did the nursing student meet the criteria? Please explain your answer.

Bladder

The urinary bladder is a smooth muscle sac that serves as a temporary reservoir for urine. It is composed of three layers of muscle tissue: the inner longitudinal layer, the middle circular layer, and the outer longitudinal layer. These three layers are called the detrusor muscle. At the base of the bladder, the middle circular layer of muscle tissue forms the internal, or involuntary, sphincter, which guards the opening between the urinary bladder and the urethra. The urethra conveys urine from the bladder to the exterior of the body.

The urinary bladder muscle is innervated by the autonomic nervous system. The sympathetic system carries inhibitory impulses to the bladder and motor impulses to the internal sphincter. These impulses cause the detrusor muscle to relax and the internal sphincter to constrict, retaining urine in the bladder. The parasympathetic system carries motor impulses to the bladder and inhibitory impulses to the internal sphincter. These impulses cause the detrusor muscle to contract and the sphincter to relax. The urinary bladder is shown in Figure 37-2.

The bladder normally contains urine under very little pressure. As the volume of urine increases, the pressure increases only slightly. The bladder wall is able to adapt to this pressure because of the muscle tissue in the bladder. This makes it

FIGURE 37-1. Frontal view of the female urinary tract (*left*) and lateral view of the male urinary tract (*right*).

possible for urine to continue to enter the bladder from the ureters against low pressure. When the pressure becomes sufficient to stimulate nerves in the bladder wall (stretch receptors), the person feels a desire to empty the bladder.

Urethra

The urethra's function is to transport urine from the bladder to the exterior of the body. The anatomy of the urethra differs in males and females. The male urethra functions in the excretory system and the reproductive system. It is about 5 1/2″ to 6 1/4″ (13.7 to 16.2 cm) long and consists of three parts: the prostatic, the membranous, and the cavernous por-

tions (Fig. 37-3). The external urethral sphincter consists of striated muscle and is located just beyond the prostatic portion of the urethra. The external sphincter is under voluntary control.

In contrast, the female urethra is about 1 1/2″ to 2 1/2″ (3.7 to 6.2 cm) long. The external, or voluntary, sphincter is located in the middle of the urethra. No portion of the female urethra is external to the body, as in the male, although the muscle at the meatus is usually called the external sphincter.

Act of Urination

The process of emptying the bladder is known as **urination, micturition,** or **voiding.** The nerve centers for urination are situated in the brain and the spinal cord. Urinating, or voiding, is largely an involuntary reflex act, but its control can be learned.

Stretch receptors in the bladder are stimulated as the urine collects. The person feels a desire to void, usually when the bladder fills to about 150 to 250 mL in an adult.

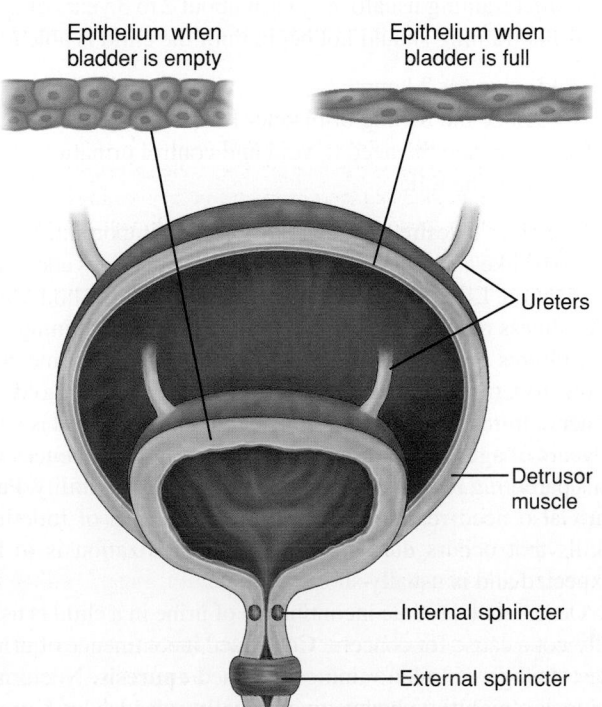

Epithelium when bladder is empty

Epithelium when bladder is full

- Ureters
- Detrusor muscle
- Internal sphincter
- External sphincter

FIGURE 37-2. The urinary bladder.

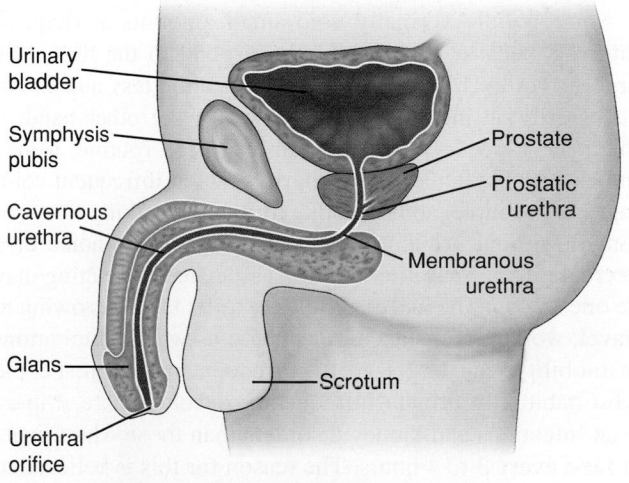

Urinary bladder
Symphysis pubis
Cavernous urethra
Glans
Urethral orifice
Prostate
Prostatic urethra
Membranous urethra
Scrotum

FIGURE 37-3. Parts of the male urethra.

The pressure within the bladder is many times greater during urination than it is during the time the bladder is filling. When urination is initiated, the detrusor muscle contracts, the internal sphincter relaxes, and urine enters the posterior urethra. The muscles of the perineum and the external sphincter relax, the muscle of the abdominal wall contracts slightly, the diaphragm lowers, and urination occurs.

The act of urination is normally painless. The voluntary control of voiding is limited to initiating, restraining, and interrupting the act.

Restraint of voiding is thought to occur subconsciously when the volume of urine in the bladder is small. If voiding is delayed, however, the bladder continues to fill. Discomfort may then be felt when undue distention occurs, and the urgency to void becomes paramount.

Sometimes increased abdominal pressure, such as occurs during coughing and sneezing, forces an involuntary escape of urine. This is a particular problem for some women because the urethra is shorter. Any involuntary loss of urine that causes such a problem is referred to as **urinary incontinence.** Strong psychological factors, such as marked fear, may also result in involuntary urination. Alternately in certain conditions, it may be difficult for a person to relax the restraining muscles sufficiently to void, such as when a shy or embarrassed person needs to give a urine specimen.

The voluntary control of urination develops as the higher nerve centers develop after infancy. Until that time, voiding is purely a reflex action. People whose bladders are no longer controlled by the brain because of injury or disease also void by reflex only. This is called **autonomic bladder.**

Frequency of Urination

The frequency of urination depends on the amount of urine being produced. The more urine produced, the more often voiding is necessary. Except when fluid intake is very large, most healthy people do not void during normal sleeping hours. The first voided urine of the day is usually more concentrated than other urine excreted during the day. Because the first urine of the day is not fresh, but rather an accumulation of a number of hours of kidney output, this urine may or may not be used as a specimen for certain tests.

Some people normally void small amounts at frequent intervals because they habitually respond to the first early urge to void. This habit usually is meaningless and is not necessarily an indication of disease. On the other hand, if this pattern occurs as a change in urination routine, it may indicate illness. Other people have habits of infrequent voiding. For example, some people go 8 to 12 waking hours or longer without urinating. A habitual low fluid intake or a decrease in the sensation of thirst associated with aging may be one reason. The inaccessibility of toilet facilities owing to travel, work circumstances, or illness, as well as limitations in mobility, can also lead to infrequent urination. People who habitually urinate infrequently develop more urinary tract infections and kidney disorders than those who urinate at least every 3 to 4 hours. The reason for this is believed to be stagnation of urine in the bladder, which serves as a good medium for bacterial growth. Newly occurring infrequent voiding can also indicate a decreased production of urine caused by a kidney or circulatory disorder. **Urinary retention** occurs when urine is produced normally but is not excreted completely from the bladder. Factors associated with urinary retention include medications, an enlarged prostate, or vaginal prolapse.

FACTORS AFFECTING URINATION

Numerous factors affect the amount and quality of urine produced by the body and the manner in which it is excreted.

Developmental Considerations

Infants are born without voluntary control of urination and with little ability to concentrate urine. An infant's urine is usually very light in color and without odor. At about 6 weeks of age, the infant's nephrons are able to control reabsorption of fluids in the tubules and effectively concentrate urine. As a child grows, the bladder gradually enlarges, with an increase in capacity. Most children develop urinary control between the ages of 2 and 5 years. Daytime control precedes nighttime control, and girls generally develop control earlier than boys. Older children and adults control urination voluntarily. They seldom wake to void at night because their kidneys are able to concentrate urine and produce less urine at night as a result of decreased renal blood flow.

Toilet Training

Voluntary control of the urethral sphincters occurs between 18 and 24 months of age. However, many other factors are required to achieve conscious control of bladder function, and toilet training usually begins at about 2 to 3 years of age.

Toilet training should not begin until the child is able to:

- Hold urine for 2 hours
- Recognize the feeling of bladder fullness
- Communicate the need to void and control urination until seated on the toilet

The child's desire to gain control is also important. Wanting to be like a parent or older sibling often provides adequate motivation. Lifelong attitudes toward urination, the body, and cleanliness may develop during the time of toilet training.

Cultures approach toilet training differently. In some cultures, toilet training begins before the child is 1 year old; in other cultures, it may not be considered until the child is near 5 years of age. Nurses must recognize cultural influences on this parenting responsibility while promoting flexibility. Parents also need reassurance that any regression of toileting skills that occurs during a child's hospitalization is to be expected and is usually short-lived.

Occasional daytime incontinence of urine in a child is usually not a cause for concern. Continued incontinence of urine past the age of toilet training is termed **enuresis.** Nocturnal enuresis (nighttime bedwetting) usually subsides by 6 years of age (Kyle, 2008).

Effects of Aging

Physiologic changes that accompany normal aging may affect urination in older adults. These changes include the following:

- The diminished ability of the kidneys to concentrate urine may result in **nocturia** (urination during the night).
- Decreased bladder muscle tone may reduce the capacity of the bladder to hold urine, resulting in increased frequency of urination.
- Decreased bladder contractility may lead to urine retention and stasis, which increase the likelihood of urinary tract infection.
- Neuromuscular problems, degenerative joint problems, alterations in thought processes, and weakness may interfere with voluntary control and the ability to reach a toilet in time.

Medications prescribed for other health problems may interfere with bladder function. Diuretics cause increased urine production, resulting in the need for increased urination and possibly urge incontinence. Sedatives and tranquilizers may diminish awareness of the need to void.

Individuals who view themselves as old, powerless, and neglected may cease to value voluntary control over urination and simply find toileting too much bother no matter what the setting. Incontinence may be the result.

> Consider Midori Morita, the wife of a 70-year-old man who has been experiencing urinary problems since his last hospitalization. The nurse would need to keep in mind these age-related changes during assessment to determine if Mrs. Morita's husband was experiencing urinary problems related to these changes or another cause. ■

Food and Fluid Intake

When the body is functioning well, the kidneys help the body maintain a careful balance of fluid intake and output, which should be about equal. When the body is dehydrated, the kidneys reabsorb fluid. The urine produced is more concentrated and is decreased in amount. Conversely, with fluid overload, the kidneys excrete a large quantity of dilute urine. Caffeine-containing beverages, such as cola, coffee, and tea, have a diuretic effect, increasing urine production. Alcohol produces the same effect by inhibiting the release of antidiuretic hormone. Foods high in water may increase urine production. Foods and beverages with high sodium content cause sodium and water reabsorption and retention, thereby decreasing urine formation. Certain foods may affect the odor of the urine (asparagus, onions) or its color (beets).

Psychological Variables

Many individual, family, and sociocultural variables influence a person's normal voiding habits. For some people, voiding is a personal and private act—something one does not talk about. Needing assistance with a bedpan or urinal provokes great embarrassment and anxiety, especially when the bedpan is offered by a nurse of the opposite gender. For others, voiding is a natural act that does not cause embarrassment, and these people readily excuse themselves to void whenever the urge presents.

Some people who experience stress void smaller amounts of urine at more frequent intervals. Stress can also interfere with the ability to relax the perineal muscles and the external urethral sphincter. When this happens, the person may feel an urge to void, but emptying the bladder completely becomes difficult or impossible.

Activity and Muscle Tone

Among the many benefits of regular exercise are increased metabolism and optimal urine production and elimination. During prolonged periods of immobility, decreased bladder and sphincter tone can result in poor urinary control and urinary stasis. People with indwelling urinary catheters lose bladder tone because the bladder muscle is not being stretched by the bladder filling with urine. Other causes of decreased muscle tone include childbearing, muscle atrophy due to decreased estrogen levels as seen with menopause, and damage to muscles from trauma.

Pathologic Conditions

Certain renal or urologic problems can affect both the quantity and the quality of urine produced. Diseases associated with renal problems include congenital urinary tract abnormalities, polycystic kidney disease, urinary tract infection, urinary calculi (kidney stones), hypertension, diabetes mellitus, gout, and certain connective tissue disorders. Renal failure is a condition in which the kidneys fail to remove metabolic end products from the blood and are unable to regulate fluid, electrolyte, and pH balance. Acute renal failure is a sudden decline in kidney function, and may be caused by conditions such as severe dehydration, anaphylactic shock, pyelonephritis, and ureteral obstruction. Chronic kidney disease is the end result of irreparable damage to the kidneys, developing slowly over many years. Chronic renal failure is caused by conditions such as diabetes, hypertension, and glomerulonephritis.

Diseases that reduce physical activity or lead to generalized weakness, such as arthritis, Parkinson's disease, and degenerative joint disease, may interfere with toileting. Cognitive deficits and certain psychiatric problems can interfere with a person's ability or desire to control urination voluntarily. Fever and diaphoresis (profuse perspiration) result in body fluid conservation by the kidneys. Urine production is decreased, and the urine is highly concentrated. Other pathologic conditions, such as congestive heart failure, may lead to fluid retention and decreased urine output. High blood glucose levels, such as with diabetes mellitus, may lead to an increase in urine output secondary to an osmotic diuretic effect.

Medications

Medications have numerous effects on urine production and elimination. Of gravest concern are the many prescription and nonprescription drugs known to be **nephrotoxic** (capable of causing kidney damage). Abuse of analgesics, such as aspirin or ibuprofen (Advil), can cause nephrotoxicity; some antibiotics, such as gentamicin, can be nephrotoxic.

Diuretics, which commonly are used in the treatment of hypertension and other disorders, prevent the reabsorption of water and certain electrolytes in the tubules. Depending on their strength, they cause moderate to severe increases in production and excretion of dilute urine. Cholinergic medications stimulate contraction of the detrusor muscle and produce urination. Some analgesics and tranquilizers suppress the central nervous system, interfering with urination by diminishing the effectiveness of the neural reflex.

Certain drugs cause urine to change color, including the following:

- Anticoagulants may cause **hematuria** (blood in the urine), leading to a pink or red color.
- Diuretics can lighten the color of urine to pale yellow.
- Phenazopyridine (Pyridium), a urinary tract analgesic, can cause orange or orange-red urine.
- The antidepressant amitriptyline (Elavil) or B-complex vitamins can turn urine green or blue-green.
- Levodopa (L-dopa), an antiparkinson drug, and injectable iron compounds can lead to brown or black urine.

THE NURSING PROCESS FOR URINARY ELIMINATION
Assessing

A comprehensive nursing assessment of the functioning of a patient's urinary system includes the following:

- Collection of data about the patient's voiding patterns, habits, and difficulties and a history of current or past urinary problems
- Physical examination of the bladder, if indicated, and urethral meatus; assessment of skin integrity and hydration; and examination of the urine
- Correlation of these findings with the results of diagnostic tests and procedures for examining the urine and the urinary tract

> *Recall Anna Galinski, the 85-year-old frail woman living in a nursing home. Initially, she was placed on a toileting regimen, but now she and other patients on the unit have indwelling catheters. In determining how to respond to the situation, it would be helpful for the nurse to perform a comprehensive assessment of the patient. Doing so would provide information to substantiate whether or not catheter insertion was indicated.* ■

Nursing History

In the initial nursing history, question the patient (or caregiver) about usual voiding habits and any current or past

> ### Box 37-1 ADDITIONAL TERMS USED TO DESCRIBE URINARY PROBLEMS
>
> **Anuria:** 24-hour urine output is less than 50 mL; synonyms are complete *kidney shutdown* or *renal failure*
> **Dysuria:** Painful or difficult urination
> **Frequency:** Increased incidence of voiding
> **Glycosuria:** Presence of sugar in the urine
> **Nocturia:** Awakening at night to urinate
> **Oliguria:** Scanty or greatly diminished amount of urine voided in a given time; 24-hour urine output is less than 400 mL
> **Polyuria:** Excessive output of urine (diuresis)
> **Proteinuria:** Protein in the urine; indication of kidney disease
> **Pyuria:** Pus in the urine; urine appears cloudy
> **Suppression:** Stoppage of urine production; normally the adult kidneys produce urine continuously at the rate of 60 to 120 mL/h
> **Urgency:** Strong desire to void
> **Urinary incontinence:** Involuntary loss of urine

voiding difficulties. Box 37-1 lists some additional terms that can be used to describe several urinary problems. When interacting with patients, use terminology that the patient and/or the caregiver understands. Focused Assessment Guide 37-1: Urinary Elimination lists elements of a urinary elimination history that should be incorporated into the initial nursing assessment.

With infants, assess the number of wet diapers per day that the infant produces. Newborns should have a minimum of six wet diapers per day (Kyle, 2008). With young children, assess whether the child has achieved bladder control during both day and nighttime. Be sure to indicate on the nursing history and care plan the words that the child uses to indicate the need to void.

With older adults, decreased bladder tone may be a problem. Note on the nursing history any problems, how the person normally handles these problems, and your judgment of the adequacy of the solution.

Patients with urinary diversions may have established individualized personal care routines. A **urinary diversion** involves the surgical creation of an alternate route for excretion of urine and is discussed later in the chapter. Assess the procedures and equipment used by patients to make sure they follow accepted guidelines and do not predispose themselves to infection or other risk. Record in both the history and the nursing plan of care any special routine, equipment, or supplies the patient uses for urinary elimination.

When a patient (or caregiver) reports a problem with voiding, explore its duration, severity, and precipitating factors. Also, note the patient's perception of the problem and the adequacy of the patient's self-care behaviors.

> *Remember Midori Morita, the wife of the 70-year-old man experiencing problems with "dribbling." The nurse*

FOCUSED ASSESSMENT GUIDE • 37-1

URINARY ELIMINATION

Factors to Assess	Questions and Approaches
Usual patterns of urinary elimination	How often do you urinate (pass your water) during the day? Do you awaken at night to empty your bladder? How would you describe your urine?
Recent changes in urinary elimination	Have you noticed any changes in your usual voiding patterns (frequency, amount, force of stream, difficulty, comfort)? Do you ever leak urine (e.g., on your way to the bathroom or when you sneeze or cough)? Do you ever notice that your undergarments are wet or damp?
Aids to elimination	Is there anything you do that helps you to urinate?
Present or past occurrence of voiding difficulties (nature of problem, onset, frequency, causes, severity, symptoms, intervention attempted, results)	Tell me about any problems you are having now when you urinate (urgency, pain or burning, difficulty starting or stopping stream, dribbling, incontinence). If there is a problem, describe what you feel like before you urinate and while you are urinating. Have you had any urinary problems in the past (any history of urinary tract infections, kidney or bladder disease or problems)? Do you use any type of absorbent pad or product to protect your clothes?
Presence of artificial orifices (normal routine, history of problems)	Tell me about your usual routine with your ileal conduit.

would need to question Mrs. Morita about the problem, obtaining specific information such as when it started, how often it occurs, how much the patient is voiding, events of the previous hospitalization, and any factors associated with it such as use of medications, increased fluid intake, or changes in mobility. ■

Physical Assessment

The physical assessment of urinary functioning includes an examination of the urinary bladder, if indicated, urethral meatus, skin, and urine. The kidneys are normally well protected by considerable fat and connective tissue, making palpation difficult. Palpation of the kidneys is usually performed as part of a more detailed assessment. This technique requires deep palpation and should be practiced only under the supervision by an advanced practitioner, such as an advanced practice nurse or physician.

BLADDER

Assessment of the bladder may be indicated when patients experience difficulty voiding or other alterations in elimination. The bladder is normally positioned below the symphysis pubis and cannot be palpated or percussed when empty. When the bladder is distended, it rises above the symphysis pubis and may reach to just below the umbilicus (Fig. 37-4). Before palpating the bladder, always ask the patient when he or she voided last. Observe the lower abdominal wall, noting any swelling, and palpate this area for tenderness. Note the smoothness and roundness of the bladder. Measure the height of the edge of the bladder above the symphysis pubis.

A bedside scanner is another way to assess the bladder. These portable bladder ultrasound devices create an image of the patient's bladder and calculate urine volume present in the bladder. This method is noninvasive and painless. A bladder scan can be performed at the bedside, poses no risk for infection, and is a safer alternative to catheterization to determine bladder urine volume. Results are most accurate when the patient is in the supine position during the scanning. Skill 37-1 outlines the procedure for assessing bladder volume using an ultrasound bladder scanner.

URETHRAL ORIFICE

Inspect the urethral orifice for any signs of inflammation, discharge, or foul odor. In females, the urethral meatus is a slit-like opening below the clitoris and above the vaginal orifice. Place female patients in the dorsal recumbent position with the inner labia retracted for good visualization of the meatus. In males, the meatus is at the tip of the penis. If the

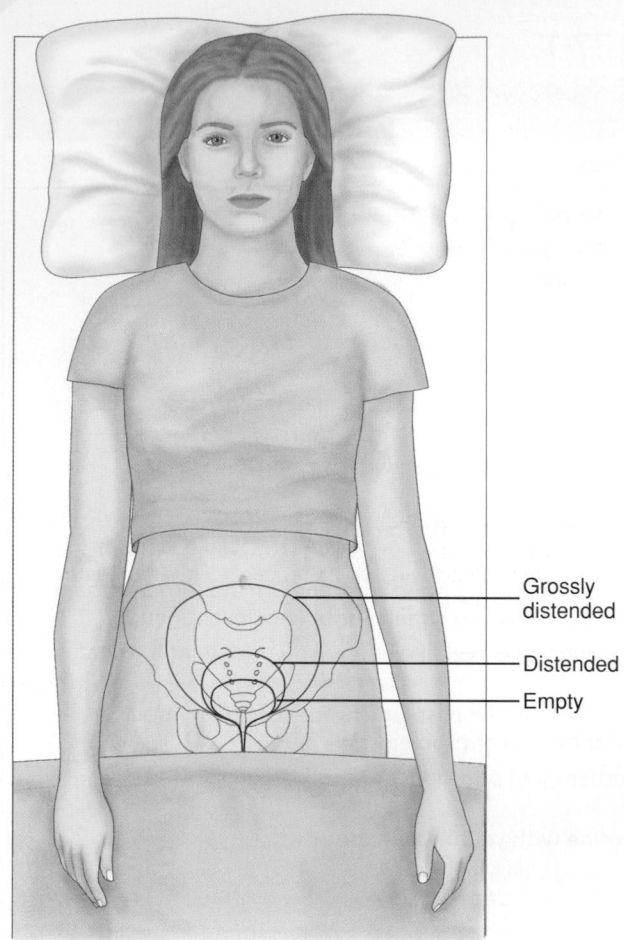

- Grossly distended
- Distended
- Empty

FIGURE 37-4. Position of bladder when empty and distended.

male patient is uncircumcised, retract the foreskin to visualize the meatus.

SKIN INTEGRITY AND HYDRATION

Because problems with urinary functioning may result in disturbances in hydration and excretion of body wastes, assess the skin carefully for color, texture, and turgor. Assess the integrity of the skin in the perineal area. Problems with incontinence may result in severe excoriation (abrasion of the epidermis).

> *Inspecting the perineal area would be extremely important when assessing Mrs. Jaspars. Her problems with urinary incontinence places the patient at risk for changes in skin integrity.* ■

URINE

Assess the patient's urine for color, odor, clarity, and the presence of any sediment. Note any abnormalities. In select patients, monitor the pH and specific gravity of the urine and check the urine for abnormal constituents such as protein, blood, glucose, ketone bodies, and bacteria (see the section, Point of Care Urine Testing). The normal characteristics of urine are detailed in Table 37-1.

Special Assessment Techniques

In addition to the nursing history and physical examination, the nurse gathers data about urinary elimination through the following assessment measures: measuring urine output, collecting urine specimens, performing point of care urine testing, and assisting with diagnostic procedures. These are discussed in the following sections.

MEASURING URINE OUTPUT

Measuring the patient's fluid intake and output is an important nursing responsibility. Accuracy of the total fluid intake and output from all sources aids in identifying potential alterations in fluid balance and is essential for planning the patient's nursing and medical care. The measurement of fluid intake and output is described further in Chapter 40. Gloves are required when handling urine to prevent exposure to pathogenic microorganisms or blood that may be present in the urine. Goggles also are worn whenever there is a concern of urine splashing. The measurement of fluid intake and output may be delegated to unlicensed personnel. However, the nurse is responsible for ensuring that staff members understand the required procedures and the nurse must validate the accuracy of the measurements.

Measuring Urine Output in Patients Who Are Continent

Patients who have self-control over urination are continent. The procedure for measuring the urine output of a patient who is continent and voiding is as follows:

1. Ask the patient to void into a bedpan, urinal, or specimen hat, either in bed or in the bathroom. Urinary devices used to collect or measure urine are shown in Figure 37-5.
2. Pour the urine from the collection device into the appropriate measuring device provided by the agency. The devices are calibrated in milliliters. Collection devices may be calibrated for measurement, eliminating the need for an additional measuring device.
3. Place the calibrated container on a flat surface, such as a shelf, for an accurate reading. Reading at eye level, note the amount of urine voided and record it on the appropriate form. Figure 37-6 shows a paper form used for recording urine output. The form is usually kept at the patient's bedside. Alternately, the information may be recorded in the patient's electronic record. Record the total amount voided during each shift and 24-hour period on the patient's permanent record.
4. Discard the urine in the toilet unless a specimen is required. If a specimen is required, pour the urine into an appropriate specimen container.

To ensure that all voided urine is measured, be sure to tell ambulatory patients when their urine output is to be measured and recorded. A specimen hat is a valuable device that can be placed under the toilet seat to collect and measure voided urine for ambulatory patients (see Fig. 37-5). Patients

TABLE 37-1	CHARACTERISTICS OF URINE	
Characteristic	Normal Findings	Special Considerations
Color	A freshly voided specimen is pale yellow, straw-colored, or amber, depending on its concentration.	Urine is darker than normal when it is scanty and concentrated. Urine is lighter than normal when it is excessive and diluted. Certain drugs, such as cascara, L-dopa, and sulfonamides, alter the color of urine. Some foods can alter the color; for example, beets can cause urine to appear red.
Odor	Normal urine smell is aromatic. As urine stands, it often develops an ammonia odor because of bacterial action.	Some foods cause urine to have a characteristic odor; for example, asparagus causes urine to have a strong, musty odor. Urine high in glucose content has a sweet odor. Urine that is heavily infected has a fetid odor.
Turbidity	Fresh urine should be clear or translucent; as urine stands and cools, it becomes cloudy.	Cloudiness observed in freshly voided urine is abnormal and may be due to the presence of red blood cells, white blood cells, bacteria, vaginal discharge, sperm, or prostatic fluid.
pH	The normal pH is about 6.0, with a range of 4.6 to 8. (Urine alkalinity or acidity may be promoted through diet to inhibit bacterial growth or urinary stone development or to facilitate the therapeutic activity of certain medications.) Urine becomes alkaline on standing when carbon dioxide diffuses into the air.	A high-protein diet causes urine to become excessively acidic. Certain foods tend to produce alkaline urine, such as citrus fruits, dairy products, and vegetables, especially legumes. Certain foods such as meats tend to produce acidic urine. Certain drugs influence the acidity or alkalinity of urine; for example, ammonium chloride produces acidic urine, and potassium citrate and sodium bicarbonate produce alkaline urine.
Specific gravity	This is a measure of the concentration of dissolved solids in the urine. The normal range is 1.015 to 1.025.	Concentrated urine will have a higher than normal specific gravity, and diluted urine will have a lower than normal specific gravity. In the absence of kidney disease, a high specific gravity usually indicates dehydration and a low specific gravity indicates overhydration.
Constituents	*Organic* constituents of urine include urea, uric acid, creatinine, hippuric acid, indican, urene pigments, and undetermined nitrogen. *Inorganic* constituents are ammonia, sodium, chloride, traces of iron, phosphorus, sulfur, potassium, and calcium.	*Abnormal constituents* of urine include blood, pus, albumin, glucose, ketone bodies, casts, gross bacteria, and bile.

who are willing and able can be taught to measure and record their own output.

Measuring Urine Output in Patients Who Are Incontinent

Urinary incontinence is the involuntary or uncontrolled loss of urine from the bladder. It is difficult to accurately measure urinary output for incontinent patients. The nurse should note the number of times the patient is incontinent and any urine characteristics that may be noted, such as color and odor. Additional nursing interventions are required to collect urine for measurement. Use of scheduled toileting (assisting the patient to the toilet to attempt to void on a regular basis, such as every 2 hours) can assist in obtaining urine for measurement, for required laboratory specimens,

and prevent incontinence. Urinary incontinence is discussed in more detail later in the chapter.

Measuring Urine Output in Patients With an Indwelling Catheter

For patients with an indwelling catheter, the procedure for measuring urine output is as follows:

1. Put on clean gloves.
2. Place a calibrated measuring device beneath the urine collection bag at the bedside. To prevent the spread of infection, each patient should have his or her own calibrated measuring device.
3. Place the drainage spout from the collection bag above, but not touching, the calibrated measuring device, and open the clamp.

Bedpan and fracture pan: containers used to collect urine from
nonambulatory patients.
Urinal container used to collect urine from nonambulatory male
patients.

Large urine collection bag with urimeter for use with
patients who have indwelling urinary catheters and require
frequent urine output measurements, such as hourly.
Small urine collection bag, commonly called a leg bag, for
use by ambulatory patients who have an indwelling
urinary catheter.
Large urine collection bag.

Specimen hat: container that is placed anteriorly on the toilet,
underneath the seat. Used to collect urine.
Specimen cup: container that holds urine.
Calibrated measuring device: makes possible the recording of an
accurate urine output.

FIGURE 37-5. Devices for collecting and measuring urine.

4. Allow the urine to flow from the collection bag into
   the measuring device.
5. Reclamp the drainage tube, wipe the spout of the
   tube with an alcohol pad, and replace the tube into
   the slot on the drainage bag. Proceed with measurement of urine as described above.

Catheterized patients who are acutely ill may require
hourly measurements of urine. This is facilitated by using a
special collection bag that has a built-in calibrated measuring chamber called an urimeter (see Fig. 37-5). After assessing and recording the amount of urine produced hourly, tilt
the measuring chamber so that this urine flows into the general collection bag. This empties the measuring chamber,
making it ready to collect the next hour's urine.

COLLECTING URINE SPECIMENS

Nurses use different techniques for collecting urine specimens. The nurse needs to understand the rationale for the
specific test ordered, as well as the correct collection procedure associated with the required test in order to ensure
obtaining the appropriate urine sample.

Routine Urinalysis

A sterile urine specimen is not required for a routine urinalysis. Collect urine by having the patient void into a clean
bedpan, urinal, or receptacle (e.g., a specimen hat in the toilet bowl). Care is taken to avoid contamination with feces. If
a woman is menstruating when a urine sample is obtained,
note this on the laboratory slip because red blood cells may
appear in the urine. When patients are voiding into a bedpan
or collection device on the toilet, instruct them not to place
toilet tissue into the urine because this makes analysis more
difficult. Using aseptic technique, pour the urine into an
appropriate container; label it with the patient's name, date,
and time of collection; package it appropriately; and send it
to the laboratory for examination. Do not leave urine standing at room temperature for a long period before sending it
to the laboratory because this may alter both the appearance
and chemistry of the urine.

Clean-Catch or Midstream Specimen

A clean-catch specimen of urine is required in some situations. Most healthcare agencies specify that a clean-catch

Intake and Output Chart

7:00 AM _11-18-12_ to 7:00 AM _11-19-12_

	Oral	I.V.	Blood	Other	Comments	Urine	Stool	Gastric tube	Drainage tubes		Vomitus	Other	Comments
7-8	250				Force fluids to 1100cc/shift	300							
8-9													
9-10	120												
10-11	60												
11-12	100					250							
12-1	300												
1-2	240												
2-3	100					200							
8 hr Tot	1170					750							voiding ē discomfort
3-4													
4-5													
5-6													
6-7													
7-8													
8-9													
9-10													
10-11													
8 hr Tot													
11-12													
12-1													
1-2													
2-3													
3-4													
4-5													
5-6													
6-7													
8 hr Tot													
24 hr Tot													
Total intake					**Total output**								

FIGURE 37-6. An example of a paper form used for recording intake and output.

specimen be collected during midstream. This means that the patient voids and discards a small amount of urine; continues voiding in a sterile specimen container to collect the urine; stops voiding into container; removes container and continues voiding; then discards the last amount of urine in the bladder. The first small amount of urine voided helps to flush away any organisms near the meatus because the findings may be inaccurate if these organisms enter the specimen. Additionally, it is generally thought that urine voided at midstream is most characteristic of the urine the body is producing.

A patient who can carry out the technique properly may collect his or her own clean-catch midstream urine specimen and often prefers to do so. The nurse provides the appropriate equipment and instructions for the procedure. Refer to Guidelines for Nursing Care 37-1: Obtaining a Clean-Catch or Midstream Urine Specimen.

Sterile Specimen

Sterile urine specimens may be obtained by catheterizing the patient's bladder (Refer to Catheterizing Patient's Bladder and Guidelines 37-2 later in the chapter), or by taking the specimen from an indwelling catheter already in place.

When it is necessary to collect a urine specimen from a patient with an indwelling catheter, always obtain it from the catheter itself using the special port for specimens. A specimen from the collecting receptacle (drainage bag) may not be fresh urine and could result in an inaccurate analysis. Always observe sterile technique while collecting a urine specimen from an indwelling catheter. Gather equipment, including a syringe, an antiseptic swab, a sterile specimen container, nonsterile gloves, and possibly a clamp. The size of the syringe for the specimen depends on the specific laboratory test. A urine culture requires about 3 mL, whereas routine urinalysis requires at least 10 mL of urine. Also, check the catheter to determine if an access port for specimen removal is present. Wearing gloves protects the nurse from any contact with the specimen.

If urine is not present in the tube, clamp the tube below the access port briefly (not to exceed 30 minutes) to allow urine to accumulate. Clean the access port with the antiseptic swab, and carefully attach the syringe to the port (Fig. 37-7).

Guidelines for Nursing Care • 37-1

OBTAINING A CLEAN-CATCH OR MIDSTREAM URINE SPECIMEN

Female

- Perform hand hygiene.
- Wear clean gloves.
- Separate the labia. Clean the area at the meatus with soap and water, or according to policy.
- Have the patient void about 30 mL into the toilet or bedpan and discard this urine.
- Position the sterile specimen container near, but not touching, the meatus, and collect at least 10 mL of urine in the container. If the specimen is being collected while the patient is lying down, ask her to void forcibly to prevent urine from dribbling across the perineum.
- Stop collecting urine before the patient empties the bladder. Allow patient to continue voiding into a bedpan or the commode and discard this urine.
- Remove gloves and perform hand hygiene.
- Label the specimen container, package it appropriately, and send the specimen to the laboratory.

Male

- Perform hand hygiene.
- Wear clean gloves.
- Retract the foreskin to expose the glans penis in the uncircumcised male patient.
- Clean the area of the external meatus with soap and water.
- Have the patient void about 30 mL into the toilet or urinal and discard this urine.
- Have the patient void directly into the sterile container and collect at least 10 mL of urine in the container.
- Stop collecting urine before the patient empties his bladder. Allow the patient to void the remaining urine into the toilet or urinal and discard it.
- Return the foreskin to its normal position in an uncircumcised patient to prevent swelling and irritation of the glans penis.
- Remove gloves and perform hand hygiene.
- Label the specimen container appropriately and send the specimen to the laboratory.

Aspirate urine into the syringe, remove the syringe, release the clamp if one was used, and transfer the specimen to the appropriate container. Place the syringe in the sharps container. Then package and transport the specimen according to facility policy.

24-Hour Urine Specimens

For some laboratory studies, 24-hour specimen collection is required. The patient and the entire nursing team must understand the importance of collecting all the urine voided in a 24-hour period. Post a sign on the patient's bathroom door as a helpful reminder not to discard urine. Initiate a collection at a specific time (which is recorded) by asking the patient to empty his or her bladder. Discard this urine and then collect all urine voided for the next 24 hours. At the end of the 24 hours, ask the patient to void. Add this urine to the previously collected urine, and then send the entire specimen to the laboratory.

Depending on the type of examination, the urine from each voiding may be kept in a separately marked container and the time of each voiding recorded, or all urine voided may be collected in a common receptacle. The laboratory usually specifies whether a preservative is used to retard decomposition and whether the specimen is to be refrigerated or kept on ice.

FIGURE 37-7. Obtaining a urine specimen from an indwelling urinary catheter. (**A**) Use an antiseptic swab to clean the access port. (**B**) Attach syringe and aspirate urine into the syringe. *(Photos by B. Proud.)*

FIGURE 37-8. Disposable urine collection device for infants and young children.

In some situations, the patient may be required to collect the specimen at home. Many laboratories have a transport service that picks up specimens from a patient's home and returns them to the laboratory within the appropriate time frame.

Specimens From Infants and Children

Plastic disposable collection bags are available for collecting urine specimens from infants and young children who have not achieved voluntary bladder control (Fig. 37-8). Follow the manufacturer's instructions and take care when applying and removing the bag to avoid irritating the sensitive perineal skin.

POINT OF CARE URINE TESTING

In some situations, the nurse may perform tests to detect abnormal constituents in urine specimens at the bedside or in the office setting. This is especially true when urine specimens are being tested repeatedly for known abnormalities, when screening tests are being used, or when laboratory facilities are not readily available. For example, a nurse may test urine for the presence of glucose, protein, bilirubin, bacteria, and blood. The results of the test are recorded on the patient's record. Many commercially prepared diagnostic kits are available for such tests and can be used in the home or the healthcare facility. Although these tests are economical and fast, laboratory analysis is recommended when precise results are needed.

Most commercially prepared diagnostic kits contain all needed equipment and the appropriate reagent (a substance used in a chemical reaction to detect another substance). Reagents are available as tablets, fluids, impregnated paper, and plastic strips with a special coating. When the urine comes in contact with the reagent, a chemical reaction occurs, causing a color change. This color is then compared with an accompanying chart that describes the significance of the color.

The precise directions for the amount of the specimen, the time allowed for the chemical reaction, and the interpretation of the color vary with the manufacturer. Therefore, always follow the directions accompanying the diagnostic kit exactly.

The nurse may also determine the **specific gravity** of urine, which is a measure of the density of urine compared with the density of water (see Table 37-1). The higher the number, the more concentrated the urine is, unless there are abnormal components, such as glucose or protein, in the urine. Specific gravity can be determined with manufactured plastic reagent strips, as described above.

ASSISTING WITH DIAGNOSTIC PROCEDURES

Nurses also assist with diagnostic procedures. Various diagnostic procedures, typically performed in a hospital operating room or outpatient facility, are used to study the urinary system. Common diagnostic procedures related to the urinary system include urodynamic studies, cystoscopy, intravenous pyelogram, retrograde pyelogram, computed tomography (CT) scans, renal biopsy, and ultrasound examination. Nurses are responsible for preparing the patient for the procedure and giving appropriate aftercare. Explaining the procedure helps reduce the patient's anxieties. The preparation and aftercare of the patient for each of these procedures are described in Box 37-2.

Diagnosing

The data collected about the patient's urinary functioning may lead to one or more nursing diagnoses. Some data are appropriately reported to the primary care provider and may contribute to the identification of a medical diagnosis.

Urinary Functioning as the Problem

Nursing diagnoses that specifically address problems in urinary functioning include problems of incontinence, pattern alteration, and urinary retention. Sample defining characteristics for these diagnoses appear in the box Examples of NANDA Nursing Diagnoses: Urinary Elimination.

Urinary Functioning as the Etiology

Difficulty with urination or changes in normal voiding patterns may affect other areas of human functioning. Examples of nursing diagnoses related to urinary problems include the following:

- Anxiety related to incontinence, diagnostic procedures
- Caregiver Role Strain related to incontinence of family member
- Risk for Infection related to indwelling urinary catheter
- Impaired Skin Integrity (Actual, Risk for) related to incontinence
- Deficient Knowledge related to any existing or new urinary disease or disorder, lack of information about personal hygiene
- Noncompliance With Medication Regimen related to misunderstanding of the need to finish all doses of medication for urinary tract infection
- Acute Pain related to bladder spasms, dysuria, urinary retention, cancer of the bladder, diagnostic procedures

Box 37-2 COMMON DIAGNOSTIC PROCEDURES USED TO STUDY THE URINARY TRACT

Urodynamic Studies

Urodynamic studies are a group of tests that measure how urine flows, is stored, and is eliminated in the lower urinary tract. They are used to identify abnormal voiding patterns in persons with incontinence or the inability to void normally.

Preparation
- Usually no fluid or food restrictions are necessary before the test.
- Bladder should be full before the test.
- Inform the patient that a catheter will be inserted during the test.

Aftercare
- Teach the patient to drink 8 to 10 glasses of water in the 24 hours after the test.
- Teach the patient the signs and symptoms of a urinary tract infection and to report any symptoms immediately.

Cystoscopy

Cystoscopy is the direct visual examination of the bladder, ureteral orifices, and urethra with a cystoscope. It is used to view, diagnose, and treat disorders of the lower urinary tract, interior bladder, urethra, male prostatic urethra, and ureteral orifices.

Preparation
- The patient is allowed liquids on the morning of the examination.
- Sedation and analgesics are usually prescribed before the procedure.
- Obtain a signed consent form (required for the procedure).
- Tell the patient that the procedure is ordinarily painless.

Aftercare
- Know that tissue swelling, dysuria, and hematuria may occur because of trauma from the procedure.
- Encourage a generous fluid intake, and observe and measure urine output for at least 24 hours.
- Observe the patient for urinary retention and for signs of infection; nosocomial infection after a cystoscopy is common.

Intravenous Pyelogram (Excretory Urography)

Intravenous pyelogram is the radiographic examination of the kidney and ureter after a contrast material is injected intravenously. It is used to diagnose kidney and ureter disease and impaired renal function.

Preparation
- Withhold or limit fluids or foods before testing. Obtain patient's allergy history, focusing on sensitivity to iodine, shellfish, or seafood (contrast may contain iodine).
- This test is contraindicated for patients with elevated BUN and creatinine levels and pregnant patients.
- Elderly, debilitated, or young patients may not tolerate this dehydration, and compromises may need to be made.
- Give a laxative the evening before the examination and an enema the morning of the examination so that stool and gas do not interfere with visualization.
- Obtain a signed consent form (required for the procedure).
- Tell the patient to void before the examination.

Aftercare
- Offer fluids and food immediately after the examination.
- Provide sufficient fluids to replace those lost during the pretest period.

- Observe the patient for signs of a reaction to the contrast material, such as a rash, nausea, and hives. Contrast may initiate acute renal failure. Monitor intake and output.

Retrograde Pyelogram

Retrograde pyelogram is the radiographic and endoscopic examination of the kidneys and ureters after a contrast material is injected into the renal pelvis through the ureter.

Preparation
- Do not give fluids or food after midnight before the examination.
- This test is contraindicated for pregnant patients and those with an iodine allergy.
- Give a laxative the evening before the examination and an enema the morning of the examination so that stool and gas do not interfere with visualization.
- Tell the patient to void before the examination.
- Obtain a signed consent form (required for the procedure).

Aftercare
- Offer foods and fluids immediately if no anesthesia has been used. If anesthesia has been used, delay offering foods and fluids for several hours.
- Check the vital signs regularly if anesthesia has been used.
- Observe the patient for signs of a reaction to the contrast material, such as a rash, nausea, and hives.
- Monitor urine output and appearance for at least 24 hours. Hematuria and dysuria can occur.
- Be aware that ureteral catheters may be in place and should be connected to drainage receptacles so that the amount and character of drainage from each catheter can be noted.

Renal Ultrasound

A renal ultrasound is a noninvasive procedure that involves the use of ultrasound to visualize the renal parenchyma and renal blood vessels. It is used to characterize renal masses and infections; visualize large calculi; detect malformed kidneys; provide guidance during other procedures, such as biopsy; and monitor the status of renal transplants and kidney development in children with congenital processes.

Preparation
- Obtain a signed consent form (required).
- Restrict food and fluids for 8 to 12 hours before renal ultrasound.
- Tell the patient not to smoke or chew gum before the procedure to prevent swallowing air.
- Inform the patient that the procedure is painless.

Aftercare
- Know that no special care is required after the test.
- Inform the patient that results are usually available 1 to 2 days after the study.

Computed Tomography (CT Scanning)

CT scanning is a noninvasive radiographic procedure whereby a body part can be scanned from different angles with an x-ray beam and a computer that calculates varying tissue densities and records a cross-sectional image on paper.

Preparation
- Obtain a signed consent form (required).
- The patient is usually NPO for 8 hours before the test if a contrast dye is used.

(continued)

> **Box 37-2** **COMMON DIAGNOSTIC PROCEDURES USED TO STUDY THE URINARY TRACT** *(continued)*

- Obtain patient's history of any allergic reaction or hypersensitivity to shellfish, iodine, or any contrast dyes (contrast may contain iodine).
- Remove all metal objects from the patient before the test.
- Medications may usually be taken until 2 hours before the test.

Aftercare
- Observe for a delayed reaction to the contrast dye (skin rash, urticaria, headache, vomiting). An oral antihistamine may be given for mild reactions.
- Be supportive to patient and family. The test can be frightening.
- Instruct the patient to resume usual diet and activity unless otherwise indicated.

Renal Biopsy
It is an invasive procedure that involves obtaining a small piece of renal tissue for microscopic examination. Tissue sample may be obtained by needle and syringe through a skin puncture or small incision, during an open surgical procedure during which

a wedge of tissue is removed, or through a cystoscope during which a brush is used to obtain a tissue fragment.

Preparation
- Obtain coagulation studies and hematocrit.
- Obtain baseline vital signs.
- Withhold food and fluid before the procedure.
- Obtain a signed consent form (required).
- Sedation may be necessary, depending on the type of procedure.

Aftercare
- Instruct the patient to lie quietly for 4 hours.
- Monitor urine for hematuria during the first 24 hours. Collect each voided specimen in a separate cup labeled with the time.
- Monitor vital signs and dressing for any indication of shock or bleeding.
- Instruct the patient to avoid strenuous activities or heavy lifting for several days and to report any flank pain, hematuria, or dizziness.

(Adapted from Collis Pellatt, G. [2007a]. Anatomy and physiology of urinary elimination. Part 1. *British Journal of Nursing, 16*[7], 406–410.; Fischbach, F., & Dunning, M. [2009]. *A manual of laboratory and diagnostic tests* [8th ed.]. Philadelphia: Wolters Kluwer Health/Lippincott Williams & Wilkins; and Porth, C., & Matfin, G. [2009]. *Pathophysiology: Concepts of altered health states* [8th ed.]. Philadelphia: Wolters Kluwer Health/Lippincott Williams & Wilkins.)

- Situational Low Self-Esteem related to urinary incontinence, urinary diversion
- Sexual Dysfunction related to urinary incontinence, urinary diversion
- Disturbed Sleep Pattern related to nocturia
- Toileting Self-Care Deficit related to parent's lack of knowledge or motivation to toilet train child, neuromuscular impairment or musculoskeletal disorders, immobility, trauma or surgical procedures, confusion, disorientation

The nurse's challenge is to identify human responses to alterations in urinary elimination that pose specific health problems for the patient and family.

Outcome Identification and Planning

When the patient is ambulatory and not experiencing difficulties with the urinary system, normal voiding is usually not a problem. Trauma or illness, however, may result in the patient's need for nursing assistance with voiding. Nursing interventions should support planned patient outcomes. The patient will:

- Produce urine output about equal to fluid intake
- Maintain fluid and electrolyte balance
- Empty the bladder completely at regular intervals
- Report ease of voiding
- Maintain skin integrity

Implementing

Nursing interventions focus on maintaining and promoting normal urinary patterns, improving or controlling urinary

incontinence, preventing potential problems associated with bladder catheterization, and assisting with care of urinary diversions. Nurses can assist the patient and family to achieve desirable outcomes for their urination needs.

> ➤ *Think back to Anna Galinski, the frail woman in a nursing home. The toileting program focused on maintaining and promoting the patient's normal urinary patterns. However, now that the patient has an indwelling catheter, the nurse needs to focus on preventing problems associated with catheterization. Weighing the risks and benefits of catheterization for this patient would be crucial.* ■

The accompanying Examples of Nursing Intervention and Nursing Outcome Classifications (NIC/NOC) box offers suggested nursing outcomes and interventions related to Functional Urinary Incontinence.

Promoting Normal Urination

Nursing care to promote normal urination includes interventions to support normal voiding habits, fluid intake, strengthening of muscle tone, stimulating urination and resolving urinary retention, and assisting with toileting. Nurses who role model good health behaviors are more effective teachers. Use Promoting Health 37-1 for yourself before using it with others.

MAINTAINING NORMAL VOIDING HABITS

If the patient's voiding habits are adequate, the nurse provides care or teaches the patient to maintain these habits to

Examples of NANDA Nursing Diagnoses

Urinary Elimination

Nursing Diagnoses	Related Factors	Sample Defining Characteristics
Impaired Urinary Elimination	Sensory motor impairment Urinary tract infection Anatomical obstruction	Postvoid residual of 450 mL via bladder scanner *"It hurts when I pass my water and I have to go every hour!"* *"I have to get up frequently at night to urinate."* Urinalysis reveals hematuria and proteinuria.
Functional Urinary Incontinence	Altered environment Sensory, cognitive, or mobility deficits	*"I don't know why Johnny started wetting since he's been hospitalized. He has been toilet trained for 6 months now."* *"When I remember to take Mother to the toilet she urinates fine. But if I don't remember, I find her wet."*
Reflex Urinary Incontinence	Neurologic impairment Age-related degenerative changes High intra-abdominal pressure Incompetent bladder outlet	Patient with spinal cord lesion reports no awareness of bladder filling, no urge to void or feelings of bladder fullness, involuntary loss of urine at somewhat regular intervals.
Stress Urinary Incontinence	Overdistention between voidings Weak pelvic muscles and structural supports	Obese mother of four reports involuntary dribbling of urine with coughs, sneezes, hearty laughter. Patient "too busy to void" during day reports involuntary leakage of urine with sudden movement, coughing, sneezing, and laughing.
Total Urinary Incontinence	Neurologic impairment Trauma or disease affecting spinal cord nerves	Constant flow of urine at unpredictable times without distention or uninhibited bladder contractions Nocturia Unawareness of incontinence
Urge Urinary Incontinence	Decreased bladder capacity Bladder spasms Increased intake of caffeine or alcohol Increased urine concentration Overdistention of bladder	*"I can never make it to the bathroom in time."* Urgency, frequency, nocturia, bladder contracture or spasm
Urinary Retention	High urethral pressure caused by weak detrusor Inhibition of reflex arc Strong sphincter Blockage	Elderly man diagnosed with benign prostatic hypertrophy complains of inability to urinate despite feeling bladder is full. Woman 6 hours after delivery has had no urine output since labor; 800 mL IV fluids infused; fundus of uterus is displaced to the right by a full bladder.

ensure comfort and satisfactory urine output. Attention to the following variables is helpful:

- *Schedule:* Some patients report urinating on demand in no apparent pattern. Others have inflexible patterns that have developed over the years and become anxious if these are interrupted. Some patients need assistance to urinate and

may experience urgency. Nursing actions should support the patient's usual urinating pattern as much as possible.

- *Urge to void:* Assist the patient to void when he or she first feels the urge to void. Routinely delaying urination may result in difficulty initiating a stream and/or urinary stasis. Urinary stasis can contribute to the development of urinary tract infections.

Examples of Nursing Interventions and Nursing Outcomes Classifications (NIC/NOC)

Functional Urinary Incontinence

Nursing Interventions	Nursing Outcomes
• Prompted Voiding	• Self-Care: Toileting
• Self-Care Assistance: Toileting	• Urinary Continence
• Urinary Elimination Management	• Urinary Elimination
• Urinary Habit Training	

From Moorhead, S., Johnson, M., Maas, M., Swanson, E. (Eds). (2008). *Nursing outcomes classification (NOC)* (4th ed.). St. Louis: Mosby Elsevier; and Bulechek, G., Butcher, H., & McCloskey Dochterman, J. (Eds.). (2008). *Nursing interventions classification (NIC)* (5th ed.). St. Louis: Mosby Elsevier. A full listing of nursing activities for each nursing outcome and intervention can be found in these books.

• *Privacy:* Many adults and children cannot urinate in the presence of another person. Unless the patient is extremely weak and requires assistance, provide privacy in the healthcare facility and in the home.

• *Position:* Helping patients assume their usual voiding position may be all that is necessary to resolve an inability to urinate. Some male patients cannot use a urinal while lying down or sitting; encourage them to void while standing at the bedside unless this is contraindicated. Similarly, some female patients cannot void easily on a bedpan but respond favorably with a bedside commode.

• *Hygiene:* Patients who are confined to bed find it difficult to perform their usual genital hygiene. Careful cleansing of the perineal and genital areas is needed for patient comfort and to prevent infection. This is easily accomplished for patients on bed rest by using a bedpan and then pouring warm soapy water over the perineal area, followed by clear water. Families providing care for ill members at home may be taught this technique.

Because many people customarily wash their hands after toileting, offer patients confined to bed a moistened towelette or soap and water to wipe their hands after removing the bedpan or urinal. Specific recommendations for urinary elimination problems that affect older adults are listed in the accompanying box Focus on the Older Adult.

PROMOTING HEALTH • 37-1

Urine Elimination

Patients view nurses as role models for achieving healthy lifestyles. Use the assessment checklist to determine how well you are meeting your needs related to urinary elimination. Then develop a prescription for self-care by choosing appropriate behaviors from the list of suggestions.

Assessment Checklist

❑ almost always   ❑ sometimes   ❑ almost never

❑ ❑ ❑   1. I urinate at regular intervals throughout the day.

❑ ❑ ❑   2. I have an adequate fluid intake.

❑ ❑ ❑   3. I limit my sodium intake.

❑ ❑ ❑   4. My urine volume remains relatively constant.

Self-Care Behaviors

1. Maintain a normal voiding pattern and volume.
2. Respond as soon as possible to the urge to void.
3. Drink 8 to 10 glasses of water daily.
4. Avoid foods that contain excess sodium.
5. Monitor use of caffeine, alcohol, or medication schedules that promote voiding and may interfere with sleep.
6. Seek medical assistance for any change in the characteristics of urine or presence of pain on urination.

Information to promote effective urinary elimination, such as information about elimination problems, urinary incontinence, and renal and bladder diseases is available online. Check out these sites: MedlinePlus at www.nlm.nih.gov/medlineplus; National Institutes of Health: Health Information at http://health.nih.gov/; and National Kidney and Urologic Diseases Information /clearinghouse (NKUDIC): http://kidney.niddk.nih.gov/.

FOCUS ON THE OLDER ADULT

NURSING STRATEGIES FOR URINARY ELIMINATION PROBLEMS AFFECTING OLDER ADULTS

Nocturia, Frequency, and Urgency

- Ensure easy access to the bathroom or commode.
- Discourage fluid intake at bedtime.
- Discourage alcohol use before bedtime.
- Evaluate medication regimen and schedule, particularly diuretics and drugs that produce sedation or confusion.
- Use a night light.
- Use clothing that is easily removed for voiding.
- Keep assistive ambulatory devices (walkers, canes, etc.) readily available.
- Provide call bell if assistance is necessary.
- Evaluate gait and ability to ambulate safely.
- Assess for urinary tract infection.

Incontinence

- Maintain a fluid intake of 1,500 to 2,000 mL/day.
- Discourage use of alcohol, NutraSweet, and caffeine.
- Provide easy access to the bathroom.
- Assess factors that influence voiding.
- Use assistive devices when necessary (raised toilet seat, grab bars, walker).

- Use collection devices when necessary (urinal or bedpan).
- Ensure safety when ambulating (e.g., skid-proof slippers).
- Encourage use of whole, unprocessed, coarse wheat bran to prevent constipation and fecal impaction.
- Perform Kegel exercises several times daily.
- Encourage participation in a bladder retraining program.
- Consider insertion of an indwelling catheter as the last resort.

Urinary Tract Infections

- Maintain a liberal fluid intake.
- Encourage shower instead of tub bath to decrease opportunity for bacteria in bath water to enter urethra.
- Void at frequent intervals; every 2 hours if possible.
- Void immediately after sexual intercourse.
- Assess for signs of urinary tract infection (may be nonspecific in elderly patient).
- Use dipstick (Microstix) if recommended to monitor bacteria count in urine.
- Continue antimicrobial therapy as ordered.

> *Recall Anna Galinski, the frail older woman in the nursing home. Ideally, before the charge nurse had inserted the catheter into Mrs. Galinski, these strategies should have been attempted to determine their effectiveness in promoting urinary elimination. In addition, when advocating for the patient, the nurse would strongly urge incorporating these strategies into the patient's plan of care to determine their effectiveness, ultimately substantiating that catheterization was not necessary.* ∎

PROMOTING FLUID INTAKE

Many people routinely drink less fluid than is optimal to promote healthy urinary functioning. Adults with no disease-related fluid restrictions should drink 2,000 to 2,400 mL (8 to 10 8-oz glasses) of fluid daily. A common misperception is that drinking this much fluid causes water retention and contributes to weight gain. If a good proportion of the daily fluid intake is water, the kidneys and urinary structures are well flushed, and waste products, including potentially harmful bacteria, are removed. Monitor fluid intake for excessive amounts of caffeine-containing beverages, high-sodium beverages, and high-sugar beverages.

Provide fresh water, juices, and fluids of preference to patients confined to bed. Patients who are confused and children may need to be reminded to drink. Fluid restrictions may be ordered by the physician for patients with certain diseases. For others, forced fluids (above-average intake of

fluids) are prescribed. Incorporate this information in the plan of care and explain it to the patient.

STRENGTHENING MUSCLE TONE

Weakening of the pelvic floor muscles is a common cause of urinary continence problems in women and men (Robinson, 2008; Yates, 2008). Pelvic floor muscle training (PFMT) can improve voluntary control of urination and significantly reduce or eliminate problems with stress incontinence by strengthening perineal and abdominal muscle tone. PFMT, more commonly called **Kegel exercises,** targets the inner muscles that lie under and support the bladder. These muscles can be toned, strengthened, and actually made larger by a regular routine of tightening and relaxing. Often patients have difficulty determining which muscles to exercise. These are the same muscles that the patient contracts to stop urinating in midstream or to control defecation. Instruct patients to contract the pelvic floor muscles for 10 seconds and to relax them for 10 seconds. Encourage the patient to perform Kegel exercises without involving the muscles in the abdomen, inner thigh, and buttocks. When the patient is familiar with these sensations, he or she should perform these exercises 30 to 80 times a day for at least 6 weeks and possibly longer, depending on the response (Karon, 2005; Specht, 2005; Yates, 2008). The exercises can be done anywhere. Assist patients to incorporate them into their daily activities.

PFMT can also be accomplished by using vaginal weights. The patient inserts a small weighted cone into her vagina. She then contracts her pelvic floor musculature to prevent the cone from falling out. The cones can be gradually increased in weight as the muscles are strengthened.

ASSISTING WITH TOILETING

The amount of assistance provided to a patient in relation to toileting varies, depending on the patient's abilities and health status.

Toilet

Even when the patient can use the bathroom toilet, the nurse may be responsible for noting any abnormalities of urinary elimination. In some instances, patients may be taught to report abnormalities to the nurse and instructed not to flush the toilet until the nurse checks the urine. In other instances, when the urine volume is to be calculated, the patient may need to urinate in a bedpan or a specimen hat placed in the toilet so that the urine can be measured before it is discarded. Although many patients can easily be taught to measure their urine output, the nurse is responsible for observing urine at least once during a shift and more frequently if warranted.

Assist weakened patients to the bathroom. If there is any danger of the patient falling, remain in attendance. Never lock the bathroom door. Also, ensure that a signal bell is within easy reach so that the patient can summon help easily if he or she feels weak and needs assistance. A handrail near the toilet also is helpful.

Commode

Commodes are chairs—straight-back chairs or wheelchairs with open seats with a shelf or a holder underneath that holds a bedpan or bucket (Fig. 37-9). They can be used for patients who can get out of bed but cannot use the bathroom toilet. The commode can be placed adjacent to the bed, and the patient can be assisted to it with minimal exertion. If the patient has a roommate, any visitors may be asked to exit the room while the patient uses the commode. Remember to pull the curtain in the room and close the door to provide for patient privacy.

Bedpan and Urinal

Male patients confined to bed usually use the urinal for voiding and the bedpan for defecation; female patients use the bedpan for both (see Fig. 37-5). Many patients find it embarrassing and difficult to use the bedpan and/or the urinal.

FIGURE 37-9. Bedside commode.

When a patient uses a bedpan or urinal, maintain the patient's privacy.

A special bedpan called a fracture bedpan is frequently used by people with fractures of the femur or lower spine. Smaller and flatter than the ordinary bedpan, it is helpful for patients who cannot easily raise themselves onto the regular bedpan. Very thin or elderly patients often find it easier and more comfortable to use the fracture bedpan. Skills 37-2 and 37-3 show how to assist a patient with using a bedpan and urinal.

Preventing Urinary Tract Infections

Urinary tract infections (UTIs) are a leading cause of morbidity and healthcare expenditures in persons of all ages. UTIs are the leading cause of systemic infections in older adults. Because the female urethra is shorter, and in closer proximity to the vagina and rectum, women are especially vulnerable to UTIs. UTIs can affect both the upper urinary tract, involving the kidneys and ureters (pyelonephritis) and/or lower urinary tract, involving the bladder and urethra (cystitis). Escherichia coli, bacteria commonly found in the gastrointestinal tract, are the most common causal organism (Griebling, 2004a, 2004b).

RISK FACTORS

Those at greatest risk for a UTI include the following:

- *Sexually active women.* During intercourse, perineal bacteria can migrate into the urethra and bladder.
- *Women who use diaphragms for contraception:* The spermicide used with a diaphragm decreases the amount of normally protective vaginal flora.
- *Postmenopausal women:* Urinary stasis, which is common at this age, provides an optimal environment for bacteria to multiply; in addition, decreased estrogen contributes to loss of protective vaginal flora.
- *Individuals with an indwelling urinary catheter in place:* About half of all patients with an indwelling catheter become infected within 1 week after its insertion. Although a break in sterile technique during placement can lead to an infection, most pathogens are introduced via handling of the catheter and drainage device after placement.
- *Individuals with diabetes mellitus:* Glucose in the urine acts as an excellent medium for bacteria to proliferate.
- *Elderly people:* The physiologic changes associated with aging (listed earlier in the chapter) predispose older people to the development of UTIs (Woods, 2005).

> ➤ *Consider Anna Galinski, the frail older adult woman in the nursing home. Her risk for developing a UTI is increased due to her age. This risk now is further increased because of the catheter insertion.* ∎

DIAGNOSTIC EVALUATION

In addition to the nursing history and physical examination, laboratory findings can identify the presence of a UTI.

A urine sample from a clean-catch or sterile specimen should be sent to the laboratory for a culture and sensitivity (C&S) test. A C&S is positive if it shows at least 100,000 organisms per milliliter of urine. Lower counts may be considered clinically significant if the patient has signs and symptoms of a UTI (Fischbach & Dunning, 2009). The presence of bacteria in a clean-catch midstream or sterile urine specimen, accompanied by symptoms (e.g., dysuria, urinary frequency or urgency, or cloudy urine with a foul odor), indicates a UTI. Red blood cells and nitrates also may be present in the urine.

TREATMENT

Various protocols are used to treat UTIs. A short-course antibiotic regimen (1 large dose versus 3 or 7 days of smaller doses) usually eradicates infections of the lower urinary tract; longer antimicrobial therapy is required for upper urinary tract infections. Patient education can help prevent UTI recurrence. Teaching the patient about measures that promote health and decrease the severity and incidence of UTIs is a major nursing responsibility. Instruct the patient to:

- Drink 8 to 10, 8-oz glasses of water daily.
- Observe the urine for color, amount, odor, and frequency. Report any sign of infection to your healthcare provider.
- Dry the perineal area after urination or defecation from the front to the back, or from the urethra toward the rectum.
- Drink two glasses of water before and after sexual intercourse and void immediately after intercourse.
- Take showers rather than baths.
- Wear underwear with a cotton crotch, and avoid clothing that is tight and restrictive on the lower half of the body.
- Drink 10 oz of cranberry or blueberry juice daily. These juices contain chemicals that may help prevent **bacteriuria** (bacteria in the urine) by inhibiting bacteria from adhering to the bladder wall and urinary catheters (Woods, 2005).

Nursing interventions to prevent UTIs for a patient with an indwelling catheter are discussed later in the chapter.

Caring for an Incontinent Patient

Urinary incontinence, any involuntary leakage of urine, is widely underreported and underdiagnosed. It is one of the most common chronic health problems. However, it is not an inevitable result of growing old or bearing children. Many people self-manage this life-altering condition for many years before seeking assistance from a healthcare provider.

Urinary incontinence is more prevalent in women and increases with age. It is a special problem for older adults who may experience decreasing control over urination and who may find it more difficult to reach a toilet in time to void because of mobility problems or dexterity problems in undressing. The discomfort, odor, and embarrassment of urine-soaked clothing can greatly diminish a person's self-concept, causing him or her to feel like a social outcast.

Age-related changes do affect urinary function, but urinary incontinence can be treated and individualized interventions can help the patient lead a normal life. Of those who seek treatment, 80% are cured or have their symptoms improved notably.

Patients frequently turn to absorbent products for protection when they are incontinent of urine if they have not had this condition properly diagnosed and treated. These products absorb or contain urine leakage. Many types of disposable and reusable products are available, including perineal pads or liners, protective underwear, guards and drip collection pouches, and adult briefs. When used improperly, such products may cause skin breakdown and place the patient at risk for a UTI. Long-term use of these products is not recommended until the following factors have been considered and discussed with a healthcare provider:

- Functional disability of the patient
- Type and severity of incontinence
- Gender
- Availability of caregivers
- Failure of previous treatment programs
- Patient preference

Advertisements for adult disposable undergarments have increased public awareness about urinary incontinence, but they fail to mention possible treatment strategies (see Focused Critical Thinking Guide 37-1).

> ➤ *Review the scenario at the beginning of the chapter describing Midori Morita and her husband. It would be important for the nurse to assess the feelings of Midori and her husband related to the problems associated with urinary dribbling and incontinence. Midori may be feeling overwhelmed and possibly upset or angry. Her husband most likely would be feeling embarrassed and possibly disgusted. Helping them resolve these feelings is essential for effective care.* ∎

TYPES OF URINARY INCONTINENCE

Specht (2005) identifies numerous types of urinary incontinence. **Transient incontinence** appears suddenly and lasts for 6 months or less. It is usually caused by treatable factors, such as confusion secondary to acute illness, infection, and as a result of medical treatment, such as the use of diuretics or intravenous fluid administration. **Stress incontinence** occurs when there is an involuntary loss of urine related to an increase in intra-abdominal pressure. This commonly occurs during coughing, sneezing, laughing, or other physical activities. Childbirth, menopause, obesity, or straining from chronic constipation can also result in urine loss. The leakage usually does not occur when the person is supine. **Urge incontinence** is the involuntary loss of urine that occurs soon after feeling an urgent need to void (urgency). These patients experience a loss of urine before getting to the toilet and an inability to suppress the need to urinate. A diagnosis of

FOCUSED CRITICAL THINKING GUIDE • 37-1

Urinary Incontinence

You have been assigned to care for an 80-year-old patient who was admitted with a recurrent leg ulcer and is due to be discharged the following day. Her nursing notes indicate that she has had two or three episodes of urinary incontinence every day while in the hospital and her plan of care states "use adult diapers." You go into the room to answer Mrs. Bartowski's call bell and help her into the bathroom. She is wearing an adult diaper, and a half-used package of diapers is on the chair. After voiding 150 mL of urine, she tearfully begs, "Please don't put that diaper back on me; I'm not a child." According to her chart, Mrs. Bartowski is mentally alert, lives at home with her daughter who visits frequently, and appears able to identify her need to urinate. You're aware that there are effective alternative therapies to resolve or minimize urinary incontinence rather than relying on absorbent products. However, the nurses have obviously made a decision to use diapers in this situation. You prefer to leave the diaper off, try some other measures, and possibly discuss this with the patient's daughter, but as a student nurse, you are here for only 2 days. You want to be a patient advocate and do the right thing. What should you do?

1. Identify Goal of Thinking

Determine whether it is more important to replace the diaper against the patient's wishes or leave it off and discuss the possibility of using behavioral strategies with the staff.

2. Assess Adequacy of Knowledge

Pertinent circumstances: Mrs. Bartowski is alert and oriented and obviously upset that diapers are being used. She has used her call bell when she feels the urge to urinate, but incontinent episodes have also been documented. The nursing staff has decided that diapers are appropriate for this patient. Her daughter, with whom she lives, appears supportive and attentive. Discharge is scheduled for tomorrow.

Prerequisite knowledge: Before you decide what to do in this situation, you need to discuss your options with your instructor. Of primary importance is whether the patient and her daughter are interested in pursuing alternatives. They can also provide invaluable information about her elimination pattern at home. The primary care provider must be consulted to determine the etiology of the incontinence and validate that her urinary tract is intact and functioning adequately. You will also need to review the various treatment options for incontinence because these will have to be communicated to the patient and her daughter before discharge.

Room for error/time constraints: Absorbent products can provide a sense of security and are widely used for incontinence. There is, however, the possibility that continence can be restored once incontinence is assessed, recognized, and addressed. Early dependence on absorbent products can remove the motivation to seek treatment and promote acceptance of the condition. The treatment options should be discussed with Mrs. Bartowski and her daughter before discharge tomorrow.

3. Address Potential Problems

Continuing to use absorbent products offers a temporary solution to the problem. They may protect the patient from embarrassment and provide a sense of security, although they do nothing to prevent incontinent episodes. Explore the patient's feelings regarding the use of these products. The use of these products can communicate expectations of an acceptance of incontinence as an inevitable part of aging, which is not true. Absorbent products can also interfere with the patient's ability to use the toilet independently. Using behavioral techniques to control incontinence will require health teaching before discharge and a long-term commitment to follow-up in the home.

4. Consult Helpful Resources

The patient's motivation to restore continence is your most valuable resource. The primary nurse or case manager, the primary care provider, and your instructor can also help you sort through your priorities in this situation. The latest research recommends use of behavioral techniques first to treat incontinence.

5. Critique Judgment/Decision

If you decide to reapply a diaper against the patient's wishes, you may, in fact, be supporting the myth that incontinence is inevitable and untreatable. Long-term use of absorbent products can place the patient at risk for skin breakdown and a urinary tract infection if used improperly. You decide to leave the diaper off and establish regular intervals for voiding for the 2 days you will be caring for Mrs. Bartowski. In this short time, you hope to demonstrate to the patient, her daughter, and the staff that it is possible for Mrs. Bartowski to maintain a pattern of continence. Because she will most likely be discharged tomorrow, you also discuss the possibility of referral to home care or a continence expert who will instruct, support, and follow through with the necessary components of care. When you discuss your situation at postconference, your clinical group supports your decision.

mixed incontinence indicates that there is urine loss with features of two or more types of incontinence. With **overflow incontinence,** the involuntary loss of urine is associated with overdistention and overflow of the bladder. The signal to empty the bladder may be underactive or absent, the bladder fills, and dribbling occurs. It may be due to a secondary effect of some drugs, fecal impaction, or neurologic conditions. **Functional incontinence** is urine loss caused by the inability to reach the toilet because of environmental barriers, physical limitations, loss of memory, or disorientation.

Patients with **reflex incontinence** experience emptying of the bladder without the sensation of the need to void. Spinal cord injuries may lead to this type of incontinence. **Total incontinence** is a continuous and unpredictable loss of urine, resulting from surgery, trauma, or physical malformation. Urination can not be controlled due to an anatomic abnormality (Specht, 2005).

Urinary incontinence is treatable. Appropriate interventions can significantly reduce the symptoms of urinary incontinence and even prevent its occurrence.

ASSESSMENT

Through careful assessment and planned interventions (see below), continence may be restored. Carefully assess environmental factors for their potential impact on urinary incontinence. Equipment that gives the person better access to toileting facilities, such as a walker, cane, wheelchair, and Velcro closings on clothing, may be necessary. Dietary habits, such as excess caffeine intake or insufficient fluid intake, both of which can irritate the bladder and contribute to incontinence, indicate the need for teaching about nutrition.

A voiding record or diary provides information about the frequency, timing, and amount of voiding. By noting any patterns to voiding, either continent or incontinent, the nurse may find correlations with medications, fluid intake, or other causes of incontinence and may be able to prevent any further incontinent episodes. Voiding diaries can also be used to evaluate the effectiveness of interventions.

Physical examination and specific diagnostic tests also aid in identifying urinary incontinence. Palpate the patient's abdomen for a distended bladder, any masses, or tenderness. The **postvoid residual (PVR)** urine (the amount of urine remaining in the bladder immediately after voiding) can be measured by the use of a portable ultrasound device that scans the bladder. Bladder ultrasound poses no risk for infection and is considered a safer alternative to catheterization. This measurement can also be obtained by catheterizing the patient. Catheterization, however, involves the increased risk for introduction of microorganisms into the bladder and resulting UTI. A PVR of less than 50 mL indicates adequate bladder emptying. A PVR of greater than 150 mL is often recommended as the guideline for catheterization because residual urine volumes of greater than 150 mL have been associated with the development of urinary tract infections (Stevens, 2005). Refer to Skill 37-1 for the procedure for assessing bladder volume using an ultrasound bladder scanner.

> ➤ *Think back to Midori Morita, the woman caring for her husband who had urinary problems at home. The nurse would need to carefully assess all aspects of the patient's current status, including the environment, and develop a patient-specific teaching plan for Midori and her husband.* ■

TREATMENT

Noninvasive, low-risk behavioral interventions are the first line of therapy for urinary incontinence (Box 37-3). The home setting is ideally suited for using these interventions. Nurses can identify patients who are incontinent and use these techniques or refer them to nurse or physician continence experts in the community. All nurses caring for older adults need to be familiar with education about urinary incontinence.

Many possible treatment interventions for urinary incontinence fall within the nurse's scope of practice. (See Box 37-3 for a summary of these treatment interventions.) Refer to the accompanying Research in Nursing display regarding one facility's experience with bladder retraining as treatment for incontinence.

Many patients incorrectly believe that surgery is the only treatment option for urinary incontinence. Surgical intervention is considered only if behavioral and pharmacologic measures prove ineffective. Nursing skills and creativity can help patients become continent again before surgery is used.

Applying an External (Condom) Catheter

When voluntary control of urination is not possible for male patients, an alternative to an indwelling catheter (see below) is the **external condom catheter.** This soft, pliable sheath made of silicone material is applied externally to the penis. Most devices are self-adhesive. The catheter is connected to drainage tubing and a collection bag, and can be used with a leg bag. The accompanying Research in Nursing display discusses the use of condom catheters related to infection risk and patient satisfaction.

> ➤ *Think back to Midori Morita, the woman described at the beginning of the chapter who is caring for her husband at home. The nurse might suggest using a condom catheter for Mrs. Morita's husband as a possible alternative, rather than an indwelling catheter, which would increase his risk for infection.* ■

Nursing care of a patient with a condom catheter includes vigilant skin care to prevent excoriation. Remove the condom daily and wash the penis with soap and water, dry it carefully, and inspect the skin for irritation. In hot and humid weather, more frequent changing may be required. Always follow the manufacturer's instructions for applying the condom because there are several variations. In all cases, care must be taken to fasten the condom securely enough to prevent leakage, yet not so tightly as to constrict the blood vessels

Box 37-3 TREATMENT OPTIONS FOR URINARY INCONTINENCE

Behavioral Techniques

- Pelvic floor exercises: Kegel exercises to strengthen pelvic floor muscles and sphincter muscles. Kegel exercises can be done alone, with weighted cones, or with biofeedback.
- Biofeedback: Measuring devices are used to help patient become aware of when pelvic floor muscles are contracting.
- Electrical stimulation: Electrodes are placed in the vagina or rectum that then stimulate nearby muscles to contract.
- Timed voiding or bladder training: May be used with biofeedback. Patient keeps track of when voiding and leaking occur so that he or she may plan when to void, with increasing length of voiding intervals. Bladder training involves biofeedback and muscle training. Urgency control is addressed using distraction and relaxation techniques.

Pharmacologic Treatment

- Treatment dependent on type of incontinence. Some medications inhibit contractions of the bladder, others may relax muscles, and some tighten muscles at the bladder neck and urethra.

- Estrogen may be used in postmenopausal women to relieve atrophy of involved muscles.
- Collagen may be injected into the tissue around the urethra to add bulk and help close the urethral opening.

Mechanical Treatment

- Pessaries: A stiff ring that is inserted into the vagina, where it helps to reposition the urethra. The pessary may be placed by the patient or by a nurse.
- External barriers: Adhere to the urethral opening to stop urine leakage. The barrier is a small foam pad placed over the urethral opening. It seals against the body to keep urine from leaking. It is removed and discarded before the patient voids.
- Urethral insert: Small device, like a plug, that fits into the urethra. Removed to void, the insert is replaced until the patient needs to void again.
- Surgical intervention: Used as a last resort. Type of surgery depends on cause of incontinence.

(Adapted from Karon, S. [2005]. A team approach to bladder retraining: A pilot study. *Urologic Nursing, 25*[4], 269–276; National Kidney and Urologic Diseases Information Clearinghouse [NKUDIC]. [2007b]. *Urinary incontinence in men.* NIH publication No. 07-5280. Available at http://kidney.niddk.nih.gov/kudiseases/pubs/uimen/; National Kidney and Urologic Diseases Information Clearinghouse [NKUDIC]. [2007c]. *Urinary incontinence in women.* NIH publication No. 08-4132. Available at http://kidney.niddk.nih.gov/kudiseases/pubs/uiwomen/.; National Kidney and Urologic Diseases Information Clearinghouse (NKUDIC). [2007a]. *Bladder control for women.* Available at http://kidney.niddk.nih.gov/kudiseases/pubs/bcw_ez/index.htm.; and Weiss, B. [2005]. Selecting medications for the treatment of urinary incontinence. *American Family Physician, 71*[2], 315–322.)

in the area. The tip of the tubing should be kept 1″ to 2″ (2.5 to 5 cm) beyond the tip of the penis to prevent irritation to the sensitive glans area. Maintaining free urinary drainage is another nursing priority. Institute measures to prevent the tubing from becoming kinked and urine from backing up in the tubing. Urine can lead to excoriation of the glans, so position the tubing that collects the urine from the condom to draw urine away from the penis. Steps for applying a condom catheter are described in Skill 37-4.

For some men, the condom catheter may not be an option because of penis retraction. For these patients, the retracted penis pouch may be appropriate. This is a bag-like appliance in which the penis is placed. The pouch can then be connected to a leg bag.

RESEARCH IN NURSING
Bridging the Gap to Evidence-Based Practice

BLADDER RETRAINING AND INCONTINENCE

Urinary incontinence is a common chronic medical condition and frequently goes undiagnosed. Patients with urinary incontinence experience behavior limitations, psychological effects, and social embarrassment, as well as potential impairment of skin integrity. Bladder training is one intervention that can reverse or reduce the symptoms of urge or stress/urge incontinence.

Related Research

Huang, J., Lin, S., Yeh, S., & Wang, C. (2007). Effects of bladder training at reducing incontinence episodes, symptom distress and incontinence impact among women with urinary incontinence. *Journal of Evidence-Based Nursing, 3*(4), 289–299.

Women with mixed or urgent urinary incontinence received a 6-week course in bladder training. Data were collected pre- and postintervention using bladder diaries and questionnaires that included demographics, a urogenital distress inventory, and questions about incontinence impact. At the end of the training course, the participants reported a statistically significant reduction of incontinence episodes, as well as a decreased degree of symptom distress and incontinence impact.

Relevance to Nursing Practice

Urinary incontinence can be managed with nonpharmacologic and nonmedical interventions. Bladder training can be an effective intervention. Nurses need to identify patients who would benefit from interventions to reverse or reduce symptoms of urinary incontinence to improve the patient's quality of life.

For additional research, visit thePoint.

RESEARCH IN NURSING
Bridging the Gap to Evidence-Based Practice

CONDOM CATHETERS VERSUS INDWELLING URINARY CATHETERS

The health risks of indwelling urinary catheterization are well known. For male patients who do not retain urine, external urine collection systems are an option. How do they compare with indwelling urinary catheters?

Related Research

Saint, S., Kaufman, S., Rogers, M., Baker, P., Ossenkop, K., Lipsky, B. (2006). Condom versus indwelling urinary catheters: A randomized trial. *Journal of the American Geriatrics Society, 54*(7), 1055–1061.

This trial compared condom and indwelling urinary catheters in terms of infection risk and patient satisfaction. Hospitalized men aged 40 and older who required a urinary collection device were included in this randomized, unblended, controlled study. The incidence of adverse outcomes, including bacteremia, symptomatic urinary tract infection, or death, and patient satisfaction were recorded. Dementia status was recorded to assess effect modification by the presence of

dementia. Seventy-five subjects were randomized, with 41 receiving an indwelling catheter and 34 a condom catheter. Condom catheter use reduced adverse outcomes. Patients without dementia who had an indwelling catheter were five times as likely to develop bacteriuria or symptomatic urinary tract infection or to die as those with a condom catheter. Patients reported that condom catheters were more comfortable and less painful than indwelling catheters.

Relevance to Nursing Practice

The use of a condom catheter for male patients without dementia who require a urine collection device may reduce the incidence of catheter-related bacteriuria and symptomatic urinary tract infections. In addition, the condom catheter may cause less discomfort than an indwelling urinary catheter. Nurses should consider discussing the use of external collection devices as part of the plan of care wherever possible.

For additional research, visit the**Point**.

Catheterizing the Patient's Bladder

Urinary catheterization is the introduction of a catheter (tube) through the urethra into the bladder for the purpose of withdrawing urine. Catheter-associated urinary tract infections are the most common hospital-acquired infection in the United States and is one reason catheterization should be avoided whenever possible (Chettle, 2008). When it is deemed necessary, it should be performed using strict aseptic technique and left in place for the shortest length of time possible. The duration of catheterization is the most important risk factor for the development of a urinary tract infection (Chettle, 2008). See the accompanying PICO in Practice box.

IMPORTANT CONSIDERATIONS ABOUT THE LOWER URINARY TRACT

When catheterization is planned, consider the following about the lower urinary tract:

- The bladder is normally a sterile cavity.
- The external opening to the urethra can never be sterilized.
- The bladder has defense mechanisms. It empties itself of urine regularly and maintains an acidic environment, which has antibacterial advantages. These help to maintain a sterile bladder under normal circumstances and also help in clearing an infection if it occurs.
- Pathogens introduced into the bladder can ascend the ureters and cause bladder and kidney infections.
- A healthy bladder is not as susceptible to infection as an injured one. A state of lowered resistance, present in many diseases and stressful situations, predisposes the patient to urinary infection.

TYPES OF CATHETERS

Intermittent urethral catheters, or straight catheters, are used to drain the bladder for shorter periods. Intermittent catheterization, performed by the patient or a caregiver in the home, may be necessary for patients with spinal cord injuries or other neurologic conditions. Although the risk for UTI is always present, most research supports the use of clean, rather than sterile, technique in this environment. Patients can be taught to insert and remove intermittent catheters themselves. The procedure for self-catheterization is essentially the same as that used by the nurse to catheterize a patient. Initially a female patient may use a mirror to locate the meatus, but eventually she can learn to insert the catheter using just touch. Self-catheterization is recommended at regular intervals to prevent overdistention of the bladder and decreased blood flow through the wall of the bladder (Smeltzer, Bare, Hinkle, & Cheever, 2010). Intermittent catheters are discussed in Guidelines for Nursing Care 37-2.

If a catheter is to remain in place for continuous drainage, an **indwelling urethral catheter** is used. Indwelling catheters are also called retention or Foley catheters. The indwelling urethral catheter is designed so that it does not slip out of the bladder. A balloon is inflated to ensure that the catheter remains in the bladder once it is inserted. Indwelling catheters are used for the gradual decompression of an overdistended bladder, for intermittent bladder drainage and irrigation, and for continuous bladder drainage. Several types of indwelling catheters are available, but the principles on which they operate are similar.

The indwelling catheter has more than one lumen or open tube within the catheter. In a double-lumen catheter, one lumen is connected directly to the balloon, which is inflated with

PICO IN PRACTICE
Asking Clinical Questions

Scenario: You are an acute care nurse practitioner who works on an orthopedic surgery service. You assess patients admitted to an orthopedics unit postoperatively and prescribe their routine postoperative treatments until they are discharged from the hospital. Your standing orders for patients who have had either total knee or total hip replacements include that the indwelling urethral catheters (i.e., Foley catheters) that are placed in the operating room are not removed until at least the second post-operative day. One day, the nurse manager of the orthopedics unit tells you that they have purchased a portable bladder scanner for use on the unit and the staff nurses have been educated in its use. She asks whether or not you may consider changing your standard postoperative orders for the total knee and hip replacement patients. In particular, she asks you to stop requiring that indwelling urethral catheters be kept in place for 48 hours postoperatively and instead write standing orders for use of intermittent catheters, based upon patients' self-reported urge to urinate but inability to do so and confirmation of at least 400 milliliters of urine in the bladder by the bladder scanner. She asserts that use of indwelling urethral catheters is associated with higher rates of urinary tract infections (UTIs) than are intermittent urethral catheters.

- POPULATION: Postoperative patients with total knee and hip replacements
- INTERVENTION: Intermittent urethral catheterization as needed

- COMPARISON: Routine use of indwelling urethral catheters
- OUTCOME: UTIs

PICO Question: Among patients who have had total knee and hip replacement surgery, is intermittent urethral catheterization on an as-needed basis associated with reduced rates of UTIs than use of indwelling urethral catheters?

Finding: From the Cochrane Collaboration: Niel-Weise, B. S., & van den Broek, P. J. (2005). Urinary catheter policies for short-term bladder drainage in adults. *Cochrane Database of Systematic Reviews, 3,* CD004203.

This systematic review found that using urethral catheters intermittently as needed rather than leaving indwelling urethral catheters in place reduced the chances of having UTIs in patients who had either knee or hip surgery.

Level of Evidence: Level I

Recommendation: You decide to rewrite your standing postoperative orders for patients who have total knee or hip replacement surgery so that their indwelling urethral catheters are removed within the first few hours postoperatively. You institute a protocol for use of intermittent catheters that follows the guidelines suggested by the orthopedics nurse manager. You and the nurse manager agree to monitor the rates of UTIs in these patients to determine if they are less after the new policy is implemented.

---

sterile water; the other is the lumen through which the urine drains. The triple-lumen catheter provides an additional lumen for the instillation of irrigating solution. Figure 37-10 illustrates a triple-lumen, double-lumen, and straight catheter.

A **suprapubic catheter** is used for long-term continuous drainage. This type of catheter is inserted surgically through a small incision above the pubic area (Fig. 37-11). Suprapubic bladder drainage diverts urine from the urethra when injury, stricture, prostatic obstruction, or gynecologic or abdominal surgery has compromised the flow of urine through the urethra. A suprapubic catheter is often preferred over indwelling urethral catheters for long-term urinary drainage. Suprapubic catheters are associated with decreased risk of contamination with organisms from fecal material, elimination of damage to the urethra, a higher rate of patient satisfaction, and lower risk of catheter-associated urinary tract infections (Mercer Smith, 2003). The drainage tube is secured with sutures or tape. Care of the patient with a suprapubic catheter includes skin care around the insertion site; care of the drainage tubing and drainage bag is the same as for an indwelling catheter (see Caring for patients with indwelling catheters later in the chapter).

Urinary catheters are available in several different types of materials, with varying benefits and problems. The newest technology involves the use of antimicrobial coatings, such as silver alloy, on the catheter to reduce bacterial attachment, colonization, and migration, with resulting catheter-associated urinary tract infections (Schumm & Lam, 2008; Mercer Smith, 2003; Newman, 2008).

REASONS FOR URINARY CATHETERIZATION
Common reasons for urinary catheterization include:

- Relieving urinary retention. Retention is often temporary and is common after surgery involving the lower abdomen, pelvis, bladder, or urethra, especially if ambulation is delayed, fluid intake is minimal, or epidural analgesia is used for pain control. Any mechanical obstruction, such as swelling at the meatus, which can occur after childbirth, or an enlarged prostate in men, may cause retention.
- Obtaining a sterile urine specimen
- Obtaining a urine specimen when a specimen cannot be secured satisfactorily by other means. Examples include

Guidelines for Nursing Care • 37-2

INTERMITTENT URETHRAL CATHETERIZATION

Female

- Identify the patient. Discuss the procedure with the patient and assess the patient's ability to assist with the procedure. Discuss any allergies with the patient, especially to iodine and latex. Review the chart for any limitations in physical activity.

- Bring the catheter kit and other necessary equipment to the bedside. Obtain assistance from another staff member, if necessary. Perform hand hygiene. Put on disposable gloves.

- Close curtains around the bed and close the door to the room if possible.

- Provide for good light. Artificial light is recommended (use of a flashlight requires an assistant to hold and position it). Place a trash receptacle within easy reach.

- Raise the bed to a comfortable working height. Stand on the patient's right side if you are right handed, the patient's left side if you are left handed.

- Assist the patient to the dorsal recumbent position with knees flexed, feet about 2 feet apart, with her legs abducted. Drape the patient. Alternately, use the Sims, or lateral, position. Place the patient's buttocks near the edge of the bed with her shoulders at the opposite edge and her knees drawn toward her chest. Slide waterproof drape under the patient.

- Put on clean gloves. Clean the perineal area with washcloth, skin cleanser, and warm water, using a different corner of the washcloth with each stroke. Wipe from above orifice downward toward sacrum (front to back). Rinse and dry. Remove gloves. Perform hand hygiene again.

- Open sterile catheterization tray on a clean overbed table using sterile technique.

- Put on sterile gloves. Grasp upper corners of the drape and unfold the drape without touching unsterile areas. Fold back a corner on each side to make a cuff over gloved hands. Ask the patient to lift her buttocks and slide the sterile drape under her with gloves protected by cuff.

- Place a fenestrated sterile drape over the perineal area, exposing the labia, if appropriate.

- Place sterile tray on drape between the patient's thighs.

- Open all the supplies. Fluff cotton balls in tray before pouring antiseptic solution over them. Alternately, open package of antiseptic swabs. Open specimen container if specimen is to be obtained.

- Lubricate 1 to 2 inches of catheter tip.

- With thumb and one finger of nondominant hand, spread labia and identify meatus. If the patient is in the side-lying position, lift the upper buttock and labia to expose the urinary meatus. Be prepared to maintain separation of labia with one hand until the catheter is inserted and urine is flowing well and continuously.

- Use your dominant hand to pick up a cotton ball. Clean one labial fold, top to bottom (from above the meatus down toward the rectum), then discard the cotton ball. Using a new cotton ball for each stroke, continue to clean the other labial fold, then directly over the meatus.

- With your uncontaminated, dominant hand, place drainage end of catheter in receptacle. If a specimen is required, place the end into the specimen container in the receptacle.

- Using your dominant hand, hold the catheter 2 to 3 inches from the tip and insert it slowly into the urethra. Advance the catheter until there is a return of urine (approximately 2 to 3 inches [4.8 to 7.2 cm]). Do not force the catheter through the urethra into the bladder. Ask the patient to breathe deeply, and rotate the catheter gently if slight resistance is met as the catheter reaches the external sphincter.

- Hold the catheter securely at the meatus with your nondominant hand while the bladder empties. If a specimen is being collected, remove the drainage end of the tubing from the specimen container after the required amount is obtained and allow urine to flow into receptacle. Set specimen container aside and place lid on container.

- Allow the bladder to empty. Withdraw the catheter slowly and smoothly after urine has stopped flowing. Remove equipment and dispose of according to facility policy. Wash and dry the perineal area as needed.

- Remove your gloves. Assist the patient to a comfortable position. Cover the patient with bed linens. Place the bed in the lowest position.

- Put on clean gloves. Secure the container lid and label specimen. Send urine specimen to the laboratory promptly or refrigerate it.

- Remove gloves. Perform hand hygiene.

Male

- Identify the patient. Discuss the procedure with the patient and assess the patient's ability to assist with the procedure. Discuss any allergies with the patient, especially to iodine and latex. Review the chart for any limitations in physical activity.

- Bring the catheter kit and other necessary equipment to the bedside. Obtain assistance from another staff member, if necessary. Perform hand hygiene. Put on disposable gloves.

- Close curtains around the bed and close the door to the room if possible.

- Provide for good light. Artificial light is recommended. Place a trash receptacle within easy reach.

- Raise the bed to a comfortable working height. Stand on the patient's right side if you are right handed, the patient's left side if you are left handed.

- Position the patient on his back with thighs slightly apart. Drape the patient so that only the area around the penis is exposed. Slide waterproof pad under the patient.

- Put on clean gloves. Clean the genital area with washcloth, skin cleanser, and warm water. Clean the tip of the penis

INTERMITTENT URETHRAL CATHETERIZATION *continued*

first, moving the washcloth in a circular motion from the meatus outward. Wash the shaft of the penis using downward strokes toward the pubic area. Rinse and dry. Remove gloves. Perform hand hygiene again.

- Open sterile catheterization tray on a clean overbed table using sterile technique.

- Put on sterile gloves. Open sterile drape and place on the patient's thighs. Place fenestrated drape with opening over penis.

- Place catheter set on or next to the patient's legs on sterile drape.

- Open all the supplies. Fluff cotton balls in tray before pouring antiseptic solution over them. Alternately, open package of antiseptic swabs. Open specimen container if specimen is to be obtained.

- Remove cap from syringe prefilled with lubricant.

- Lift penis with nondominant hand. Retract foreskin in uncircumcised patient. Be prepared to keep this hand in this position until the catheter is inserted and urine is flowing well and continuously.

- Using your dominant hand and the forceps, pick up a cotton ball. Using a circular motion, clean the penis, moving from the meatus down the glans of the penis. Repeat this cleansing motion two more times, using a new cotton ball each time. Discard each cotton ball after one use.

- Hold penis with slight upward tension and perpendicular to the patient's body. Use your dominant hand to pick up the lubricant syringe. Gently insert tip of syringe with lubricant into urethra and instill the 10 mL of lubricant.

- With your uncontaminated, dominant hand, place drainage end of catheter in receptacle. If a specimen is required, place the end into the specimen container in the receptacle.

- Use your dominant hand to pick up the catheter and hold it an inch or two from the tip. Ask patient to bear down as if voiding. Insert catheter tip into meatus. Ask the patient to take deep breaths as you advance the catheter 6 to 8 inches (14.4 to 19.2 cm) or until urine flows.

- Hold the catheter securely at the meatus with your nondominant hand while the bladder empties. If a specimen is being collected, remove the drainage end of the tubing from the specimen container after the required amount is obtained and allow urine to flow into receptacle. Set specimen container aside.

- Allow the bladder to empty. Withdraw the catheter slowly and smoothly after urine has stopped flowing. Remove equipment and dispose of according to facility policy. Wash and dry the genital area as needed. Replace foreskin in forward position if necessary.

- Remove your gloves. Assist the patient to a comfortable position. Cover the patient with bed linens. Place the bed in the lowest position.

- Put on clean gloves. Cover and label specimen. Send urine specimen to the laboratory promptly or refrigerate it.

- Remove gloves. Perform hand hygiene.

FIGURE 37-10. (**A**) Triple-lumen indwelling catheter. (**B**) Double-lumen indwelling catheter. (**C**) Straight catheter.

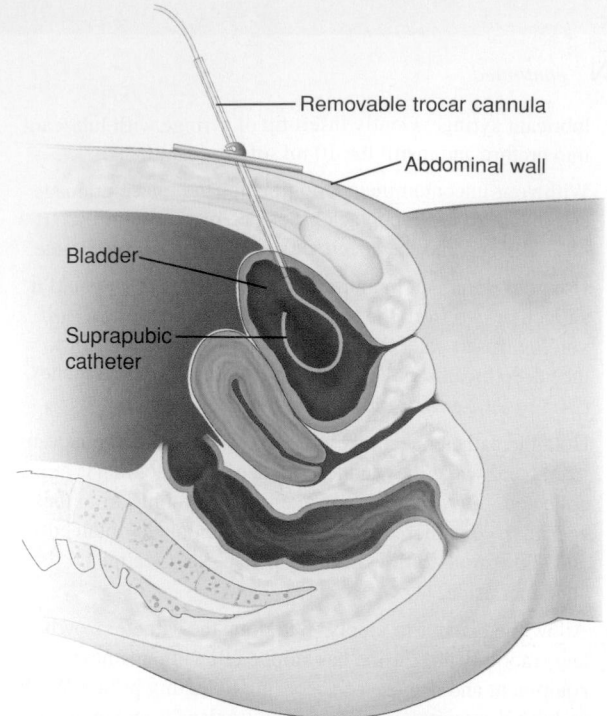

— Removable trocar cannula

— Abdominal wall

Bladder

Suprapubic
catheter

FIGURE 37-11. A suprapubic catheter positioned in the bladder.

collecting an uncontaminated specimen from a woman who is menstruating or from an incontinent patient.
- Emptying the bladder before, during, or after surgery and before certain diagnostic examinations.
- Monitoring of critically ill patients

HAZARDS OF URETHRAL CATHETERIZATION

Sepsis and trauma are the two major hazards of introducing an instrument such as a catheter into the bladder. The male urethra is especially vulnerable to injury because of its longer length. An object forced through a stricture or an irregular opening from the wrong angle can seriously damage the urethra. Although the female urethra is shorter than the male urethra, it is also susceptible to damage if a catheter is forced through it. The mucous membrane lining the urethra is delicate and damaged easily by the friction resulting from the insertion of a catheter. Bacteria can enter the bladder when the catheter is inserted. When the catheter is left in place, the organisms may move up the catheter lumen or the space between the catheter and the urethral wall. This asymptomatic condition in which bacteria is present in the urine is known as **bacteriuria.**

EQUIPMENT

The equipment used for catheterization is usually prepackaged in a sterile, disposable tray and are the same for both male and female patients. Most kits already contain a standard-sized catheter. Catheters are graded on the French (F) scale according to lumen size. For long-term use in an adult, a 14F to 16F catheter with a 5- to 10-mL balloon is commonly used (Mercer Smith, 2009; Newman, 2008). Smaller catheters usually are not necessary. A smaller lumen would be so small

that it would increase the time necessary for emptying the bladder. Larger catheters distend the urethra and increase the discomfort of the procedure. Size 5F to 8F are used for infants and young children. Size 8F to 12F catheters are commonly used for older children (Hockenberry & Wilson, 2008).

PATIENT PREPARATION

Before the catheterization, explain to the patient the procedure and the reason for it. Tell the patient that catheter insertion produces a sensation of pressure and some discomfort. Explain that measures will be taken to avoid exposure and embarrassment. The more relaxed the patient is, the easier it will be to insert the catheter.

The most common patient position for catheter insertion is the dorsal recumbent position, with the patient preferably on a solid surface, such as a firm mattress or a treatment table. Catheterizing a patient in a bed with a soft mattress, especially a female patient, is not as satisfactory because the patient's pelvic surfaces are not firmly supported and visualization of the meatus is difficult. Also, the patient may sink into the bed, causing the bladder to be lower than the outlet of the catheter. If the patient is in bed, supporting the buttocks on a firm cushion is helpful.

The Sims, or lateral, position is an alternate position for catheter insertion in female patients. This position may allow better visualization and be more comfortable for the patient, especially if hip and knee movements are difficult. The smaller area of exposure is also less stressful for the patient. Allow the patient to lie on either side, depending on which position is easiest for the nurse and best for the patient's comfort. Place the patient's buttocks near the edge of the bed with her shoulders at the opposite edge and her knees drawn toward her chest. Lift the upper buttock and labia to expose the urinary meatus (Fig. 37-12).

URETHRAL CATHETER INSERTION

Nurses are responsible for inserting indwelling catheters and caring for the patient. Skill 37-5 describes Catheterizing the Female Urinary Bladder, and Skill 37-6 describes Catheterizing the Male Urinary Bladder. Adhering to surgical asepsis is of utmost importance to help prevent urinary tract infections. An inflated balloon holds the indwelling catheter in position in the bladder. The prefilled syringe included in the catheter kit contains the amount of sterile water needed to inflate the balloon to the desired spherical shape. It is important to use the entire amount provided by the manufacturer to avoid under inflation of the catheter balloon. A balloon that is only partially inflated could cause irritation and erosion to the mucosa in the bladder.

The practice of inserting an indwelling catheter in a male patient just until there is urine return is also no longer recommended. Indwelling catheters for male patients should be inserted to the catheter bifurcation to avoid inadvertent inflation of the balloon in the urethra. In addition, the technique of applying lubricant to the catheter before inserting it in a male patient is not recommended. Lubricant applied externally to the catheter remains at the meatus, essentially allowing an

FIGURE 37-12. Demonstration of the side-lying position (*left*) and of how to expose the urinary meatus when catheterizing a female patient in the side-lying position (*right*).

unlubricated catheter to cause trauma to the lining of the urethra. Currently, the recommendation is to gently insert the tip of a syringe prefilled with lubricant into the male urethra before inserting the catheter (see Skill 37-6). If the prepackaged kit does not contain a syringe with lubricant, the nurse may need assistance in filling a syringe while keeping the lubricant sterile. Some institutions use lidocaine jelly for lubrication before insertion of the catheter. The jelly comes prepackaged in a sterile syringe and serves a dual purpose of lubricating and numbing the urethra. A medical order is necessary for the use of lidocaine jelly.

An indwelling catheter must be properly secured to prevent injury and friction and the indwelling catheter is connected to a drainage and collection system that must be properly positioned and secured to minimize the risk for infection. The following technique is used to complete the closed urinary drainage system:

- Check to see that the patient is not lying on the drainage tubing and compressing it.
- Keep the catheter drainage bag below the level of the bladder at all times.
- Keep the drainage bag off the floor at all times to reduce the risk of infection. The floor is grossly contaminated.
- Check that all connections are secure and that no leakage is occurring.

See the accompanying Through the Eyes of a Student for a student's account of their experience with urinary catheterization.

CARING FOR PATIENTS WITH AN INDWELLING CATHETER

The following are nursing measures used to care for patients with an indwelling catheter:

- Wash hands before and after caring for a patient with an indwelling catheter.
- Clean the perineal area thoroughly, especially around the meatus, daily and after each bowel movement.
- Cleanse the catheter by cleaning gently from the meatus outward.
- Use mild soap and water or a perineal cleanser to clean the perineal area; rinse the area well. Do not use powders and lotions after cleaning. Do not use antibiotic or other antimicrobial cleaners or Betadine at the urethral meatus (Society of Urologic Nurses and Associates [SUNA], 2005a).
- Make sure that the patient maintains a generous fluid intake, unless contraindicated by other health concerns. This helps prevent infection and irrigates the catheter naturally by increasing urine output.
- Encourage the patient to be up and about, as ordered.
- Note the volume and character of urine, and record observations carefully. Observe the urine through the drainage tubing and in the collecting container. Note and record the amount of urine on the patient's intake-and-output record every 8 hours. The collecting container is calibrated, but the volume markings are only approximations. Empty the urine into a graduated container that is calibrated accurately for correct determination of output.
- Do not open the drainage system to obtain urine specimens or to measure urine. If the tubing becomes disconnected and the sterile closed drainage system has been compromised, replace the collecting system (SUNA, 2005a). Wipe the end of the catheter with antiseptic solution before connecting it to the new system. When emptying the drainage bag, make sure the drainage spout does not touch a contaminated surface.

Through the Eyes of a Student

Remembering my first hospital experiences, I would have to say that doing my first catheterization was the scariest. I was working with a nurse on the maternity floor. Our patient had not voided in more than 8 hours and seemed to be in great discomfort. We palpated her abdomen to see if her bladder was distended, and it was. Because she didn't have an urge to void, we decided to straight cath her to lessen her discomfort. The nurse I was working with turned and handed me the kit. She said, "You know what to do, right?" Automatically I replied, "Sure."

My heart began to race. Of course, I knew the procedure, but I never actually did it on a real person. Not only was I nervous about doing the procedure, but I also didn't want to make her labor more painful. The nurse, out of courtesy, asked the patient if she minded if I did the procedure. Thank God, the patient had a soft side for a beginner. Smiling, she looked at me and said, "You know what you're doing, right?" Again, I said, "Sure." I began setting up to begin my mission. To my amazement, I really did remember how to prepare for a catheterization. I even

was amazed that my sterile procedure wasn't bad for the first time. When it was time to insert the catheter, I took a deep breath. Thankfully, it went in nice and smooth, and I reached the bladder in seconds. The urine began flowing through rapidly. It seemed like it would never stop. Amazingly, it filled the container. I removed the catheter, cleaned up, and let out my breath.

In summary, I was glad that I had the experience to do a catheterization. The nurse told me that I did a good job, which made me feel good. Also, my patient thanked me for relieving some of her discomfort and gave me a reassuring smile. As I look back now, it wasn't as bad as I had myself believed it would be. Even though it's invasive to the patient, sometimes it's necessary. I want to do everything I can to help my patients. Now, I look at all my new adventures as helping my patients feel better.

—*Alysia Paxson*
Holy Family College, Philadelphia

- Teach the patient the importance of personal hygiene, especially the importance of careful cleaning after having a bowel movement and thorough, frequent hand hygiene.
- Promptly report any signs or symptoms of infection. These include a burning sensation and irritation at the meatus, cloudy urine, a strong odor to the urine, an elevated temperature, and chills.
- Help the patient take a tub or shower bath if possible. Remember to keep the collecting bag lower than the bladder to promote drainage.
- Change indwelling catheters only as necessary. Refer to manufacturers' recommendations (Toughill, 2005). The interval between catheter changes varies and should be individualized for the patient, based on clinical symptoms: catheter encrustations, leakage, bleeding, and catheter-associated UTIs (SUNA, 2005a).

PATIENT EDUCATION

Teach patients who have an indwelling catheter how the system functions and how they can assist with their care. Teaching points include keeping the tubing free of kinks, maintaining a constant downward flow of urine, maintaining an adequate fluid intake, and promptly reporting any unusual symptoms.

If the patient is ambulatory, connect the indwelling catheter to a smaller drainage bag that can be secured to the leg. Instruct the patient to do the following:

- Empty the leg bag at regular intervals. A full drainage bag may cause reflux of urine into the bladder or may pull away from its attachment on the leg.
- Wash hands before and after emptying the leg bag. Use an antiseptic solution to cleanse the connections.

- Care for the drainage bag daily, using a vinegar solution (1 part vinegar to 3 parts water). Clean the tubing and bag and allow to air dry before using again (SUNA, 2005a).

IRRIGATING THE INDWELLING CATHETER OR BLADDER

The flushing of a tube, canal, or area with solution is called irrigation. Natural irrigation of the catheter through increased fluid intake by the patient is preferred. The purpose of an external catheter irrigation is to restore or maintain its patency. A bladder irrigation rinses out the bladder and can also instill medication that acts directly on the bladder wall. Routine intermittent irrigation of long-term catheters is not recommended (SUNA, 2005a). Catheter irrigation should be avoided unless necessary to relieve or prevent obstruction. Skill 37-7 describes the procedure to perform an intermittent irrigation for an indwelling catheter using a closed system.

Continuous or frequent irrigations may be ordered when a blood clot or other debris threatens to block the catheter. Closed system irrigation is recommended to prevent the introduction of pathogens into the bladder. Preferably, the patient who needs frequent irrigation so that the catheter and tubing remain patent will have a triple-lumen catheter using continuous irrigation (Fig. 37-13). Skill 37-8 describes continuous bladder irrigation.

REMOVING THE INDWELLING CATHETER

The removal of an indwelling catheter and the aftercare of the patient should include the following nursing measures:

- Wash hands before and after the procedure and wear gloves.
- Deflate the balloon before attempting to remove the catheter by inserting a syringe into the balloon valve

FIGURE 37-13. A continuous bladder irrigation (CBI) setup.

Labels on figure:
- Irrigation bag
- Drip chamber
- Clamp
- Bladder
- Tubing to irrigation port
- Port for inflation of catheter balloon
- Drainage bag
- Tubing from bladder

and aspirating all of the sterile water used to inflate it. Do not cut the tubing with scissors.

- Ask the patient to take several deep breaths to relax while you gently remove the catheter. Wrap the catheter in a towel or disposable waterproof drape.
- Clean the perineal area after the catheter is removed.
- Ensure that the patient's fluid intake is generous, and record the patient's fluid intake as well as time and amount of fluid output for at least 24 hours (or according to agency policy) following catheter removal. Instruct the patient to void into the bedpan or urinal. If patient does not void within 8 to 10 hours of removal of the indwelling catheter, notify the primary care provider.
- Inform the patient that it may take a little while for the bladder to reestablish voluntary control and that an accident now is not unusual.

- Tell the patient that there may be a slight burning sensation when voiding the first one or two times after catheter removal.
- Observe the urine carefully for any abnormalities.
- Record and report any unusual signs or symptoms, such as discomfort, a burning sensation when voiding, bleeding, or changes in vital signs, especially the patient's temperature. Be alert to any signs or symptoms of infection, and report them promptly.

Caring for a Patient With a Urologic Stent

When a patient has a urinary tract obstruction, a urologic stent may be inserted. The stent may be temporary (when placed in the ureters) or permanent (when positioned in the urethra). Temporary stents are usually made of a pliable material such as radiopaque silicone. Permanent stents are stronger and typically are made of a flexible metal mesh. They are commonly inserted during a cystoscopic procedure, and in most cases, the patient receives only a local anesthetic and sedation. Urologic stents relieve urinary obstructions and provide a path for the flow of urine. Major nursing responsibilities include assessment, measurement, and documentation of urinary output. Never irrigate a blocked stent. Instruct the patient with a urologic stent to notify the primary care provider immediately if the urine becomes bright red, severe pain occurs, the drainage pattern changes, or any sign of infection is present. Also, encourage the patient to wear a medical alert bracelet at all times.

Caring for a Patient With a Urinary Diversion

Obstructions or tumors in the urinary tract may require some patients to have urinary flow diverted surgically. An **ileal conduit** is a cutaneous urinary diversion. An ileal conduit involves a surgical resection of the small intestine, with transplantation of the ureters to the isolated segment of small bowel. This separated section of the small intestine is then brought to the abdominal wall, where urine is excreted through a stoma, a surgically created opening on the body surface. Figure 37-14 shows how the ureters are diverted in an ileal conduit. Such diversions are usually permanent, and the patient wears an external appliance to collect the urine because elimination of the urine from the stoma cannot be controlled voluntarily.

Another option is a continent urostomy (e.g., the Kock continent ileal reservoir). This is a surgical alternative that uses a section of the intestine to create an internal reservoir that holds urine. The external stoma or outlet must be catheterized at regular intervals to drain the urine that has collected in this reservoir.

Another type of surgical intervention is the Mitrofanoff procedure. The bladder neck is closed, and the appendix is used to gain access to the bladder from the skin surface. One end of the appendix is brought to the skin surface and used as a stoma; the other end is tunneled into the bladder (Smeltzer et al., 2010). The patient must intermittently

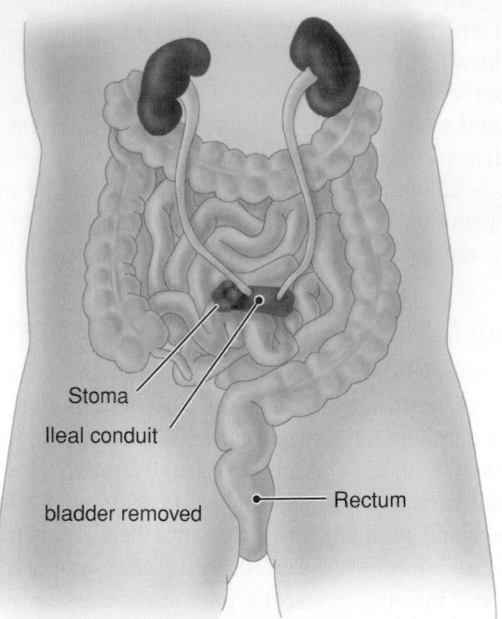

FIGURE 37-14. Location of an ileal conduit. The ureters are brought to the separated segment of the ileum of the small intestine and a stoma is made where the urine is excreted.

catheterize the bladder via the stoma. This type of diversion allows patients who normally could not intermittently catheterize themselves through the urethra to provide self-care. It also helps to decrease the embarrassment associated with needing a second person to perform the catheterization.

GENERAL CARE GUIDELINES

Creation of a urinary diversion is a surgical procedure. Therefore, the patient needs physical and psychological support before and after surgery. This support can come from the patient's significant others, as well as from members of the healthcare team and from people who have had similar experiences. The ostomy created for the diversion requires specific physical care for which the nurse is initially responsible. The following guidelines help to promote the patient's physical and psychological comfort:

- Inspect the patient's stoma regularly. It should be dark pink to red and moist (Fig. 37-15). A pale stoma may indicate anemia, and a dark or purple-blue stoma may reflect compromised circulation or ischemia. Bleeding around the stoma and its stem should be minimal. Notify the primary care provider promptly if bleeding persists or is excessive or if color changes occur in the stoma.
- Note the size of the stoma, which usually stabilizes within 6 to 8 weeks. Most stomas protrude 1/2″ to 1″ from the abdominal surface and may initially appear swollen and edematous. The edema usually subsides after 6 weeks. If an abdominal dressing is in place over the

surgical incision, check it frequently for drainage and bleeding. The dressing is usually removed after 24 hours.
- Keep the skin around the stoma site (peristomal area) clean and dry. If care is not taken to protect the skin around the stoma, irritation or infection may occur. A leaking appliance frequently causes skin erosion. Candida or yeast infections can also occur around the stoma if the area is not kept dry.
- Measure the patient's fluid intake and output. Careful monitoring of the patient's urinary output is necessary to detect fluid imbalances and adequate functioning of diversion.
- Keep the patient as free of odors as possible. Empty the appliance frequently.
- Monitor the return of intestinal function and peristalsis. Initially after surgery, peristalsis is inhibited. Remember, the patient had a bowel resection as part of the urinary diversion procedure.
- If the patient has an ileal conduit, mucus may appear in the urine as a normal finding because the isolated segment of small intestine continues to produce mucous, as part of its normal functioning.
- Explain each aspect of care to the patient and explain what his or her role will be when he or she begins self-care. Patient teaching is one of the most important aspects of care and should include family members when appropriate. Teaching can begin before surgery so that the patient has adequate time to absorb information.
- Encourage the patient to participate in care and to look at the stoma. Patients normally experience emotional depression during the early postoperative period. Help

FIGURE 37-15. The appearance of a normal stoma is red and smooth with a mucous membrane surface.

the patient to cope by listening, explaining, and being available and supportive. A visit from a representative of the local ostomy support group may be helpful. Patients usually begin to accept their altered body image when they are willing to look at the stoma, make neutral or positive statements concerning the ostomy, and express interest in learning self-care.

EXTERNAL APPLIANCES

With an ileal conduit, the external appliance to collect the urine is typically a soft pouch that is either reusable or disposable. The upper part of the pouch has a firm faceplate several inches in diameter, with an opening the size of the stoma. Some faceplates are detachable from the pouch, while other appliances are one piece. The plate surface is secured firmly around the stoma opening with a moisture-proof adherent so that no urine leakage occurs. Many patients also wear an elasticized belt that goes around the waist and connects to each side of the faceplate for added support. The lower end of the pouch has a drainage valve, which is used for emptying.

The patient needs to empty the pouch frequently. This is to prevent the pouch from becoming heavy with the weight of urine, causing tension on the faceplate, and possibly loosening the seal. For most people, this means emptying the appliance several times a day. The pouch can also be attached to drainage tubing and a large collection bag to avoid having to frequently empty the appliance, such as during the night or when confined to bed. In home situations, urine collection tubing and receptacles designed to be placed under the bed can be used at night.

URINARY APPLIANCE APPLICATION AND REMOVAL

The frequency of changing the appliance depends on the type being used. The appliance usually is changed after a time of low fluid intake, such as in the early morning. Urine production is less at this time, making changing the appliance easier. Skill 37-9 describes how to change an appliance worn over an ileal conduit.

PATIENT EDUCATION

Patient education is essential for independence in self-care. As the patient assumes responsibility for self-care, teach the patient how to make the necessary observations, to be aware of indications of problems, and to recognize when to seek assistance. For these goals to be met, the patient needs to be able to do the following:

- Explain the reason for the urinary diversion and the rationale for treatment.
- Demonstrate self-care behaviors that effectively manage the diversion.
- Describe follow-up care and existing support resources.
- Report where supplies may be obtained in the community.
- Verbalize related fears and concerns.
- Demonstrate a positive body image.

The assistance of a wound, ostomy, and continence nurse (WOCN) can help the patient achieve these outcomes. Also, refer the patient to the United Ostomy Association for further information and helpful periodicals.

Caring for a Patient Receiving Dialysis

Dialysis is used to treat patients who experience severely decreased or total loss of kidney function. Dialysis is a mechanical way of filtering waste from the blood. There are two categories of dialysis: hemodialysis and peritoneal dialysis.

Hemodialysis involves a machine that does the work healthy kidneys normally perform by filtering harmful wastes, electrolytes, and fluid from the blood that would normally be eliminated in the patient's urine. Patients receive a vascular access. This vascular access, an arteriovenous (AV) fistula (a surgically created connection between an artery and a vein) or AV graft (a surgically created path between an artery and a vein using a flexible, synthetic tube) allows for easy access to the bloodstream. It is the point where blood is removed from the patient's body for dialysis and then returned (Mayo, 2008).

Peritoneal dialysis involves using blood vessels in the abdominal lining (peritoneum) to fill in for your kidneys, with the help of a fluid (dialysate) washed in and out of the peritoneal space. Patients receive a catheter (a thin, soft plastic tube) surgically placed through the abdomen into the peritoneal cavity. It is used to carry the dialysis solution in and out of the patient's abdomen (Mayo, 2008a).

Care of either catheter site is a nursing responsibility. Care involves assessment of the catheter sites. Skill 37-10 outlines nursing care related to caring for a hemodialysis access. Refer to Skill 37-11 for nursing care related to caring for a patient with a peritoneal dialysis catheter.

Evaluating

The nurse evaluates the effectiveness of a plan of care to promote healthy urinary functioning by checking whether the patient has met the individualized patient goals specified in the plan. See the Nursing Plan of Care 37-1 for Mrs. Jaspers. Nursing care is considered effective if the patient expresses satisfaction with the regular voiding pattern and is able to:

- Produce a sufficient quantity of urine to maintain fluid, electrolyte, and acid–base balance
- Empty the bladder completely at regular intervals without discomfort
- Provide care for urinary diversion and know when to notify the physician
- Develop a plan to modify any factors that contribute to current urinary problems or that might impair urinary functioning in the future
- Correct unhealthy urinary habits, such as delaying voiding, drinking insufficient fluids, or abusing diuretics

NURSING PLAN OF CARE • 37-1

For Elana Jaspers

Mrs. Elana Jaspers is an alert, 83-year-old woman whose husband of 59 years died 6 months ago. Although Mrs. Jaspers was adamant about wanting to live independently in her own home, arthritis severely restricted her movement and ability to manage. After a hospitalization for pneumonia, she was transferred to a nursing home 1 month ago. The admitting medical diagnoses included hypertension, osteoarthritis, and depression. A comprehensive nursing assessment of Mrs. Jaspers performed 1 month after her admission to the nursing home included the following notations:

- Continent of urine on admission
- At present, incontinent of urine one or two times a day; often found wet in the morning; states it is "too much bother to get into the bathroom"
- Sits in chair in room unless encouraged and assisted to walk, although capable of independent ambulation with care; progressive muscle atrophy and joint stiffness
- No identifiable pathology underlying incontinence
- Medications include a diuretic for hypertension and a tricyclic antidepressant
- Reddened skin in the perineal area

NURSING DIAGNOSIS   Functional Urinary Incontinence related to difficult transition to nursing home and mobility deficit as manifested by incontinence of urine one or two times a day; feeling toileting is too much bother; mobility deficits secondary to osteoarthritis; diuretic and antidepressant therapy.

EXPECTED OUTCOME   By the next monthly assessment, 5/1/12, the patient will:

- Verbalize the importance of getting to bathroom or toilet when she first feels the need to void.

Nursing Interventions	Rationale	Evaluative Statement
Assess the value the patient attaches to voluntary control of urination and urinary continence; counsel appropriately.	Unless the patient is committed to the plan of care, goal achievement is impossible.	5/1/12 Outcome partially met. Patient has commented on the importance of regular toileting but still finds this "too much trouble" some days.
Teach the importance of complete bladder emptying at regular intervals and the harmful effects of ignoring the urge to void.	Patient understanding of the causes and harmful effects of urinary incontinence may motivate desire for reestablishment of voluntary control.	*Revision:* Reinforce value. *D. Mora, RN*
Assess patient's normal voiding habits at home and assist her to reestablish these. Initial reminders to toilet herself may be necessary.	Respect for the patient's normal voiding schedule and patterns communicates nursing's sincere concern for the individual and encourages patient achievement of goals.	

EXPECTED OUTCOME   By the next monthly assessment, 5/1/12, the patient will:

- Demonstrate the ability to walk to the bathroom using cane to toilet herself.

(continued)

NURSING PLAN OF CARE · 37-1

For Elana Jaspers (continued)

Nursing Interventions	Rationale	Evaluative Statement
Assess the patient's ability to toilet herself independently. Work consistently with her to increase activity tolerance: encourage short walks throughout the day to increase mobility.	One response to experiencing the multiple losses associated with aging is to surrender all control and become increasingly dependent. Nonpathology-based incontinence is less likely to occur if the daily living of the person keeps her more mobile, flexible, oriented, and motivated. An older person who seeks to take control and has a positive self-image is more continent.	5/1/12 Outcome met. Patient can safely walk to bathroom using cane and toilet herself when she wants to. *D. Mora, RN*
Refer patient to occupational therapy for assistance with diagnosis and treatment if necessary.	The specialized skills of the occupational therapist may facilitate relearning toileting skills.	5/1/12 Outcome not met. Patient repeatedly neglects a.m. perineal care.
Communicate clearly that the patient is expected to use the toilet to urinate. Refrain from using incontinent briefs or pads. Talk with family about patient's having sufficient undergarments to allow changes as needed until control is reestablished.	Understanding that the staff expects continence and is committed to working with the patient to achieve it is a powerful patient motivator.	*Revision:* Reteach both the importance and procedure of perineal care. Assess each a.m. *D. Mora, RN*
Assess patient's motivation and ability to be clean, dry, and comfortable.	Patient may not understand how easily skin irritation can occur and danger of pressure ulcers.	
Teach perineal hygiene.	Keeping the perineal area clean and dry promotes intact skin around the urinary meatus and the perineal area. Proper hygiene measures also decrease the possibility of bacteria or organisms migrating into the bladder.	

EXPECTED OUTCOME   By the next monthly assessment, 5/1/12, the patient will:

• Decrease urinary incontinent episodes to less than three or four per week

(continued)

NURSING PLAN OF CARE · 37-1

For Elana Jaspers (continued)

Nursing Interventions	Rationale	Evaluative Statement
Communicate to patient that the nurses *care* about her reestablishing urinary continence and believe she can do this. Use verbal reinforcement to reward "dry" days.	A common feeling of recently institutionalized elderly people is *abandonment* and the sense that no one cares; response: "Why should I?" Communicating that the patient's progress toward goal achievement is valued by the nurses is an excellent encouragement to continue progress.	5/1/12 Outcome met. Patient in last week was completely dry for 4 of 7 days. Recorded four incontinent episodes.

D. Mora, RN |
| Chart incontinent episodes and monitor progress; discuss this with patient. | This records progress with incontinent episodes and provides positive reinforcement. | |

NURSING DIAGNOSIS	Impaired Skin Integrity related to functional urinary incontinence as manifested by reddened perineal area (skin still intact)
EXPECTED OUTCOME	By the next monthly assessment, 5/1/12, the patient will:
	• Demonstrate healing of reddened perineal area

Nursing Interventions	Rationale	Evaluative Statement
Assess skin for breakdown each a.m. and p.m. and after each incontinent episode.	Perineal care is often neglected or assigned to the least trained personnel in care settings. Skin irritation not detected and treated early may progress to serious pressure ulcers.	5/1/12 Outcome partially met. Perineal area is less inflamed. *Revision:* Continue to monitor perineal hygiene. No need for protective ointment.

D. Mora, RN |
| Teach the patient the importance of washing this area carefully with soap and water each a.m. and after incontinent episodes. Teach the importance of always cleaning and wiping the perineum from front to back to prevent autoinfection. Until incontinent episodes are eliminated, a protective waterproof ointment may be indicated. | The woman who is doing self-care may neglect it entirely or use incorrect technique. | |
| Encourage use of cotton underwear and avoidance of nylon pantyhose, girdles, tight-fitting pants. | Nylon products tend to hold moisture and may minimize airflow to the perineal area. | |

SAMPLE DOCUMENTATION	4/3/12 Nursing
	This a.m., after an incontinent episode, Mrs. Jaspers began to talk about how hard it is to get adjusted to living here, and commented, "I feel like just giving up." We talked about the importance of being as independent as possible and the dangers of becoming passively dependent. Nursing teaching and counseling included values of independently adhering to usual toileting schedule and importance of perineal hygiene. Two hours later, after lunch, Mrs. Jaspers walked to bathroom and toileted herself. Progress with urinary incontinence will continue to be monitored. Ability definitely present but encouragement needed.
	D. Mora, RN

Skill · 37-1   Assessing Bladder Volume Using an Ultrasound Bladder Scanner

EQUIPMENT

- Bladder scanner
- Ultrasound gel or bladder scan gel pad
- Alcohol wipe or other sanitizer recommended by the scanner manufacturer and/or facility policy
- Clean gloves
- Additional PPE, as indicated
- Paper towel or washcloth

IMPLEMENTATION

ACTION	RATIONALE
1. Review the patient's chart for any limitations in physical activity.	Physical limitations may require adaptations in performing the skill.
2. Bring the bladder scanner and other necessary equipment to the bedside.	Bringing everything to the bedside conserves time and energy. Arranging items nearby is convenient, saves time, and avoids unnecessary stretching and twisting of muscles on the part of the nurse.
3. Perform hand hygiene and put on PPE, if indicated.	Hand hygiene and PPE prevent the spread of microorganisms. PPE is required based on transmission precautions.
4. Identify the patient.	Identifying the patient ensures the right patient receives the intervention and helps prevent errors.
5. Close curtains around bed and close door to room if possible. Discuss the procedure with the patient and assess patient's ability to assist with the procedure, as well as personal hygiene preferences.	This ensures the patient's privacy. This discussion promotes reassurance and provides knowledge about the procedure. Dialogue encourages patient participation and allows for individualized nursing care.
6. Adjust the bed to a comfortable working height, usually elbow height of the caregiver (VISN 8, 2009). Place the patient in a supine position. Drape patient. Stand on the patient's right side if you are right-handed, patient's left side if you are left-handed.	Having the bed at the proper height prevents back and muscle strain. Proper positioning allows accurate assessment of bladder volume. Keeping the patient covered as much as possible promotes patient comfort and privacy. Positioning allows for ease of use of dominant hand for the procedure.
7. Put on clean gloves.	Gloves prevent contact with blood and body fluids.
8. Press the "On" button. Wait until the device warms up. Press the "Scan" button to turn on the scanning screen.	Many devices require a few minutes to prepare the internal programs.
9. Press the appropriate gender button. The appropriate icon for male or female will appear on the screen (Figure 1).	The device must be programmed for the gender of the patient by pushing the correct button on the device. If a female patient has had a hysterectomy, the male button is pushed (Altschuler & Diaz, 2006).
10. Clean the scanner head with the appropriate cleaner (Figure 2).	Cleaning the scanner head deters transmission of microorganisms.

FIGURE 1. Identifying the icon for the patient's gender. *(Photo by B. Proud.)*

FIGURE 2. Cleaning scanner head. *(Photo by B. Proud.)*

(continued)

Skill · 37-1   Assessing Bladder Volume Using an Ultrasound Bladder Scanner *continued*

ACTION

11. **Gently palpate the patient's symphysis pubis. Place a generous amount of ultrasound gel or gel pad midline on the patient's abdomen, about 1″ to 1 1/2″ above the symphysis pubis (anterior midline junction of pubic bones) (Figure 3).**

RATIONALE

Palpation identifies the proper location and allows for correct placement of scanner head over the patient's bladder.

FIGURE 3. (**A**) Placing ultrasound gel about 1″ to 1 1/2″ above symphysis pubis. *(Photo by B. Proud.)* (**B**) Gel pad. (From Patraca, K. [2005]. Measure bladder volume without catheterization. *Nursing, 35*[4], 47.)

12. **Place the scanner head on the gel or gel pad, with the directional icon on the scanner head toward the patient's head. Aim the scanner head toward the bladder (point the scanner head slightly downward toward the coccyx) (Patraca, 2005). Press and release the "Scan" button (Figure 4).**

Proper placement allows for accurate reading of urine in bladder.

FIGURE 4. (**A**) Positioning the scanner head with directional icon toward the patient's head. (**B**) Pressing the scan button. *(Photos by B. Proud.)*

13. Observe the image on the scanner screen. **Adjust the scanner head to center the bladder image on the crossbars (Figure 5).**

This action allows for accurate reading of urine in bladder.

14. Press and hold the "Done" button until it beeps. Read the volume measurement on the screen. Print the results, if required, by pressing "Print."

This action provides for accurate documentation of reading.

ACTION

RATIONALE

Aiming icon

BladderScan

FIGURE 5. Centering the image on the crossbars. (From Patraca, K. [2005]. Measure bladder volume without catheterization. *Nursing, 35*[4], 47.)

ACTION	RATIONALE
15. Use a washcloth or paper towel to remove remaining gel from the patient's skin. Alternately, gently remove gel pad from patient's skin. Return the patient to a comfortable position. Remove your gloves and ensure that the patient is covered.	Removal of the gel promotes patient comfort. Removing contaminated gloves prevents spread of microorganisms.
16. Lower bed height and adjust head of bed to a comfortable position. Reattach call bell if necessary.	These actions promote patient safety.
17. Remove additional PPE, if used. Perform hand hygiene.	Removing PPE properly reduces the risk for infection transmission and contamination of other items. Hand hygiene prevents the spread of microorganisms.

DOCUMENTATION

Guidelines

Document the assessment data that led to the use of the bladder scanner, the urine volume measured, and the patient's response.

Sample Documentation

7/06/12 1130 Patient has not voided 8 hours post catheter removal. Patient denies feelings of discomfort, pressure, and pain. Bladder not palpable. Bladder scanned for 120 mL of urine. Patient encouraged to increase oral fluid intake to eight 6-oz. glasses today. Dr. Liu notified of assessment. Orders received to rescan in 4 hours if patient does not void.

—B. Clapp, RN

UNEXPECTED SITUATIONS AND ASSOCIATED INTERVENTIONS

• *Nurse presses wrong icon for patient's gender when initiating scanner:* Turn scanner off and back on. Reenter information using correct gender button.

• *Nurse has reason to believe bladder is full, based on assessment data, but scanner reveals little to no urine in bladder:* Ensure proper positioning of scanner head. Place a generous amount of ultrasound gel or gel pad midline on the patient's abdomen, about 1″ to 1 1/2″ above the symphysis pubis. Place the scanner head on the gel or gel pad, with the directional icon on the scanner head toward the patient's head. Aim the scanner head toward the bladder (point the scanner head slightly downward toward the coccyx). Ensure that the bladder image is centered on the crossbars.

Skill · 37-2 Assisting With the Use of a Bedpan

EQUIPMENT

- Bedpan (regular or fracture)
- Toilet tissue
- Disposable clean gloves
- Additional PPE, as indicated
- Cover for bedpan or urinal (disposable waterproof pad or cover)

IMPLEMENTATION

ACTION	RATIONALE
1. Review the patient's chart for any limitations in physical activity.	Activity limitations may contraindicate certain actions by the patient.
2. Bring bedpan and other necessary equipment to the bedside stand or overbed table.	Bringing everything to the bedside conserves time and energy. Arranging items nearby is convenient, saves time, and avoids unnecessary stretching and twisting of muscles on the part of the nurse.
3. Perform hand hygiene and put on PPE, if indicated.	Hand hygiene and PPE prevent the spread of microorganisms. PPE is required based on transmission precautions.
4. Identify the patient.	Identifying the patient ensures the right patient receives the intervention and helps prevent errors.
5. Close curtains around bed and close door to room if possible. Discuss the procedure with the patient and assess the patient's ability to assist with the procedure, as well as personal hygiene preferences.	This ensures the patient's privacy. This discussion promotes reassurance and provides knowledge about the procedure. Dialogue encourages patient participation and allows for individualized nursing care.
6. Unless contraindicated, apply powder to the rim of the bedpan. Place bedpan and cover on chair next to bed. Put on gloves.	Powder helps keep the bedpan from sticking to the patient's skin and makes it easier to remove. Powder is not applied if the patient has respiratory problems or is allergic to powder or if a urine specimen is needed (could contaminate the specimen). The bedpan on the chair allows for easy access. Gloves prevent contact with blood and body fluids.
7. Adjust bed to comfortable working height, usually elbow height of the caregiver (VISN 8, 2009). Place the patient in a supine position, with the head of the bed elevated about 30 degrees, unless contraindicated.	Having the bed at the proper height prevents back and muscle strain. Supine position is necessary for correct placement of patient on bedpan.
8. Fold top linen back just enough to allow placement of bedpan. If there is no waterproof pad on the bed and time allows, consider placing a waterproof pad under patient's buttocks before placing bedpan.	Folding back the linen in this manner minimizes unnecessary exposure while still allowing the nurse to place the bedpan. The waterproof pad will protect the bed should there be a spill.
9. Ask the patient to bend the knees. Have the patient lift his or her hips upward. Assist patient, if necessary, by placing your hand that is closest to the patient palm up, under the lower back, and assist with lifting. Slip the bedpan into place with other hand (Figure 1).	The nurse uses less energy when the patient can assist by placing some of his or her weight on the heels.
10. **Ensure that bedpan is in proper position and patient's buttocks are resting on the rounded shelf of the regular bedpan or the shallow rim of the fracture bedpan.**	Having the bedpan in the proper position prevents spills onto the bed, ensures patient comfort, and prevents injury to the skin from a misplaced bedpan.
11. Raise head of bed as near to sitting position as tolerated, unless contraindicated. Cover the patient with bed linens.	This position makes it easier for the patient to void or defecate, avoids strain on the patient's back, and allows gravity to aid in elimination. Covering promotes warmth and privacy.
12. **Place call bell and toilet tissue within easy reach. Place the bed in the lowest position.** Leave patient if it is safe to do so. Use side rails appropriately (Figure 2).	Falls can be prevented if the patient does not have to reach for items he or she needs. Placing the bed in the lowest position promotes patient safety. Leaving patient alone, if possible, promotes self-esteem and shows respect for privacy. Side rails assist the patient in repositioning.
13. Remove gloves and additional PPE, if used. Perform hand hygiene.	Proper removal of PPE prevents transmission of microorganisms. Hand hygiene deters the spread of microorganisms.

FIGURE 1. Assisting patient to raise self in bed to position the bedpan. *(Note: Covers should only be folded back just enough to work, not expose patient unnecessarily. Covers in this series of photos have been pulled back to show action.)*

FIGURE 2. Placing call bell within patient's reach and handing patient toilet tissue.

ACTION	RATIONALE

Removing the Bedpan

14. Perform hand hygiene and put on gloves and additional PPE, as indicated. Adjust bed to comfortable working height, usually elbow height of the caregiver (VISN 8, 2009). Have a receptacle, such as plastic trash bag, handy for discarding tissue.

Hand hygiene deters the spread of microorganisms. Gloves prevent exposure to blood and body fluids. Having the bed at the proper height prevents back and muscle strain. Proper disposal of soiled tissue prevents transmission of microorganisms.

15. Lower the head of the bed, if necessary, to about 30 degrees. Remove bedpan in the same manner in which it was offered, being careful to hold it steady. Ask the patient to bend the knees and lift the buttocks up from the bedpan. Assist patient, if necessary, by placing your hand that is closest to the patient palm up, under the lower back, and assist with lifting. Place the bedpan on the bedside chair and cover it.

Holding the bedpan steady prevents spills. The nurse uses less energy when the patient can assist by placing some of his or her weight on the heels. Covering the bedpan helps to prevent the spread of microorganisms.

16. If patient needs assistance with hygiene, wrap tissue around the hand several times, and wipe patient clean, using one stroke from the pubic area toward the anal area. Discard tissue, and use more until patient is clean. Place patient on his or her side and spread buttocks to clean anal area.

Cleaning area from front to back minimizes fecal contamination of the vagina and urinary meatus. Cleaning the patient after he or she has used the bedpan prevents offensive odors and irritation to the skin.

17. Do not place toilet tissue in the bedpan if a specimen is required or if output is being recorded. Place toilet tissue in appropriate receptacle.

Mixing toilet tissue with a specimen makes laboratory examination more difficult and interferes with accurate output measurement.

18. Return the patient to a comfortable position. Make sure the linens under the patient are dry. Replace or remove pad under the patient as necessary. Remove your gloves and ensure that the patient is covered.

Positioning helps to promote patient comfort. Removing contaminated gloves prevents spread of microorganisms.

19. Raise side rail. Lower bed height and adjust head of bed to a comfortable position. Reattach call bell.

These actions promote patient safety.

20. Offer patient supplies to wash and dry his or her hands, assisting as necessary.

Washing hands after using the urinal helps prevent the spread of microorganisms.

21. Put on clean gloves. Empty and clean the bedpan, measuring urine in graduated container, as necessary. Discard trash receptacle with used toilet paper per facility policy.

Gloves prevent exposure to blood and body fluids. Cleaning reusable equipment helps prevent the spread of microorganisms.

22. Remove additional PPE, if used. Perform hand hygiene.

Removing PPE properly reduces the risk for infection transmission and contamination of other items. Hand hygiene prevents the spread of microorganisms.

(continued)

Skill · 37-2   Assisting With the Use of a Bedpan   *continued*

DOCUMENTATION

Guidelines

Document the patient's tolerance of the activity. Record the amount of urine voided on the intake and output record, if appropriate. Document any other assessments, such as unusual urine characteristics or alterations in the patient's skin.

Sample Documentation

> 12/06/12 0730 Patient placed on fracture bedpan with a 2-person assist. Voided 400 mL dark yellow urine, strong odor noted. Specimen sent for urinalysis as ordered.
>
> —S. Barnes, RN

SPECIAL CONSIDERATIONS

- A fracture bedpan is usually more comfortable for the patient, but it does not hold as large a volume as the regular bedpan.
- Bedpan should not be left in place for extended periods of time as this can result in excessive pressure and irritation to the patient's skin.

Skill · 37-3   Assisting With the Use of a Urinal

EQUIPMENT

- Urinal with end cover (usually attached)
- Toilet tissue
- Clean gloves
- Additional PPE, as indicated

IMPLEMENTATION

ACTION	RATIONALE
1. Review the patient's chart for any limitations in physical activity.	Activity limitations may contraindicate certain actions by the patient.
2. Bring urinal and other necessary equipment to the bedside stand or overbed table.	Bringing everything to the bedside conserves time and energy. Arranging items nearby is convenient, saves time, and avoids unnecessary stretching and twisting of muscles on the part of the nurse.
3. Perform hand hygiene and put on PPE, if indicated.	Hand hygiene and PPE prevent the spread of microorganisms. PPE is required based on transmission precautions.
4. Identify the patient.	Identifying the patient ensures the right patient receives the intervention and helps prevent errors.
5. Close the curtains around the bed and close the door to the room if possible. Discuss procedure with patient and assess the patient's ability to assist with the procedure, as well as personal hygiene preferences.	This ensures the patient's privacy. This discussion promotes reassurance and provides knowledge about the procedure. Dialogue encourages patient participation and allows for individualized nursing care.
6. Put on gloves.	Gloves prevent exposure to blood and body fluids.
7. Assist the patient to an appropriate position as necessary: standing at the bedside, lying on one side or back, sitting in bed with the head elevated, or sitting on the side of the bed.	These positions facilitate voiding and emptying of the bladder.
8. If the patient remains in the bed, fold the linens just enough to allow for proper placement of the urinal.	Folding back the linen in this manner minimizes unnecessary exposure while still allowing the nurse to place the urinal.
9. If the patient is not standing, have him spread his legs slightly. **Hold the urinal close to the penis and position the penis completely within the urinal (Figure 1). Keep the bottom of the urinal lower than the penis. If necessary, assist the patient to hold the urinal in place.**	Slight spreading of the legs allows for proper positioning of the urinal. Placing penis completely within the urinal and keeping the bottom lower than the penis avoids urine spills.
10. Cover the patient with the bed linens.	Covering promotes warmth and privacy.

ACTION

RATIONALE

FIGURE 1. Positioning urinal in place for a male patient. (*Note: Covers should only be folded back just enough to work, not expose patient unnecessarily. Covers have been pulled back to show action.*)

11. Place call bell and toilet tissue within easy reach. Have a receptacle, such as plastic trash bag, handy for discarding tissue. Ensure the bed is in the lowest position. Leave patient if it is safe to do so. Use side rails appropriately.

Falls can be prevented if the patient does not have to reach for items he or she needs. Placing the bed in the lowest position promotes patient safety. Leaving patient alone, if possible, promotes self-esteem and shows respect for privacy. Side rails assist the patient in repositioning.

12. Remove gloves and additional PPE, if used. Perform hand hygiene.

Proper removal of PPE reduces transmission of microorganisms. Hand hygiene deters the spread of microorganisms.

Removing the Urinal

13. Perform hand hygiene. Put on gloves and additional PPE, as indicated.

Hand hygiene and PPE prevent the spread of microorganisms. Gloves prevent exposure to blood and body fluids. PPE is required based on transmission precautions.

14. Pull back the patient's bed linens just enough to remove the urinal. Remove the urinal. Cover the open end of the urinal. Place on the bedside chair. If patient needs assistance with hygiene, wrap tissue around the hand several times, and wipe patient clean. Place tissue in receptacle.

Covering the end helps to prevent the spread of microorganisms.

15. Return the patient to a comfortable position. Make sure the linens under the patient are dry. Remove your gloves and ensure that the patient is covered.

Proper positioning promotes patient comfort. Removing contaminated gloves prevents spread of microorganisms.

16. Ensure patient call bell is in reach.

Promotes patient safety.

17. Offer patient supplies to wash and dry his hands, assisting as necessary.

Washing hands after using the urinal helps prevent the spread of microorganisms.

18. Put on clean gloves. Empty and clean the urinal, measuring urine in graduated container, as necessary. Discard trash receptacle with used toilet paper per facility policy.

Measurement of urine volume is required for accurate intake and output records.

19. Remove gloves and additional PPE, if used and perform hand hygiene.

Gloves prevent exposure to blood and body fluids. Removing PPE properly reduces the risk for infection transmission and contamination of other items. Hand hygiene prevents the spread of microorganisms.

DOCUMENTATION

Guidelines

Document the patient's tolerance of the activity. Record the amount of urine voided on the intake and output record, if appropriate. Document any other assessments, such as unusual urine characteristics or alterations in the patient's skin.

(*continued*)

Skill · 37-3   Assisting With the Use of a Urinal *continued*

Sample Documentation

12/06/12 0730 Patient using urinal at bedside to void. Voided 600 mL yellow urine. Reinforced need for continued use of urinal for recording accurate output. Patient verbalized an understanding of instructions.

—S. Barnes, RN

SPECIAL CONSIDERATIONS

• Urinal should not be left in place for extended periods of time, as pressure and irritation to the patient's skin can result. If patient is unable to use alone or with assistance, consider other interventions, such as commode or external condom catheter.

• It may be necessary to assist patients who have difficulty holding urinal in place, such as those with limited upper extremity movement or alteration in mentation, to prevent spillage of urine.

• The urinal may also be used standing or sitting at the bedside or in the patient's bathroom, if patient is able to do so.

Skill · 37-4   Applying an External Condom Catheter

EQUIPMENT

• Condom sheath in appropriate size
• Skin protectant, such as 3M or Skin Prep
• Bath blanket
• Reusable leg bag with tubing or urinary drainage setup
• Basin of warm water and soap
• Disposable gloves
• Additional PPE, as indicated
• Washcloth and towel
• Scissors

IMPLEMENTATION

ACTION	RATIONALE
1. Bring necessary equipment to the bedside.	Bringing everything to the bedside conserves time and energy. Arranging items nearby is convenient, saves time, and avoids unnecessary stretching and twisting of muscles on the part of the nurse.
2. Perform hand hygiene and put on PPE, if indicated.	Hand hygiene and PPE prevent the spread of microorganisms. PPE is required based on transmission precautions.
3. Identify the patient.	Identifying the patient ensures the right patient receives the intervention and helps prevent errors.
4. Close curtains around bed and close door to room if possible. Discuss procedure with patient. Ask the patient if he has any allergies, especially to latex.	This ensures the patient's privacy. This discussion promotes reassurance and provides knowledge about the procedure. Dialogue encourages patient participation and allows for individualized nursing care. Some condom catheters are made of latex.
5. Adjust bed to comfortable working height, usually elbow height of the caregiver (VISN 8, 2009). Stand on the patient's right side if you are right-handed, patient's left side if you are left-handed.	Having the bed at the proper height prevents back and muscle strain. Positioning on one side allows for ease of use of dominant hand for catheter application.
6. Prepare urinary drainage setup or reusable leg bag for attachment to condom sheath.	Provides for an organized approach to the task.
7. Position patient on his back with thighs slightly apart. Drape patient so that only the area around the penis is exposed. Slide waterproof pad under patient.	Positioning allows access to site. Draping prevents unnecessary exposure and promotes warmth. The waterproof pad will protect bed linens from moisture.
8. Put on disposable gloves. Trim any long pubic hair that is in contact with penis.	Gloves prevent contact with blood and body fluids. Trimming pubic hair prevents pulling of hair by adhesive without the risk of infection associated with shaving.

ACTION	**RATIONALE**
9. Clean the genital area with washcloth, skin cleanser, and warm water. If patient is uncircumcised, retract foreskin and clean glans of penis. Replace foreskin. Clean the tip of the penis first, moving the washcloth in a circular motion from the meatus outward. Wash the shaft of the penis using downward strokes toward the pubic area. Rinse and dry. Remove gloves. Perform hand hygiene again.	Washing removes urine, secretions, and microorganisms. The penis must be clean and dry to minimize skin irritation. If the foreskin is left retracted, it may cause venous congestion in the glans of the penis, leading to edema.
10. Apply skin protectant to penis and allow to dry.	Skin protectant minimizes the risk of skin irritation from adhesive and moisture and increases adhesive's ability to adhere to skin.
11. Roll condom sheath outward onto itself. Grasp penis firmly with nondominant hand. **Apply condom sheath by rolling it onto penis with dominant hand (Figure 1). Leave 1″ to 2″ (2.5–5 cm) of space between tip of penis and end of condom sheath.**	Rolling the condom sheath outward allows for easier application. The space prevents irritation to tip of penis and allows free drainage of urine.
12. **Apply pressure to sheath at the base of penis for 10 to 15 seconds.**	Application of pressure ensures good adherence of adhesive with skin.
13. Connect condom sheath to drainage setup (Figure 2). Avoid kinking or twisting drainage tubing.	The collection device keeps the patient dry. Kinked tubing encourages backflow of urine.

FIGURE 1. Unrolling sheath onto penis.

FIGURE 2. Connecting condom sheath to drainage setup.

14. Remove gloves. Secure drainage tubing to the patient's inner thigh with Velcro leg strap or tape. Leave some slack in tubing for leg movement.	Proper attachment prevents tension on the sheath and potential inadvertent removal.
15. Assist the patient to a comfortable position. Cover the patient with bed linens. Place the bed in the lowest position.	Positioning and covering provide warmth and promote comfort. Bed in the lowest position promotes patient safety.
16. Secure drainage bag below the level of the bladder. Check that drainage tubing is not kinked and that movement of side rails does not interfere with the drainage bag.	This facilitates drainage of urine and prevents the backflow of urine.
17. Remove equipment. Remove gloves and additional PPE, if used. Perform hand hygiene.	Proper disposal of equipment prevents transmission of microorganisms. Removing PPE properly reduces the risk for infection transmission and contamination of other items. Hand hygiene prevents the spread of microorganisms.

DOCUMENTATION

Guidelines   Document the application of the condom catheter and the condition of the patient's skin. Record urine output on the intake and output record.

(continued)

Skill · 37-4   Applying an External Condom Catheter   *continued*

Sample Documentation

> 7/12/12 1910 Patient incontinent of urine; states, "It just comes too fast. I can't get to the bathroom in time." Perineal skin slightly reddened. Discussed rationale for use of condom catheter. Patient and wife agreeable to trying condom catheter. Medium-sized condom catheter applied. 200 mL of clear urine returned. Leg bag in place for daytime use. Patient verbalized understanding of need to call for assistance to empty drainage bag.
>
> —B. Clapp, RN

UNEXPECTED SITUATIONS AND ASSOCIATED INTERVENTIONS

- *Condom catheter leaks with every voiding:* Check size of condom catheter. If it is too big or too small, it may leak. Check space between tip of penis and end of condom sheath. If this space is too small, the urine has no place to go and will leak out.

- *Condom catheter will not stay on patient:* Ensure that condom catheter is correct size and that penis is thoroughly dried before applying condom catheter. Remind patient that condom catheter is in place, so that patient does not tug at tubing. If the patient has a retracted penis, a condom catheter may not be the best choice; there are pouches made for patients with a retracted penis.

- *When assessing patient's penis, nurse finds a break in skin integrity:* Do not reapply condom catheter. Allow skin to be open to air as much as possible. If institution has a wound, ostomy, and continence nurse, a consult would be appropriate.

Skill · 37-5   Catheterizing the Female Urinary Bladder

EQUIPMENT

- Sterile catheter kit that contains:
  - Sterile gloves
  - Sterile drapes (one of which is fenestrated [having a window-like opening])
  - Sterile catheter (use the smallest appropriate-size catheter, usually a 14F to 16F catheter with a 5- to 10-mL balloon [Mercer Smith, 2003; Newman, 2008]).
  - Antiseptic cleansing solution and cotton balls or gauze squares; antiseptic swabs
- Lubricant
- Forceps
- Prefilled syringe with sterile water (sufficient to inflate indwelling catheter balloon)
- Sterile basin (usually base of kit serves as this)
- Sterile specimen container (if specimen is required)
- Flashlight or lamp
- Waterproof disposable pad
- Sterile disposable urine collection bag and drainage tubing (may be connected to catheter in catheter kit)
- Velcro leg strap or tape
- Disposable gloves
- Additional PPE, as indicated
- Washcloth and warm water to perform perineal hygiene before and after catheterization

IMPLEMENTATION

ACTION	RATIONALE
1. Review the patient's chart for any limitations in physical activity. Confirm the medical order for indwelling catheter insertion.	Physical limitations may require adaptations in performing the skill. Verifying the medical order ensures that the correct intervention is administered to the right patient.
2. Bring the catheter kit and other necessary equipment to the bedside. Obtain assistance from another staff member, if necessary.	Bringing everything to the bedside conserves time and energy. Arranging items nearby is convenient, saves time, and avoids unnecessary stretching and twisting of muscles on the part of the nurse. Assistance from another person may be required to safely perform the intervention.
3. Perform hand hygiene and put on PPE, if indicated.	Hand hygiene and PPE prevent the spread of microorganisms. PPE is required based on transmission precautions.

ACTION

4. Identify the patient.

5. Close curtains around bed and close door to room if possible. Discuss procedure with the patient and assess patient's ability to assist with the procedure. Ask the patient if she has any allergies, especially to latex or iodine.

6. Provide good lighting. Artificial light is recommended (use of a flashlight requires an assistant to hold and position it). Place a trash receptacle within easy reach.

7. Adjust the bed to a comfortable working height, usually elbow height of the caregiver (VISN 8, 2009). Stand on the patient's right side if you are right-handed, patient's left side if you are left-handed.

8. Assist the patient to a dorsal recumbent position with knees flexed, feet about 2 feet apart, with her legs abducted. Drape patient (Figure 1). Alternately, the Sims', or lateral, position can be used. Place the patient's buttocks near the edge of the bed with her shoulders at the opposite edge and her knees drawn toward her chest (refer back to Figure 37-12). Allow the patient to lie on either side, depending on which position is easiest for the nurse and best for the patient's comfort. Slide waterproof pad under patient.

9. Put on clean gloves. Clean the perineal area with washcloth, skin cleanser, and warm water, using a different corner of the washcloth with each stroke. Wipe from above orifice downward toward sacrum (front to back). Rinse and dry. Remove gloves. Perform hand hygiene again.

10. Prepare urine drainage setup if a separate urine collection system is to be used. Secure to bed frame according to manufacturer's directions.

11. Open sterile catheterization tray on a clean overbed table using sterile technique.

RATIONALE

Identifying the patient ensures the right patient receives the intervention and helps prevent errors.

This ensures the patient's privacy. This discussion promotes reassurance and provides knowledge about the procedure. Dialogue encourages patient participation and allows for individualized nursing care. Some catheters and gloves in kits are made of latex. Some antiseptic solutions contain iodine.

Good lighting is necessary to see the meatus clearly. A readily available trash receptacle allows for prompt disposal of used supplies and reduces the risk of contaminating the sterile field.

Having the bed at the proper height prevents back and muscle strain. Positioning allows for ease of use of dominant hand for catheter insertion.

Proper positioning allows adequate visualization of the urinary meatus. Embarrassment, chilliness, and tension can interfere with catheter insertion; draping the patient will promote comfort and relaxation. The Sims' position may allow better visualization and be more comfortable for the patient, especially if hip and knee movements are difficult. The smaller area of exposure is also less stressful for the patient. The waterproof pad will protect bed linens from moisture.

FIGURE 1. Patient in dorsal recumbent position and draped properly.

Gloves reduce the risk of exposure to blood and body fluids. Cleaning reduces microorganisms near the urethral meatus and provides opportunity to visualize perineum and landmarks before procedure. Hand hygiene reduces the spread of microorganisms.

This facilitates connection of the catheter to the drainage system and provides for easy access.

Placement of equipment near worksite increases efficiency. Sterile technique protects patient and prevents transmission of microorganisms.

(continued)

Skill · 37-5   Catheterizing the Female Urinary Bladder   *continued*

ACTION	RATIONALE
12. Put on sterile gloves. Grasp upper corners of drape and unfold drape without touching unsterile areas. Fold back a corner on each side to make a cuff over gloved hands. Ask patient to lift her buttocks and slide sterile drape under her with gloves protected by cuff.	The drape provides a sterile field close to the meatus. Covering the gloved hands will help keep the gloves sterile while placing the drape.
13. Based on facility policy, position the fenestrated sterile drape. Place a fenestrated sterile drape over the perineal area, exposing the labia (Figure 2). (Please note that the fenestrated drape is not shown in the remaining illustrations in order to provide a clear view of the procedure.)	The drape expands the sterile field and protects against contamination. Use of a fenestrated drape may limit visualization and is considered optional by some practitioners and/or facility policies.
14. Place sterile tray on drape between patient's thighs.	This provides easy access to supplies.
15. Open all the supplies. Fluff cotton balls in tray before pouring antiseptic solution over them. Alternately, open package of antiseptic swabs. Open specimen container if specimen is to be obtained.	It is necessary to open all supplies and prepare for the procedure while both hands are sterile.
16. Lubricate 1″ to 2″ of catheter tip.	Lubrication facilitates catheter insertion and reduces tissue trauma.
17. With thumb and one finger of nondominant hand, spread labia and identify meatus. **Be prepared to maintain separation of labia with one hand until catheter is inserted and urine is flowing well and continuously (Figure 3).** If the patient is in the side-lying position, lift the upper buttock and labia to expose the urinary meatus.	Smoothing the area immediately surrounding the meatus helps to make it visible. Allowing the labia to drop back into position may contaminate the area around the meatus, as well as the catheter. The nondominant hand is now contaminated.

FIGURE 2. Patient with fenestrated drape in place over perineum.

FIGURE 3. Using dominant hand to separate and hold labia open.

18. Use the dominant hand to pick up a cotton ball or antiseptic swab. **Clean one labial fold, top to bottom (from above the meatus down toward the rectum), then discard the cotton ball. Using a new cotton ball/swab for each stroke, continue to clean the other labial fold, then directly over the meatus (Figure 4).**	Moving from an area where there is likely to be less contamination to an area where there is more contamination helps prevent the spread of microorganisms. Cleaning the meatus last helps reduce the possibility of introducing microorganisms into the bladder.
19. With your uncontaminated, dominant hand, place drainage end of catheter in receptacle. If the catheter is preattached to sterile tubing and drainage container (closed drainage system), position catheter and setup within easy reach on sterile field. Ensure that clamp on drainage bag is closed.	This facilitates drainage of urine and minimizes risk of contaminating sterile equipment.

ACTION

RATIONALE

FIGURE 4. Wiping perineum with cotton ball held by forceps. Wipe in one direction from top to bottom.

20. **Using your dominant hand, hold the catheter 2″ to 3″ from the tip and insert slowly into the urethra (Figure 5). Advance the catheter until there is a return of urine (approximately 2″ to 3″ [4.8–7.2 cm]). Once urine drains, advance catheter another 2″ to 3″ (4.8–7.2 cm). Do not force catheter through urethra into bladder.** Ask patient to breathe deeply, and rotate catheter gently if slight resistance is met as catheter reaches external sphincter.

21. Hold the catheter securely at the meatus with your nondominant hand. Use your dominant hand to inflate the catheter balloon (Figure 6). Inject entire volume of sterile water supplied in prefilled syringe.

The female urethra is about 1.5″ to 2.5″ (3.6–6.0 cm) long. Applying force on the catheter is likely to injure mucous membranes. The sphincter relaxes and the catheter can enter the bladder easily when the patient relaxes. Advancing an indwelling catheter an additional 2″ to 3″ (4.8–7.2 cm) ensures placement in the bladder and facilitates inflation of the balloon without damaging the urethra.

Bladder or sphincter contraction could push the catheter out. The balloon anchors the catheter in place in the bladder. Manufacturer provides appropriate amount of sterile water for the size of catheter in the kit; as a result, use entire syringe provided in the kit.

FIGURE 5. Inserting catheter with dominant hand while nondominant hand holds labia apart.

FIGURE 6. Inflating balloon of indwelling catheter.

22. Pull gently on catheter after balloon is inflated to feel resistance.

23. Attach catheter to drainage system if not already preattached (Figure 7).

24. Remove equipment and dispose of it according to facility policy. Discard syringe in sharps container. Wash and dry the perineal area, as needed.

Improper inflation can cause patient discomfort and malpositioning of catheter.

Closed drainage system minimizes the risk for microorganisms being introduced into the bladder.

Proper disposal prevents the spread of microorganisms. Placing syringe in sharps container prevents reuse. Cleaning promotes comfort and appropriate personal hygiene.

(continued)

Skill · 37-5   Catheterizing the Female Urinary Bladder   *continued*

ACTION	RATIONALE
25. Remove gloves. **Secure catheter tubing to the patient's inner thigh with Velcro leg strap or tape (Figure 8).** Leave some slack in catheter for leg movement.	Proper attachment prevents trauma to the urethra and meatus from tension on the tubing. Whether to tape the drainage tubing over or under the leg depends on gravity flow, patient's mobility, and comfort of the patient.

FIGURE 7. Attaching catheter to drainage bag.

FIGURE 8. Catheter attached to leg.

26. Assist the patient to a comfortable position. Cover the patient with bed linens. Place the bed in the lowest position.	Positioning and covering provides warmth and promotes comfort.
27. Secure drainage bag below the level of the bladder. Check that drainage tubing is not kinked and that movement of side rails does not interfere with catheter or drainage bag.	This facilitates drainage of urine and prevents the backflow of urine.
28. Put on clean gloves. Obtain urine specimen immediately, if needed, from drainage bag. Label specimen. Send urine specimen to the laboratory promptly or refrigerate it.	Catheter system is sterile. Obtaining specimen immediately allows access to sterile system. Keeping urine at room temperature may cause microorganisms, if present, to grow and distort laboratory findings.
29. Remove gloves and additional PPE, if used. Perform hand hygiene.	Removing PPE properly reduces the risk for infection transmission and contamination of other items. Hand hygiene prevents the spread of microorganisms.

DOCUMENTATION

Guidelines

Document the type and size of catheter and balloon inserted, as well as the amount of fluid used to inflate the balloon. Document the patient's tolerance of the activity. Record the amount of urine obtained through the catheter and any specimen obtained. Document any other assessments, such as unusual urine characteristics or alterations in the patient's skin. Record urine amount on intake and output record, if appropriate.

Sample Documentation

> 7/14/12 0915 Primary care provider notified of palpable bladder (3 cm below umbilicus) and patient's inability to void; 750 mL of urine noted with bladder scan. 16F Foley catheter inserted without difficulty. 10 mL of sterile water injected into balloon port. 700 mL clear yellow urine returned. Patient states, "Oh, I feel much better now." Bladder is no longer palpable. Patient tolerated procedure without adverse event.
>
> —B. Clapp, RN

UNEXPECTED SITUATIONS AND ASSOCIATED INTERVENTIONS

- *No urine flow is obtained, and nurse notes that catheter is in vaginal orifice:* Leave catheter in place as a marker. Obtain new sterile gloves and catheter kit. Start the procedure over and attempt to place new catheter directly above misplaced catheter. Once the new catheter is correctly in place, remove the catheter in the vaginal orifice. Because of the risk of cross-infection, never remove a catheter from the vagina and insert it into the urethra (Robinson, 2004).

- *Patient moves legs during procedure:* If no supplies have been contaminated, ask patient to hold still and continue with procedure. If supplies have been contaminated, stop procedure and start over. If necessary, get an assistant to remind the patient to hold still.

- *Urine flow is initially well established and urine is clear, but after several hours, flow dwindles:* Check tubing for kinking. If patient has changed position, the tubing and drainage bag may need to be moved to facilitate drainage of urine.

- *Patient complains of extreme pain when nurse is inflating balloon:* Stop inflation of balloon. Balloon is most likely still in urethra. Withdraw the solution from the balloon. Insert catheter an additional 1/2" to 1" (1.2–2.4 cm) and slowly attempt to inflate balloon again.

- *Urine leaks out of meatus around the catheter:* Do not increase the size of the indwelling catheter. Make sure the smallest sized catheter with a 10-mL balloon is used. Large catheters cause bladder and urethral irritation and trauma. Large balloon-fill volumes occupy more space inside the bladder and put added weight on the base of the bladder. Irritation of the bladder wall and detrusor muscle can cause leakage. If leakage persists, consider an evaluation for urinary tract infection. Ensure that the correct amount of solution was used to inflate the balloon. Under filling the balloon can cause the catheter to dislodge into the urethra, causing urethral spasm, pain, and discomfort. If you suspect under fill, do not attempt to push the catheter further into the bladder. Remove the catheter and replace. Assess the patient for constipation. Bowel full of stool can cause pressure on the catheter lumen and prevent the drainage of urine. Implement interventions to prevent/treat constipation (Mercer Smith, 2003; Robinson, 2004).

SPECIAL CONSIDERATIONS
General Considerations

- In the past, pretesting of the catheter balloon was recommended to prevent insertion of a defective catheter. Most catheter manufacturers in the United States no longer recommend pretesting because the balloons are pretested during the manufacturing process. Pretesting silicone balloons is not recommended; the silicone can form a cuff or crease at the balloon area that can cause trauma to the urethra during catheter insertion (Mercer Smith, 2003).

- Be familiar with facility policy and/or primary practitioner guidelines for the maximum amount of urine to remove from bladder at the time of insertion.

- If patient is unable to lift buttocks or maintain required position for the procedure, the assistance of another staff member may be necessary to place the drape under the patient and to help the patient maintain the required position.

- Supplies can be opened and prepared on the overbed table, moving the tray onto the bed just before cleansing the patient.

- If there is not an immediate flow of urine after the catheter has been inserted, several measures may prove helpful:
  - Have the patient take a deep breath, which helps to relax the perineal and abdominal muscles.
  - Rotate the catheter slightly, because a drainage hole may be resting against the bladder wall.
  - Raise the head of the patient's bed to increase pressure in the bladder area.
  - Assess the patient's intake to ensure adequate fluid intake for urine production.
  - Assess the catheter and drainage tubing for kinks and occlusion.

- If the catheter cannot be advanced, have the patient take several deep breaths. Rotate the catheter half a turn and try to advance. If you are still unable to advance, remove the catheter. Notify the primary care provider.

- Some catheter kits do not contain the catheter. This allows you to select a catheter and balloon size separately.

(continued)

Skill · 37-5 **Catheterizing the Female Urinary Bladder** *continued*

Infant and Child Considerations

• Size 5F to 8F is used for infants and young children. Size 8F to 12F catheters are commonly used for older children (Hockenberry & Wilson, 2008).

• Distraction, such as blowing bubbles, deep breathing, or singing a song, can help the child relax.

• Lidocaine jelly is often used to anesthetize and lubricate the area before insertion of the catheter, decreasing the child's discomfort and anxiety.

Skill · 37-6 **Catheterizing the Male Urinary Bladder**

EQUIPMENT

• Sterile catheter kit that contains:
  • Sterile gloves
  • Sterile drapes (one of which is fenestrated [having a window-like opening])
  • Sterile catheter (use the smallest appropriate-size catheter, usually a 14F to 16F catheter with a 5- to 10-mL balloon [Mercer Smith, 2003; Newman, 2008]).
  • Antiseptic cleansing solution and cotton balls or gauze squares; antiseptic swabs

• Lubricant
• Forceps
• Prefilled syringe with sterile water (sufficient to inflate indwelling catheter balloon)
• Sterile basin (usually base of kit serves as this)
• Sterile specimen container (if specimen is required)
• Flashlight or lamp
• Waterproof disposable pad

• Sterile disposable urine collection bag and drainage tubing (may be connected to catheter in catheter kit)
• Velcro leg strap or tape
• Disposable gloves
• Additional PPE, as indicated
• Washcloth and warm water to perform perineal hygiene before and after catheterization

IMPLEMENTATION

ACTION	RATIONALE
1. Review chart for any limitations in physical activity. Confirm the medical order for indwelling catheter insertion.	Physical limitations may require adaptations in performing the skill. Verifying the medical order ensures that the correct intervention is administered to the right patient.
2. Bring catheter kit and other necessary equipment to the bedside. Obtain assistance from another staff member, if necessary.	Bringing everything to the bedside conserves time and energy. Arranging items nearby is convenient, saves time, and avoids unnecessary stretching and twisting of muscles on the part of the nurse. Assistance from another person may be required to safely perform the intervention.
3. Perform hand hygiene and put on PPE, if indicated.	Hand hygiene and PPE prevent the spread of microorganisms. PPE is required based on transmission precautions.
4. Identify the patient.	Identifying the patient ensures the right patient receives the intervention and helps prevent errors.
5. Close curtains around bed and close door to room if possible. Discuss the procedure with the patient and assess patient's ability to assist with the procedure. Ask the patient if he has any allergies, especially to latex or iodine.	This ensures the patient's privacy. This discussion promotes reassurance and provides knowledge about the procedure. Dialogue encourages patient participation and allows for individualized nursing care. Some catheters and gloves in kits are made of latex. Some antiseptic solutions contain iodine.
6. Provide good lighting. Artificial light is recommended (use of a flashlight requires an assistant to hold and position it). Place a trash receptacle within easy reach.	Good lighting is necessary to see the meatus clearly. A readily available trash receptacle allows for prompt disposal of used supplies and reduces the risk of contaminating the sterile field.
7. Adjust the bed to a comfortable working height, usually elbow height of the caregiver (VISN 8, 2009). Stand on the patient's right side if you are right-handed, patient's left side if you are left handed.	Having the bed at the proper height prevents back and muscle strain. Positioning allows for ease of use of dominant hand for catheter insertion.

ACTION

8. Position patient on his back with thighs slightly apart. Drape patient so that only the area around the penis is exposed. Slide waterproof pad under patient.

9. Put on clean gloves. Clean the genital area with washcloth, skin cleanser, and warm water. Clean the tip of the penis first, moving the washcloth in a circular motion from the meatus outward. Wash the shaft of the penis using downward strokes toward the pubic area. Rinse and dry. Remove gloves. Perform hand hygiene again.

10. Prepare urine drainage setup if a separate urine collection system is to be used. Secure to bed frame according to manufacturer's directions.

11. Open sterile catheterization tray on a clean overbed table, using sterile technique.

12. Put on sterile gloves. Open sterile drape and place on patient's thighs. Place fenestrated drape with opening over penis (Figure 1).

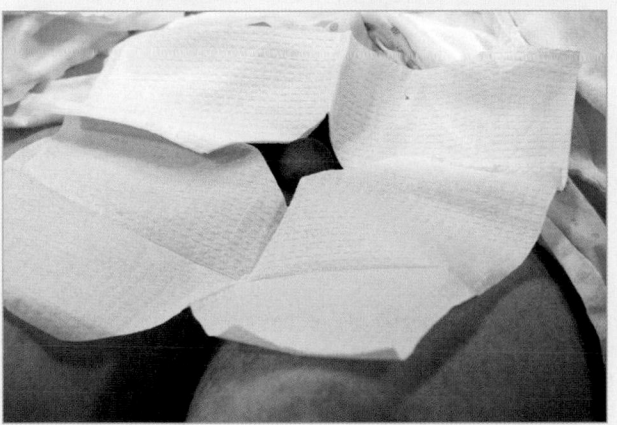

RATIONALE

This prevents unnecessary exposure and promotes warmth. The waterproof pad will protect bed linens from moisture.

Gloves reduce the risk of exposure to blood and body fluids. Cleaning the penis reduces microorganisms near the urethral meatus. Hand hygiene reduces the spread of microorganisms.

This facilitates connection of the catheter to the drainage system and provides for easy access.

Placement of equipment near worksite increases efficiency. Sterile technique protects patient and prevents spread of microorganisms.

This maintains a sterile working area.

FIGURE 1. Patient lying supine with fenestrated drape over penis.

13. Place catheter set on or next to patient's legs on sterile drape.

14. Open all the supplies. Fluff cotton balls in tray before pouring antiseptic solution over them. Alternately, open package of antiseptic swabs. Open specimen container if specimen is to be obtained. Remove cap from syringe prefilled with lubricant.

15. Place drainage end of catheter in receptacle. If the catheter is preattached to sterile tubing and drainage container (closed drainage system), position catheter and setup within easy reach on sterile field. Ensure that clamp on drainage bag is closed.

16. Lift penis with nondominant hand. Retract foreskin in uncircumcised patient. **Be prepared to keep this hand in this position until catheter is inserted and urine is flowing well and continuously. Using the dominant hand and the forceps, pick up a cotton ball or antiseptic swab. Using a circular motion, clean the penis, moving from the meatus down the glans of the penis (Figure 2). Repeat this cleansing motion two more times, using a new cotton ball/swab each time. Discard each cotton ball/swab after one use.**

Sterile setup should be arranged so that nurse's back is not turned to it, nor should it be out of the nurse's range of vision.

It is necessary to open all supplies and prepare for the procedure while both hands are sterile.

This facilitates drainage of urine and minimizes risk of contaminating sterile equipment.

The hand touching the penis becomes contaminated. Cleansing the area around the meatus and under the foreskin in the uncircumcised patient helps prevent infection. Moving from the meatus toward the base of the penis prevents bringing microorganisms to the meatus.

(continued)

Skill · 37-6   Catheterizing the Male Urinary Bladder   *continued*

ACTION

17. Hold penis with slight upward tension and perpendicular to patient's body. Use the dominant hand to pick up the lubricant syringe. **Gently insert tip of syringe with lubricant into urethra and instill the 10 mL of lubricant** (SUNA, 2005c) (Figure 3).

RATIONALE

The lubricant causes the urethra to distend slightly and facilitates passage of the catheter without traumatizing the lining of the urethra (Mercer Smith, 2003; SUNA, 2005c). If the prepackaged kit does not contain a syringe with lubricant, the nurse may need assistance in filling a syringe while keeping the lubricant sterile. Some institutions use lidocaine jelly for lubrication before insertion of the catheter. The jelly comes prepackaged in a sterile syringe and serves a dual purpose of lubricating and numbing the urethra. A medical order is necessary for the use of lidocaine jelly.

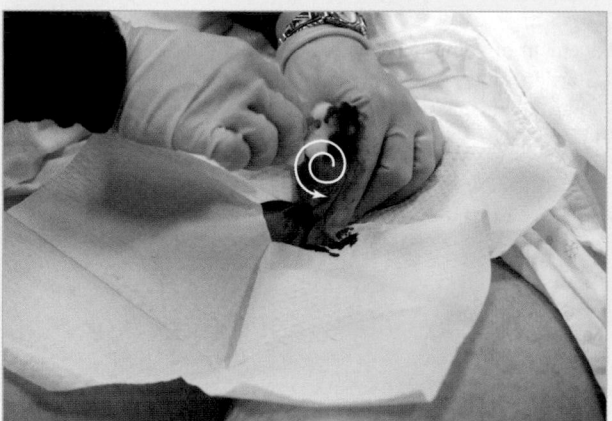

FIGURE 2. Lifting penis with gloved nondominant hand and cleaning meatus with cotton ball held with forceps in gloved dominant hand.

FIGURE 3. Inserting syringe with lubricant into urethra.

18. Use the dominant hand to pick up the catheter and hold it an inch or two from the tip. Ask patient to bear down as if voiding. **Insert catheter tip into meatus (Figure 4). Ask the patient to take deep breaths. Advance the catheter to the bifurcation or "Y" level of the ports. Do not use force to introduce catheter.** If catheter resists entry, ask patient to breathe deeply and rotate catheter slightly.

Bearing down eases the passage of the catheter through the urethra. The male urethra is about 20 cm long. Having the patient take deep breaths or twisting the catheter slightly may ease the catheter past resistance at the sphincters. Advancing an indwelling catheter to the bifurcation ensures its placement in the bladder and facilitates inflation of the balloon without damaging the urethra.

FIGURE 4. Inserting catheter with dominant hand.

ACTION

RATIONALE

19. Hold the catheter securely at the meatus with your nondominant hand. Use your dominant hand to inflate the catheter balloon. **Inject entire volume of sterile water supplied in prefilled syringe. Once balloon is inflated, catheter may be gently pulled back into place. Replace foreskin over catheter.** Lower penis.

Bladder or sphincter contraction could push the catheter out. The balloon anchors the catheter in place in the bladder. Manufacturer provides appropriate amount of solution for the size of catheter in the kit; as a result, use entire syringe provided in the kit.

20. Pull gently on catheter after balloon is inflated to feel resistance.

Improper inflation can cause patient discomfort and malpositioning of catheter.

21. Attach catheter to drainage system, if necessary.

Closed drainage system minimizes the risk for microorganisms being introduced into the bladder.

22. Remove equipment and dispose of according to facility policy. Discard syringe in sharps container. Wash and dry the perineal area as needed.

Proper disposal prevents the spread of microorganisms. Placing syringe in sharps container prevents reuse. Promotes comfort and appropriate personal hygiene.

23. Remove gloves. Secure catheter tubing to the patient's inner thigh or lower abdomen (with the penis directed toward the patient's chest) with Velcro leg strap or tape. Leave some slack in catheter for leg movement.

Proper attachment prevents trauma to the urethra and meatus from tension on the tubing. Whether to take the drainage tubing over or under the leg depends on gravity flow, patient's mobility, and comfort of the patient.

24. Assist the patient to a comfortable position. Cover the patient with bed linens. Place the bed in the lowest position.

Positioning and covering provides warmth and promotes comfort.

25. Secure drainage bag below the level of the bladder. Check that drainage tubing is not kinked and that movement of side rails does not interfere with catheter or drainage bag.

This facilitates drainage of urine and prevents the backflow of urine.

26. Put on clean gloves. Obtain urine specimen immediately, if needed, from drainage bag. Label specimen. Send urine specimen to the laboratory promptly or refrigerate it.

Catheter system is sterile. Obtaining specimen immediately allows access to sterile system. Keeping urine at room temperature may cause microorganisms, if present, to grow and distort laboratory findings.

27. Remove gloves and additional PPE, if used. Perform hand hygiene.

Removing PPE properly reduces the risk for infection transmission and contamination of other items. Hand hygiene prevents the spread of microorganisms.

DOCUMENTATION

Guidelines

Document the type and size of catheter and balloon inserted, as well as the amount of fluid used to inflate the balloon. Document the patient's tolerance of the activity. Record the amount of urine obtained through the catheter and any specimen obtained. Document any other assessments, such as unusual urine characteristics or alterations in the patient's skin. Record urine amount on intake and output record, if appropriate.

Sample Documentation

7/14/12 1830 Patient unable to void × 8 hours and reports, "I feel like I have to go to the bathroom." Bladder scanned for 540 mL urine. Primary care provider notified. 10 mL 2% lidocaine jelly instilled before catheterization per order. 14F Foley catheter inserted without difficulty. 10 mL of sterile water injected into 5-mL balloon port. 525 mL clear yellow urine returned. Patient reports decreased bladder pressure. Patient tolerated procedure without adverse event.

—B. Clapp, RN

UNEXPECTED SITUATIONS AND ASSOCIATED INTERVENTIONS

• *Patient complains of intense pain when nurse begins to inflate balloon:* Stop inflation. Be sure to insert catheter all the way into the bifurcation. The balloon is probably still in the urethra. Damage to the urethra can result if balloon is inflated in urethra.

• *Nurse cannot insert catheter past 3" to 4"; rotating the catheter and having patient breathe deeply are of no help:* If still unable to place catheter, notify primary care provider. Repeated catheter placement attempts can traumatize the urethra. Primary care provider may order and insert a Coude catheter.

(continued)

Skill · 37-6   Catheterizing the Male Urinary Bladder   *continued*

- *Patient is obese or has retracted penis:* Have assistant available to place fingers on either side of the pubic area and press backward to bring the penis out of the pubic cavity. Hold patient's penis up and forward. The catheter still needs to be inserted to the bifurcation; the length of the urethra has not changed.

- *Urine flow initially contains a large amount of sediment (precipitate) and then suddenly stops; bladder remains palpable:* Catheter may be plugged with sediment. After obtaining an order from the primary care provider, gently irrigate the catheter to restore flow.

- *Urine leaks out of meatus around the catheter:* Do not increase the size of the indwelling catheter. Make sure the smallest sized catheter with a 10-mL balloon is used. Large catheters cause bladder and urethral irritation and trauma. Large balloon-fill volumes occupy more space inside the bladder and put added weight on the base of the bladder. Irritation of the bladder wall and detrusor muscle can cause leakage. If leakage persists, consider an evaluation for urinary tract infection. Ensure that the correct amount of solution was used to inflate the balloon. Under filling the balloon can cause the catheter to dislodge into the urethra, causing urethral spasm, pain, and discomfort. If under fill is suspected, do not attempt to push the catheter further into the bladder. Remove the catheter and replace. Assess the patient for constipation. Bowel full of stool can cause pressure on the catheter lumen and prevent the drainage of urine. Implement interventions to prevent/treat constipation (Mercer Smith, 2003; Robinson, 2004).

- *Urine flow is initially well established and urine is clear, but after several hours, urine flow dwindles:* Check tubing for kinking. If patient has changed position, the tubing and drainage bag may need to be moved to facilitate drainage of urine.

SPECIAL CONSIDERATIONS
General Considerations

- In the past, pretesting of the catheter balloon was recommended to prevent insertion of a defective catheter. Most catheter manufacturers in the United States no longer recommend pretesting because the balloons are pretested during the manufacturing process. Pretesting silicone balloons is not recommended; the silicone can form a cuff or crease at the balloon area that can cause trauma to the urethra during catheter insertion (Mercer Smith, 2003).

- Be familiar with facility policy and/or primary practitioner guidelines for the maximum amount of urine to remove from bladder at the time of insertion.

- Supplies can be opened and prepared on the overbed table, moving the tray onto the bed just before cleansing the patient.

- If there is not an immediate flow of urine after the catheter has been inserted, several measures may prove helpful:
  - Have the patient take a deep breath, which helps to relax the perineal and abdominal muscles.
  - Rotate the catheter slightly, because a drainage hole may be resting against the bladder wall.
  - Raise the head of the patient's bed to increase pressure in the bladder area.
  - Assess the patient's intake to ensure adequate fluid intake for urine production.
  - Assess the catheter and drainage tubing for kinks and occlusion.
  - Urethral strictures, false passages, prostatic enlargement, and postsurgical bladder-neck contractures can make urethral catheterization difficult and may require the services of a urologist. If there is any question as to the location of the catheter, such as no return of urine, do not inflate the balloon. Remove the catheter and notify the physician (SUNA, 2005c).

- If the catheter cannot be advanced, having the patient take several deep breaths may be helpful. Rotate the catheter half a turn, and try to advance. If you are still unable to advance, remove the catheter. Notify the physician.

- Some catheter kits do not contain the catheter. This allows you to select a catheter and balloon size separately.

Infant and Child Considerations

- Size 5F to 8F is used for infants and young children. Size 8F to 12F catheters are commonly used for older children (Hockenberry & Wilson, 2008).
- Distraction, such as blowing bubbles, deep breathing, or singing a song, can be used to help the child relax.
- Lidocaine jelly is often used to anesthetize and lubricate the area before insertion of the catheter, decreasing the child's discomfort and anxiety.

Older Adult Considerations

- If resistance is met while inserting catheter and rotating does not help, the catheter is never forced. Enlargement of the prostate gland is commonly seen in men over age 50. A special crook-tipped catheter called a Coude catheter, inserted by the physician or advanced practice nurse, may be required to maneuver past the prostate gland.

Skill · 37-7 Performing Intermittent Closed Catheter Irrigation

EQUIPMENT

- Sterile basin or container
- Sterile irrigating solution (at room temperature or warmed to body temperature)
- 30- to 60-mL syringe (with 18- or 19-gauge blunt-end needle, if catheter access port is not a needleless system)
- Clamp for drainage tubing
- Bath blanket
- Disposable gloves
- Additional PPE, as indicated
- Waterproof pad

IMPLEMENTATION

ACTION	RATIONALE
1. Confirm the order for catheter irrigation in the medical record.	Verifying the medical order ensures that the correct intervention is administered to the right patient.
2. Bring necessary equipment to the bedside.	Bringing everything to the bedside conserves time and energy. Arranging items nearby is convenient, saves time, and avoids unnecessary stretching and twisting of muscles on the part of the nurse.
3. Perform hand hygiene and put on PPE, if indicated.	Hand hygiene and PPE prevent the spread of microorganisms. PPE is required based on transmission precautions.
4. Identify the patient.	Identifying the patient ensures the right patient receives the intervention and helps prevent errors.
5. Close curtains around bed and close door to room if possible. Discuss procedure with patient.	This ensures the patient's privacy. This discussion promotes reassurance and provides knowledge about the procedure. Dialogue encourages patient participation and allows for individualized nursing care.
6. Adjust bed to comfortable working height, usually elbow height of the caregiver (VISN 8, 2009).	Having the bed at the proper height prevents back and muscle strain.
7. Put on gloves. Empty the catheter drainage bag and measure the amount of urine, noting the amount and characteristics of the urine. Remove gloves.	Gloves prevent contact with blood and body fluids. Emptying the drainage bag allows for accurate assessment of drainage after the irrigation solution is instilled. Assessment of urine provides baseline for future comparison. Proper removal of PPE prevents transmission of microorganisms.
8. Assist patient to comfortable position and expose access port on catheter setup. Place waterproof pad under catheter and aspiration port. Remove catheter from device or tape anchoring catheter to the patient.	This provides adequate visualization. Waterproof pad protects patient and bed from leakage. Removing the catheter from the anchoring device or tape allows for manipulation of catheter.
9. Open supplies, using aseptic technique. Pour sterile solution into sterile basin. Aspirate the prescribed amount of irrigant (usually 30–60 mL) into sterile syringe. Put on gloves.	Use of aseptic technique ensures sterility of irrigating fluid and prevents spread of microorganisms. Gloves prevent contact with blood and body fluids.

(continued)

Skill · 37-7   Performing Intermittent Closed Catheter Irrigation   *continued*

ACTION	RATIONALE
10. **Cleanse the access port on catheter with antimicrobial swab (Figure 1).**	Cleaning the port reduces the risk of introducing organisms into the closed urinary system.
11. Clamp or fold catheter tubing below the access port (Figure 2).	This directs the irrigating solution into the bladder, preventing flow into the drainage bag.

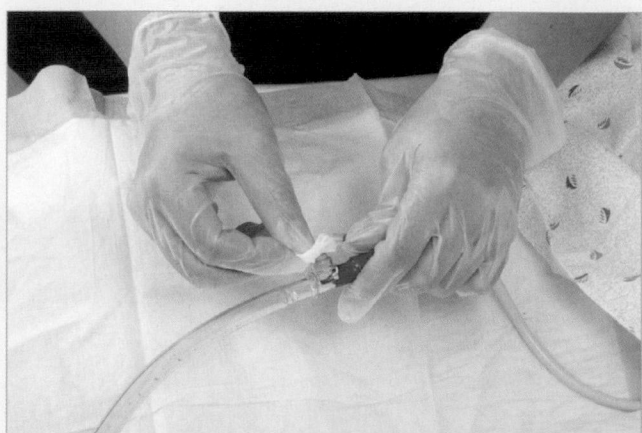

FIGURE 1. Cleansing access port on catheter.

FIGURE 2. Clamping catheter below access port.

12. Attach the syringe to the access port on catheter using a twisting motion (Figure 3). **Gently instill solution into catheter (Figure 4).**	Gentle irrigation prevents damage to bladder lining. Instillation of fluid dislodges material blocking catheter.

FIGURE 3. Attaching syringe to access port with twisting motion.

FIGURE 4. Gently instilling irrigation solution.

13. Remove syringe from access port (Figure 5). **Unclamp or unfold tubing and allow irrigant and urine to flow into the drainage bag.** Repeat procedure as necessary.	Gravity aids drainage of urine and irrigant from the bladder.
14. Remove gloves. Secure catheter tubing to the patient's inner thigh or lower abdomen (if a male patient) with anchoring device or tape. Leave some slack in catheter for leg movement.	Proper attachment prevents trauma to the urethra and meatus from tension on the tubing. Whether to take the drainage tubing over or under the leg depends on gravity flow, patient's mobility, and comfort of the patient.
15. Assist the patient to a comfortable position. Cover the patient with bed linens. Place the bed in the lowest position.	Positioning and covering provide warmth and promote comfort. Lowering bed contributes to patient safety.

ACTION

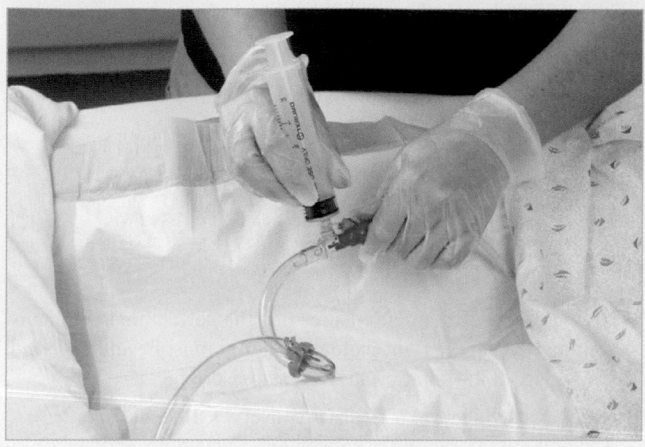

RATIONALE

FIGURE 5. Removing syringe from access port.

16. Secure drainage bag below the level of the bladder. Check that drainage tubing is not kinked and that movement of side rails does not interfere with catheter or drainage bag.

This facilitates drainage of urine and prevents the backflow of urine.

17. Remove equipment and discard syringe in appropriate receptacle. Remove gloves and additional PPE, if used. Perform hand hygiene.

Proper disposal of equipment prevents transmission of microorganisms. Removing PPE properly reduces the risk for infection transmission and contamination of other items. Hand hygiene prevents the spread of microorganisms.

18. Assess patient's response to procedure and quality and amount of drainage after the irrigation.

This provides accurate assessment of the patient's response to the procedure.

DOCUMENTATION

Guidelines

Document baseline assessment of patient. Document the amount and type of irrigation solution used and the amount and characteristics of drainage returned after the procedure. Document the ease of irrigation and the patient's tolerance of the procedure. Record urine amount emptied from the drainage bag before the procedure and the amount of irrigant used on intake and output record. Subtract irrigant amount from the urine output when totaling output to provide accurate recording of urine output.

Sample Documentation

7/22/12 1630 Urinary catheter irrigated with 60 mL of normal saline without difficulty. All of irrigation returned plus 200 mL of cloudy yellow urine. Patient tolerated procedure without adverse effect. Order received to notify physician if urine output <30 mL per hour.

—B. Clapp, RN

UNEXPECTED SITUATIONS AND ASSOCIATED INTERVENTIONS

- *Irrigation solution will not enter the catheter:* Do not force the solution into the catheter. Notify primary care provider. Prepare to change catheter.

- *Tubing was not clamped before introducing irrigation solution:* Repeat irrigation. If the tubing is not clamped, the irrigation solution will drain into the urinary drainage bag and not enter the catheter.

SPECIAL CONSIDERATIONS

- If irrigant is a medication intended for action in bladder, be aware of specific dwell time included in the order or determined by the action of the medication. Allow the appropriate amount of time to lapse before unclamping drainage tubing after instillation of irrigant.

Skill · 37-8   Administering a Continuous Closed Bladder Irrigation

EQUIPMENT

- Sterile irrigating solution (at room temperature or warmed to body temperature)
- Sterile tubing with drip chamber and clamp for connection to irrigating solution
- IV pole
- IV pump (if bladder is being irrigated with a solution containing medication)
- Three-way indwelling catheter in place in patient's bladder
- Indwelling catheter drainage setup (tubing and collection bag)
- Alcohol swabs
- Bath blanket
- Disposable gloves
- Additional PPE, as indicated

IMPLEMENTATION

ACTION	RATIONALE
1. Confirm the order for catheter irrigation in the medical record. Calculate the drip rate via gravity infusion for prescribed infusion rate.	Verifying the medical order ensures that the correct intervention is administered to the right patient. Solution must be administered via gravity at the appropriate rate, as prescribed.
2. Bring necessary equipment to the bedside.	Bringing everything to the bedside conserves time and energy. Arranging items nearby is convenient, saves time, and avoids unnecessary stretching and twisting of muscles on the part of the nurse.
3. Perform hand hygiene and put on PPE, if indicated.	Hand hygiene and PPE prevent the spread of microorganisms. PPE is required based on transmission precautions.
4. Identify the patient.	Identifying the patient ensures the right patient receives the intervention and helps prevent errors.
5. Close curtains around the bed and close the door to the room if possible. Discuss the procedure with patient.	This ensures the patient's privacy. This discussion promotes reassurance and provides knowledge about the procedure. Dialogue encourages patient participation and allows for individualized nursing care.
6. Adjust bed to comfortable working height, usually elbow height of the caregiver (VISN 8, 2009).	Having the bed at the proper height prevents back and muscle strain.
7. Empty the catheter drainage bag and measure the amount of urine, noting the amount and characteristics of the urine.	Emptying the drainage bag allows for accurate assessment of drainage after the irrigation solution is instilled. Assessment of urine provides baseline for future comparison.
8. Assist patient to comfortable position and expose the irrigation port on the catheter setup. Place waterproof pad under catheter and aspiration port.	This provides adequate visualization. Waterproof pad protects the patient and bed from leakage.
9. Prepare sterile irrigation bag for use as directed by manufacturer. Clearly label the solution as "Bladder Irrigant." Include the date and time on the label. Hang bag on IV pole 2 1/2′ to 3′ above level of patient's bladder. Secure tubing clamp and insert sterile tubing with drip chamber to container using aseptic technique (Figure 1). Release clamp and remove protective cover on end of tubing without contaminating it. Allow solution to flush tubing and remove air (Figure 2). Clamp tubing and replace end cover.	Proper labeling provides accurate information for caregivers. Sterile solution not used within 24 hours of opening should be discarded. Aseptic technique prevents contamination of solution irrigation system. Priming the tubing before attaching irrigation clears air from the tubing that might cause bladder distention.
10. Put on gloves. **Cleanse the irrigation port on the catheter with an alcohol swab. Using aseptic technique, attach irrigation tubing to irrigation port of three-way indwelling catheter (Figure 3).**	Aseptic technique prevents the spread of microorganisms into the bladder.
11. Check the drainage tubing to make sure clamp, if present, is open.	An open clamp prevents accumulation of solution in the bladder.
12. **Release clamp on irrigation tubing and regulate flow at determined drip rate, according to the ordered rate (Figure 4).** If the bladder irrigation is to be done with a medicated solution, use an electronic infusion device to regulate the flow.	This allows for continual gentle irrigation without causing discomfort to the patient. An electronic infusion device regulates the flow of the medication.

ACTION

FIGURE 1. Inserting tubing into solution bag.

FIGURE 3. Attaching irrigation tubing to irrigation port on catheter.

RATIONALE

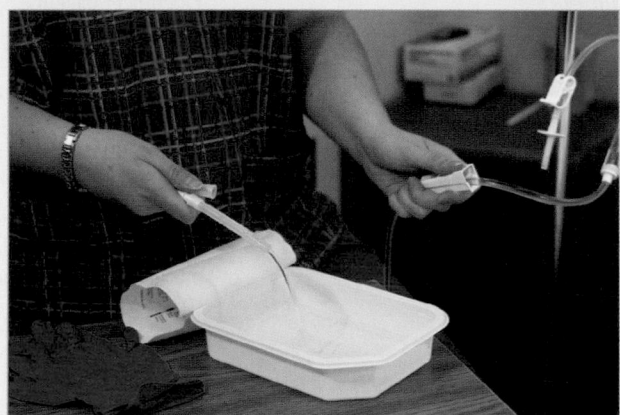

FIGURE 2. Removing air from irrigation tubing.

FIGURE 4. Regulating irrigation flow rate using flow clamp.

13. Remove gloves. Assist the patient to a comfortable position. Cover the patient with bed linens. Place the bed in the lowest position.

14. Assess patient's response to procedure and quality and amount of drainage.

15. Remove equipment. Remove gloves and additional PPE, if used. Perform hand hygiene.

16. As irrigation fluid container nears empty, clamp the administration tubing. Do not allow drip chamber to empty. Disconnect empty bag and attach a new full irrigation solution bag.

17. Put on gloves and empty drainage collection bag as each new container is hung and recorded.

Positioning and covering provide warmth and promote comfort and safety.

Assessment is necessary to determine effectiveness of intervention and detection of adverse effects.

Proper disposal of equipment prevents transmission of microorganisms. Removing PPE properly reduces the risk for infection transmission and contamination of other items. Hand hygiene prevents the spread of microorganisms.

This eliminates the need to separate tubing from the catheter and clear air from the tubing. Opening the drainage system provides access for microorganisms.

Gloves protect against exposure to blood, body fluids, and microorganisms.

(continued)

Skill · 37-8 Administering a Continuous Closed Bladder Irrigation *continued*

DOCUMENTATION

Guidelines

Document baseline assessment of patient. Document the amount and type of irrigation solution used and the patient's tolerance of the procedure. Record urine amount emptied from the drainage bag before the procedure and the amount of irrigant used on intake and output record. Record the amount of urine and irrigant emptied from the drainage bag. **Subtract the amount of irrigant instilled from the total volume of drainage to obtain the volume of urine output.**

Sample Documentation

> 12/14/12 1330 Foley catheter replaced with 3-way Foley catheter. Bladder nonpalpable. Continuous bladder irrigation with normal saline initiated at 100 mL/hour. Patient tolerated procedure without adverse effect. Drainage from bladder slightly cloudy, light cherry colored. No evidence of clots.
>
> —B. Clapp, RN

UNEXPECTED SITUATIONS AND ASSOCIATED INTERVENTIONS

- *Continuous bladder irrigation begins and hourly drainage is less than amount of irrigation being given:* Palpate for bladder distention. If patient is lying supine, rolling the patient onto side may help increase the amount of drainage. Check to make sure that the tubing is not kinked. If return flow remains decreased, notify physician.

- *Bladder irrigation is not flowing at ordered rate, even with clamp wide open:* Check the tubing for kinks or pressure points. Raise the bag 3″ to 6″ and then check flow of irrigation solution. Frequently check flow rate of irrigation solution.

Skill · 37-9 Emptying and Changing a Stoma Appliance on an Ileal Conduit

EQUIPMENT

- Basin with warm water
- Skin cleanser, towel, washcloth
- Silicone-based adhesive remover
- Gauze squares
- Washcloth or cotton balls
- Skin protectant
- Ostomy appliance
- Stoma measuring guide
- Graduated container
- Ostomy belt (optional)
- Disposable gloves
- Additional PPE, as indicated
- Waterproof disposable pad
- Small plastic trash bag

IMPLEMENTATION

ACTION	RATIONALE
1. Bring necessary equipment to the bedside stand or overbed table.	Bringing everything to the bedside conserves time and energy. Arranging items nearby is convenient, saves time, and avoids unnecessary stretching and twisting of muscles on the part of the nurse.
2. Perform hand hygiene and put on PPE, if indicated.	Hand hygiene and PPE prevent the spread of microorganisms. PPE is required based on transmission precautions.
3. Identify the patient.	Identifying the patient ensures the right patient receives the intervention and helps prevent errors.
4. Close curtains around bed and close door to room if possible. Explain what you are going to do and why you are going to do it to the patient. Encourage patient to observe or participate if possible.	This ensures the patient's privacy. Explanation relieves anxiety and facilitates cooperation. Discussion promotes cooperation and helps to minimize anxiety. Having the patient observe or assist encourages self-acceptance.

5. Assist patient to a comfortable sitting or lying position in bed or a standing or sitting position in the bathroom. If the patient is in bed, adjust the bed to a comfortable working height, usually elbow height of the caregiver (VISN 8, 2009). Place waterproof pad under the patient at the stoma site.

Emptying the Appliance

6. Put on gloves. Hold end of appliance over a bedpan, toilet, or measuring device. Remove the end cap from the spout. Open spout and empty contents into the bedpan, toilet, or measuring device (Figure 1).

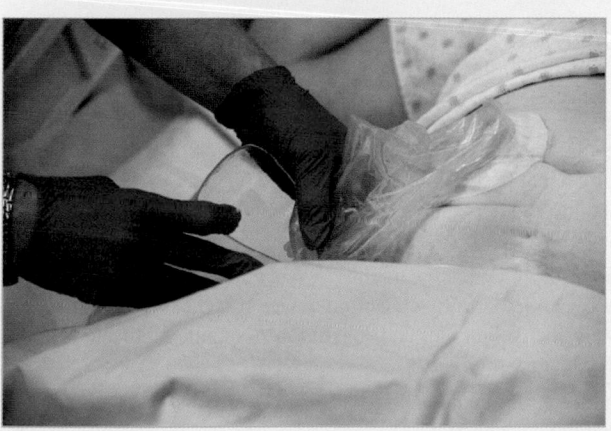

7. Close the spout. Wipe the spout with toilet tissue. Replace the cap.

8. Remove equipment. Remove gloves. Assist patient to comfortable position.

9. If appliance is not to be changed, place bed in lowest position. Remove additional PPE, if used. Perform hand hygiene.

Changing the Appliance

10. Place a disposable waterproof pad on the overbed table or other work area. Set up the washbasin with warm water and the rest of the supplies. Place a trash bag within reach.

11. Put on clean gloves. Place waterproof pad under the patient at the stoma site. Empty the appliance if necessary as described in Steps 6 to 8.

12. Gently remove appliance faceplate from skin by pushing skin from appliance rather than pulling appliance from skin. Start at the top of the appliance, while keeping the skin taut (Figure 2). Apply a silicone-based adhesive remover by spraying or wiping with the remover wipe. Push the skin from the appliance rather than pulling the appliance from the skin (Figure 3).

13. Place the appliance in the trash bag, if disposable. If reusable, set aside to wash in lukewarm soap and water and allow to air dry after the new appliance is in place.

Either position should allow the patient to view the procedure in preparation for learning to perform it independently. Lying flat or sitting upright facilitates smooth application of the appliance. Having the bed at the proper height prevents back and muscle strain. A waterproof pad protects linens and patient from moisture.

Gloves protect nurse from exposure to blood and body fluids. Emptying the pouch before handling it reduces the likelihood of spilling the excretions.

FIGURE 1. Emptying urine into graduated container.

Drying the spout removes any urine.

Proper removal of PPE prevents the transmission of microorganisms. Ensures patient comfort.

Lowering bed promotes patient safety. Removing PPE properly reduces the risk for infection transmission and contamination of other items. Hand hygiene prevents the spread of microorganisms.

The pad protects the surface. Organization facilitates performance of procedure.

Waterproof pad protects linens and patient from moisture. Emptying the contents before removal prevents accidental spillage of fecal material.

The seal between the surface of the faceplate and the skin must be broken before the faceplate can be removed. Harsh handling of the appliance can damage the skin and impair the development of a secure seal in the future. Silicone-based adhesive remover allows for the rapid and painless removal of adhesives and prevents skin stripping (Rudoni, 2008; Stephen-Haynes, 2008).

Thorough cleaning and airing of the appliance reduces odor and deterioration of appliance. For aesthetic and infection-control purposes, used appliances should be discarded appropriately.

(continued)

Skill · 37-9   **Emptying and Changing a Stoma Appliance on an Ileal Conduit**   *continued*

ACTION

FIGURE 2. Removing appliance faceplate from skin.

RATIONALE

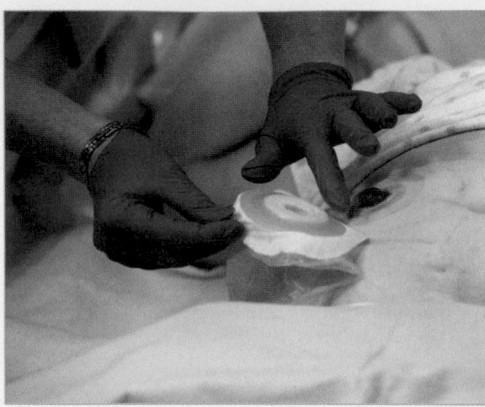

FIGURE 3. Pushing skin from appliance rather than pulling appliance from skin.

14. Clean skin around stoma with mild soap and water or a cleansing agent and a washcloth (Figure 4). Remove all old adhesive from skin; additional adhesive remover may be used. Do not apply lotion to peristomal area.

15. Gently pat area dry. **Make sure skin around stoma is thoroughly dry.** Assess stoma and condition of surrounding skin.

16. Place one or two gauze squares over stoma opening (Figure 5).

Cleaning the skin removes excretions and old adhesive and skin protectant. Excretions or a buildup of other substances can irritate and damage the skin. Lotion will prevent a tight adhesive seal.

Careful drying prevents trauma to skin and stoma. An intact, properly applied urinary collection device protects skin integrity. Any change in color and size of the stoma may indicate circulatory problems.

Continuous drainage must be absorbed to keep skin dry during appliance change.

FIGURE 4. Cleaning stoma with cleansing agent and water and washcloth.

FIGURE 5. Placing one or two gauze squares over opening.

17. Apply skin protectant to a 2″ (5-cm) radius around the stoma, and allow it to dry completely, which takes about 30 seconds.

18. Lift the gauze squares for a moment and measure the stoma opening, using the measurement guide. Replace the gauze. Trace the same size opening on the back center of the appliance. Cut the opening 1/8″ larger than the stoma size (Figure 6). Check that the spout is closed and the end cap is in place.

Skin protectant minimizes the risk of skin irritation from adhesive and moisture and increases adhesive's ability to adhere to skin.

The appliance should fit snugly around the stoma, with only 1/8″ of skin visible around the opening. A faceplate opening that is too small can cause trauma to the stoma. If the opening is too large, exposed skin will be irritated by urine. A closed spout and secured end cap prevent urine from leaking from the appliance.

ACTION

19. Remove the backing from the appliance. Quickly remove the gauze squares and discard appropriately; ease the appliance over the stoma. **Gently press onto the skin while smoothing over the surface (Figure 7). Apply gentle pressure to appliance for a few minutes.**

RATIONALE

The appliance is effective only if it is properly positioned and adhered securely.

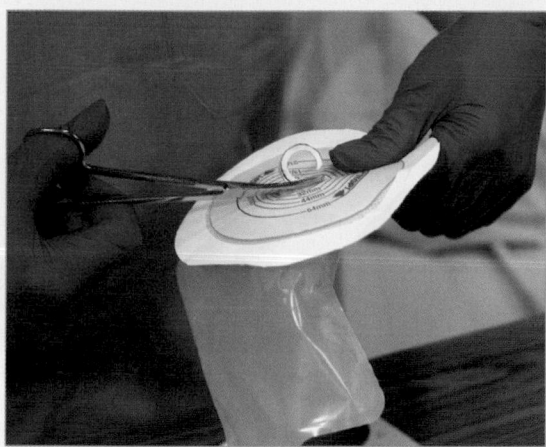

FIGURE 6. Cutting the faceplate opening 1/8" larger than stoma size.

FIGURE 7. Applying faceplate over stoma.

20. Secure optional belt to appliance and around patient.

An elasticized belt helps support the appliance for some people.

21. Remove gloves. Assist the patient to a comfortable position. Cover the patient with bed linens. Place the bed in the lowest position.

Removing gloves reduces risk of transmission of microorganisms. Positioning and covering provide warmth and promote comfort. Bed in lowest position promotes patient safety.

22. Put on clean gloves. Remove or discard any remaining equipment and assess patient's response to procedure.

The patient's response may indicate acceptance of the ostomy as well as the need for health teaching.

23. Remove gloves and additional PPE, if used. Perform hand hygiene.

Removing PPE properly reduces the risk for infection transmission and contamination of other items. Hand hygiene prevents the spread of microorganisms.

DOCUMENTATION

Guidelines

Document the procedure, including the appearance of the stoma, condition of the peristomal skin, characteristics of the urine, and the patient's response to the procedure.

Sample Documentation

7/23/12 1245 Ileal conduit appliance changed. Mr. Jones present. Mrs. Jones asking questions about care for ileal conduit, states, "I don't know if I'll ever be able to care for this thing at home." Tearful at times. Patient encouraged to express feelings. Patient agreed to talk with wound, ostomy, and continence nurse about concerns. Mr. Jones very supportive, also asking appropriate questions. Patient states would like to watch change one more time before she attempts to do it. Stoma is moist and red, peristomal skin intact, draining yellow urine with small amount of mucus.

—B. Clapp, RN

(continued)

Skill · 37-9 Emptying and Changing a Stoma Appliance on an Ileal Conduit *continued*

UNEXPECTED SITUATIONS AND ASSOCIATED INTERVENTIONS

- *Nurse removes appliance and finds area of skin excoriated:* If institution has a wound, ostomy, and incontinence nurse, consider a consultation. Cleanse the skin thoroughly and pat dry. Apply products made for excoriated skin before placing appliance over stoma. Frequently check faceplate to ensure that a seal has formed and that there is no leakage. Document the excoriation in the patient's chart.

- *Faceplate is leaking after applying new appliance:* Remove appliance, clean the skin, and start over.

- *Nurse is ready to place faceplate and notices that opening is cut too large:* Discard appliance and begin over. A faceplate that is cut too big may lead to excoriation of the skin.

SPECIAL CONSIDERATIONS

- If using a two-piece appliance, after applying faceplate, snap the appliance pouch in place. Lay the pouch flange over the flange on the faceplate. Start at the bottom, and push as you run your fingers around the flange, snapping the pouch onto the flange.

Skill · 37-10 Caring for a Hemodialysis Access (Arteriovenous Fistula or Graft)

EQUIPMENT

- Stethoscope
- PPE, as indicated

IMPLEMENTATION

ACTION	RATIONALE
1. Perform hand hygiene and put on PPE, if indicated.	Hand hygiene and PPE prevent the spread of microorganisms. PPE is required based on transmission precautions.
2. Identify the patient.	Identifying the patient ensures the right patient receives the intervention and helps prevent errors.
3. Close curtains around bed and close door to room if possible. Explain what you are going to do, and why you are going to do it, to the patient.	This ensures the patient's privacy. Explanation relieves anxiety and facilitates cooperation. Discussion promotes cooperation and helps to minimize anxiety.
4. **Inspect area over access site for any redness, warmth, tenderness, or blemishes. Palpate over access site, feeling for a thrill or vibration (Figure 1). Palpate pulses distal to the site. Auscultate over access site with bell of stethoscope, listening for a bruit or vibration.**	Inspection, palpation, and auscultation aid in determining the patency of the hemodialysis access. Assessment of distal pulse aids in determining the adequacy of circulation.

FIGURE 1. Palpating access site for thrill.

ACTION	RATIONALE
5. Ensure that a sign is placed over head of bed informing the healthcare team which arm is affected. **Do not measure blood pressure, perform a venipuncture, or start an IV on the access arm.**	The affected arm should not be used for any other procedures such as obtaining blood pressure, which could lead to clotting of the graft or fistula. Venipuncture or IV access could lead to an infection of the affected arm and could cause the loss of the graft or fistula.
6. Instruct patient not to sleep with the arm with the access site under head or body.	This could lead to clotting of the fistula or graft.
7. Instruct patient not to lift heavy objects with, or put pressure on, the arm with the access site. Advise the patient not to carry heavy bags (including purses) on the shoulder of that arm.	This could lead to clotting of the fistula or graft.
8. Remove PPE, if used. Perform hand hygiene.	Removing PPE properly reduces the risk for infection transmission and contamination of other items. Hand hygiene prevents the spread of microorganisms.

DOCUMENTATION

Document assessment findings, including the presence or absence of a bruit and thrill. Document any patient education and patient response.

Sample Documentation

> <u>5/10/12</u> 0830 Arteriovenous fistula patent in left upper arm. Area without redness, pain, and edema; skin at site similar to surrounding skin tone. Patient denies pain and tenderness. Positive bruit and thrill noted. Patient verbalized understanding of importance of avoiding venipuncture in left arm.
>
> —B. Clapp, RN

UNEXPECTED SITUATIONS AND ASSOCIATED INTERVENTIONS

- *Thrill is not palpable and/or bruit is not audible:* Notify the primary care provider immediately. The thrill and bruit are caused by arterial blood flowing into the vein. If these signs are not present, the access may be clotting off.

- *Site is warm to touch, erythematous, or painful or has a skin blemish:* Notify the primary care provider. These signs can indicate a site infection.

Skill · 37-11 Caring for a Peritoneal Dialysis Catheter

EQUIPMENT

- Face masks (2)
- Sterile gloves
- Nonsterile gloves
- Additional PPE, as indicated
- Antimicrobial cleansing agent, per facility policy
- Sterile gauze squares (4)
- Sterile basin
- Sterile drain sponge
- Topical antibiotic, such as mupirocin or gentamicin, depending on order and policy
- Sterile applicator
- Plastic trash bag
- Bath blanket

IMPLEMENTATION

ACTION	RATIONALE
1. Bring necessary equipment to the bedside stand or overbed table.	Bringing everything to the bedside conserves time and energy. Arranging items nearby is convenient, saves time, and avoids unnecessary stretching and twisting of muscles on the part of the nurse.
2. Perform hand hygiene and put on PPE, if indicated.	Hand hygiene and PPE prevent the spread of microorganisms. PPE is required based on transmission precautions.

(continued)

Skill · 37-11 Caring for a Peritoneal Dialysis Catheter *continued*

ACTION	RATIONALE
3. Identify the patient.	Identifying the patient ensures the right patient receives the intervention and helps prevent errors.
4. Close curtains around bed and close door to room if possible. Explain what you are going to do and why you are going to do it to the patient. Encourage patient to observe or participate if possible.	This ensures the patient's privacy. Explanation relieves anxiety and facilitates cooperation. Discussion promotes cooperation and helps to minimize anxiety. Having the patient observe or assist encourages self-acceptance.
5. Adjust bed to comfortable working height, usually elbow height of the caregiver (VISN 8, 2009). Assist patient to a supine position. Expose the abdomen, draping the patient's chest with the bath blanket, exposing only the catheter site.	Having the bed at the proper height prevents back and muscle strain. The supine position is usually the best way to gain access to the peritoneal dialysis catheter. Use of bath blanket provides patient warmth and avoids unnecessary exposure.
6. Put on unsterile gloves. Put on one of the face masks; have patient put on the other mask.	Gloves protect nurse from contact with blood and bodily fluids. Use of face masks deters the spread of microorganisms.
7. Gently remove old dressing, noting odor, amount, and color of drainage; leakage; and condition of skin around catheter. Discard dressing in appropriate container.	Drainage, leakage, and skin condition can indicate problems with the catheter, such as infection.
8. Remove gloves and discard. Set up sterile field. Open packages. Using aseptic technique, place two sterile gauze squares in basin with antimicrobial agent. Leave two sterile gauze squares opened on sterile field. Alternately (based on facility's policy), place sterile antimicrobial swabs on the sterile field. Place sterile applicator on field. Squeeze a small amount of the topical antibiotic on one of the gauze squares on the sterile field.	Until catheter site has healed, aseptic technique is necessary for site care to prevent infection.
9. Put on sterile gloves. Pick up dialysis catheter with nondominant hand. **With the antimicrobial-soaked gauze or swab, cleanse the skin around the exit site using a circular motion, starting at the exit site and then slowly going outward 3″ to 4″. Gently remove crusted scabs if necessary.**	Aseptic technique is necessary to prevent infection. The antimicrobial cleanses the skin and removes any drainage or crust from the wound, reducing the risk for infection.
10. **Continue to hold catheter with nondominant hand. After skin has dried, clean the catheter with an antimicrobial-soaked gauze, beginning at exit site, going around catheter, and then moving up to end of catheter. Gently remove crusted secretions on the tube if necessary.**	Antimicrobial cleanses the catheter and removes any drainage or crust from the tube, reducing the risk for infection.
11. Using the sterile applicator, apply the topical antibiotic to the catheter exit site, if prescribed.	Application of mupirocin and gentamicin at catheter exit site prevents exit site infection and peritonitis (Bernardini et al., 2005; The Joanna Briggs Institute, 2004).
12. Place sterile drain sponge around exit site. Then place a 4 × 4 gauze over exit site. Remove your gloves and secure edges of gauze pad with tape. Some institutions recommend placing a transparent dressing over the gauze pads instead of tape. Remove masks.	The drain sponge and 4 × 4 gauze are used to absorb any drainage from the exit site. Occlusion of the site with a dressing deters contamination of site. Once the site is covered, masks are no longer necessary.
13. Coil the exposed length of tubing and secure to the dressing or patient's abdomen with tape.	Anchoring the catheter absorbs any tugging, preventing tension on and irritation to the skin or abdomen.
14. Assist the patient to a comfortable position. Cover the patient with bed linens. Place the bed in the lowest position.	Positioning and covering provide warmth and promote comfort. A bed in the low position promotes patient safety.
15. Put on clean gloves. Remove or discard equipment and assess patient's response to procedure.	These actions deter the spread of microorganisms. The patient's response may indicate acceptance of the catheter or the need for health teaching.
16. Remove gloves and additional PPE, if used. Perform hand hygiene.	Removing PPE properly reduces the risk for infection transmission and contamination of other items. Hand hygiene prevents the spread of microorganisms.

DOCUMENTATION

Guidelines

Document the dressing change, including condition of skin surrounding exit site, drainage, or odor, as well as patient's reaction to procedure, and any patient teaching provided.

Sample Documentation

8/22/12 1530 Peritoneal dialysis catheter dressing changed; skin surrounding catheter slightly erythematous but remains intact. Small amount of clear drainage approximately the size of a dime without odor noted on drain sponge. Pt asking appropriate questions regarding dressing change. Verbalized an understanding of explanations.

—B. Clapp, RN

UNEXPECTED SITUATIONS AND ASSOCIATED INTERVENTIONS

- *Patient complains of pain when nurse palpates abdomen; purulent or cloudy drainage is present, or foul odor is noted when old dressing is removed:* Notify primary care provider immediately. Any of these signs could indicate a site infection or peritonitis.

- *Nurse notes that old dressing is saturated with clear fluid:* Replace dressing to prevent skin breakdown. Notify primary care provider. A frequent complication is leaking from exit site. Frequently check dressing, especially after patient has had solution placed in the abdominal cavity.

SPECIAL CONSIDERATIONS

General Considerations

- Patients with a peritoneal dialysis catheter should avoid baths and public pools.

- Patients performing own site care should be reminded of the importance of good handwashing before self-care.

- Once site is healed, some primary care providers do not require patients to wear a dressing unless the site is leaking. The patient may shower with an occlusive dressing over the exit site. The catheter exit site should be cleansed after showering.

Home Care Considerations

- Often, clean technique, instead of sterile technique, is used by the patient and caregivers in the home.

● Developing Critical Thinking Skills

1. The daughter of an older patient who is about to be discharged to the daughter's home requests that a catheter be inserted in her mother to make home care easier. The mother knows when she needs to void but needs assistance to get to the bathroom. How do you respond to the daughter's request?

2. If you noted the following when assessing a patient, what would you do?
   - A 6-year-old refuses to give a urine sample.
   - Frank blood appears in urine of a patient who has no history of urinary problems.
   - When you ask for a urine sample, a teenager asks, "This won't reveal drugs, will it?"
   - A young woman complains of painful urination with burning.
   - An older man reports frequency and pain when voiding.

● Practicing for the NCLEX

1. When collecting a urine specimen for routine urinalysis from a patient, the nurse keeps in mind which of the following?
   a. A sterile specimen is required for collection.
   b. Results may be altered if a sample is left standing at room temperature for a long time.
   c. The external meatus requires cleaning with antiseptic soap and water before voiding.
   d. A clean-catch midstream specimen is necessary.

2. Which of the following would the nurse incorporate into the teaching plan for a patient to promote healthy urinary functioning?
   a. Drinking more than 2,000 mL of fluid per day will cause fluid retention.
   b. The healthy adult should drink four to six 8-ounce glasses of water per day.

c. Children need fewer reminders to drink because of greater thirst sensitivity.

d. Caffeine-containing beverages should be monitored to prevent excess intake.

3. When a person has a fever or diaphoresis, how would the urine output be described?
   a. Decreased and highly concentrated
   b. Decreased and highly dilute
   c. Increased and concentrated
   d. Increased and dilute

4. The physician has ordered an indwelling catheter inserted in a hospitalized male patient. The nurse is aware of which of the following considerations?
   a. The male urethra is more vulnerable to injury during insertion.
   b. In the hospital, a clean technique is used for catheter insertion.
   c. The catheter is inserted 2″ to 3″ into the meatus.
   d. Since it uses a closed system, the risk for urinary tract infection is absent.

5. Nursing care for a patient with an indwelling catheter includes which of the following?
   a. Irrigation of the catheter with 30 mL of normal saline solution every 4 hours
   b. Disconnecting and reconnecting the drainage system quickly to obtain a urine specimen
   c. Encouraging a generous fluid intake if not contraindicated by the patient's condition.
   d. Telling the patient that burning and irritation are normal, subsiding within a few days

6. After surgery, Ms. Young is having difficulty voiding. Which nursing action would most likely lead to an increased difficulty with voiding?
   a. Pouring warm water over Ms. Young's fingers
   b. Having Ms. Young ignore the urge to void until her bladder is full
   c. Using a warm bedpan when Ms. Young feels the urge to void
   d. Stroking Ms. Young's leg or thigh

7. Mr. Cheng, a hospitalized patient with diabetes mellitus, has developed a UTI. He is 80 years old and has an indwelling catheter in place. Which factor is most likely the cause of his UTI?
   a. The close proximity of the male genitalia to the rectum
   b. Decreased immunity
   c. A high urine glucose level
   d. The indwelling urinary catheter

8. Which of the following terms denotes a patient's inability to void even though the kidneys are producing urine that enters the bladder?
   a. Urgency
   b. Retention
   c. Oliguria
   d. Dysuria

9. Mrs. D'Ambrosia, an alert, ambulatory, older nursing home resident, voids frequently and has difficulty making it to the bathroom in time. The nurse planning her care is aware of which of the following?
   a. Incontinence is to be expected in a woman Mrs. D'Ambrosia's age.
   b. One of every 10 nursing home residents is incontinent.
   c. Kegel exercises performed at regular intervals throughout the day may be helpful.
   d. An indwelling catheter should be inserted as soon as possible.

10. The priority treatment option for Mrs. D'Ambrosia would most likely involve which of the following?
    a. Behavioral techniques
    b. Pharmacologic measures
    c. Surgical intervention
    d. Use of absorbent products

11. A patient taking phenazopyridine (Pyridium, a urinary tract analgesic) should be cautioned that her urine may change to what color?
    a. Pale yellow
    b. Green
    c. Orange-red
    d. Brown

12. Mr. Bales is 60 years old and alert. He is timid and reluctant to talk about his urinary retention problem. Which part of this plan could create stress for Mr. Bales and possibly increase his inability to urinate?
    a. Assisting him in assuming his normal voiding position
    b. Pulling curtains around him to provide privacy during voiding
    c. Staying with him while voiding
    d. Offering the urinal on a regular schedule

13. Which of the following is a nursing priority when caring for a male patient with a condom catheter?
    a. Preventing the tubing from kinking to maintain free urinary drainage
    b. Not removing the catheter for any reason
    c. Fastening the condom tightly to prevent the possibility of leakage
    d. Maintaining bed rest at all times to prevent the catheter from slipping off

14. A patient has a nursing diagnosis of Impaired Urinary Elimination related to maturational enuresis. You recognize that your patient is which of the following?
    a. An adult older than 65 years of age who is incontinent
    b. A child older than 4 years of age who has involuntary urination
    c. A 12-month-old child who has involuntary urination
    d. A patient with neurologic damage resulting in bladder dysfunction

15. Data must be collected to evaluate the effectiveness of a plan to reduce urinary incontinence in an older adult patient. Of the information below, which is least important for the evaluation process?
    a. The incontinence pattern
    b. State of physical mobility
    c. Medications being taken
    d. Age of the patient

● Answers with Rationale

1. *b.* Urine chemistry is altered after urine stands at room temperature for a long period of time. For a routine urinalysis, a clean specimen is adequate. The external meatus does not need to be cleaned with an antiseptic, as is required for a clean-catch midstream specimen.

2. *d.* Caffeine intake should be limited because it is irritating to the bladder mucosa. It is recommended that a healthy adult drink 8 to 10 8-oz glasses of fluid daily. Unless a disease process is present, this will not cause fluid retention. Children frequently need to be reminded to drink fluids.

3. *a.* Fever and diaphoresis cause the kidneys to conserve body fluids. Thus, the urine is concentrated and decreased in amount.

4. *a.* Because of its length, the male urethra is more prone to injury and requires that the catheter be inserted 6″ to 8″. This procedure requires surgical asepsis to prevent introducing bacteria into the urinary tract. The presence of an indwelling catheter places the patient at risk for a UTI.

5. *c.* A generous fluid intake promotes healthy urinary tract functioning. Irrigation may introduce bacteria into the urinary tract and is not routinely ordered. The drainage system should never be disconnected to obtain a specimen because this may allow bacteria to enter the urinary tract. Burning and irritation may indicate that an infection is present and should never be disregarded.

6. *b.* Ignoring the urge to void makes urination even more difficult and should be avoided. The other activities are all recommended nursing activities to promote voiding.

7. *d.* Most UTIs in hospitalized patients are caused by the presence of an indwelling catheter. Additional, although less significant, causes of UTI include a decrease in immunity common in elderly people and the presence of glucose in the urine, as seen in diabetes.

8. *b.* Urgency is a strong desire to void. Oliguria is scanty or a greatly diminished amount of urine voided in a given time. Dysuria is difficulty urinating.

9. *c.* Kegel exercises may help a patient regain control of the micturition process. Incontinence is not a normal consequence of aging, and at least half of nursing home residents may be incontinent. An indwelling catheter is the last choice of treatment.

10. *a.* The least invasive interventions should be attempted first. Pharmacologic and surgical interventions are not recommended until behavioral techniques have been attempted. Using absorbent products may remove motivation from the patient and caregiver to seek evaluation and treatment of the incontinence. They should be used only after careful evaluation by a healthcare provider.

11. *c.* Pyridium is noted for turning the urine orange-red, and the patient needs to be aware of this.

12. *c.* Mr. Bales will probably be embarrassed if the nurse remains with him as he attempts to void and is more likely to have difficulty voiding.

13. *a.* The catheter should be allowed to drain freely through tubing that is not kinked. It also should be removed daily to prevent skin excoriation and should not be fastened too tightly or restriction of blood vessels in the area is likely. Confining a patient to bed rest increases the risk for other hazards related to immobility.

14. *b.* Maturational enuresis is involuntary urination after an age when continence should be present. A 12-month-old child is not expected to be continent, and incontinence and neurologic damage are not maturational problems.

15. *d.* Incontinence is not a natural consequence of the aging process. All the other factors are necessary information for the plan of care.

Taylor Suite Resources

The Taylor Suite offers these additional resources to enhance learning and facilitate understanding of this chapter:

- thePoint online resource, http://thepoint.lww.com/Taylor7E
- Student DVD-ROM included with the book
- Study Guide for Taylor's Fundamentals of Nursing
- Skill Checklists for Taylor's Fundamentals of Nursing
- Taylor's Video Guide to Clinical Nursing Skills: *Urinary Elimination* and *Urinary Catheters*
- Taylor's Clinical Nursing Skills: *Chapter 12, Urinary Elimination*

BIBLIOGRAPHY

Altschuler, V., & Diaz, L. (2006). Bladder ultrasound. *MEDSURG Nursing, 15*(5), 317–318.

Andrews, M., & Boyle, J. (2008). *Transcultural concepts in nursing care* (5th ed.). Philadelphia: Wolters Kluwer Health/ Lippincott Williams & Wilkins.

Aschenbrenner, D., & Venable, S. (2009). *Drug therapy in nursing* (3rd ed.). Philadelphia: Wolters Kluwer Health/Lippincott Williams & Wilkins.

Bernardini, J., Bender, F., Florio, T., Sloand, L., PalmMontalbano, L., Fried, L., et al. (2005). Randomized, double-blind trial of antibiotic exit site cream for prevention of exit site infection in peritoneal dialysis patients. *Journal of the American Society of Nephrology, 16*(2), 539–545.

Best Practices: Evidence-based nursing procedures. (2007). (2nd ed.). Philadelphia: Wolters Kluwer Health/Lippincott Williams & Wilkins.

Bulechek, G., Butcher, H., & McCloskey Dochterman, J. (Eds.). (2008). *Nursing interventions classification (NIC)* (5th ed.). St. Louis: Mosby Elsevier.

Carpenito-Moyet, L. (2008). *Nursing diagnosis: Application to clinical practice* (12th ed.). Philadelphia: Wolters Kluwer Health/Lippincott Williams & Wilkins.

Chettle, C. (2008). Nurses critical as reimbursement dries up for catheter-associated UTIs. *Nursing Spectrum, 17*(16), 24–28.

Cohen, B., & Taylor, J. (2009). *Memmler's structure and function of the human body* (9th ed.). Philadelphia: Wolters Kluwer Health/Lippincott Williams & Wilkins.

Collis Pellatt, G. (2007a). Anatomy and physiology of urinary elimination. Part 1. *British Journal of Nursing, 16*(7), 406–410.

Collis Pellat, G. (2007b). Urinary elimination: Part 2- retention, incontinence and catheterization. *British Journal of Nursing, 16*(8), 480–485.

Crosby, C. (2005). Securing Foley catheters; controlling biofilm. *HEALTHCARE Purchasing NEWS, 29*(10), 34.

Fischbach, F., & Dunning, M. (2006). *Common laboratory & diagnostic tests* (4th ed.). Philadelphia: Lippincott Williams & Wilkins.

Fischbach, F., & Dunning, M. (2009). *A manual of laboratory and diagnostic tests* (8th ed.). Philadelphia: Wolters Kluwer Health/ Lippincott Williams & Wilkins.

Gotelli, J., Merryman, P., Carr, C., McElveen, L., Epperson, C., & Bynum, D. (2008). A quality improvement project to reduce the complications associated with indwelling urinary catheters. *UROLOGIC NURSING, 28*(6), 465–473.

Griebling, T. (2004a). Urinary tract infection in men. In M. Litwin & C. Saigal (Eds.), *Urologic diseases in America* (pp. 187–212). US Department of Health and Human Services, Public Health Service, National Institutes of Health, National Institute of Diabetes and Digestive and Kidney Diseases, Washington, DC: US Government Publishing Office; NIH publication no. 04-5512.

Griebling, T. (2004b). Urinary tract infection in women. In M. Litwin & C. Saigal (Eds.), *Urologic diseases in America* (pp. 153–186). US Department of Health and Human Services, Public Health Service, National Institutes of Health, National Institute of Diabetes and Digestive and Kidney Diseases, Washington, DC: US Government Publishing Office; NIH publication no. 04-5512.

Hockenberry, M., & Wilson, D. (2008). *Wong's essentials of pediatric nursing* (8th ed.). St. Louis: Elsevier Mosby.

Huang, J., Lin, S., Yeh, S., & Wang, C. (2007). Effects of bladder training at reducing incontinence episodes, symptom distress and incontinence impact among women with urinary incontinence. *Journal of Evidence-Based Nursing, 3*(4), 289–99.

Jarvis, C. (2008). *Physical examination & health assessment* (5th ed.). St. Louis: Saunders/Elsevier.

The Joanna Briggs Institute. (2004). Clinical effectiveness of different approaches to peritoneal dialysis catheter exit-site care. *BestPractice, 8*(1), 1–7.

Karon, S. (2005). A team approach to bladder retraining: A pilot study. *Urologic Nursing, 25*(4), 269–276.

Kassler, J., & Barnett, J. (2008). A rehabilitation hospital's experience with ionic silver Foley catheters. *Urologic Nursing, 28*(2), 97–99.

Kyle, T. (2008). *Essentials of pediatric nursing.* Philadelphia: Wolters Kluwer/Lippincott Williams & Wilkins.

The Mayo Clinic. (2008a). Hemodialysis. Available at www.mayoclinic.com/health/hemodialysis/MY00281.

The Mayo Clinic. (2008b). Peritoneal dialysis. Available at http://www.mayoclinic.com/health/peritoneal-dialysis/MY00282.

Mercer Smith, J. (2003). Indwelling catheter management: From habit-based to evidence-based practice. *OstomyWound Management, 49*(12), 34–45.

Moorhead, S., Johnson, M., Maas, M., Swanson, E. (Eds). (2008). *Nursing outcomes classification (NOC)* (4th ed.). St. Louis: Mosby Elsevier.

National Kidney and Urologic Diseases Information Clearinghouse (NKUDIC). (2007a). *Bladder control for women.* Available at http://kidney.niddk.nih.gov/kudiseases/pubs/bcw_ez/index.htm.

National Kidney and Urologic Diseases Information Clearinghouse (NKUDIC). (2007b). *Urinary incontinence in men.* NIH publication No. 07-5280. Available at http://kidney.niddk.nih.gov/kudiseases/pubs/uimen/.

National Kidney and Urologic Diseases Information Clearinghouse (NKUDIC). (2007c). *Urinary incontinence in women.* NIH publication No. 08-4132. Available at http://kidney.niddk.nih.gov/kudiseases/pubs/uiwomen/.

National Kidney and Urologic Diseases Information Clearinghouse (NKUDIC). (2007d). *Urinary tract infections.* Available at http://kidney.niddk.nih.gov/kudiseases/pubs/uti_ES/index.htm.

Nazarko, L. (2008a). Caring for a patient with a urostomy in a community setting. *British Journal of Community Nursing, 13*(8), 354, 356, 358.

Nazarko, L. (2008b). Effective evidence based catheter management. *British Journal of Community Nursing, 13*(3), 110, 112–114.

Newman, D. (2008). Internal and external urinary catheters: A primer for clinical practice. *Ostomy Wound Management, 54*(12), 18–20, 22–26, 28–38.

NANDA-I. (2009). *Nursing diagnoses: Definitions and classification 2009–2011.* West Sussex, UK: Wiley-Blackwell.

Patraca, K. (2005). Measure bladder volume without catheterization. *Nursing, 35*(4), 46–47.

Porth, C., & Matfin, G. (2009). *Pathophysiology: Concepts of altered health states* (8th ed.). Philadelphia: Wolters Kluwer Health/Lippincott Williams & Wilkins.

Redmond, A., & Doherty, E. (2005). Peritoneal dialysis. *Nursing Standard, 19*(40), 55–65.

Rigby, D., & Gray, K. (2005). Understanding urine testing. *Nursing Times, 101*(12), 60–62.

Robinson, J. (2004). A practical approach to catheter-associated problems. *Nursing Standard, 14*(18), 38–42.

Robinson, J. (2007). Intermittent self-catheterisation: Teaching the skill to patients. *Nursing Standard, 21*(29), 48–56.

Robinson, J. (2008). Post micturition dribble in men: Causes and treatment. *Nursing Standard, 22*(30), 43–46.

Roy-Chaudhury, P., Kelly, B., Melhem, M., Zhang, J., Li, J., Desai, P., et al. (2005). Vascular access in hemodialysis: Issues, management, and emerging concepts. *Cardiology Clinics, 23*(3), 249–273.

Rudoni, C. (2008). A service evaluation of the use of silicone-based adhesive remover. *British Journal of Nursing, Stoma Care Supplement, 17*(2), 54, 56, 58–59.

Saint, S., Kaufman, S., Rogers, M., Baker, P., Ossenkop, K., & Lipsky, B. (2006). Condom versus indwelling urinary catheters: A randomized trial. *Journal of the American Geriatrics Society, 54*(7), 1055–1061.

Schumm, K., & Lam, T. (2008). Types of urethral catheters for management of short-term voiding problems in hospitalised adults. *Cochrane Database of Systematic Reviews 2008,* Issue 2. Art. No,: CD004013. DOI: 1002/14651858. CD0044013.pub3.

Seymour, C. (2006). Audit of catheter-associated UTI using silver alloy-coated Foley catheters. *British Journal of Nursing, 15*(11), 598, 600–603.

Smeltzer, S., Bare, B., Hinkle, J., & Cheever, K. (2010). *Brunner & Suddarth's textbook of medical-surgical nursing* (12th ed.). Philadelphia: Wolters Kluwer Health/Lippincott Williams & Wilkins.

Society of Urologic Nurses and Associates (SUNA). (2005a). *Care of the patient with an indwelling catheter: Clinical practice guideline.* Available at http://www.suna.org/resources/indwellingCatheter.pdf.

Society of Urologic Nurses and Associates. (2005b). *Female urethral catheterization: Clinical practice guideline.* Available at http://www.suna.org/resources/femaleCatheterization.pdf.

Society of Urologic Nurses and Associates. (2005c). *Male urethral catheterization: Clinical practice guideline.* Available at http://www.suna.org/resources/maleCatheterization.pdf.

Specht, J. (2005). 9 myths of incontinence in older adults. *American Journal of Nursing, 105*(6), 58–69.

Stephen-Hayes, J. (2008). Skin integrity and silicone: APPEEL 'nosting' medical adhesive remover. *British Journal of Nursing, 17*(2), 792–795.

Stevens, E. (2005). Bladder ultrasound: Avoiding unnecessary catheterizations. *Medsurg Nursing, 14*(4), 249–253.

Tabloski, P. (2006). *Gerontological nursing.* Upper Saddle River, NJ: Pearson Prentice Hall.

Toughill, E. (2005). Bladder matters. Indwelling urinary catheters: Common mechanical and pathogenic problems. *American Journal of Nursing, 105*(5), 35–37.

Ünlü, H., Çetinkaya Şardan, Y., & Ülker, S. (2007). Comparison of sampling methods for urine cultures. *Journal of Nursing Scholarship, 39*(4), 325–329.

Uttley, L., Vardhan, A., Mahajan, S., Smart, B., Hutchison, A., & Gokal, R. (2004). Decrease in infections with the introduction of mupirocin cream at the peritoneal dialysis catheter exit site. *Journal of Nephrology, 17*(2), 242–245.

VISN 8 Patient Safety Center. (2009). *Safe patient handling and measurement algorithms.* Tampa, FL: Author. Available at www.visn8.va.gov/patientsafetycenter/safePtHandling. Accessed April 23, 2010.

Weber, J., & Kelley, J. (2007). *Health assessment in nursing* (3rd ed.). Philadelphia: Wolters Kluwer/Lippincott Williams & Wilkins.

Weiss, B. (2005). Selecting medications for the treatment of urinary incontinence. *American Family Physician, 71*(2), 315–322.

Wilson, L. (2005). Urinalysis. *Nursing Standard, 19*(35), 51–54.

Woods, A. (2005). Managing UTIs in older adults. *Nursing, 35*(3), 12.

Yates, A. (2008). Identifying and managing urinary continence problems. *Practice Nurse, 36*(9), 31–32, 34, 36.

38 Bowel Elimination

JEREMY GREEN

Jeremy, age 4, has been attending daycare since his mother returned to work 6 months ago. He presents at the hospital with a history of liquid stools, six to seven times a day, for the last 3 days.

ALBERTA FRANKLIN

Alberta, age 55, has recently undergone abdominal surgery and creation of a sigmoid colostomy. Her stoma is bright red and moist and draining semisoft brown stool. Her ostomy appliance needs to be changed.

LEROY COBBS

Leroy, newly diagnosed with cancer, is taking acetaminophen (Tylenol) with codeine for pain. He is hospitalized for fecal impaction. "Nobody told me I would get so constipated," he says. "It's been almost a week and I'm still not moving my bowels normally. I didn't know anything could hurt so bad. I'll take my chances with the cancer pain in the future rather than take more pain meds and have this happen again."

After completing the chapter, you will be able to accomplish the following:

1. Describe the physiology of bowel elimination.

2. Identify variables that influence bowel elimination.

3. Assess bowel elimination using appropriate interview questions and physical assessment skills.

4. Assist with stool collection for laboratory analysis and direct and indirect visualization studies of the gastrointestinal tract.

5. Develop nursing diagnoses that identify bowel elimination problems amenable to nursing intervention.

6. Identify appropriate nursing interventions to promote regular bowel habits.

7. Identify appropriate nursing interventions when administering cathartics, laxatives, and antidiarrheals.

8. Identify appropriate nursing interventions when administering enemas, rectal suppositories, rectal catheters, and performing digital removal of stool.

9. Design and implement bowel training programs.

10. Identify appropriate nursing interventions to use comfort measures to ease defecation.

11. Plan nursing care for a patient with an ostomy.

12. Plan, implement, and evaluate nursing care related to select nursing diagnoses that involve bowel problems.

KEY TERMS

anus	flatulence
bowel incontinence	flatus
bowel training program	hemorrhoids
cathartic	ileostomy
colostomy	laxative
constipation	occult blood
defecation	ostomy
diarrhea	paralytic ileus
endoscopy	peristalsis
enema	stoma
fecal impaction	stool
fecal incontinence	suppository
feces	Valsalva maneuver

Patients differ widely in their expectations about bowel elimination, their usual pattern of defecation, and the ease with which they speak of bowel problems. Although most people have experienced minor acute bouts of diarrhea or constipation, some patients experience severe or chronic alterations in bowel elimination that affect their fluid and electrolyte balance, hydration, nutritional status, skin integrity, comfort, and self-concept. Moreover, many illnesses, diagnostic tests, medications, and surgical treatments can affect bowel elimination.

This chapter discusses the physiology of bowel elimination and the multiple factors that influence this process. A guide for assessing bowel elimination, including diagnostic studies of the gastrointestinal tract and their associated nursing responsibilities, is presented. Numerous examples of nursing diagnoses are included.

The chapter describes goals for both the nurse and the patient and nursing strategies to meet those goals. The accompanying Reflective Practice display illustrates nursing strategies addressing bowel diversions. The concluding nursing plan of care illustrates the use of specific nursing interventions to resolve bowel elimination problems.

ANATOMY AND PHYSIOLOGY

The gastrointestinal tract, also known as the alimentary tract or canal, extends from the mouth to the anus. The anatomy of the gastrointestinal tract is shown in Figure 38-1. The stomach and small intestine are discussed briefly. However, the major organ involved with bowel elimination is the large intestine.

Stomach

The stomach is a hollow, J-shaped, muscular organ located in the left upper portion of the abdomen. The stomach stores food during eating, secretes digestive fluids, churns food to aid in digestion, and pushes the partially digested food, called chyme, into the small intestine. The pyloric sphincter, a muscular ring that regulates the size of the opening at the end of the stomach, controls the movement of chyme from the stomach into the small intestine.

Small Intestine

The small intestine is about 20 feet (6 m) long and about 1 inch (2.2 cm) wide. The small intestine is made up of three parts: the first is the duodenum, the middle section is the jejunum, and the distal section that connects with the large intestine is the ileum (Fig. 38-2). The small intestine secretes enzymes that digest proteins and carbohydrates. Digestive juices from the liver and pancreas enter the small intestine through a small opening in the duodenum. The small intestine is responsible for digestion of food and absorption of nutrients into the bloodstream.

Large Intestine

The connection between the ileum of the small intestine and the large intestine is the ileocecal, or ileocolic, valve. This

REFLECTIVE PRACTICE

Challenge to Technical Skills

Although nursing students learn the technologies in the simulation practice laboratory, it is often quite a different situation when they are asked to perform the technology for the first time independently. I found this to be true the first time that I had to perform colostomy care independently.

I met Alberta Franklin while working as a nursing extern this summer. She was a 55-year-old woman who had recently undergone abdominal surgery and creation of a sigmoid colostomy. She required a new colostomy bag, and I was asked to change the bag. Although colostomies do not require the computerized technology found in an ICU, they do require technical skills. I had practiced changing colostomy bags in the nursing skills lab and had observed nurses changing the colostomy bag in the hospital. I had even previously changed a colostomy bag while being supervised by a nurse. Although I was not completely comfortable with the situation, I agreed to change the bag. I quickly reviewed the steps in the protocol book and went into the patient's room. I measured the colostomy and then cut the bag to the appropriate size. Unfortunately, I had measured the colostomy incorrectly, and the bag was too large, so I had to leave the room and get more supplies. After a few more obstacles, I was able to adhere a properly fitting bag to the patient—but not before the patient correctly guessed that this was the first time I had performed this skill! Her ability to guess that I had never performed this skill before illustrates my technical incompetence.

Thinking Outside the Box: Possible Courses of Action

- Refuse to provide the care and ask another nurse to change the colostomy bag.
- Observe a nurse performing the care one more time.
- Check protocol and perform the care, knowing that I could call a nurse if needed.

- "Wing it" and hope that I remember what I had learned in lab.

Evaluating a Good Outcome: How Do I Define Success?

- Patient receives safe care.
- Patient's needs are met.

- Nurse demonstrates technical competency with the skill.

Personal Learning: Here's to the Future!

I think that my actions were appropriate. Although I was unsure about my technical skills regarding colostomy care, I performed the skill adequately. In addition, I reviewed the appropriate steps and I knew that I could summon the assistance of a nurse in case I needed to do so. I also made sure that I knew where the nurse was so that if I did need help, I wouldn't waste any time looking for help. Therefore, I ensured that the patient's safety would not be compromised. Although at that time I would have preferred to have another nurse perform the colostomy change, I am glad that I completed this technical skill independently. Observing another person performing a skill can be beneficial, but there comes a point when you must "spread your wings" and complete the skill on your own. Of course, this philosophy regarding spreading your wings applies only to certain technologies: It would be inappropriate to use this philosophy if it compromised patient safety. However, in incidences like this one, where patient safety is not compromised and the appropriate teaching and training have been completed, I think it is appropriate to take action. If you don't, the various technologies in the hospital can become extremely intimidating and overwhelming. As a result, fear increases, which can possibly threaten a patient's safety and lead to injury.

Elizabeth Nalli, Georgetown University

Reflection

How do you think you would respond in a similar situation? Why? What does this tell you about yourself and about the adequacy of your skills for professional practice? Did the nursing student's actions adhere to ethical and legal principles? If not, describe what principles were violated. Could the nursing student have done anything more to deal with this situation? Explain your answer. What actions or behaviors by the nursing student might have provided clues to the patient that this was the nursing student's first independent attempt at the skill? Can you think of other ways to respond? What other skills (cognitive, interpersonal, technical, ethical/legal) would you need to respond well in this situation? Do you agree with the criteria to evaluate a successful outcome? Are there any other criteria that would need to be included? If so, specify these criteria. Did the nursing student meet the criteria listed?

valve normally prevents contents from entering the large intestine prematurely and prevents waste products from returning to the small intestine.

The large intestine, the primary organ of bowel elimination, is the lower, or distal, part of the gastrointestinal tract. The large intestine, also known as the colon, extends from the ileocecal valve to the anus. The colon in adults is about 5 feet (1.5 m) long, but variations in length are normal. Width also varies; at its narrowest point, the colon is about 1 inch (2.5 cm) wide; at its widest point, it is about 3 inches (7.5 cm). The diameter of the colon decreases from the cecum to the anus (see Fig. 38-2).

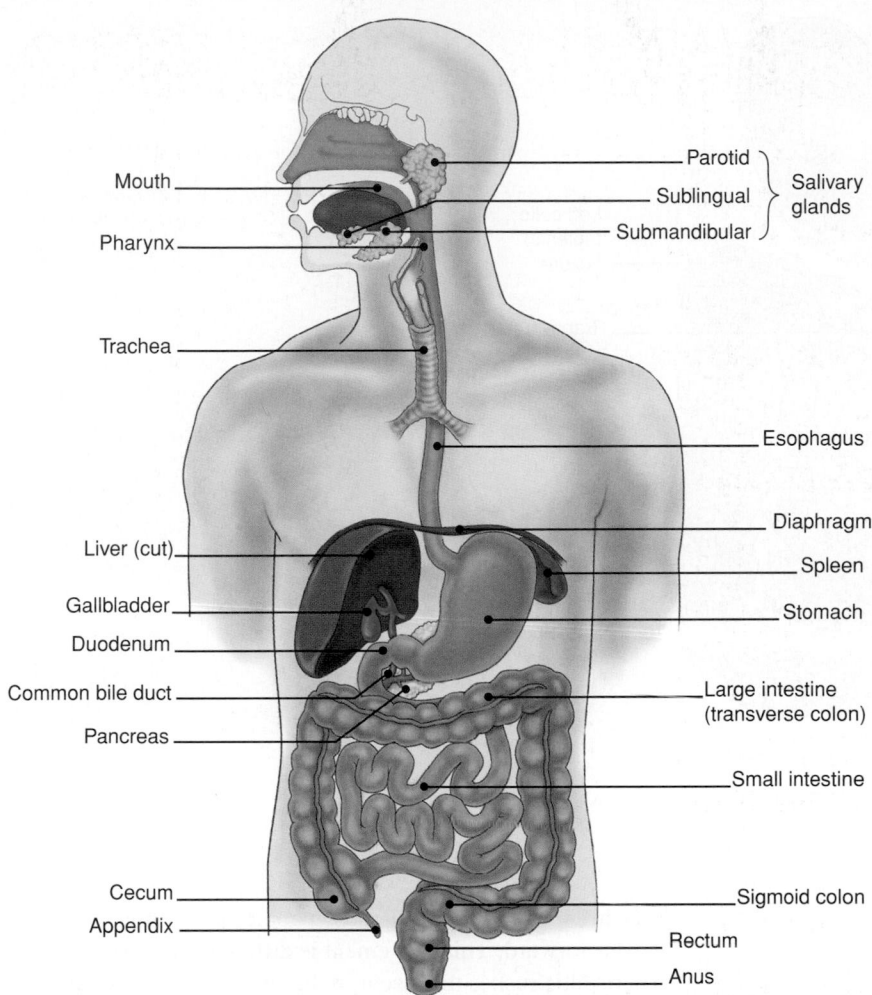

Mouth

Pharynx

Trachea

Liver (cut)

Gallbladder

Duodenum

Common bile duct

Pancreas

Cecum

Appendix

Parotid ⎫
Sublingual ⎬ Salivary glands
Submandibular ⎭

Esophagus

Diaphragm

Spleen

Stomach

Large intestine (transverse colon)

Small intestine

Sigmoid colon

Rectum

Anus

FIGURE 38-1. Organs of the gastrointestinal tract.

From the cecum, the first part of the large intestine, the digestive contents enter the colon, which consists of several segments. The ascending colon extends from the cecum upward toward the liver, where it turns to cross the abdomen. This turn is called the hepatic flexure. Upon turning, this portion of the colon becomes the transverse colon, crossing the abdomen from right to left. The colon then turns at the splenic flexure to become the descending colon. The descending colon passes down the left side of the body to the sigmoid, or pelvic, colon.

The sigmoid colon contains **feces,** solid waste products that have reached the distal end of the colon and are ready for excretion. Once excreted, feces are called **stool.** The sigmoid colon empties into the rectum, the last part of the large intestine. The rectum is about 12 cm (5 inches) long, 2.5 cm (1 inch) of which is the anal canal. In the rectum, three transverse folds of tissue are present that may help to hold the fecal material in the rectum temporarily. Vertical folds also are present, each of which contains an artery and a vein. If the veins become abnormally distended, **hemorrhoids** occur.

The rectum is empty except immediately before and during **defecation** (the process of bowel elimination; a bowel movement). Feces are excreted from the rectum through the anal canal, which is approximately 2.5 to 3.8 cm (1 to 1.5 inches) long, and out an opening called the **anus.**

Functions of the large intestine include the absorption of water, the formation of feces, and the expulsion of feces from the body. Bacteria that reside in the large intestine act on food residue while it makes its way through the large intestine. Bacterial action produces vitamin K and some of the B-complex vitamins. The products of digestion, chyme, move from the small intestine, passing through the ileocecal valve, and enter the cecum. Approximately 1,500 mL of chyme enters the large intestine daily. Its contents are liquid or watery. While passing through the large intestine, most water is absorbed. About 800 to 1,000 mL of liquid is absorbed daily by the intestinal tract, allowing for the formed, semisolid consistency of the normal stool. When absorption does not occur properly, such as when the waste products pass through the large intestine rapidly, the stool is soft and watery. Conversely, if the stool remains in the large intestine too long, or if too much water is absorbed, the stool becomes dry and hard.

▶ *Recall Alberta Franklin, the woman who had surgery that resulted in the creation of a sigmoid colostomy, described at the beginning of the chapter. Knowledge of normal gastrointestinal function would help the nurse in developing a teaching plan for this patient about her ostomy and what to expect in relation to bowel function.* ■

FIGURE 38-2. The small and large intestines.

Nervous System Control

The autonomic nervous system innervates the muscles of the colon. The parasympathetic nervous system stimulates movement, while the sympathetic system inhibits movement. Contractions of the circular and longitudinal muscles of the intestine, **peristalsis,** occur every 3 to 12 minutes, moving waste products along the length of the intestine continuously (Fig. 38-3). Mass peristaltic sweeps occur one to four times

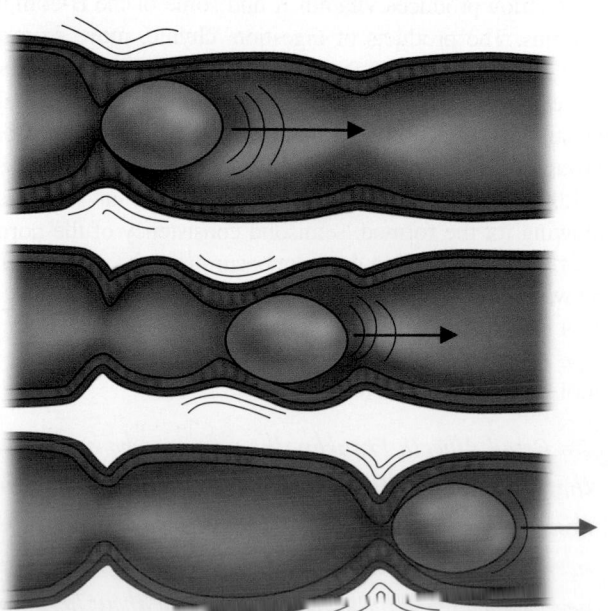

FIGURE 38-3. Peristaltic movements in the intestine.

each 24-hour period in most people, propelling the fecal mass forward. This movement is different from the frequent peristaltic rushes that occur in the small intestine. Mass peristalsis often occurs after food has been ingested, accounting for the urge to defecate that often occurs after meals. Timing nursing interventions to evacuate bowel contents with this natural urge to defecate is helpful. One third to one half of ingested food waste is normally excreted in the stool within 24 hours, and the remainder within the next 24 to 48 hours.

After passing through the sigmoid colon, the waste products enter the rectum, where they are stopped from exiting by the anal sphincters. The internal sphincter in the anal canal and the external sphincter at the anus control the discharge of feces and **flatus** (intestinal gas). The internal sphincter consists of involuntary smooth muscle tissue that is innervated by the autonomic nervous system. Motor impulses are carried by the sympathetic system (thoracolumbar) and inhibitory impulses by the parasympathetic system (craniosacral). These two divisions of the autonomic nervous system function antagonistically in a dynamic equilibrium. The external sphincter at the anus has striated muscle tissue and is under voluntary control. The levator ani muscle reinforces the action of the external sphincter and is controlled voluntarily (Fig. 38-4).

Defecation

Defecation refers to the emptying of the large intestine. Two centers govern the reflex to defecate, one in the medulla and a subsidiary one in the spinal cord. When parasympathetic

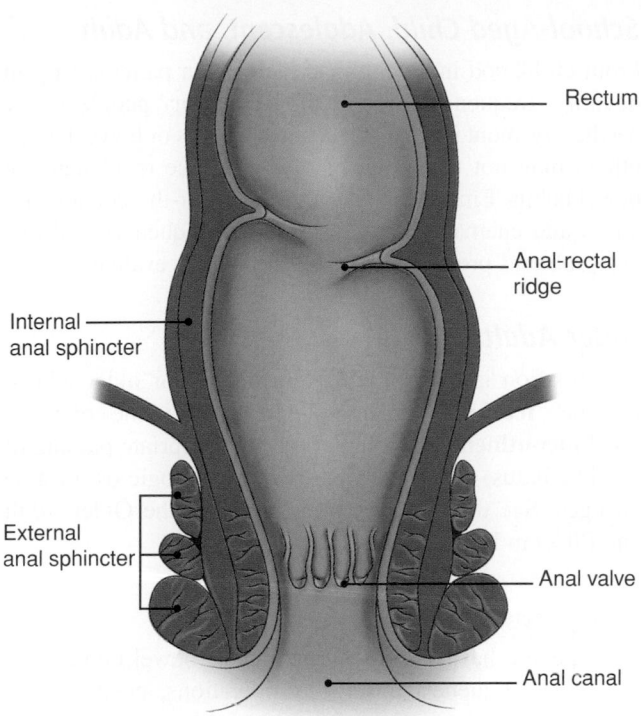

FIGURE 38-4. Interior view of the rectum and anal canal.

stimulation occurs, the internal anal sphincter relaxes and the colon contracts, allowing the fecal mass to enter the rectum.

The rectum becomes distended by the fecal mass, the primary stimulus for the defecation reflex. Rectal distention leads to an increase in intrarectal pressure, causing the muscles to stretch and thereby stimulating the defecation reflex and subsequently the urge to eliminate.

The external anal sphincter, which is under voluntary control, is constricted or relaxed at will. If the urge to defecate is ignored, defecation often can be delayed voluntarily. During the act of defecation, several additional muscles aid in the process. Voluntary contraction of the muscles of the abdominal wall by holding one's breath, contracting the diaphragm, and closing the glottis increases intra-abdominal pressure up to four or five times the normal pressure, which helps expel feces. Simultaneously, the muscles on the pelvic floor contract and aid in expulsion of the fecal mass. Defecation is eased by flexing the thigh muscles, which increases abdominal pressure, and by the sitting position, which increases downward pressure on the rectum.

When an individual bears down to defecate, the increased pressures in the abdominal and thoracic cavities result in a decreased blood flow to the atria and ventricles, thus temporarily lowering cardiac output. Once bearing down ceases, the pressure is lessened, and a larger than normal amount of blood returns to the heart. This act may dangerously elevate the blood pressure in an already hypertensive individual (Smeltzer, Bare, Hinkle, & Cheever, 2010). Therefore, this technique of bearing down, termed the **Valsalva maneuver,** may be contraindicated in people with cardiovascular problems and other illnesses.

The act of defecation is usually painless. If the bowels move at regular intervals and the stools are formed and soft, functional problems involving frequency of elimination seldom occur. Many people become concerned if they do not have a daily bowel movement. Normal elimination patterns can vary widely among individuals. Although many adults pass one stool each day, other healthy people have more frequent or less frequent bowel movements. Some people have a bowel movement two or three times a week; others, two or three times a day.

FACTORS AFFECTING BOWEL ELIMINATION

Various factors can affect bowel elimination. Interference with the normal functioning of elimination from the intestines can occur in health as well as during illness. Elimination can be affected by a person's developmental stage, daily patterns, the amount and quality of fluid or food intake, the level of activity, lifestyle, emotional states, pathologic processes, medications, and procedures, such as diagnostic tests and surgery.

Developmental Considerations

Age affects what a person eats and the body's ability to digest nutrients and eliminate wastes. The stools of an infant are markedly different from those of an older person. Because patients are often reluctant to discuss their bowel habits and stool characteristics, nurses need to be familiar with bowel concerns pertinent to each developmental group.

Infant

The stool characteristics depend on whether the infant is being fed breast milk or formula. Breast milk is easier for the intestines to break down and absorb. Breastfed babies have more frequent stools, and the stools are yellow to golden and loose and usually have little odor. With formula or cow's milk feedings, the infant's stools vary from yellow to brown, are paste-like in consistency, and have a stronger odor because of the decomposition of protein. Both stools may have curds and mucus. Infants have no voluntary control over bowel elimination.

The number of stools infants pass varies greatly. For example, breastfed infants can pass from 2 to 10 stools daily, whereas bottle-fed infants typically pass 1 or 2 stools daily. At the age of 1 year, all infants commonly pass one or two stools a day. Parents may mistakenly interpret the infant's liquid stool as **diarrhea** (passage of more than three loose stools a day). Loose stools may be related to overfeeding or too much corn syrup in formula. Diarrhea is an increase in frequency, and a change in consistency, of stools. True diarrhea requires evaluation. Some children have bowel movements only once every 2 to 3 days. Teach parents that as long as the stools are soft, the child is not constipated. If **constipation** (dry, hard stool; persistently difficult passage of stool; and/or the incomplete passage of stool) occurs, dietary manipulation is the initial treatment. The consistent use of suppositories and laxatives is discouraged. Infants with persistent constipation require evaluation for structural defects.

Toddler

Between the ages of 18 and 24 months, the nerve fibers innervating the internal and external anal sphincters become fully developed, and voluntary control of defecation becomes possible. Voluntary defecation requires intact muscular, sensory, and nervous structures. Successful bowel training also includes awareness by the toddler of the need to defecate, the ability to communicate this need, the wish to please the significant person involved in bowel training, and praise and reinforcement for the toddler's successful behavior. Daytime bowel control is normally attained by 30 months of age, but the age varies with each child.

Help parents to understand that physiologic maturity is the first priority for successful bowel training. Discourage the use of punishment or shame for a lack of readiness to become toilet-trained or for elimination accidents. Toddlers who are toilet-trained often regress and experience soiling when hospitalized; scolding or acting disgusted only reinforces this behavior. Use a constructive approach by seeking the underlying cause.

School-Aged Child, Adolescent, and Adult

From childhood into adulthood, defecation patterns vary in quantity, frequency, and rhythmicity. Many people worry needlessly about normal stool characteristics or bowel habits; others may not understand the significance of changes in bowel habits. Emphasize that the use of over-the-counter laxatives and enemas can have serious consequences and that any problems prompting such use need to be evaluated.

Older Adult

Constipation is often a chronic problem for older adults. Diarrhea, **fecal impaction** (build up of stool in the colon), or **fecal incontinence** (involuntary or inappropriate passing of stool or flatus) can also result from physiologic or lifestyle changes. See the accompanying Focus on the Older Adult and PICO in Practice boxes.

Daily Patterns

Most people have individual patterns of bowel elimination involving frequency, timing considerations, position, and place. Changes in any of these patterns may upset a person's routine and lead to constipation. For example, many people defecate after breakfast, when the gastrocolic and duodenocolic reflexes cause mass propulsive movements in the large

FOCUS ON THE OLDER ADULT

BOWEL ELIMINATION PROBLEMS

Older adults frequently experience problems with bowel elimination. These can be due to a variety of causes and can have serious implications for the elderly patient. Refer to the appropriate chapter sections for related nursing interventions.

Bowel Elimination Problem	Related Factors and Implications

Chronic constipation	Can be caused by:
	    Decreased gastrointestinal motility
	    Effect of medications (e.g., antacids, opioids, antihypertensives)
	    Decreased fluid intake
	    Less active lifestyle
	    Inadequate fiber intake
	    Incomplete emptying of the bowel
	Can lead to laxative abuse

Diarrhea	Can be caused by:
	    Laxative abuse
	    Effect of medications/tube feedings
	Can lead to life-threatening dehydration and electrolyte imbalance

Fecal impaction	Can result from chronic constipation May be preceded by oozing of liquid feces—often mistaken for diarrhea Can lead to distended abdomen, abdominal pain, and complete bowel obstruction

Fecal incontinence	Can be caused by:
	    Decreased muscle tone
	    Alteration in nervous system innervation to rectum
	    Altered cognition
	Can lead to skin breakdown and depression

PICO IN PRACTICE
Asking Clinical Questions

Scenario: You are the nurse manager of an assisted-living facility. You know all of the 50 elderly residents of this facility quite well. Knowing that you are a nurse, they are very comfortable confiding in you their various physical ailments. You begin to note a trend among them. It seems to you that those elderly residents who are more active physically tend to voice fewer complaints of chronic constipation than those who are more sedentary. You wonder if encouraging those elderly residents who voice concerns of chronic constipation to join in structured exercise classes led by the activity aide three times weekly may relieve their symptoms.

- POPULATION: Elderly residents of an assisted-living facility
- INTERVENTION: Participation in a structured exercise class three times weekly
- COMPARISON: Sedentary lifestyle without regular exercise
- OUTCOME: Chronic constipation

PICO Question: Can participation in a structured exercise class three times weekly result in reduced rates of self-reported chronic constipation in elderly residents of an assisted-living facility?

Finding: From the Joanna Briggs Institute: Joanna Briggs Institute. (2008). Management of constipation in older adults. *Best Practice, 12*(7).

This evidence-based guideline recommends several effective first-line interventions that nurses may implement to relieve older adults' chronic constipation, including encouraging older adults to modify their diets as needed to include fiber, increasing their intake of fluids, and encouraging them to exercise regularly, if advisable.

Level of Evidence: Level I

Recommendation: You think that it is worthwhile to encourage sedentary elderly residents who voice concerns of chronic constipation to join in the regularly scheduled exercises led by the activity aide. You intend to follow-up with them 3 weeks after they join the exercise class to find whether or not their symptoms improve.

---

intestine. If this urge to defecate is ignored because the person finds the time or place inconvenient, the feces remain in the rectum until the defecation reflex is again initiated. Meanwhile, water continues to be absorbed from the unexpelled feces, which makes the stool dry, hard, and painful to pass.

Most people assume the squatting or slightly forward-sitting position with the thighs flexed. In either position, increased pressure is placed on the abdomen, as well as downward pressure on the rectum; both facilitate defecation. Obtaining the same results when seated on a bedpan is difficult. Embarrassment may further inhibit defecation. In addition, for most people, defecation is a private affair experienced easily only in the comfort of one's own bathroom. Defecation may be difficult in a shared hospital room with only a curtain for privacy.

Food and Fluid

Both the type and the amount of foods eaten and the amount of fluids ingested affect elimination. A high-fiber diet and a daily fluid intake of 2,000 to 3,000 mL facilitate bowel elimination. High-fiber foods, such as whole grains and bran, dried peas and beans, and fresh fruits and vegetables, increase the bulk in fecal material. Bulkier feces increase pressure on the intestinal wall, which serves as a stimulus for peristalsis. As a result, feces move more quickly through the colon, allowing less time for water to be reabsorbed. Subsequently, the stool is soft and easy to pass. When the stool moves quickly through the colon there is also less time for toxins to be absorbed from

feces by the colon. Many believe that these toxins play an important role in promoting the development of colon cancer. Therefore, preventing their absorption by the colon is a key part of colon cancer prevention.

People digest and tolerate foods differently. This variation is determined in part by one's culture. For example, travelers to a foreign country who eat native foods or drink the water may suffer severe indigestion and elimination problems, such as diarrhea.

Food intolerance may alter bowel elimination, possibly resulting in diarrhea, gaseous distention, and cramping. For example, people who lack the enzyme lactase, which helps to break down the simple sugar lactose found in milk and milk products, cannot digest milk; this is called lactose intolerance. These people often experience excessive intestinal gas and diarrhea when they ingest milk.

Certain foods have been associated with specific effects on bowel elimination. These include:

- Constipating foods: processed cheese, lean meat, eggs, pasta
- Foods with laxative effect: certain fruits and vegetables (e.g., prunes), bran, chocolate, spicy foods, alcohol, coffee
- Gas-producing foods: onions, cabbage, beans, cauliflower

Activity and Muscle Tone

Regular exercise improves gastrointestinal motility and muscle tone, whereas inactivity decreases both. Adequate tone in the abdominal muscles, the diaphragm, and the perineal muscles is essential for ease of defecation. Patients on prolonged bed rest are prime candidates for constipation.

Lifestyle

Many individual, family, and sociocultural variables influence a person's usual elimination habits. The long-term effects of bowel training may result in a person's (1) acceptance of bowel elimination as a normal life process, (2) preoccupation with bowel elimination, or (3) feeling that bowel elimination is a "dirty" process. Rituals associated with bowel elimination, cleanliness considerations, the language used to talk about bowel elimination or reluctance to discuss it, individual responses to involuntary passage of flatus (gas), and so on vary widely among people. A person's daily schedule, occupation, and leisure activities may contribute to a habit of defecating at regular times or to an irregular pattern. Nurses who role model good health behaviors are more effective teachers. Use the Promoting Health 38-1 display for yourself before using it with others.

Psychological Variables

Psychological stress affects the body in many ways. In some people, anxiety seems to have a direct effect on gastrointestinal motility, and diarrhea accompanies periods of high anxiety. In the fight-or-flight response, when the body mobilizes itself for intense action, blood is shunted away from the stomach and intestines, resulting in a slowing of gastrointestinal motility. Persons who chronically worry and those with certain personality types who tend to hold onto problems and negative feelings may experience frequent constipation.

Pathologic Conditions

Numerous pathologic processes may change a person's usual bowel elimination habits. Changes in stool characteristics or frequency may be one of the first clinical manifestations of a disease, and their evaluation may lead to the diagnosis of the disease. For example, when a patient reports that his or her stool has become narrower or ribbon-like, a tumor may be obstructing normal stool passage through the colon. The nurse should report this finding to the physician. Similarly, a parent's report that a child's stools are frequent, bulky, greasy, and foul smelling suggests cystic fibrosis and would require further evaluation, especially if other clinical manifestations are present.

Diarrhea may result from pathologic conditions such as diverticulitis (inflammation of a diverticulum from obstruction [by fecal matter], resulting in abscess formation), infection, malabsorption syndromes (the inability of the digestive system to absorb one or more of the major vitamins, minerals, or nutrients), neoplastic diseases (tumors), diabetic neuropathy

---

PROMOTING HEALTH • 38-1

Bowel Elimination

Patients view nurses as role models for achieving healthy lifestyles. Use the assessment checklist to determine how well you are meeting your needs related to bowel elimination. Then develop a prescription for self-care by choosing appropriate behaviors from the list of suggestions.

Assessment Checklist

❏ almost always   ❏ sometimes   ❏ almost never

❏ ❏ ❏   1. I have a regular bowel elimination pattern, satisfactory to support comfort and activities of daily living.

❏ ❏ ❏   2. I eat a diet high in fiber.

❏ ❏ ❏   3. I exercise regularly.

❏ ❏ ❏   4. I have an adequate intake of fluids.

Self-Care Behaviors

1. Accept individual patterns of defecation as normal.
2. Eat a balanced diet, including high fiber foods, such as fruits, vegetables, and nuts.

3. Follow a regular exercise program with 30 to 45 minutes of activity three to four times a week.
4. Do not ignore the urge to defecate.
5. Establish a routine, if needed (1 hour after meals is usually best).
6. Avoid prolonged use of over-the-counter medications or enemas to treat constipation.
7. Drink 8–10 glasses of water per day.
8. Seek medical assistance for any change in the characteristics of stool or presence of blood in stool.

Information to promote effective bowel elimination, such as information about elimination problems, bowel incontinence, ostomies, and anal and rectal diseases is available online. Check out these sites: NDDIC (National Digestive Diseases Information Clearinghouse) at http://digestive.niddk.nih.gov/index.htm; Medline Plus available at www.nlm.nih.gov/medlineplus; and UOAA (United Ostomy Associations of America) at www.uoaa.org.

(damage to nerve cells), hyperthyroidism, and uremia (retention of urea in the blood).

Constipation may be the result of conditions such as diseases within the colon or rectum and injury to, or degeneration of, the spinal cord and megacolon (extremely dilated colon). Changes in color, contents, odor, and appearance of stool may be related to conditions that traumatize the stomach or intestines, or that interfere with normal digestion. Thus, stool assessment is an important diagnostic task for the nurse.

Outbreaks of food poisoning can result in severe gastrointestinal symptoms, including diarrhea. For example, infections caused by certain types of *Escherichia coli,* particularly dangerous for young children (under 10 years of age) and older adults, can progress quickly to life-threatening hematologic and renal complications (Porth & Matfin, 2009). Severe abdominal cramping followed by watery or bloody diarrhea may signal a microbial infection, which can be confirmed by a stool sample. Supportive treatment, careful monitoring, and attentive nursing care are essential.

Intestinal obstruction occurs when blockage prevents the normal flow of intestinal contents through the intestinal tract (Smeltzer et al., 2010). Mechanical obstructions result from pressure on the intestinal walls. Examples of causes of mechanical obstruction include tumors, stenosis, adhesions, hernias, and strictures. Functional obstructions result from an inability of the intestinal musculature to move the contents through the bowel. Examples of causes of functional obstruction include muscular dystrophy, diabetes mellitus, Parkinson's disease, and manipulation of the bowel during surgery. The effects of surgery are further detailed below.

Medications

Medications are available that can promote peristalsis (cathartics and laxatives) or inhibit peristalsis (antidiarrheal medications). These are discussed later in the chapter.

Other types of medications may affect bowel elimination and stool characteristics. Opioids, antacids containing aluminum, iron sulfate, and anticholinergic medications decrease gastrointestinal motility, with the potential to cause constipation.

> Remember Leroy Cobbs, the patient described at the beginning of the chapter who developed fecal impaction resulting from the narcotic analgesics he was using to control his cancer pain. Had the possible adverse effects of narcotics for pain control been addressed in the patient's medication teaching plan when the drug was first prescribed, the risk for fecal impaction could have been reduced. Additionally, the teaching plan could have addressed measures to counteract the effects of the medication. ■

Many medications can cause diarrhea as a side effect. For example, diarrhea is a potential adverse effect of treatment with amoxicillin clavulanate (Augmentin), an antibiotic. In this situation, using antidiarrheal drugs is not recommended because their use would prolong the exposure of the intestinal mucosa to the irritating effect of the antibiotic or bacterial toxin. Medications with magnesium, such as over the counter antacids, can cause diarrhea. If diarrhea is severe enough, the drug may need to be discontinued.

Medications may also influence the appearance of the stool, for a variety of reasons. Any drug with the potential to cause gastrointestinal bleeding (e.g., anticoagulants, aspirin products) may cause the stool to appear pink to red to black. Iron salts result in a black stool from the oxidation of iron. Antacids may cause a white discoloration or speckling in the stool. Antibiotics may cause a green-gray color related to impaired digestion.

Patients receiving treatment with antibiotics are at risk for a healthcare acquired infection with *clostridium difficile (C. difficile)*, which causes intestinal mucosal damage and inflammation, resulting in diarrhea and abdominal cramping. Treatment with broad-spectrum antibiotics disrupts the normal intestinal flora and allows microorganism to flourish within the intestine. *C. difficile* spores are relatively resistant to disinfectants and can be spread on the hands of healthcare providers after contact with equipment or surfaces contaminated with the microorganism. Because antibiotics are used so extensively in the healthcare setting, many patients are at risk for infection with *C. difficile* (Smeltzer et al., 2010). Institute contact precautions for infected patients. Environmental surfaces and items close to the patient, such as the side rails and overbed table, should be considered contaminated and intensified environmental cleaning is required (Smeltzer et al., 2010; Centers for Disease Control and Prevention [CDC], 2004).

Diagnostic Studies

A patient's usual bowel elimination pattern may be affected by diagnostic studies. For example, patients may need to fast for diagnostic studies. The ingestion of barium during diagnostic procedures, such as a barium enema, is a common and often overlooked reason for constipation (Bisanz, 2007). Additionally, the stress of hospitalization and waiting for the results of studies, combined with changes in food intake, can severely alter a patient's usual elimination patterns. The cathartics or enemas used for bowel cleansing before certain diagnostic studies of the gastrointestinal tract can interfere with the normal timing of a patient's bowel movements. Refer to Table 38-2 later in this chapter for additional information related to laxatives.

Surgery and Anesthesia

Direct manipulation of the bowel during abdominal surgery inhibits peristalsis, causing a condition termed **paralytic ileus.** This temporary stoppage of peristalsis normally lasts 24 to 48 hours; during this time, food and fluids are withheld. Many times, the patient is receiving narcotics for pain relief, which can exacerbate the situation. If this condition persists, distention and symptoms of acute obstruction may occur, possibly resulting in the need for surgical intervention. Inhaled general anesthetic agents also inhibit peristalsis by blocking the parasympathetic impulses to the intestinal musculature. However, local and regional anesthetics have little effect on peristalsis.

THE NURSING PROCESS FOR PATIENTS WITH BOWEL ELIMINATION DISTURBANCES
Assessing

Assessment of gastrointestinal tract and bowel elimination includes pertinent patient history, physical assessment, and diagnostic studies.

Nursing History

Because many patients are reluctant to initiate a conversation about their bowel status, include pertinent bowel elimination questions in each comprehensive nursing history. See Focused Assessment Guide 38-1.

If the patient is experiencing any disturbance in bowel elimination, conduct a more detailed assessment, directing attention to the factors described earlier that may influence bowel elimination.

Patients who are critically ill or who have impaired cognition may be incapable of reporting their bowel status accurately. Record the patient's daily bowel status to look for clues to impending problems. While making daily rounds, ask patients who can give reliable answers, "When did you move your bowels last?" and chart the response. If the patient cannot provide this information, the nurse or ancillary staff who assists the patient with bowel elimination records any bowel movement.

Physical Assessment

Assessment of bowel elimination includes physical assessment of the abdomen, anus, and rectum, which are discussed in Chapter 25, Health Assessment. Described below are examination techniques that may be helpful when assessing the functioning of the gastrointestinal tract.

FOCUSED ASSESSMENT GUIDE • 38-1

BOWEL ELIMINATION

Factors to Assess	Questions and Approaches
Usual patterns of bowel elimination	How often do you move your bowels? Any special time of the day? What does your stool look like: • Frequency • Time of day • Description of usual stool characteristics (amount, consistency, shape, color, odor)
Aids to elimination	Do you use anything to help move your bowels? • Natural aids (liquids, food) • Pharmacologic aids (laxatives) • Enemas
Recent changes in bowel elimination	Have you noticed any changes in your stool recently? Have you noticed any blood in your stool? (May need to ask patient about color blindness) Have you noted a difference in the appearance of your stool (narrowing, presence of mucus)?
Problems with bowel elimination	Are your bowels causing you any problem now? • Nature of disturbance • Onset and frequency • Causes (*physical:* food and fluid intake, exercise status, history of surgery or illnesses influencing gastrointestinal tract; psychosocial; medicine related) • Severity • Symptoms • Interventions attempted and results
Presence of artificial orifices	What is your usual routine with your colostomy or ileostomy? Do you have any problems with it?

ABDOMEN

The sequence for abdominal assessment proceeds from inspection, auscultation, and percussion to palpation. Inspection and auscultation are performed before palpation because palpation may disturb normal peristalsis and bowel motility. Place the patient comfortably in the supine position with the abdomen exposed, the chest and pubic area draped, and the knees slightly flexed. Encourage the patient to urinate prior to the examination so that the bladder is empty.

Inspection

First, observe the contour of the abdomen, noting any masses, scars, or areas of distention. Peristalsis is usually not visible except in very thin patients. When an intestinal obstruction is present, the visible waves of peristalsis to the point of the obstruction may be observed on the abdomen. Observe the contour of the abdomen. Significant findings may include the presence of distention (inflation) or protrusion (projection).

Auscultation

Using the diaphragm of a warmed stethoscope, listen for bowel sounds in all abdominal quadrants, using a systematic, clockwise approach. If the patient has a nasogastric tube in place, disconnect it from suction during this assessment to allow for accurate interpretation of sounds. Keep in mind that the timing of the patient's most recent meal or a full bladder may also affect the examination.

Note the frequency and character of bowel sounds, audible clicks, and gurgles produced by the movement of air and flatus in the gastrointestinal tract. They are usually high-pitched, gurgling, and soft. Their frequency may range from 5 to 34 bowel sounds per minute, depending on the rate of peristalsis (Weber & Kelly, 2007). Significant findings include hypoactive bowel sounds, a diminished rate of sounds; hyperactive bowel sounds, intense with increased frequency; and absent or infrequent bowel sounds. Hypoactive bowel sounds indicate diminished bowel motility, commonly caused by abdominal surgery or late bowel obstruction. Hyperactive bowel sounds indicate increased bowel motility, commonly caused by diarrhea, gastroenteritis, or early bowel obstruction. Decreased or absent bowel sounds (evidenced only after listening for 5 minutes) signify the absence of bowel motility, commonly associated with peritonitis, paralytic ileus, and/or prolonged immobility (Weber & Kelly, 2007). Describe bowel sounds as audible, hyperactive, hypoactive, or inaudible.

Percussion

Percuss all quadrants of the abdomen in a systematic, clockwise manner to identify any masses, fluid, or air in the abdomen. Expect a resonant sound or tympany over the abdomen and stomach because these are hollow organs. With practice, learn to distinguish normal resonance from the hyperresonance that occurs when excess flatus is trapped in the intestines. An intestinal obstruction sounds dull on percussion. Areas of increased dullness may be caused by fluid, a mass, or a tumor.

Palpation

Both light palpation and deep palpation in each quadrant are performed next. Note any muscular resistance, tenderness, enlargement of organs, and masses. If the patient's abdomen is distended, note the presence of firmness or tautness. If the patient is in pain, administer medication before proceeding with the palpation.

ANUS AND RECTUM

Perform a superficial examination each time you wash a patient's anal area or assist with bowel evacuation. The nurse's skill level determines the extent of further rectal examination. If a rectal exam is to be performed, position the patient in the left Sims position.

Inspection and Palpation

First, examine the anal area for cracks, nodules, hemorrhoids (distended veins), masses, or polyps. Observe for a fecal mass, which may distend the anus. Inspect the perineal area for areas of skin irritation or breakdown secondary to diarrhea or fecal incontinence. Insert a gloved, lubricated finger through the anus into the rectum to assess sphincter tone and smoothness of the mucosal lining; note any masses, polyps, hardened stool, bleeding, pain, or abnormal discharge.

STOOL CHARACTERISTICS

Nurses are responsible for observing and recording information about the patient's stool. Table 38-1 describes the characteristics of a normal stool, along with special considerations used when observing a stool. Report and record anything unusual, including the passage of little or no gas or unusual amounts.

Note and record, usually on the patient's bedside flow sheet, the frequency, amount, and characteristics of the patient's bowel movements. Describe any additional unusual observations, such as lightheadedness or straining, on the patient's medical record. When assistive personnel or the patient assumes this responsibility, check with the patient at regular intervals to see that the recording is accurate.

Ideally, populations at high risk for bowel elimination problems are identified before problems occur, and such problems are prevented or minimized through vigilant nursing care. Be aware of the clinical manifestations of colon cancer because early detection significantly improves survival. Refer to Box 38-1, Warning Signs of Colon Cancer.

Box 38-1   WARNING SIGNS OF COLON CANCER

- Change in the bowel elimination pattern
- Blood in the stools
- Rectal or abdominal pain
- Change in the character of the stool
- Sensation of incomplete emptying after bowel movement

TABLE • 38-1	THE STOOL: NORMAL CHARACTERISTICS AND SPECIAL CONSIDERATIONS FOR OBSERVATION	
Characteristic	**Normal Finding**	**Special Considerations for Observation**
Volume	Variable	The volume of the stool depends on the amount the person eats and the nature of the diet. For example, a diet high in roughage produces more feces than a soft, bland diet. Consistently large diarrheal stools suggest a disorder in the small bowel or proximal colon; small, frequent stools with urgency to pass them suggest a disorder of the left colon or rectum.
Color	Infant: Yellow to brown Adult: Brown	The brown color of the stool is due to stercobilin, a bile pigment derivative. The rapid rate of peristalsis in the breastfed infant causes the stool to be yellow. The color of the stool is influenced by diet. For example, the stool will be almost black if the person eats red meat and dark green vegetables, such as spinach. The stool will be light brown if the diet is high in milk and milk products and low in meat. The absence of bile may cause the stool to appear white or clay-colored. Certain drugs influence the color of the stool. For example, iron salts cause the stool to be black. Antacids cause it to be whitish. Bleeding high in the intestinal tract causes a stool to be black owing to the digestion of the blood. Bleeding low in the intestinal tract results in fresh blood in the stool. The stool darkens with standing.
Odor	Pungent; may be affected by foods ingested	The characteristic odor of the stool is due to indole and skatole, caused by putrefaction and fermentation in the lower intestinal tract. The odor of the stool is influenced by its pH value, which normally is neutral or slightly alkaline. Excessive putrefaction causes a strong odor. The presence of blood in the stool causes a unique odor.
Consistency	Soft, semisolid, and formed	The consistency of the stool is influenced by fluid and food intake and gastric motility. The less time stool spends in the intestine (or the shorter the intestine), the more liquid the stool. Many pathologic conditions influence consistency.
Shape	Formed stool is usually about 1 inch (2.5 cm) in diameter and has the tubular shape of the colon, but may be larger or smaller, depending on the condition of the colon.	A gastrointestinal obstruction may result in a narrow, pencil-shaped stool. Rapid peristalsis thins the stool. Increased time spent in the large intestine may result in a hard, marble-like fecal mass.
Constituents	Waste residues of digestion: bile, intestinal secretions, shed epithelial cells, bacteria, and inorganic material (chiefly calcium and phosphates); seeds, meat fibers, and fat may be present in small amounts	Internal bleeding, infection, inflammation, and other pathologic conditions may result in abnormal constituents. These include blood, pus, excessive fat, parasites, ova, and mucus. Foreign bodies also may be found in the stool.

Diagnostic Studies

The nurse is often responsible for caring for patients with elimination problems who are undergoing diagnostic testing. Following are specific guidelines for the nurse's role in stool collection and direct and indirect visualization studies.

STOOL COLLECTION

The nurse is responsible for obtaining the specimen according to agency procedure, labeling the specimen, and ensuring that the specimen is transported to the laboratory in a timely manner. The institution's policy and procedure manual or laboratory manual identifies specific information about the amount of stool needed, the time frame during which stool is to be collected, and the type of specimen container to use.

Use of medical aseptic techniques is imperative. Always wear disposable gloves when any contact or handling of a stool specimen is likely. Hand hygiene, before and after glove use, is essential. Also, take care not to contaminate the outside of the specimen container with stool. To ensure that no leakage of the specimen occurs, package, label, and transport specimens according to agency policy. Patients may

Guidelines for Nursing Care • 38-1

TESTING FOR FECAL OCCULT BLOOD

- Instruct the patient about food and drug restrictions for at least 4 days before the test, if they apply.
- Review manufacturer's directions for collecting the specimen. Equipment may include a specimen card, collection tissues, or test paper.
- Avoid mixing the specimen with urine or water.
- Inform the patient that multiple or serial specimens are usually collected from different bowel movements to verify results.
- Collect the amount recommended for the particular test (usually only a small amount is required).

- Wear gloves and perform thorough hand hygiene if collecting a specimen from a bedpan, commode, or plastic receptacle.
- Use tongue blades to transfer the stool to the test tape or folder.
- Follow instructions based on type of test. Hemoccult slide test requires placing 2 drops of developer solution on the backside of the specimen paper. The tablet test directions include placing 2 to 3 drops of tap water on the tablet, which is centered on the stool specimen.
- Document the test results according to agency policy. *A blue color is a positive result and needs to be reported.*
- Inform the patient of the test results.

---

need specific instructions about collecting a stool specimen. These instructions may include the following:

- Void first, because the laboratory study may be inaccurate if the stool contains urine.
- Defecate into the required container, such as clean or sterile bedpan or the bedside commode (depending on the specimen required), rather than the toilet, because the analysis results may be affected by the water in the toilet bowl.
- Do not place toilet tissue in the bedpan or specimen container because contents in the paper may influence laboratory results.
- Notify the nurse when the specimen is available, so that it may be collected and transported to the laboratory as required.

When placing a specimen in a laboratory container, put on gloves and use two clean tongue blades. Usually, 1 inch (2.5 cm) of formed stool or 15 to 30 mL of liquid stool is sufficient. If portions of the stool include visible blood, mucus, or pus, include these with the specimen. Also, be sure that the specimen is free of any barium or enema solution. Because a fresh specimen produces the most accurate results, send the specimen to the laboratory immediately. If this is not possible, refrigerate it unless contraindicated.

To test the stool for pH or blood, use a commercial tape, dipstick, or solution according to the manufacturer's directions. **Occult blood** in the stool (blood that is hidden in the specimen or cannot be seen on gross examination) can be detected with screening tests. Certain conditions, such as ulcer disease, inflammatory bowel disorders, and colon cancer, place the patient at high risk for intestinal bleeding. The color of the stool may reflect the source of the bleeding. Generally, black stools indicate upper gastrointestinal bleeding, such as from a peptic ulcer, due to a reaction between hemoglobin and gastric acid. Lower gastrointestinal bleeding, such as from hemorrhoids or a polyp, may produce bright-red blood in the stool. Certain foods and medications can also cause a black or reddish stool.

Tests for occult blood in the stool may be performed by nurses at the bedside within an institution or by patients at home. These simple tests use reagent substances to detect the enzyme peroxidase in the hemoglobin molecule. The Hematest and guaiac test are chemical tests commonly used to determine occult blood in the stool. Guidelines for Nursing Care 38-1 gives additional nursing considerations for fecal occult blood testing. Figure 38-5 demonstrates the procedure for a Hemoccult test.

Ingestion of certain substances before the specimen collection can result in false-positive results. These substances

FIGURE 38-5. Testing a stool specimen for occult blood. (**A**) Applying a stool specimen to the test paper. (**B**) Adding developing solution to the backside of the paper according to directions. (**C**) Blue coloration indicating positive results. (*Photos by B. Proud.*)

include red meat, animal liver and kidneys, salmon, tuna, mackerel and sardines, tomatoes, cauliflower, horseradish, turnips, melon, bananas, and soybeans. Certain medications, such as a salicylate intake of more than 325 mg daily, steroids, iron preparations, and anticoagulants, also may lead to false-positive readings (Fischbach & Dunning, 2009). The ingestion of vitamin C can produce false-negative results even if bleeding is present. The following are recommendations for the patient preparing for a fecal occult blood test:

- Before stool testing, avoid the foods (for 4 days) and drugs (for 7 days) that may alter test results.
- In a woman who is menstruating, postpone the test until 3 days after her period has ended.
- Postpone the test if hematuria or bleeding hemorrhoids are present.
- Postpone the test if the patient has had a recent nose or throat bleed.
- Caution a person who is color-blind to the color blue not to attempt to interpret the test results.

In clinical settings, these restrictions are usually not practical. It is important to note the presence of any of the aforementioned conditions in the clinical setting.

Timed Specimens

Consider the first stool passed by the patient as the start of the collection period. Depending on the test, it may require saving the entire stool passed or only a sample. Collect the required volume of every stool passed within the designated period. Follow laboratory instructions for sending stools to the laboratory.

Specimens for Pinworms

Adult pinworms, parasitic intestinal worms, live in the cecum. Pinworms migrate to the anal area during the night to deposit eggs and retreat into the anal canal during the day. The most common symptom of a pinworm infection is perianal itching. Collect this specimen in the morning, immediately after the patient awakens and before the patient urinates, has a bowel movement, or a bath. Use clear cellophane tape to collect a specimen for pinworms; frosted tape makes examination difficult. Apply gloves and press the tape against the anal opening, remove it immediately, and then place it on a slide. Pinworm eggs can usually be detected on the tape under a microscope. For accurate results, this test may need to be repeated on consecutive days.

DIRECT VISUALIZATION STUDIES

Endoscopy is the direct visual examination of body organs or cavities. Most commonly, this is done using a fiber-optic endoscope, a long, flexible tube containing glass fibers that transmit light into the organ and return an image that can be viewed. Pincers may be inserted through the tube to obtain a tissue sample for biopsy. An endoscope enables the physician to view the integrity of the mucosa, blood vessels, and specific organ parts and is helpful for diagnosing inflammatory, ulcerative, and infectious diseases; benign and malignant

neoplasms; and other lesions of the esophageal, gastric, and intestinal mucosa. Endoscopic studies include the following:

- Esophagogastroduodenoscopy: visual examination of the esophagus, the stomach, and the duodenum
- Colonoscopy: visual examination of the large intestine from the anus to the ileocecal valve
- Sigmoidoscopy: visual examination of the sigmoid colon, the rectum, and the anal canal.

Nursing responsibilities before and after these studies are described in Box 38-2.

A newer procedure is wireless capsule endoscopy. In this procedure, the patient swallows a capsule, about the size of a vitamin, which contains a small camera that emits a radio signal. The capsule is propelled through the small intestine via peristalsis, taking two pictures per second. Several wires on the patient's abdomen pick up the radio signal from the capsule, and the data are recorded on a data recorder, which the patient wears on a belt. The system captures about 55,000 images in an 8-hour exam. The patient returns to the facility after 8 hours, and the external sensors and data recorder are removed. The information is downloaded from the recorder to a computer and can be transferred to a videotape for easy viewing by the physician. The capsule is excreted during the process of normal defecation in 24 to 48 hours and is intended for one-time use only (Fischbach & Dunning, 2009; Jungles, 2004).

The patient is normally NPO (fasting) for 10 to 12 hours the evening before capsule ingestion. During the first 2 hours of the study, the patient is not allowed to eat or drink anything. After the first 2 hours, the patient may consume small amounts of liquids. After 4 hours, the patient may have a small meal. The patient may resume normal activities while the camera is passing through the small intestine. Because there is no sedation or discomfort and a normal day can be planned, many patients prefer this method of endoscopy. Additionally, no air is needed to expand the small intestine, as it is in traditional endoscopy; therefore, the patient does not feel uncomfortable and bloated. This method, however, does not allow for obtaining biopsies of any suspicious area, so additional endoscopic studies may be required, based on the results.

INDIRECT VISUALIZATION STUDIES

Indirect visualization of the gastrointestinal tract is commonly performed through radiography. The passage of x-rays through the patient creates a radiograph or film depicting body structures. This technique is useful for detecting obstructions, strictures, inflammatory disease, tumors, ulcers, and other lesions and for diagnosing hiatal hernia and other structural changes in the gastrointestinal tract. Use of a radiopaque contrast medium, such as barium sulfate, accentuates the body structures being visualized. In the upper gastrointestinal examination and small bowel series, the patient drinks the barium sulfate like a milkshake. The barium coats the esophagus, stomach, and small intestine to enhance visualization. In the barium enema or lower gastrointestinal examination, barium sulfate is instilled into the large intestine through a rectal tube inserted through the anus. Fluoroscopy

Box 38-2   COMMON DIAGNOSTIC STUDIES FOR THE GASTROINTESTINAL TRACT

Esophagogastroduodenoscopy

It allows visual examination of the esophagus, stomach, and upper duodenum by means of a long, flexible, fiber-optic–lighted scope.

Preparation
- A signed consent form is required for this procedure.
- Fasting is required 6 to 12 hours before the test (check agency policy).
- Dentures need to be removed before the test.
- Remind the patient that he will be awake but sedated and that a local anesthetic will be sprayed into the mouth and throat to depress the gag reflex.

Aftercare
- Withhold food and fluids until the gag reflex returns.
- Check vital signs according to the protocol.
- Observe for signs of perforation: pain, persistent difficulty swallowing, vomiting blood, or black, tarry stools.
- Explain to the patient that it is normal to sense throat soreness and hoarseness for several days; saline gargles and lozenges may be helpful.

Colonoscopy

It allows visual examination of the rectum, colon, and distal small bowel using a long, flexible, fiber-optic–lighted scope.

Preparation
- Ensure that an informed consent is signed.
- Preparation prior to test may involve:
  - Clear liquid diet (24–48 h before test)
  - 2 day bowel preparation—strong cathartic and Dulcolax on day 1 and enema the day of the test, *or*
  - 1 day bowel preparation—ingestion of a gallon of bowel cleanser, such as GoLytely, in a short period of time
- Sedation will be given before the test.

Aftercare
- Patient may experience flatulence or gas pains because air was used to distend the intestines for better visibility.
- Usual diet may be resumed once patient recovers from the sedation.
- Check vital signs according to agency protocol.
- Observe for signs of bowel perforation: rectal bleeding, abdominal pain and distention, fever, malaise.

Sigmoidoscopy

It allows visual examination of the distal sigmoid colon, the rectum, and the anal canal through a flexible or rigid sigmoidoscope.

Preparation
- Ensure that an informed consent is signed.
- Preparation usually consists of light meal before the test and two Fleet enemas.
- Sedation is not usually required.

Aftercare
- Patient may experience flatulence or gas pains because air was used to distend the intestines for better visibility.
- Observe for signs of bowel perforation.
- If biopsy was performed, patient should be informed that slight rectal bleeding may occur.

Upper Gastrointestinal (UGI) and Small Bowel Series

This involves fluoroscopic examination of the esophagus, stomach, and small intestine after ingestion of barium sulfate.

Preparation
- Ensure that an informed consent is signed.
- Keep patient NPO after midnight the day of the test.
- Inform patient that a chalky-tasting barium contrast mixture will be given to drink before the test.

Aftercare
- A post-test cathartic (e.g., Milk of Magnesia) is usually prescribed to prevent fecal impaction from barium sulfate that has hardened. Notify the physician or primary medical provider if barium is not passed, usually within 2 days.
- Explain that the barium may lighten the color of stools for the next several days. After the barium is expelled, the stool color will return to normal.

Barium Enema

This involves a series of radiographs that examine the large intestine after rectal instillation of barium sulfate.

Preparation
- An informed consent must be signed.
- Preparation may consist of dietary modifications, increased fluid intake, a cathartic, NPO after midnight, and enemas until clear before the test.
- Review the patient's history for any history of ulcerative colitis or active GI bleeding that would prohibit the use of the standard bowel preparation.

Aftercare
- Encourage fluids to prevent dehydration.
- Inform the patient that the barium may lighten the color of the stools. A cathartic may be prescribed. Notify the physician or primary medical provider if barium is not passed, usually within 2 days.
- Encourage rest because the bowel preparation and the test exhaust many patients.

Abdominal Ultrasound

Uses ultrasound waves to visualize organs via a small transducer placed against the skin.

Preparation
- Assure the patient that no radiation is employed and that the test is painless.
- Patient must be NPO for a minimum of 8 hours before the examination.
- Explain that gel will be applied to the skin and that a sensation of warmth or wetness may be felt. The gel does not stain, but avoid wearing nonwashable clothing.
- Abdominal ultrasound must be performed before studies involving barium, as retained barium may compromise the study.

Aftercare
- Ensure any residual gel is removed from the skin.
- Normal diet and fluids may be resumed, unless contraindicated by the test results.

Magnetic Resonance Imaging (MRI)

This test provides physiologic information and detailed anatomic views of tissues using a superconducting magnet and radiofrequency signals.

Preparation
- Evaluate the patient for need for sedation. Patients who are claustrophobic or unable to lie still during study may benefit from sedation.

(continued)

Box 38-2 **COMMON DIAGNOSTIC STUDIES FOR THE GASTROINTESTINAL TRACT** *(continued)*

- Patient may need to fast or consume only clear liquids prior to study. Patient should avoid alcohol, nicotine, caffeine, and iron supplements prior to the study.
- Patients with implanted surgical clips or other metallic structures and those with implanted electromechanical devices, such as cardiac pacemakers, drug infusion pumps, and cochlear implants, should not be exposed to MRI procedures.
- An informed consent is required.
- Pregnant patients are not routinely scanned because an increase in amniotic fluid/fetal temperature may be harmful.

Aftercare
- If intravenous contrast is used during study, monitor for sensitivity and adverse reactions.
- Monitor contrast injection site for signs of irritation, infection, and bruising.
- If prestudy sedation was given, monitor patient closely until sedation wears off to prevent injury.

Abdominal CT Scan
Thin beams of x-rays are directed at and move around the abdomen, resulting in computer-manipulated pictures that are not obscured by overlying anatomy.

Preparation
- An oral contrast is consumed before the study if the upper gastrointestinal tract is to be examined.
- Intravenous iodine contrast is usually administered.
- Assess for patient allergies to iodine, IV contrast, and/or shellfish. Prestudy preparation may be required if allergies are present.
- Assess for renal impairment; check laboratory values for elevated BUN and creatinine levels.
- Patient should be NPO for at least 4 hours before study.
- CT scan is contraindicated for pregnant patients.
- An informed consent is required.
- Metformin (Glucophage) must be discontinued prior to study and held after study to prevent renal failure. Consult with physician for patient medication modifications.

Aftercare
- If intravenous contrast is used during study, monitor for sensitivity and adverse reactions.
- Monitor contrast injection site for signs of irritation, infection, and bruising.
- If prestudy sedation was given, monitor patient closely until sedation wears off to prevent injury.

Adapted from Fischbach, F., & Dunning, M. (2009). *A manual of laboratory and diagnostic tests* (8th ed.). Philadelphia: Wolters Kluwer Health/Lippincott Williams & Wilkins; Fischbach, F., & Dunning, M. (2006). *Common laboratory & diagnostic tests* (4th ed.). Philadelphia: Lippincott Williams & Wilkins.

projects consecutive x-ray images onto a screen for continuous observation of the flow of the barium. During a CT (computerized axial tomography) scan, thin beams of x-rays are directed at and move around the abdomen, resulting in computer-manipulated pictures that are not obscured by overlying anatomy. Contrast may be given orally or intravenously to enhance the images. MRI (magnetic resonance imaging) provides physiologic information and detailed anatomic views of tissues using a superconducting magnet and radiofrequency signals. Computers use the signals to construct detailed sectional images of the abdomen. Intravenous contrast can be given to enhance the images. Abdominal ultrasound visualizes all solid upper abdominal organs, including the liver, bile ducts, gallbladder, appendix, pancreas, kidneys, adrenals, spleen, and the abdominal aorta and vena cava. The specific nursing responsibilities related to these studies are included in Box 38-2.

SCHEDULING FOR DIAGNOSTIC STUDIES

Nurses are commonly involved in scheduling diagnostic studies when a patient is to undergo multiple studies. Use the following guidelines for scheduling studies of the gastrointestinal tract:

1. Follow a logical sequence when more than one test is required for accurate diagnosis:
   Fecal occult blood tests: to detect gastrointestinal bleeding
   Barium studies: to visualize gastrointestinal structures and reveal any inflammation, ulcers, tumors, strictures, or other lesions

   Endoscopic examinations: to visualize an abnormality, locate a source of bleeding, and if necessary provide biopsy tissue samples
2. A barium enema and routine radiography should precede an upper gastrointestinal series because retained barium from an upper gastrointestinal series could take several days to pass through the gastrointestinal tract and cloud anatomic detail on the barium enema studies.
3. Noninvasive procedures usually take precedence over invasive procedures, such as endoscopic studies, when sufficient diagnostic data can be obtained from them. (In some instances, endoscopic studies may be done before barium studies to ensure visualization.)

Diagnosing

Nursing Diagnoses for bowel elimination can be divided into two categories: Bowel elimination as the problem and bowel elimination as the etiology.

Bowel Elimination as the Problem

When the analysis of assessment data points to a bowel elimination problem that can be prevented or resolved by independent nursing intervention, a nursing diagnosis is developed. If alterations in bowel elimination require new self-care behaviors, for example colostomy management, Deficient Knowledge may be an appropriate nursing diagnosis. See the accompanying box, Examples of NANDA Nursing Diagnoses: Bowel Elimination

Examples of NANDA Nursing Diagnoses
Bowel Elimination

Nursing Diagnoses	Related Factors	Sample Defining Characteristics
Constipation	Decreased fiber in diet Decreased fluid intake Inactivity Delaying defecation when urge is present Abuse of laxatives Use of constipating medications (antacids, narcotic analgesics [opioids], anticholinergics) Change in routine Pain associated with defecation	*"I feel bloated and know I have to move my bowels but I can't."* *"Whenever I'm constipated I feel lethargic and lose my appetite."* • Reports straining during defecation with little result • Passes small "marbles" of dry, hard stool • Decreased frequency • Decreased frequency of bowel sounds or changes in abdominal growling • Straining often results in small amount of bleeding from swollen external hemorrhoids • Reports feeling rectal fullness or pressure in rectum • Headache
Risk for Constipation	Habitually ignores urge to defecate Inactivity Decreased fiber in diet Inadequate fluid intake Use of pharmacologic agents that can result in constipation (iron, opioids, anticholinergics) Stress, confusion	• *"I'm in such a rush in the morning that I never take time to go to the bathroom."* • Reports straining during defecation • Passes small, hard, dry stool • Reports feeling bloated
Perceived Constipation	Culture Family health beliefs Faulty appraisal Impaired thought processes	• Expectation of daily bowel movement with resulting abuse of laxatives, enemas, suppositories • Expected passage of stool at the same time every day
Diarrhea	Food intolerance (coarse, greasy, or spicy foods) Food or drug allergies Abuse of laxatives Alteration in normal bacterial flora of the intestine (antibiotic therapy) Emotional stress Intestinal infection Colon disease and other diseases Surgical alterations	• Loose liquid stools, increased frequency • Urgency with soiling • Reports of abdominal pain and cramping • Increased frequency of bowel sounds
Bowel Incontinence	Gross constipation with impaction and subsequent overflow Organic changes in neural innervation of the rectum Local causes (inflammation, cancer of rectum, prolapsed anus, semifluid stool) Extreme debilitation Cognitive impairment	• Involuntary passage of stool (stool characteristics vary) • *"I'm sorry, I couldn't get into the bathroom (or onto the bedpan) quickly enough."* • *"It came so fast I couldn't hold it back."* • History of constipation with sudden development of oozing diarrheal stool

Bowel Elimination as the Etiology

Problems of bowel elimination may also affect other areas of human functioning. In the nursing diagnoses that follow, problems of bowel elimination are the etiology for other problems:

- Delayed Growth and Development related to child's inability to attain bowel control secondary to inconsistency and lack of adequate parental knowledge
- Imbalanced Nutrition: Less Than Body Requirements related to loss of appetite from flatulence or impaction, prolonged diarrhea
- Anxiety related to lack of voluntary control of fecal elimination and significant others' response to ostomy
- Disturbed Body Image related to ostomy, need to wear disposable adult briefs, continuous episodes of diarrhea
- Deficient Fluid Volume related to prolonged diarrhea
- Impaired Skin Integrity related to prolonged diarrhea, fecal incontinence
- Ineffective Coping related to inability to accept permanent ostomy
- Deficient Knowledge: Bowel Training related to no previous experience
- Pain related to intestinal distention, prolonged constipation or impaction, fecal incontinence, hemorrhoids
- Toileting Self-Care Deficit related to mobility deficit, weakness, confusion
- Low Self-Esteem related to need for assistance with toileting, fecal incontinence
- Sexual Dysfunction related to perceived change in body image, lack of interest, loss of self-esteem

Outcome Identification and Planning

Interventions for patients without specific bowel elimination problems are directed toward the patient's achievement of the following outcomes. The patient will:

- Have a soft, formed bowel movement every 1 to 3 days without discomfort
- Explain the relationship between bowel elimination and dietary fiber, fluid intake, and exercise
- Relate the importance of seeking medical evaluation if changes in stool color or consistency persist

Interventions for patients with specific bowel elimination problems are directed to appropriate outcomes based on the specific problem. Examples of problem-based outcomes include the following: The patient will:

- Describe the functioning and purpose of his ostomy
- Ingest an adequate amount of fiber
- Monitor the amount and consistency of stools
- Express acceptance of his ostomy
- Demonstrate skin care for ostomy
- Respond to the urge to defecate in a timely manner
- Maintain the integrity of perineal skin

Implementing

Nursing care related to bowel elimination includes interventions related to promotion of regular bowel habits, prevention and treatment of constipation, prevention and treatment of diarrhea, decreasing flatulence, promoting elimination of feces, managing bowel incontinence, and implementing bowel training programs. Nursing care related to caring for a patient with a nasogastric tube for gastric decompression is also discussed in the following sections.

Promoting Regular Bowel Habits

Promote regular bowel habits in well and ill patients by attention to timing, positioning, privacy, nutrition, and exercise.

TIMING

Encourage toileting at the patient's usual time during the day. Offer whatever assistance is needed to help the patient to the bathroom, commode, or bedpan at the time that a patient usually experiences the urge to defecate. This is often about an hour after meals, when mass colonic peristalsis occurs. Do not schedule nursing care or treatments during this time. Because many patients feel uncomfortable about requesting time for elimination, inform all patients about the importance of heeding this natural urge, explaining that postponing it could result in constipation and other problems.

POSITIONING

Sitting upright on a toilet or commode promotes defecation. Most patients who are able to use the bedside commode or bathroom toilet have little difficulty assuming this position, although they may need support. An elevated toilet seat may be ordered for patients with orthopedic problems who cannot lower themselves to a toilet seat. Sitting upright promotes a sense of normalcy and the effects of gravity help to promote regular bowel movements.

Patients who need to use a bedpan in bed often benefit from having the head of the bed elevated 30 degrees, unless this is contraindicated. This eliminates the hyperextension of the back that occurs when a patient who is lying flat attempts to lift his or her hips onto the pan. After the head of the bed is elevated, the patient raises the hips by bending the knees, digging in the heels, and lifting the hips upward. An overhead trapeze may be helpful for patients with weak lower extremities. Do not raise the head of the bed more than 45 degrees because this makes it harder for the patient to lift the hips straight up. Refer to Skill 37-1 for more information about positioning a patient on a bedpan. Offer the patient moistened hand wipes at the bedside to substitute for handwashing after toileting. Always empty, clean, and return bedpans to the patient's bedside stand promptly.

PRIVACY

Because most people consider elimination a private act, always respect the patient's need to be alone while defecating, unless the patient's condition makes this impossible. Pull the bedside drapes around a patient who is using a bedside commode or bedpan. If any visitors are present, ask them to step outside for a few minutes. For well patients who cannot defecate in a public restroom (with multiple toilets) or strange environment, suggest that they use a private restroom with only one toilet.

NUTRITION

Patients with bowel elimination problems may need a dietary analysis to determine which foods and fluids are contributing to their problem and which may help in its treatment. General dietary recommendations to promote regular defecation include a fluid intake of 2,000 to 3,000 mL and high fiber intake. Water is recommended as the fluid of choice because fluids containing large amounts of caffeine and sugar may have a diuretic effect. Increasing fiber intake without sufficient fluid intake can result in severe gastrointestinal problems, including fecal impaction. Specific recommendations for treating constipation, diarrhea, and excessive flatulence are discussed below.

EXERCISE

Regular exercise improves gastrointestinal motility and aids in defecation. Encourage well patients to exercise regularly three to five times a week. Ambulate patients who are ill as soon as possible, instructing them about how inactivity can lead to constipation, distention, and impaction. Bedside exercises may be helpful for patients who are immobile.

The following exercises may help patients with weak abdominal and perineal muscles who are using a bedpan:

- Abdominal setting: The patient, lying in a supine position, tightens and holds the abdominal muscles for 6 seconds and then relaxes them. Repeat several times each waking hour.
- Thigh strengthening: The thigh muscles are flexed and contracted by slowly bringing the knees up to the chest one at a time and then lowering them to the bed. Perform this exercise several times for each knee each waking hour.

Providing Comfort Measures

Comfort measures related to defecation include working with the patient to develop a bowel elimination routine that results in the easy passage of a soft, formed stool; being attentive to perineal hygiene and the maintenance of skin integrity; and using warm moist heat (sitz bath or tub bath) to soothe the perineal area. Additional nonsurgical treatment options include the following (Smeltzer et al., 2010):

- Encouraging recommended diet (if pertinent) and exercise
- Using medications, such as laxatives and antidiarrheals, only as needed
- Applying ointments or astringents (witch hazel)
- Using suppositories that contain anesthetics

Preventing and Treating Constipation

Constipation is dry, hard stool; persistently difficult passage of stool; and/or the incomplete passage of stool. Decreased gastric motility slows the passage of feces through the large intestine, resulting in increased fluid absorption from the fecal mass and causing dry, hard stool. Straining often accompanies defecation. Some people may be constipated and yet have a daily bowel movement, whereas others who regularly defecate no more than three times a week are not constipated. Individuals at high risk for constipation include (1) patients on bed rest who take constipating medications (opioids, anticholinergics), (2) patients with reduced fluids or bulk in their diet, (3) people who are depressed, and (4) patients with central nervous system disease or local lesions that cause pain.

TEACHING ABOUT NUTRITION

Promoting healthy behaviors can assist the patient and family to achieve mutually desirable outcomes for preventing constipation. A combination of high-fiber foods (20 to 35 g of fiber), eight 8-oz. glasses of water daily, and exercise has been shown to be effective in controlling constipation (Bisanz, 2007). Caution the patient to avoid increasing fiber intake without drinking enough fluids; this can lead to a bowel obstruction. Foods that contain high amounts of fiber include bran, fruits, vegetables, and whole grains. See the accompanying Research in Nursing box.

> *Think back to Leroy Cobbs, the patient who developed fecal impaction from using narcotic analgesics. The nurse should list in the teaching plan foods that stimulate peristalsis to prevent future episodes of constipation. If the patient knows to include these foods in his diet, he will be less worried about future problems and may be more amenable to using the medication to control his pain.* ∎

TEACHING ABOUT LAXATIVES

Cathartics and **laxatives** are drugs that induce emptying of the intestinal tract. Although these terms are sometimes used interchangeably, cathartics exert a stronger effect on the intestines than do laxatives. Some of these drugs, such as castor oil, cascara, senna, and phenolphthalein, and bisacodyl (Dulcolax), act chemically by stimulating peristalsis. Others, such as psyllium hydrophilic mucilloid (Metamucil), act by increasing the intestinal bulk, which promotes additional mechanical stimulation on the intestine. Still others, such as mineral oil and docusate sodium (Colace), soften the fecal material. Other frequently used laxatives are the saline-osmotics, such as magnesium hydroxide (Milk of Magnesia [MOM]) and sodium phosphate (Phospho-Soda). These act by drawing water into the intestines, stimulating peristalsis. Magnesium hydroxide has antacid properties in small dosages and laxative properties in larger doses. Table 38-2 summarizes the types of laxatives.

Laxatives are sometimes necessary for people with limited activity or poor food intake. They are also used to empty the intestinal tract in preparation for surgery or diagnostic tests. Laxatives such as docusate sodium (Colace) may be used in conjunction with some prescribed medications to counteract

RESEARCH IN NURSING
Bridging the Gap to Evidence-Based Practice

BRAN SUPPLEMENTS AND CONSTIPATION

Constipation is a common problem, particularly among older people. Diet, exercise, and daily routine are important factors in maintaining normal bowel patterns. Nursing interventions, such as increasing daily fluid intake, increasing fiber in the diet, encouraging physical activity and regular exercise, timing, and privacy are important aspects of patient care.

Related Research

Kaçmaz, Z., & Kaşikçi, M. (2007). Effectiveness of bran supplement in older orthopaedic patients with constipation. *Journal of Clinical Nursing, 16*(5), 928–936.

The purpose of this study was to evaluate the effectiveness of planned nursing interventions, including bran supplement, on the bowel management of older postoperative orthopedic patients. Patients in the control group received routine nursing care according to clinic routine. Patients in the experimental group received bran supplement together with planned nursing interventions. Patients in the experimental group showed

significant improvements in most characteristics of bowel elimination, such as time interval between defecation, intensity of elimination, color of feces, and amount of feces. The control group showed a significant improvement only in duration of time required for defecation. Nursing interventions including bran supplement were more effective than routine nursing interventions for management of constipation in postoperative orthopedic patients.

Relevance to Nursing Practice

Nurses have an important part to play in both prevention and management of constipation. Constipation is a problem especially for older orthopedic patients. Bran supplementation is an inexpensive and simple intervention. Planned nursing interventions that include bran supplements, with corresponding adequate fluid intake, may be more effective than routine nursing interventions for management of constipation problems in older orthopedic patients.

For additional research, visit thePoint.

TABLE • 38-2   CLASSIFICATION OF LAXATIVES

Type	Action	Advantages	Caution
Bulk-forming (e.g., Metamucil)	Psyllium, grain, or synthetic product that causes stool to absorb water and swell, thus stimulating peristalsis	Usually acts within 24 hours	May interfere with absorption of calcium and iron and certain drugs Should not be given to bedridden patients or those with intestinal strictures May be expensive
Stool softener (e.g., Colace)	Agents with detergent activity that allow water and fat to penetrate and lubricate the stool	Recommended for those who must avoid straining	Has lubricant component of drug that may interfere with absorption of fat-soluble vitamins
Emollient (lubricant) (e.g., mineral oil)	Lubricates the intestinal tract and retards colonic absorption of water, softening the stool, making it easier to pass.	Usually effective within 8 hours	May interfere with absorption of fat-soluble vitamins Can be aspirated, possibly resulting in a lipid pneumonia
Stimulant (e.g., Dulcolax)	Drug promotes peristalsis by irritating the intestinal mucosa or stimulating nerve endings in intestinal wall.	Works more quickly than bulking agents	Are the most abused laxatives on the market Causes lazy bowel syndrome May affect absorption of vitamin D and calcium Not recommended for elderly patients because of prolonged action Alters electrolyte transport
Saline-osmotic (e.g., MOM)	Drug draws water into intestine and stimulates peristalsis.	Is used when rapid cleansing desired	Should not be used by elderly people Can produce dehydration Not recommended in patients with kidney disease or heart failure

the medications' constipating properties. Occasional use of laxatives is not harmful for most people, but people should not become dependent on them. Because many laxatives are available as nonprescription drugs, and advertising promotes their use, many people take them frequently on their own initiative, whether they need them or not.

Because of their chemical action, laxatives should not be taken when there is abdominal pain because an intestinal pathologic condition could be harmed by the increased peristalsis. Although many people take laxatives because they believe they are constipated, most are unaware that habitual use of laxatives is the most common cause of chronic constipation.

Nurses play a key role in helping patients who abuse laxatives. Breaking the physical and psychological habit of using laxatives is not easy for a person who has come to depend on them; it often requires much patience, support, and teaching. The person also frequently needs assistance with his or her diet, fluid intake, activity, and regularity of habits.

Preventing and Treating Diarrhea

Diarrhea is the passage of more than three loose stools a day. Frequent bowel movements are not always indicative of diarrhea, but patients with diarrhea usually pass stools more frequently. Diarrhea is often associated with intestinal cramps. Nausea and vomiting may occur; blood also may be noted. Diarrhea is a protective response when the cause is irritants in the intestinal tract. Regardless of the cause, however, large amounts of fluids and electrolytes may be lost relatively quickly through diarrhea, especially in infants, young children, and older adults. If diarrhea is untreated, this loss of fluids and electrolytes places the person at high risk for life-threatening complications. If oral intake is possible, teach patients to avoid cold fluids and rich foods, especially sweets.

Additional nursing measures for the patient with diarrhea include the following:

- Answer the patient's call bell immediately or ensure that a bedpan or commode is within easy reach. Diarrhea can be embarrassing, and the patient needs to know that the nurse is there to help.
- Whenever possible, remove the cause of the diarrhea. Discontinuing medications that cause diarrhea usually results in a return to normal defecation within 1 to 3 days.
- If there is any indication of an impaction, obtain a physician's order for a rectal examination before using antidiarrheal medications.
- Give special care to the region around the anus, where skin irritation is common. Keep the area clean and dry. Use skin creams, moisture barriers, ointments, or powders as necessary.

> *Skin care measures would be important to include in the plan of care for Jeremy Green, the young boy experiencing episodes of diarrhea. Doing so reduces his risk for perianal excoriation and breakdown, which could further*

impair his body image and cause additional discomfort and pain. ∎

TEACHING ABOUT FOOD SAFETY

The first precaution is to ensure that food is safe for consumption and prepared and stored properly. Food poisoning, and the diarrhea that frequently accompanies it, can be prevented by these common measures:

- Never purchase food with damaged packaging.
- Take items that require refrigeration home immediately.
- Never use raw eggs in any form because of the danger of infection with the Salmonella bacillus. When cooking eggs, use only fresh ones that have been purchased within 3 to 5 weeks and kept in the refrigerator.
- Cook ground meat thoroughly. It should not have a pink center and should not drain pink juices. Avoid placing cooked meat on platters or cutting boards that held uncooked meat. Do not use knives previously used to cut uncooked meat.
- Never cut meat on a wooden surface.
- Do not eat seafood raw. Do not eat seafood if it has a strong, unpleasant odor.
- Thoroughly clean all vegetables and fruit before eating.
- Refrigerate leftovers within 2 hours of preparation.
- Give only pasteurized fruit juices to small children.

Additional measures for preventing or treating diarrhea include avoiding highly spiced foods and foods with laxative effects, such as raw fruits and vegetables. Encourage the patient to eat foods with low fiber content. Foods low in fiber include eggs; well-cooked meat, fish, and poultry; juices without pulp; refined bread and cereal products; and well-cooked fruits and vegetables. Replace lost fluids and electrolytes with weak tea, water, bouillon, clear soup, and gelatin. If diarrhea is severe, intravenous therapy may be needed.

PREVENTING AND MANAGING TRAVELER'S DIARRHEA

There has been a significant increase in the numbers of people traveling outside their native countries, including overseas travel. Traveler's diarrhea, caused by bacterial enteropathogens, viruses, or parasites, is the most common illness among persons traveling from developed to underdeveloped countries (Huntzinger, 2007). Symptoms include more than three loose stools in a 24-hour period, fever, nausea, vomiting, and abdominal cramps.

Management includes education about prevention and self-treatment strategies. Advise patients to peel fruits and vegetables, and consume dry foods and foods that are piping hot and cooked thoroughly. Travelers should avoid tap water, ice cubes, fruit juice, fresh salads, unpasteurized dairy products, cold sauces and toppings, open buffets, and undercooked or reheated foods.

Treatment strategies include maintaining hydration with bottled water and/or fluids containing oral rehydration salts, use of antimotility agents, such as loperamide (Imodium), and antibiotics. Encourage patients considering travel to underdeveloped countries to discuss their personal risks and the provision of prescription medication with their physician or healthcare provider before beginning their travels (Huntzinger, 2007).

TEACHING ABOUT TREATMENT FOR DIARRHEA

Treatment for diarrhea typically depends on whether the problem is acute or chronic. Acute diarrhea may result from a viral or bacterial infection, a reaction to medication, or alterations in diet. It is characterized by its sudden onset and lasts several hours to several days. Rehydration is key with acute diarrhea. Oral liquids may be used if the patient can tolerate them; otherwise, intravenous fluid replacement may be necessary. Stress the importance of hand hygiene with the patient and family. Antidiarrheal agents are avoided in acute diarrhea until a bacterial causative agent has been ruled out.

Chronic diarrhea typically lasts for more than 3 to 4 weeks. Investigate chronic diarrhea to determine the underlying cause. Chronic diarrhea has many possible causes, such as irritable bowel syndrome (e.g., Crohn's disease, ulcerative colitis), malabsorption syndromes, bowel tumor, metabolic disease (diabetes, hyperthyroidism), parasitic infection, side effects of drugs, laxative abuse, surgery, alcohol abuse, and radiation and chemotherapeutic agents. Chronic diarrhea usually necessitates pharmacologic intervention along with

fluid and electrolyte replacement. Antidiarrheal medications are usually reserved for treatment of chronic diarrhea. Whatever the type of diarrhea, every effort must be made to identify and eliminate the underlying cause.

Several types of antidiarrheal medications are available. Medications such as camphorated opium tincture (Paregoric), loperamide (Imodium), and diphenoxylate hydrochloride (Lomotil) act directly on the smooth muscle of the gastrointestinal tract. Kaolin and pectin (Kaopectate) is thought to act as an absorbent and demulcent. Bismuth subsalicylate (Pepto-Bismol) has an antimicrobial action and an antisecretory effect. Table 38-3 highlights the major antidiarrheal agents.

The focus of nursing care is on eliminating the cause of the diarrhea and replacing lost fluids as well as treating the symptoms. Some commercial fluid and electrolyte replacement products, such as Gatorade, may be helpful. Oral rehydration therapy using fluid and electrolyte replacement and water for adults is cost-effective and replaces fluid loss without the challenges associated with intravenous fluid therapy. It is particularly important that fluid balance be maintained in older patients because of their increased risk for dehydration, fluid overload, and electrolyte imbalances.

Infants and children require more water than do adults. Alterations in fluid and electrolyte balance occur faster and more often in infants and children than in adults (Hockenberry, 2005). Encourage fluids, especially soy formula and

TABLE • 38-3   CLASSIFICATION OF ANTIDIARRHEAL MEDICATIONS

Category	Name	Action	Advantages	Cautions
Action on gastrointestinal smooth muscle	Opium (Paregoric)	Increases smooth muscle tone Decreases GI motility Diminishes GI secretions	Effective	May be addictive due to morphine content May cause drowsiness and lightheadedness Should be discontinued as soon as diarrhea has diminished
	Diphenoxylate and atropine (Lomotil)	Slows gastric motility through local effect on gastrointestinal wall	Effective	Is chemically related to morphine; atropine added to prevent addiction but in high doses can become addictive May cause drowsiness
	Loperamide (Imodium)	Inhibits peristalsis via direct effect on gastrointestinal wall muscles	Not addictive Longer duration than Lomotil	May cause drowsiness Must be discontinued if no improvement in 48 hours with acute cases
Absorbent	Kaolin-pectin (Kaopectate)	Absorbs and soothes	No drowsiness	May interfere with absorption of other oral medications May interfere with absorption of nutrients with prolonged use
Antisecretory/antimicrobial	Bismuth subsalicylate (Pepto-Bismol)	Decreases gastrointestinal tract secretion Has antimicrobial action against bacterial and viral pathogens	No drowsiness	Contains salicylates, so check with physician before giving to children or administering with aspirin May decrease absorption of some medications

Pedialyte (an oral electrolyte solution for children that is low in sugar), and make them accessible for the child. Special diets for dehydration such as the BRAT diet (bananas, rice cereal, applesauce, and toast) are no longer recommended because they lack sufficient calories.

Decreasing Flatulence

Excessive formation of gases in the stomach or intestines is known as **flatulence.** When the gas is not expelled but accumulates in the intestinal tract, the condition is referred to as intestinal distention or tympanites. Gas-producing foods, such as beans, cabbage, onions, cauliflower, and beer, often predispose a person to flatulence and distention.

> *Recall Alberta Franklin, the patient described in the Reflective Practice display. The nurse should include information about gas-producing foods in this patient's teaching plan to avoid excess gas formation and accumulation, which could cause her colostomy bag to overfill and possibly lead to detachment and leakage.* ■

In addition to teaching about the avoidance of irritating foods, explain to the patient that he or she should avoid reclining after meals and should move around in bed and ambulate in order to promote peristalsis and the escape of flatus.

Emptying the Colon of Feces

Several methods are used to help promote elimination of feces: enemas, suppositories, oral intestinal lavage, and digital removal of stool. Each of these methods is discussed below.

ENEMAS

An **enema** is the introduction of a solution into the large intestine, usually to remove feces. The instilled solution distends the intestine and irritates the intestinal mucosa, thus increasing peristalsis. Enemas are classified as cleansing, retention, or return-flow enemas.

Cleansing Enemas

Cleansing enemas are given to remove feces from the colon, commonly to:

- Relieve constipation or fecal impaction
- Prevent involuntary escape of fecal material during surgical procedures
- Promote visualization of the intestinal tract by radiographic or instrument examination
- Help establish regular bowel function during a bowel training program

The most common types of solutions used for cleansing enemas are tap water, normal saline solution, soap solution, and hypertonic solution. Commonly used enema solutions are described in Table 38-4.

Hypotonic (tap water) and isotonic (normal saline solution) enemas are large-volume enemas that result in rapid colonic emptying. However, using such large volumes of solution (adults, 500 to 1,000 mL; infants, 150 to 250 mL) may be dangerous for patients with weakened intestinal walls. These solutions often require special preparation and equipment.

Hypertonic solution preparations are available commercially and are administered in smaller volumes (adult, 70 to 130 mL). These solutions draw water into the colon, which stimulates the defecation reflex. They may be contraindicated in patients for whom sodium retention is a problem. They are also contraindicated for patients with renal impairment or reduced renal clearance because such patients have compromised ability to excrete phosphate adequately, with resulting hyperphosphatemia (Bowers, 2006).

TABLE • 38-4 **COMMONLY USED ENEMA SOLUTIONS**

Solution	Amount	Action	Time to Take Effect	Adverse Effects
Tap water (hypotonic)	500–1,000 mL	Distends intestine, increases peristalsis, softens stool	15 min	Fluid and electrolyte imbalance, water intoxication
Normal saline (isotonic)	500–1,000 mL	Distends intestine, increases peristalsis, softens stool	15 min	Fluid and electrolyte imbalance, sodium retention
Soap	500–1,000 mL (concentrate at 3–5 mL/1,000 mL)	Distends intestine, irritates intestinal mucosa, softens stool	10–15 min	Rectal mucosa irritation or damage
Hypertonic	70–130 mL	Distends intestine, irritates intestinal mucosa	5–10 min	Sodium retention
Oil (mineral, olive, or cottonseed oil)	150–200 mL	Lubricates stool and intestinal mucosa	30 min	

Retention Enemas

Retention enemas are retained in the bowel for a prolonged period for different reasons:

- Oil-retention enemas: lubricate the stool and intestinal mucosa, making defecation easier. About 150 to 200 mL of solution is administered to adults.
- Carminative enemas: help to expel flatus from the rectum and provide relief from gaseous distention. Common solutions include the milk and molasses enema (equal parts) and the magnesium sulfate–glycerin–water (MGW) enema (30 mL of magnesium sulfate, 60 mL of glycerin, and 90 mL of warm water).
- Medicated enemas: provide medications that are absorbed through the rectal mucosa.
- Anthelmintic enemas: destroy intestinal parasites.

Equipment

Commercially prepared enema kits include a flexible bottle containing hypertonic solution with an attached prelubricated firm tip about 5 to 7.5 cm (2 to 3 inches) long. Its ease of use makes it particularly convenient in the home. Patients can readily administer their own enema in many instances.

For tap water, saline solution, or soap solution enema, a container, rubber or plastic tubing with side openings near its distal end, a tubing clamp, lubricant, and the solution are necessary. Regardless of the type of enema to be given, clean or medically aseptic technique is used. Always wear or have the caregiver wear disposable gloves to protect from exposure to blood, body fluids, and microorganisms.

Patient Preparation

Because enemas are a common procedure, some patients already know why they are used and how they are administered. Reinforce this information and correct any misconceptions that they may have. For patients who have not previously had an enema, explain the purpose, what they can expect, and how they can participate. In all cases, provide for patient privacy. The procedure offers an excellent opportunity for health teaching because many people are unfamiliar with or uncomfortable talking about the functioning of the intestinal tract. Failure to provide explanations and protect privacy may result in an uncomfortable and disagreeable situation for the patient.

A reclining position for enema administration, specifically left side-lying or the knee-chest position, is recommended, but if the patient has a respiratory disorder or is having difficulty breathing, elevate the head of the bed slightly. Avoid the Fowler's position because the solution will remain in the rectum and expulsion will occur rapidly, resulting in minimal cleansing. Some patients think the solution should be expelled as soon as possible. Reinforce the need to retain the solution to achieve the desired results.

Administration Using a Large Volume of Solution

The procedure for administering a cleansing enema using a large volume of solution is described in Skill 38-1.

Administration Using a Hypertonic (small volume) Solution

Administering a cleansing enema using a hypertonic solution differs from the procedure described in Skill 38-1 in the following ways:

- The equipment is included in the commercially prepared set. The only additional equipment needed is a bedpan for a bedridden patient and a disposable waterproof pad to protect bed linens.
- Do not warm the hypertonic solution. Administer it at room temperature, and warm it only if it is very cold.
- Place the patient in the left side-lying position or the knee-chest position, which helps to distribute the solution throughout the lower intestinal tract and is recommended if the patient can assume it. Additional lubrication of the rectal tip is recommended, even though it is prelubricated.
- Instill the solution into the rectum by applying gentle pressure on the collapsible solution container (Fig. 38-6). It should take 1 to 2 minutes to administer the enema.
- Administer the hypertonic enema solution (Fleet enema) cautiously to a patient with hemorrhoids. The rigid tip may tear fragile rectal mucosa that is enlarged and inflamed, causing pain, torn rectal tissue, and necrosis. A rectal examination and generous lubrication are recommended before inserting the enema tip.

Administration of an Oil-Retention Enema

The procedure for giving an oil-retention enema differs from that for giving a cleansing enema in the following respects:

- A small rectal tube is used. The small size helps to reduce intestinal contractions so that the patient can retain the oil more easily. Oil enemas are available in commercial kits similar to those for hypertonic solution enemas. The kits contain a small rectal tube.
- Administer the oil-retention enema at body temperature to minimize muscle contractions caused by a warmer or cooler solution.
- Instruct the patient to retain the oil for at least 30 minutes for best cleansing results.

FIGURE 38-6. Technique for compressing Fleet enema container.

• A cleansing enema is often ordered after an oil-retention enema to facilitate emptying of the bowel.

RECTAL SUPPOSITORIES

A **suppository** is a conical or oval solid substance shaped for easy insertion into a body cavity and designed to melt at body temperature. Various rectal suppositories are available. Some are fecal softeners, others have a direct action on the nerve endings in the rectal mucosa, and some liberate carbon dioxide when moistened. Fecal softeners are useful when the stool is very hard. Substances that stimulate the rectal nerves are helpful for people with weak muscle tone or poor innervation. The carbon dioxide suppositories liberate about 200 mL of gas, which causes distention, causing stimulation and elimination impulses. Refer to Chapter 29 for Guidelines for Nursing Care 29-10, Inserting a Rectal Suppository.

ORAL INTESTINAL LAVAGE

An oral solution, such as GoLYTELY or Colyte, can be used to cleanse the intestine of feces. This solution is prescribed by the physician and can be administered before diagnostic tests that require a clear bowel for visualization purposes or as a "bowel prep" before intestinal surgery. Evacuation of feces usually begins within 1 hour after the first glass and is completed within 4 to 6 hours. As with an enema, a clear return indicates that the bowel preparation is complete. A clear diet for 24 hours before taking this solution lessens the time needed for completion of the bowel prep, but potassium replacement may be required before surgery because of the limited potassium in a clear diet. The solution has a slightly salty taste and is easier to tolerate if it is cold and consumed quickly. Older patients require careful assessment because they are more prone to electrolyte imbalances.

DIGITAL REMOVAL OF STOOL

Fecal impaction often prevents the passage of normal stools. Small amounts of fluid may pass around the impacted mass; liquid fecal seepage with no passage of normal feces is a sign of an impaction.

Dietary interventions, adequate fluids, and adjustment of medication should be included in the patient's plan of care before digital removal of feces is considered (Kyle, Prynn, & Oliver, 2004). If a patient with a fecal impaction cannot expel the fecal mass voluntarily and oil and cleansing enemas fail to break up the mass, the impaction must be broken up manually. A physician's order is required. This procedure is very uncomfortable and may cause great discomfort to the patient as well as irritation of the rectal mucosa and bleeding. Digital removal of a fecal mass can stimulate the vagus nerve, resulting in a slowed heart rate. If this occurs, stop the procedure immediately, monitor the patient's heart rate and blood pressure, and notify the physician. Many patients find that a sitz bath or tub bath after this procedure soothes the irritated perineal area. An oil-retention enema may be ordered to be given before the procedure to soften stool. The procedure for digital (manual) removal of a fecal impaction is outlined in the Guidelines for Nursing Care 38-2 Digital Removal of Fecal Impaction.

> *It is important for the nurse caring for Leroy Cobbs, the patient with fecal impaction described at the beginning of the chapter, to demonstrate competency and care when performing manual disimpaction to decrease the patient's discomfort and embarrassment. Additionally, the nurse may need to adapt the procedure to ensure that the patient experiences relief as quickly as possible without any undue harm or injury.* ∎

Managing Bowel Incontinence

Bowel incontinence is the inability of the anal sphincter to control the discharge of fecal and gaseous material. The cause of incontinence is usually an organic disease, resulting either in a mechanical condition that hinders the proper functioning of the anal sphincter or an impairment in the nerve supply to the anal sphincter. Mental illness may also cause a patient to be indifferent to the passage of stool. Although bowel incontinence is seldom life-threatening, patients with bowel incontinence suffer embarrassment, may become depressed, and pose a challenge for nurses because of the risk for skin breakdown.

The following nursing interventions are helpful for a patient who suffers from bowel incontinence:

• Note when incontinence is most likely to occur, and place the patient on a bedpan at those times. If there is no pattern, offer a bedpan at regular intervals, such as every few hours.
• Keep the skin clean and dry by using proper hygienic measures. Apply a protective skin barrier after cleaning the skin, according to manufacturer's directions. Impaired skin integrity may develop when such measures are overlooked.
• Change bed linens and clothing as necessary to avoid odor, skin irritation, and embarrassment. Disposable bed pads and moisture-proof undergarments can be considered but should not be used until other measures have been tried. These materials often worsen any skin irritation or breakdown present as a result of skin contact with stool by retaining moisture against the skin, raising the pH of the skin, and prolonging contact of the stool against the skin, increasing damage from digestive enzymes present in the stool (Gray, 2007).
• Confer with the physician about using a suppository or a daily cleansing enema. These measures empty the lower colon regularly and often help to decrease incontinence. Bowel training programs may be helpful.

RECTAL INDWELLING CATHETER

In some healthcare agencies, a rectal indwelling catheter is used for patients with uncontrollable diarrhea, but relatively little research supports the safety of this procedure. Some nurses think that the rectal indwelling catheter stimulates sensory nerve fibers in the rectum, thus increasing peristalsis and worsening the diarrhea. Others are concerned about the danger of rectal perforation and the development of mucosal

Guidelines for Nursing Care • 38-2

DIGITAL REMOVAL OF FECAL IMPACTION

To manually remove a fecal impaction, the following technique is recommended:

- Have a second person assist with the procedure. The second person can reassure and comfort the patient while the first person works to break up the mass.

- Place the patient in a side-lying position.

- Place a bedpan on the bed for depositing removed feces. Have toilet paper and personal cleaning supplies on hand for use after the procedure is completed.

- Drape the patient to preserve privacy yet provide easy access.

- Use clean gloves for the procedure because the intestinal tract is not sterile.

- Lubricate the index finger generously to reduce irritating the rectum, and insert the finger gently into the anal canal

(Figure A). The presence of the finger added to the mass tends to cause discomfort for the patient if the work is not done slowly and gently.

- Slowly and gently, work the finger around and into the hardened mass to break it up (Figures B and C) and then remove pieces of it (Figure D). Instruct the patient to bear down, if possible, while extracting feces to ease in removal.

- Remove the impaction at intervals if it is severe. This helps to avoid discomfort as well as irritation, which can injure intestinal mucosa.

- Use an oil-retention enema if necessary. The enema may be given before attempts are made to break up and remove the impaction digitally, or it may be ordered after digital attempts fail. A cleansing enema is often ordered after an oil-retention enema.

A

Inserting the gloved, lubricated finger into the fecal mass.

B

Slowly and gently, using the finger to break up some of the hardened mass.

C

Breaking off a section of the impaction.

D

Removing a section of the impaction.

necrosis. Indwelling rectal catheters should not be used to manage large volumes of diarrhea. The fecal incontinence pouch is a safer alternative and is discussed below.

FECAL INCONTINENCE POUCH

An alternative measure to protect perianal skin from repeated episodes of fecal incontinence is the fecal incon-

tinence pouch. This device can be secured via adhesive around the anal opening and attached to gravity drainage, allowing liquid stool to accumulate in a collection bag. See Figure 38-7. It is best applied before the perianal area becomes excoriated. If excoriation is already present, application of a skin barrier prior to applying the pouch can be effective.

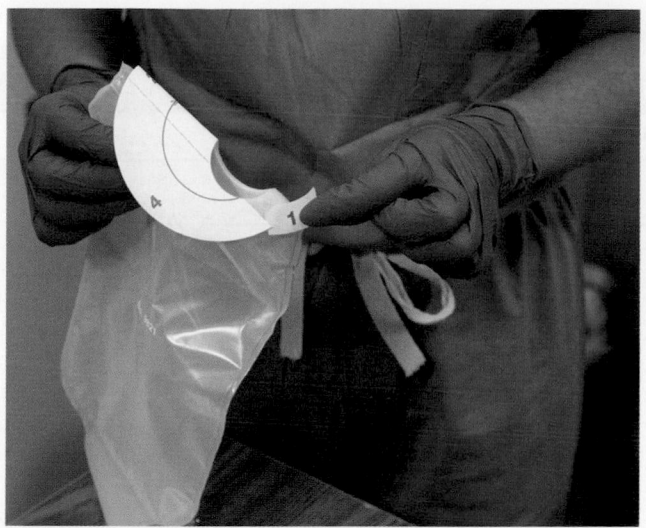

Removing paper backing from adhesive of rectal pouch.

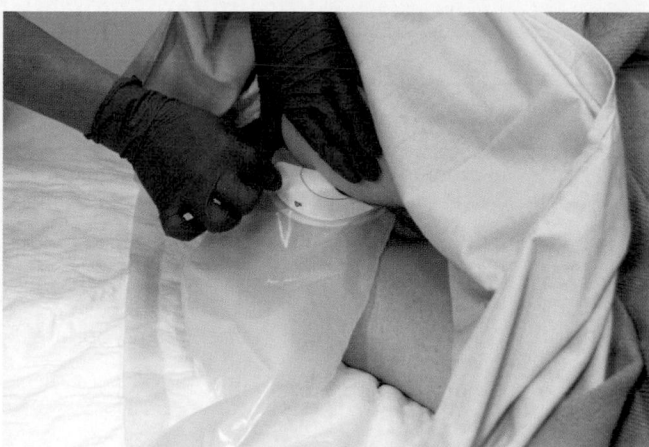

Applying pouch over anal opening.

Attaching connector of fecal pouch to tubing of drainage bag.

FIGURE 38-7. Applying a fecal incontinence pouch.

Nursing responsibilities include careful regular assessment and documentation of the perianal skin condition and attentive management of the drainage system. Change the pouch at least every 72 hours, or sooner if it is not intact or leakage has occurred. Provide explanations and support to the patient and family members so that they understand the benefits of this system.

Designing and Implementing Bowel Training Programs

Patients with a history of chronic constipation and impaction and those who are incontinent of stool may benefit from a **bowel training program.** The purpose of this program is to manipulate factors within the person's control (food and fluid intake, exercise, time for defecation) to produce the elimination of a soft, formed stool at regular intervals without a laxative. This effort to regain bowel control may be initiated in the healthcare setting or the patient's home. The accompanying Nursing Intervention and Nursing Outcome Classifications (NIC/NOC) box lists standardized nursing interventions and corresponding outcomes related to bowel management and training. When the patient has established

a regular pattern of defecation, continue to offer assistance with toileting at the successful time.

Maintaining a Nasogastric Tube

Nasogastric tubes may be inserted to decompress or drain the stomach of fluid or unwanted stomach contents such as poison or medication and air, and when conditions are present in which peristalsis is absent. Several of these conditions are detailed previously in the chapter. Examples include paralytic ileus and intestinal obstruction by tumor or hernia. Nasogastric tubes are also used to allow the gastrointestinal tract to rest before or after abdominal surgery to promote healing and are inserted to monitor gastrointestinal bleeding. Historically, a nasogastric tube has often been used postoperatively as a routine part of care after major abdominal surgery, to rest the intestinal tract and promote healing. Some research has suggested that the routine use of NGT after abdominal surgery may serve no beneficial purpose and may actually delay the patient's progress, increasing the time required for flatus to occur and increasing pulmonary complications. It is suggested that selective decompression should be reserved for patients with nausea, vomiting, and

Examples of Nursing Interventions and Nursing Outcomes Classifications (NIC/NOC)

Bowel Management

Nursing Interventions	Nursing Outcomes
• Plan bowel program with patient and appropriate others • Monitor bowel movements including frequency, consistency, shape, volume, and color, as appropriate • Monitor bowel sounds • Teach patient about specific foods that are assistive in promoting bowel regularity • Instruct patient on foods high in fiber, as appropriate • Monitor hydration status • Encourage fluids, as appropriate • Ensure privacy	• Bowel Elimination • Symptom Control • Hydration • Gastrointestinal Function

From Bulechek, G., Butcher, H., & McCloskey Dochterman, J. (Eds.). (2008). *Nursing interventions classification (NIC)* (5th ed., p. 336). St. Louis: Mosby Elsevier; and Moorhead, S., Johnson, M., Maas, M., Swanson, E. (Eds.). (2008). *Nursing outcomes classification (NOC)* (5th ed., p. 746). A full listing of nursing activities for each nursing intervention and outcomes can be found in these books.

abdominal distention after surgery (Brennan, 2008; Gannon, 2007; Nelson, Edwards, & Tse, 2007; Vermeulen, Storm-Versloot, Busch, & Ubbink, 2006).

A nasogastric tube is a pliable single- or double-lumen (inner open space) tube that is hollow, allowing for the removal of gastric secretions and instillation of solutions into the stomach. The tube is passed through the nasopharynx into the stomach. See Figure 38-8. Refer to Chapter 36, Nutrition, Skill 36-1 for the procedure for nasogastric tube insertion and Skill 36-3 for the procedure for removal of a nasogastric tube.

Tubes for decompression typically are attached to suction. Suction can be applied intermittently or continuously.

The Levin tube is a common single-lumen tube. It lacks a venting system, and mucosal damage can occur when suction is applied continuously. Therefore, suction usually is applied intermittently. Salem sump nasogastric tubes are double-lumen tubes. One lumen empties the stomach, and the other provides for a continuous flow of air. The airflow lumen controls suction by preventing the drainage lumen from pulling stomach mucosa into the tube's openings and

FIGURE 38-8. Levine tube and Salem sump nasogastric tubes. Insert on right shows close up of a one-way antireflux valve for Salem sump tube.

irritating the stomach lining. A one-way antireflux valve may be used in the airflow lumen to prevent reflux of gastric contents through the airflow lumen (see Fig. 38-8). When pressure from gastric contents enters the airflow tubing, the valve closes to prevent secretions from exiting the tube.

Nasogastric tubes used for decompression require irrigation with 30 to 60 mL of normal saline solution to maintain patency. Skill 38-2 describes the procedure for irrigating a nasogastric tube connected to suction.

To promote patient safety when instilling solutions into a nasogastric tube, tube placement must be verified before administration of any fluids or medications. Radiographic examination to confirm placement is the most accurate method for checking if the NG tube is in the stomach, but is often only ordered on initial placement, and many times is not prescribed for nasogastric tubes inserted for decompression. Two methods recommended for checking placement, other than radiograph, are visual assessment of aspirated gastric contents and measuring the pH of the aspirate (Higgins, 2008a; Smeltzer et al., 2010; May, 2007; Grindel, 2007; American Association of Critical-Care Nurses [AACN], 2005). Refer to Guidelines for Nursing Care 36-1 Visual Assessment and pH Measurement of Gastric Contents (Chapter 36, Nutrition). In addition, the length of the exposed tube is measured and marked after insertion and documented. Check and compare tube length with this initial measurement, in conjunction with the previous two methods for checking tube placement. An increase in the length of the exposed tube may indicate dislodgement (Smeltzer et al., 2010).

Patients with nasogastric tubes often experience discomfort related to irritation to nasal and throat mucosa, and drying of the oral mucous membranes. Administer oral hygiene frequently, as often as every 2 to 4 hours, to prevent drying of tissues and to relieve thirst. Frequently offer the patient the opportunity to rinse the mouth with warm water and mouthwash solution. Lubricate the lips generously. Keep the nares clean, especially around the tube, where secretions tend to accumulate. Use a lubricant after cleaning the nares. Help control local irritation from the tube in the throat by offering analgesic throat lozenges or anesthetic sprays, as prescribed. Ensure the tube is secured to the patient's nose and gown to prevent tension and tugging on the tube, causing trauma to the nares and potential displacement.

Meeting the Needs of Patients With Bowel Diversions

Sometimes patients undergo surgical procedures to create an opening into the abdominal wall for fecal elimination. The word **ostomy** is a term for a surgically formed opening from the inside of an organ to the outside. The intestinal mucosa is brought out to the abdominal wall, and a **stoma,** the part of the ostomy that is attached to the skin, is formed by suturing the mucosa to the skin. An **ileostomy** allows liquid fecal content from the ileum of the small intestine to be eliminated through the stoma. A **colostomy** permits formed feces in the colon to exit through the stoma. Colostomies are further classified by the part of the colon from which they originate.

Figure 38-9 shows the location of an ileostomy and various colostomies.

In many institutions, if the ostomy surgery is not emergent, patients meet with a specially trained registered nurse called a wound, ostomy, and continence nurse (WOCN). Together, they determine the ideal location for the stoma.

An ileostomy or colostomy may be either temporary or permanent. Temporary ostomies are performed to allow the

A. Sigmoid colostomy

B. Descending colostomy

C. Transverse colostomy

D. Ascending colostomy

E. Ileostomy

FIGURE 38-9. (**A–D**) Location of various colostomies, and (**E**) location of an ileostomy. The shaded portions represent the sections of the bowel that have been removed or are currently inactive.

Loop
ileostomy

Ileal-reservoir
"S" pouch

Ileal-anal
anastomosis

FIGURE 38-10. Ileoanal reservoir.

intestine to repair itself after inflammatory disease, some types of intestinal surgery, or injury. The patient returns for a second surgery in several weeks, and the intestine is reconnected. Permanent ostomies are performed for debilitating intestinal diseases or cancer of the colon or rectum. The patient will have this ostomy for the rest of his life.

A continent ileostomy is an alternative to the traditional surgical procedure. An internal pouch is created that the patient accesses through a nipple-like valve constructed from the ileum on the abdominal wall. The patient does not need to wear an external collection device, but because the valve malfunctions frequently, this procedure has limited use at this time. Another surgical alternative that does not involve an external stoma is the creation of an ileoanal reservoir. The terminal ileum is sutured directly to the anus, a pouch is created, and the patient is able to control expulsion

of feces through the intact anal sphincter (Fig. 38-10). This procedure also has complications, and candidates are carefully selected for this surgery.

COLOSTOMY AND ILEOSTOMY CARE

The patient with an ostomy needs physical and psychological support both preoperatively and postoperatively. This support can come from the patient's significant others, members of the healthcare team, and from people who have had similar experiences. The ostomy requires specific physical care for which the nurse is responsible initially. The following guidelines help to promote the ostomy patient's physical and psychological comfort:

- Keep the patient as free of odors as possible. Empty the ostomy appliance frequently.
- Inspect the patient's stoma regularly. It should be dark pink to red and moist. A pale stoma may indicate anemia, and a dark or purple-blue stoma may reflect compromised circulation or ischemia (Fig. 38-11). Bleeding around the stoma and its stem should be minimal. Notify the physician promptly if bleeding persists or is excessive or if color changes occur in the stoma.
- Note the size of the stoma, which usually stabilizes within 6 to 8 weeks. Most stomas protrude ½ to 1 inch from the abdominal surface and may initially appear swollen and edematous. After 6 weeks, the edema has usually subsided. Depending on the surgical technique, the final stoma may be flush with the skin. Erosion of skin around the stoma area can also lead to a flush stoma (Fig. 38-11). If an abdominal dressing is in place, check it frequently for drainage and bleeding.
- Keep the skin around the stoma site (peristomal area) clean and dry. If care is not taken to protect the skin around the stoma, irritation or infection may occur. A leaking appliance frequently causes skin erosion.

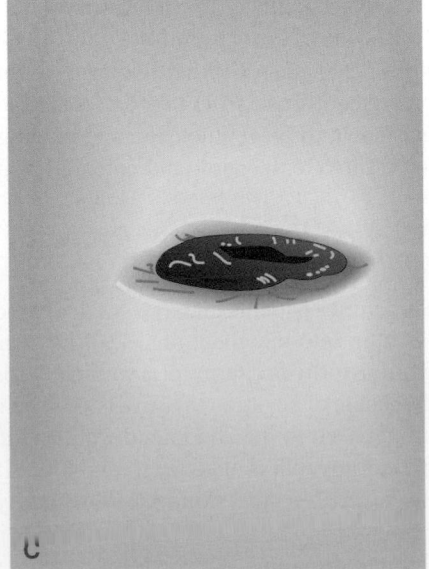

A

B

C

FIGURE 38-11. Comparison of stomal appearance. (**A**) Normal-appearing stoma is bright red, moist, and perfectly round. (**B**) A pale stoma indicates severe anemia. (**C**) Eroded skin around the area may lead to a flush stoma.

Candida or yeast infections can also occur around the stoma if the area is not kept dry.

- Measure the patient's fluid intake and output. Check the ostomy appliance for the quality and quantity of discharge. Initially after surgery, peristalsis may be inhibited. As peristalsis returns, stool will be eliminated from the stoma. Record intake and output every 4 hours for the first 3 days after surgery. If the patient's output decreases while intake remains stable, report the condition promptly.

- Explain each aspect of care to the patient and explain what his or her role will be when he or she begins self-care. Patient teaching is one of the most important aspects of colostomy care and should include family members when appropriate. Teaching can begin before surgery so that the patient has adequate time to absorb information.

- Encourage the patient to participate in care and to look at the ostomy. Patients normally experience emotional depression during the early postoperative period. Help the patient cope by listening, explaining, and being available and supportive. A visit from a representative of the local ostomy support group may be helpful. Patients usually begin to accept their altered body image when they are willing to look at the stoma, make neutral or positive statements concerning the ostomy, and express interest in learning self-care.

Changing the Ostomy Appliance

The ostomy appliance should protect the skin, collect the fecal discharge, and control odor. Typically, a colostomy does not produce drainage until normal peristalsis returns, usually within 2 to 5 days. An ileostomy drains within 24 to 48 hours because of the liquid contents in the small intestine.

For the first few days after surgery, most patients wear an open-ended appliance that allows for drainage of fecal material without removing the appliance. The skin barrier has an adhesive barrier that protects the surrounding skin from the stoma output. Appliances are either one-piece (barrier backing already attached to the pouch) or two-piece (separate pouch that fastens to the barrier backing). A transparent one-piece appliance is used in the initial postoperative period to allow for visualization of the stoma.

Appliances can be either drainable or closed. A pouch that can be drained is emptied when it is one-third full and replaced every 3 to 7 days, or whenever the seal comes away from the skin. Nondrainable pouches require removal and changing when they are half full. Types of ostomy equipment are illustrated in Figure 38-12 and include various types of one-piece and two-piece pouches (drainable and nondrainable) and clamps that securely close drainable pouches.

> *Recall Alberta Franklin, the patient with the new colostomy requiring a change of her appliance. The nurse needs to demonstrate competence and dexterity when changing this patient's bag by being adequately prepared and organized. Additionally, the nurse can use the time during bag changes to teach the patient about self-care measures and to assess the patient's acceptance of the colostomy.* ■

One-piece pouch with clamp

Two-piece pouches

Cut-to-fit pouch

FIGURE 38-12. Examples of ostomy pouches and closures. This equipment comes in various models and sizes. Convex pouches, belts, and other devices to prevent leaks and irritation are also available. *(Second and third photos copyright Hollister Inc. Used with permission.)*

If an appliance is leaking from underneath the skin barrier, ring, or wafer, the bag will have to be removed, the skin cleaned, and a new bag applied. Changing or emptying an ostomy appliance is shown in Skill 38-3. The act of removing an appliance from the skin can result in skin stripping, removal of the outer, loosely bound, epidermal cell layers. This can be uncomfortable or even very painful for the patient. The cumulative effects of skin stripping over time can result in peristomal skin breakdown. The use of a silicone-based adhesive remover allows for the easy, rapid, and painless removal of a stoma pouch without the associated problems of skin stripping (Rudoni, 2008; Stephen-Haynes, 2008).

Irrigating a Colostomy

Irrigations are infrequently used to promote regular evacuation of some colostomies. Various factors, such as the site of the colostomy in the colon (sigmoid colostomy) and the patient's and physician's preferences, determine whether a colostomy is irrigated. Ileostomies are not irrigated because the fecal content of the ileum is liquid and cannot be controlled.

Water is inserted into the colostomy, and the water and feces are expelled from the colostomy into the irrigation sleeve and then the toilet. Following a colostomy irrigation, no feces or flatus should pass from the colostomy until the next irrigation (Burch & Sica, 2007). If a colostomy irrigation is to be implemented, the nurse should consult facility policy regarding the accepted procedure.

LONG-TERM OSTOMY CARE

The patient can return to an active and full life with an ostomy. He or she should be aware of community resources available for assistance, such as home healthcare nurses, special clinics, and ostomy support groups. Encourage the patient to seek medical follow-up care on a regular basis.

During the first 6 to 8 weeks after surgery, encourage the patient with an ostomy to avoid foods high in fiber (e.g., foods with skins, seeds, shells) as well as any other foods that cause diarrhea or excessive flatus. By gradually adding new foods, the ostomy patient can progress to a normal diet. Urge patients to drink at least 2 quarts of fluids, preferably water, daily. Additional dietary considerations for patients with an ileostomy or colostomy are outlined in Box 38-3.

Patients with ileostomies need to be aware they may experience a tendency to develop food blockages, especially when high-fiber foods are consumed. This is because scar tissue from the place where the intestine passes through the abdominal muscle tightens the inside diameter of the ileum and can narrow it to much less than its normal 1 inch diameter. Fiber

blockages can cause foul-smelling watery output, abdominal cramping, and distention, along with nausea and vomiting.

Health teaching about medication use is frequently overlooked for patients with ostomies. Some medications may discolor the stool and cause unusual odors, some may cause constipation, and some may not dissolve or be absorbed completely because the small bowel is where most absorption occurs. The use of liquid, chewable, or injectable forms rather than long-acting, enteric-coated, or sustained-release medications is recommended. Laxatives and enemas are dangerous because they may cause severe fluid and electrolyte imbalance.

Many times, patients are embarrassed when they have to use public restrooms to empty their bag. Teach patients with ostomies about the various methods of odor control. Remind them that if the bag is clean and sealed well, odor usually is not a problem during normal activity. Encourage the intake of dark green vegetables. These vegetables contain chlorophyll, which helps to deodorize the feces. Buttermilk, cranberry juice, parsley, and yogurt can also prevent odor. Crackers, toast, and yogurt can help to reduce gas, which in turn aids in odor control. Commercial odor-control products also are available for purchase. The Wound, Ostomy, and Continence Nurse (WOCN) can help with the selection of odor-control strategies.

The patient with an ostomy can resume normal activity, including work and sexual relations. However, direct physical contact sports and heavy lifting should be avoided. The patient can go swimming. When traveling, the patient should carry a 1- to 2-day supply of equipment in a carry-on bag in case checked luggage is lost. Nurses play a significant role in helping patients, their families, and significant others adjust to this major life change. These surgeries result in physical

---

Box 38-3   DIETARY CONSIDERATIONS FOR PATIENTS WITH AN ILEOSTOMY OR COLOSTOMY

Foods That May Cause Gas

Alcohol and beer	Fried food (some)
Carbonated beverages	Melon
Chewing gum	Onions
Chives	Peppers
Cucumbers	Pickles
Dried peas, beans, and lentils	Sauerkraut
Eggs	

Vegetables from the cabbage family such as broccoli, Brussels sprouts, cabbage, cauliflower, and turnip

Foods That May Cause Stomal Blockage

Bean sprouts	Nuts
Cabbage	Olives
Carrots (raw)	Peas
Celery	Pickles
Coconut	Pineapple
Corn	Popcorn
Cucumbers	Seeds
Dried fruit	Skins and seeds from
Green pepper skin	fruits and vegetables
Lettuce	Spinach
Mushrooms	

Foods That May Help To Control Diarrhea

Applesauce	Soda crackers
Bananas	Starchy foods (rice, pasta,
Cheese	barley)
Creamy peanut butter	Tapioca
Oatmeal or oatbran	Yogurt
Potatoes	

Foods That Produce Odor

Asparagus	Garlic
Dried peas, beans, and lentils	Onions
Eggs	Some spicy foods
Fish	Turnip

Foods That Are Natural Intestinal Deodorizers

Buttermilk
Parsley
Yogurt

From Dudek, S. (2006). *Nutrition essentials for nursing practice* (5th ed). Philadelphia: Lippincott Williams & Wilkins, p. 511.

RESEARCH IN NURSING
Bridging the Gap to Evidence-Based Practice

ADJUSTMENT TO A COLOSTOMY

A stoma operation causes major changes in a patient's life because of the resulting physical damage, disfigurement, loss of bodily function, and change in personal hygiene. Such changes are a cause of major concern for patients and raise important issues for the provision of quality care.

Related Research

Simmons, K., Smith, J., Bobb, K., & Liles, L. (2007). Adjustment to colostomy: stoma acceptance, stoma care self-efficacy, and interpersonal relationships. *Journal of Advanced Nursing, 60*(6), 627–635.

This study examined the adjustment of patients with a new colostomy and its relationship with stoma acceptance and social interaction. In addition, it looked at the relationship between stoma care self-efficacy and adjustment in the presence of acceptance and social interactions. Patients with new colostomies provided demographic and clinical data for this study, as well as completing questionnaires to measure acceptance of their stoma, their relationships with others, and stoma

care self-efficacy, 6 months after their surgery. Multiple regression analysis showed that stoma self-care efficacy, stoma acceptance, interpersonal relationships, and the location of the stoma were strongly associated with adjustment.

Relevance to Nursing Practice

Patients experiencing life-altering surgeries, such as colostomies and ileostomies, require much information and support to adapt and achieve an adequate standard of living. Nurses are the members of the healthcare team who typically spend the most time in direct contact with these patients. Nurses have a unique opportunity to provide the education and support these patients need, and improve the care provided to these patients. In addition to assisting patients to learn the physical care needs related to a stoma, nurses must address the psychosocial concerns of patients with ostomies as part of their nursing interventions. Assisting patients to adjust and encouraging social interactions should be part of the care routinely given to stoma patients.

For additional research, visit the Point.

discomfort, changes in body image, loss of body function, and changes in personal hygiene. Patients need significant physical and psychological support to adjust to these changes. See the accompanying Research in Nursing Display, Adjustment to Colostomy.

Evaluating

The nurse evaluates the effectiveness of the plan of care to promote regular bowel elimination by checking to see if the patient has met the individualized patient outcomes specified in the plan. Nursing care is considered effective if the patient

expresses satisfaction with his or her regular pattern of defecation and the ability to pass a soft, formed stool comfortably without the use of medications or laxatives. The plan of care is most successful when the patient is able to accomplish the following:

- Verbalize the relationships among bowel elimination and nutrition, fluid intake, exercise, and stress management.
- Develop a plan to modify any factors that contribute to current bowel problems or that might adversely affect bowel functioning in the future.

See the accompanying Nursing Plan of Care 38-1.

NURSING PLAN OF CARE · 38-1

For Jeremy Green

Jeremy Green, 4 years of age, was placed in daycare when his mother returned to work 6 months ago. He presents at the hospital with a diagnosis of viral gastroenteritis. A comprehensive nursing assessment included the following notations:

- Admitted with complaints of diarrhea beginning 3 days ago
- Seen today by pediatrician who recommended admission and work-up to exclude causes other than viral
- Mother reports liquid stools (no observable blood, pus, or mucus) six to seven times daily beginning 3 days ago with amounts of "one to two cups."
- Urgency results in soiling of pants.

- Child has sipped boiled skim milk and cola and eaten a small amount of broth and a few pretzels but has no appetite.
- Complained of nausea and vomited twice 3 days ago
- Child is pale and eyes are sunken.
- Skin is warm and dry with decreased turgor, dry mucous membranes.
- Hyperactive bowel sounds (52/minute)
- Height, 45 inches; weight, 36 lb; temperature, 99.8°F (rectally); pulse, 88 beats/min; respiratory rate, 18 breaths/min
- Mother reported several other children in same daycare center are out sick with diarrhea.

(continued)

NURSING PLAN OF CARE · 38-1

For Jeremy Green *(continued)*

NURSING DIAGNOSIS   Diarrhea related to unknown cause (possibly viral, rule out malabsorption of lactose and other causes) as manifested by passage of liquid stools (1–2 cups) for 3 days; urgency with fecal soiling.

EXPECTED OUTCOME   At the time of discharge, the patient will:

- Voluntarily pass a formed stool of usual consistency (experience less or no diarrhea)

Nursing Interventions	Rationale	Evaluative Statement
Assess and chart frequency and amount of diarrhea, stool characteristics, precipitating factors, and accompanying manifestations (gastrointestinal symptoms, hyperactive bowel sounds).	This assists in identifying the cause of the diarrhea.	5/8/12 Outcome partially met. No recurrence of liquid stools for 24 hours. Revision: Continue to monitor. *D. Lentsky, RN*

EXPECTED OUTCOME   At the time of discharge, the patient will:

- Exhibit decreased bowel sounds (5 to 34/min)

Nursing Interventions	Rationale	Evaluative Statement
Work collaboratively with the physician to identify the cause of the diarrhea. Obtain stool specimens and send to laboratory.	Correct treatment depends on identification of the cause of the diarrhea. Viral diarrhea is usually self-limiting and lasts 24 to 72 hours. Prolonged diarrhea after acute viral illness may be from temporary malabsorption of lactose or other simple sugars.	5/8/12 Outcome met. Bowel sounds are normal. *D. Lentsky, RN*
Instruct Jeremy and his parents (if they want to participate in care) on correct infection control precautions for handling stool.	Proper precautions prevent transmissions of infectious diarrhea to others.	
Increase frequency and length of rest periods and discourage strenuous activity.	Exercise and activity stimulate peristalsis.	
Administer prescribed antidiarrheal medication and observe for adverse effects.	Antidiarrheal medications may cause drowsiness and dizziness. These agents may be used in diarrhea due to viruses to slow peristalsis and passage of stool.	

SAMPLE DOCUMENTATION   5/7/12 Nursing
Liquid stools have decreased to two in the past 24 hours. Negative report on stool culture. Normal bowel sounds auscultated in all four quadrants.

D. Lentsky, RN

Skill · 38-1   Administering a Large-Volume Cleansing Enema

EQUIPMENT

- Solution as ordered by the physician at a temperature of 105°F to 110°F (40°C to 43°C) for adults in the prescribed amount. (Amount will vary depending on type of solution, patient's age, and patient's ability to retain the solution. Average cleansing enema for an adult may range from 750 to 1,000 mL.)
- Disposable enema set, which includes a solution container and tubing
- Water-soluble lubricant
- IV pole
- Necessary additives as ordered
- Waterproof pad
- Bath thermometer (if available)
- Bath blanket
- Bedpan and toilet tissue
- Disposable gloves
- Additional PPE, as indicated
- Paper towel
- Washcloth, soap, and towel

IMPLEMENTATION

ACTION

1. Verify the order for the enema. Bring necessary equipment to the bedside stand or overbed table.

2. Perform hand hygiene and put on PPE, if indicated.

3. Identify the patient.

4. Close curtains around the bed and close door to room if possible. Explain what you are going to do and why you are going to do it to the patient. Discuss where the patient will defecate. Have a bedpan, commode, or nearby bathroom ready for use.

5. Warm solution in amount ordered, and check temperature with a bath thermometer if available. If bath thermometer is not available, warm to room temperature or slightly higher, and test on inner wrist. If tap water is used, adjust temperature as it flows from faucet (Figure 1).

RATIONALE

Verifying the physician's order is crucial to ensuring that the proper enema is administered to the right patient. Bringing everything to the bedside conserves time and energy. Arranging items nearby is convenient, saves time, and avoids unnecessary stretching and twisting of muscles on the part of the nurse.

Hand hygiene and PPE prevent the spread of microorganisms. PPE is required based on transmission precautions.

Identifying the patient ensures the right patient receives the intervention and helps prevent errors.

This ensures the patient's privacy. Explanation relieves anxiety and facilitates cooperation. The patient is better able to relax and cooperate if he or she is familiar with the procedure and knows everything is ready when the urge to defecate is felt. Defecation usually occurs within 5 to 15 minutes.

Warming the solution prevents chilling the patient, adding to the discomfort of the procedure. Cold solution could cause cramping; solution that is too warm could cause trauma to intestinal mucosa.

FIGURE 1. Preparing enema bag.

6. Add enema solution to container. Release clamp and allow fluid to progress through tube before reclamping.

This causes any air to be expelled from the tubing. Although allowing air to enter the intestine is not harmful, it may further distend the intestine.

(continued)

Skill · 38-1   Administering a Large-Volume Cleansing Enema   *continued*

ACTION

7. Adjust bed to comfortable working height, usually elbow height of the caregiver (VISN 8, 2009). Position the patient on the left side (Sims' position), as dictated by patient comfort and condition. Fold top linen back just enough to allow access to the patient's rectal area. Place a waterproof pad under the patient's hip.

8. Put on nonsterile gloves.

9. Elevate solution so that it is no higher than 18″ (45 cm) above level of anus (Figure 2). Plan to give the solution slowly over a period of 5 to 10 minutes. Hang the container on an IV pole or hold it at the proper height.

10. Generously lubricate end of rectal tube 2″ to 3″ (5–7 cm). A disposable enema set may have a prelubricated rectal tube.

11. Lift buttock to expose anus. Slowly and gently insert the enema tube 3″ to 4″ (7–10 cm) for an adult. Direct it at an angle pointing toward the umbilicus, not bladder (Figure 3). Ask patient to take several deep breaths.

RATIONALE

Having the bed at the proper height prevents back and muscle strain. Sims' position facilitates flow of solution via gravity into the rectum and colon, optimizing retention of solution. Folding back the linen in this manner minimizes unnecessary exposure and promotes the patient's comfort and warmth. The waterproof pad will protect the bed.

Gloves prevent contact with contaminants and body fluids.

Gravity forces the solution to enter the intestine. The amount of pressure determines the rate of flow and pressure exerted on the intestinal wall. Giving the solution too quickly causes rapid distention and pressure, poor defecation, or damage to the mucous membrane.

Lubrication facilitates passage of the rectal tube through the anal sphincter and prevents injury to the mucosa.

Good visualization of the anus helps prevent injury to tissues. The anal canal is about 1″ to 2″ (2.5–5 cm) long. The tube should be inserted past the external and internal sphincters, but further insertion may damage intestinal mucous membrane. The suggested angle follows the normal intestinal contour and thus will help to prevent perforation of the bowel. Slow insertion of the tube minimizes spasms of the intestinal wall and sphincters. Deep breathing helps relax the anal sphincters.

FIGURE 2. Adjusting the height of the solution container until it is no more than 18″ above the patient.

FIGURE 3. Inserting enema tip into anus, directing tip toward umbilicus.

12. If resistance is met while inserting tube, permit a small amount of solution to enter, withdraw tube slightly, and then continue to insert it. **Do not force entry of the tube.** Ask patient to take several deep breaths.

13. Introduce solution slowly over a period of 5 to 10 minutes. Hold tubing all the time that solution is being instilled.

14. Clamp tubing or lower container if patient has desire to defecate or cramping occurs (Figure 4). Instruct the patient to take small, fast breaths or to pant.

Resistance may be due to spasms of the intestine or failure of the internal sphincter to open. The solution may help to reduce spasms and relax the sphincter, thus making continued insertion of the tube safe. Forcing a tube may injure the intestinal mucosa wall. Taking deep breaths helps relax the anal sphincter.

Introducing the solution slowly helps prevent rapid distention of the intestine and a desire to defecate.

These techniques help relax muscles and prevent premature expulsion of the solution.

ACTION

15. After solution has been given, clamp tubing (Figure 5) and remove tube. Have paper towel ready to receive tube as it is withdrawn.

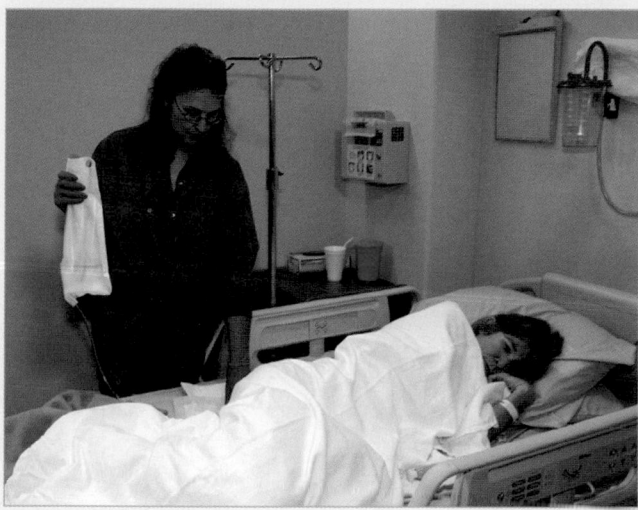

FIGURE 4. Holding bag lower to slow flow of enema solution.

16. Return the patient to a comfortable position. Encourage the patient to hold the solution until the urge to defecate is strong, usually in about 5 to 15 minutes. Make sure the linens under the patient are dry. Remove your gloves and ensure that the patient is covered.

17. Raise side rail. Lower bed height and adjust head of bed to a comfortable position.

18. Remove additional PPE, if used. Perform hand hygiene.

19. When patient has a strong urge to defecate, place him or her in a sitting position on a bedpan or assist to commode or bathroom (Figure 6). Offer toilet tissue, if not in patient's reach. Stay with patient or have call bell readily accessible.

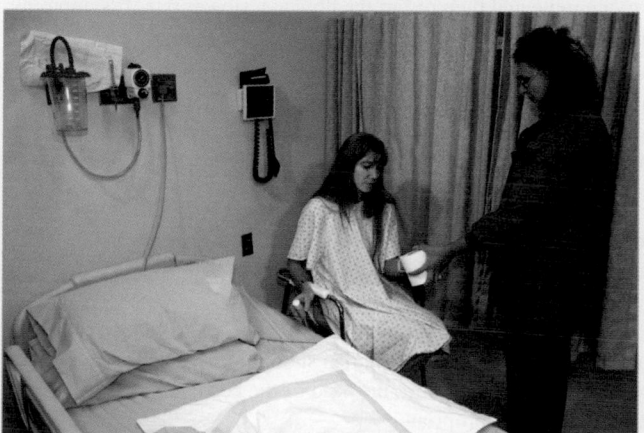

RATIONALE

Wrapping tube in paper towel prevents dripping of solution.

FIGURE 5. Clamping tubing before removing.

This amount of time usually allows muscle contractions to become sufficient to produce good results. Promotes patient comfort. Removing contaminated gloves prevents spread of microorganisms.

Promotes patient safety.

Removing PPE properly reduces the risk for infection transmission and contamination of other items. Hand hygiene prevents the spread of microorganisms.

The sitting position is most natural and facilitates defecation. Fall prevention is a high priority due to the urgency of reaching the commode.

FIGURE 6. Offering toilet tissue to patient on bedside commode.

(continued)

Skill · 38-1 Administering a Large-Volume Cleansing Enema *continued*

ACTION

20. Remind patient not to flush commode before nurse inspects results of enema.

21. Put on gloves and assist patient if necessary with cleaning of anal area. Offer washcloths, soap, and water for handwashing. Remove gloves.

22. Leave the patient clean and comfortable. Care for equipment properly.

23. Perform hand hygiene.

RATIONALE

The nurse needs to observe and record the results. Additional enemas may be necessary if physician has ordered enemas "until clear."

Gloves prevent contact with contaminants and body fluids. Cleaning the anal area and proper hygiene deter the spread of microorganisms.

Bacteria that grow in the intestine can be spread to others if equipment is not properly cleaned.

Hand hygiene deters the spread of microorganisms.

DOCUMENTATION

Guidelines

Document the amount and type of enema solution used; amount, consistency, and color of stool; pain assessment rating; assessment of perineal area for any irritation, tears, or bleeding; and patient's reaction to procedure.

Sample Documentation

7/22/12 1310 800 mL warm tap water enema given via rectum. Large amount of soft, brown stool returned. No irritation, tears, or bleeding noted in perineal area. Patient complained of "stomach cramping" relieved when enema was released. Rates pain as 0 after evacuation of enema.

—K. Sanders, RN

UNEXPECTED SITUATIONS AND ASSOCIATED INTERVENTIONS

- *Solution does not flow into rectum:* Reposition rectal tube. If solution will still not flow, remove tube and check for any fecal contents.

- *Patient cannot retain enema solution for adequate amount of time:* Patient may need to be placed on bedpan in the supine position while receiving enema. The head of the bed may be elevated 30 degrees for the patient's comfort.

- *Patient cannot tolerate large amount of enema solution:* Amount and length of administration may have to be modified if patient begins to complain of pain.

- *Patient complains of severe cramping with introduction of enema solution:* Lower solution container and check temperature and flow rate. If the solution is too cold or flow rate too fast, severe cramping may occur.

SPECIAL CONSIDERATIONS

General Considerations

- Rectal agents and rectal manipulation, including enemas, should not be used with myelosuppressed patients and/or patients at risk for myelosuppression and mucositis. These interventions can lead to development of bleeding, anal fissures, or abscesses, which are portals for infection.

- If the patient experiences fullness or pain or if fluid escapes around the tube, stop administration. Wait 30 seconds to a minute and then restart the flow at a slower rate. If symptoms persist, stop administration and contact the patient's physician.

- If enema has been ordered to be given "until clear," check with the physician before administering more than three enemas. Severe fluid and electrolyte imbalances may occur if the patient receives more than three cleansing enemas. Results are considered clear whenever there are no more pieces of stool in enema return. The solution may be colored but still considered a clear return.

Infant and Child Considerations

- When administering an enema to a child, ensure that the volume of solution is appropriate and the solution is at a temperature of 100°F (37.7°C).

- Insert tubing into the rectum 2″ to 3″ for children, 1″ to 1½″ for infants.

Older Adult Considerations

- Older adult patients who cannot retain the enema solution should receive the enema while on the bedpan in the supine position. For comfort, the head of the bed can be elevated 30 degrees if necessary and pillows used appropriately.

Skill 38-2 Irrigating a Nasogastric Tube Connected to Suction

EQUIPMENT

- NG tube connected to continuous or intermittent suction
- Normal saline solution for irrigation
- Nonsterile gloves
- Additional PPE, as indicated
- Irrigation set (or a 60-mL catheter-tip syringe and cup for irrigating solution)
- Clamp
- Disposable pad or bath towel
- Emesis basin
- Tape measure, or other measuring device
- pH paper and measurement scale

IMPLEMENTATION

ACTION	RATIONALE
1. Assemble equipment. Verify the medical order or facility policy and procedure regarding frequency of irrigation, solution type, and amount of irrigant. Check expiration dates on irrigating solution and irrigation set.	Assembling equipment provides for organized approach to task. Verification ensures patient receives correct intervention. Agency policy dictates safe interval for reuse of equipment.
2. Perform hand hygiene and put on PPE, if indicated.	Hand hygiene and PPE prevent the spread of microorganisms. PPE is required based on transmission precautions.
3. Identify the patient.	Identifying the patient ensures the right patient receives the intervention and helps prevent errors.
4. Explain the procedure to the patient and why this intervention is needed. Answer any questions as needed. Perform key abdominal assessments as described above.	Explanation facilitates patient cooperation. Due to potential changes in patient's condition, assessment is vital before initiating intervention.
5. Pull the patient's bedside curtain. Raise bed to a comfortable working position, usually elbow height of the caregiver (VISN 8, 2009). Assist patient to 30- to 45-degree position, unless this is contraindicated. Pour the irrigating solution into container.	Provide for privacy. Appropriate working height facilitates comfort and proper body mechanics for the nurse. This position minimizes risk for aspiration. Preparing the irrigation provides for organized approach to the task.
6. Put on gloves. **Check placement of NG tube.**	Checking placement before the instillation of fluid is necessary to prevent accidental instillation into the respiratory tract if the tube has become dislodged.
7. Draw up 30 mL of saline solution (or amount indicated in the order or policy) into syringe (Figure 1).	This delivers measured amount of irrigant through tube. Saline solution (isotonic) compensates for electrolytes lost through nasogastric drainage.

FIGURE 1. Drawing up saline solution.

(continued)

Skill · 38-2   **Irrigating a Nasogastric Tube Connected to Suction**   *continued*

ACTION

8. Clamp suction tubing near connection site (Figure 2). If needed, disconnect tube from suction apparatus and lay on disposable pad or towel, or hold both tubes upright in nondominant hand (Figure 3).

FIGURE 2. Clamping suction tube while disconnecting it from NG tube.

9. Place tip of syringe in tube. **If Salem sump or double-lumen tube is used, make sure that the syringe tip is placed in drainage port and not in blue air vent.** Hold syringe upright and gently insert the irrigant (or allow solution to flow in by gravity if agency policy or physician indicates) (Figure 4). **Do not force solution into tube.**

10. **If unable to irrigate tube, reposition patient and attempt irrigation again. Inject 10 to 20 mL of air and aspirate again (Figure 5). Check with physician or follow agency policy if repeated attempts to irrigate tube fail.**

FIGURE 4. Gently instilling irrigation.

11. After irrigant has been instilled, hold end of NG tube over irrigation tray or emesis basin. Observe for return flow of NG drainage into available container. Alternately, the nurse may reconnect the NG tube to suction and observe the return drainage as it drains into the suction container.

RATIONALE

Clamping protects patient from leakage of nasogastric drainage.

FIGURE 3. Holding both tubes upright to prevent backflow.

Gentle insertion of saline solution (or gravity insertion) is less traumatic to gastric mucosa.

The blue air vent acts to decrease pressure built up in the stomach when the Salem sump is attached to suction. It is not to be used for irrigation.

Tube may be positioned against gastric mucosa, making it difficult to irrigate. Injection of air may reposition end of tube.

FIGURE 5. Injecting 10–20 mL of air into tube.

Return flow may be collected in an irrigating tray or other available container and measured. This amount will need to be subtracted from the irrigant to record the true NG drainage. A second method involves subtracting the total irrigant from the shift from the total NG drainage emptied over the entire shift, to find the true NG drainage. Check agency policy for guidelines. Observation determines patency of tube and correct operation of suction apparatus.

ACTION	RATIONALE

12. **If not already done, reconnect drainage port to suction, if ordered.**

Allows for continued removal of gastric contents, as ordered.

13. **Inject air into blue air vent after irrigation is complete. Position the blue air vent above the patient's stomach.**

Following irrigation, the blue air vent is injected with air to keep it clear. Positioning the blue air vent above the stomach prevents the stomach contents from leaking from the NG tube.

14. Remove gloves. Lower the bed and raise side rails, as necessary. Assist the patient to a position of comfort. Perform hand hygiene.

Lowering bed and assisting patient to a comfortable position promote safety and comfort.

15. Put on gloves. Measure returned solution, if collected outside of suction apparatus. Rinse equipment if it will be reused. Label with the date, patient's name, room number, and purpose (for NG tube/ irrigation).

Gloves prevent contact with blood and body fluids. Irrigant placed in tube is considered intake; solution returned is recorded as output. Record on the intake and output record. Rinsing promotes cleanliness, infection control, and prepares equipment for next irrigation.

16. Remove gloves and additional PPE, if used. Perform hand hygiene.

Removing PPE properly reduces the risk for infection transmission and contamination of other items. Hand hygiene prevents transmission of microorganisms.

DOCUMENTATION

Guidelines

Document assessment of the patient's abdomen. Record if the patient's NG tube is clamped or connected to suction, including the type of suction. Document the color and consistency of the NG drainage. Record the solution type and amount used to irrigate the NG tube, as well as ease of irrigation or if there was any difficulty related to the procedure. Record the amount of returned irrigant, if collected outside of suction apparatus. Alternately, record irrigant amount so it can be subtracted from total NG drainage amount at the end of the shift. Record the patient's response to the procedure and any pertinent teaching points that were reviewed, such as instructions for the patient to contact the nurse for any feelings of nausea, bloating, or abdominal pain.

Sample Documentation

10/15/12 1100 Abdomen slightly distended but soft, absent bowel sounds, denies nausea. NG tube placement confirmed; gastric contents clear with brown flecks, pH-4; exposed NG tube 20 cm, consistent with documented length. NG irrigated with 30 mL of NS. NG reconnected to low intermittent suction. Clear drainage with brown flecks noted from tube. Patient tolerated irrigation without incident.

—S. Essner, RN

UNEXPECTED SITUATIONS AND ASSOCIATED INTERVENTIONS

• *Flush solution is meeting a lot of force when plunger is pushed:* Inject 20 to 30 mL of free air into the abdomen in attempt to reposition the tube and enable the nurse to flush the tube.

• *Tube is connected to suction as ordered, but nothing is draining from tube:* First check the suction canister to ensure that the suction is working appropriately. Disconnect the NG tube from suction and place your gloved thumb over the end of the suction tubing. If there is suction present, the problem lies in the NG tube itself. Next, attempt to flush the tube to ensure patency of the tube.

• *After flushing the tube, the tube is not reconnected to suction as ordered:* Reconnect the tube to suction as soon as error is noticed. Assess the abdomen for distention and ask patient if he/she is experiencing any nausea or any abdominal discomfort. Complete any paperwork per institutional policy, such as an incident report.

SPECIAL CONSIDERATIONS

A one-way antireflux valve may be used in the airflow lumen to prevent reflux of gastric contents through the airflow lumen (see Figure 5.). When pressure from gastric contents enters the airflow tubing, the valve closes to prevent secretions from exiting the tube. This valve is removed prior to flushing the lumen with air and then replaced.

Skill · 38-3   Changing and Emptying an Ostomy Appliance

EQUIPMENT

- Basin with warm water
- Skin cleanser, towel, washcloth
- Silicone-based adhesive remover
- Gauze squares
- Washcloth or cotton balls

- Skin protectant, such as SkinPrep
- One-piece ostomy appliance
- Closure clamp, if required for appliance
- Stoma measuring guide
- Graduated container, toilet or bedpan

- Ostomy belt (optional)
- Disposable gloves
- Additional PPE, as indicated
- Small plastic trash bag
- Waterproof disposable pad

IMPLEMENTATION

ACTION	RATIONALE
1. Bring necessary equipment to the bedside stand or overbed table.	Bringing everything to the bedside conserves time and energy. Arranging items nearby is convenient, saves time, and avoids unnecessary stretching and twisting of muscles on the part of the nurse.
2. Perform hand hygiene and put on PPE, if indicated.	Hand hygiene and PPE prevent the spread of microorganisms. PPE is required based on transmission precautions.
3. Identify the patient.	Identifying the patient ensures the right patient receives the intervention and helps prevent errors.
4. Close curtains around bed and close door to room if possible. Explain what you are going to do and why you are going to do it to the patient. Encourage patient to observe or participate if possible.	This ensures the patient's privacy. Explanation relieves anxiety and facilitates cooperation. Discussion promotes cooperation and helps to minimize anxiety. Having the patient observe or assist encourages self-acceptance.
5. Assist patient to a comfortable sitting or lying position in bed or a standing or sitting position in the bathroom.	Either position should allow the patient to view the procedure in preparation for learning to perform it independently. Lying flat or sitting upright facilitates smooth application of the appliance.

Emptying an Appliance

6. Put on disposable gloves. Remove clamp and fold end of pouch upward like a cuff (Figure 1).	Gloves prevent contact with blood, body fluids, and microorganisms. Creating a cuff before emptying prevents additional soiling and odor.
7. Empty contents into bedpan, toilet, or measuring device (Figure 2).	Appliances do not need rinsing because rinsing may reduce appliance's odor barrier.

FIGURE 1. Removing clamp, getting ready to empty pouch.

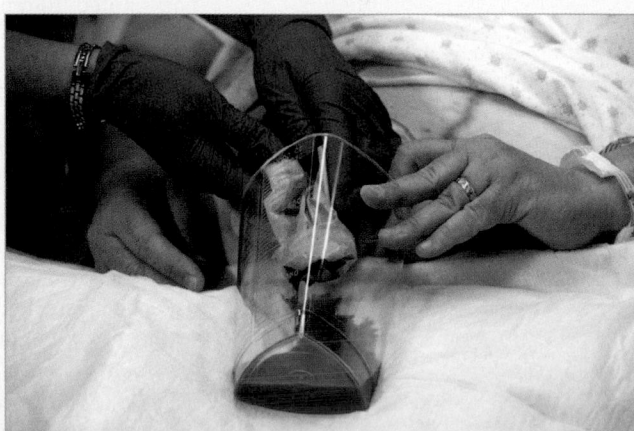

FIGURE 2. Emptying pouch into a measuring device.

8. Wipe the lower 2″ of the appliance or pouch with toilet tissue (Figure 3).

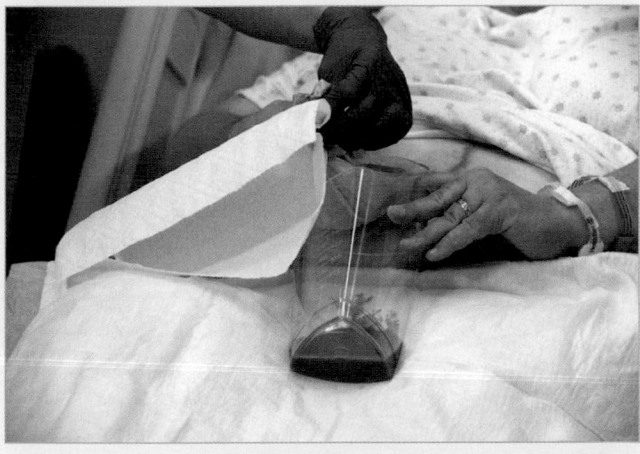

9. Uncuff edge of appliance or pouch and apply clip or clamp, or secure Velcro closure. Ensure the curve of the clamp follows the curve of the patient's body. Remove gloves. Assist patient to a comfortable position.

10. If appliance is not to be changed, remove additional PPE, if used. Perform hand hygiene.

Changing an Appliance

11. Place a disposable pad on the work surface. Set up the washbasin with warm water and the rest of the supplies. Place a trash bag within reach.

12. Put on clean gloves. Place waterproof pad under the patient at the stoma site. Empty the appliance, as described previously.

13. Gently remove pouch faceplate from skin by pushing skin from appliance rather than pulling appliance from skin. Start at the top of the appliance, while keeping the abdominal skin taut. Apply a silicone-based adhesive remover by spraying or wiping with the remover wipe (Figure 4).

FIGURE 4. Removing appliance.

Drying the lower section removes any additional fecal material, thus decreasing odor problems.

FIGURE 3. Wiping lower 2″ of pouch with toilet tissue.

The edge of the appliance or pouch should remain clean. The clamp secures closure. Hand hygiene deters spread of microorganisms. Ensures patient comfort.

Removing PPE properly reduces the risk for infection transmission and contamination of other items. Hand hygiene prevents the spread of microorganisms.

Protects surface. Organization facilitates performance of procedure.

Protects linens and patient from moisture. Emptying the contents before removal prevents accidental spillage of fecal material.

The seal between the surface of the faceplate and the skin must be broken before the faceplate can be removed. Harsh handling of the appliance can damage the skin and impair the development of a secure seal in the future. Silicone-based adhesive remover allows for the rapid and painless removal of adhesives and prevents skin stripping (Rudoni, 2008; Stephen-Haynes, 2008).

(continued)

Skill · 38-3 Changing and Emptying an Ostomy Appliance *continued*

ACTION	RATIONALE
14. Place the appliance in the trash bag, if disposable. If reusable, set aside to wash in lukewarm soap and water and allow to air dry after the new appliance is in place.	Thorough cleaning and airing of the appliance reduce odor and deterioration of appliance. For esthetic and infection-control purposes, discard used appliances appropriately.
15. Use toilet tissue to remove any excess stool from stoma (Figure 5). Cover stoma with gauze pad. Clean skin around stoma with mild soap and water or a cleansing agent and a washcloth. Remove all old adhesive from skin; use an adhesive remover as necessary. Do not apply lotion to peristomal area.	Toilet tissue, used gently, will not damage the stoma. The gauze absorbs any drainage from the stoma while the skin is being prepared. Cleaning the skin removes excretions and old adhesive and skin protectant. Excretions or a buildup of other substances can irritate and damage the skin. Lotion will prevent a tight adhesive seal.
16. Gently pat area dry. Make sure skin around stoma is thoroughly dry. Assess stoma and condition of surrounding skin (Figure 6).	Careful drying prevents trauma to skin and stoma. An intact, properly applied urinary collection device protects skin integrity. Any change in color and size of the stoma may indicate circulatory problems.

FIGURE 5. Using toilet tissue to wipe around stoma.

FIGURE 6. Assessing stoma and peristomal skin.

17. Apply skin protectant to a 2″ (5-cm) radius around the stoma, and allow it to dry completely, which takes about 30 seconds.	The skin needs protection from the excoriating effect of the excretion and appliance adhesive. The skin must be perfectly dry before the appliance is placed to get good adherence and to prevent leaks.
18. Lift the gauze squares for a moment and measure the stoma opening, using the measurement guide (Figure 7). Replace the gauze. Trace the same-size opening on the back center of the appliance (Figure 8). Cut the opening 1/8″ larger than the stoma size (Figure 9).	The appliance should fit snugly around the stoma, with only 1/8″ of skin visible around the opening. A faceplate opening that is too small can cause trauma to the stoma. If the opening is too large, exposed skin will be irritated by stool.
19. Remove the backing from the appliance (Figure 10). Quickly remove the gauze squares and ease the appliance over the stoma (Figure 11). Gently press onto the skin while smoothing over the surface. Apply gentle pressure to appliance for 5 minutes.	The appliance is effective only if it is properly positioned and adhered securely.
20. Close bottom of appliance or pouch by folding the end upward and using clamp or clip that comes with product, or secure Velcro closure (Figure 12). Ensure the curve of the clamp follows the curve of the patient's body.	A tightly sealed appliance will not leak and cause embarrassment and discomfort for the patient.
21. Remove gloves. Assist the patient to a comfortable position. Cover the patient with bed linens. Place the bed in the lowest position.	Provides warmth and promotes comfort and safety.

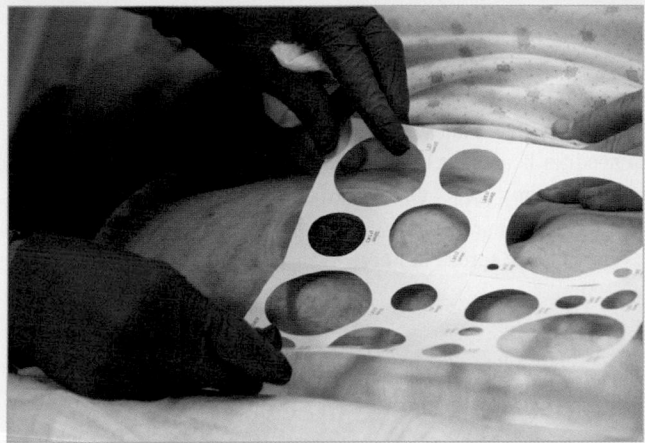

FIGURE 7. Using template to measure size of stoma.

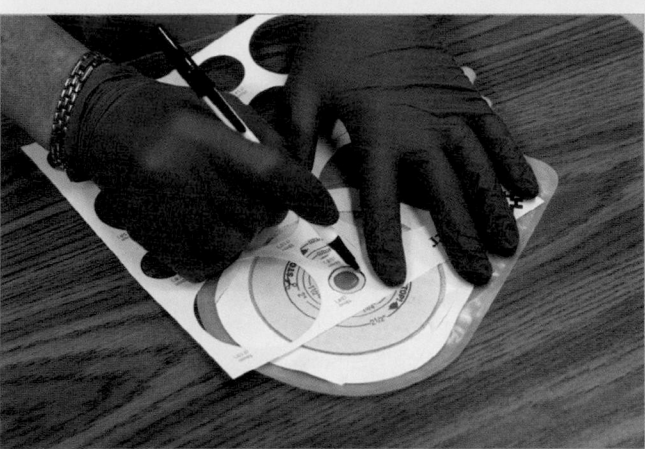

FIGURE 8. Tracing the same-sized circle on the back and center of skin barrier.

FIGURE 9. Cutting the opening 1/8″ larger than the stoma size.

FIGURE 10. Removing paper backing on faceplate.

FIGURE 11. Easing appliance over the stoma.

FIGURE 12. Closing bottom of pouch.

(continued)

Skill · 38-3 Changing and Emptying an Ostomy Appliance *continued*

ACTION	RATIONALE
22. Put on clean gloves. Remove or discard equipment and assess patient's response to procedure.	Gloves prevent contact with blood, body fluids, and microorganisms that contaminate the used equipment. The patient's response may indicate acceptance of the ostomy as well as the need for health teaching.
23. Remove gloves and additional PPE, if used. Perform hand hygiene.	Removing PPE properly reduces the risk for infection transmission and contamination of other items. Hand hygiene prevents the spread of microorganisms.

DOCUMENTATION

Guidelines

Document appearance of stoma, condition of peristomal skin, characteristics of drainage (amount, color, consistency, unusual odor), and patient's reaction to procedure.

Sample Documentation

7/22/12 1630 Colostomy appliance changed due to leakage. Stoma is pink, moist, and flat against abdomen. No erythema or excoriation of surrounding skin. Moderate amount of pasty, brown stool noted in bag. Patient asking appropriate questions during appliance application. States, "I'm ready to try the next one."

—B. Clapp, RN

UNEXPECTED SITUATIONS AND ASSOCIATED INTERVENTIONS

- *Peristomal skin is excoriated or irritated:* Make sure that the appliance is not cut too large. Skin that is exposed inside of the ostomy appliance will become excoriated. Assess for the presence of a fungal skin infection. If present, consult with prescriber to obtain appropriate treatment. Thoroughly cleanse skin and apply skin barrier. Allow to dry completely. Reapply pouch. Monitor pouch adhesion and change pouch as soon as there is a break in adhesion.

- *Patient continues to notice odor:* Check system for any leaks or poor adhesion. Clean outside of bag thoroughly when emptying.

- *Bag continues to come loose or fall off:* Thoroughly cleanse skin and apply skin barrier. Allow to dry completely. Reapply pouch. Monitor pouch adhesion and change pouch as soon as there is a break in adhesion.

- *Stoma is protruding into bag:* This is called a prolapse. Have patient rest for 30 minutes. If stoma is not back to normal size within that time, notify physician. If stoma stays prolapsed, it may twist, resulting in impaired circulation to the stoma.

● Developing Critical Thinking Skills

1. Discuss the appropriate nursing intervention if an assessment revealed the following:
   - Patient has frank blood in stool.
   - Parent reports that child's stool is unusually foul smelling and greasy.
   - Patient's stool is ribbon-like.
   - Patient receiving cancer pain medication reports chronic constipation.
   - Teenager reports frequent episodes of diarrhea that leave her weak and dehydrated.

2. A 52-year-old man presents with acute stomach pain and altered bowel elimination: diarrhea. Role-play with another student the interview you would use to assess his bowel elimination status. Identify variables that make you, as either the nurse or patient, uncomfortable talking about elimination. Discuss how you can best address your discomfort.

● Practicing for NCLEX

1. If a patient was instructed to avoid foods that may have a laxative effect, the nurse would advise the patient to avoid which of the following foods?
   a. Cheese
   b. Alcohol
   c. Eggs
   d. Pasta

2. Which of the following is a true statement about the effects of medication on bowel elimination?
   a. Diarrhea commonly occurs with amoxicillin clavulanate use.
   b. Anticoagulants cause a white discoloration of the stool.
   c. Narcotic analgesics increase gastrointestinal motility.
   d. Iron salts impair digestion and cause a green stool.

3. Mr. J. has a fecal impaction. The nurse correctly administers an oil-retention enema by doing which of the following?
   a. Administering a large volume of solution (500–1,000 mL)
   b. Mixing milk and molasses in equal parts for an enema
   c. Instructing the patient to retain the enema for at least 30 minutes
   d. Administering the enema while the patient is sitting on the toilet

4. As the nurse prepares to assist Mrs. P. with her newly created ileostomy, she is aware of which of the following?
   a. An appliance will not be required on a continual basis
   b. The size of the stoma stabilizes within 2 weeks
   c. Irrigation is necessary for regulation
   d. Fecal drainage will be liquid

5. Which class of laxative acts by causing the stool to absorb water and swell?
   a. Bulk-forming
   b. Emollient
   c. Lubricant
   d. Stimulant

6. Mr. T. is nervous about a colonoscopy scheduled for tomorrow. The nurse describes the test by explaining that it allows which of the following?
   a. Visual examination of the esophagus and stomach
   b. Visual examination of the large intestine
   c. Radiographic examination of the large intestine
   d. Fluoroscopic examination of the small intestine

7. A bowel training program includes which of the following?
   a. Using a diet that is low in bulk
   b. Decreasing fluid intake to 1,000 mL
   c. Administering an enema once a day to stimulate peristalsis
   d. Allowing ample time for evacuation

8. Your patient complains of excessive flatulence. When reviewing the patient's dietary intake, which food, if eaten regularly, would you identify as possibly responsible?
   a. Meat
   b. Cauliflower

c. Potatoes
d. Ice cream

9. A barium enema should be done before an upper gastrointestinal series because of which of the following?
   a. Retained barium may cloud the colon.
   b. Barium can cause lower gastrointestinal bleeding.
   c. The physician's orders are in that sequence.
   d. Barium is absorbed readily in the lower intestine.

10. Nurses should recommend avoiding the habitual use of laxatives. Which of the following is the rationale for this?
    a. They will cause a fecal impaction.
    b. They will cause chronic constipation.
    c. They change the pH of the gastrointestinal tract.
    d. They inhibit the intestinal enzymes.

11. When explaining the action of a hypertonic solution enema, the nurse incorporates which of the following as the basis for action?
    a. Bowel mucosa irritation
    b. Diffusion of water out of colon
    c. Osmosis of water into colon
    d. Softening of fecal contents

12. Which of the following are included in the nursing plan of care to prevent adverse effects when caring for a patient with a nasogastric tube in place for gastric decompression? Select all that apply.
    a. Irrigate with saline.
    b. Measure the length of the exposed tube.
    c. Measure the pH of the aspirated tube contents.
    d. Administer frequent oral hygiene.

13. During removal of a fecal impaction, which of the following could occur because of vagal stimulation?
    a. Bradycardia
    b. Atelectasis
    c. Tachycardia
    d. Cardiac tamponade

14. Which of the following would be a common nursing diagnosis for the patient with an ileostomy?
    a. Disturbed Body Image
    b. Constipation
    c. Delayed Growth and Development
    d. Excess Fluid Volume

15. Which of the following is an appropriate nursing action to promote regular bowel habits?
    a. encouraging the patient to avoid moving his bowels until a certain time of the day
    b. encouraging the patient to avoid excess fluid intake and too much fiber
    c. avoiding strenuous exercise to limit stress on abdominal muscles and impair peristalsis
    d. assisting the patient to as normal position as possible to defecate

Answers With Rationale

1. **b.** All the foods listed except alcohol have a constipating effect.

2. **a.** Anticoagulants may result in the stool having a pink to red to black appearance, whereas iron salts also cause a black stool. Narcotic analgesics decrease gastric motility.

3. **c.** The usual amount of solution administered with a retention enema is 150 to 200 mL for an adult. The milk and molasses mixture is a carminative enema that helps to expel flatus, as does the Harris flush procedure.

4. **d.** An appliance is usually required on a continual basis because the fecal drainage is liquid. Stoma size usually stabilizes within 4 to 6 weeks, and ileostomy irrigation is not necessary because fecal matter is liquid.

5. **a.** Emollients lubricate the stool; lubricants soften the stool, making it easier to pass; and stimulants promote peristalsis by irritating the intestinal mucosa or stimulating nerve endings in the intestinal wall.

6. **b.** An esophagogastroduodenoscopy allows visual examination of the esophagus and stomach. The radiographic examination of the large intestine refers to a barium enema, and a fluoroscopic examination of the small intestine refers to an upper gastrointestinal series.

7. **d.** For a bowel training program to be effective, the patient must have ample time for evacuation (usually 20 to 30 minutes). Fluid intake is increased to 2,500 to 3,000 mL; food high in bulk is recommended as part of the program; and a daily enema is not administered in a bowel training program. A cathartic suppository may be used 30 minutes before the patient's usual defecation time to stimulate peristalsis.

8. **b.** Cauliflower is a gas-producing food that results in flatulence.

9. **a.** The barium enema should always precede the upper gastrointestinal series because retained barium from the latter may take several days to pass through the gastrointestinal tract and may cloud anatomic detail on the barium enema studies.

10. **b.** Habitual use of laxatives is the most common cause of chronic constipation.

11. **c.** Hypertonic solutions draw water into the colon by osmosis, thus stimulating the defecation reflex. Oil solutions soften fecal contents, and soap solutions distend the intestine and irritate the bowel mucosa.

12. **a, b, c, d.** After checking placement, the NGT should be irrigated with 30 to 60 mL of normal saline to maintain patency. The frequency is determined by facility policy, medical order, and nursing judgment. The length of the exposed tube should be measured after insertion and routinely thereafter, as part of the assessment to verify placement and ensure the tube has not dislodged. Measuring the pH of aspirated tube contents is one way to validate tube placement in the intestinal tract. The other method is to visually assess aspirate to confirm gastric contents. Patients with NGTs often experience discomfort related to irritation to nasal and throat mucosa and drying of the mucous membranes. Frequent oral hygiene should be administered, as well as applying lubricant to the lips.

13. **a.** Removing a fecal impaction manually may result in stimulation of the vagal nerve and resulting bradycardia.

14. **a.** Constipation does not occur with an ileostomy because the drainage is liquid. Growth and development are not affected by the formation of an ileostomy. Excess fluid volume is unlikely to occur because the drainage is liquid and probably continual.

15. **d.** Sitting upright on a toilet or commode promotes defecation. If the patient must use a bedpan, raise the head of the bed 30 to 45 degrees. Patients should be encouraged to move their bowels at their usual time of the day. However, the patient should not be encouraged to put off defecation if the urge arises before or after their "usual time." Patients should be encouraged to consume 2,000 to 3,000 mL of fluid, preferably water, and increased fiber, to promote regular defecation. Regular exercise improves gastrointestinal activity and aids in defecation.

Taylor Suite Resources

The Taylor Suite offers these additional resources to enhance learning and facilitate understanding of this chapter:

- thePoint online resource, http://thepoint.lww.com/Taylor7E
- Student DVD-ROM included with the book
- Study Guide for Taylor's Fundamentals of Nursing
- Skill Checklists for Taylor's Fundamentals of Nursing
- Taylor's Video Guide to Clinical Nursing Skills: *Bowel Elimination*
- Taylor's Clinical Nursing Skills: *Chapter 13, Bowel Elimination*

BIBLIOGRAPHY

Addison, R., & Smith, M. (2006). Royal College of Nursing. Digital rectal examination and manual removal of faeces. Guidance for nurses. London: Royal College of Nursing. Publication code 000934. Available at www.bwd.nhs.uk/policies-and-procedures/?assetesct/223605=1626. Accessed June 2, 2010.

American Association of Critical-Care Nurses (AACN). (2005). *AACN practice alert. Verification of feeding tube placement.* Available at www.aacn.org/WD/Practice/Content/practicealerts.pcms?pid=1&&menu=.

Aschenbrenner, D., & Venable, S. (2009). *Drug therapy in nursing* (3rd ed.). Philadelphia: Wolters Kluwer Health/Lippincott Williams & Wilkins.

Banks, N., & Razor, B. (2003). Preoperative stoma site assessment and marking: Trained RNs can improve ostomy outcomes. *American Journal of Nursing, 103*(3), 64A–64B, 64E.

Bisanz, A. (2007). Chronic constipation. *American Journal of Nursing, 107*(4), 72B–72I.

Bowers, B. (2006). Evaluating the evidence for administering phosphate enemas. *British Journal of Nursing, 15*(7), 378–381.

Brennan, M. (2008). Review: Routine NG decompression after abdominal surgery delays return of bowel function and increases pulmonary complications. *Evidence-Based Nursing, 11*(2), 55.

Bulechek, G., Butcher, H., & McCloskey Dochterman, J. (Eds.). (2008). *Nursing interventions classification (NIC)* (5th ed.). St. Louis: Mosby Elsevier.

Burch, J., & Sica, J. (2007). One- and two-piece colostomy appliances: Merits and indications. *British Journal of Nursing, 16*(17), 1042–1047.

Carpenito-Moyet, L. (2008). *Nursing diagnosis: Application to clinical practice* (12th ed.). Philadelphia: Wolters Kluwer Health/Lippincott Williams & Wilkins.

Centers for Disease Control and Prevention (CDC). (2004). *Clostridium difficile* – Information for healthcare providers. Available at www.cdc.gov/ncidod/dhqp/id_CdiffFAQ_HCP.html.

Cesaretti, I., Santos, V., Schiftan, S., & Vianna, L. (2008). Colostomy irrigation: Review of a number of technical aspects. *Acto Paulista de Enfermagem* [online], *21*(2), 338–344. Available www.scielo.br/scielo.php?.

Clinical Center. National Institutes of Health. (2007). Patient education. Managing bowel dysfunction. Available at www.cc.nih.gov/ccc/patient-education/pepubs/bowel.pdf

Cohen, B., & Taylor, J. (2005). *Memmler's structure and function of the human body* (8th ed.). Philadelphia: Lippincott Williams & Wilkins.

Collis Pellatt, G. (2007). Clinical skills: Bowel elimination and management of complications. *British Journal of Nursing, 16*(6), 351–355.

Cronin, E. (2008). Colostomies and the use of colostomy appliances. *British Journal of Nursing, 17*(17), S12–19.

Dudek, S. (2006). *Nutrition essentials for nursing practice* (5th ed.). Philadelphia: Lippincott Williams & Wilkins.

Ellett, M. (2004). What is known about methods of correctly placing gastric tubes in adults and children. *Gastroenterology Nursing, 27*(6), 253–261.

Fischbach, F., & Dunning, M. (2009). *A manual of laboratory and diagnostic tests* (8th ed.). Philadelphia: Wolters Kluwer Health/Lippincott Williams & Wilkins.

Fischbach, F., & Dunning, M. (2006). *Common laboratory & diagnostic tests* (4th ed.). Philadelphia: Lippincott Williams & Wilkins.

Gannon, R. (2007). Current strategies for preventing or ameliorating postoperative ileus: A multimodal approach. *American Journal of Health-System Pharmacy, 64*(20), S8–12.

Gray, M. (2007). Incontinence-related skin damage: Essential knowledge. *Ostomy Wound Management, 53*(12), 28–32.

Grindel, M. (2007). Nasogastric tube placement verification: What is best practice? *Med-Surg Matters, 16*(3), 5.

Higgins, D. (2008a). Patient assessment Part 3 – Measurement of gastric fluid pH. *Nursing Times, 104*(9), 26–27.

Higgins, D. (2008d). Specimen collection Part 3 – Collecting a stool specimen. *Nursing Times, 104*(19), 22–23.

Hockenberry, M. (2005). *Wong's essentials of pediatric nursing* (7th ed.). St. Louis: Elsevier Mosby.

Huntzinger, A. (2007). Practice guidelines. IDSA (Infectious Diseases Society of America) released guidelines on travel medicine. Available at www.aafp.org/afp/2007/0601/p1712.html.practice.html#p1.

Irwin, K. (2002). Digital rectal examination/manual removal of faeces in adults. *Journal of Community Nursing, 16*(4), 16, 18, 20.

Jarvis, C. (2008). *Physical examination & health assessment.* (5th ed.). St. Louis: Saunders/Elsevier.

Jungles, S. (2004). Video wireless capsule endoscopy. *Gastroenterology Nursing, 27*(4), 170–175.

Kaçmaz, Z., & Kaşikçi, M. (2007). Effectiveness of bran supplement in older orthopaedic patients with constipation. *Journal of Clinical Nursing, 16*(5), 928–936.

Karadag, A., Mentes, B., & Ayaz, S. (2005). Colostomy irrigation: Results of 25 cases with particular reference to quality of life. *Journal of Clinical Nursing, 14*(4), 479–485.

Kyle, G., Prynn, P., & Oliver, H. (2004). An evidence-based procedure for the digital removal of feces. *Nursing Times, 100*(48), 71.

Kyle, T. (2008). *Essentials of pediatric nursing.* Philadelphia: Wolters Kluwer Health/Lippincott Williams & Wilkins.

Laxatives: Dealing with irregularity. (2005). *Mayo Clinic Health Letter, 23*(6), 4–5.

Levin, B., Lieberman, D., McFarland, B., Smith, R., Brooks, D., Andrews, K., et al. (2008). Screening and surveillance for the early detection of colorectal cancer and adenomatous polyps, 2008: A joint guideline from the American Cancer Society, the US Multi-Society Task Force on Colorectal Cancer, and the American College of Radiology. *CA – A Cancer Journal for Clinicians, 58*(3), 130–160.

Mandel, J. (2008). Screening for colorectal cancer. *Gastroenterology Clinics, 37*(1), 97–115.

Mauk, K. (2005). Preventing constipation in older adults. *Nursing, 35*(6), 22–23.

May, S. (2007). Testing nasogastric tube positioning in the critically ill: Exploring the evidence. *British Journal of Nursing, 16*(7), 414–418.

McCloskey Dochterman, J., & Bulechek, G. (2004). *Nursing interventions classification (NIC)* (4th ed.). St. Louis: C. V. Mosby.

McConnell, E. (2000). Myths & facts about rectal catheters. *Nursing, 30*(1), 73.

Mitchell, S., Schaefer, D., & Dubagunta, S. (2004). A new view of occult and obscure gastrointestinal bleeding. *American Family Physician, 69*(4), 875–881.

Moorhead, S., Johnson, M., Maas, M., & Swanson, E. (Eds). (2008). *Nursing outcomes classification (NOC)* (4th ed.). St. Louis: Mosby Elsevier.

Nazarko, L. (2007). Managing diarrhoea in the home to prevent admission. *British Journal of Community Nursing, 12*(11), 508, 10–12.

Nelson, R., Edwards, S., & Tse, B. (2007). Prophylactic nasogastric decompression after abdominal surgery. *Cochrane Database Systematic Review,* Issue 3. Art. No.: DOI: 10.1002/14651858.CD004929.pub3.

NANDA International. (2009). *Nursing diagnoses: Definitions and classification 2009–2011.* West Sussex, UK: Wiley-Blackwell.

Norton, C. (2006). Constipation in older patients: Effects on quality of life. *British Journal of Nursing, 15*(4), 188–192.

Pegram, A., Bloomfield, J., & Jones, A. (2008). Safe use of rectal suppositories and enemas with adult patients. *Nursing Standard, 22*(38), 38–40.

Persson, E., Gustavsson, R., Hellstrom, A., Lappas, G., & Hulten, L. (2005). Ostomy patients' perceptions of quality care. *Journal of Advanced Nursing, 49*(1), 51–58.

Porth, C., & Matfin, G. (2009). *Pathophysiology. Concepts of altered health states* (8th ed.). Philadelphia: Wolters Kluwer Health/Lippincott Williams & Wilkins.

Rudoni, C. (2008). A service evaluation of the use of silicone-based adhesive remover. *British Journal of Nursing, Stoma Care Supplement, 17*(2), S4, S6, S8–9.

Simmons, K., Smith, J., Bobb, K., & Liles, L. (2007). Adjustment to colostomy: Stoma acceptance, stoma care self-efficacy and interpersonal relationships. *Journal of Advanced Nursing, 60*(6), 627–635.

Smeltzer, S., Bare, B., Hinkle, J. H., & Cheever, K. H. (2010). *Brunner and Suddarth's textbook of medical–surgical nursing* (12th ed.). Philadelphia: Lippincott Williams & Wilkins.

Snow, M. (2006). Pinning down pinworms. *Nursing, 36*(5), 17.

Stephen-Haynes, J. (2008). Skin integrity and silicone: APPEEL 'no-sting' medical adhesive remover. *British Journal of Nursing, 17*(12), 792–795.

Vermeulen, H., Storm-Versloot, M., Busch, O., & Ubbink, D. (2006). Nasogastric intubation after abdominal surgery. *Archives of Surgery, 141*(3), 307–314.

VISN 8 Patient Safety Center. (2009). *Safe patient handling and movement algorithms.* Tampa, FL: Author. Available at www.VISN8.va.gov/patientsafetycenter/SafePtHandling. Accessed April 23, 2010.

Weber, J., & Kelley, J. (2007). *Health assessment in nursing* (3rd ed.). Philadelphia: Lippincott Williams & Wilkins.

Williams, J. (2008). Flatus, odour and the ostomist: Coping strategies and interventions. *British Journal of Nursing, 17*(2), S10–14.

Williams, J. (2007). Stoma care nursing: What the community nurse needs to know. *British Journal of Community Nursing, 12*(8), 342, 344, 346.

Oxygenation

TYRONE JACOBS

Tyrone, age 12, is brought to the emergency room gasping for breath. His parents are frantic. "It just seemed like he had a really bad cold," his mother says. An acute asthma attack is suspected, and measures are instituted immediately to protect the child's airway.

YAN KIM

Yan, age 57, developed respiratory failure from complications associated with pulmonary surgery. He is receiving oxygen therapy and mechanical ventilation via an endotracheal tube and undergoing continuous cardiac monitoring.

JOAN McINTYRE

Joan, age 72, has been admitted to your medical unit with an acute exacerbation of chronic obstructive pulmonary disease (COPD). This is the fifth time she has been in the hospital this year. She is receiving supplemental oxygen and multiple medications to support her breathing. She is very weak, unable to perform ADLs for herself, and becomes extremely short of breath with minimal exertion. She has verbalized feelings of despair and has asked the staff, "to let me go if I should stop breathing."

KEY TERMS

adventitious	internal respiration
alveoli	metered-dose inhaler
atelectasis	(MDI)
atria	nasal cannula
bradypnea	nebulizer
bronchial	perfusion
bronchodilator	pleural effusion
bronchovesicular	pleural friction rub
cilia	pneumothorax
crackles	pulmonary ventilation
diffusion	pulse oximetry
dry powder inhaler	respiration
(DPI)	spirometer
dyspnea	sputum
endotracheal tube	surfactant
expiration	tachypnea
hemothorax	thoracentesis
hyperventilation	tracheostomy
hypoventilation	ventricles
hypoxemia	vesicular
hypoxia	wheezes
inspiration	

This chapter describes the respiratory system's anatomy and physiology and those parts of the anatomy and physiology of the cardiovascular system that relate to respiration. In addition, this chapter explores general factors affecting respiratory functioning and oxygenation, the process of providing cells life-sustaining oxygen. Suggestions for performing a comprehensive respiratory assessment are presented, including sample interview questions for both a general and focused respiratory history, a description of the nursing examination, and laboratory and radiologic studies. After analyzing the data collected, nurses decide whether the respiratory data lead to a problem statement, indicate another problem, or are the possible cause of a problem. The chapter provides numerous examples of nursing diagnoses. Expected patient outcomes and specific nursing strategies for implementation are described. The concluding patient care study illustrates how, with knowledge of respiratory functioning and skilled nursing interventions, the nurse cares for a patient with respiratory problems. Refer also to the accompanying Reflective Practice box.

ANATOMY AND PHYSIOLOGY OF RESPIRATION

The respiratory system performs its functions through pulmonary ventilation, respiration, and perfusion. Normal functioning depends on essentially three factors:

- The integrity of the airway system to transport air to and from the lungs
- A properly functioning alveolar system in the lungs to oxygenate venous blood and to remove carbon dioxide from the blood
- A properly functioning cardiovascular and hematologic system to carry nutrients and wastes to and from body cells

Knowledge of the basic anatomy and physiology of the respiratory system and an understanding of the role of the cardiovascular system in the exchange of gasses during respiration provides a firm foundation for assessing oxygenation in patients and for planning and implementing interventions to promote optimal respiratory function. This knowledge also helps nurses understand, interpret, and analyze assessment findings and provides the rationale for sound nursing interventions.

Structures of the Respiratory System

The airway, which begins at the nose and ends at the terminal bronchioles, is a pathway for the transport and exchange of oxygen and carbon dioxide. The airway is divided into the upper and the lower airways.

The upper airway is composed of the nose, pharynx, larynx, and epiglottis. Its main function is to warm, filter, and humidify inspired air. The lower airway, known as the tracheobronchial tree, includes the trachea, right and left main stem bronchi, segmental bronchi, and terminal bronchioles

REFLECTIVE PRACTICE
Challenge to Technical Skills

Ventilators and telemetry have always intimidated me, so having a patient like Yan Kim was overwhelming. Mr. Kim was a 57-year-old man who had developed respiratory failure from complications secondary to pulmonary surgery. He was receiving oxygen therapy and mechanical ventilation via an endotracheal tube and was also undergoing continuous cardiac monitoring. Providing care for him with all his equipment and so many alarms that could sound seemed insurmountable. The monitor had several different values on it and the continuous electrocardiogram (ECG) monitor always made me feel like the patient was on the verge of dying. We had not covered these skills yet in class, and I felt incompetent for the first 2 weeks of my critical care clinical experience. I could have voiced my concerns with these two machines, and I should have asked the first day what I should and shouldn't be worried about with critical care patients. But I didn't.

Thinking Outside the Box: Possible Course of Action

- Ask my instructor if there was any danger in having a patient who was receiving mechanical ventilation and being monitored by telemetry.
- Ask for someone to explain the ECG waveforms on the monitor and what to be concerned with when looking at them.

- Avoid caring for patients on ventilators and undergoing telemetry.

Evaluating a Good Outcome: How Do I Define Success?

- Patient is safe and receives care by a competent care provider promoting his health.
- I am confident in my technical skills and able to use technology to deliver the most helpful care.

- I continue to ask questions, challenge my practice, and learn to contribute to improved care, which will lead to enhanced nursing.

Personal Learning: Here's To the Future!

Fortunately, our clinical rotations are planned so that we do not take care of critical care patients until we learn the necessary skills (telemetry and ventilation). This semester in my critical care clinical experiences, my fears have dissipated. I have learned that having patients that are being monitoring continuously via telemetry is quite reassuring. It serves as a constant monitor for me. Although I still assess the patient on my own, having continuous values to check is reassuring. As for the ventilator, I realized I knew a lot more than I thought. My instructor gave me a lesson on the ventilator during my clinical experience and connected the class lectures and bookwork with what I was seeing with my patient. I asked many questions and checked to see if I knew which settings would change with different scenarios. There are several settings and several values constantly being measured with the machine. Once I was able to see what all of these numbers meant and realized that I understood what each was for, I felt much more comfortable with patients on a ventilator. I realized my concerns and made sure that I provided unbiased care so that my concerns did not force me to neglect a patient.

Before, I would have been scared to get too close to the machine for fear of hitting the wrong button, fearing I would harm the patient. Now I am learning how the settings are specific to each patient. I feel comfortable reading the values and setting the controls. Still, I ask questions about the ventilator and telemetry readings because I want to know that I am interpreting them correctly. I feel it is my responsibility to obtain as much understanding and knowledge as I can so that I can provide the best care to these patients. This is very relieving and rewarding: now critical care patients don't seem so critical! My care for these patients is enhanced since I am more confident in my skills, and this enhances the care I deliver. Next time there is something new to me, I will voice my concern early on even if I am not "supposed to know" it yet.

Overall, although I still do not have much experience, I feel technically competent as a senior nursing student. I am confident because I challenge myself and I am self-motivated when it comes to searching for more information when needed.

Carrie Staines, Georgetown University

Reflection

How would you respond in a similar situation? Why? What does this tell you about yourself and about the adequacy of your skills for professional practice? How did the nursing student apply the knowledge obtained through the lessons given by the instructor? How do you think the nursing student would have responded if the clinical experience was strictly observational? What information did the nursing student receive from the monitors? How did the nursing student use this information? What interventions did the nursing student implement to care for the patient's psychosocial status? Can you think of other ways to respond? What other skills (cognitive, interpersonal, technical, ethical/legal) would you need to respond well in this situation? Do you agree with the criteria to evaluate a successful outcome? Are there any other criteria that would be appropriate to use? Did the nursing student meet the criteria? Why or why not?

FIGURE 39-1. The organs of the respiratory tract. (**A**) Overview. (**B**) Alveoli (air sacs) of the lungs and the blood capillaries. (**C**) Transverse section through the lungs.

(Fig. 39-1). Its major functions are conduction of air, mucociliary clearance, and production of pulmonary surfactant.

The airways are lined with mucus, which traps cells, particles, and infectious debris. This mucus covering also helps to protect the underlying tissues from irritation and infection. **Cilia,** which are microscopic hair-like projections, propel trapped material and accompanying mucus toward the upper airway so they can be removed by coughing. Removal is facilitated when mucus is watery in consistency. An adequate fluid intake is necessary for the production of watery mucus normally present in the respiratory tract and for ciliary action.

The lungs, the main organs of respiration, are located within the thoracic cavity on the right and left sides (see Fig. 39-1). The lungs extend from the base at the level of the diaphragm to the apex (top), which is above the first rib. The heart lies between the right and left lung.

Each lung is divided into lobes. The right lung has three lobes; the left has two. Each lobe is subdivided into segments or lobules. The right lung has 10 bronchopulmonary segments; the left has 8. The main bronchus branches to each lung from the trachea. It immediately subdivides into secondary bronchi, one to each lobe. The bronchi subdivide again and again, becoming smaller and smaller as they branch through the lung. The smallest of these branches are the bronchioles, ending at the terminal bronchioles. The lungs are composed of elastic tissue that can stretch or recoil. Normally,

the elastic fibers are partially stretched at all times, thus partially filling the thoracic cavity.

At the end of the terminal bronchioles there are clusters of **alveoli** (singular, alveolus), small air sacs. The alveoli are the site of gas exchange. The wall of each alveolus is made of a single-cell layer of squamous epithelium (see Fig. 39-1). This thin wall allows for exchange of gases with the capillaries covering the alveoli. The average adult has more than 300 million alveoli. **Surfactant,** a detergent-like phospholipid, reduces the surface tension between the moist membranes of the alveoli, preventing their collapse. When surfactant production is reduced, the lung becomes stiff and the alveoli collapse.

The lungs and thoracic cavity are lined with a serous membrane called the pleura. The visceral pleura covers the lungs, and the parietal pleura lines the thoracic cavity. These two membranes are continuous with each other and form a closed sac. The pleural space lies between the two layers. Pleural fluid between the membranes acts as a lubricant and as an adhesive agent to hold the lungs in an expanded position. A few milliliters of fluid between the pleural surfaces allows the lungs to move easily along the chest wall as they expand and contract. Without this fluid, filling and emptying of the lungs are difficult.

Pressure within the pleural space (intrapleural pressure) is always subatmospheric (a negative pressure). This constant negative intrapleural pressure, along with the pleural fluid, holds the lungs in an expanded position.

Physiology of the Respiratory System

Living cells require oxygen and the removal of carbon dioxide, a byproduct of oxidation. Gas exchange, the intake of oxygen and the release of carbon dioxide, is made possible by pulmonary ventilation, respiration, and perfusion. **Pulmonary ventilation** refers to the movement of air into and out of the lungs. **Respiration** involves gas exchange between the atmospheric air in the alveoli and blood in the capillaries. **Perfusion** is the process by which oxygenated capillary blood passes through body tissues.

Pulmonary Ventilation

Pulmonary ventilation (breathing) is the movement of air into and out of the lungs. The process of ventilation has two phases: inspiration (inhalation) and expiration (exhalation). **Inspiration,** the active phase, involves movement of muscles and the thorax to bring air into the lungs. **Expiration,** the passive phase, is the movement of air out of the lungs.

Immediately before inspiration, the air pressure in the lungs is equal to that of the surrounding atmospheric pressure.

According to Boyle's law, the volume of a gas at a constant temperature varies inversely with the pressure. This means that less pressure in the lungs facilitates the movement of more air into the lungs. The pressure within the lungs (intrapulmonic pressure) decreases as the volume of the lungs increases.

During inspiration, the following events occur: the diaphragm contracts and descends, lengthening the thoracic cavity; the external intercostal muscles contract, lifting the ribs upward and outward; and the sternum is pushed forward, enlarging the chest from front to back. This combination of an increased lung volume and decreased intrapulmonic pressure allows atmospheric air to move from an area of greater pressure (outside air) into an area of lesser pressure (within the lungs). The relaxation, or recoil, of these structures then results in expiration. The diaphragm relaxes and moves up, the ribs move down, and the sternum drops back into position. This causes a decreased volume in the lungs and an increase in intrapulmonic pressure. As a result, air in the lungs moves from an area of greater pressure to one of lesser pressure and is expired (Fig. 39-2).

Other physical factors contribute to airflow in and out of the lungs. These factors include the condition of the musculature,

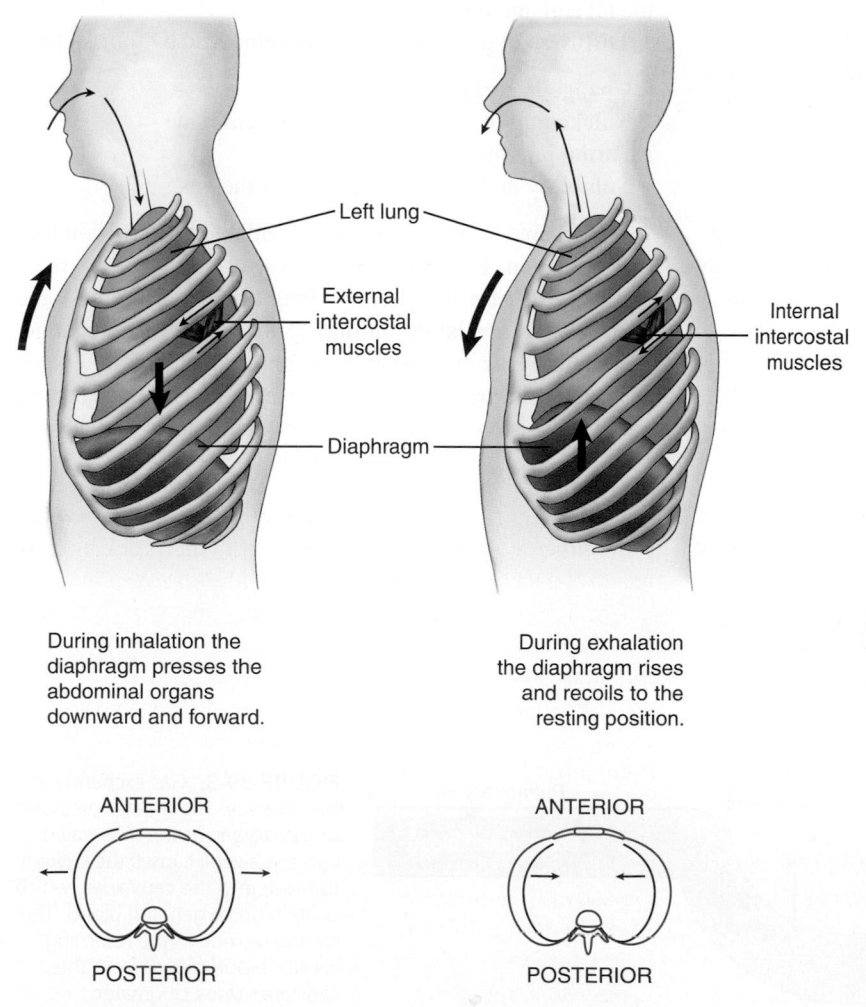

Left lung

External intercostal muscles

Internal intercostal muscles

Diaphragm

During inhalation the diaphragm presses the abdominal organs downward and forward.

During exhalation the diaphragm rises and recoils to the resting position.

ANTERIOR

POSTERIOR

Action of rib cage in inhalation

ANTERIOR

POSTERIOR

Action of rib cage in exhalation

FIGURE 39-2. Pulmonary ventilation.

compliance of lung tissue, and airway resistance. The condition of the body's musculature can affect the process of respiration. The accessory muscles of the abdomen, neck, and back are used to maintain respiratory movements at times when breathing is difficult. These muscles are used to facilitate breathing; the movement is called retractions. The most common retractions involve the intercostal, scalene, sternocleidomastoid, trapezius, and pectoralis muscles.

Lung compliance refers to the ease with which the lungs can be inflated. The compliance of lung tissue affects lung volume. The ability of the lungs to adequately fill with air during inhalation is achieved by the normal elasticity of lung tissue, aided by the presence of surfactant. The varying changes in lung pressure and resulting lung compliance can be compared to differences in blowing up a new, noncompliant balloon versus one that was inflated previously. A stiff, noncompliant lung (like a new balloon) requires a greater inspiratory effort to inflate it. Emphysema, a chronic lung condition, and the normal changes associated with aging are examples of conditions that result in decreased elasticity of lung tissue, which, in turn, decreases compliance.

Airway resistance is the result of any impediment or obstruction that air meets as it moves through the airway. Any process that changes the bronchial diameter or width causes airway resistance. Obstruction in any part of the normal passageways impedes respiration. Obstruction can be caused by a foreign substance, such as a piece of food, a coin, or a toy, or by liquids, as in the case of a drowning victim. Obstruction can also result from secretions (e.g., excessive or thickened secretions) or tissues (e.g., tumors or edema of the respiratory tract). A decrease in the size of air passages resulting from constriction or poor neck positioning can also impede respiration. Bronchial constriction in asthma is an example of airway resistance related to a decrease in the size of air passages.

> *Consider Tyrone Jacobs, the 12-year-old boy with suspected asthma. An understanding of the underlying* *pathophysiologic processes involved with this disorder would provide the basis for the nurse's actions to protect the child's airway.* ■

Respiration

Respiration, gas exchange, occurs at the terminal alveolar capillary system. Gases are exchanged between the air and blood via the dense network of capillaries in the respiratory portion of the lungs and the thin alveolar walls (see Fig. 39-1, Fig. 39-3). Gas exchange occurs via **diffusion.** Diffusion is the movement of gas or particles from areas of higher pressure or concentration to areas of lower pressure or concentration. In respiration, diffusion refers to the movement of oxygen and carbon dioxide between the air (in the alveoli) and the blood (in the capillaries). These gases move passively from an area of higher concentration to an area of lower concentration. The greater pressure of oxygen in the alveoli causes the oxygen to move from the alveoli into the capillaries containing the unoxygenated venous blood. Likewise, the carbon dioxide in the returning venous blood exerts a greater pressure than the carbon dioxide in the alveoli. Therefore, carbon dioxide diffuses across the capillary into the alveoli and ultimately is exhaled.

Diffusion of gases in the lung is influenced by four factors:

- Change in surface area available
- Thickening of alveolar–capillary membrane
- Partial pressure
- Solubility and molecular weight of the gas

Any change in the surface area available for diffusion hinders diffusion. For example, removal of a lung or the presence of a disease that destroys lung tissue can decrease the surface area available, ultimately affecting gas exchange. Incomplete lung expansion or the collapse of alveoli, known as **atelectasis,** prevents pressure changes and the exchange of gas by diffusion in the lungs. Atelectatic areas of the lung

FIGURE 39-3. Gas exchange in the alveolus. The greater pressure of the oxygen in the air inhaled into the alveoli causes the oxygen to move into the capillaries, which contain unoxygenated blood. The carbon dioxide in the returning venous blood moves from the capillaries (area of greater concentration) into the alveoli (area of lesser concentration).

cannot fulfill the function of respiration. Examples of conditions that predispose a patient to atelectasis are obstructions of the airway by foreign bodies, mucus, airway constriction, external compression by tumors or enlarged blood vessels, and immobility. Any disease or condition that results in thickening of the alveolar–capillary membrane, such as pneumonia or pulmonary edema, makes diffusion more difficult.

The partial pressure, or pressure resulting from any gas in a mixture depending on its concentration, can also affect diffusion. If environmental oxygen is reduced, such as when a person is at higher altitudes or in the presence of toxic fumes, less oxygen is available for diffusion. When oxygen is administered, an increased amount of oxygen is available, resulting in greater diffusion across capillary membranes.

Finally, the solubility and molecular weight of the gas are factors in diffusion. Carbon dioxide has greater solubility in the respiratory membranes and diffuses more rapidly than oxygen. This allows for carbon dioxide to be released from the lungs with each exhalation.

Perfusion

Oxygenated capillary blood passes through the tissues of the body in the process called perfusion. The amount of blood flowing through the lungs is a factor in the amount of oxygen and other gases that are exchanged. The amount of blood present in any given area of lung tissue depends partially on whether the person is sitting, standing, or lying down. Perfusion is greater in dependent areas. The perfusion of lung tissue also depends on the person's activity level. Greater activity results in an increased need for cellular oxygen by the body's tissues and a subsequent increase in cardiac output and consequently in increased blood return to the lungs. In addition, perfusion to the body's tissues depends on an adequate blood supply and proper cardiovascular functioning to carry oxygen and carbon dioxide to and from the lungs (see below).

If a problem exists in ventilation, respiration, or perfusion, **hypoxia** may occur. Hypoxia is a condition in which an inadequate amount of oxygen is available to cells. The most common symptoms of hypoxia are **dyspnea** (difficulty breathing), an elevated blood pressure with a small pulse pressure, increased respiratory and pulse rates, pallor, and cyanosis. Anxiety, restlessness, confusion, and drowsiness also are common signs of hypoxia. Hypoxia is often caused by **hypoventilation** (decreased rate or depth of air movement into the lungs). Hypoxia can also be a chronic condition. The effects of chronic hypoxia can be detected in all body systems and are manifested as altered thought processes, headaches, chest pain, enlarged heart, clubbing of the fingers and toes, anorexia, constipation, decreased urinary output, decreased libido, weakness of extremity muscles, and muscle pain.

Regulation of Respiration

The respiratory center is located in the medulla in the brainstem, immediately above the spinal cord. It is stimulated by an increased concentration of carbon dioxide and hydrogen ions and, to a lesser degree, by the decreased amount of oxygen in the arterial blood. In addition, chemoreceptors in the aortic arch and carotid bodies are sensitive to the same arterial blood gas levels and blood pressure and can activate the medulla. Proprioceptors in the muscles and joints respond to body movements, such as exercise, and cause an increase in ventilation.

Stimulation of the medulla increases the rate and depth of ventilation (both inspiration and expiration) to blow off carbon dioxide and hydrogen and increase oxygen levels (the patient is breathing faster and more deeply). The medulla sends an impulse down the spinal cord to the respiratory muscles to stimulate a contraction leading to inhalation. If a condition causes a chronic change in the oxygen and carbon dioxide levels, these chemoreceptors may become desensitized and not regulate ventilation adequately.

The Cardiovascular System and Transport of Respiratory Gases

This section focuses on the relationship between the function of the cardiovascular system and the respiratory system. Additional information related to the cardiovascular system, including pulse, pulse physiology, blood pressure, and the physiology of blood pressure is discussed in Chapter 24, Vital Signs.

Oxygen and carbon dioxide must move through the alveoli and be carried to and from body cells by the blood. Thus, an adequately functioning cardiovascular system is vital for exchange of gases. The cardiovascular system is composed of the heart and the blood vessels. The heart is a cone shaped, muscular pump, divided into four hollow chambers. The upper chambers, the **atria** (singular, atrium), receive blood from the veins (the superior and inferior vena cava and the left and right pulmonary veins). The lower chambers, the **ventricles,** force blood out of the heart through the arteries (the left and right pulmonary arteries and the aorta). One-way valves that direct blood flow through the heart are located at the entrance (tricuspid and mitral valves) and exit (pulmonary and aortic valves) of each ventricle. Refer to Figure 39-4. The blood vessels form a closed circuit of tubes that carry blood between the heart and the body cells. Arteries and arterioles conduct blood away from the ventricles to the capillaries and the venules and veins and return blood from the capillaries to the atria. Capillaries function in the exchange of substances between the blood and the body cells.

Deoxygenated blood (low in oxygen; high in carbon dioxide) is carried from the right side of the heart to the lungs, where oxygen is picked up and carbon dioxide is released, then returned to the left side of the heart. This oxygenated blood (high in oxygen; low in carbon dioxide) is pumped out to all other parts of the body and back again (refer to Fig. 39-5). Oxygen is carried via plasma and red blood cells. It is dissolved in plasma, but because oxygen is insoluble in liquids, little oxygen is carried in this way. The majority of oxygen is carried by the red blood cells. The hemoglobin in red blood cells has a strong affinity for oxygen. Therefore, most oxygen (97%) is carried in the body

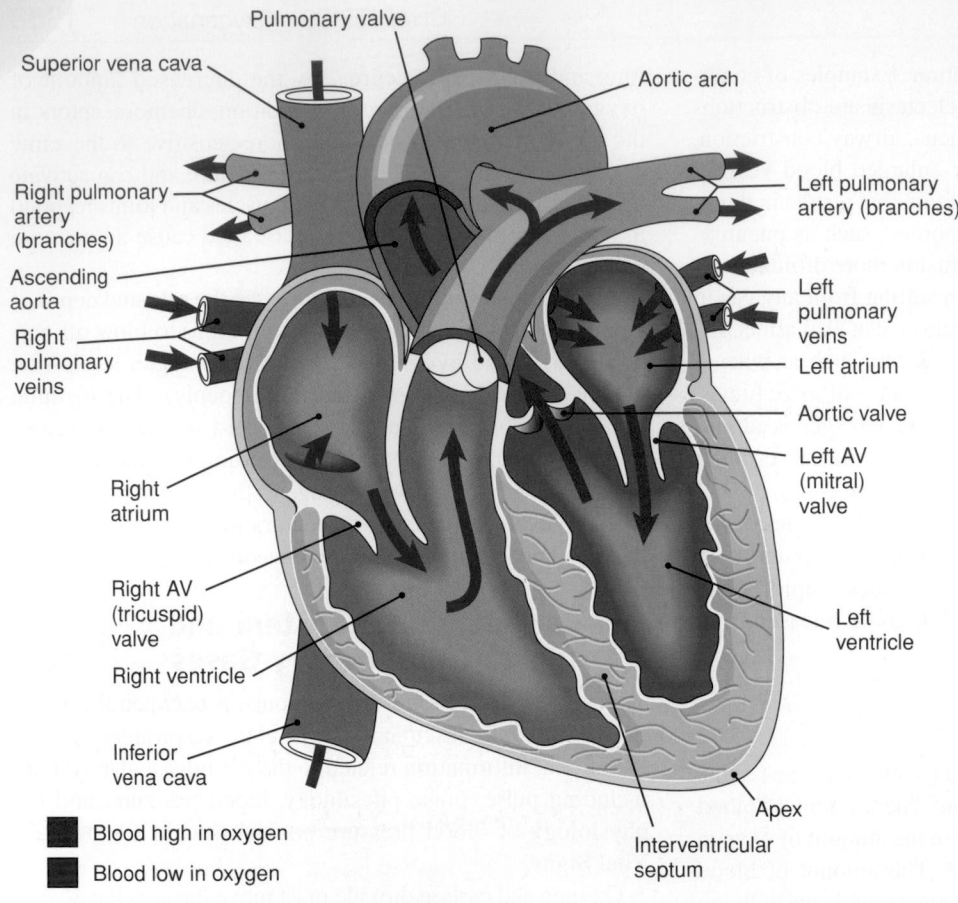

Pulmonary valve

Superior vena cava

Aortic arch

Right pulmonary artery (branches)

Left pulmonary artery (branches)

Ascending aorta

Left pulmonary veins

Right pulmonary veins

Left atrium

Aortic valve

Left AV (mitral) valve

Right atrium

Right AV (tricuspid) valve

Right ventricle

Left ventricle

Inferior vena cava

Apex

■ Blood high in oxygen
■ Blood low in oxygen

Interventricular septum

FIGURE 39-4. The heart, valves, and vessels. (Adapted from Cohen, B. J. & Taylor, J. J. [2009]. *Memmler's structure and function of the human body* [9th ed.]. Philadelphia: Lippincott Williams & Wilkins.)

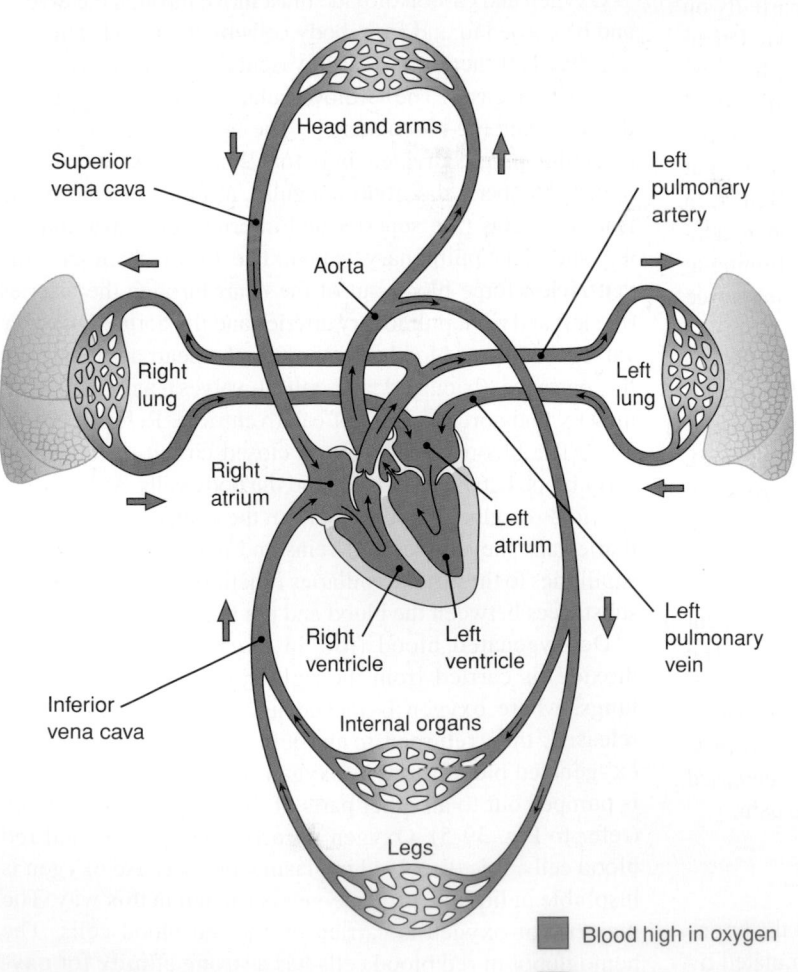

Head and arms

Superior vena cava

Left pulmonary artery

Aorta

Right lung

Left lung

Right atrium

Left atrium

Left pulmonary vein

Inferior vena cava

Right ventricle

Left ventricle

Internal organs

Legs

■ Blood high in oxygen
■ Blood low in oxygen

FIGURE 39-5. The right side of the heart pumps deoxygenated blood to the lungs, where oxygen is picked up and carbon dioxide released. The left side of the heart pumps oxygenated blood out to all other parts of the body. (From Cohen, B. J. & Taylor, J. J. [2009]. *Memmler's structure and function of the human body* [9th ed.]. Philadelphia: Lippincott, Williams & Wilkins.)

by red blood cells as part of hemoglobin in the form of oxyhemoglobin. Hemoglobin also carries carbon dioxide easily in the form of carboxyhemoglobin.

Once the red blood cells reach the tissues, **internal respiration** must occur. Internal respiration is the exchange of oxygen and carbon dioxide between the circulating blood and the tissue cells. Any abnormality in the blood's constituents affects internal respiration. For example, hemorrhage or loss of blood can cause a decrease in cardiac output. A decrease in cardiac output causes a reduction in the amount of circulating blood that is available to deliver oxygen to the tissues. Anemia, a decrease in the amount of red blood cells or erythrocytes, results in insufficient hemoglobin available to transport oxygen. This may lead to an inadequate supply of oxygen to the tissues of the body. Alternately, exercise can improve the transport of oxygen. Regular exercise contributes to more effective pumping of the heart muscle, and improved oxygen transport to cells.

FACTORS AFFECTING RESPIRATORY FUNCTIONING

A variety of factors affect adequate respiratory functioning. Seven important factors are discussed in the following sections.

Level of Health

Acute and chronic illnesses can affect a person's respiratory function dramatically. For example, people with renal or cardiac disorders often have compromised respiratory functioning because of fluid overload and impaired tissue perfusion. People with chronic illnesses often have muscle wasting and poor muscle tone. These problems affect all the muscles, including those of the respiratory system. Alterations in muscle function contribute to inadequate pulmonary ventilation and respiration. Anemia can result in

impaired respiratory function. As discussed previously, anemia may lead to an inadequate supply of oxygen to the tissues of the body. Because hemoglobin also carries carbon dioxide to the lungs, anemia results in diminished carbon dioxide exchange. Myocardial infarction (heart attack) causes a lack of blood supply to the heart muscle. Damage to the heart muscle interferes with effective contractions of the heart muscle, leading to decreased perfusion of tissues and decreased gas exchange. Physical changes such as scoliosis (curvature of the spine) influence breathing patterns and may cause air trapping. Research reveals a statistically significant correlation between obesity and chronic bronchitis. Moreover, people who are obese are often short of breath during activity, ultimately leading to less participation in exercise. As a result, the alveoli at the base of the lungs are rarely stimulated to expand fully.

> ➤ *Recall Yan Kim, the 57-year-old patient who developed respiratory failure from complications associated with pulmonary surgery. The acuity of the situation played a major role in the patient's current condition. The pulmonary surgery most likely reduced his respiratory function. The effects of anesthesia on his lungs and subsequently the development of complications compounded his situation.* ■

Developmental Considerations

There are many age-related developmental considerations affecting respiratory function. Table 39-1 summarizes respiratory variations in the life cycle.

Neonates and Infants

Birth necessitates many adaptations by a newborn. The most obvious changes occur in the lungs, which are transformed

TABLE • 39-1	RESPIRATORY VARIATIONS IN THE LIFE CYCLE			
	Infant (Birth–1 year)	Early Childhood (1–5 years)	Late Childhood (6–12 years)	Aged Adult (65+ years)
Respiratory rate	30–60 breaths/min	20–40 breaths/min	15–25 breaths/min	16–20 breaths/min
Respiratory pattern	Abdominal breathing, irregular in rate and depth	Abdominal breathing, irregular	Thoracic breathing, regular	Thoracic, regular
Chest wall	Thin, little muscle, ribs and sternum easily seen	Same as infant's but with more subcutaneous fat	Further subcutaneous fat deposited, structures less prominent	Thin, structures prominent
Breath sounds	Loud, harsh crackles at end of deep inspiration	Loud, harsh expiration longer than inspiration	Clear inspiration is longer than expiration	Clear
Shape of thorax	Round	Elliptical	Elliptical	Barrel shaped or elliptical

from fluid-filled structures to air-filled organs. The normal infant's chest is small, the airways are short, and aspiration is a potential problem. The respiratory rate is more rapid in infants than at any other age (see Table 39-1). As the alveoli increase in number and size, adequate oxygenation is accomplished at lower respiratory rates. Surfactant is formed in utero between 34 and 36 weeks. An infant born before 34 weeks may not have produced sufficient surfactant, leading to collapse of the alveoli and poor alveolar exchange. Synthetic surfactant can be given to the infant to help reopen the alveoli. Respiratory activity is primarily abdominal in infants.

Toddlers, Preschoolers, School-aged Children, and Adolescents

The preschool child's eustachian tubes, bronchi, and bronchioles are elongated and less angular. Thus, the average number of routine colds and infections decreases until the child enters daycare or school and is exposed more frequently to pathogens. Young children who are not placed in daycare usually have not had the opportunity to develop antibodies for the variety of viruses and bacteria they may encounter in a school setting. Encourage good hand hygiene and tissue etiquette. Most children at this age have colds or upper respiratory infections, but some have more serious problems of otitis media, bronchitis, and pneumonia. By the end of late childhood and during adulthood, the immune system is prepared to protect the person from most infections.

Older Adults

Specific physical changes occur in older adults that are unrelated to any pathology. Refer to the Focus on the Older Adult box. The tissues and airways of the respiratory tract (including the alveoli) become less elastic. The power of the respiratory and abdominal muscles is reduced, and therefore the diaphragm moves less efficiently. The chest is unable to stretch as much, resulting in a decline in maximum inspiration and expiration. Airways collapse more easily. These alterations increase the risk for disease, especially pneumonia and other chest infections.

> ➤ *Think back to Joan McIntyre, the 72-year-old woman who is having an exacerbation of her chronic COPD. The nurse needs to incorporate information about age-related changes when planning the patient's care. The nurse also needs to consider that some of these age-related changes may be intensifying some of her symptoms and contributing to her decreased ability to care for herself.* ∎

Medications

Many medications affect the function of the respiratory system. Patients receiving drugs that affect the central nervous system need to be monitored carefully for respiratory complications. For example, opioids are chemical agents that

---

FOCUS ON THE OLDER ADULT

NURSING STRATEGIES FOR OXYGEN PROBLEMS AFFECTING OLDER ADULTS

Age-Related Changes	Nursing Strategies
Decreased Gas Exchange and Increased Work of Breathing	
• Decreased elastic recoil of the lungs • Expiration requiring use of accessory muscles • Fewer functional capillaries and more fibrous tissue in alveoli • Decreased skeletal muscle strength in thorax • Reduction in vital capacity and increase in residual volume	• Encourage rest periods, as necessary. • Encourage cessation or moderation of smoking and second-hand smoke exposure. • Teach breathing exercises. • Remind about avoiding air pollutants. • Caution about effect of extreme weather conditions. • Instruct to avoid narcotics and sleeping pills. • Discuss home management with patient and family. • Teach avoidance of infection and preventive measures (i.e., flu vaccination). • Use pillows as necessary to sleep.
Decreased Ventilation and Ineffective Cough	
• Less air exchange; more secretions remain in lungs • Drier mucous membranes • Altered pain sensation • Different norms for body temperature; fever may be atypical • Greater risk for aspiration due to slower gastric motility • Impaired mobility and inactivity, effects of medication	• Encourage increased fluid intake, especially water, as allowed. • Use cool-mist humidifier (teach proper cleaning technique). • Encourage attendance at pulmonary exercise rehabilitation program. • Discourage use of over-the-counter medications. • Teach how to splint thorax and cough effectively. • Instruct in use of supplemental oxygen. • Teach avoidance of milk products if they are troublesome.

PROMOTING HEALTH • 39-1

Oxygenation

Patients view nurses as role models for achieving healthy lifestyles. Nurses dealing with stresses from professional and personal aspects of their own lives sometimes channel their energies into destructive behaviors. If the nurse wishes to encourage optimal respiratory functioning, he or she must demonstrate behaviors that support a healthy lifestyle.

Use the assessment checklist to determine how well you are meeting your oxygenation needs. Then develop a prescription for self-care by choosing appropriate behaviors from the list of suggestions.

Assessment Checklist

❏ almost always   ❏ sometimes   ❏ almost never

❏ ❏ ❏ 1. I breathe easily, without discomfort and without feeling short of breath.

❏ ❏ ❏ 2. I exercise regularly.

❏ ❏ ❏ 3. I maintain normal weight for my height and body frame.

❏ ❏ ❏ 4. I live in an environment free of pollution.

❏ ❏ ❏ 5. I avoid substances (tobacco, chemicals) that cause respiratory problems.

❏ ❏ ❏ 6. I arrange to receive recommended immunizations.

Self-Care Behaviors

1. Follow a regular exercise program with at least 30 minutes a day of at least moderate-intensity physical activity on most, and preferably all, days of the week (Marcus, Williams, Dubbert, Sallis, King, Yancey, et al., 2006).
2. Maintain normal body weight.
3. Obtain medical evaluation for chest pain, problems with breathing, and/or chronic cough with sputum or blood.
4. Evaluate personal use of nicotine.
5. Incorporate a plan to reduce smoking and then stop smoking on a specific target date.
6. Avoid exposure to second-hand smoke when possible.
7. Arrange to have a tuberculin test (PPD) done annually.
8. Receive a yearly influenza immunization.
9. Avoid chemical substances that cause respiratory depression.
10. Maintain a pollution-free environment (as much as possible).
11. Support federal and community efforts to keep the air free of pollution.

Information to promote respiratory health, such as information about asthma, allergies, air quality, smoking cessation, lung cancer, and chronic lung diseases is available online. Check out these sites: American Lung Association at www.lungusa.org; the National Lung Health Education Program at www.nlhep.org; and Air Pollution and Respiratory Health Program at www.cdc.gov/nceh/airpollution/.

depress the medullary respiratory center. As a result, the rate and depth of respirations decrease. Be alert for the possibility of respiratory depression or arrest when administering any narcotic or sedative.

Lifestyle

Activity levels and habits can dramatically affect a person's respiratory status. For example, sedentary activity patterns do not encourage the expansion of alveoli and the development of pulmonary exercise patterns (deep breathing). People who exercise (e.g., aerobics, walking, swimming) three to six times per week can better respond to stressors to respiratory health.

Cigarette smoking (active or passive) is a major contributor to lung disease and respiratory distress. Cigarette smoking is the most important risk factor for chronic COPD (Macnee, 2007).

Nurses working with patients to initiate changes in health habits that affect respiration must also examine themselves

as a factor in the success of the plan. Nurses who role model good health behaviors are more effective teachers. Use the Promoting Health Display 39-1: Oxygenation for yourself before using it with others.

Environment

Although it is impossible to pinpoint all the effects of air pollution, researchers have demonstrated a high correlation between air pollution and cancer and lung diseases. For example, a person with adequate respiratory functioning who is exposed to air pollution may experience stinging of eyes and nasal passages, coughing, choking, headache, and dizziness. Occupational exposure to asbestos, silica, or coal dust, as well as environmental pollution, can lead to chronic pulmonary disease. Chronic exposure to radon, radiation, asbestos, and arsenic can lead to lung cancer. Additionally, people who have experienced an alteration in respiratory functioning in the past often have difficulty continuing to perform self-care activities in a polluted environment.

Psychological Health

Many psychological factors and conditions can affect the respiratory system. Individuals responding to stress may sigh excessively or exhibit **hyperventilation** (increased rate and depth of ventilation, above the body's normal metabolic requirements). Hyperventilation can lead to a lowered level of arterial carbon dioxide. Generalized anxiety has been shown to cause enough bronchospasm to produce an episode of bronchial asthma. In addition, patients with respiratory problems often develop some anxiety as a result of the hypoxia caused by the respiratory problem.

> ➤ *Think back to Tyrone Jacobs, the young boy described at the beginning of the chapter. The patient is gasping for breath, which is extremely frightening and anxiety producing. In addition, his parents are frantic; this would increase Tyrone's anxiety level, further limiting his ability to breathe. The nurse needs to incorporate an understanding of this situation and plan interventions that promote oxygenation while reducing anxiety.* ∎

THE NURSING PROCESS FOR OXYGENATION
Assessing

The patient's health history is an essential component for assessing respiratory functioning. Either the patient or a family member can provide this information. The nursing examination combined with laboratory findings can provide information to identify a patient's strengths, the nature of the problem, its course, related signs and symptoms, and its onset, frequency, and effects on activities of daily living. The nurse decides, based on these findings, what problems can be treated independently by nursing. Other problems are referred to a physician and/or other collaborative professionals for decisions on treatment.

Nursing History

The nursing history, an important clinical tool in the early steps of the nursing process, always includes a respiratory component. The information gained provides data about why the patient needs nursing care and what kind of care is required to maintain a sufficient intake of air. Interview questions help identify current or potential health deviations, actions performed by the patient for meeting respiratory needs and the effects of such actions, contributing factors, the use of any aids to improve the intake of air, and effects on the patient's lifestyle and relationships with others.

Before starting the interview, ascertain that the patient is not in acute distress. If the patient is experiencing any respiratory distress, initiate appropriate actions immediately to help relieve symptoms. Enlist the aid of family members or others to help answer questions. When the patient is able, interview the patient to expand the initial database. If no emergency interventions are necessary for the patient's clinical condition, obtain a comprehensive history at this time.

When a health deviation is noted during the data collection, collect as much descriptive information as possible, including whether the problem evolved suddenly or slowly. The accompanying Focused Assessment Guide 39-1 provides some appropriate questions for health history assessment related to oxygenation.

Physical Assessment

The basic examination of the lungs and respiratory status is discussed in Chapter 25, Health Assessment. Always proceed in a well-organized manner through a sequence of inspection, palpation, percussion, and auscultation.

> ➤ *Recall Mr. Kim, the 57-year-old man who is receiving oxygen therapy and mechanical ventilation via an endotracheal tube. A complete assessment is necessary to identify specific problems related to oxygenation as well as to determine the effectiveness of current treatments.* ∎

INSPECTION

Inspect the chest contour and shape. Normally, the adult chest contour is slightly convex, with no sternal depression. The anteroposterior diameter should be less than the transverse diameter. The infant's chest wall is so thin and has so little musculature that the ribs, sternum, and xiphoid process are seen easily. Infants have a rounded chest wall in which the anteroposterior diameter (the measurement from the front to the back of the thorax) equals the transverse diameter. In preschool-aged and school-aged children, some subcutaneous fat is deposited on the chest wall, making landmarks less prominent than they were in infants. Muscular development is also more noticeable. The ratio of the transverse diameter to the anteroposterior diameter reaches the adult configuration of 1:2 by age 6 years. Bony landmarks are more prominent because of the loss of subcutaneous fat. Kyphosis (curvature of the spine) contributes to the older person's appearance of leaning forward. Barrel chest deformity (see Fig. 25-25 in Chap. 25) may result in an increased anteroposterior diameter.

Describe or sketch any abnormalities in thoracic structure (see Fig. 25-30 in Chap. 25 for structures). Note the contour of the intercostal spaces, which should be flat or depressed, and the movement of the chest, which should be symmetrical. Inspect the skin over the thorax for temperature and color. It should be warm and dry and even in color, with no cyanosis or pallor, which could indicate less than optimal oxygenation. Note any scars, recording the origin of such in the history under previous surgery or accidents.

Observe the respiratory rate and rhythm for one full minute. Normally, respirations are quiet and nonlabored. Note any flaring of the nostrils, muscular retractions, **tachypnea** (rapid breathing), or **bradypnea** (slow breathing), which are suggestive of a health deviation requiring further evaluation.

FOCUSED ASSESSMENT GUIDE • 39-1

RESPIRATION AND OXYGENATION

Factors to Assess	Questions and Approaches
Usual patterns of respiration	How would you describe your breathing? Do you have allergies? What type(s) of allergies do you have? What relief measures do you use?
Medications	Are you taking any medications for your breathing?
Health history	Do you have any heart, lung, or breathing conditions? Does any one in your family/home have any breathing conditions or respiratory infections?
Recent changes	Have you noticed any changes in your breathing (out of breath, cough, wheezing, pain)? Do you have chest pain? Do you have a respiratory infection? If so, what type? What relief measures are you using?
Lifestyle and environment	Do you smoke? If so, how many years have you smoked? How much do you smoke (i.e., how many packs per day or year)? Do you live with a smoker or are there smokers in your workplace? Are you exposed to respiratory irritants in your workplace? Are there other pollutants in your workplace?
Cough	How much and how often do you cough? Is the cough related to the time of day or any activity? What is it like (dry, bubbly, hoarse)? Do you cough up mucus? If so, how much and what does it look like? Do you have a history of allergies? Do you ever wheeze? Are you exposed to dust? Fumes? Where do you work? What kind of work? How are you treating the cough?
Sputum	Do you ever cough up and spit out mucus? How much do you spit out and do you associate it with anything (time of day, environment)? What color is it? Is it ever blood tinged? What is its odor?
Chest pain	Do you have pain with breathing? When did it start? On a scale of 0 to 10 (10 being very painful), how severe is the pain? Where is the pain? Is the pain worse with inspiration? Expiration? Cough? Does the pain radiate? What measures are you using to relieve the pain?

(continued)

FOCUSED ASSESSMENT GUIDE • 39-1

RESPIRATION AND OXYGENATION *(continued)*

Factors to Assess	Questions and Approaches
Dyspnea	Is it constant or remittent or related to any activity?
	How do different positions affect it?
	How does it affect your daily activities?
	Is any part of your body bluish during the breathing problem?
	What do you do during and after the breathing attack?
	Have you ever been told that you have asthma? Emphysema? Tuberculosis? Heart disease?
	Do you think the problem is getting worse or staying the same?
Fever	Have you had pneumonia recently?
	Do you have any contact with people who have tuberculosis?
	Do you have night sweats?
	Are others in your household well or ill?
	Have you traveled anywhere recently?
	What medications are you using?
Fatigue	Have you noticed you feel more tired lately?
	Are you getting your normal amount of sleep at night?
	Has your sleep at night been affected by any difficulty breathing?
	Do you become easily fatigued when you climb stairs?
	Has your pattern of daily activity changed lately?
	Can you sleep lying flat? How many pillows do you use?

Always be alert for common clinical manifestations that may indicate an airway emergency. Specific disease processes and conditions leading to acute respiratory failure, and their associated clinical manifestations, are discussed in medical–surgical nursing textbooks.

PALPATION

Palpate the trachea, which should lie equidistant from each clavicle. Skin temperature in this area is typically the same as the rest of the body.

Measure thoracic excursion by placing your hands on the patient's posterior thorax at the 10th rib, with both thumbs almost touching the vertebrae. Ask the patient to take a few deep breaths, and watch the movement of the hands. Usually the thumbs move 5 to 8 cm symmetrically at maximal inspiration (see Fig. 25-28 in Chapter 25).

Assess tactile fremitus (the capacity to feel sound on the chest wall) by placing your palm to the patient's chest wall, avoiding bony areas (e.g., scapulae). Ask the patient to repeat some multi-syllable word (e.g., "ninety-nine") and feel for the vibration. Normally the vibrations are equal bilaterally in different areas on the chest wall. The greatest intensity is noted at the anterior and posterior base of the neck and along the trachea and large bronchi. Increased fremitus occurs in patients with pneumonia because solid tissue conducts sound well. Conversely, patients with COPD have decreased fremitus

because air does not conduct sound as well. Note the presence or absence of masses, edema, or tenderness on palpation.

PERCUSSION

Percussion is used to assess the position of the lungs, density of lung tissue, and identify changes in the tissue. This assessment skill is not used frequently. When used, it is usually included in examinations performed by advanced practice nurses and other advanced practice professionals. It is discussed in Chapter 25, Health Assessment.

AUSCULTATION

Using the diaphragm of a stethoscope, move from apex to base of the lungs, comparing one side with the other side while listening to a complete respiratory cycle: inspiration and expiration. Normal breath sounds include **vesicular** (low-pitched, soft sounds heard over peripheral lung fields), **bronchial** (loud, high-pitched sounds heard primarily over the trachea and larynx), and **bronchovesicular** (medium-pitched blowing sounds heard over the major bronchi) sounds (see Table 25-8 in Chapter 25). Auscultate as the patient breathes slowly through an open mouth. Breathing through the nose can produce falsely abnormal breath sounds. Breathing too quickly, such as with hyperventilation, may cause syncope and patient distress. If abnormal breath sounds are detected, instruct the patient to cough and auscultate again for at least two complete respiratory cycles. Record location, change in breath sounds after coughing, and the phase of respiration in which any abnormal sound is heard (e.g., wheezing on expiration).

Adventitious breath sounds, or abnormal lung sounds, are categorized as either discontinuous or continuous sounds (see Table 25-9 in Chapter 25). **Crackles,** frequently heard on inspiration, are soft, high-pitched discontinuous (intermittent) popping sounds. They are produced by fluid in the airways or alveoli and delayed reopening of collapsed alveoli. They occur due to inflammation or congestion and are associated with pneumonia, congestive heart failure, bronchitis, and COPD. Crackles can be further classified as fine or coarse. Fine crackles are brief sounds, similar to the sound of hair rubbing together between the fingers. Coarse crackles are somewhat louder, moist, bubbling sounds (Jarvis, 2008; Smeltzer, Bare, Hinkle, & Cheever, 2010). Occasional fine crackles at the end of deep inspiration heard on auscultation of the infant's thorax are normal.

Wheezes are continuous, musical sounds, produced as air passes through airways constricted by swelling, narrowing, secretions, or tumors. They can be further classified as sibilant wheezes or sonorous wheezes. Sibilant wheezes originate in smaller airways and are high pitched and whistling, whereas sonorous wheezes can be heard over larger airways and sound like a snore (Jarvis, 2008; Smeltzer et al., 2010). They are often heard in patients with asthma, tumors, or a buildup of secretions.

A **pleural friction rub** is a continuous, dry grating sound. Pleural friction rub is caused by inflammation of pleural surfaces and loss of lubricating pleural fluid. It resembles the sound made by rubbing two leather surfaces together.

Common Diagnostic Tests

In addition to the nursing history and physical examination, the laboratory and radiologic tests described in Box 39-1 provide further assessment data that can aid in the formation of nursing diagnoses.

> *The nurse might anticipate diagnostic procedures such as arterial blood gas and pH analysis (ABG) for Joan McIntyre, the older woman with the acute exacerbation of COPD. This diagnostic test would provide information regarding the adequacy of her oxygenation and ventilation and to help titrate (adjust) the administration of supplemental oxygen. It would also be used to evaluate her response to treatment and therapies.* ∎

The tests described in the next sections are not distinctive for a particular disease but reflect how well the respiratory system is functioning.

PULMONARY FUNCTION STUDIES

Pulmonary function studies encompass a group of tests used to evaluate patients with respiratory disorders and are performed routinely to evaluate pulmonary status and detect

abnormalities. They provide an evaluation of lung dysfunction, diagnose disease, assess disease severity, assist in management of disease, and evaluate respiratory interventions. Most tests are administered by a respiratory therapist, technician, nurses with specialized training, or physicians. Several tests commonly encountered are described below. More specialized tests and their purposes include:

- Inert gas dilution, nitrogen washout, and body plethysmography measure lung volumes.
- Diffusion capacity estimates the patient's ability to absorb alveolar gases and determine if a gas exchange problem exists.
- Maximal respiratory pressures help evaluate neuromuscular causes of respiratory dysfunction.
- Exercise testing helps evaluate dyspnea during exertion.

Refer to Box 39-2 for Commonly Measured Values From Pulmonary Function Tests.

Spirometry

Spirometry measures the volume of air in liters exhaled or inhaled by a patient over time. It evaluates lung function and airway obstruction through respiratory mechanics. Spirometry can be used to measure the degree of airway obstruction and evaluates response to inhaled medications. The patient inhales deeply and exhales forcefully into a **spirometer,** an instrument that measures lung volumes and airflow.

Peak Expiratory Flow Rate

Peak expiratory flow rate (PEFR) refers to the point of highest flow during forced expiration. PEFR reflects changes in the size of pulmonary airways and is measured using a peak flow meter. It is routinely used for patients with moderate or severe asthma to measure the severity of the disease and degree of disease control. With the patient standing or sitting with the back positioned as straight as possible, the patient takes a deep breath and places the peak flow meter in his or her mouth, closing the lips tightly around the mouthpiece. The patient forcibly exhales into the peak flow meter, and an indicator on the meter rises to a number. The patient is asked to repeat this three times, and the highest number is recorded. This produces a measurement in liters indicating the maximum flow rate during a forced expiration. Normal values are established in regard to height, age, and gender, as well as individual baseline values for patients with disease. Patients commonly measure PEFR at home to monitor airflow. The results are used to track disease progression and regulate treatment by the patient and clinician.

PULSE OXIMETRY

Pulse oximetry is a noninvasive technique that measures the arterial oxyhemoglobin saturation (SaO_2 or SpO_2) of arterial blood. Pulse oximetry is useful for monitoring patients receiving oxygen therapy, titrating oxygen therapy, monitoring those at risk for hypoxia, and monitoring postoperative patients. Pulse oximetry does not replace arterial blood gas analysis. Desaturation indicates gas exchange abnormalities.

Box 39-1   COMMON DIAGNOSTIC PROCEDURES USED TO ASSESS RESPIRATORY FUNCTIONING

Arterial Blood Gas and pH Analysis

These examine arterial blood to determine the pressure exerted by oxygen and carbon dioxide in the blood and the blood pH. This test measures the adequacy of oxygenation, ventilation, and perfusion. Normal results are: pH (7.35–7.45), PCO_2 (35–45 mm Hg), PO_2 (80–100 mm Hg), HCO_3 (22–26 mEq/L), and base excess or deficit (-2 to $+2$ mmol/L).

Preparation

- Explain to the patient that this test requires an arterial puncture and collection of a blood specimen.
- The radial, brachial, or femoral arteries are usually the sites of choice.
- Perform Allen's test to ensure adequate ulnar blood flow when using radial artery.

Aftercare

- Record supplemental oxygen or respirator settings on laboratory slip.
- The arterial specimen is immediately placed on ice and taken to the laboratory.
- Apply pressure for 5 to 10 minutes and watch for evidence of bleeding. If patient is taking anticoagulants, pressure must be applied for a longer interval.

Cytologic Study

This involves a microscopic examination of sputum and the cells it contains. It is done primarily to detect cells that may be malignant, determine organisms causing infection, and identify blood or pus in the sputum.

Preparation

- Collect the specimen, if possible, in the morning before breakfast. The test usually involves 3 successive days of sputum collection. About 1 teaspoon of sputum is needed for a specimen.
- Instruct the patient that saliva is not a satisfactory specimen.
- Patient should take a deep breath and then expel the air with a deep cough.
- Expectorate the specimen into a sterile specimen container with the appropriate preservative, if indicated.
- Close the container with a tight-fitting lid.

Aftercare

- Advise the patient to inform the nurse when the specimen has been obtained.
- Label and package the specimen and send it to the laboratory as soon as possible.

Endoscopic Studies

These involve direct visualization of a body cavity. A bronchoscope is used to examine the larynx, bronchi, and trachea. Bronchoscopy is used to view lesions, obtain a biopsy, improve drainage, remove foreign substances, evaluate trauma, and drain abscesses.

Preparation

- Verify that an informed consent was obtained.
- The patient should be NPO for 6 to 8 hours before the test.
- An analgesic, sedative, and/or anticholinergic may be administered before the test.
- Local anesthetic is sprayed into the throat.

Aftercare

- Withhold food and fluids until the gag reflex returns.
- Check vital signs according to the protocol.
- Observe carefully for signs of respiratory impairment. Emergency resuscitation equipment should be available.
- Warm saline gargles may relieve throat irritation once the gag reflex has returned.

Skin Tests

These determine antigen–antibody reactions. In intradermal tests, antigens (to which the patient may have previously been exposed) are injected into the superficial layer of the skin with a needle and syringe to evaluate immune response.

Preparation

- Check patient's history for hypersensitivity to any of the test antigens. If positive, notify the physician before performing test.
- Cleanse the test area with alcohol and allow it to dry.

Aftercare

- Instruct the patient to have the test results read at the appropriate time.
- After reading the results, document the reaction, noting the amount of erythema or induration. Record the test, time, date, method, and site of administration on the patient record.

Radiography

Radiography is an x-ray examination of the lungs and the thoracic cavity. Radiographic examinations of the lungs are done to help diagnose pulmonary diseases and to determine the progress or development of disease.

Preparation

- Instruct patient to remove clothing to the waist and put on gown. All metal jewelry should be removed.
- The patient will be required to take a deep breath and hold it during the radiograph.

Aftercare

- No special care is required after chest radiograph.

Lung Scan

Lung scan is the recording on a photographic plate of the emissions of radioactive waves from a substance injected into a vein as it circulates through the lung. A *perfusion scan* (Q scan) is done to measure integrity of pulmonary blood vessels and evaluate blood flow abnormalities (e.g., pulmonary emboli). A *ventilation scan* (V scan) is done to detect ventilation abnormalities (especially in patients with emphysema). Both scans used together provide greater and more accurate diagnostic information than either test used solely.

Preparation

- Verify that an informed consent was obtained, if required by agency.
- Explain that no fasting is required.
- Patient should be told to remove jewelry from the chest area.

Aftercare

- No special care is required after the lung scan.
- Reassure patient that no radiation precautions are necessary.

Adapted from Fischbach, F., & Dunning, M. (2009). *A manual of laboratory and diagnostic tests* (8th ed.). Philadelphia: Wolters Kluwer/Lippincott Williams & Wilkins; Smeltzer, S., Bare, B., Hinkle, J., & Cheever, K. (2010). *Brunner & Suddarth's textbook of medical-surgical nursing* (12th ed.). Philadelphia: Wolters Kluwer Health/Lippincott Williams & Wilkins; Fischbach, F., & Dunning, M. (2006). *Common laboratory and diagnostic tests* (4th ed.). Philadelphia: Lippincott Williams & Wilkins.

COMMONLY MEASURED VALUES FROM PULMONARY FUNCTION TESTS

- Vital Capacity (VC): The amount of air displaced by maximal exhalation
- Forced Expiratory Vital Capacity (FEVC): The amount of air expelled from a point of maximal inspiration to a point of maximal inspiration
- Forced Inspiratory Vial Capacity (FIVC): The amount of air inhaled from a point of maximal exhalation to a point of maximal expiration
- Forced Expiratory Volume (FEV): The forced expiratory volume that can be expressed in 1, 2, or 3 seconds in the first second of the FEVC maneuver
- Total Lung Capacity (TLC): The amount of air contained within the lungs at maximum inspiration
- Residual Volume (RV): The amount of air left in the lungs at maximal expiration
- Peak Expiratory Flow Rate (PEFR): The maximum flow attained during the forced expiratory maneuver

Adapted from Fischbach, F., & Dunning M. (2009). *A manual of laboratory and diagnostic tests* (8th ed.). Philadelphia: Wolters Kluwer/Lippincott Williams & Wilkins; Schultz, N. (2007). Spirometry essentials for medical assistants Part II: The important test variables and predicted values. *Journal of Continuing Education Topics & Issues, 9*(1), 18–21.

FIGURE 39-6. Portable pulse oximetry unit, used to measure oxygen saturation (SpO₂) of arterial blood.

Be aware of the patient's hemoglobin level before evaluating oxygen saturation because the test measures only the percentage of oxygen carried by the available hemoglobin. Thus, even a patient with a low hemoglobin could appear to have a normal SpO₂ because most of that hemoglobin is saturated. However, the patient may not have enough oxygen to meet body needs. A range of 95% to 100% is considered normal SpO₂; values ≤90% are abnormal, indicate that oxygenation to the tissues is inadequate, and should be investigated for potential hypoxia or technical error (Booker, 2008a; DeMeulenaere, 2007). Refer to the accompanying Research in Nursing Box.

> *Consider Tyrone Jacobs, the young boy with asthma described at the beginning of the chapter. The nurse would use pulse oximetry initially to obtain baseline information about the patient's oxygen saturation level and then as a means to evaluate the effectiveness of therapy.* ■

Figure 39-6 shows a nurse using a pulse oximetry unit, and Skill 39-1 outlines nursing responsibilities when using a pulse oximetry unit.

THORACENTESIS

Thoracentesis is the procedure of puncturing the chest wall and aspirating pleural fluid. The pleural cavity is a

RESEARCH IN NURSING
Bridging the Gap to Evidence-Based Practice

FINGERNAIL POLISH AND PULSE OXIMETRY

Pulse oximetry is a commonly used, noninvasive technique for assessing arterial oxygenation. The fingers are usually the first choice of site for this measurement. Patients routinely present with fingernail polish in place. Removal of the polish requires additional supplies, patient consent for removal, and valuable time for removal by the healthcare staff.

Related Research

Rodden, A., Spicer, L., Diaz, V., & Steyer, T. E. (2007). Does fingernail polish affect pulse oximeter readings? *Intensive and Critical Care Nursing, 23*(1), 51–55.

The objective of this study was to determine if fingernail polish affects oxygen saturation, as measured by two different pulse oximeter machines. Results from previous studies evaluating the effects of nail polish on oxygen saturation determined by pulse oximeter monitors were inconsistent. Ten nail polish colors were used in the study. Participants were healthy and had baseline oxygen saturation readings ≥95%. Each participant had their oxygen saturation measured on each of their 10 nails with and without nail polish. All 10 colors that were studied had a less than 1% change in pulse oximetry reading. The presence of nail polish was determined to not be clinically significant.

Relevance to Nursing Practice

Fingernail polish colors do not appear to cause a clinically significant change in pulse oximeter readings in healthy people. Therefore, the time and expense needed to remove fingernail polish in clinical practice may not be warranted.

For additional research, visit thePoint.

potential cavity because it is normally not distended with fluid or air. The physician can perform a thoracentesis at the bedside with the nurse assisting. The patient is required to sign a permit for this procedure. A thoracentesis may be performed to obtain a specimen for diagnostic purposes or to remove fluid that has accumulated in the pleural cavity and is causing respiratory difficulty and discomfort. Because the cavity being entered is sterile, surgical asepsis is required. Standard precautions also are used.

Procedure

A thoracentesis is usually carried out with the patient sitting on a chair or the edge of the bed with the legs supported and the arms folded and resting on a pillow on the bedside table (Fig. 39-7). If unable to sit up, the patient may lie on the unaffected side with the hand of the affected side raised above the shoulder.

The location where the needle is inserted depends on where the fluid is present and where the physician can best aspirate it. Once this spot is identified by the physician, the skin is prepared over the area. A local anesthetic is administered and then the needle is inserted between the ribs through the intercostal muscles and fascia and into the pleura. After the procedure, the needle or plastic catheter is removed and a small sterile dressing is placed over the entry site.

During thoracentesis, fluid or air can be removed from the pleural cavity with a syringe. Another method for removing fluid is to drain the fluid into a bottle in which a partial vacuum has been created. With this technique, a small plastic catheter may be threaded through the needle, allowing the needle to be withdrawn. This catheter reduces the possibility of puncturing the lung. When this method is used, the tubing connecting the needle and the bottle must be sterile. Commonly, a calibrated bottle is used to collect the drainage, allowing the amount of fluid removed to be determined. The maximum amount of fluid removed is generally 1,000 mL.

Nursing Responsibilities

The nurse is responsible for collecting baseline data before the procedure and preparing the patient physically and emotionally for the procedure. Instruct the patient not to cough or breathe deeply during the procedure. Urge the patient to remain as still as possible to diminish the risk for accidental injury to the lung. Administer analgesics before the procedure as ordered.

During the procedure, observe the patient's reactions. Monitor the patient's color, pulse, and respiratory rates, reporting immediately to the physician any deviation from the patient's baseline. Fainting, nausea, and vomiting may occur. Ensure that specimens, if obtained, are taken to the laboratory immediately.

After the procedure, assess the patient for changes in vital signs, particularly respirations. If a large amount of fluid was removed, respirations usually become easier. If the lung was punctured, respiratory distress becomes acute. If blood appears in the sputum or the patient has severe coughing, notify the physician promptly. A chest radiograph is usually done after the procedure to verify the absence of complications.

Diagnosing

Each nursing diagnosis statement identifies an actual or potential patient problem and suggests expected patient outcomes. The etiology of the problem directs nursing interventions. In analyzing the assessment data, determine whether the alteration in respiratory function:

- Is the problem
- Is contributing to a different problem or a sign or symptom of a problem

Alterations in Respiratory Function as the Problem

After the assessment is completed and the data are examined, the nurse concludes either that there is no problem at this time or that there is an actual or potential respiratory problem that is amenable to independent or interdependent nursing actions. Nursing diagnoses indicating alterations in respiratory function are:

- Ineffective Airway Clearance
- Ineffective Breathing Pattern
- Impaired Gas Exchange

Common etiologies for these diagnoses include an inability to maintain proper position, pain or fear of pain, viscous secretions, fatigue, decreased level of consciousness, lack of knowledge, smoking, allergy, mechanical obstruction, medications, and decreased elasticity of the lungs. Examples of these diagnoses, etiologic factors, and defining characteristics appear in Examples of NANDA Nursing Diagnoses: Oxygenation.

FIGURE 39-7. Position of the patient for thoracentesis.

Examples of NANDA Nursing Diagnoses

Oxygenation

Nursing Diagnoses	Related Factors	Sample Defining Characteristics
Ineffective Airway Clearance	Thick yellow secretions, fever, fatigue, dehydration, poor nutrition	• *"I never feel as though I am getting enough air."* • A 20-year history of COPD, with recent development of pneumonia. • Pale skin with circumoral cyanosis; respiratory rate is 40 breaths/min and shallow. Coarse crackles are auscultated bilaterally. • Cannot sit quietly in chair or on bed. Inability to walk length of room without coughing episode, which produces little sputum.
Impaired Gas Exchange	Smokes one pack per day; works with asbestos in auto factory; has had a cold for 7 days	• Cyanosis; using pursed-lip breathing • Sitting hunched forward with overbed table supporting arms. • Altered blood gases show respiratory acidosis. • Reports shortness of breath, nausea, and ankle edema for 1 week.
Ineffective Breathing Pattern	Anxious about results of cardiac catheterization and possible cardiac surgery	• Hyperventilating, tachypneic (40 breaths/minute). • *"I have a tingling feeling in my fingers."*

Alterations in Respiratory Function as the Etiology

An alteration in respiratory functioning may affect other areas of human functioning. Nursing diagnoses resulting from alterations in respiratory functioning include:

• Activity Intolerance related to shortness of breath
• Anxiety related to feeling of suffocation
• Acute Pain related to pleural inflammation
• Acute Confusion related to impaired ventilation
• Ineffective Coping related to frequent hospitalization resulting from acute symptoms of COPD
• Deficient Diversional Activity related to loss of ability to perform specific activities because of shortness of breath
• Fatigue related to impaired oxygen transport system
• Dysfunctional Grieving related to loss of normal respiratory functioning
• Ineffective Health Maintenance related to smoking
• Noncompliance (e.g., with performance of daily respiratory exercises) related to side effects of therapy
• Imbalanced Nutrition: Less Than Body Requirements, related to difficulty breathing
• Impaired Oral Mucous Membrane related to presence of endotracheal tube
• Chronic/Situational Low Self-Esteem related to loss of normal respiratory function
• Disturbed Sleep Pattern related to orthopnea and bronchodilators
• Social Isolation related to inability to walk to usual "people places"

• Risk for Suffocation related to child playing with a plastic bag
• Risk for Activity Intolerance related to COPD

Outcome Identification and Planning

When caring for patients with an alteration in respiratory function, nursing measures support the following general expected outcomes. The patient will:

• Demonstrate improved gas exchange in the lungs by an absence of cyanosis or chest pain and a pulse oximetry reading more than 95%
• Relate the causative factors, if known, and demonstrate a method of coping with these factors
• Preserve pulmonary function by maintaining an optimal level of activity
• Demonstrate self-care behaviors that provide relief from symptoms and prevent further pulmonary problems

When the patient's physical, psychosocial, and spiritual dimensions contribute to alterations in respiratory function, individualized expected outcomes are developed with the patient's input (e.g., "By March 15, the patient will be able to walk up one flight of steps at home without dyspnea.").

Implementing

Oxygen deficits, particularly in older people, impair all aspects of daily living. Going to get the mail or cleaning the house may become a monumental task for people with oxygen deficits.

Nursing interventions related to oxygenation aim to promote optimal functioning of the respiratory system, to promote comfort, and to promote and control coughing. Nurses may also need to intervene by performing chest physiotherapy, suctioning the airway, meeting respiratory needs with medications, providing supplemental oxygen, managing chest tubes, using artificial airways, clearing an obstructed airway, and administering CPR.

Promoting Optimal Function

Teaching patients with respiratory disorders about pollution-free environments is an important part of respiratory management. Most people with altered respiratory functioning experience anxiety as a result of their symptoms and the actual or potential loss of independence. It is important to minimize anxiety in patients with respiratory disorders in order to promote optimal functioning. Promoting good nutrition is another vital part of promoting optimal respiratory functioning.

Nurses should teach patients about their health conditions and provide information and support to improve health literacy by their patients. Refer to the accompanying Promoting Health Literacy box.

TEACHING ABOUT POLLUTION-FREE ENVIRONMENTS

A pollution-free environment is particularly important for individuals with respiratory problems. Teach the patient to assess the environment and make adjustments, whenever possible, to factors that impair respiratory functioning or "triggers." The patient must actively plan to prevent exposure to pollutants and triggers. This might involve a job change, use of protective equipment, requesting enforcement of laws by government agencies, or subcontracting jobs. In order to minimize triggers in the home, dusting and vacuuming the office and home must be done at least twice per week. In some situations, the patient may be asked to wear a mask to prevent some symptoms of respiratory distress. Exposure to industrial or occupational hazards (e.g., paint, varnish, gaseous fumes, asbestos) must be restricted.

In the United States, fine pollutants, including carbon monoxide, sulfur dioxide, total suspended particulates, ozone, and nitrogen dioxide that pose a hazard to health, are monitored closely. On days when pollutant levels are elevated significantly, morbidity and mortality rates among people with pre-existing pulmonary disease are increased greatly. Thus, on days when pollution alerts are announced, people with altered respiratory function should reduce their activities, stay indoors, and use an air conditioner, electronic air cleaner, or air filter. If pollen alters the patient's respiratory function, the same principles apply.

Cigarette smoking is the most important risk factor in pulmonary disease. The inhalation of cigarette smoke increases airway resistance, reduces ciliary action, increases mucus production, causes thickening of the alveolar–capillary membrane, and causes bronchial walls to thicken and lose

---

Promoting Health Literacy

IN PATIENTS WITH COPD

Patient Scenario

Nickoli Romanov, age 69, has been experiencing a morning cough for "several years," but states, "It wasn't too bad, so I lived with it." He reports increasing shortness of breath and fatigue over the last few months, with mucous production. States he has noticed increased amounts of mucous during last few weeks, and significantly increased difficulty breathing with activity. Mr. Romanov reports smoking cigarettes for 40 years, but has recently been thinking about quitting. After having a medical workup, including pulmonary function studies, Mr. Romanov was diagnosed with chronic obstructive pulmonary disease (COPD). He tells the nurse that he doesn't really think that he can use "all these medications, especially that breathing thing," and doesn't really understand what COPD is. He asks, "Do you think my smoking is making me worse?"

Nursing Considerations: *Tips for Improving Health Literacy*

Provide Mr. Romanov with easy to read information about COPD. Encourage him to ask his primary care provider as many questions as needed to understand his condition. Explain that it is a breathing problem that comes on over a long time, but there are things he can do to feel better and help keep from getting worse. Reinforce that it is important to take the medications every day and learn the right way to use inhaled medications. Provide information and resources to aid him to quit smoking. Encourage Mr. Romanov to ask his primary care provider the following three questions:

- What is my main problem?
- What do I need to do?
- Why is it important for me to do this?

What additional measures can you take to help increase health literacy in this patient? What other measures would be helpful for Mr. Romanov if he did not speak English, could not read, or had other learning deficits?

their elasticity. These effects occur in both smokers and nonsmokers (children and adults) who live with smokers. Habitual smokers usually have great difficulty quitting or reducing their smoking and need much encouragement. The American Lung Association and the American Heart Association offer many free educational materials to aid and support patients who are trying to stop smoking. Their addresses and phone numbers are listed in local telephone directories, and both agencies offer extensive information online. As a nurse, it is important to play a key role in presenting accurate information about the negative effects of smoking. Encourage the decision to stop smoking or to never start smoking.

REDUCING ANXIETY

It is important to create an environment that is likely to reduce anxiety. Help institute measures to alleviate discomfort immediately. Use effective listening skills and accurate observation to display a caring attitude. Attempt to understand the patient's life experiences and habits without judging them. Patients with harmful health habits often fear they will be judged, and this impedes the use of nursing interventions. Patients who believe nurses are genuinely concerned about them and their families are more willing to work toward achieving mutually desirable outcomes.

> ➤ *Think back to Joan McIntyre, the woman requesting to be "let go" if she should stop breathing. The nurse needs to provide support to the patient, showing genuine concern for her welfare. In addition, the nurse needs to act ethically and legally to ensure the patient's rights.* ∎

MAINTAINING GOOD NUTRITION

People who work hard at breathing often do not have much energy for eating. Many of the medications used for treatment can cause anorexia and nausea. However, maintaining an adequate nutritional intake is crucial. Assess nutritional status by measuring the patient's height, weight, upper arm circumference, serum protein levels, and nitrogen balance. Interventions should focus on ensuring an adequate intake of proteins, vitamins, and minerals. Consider the use of six small meals distributed over the course of the day instead of the usual three larger meals. Provide frequent oral hygiene and rest periods before eating to help improve the patient's intake. Meals should be eaten 1 to 2 hours after breathing treatments and exercises.

Patients who have COPD require a high protein/high calorie diet to counter malnutrition. Encourage obese patients to lose weight using a calorie-controlled diet. Diets should be 40% to 55% carbohydrates, 30% to 40% fat, and 12% to 20% protein. A diet rich in antioxidants, vitamins A and C, and the B vitamins is important. If supplemental oxygen is used, reinforce the importance of wearing the cannula during and after meals. Eating and digestion require energy, which causes the body to use more oxygen (Dudek, 2006).

Promoting Comfort

Interventions to promote patient comfort are an important part of nursing care for patients with alterations in respiratory function. Promoting proper positioning, adequate fluid intake, humidification of inspired air, and appropriate breathing techniques are used to maximize the patient's sense of well-being.

POSITIONING

Proper positioning is important to ease respirations. A proper position for breathing is a position that allows free movement of the diaphragm and expansion of the chest wall. Alternately, sitting in a slumped position permits the abdominal contents to push upward on the diaphragm, decreasing lung expansion during inspiration. People with dyspnea and orthopnea are most comfortable in a high Fowler's position because accessory muscles can easily be used to promote respiration. Research has demonstrated that, in patients with pulmonary disease who are acutely ill, turning to the prone position on a regular basis promotes oxygenation (Alsaghir & Martin, 2008; Pruitt, 2007b). In this position, the posterior dependent sections of the lungs are better ventilated and perfused. A partially prone position appears to be sufficient to achieve better ventilation while allowing access to invasive lines and the airway.

MAINTAINING ADEQUATE FLUID INTAKE

Patients can help keep their secretions thin by drinking 2 to 3 quarts (1.9 to 2.9 L) of clear fluids daily. Fluid intake should be increased to the maximum that the patient's health state can tolerate. Increased fluids are needed by patients who have an elevated temperature, who are breathing through the mouth, who are coughing, or who are losing excessive body fluids in other ways.

PROVIDING HUMIDIFIED AIR

Inspiring dry air removes the normal moisture in the respiratory passages that protect against irritation and infection. This is especially troublesome for patients who cannot breathe through their nose. When air humidity is low, it may be necessary to humidify the air with room humidifiers or vaporizers. Electric vaporizers that produce steam or cool mist are also useful, but neither device has been demonstrated to have greater therapeutic value than the other. Although a cool-mist vaporizer reduces the danger of burns because it does not generate heat or hot water, it can be a medium for pathogen growth if it is not cleaned adequately. A steam vaporizer does not present this risk for infection because the heat kills most pathogens.

Promoting Proper Breathing

Many people, both well and ill, have breathing habits that are not conducive to maximal respiratory functioning. Some people develop a pattern of shallow breathing or walk with a posture that makes the chest wall appear caved in, affecting chest expansion. Ill people may limit their respiratory efforts to compensate for disease symptoms or an illness. Breathing

Examples of Nursing Interventions and Nursing Outcomes Classifications (NIC/NOC)
Ventilation Assistance

Nursing Interventions

- Maintain a patent airway
- Auscultate breath sounds, noting areas of decreased or absent ventilation, and presence of adventitious sounds
- Initiate and maintain supplemental oxygen, as prescribed
- Administer appropriate pain medication to prevent hypoventilation
- Ambulate three to four times per day, as appropriate
- Monitor respiratory and oxygenation status
- Administer medications (e.g., bronchodilators and inhalers) that promote airway patency and gas exchange
- Teach pursed-lip breathing techniques, as appropriate
- Initiate a program of respiratory muscle strength and/or endurance training, as appropriate

Nursing Outcomes

- Respiratory Status: Gas Exchange
- Tissue Perfusion: Pulmonary
- Respiratory Status: Ventilation
- Vital Signs
- Cardiopulmonary Status
- Tissue Perfusion: Cellular

From Bulechek, G., Butcher, H., & McCloskey Dochterman, J. (Eds.). (2008). *Nursing interventions classification (NIC)* (5th ed., p. 336). St. Louis: Mosby Elsevier; and Moorhead, S., Johnson, M., Maas, M., & Swanson, E. (Eds.). (2008). *Nursing outcomes classification (NOC)* (5th ed., p. 746). A full listing of nursing activities for each nursing intervention and outcomes can be found in these books.

exercises are designed to help patients achieve more efficient and controlled ventilations, to decrease the work of breathing, and to correct respiratory deficits. The accompanying Nursing Intervention and Nursing Outcome Classifications (NIC/NOC) box lists standardized nursing interventions and corresponding outcomes related to maximizing oxygen and carbon dioxide exchange in the lungs. Specific techniques are described below.

DEEP BREATHING

When hypoventilation occurs, a decreased amount of air enters and leaves the lungs. However, deep-breathing exercises can be used to overcome hypoventilation.

Instruct the patient to make each breath deep enough to move the bottom ribs. Unless the patient has a nasal condition that prohibits or prevents normal breathing, have the patient start slowly taking deep ventilations nasally and then expiring slowly through the mouth. Breathing through the nose warms, filters, and humidifies the air. The patient's respiratory status, motivation, and general clinical condition dictate the timing of this exercise, which should be done hourly while awake or four times daily.

USING INCENTIVE SPIROMETRY

Incentive spirometry provides visual reinforcement for deep breathing by the patient. An incentive spirometer assists the patient to breathe slowly and deeply and to sustain maximal inspiration. The gauge on the spirometer allows the patient to measure her own progress, providing immediate positive reinforcement. It encourages the patient to maximize lung inflation and prevent or reduce atelectasis. Optimal gas exchange is supported Promoting secretions can be cleared and expectorated. Before using incentive spirometry equipment,

the patient needs instructions on using the equipment properly. Validate the patient's correct use of this equipment in both healthcare and home environments. See Guidelines for Nursing Care 39-1, for teaching patients to use this device.

PURSED-LIP BREATHING

Patients who experience dyspnea and feelings of panic can often reduce these symptoms by using pursed-lip breathing. Exhaling through pursed lips creates a smaller opening for air movement, effectively slowing and prolonging expiration. Prolonged expiration is thought to result in decreased airway narrowing during expiration and prevent the collapse of small airways. This results in improved air exchange and decreased dyspnea. Pursed-lip breathing also helps the patient to control the rate and depth of respiration, helping to reduce feelings of dyspnea. It also encourages relaxation, which aids the patient to gain control of dyspnea and reduce feelings of panic. Encourage patients with COPD to try this breathing technique to help manage their daily activities (Smeltzer et al., 2010).

While sitting upright, the patient inhales through the nose while counting to three and then exhales slowly and evenly against pursed lips while tightening the abdominal muscles. During exhalation, the patient counts to seven. To purse the lips, the patient should position the lips as though he or she was sucking through a straw or whistling. When walking and using pursed lip breathing, the patient should inhale while taking two steps and then exhale through pursed lips while taking the next four steps, and then repeat the cycle. Before teaching these techniques, practice them alone and then with a partner.

ABDOMINAL OR DIAPHRAGMATIC BREATHING

Many people with COPD breathe in a shallow, rapid, and exhausting pattern. Teach the patient with COPD to change

Guidelines for Nursing Care • 39-1

TEACHING PATIENTS TO USE AN INCENTIVE SPIROMETER

- Assist the patient to an upright position if possible.
- Remove dentures if they fit poorly.
- Administer ordered pain medication if needed.
- Demonstrate how to steady device with one hand and hold mouthpiece with other hand.
- Instruct the patient to exhale normally and then place lips securely around mouthpiece.
- Instruct the patient not to breathe through his or her nose. Use a nose clip if necessary.
- Instruct the patient to inhale slowly, and as deeply as possible, through the mouthpiece.
- Tell the patient to hold breath and count to three. Check position of gauge to determine progress and level attained.
- Instruct the patient to remove lips from mouthpiece and exhale normally.

- Tell the patient to complete breathing exercises about 10 times every hour if possible. Rest in between breaths as necessary.

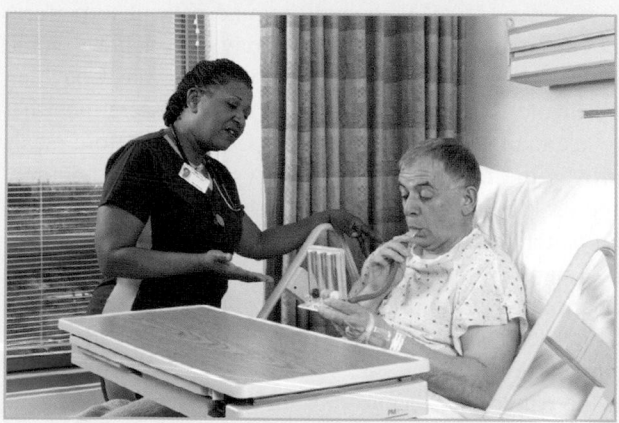

this type of upper chest breathing to another form of breathing, diaphragmatic breathing. Diaphragmatic breathing reduces the respiratory rate, increases tidal volume, and reduces functional residual capacity.

To do this, the patient places one hand on the stomach and the other on the middle of the chest. He or she breathes in slowly through the nose, letting the abdomen protrude as far as it will go. Then the patient breathes out through pursed lips while contracting the abdominal muscles, with one hand pressing inward and upward on the abdomen. He or she repeats these steps for 1 minute, followed by a rest for 2 minutes. Encourage the patient to practice this breathing pattern several times during the day, so that eventually it becomes automatic.

Promoting and Controlling Coughing

A cough is a cleansing mechanism of the body. It is a means of helping to keep the airway clear of secretions and other debris. A cough that is dry is termed a nonproductive cough. A cough that produces respiratory secretions is termed a productive cough. The respiratory secretion expelled by coughing or clearing the throat is called **sputum.**

When the patient has excessive fluids or secretions in an organ or body tissue, the patient is said to be congested. Thus, a person with secretions or fluid in the lungs is said to have congested lungs. If the cough is dry, the patient is said to be congested with a nonproductive cough. If the cough produces sputum, the patient is said to be congested with a productive cough. Thick respiratory secretions are sometimes called phlegm. A patient who is coughing and does not have any congestion or secretions produced is said to be noncongested with a nonproductive cough.

A series of events produce a cough. The cough mechanism (Fig. 39-8) consists of an initial irritation; a deep

inspiration; a quick, tight closure of the glottis together with a forceful contraction of the expiratory intercostal muscles; and an upward push of the diaphragm. This causes an explosive movement of air from the lower to the upper respiratory tract. To be effective, a cough should have enough muscle contraction to force air to be expelled and to propel a liquid or a solid on its way out of the respiratory tract. Coughing is most effective when the patient is sitting upright with feet flat on the floor. Coughing can be voluntary or involuntary.

VOLUNTARY COUGHING

When a cough does not occur as a result of reflex stimulation of the cough-sensitive areas, it can be induced voluntarily.

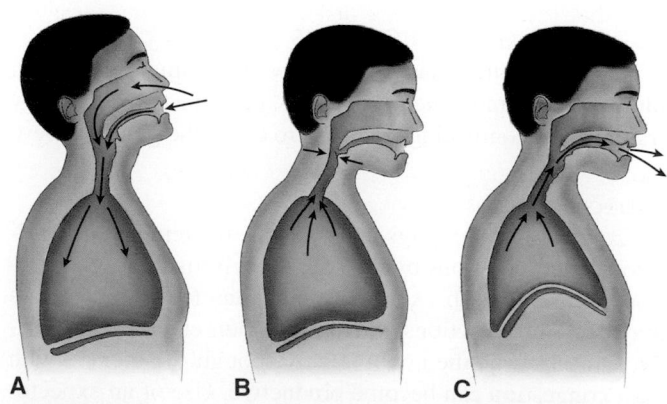

FIGURE 39-8. (**A**) A cough begins with a deep inspiration, distending the trachea and hyperinflating the lungs. (**B**) After inspiration, the glottis closes while intercostal and abdominal muscles contract forcibly. (**C**) When intrathoracic pressure reaches a high level, the glottis opens slightly, and the diaphragm is pushed up, producing an explosive movement of air.

Teaching the patient to cough voluntarily is an important aspect of preoperative and postoperative care. Coughing is more effective when combined with deep breathing. Although teaching a patient to cough and deep breathe is relatively easy, experience has shown that it is difficult to motivate patients to follow through and perform coughing on their own. Refer to Guidelines for Nursing Care 30-2 (Chapter 30), Effective Coughing, for detailed instructions for teaching this intervention. Frequently remind patients to perform effective coughing throughout the day. Develop a specific schedule for coughing on the patient's plan of care. Coughing early in the morning after rising removes secretions that have accumulated during the night. Coughing before meals improves the taste of food and oxygenation. At bedtime, coughing removes any buildup of secretions and improves sleep patterns. For a patient who is unable to cough voluntarily, manual stimulation over the trachea and prolonged exhalation can be helpful. If neither of these methods is successful, mechanical endotracheal suctioning with a catheter may be necessary.

If the patient has a neuromuscular disorder and is unable to cough physically, an assisted cough may be used. For an assisted cough, firm pressure is placed on the abdomen below the diaphragm in rhythm with exhalation. This pressure is similar to the Heimlich maneuver but with less force. This pressure is used to substitute for the weakened or paralyzed abdominal muscles.

INVOLUNTARY COUGHING

Involuntary coughing often accompanies respiratory tract infections and irritations. Many times respiratory infections lead to the production of respiratory secretions. These secretions can trigger the cough mechanism. When the cough is productive, it helps clear the airway. However, when the cough is nonproductive, it can be fatiguing and irritating. Medications may control involuntary coughing. Refer to the section below, Cough Suppressants. Observation of the patient's breathing and coughing characteristics is necessary to determine the appropriate type of medication.

USING COUGH MEDICATIONS

Various medications can be used to promote coughing, aiding in the movement of mucus through the respiratory tract, and in controlling coughing to allow the patient to rest.

Expectorants

Expectorants are drugs that facilitate the removal of respiratory tract secretions by reducing the viscosity of the secretions. Patients with extremely tenacious (thick) secretions may need the secretions liquefied for their cough to be effective. In that way, the nonproductive cough of a person with lung congestion can become productive. Use of an expectorant by a person without congestion is inappropriate. Guaifenesin is widely used as an expectorant in cold and cough medications (e.g., Robitussin). Adequate fluid intake and air humidification are considered effective expectorants by some authorities.

Cough Suppressants

Suppressants are drugs that depress a body function—in this case, the cough reflex. Codeine, which is present in many cough preparations, is generally considered the preferred cough suppressant ingredient. However, codeine can be addictive, and because of possible abuse, many states require a prescription for its use. Drowsiness (also common with antihistamines) is a side effect, so it may not be safe to use codeine when the person must remain alert, such as when driving a car. A suppressant that is not addictive is dextromethorphan, which can be found in many over-the-counter cold and cough remedies.

An irritating, nonproductive cough in people without congestion may be treated appropriately with suppressants. Suppression of the productive cough is usually not recommended unless the patient is trying to sleep. If a productive cough is suppressed, secretions can be retained, leading to a pulmonary infection.

Lozenges

Cough lozenges can often relieve mild, nonproductive coughs in people without congestion. A lozenge is a small, solid medication intended to be held in the mouth until it dissolves. Lozenges generally control coughs by the local anesthetic effect of benzocaine. The local anesthetic acts on sensory and motor nerves, controlling the primary irritation and inhibiting afferent and efferent impulses.

Teaching About Cough Medications

Cough medications are readily available, and people who purchase them are usually eager for relief. Often, consumers take excessive amounts of more than one type. Teach about the appropriate choice of expectorants and suppressants and about misuse of cough mixtures. For example, cough syrups with a high sugar or alcohol content can disturb the metabolic balance of patients with diabetes mellitus or can trigger a relapse for recovering alcoholics. Preparations containing antihistamines have an anticholinergic action, which can cause serious problems for people with glaucoma or cause urinary retention in men with prostate enlargement. Other cough preparations can be detrimental to people with hypertension or thyroid or cardiac diseases. In addition, prolonged use of self-prescribed cough preparations can conceal more serious health problems. If a cough lasts more than 7 days, urge the person to contact a physician. In addition, encourage the person to increase fluid intake if the secretions become too thick to expectorate.

Performing Chest Physiotherapy

Chest physiotherapy helps loosen and mobilize secretions, increasing mucous clearance. This is especially helpful for patients with large amounts of secretions or an ineffective cough. Chest physiotherapy includes percussion, vibration, and postural drainage.

PERCUSSION

Percussion of lung areas involves the use of a cupped palm to loosen pulmonary secretions so that they can be

FIGURE 39-9. (**A**) The cupping position and action of the hand on manual percussion of the lung area. (**B**) The position and action of the hands necessary to use vibration to loosen respiratory secretions in the lungs. *(Photos by B. Proud.)*

expectorated with greater ease. With the hand held in a rigid, dome-shaped position (Fig. 39-9), strike the area over the lung lobes to be drained in a rhythmic pattern. Position the patient in a lateral, supine, or prone position, based on the lobes to be treated. Proper hand and patient positioning will ensure that the patient does not experience any pain with this procedure. Percussion is never done on bare skin or performed over surgical incisions, below the ribs, or over the spine or breasts because of the danger of tissue damage. Typically, each area is percussed for 30 to 60 seconds several times a day. If the patient has tenacious secretions, the area may be percussed for up to 3 to 5 minutes several times per day. Patients may learn how to percuss the anterior surfaces of their own chest wall. In addition, it is a good idea to teach family members how to percuss posterior surfaces. Mechanical devices as well as manual handheld cupping devices also are available for percussion on the chest wall.

VIBRATING

Vibration uses manual compression and tremor on the patient's chest wall to help loosen respiratory secretions. Loosened secretions can be expectorated more easily. The practitioner uses rhythmic contraction and relaxation of arm and shoulder muscles while holding the hands flat on the patient's chest wall as the patient exhales. Vibration can be done for several minutes, several times a day. To avoid causing patient discomfort, vibration is never done over the patient's breasts, spine, sternum, and lower rib cage. Vibration (see Fig. 39-9) can also be taught to family members or accomplished using a mechanical device.

PROVIDING POSTURAL DRAINAGE

Postural drainage makes use of gravity to drain secretions from the lungs. Position the patient in a way that promotes the drainage of secretions from smaller pulmonary branches into larger ones, where they can be removed by coughing (Fig. 39-10). Vibration, percussion, or both often precede postural drainage.

When implementing postural drainage, have tissues and an emesis basin close at hand for the patient to use when coughing and expectorating secretions. Place the patient in

an appropriate position to promote drainage from the lobes of the lungs. Postural drainage should be done two to four times a day for 20 to 30 minutes. Discontinue the drainage if the patient begins to feel weak or faint. Delay postural drainage for 1 to 2 hours after meals to avoid provoking vomiting. Appropriate positioning to achieve postural drainage is as follows:

- Use high Fowler's position to drain the apical sections of the upper lobes of the lungs.
- Place the patient in a lying position, half on the abdomen and half on the side, right and left, to drain the posterior sections of the upper lobes of the lungs.
- Place the patient lying on the left side with a pillow under the chest wall to drain the right lobe of the lung.
- Place the patient in the Trendelenburg position to drain the lower lobes of the lungs.

Suctioning the Airway

If a patient is unable to remove secretions with coughing, aspirate secretions with a suctioning device. If the patient is able to raise secretions from the airways but unable to clear from the mouth, suctioning of the oropharynx or nasopharynx may be indicated, as demonstrated in Skill 39-2. If the patient is unable to raise secretions from the airways, tracheal suctioning may be indicated. Tracheal suctioning may be performed by passing a sterile catheter through the mouth (orotracheal) or through the nose (nasotracheal). It may also be passed through a tracheostomy or endotracheal tube (discussed later in the chapter). Suctioning to remove secretions is performed using the sterile technique as described in Chapter 27, Asepsis and Infection Control. The frequency of suctioning varies with the amount of secretions present but should be done often enough to keep ventilation effective and as effortless as possible. The suction catheter should be small enough not to occlude the airway being suctioned but large enough to remove secretions. Several sizes of catheters are available.

Suctioning irritates the mucosa and removes oxygen from the respiratory tract, possibly causing **hypoxemia** (insufficient oxygen in the blood). Thus, it is important to pre-oxygenate the

FIGURE 39-10. Postural drainage. Shown are four positions that use the force of gravity to assist the drainage of secretions from the smaller bronchial airways into the main bronchi and trachea so the patient is able to cough them up.

patient before suctioning. This is accomplished by applying or increasing supplemental oxygen and having the patient take several deep breaths before inserting the catheter.

When performed correctly, suctioning provides comfort by relieving respiratory distress. When performed incorrectly, it can increase anxiety and pain and cause respiratory arrest. At minimum, it is an uncomfortable procedure and it can be a very painful and/or distressing experience. Individualized pain management must be performed in response to the patient's needs (Arroyo-Novoa et al., 2007). Anticipate the administration of analgesic medication to a patient who has had surgery or other trauma before suctioning, because the cough reflex will be stimulated. Possible complications of suctioning include infection, cardiac arrhythmias, hypoxia, mucosal trauma, and death.

Wear gloves on both hands, goggles, and a mask, and a gown, if necessary, for protection from microorganisms. Continuously monitor the patient's color and heart rate and the color, amount, and consistency of secretions. If cyanosis, an excessively slow or rapid heart rate, or suddenly bloody secretions are noted, stop suctioning immediately, administer oxygen, and notify the physician. Cyanosis and a change in heart rate can indicate hypoxemia. Blood can indicate damage to the mucosa.

Meeting Respiratory Needs With Medications

Although treating patients with medications is a dependent nursing intervention, monitoring the patient's response and

development of side effects to medications is an independent nursing action. Table 39-2 lists some common medications for improving respiratory functioning, their side effects, and nursing implications. Many of the drugs used to dilate bronchial airways interact with caffeine. Encourage patients to avoid caffeine, which may potentiate the side effects of bronchodilators.

ADMINISTERING INHALED MEDICATIONS

Inhaled medications may be administered to open narrowed airways (**bronchodilators**), to liquefy or loosen thick secretions (mucolytic agents), or to reduce inflammation in airways (corticosteroids). These medications typically are administered via nebulizer, metered-dose inhaler, or dry powder inhaler.

Nebulizers disperse fine particles of liquid medication into the deeper passages of the respiratory tract, where absorption occurs. The treatment continues until all the medication in the nebulizer cup has been inhaled.

A **metered-dose inhaler (MDI)** delivers a controlled dose of medication with each compression of the canister. Common mistakes that patients make when using MDIs include the following:

- Failing to shake the canister
- Holding the inhaler upside down
- Inhaling through the nose rather than the mouth
- Inhaling too rapidly
- Stopping the inhalation when the cold propellant is felt in the throat

Medications	Activity	Route	Side Effects	Nursing Implications
TABLE • 39-2 SELECTED MEDICATIONS USED TO IMPROVE RESPIRATORY FUNCTION				
Zafirlukast (Accolate)	Bronchodilator	PO	Headache, dizziness, nausea, vomiting	Not used to treat acute attacks.
Montelukast (Singulair)	Also inhibits leukotriene release as well as inflammatory reaction			Do not give Accolate with meals. Singulair should be given before bedtime.
Albuterol	Bronchodilator	PO, inhalation	Tremors, anxiety, insomnia, headache, palpitations, hypertension, vomiting	Caution patient not to increase dosage without consulting physician. Be aware that children 2–6 years of age more frequently exhibit CNS stimulation.
Theophylline (Aminophylline)	Bronchodilator	PO, IV, rectally	Nausea, vomiting, tachycardia, diuresis, irritability, vertigo, convulsions, nervousness	Monitor vital signs closely. Force fluids as clinical status allows. Monitor serum theophylline levels, especially if patient does not respond to drug or if severe side effects develop.
Corticosteroids (prednisone, dexamethasone, budesonide, triamcinolone acetonide)	Reduces inflammation	PO, IV, inhalation, intranasal	Fluid retention, hypertension, mood swings, weight gain, gastritis hyperglycemia, insomnia	Reduce sodium intake. Make patient and family aware of potential for labile emotions. Weigh daily in morning. Monitor blood pressure and blood sugar.
Diphenhydramine (Benadryl)	Antihistamine H₁-, receptor antagonist	PO	Drowsiness, anorexia, dry mouth, constipation, blurred vision, urinary retention	Warn patient to use only with physician's advice in presence of bronchial asthma.
Cetirizine (Zyrtec)	Antihistamine H₁-, receptor antagonist	PO	Headache with limited sedative effect, not associated with anticholinergic effects	Monitor effectiveness of drug. Contraindicated while breastfeeding.
Fexofenadine (Allegra)	Antihistamine H₁-, receptor antagonist	PO	Headache, not associated with anticholinergic or sedative effects	
Cromolyn sodium (Intal)	Mast cell stabilizer Asthma prophylactic agent—no bronchodilator, antihistamine, or vasoconstrictor properties	Inhalation—MDI or nasal solution	Cough, nausea, nasal stinging and burning, throat irritation	Remind patient this is used to prevent asthma attacks, not to treat acute episodes. Inform patient that drug is effective only if taken routinely (2–4 times per week). Safety not established during pregnancy and breastfeeding.

CNS, central nervous system; PO, orally; IV, intravenously.

- Failing to hold their breath after inhalation
- Inhaling two sprays with one breath

To use an MDI, the patient must activate the device while continuing to inhale. For some patients, especially young children and older adults, a spacer or extender device may be necessary to aid delivery of medication by the inhalation route. The spacer acts as a reservoir. When the MDI is compressed, the medication is deposited in the reservoir, and the patient then inhales the medication from the spacer device. This makes administration less complicated and the dose more predictable.

Dry powder inhalers (DPI) are another type of delivery method for inhaled medications. DPIs are breath activated. A quick deep breath by the patient activates the flow of medication, eliminating the need to coordinate activating the inhaler (spraying the medicine) while inhaling the medicine at the same time. DPIs require less manual dexterity than does an MDI. DPIs are actuated by the patient's inspiration, so there is no need to coordinate the delivery of puffs with inhalation. Many types of DPIs are available with distinctive operating instructions. Some have to be loaded with a dose of medication each time they are used. Some hold a preloaded number of doses. It is important to understand the particular instructions for the medication being used. One disadvantage of DPIs is that the medication in DPIs will clump if exposed to humidity.

> ➤ *Remember Tyrone, the 12-year-old boy with suspected asthma. During this acute attack, the nurse would anticipate administering bronchodilators via a nebulizer. The physician may order bronchodilators to be administered at home using a nebulizer or possibly an MDI with a spacer or dry powder inhaler.* ■

TEACHING PATIENTS ABOUT INHALED MEDICATIONS

Patients need repeated instruction on how to use inhalers and nebulizers effectively and safely. Overuse may result in serious side effects and eventual ineffectiveness of the medication. Information about how to use MDIs, DPIs, and small-volume nebulizers properly, including patient teaching information, is provided in Chapter 29, Guidelines for Nursing Care 29-11. Package inserts with the medication also reinforce correct technique for using inhalers.

To ensure correct administration when a spacer is used, slow, deep inspirations are necessary. To prevent inhaling too quickly, some spacers are equipped with a whistle device that sounds if inhalation is too rapid. A spacer is also recommended for patients using corticosteroid inhaled agents because it reduces the risk of acquiring an oral fungal infection.

Providing Supplemental Oxygen

Providing a supplemental oxygen supply via oxygen therapy can increase the amount of oxygen transported in the blood.

Oxygen is considered a medication and must be ordered by a healthcare provider. Oxygen therapy can be intimidating or frighten patients. Therefore, provide clear explanations about the procedures and purpose to help reduce anxiety. Encourage patients to discuss concerns. If oxygen is given in an emergency, explanations concurrent with administration are appropriate.

SOURCES OF OXYGEN

Therapeutic oxygen is supplied from a wall outlet or a portable cylinder. A specially designed flow meter is attached to the wall outlet (see Skill 39-3 for an illustration of a flow meter). A valve regulates the oxygen flow in liters per minute. To release oxygen safely and at the desired rate from a cylinder or tank, a regulator is used. The regulator has two gauges. The one nearest the tank shows the pressure or amount of oxygen in the tank. The other gauge indicates the number of liters per minute of oxygen being released. In patients with chronic respiratory insufficiency who use oxygen on a daily basis at home, having to transport an oxygen canister can impede their functional exercise capacity. The portable canister's weight and increased respiratory and skeletal muscle load contributes an additional burden for these patients. A small walking aid may be suggested to reduce the patient's burden. Refer to the accompanying Research in Nursing box.

Oxygen concentrators are another way to provide oxygen. This oxygen delivery system concentrates room air to provide the appropriate concentration of oxygen to the patient. They are used frequently in home situations.

OXYGEN FLOW RATE

The flow rate of oxygen, measured in liters per minute, determines the amount of oxygen delivered to the patient. The rate varies depending on the condition of the patient and the route of administration of the oxygen. The flow rate does not necessarily reflect the oxygen concentration actually inspired by the patient because there is leaking and mixing with atmospheric air. If more precise doses are necessary, they are usually prescribed in terms of percentage of inspired oxygen. To regulate the oxygen percentage concentration accurately, samples of the air mixture the patient is actually inhaling should be analyzed every 4 hours. Several types of commercial oxygen analyzers are available.

The physician's written order prescribes the rate of oxygen administration. Closely monitor the flow rate for patients with chronic lung conditions, such as emphysema. Normally, excessive levels of carbon dioxide in the blood stimulate the patient to breathe. However, the chemoreceptors of some, but not all, patients with chronic lung disease become insensitive to carbon dioxide and respond to hypoxia to stimulate breathing (McGlolin, 2008). If excessive oxygen is given, the stimulus to breathe is removed; as a result, the patient may stop breathing completely. Monitor arterial blood gas results closely for changes. Many times, continuous pulse oximetry also is used to monitor the patient receiving oxygen.

RESEARCH IN NURSING
Bridging the Gap to Evidence-Based Practice

THE EFFECTS OF A WALKING AID FOR PATIENTS USING PORTABLE OXYGEN AT HOME

Patients with COPD have reduction in functional exercise capacity as their disease progresses. The patient's dyspnea may become so disabling that they reduce exercise and activity, becoming increasingly sedentary. Even participation in activities of daily living is affected. It is very important to preserve the ability to participate in walking, the preferred exercise for patients with COPD, and the ability to maintain self-care. The use of a heavy portable oxygen canister can produce a limitation of functional exercise due to its weight and the increased demand on the respiratory and skeletal muscles related to pulling it.

Related Research

Crisafulli, E., Costi, S., DeBlasio, F., Biscione, G., Americi, F., Penza, S., et al. (2007). Effects of a walking aid in COPD patients receiving oxygen therapy. *CHEST, 131*(4), 1068–1074.

This study looked at whether a simple walking aid may improve the physical performance in COPD patients with chronic respiratory insufficiency who usually carry their own heavy oxygen canister. Sixty stable COPD patients with chronic respiratory

insufficiency randomly performed a standardized 6-minute walking test on two consecutive days. The patients were asked to walk using two different modalities: with a full-weight oxygen canister transported using a small wheeled cart and pulled by the patient (Aid modality) and with a full-weight oxygen canister carried on the patient's shoulder (No-aid modality). The distance walked, peak effort dyspnea, and leg fatigue for each patient, as well as cardiorespiratory parameters were recorded during both tests. A significant difference between the two tests occurred for all the measured outcomes in favor of the Aid modality.

Relevance to Nursing Practice

A simple walking aid may be helpful in COPD patients receiving long-term outpatient oxygen therapy. The use of this type of device could help improve patients' tolerance for activity, exercise, and participation in activities of daily living, improving their quality of life. Nurses engage in patient teaching as a part of patient care and could incorporate this simple intervention as part of that teaching for patients with chronic lung disease.

For additional research, visit thePoint.

HUMIDIFICATION

Most institutions do not require humidification with very low-flow oxygen (2 L/min or less) delivered by nasal cannula (see oxygen delivery systems below) when administered to adults. However, because oxygen dries and dehydrates the respiratory mucous membranes, humidifying devices (supplying 20% to 40% humidity) are commonly used when oxygen is delivered at higher flow rates. Distilled or sterile water is commonly used to humidify oxygen. When moving patients receiving humidified oxygen, make sure that water from the humidifier does not enter the tubing through which the oxygen is flowing. Additional suggestions for transporting a patient with a portable oxygen tank are given in Guidelines for Nursing Care 39-2.

PRECAUTIONS FOR OXYGEN ADMINISTRATION

Oxygen, which constitutes 21% of normal air, is a tasteless, odorless, and colorless gas. It supports combustion. To prevent fires and injuries, take the following precautions:

- Avoid open flames in the patient's room.
- Place "no smoking" signs in conspicuous places in the patient's home. Instruct the patient and visitors about the hazard of smoking when oxygen is in use.
- Check to see that electrical equipment used in the room, such as electric bell cords, razors, radios, and suctioning equipment, is in good working order and emits no sparks.
- Avoid wearing and using synthetic fabrics that build up static electricity.
- Avoid using oils in the area. Oil can ignite spontaneously in the presence of oxygen.

OXYGEN DELIVERY SYSTEMS

Oxygen can be administered by many different delivery systems: nasal cannula, nasopharyngeal catheter, transtracheal catheter, simple mask, partial rebreather mask, nonrebreather mask, Venturi mask, and tent. Table 39-3 compares several oxygen delivery systems.

Nasal Cannula

A **nasal cannula,** also called nasal prongs, is the most commonly used oxygen delivery device. The cannula is a disposable plastic device with two protruding prongs that are inserted into the nostrils. The cannula is connected to an oxygen source with a flow meter and, many times, a humidifier. The cannula does not impede eating or speaking and is used easily in the home. Disadvantages of this system are that it can be dislodged easily and can cause dryness of the nasal mucosa. Skill 39-3 describes oxygen administration by nasal cannula.

Nasopharyngeal Catheter

A nasopharyngeal catheter is another efficient means for administering oxygen, but it is infrequently used because it is uncomfortable for the patient and may cause trauma to respiratory mucous membranes. It is inserted into the nose through one nostril, with the end of the catheter resting in the oropharynx. The catheter must be removed for cleaning and changed to the other nostril every 12 to 24 hours (Eastwood, Gardner, & O'Connell, 2007). Gastric distention often occurs because the gas flow can be misdirected into the stomach.

Face Masks

Disposable and reusable face masks are available. The mask is fitted carefully to the patient's face to avoid leakage of

Guidelines for Nursing Care • 39-2

TRANSPORTING A PATIENT WITH A PORTABLE OXYGEN CYLINDER

Before the Transfer

- Check that an additional oxygen source is available where the patient is being transferred.
- Check the amount of oxygen in the cylinder (place cylinder key or wrench on valve stem and turn fully counterclockwise until needle on gauge indicates amount of available oxygen; turn the key back a half turn; use cylinder only if gauge indicates more than 500 psi).
- If available, use a table that gives the estimated minutes of available oxygen according to the amount of oxygen in the cylinder and the rate of flow ordered for the patient. This can help to determine whether the supply of oxygen is adequate for the transfer (Davis & Johnston, 2008).
- Connect the oxygen tubing or a humidifier bottle with tubing to the flow meter adapter and adjust the flow-control dial to the prescribed setting.
- Attach the patient's oxygen cannula to transport oxygen.
- Ensure that the cylinder is secured in a holder before transporting the patient (it is a dangerous practice to place the cylinder between the patient's legs or next to the patient during transfer because injury to the patient may result). If a humidifier is used, ensure that cylinder remains upright.
- Place coiled tubing under a pillow or attach it to linen or a patient's gown.

After the Transfer

- Attach the patient's oxygen cannula to wall oxygen.
- Turn off the oxygen flow from the cylinder by turning the cylinder key clockwise until it is tight.
- Remove any excess oxygen in the pressure gauge by "bleeding" it. Turn the flow-control dial back on until hissing sound stops and needle on gauge has fallen to zero. Turn flow-control dial off.

oxygen and should be comfortably snug but not tight against the face. The most commonly used types of masks are the simple face mask, the partial rebreather mask, the nonrebreather mask, and the Venturi mask. Skill 39-4 describes the actions and rationales involved in using face masks.

The simple face mask is connected to oxygen tubing, a humidifier, and a flow meter, just like the nasal cannula. This mask has vents on its sides that allow room air to leak in at many places, thereby diluting the source oxygen. The vents also allow exhaled carbon dioxide to escape. Often a simple mask is used when an increased delivery of oxygen is needed for short periods (e.g., less than 12 hours). The mask should fit closely to the face to deliver this higher concentration of oxygen effectively. Patients may have difficulty keeping the mask in position over the nose and mouth, and because of this pressure and the presence of moisture, skin

breakdown is a possibility. Eating or talking with the mask in place can be difficult. Because of the risk of retaining carbon dioxide, never apply the simple face mask with a delivery flow rate of less than 5 liters per minute.

The partial rebreather mask is similar to a simple face mask, but is equipped with a reservoir bag for the collection of the first part of the patient's exhaled air. The remaining exhaled air exits through vents. The air in the reservoir is mixed with 100% oxygen for the next inhalation. Thus, the patient rebreathes about one third of the expired air from the reservoir bag. This type of mask permits the conservation of oxygen. An additional advantage is that the patient can inhale room air through openings in the mask if the oxygen supply is briefly interrupted. The disadvantages are those of any mask: eating and talking are difficult, a tight seal is required, and there is the potential for skin breakdown. Monitor the

TABLE • 39-3   OXYGEN DELIVERY SYSTEMS

Method	Amount Delivered FiO₂ (Fraction Inspired Oxygen)	Priority Nursing Interventions
Nasal cannula	*Low Flow* 1 L/min = 24% 2 L/min = 28% 3 L/min = 32% 4 L/min = 36% 5 L/min = 40% 6 L/min = 44%	Check frequently that both prongs are in patient's nares. May be no more than 2–3 L/min to patient with chronic lung disease.
Simple mask	*Low Flow* 6–10 L/min = 35%–60% (5 L/min is minimum setting)	Monitor patient frequently to check placement of the mask. Support patient if claustrophobia is a concern. Secure physician's order to replace mask with nasal cannula during mealtime.
Partial rebreather mask	*Low Flow* 6–15 L/min = 70%–90%	Set flow rate so that mask remains two-thirds full during inspiration. Keep reservoir bag free of twists or kinks.
Nonrebreather mask	*Low Flow* 6–15 L/min = 60%–100%	Maintain flow rate so reservoir bag collapses only slightly during inspiration. Check that valves and rubber flaps are functioning properly (open during expiration and closed during inhalation). Monitor SaO₂ with pulse oximeter.
Venturi mask	*High Flow* 4–10 L/min = 24%–55%	Requires careful monitoring to verify FiO₂ at flow rate ordered. Check that air intake valves are not blocked.

reservoir bag carefully. It should deflate slightly with inspiration; if it deflates completely, the flow rate should be increased until only a slight deflation is noted.

The nonrebreather mask delivers the highest concentration of oxygen via a mask to a spontaneously breathing patient. It is similar to the partial rebreather mask except two one-way valves prevent the patient from rebreathing exhaled air. The reservoir bag is filled with oxygen that enters the mask on inspiration. Exhaled air escapes through side vents. A malfunction of the bag could cause carbon dioxide buildup and suffocation. This mask can also be used to administer other gases, such as heliox. Heliox is a mixture of helium and oxygen, used to reduce the work of breathing, deliver aerosols, and reduce fear and anxiety for patients in respiratory distress. Helium has a very low density that allows it to flow easily into narrow or twisty air passages, delivering nebulized medications into the lower airways. In addition, carbon dioxide diffuses through helium at four to five times the rate it diffuses through room air, so it can exit the body faster and easier (Pruitt, 2007a).

The Venturi mask gets its name from the Venturi effect, which allows the mask to deliver the most precise concentrations of oxygen. This mask has a large tube with an oxygen inlet. As the tube narrows, the pressure drops, causing air to be pulled in through side ports. These ports are adjusted according to the prescription for oxygen concentration. Be sure that the ports are always open. If these are occluded by linens, clothing, or a patient rolling on the mask, the oxygen delivered might be at an unsafe (too high or too low) concentration.

Oxygen Tent

Oxygen also can be administered by way of an oxygen tent. An oxygen tent is a light, portable structure made of clear plastic and attached to a motor-driven unit. The motor helps to circulate and cool the air in the tent. The cooling device functions like an electric refrigeration unit. A thermostat in the unit keeps the tent at the temperature considered most comfortable for the patient. The tent fits over the top part of the bed so that the patient's head and thorax are inside. It has side openings through which nursing care can be administered. Because the tent is highly humidified and covers most of the patient's gown and linens, check the patient frequently to prevent the patient from lying in a wet bed. Although an oxygen tent is commonly used with children who need a cool and highly humidified airflow (e.g., children with pneumonia), the tent does not allow the maintenance of a satisfactory or precise oxygen concentration, so it is rarely used with other patients.

OXYGEN THERAPY IN THE HOME

Liquid oxygen and oxygen concentrators, rather than cylinders, are used more commonly in the home setting. Liquid oxygen is kept inside a small thermal container that can be refilled from a larger storage tank kept in the home. An oxygen concentrator removes nitrogen from the room air and concentrates the oxygen left in the air. The oxygen concentrator needs a power source such as an electrical outlet or battery pack. Oxygen concentrators are portable, cost-effective, and easy to use but cannot deliver oxygen flow at greater than 4 L/min (fraction of inspired oxygen [FiO_2] of about 36%).

Patients using continuous supplemental oxygen therapy in the home have another alternative: transtracheal oxygen delivery (Fig. 39-11). With this type of delivery system, a small catheter is inserted into the trachea under local anesthesia, and then the catheter is attached to the oxygen source. A transtracheal catheter does not interfere with talking, eating, or drinking and delivers oxygen throughout the respiratory cycle rather than just at inspiration. The patient or family must assume responsibility for daily catheter care. Patients usually report improved mobility, comfort, and appearance, and lower cost with this delivery system.

Patients using oxygen at home need instruction regarding safety precautions. See Teaching Tips 39-1 for information regarding the use of oxygen in the home setting.

Managing Chest Tubes

Patients with fluid (**pleural effusion**), blood (**hemothorax**), or air (**pneumothorax**) in the pleural space require a chest tube to drain these substances and allow the compressed lung to reexpand. A chest tube is a firm plastic tube with drainage holes in the proximal end that is inserted in the pleural space. Once inserted, the tube is secured with a suture and tape, covered with an airtight dressing, and attached to a drainage system that may or may not be attached to suction. Other

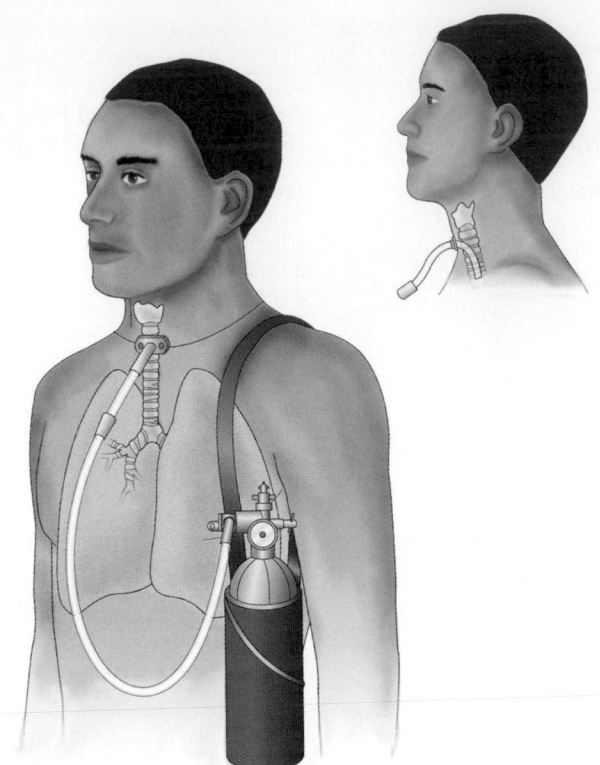

FIGURE 39-11. A transtracheal oxygen setup.

components of the system may include a closed water-seal drainage system that prevents air from reentering the chest once it has escaped and a suction control chamber that prevents excess suction pressure from being applied to the

---

Tips ### TEACHING TIPS • 39-1

USING OXYGEN AT HOME

Health Topic	Teaching Tip	Why Is This Important?
Safety	• No smoking or open flames are allowed within 10 feet of the oxygen source. • Do not use electrical equipment near oxygen administration set (e.g., space heaters, blow dryers). • Use caution with gas or electric appliances. • Ground oxygen concentrators. • Secure the oxygen tank in a holder and away from direct sunlight or heat. • Allow adequate airflow around the oxygen concentrator (avoid placing flush against the wall). • Notify local fire department of the oxygen in the home.	Oxygen is a combustible gas; a spark may ignite the oxygen.
Administration	• Follow the physician's prescription for the oxygen flow rate. • Have the physician's and nurse's phone number readily available. • Ensure enough available oxygen prior to leaving house for errands or trips. • Know how to reach the oxygen equipment vendor and the reasons for contacting the vendor. • Know signs and symptoms that indicate the need to call for emergency assistance.	Too much or too little oxygen may be detrimental to the patient.

pleural cavity. The suction chamber may be a water-filled or a dry chamber. A water-filled suction chamber is regulated by the amount of water in the chamber, whereas dry suction has a one-way mechanical valve system that allows air to leave the chest and prevents air from moving back into the chest and is automatically regulated to changes in the patient's pleural pressure. Most healthcare agencies use a molded plastic, three-compartment disposable chest drainage unit for management of chest tubes (Fig. 39-12). There are also portable drainage systems that utilize gravity for drainage.

The placement of the chest tube is determined by the type of drainage. When air is to be drained, the tube is placed higher in the chest. If fluid needs to be drained, the tube is inserted lower in the lung because fluids settle at the base of the lung.

Nursing responsibilities include assisting with insertion and removal of a chest tube. Once the tube is in place, monitor the patient's respiratory status and vital signs, check the dressing, and maintain the patency and integrity of the drainage system. Guidelines for monitoring a patient with a chest tube are shown in Guidelines for Nursing Care 39-3.

Using Artificial Airways

Artificial airways are used to preserve a functioning airway in patients who are unable to maintain a patent airway without assistance.

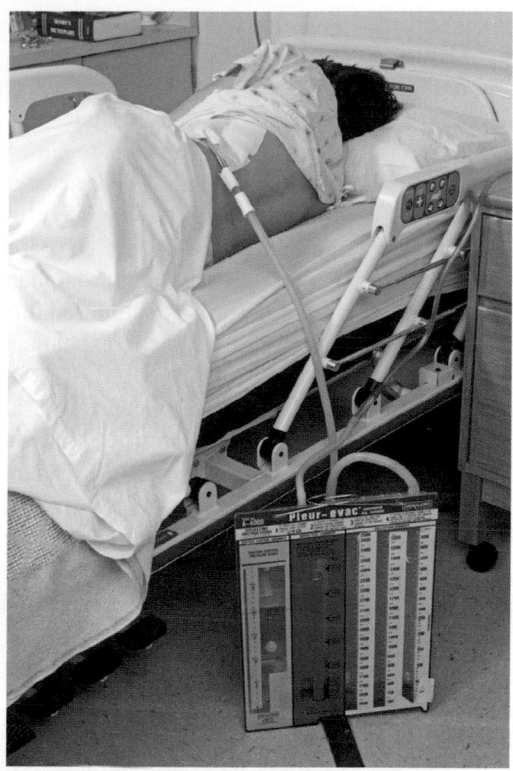

FIGURE 39-12. A chest drainage system attached to a patient. *(Photo by Rick Brady.)*

Guidelines for Nursing Care • 39-3

MONITORING A PATIENT WITH A CHEST TUBE

- Assess the patient's respiratory status, vital signs, and breath sounds. Monitor for any indication of change in respiratory status.

- Observe the dressing around the chest tube insertion site and ensure that it is occlusive. All connections should also be taped securely.

- Check that the drainage tube has no dependent loops or kinks. The drainage collection device must be positioned below the tube insertion site to facilitate drainage.

- Keep drainage collection device secure so that it does not tip over.

- Check that two padded Kelly clamps are available and secured at the bedside. If the drainage unit requires changing, position one clamp 1½ to 2½ inches from the insertion site; position the second clamp 1 inch down from the first one until the unit has been switched. Alternately, many systems have integrated clamps on the tubing. The physician may order a chest tube clamped before its removal to observe the patient's tolerance when it is discontinued or the chest tube may be clamped to assess for an air leak.

- Keep bottle of sterile saline or water at bedside. If chest tube disconnects from drainage unit, submerge end in water. This is done instead of clamping to prevent another pneumothorax. Air is still allowed to escape.

- Never clamp the tube if the patient leaves the unit for a test or moves away from the bed. Disconnect the suction tubing from the drainage system, allowing the unit to continue to collect drainage by gravity.

- Avoid milking or stripping the tube to promote drainage. This creates excessive negative pressure that can damage delicate lung tissue.

- Assess the suction control chamber if suction is in use. If water suction is used, ensure that water is at the appropriate level (fluid can evaporate); add water to ensure that suction is adequate. Gentle bubbling in the suction chamber indicates that suction is being applied to assist drainage.

- Assist the patient to remain in high Fowler's position (if hemothorax is present) or semi-Fowler's position (for pneumothorax) for improved drainage or evacuation.

- Measure drainage output at the end of each shift by marking the level on the container or placing a small piece of tape at the drainage level to indicate date and time. Drainage is never emptied from the collection chamber. Document color and consistency of drainage. Drainage exceeding 100 mL/hr or a change in drainage to a bright-red color that indicates fresh bleeding requires immediate notification of the physician.

OROPHARYNGEAL AND NASOPHARYNGEAL AIRWAYS

An oropharyngeal or nasopharyngeal airway is a semicircular tube of plastic or rubber inserted into the back of the pharynx through the mouth (oro) or nose (naso) in a patient who is breathing spontaneously. The oropharyngeal airway is used to keep the tongue clear of the airway. It is often used for postoperative patients until they regain consciousness. Once the patient regains consciousness, the oropharyngeal airway is removed. Tape is not used to hold the airway in place because the patient should be able to expel the airway once he or she becomes alert.

A nasopharyngeal airway, commonly called a nasal trumpet, is inserted through the nare and protrudes into the back of the pharynx. The nasal trumpet allows for frequent nasotracheal suctioning without trauma to the nasal passageway. This airway may be left in place, without much discomfort, in the patient who is alert and conscious. Techniques to use when inserting an artificial airway are given in Guidelines for Nursing Care 39-4.

ENDOTRACHEAL TUBE

An **endotracheal tube** is a polyvinylchloride airway that is inserted through the nose or the mouth into the trachea, using a laryngoscope as a guide. It is used to administer oxygen by mechanical ventilator, to suction secretions easily, or to bypass upper airway obstructions (e.g., tongue or tracheal edema). Although uncomfortable and easy to manipulate with the tongue, orotracheal insertion is often the method of choice, especially in an emergency, because insertion is easier and a larger tube can be used, making ventilation easier. Placement of the tube through the nasotracheal route, although tolerated better by patients, is more difficult and requires the use of a narrower tube. Most commonly, a cuffed endotracheal tube is used (Fig. 39-13). This type of tube prevents air leakage and bronchial aspiration of foreign material while allowing more precise control of oxygen and mechanical ventilation. However, careful monitoring of cuff pressure is necessary to decrease the risk for tracheal necrosis. The smallest amount of air that results in an airtight seal between the trachea and the tube is desirable and less likely to result in complications.

Guidelines for Nursing Care • 39-4

INSERTING AN ARTIFICIAL AIRWAY

Inserting an Oropharyngeal Airway

- Use an airway that is the correct size (size 90 mm is appropriate for the average adult). Airway should reach from opening of mouth to the back angle of the jaw.

- Explain what you are doing to the patient, even though the patient appears unconscious.

- Wash your hands and don gloves (if patient is coughing, wear mask and goggles or face shield).

- Remove dentures if they are present.

- Position patient on his or her back with neck hyperextended (unless this is inappropriate).

- Open patient's mouth by using your thumb and index finger to gently pry teeth apart.

- Insert the airway with the curved tip pointing up toward the roof of the mouth.

- Slide the airway across the tongue to the back of the mouth.

- Rotate the airway 180 degrees as it passes the uvula (a flashlight can confirm the position of the airway with the curve fitting over the tongue).

- Ensure adequate ventilation by auscultating breath sounds.

- Position patient on his or her side when airway is in place.

- Remove airway for a brief period every 4 hours. Provide mouth care and rinse airway before reinserting it.

Inserting a Nasopharyngeal Airway (Nasal Trumpet)

- Use an airway that is the correct size (size 28 French is an average adult size). Airway should reach from the tragus of the ear to the nostril plus 1 inch.

- Perform hand hygiene and don gloves (wear mask and goggles if patient is coughing).

- Explain the procedure to the patient.

- Lubricate the airway with the water-soluble lubricant.

- Position the patient on his or her back or in a side-lying position.

- Gently insert the airway into the naris. If resistance is met, stop and try inserting in the other naris.

- Remove the airway and place it in the other naris at least every 24 hours. Assess for any evidence of skin breakdown.

- Be aware that the airway may be used for suctioning to prevent trauma to the mucosa.

Airway
Tongue
Epiglottis
Trachea
Esophagus

FIGURE 39-13. Endotracheal tube. (**A**) (*1*) Parts of a cuffed endotracheal tube; (*2*) tube in place with the cuff inflated; (*3*) tube in place with the cuff deflated. (**B**) Endotracheal tube in place.

For a patient with an endotracheal tube who is receiving continuous mechanical ventilation, a closed airway suction system can be used to keep the airway patent and reduce the risk of hypoxia or, possibly, infection (Fig. 39-14). The catheter, encased in a plastic sleeve, remains connected to the patient's airway or ventilator tubing for up to 24 hours. This closed system is cost-effective because only one catheter is used daily, and the caregiver has additional protection from exposure to the patient's secretions. Some systems have an access valve, a safety feature that completely closes off access between the suction catheter and the endotracheal tube.

> *Consider Mr. Kim, the 57-year-old man receiving oxygen therapy and mechanical ventilation via an endotracheal tube. When developing the patient's plan of care, the nurse needs to assess the patient closely and frequently for signs and symptoms indicating an increase in secretions. If secretions increase, the nurse needs to suction the patient*

to maintain a patent airway and minimize his risk for hypoxemia and infection. ∎

TRACHEOSTOMY

A tracheostomy tube is inserted for a variety of reasons. It may be used to replace an endotracheal tube, to provide a method for mechanical ventilation of the patient, to bypass an upper airway obstruction, or to remove tracheobronchial secretions.

Tracheostomy Procedure and Tubes

A **tracheostomy** is an artificial opening made into the trachea, usually at the level of the second or third cartilaginous ring. A curved tube, called a tracheostomy tube, is inserted through the opening. It is inserted in the operating room or intensive care unit under sterile conditions using local anesthesia, and can be temporary or permanent.

The tube is made of semiflexible plastic (polyurethane or silicone), rigid plastic, or metal and is available in different

FIGURE 39-14. Closed airway suction system. (**A**) Closed tracheal suction system. (**B**) Closed system connected by a T-piece to the endotracheal tube and ventilator.

Cuffless

Cuffed

FIGURE 39-15. Two types of tracheostomy sets: cuffless and cuffed.

sizes with varied angles. The condition and needs of the patient determine the selection of either a metal or plastic tracheostomy tube. Although metal tubes are more cost-effective for long-term use, most do not have an adapter at the neckplate that permits connection to respiratory therapy equipment (e.g., an oxygen delivery system, Ambu bag, or mechanical ventilator).

A tracheostomy tube consists of an outer cannula or main shaft, an inner cannula, and an obturator. An obturator, which guides the direction of the outer cannula, is inserted into the tube during placement and removed once the outer cannula of the tube is in place (Fig. 39-15). Many tubes also have inner cannulas that may or may not be disposable. The outer cannula remains in place in the trachea, and the inner cannula is removed for cleaning or replaced with a new one. Periodic cleaning or replacement of the inner cannula prevents airway obstruction from secretions that have accumulated on the tube's inner surface. A tube with an inner cannula is necessary when patients have excessive secretions or have difficulty clearing their secretions. It also may be recommended for a patient who will be discharged with a tracheostomy tube in place.

Tracheostomy tubes may be either cuffed or cuffless (see Fig. 39-15). The inflated cuff seals the opening around the tube to create a tight fit in the trachea. This prevents air leakage and aspiration, and permits mechanical ventilation. Newer tracheal cuffs are low pressure, do not require deflating for short intervals every few hours, and can be maintained at lower than tracheal capillary pressure. If a cuffed tube is used, always deflate it before oral feeding unless the patient is at high risk for aspiration. If left cuffed, the balloon can cause pressure that extends through the trachea and onto the esophagus, possibly impeding swallowing or causing erosion of the tissue.

A fenestrated tracheostomy tube has one large or several small openings or windows on its outer curve, has an inner cannula, and can be cuffed or cuffless. When the patient is being mechanically ventilated, the inner cannula is in place, blocking the small openings. After the patient is no longer connected to the ventilator, the inner cannula can be removed,

the cuff deflated, and the tube plugged, allowing the patient to speak. Because the tube has these openings, it is not recommended for use in patients with a history of aspiration.

The tracheostomy tube is held in place by twill tapes or a Velcro strip fastened around the patient's neck. When the tracheostomy is new, a sterile, square gauze pad that has been precut by the manufacturer may be placed between the skin and outer wings of the tube. This tracheostomy dressing must be kept dry to prevent infection and skin irritation.

Regularly check cuff pressure, although some tubes have a pressure-release valve that prevents pressure from increasing to damaging levels. Also, because the tracheostomy tube bypasses the natural humidifying and heating mechanisms in the nose and mouth, administer heated, humidified oxygen to prevent secretions from becoming dry. Also, keep the tracheostomy tube free from foreign objects and nonsterile materials, such as cotton balls, loose threads from dressings, needles, and other small objects, to reduce the risk of obstruction and infection. Artificial noses, small pieces that attach over the end of the tracheostomy tube, are available to filter and warm the air before it enters the trachea.

Preparation for emergency situations is an important part of nursing care for these patients. The tracheostomy is the patient's only airway, and measures to maintain its patency need to be readily available. Standard bedside equipment for emergency use should include the obturator from the current tube, suction equipment, oxygen, a spare tracheostomy tube of the same size, and one a size smaller (Roman, 2005).

A patient who has a tracheostomy is unable to speak. Consider his or her impaired ability to communicate and keep communication tools (e.g., writing board, letters, vocabulary cards) close at hand along with the call light or bell. To prevent anxiety, offer frequent reassurance and explanations and anticipate his or her needs.

Suctioning the Tracheostomy

Patients with tracheostomies frequently have an ineffective cough mechanism and copious secretions, which necessitate tracheal suctioning to remove secretions. Tracheal suctioning is an uncomfortable procedure at the minimum, and it can be a very painful and/or distressing experience. Therefore, anticipate assessing for the need for the administration of analgesic medication to a patient before suctioning (Arroyo-Novoa et al., 2007). However, only perform suctioning when clinically necessary because there are many potential risks. Risks include hypoxia, infection, tracheal tissue damage, dysrhythmias, and atelectasis. Closely assess the patient before, during, and after the procedure to limit negative effects. In order to prevent hypoxia, hyperoxygenate the patient before and after suctioning and limit the application of suction to 10 to 20 seconds. Monitor the patient's pulse frequently to detect potential effects of hypoxia and stimulation of the vagus nerve. Using an appropriate suction pressure (80–120 mm Hg) will help prevent atelectasis related to the use of high negative pressure (Roman, 2005). Research suggests that insertion of the suction catheter should be limited to a predetermined length (no further than 1 cm past the length of the tracheal or endotracheal tube) to avoid tracheal mucosal damage, including epithelial denudement, loss of cilia, edema, and fibrosis (Pate, 2004). Skill 39-5 describes suctioning a tracheostomy. For a patient with a tracheostomy tube who is receiving continuous mechanical ventilation, a closed airway suction system can be used to keep the airway patent and reduce the risk of hypoxemia or infection. See the previous description of this closed suction system (Endotracheal Tube).

Providing Tracheostomy Care

In addition to suctioning the tracheostomy, the nurse is responsible for either cleaning a nondisposable inner cannula or replacing a disposable one. The inner cannula requires cleaning or replacement to prevent accumulation of secretions that can interfere with respiration and occlude the airway. Because soiled tracheostomy dressings place the patient at risk for the development of skin breakdown and infection, regularly change dressings and ties. Use gauze dressings that are not filled with cotton to prevent aspiration of foreign bodies (e.g., lint or cotton fibers) into the trachea. Clean the skin around a tracheostomy to prevent buildup of dried secretions and skin breakdown. Exercise care when changing the tracheostomy ties to prevent accidental decannulation or expulsion of the tube. Have an assistant hold the tube in place during the change or keep the soiled tie in place until a clean one is securely attached. Agency policy and patient condition determine specific procedures and schedules, but a newly inserted tracheostomy may require attention every 1 to 2 hours. Skill 39-6 outlines tracheostomy care.

ASSISTING VENTILATION

Mechanical ventilators are used to assist or completely control ventilation. These machines are used with patients who have endotracheal or tracheostomy tubes in place. Mechanical ventilation can be performed in acute care facilities, in extended care settings, and in the home. Mechanical ventilation improves oxygenation and ventilation and supports the patient's breathing function during emergency or acute care episodes as well as long-term situations.

Many types of ventilators are available. The nurse is responsible for addressing the physical and psychological concerns of the patient and family. In addition, key interventions include evaluating the patient's response to ventilation therapy, using safe practices and techniques, and monitoring the patient carefully for complications. (See specific clinical texts and literature that discuss the use of mechanical ventilators in greater detail.)

Another mechanical device used to assist ventilation is intermittent positive-pressure breathing (IPPB). This is a method of providing a specific amount of air, oxygen, and aerosolized medication under increased pressure to the respiratory tract. The patient receiving IPPB inhales the aerosol therapy through a mouthpiece or face mask. IPPB forces deeper inspiration by positive-pressure inhalation and then permits passive exhalation. The amount of pressure varies with each patient. It is now recognized as an alternative therapy when the patient is unable or unwilling to make the effort to ventilate his or her lungs. However, conservative methods must be attempted first, such as deep-breathing and coughing exercises, percussion, vibration, and postural drainage.

In emergency situations, the manual resuscitation bag (or Ambu bag) can be used to assist ventilation in patients whose respirations have ceased. With the patient's head tilted back, jaw pulled forward, and airway cleared, the mask is held tightly over the patient's nose and mouth. The bag also fits easily over tracheostomy and endotracheal tubes. The operator's other hand compresses the bag at a rate that approximates normal respiratory rate (e.g., 16 to 20 breaths/minute in adults). The one-way valve in the mask allows exhaled air to escape. Artificial ventilation can be sustained until spontaneous breathing starts, until other mechanical assistance is available, or until death is confirmed. The bag is self-inflating and may be attached to supplemental oxygen if needed.

Clearing an Obstructed Airway

Foreign-body obstruction of the airway often occurs during eating. In adults, meat is the most common food-related cause. In children, any variety of foods or objects can obstruct the upper airway. A patient who is semiconscious or unconscious develops airway obstruction as the tongue falls back, covering the pharynx. In fact, the tongue is the most common cause of airway obstruction.

Foreign bodies can cause a partial or complete airway obstruction. In partial airway obstruction with good air exchange, the patient can cough forcefully. Allow the person to cough, and encourage spontaneous breathing. Do not interfere with the patient's efforts to expel the object. With a partial airway obstruction, good air exchange can progress to poor air exchange. Poor air exchange may be indicated by a weak, ineffective cough, high-pitched noises while inhaling, increased breathing difficulties, and cyanosis. When this occurs, it is managed in the same way as complete airway obstruction.

With a complete airway obstruction, the victim is unable to speak or cough and may demonstrate the universal distress signal (clutching his or her throat with both hands). Immediate action is necessary, or the patient will become unconscious as the brain becomes hypoxic. After complete

FIGURE 39-16. Placement of the automated external defibrillator (AED). (**A**) AED device. (**B**) Place the AED pad attached to the red cable connector to the left of the heart apex. To help remember where to place the pads, think "white right, red ribs." Placement of both electrode pads is the same as it is for manual defibrillation or cardioversion. *(Photo by B. Proud.)*

airway obstruction has been determined, perform the Heimlich maneuver (abdominal thrusts). Follow the American Heart Association protocols for cardiopulmonary resuscitation (see below) and obstructed airways. These protocols are continually being developed and updated.

Administering Cardiopulmonary Resuscitation

Cardiopulmonary resuscitation (CPR) is the combination of mouth-to-mouth breathing, which supplies oxygen to the lungs, and chest compressions, which circulate blood. It is often described in terms of the ABCDs of basic life support:

Airway: Tip the head and check for breathing. The respiratory tract must be opened so that air can enter.

Breathing: If the victim does not start to breathe spontaneously after the airway is opened, give two breaths lasting 1.5 to 2 seconds.

Circulation: Check the pulse. If the victim has no pulse, chest compressions are initiated to provide artificial circulation.

Defibrillation: Apply the AED as soon as it is available.

Start CPR in any situation in which either breathing alone or breathing and a heartbeat are absent. The brain is sensitive to hypoxia and will sustain irreversible damage after 4 to 6 minutes of no oxygen. The faster CPR is initiated, the greater the chance of survival.

During CPR, standard precautions are followed even though contact with a patient's blood or body fluids does not always occur. Occupational Safety and Health Administration (OSHA) standards require healthcare facilities to provide an ample supply of ventilation masks along with other protective barriers for staff to use during resuscitation efforts.

Another device, the automated external defibrillator (AED), has also proved effective in reducing deaths attributed to cardiac arrest. This easy-to-use, computer-based device is designed to deliver a shock to the heart muscle quickly to interrupt ventricular fibrillation, the most common initial rhythm occurring in cardiac arrest. The AED has the ability to analyze the heart's rhythm, direct the operator to deliver a shock when

appropriate or deliver one automatically, and then reanalyze the rhythm to determine whether it has returned to normal (Fig. 39-16). Using the AED is an integral part of resuscitation.

Most professional organizations recommend and support widespread efforts to teach CPR to lay people and all health professionals. Mannequins for practice can be obtained from the American Heart Association, the American Red Cross, and health agencies. The nurse is professionally responsible for maintaining proficiency in CPR skills. This necessitates periodic practice with mannequins (adult and infant). CPR must be administered quickly and accurately, without hesitation, when cardiac or pulmonary arrest occurs. In 2008, the American Heart Association (AHA) instituted changes in their suggestions regarding emergency interventions outside of healthcare facilities. Learning conventional CPR is still recommended. However, the AHA alternately recommends that when an adult suddenly collapses, persons near the victim should call 911 (activate the emergency response system) and push hard and fast in the center of the victim's chest. Studies of real emergencies that have occurred in homes, at work, or in public locations, show that these two steps, called Hands-Only CPR, can be as effective as conventional CPR. Providing Hands-Only CPR to an adult who has collapsed from a sudden cardiac arrest can more than double that person's chance of survival (AHA, 2008).

Evaluating

Evaluation is the final step of the nursing process; the accompanying concept map illustrates the nursing process for the care of Tyrone Jacobs. Evaluation is an ongoing and deliberate part of the nursing process that involves the nurse, patient, family, and other healthcare team members. It compares the patient's health status with previously defined expected outcomes and examines the patient's projected progress in meeting those outcomes. Everyone involved in the evaluation process needs to identify effective interventions and reasons for any failures in achieving the expected outcomes. Adjustments in the nursing plan of care are made accordingly. See Nursing Plan of Care 39-1 for Joan McEntyre.

Tyrone Jacobs, age 12, is admitted to the pediatric unit after having a cold for 4 days. He is diagnosed with acute asthma and upper respiratory infection. His vital signs are as follows: BP 100/60 mm Hg, pulse 140 beats per minute, respiratory rate 40 breaths/minute, temperature of 101° F, and oxygen saturation of 90%. While listening to his lungs, you hear diffuse inspiratory and expiratory wheezes and scattered coarse crackles. You note an occasional cough, productive for thick yellow mucus. He is sitting upright in bed in a tripod position. He states, "Help me I can't breathe." Tyrone is placed on O₂ 2 liters/minute via nasal cannula and is receiving albuterol nebulizer treatments and IV antibiotics. His sputum culture reveals Gram-positive cocci. His mother appears very anxious and is pacing in the room. Tyrone is not making eye contact with mother or caregivers.

Priority 1

Nursing Diagnosis: Impaired Gas Exchange related to bronchoconstriction and inflammation of airways.
Supporting Data:
- Oxygen saturation is 90%
- O₂ @ 2 L/min via nasal cannula
- Respiratory rate is 40 breaths/min
- Sitting in tripod position
- Had cold for 4 days prior to admission
- Wheezes and coarse crackles auscultated
- Receiving albuterol nebulizer treatments

Outcome:
Patient will maintain oxygen saturation within normal limits on supplemental oxygen.

Nursing Interventions:
- Monitor pulse oximetry every 4 hrs
- Monitor and evaluate vital signs every 4hrs
- Maintain patient in position of comfort (tripod position)
- Evaluate effectiveness of albuterol nebulizer treatments
- Auscultate lungs every 4 hrs

Evaluation: Tyrone continues to have oxygen saturation below normal limits, tachypnea, and wheezing. Continue to monitor response to collaborative interventions. Notify physician for an increase in respiratory distress and a decrease in pulse oximetry.

Priority 2

Nursing Diagnosis: Ineffective Airway Clearance related to increased mucous production due to upper respiratory infection and asthma.
Supporting Data:
- Expectorating yellow mucus
- Temperature is 101° F
- Receiving IV antibiotics
- Sputum culture reveals Gram-positive cocci
- Receiving albuterol nebulizer treatments
- Has frequent bouts of coughing
- Wheezing and coarse crackles auscultated

Outcome:
Patient will readily expectorate secretions; lung sounds will clear.

Nursing Interventions:
- Encourage and instruct in coughing and pursed-lip breathing techniques
- Monitor effectiveness of bronchodilators in increasing expectoration of secretions
- Note characteristics of sputum
- Evaluate respiratory rate and effort
- Encourage increased fluid intake
- Auscultate breath sounds every 4 hrs

Evaluation: Tyrone continues to have audible adventitious sounds. He is readily expectorating secretions. Continue to monitor.

Priority 3

Nursing Diagnosis: Anxiety related to difficulty breathing and parental reaction to acute illness of child.
Supporting Data:
- Tyrone states, "Help me. I can't breathe."
- Mother pacing back and forth in room
- Heart rate is 140 beats/min
- Respiratory rate is 40 breaths/min
- Tyrone is not making eye contact with mother or caregivers

Outcome:
Patient will appear relaxed with reduced heart rate and respiratory rate; will interact with family and caregivers.

Nursing Interventions:
- Assess level of anxiety
- Provide calm, reassuring presence
- Utilize Therapeutic Touch
- Keep patient and family informed of actions taken to improve breathing
- Use brief, simple explanations
- Maintain quiet, calm environment
- Encourage pursed-lip breathing to manage dyspnea

Evaluation: Tyrone made eye contact with nurse as she explained the actions of his bronchodilators. Mother stopped pacing and sat beside son to provide comfort and reassurance. Continue interventions.

- - - - - **Relationship** ■ **Assesment** ■ **Nursing Diagnosis** ■ **Outcome Identification** ■ **Interventions** ■ **Evaluation**

Concept map displaying the nursing process for Tyrone Jacobs.

NURSING PLAN OF CARE • 39-1

For Joan McIntyre

Joan, age 72, has been admitted to your medical unit with an acute exacerbation of chronic obstructive pulmonary disease (COPD). This is the fifth time she has been in the hospital this year. She is receiving supplemental oxygen and multiple medications to support her breathing. She is very weak, unable to perform ADLs for herself, and becomes extremely short of breath with minimal exertion. Mrs. McIntyre has been eating only small amounts and states, "It is just too much!" She has verbalized feelings of despair and has asked the staff "to let me go if I should stop breathing." A comprehensive assessment revealed the following findings:

Respiratory rate, 32 breaths/min

Frequent weak cough, difficulty raising secretions, occasionally productive for yellow sputum; patient states, "I just can't get it out."

Dyspnea with minimal exertion; patient states, "I can't even eat or brush my teeth without feeling like I can't catch my breath!"

Lungs with decreased breath sounds, scattered sonorous wheezing

Oxygen saturation on oxygen at 3 liters/min = 90–92%

Picks at breakfast; consumes less than ¼ of breakfast tray

NURSING DIAGNOSIS	Ineffective Airway Clearance related to bronchoconstriction, increased mucous production, and ineffective cough as manifested by frequent weak cough, inability to consistently expectorate sputum, presence of sonorous wheezes (rhonchi)
EXPECTED OUTCOME	By 3/20/12, the patient will: • cough effectively and expectorate sputum

Nursing Interventions	Rationale	Evaluative Statement
Assess respiratory status at least every 4 hours	Establish standards to detect early signs of compromise	3/19/12 Outcome met. Mrs. McIntyre is able to consistently cough up and expectorate sputum. Patient states feelings of improved ability to clear sputum.
Teach importance of adequate hydration	Patient understanding increases compliance and involve the patient in care	
Offer patient a choice of preferred liquids every 2 hours	Liquids help to liquefy secretions and prevent dehydration.	*M. Jones, RN*
Teach and encourage the use of diaphragmatic breathing and coughing techniques.	Helps to improve ventilation and mobilize secretions without causing breathlessness and fatigue.	

NURSING DIAGNOSIS	Self-care deficit: hygiene, related to fatigue secondary to increased work of breathing
EXPECTED OUTCOME	By 3/20/12, the patient will: • Patient's self-care needs are met and patient has improved ability to participate in bathing and personal hygiene measures

(continued)

NURSING PLAN OF CARE · 39-1

For Joan McIntyre   (continued)

Nursing Interventions	Rationale	Evaluative Statement
Observe patient's functional level every shift	Careful assessment guides adjustment of actions to meet patient's needs	3/19/12 Continue interventions. Patient able to perform ¾ of bath before becoming too fatigued and weak. Patient requires continued rein-forcement regarding diaphragmatic breathing during activity. Continue guidance to break activity into smaller tasks and utilize rest between activi-ties. Patient states frustration with inability to accomplish entire personal care tasks in short period of time.

M. Jones, RN |
Encourage patient to voice feelings and concerns about self-care deficits	Assists patient to achieve highest functional level possible	
Teach patient to coordinate diaphrag-matic breathing with activity	Helps avoid excessive fatigue and dyspnea during activity	
Group personal care activities into smaller steps; allow rest periods between activities	Promotes energy conservation and helps avoid excessive fatigue and dyspnea	
Assist with bathing and hygiene tasks as needed and only when patient has difficulty	Promotes feeling of independence	

SAMPLE DOCUMENTATION

3/17/12 1500 Nursing
Patient verbalizes frustration with length of time required to complete personal care activi-ties. Patient states, "I just want to be able to take care of myself without having to take an entire day to do it." Possible consult with occupational therapy/physical therapy discussed with patient, husband, and Dr. Miller. Patient expresses an interest in working with the occupational/physical therapist.

M. Jones, RN

Skill · 39-1   Using a Pulse Oximeter

EQUIPMENT

- Pulse oximeter with an appropriate sensor or probe
- Alcohol wipe(s) or disposable cleansing cloth
- Nail polish remover (if necessary)
- PPE, as indicated

IMPLEMENTATION

ACTION	RATIONALE
1. Review chart for any health problems that would affect the patient's oxygenation status.	Identifying influencing factors aids in interpretation of results.
2. Bring necessary equipment to the bedside stand or overbed table.	Bringing everything to the bedside conserves time and energy. Arranging items nearby is convenient, saves time, and avoids unnecessary stretching and twisting of muscles on the part of the nurse.
3. Perform hand hygiene and put on PPE, if indicated.	Hand hygiene and PPE prevent the spread of microorganisms. PPE is required based on transmission precautions.

(continued)

Skill · 39-1   **Using a Pulse Oximeter**   *continued*

ACTION

4. Identify the patient.

5. Close curtains around bed and close door to room if possible. Explain what you are going to do and why you are going to do it to the patient.

6. Select an adequate site for application of the sensor.

   a. Use the patient's index, middle, or ring finger (Figure 1).

   b. Check the proximal pulse (Figure 2) and capillary refill (Figure 3) at the pulse closest to the site.

   c. If circulation at site is inadequate, consider using the earlobe, forehead, or bridge of nose.

   d. Use a toe only if lower extremity circulation is not compromised.

RATIONALE

Identifying the patient ensures the right patient receives the intervention and helps prevent errors.

This ensures the patient's privacy. Explanation relieves anxiety and facilitates cooperation.

Inadequate circulation can interfere with the oxygen saturation (SpO_2) reading.

Fingers are easily accessible.

Brisk capillary refill and a strong pulse indicate that circulation to the site is adequate.

These alternate sites are highly vascular alternatives.

Peripheral vascular disease is common in lower extremities.

FIGURE 1. Selecting an appropriate finger.

FIGURE 2. Assessing pulse.

FIGURE 3. Assessing capillary refill.

ACTION	RATIONALE

7. Select proper equipment:

a. If one finger is too large for the probe, use a smaller one. A pediatric probe may be used for a small adult.

Inaccurate readings can result if probe or sensor is not attached correctly.

b. Use probes appropriate for patient's age and size.

Probes come in adult, pediatric, and infant sizes.

c. Check if patient is allergic to adhesive. A nonadhesive finger clip or reflectance sensor is available.

A reaction may occur if patient is allergic to adhesive substance.

8. Prepare the monitoring site. Cleanse the selected area with the alcohol wipe or disposable cleansing cloth (Figure 4). Allow the area to dry. If necessary, remove nail polish and artificial nails after checking pulse oximeter's manufacturer instructions.

Skin oils, dirt, or grime on the site can interfere with the passage of light waves. Research is conflicting regarding the effect of dark color nail polish and artificial nails; refer to facility policy and pulse oximeter's manufacturer instructions (Collins & Andersen, 2007; DeMeulenaere, 2007).

9. **Apply probe securely to skin (Figure 5). Make sure that the light-emitting sensor and the light-receiving sensor are aligned opposite each other (not necessary to check if placed on forehead or bridge of nose).**

Secure attachment and proper alignment promote satisfactory operation of the equipment and accurate recording of the SpO_2.

FIGURE 4. Cleaning the area.

FIGURE 5. Attaching probe to patient's finger.

10. Connect the sensor probe to the pulse oximeter (Figure 6), turn the oximeter on, and check operation of the equipment (audible beep, fluctuation of bar of light or waveform on face of oximeter).

Audible beep represents the arterial pulse, and fluctuating waveform or light bar indicates the strength of the pulse. A weak signal will produce an inaccurate recording of the SpO_2. Tone of beep reflects SpO_2 reading. If SpO_2 drops, tone becomes lower in pitch.

11. Set alarms on pulse oximeter. Check manufacturer's alarm limits for high and low pulse rate settings (Figure 7).

Alarm provides additional safeguard and signals when high or low limits have been surpassed.

12. Check oxygen saturation at regular intervals, as ordered by primary care provider, nursing assessment, and signaled by alarms. Monitor hemoglobin level.

Monitoring SpO_2 provides ongoing assessment of patient's condition. A low hemoglobin level may be satisfactorily saturated yet inadequate to meet a patient's oxygen needs.

13. Remove sensor on a regular basis and check for skin irritation or signs of pressure (every 2 hours for spring tension sensor or every 4 hours for adhesive finger or toe sensor).

Prolonged pressure may lead to tissue necrosis. Adhesive sensor may cause skin irritation.

14. Clean nondisposable sensors according to the manufacturer's directions. Remove PPE, if used. Perform hand hygiene.

Cleaning equipment between patient use reduces the spread of microorganisms. Removing PPE properly reduces the risk for infection transmission and contamination of other items. Hand hygiene prevents the spread of microorganisms.

(continued)

Skill · 39-1   Using a Pulse Oximeter   *continued*

FIGURE 6. Connecting sensor probe to unit.

FIGURE 7. Checking alarms.

DOCUMENTATION

Guidelines

Documentation should include the type of sensor and location used; the assessment of the proximal pulse and capillary refill; pulse oximeter reading; the amount of oxygen and delivery method if the patient is receiving supplemental oxygen; lung assessment, if relevant; and any other relevant interventions required as a result of the reading.

Sample Documentation

> 9/03/12 Pulse oximeter placed on patient's index finger on right hand. Radial pulse present with brisk capillary refill. Pulse oximeter reading 98% on oxygen at 2 L via nasal cannula. Heart rate measured by oximeter correlates with the radial pulse measurement.
> —*C. Bausler, RN*

UNEXPECTED SITUATIONS AND ASSOCIATED INTERVENTIONS

- *Absent or weak signal:* Check vital signs and patient condition. If satisfactory, check connections and circulation to site. Hypotension makes an accurate recording difficult. Equipment (restraint, blood pressure cuff) may compromise circulation to site and cause venous blood to pulsate, giving an inaccurate reading. If extremity is cold, cover with a warm blanket.

- *Inaccurate reading:* Check prescribed medications and history of circulatory disorders. Try device on a healthy person to see if problem is equipment-related or patient-related. Drugs that cause vasoconstriction interfere with accurate recording of oxygen saturation.

- *A bright light (sunlight or fluorescent light) is suspected of causing equipment malfunction:* Turn off light or cover probe with a dry washcloth. Bright light can interfere with operation of light sensors and cause unreliable report.

SPECIAL CONSIDERATIONS

General Considerations

- Accuracy of readings can be influenced by conditions that decrease arterial blood flow, such as peripheral edema, hypotension, and peripheral vascular disease.

- Correlate the pulse reading on the pulse oximeter with the patient's heart rate. Variation between pulse and heart rate may indicate that not all pulsations are being detected and another sensor site may be required (Moore, 2007).

- Excessive motion of sensor probe site, such as with extremity tremors or shivering, can also interfere with obtaining an accurate reading.

- Bradycardia and irregular cardiac rhythms may also cause inaccurate readings.

- In patients with low cardiac index (cardiac output in liters per minute divided by body surface area in square meters), the forehead sensor may be better than the digit sensor for pulse oximetry (Fernandez et al., 2007).

Infant and Child Considerations	• For infants, the oximeter probe may be placed on the toe or foot.
Older Adult Considerations	• Careful attention to the patient's skin integrity and condition is necessary to prevent injury. Pressure or tension from the probe, as well as any adhesive used, can damage older, dry, thin skin.
Home Care Considerations	• Portable units are available for use in the home or an outpatient setting.

Skill · 39-2   Suctioning the Nasopharyngeal and Oropharyngeal Airways

EQUIPMENT

- Portable or wall suction unit with tubing
- A commercially prepared suction kit with an appropriate-sized catheter or
  - Sterile suction catheter with Y-port in the appropriate size (Adult: 10 Fr–16 Fr)
- Sterile disposable container
- Sterile gloves
- Sterile water or saline
- Towel or waterproof pad
- Goggles and mask or face shield
- Disposable, clean gloves
- Water-soluble lubricant
- Additional PPE, as indicated

IMPLEMENTATION

ACTION	**RATIONALE**
1. Bring necessary equipment to the bedside stand or overbed table.	Bringing everything to the bedside conserves time and energy. Arranging items nearby is convenient, saves time, and avoids unnecessary stretching and twisting of muscles on the part of the nurse.
2. Perform hand hygiene and put on PPE, if indicated.	Hand hygiene and PPE prevent the spread of microorganisms. PPE is required based on transmission precautions.
3. Identify the patient.	Identifying the patient ensures the right patient receives the intervention and helps prevent errors.
4. Close curtains around bed and close door to room if possible.	This ensures the patient's privacy.
5. Determine the need for suctioning. Verify the suction order in the patient's chart, if necessary. **For postoperative patient, administer pain medication before suctioning.**	To minimize trauma to airway mucosa, suctioning should be done only when secretions have accumulated or adventitious breath sounds are audible. Some facilities require an order for naso- and oropharyngeal suctioning. Suctioning stimulates coughing, which is painful for patients with surgical incisions.
6. Explain what you are going to do and the reason for suctioning to the patient, even if the patient does not appear to be alert. Reassure patient you will interrupt procedure if he or she indicates respiratory difficulty.	Explanation alleviates fears. Even if patient appears unconscious, explain what is happening. Any procedure that compromises respiration is frightening for the patient.
7. Adjust bed to comfortable working height, usually elbow height of the caregiver (VISN 8, 2009). Lower side rail closest to you. **If patient is conscious, place him or her in a semi-Fowler's position. If patient is unconscious, place him or her in the lateral position, facing you.** Move the bed table close to your work area and raise to waist height.	Having the bed at the proper height prevents back and muscle strain. A sitting position helps the patient to cough and makes breathing easier. Gravity also facilitates catheter insertion. The lateral position prevents the airway from becoming obstructed and promotes drainage of secretions. The bed table provides a work surface and helps maintain sterility of objects on the work surface.
8. Place towel or waterproof pad across the patient's chest.	This protects bed linens.

(continued)

Skill · 39-2   Suctioning the Nasopharyngeal and Oropharyngeal Airways *continued*

ACTION

RATIONALE

9. **Adjust suction to appropriate pressure (Figure 1).**

For a wall unit for an adult: 100–120 mm Hg (Roman, 2005); neonates: 60–80 mm Hg; infants: 80–100 mm Hg; children: 80–100 mm Hg; adolescents: 80–120 mm Hg (Ireton, 2007).

For a portable unit for an adult: 10–15 cm Hg; neonates: 6–8 cm Hg; infants: 8–10 cm Hg; children: 8–10 cm Hg; adolescents: 8–10 cm Hg.

Put on a disposable, clean glove and occlude the end of the connecting tubing to check suction pressure. Place the connecting tubing in a convenient location.

Higher pressures can cause excessive trauma, hypoxemia, and atelectasis.

FIGURE 1. Adjusting wall suction.

10. Open sterile suction package using aseptic technique. The open wrapper or container becomes a sterile field to hold other supplies. Carefully remove the sterile container, touching only the outside surface. Set it up on the work surface and pour sterile saline into it.

Sterile normal saline or water is used to lubricate the outside of the catheter, minimizing irritation of mucosa during introduction. It is also used to clear the catheter between suction attempts.

11. Place a small amount of water-soluble lubricant on the sterile field, taking care to avoid touching the sterile field with the lubricant package.

Lubricant facilitates passage of the catheter and reduces trauma to mucous membranes.

12. Increase the patient's supplemental oxygen level or apply supplemental oxygen per facility policy or primary care provider order.

Suctioning removes air from the patient's airway and can cause hypoxemia. Hyperoxygenation can help prevent suction-induced hypoxemia.

13. Put on face shield or goggles and mask. Put on sterile gloves. **The dominant hand will manipulate the catheter and must remain sterile. The nondominant hand is considered clean rather than sterile and will control the suction valve (Y port) on the catheter.**

Handling the sterile catheter using a sterile glove helps prevent introducing organisms into the respiratory tract; the clean glove protects the nurse from microorganisms.

14. With dominant gloved hand, pick up sterile catheter. Pick up the connecting tubing with the nondominant hand and connect the tubing and suction catheter (Figure 2).

Sterility of the suction catheter is maintained.

15. Moisten the catheter by dipping it into the container of sterile saline (Figure 3). Occlude Y-tube to check suction.

Lubricating the inside of the catheter with saline helps move secretions in the catheter. Checking suction ensures equipment is working properly.

CHAPTER 39 Oxygenation **1393**

ACTION

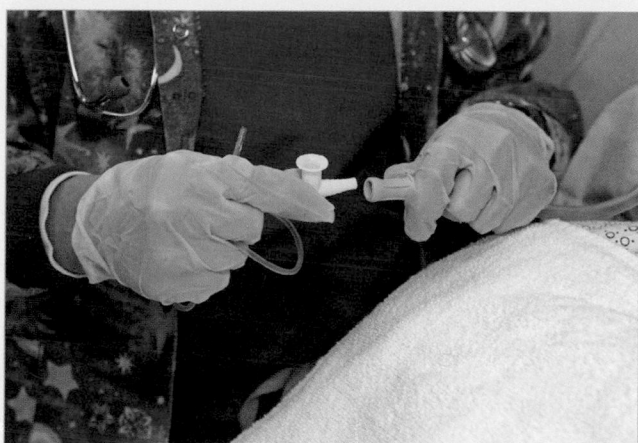

FIGURE 2. Connecting catheter to tubing.

16. Encourage the patient to take several deep breaths.

17. Apply lubricant to the first 2″ to 3″ of the catheter, using the lubricant that was placed on the sterile field.

18. Remove the oxygen delivery device, if appropriate. Do not apply suction as the catheter is inserted. Hold the catheter between your thumb and forefinger.

19. Insert the catheter:

a. For nasopharyngeal suctioning, gently insert catheter through the naris and along the floor of the nostril toward the trachea (Figure 4). Roll the catheter between your fingers to help advance it. Advance the catheter approximately 5″ to 6″ to reach the pharynx.

b. For oropharyngeal suctioning, insert catheter through the mouth, along the side of the mouth toward the trachea. Advance the catheter 3″ to 4″ to reach the pharynx.

RATIONALE

FIGURE 3. Dipping catheter into sterile saline.

Suctioning removes air from the patient's airway and can cause hypoxemia. Hyperventilation can help prevent suction-induced hypoxemia.

Lubricant facilitates passage of the catheter and reduces trauma to mucous membranes.

Using suction while inserting the catheter can cause trauma to the mucosa and removes oxygen from the respiratory tract. Correct distance for insertion ensures proper placement of the catheter. The general guideline for determining insertion distance for nasopharyngeal suctioning for an individual patient is to estimate the distance from the patient's earlobe to the nose.

FIGURE 4. Inserting catheter into naris.

(continued)

Skill · 39-2 Suctioning the Nasopharyngeal and Oropharyngeal Airways *continued*

ACTION

20. Apply suction by intermittently occluding the Y port on the catheter with the thumb of your nondominant hand and gently rotate the catheter as it is being withdrawn (Figure 5). **Do not suction for more than 10 to 15 seconds at a time.**

21. Replace the oxygen-delivery device using your nondominant hand, if appropriate, and have the patient take several deep breaths.

22. Flush catheter with saline (Figure 6). Assess effectiveness of suctioning and repeat as needed and according to patient's tolerance. Wrap the suction catheter around your dominant hand between attempts.

RATIONALE

Turning the catheter as it is withdrawn minimizes trauma to the mucosa. Suctioning for longer than 10 to 15 seconds robs the respiratory tract of oxygen, which may result in hypoxemia. Suctioning too quickly may be ineffective at clearing all secretions.

Suctioning removes air from the patient's airway and can cause hypoxemia. Hyperventilation can help prevent suction-induced hypoxemia.

Flushing clears catheter and lubricates it for next insertion. Reassessment determines the need for additional suctioning. Wrapping prevents inadvertent contamination of catheter.

FIGURE 5. Suctioning nasopharynx.

FIGURE 6. Rinsing catheter.

23. **Allow at least a 30-second to 1-minute interval if additional suctioning is needed. No more than three suction passes should be made per suctioning episode. Alternate the nares, unless contraindicated, if repeated suctioning is required.** Do not force catheter through the nares. Encourage patient to cough and deep breathe between suctioning. Suction the oropharynx after suctioning the nasopharynx.

24. When suctioning is completed, remove gloves from dominant hand over the coiled catheter, pulling it off inside out. Remove glove from nondominant hand and dispose of gloves, catheter, and container with solution in the appropriate receptacle. Assist patient to a comfortable position. Raise bed rail and place bed in the lowest position.

25. Turn off suction. Remove supplemental oxygen placed for suctioning, if appropriate. Remove face shield or goggles and mask. Perform hand hygiene.

26. Offer oral hygiene after suctioning.

27. Reassess patient's respiratory status, including respiratory rate, effort, oxygen saturation, and lung sounds.

28. Remove additional PPE, if used. Perform hand hygiene.

The interval allows for reventilation and reoxygenation of airways. Excessive suction passes contribute to complications. Alternating nares reduces trauma. Suctioning the oropharynx after the nasopharynx clears the mouth of secretions. More microorganisms are usually present in the mouth, so it is suctioned last to prevent transmission of contaminants.

This technique reduces transmission of microorganisms. Proper positioning with raised side rails and proper bed height provides for patient comfort and safety.

Proper removal of PPE and hand hygiene reduces risk of transmission of microorganisms.

Respiratory secretions that are allowed to accumulate in the mouth are irritating to mucous membranes and unpleasant for the patient.

This assesses effectiveness of suctioning and the presence of complications.

Removing PPE properly reduces the risk for infection transmission and contamination of other items. Hand hygiene prevents the spread of microorganisms.

DOCUMENTATION

Guidelines

Document the time of suctioning, your pre- and post-intervention assessment, reason for suctioning, route used, and the characteristics and amount of secretions.

Sample Documentation

9/17/12 1440 Patient with gurgling on inspiration and weak cough; unable to clear secretions. Lungs with sonorous wheezes in upper airways. Nasopharyngeal suction completed with 12F catheter. Large amount of thick, yellow secretions obtained. After suctioning lung sounds clear in all lobes, respirations 18 breaths per min, no gurgling noted.

—*C. Bausler, RN*

UNEXPECTED SITUATIONS AND ASSOCIATED INTERVENTIONS

- *The catheter or sterile glove touches an unsterile surface:* Stop the procedure. If the gloved hand is still sterile, call for assistance and have someone open another catheter or remove the gloves and start the procedure over.
- *Patient vomits during suctioning:* If the patient gags or becomes nauseated, remove the catheter; it has probably entered the esophagus inadvertently. If the patient needs to be suctioned again, change catheters, as it is probably contaminated. Turn patient to the side and elevate the head of the bed to prevent aspiration.
- *Secretions appear to be stomach contents:* Ask the patient to extend the neck slightly. This helps to prevent the tube from passing into the esophagus.
- *Epistaxis is noted with continued suctioning:* Notify physician and anticipate the need for a nasal trumpet. The nasal trumpet will protect the nasal mucosa from further trauma related to suctioning.

SPECIAL CONSIDERATIONS

Infant and Child Considerations

- For infants, use a 5 Fr to 6 Fr catheter.
- For children, use a 6 Fr to 10 Fr catheter.

Skill · 39-3   Administering Oxygen by Nasal Cannula

EQUIPMENT

- Flow meter connected to oxygen supply
- Humidifier with sterile distilled water (optional for low-flow system)
- Nasal cannula and tubing
- Gauze to pad tubing over ears (optional)
- PPE, as indicated

IMPLEMENTATION

ACTION	RATIONALE
1. Bring necessary equipment to the bedside stand or overbed table.	Bringing everything to the bedside conserves time and energy. Arranging items nearby is convenient, saves time, and avoids unnecessary stretching and twisting of muscles on the part of the nurse.
2. Perform hand hygiene and put on PPE, if indicated.	Hand hygiene and PPE prevent the spread of microorganisms. PPE is required based on transmission precautions.
3. Identify the patient.	Identifying the patient ensures the right patient receives the intervention and helps prevent errors.
4. Close curtains around bed and close door to room if possible.	This ensures the patient's privacy.

(continued)

Skill · 39-3   Administering Oxygen by Nasal Cannula   *continued*

ACTION	RATIONALE
5. Explain what you are going to do and the reason for doing it to the patient. Review safety precautions necessary when oxygen is in use. Place "No Smoking" signs in appropriate areas.	Explanation relieves anxiety and facilitates cooperation. Oxygen supports combustion; a small spark could cause a fire.
6. Connect nasal cannula to oxygen setup with humidification, if one is in use (Figure 1). Adjust flow rate as ordered (Figure 2). Check that oxygen is flowing out of prongs.	Oxygen forced through a water reservoir is humidified before it is delivered to the patient, thus preventing dehydration of the mucous membranes. Low-flow oxygen does not require humidification.

FIGURE 1. Connecting cannula to oxygen source.

FIGURE 2. Adjusting flow rate.

7. Place prongs in patient's nostrils (Figure 3). Place tubing over and behind each ear with adjuster comfortably under chin. Alternately, the tubing may be placed around the patient's head, with adjuster at the back or base of the head. Place gauze pads at ear beneath the tubing as necessary (Figure 4).	Correct placement of the prongs and fastener facilitates oxygen administration and patient comfort. Pads reduce irritation and pressure and protect the skin.

FIGURE 3. Applying cannula to nares.

FIGURE 4. Placing gauze pad at ears.

8. Adjust the fit of the cannula as necessary (Figure 5). Tubing should be snug but not tight against the skin.	Proper adjustment maintains the prongs in the patient's nose. Excessive pressure from tubing could cause irritation and pressure to the skin.
9. **Encourage patients to breathe through the nose, with the mouth closed.**	Nose breathing provides for optimal delivery of oxygen to patient. The percentage of oxygen delivered can be reduced in patients who breathe through the mouth.

ACTION	RATIONALE

10. Reassess patient's respiratory status, including respiratory rate, effort, and lung sounds. Note any signs of respiratory distress, such as tachypnea, nasal flaring, use of accessory muscles, or dyspnea.

These assess the effectiveness of oxygen therapy.

11. Remove PPE, if used. Perform hand hygiene.

Removing PPE properly reduces the risk for infection transmission and contamination of other items. Hand hygiene prevents the spread of microorganisms.

12. Put on clean gloves. Remove and clean the cannula and assess nares at least every 8 hours, or according to agency recommendations (Figure 6). Check nares for evidence of irritation or bleeding.

The continued presence of the cannula causes irritation and dryness of the mucous membranes.

FIGURE 5. Adjusting cannula if needed.

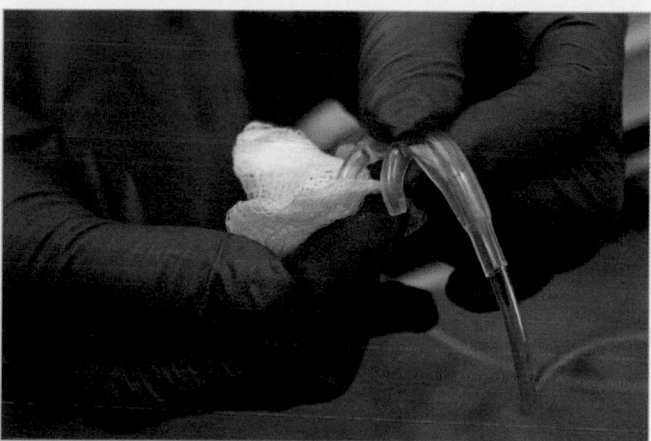

FIGURE 6. Cleaning cannula when indicated.

DOCUMENTATION

Guidelines

Document your assessment pre- and post-intervention. Document the amount of oxygen applied, the patient's respiratory rate, oxygen saturation, and lung sounds.

Sample Documentation

9/17/12 1300 Oxygen via nasal cannula applied at 2 L/min. Humidification in place. Pulse oximeter before placing oxygen 92%; after oxygen at 2 L/min 98%. Respirations even and unlabored. Chest rises symmetrically. No nasal flaring or retractions noted. Lung sounds clear and equal all lobes.

—C. Bausler, RN

UNEXPECTED SITUATIONS AND ASSOCIATED INTERVENTIONS

• *Patient was fine on oxygen delivered by nasal cannula but now is cyanotic, and the pulse oximeter reading is <93%:* Check to see that the oxygen tubing is still connected to the flow meter and the flow meter is still on the previous setting. Someone may have stepped on the tubing, pulling it from the flow meter, or the oxygen may have accidentally been turned off. Assess lung sounds to note any changes.

• *Areas over ear or back of head are reddened:* Ensure that areas are adequately padded and that tubing is not pulled too tight. If available, a skin care team may be able to offer some suggestions.

• *When dozing, patient begins to breathe through the mouth:* Temporarily place the nasal cannula near the mouth. If this does not raise the pulse oximeter reading, you may need to obtain an order to switch the patient to a mask while sleeping.

(continued)

Skill · 39-3 Administering Oxygen by Nasal Cannula *continued*

SPECIAL CONSIDERATIONS

Home Care Considerations

- Oxygen administration may need to be continued in the home setting. Portable oxygen concentrators are used most frequently. Caregivers require instruction concerning safety precautions with oxygen use and need to understand the rationale for the specific liter flow of oxygen.

- To prevent fires and injuries, take the following precautions:
  - Avoid open flames.
  - Place "No Smoking" signs in conspicuous places in the patient's home. Instruct the patient and visitors about the hazard of smoking when oxygen is in use.
  - Check to see that electrical equipment used in the room is in good working order and emits no sparks.
  - Avoid using oils in the area. Oil can ignite spontaneously in the presence of oxygen.

Skill · 39-4 Administering Oxygen by Mask

EQUIPMENT

- Flow meter connected to oxygen supply
- Humidifier with sterile distilled water, if necessary, for the type of mask prescribed
- Face mask, specified by physician
- Gauze to pad elastic band (optional)
- PPE, as indicated

IMPLEMENTATION

ACTION	RATIONALE
1. Bring necessary equipment to the bedside stand or overbed table.	Bringing everything to the bedside conserves time and energy. Arranging items nearby is convenient, saves time, and avoids unnecessary stretching and twisting of muscles on the part of the nurse.
2. Perform hand hygiene and put on PPE, if indicated.	Hand hygiene and PPE prevent the spread of microorganisms. PPE is required based on transmission precautions.
3. Identify the patient.	Identifying the patient ensures the right patient receives the intervention and helps prevent errors.
4. Close curtains around bed and close door to room if possible.	This ensures the patient's privacy.
5. Explain what you are going to do and the reason for doing it to the patient. Review safety precautions necessary when oxygen is in use. Place "No Smoking" signs in appropriate areas.	Explanation relieves anxiety and facilitates cooperation. Oxygen supports combustion; a small spark could cause a fire.
6. Attach face mask to oxygen source (with humidification, if appropriate, for the specific mask) (Figure 1). Start the flow of oxygen at the specified rate. For a mask with a reservoir, be sure to allow oxygen to fill the bag (Figure 2) before proceeding to the next step.	Oxygen forced through a water reservoir is humidified before it is delivered to the patient, thus preventing dehydration of the mucous membranes. A reservoir bag must be inflated with oxygen because the bag is the source of oxygen supply for the patient.

ACTION

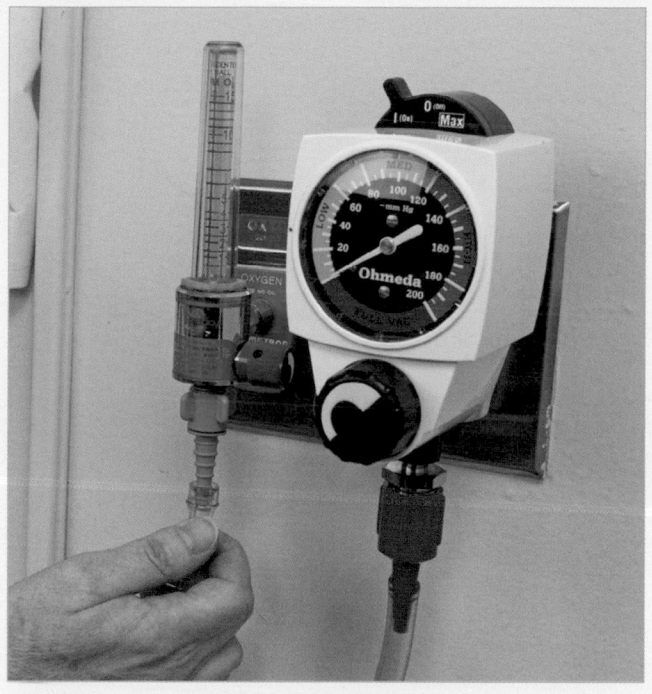

FIGURE 1. Connecting face mask to oxygen source.

RATIONALE

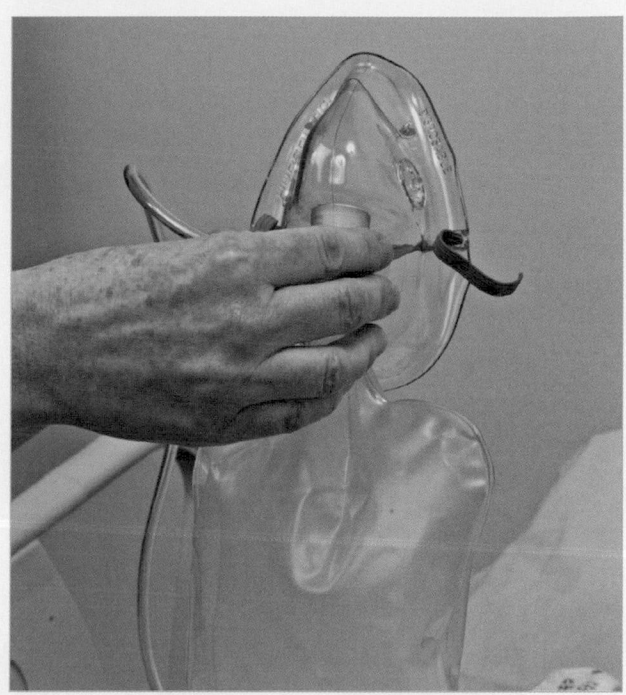

FIGURE 2. Allowing oxygen to fill the bag.

7. Position face mask over patient's nose and mouth (Figure 3). Adjust the elastic strap so that the mask fits snugly but comfortably on the face (Figure 4). Adjust the flow rate to the prescribed rate (Figure 5).

8. If the patient reports irritation or redness is noted, use gauze pads under the elastic strap at pressure points to reduce irritation to ears and scalp.

A loose or poorly fitting mask will result in oxygen loss and decreased therapeutic value. Masks may cause a feeling of suffocation, and the patient needs frequent attention and reassurance.

Pads reduce irritation and pressure and protect the skin.

FIGURE 3. Applying face mask over nose and mouth.

FIGURE 4. Adjusting elastic straps.

(continued)

Skill · 39-4 Administering Oxygen by Mask *continued*

ACTION

FIGURE 5. Adjusting flow rate.

RATIONALE

9. Reassess patient's respiratory status, including respiratory rate, effort, and lung sounds. Note any signs of respiratory distress, such as tachypnea, nasal flaring, use of accessory muscles, or dyspnea.

This helps assess the effectiveness of oxygen therapy.

10. Remove PPE, if used. Perform hand hygiene.

Removing PPE properly reduces the risk for infection transmission and contamination of other items. Hand hygiene prevents the spread of microorganisms.

11. **Remove the mask and dry the skin every 2 to 3 hours if the oxygen is running continuously. Do not use powder around the mask.**

The tight-fitting mask and moisture from condensation can irritate the skin on the face. There is a danger of inhaling powder if it is placed on the mask.

DOCUMENTATION

Guidelines

Document type of mask used, amount of oxygen used, oxygen saturation level, lung sounds, and rate/pattern of respirations. Document your assessment pre- and post-intervention.

Sample Documentation

9/22/12 Patient reports feeling short of breath. Skin pale, respirations 30 breaths per minute and labored. Lung sounds decreased throughout. Oxygen saturation via pulse oximeter 88%. Findings reported to Dr. Lu. Oxygen via nonrebreather face mask applied at 12 L/min as ordered. Patient's skin is pink after O_2 applied. Oxygen saturation increased to 98%. Respirations even and unlabored. Chest rises symmetrically. Respiratory rate 18 breaths per min. Lungs remain with decreased breath sounds throughout. Patient denies dyspnea.

—C. Bausler, RN

UNEXPECTED SITUATIONS AND ASSOCIATED INTERVENTIONS	• *Patient was previously fine but now is cyanotic, and the pulse oximeter reading is <93%:* Check to see that the oxygen tubing is still connected to the flow meter and the flow meter is still on the previous setting. Someone may have stepped on the tubing, pulling it from the flow meter, or the oxygen may have accidentally been turned off. Assess lung sounds for any changes.
	• *Areas over ear or back of head are reddened:* Ensure that areas are adequately padded and that tubing is not pulled too tight. If available, a skin care team may be able to offer some suggestions.
SPECIAL CONSIDERATIONS	• Different types of face masks are available for use.
	• It's important to ensure the mask fits snugly around the patient's face. If it's loose, it will not effectively deliver the right amount of oxygen.
	• The mask must be removed for the patient to eat, drink, and take medications. Obtain an order for oxygen via nasal cannula for use during mealtimes and limit the amount of times the mask is removed to maintain adequate oxygenation.

Skill · 39-5   Suctioning the Tracheostomy: Open System

EQUIPMENT

- Portable or wall suction unit with tubing
- A commercially prepared suction kit with an appropriate size catheter (See General Considerations) or
  - Sterile suction catheter with Y-port in the appropriate size
- Sterile disposable container
- Sterile gloves
- Towel or waterproof pad
- Goggles and mask or face shield
- Additional PPE, as indicated
- Disposable, clean gloves
- Resuscitation bag connected to 100% oxygen

IMPLEMENTATION

ACTION	RATIONALE
1. Bring necessary equipment to the bedside stand or overbed table.	Bringing everything to the bedside conserves time and energy. Arranging items nearby is convenient, saves time, and avoids unnecessary stretching and twisting of muscles on the part of the nurse.
2. Perform hand hygiene and put on PPE, if indicated.	Hand hygiene and PPE prevent the spread of microorganisms. PPE is required based on transmission precautions.
3. Identify the patient.	Identifying the patient ensures the right patient receives the intervention and helps prevent errors.
4. Close curtains around bed and close door to room if possible.	This ensures the patient's privacy.
5. Determine the need for suctioning. Verify the suction order in the patient's chart. **Assess for pain or the potential to cause pain. Administer pain medication as prescribed before suctioning.**	To minimize trauma to airway mucosa, suctioning should be done only when secretions have accumulated or adventitious breath sounds are audible. Suctioning can cause moderate to severe pain for patients. Individualized pain management is imperative (Arroyo-Novoa et al., 2007). Suctioning stimulates coughing, which is painful for patients with surgical incisions.
6. Explain to the patient what you are going to do and the reason for doing it, even if the patient does not appear to be alert. Reassure patient you will interrupt procedure if he or she indicates respiratory difficulty.	Explanation alleviates fears. Even if patient appears unconscious, the nurse should explain what is happening. Any procedure that compromises respiration is frightening for the patient.

(continued)

Skill · 39-5   Suctioning the Tracheostomy: Open System   *continued*

ACTION	**RATIONALE**
7. Adjust bed to comfortable working position, usually elbow height of the caregiver (VISN 8, 2009). Lower side rail closest to you. **If patient is conscious, place him or her in a semi-Fowler's position (Figure 1). If patient is unconscious, place him or her in the lateral position, facing you.** Move the overbed table close to your work area and raise to waist height.	Having the bed at the proper height prevents back and muscle strain. A sitting position helps the patient to cough and makes breathing easier. Gravity also facilitates catheter insertion. The lateral position prevents the airway from becoming obstructed and promotes drainage of secretions. The overbed table provides work surface and maintains sterility of objects on work surface.
8. Place towel or waterproof pad across patient's chest.	This protects bed linens and the patient.
9. **Turn suction to appropriate pressure (Figure 2).**	Higher pressures can cause excessive trauma, hypoxemia, and atelectasis. Glove prevents contact with blood and body fluids. Checking pressure ensures equipment is working properly. Allows for an organized approach to procedure.
For a wall unit for an adult: 100–120 mm Hg (Roman, 2005); neonates: 60–80 mm Hg; infants: 80–100 mm Hg; children: 80–100 mm Hg; adolescents: 80–120 mm Hg (Ireton, 2007).	
For a portable unit for an adult: 10–15 cm Hg; neonates: 6–8 cm Hg; infants: 8–10 cm Hg; children: 8–10 cm Hg; adolescents: 8–10 cm Hg.	
Put on a disposable, clean glove and occlude the end of the connecting tubing to check suction pressure. Place the connecting tubing in a convenient location. If using, place resuscitation bag connected to oxygen within convenient reach.	

FIGURE 1. Patient in semi-Fowler's position.

FIGURE 2. Turning suction device to the appropriate pressure.

10. Open sterile suction package using aseptic technique. The open wrapper or container becomes a sterile field to hold other supplies. Carefully remove the sterile container, touching only the outside surface. Set it up on the work surface and pour sterile saline into it.	Sterile normal saline or water is used to lubricate the outside of the catheter, minimizing irritation of mucosa during introduction. It is also used to clear the catheter between suction attempts.
11. Put on face shield or goggles and mask (Figure 3). Put on sterile gloves. **The dominant hand will manipulate the catheter and must remain sterile. The nondominant hand is considered clean rather than sterile and will control the suction valve (Y port) on the catheter.**	Handling the sterile catheter using a sterile glove helps prevent introducing organisms into the respiratory tract; the clean glove protects the nurse from microorganisms.

ACTION

12. With dominant gloved hand, pick up sterile catheter. Pick up the connecting tubing with the nondominant hand and connect the tubing and suction catheter (Figure 4).

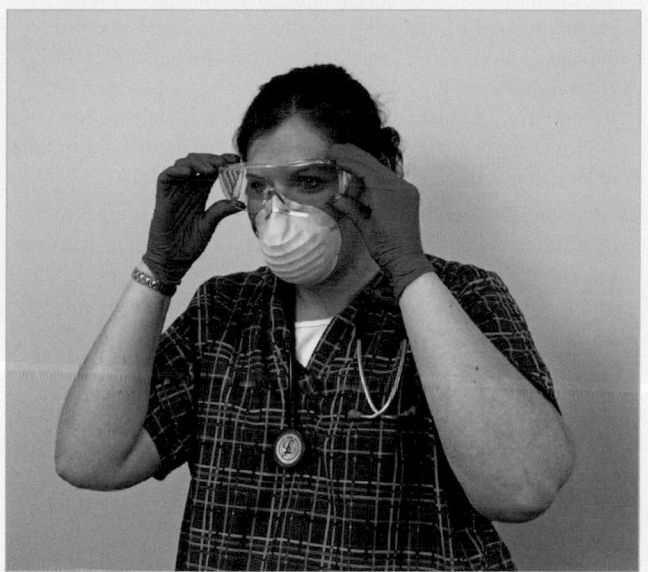

FIGURE 3. Putting on goggles and mask.

13. Moisten the catheter by dipping it into the container of sterile saline, unless it is a silicone catheter (Figure 5). Occlude Y-tube to check suction (Figure 6).

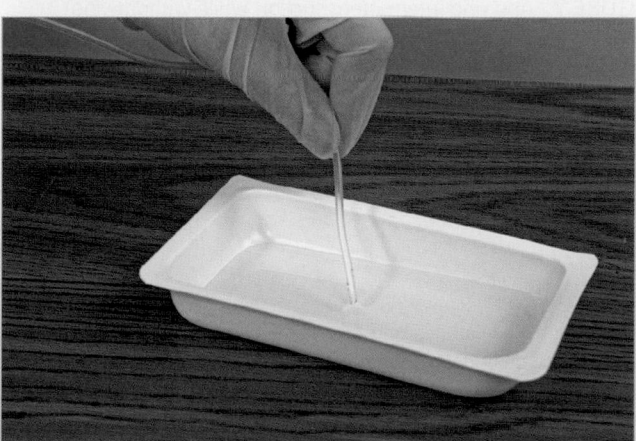

FIGURE 5. Moistening catheter in saline solution.

14. Using your nondominant hand and a manual resuscitation bag, hyperventilate the patient, delivering 3 to 6 breaths or use the sigh mechanism on a mechanical ventilator.

15. Open the adapter on the mechanical ventilator tubing or remove oxygen delivery setup with your nondominant hand.

RATIONALE

Sterility of the suction catheter is maintained.

FIGURE 4. Connecting suction catheter to the suction tubing.

Lubricating the inside of the catheter with saline helps move secretions in the catheter. Silicone catheters do not require lubrication. Checking ensures equipment is working properly.

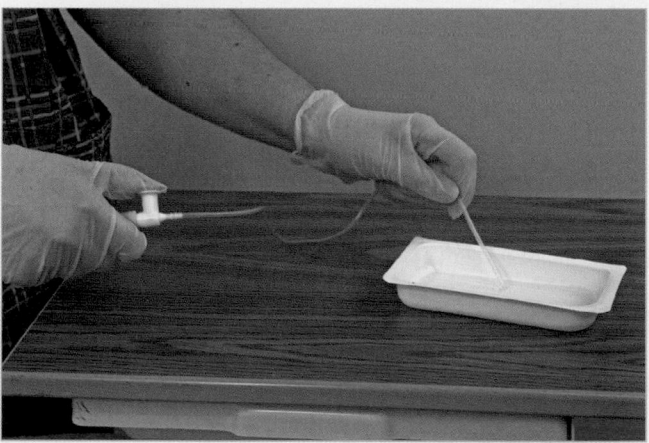

FIGURE 6. Occluding Y-port to check for proper suction.

Hyperoxygenation and hyperventilation aid in preventing hypoxemia during suctioning.

This exposes tracheostomy tube without contaminating sterile gloved hand.

(continued)

Skill · 39-5   Suctioning the Tracheostomy: Open System   *continued*

ACTION	RATIONALE
16. Using your dominant hand, gently and quickly insert catheter into trachea. **Advance the catheter to the predetermined length. Do not occlude Y-port when inserting catheter.**	Catheter contact and suction cause tracheal mucosal damage, loss of cilia, edema, and fibrosis, as well as increasing the risk of infection and bleeding for the patient. Insertion of the suction catheter to a predetermined distance, no more than 1 cm past the length of the endotracheal tube, avoids contact with the trachea and carina, reducing the effects of tracheal mucosal damage (Ireton, 2007; Pate, 2004; Pate & Zapata, 2002). If resistance is met, the carina or tracheal mucosa has been hit. Withdraw the catheter at least 1/2″ before applying suction. Suctioning when inserting catheter increases the risk for trauma to airway mucosa and increases risk of hypoxemia.
17. Apply suction by intermittently occluding the Y port on the catheter with the thumb of your nondominant hand, and gently rotate the catheter as it is being withdrawn (Figure 7). **Do not suction for more than 10 to 15 seconds at a time.**	Turning the catheter as it is withdrawn minimizes trauma to the mucosa. Suctioning for longer than 10 to 15 seconds robs the respiratory tract of oxygen, which may result in hypoxemia. Suctioning too quickly may be ineffective at clearing all secretions.

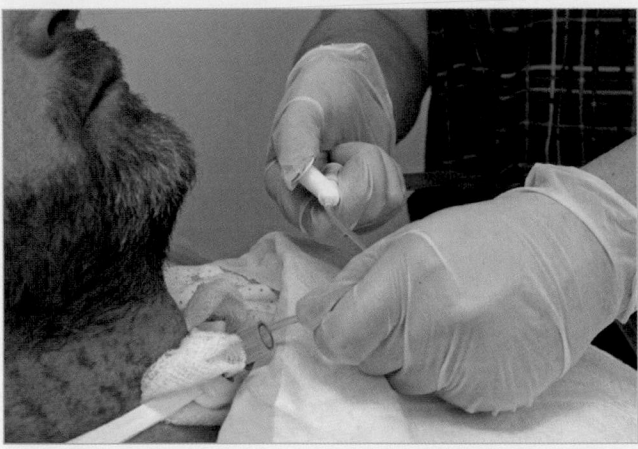

FIGURE 7. Applying intermittent suction while withdrawing catheter.

18. Hyperventilate the patient using your nondominant hand and a manual resuscitation bag, delivering 3 to 6 breaths. Replace the oxygen delivery device, if applicable, using your nondominant hand and have the patient take several deep breaths. If the patient is mechanically ventilated, close the adapter on the mechanical ventilator tubing and use the sigh mechanism on a mechanical ventilator.	Suctioning removes air from the patient's airway and can cause hypoxemia. Hyperventilation can help prevent suction-induced hypoxemia.
19. Flush catheter with saline. Assess effectiveness of suctioning and repeat as needed and according to patient's tolerance. Wrap the suction catheter around your dominant hand between attempts.	Flushing clears catheter and lubricates it for next insertion. Reassessment determines need for additional suctioning. Prevents inadvertent contamination of catheter.
20. **Allow at least a 30-second to 1-minute interval if additional suctioning is needed. No more than three suction passes should be made per suctioning episode. Encourage patient to cough and deep breathe between suctionings.** Suction the oropharynx after suctioning the trachea. Do not reinsert in the tracheostomy after suctioning the mouth.	The interval allows for reventilation and reoxygenation of airways. Excessive suction passes contribute to complications. Alternating nares reduces trauma. Clears the mouth of secretions. More microorganisms are usually present in the mouth, so it is suctioned last to prevent transmission of contaminants.

21. When suctioning is completed, remove gloves from dominant hand over the coiled catheter, pulling it off inside out (Figure 8). Remove glove from nondominant hand and dispose of gloves, catheter, and container with solution in the appropriate receptacle. Assist patient to a comfortable position. Raise bed rail and place bed in the lowest position.

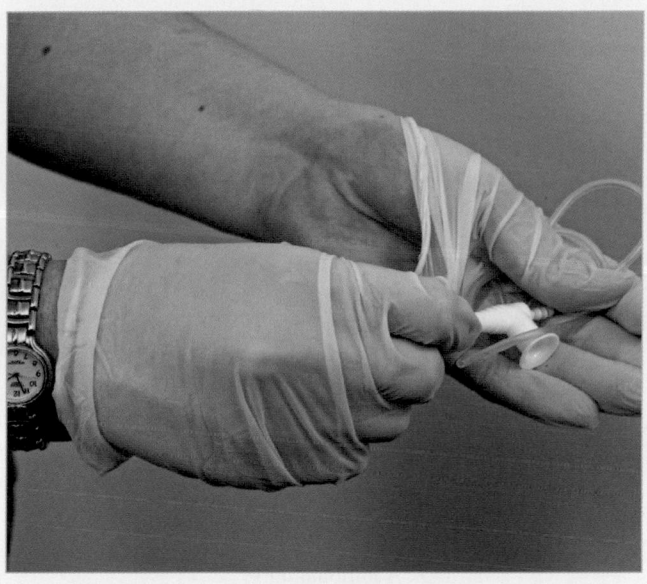

FIGURE 8. Removing gloves while keeping catheter inside.

22. Turn off suction. Remove supplemental oxygen placed for suctioning, if appropriate. Remove face shield or goggles and mask. Perform hand hygiene.

23. Offer oral hygiene after suctioning.

24. Reassess patient's respiratory status, including respiratory rate, effort, oxygen saturation, and lung sounds.

25. Remove additional PPE, if used. Perform hand hygiene.

This technique reduces transmission of microorganisms. Ensures patient comfort. Proper positioning with raised side rails and proper bed height provides for patient comfort and safety.

Removing PPE properly reduces the risk for infection transmission and contamination of other items. Hand hygiene prevents transmission of microorganisms.

Respiratory secretions that are allowed to accumulate in the mouth are irritating to mucous membranes and unpleasant for the patient.

These assess effectiveness of suctioning and the presence of complications.

Removing PPE properly reduces the risk for infection transmission and contamination of other items. Hand hygiene prevents the spread of microorganisms.

DOCUMENTATION

Guidelines

Document the time of suctioning, your pre- and post-intervention assessment, reason for suctioning, and the characteristics and amount of secretions.

Sample Documentation

9/1/12 1515 Lungs auscultated for wheezes in upper and lower lobes bilaterally. Respirations at 24 breaths per min. Weak, ineffective cough noted. Tracheal suction completed with 12F catheter. Large amount of thick, yellow secretions obtained. Specimen for culture collected and sent as ordered. After suctioning, lung sounds clear all lobes, oxygen saturation at 97%, respirations 18 breaths per min.

—*C. Bausler, RN*

(continued)

Skill · 39-5 Suctioning the Tracheostomy: Open System *continued*

UNEXPECTED SITUATIONS AND ASSOCIATED INTERVENTIONS	• *Patient coughs hard enough to dislodge tracheostomy:* Keep a spare tracheostomy and obturator at the bedside. Insert obturator into tracheostomy tube and reinsert tracheostomy into stoma. Remove obturator. Secure ties and auscultate lung sounds. Palpate for any subcutaneous emphysema. • *Lung sounds do not improve greatly and oxygen saturation remains low after three suctionings:* Allow patient time to recover from previous suctioning. If needed, hyperoxygenate again. Suction the patient again and assess whether the oxygen saturation increases, lung sounds improve, and secretion amount decreases.
SPECIAL CONSIDERATIONS	• Determine the size catheter to use by the size of the tracheostomy. The external diameter of the suction catheter should not exceed half of the internal diameter of the tracheostomy. Larger catheters can contribute to trauma and hypoxemia. • Emergency equipment should be easily accessible at the bedside. Keep bag-valve mask, oxygen, and suction equipment at the bedside of a patient with a tracheostomy tube at all times.

Skill · 39-6 Providing Tracheostomy Care

EQUIPMENT

- Disposable gloves
- Sterile gloves
- Goggles and mask or face shield
- Additional PPE, as indicated
- Sterile normal saline
- Sterile cup or basin

- Sterile cotton-tipped applicators
- Sterile gauze sponges
- Disposable inner tracheostomy cannula, appropriate size for patient
- Sterile suction catheter and glove set

- Commercially prepared tracheostomy or drain dressing
- Commercially prepared tracheostomy holder
- Plastic disposal bag
- Additional nurse

IMPLEMENTATION

ACTION	RATIONALE
1. Bring necessary equipment to the bedside stand or overbed table.	Bringing everything to the bedside conserves time and energy. Arranging items nearby is convenient, saves time, and avoids unnecessary stretching and twisting of muscles on the part of the nurse.
2. Perform hand hygiene and put on PPE, if indicated.	Hand hygiene and PPE prevent the spread of microorganisms. PPE is required based on transmission precautions.
3. Identify the patient.	Identifying the patient ensures the right patient receives the intervention and helps prevent errors.
4. Close curtains around bed and close door to room if possible.	This ensures the patient's privacy.
5. Determine the need for tracheostomy care. **Assess patient's pain and administer pain medication, if indicated.**	If tracheostomy is new, pain medication may be needed before performing tracheostomy care.
6. Explain what you are going to do and the reason to the patient, even if the patient does not appear to be alert. Reassure patient you will interrupt procedure if he or she indicates respiratory difficulty.	Explanation alleviates fears. Even if patient appears unconscious, the nurse should explain what is happening. Any procedure that compromises respiration is frightening for the patient.
7. Adjust bed to comfortable working position, usually elbow height of the caregiver (VISN 8, 2009). Lower side rail closest to you. **If patient is conscious, place him or her in a semi-Fowler's position. If patient is unconscious, place him or her in the lateral position, facing you.** Move the overbed table close to your work area and raise to waist height. Place a trash receptacle within easy reach of work area.	Having the bed at the proper height prevents back and muscle strain. A sitting position helps the patient to cough and makes breathing easier. Gravity also facilitates catheter insertion. The lateral position prevents the airway from becoming obstructed and promotes drainage of secretions. The overbed table provides work surface and maintains sterility of objects on work surface. Trash receptacle within reach prevents reaching over sterile field or turning back to field to dispose of trash.

ACTION

8. Put on face shield or goggles and mask. Suction tracheostomy if necessary. If tracheostomy has just been suctioned, remove soiled site dressing and discard before removal of gloves used to perform suctioning.

Cleaning the Tracheostomy: Disposable Inner Cannula

9. Carefully open the package with the new disposable inner cannula, taking care not to contaminate the cannula or the inside of the package (Figure 1). Carefully open the package with the sterile cotton-tipped applicators, taking care not to contaminate them. Open sterile cup or basin and fill 0.5 inches deep with saline. Open the plastic disposable bag and place within reach on work surface.

10. Put on disposable gloves.

11. Remove the oxygen source if one is present. Stabilize the outer cannula and faceplate of the tracheostomy with your nondominant hand. Grasp the locking mechanism of the inner cannula with your dominant hand. Press the tabs and release lock (Figure 2). Gently remove inner cannula and place in disposal bag. If not already removed, remove site dressing and dispose of in the trash.

RATIONALE

Personnel protective equipment prevents contact with contaminants. Suctioning removes secretions to prevent occluding outer cannula while the inner cannula is removed.

Inner cannula must remain sterile. Saline and applicators will be used to clean tracheostomy site. Plastic disposable bag will be used to discard removed inner cannula.

Gloves protect against exposure to blood and body fluids.

Stabilizing base plate prevents trauma to and pain from stoma. Releasing the lock permits removal of the inner cannula.

FIGURE 1. Carefully opening package with new disposable inner cannula. *(Photo by B. Proud.)*

FIGURE 2. Releasing lock on inner cannula.

12. Discard gloves and put on sterile gloves. Pick up the new inner cannula with your dominant hand, stabilize the faceplate with your nondominant hand, and gently insert the new inner cannula into the outer cannula. Press the tabs to allow the lock to grab the outer cannula (Figure 3). Reapply oxygen source if needed.

Applying Clean Dressing and Holder

13. Remove oxygen source, if necessary. Dip cotton-tipped applicator or gauze sponge in cup or basin with sterile saline and clean stoma under faceplate. **Use each applicator or sponge only once, moving from stoma site outward (Figure 4).**

Sterile gloves are necessary to prevent contamination of the new inner cannula. Locking to outer cannula secures the inner cannula in place. Maintains oxygen supply to the patient.

Saline is nonirritating to tissue. Cleansing from stoma outward and using each applicator only once promotes aseptic technique.

(continued)

Skill · 39-6 **Providing Tracheostomy Care** *continued*

ACTION

FIGURE 3. Locking new inner cannula in place.

14. Pat skin gently with dry 4″ × 4″ gauze sponge.

15. Slide commercially prepared tracheostomy dressing or prefolded noncotton-filled 4″ × 4″ dressing under the faceplate.

16. Change the tracheostomy holder:

   a. **Obtain the assistance of a second individual to hold the tracheostomy tube in place while the old collar is removed and the new collar is placed.**

   b. Open the package for the new tracheostomy collar.

   c. Both nurses should put on clean gloves.

   d. One nurse holds the faceplate while the other pulls up the Velcro tabs. Gently remove the collar.

   e. The first nurse continues to hold the tracheostomy faceplate.

   f. The other nurse places the collar around the patient's neck and inserts first one tab, then the other, into the openings on the faceplate and secures the Velcro tabs on the tracheostomy holder (Figure 5).

   g. Check the fit of the tracheostomy collar. You should be able to fit one finger between the neck and the collar. Check to make sure that the patient can flex neck comfortably. Reapply oxygen source if necessary (Figure 6).

RATIONALE

FIGURE 4. Cleaning from stoma site, outward.

Gauze removes excess moisture.

Lint or fiber from a cut cotton-filled gauze pad can be aspirated into the trachea, causing respiratory distress, or can embed in the stoma and cause irritation or infection.

Holding the tracheostomy tube in place ensures that the tracheostomy will not inadvertently be expelled if the patient coughs or moves. Doing so provides attachment for one side of the faceplate.

Allows access to the new collar.

Gloves prevent contact with blood, body fluids, and contaminants.

Holding the tracheostomy tube in place ensures that the tracheostomy will not inadvertently be expelled if patient coughs or moves. Pulling up the Velcro tabs loosens the collar.

Prevents accidental extubation.

Securing the Velcro tabs holds the tracheostomy in place and prevents accidental expulsion of the tracheostomy tube.

Allowing one fingerbreadth under collar permits neck flexion that is comfortable and ensures that collar will not compromise circulation to the area. Maintains oxygen supply to the patient.

FIGURE 5. Securing tabs on tracheostomy holder.

FIGURE 6. Reapplying oxygen source.

ACTION

17. Remove gloves. Assist patient to a comfortable position. Raise the bed rail and place the bed in the lowest position.

18. Remove face shield or goggles and mask. Remove additional PPE, if used. Perform hand hygiene.

19. Reassess patient's respiratory status, including respiratory rate, effort, oxygen saturation, and lung sounds.

RATIONALE

Removing PPE properly reduces the risk for infection transmission and contamination of other items. Ensures patient comfort. Proper positioning with raised side rails and proper bed height provides for patient comfort and safety.

Removing PPE properly reduces the risk for infection transmission and contamination of other items. Hand hygiene prevents the spread of microorganisms.

Assessments determine the effectiveness of interventions and for the presence of complications.

DOCUMENTATION

Guidelines

Document pre- and post-assessments, including site assessment, presence of pain, lung sounds, and oxygen saturation levels. Document presence of skin breakdown that may result from irritation or pressure from tracheostomy collar. Document care given.

Sample Documentation

> 9/26/12 1300 Tracheostomy care completed; lung sounds clear in all lobes; respirations even/unlabored; site without erythema or edema; small amount of thick yellow secretions noted at site.
>
> —C. Bausler, RN

UNEXPECTED SITUATIONS AND ASSOCIATED INTERVENTIONS

- *Patient coughs hard enough to dislodge tracheostomy:* A spare tracheostomy and obturator should be kept at bedside. Insert obturator into the new tracheostomy and insert tracheostomy into stoma. Remove obturator. Secure ties and auscultate lung sounds. Palpate for any subcutaneous emphysema.

- *On palpating around insertion site, you note a moderate amount of subcutaneous emphysema in tissue:* Assess for dislodgement of the tracheostomy tube. If the tube becomes displaced, a buildup of air in the subcutaneous portion of the skin is likely. Notify physician if the subcutaneous emphysema is a change in the status of the tracheostomy.

SPECIAL CONSIDERATIONS

General Considerations

- One nurse working alone should always place new tracheostomy ties in place before removing old ties to prevent accidental extubation of tracheostomy. If it is necessary to remove old ties first, obtain the assistance of a second person to hold the tracheostomy tube in place while the old tie is removed and the new tie is replaced.

- Emergency equipment should be easily accessible at the bedside. Keep a bag-valve mask, oxygen, the obturator from the current tracheostomy, spare tracheostomy of the same size, spare tracheostomy one size smaller, and suction equipment at the bedside of a patient with an endotracheal tube at all times.

- If the patient is currently using a tracheostomy without a cuff, keep a spare tracheostomy of the same size with a cuff at the bedside for emergency use.

Home Care Considerations

- Instruct the patient and home caregiver on how to perform tracheostomy care. Observe a return demonstration and provide feedback.

- Clean rather than sterile technique can be used in the home setting.

- Sterile saline can be made by mixing 1 teaspoon of table salt in 1 quart of water and boiling for 15 minutes. The solution is cooled and stored in a clean, dry container. Discard saline at the end of each day to prevent growth of bacteria.

- The patient who is performing self-care should use a mirror to view the steps in the procedure.

● Developing Critical Thinking Skills

1. Using the Focused Assessment Guide in this chapter, work with a partner to assess the respiratory functioning of the following patients. Discuss ways in which you would modify your assessment to meet the specific needs of individual patients:
   - A 6-year-old who presents with asthma and is experiencing difficulty breathing
   - A 12-year-old who is brought to emergency room after illicit use of inhalants ("huffing")
   - An adult dying of cancer who is receiving increasing doses of narcotics, which depress respiratory functioning
   - A hospitalized young adult with a 24-pack/year history of smoking who is noted to have a persistent, hacking cough

2. A postoperative patient who is at high risk for pulmonary complications because of a long history of smoking refuses to use the incentive spirometer or to cooperate with instructions to deep breathe. How would you respond to this patient? Discuss with other students what nursing response is most likely to secure his cooperation in necessary self-care measures.

● Practicing for NCLEX

1. A patient has a fractured rib and is breathing less often and with less depth because of the pain. The nurse would document this finding using which term?
   a. Fremitus
   b. Hyperventilation
   c. Pleural friction rub
   d. Hypoventilation

2. When auscultating Mr. Chang's breath sounds, the nurse detects a continuous, musical sound heard on expiration. The nurse identifies this sound as which of the following?
   a. Crackles
   b. Wheezes
   c. Bronchial sounds
   d. Pleural friction rub

3. Air that develops in the pleural space is referred to as:
   a. Pneumothorax
   b. Pleural effusion
   c. Hemothorax
   d. Atelectasis

4. When planning care for a patient with chronic lung disease who is receiving oxygen through a nasal cannula, what does the nurse expect?
   a. The oxygen must be humidified.
   b. The rate will be 2 L/min or less.
   c. Arterial blood gases will be drawn every 4 hours to assess flow rate.
   d. The rate will be 6 L/min or more.

5. Which oxygen delivery device would the nurse expect to use to provide the highest concentration of oxygen to a patient who is breathing spontaneously?
   a. Partial rebreather mask
   b. Nonrebreather mask
   c. Simple mask
   d. Venturi mask

6. When teaching a patient about pulse oximetry, which statement would the nurse most likely include in the discussion?
   a. A range of 95% to 100% is considered normal oxygen saturation.
   b. Oximetry measures the oxygen saturation of venous blood.
   c. Fasting is required for 12 hours before the test.
   d. Pulse oximetry is a replacement for arterial blood gas analysis.

7. Which action would the nurse include when performing oropharyngeal suctioning on a patient?
   a. Use clean technique.
   b. Apply suction as the catheter is introduced.
   c. Flush the catheter with saline between catheter insertions.
   d. Limit suctioning to 25- to 30-second intervals at one time.

8. Effective use of a metered-dose inhaler requires that the patient accomplish which action?
   a. Breathe in through the nose.
   b. Inhale two sprays with one breath.
   c. Hold the breath for 5 to 10 seconds after inspiration.
   d. Exhale quickly through an open mouth.

9. Mr. Parks has chronic obstructive pulmonary disease (COPD). The nurse has taught him that pursed-lip breathing helps him by:
   a. Increasing carbon dioxide, which stimulates breathing
   b. Prolonging inspiration and shortening expiration
   c. Liquefying his secretions
   d. Decreasing the amount of air trapping and resistance

10. A patient develops sudden cardiac arrest. It is imperative to begin CPR as soon as possible. What is the critical time that the nurse must keep in mind before irreversible brain damage occurs?
    a. 1 to 3 minutes
    b. 2 to 4 minutes
    c. 4 to 6 minutes
    d. 8 to 10 minutes

11. David White is in the hospital with a medical diagnosis of viral pneumonia. He is receiving oxygen through a simple face mask. The nurse ensures that the mask fits snugly over the patient's face for which reason?
    a. To prevent mask movement and consequent skin breakdown
    b. To help the patient feel secure
    c. To maintain carbon dioxide retention
    d. To aid in maintaining expected oxygen delivery

12. When suctioning a patient through a tracheostomy tube, the nurse was careful not to occlude the Y port when inserting the suction catheter because this would do which of the following?
    a. Prevent suctioning from occurring
    b. Cause trauma to the tracheal mucosa
    c. Break the sterile technique
    d. Suction out all the carbon dioxide

13. What action does the nurse use to follow safe technique when using a portable oxygen cylinder?
    a. Checking the amount of oxygen in the cylinder before using it
    b. Using a cylinder for a patient transfer that indicates available oxygen is 500 psi
    c. Placing the oxygen cylinder on the stretcher next to the patient
    d. Discontinuing oxygen flow by turning cylinder key counterclockwise until tight

14. Which of the following assessments should the nurse consider when performing tracheal suctioning? Select all that apply.
    a. Close assessment of the patient before, during, and after the procedure.
    b. Hyperoxygenate the patient before and after suctioning.
    c. Limit the application of suction to 20 to 30 seconds.
    d. Monitor the patient's pulse frequently to detect potential effects of hypoxia and stimulation of the vagus nerve.
    e. Using an appropriate suction pressure (80–120 mm Hg).
    f. Insert the suction catheter as far as it will go before applying suction. This will help prevent atelectasis related to the use of high negative pressure.

15. Abdominal breathing at 30 to 60 breaths/minute with an irregular pattern of rate and depth would closely describe the breathing patterns of what age group?
    a. Aged adult
    b. Infant
    c. Early childhood
    d. Late childhood

● Answers With Rationale

1. *d.* Hypoventilation is a decreased rate or depth of air movement into the lungs. Hyperventilation is an increased rate and depth of ventilation. Fremitus is the vibration of the chest wall that can be palpated. A pleural friction rub is a dry grating sound caused by inflammation of pleural surfaces.

2. *b.* Wheezes are a continuous sound heard on expiration. Crackles are not described as squeaky. The pleural friction rub is a dry, grating sound. Bronchial breath sounds are normal sounds heard over the trachea.

3. *a.* Air in the pleural space is termed pneumothorax. Fluid in the pleural space is referred to as a pleural effusion. Blood collection in the pleural space is referred to as a hemothorax. Atelectasis refers to an incomplete expansion or collapse of the alveoli.

4. *b.* A rate higher than 2 L/min may destroy the hypoxic drive that stimulates respirations in the medulla in a patient with chronic lung disease. Oxygen delivered at low rates does not necessarily have to be humidified, and arterial blood gases are not required at regular intervals to determine the flow rate.

5. *b.* The nonrebreather mask provides the highest concentration of oxygen to a spontaneously breathing patient. None of the other devices would provide this.

6. *a.* Pulse oximetry measures oxygen saturation levels of arterial blood, which normally range from 95% to 98%. Fasting is not required before the test. Pulse oximetry is an adjunct therapy, not a replacement for arterial blood gas analysis.

7. *c.* Flushing the catheter with saline between insertions is important to clear the catheter of secretions. The nurse should use sterile technique and should not apply suction as the catheter is being introduced; suctioning should be limited to 10- to 15-second intervals to avoid causing hypoxia.

8. *c.* Holding one's breath for 5 to 10 seconds after inspiration of the medication allows the drug to reach the alveoli. Correct technique for using an MDI includes breathing in through the mouth so that all the medication is properly delivered to the lungs, using one spray of medication for each breath to receive the correct dose, and exhaling slowly through pursed lips to minimize airway trapping and resistance.

9. *d.* Doing pursed-lip breathing correctly diminishes carbon dioxide retention. It also prolongs expiration, increases airway pressure, and lessens the amount of airway trapping and resistance.

10. *c.* After 4 to 6 minutes without oxygen, irreversible brain damage can occur.

11. *d.* A snug-fitting mask is necessary to deliver the expected rate of oxygen. A simple face mask does not trap carbon dioxide or cause retention. Patients often complain that an oxygen mask is uncomfortable. A snug fit may limit but not prevent movement of the mask.

12. *b.* Occluding the Y port causes suction and may traumatize the tracheal mucosa if applied when the catheter is inserted. Occluding the Y port does not prevent suction.

13. *a.* The cylinder must always be checked before use to ensure that enough oxygen is available for the patient. It is unsafe to use a cylinder that reads 500 psi or less because not enough oxygen remains for a patient transfer. A cylinder that is not secured properly may result in injury to the patient. Oxygen flow is discontinued by turning the valve clockwise until it is tight.

14. **a, b, d, e.** Close assessment of the patient before, during, and after the procedure is necessary to limit negative effects. Risks include hypoxia, infection, tracheal tissue damage, dysrhythmias, and atelectasis. Hyperoxygenate the patient before and after suctioning. Limit the application of suction to 10 to 20 seconds. These interventions help prevent hypoxia. Monitor the patient's pulse frequently to detect potential effects of hypoxia and stimulation of the vagus nerve. Using an appropriate suction pressure (80–120 mm Hg) will help prevent atelectasis related to the use of high negative pressure. Research suggests that insertion of the suction catheter should be limited to a predetermined length (no further than 1 cm past the length of the tracheal or endotracheal tube) to avoid tracheal mucosal damage, including epithelial denudement, loss of cilia, edema, and fibrosis (Roman, 2005).

15. **b.** Respirations in the infant are more rapid and have not stabilized. As alveoli increase in number and size, the respiratory rate decreases.

Taylor Suite Resources

The Taylor Suite offers these additional resources to enhance learning and facilitate understanding of this chapter:

- thePoint online resource, http://thepoint.lww.com/Taylor7E
- Student DVD-ROM included with the book
- Study Guide for Taylor's Fundamentals of Nursing
- Skill Checklists for Taylor's Fundamentals of Nursing
- Taylor's Clinical Nursing Skills: *Chapter 14, Oxygenation*
- Taylor's Video Guide to Clinical Nursing Skills: *Oxygenation* and *Tracheostomy Care*

BIBLIOGRAPHY

AARC Clinical Practice Guideline. (2004). Nasotracheal suctioning—2004 revision & update. *Respiratory Care, 49*(9), 1080–1084.

American Heart Association (AHA). (2008). *Hands-only CPR.* Available at http://handsonlycpr.eisenberginc.com.

Alsaghir, A., & Martin, C. (2008). Effect of prone positioning in patients with acute respiratory distress syndrome: A meta-analysis. *Critical Care, 36*(2), 603–609.

American Heart Association (AHA). (2005). Highlights of the 2005 American Heart Association guidelines for cardiopulmonary resuscitation and emergency cardiovascular care. *Currents in Emergency Cardiovascular Care, 16*(4), 1–27.

Arroyo-Novoa, C., Figueroa-Ramos, M., Puntillo, K., Stanik-Hutt, J., Thompson, C. L., White, C., et al. (2007). Pain related to tracheal suctioning in awake acutely and critically ill adults: A descriptive study. *Intensive & Critical Care Nursing, 24*(1), 20–27.

Aschenbrenner, D., & Venable, S. (2009). *Drug therapy in nursing* (3rd ed.). Philadelphia: Wolters Kluwer Health/Lippincott Williams & Wilkins.

Björling, G., Belink, A. L., Hellström, C., Schedin, U., Ransjö, U., Alenius, M., et al. (2007). Tracheostomy inner cannula care: A randomized crossover study of two decontamination procedures. *American Journal of Infection Control, 35*(9), 600–605.

Booker, R. (2008a). Pulse oximetry. *Nursing Standard, 22*(30), 39–41.

Booker, R. (2008b). Simple spirometry measurement. *Nursing Standard, 22*(32), 35–39.

Bulechek, G., Butcher, H., & McCloskey Dochterman, J. (Eds.). (2008). *Nursing interventions classification (NIC)* (5th ed.). St. Louis: Mosby Elsevier.

Carpenito-Moyet, L. (2008). *Nursing diagnosis: Application to clinical practice* (12th ed.). Philadelphia: Wolters Kluwer Health/Lippincott Williams & Wilkins.

Cohen, B., & Taylor J. (2009). *Memmler's structure and function of the human body* (9th ed.). Philadelphia: Wolters Kluwer Health/Lippincott Williams & Wilkins.

Collins, C. L., & Andersen, C. C. (2007). Deceptive simplicity: systemic oxygen delivery and pulse oximetry. *Journal of Pediatrics & Child Health, 43*(7–8), 510–512.

Crisafulli, E., Costi, S., DeBlasio, F., Biscione, G., Americi, F., Penza, S., et al. (2007). Effects of a walking aid in COPD patients receiving oxygen therapy. *CHEST, 131*(4), 1068–1074.

Davis, M., & Johnston, J. (2008). Maintaining supplemental oxygen during transport. *American Journal of Nursing, 108*(1), 35–36.

DeMeulenaere, S. (2007). Pulse oximetry: Uses and limitations. *The Journal for Nurse Practitioners, 3*(5), 312–317.

Dudek, S. (2006). *Nutrition essentials for nursing practice* (5th ed.). Philadelphia: Lippincott Williams & Wilkins.

Dulak, S. (2005). Hands-on help: Placing an oropharyngeal airway. *RN, 68*(2), 20ac1–20ac3.

Eastwood, G., Gardner, A., & O'Connell, B. (2007). Low-flow oxygen therapy: Selecting the right device. *Australian Nursing Journal, 15*(4), 27–30.

Fernandez, M., Burns, K., Calhoun, B., George, S., Martin, B., & Weaver, C. (2007). Evaluation of a new pulse oximeter sensor. *American Journal of Critical Care, 16*(2), 146–152.

Ferns, T., & West, S. (2008). The art of auscultation: Evaluating a patient's respiratory pathology. *British Journal of Nursing, 17*(12), 772–777.

Fischbach, F., & Dunning, M. (2006). *Common laboratory and diagnostic tests* (4th ed.). Philadelphia: Lippincott Williams & Wilkins.

Fischbach, F., & Dunning M. (2009). *A manual of laboratory and diagnostic tests* (8th ed.). Philadelphia: Wolters Kluwer/ Lippincott Williams & Wilkins.

Friesner, S., Curry, D., & Moddeman, G. (2006). Comparison of two pain-management strategies during chest tube removal: Relaxation exercise with opioids and opioids alone. *Issues in Pain Management, 35*(4), 269–276.

Halm, M. (2007). To strip or not to strip? Physiological effects of chest tube manipulation. *American Journal of Critical Care, 16*(6), 609–612.

Ireton, J. (2007). Tracheostomy suction: A protocol for practice. *Paediatric Nursing, 19*(10), 14–18.

Jarvis, C. (2008). *Physical examination & health assessment* (5th ed.). St. Louis: Saunders/Elsevier.

Jongerden, I., Rovers, M., Grypdonck, M., & Bonten, M. J. (2007). Open and closed endotracheal suction systems in mechanically ventilated intensive care patients: A meta-analysis. *Critical Care Medicine, 35*(1), 260–270.

Kara, M. (2005). Preparing nurses for the global pandemic of chronic obstructive pulmonary disease. *Journal of Nursing Scholarship, 37*(2), 127–133.

Kyle, T. (2008). *Essentials of pediatric nursing*. Philadelphia: Wolters Kluwer Health/Lippincott Williams & Wilkins.

Lannefors, L. (2006). Inhalation therapy: Practical considerations for nebulisation therapy. *Physical Therapy Reviews, 11*(1), 21–27.

Macnee, W. (2007). Pathogenesis of chronic obstructive pulmonary disease. *Clinics in Chest Medicine, 28*(3), 479–513.

Marcus, B., Williams, D., Dubbert, P., Sallis, J. F., King, A. C., Yancey, A. K., et al. (2006). Physical activity intervention studies: What we know and what we need to know: A scientific statement from the American Heart Association Council on nutrition, physical activity, and metabolism. *Circulation, 114*(24), 2739–2752.

McCool, F., & Rosen, M. (2006). Nonpharmacologic airway clearance therapies: ACCP evidence-based clinical practice guidelines. *Chest, 129*(1): Supplement, 250S–259S.

McGloin, S. (2008). Administration of oxygen therapy. *Nursing Standard, 22*(21), 46–48.

Moore, T. (2007). Respiratory assessment in adults. *Nursing Standard, 21*(49), 48–56.

Moorhead, S., Johnson, M., Maas, M., & Swanson E. (Eds). (2008). *Nursing outcomes classification (NOC)* (4th ed.). St. Louis: Mosby Elsevier.

NANDA International. (2009). *Nursing diagnoses: Definitions and classification 2009–2011.* West Sussex, UK: Wiley-Blackwell.

Pate, M. (2004). Placement of endotracheal and tracheostomy tubes. *Critical Care Nurse, 24*(3), 13–14.

Pate, M., & Zapata, T. (2002). Ask the experts: How deeply should I go when I suction an endotracheal or tracheostomy tube? *Critical Care Nurse, 22*(2), 130–131.

Porth, C., & Matfin, G. (2008). *Pathophysiology: Concepts of altered health states* (8th ed.). Philadelphia: Wolters Kluwer Health/Lippincott Williams & Wilkins.

Pruitt, B. (2007a). Latest advances in respiratory care. *Nursing, 37*(7), 56cc1, 56cc3.

Pruitt, B. (2007b). Take an evidence-based approach to treating acute lung injury. *Nursing, 37*(Supplement), 14–18.

Rodden, A., Spicer, L., Diaz, V., & Steyer, T. E. (2007). Does fingernail polish affect pulse oximeter readings? *Intensive and Critical Care Nursing, 23*(1), 51–55.

Roman, M. (2005). Tracheostomy tubes. *MEDSURG Nursing, 14*(2), 143–144.

Rushing, J. (2007). Clinical do's and don'ts: Managing a water-seal chest drainage unit. *Nursing, 37*(12), 12.

Schultz, N. (2007a). Spirometry essentials for medical assistants Part II: The important test variables and predicted values. *Journal of Continuing Education Topics & Issues, 9*(1), 18–21.

Schultz, N. (2007b). Spirometry essentials for medical assistants Part III: Standards for the test procedure. *Journal of Continuing Education Topics & Issues, 9*(1), 22–25.

Simpson, H. (2006). Respiratory assessment. *British Journal of Nursing, 15*(9), 484–488.

Smeltzer, S., Bare, B., Hinkle, J., & Cheever, K. (2010). *Brunner & Suddarth's textbook of medical-surgical nursing* (12th ed.). Philadelphia: Lippincott Williams & Wilkins.

Subirana, M., Solà, I., & Benito, S. (2007). Closed tracheal suction systems versus open tracheal suction systems for mechanically ventilated adult patients. *Cochrane Database of Systematic Reviews, Issue 4.* Art. No.: CD004581.DOI: 10.1002/14651858.CD004581.pub2.

Sullivan, B. (2008). Nursing management of patients with a chest drain. *British Journal of Nursing, 17*(6), 388–393.

VISN 8 Patient Safety Center. (2009). *Safe patient handling and movement algorithms.* Tampa, FL: Author. Available at www.visn8.va.gov/patientsafetycenter/SafePtHandling. Accessed April 23, 2010.

Walters, T. (2007). Pulse oximetry knowledge and its effects on clinical practice. *British Journal of Nursing, 16*(21), 1332–1340.

Weber, J., & Kelley, J. (2007). *Health assessment in nursing* (3rd ed.). Philadelphia: Lippincott Williams & Wilkins.

40 Fluid, Electrolyte, and Acid–Base Balance

JEREMIAH STEIN

Jeremiah, a 22-year-old young adult, comes to the campus health center because he has been having two or three loose bowel movements a day for the past week. "I've been trying to control this problem myself. I am really working hard at school and I didn't want to take the time to take care of this. Now I am at the point where I just don't feel good." Dehydration and electrolyte imbalances are a concern.

JACK SOO PARK

Jack, a 78-year-old man receiving intravenous (IV) therapy with antibiotics, states, "I'm having trouble breathing. It just started a little while ago." Physical examination reveals a bounding pulse, distended neck veins, and crackles and wheezes in the lungs. Excess fluid volume is suspected. Further checking reveals an IV fluid-administration error that has resulted in overhydration.

GRACE GILLIGAN

Grace, a 28-year-old woman, arrives at the emergency department with complaints of severe bouts of nausea and vomiting. She has a past medical history of gastrointestinal (GI) problems, for which she underwent abdominal surgery several months ago. "I thought my problems were over once I had the surgery." IV therapy was ordered to restore her fluid balance.

LEARNING OBJECTIVES

After completing the chapter, you will be able to accomplish the following:

1. Describe the location and functions of body fluids, including the factors that affect variations in fluid compartments.

2. Describe the functions, regulation, sources, and losses of the main electrolytes of the body.

3. Explain the principles of osmosis, diffusion, active transport, and filtration.

4. Describe how thirst and the organs of homeostasis (kidneys, heart and blood vessels, lungs, adrenal glands, pituitary gland, parathyroid glands) function to maintain fluid homeostasis.

5. Describe the role of buffer systems and respiratory and renal mechanisms in achieving and maintaining acid–base balance.

6. Identify the etiologies, defining characteristics, and treatment modalities for common fluid, electrolyte, and acid–base imbalances.

7. Perform a fluid, electrolyte, and acid–base balance assessment.

8. Describe the role of dietary modification, modification of fluid intake, medication administration, IV therapy, blood replacement, and total parenteral nutrition (TPN) in resolving fluid, electrolyte, and acid–base imbalances.

9. Assess, plan, implement, and evaluate nursing care related to select nursing diagnoses involving fluid, electrolyte, and acid–base imbalances.

KEY TERMS

acid	cross-matching
acidosis	diffusion
active transport	edema
agglutinin	electrolytes
alkalosis	filtration
anions	hydrostatic pressure
antibody	hypercalcemia
antigen	hyperkalemia
autologous transfusion	hypermagnesemia
base	hypernatremia
buffer	hyperphosphatemia
cation	hypertonic
colloid osmotic pressure	hypervolemia
hypocalcemia	isotonic
hypokalemia	osmolarity
hypomagnesemia	osmosis
hyponatremia	pH
hypophosphatemia	solutes
hypotonic	solvents
hypovolemia	typing
ion	

This chapter discusses the principles of fluid, electrolyte, and acid–base balance and common disturbances. Sample interview questions for performing a fluid-balance assessment are included, with information on specific physical assessment techniques and laboratory studies. Numerous examples of nursing diagnoses are provided. Expected outcomes and specific nursing interventions to promote fluid and electrolyte balance are described. These interventions include ongoing assessments, modifying dietary and fluid intake, administering medications, assisting with IV therapy, and blood replacement. The concluding plan of care illustrates how nurses combine their knowledge of fluid, electrolyte, and acid–base balance with skilled nursing assessments and interventions to resolve alterations in health status and to improve patient outcomes. Refer to the accompanying Reflective Practice box for an illustration of nursing care related to IV fluid therapy.

ANATOMY AND PHYSIOLOGY

Fluids and electrolytes are vital to life and adequate balance is imperative to maintain healthy functioning of the body. Fluids and electrolytes are involved in almost every cellular reaction and function. Chemical reactions that occur in the body depend upon a careful acid and base balance.

Body Fluids

As the primary body fluid, water is the most important nutrient of life. Although life can be sustained for many days without food, humans can survive for only a few days without water. Water in the body functions primarily to:

- Provide a medium for transporting nutrients to cells and wastes from cells
- Provide a medium for transporting substances such as hormones, enzymes, blood platelets, and red and white blood cells throughout the body
- Facilitate cellular metabolism and proper cellular chemical functioning
- Act as a solvent for electrolytes and nonelectrolytes
- Help maintain normal body temperature
- Facilitate digestion and promote elimination
- Act as a tissue lubricant

REFLECTIVE PRACTICE

Challenge to Interpersonal Skills

During my clinical rotation in the emergency department, I met Grace Gilligan. She was a 28-year-old woman who came to the emergency department with complaints of severe nausea and vomiting. She has a past medical history of gastrointestinal (GI) problems, for which she underwent abdominal surgery several months ago. "I thought my problems were over once I had the surgery." The patient was dehydrated and needed IV fluid therapy.

My coassigned nurse attempted to start a peripheral venous access not once, but six times. The patient was already upset by her recurrent abdominal symptoms, but now had to deal with the continuous painful stick of a needle. During the course of attempts to start the IV, the patient stated that a nurse on the IV team always had to be called to insert her IVs. Although my nurse acknowledged the information, she continued trying to start the IV. Finally, on the sixth try, as the patient was in tears, the nurse was successful. It seemed as if the nurse was out to prove her abilities without caring for the patient. By the end, I had difficulty even watching.

Thinking Outside the Box: Possible Courses of Action

- While assisting the nurse to obtain more supplies (outside the patient's room), mention to the nurse that maybe the IV team should be called, since "enough is enough!"
- Tell my clinical instructor that the patient is being abused.
- Ask the doctor if he or she could address the situation.
- Tell the patient when the nurse was out of the room to refuse any more sticks until the IV team was called.

Evaluating a Good Outcome: How Do I Define Success?

- Patient is benefited by my actions. . . . or at least not harmed.
- All actions are supported by rationale.
- The patient's wishes are respected.
- Personal integrity is not compromised.

Personal Learning: Here's to the Future!

Unfortunately, I did not take any actions to protect this patient. This was my first time in the emergency room as well as my first introduction to the nurse. I was intimidated by her. Furthermore, I was scared when she continued to attempt the catheter insertion with the patient in tears. I know that it is my responsibility to advocate for the needs of my patients. In the future, I hope that I will never compromise my integrity, beliefs, and values to prove something to a student. If I fail or am not confident in my skills, I will admit this and stop before my patient is put at risk.

Amy Persinger, Georgetown University

Reflection

How do you think you would respond in a similar situation? Why? What does this tell you about yourself and about the adequacy of your skills for professional practice? What might have prompted the emergency room nurse to act as she did? The nursing student? How could the nursing student have advocated for the patient? What other barriers (other than those listed above) might have interfered with the nursing student acting as an advocate? Can you think of other ways to respond? What other skills (cognitive, interpersonal, technical, ethical/legal) would you need to respond well in this situation? Do you agree with the criteria to evaluate a successful outcome? Were any of the criteria met?

Body Water and Fluid Compartments

The term *total body water* or *fluid* refers to the total amount of water, which is approximately 50% to 60% of body weight in a healthy person. Fluid is located in two fluid compartments—the intracellular fluid (ICF) or extracellular fluid (ECF), based on its location in the body. ICF is the fluid within cells, constituting about 70% of the total body water or 40% of the adult's body weight. ECF is all the fluid outside the cells, accounting for about 30% of the total body water or 20% of the adult's body weight. ECF includes two major areas, the intravascular and interstitial compartments. A third, usually minor, compartment is the transcellular fluids. Intravascular fluid, or plasma, is the liquid component of the blood (i.e., fluid found within the vascular system). Interstitial

fluid is the fluid that surrounds tissue cells and includes lymph (Smeltzer, Bare, Hinkle, & Cheever, 2008). Transcellular fluids include cerebrospinal, pericardial, synovial, intraocular, and pleural fluids, as well as sweat and digestive secretions. The capillary walls and cell membranes separate the intracellular and extracellular compartments. Figure 40-1 illustrates the components of total body fluid and the primary fluid compartments.

Variations in Fluid Content

Variations in the fluid content from the normal 50% to 60% of the body's weight can occur, depending on such factors as the person's age, body fat, and gender. Table 40-1 illustrates age-related differences in total body water and in the various

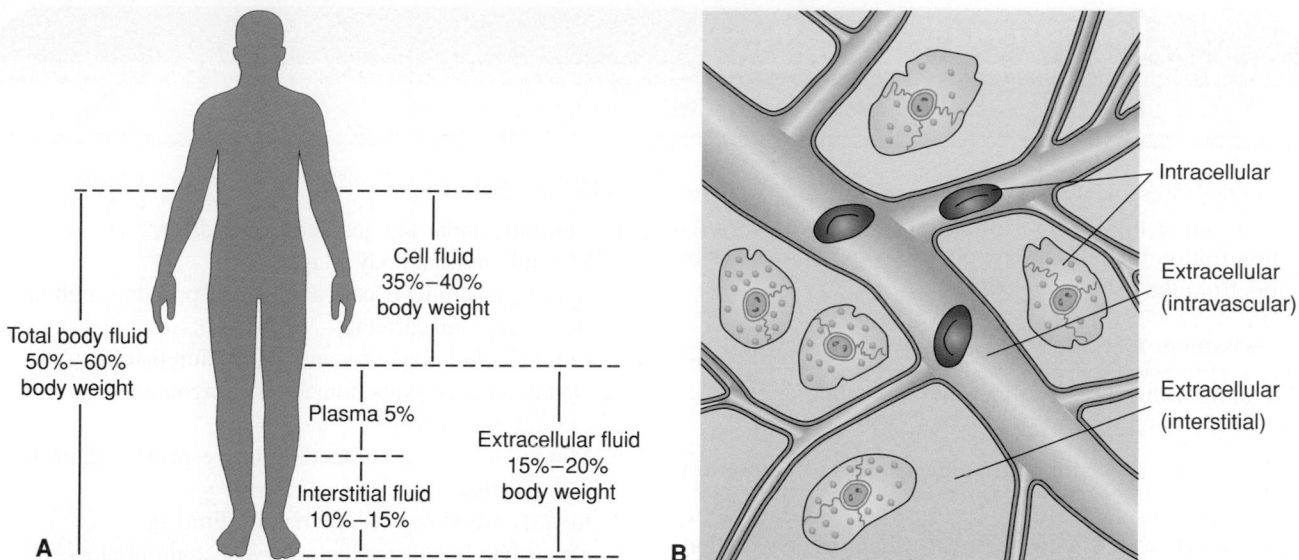

FIGURE 40-1. (**A**) Total body fluid represents 50% to 60% of body weight of a normal adult. (**B**) Primary fluid compartments.

water compartments of the body. Infants have considerably more total body fluid and ECF than adults. Because ECF is more easily lost from the body than ICF, infants are more prone to fluid volume deficits.

Total body water also differs by gender and the amount of fat cells in the body. Fat cells contain little water, whereas lean tissue is rich in water. Thus, the more obese a person is, the smaller the person's percentage of total body water is when compared with body weight. Because women tend to have proportionally more body fat than men do, they also have less body fluid than men. Similarly, the decreasing percentage of body fluid in older people is related to an increase in fat cells. In addition, older adults lose muscle mass as a part of aging. The combined increase of fat and loss of muscle results in reduced total body water; after the age of 60, total body water is about 45% of a person's body weight. This decrease in water increases the risk for fluid imbalance in older adults.

Fluid Balance

The desirable amount of fluid intake and loss in adults ranges from 1,500 to 3,500 mL each 24 hours, with most people averaging 2,500 to 2,600 mL per day. Although these figures are helpful guidelines, the individual's health state as well as balance between actual intake and loss must be considered when assessing nursing needs. A person's intake should normally be approximately balanced by output or fluid loss. A general rule is that in healthy adults, the output of urine normally approximates the ingestion of liquids, and the water from food and oxidation is balanced by the water loss through the feces, the skin, and the respiratory process. The intake–output balance may not always occur in a single 24-hour period but should normally be achieved within 2 to 3 days.

Any deviations from normal ranges for a balanced water intake and output should alert the nurse to potential imbalances. The accompanying Promoting Health 40-1: Fluid and Electrolyte Balance reflects on self-care behaviors vital for maintaining a healthy fluid and electrolyte balance. Nurses who role model good health behaviors are more effective teachers. Use the Promoting Health Display for yourself before using it with others.

FLUID SOURCES

The human body obtains water from several sources, including ingested liquids, food, and as a by-product of metabolism. The ingestion of liquids provides the largest amount of water normally taken into the body. Fluid intake is regulated primarily by the thirst mechanism. Located within the hypothalamus, the thirst control center is stimulated by intracellular dehydration and decreased blood volume. The water contained in food is the second largest source of water for the body. The amount of water ingested depends on the diet. For example, melons and citrus fruit are high in water content, whereas cereal and dried fruits have relatively low water content. Water is an end product of the oxidation that occurs during the metabolism of food substances, specifically carbohydrates, fats, and protein. This amount of water obtained varies among the different types

TABLE • 40-1	WATER AS A PERCENTAGE OF BODY WEIGHT			
Water Compartment	Infant (%)	Adult (%) Man	Adult (%) Woman	Elderly Person (%)
Extracellular				
Intravascular	4	4	5	5
Interstitial	25	11	10	15
Intracellular	48	45	35	25
Total body water	77	60	50	45

PROMOTING HEALTH • 40-1

Fluid and Electrolyte Balance

Use the assessment checklist to determine how well you are meeting fluid and electrolyte needs. Then develop a prescription for self-care by choosing appropriate behaviors from the list of suggestions.

Assessment Checklist

❏ almost always	❏ sometimes	❏ almost never

❏ ❏ ❏   1. I drink six to eight glasses of water every day.

❏ ❏ ❏   2. I am aware of early signs of dehydration or fluid retention.

❏ ❏ ❏   3. I limit sugar, alcohol, and caffeine in my diet.

❏ ❏ ❏   4. I am alert for any sudden variations in my weight.

❏ ❏ ❏   5. I am aware of fluid and electrolyte imbalances that may be associated with intake of certain medications.

❏ ❏ ❏   6. I diet sensibly when I need to lose weight.

Self-Care Behaviors

1. Consume about 1½ quarts of water daily.
2. Maintain normal body weight.
3. Avoid consuming excess amounts of products high in salt, sugar, and caffeine.
4. Limit alcohol intake because of its diuretic effect.
5. Obtain medical evaluation for any ongoing indications of fluid imbalance.
6. Monitor side effects of medications, especially diuresis and diarrhea.
7. Identify situations of high risk for fluid and electrolyte imbalance and intervene appropriately.

Information to promote fluid and electrolyte balance, such as information about dehydration, overhydration, food and nutrition, dietary supplements, and minerals and electrolytes is available online. Check out these sites: Medline Plus: Fluid and Electrolyte Balance www.nlm.nih.gov/medlineplus/fluidandelectrolytebalance.html; Dietary Supplements. U.S. Food and Drug Administration www.fda.gov/AboutFDA/Basics/ucm193949.htm

of nutrients. Generally, fluid intake averages 2,600 mL per day, with approximately 1,300 mL coming from ingested water, 1,000 mL coming from ingested food, and 300 mL from metabolic oxidation. Figure 40-2 illustrates daily fluid balance in a healthy individual.

FLUID LOSSES

Fluid is lost from the body through *sensible* and *insensible* losses. Sensible losses can be measured and include fluid lost during urination, defecation, and wounds. Insensible losses can't be measured or seen and include fluid lost from evaporation through the skin and as water vapor from the lungs during respiration. Water losses vary according to the person and the circumstances.

Fluid output averages 2,500 to 2,900 mL per day (average 2,600 mL), with approximately 1,500 mL as urine from the kidneys, 600 mL fluid loss from the skin, 300 mL from the lungs, and 200 mL in feces via the gastrointestinal tract (see Fig. 40-2).

HOMEOSTATIC MECHANISMS

Fluid homeostasis normally functions automatically and effectively. Almost every organ and system in the body helps in some way to maintain fluid homeostasis. The following sections describe the primary organs and systems of homeostasis. Their functions are highlighted in Table 40-2.

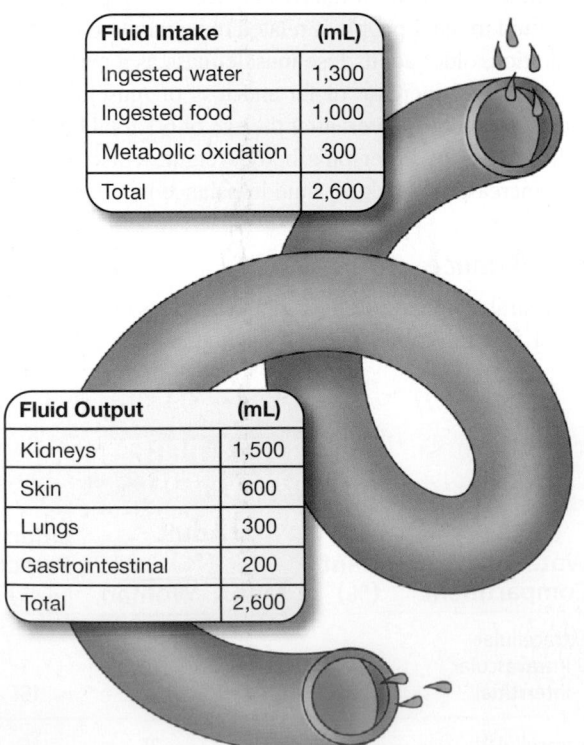

Fluid Intake	(mL)
Ingested water	1,300
Ingested food	1,000
Metabolic oxidation	300
Total	2,600

Fluid Output	(mL)
Kidneys	1,500
Skin	600
Lungs	300
Gastrointestinal	200
Total	2,600

FIGURE 40-2. In health, fluid intake and fluid losses are about equal. The amounts indicated are average adult daily fluid sources and losses.

TABLE • 40-2   HOMEOSTATIC MECHANISMS THAT MAINTAIN THE COMPOSITION AND VOLUME OF BODY FLUID WITHIN NARROW LIMITS OF NORMAL

Organs of Homeostasis	Functions
Kidneys	• Regulate extracellular fluid (ECF) volume and osmolality by selective retention and excretion of body fluids • Regulate electrolyte levels in the ECF by selective retention of needed substances and excretion of unneeded substances • Regulate pH of ECF by excretion or retention of hydrogen ions • Excrete metabolic wastes (primarily acids) and toxic substances
Heart and blood vessels	• Circulate blood through the kidneys under sufficient pressure for urine to form (pumping action of the heart) • React to hypovolemia by stimulating fluid retention (stretch receptors in the atria and blood vessels)

Lungs	• Eliminate about 13,000 mEq of hydrogen ions (H^+) daily, as opposed to only 40 to 80 mEq excreted daily by the kidneys
	• Act promptly to correct metabolic acid–base disturbances; regulate H^+ concentration (pH) by controlling the level of carbon dioxide (CO_2) in the extracellular fluid as follows:
	  1. Metabolic alkalosis causes compensatory hypoventilation, resulting in CO_2 retention (increases acidity of the extracellular fluid).
	  2. Metabolic acidosis causes compensatory hyperventilation, resulting in CO_2 excretion (decreases acidity of the extracellular fluid).
	• Remove approximately 300 mL of water daily through exhalation (insensible water loss) in the normal adult

Adrenal glands	• Regulate blood volume and sodium and potassium balance by secreting aldosterone, a mineral corticoid secreted by the adrenal cortex
	  1. The primary regulator of aldosterone appears to be angiotensin II, which is produced by the renin–angiotensin system. A decrease in blood volume triggers this system and increases aldosterone secretion, which causes sodium retention (and thus water retention) and potassium loss.
	  2. Decreased secretion of aldosterone causes sodium and water loss and potassium retention.
	• Cortisol, another adrenocortical hormone, has only a fraction of the potency of aldosterone.
	• However, secretion of cortisol in large quantities can produce sodium and water retention and potassium deficit.

Pituitary gland	• Stores and releases the antidiuretic hormone (ADH), which makes the body retain water; functions of ADH include:
	  1. Maintains osmotic pressure of the cells by controlling renal water retention or excretion
	    a. When osmotic pressure of the ECF is greater than that of the cells (as in hypernatremia—excess sodium—or hyperglycemia), ADH secretion is increased, causing renal retention of water.
	    b. When osmotic pressure of the ECF is less than that of the cells (as in hyponatremia), ADH secretion is decreased, causing renal excretion of water.
	  2. Controls blood volume (less influential than aldosterone)
	    a. When blood volume is decreased, an increased secretion of ADH results in water conservation.
	    b. When blood volume is increased, a decreased secretion of ADH results in water loss.

Nervous system	• Inhibits and stimulates mechanisms influencing fluid balance; acts chiefly to regulate sodium and water intake and excretion • Regulates oral intake by sensing intracellular dehydration, which triggers thirst (thirst center located in hypothalamus)

Parathyroid glands	• Regulate calcium (Ca^{2+}) and phosphate (HPO_4^{2-}) balance by means of parathyroid hormone (PTH); PTH influences bone reabsorption, calcium absorption from the intestines, and calcium reabsorption from the renal tubules.
	  1. Increased secretion of PTH causes:
	    a. Elevated serum calcium concentration
	    b. Lowered serum phosphate concentration
	  2. Conversely, decreased secretion of PTH causes:
	    a. Lowered serum calcium concentration
	    b. Elevated serum phosphate concentration

Data from *Fluids & electrolytes: A 2-in-1 reference for nurses.* (2006). Philadelphia: Wolters Kluwer Health/Lippincott Williams & Wilkins; Porth, C., & Matfin, G. (2009). *Pathophysiology: Concepts of altered health states* (8th ed.). Philadelphia: Wolters Kluwer Health/Lippincott Williams & Wilkins.

Fluid balance is threatened when any organ or system fails to function properly.

- The kidneys, frequently referred to as the *master chemists* of the body, normally filter 180 L of plasma daily in the adult, while excreting only 1.5 L of urine. The kidneys selectively retain electrolytes and water and excrete wastes and excesses according to the body's needs.
- The cardiovascular system is responsible for pumping and carrying nutrients and water throughout the body.
- The lungs regulate oxygen and carbon dioxide levels of the blood. Regulation of the carbon dioxide level is especially crucial in maintaining acid–base balance (see discussion later in this chapter).
- The adrenal glands secrete aldosterone, a mineralocorticoid hormone that helps the body conserve sodium, helps save chloride and water, and causes potassium to be excreted.
- Thyroxine, released by the thyroid gland, increases blood flow in the body, leading to increased renal circulation and resulting in increased glomerular filtration and urinary output.
- The parathyroid glands secrete parathyroid hormone, which regulates the level of calcium and phosphorus. Parathyroid hormone draws calcium into the blood from the bones, kidneys, and intestines. It also facilitates the movement of phosphorus from the blood to the kidneys, where it is excreted in the urine.
- The gastrointestinal tract absorbs water and nutrients that enter the body through this route.
- The nervous system, acting as a switchboard to inhibit and stimulate mechanisms that influence fluid balance, functions chiefly as the regulator of sodium and water intake and excretion.
- The thirst center is located in the hypothalamus of the brain. Antidiuretic hormone (ADH) is manufactured in the hypothalamus and is stored in the posterior lobe of the pituitary gland.
- Neurons, called osmoreceptors, are sensitive to changes in the concentration of ECF, sending appropriate impulses to the pituitary gland to release ADH or inhibit its release to maintain ECF volume concentration.

Electrolytes

Electrolytes are substances that are capable of breaking into particles called ions. An **ion** is an atom or molecule carrying an electrical charge. Some ions develop a positive charge and are called **cations.** The major cations in body fluid are sodium, potassium, calcium, hydrogen, and magnesium ions. Other ions develop a negative charge and are called **anions.** The major anions in body fluid are chloride, bicarbonate, and phosphate. These charged particles are the basis of chemical interactions in the body necessary for metabolism and other functions. Molecules in the body that remain intact, without a charge, are called nonelectrolytes. In the human body, urea and glucose are examples of nonelectrolytes. **Solvents** are liquids that hold a substance in solution; **solutes** are substances that are dissolved in a solution. Water is the primary solvent in the body. The solutes are electrolytes and nonelectrolytes.

Fluids in various compartments of the body differ in their constituents. Major electrolytes in the ECF include sodium, chloride, calcium, and bicarbonate. Major electrolytes in the ICF include potassium, phosphorus, and magnesium. The functions, sources, means of loss, and regulation of these electrolytes are highlighted in Table 40-3 (hydrogen is discussed as part of acid–base balance). Figure 40-3 illustrates differences in the electrolyte composition of body fluids according to the compartments in which the fluids are found.

Electrolytes are measured in terms of their chemical combining power, or chemical activity. The milliequivalent (mEq) is the unit of measure that describes the chemical activity of electrolytes. One milliequivalent of either a cation or an anion is chemically equivalent to the activity of 1 mg of hydrogen. Therefore, 1 mEq of any cation is equivalent to 1 mEq of any anion.

The total cations in the body are normally equal to the total anions, maintaining homeostasis (balanced state). In healthy people, the milliequivalents per liter for electrolytes

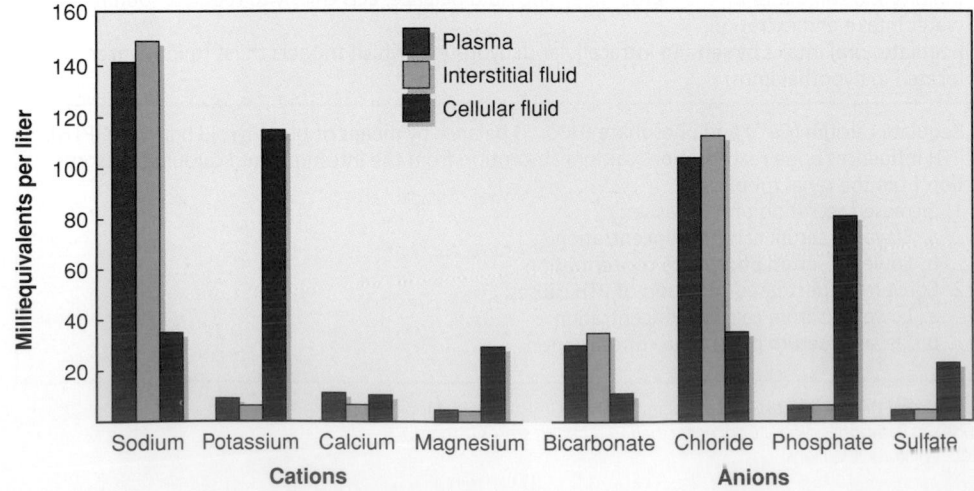

FIGURE 40-3. Electrolyte composition of body fluids according to compartment.

T ABLE • 40-3   **MAJOR ELECTROLYTES**

Electrolyte	Functions	Sources and Losses	Regulation
Sodium (Na$^+$): chief electrolyte of ECF; primary influence outside cell; the normal serum concentration of sodium: 135–145 mEq/L	Controls and regulates extracellular fluid volume Affects serum osmolality Participates in muscle contraction and transmission of nerve impulses Important in regulation of acid–base balance as sodium bicarbonate Loss or gain of sodium usually accompanied by a loss or gain of water	Normally enters the body through the gastrointestinal tract Derived easily from dietary sources, such as salt added to processed foods, sodium preservatives added to processed foods Lost from gastrointestinal tract, kidneys, and skin	Transported out of the cell by the sodium-potassium pump Sodium concentrations affected by salt, as well as water, intake Regulated by renin-angiotensin-aldosterone system Elimination and reabsorption regulated by the kidneys
Potassium (K$^+$): major cation of ICF; primary influence inside cell; the normal serum concentration of potassium: 3.5–5.0 mEq/L	Helps control intracellular osmolality Is the chief regulator of cellular enzyme activity Plays a vital role in such processes as the transmission of electric impulses, particularly in nerve, heart, skeletal, intestinal, and lung tissue; protein and carbohydrate metabolism; and cellular building Assists in regulation of acid–base balance by cellular exchange with H$^+$	Adequate quantities usually in a well-balanced diet Leading food sources: fruits and vegetables, dried peas and beans, whole grains, milk, meats Lost via kidneys, stool, sweat Gastrointestinal (GI) secretions contain potassium in large quantities, so can be lost through vomitus	Regulated by aldosterone Eliminated by the kidneys (no effective method of conserving potassium) Additional regulation via transcellular shift between the ICF and ECF compartments
Calcium (Ca^{2+}): most abundant electrolyte in the body; major component of bones and teeth; 99% of body calcium is stored in bone; 1% is located inside cells; 0.1% is located in the extracellular fluid; normal total serum calcium level: 8.6–10.2 mg/dL; normal ionized serum calcium level: 4.5–5.1 mg/dL	Major role in transmitting nerve impulses Helps regulate muscle contraction and relaxation Role in blood coagulation Activates enzymes that stimulate essential chemical reactions in the body	Absorbed from foods in the presence of normal gastric acidity and vitamin D Lost via feces and urine Sources include milk, milk products, cheese, and dried beans; fortified orange juice; green leafy vegetables, small fish with bones, and dried peas and beans	Primarily excreted by gastrointestinal tract; lesser extent by kidneys Regulated by parathyroid hormone and calcitonin High serum phosphate results in decreased serum calcium level; low serum phosphate leads to increased serum calcium
Magnesium (Mg^{2+}): second most abundant ICF cation after potassium; the normal serum concentration of magnesium: 1.3–2.3 mEq/L	Is important for the metabolism of carbohydrates and proteins Activator for many intracellular enzyme systems Role in neuromuscular function Acts on cardiovascular system, producing vasodilation	Enters the body via gastrointestinal tract Magnesium found in green leafy vegetables, nuts, seafood, whole grains, dried peas and beans; cocoa Lost via urine with use of loop diuretics	Eliminated by kidneys Regulated by parathyroid hormone
Chloride (Cl$^-$): major extracellular anion; normal serum level of chloride: 97–107 mEq/L	Major component of interstitial and lymph fluid; gastric and pancreatic juices, sweat, bile, and saliva Acts with sodium to maintain the osmotic pressure Plays a role in the body's acid–base balance; combines with hydrogen ions to produce hydrochloric acid	Enters body via gastrointestinal tract Almost all chloride in diet comes from salt Found in foods high in sodium, processed foods	Normally paired with sodium; excreted and conserved with sodium by the kidneys Regulated by aldosterone alongside sodium Low potassium level leads to low chloride level

(continued)

Table • 40-3	MAJOR ELECTROLYTES	(continued)	
Electrolyte	**Functions**	**Sources and Losses**	**Regulation**
Bicarbonate (HCO_3^-): an anion that is the major chemical base buffer within the body; found in both ECF and ICF; normal serum bicarbonate level: 25–29 mEq/L	Regulates acid–base balance	Losses possible via diarrhea, diuretics, and early renal insufficiency; excess possible via over ingestion of acid neutralizers, such as sodium bicarbonate	Bicarbonate levels regulated primarily by the kidneys Bicarbonate readily available as a result of carbon dioxide formation during metabolism
Phosphate (PO_4^-): major ICF anion; a buffer anion in both ICF and ECF; normal serum phosphate level: 2.5–4.5 mg/dL	Helps maintain the body's acid–base balance as a hydrogen buffer Promotes energy storage; carbohydrate, protein, and fat metabolism Bone and teeth formation Regulation of hormone and coenzyme activity Role in muscle and red blood cell function	Enters body via gastrointestinal tract Sources include all animal products (meat, poultry, eggs, milk, bread, ready-to-eat cereal) Absorption is diminished by concurrent ingestion of calcium, magnesium, and aluminum	Eliminated by kidneys Regulation by parathyroid hormone and by activated vitamin D Phosphate and calcium are inversely proportional; an increase in one results in a decrease in the other

in the body vary within a relatively narrow range. When electrolytes are not in balance, the person is at risk for alterations in health.

> *Consider Grace Gilligan, the young woman described in one of the beginning chapter scenarios. The nurse would need to be alert for electrolyte imbalances and possible acid–base imbalance due to the loss of gastric secretions from vomiting.* ∎

Fluid and Electrolyte Regulation

Maintaining homeostasis of fluid volume and electrolytes is essential to healthy body functioning (Kear, 2005). The body produces this balance by shifting fluids between the ECF and the ICF. The mechanisms responsible for regulating this shift of fluids and transporting materials to and from intracellular compartments are osmosis, diffusion, active transport, and filtration, described in the following sections.

Osmosis

Cell membranes are semipermeable, allowing some, but not all, solutes to pass through the cell membranes. The cell membrane is permeable to water or fluids. **Osmosis** is the major method of transporting body fluids. Water shifts and balance depend heavily on this route of transport (Fig. 40-4).

Through the process of osmosis, water (the solvent) passes from an area of lesser solute concentration and more water to an area of greater solute concentration and less water until equilibrium is established. As a result, the volume of the more concentrated solution increases, and the volume of the weaker solution decreases. The process of

osmosis stops when the concentration of solutes has been equalized on both sides of the cell membrane. The greater the difference in the concentration of the two solutions on each side of a semipermeable membrane, the greater the osmotic pressure or drawing power of water.

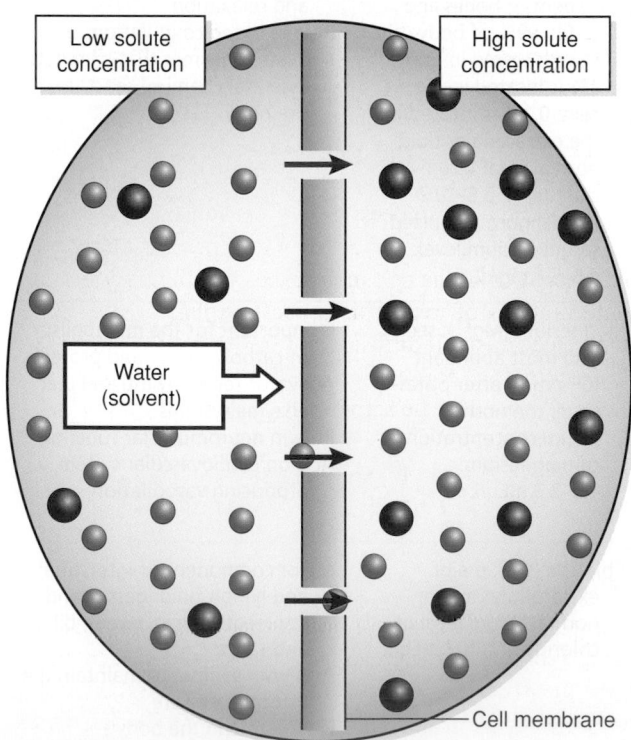

FIGURE 40-4. Body fluids are transported through cell membranes through the process of osmosis. Water, a solvent, moves from an area of lesser solute concentration to one of greater solute concentration, until equilibrium is established.

The concentration of particles in a solution, or its pulling power, is referred to as the **osmolarity** of a solution. A solution that has about the same concentration of particles, or osmolarity, as plasma (between 275 and 295 mOsm/L) is considered an **isotonic** solution.

An isotonic fluid remains in the intravascular compartment without any net flow across the semipermeable membrane. In contrast, a **hypertonic** solution has a greater osmolarity than plasma (>295 mOsm/L). Because a hypertonic solution has a greater osmolarity, water moves out of the cells and is drawn into the intravascular compartment, causing the cells to shrink. A **hypotonic** solution has less osmolarity than plasma (<275 mOsm/L). Because of a lower osmolarity, a hypotonic solution in the intravascular space moves out of the intravascular space and into intracellular fluid, causing cells to swell and possibly burst. In addition, electrolytes have "osmotic potential," which refers to the electrolytes' affinity for water (i.e., the capacity to pull water into a fluid compartment). Sodium, for example, has a high osmotic potential.

Diffusion

Diffusion is the tendency of solutes to move freely throughout a solvent. The solute moves from an area of higher concentration to an area of lower concentration (i.e., "downhill") until equilibrium is established. Gases also move by diffusion. Oxygen and carbon dioxide exchange in the lung's alveoli and capillaries occurs by diffusion.

Active Transport

Active transport is a process that requires energy for the movement of substances through a cell membrane from an area of lesser solute concentration to an area of higher solute concentration. Adenosine triphosphate or ATP, stored in all cells, supplies energy for solute movement in and out of the cell. Although this process is not entirely understood, the energy requirements for active transport are affected by characteristics of the cell membrane, specific enzymes, and concentrations of ions. This process explains the so-called pump mechanism. If diffusion can be called "coasting downhill," active transport can be called "pumping uphill." Substances believed to use active transport include amino acids, glucose (in certain places only, such as in the kidneys and intestines), and ions of sodium, chloride, potassium, hydrogen, and calcium (*Portable fluids & electrolytes,* 2008).

Filtration

Filtration is the passage of fluid through a permeable membrane. Fluids move from an area of high pressure to one of lower pressure. Capillary filtration results from the force of blood "pushing" against the walls of the capillaries. At the arterial end of the capillaries, filtration is dependent primarily on arterial blood pressure; at the venular side of the capillaries, filtration is dependent on venous blood pressure. The "pushing" force is referred to as **hydrostatic pressure.** When the hydrostatic pressure inside the capillary exceeds the surrounding interstitial space, fluids and solutes are forced out of the capillary wall into the interstitial space. In contrast, when the pressure inside the capillary is less than the pressure in the interstitial space, the fluids and solutes will move back into the capillary. Reabsorption is the process that acts to prevent too much fluid from leaving the capillaries no matter how high the hydrostatic pressure. Plasma proteins, particularly albumin, concentrated in the intravascular space or plasma facilitate this reabsorption process by "pulling" the fluid back into the capillaries. This "pulling" force is known as **colloid osmotic pressure,** or oncotic pressure. Under normal conditions, hydrostatic pressure in the arteriole end of a capillary exceeds plasma colloid pressure. Hydrostatic pressure at the venule end of the capillary is less than plasma colloid pressure. As a result, capillary filtration occurs along the first half of the vessel, and reabsorption occurs along the second half (*Portable fluids & electrolytes,* 2008). Filtration pressure is the difference between colloid osmotic pressure and blood hydrostatic pressure.

These pressures are important in understanding how fluid leaves arterioles, enters the interstitial compartment, and eventually returns to the venules. The filtration pressure is positive in the arterioles, helping to force or filter fluids into interstitial spaces; it is negative in the venules and thus helps fluid enter the venules. This is illustrated in Figure 40-5. Filtration is also involved in the proper functioning of the glomeruli of the kidneys.

Acid–Base Balance

Body fluids must maintain an acid–base balance to sustain health, homeostasis, and life. Specific chemical reactions are constantly occurring within the body that influence metabolism and the functions of various bodily systems. These chemical reactions are dependent on a balance of acids and bases. Conditions such as infection or trauma may alter this delicate acid–base balance. Acidity or alkalinity of a solution is determined by its concentration of hydrogen ions (H^+). An **acid** is a substance containing H^+ that can be liberated or released, such as carbonic acid. An alkali, or **base,** is a substance that can accept or trap H^+ ions, such as the bicarbonate ion.

An acid releases H^+, as follows:

$$\underset{\substack{\text{Carbonic} \\ \text{acid}}}{H_2CO_3} \quad \underset{\text{releases}}{\rightarrow} \quad \underset{\substack{\text{hydrogen} \\ \text{ion}}}{H^+} \quad \underset{\text{to form}}{+} \quad \underset{\substack{\text{bicarbonate} \\ \text{base}}}{HCO_3^-}$$

A base traps H^+, as follows:

$$\underset{\substack{\text{bicarbonate} \\ \text{base}}}{HCO_3^-} \quad \underset{\text{traps}}{+} \quad \underset{\substack{\text{hydrogen} \\ \text{ion}}}{H^+} \quad \underset{\text{to form}}{\rightarrow} \quad \underset{\substack{\text{Carbonic} \\ \text{acid}}}{H_2CO_3}$$

A strong acid dissociates (separates) completely in solution and releases all of its H^+ ions, whereas a weak acid releases only a small number. A base that binds or accepts H^+ ions easily is considered a strong base, whereas one that accepts H^+ ions less readily is considered weak.

The unit of measure used to describe acid–base balance is **pH,** which is an expression of H^+ ion concentration and the

FIGURE 40-5. Capillary filtration.

resulting acidity or alkalinity of a substance. The pH scale ranges from 1 to 14. A neutral solution measures 7; an example is pure water. Because pH is based on a negative logarithm, as the H$^+$ ions increase and a solution becomes more acid, the pH becomes less than 7. When the concentration of H$^+$ ions in a solution is reduced or accepted by another substance and the solution contains more base than acid, it is alkaline, and the pH is greater than 7. Gastric secretions that are strongly acidic have an approximate pH of 1 to 1.3, whereas strongly alkaline pancreatic secretions have an approximate pH of 10.

Normal blood plasma is slightly alkaline and has a normal pH range of 7.35 to 7.45. When the blood plasma pH exceeds the normal pH range in either direction, signs and symptoms of illness develop, and if the condition goes on unabated, death results. **Acidosis** is the condition characterized by an excess of H ions or loss of base ions (bicarbonate) in ECF in which the pH falls below 7.35. **Alkalosis** occurs when there is a lack of H ions or a gain of base (bicarbonate) and the pH exceeds 7.45 (see the section, Acid–Base Imbalance). Figure 40-6 illustrates normal pH, acidosis, and alkalosis and shows the points at which death typically occurs. The narrow range of normal pH is achieved through three major homeostatic regulators of hydrogen ions: (1) chemical buffer systems, (2) respiratory mechanisms, and (3) renal mechanisms. There are alterations in these systems related to the developmental stage of an individual. Newborns are not able to acidify urine as well as older individuals. As individuals age, the effectiveness of both the lungs and kidneys can vary. In an older adult, if there is underlying lung disease, the regulation of acid–base balance may be less efficient. In addition, the kidneys of the older adult can have difficulty handling excess amounts of acid (*Fluids & electrolytes made incredibly easy*, 2008).

Chemical Buffer Systems

A **buffer** is a substance that prevents body fluids from becoming overly acidic or alkaline. They combine with excess acids or bases to prevent major changes in pH, keeping the pH of body fluids as close as possible to normal (7.35–7.45).

Buffers work in one of two ways. A buffer can function like a base and bind or soak up free hydrogen ions. Alternately, a buffer may function like an acid and release hydrogen ions when too few are present in a solution. The body has three buffer systems: (1) the carbonic acid–sodium bicarbonate buffer system, (2) the phosphate buffer system, and (3) the protein buffer system, as described in the following sections.

CARBONIC ACID–SODIUM BICARBONATE BUFFER SYSTEM

The ratio of carbonic acid (H_2CO_3), the most common acid in human body fluid, to the body's most common base, bicarbonate (HCO_3^-), is important for acid–base balance and is the most important buffer system of the body. Normal ECF has a

FIGURE 40-6. Acid–base balance. Note that acidosis is used to describe the condition when the pH falls below 7.35, and alkalosis describes a pH above 7.45. When the normal pH is exceeded in either direction, death can occur.

ratio of 20 parts bicarbonate to 1 part carbonic acid. The exact quantities are unimportant for acid–base balance as long as they remain in a 20:1 ratio. Carbonic acid and bicarbonate must be carefully controlled to maintain this ratio; if either is increased or decreased, the 20:1 ratio is no longer in effect and pH will change. This system buffers as much as 90% of the H^+ of ECF. The lungs help by regulating the production of carbonic acid resulting from the combination of carbon dioxide and water. The kidneys assist the bicarbonate system by regulating the production of bicarbonate.

PHOSPHATE BUFFER SYSTEM

The phosphate buffer system is active in intracellular fluids, especially in the renal tubules. It converts alkaline sodium phosphate (Na_2HPO_4), a weak base, to acid–sodium phosphate (NaH_2PO_4) in the kidneys.

PROTEIN BUFFER SYSTEM

The third buffer system is a mixture of plasma proteins and the globin portion of hemoglobin in red blood cells. Because plasma proteins and hemoglobin possess chemical groups that can combine with or liberate hydrogen ions, they tend to minimize changes in pH and serve as excellent buffering agents over a wide range of pH values working both inside and outside the cells. For example, excess hydrogen ions in the blood cross over the plasma membrane of red blood cells and bind to the hemoglobin molecules that are plentiful in each red blood cell.

Respiratory Regulation of Hydrogen Ions

Due to the huge surface area from which CO_2 can readily diffuse, the lungs can bring about rapid changes in H^+ when needed. Carbon dioxide, constantly produced by cellular metabolism (carbonic acid [H_2CO_3] yields CO_2 and H_2O), is excreted by exhalation. When the amount of CO_2 in the blood increases, the sensitive chemoreceptors in the respiratory center in the medulla are stimulated to increase the rate and depth of respirations to eliminate more CO_2. As more CO_2 is exhaled, the H_2CO_3 level in the blood decreases, and the pH of the blood becomes more alkaline. When the blood level of CO_2 decreases, the respiratory center decreases the rate and depth of respirations to retain the CO_2 so that carbonic acid can be formed, thereby maintaining the delicate balance. As a result, the lungs are the primary controller of the body's carbonic acid supply. This total respiratory process occurs almost as rapidly as the buffering action in the carbonic acid–sodium bicarbonate system. The respiratory system is able to respond quickly in a healthy individual to restore the normal pH. However, this response is short term, and the response of the kidneys is needed for long-term adjustment (*Fluids & electrolytes*, 2006).

Renal Regulation of Hydrogen Ions

Essentially, the kidneys excrete or retain hydrogen ions and form or excrete bicarbonate ions in response to the pH of the blood. In the presence of acidosis, the kidneys excrete hydro-

gen ions and form and conserve bicarbonate ions, thus raising the pH to the normal range. If alkalosis is present, the kidneys retain hydrogen ions and excrete bicarbonate ions in an effort to return to a balanced state. As a result, the concentration of bicarbonate in the plasma is regulated by the kidneys.

Acid–base regulation by the kidneys occurs more slowly than that which occurs by the carbonic acid–sodium bicarbonate system or by respiratory regulation. It may take as long as 3 days for a normal fluid pH to be restored by the kidneys. The pH of urine varies, depending on the ions that are being excreted, but it is generally between 4.5 and 8.2.

DISTURBANCES IN FLUID, ELECTROLYTE, AND ACID–BASE BALANCE

Nurses commonly encounter disturbances in fluid, electrolyte, and acid–base balance while caring for acutely or chronically ill patients. Although many of these disturbances are interrelated and may occur together, they are described here separately for learning purposes.

Fluid Imbalances

Fluid imbalances occur when the body's compensatory mechanisms are unable to maintain a homeostatic state. Fluid imbalances involve either the volume or distribution of water or electrolytes. Nursing implications, related to fluid volume disturbances, including risk factors, nursing assessments, and interventions are discussed later in the chapter.

Fluid Volume Deficit

Fluid volume deficit can be caused by a loss of both water and solutes in the same proportion from the ECF space. The state is commonly known as **hypovolemia** or isotonic fluid loss. Both osmotic and hydrostatic pressure changes force the interstitial fluid into the intravascular space in an effort to compensate for the loss of volume in the blood vessels. As the interstitial space is depleted, its fluid becomes hypertonic, and cellular fluid is then drawn into the interstitial space, leaving cells without adequate fluid to function properly. Fluid volume deficits result from the loss of body fluids, especially if fluid intake is decreased simultaneously.

Young children, elderly people, and people who are ill are especially at risk for hypovolemia. Fluid volume deficit can rapidly result in a weight loss of 5% in adults and 10% in infants. A 5% weight loss is considered a pronounced fluid deficit; an 8% loss or more is considered severe. A 15% weight loss caused by fluid deficiency usually is life threatening.

> *Recall Jeremiah Stein, the college student with an increased number of loose stools for a week. His assessment reveals that he has been limiting his oral intake, further compounding his risk for deficient fluid volume. Weighing Jeremiah would be an important intervention to include as part of the nursing assessment to help determine the extent of fluid loss.* ∎

Third-space fluid shift refers to a distributional shift of body fluids into the transcellular compartment, such as the pleural, peritoneal (ascites), or pericardial areas; joint cavities; the bowel; or an excess accumulation of fluid in the interstitial space. The fluid moves out of the intravascular spaces (plasma) to any of these spaces. Once trapped in these spaces, the fluid is not easily exchanged with ECF. With third-space fluid shift, a deficit in ECF volume occurs. The fluid has not been lost but is trapped in another body space for a period of time and is essentially unavailable for use. These fluid shifts may be related to a disruption in the colloid osmotic pressure (decreased albumin), increased fluid volume (excess IV fluid replacement, renal dysfunction), increased capillary hydrostatic pressure (heart failure), hyponatremia, or an increase in the permeability of the capillary membrane (gross tissue trauma). A third-space shift may occur as a result of a severe burn, a bowel obstruction, or hypoalbuminemia (*Fluids & electrolytes made incredibly easy*, 2008; Holcomb, 2008). Decreased body weight does not occur as it does with an ECF volume deficit (vomiting or diarrhea), and the fluid loss cannot be measured.

Fluid Volume Excess

Excessive retention of water and sodium in ECF in near-equal proportions results in a condition termed *fluid volume excess*. It is also called **hypervolemia** or excess of isotonic fluid (*Fluids & electrolytes made incredibly easy*, 2008). Common causes include malfunction of the kidneys, causing an inability to excrete the excesses, and failure of the heart to function as a pump, resulting in accumulation of fluid in the lungs and dependent parts of the body.

Due to the increased extracellular osmotic pressure from the retained sodium and water, fluid is pulled from the cells to equalize the tonicity. By the time the intracellular and extracellular spaces are isotonic to each other, an excess of both water and sodium is in the ECF, whereas the cells are nearly depleted. The excessive ECF may accumulate in either the intravascular compartments or interstitial spaces. Accumulation of fluid in the interstitial space is known as **edema.** Edema can be observed around the eyes, fingers, ankles, and sacral space, and can also accumulate in or around body organs. Accumulation of fluid may result in a weight gain in excess of 5%. The amount or severity of edema is typically graded (Fig. 40-7). Interstitial-to-plasma shift is the movement of fluid from the space surrounding the cells to the blood. Although the body attempts to maintain normal balance in all fluid spaces, the intravascular fluid is usually protected at the expense of interstitial fluid and ICF.

> ➤ *Remember Jack Soo Park, the patient who inadvertently received too much IV fluid? In Mr. Park's case, fluid accumulation involved his lungs and heart, exhibited by his bounding pulse, distended neck veins, and abnormal lung sounds.* ■

Electrolyte Imbalances

Electrolyte imbalances commonly involve a deficit or excess of the electrolyte. Abnormalities in electrolyte levels can indicate fluid or acid–base imbalance, or neuromuscular, cardiac, renal endocrine, or skeletal dysfunction. Results from venous blood will provide essential information related to possible electrolyte imbalances. When patients present with deficits or excesses of sodium, potassium, calcium, magnesium, phosphate, or chloride, careful nursing assessment depends on an understanding of the effects of these imbalances.

Hyponatremia and Hypernatremia

Sodium is the most abundant electrolyte in the ECF. Refer to Table 40-3. **Hyponatremia** refers to a sodium deficit in ECF

RESEARCH IN NURSING
Bridging the Gap to Evidence-Based Practice

HYPONATREMIA

Hyponatremia is the most common electrolyte disturbance as a result of dysregulation of water balance in hospitalized or institutionalized patients. What is the appropriate assessment and management related to hyponatremia?

Related Research

Haskal, R. (2007). Current issues for nurse practitioners: Hyponatremia. *Journal of the American Academy of Nurse Practitioners*, *19*(11), 563–579.

A comprehensive search was conducted via PubMed, as well as review of meeting abstracts from scientific sessions, including those of the American Society of Nephrology and the Endocrine

Society. The author concluded that elderly patients, and those with certain conditions such as heart failure, tuberculosis, cirrhosis, and head injury, may be at increase risk for hyponatremia. Hospitalized surgical patients prescribed certain medications are also at increased risk.

Relevance to Nursing Practice

Nurses can use knowledge of risk factors to aid in early identification of patients with increased risk of electrolyte imbalances. Nurses need a thorough understanding of the physiology of water balance and the risk factors associated with hyponatremia to ensure prompt and effective intervention.

For additional research, visit thePoint.

1+ Pitting Edema

- Slight indentation (2 mm)
- Normal contours
- Associated with interstitial fluid volume 30% above normal

2 mm

2+ Pitting Edema

- Deeper pit after pressing (4 mm)
- Lasts longer than 1+
- Fairly normal contour

4 mm

3+ Pitting Edema

- Deep pit (6 mm)
- Remains several seconds after pressing
- Skin swelling obvious by general inspection

6 mm

4+ Pitting Edema

- Deep pit (8 mm)
- Remains for a prolonged time after pressing, possibly minutes
- Frank swelling

8 mm

Brawny Edema

- Fluid can no longer be displaced secondary to excessive interstitial fluid accumulation
- No pitting
- Tissue palpates as firm or hard
- Skin surface shiny, warm, moist

FIGURE 40-7. System for grading edema.

(serum sodium <135 mEq/L) caused by a loss of sodium or a gain of water. Sodium may be lost through vomiting, diarrhea, fistulas, sweating, or as the result of the use of diuretics. The decrease in sodium causes fluid to move by osmosis from the less concentrated ECF compartment to the ICF space. This shift of fluid leads to swelling of the cells, with resulting confusion, hypotension, edema, muscle cramps and weakness, and dry skin. Cerebral edema can lead to seizures. Permanent neurological damage can result from severe hyponatremia (Smeltzer et al., 2010). The accompanying Research in Nursing box discusses implications for practice related to hyponatremia.

Hypernatremia refers to a surplus of sodium in ECF (serum sodium >145 mEq/L) caused by excess water loss or an overall excess of sodium. Fluid deprivation, lack of fluid consumption (such as in patients who cannot perceive, respond to, or communicate thirst [Porth & Matfin, 2009]), diarrhea, and excess insensible water loss (hyperventilation, burns) lead to excess sodium. Fluids move from the cells because of the increased extracellular osmotic pressure, causing them to

shrink and leaving them without sufficient fluid. The cells of the central nervous system are especially affected, resulting in signs of neurological impairment, including restlessness, weakness, disorientation, delusion, and hallucinations. Permanent brain damage can occur (Smeltzer et al., 2010).

Hypokalemia and Hyperkalemia

Potassium is the major intracellular electrolyte. Refer to Table 40-3. **Hypokalemia** refers to a potassium deficit in ECF (serum potassium <3.5 mEq/L) and is a common electrolyte abnormality. Potassium may be lost through vomiting, gastric suction, alkalosis, diarrhea, or as the result of the use of diuretics. When the extracellular potassium level falls, potassium moves from the cell, creating an intracellular potassium deficiency. Sodium and hydrogen ions are then retained by the cells to maintain isotonic fluids. These electrolyte shifts influence normal cellular functioning, the pH of ECF, and the functions of most body systems, including the cardiovascular system. Skeletal muscles are generally the first to demonstrate a potassium deficiency. Typical signs of hypokalemia include muscle weakness and leg cramps, fatigue, paresthesias, and dysrhythmias.

Hyperkalemia refers to an excess of potassium in ECF (serum potassium >5 mEq/L). Excess potassium may result from renal failure, hypoaldosteronism, or the use of certain medications such as potassium chloride, heparin, ACE inhibitors, NSAIDs, and potassium-sparing diuretics. Although this condition occurs less frequently than hypokalemia, it can be much more dangerous. Nerve conduction as well as muscle contractility can be affected. Skeletal muscle weakness and paralysis may occur. A variety of cardiac irregularities may result, including cardiac arrest if hyperkalemia is not corrected.

Hypocalcemia and Hypercalcemia

Calcium is a major component of bones and teeth. Refer to Table 40-3. **Hypocalcemia** refers to a calcium deficit in ECF (serum calcium <8.9 mg/dL, ionized calcium <4.5 mg/dL). Common causes related to a calcium deficit involve inadequate calcium intake, impaired calcium absorption, and excessive calcium loss. Manifestations of hypocalcemia include numbness and tingling of fingers, mouth, or feet; tetany; muscle cramps; and seizures.

Hypercalcemia refers to an excess of calcium in ECF (serum calcium >10.1 mg/dL, ionized calcium >5.1 mg/dL). Two major causes of hypercalcemia are cancer and hyperparathyroidism. Manifestations of hypercalcemia include nausea, vomiting, constipation, bone pain, excessive urination, thirst, confusion, lethargy, and slurred speech. Severe hypercalcemia (serum calcium ≥17 mg/dL) is an emergency situation because cardiac arrest may result.

Hypomagnesemia and Hypermagnesemia

Magnesium is the most abundant intracellular cation after potassium. Refer to Table 40-3. **Hypomagnesemia** refers to a magnesium deficit in the ECF (serum magnesium <1.5 mEq/L). Magnesium loss may occur with nasogastric suction, diarrhea, withdrawal from alcohol, administration of tube feedings or parenteral nutrition, sepsis, or burns. This abnormality may lead to muscle weakness, tremors, tetany, seizures, heart block, change in mental status, hyperactive deep tendon reflexes (DTRs), and respiratory paralysis.

Hypermagnesemia refers to a magnesium excess in the ECF (serum magnesium >2.5 mEq/L). It usually occurs with renal failure when the kidneys fail to excrete magnesium or from excessive magnesium intake (use of magnesium-containing antacids or laxatives). Clinical manifestations include nausea, vomiting, weakness, flushing, lethargy, loss of DTRs, respiratory depression, coma, and cardiac arrest.

Hypophosphatemia and Hyperphosphatemia

Phosphorus is a critical element of all the body's tissues. Refer to Table 40-3. **Hypophosphatemia** refers to a below-normal concentration of phosphorus in the ECF (serum phosphate <2.5 mg/dL or 1.8 mEq/L). Although this may indicate phosphorus deficiency, multiple factors may lower serum phosphate levels while total body phosphorus stores are normal. Hypophosphatemia can result from administration of calories to malnourished patients, alcohol withdrawal, diabetic ketoacidosis, hyperventilation, insulin release, absorption problems, and diuretic use. Manifestations include irritability, fatigue, weakness, paresthesias, confusion, seizures, and coma.

Hyperphosphatemia refers to above-normal concentrations of phosphorus in the ECF (serum phosphate >4.5 mg/dL or 2.6 mEq/L). Common causes are impaired kidney excretion and hypoparathyroidism. Hyperphosphatemia can result in tetany, anorexia, nausea, muscle weakness, and tachycardia.

Hypochloremia and Hyperchloremia

Chloride is the major anion of the ECF. Refer to Table 40-3. **Hypochloremia** refers to below-normal level of chloride in the ECF (serum chloride <96 mEq/L). A low level of chloride can result from severe vomiting and diarrhea, drainage of gastric fluid (GI tube), metabolic alkalosis, diuretic therapy, and burns. Manifestations include hyperexcitability of muscles, tetany, hyperactive DTRs, weakness, and muscle cramps.

Hyperchloremia refers to an above-normal level of chloride in the ECF (serum chloride >106 mEq/L). Hyperchloremia can result from metabolic acidosis, head trauma, increased perspiration, excess adrenocortical hormone production, and decreased glomerular filtration. Signs and symptoms include tachypnea, weakness, lethargy, diminished cognitive ability, hypertension, decreased cardiac output, dysrhythmias, and coma.

Acid–Base Imbalances

Acid–base imbalances occur when the carbonic acid or bicarbonate levels become disproportionate. When there is a single primary cause, these disturbances are known as respiratory acidosis or alkalosis and metabolic acidosis or alkalosis, which are described in the sections that follow. Some references use the term *nonrespiratory* to refer to metabolic disturbances (Fischbach & Dunning, 2006). Although these disturbances are discussed separately, combined disturbances frequently occur. Complicated clinical situations may occur when respiratory and metabolic imbalances coexist.

Metabolic Acidosis and Alkalosis

Metabolic acidosis and alkalosis occur as the result of metabolic processes. A metabolic or nonrespiratory disturbance alters the bicarbonate level in the ECF. It is reflected in the HCO_3^- level of an ABG. Both the lungs and the kidneys attempt to compensate for this disorder by either excreting or retaining $PaCO_2$ (the lungs) and/or HCO_3^- and H^+ ions (the kidneys).

METABOLIC ACIDOSIS

Metabolic acidosis or nonrespiratory acidosis is a proportionate deficit of bicarbonate in ECF. The deficit can occur as the result of an increase in acid components or an excessive loss of bicarbonate. It can be produced by a gain of hydrogen ion or loss of bicarbonate. The lungs attempt to increase the carbon dioxide excretion by increasing the rate and depth of respirations, which occurs within a short time. However, respiratory compensation is generally not adequate, and the kidneys attempt to compensate by retaining bicarbonate and by excreting more hydrogen. In summary: Metabolic acidosis = low pH (increased hydrogen ion concentration) and a low plasma bicarbonate concentration due to a gain of hydrogen or loss of bicarbonate.

METABOLIC ALKALOSIS

Metabolic alkalosis or nonrespiratory alkalosis is associated with an excess of HCO_3, a decrease in H^+ ions, or both, in the ECF. This may be the result of excessive acid losses or increased base ingestion or retention. The body attempts to compensate by retaining carbon dioxide. The respirations become slow and shallow, and periods of no breathing may occur. The kidneys attempt to excrete excess H_2O and NA ions with the excessive bicarbonate and retain H^+ ions. In summary: Metabolic alkalosis = high pH and a high plasma bicarbonate concentration due to a gain of bicarbonate or a loss of hydrogen

Respiratory Acidosis and Alkalosis

Respiratory acidosis and alkalosis occur as a result of respiratory disturbances. A respiratory disturbance alters the carbonic acid level in the ECF. It is reflected in the $PaCO_2$ level of an ABG. Compensation for a respiratory disturbance occurs when the lungs attempt to either retain or eliminate $PaCO_2$ from the body or when the kidneys attempt to restore balance through the conservation, formation, or excretion of bicarbonate (HCO_3).

RESPIRATORY ACIDOSIS

Respiratory acidosis is a primary excess of carbonic acid in the ECF. It is produced by inadequate excretion of CO_2 with inadequate ventilation, resulting in elevated plasma CO_2 and increased levels of carbonic acid. Any decrease in alveolar ventilation that results in retention of carbon dioxide can cause respiratory acidosis. Initially, the increased amounts of CO_2 stimulate the medulla in the respiratory center to increase the respiratory rate. Due to the increase in respiratory rate, CO_2 is expelled and the CO_2 level of the blood is reduced. If the respiratory response is not effective, the increasing CO_2 levels will stimulate the kidneys to eliminate H^+ ions (acids) and conserve bicarbonate and sodium ions. The $NaHCO_3$ acts to buffer the free acids and ultimately reduce the CO_2 levels and restore acid–base balance (*Fluids & electrolytes,* 2006). In summary: Respiratory acidosis = high $PaCO_2$ due to alveolar hypoventilation.

RESPIRATORY ALKALOSIS

Respiratory alkalosis is a primary deficit of carbonic acid in the ECF. It is the result of alveolar hyperventilation, breathing that is faster and deeper, and the consequent increase in the elimination of CO_2. This loss of CO_2 leads to a decrease in the carbonic acid level in the plasma and an increase in the pH. The chemoreceptors in the medulla sense the increase in pH and the presence of less carbonic acid and stimulate the body to breathe either more slowly or less deeply. If this condition lasts for about 6 hours or longer, the kidneys attempt to alleviate the imbalance by increasing the bicarbonate excretion and by retaining more hydrogen to correct the imbalance. In summary: Respiratory alkalosis = low $PaCO_2$ due to alveolar hyperventilation.

THE NURSING PROCESS FOR FLUID, ELECTROLYTE, AND ACID–BASE BALANCE
Assessing

Acute and chronic illness, trauma, and certain therapeutic interventions may place a patient at high risk for fluid, electrolyte, and acid–base imbalances. Such imbalances can seriously compromise the patient's health status and may prove life threatening. The nursing assessment is directed toward the following:

- Identifying patients at high risk for fluid, electrolyte, and acid–base imbalances
- Determining that a specific imbalance is present and identifying the nature of the imbalance along with its severity, etiology, and defining characteristics or assessment findings
- Determining the plan of care, including the appropriate nursing diagnoses or collaborative problems, followed by the identification of specific outcomes, associated interventions, and the evaluation of the effectiveness of the plan of care

Physical assessment and clinical assessment parameters, nursing considerations, normal findings in a healthy adult, and possible abnormal or significant findings are outlined in Tables 40-4 and 40-5.

When an imbalance in fluid, particular electrolytes, or acid–base balance is suspected, the nurse needs to incorporate the associated assessments into the patient's care. The nursing assessment related to fluid, electrolyte, and acid–base balance should include a nursing history, physical assessment, fluid intake and output, daily weights, and laboratory studies.

Nursing History

A comprehensive nursing history includes questions related to the patient's fluid, electrolyte, and acid–base balance. The accompanying Focused Assessment Guide 40-1 includes interview questions helpful in identifying the patient's usual pattern of fluid intake and elimination and the patient's evaluation of his or her hydration status and awareness of particular problems.

Interview questions are also directed toward identifying patients with health conditions that increase the risk for imbalances. Risk factors include the following:

- Acute and chronic illnesses (e.g., diabetes mellitus, congestive heart failure, renal failure)

(text continues on page 1434)

TABLE • 40-4	PARAMETERS TO BE CONSIDERED IN PHYSICAL ASSESSMENT FOR FLUID, ELECTROLYTE, AND ACID–BASE BALANCE		
Assessment Parameters	**Nursing Considerations**	**Findings in Healthy Adult**	**Significant Findings**
Skin turgor (elasticity)	• The patient's skin over the sternum, inner aspect of the thighs, or forehead is pinched. • Some prefer to test skin turgor in children over the abdominal area and on the medial aspect of the thighs. • Skin turgor can vary with age, nutritional state, ethnicity, and complexion.	• Pinched skin immediately falls back to its normal position when released. • Reduced skin turgor is common in older patients (those more than 55–60 years of age) because of a primary decrease in skin elasticity.	• In a person with a fluid volume deficit, the skin flattens more slowly after the pinch is released; the skin may remain elevated for many seconds. • Severe malnutrition, particularly in infants, can cause depressed skin turgor even in the absence of fluid depletion.
Tongue turgor	• Unlike skin turgor, tongue turgor is not affected appreciably by age and thus is a useful assessment for all age groups. (In an arid climate, this may not be a reliable parameter.)	• Tongue has one longitudinal furrow.	• In the person with fluid volume deficit, there are additional longitudinal furrows and the tongue is smaller. • Sodium excess causes the tongue to look red and swollen.
Moisture and oral cavity	• A dry mouth may be the result of fluid volume deficit or of mouth breathing. (Exposure to an arid climate may result in a dry mouth.)	• Mucous membranes in oral cavity are moist.	• Dryness of the membrane where the cheek and gum meet indicates fluid volume deficit. • Dry sticky mucous membranes are noted in sodium excess. (The oral cavity feels like flypaper.)
Tearing and salivation		• Tearing and salivation decrease normally with age.	• The absence of tearing and salivation in a child is a sign of fluid volume deficit; it becomes obvious with a fluid loss of 5% of TBW.
Appearance of skin and skin temperature			• Metabolic acidosis can cause warm, flushed skin (due to peripheral vasodilation).
Facial appearance			• A person with a severe fluid volume deficit may have a pinched and drawn facial expression. • A fluid volume deficit of 10% of body weight causes decreased intraocular pressure, causing the eyes to appear sunken and to feel soft to the touch.
Edema (excessive accumulation of interstitial fluid)	• Pitting edema (see Fig. 40-7) • Measurement of an extremity or body part with a millimeter tape, in the same area each day, is a more exact method of measurement. • An excess of interstitial fluid may accumulate predominantly in the lower extremities of ambulatory patients and in the presacral region of bedridden patients. • The presence of periorbital (around the eyes) edema or pedal edema should prompt one to look for edema in other parts of the body.	• No edema	• Clinically, edema is not usually apparent in the adult until the retention of 5–10 lb of excess fluid occurs. • Pitting edema is not evident until at least a 10% increase in weight has occurred. • Formation of edema may be localized (as in thrombophlebitis) or generalized (as in heart failure, cirrhosis of liver, or nephrotic syndrome). Edema of congestive heart failure, liver cirrhosis, or nephrotic syndrome is the result of sodium retention.

(continued)

TABLE • 40-4	PARAMETERS TO BE CONSIDERED IN PHYSICAL ASSESSMENT FOR FLUID, ELECTROLYTE, AND ACID–BASE BALANCE *(continued)*		
Assessment Parameters	**Nursing Considerations**	**Findings in Healthy Adult**	**Significant Findings**
Body temperature	• Because fever increases the loss of body fluids, it is important that temperature elevations be detected early and appropriate interventions be taken. • Body temperature and other vital signs should be assessed as ordered and at the nurse's discretion.	• Baseline temperature: diurnal variations	• There is an elevation of body temperature in hypernatremia (dehydration) probably related to lack of available fluid for sweating. • There is a decrease in body temperature in fluid volume deficit, when uncomplicated by infection. • Fever increases the loss of body fluids. • A temperature elevation between 101°F (38.3°C) and 103°F (39.4°C) increases the 24-hour fluid requirement by at least 500 mL, and a temperature above 103°F increases it by at least 1,000 mL.
Pulse		• Baseline pulse rate, rhythm, and volume	• Tachycardia is usually the earliest sign of the decreased vascular volume associated with fluid volume deficit. • Irregular pulse rates also occur with potassium imbalances and magnesium deficit. • Pulse volume is decreased in fluid volume deficit and increased in fluid volume excess.
Respirations		• Baseline respiratory rate, rhythm, and qualities	• Deep, rapid respirations may be a compensatory mechanism for metabolic acidosis or a primary disorder causing respiratory alkalosis. • Slow, shallow respirations may be a compensatory mechanism for metabolic alkalosis or a primary disorder causing respiratory acidosis. • Moist crackles, in the absence of cardiopulmonary disease, indicate fluid volume excess.
Blood pressure	• Whenever a fluid imbalance is suspected, the patient's blood pressure is checked while he or she is lying down, sitting, and standing (orthostatic).	• Baseline blood pressure	• A fall in systolic pressure greater than 15 mm Hg from the lying to the sitting or standing position (postural hypotension) usually indicates fluid volume deficit.

(continued)

TABLE • 40-4	PARAMETERS TO BE CONSIDERED IN PHYSICAL ASSESSMENT FOR FLUID, ELECTROLYTE, AND ACID–BASE BALANCE *(continued)*		
Assessment Parameters	**Nursing Considerations**	**Findings in Healthy Adult**	**Significant Findings**
Neck veins and central venous pressure (CVP)	• The jugular veins provide a built-in manometer for following changes in CVP. • To estimate CVP: 1. Position the patient in a semi-Fowler's position (head of bed elevated to a 30- to 45-degree angle), keeping the neck straight 2. Remove any of the patient's clothing that could constrict the neck or upper chest 3. Provide adequate lighting to visualize effectively the external jugular veins on each side of the neck 4. Measure the levels to which the veins are distended on the neck or above the level of the manubrium • More accurate assessments of blood volume are obtained by measuring CVP by hemodynamic monitoring.	• Normally, when the patient is supine, the external jugular veins fill to the anterior border of the sternocleidomastoid muscle. With the patient positioned sitting at a 45-degree angle, venous distention normally should not extend higher than 2 cm above the sternal angle. • Pressure in the right atrium is usually 0–4 cm H_2O; pressure in the vena cava is about 4–11 cm H_2O.	• A low CVP may indicate: 1. Decreased blood volume 2. Drug-induced vasodilation (causing pooling of blood in peripheral veins) • A high CVP may indicate: 1. Increased blood volume 2. Heart failure 3. Vasoconstriction
Neuromuscular irritability	• When imbalances in calcium, magnesium, and sodium are suspected it is important to assess patients for increased or decreased neuromuscular irritability. • To test for *Chvostek's sign*, the facial nerve should be percussed about 2 cm anterior to the ear lobe. • To test for *Trousseau's sign*, a blood pressure cuff is placed on the arm and inflated above systolic pressure for 3 minutes. • A deep tendon reflex is elicited by briskly tapping a partially stretched tendon with a rubber percussion hammer, preferably over the tendon insertion of the muscle. • The muscle being tested should be slightly stretched, and the patient should be relaxed.	• Negative response • Negative response • The response in the prospective muscle is a sudden contraction (2+). • Reflexes usually are graded on a 0 to 4+ scale. 0 = no response 1+ = somewhat diminished, but present 2+ = **normal** 3+ = brisker than average and possibly but not necessarily indicative of disease 4+ = hyperactive	• Patients with hypocalcemia or hypomagnesemia respond positively with a unilateral twitching of the facial muscles, including the eyelid and lips. • A positive response is the development of carpal spasm. • Deep tendon reflexes may be hyperactive in the presence of hypocalcemia, hypomagnesemia, hypernatremia, and alkalosis. • Deep tendon reflexes may be hypoactive in the presence of hypercalcemia, hypermagnesemia, hyponatremia, hypokalemia, and acidosis.
Behavior Sensation Fatigue level	• Because these changes are often vague, they are best evaluated in context with specific imbalances.		

Data from Smeltzer, S., Bare, B., Hinkle, J., & Cheever, K. (2010) *Brunner and Suddarth's textbook of medical-surgical nursing* (12th ed.). Philadelphia: Wolters Kluwer Health/Lippincott Williams & Wilkins; Portable fluids & electrolytes. (2008). Philadelphia: Wolters Kluwer Health/Lippincott Williams & Wilkins; and Porth, C., & Matfin, G. (2009). *Pathophysiology: Concepts of altered health states* (8th ed.). Philadelphia: Wolters Kluwer Health/Lippincott Williams & Wilkins.

T ABLE • 40-5	PARAMETERS TO BE CONSIDERED IN CLINICAL ASSESSMENT FOR FLUID, ELECTROLYTE, AND ACID–BASE BALANCE		
Assessment Parameters	**Nursing Considerations**	**Findings in Healthy Adult**	**Significant Findings**
Comparison of total intake and output of fluids	• Records may be initiated by the nurse for any patient with a real or potential water or electrolyte problem. • Intake should include all fluids taken into the body. • Output should include urine, vomitus, diarrhea, drainage from fistulas, and drainage from suction apparatus. Perspiration and drainage from lesions should be noted and estimated. Prolonged hyperventilation should also be noted because it is an important route of water vapor loss.	• Fluid intake approximately equals fluid output—when averaged over 2 or 3 days. • Range of 1,500–3,500 mL fluid intake and loss; 2,000 mL is average adult intake and loss per day. • Output of urine normally approximates the ingestion of liquids; water from food and oxidation is balanced by the water loss through feces, the skin, and the respiratory process.	• When the total intake is substantially less than the total output, the patient is in danger of fluid volume deficit. • When the total intake is substantially more than the total output, the patient is in danger of fluid volume excess.
Urine volume and concentration	• All fluid losses are measured according to routes. • A device calibrated for small volumes of urine is used when hourly urine volumes need to be measured. • Factors that can alter urinary output must be accounted for: 1. Amount of fluid intake 2. Losses from skin, lungs, and GI tract 3. Amount of waste products for excretions 4. Renal concentrating ability 5. Blood volume 6. Hormonal influences (primarily aldosterone and ADH)	• Normal urinary output is about 1 mL/kg of body weight per hour (for the average adult: 1,500 mL/24 hr, which is equivalent to about 40–80 mL/hr). • Stress may diminish the 24-hour urine volume in the adult to 750–1,000 mL (or 30–50 mL/hr) because of increased aldosterone and ADH secretion. • The range of specific gravity is from 1.003 to 1.035. Urine osmolality ranges between 500 and 800 mOsm/kg (mmol/kg).	• A low urine volume with a high specific gravity indicates fluid volume deficit. • A low urine volume with a low specific gravity indicates renal disease. • A high urine volume suggests fluid volume excess. • Urine volume is increased in conditions with high solute loads, such as diabetes mellitus. • Hypovolemia causes decreased renal perfusion and thus oliguria; hypervolemia causes increased urinary volume if the kidneys are functioning normally.
Body weight	• Because of the common inaccuracies in recording intake and output, body weight is believed to be a more accurate indicator of fluid gained and lost. • Guidelines for weighing a patient: 1. Use the same scale each time. 2. Measure weight at the same time each day: in the morning before breakfast and after voiding. 3. Ensure the patient is wearing the same or similar clothing (clothing should be dry). 4. Use a bed scale if the patient is unable to stand on a small, portable scale. • A patient may have a severe fluid volume deficit even though body weight is essentially unchanged when there is a third-space loss of body fluid.	• A patient's dry weight should remain relatively stable.	• Rapid variations in weight closely reflect changes in body fluid volume. • A rapid loss of body weight occurs when the total fluid intake is less than the total fluid output. 1. Rapid loss of 2% total body weight (TBW) indicates mild fluid volume deficit. 2. Rapid loss of 5% TBW indicates moderate fluid volume deficit. 3. Rapid loss of 8% or more of TBW indicates severe fluid volume deficit. • A rapid gain of body weight occurs when the total fluid intake is greater than the total fluid output. 1. Rapid gain of 2% TBW indicates mild fluid volume excess. 2. Rapid gain of 5% TBW indicates moderate fluid volume excess. 3. Rapid gain of 8% or more of TBW indicates severe fluid volume excess. • A rapid gain or loss of 1 kg (2.2 lb) of body weight is about equal to the gain or loss of 1 L of fluid.

Data from Smeltzer, S., Bare, B., Hinkel, J., Cheever, K. (2010) *Brunner and Suddarth's textbook of medical-surgical nursing* (12th ed.). Philadelphia: Wolters Kluwer Health/Lippincott Williams & Wilkins; Portable fluids & electrolytes. (2008). Philadelphia: Wolters Kluwer Health/Lippincott Williams & Wilkins; and Porth, C., & Matfin, G. (2009). *Pathophysiology: Concepts of altered health states* (8th ed.). Philadelphia: Wolters Kluwer Health/Lippincott Williams & Wilkins.

FOCUSED ASSESSMENT GUIDE • 40-1

FLUID, ELECTROLYTE, AND ACID–BASE BALANCE

Factors to Assess	Questions and Approaches
Usual patterns of fluid intake	Describe the amount and types of fluids you usually drink in a 24-hour period. Have there been any recent changes?
Usual pattern of fluid elimination	Describe your usual voiding/urination habits. Any recent changes in frequency or amount? Is your body losing fluids in any other major way? • Vomiting • Diarrhea • Excessive perspiration • Fistula
Patient's evaluation of hydration status	Do you think there is an approximate balance between your fluid intake and output? Have you noticed any signs that your body is experiencing too much or too little hydration (difficulty breathing, edema, dry skin and mucous membranes, thirst)?
History of disease process	Is there any history of disease process or injury that might disrupt fluid and electrolyte balance (e.g., diabetes mellitus, cancer, burns)?
Medication/nutrition history	Do you take any medications or treatments that might disrupt fluid and electrolyte balance (e.g., steroids, diuretics, total parenteral nutrition, dialysis)? Have you been trying to lose weight by dieting, using diuretics, laxatives, or diet aids? Have you been following a high-protein, low-carbohydrate diet?
Fluid, electrolyte, and acid–base imbalances and contributing factors	Are you aware of any other fluid balance problems you may be experiencing? • Nature • Onset of problem and frequency • Causes • Severity • Symptoms • Intervention attempted and results

• Abnormal losses of body fluids (e.g., prolonged or severe vomiting or diarrhea, draining wounds, fistulas. Table 40-6 lists imbalances that result from loss of specific body fluids.
• Burns
• Trauma
• Therapies that may disrupt fluid and electrolyte balance (e.g., medications such as diuretics and steroids, treatments such as IV therapy and TPN)
• Surgery

Physical Assessment

Physical assessment related to fluid, electrolyte, and acid–base balance includes the assessment of multiple body systems. Include assessment of the skin and mucous membranes, vital signs, and a neurological assessment, as well as identification of relative symptoms or conditions such as excessive thirst, nausea, vomiting, diarrhea, draining wounds, or other fluid

losses. Assessment of other body systems is included based on the patient's underlying health conditions.

Fluid Intake and Output

If monitoring of a patient's intake and output is required, the patient, family, and all caregivers must be alert to the need to measure all fluids entering and leaving the body. Refer to Guidelines for Nursing Care 40-1: Measuring Fluid Intake and Output for an explanation of correct measurement of a patient's intake and output.

Daily Weights

The record of a patient's daily weight may more accurately depict fluid balance status, due to possible numerous sources of inaccuracies in fluid intake and output measurement. Weigh the patient at the same time every day. Be alert for other factors that may affect a patient's weight, such as using

TABLE • 40-6	IMBALANCES RESULTING FROM LOSS OF SPECIFIC BODY FLUID
Fluid Lost	**Imbalances Likely to Occur**
Gastric juice	Extracellular fluid volume deficit Metabolic alkalosis Sodium deficit Potassium deficit Tetany (if metabolic alkalosis is present) Ketosis of starvation Magnesium deficit
Intestinal juice	Extracellular fluid volume deficit Metabolic acidosis Sodium deficit Potassium deficit
Bile	Sodium deficit Metabolic acidosis
Pancreatic juice	Metabolic acidosis Sodium deficit Calcium deficit Extracellular fluid volume deficit
Sensible perspiration	Extracellular fluid volume deficit Sodium deficit
Insensible water loss	Water deficit (dehydration) Sodium excess
Wound exudate	Protein deficit Sodium deficit Extracellular fluid volume deficit
Ascites	Protein deficit Sodium deficit Plasma-to-interstitial fluid shift Extracellular fluid volume deficit

a different scale and weighing with the patient wearing different clothing.

Laboratory Studies

Laboratory tests are helpful in determining whether fluid, electrolyte, and acid–base balance exist. Standard tests are described below; tables of normal values are given in Appendix B.

COMPLETE BLOOD COUNT

The complete blood count determines the total number of red blood cells and values for hemoglobin and hematocrit. Significant values include the following:

- Increased hematocrit values: found in severe fluid volume deficit and shock (when hemoconcentration rises considerably)
- Decreased hematocrit values: found with acute, massive blood loss, and with hemolytic reaction after transfusion of incompatible blood or with fluid overload

- Increased levels of hemoglobin: found in hemoconcentration of the blood
- Decreased levels of hemoglobin: found with anemia states, severe hemorrhage, and after a hemolytic reaction

SERUM ELECTROLYTES, BUN, AND CREATININE LEVELS

This screening test determines plasma levels of certain electrolytes such as sodium, potassium, chloride, and bicarbonate ions. In addition, the BUN and creatinine levels can provide information related to the fluid status and the renal function of the patient. Significant values include the following:

- Below normal or above normal levels of sodium, potassium, calcium, magnesium, phosphate, and chloride. Refer to the electrolyte imbalance discussion earlier in the chapter.
- Below normal or above normal levels of bicarbonate ions. Refer to the acid–base discussion earlier in the chapter.
- Increased BUN: found with impaired renal function (such as associated with shock, heart failure, salt and water depletion), diabetic ketoacidosis, burns
- Increased creatinine: found with impaired renal function, heart failure, shock, dehydration

> ➤ *Recall Grace Gilligan, the woman described in one of the beginning scenarios. Although she needs IV therapy, it would be important for the nurse to determine the patient's electrolyte levels to establish a baseline to aid in determining the best IV solution for the patient and her need for possible electrolyte replacement.* ■

URINE PH AND SPECIFIC GRAVITY

Both the urine pH and specific gravity may be obtained by dipstick measurement, using a fresh voided specimen or through laboratory analysis. The pH of urine usually ranges between 4.6 and 8.2. Lower than normal urinary pH can occur with metabolic acidosis, diabetic ketosis, and diarrhea. Higher than normal urinary pH can occur with respiratory alkalosis, potassium depletion, and chronic renal failure. Specific gravity is a measure of the urine's concentration. The range depends on the patient's state of hydration and varies with urine volume and the load of solutes to be excreted. Normal values range from 1.005 to 1.030 (concentrated urine: ≥ 1.025, dilute urine: $\leq 1.001–1.010$). Increased urine specific gravity can occur with dehydration, vomiting, diarrhea, and heart failure. Decreased urine specific gravity can occur with renal damage.

ARTERIAL BLOOD GASES

Arterial blood gases (ABGs) are laboratory tests commonly used to determine the adequacy of oxygenation and ventilation, as well as in the assessment and treatment of acid–base imbalance. The ABG findings are obtained through analysis of an arterial blood sample. The pH of the plasma or blood indicates balance or impending acidosis or alkalosis.

Guidelines for Nursing Care • 40-1

MEASURING FLUID INTAKE AND OUTPUT

- Instruct the patient and family regarding the need for a record of all fluids entering the body and all fluid output. Provide an explanation of the rationale along with instructions for how the patient can help keep measurements accurate. Some patients may need to be reminded each morning that this measurement will continue.

- Use the patient's plan of care to communicate to other nursing personnel the need to measure fluid intake and output. A sign posted in the patient's room and a bedside form for recording intake and output are helpful reminders for both the patient and nurses.

- Measure both intake and output whenever possible, rather than estimate.

- Record intake and output totals for each 8-hour shift and total each 24 hours. If the nurse suspects a large difference between intake and output, total the columns earlier so that the primary care provider can be notified.

The Patient's Fluid Intake Includes the Following

- All fluids and foods that are liquid at room temperature (ice cream, gelatin dessert [Jell-O], etc.)

- Use the agency's designation of specific volumes for common food containers (e.g., juice glass = 90 mL;

milk carton = 240 mL). Remind the patient that sips of water or other fluids in between meals need to be recorded; small, disposable calibrated cups at the bedside facilitate accurate measurement. Remember that liquid medications or water taken with pills may significantly increase the fluid intake of some patients.

- All parenteral fluids

- Other fluids taken into the body: subcutaneous fluids, gastrointestinal tube feedings and flushes; IV flushes

The Patient's Fluid Output Includes the Following

- Urine; vomitus; diarrhea; drainage from fistulas, wounds, and ulcers; and drainage from suctioning devices or other tubes. Calibrated measuring devices should be readily available for accurate measurement. Disposable, calibrated urine collection containers that fit under the toilet seat are available for ambulatory patients. Urine or liquid feces in diapers or bed clothes, vomitus on clothing or bed linens, wound drainage saturating dressings, and so forth, need to be estimated.

- Heavy perspiration, noted on the output record, especially when the patient's clothing or bed linens are soaked

- Hyperventilation (water vapor loss) also noted on the output record. Record the rate and depth of respirations.

The blood's oxygen and carbon dioxide gas values are also reported, providing information regarding the effectiveness of the respiratory system. The partial pressures (indicated by "P") of these gases, or their tensions, are determined by the use of a nomogram, which reflects the chemical and physical activities of the two gases. The partial pressure of carbon dioxide is abbreviated $PaCO_2$; for oxygen, it is PaO_2. The "a" indicates an arterial specimen. When the PaO_2 is low, hemoglobin carries less than normal amounts of oxygen; when the PaO_2 is high, the hemoglobin carries more oxygen. The $PaCO_2$ is influenced almost entirely by respiratory activity. When the $PaCO_2$ is low, carbonic acid leaves the body in excessive amounts; when the $PaCO_2$ is high, there are excessive amounts of carbonic acid in the body. Oxygen saturation readings (SaO_2) reveal the percentage of oxygen in the blood that combines with hemoglobin.

The bicarbonate level (HCO_3^-) of the ABG report reflects the bicarbonate level of the body. The kidneys are involved in either reabsorbing bicarbonate or excreting bicarbonate, depending upon what is needed to maintain the delicate acid–base balance.

Although compensation is the body's natural attempt to restore balance, correction may also be required. Correction involves using medical and nursing interventions to promote a return to homeostasis (e.g., pharmacologic agents, mechanical ventilation, monitor intake/output, dietary teaching).

Table 40-7 outlines acid–base parameters for arterial blood gas studies.

Additional ABG values exist but are not included in this simple interpretation of acid–base imbalances. Partial pressure of oxygen (PaO_2) and oxygen saturation (SaO_2) results also directly reflect the adequacy of oxygenation and ventilation. When interpreting ABGs, follow these necessary steps:

1. Determine whether the pH is alkalotic or acidotic.
2. Check for the cause of the change in pH. Is it respiratory ($PaCO_2$) or metabolic (HCO_3^-)? In respiratory acid–base imbalances, the pH and $PaCO_2$ values are inversely abnormal (move in opposite directions):

   Respiratory acidosis:
   $\downarrow$ pH <7.35 $\uparrow$ $PaCO_2$ Normal HCO_3^-

   Respiratory alkalosis:
   $\uparrow$ pH >7.45 $\downarrow$ $PaCO_2$ Normal HCO_3^-

   In metabolic acid–base imbalances, the pH and HCO_3^- values are both high or both low:

   Metabolic acidosis:
   $\downarrow$ pH <7.35 $\downarrow$ HCO_3^- Normal $PaCO_2$

   Metabolic alkalosis:
   $\uparrow$ pH >7.45 $\uparrow$ HCO_3^- Normal $PaCO_2$

Table • 40-7	ACID–BASE PARAMETERS FOR ARTERIAL BLOOD GAS STUDIES		
	Normal	**Acid**	**Base**
pH	7.35–7.45	<7.35	>7.45
$PaCO_2$	35–45 mm Hg	>45 mm Hg	<35 mm Hg
HCO_3^-	22–26 mEq/L	<22 mEq/L	>26 mEq/L

3. Determine whether the body is compensating for the pH change. When the problem is respiratory, the renal system assists in compensation either by increasing or by decreasing HCO_3^-. In contrast, the respiratory system assists in compensating for a metabolic acid–base imbalance by regulating CO_2 levels. When compensation occurs, the $PaCO_2$ and the HCO_3^- will always point in the same direction. The focus of compensation efforts is to return the pH to the normal range:

Respiratory acidosis:
↓ pH <7.35 ↑ $PaCO_2$ ↑ HCO_3^-
(compensation attempt)

Respiratory alkalosis:
↑ pH >7.45 ↓ $PaCO_2$ ↓ HCO_3^-
(compensation attempt)

Metabolic acidosis:
↓ pH <7.35 ↓ HCO_3^- ↓ $PaCO_2$
(compensation attempt)

Metabolic alkalosis:
↑ pH >7.45 ↑ HCO_3^- ↑ $PaCO_2$
(compensation attempt)

4. Look at the total picture and determine whether compensation has occurred. Compensation is classified as follows:
   Absent if:
   pH abnormal
   One component abnormal
   Second component within normal range
   Partial if:
   pH abnormal
   One component abnormal
   Second component beginning to change
   Complete if:
   pH within normal range
   One component abnormal
   Second changed to move pH within normal range

Table 40-8 lists assessments and nursing interventions related to these acid–base disturbances.

Diagnosing

Nursing diagnoses related to fluid, electrolyte, and acid–base balance can reflect a disturbance as the problem and result in nursing diagnoses that identify a fluid volume problem. Nursing diagnoses may also reflect the impact the imbalance has on other areas of functioning for the patient.

Fluid, Electrolyte, and Acid–Base Disturbances as the Problem

When assessment data point to fluid and electrolyte problems amenable to nursing therapy, appropriate nursing diagnoses include:

- Excess Fluid Volume
- Deficient Fluid Volume
- Risk for Deficient Fluid Volume
- Risk for Imbalanced Fluid Volume

Excess fluid volume may result from greatly increased fluid intake or, more frequently, from decreased excretion, such as occurs with progressive renal disease, dysfunctions of the heart, and certain cancers. Fluid volume deficits may result from decreased intake or increased excretion of fluids as well as fluid shifts. In addition, fluid and electrolyte deficiencies may be related to situations involving strenuous exercise, extreme heat or dryness, and conditions (e.g., fever) that increase the metabolic rate. The accompanying Examples of NANDA Nursing Diagnoses: Fluid and Electrolyte Balance presents contributing factors and defining characteristics for these diagnoses.

If nursing assessments indicate that fluid volume balance currently exists, the nursing diagnosis Readiness for Enhanced Fluid Balance may be appropriate. Fluid balance would be evident, but certain nursing measures might contribute to maintenance or improvement of fluid volume balance (NANDA International, 2009).

The nurse's analysis of assessment data may also lead to the diagnosis of specific electrolyte or acid–base disturbances that are collaborative problems because they require joint intervention by such healthcare professionals as the nurse, the physician, the dietitian, and the respiratory therapist.

Fluid and Electrolyte Disturbances as the Etiology

Disturbances in fluid, electrolyte, and acid–base balance may affect many other areas of human functioning. Examples of nursing diagnoses that may be appropriate include the following:

- Activity Intolerance related to imbalance between oxygen supply and demand
- Ineffective Breathing Pattern related to compensatory mechanism by lungs (hypoventilation or hyperventilation)
- Anxiety related to hyperventilation
- Decreased Cardiac Output related to decreased blood volume, shock
- Risk for Injury related to neuromuscular irritability, cardiac arrhythmia
- Deficient Knowledge: Harmful Effects of Abuses of Dieting, Alcohol, Diuretics, Laxatives, and Enemas related to no previous experience

TABLE • 40-8 ACID–BASE DISTURBANCES

Risk Factors	Assessments	Nursing Interventions
Respiratory Acidosis (Carbonic Acid Excess)		

Acute respiratory disease:
  Pulmonary edema
  Aspiration of a foreign body
  Atelectasis
  Overdose of sedative or anesthetic
  Cardiac arrest
Chronic respiratory disease:
  Emphysema
  Bronchial asthma
  Cystic fibrosis
Inadequate mechanical ventilation
CNS depression
Neuromuscular disease
	Acute respiratory acidosis
	  Mental cloudiness
	  Dizziness
	  Muscular twitching
	  Unconsciousness
	  ABGs
	    pH <7.35
	    $PaCO_2$ >45 mm Hg (primary)
	    HCO_3^- normal or only slightly
	     elevated
	Chronic respiratory acidosis
	  Weakness
	  Dull headache
	  ABGs
	    pH <7.35 or low N
	    $PaCO_2$ >45 mm Hg (primary)
	    HCO_3^- >26 mEq/L (compensatory)
		Treatment is directed at improving
		  ventilation:
		  Pharmacologic measures
		  Pulmonary hygiene measures
		  Adequate hydration
		  Supplemental oxygen
		Mechanical ventilation may be necessary to
		  correct disorder but must be used
		  cautiously to decrease $PaCO_2$ slowly.

Respiratory Alkalosis (Carbonic Acid Deficit)		

Hyperventilation
Extreme anxiety (most common cause)
Hypoxemia
High fever
Early sepsis
Excessive ventilation by mechanical
  ventilator
CNS lesion involving the respiratory
  center
Thyrotoxicosis
	Lightheadedness
	Inability to concentrate
	Hyperventilation syndrome
	  Tinnitus
	  Palpitations
	  Sweating
	  Dry mouth
	  Tremulousness
	  Convulsions and loss of
	    consciousness
	ABGs
	  pH >7.45
	  $PaCO_2$ <35 mm Hg (primary)
	  HCO_3^- <22 mEq/L (compensatory)
		If anxiety is the cause, encourage the patient
		  to breathe more slowly (causes accumula-
		  tion of CO_2) or breathe into a closed sys-
		  tem (paper bag). Sedative may also be
		  necessary in extreme anxiety.
		Treatment of other causes is directed at cor-
		  recting the underlying problem.

Metabolic Acidosis (Base Bicarbonate Deficit)		

Diarrhea
Intestinal fistulas
Ureterosigmoidostomy
Hyperalimentation
Excessive intake of acids, such
  as salicylates
Diabetic ketoacidosis
Renal failure
Starvational ketoacidosis
	Headache
	Confusion
	Drowsiness
	Increased respiratory rate and depth
	Nausea and vomiting
	Peripheral vasodilation
	ABGs
	  pH <7.35
	  HCO_3^- <22 mEq/L (primary)
	  $PaCO_2$ <35 mm Hg
	Hyperkalemia frequently present
		Treatment is directed toward correcting the
		  metabolic deficit. If the cause of the prob-
		  lem is excessive intake of chloride, treat-
		  ment obviously focuses on eliminating the
		  source. When necessary, bicarbonate is
		  administered.

Metabolic Alkalosis (Base Bicarbonate Excess)		

Vomiting or gastric suction
Hypokalemia
Potassium-wasting diuretics
Alkali ingestion (bicarbonate-
  containing antacids)
Renal loss of H^+ (e.g., from steroid
  or diuretic use)
	Dizziness
	Tingling of fingers and toes
	Hypertonic muscles
	Depressed respirations
	  (compensatory)
	ABGs
	  pH >7.45
	  HCO_3^- >26 mEq/L (primary)
	  $PaCO_2$ >45 mm Hg
	    (compensatory)
	Hypokalemia may be present
		Treatment is aimed at reversal of the under-
		  lying disorder. Sufficient chloride must be
		  supplied for the kidney to absorb sodium
		  with chloride (allowing the excretion of
		  excess bicarbonate). Treatment also
		  includes administration of NaCl fluids to
		  restore normal fluid volume.

Adapted from *Fluids & electrolytes: A 2-in-1 reference for nurses.* (2006). Philadelphia: Wolters Kluwer Health/Lippincott Williams & Wilkins.

Examples of NANDA Nursing Diagnoses
Fluid and Electrolyte Balance

Nursing Diagnoses	Related Factors	Sample Defining Characteristics
Excess Fluid Volume	Pathophysiologic factors: renal failure, decreased cardiac output, liver disease, abnormal fluid accumulations, hormonal problems	• "I've noticed that my wedding ring is tight . . . also my clothes don't fit as well as they used to. I guess I've gained some weight." • Reports dyspnea with exertion, feeling weak and fatigued • Pitting edema in feet, ankles, lower legs • Taut, shiny skin • Jugular venous distention
	Situational factors: excessive IV infusion Nutritional factors: excessive sodium intake, low protein intake	• Bounding pulse, increased from baseline • Shallow, rapid respirations, crackles • Increased blood pressure • 10-lb (4.5-kg) weight gain over past month • Fluid intake greater than output • "Sometimes I can't catch my breath and I feel like my heart is pounding away." • "I feel bloated."
Deficient Fluid Volume; Risk for Deficient Fluid Volume	Decreased fluid intake: imposed fluid restrictions, inability to obtain or swallow fluids (debilitation, oral pain), depression	• "After I got the flu, I got so weak I couldn't get out of bed . . . I think I was out of it for a couple of days." • Increased pulse and respirations • Dry oral mucosa, cracked lips, furrowed tongue • Scanty, dark urine output • "I'm thirsty all the time."
	Abnormal fluid loss: vomiting; diarrhea; abnormal drainage; excessive use of laxative, enemas, diuretics; blood loss; diaphoresis; burns	• "I've been vomiting and I have diarrhea—several times a day." • Weight loss: 5 lb (2–3 kg) • Urine is concentrated (specific gravity, 1.035) • Fluid output greater than fluid intake • Neck veins collapsed when lying flat • Decreased skin turgor
	Increased need for fluids: strenuous exercise, extreme heat or dryness, fever (increased metabolic rate)	• Skin is warm to touch, moist, and flushed • Increased temperature, pulse, respirations • Decreased blood pressure

• Impaired Oral Mucous Membrane related to fluid volume deficit
• Impaired Skin Integrity related to fluid volume deficit or fluid volume overload
• Disturbed Thought Processes related to cerebral edema, mental confusion or disorientation, or convulsions
• Ineffective Tissue Perfusion: (specify type) related to decreased cardiac output
• Impaired Urinary Elimination related to decreased kidney perfusion secondary to decreased plasma volume

Outcome Identification and Planning

Nursing care supports the following expected outcomes. The healthy adult patient will:

• Maintain an approximate balance between fluid intake and fluid output (average about 2,500 mL fluid intake and output over 3 days)
• Maintain a urine specific gravity within normal range (1.005 to 1.030)
• Practice self-care behaviors to promote fluid, electrolyte, and acid–base balance; maintain adequate intake of fluid and electrolytes; respond appropriately to the body's signals of impending fluid, electrolyte, or acid–base imbalance

When an imbalance exists, the patient will:

• Relate relief of symptoms (specify) after implementation of treatment regimen (e.g., 1 month after decreasing sodium intake patient reports weight loss of 4 lb [1.8 kg])

Examples of Nursing Interventions and Nursing Outcomes Classifications (NIC/NOC)

Deficient Fluid Volume

Nursing Interventions	Nursing Outcomes
• Acid–base management • Electrolyte management • Electrolyte monitoring • Fluid management • Fluid monitoring • Hypovolemia management • Intravenous therapy • Nutrition management • Nutritional monitoring	• Electrolyte and acid–base balance • Fluid balance • Hydration • Nutritional status: Food and fluid intake

- Exhibit signs and symptoms of restored balance or homeostasis after initiation of treatment
- Identify signs and symptoms of recurrence of imbalance with need to notify the primary healthcare provider

Implementing

Nursing interventions to prevent or correct fluid, electrolyte, and acid–base imbalances include dietary modification, modification of fluid intake, medication administration, IV therapy, blood and blood products replacement, administration of total parenteral nutrition (TPN), allaying of anxiety as needed, and appropriate patient and family teaching. The accompanying Nursing Intervention and Nursing Outcome Classifications (NIC/NOC) box offers suggested nursing interventions and outcomes related to Deficient Fluid Volume.

Preventing Fluid Imbalances

An adequate fluid intake and a well-balanced, nutritious diet with appropriate adjustments throughout the life cycle are essential to promoting fluid balance. The following are general measures to consider to help prevent fluid imbalances:

- Be familiar with common life events that can lead to fluid imbalances, and observe the patient carefully. Infants are particularly vulnerable to fluid imbalances because body water accounts for a greater percentage of their weight, and fluid fluctuations are more common. Loss of fluid because of an illness can cause serious and life-threatening problems in infants.
- Note the patient's present fluid and food intake, and learn what his or her previous eating and drinking patterns have been. Learn whether the patient has been using a fad diet, which may lead to imbalances.
- Note whether the patient experiences excessive thirst or little or no thirst. Thirst, a subjective sensation, is an important factor determining water intake and, eventually, output through the kidneys. Although the thirst mechanism is poorly understood, both psychological and physiologic factors appear to be involved. An elderly patient is more susceptible to fluid-deficient conditions related to a less

effective thirst mechanism (Tabloski, 2006). Be aware of excessive losses of fluids from the body, and attempt to prevent losses when possible. Vomiting, pronounced perspiration, diarrhea, draining wounds, and excessive urinary output, for example, may cause excessive losses.

- Consider ways in which the patient's medical regimen may lead to fluid and electrolyte imbalances. For example, diuretics that stimulate urine formation may increase the elimination of both fluid and potassium. If food supplements high in potassium are not included in the diet or if potassium supplement drug therapy is not started, hypokalemia often follows.
- Learn whether the patient has been "treating" himself or herself in some way that may threaten fluid balance. Common practices that threaten fluid balance include the indiscriminate use of enemas, laxatives, antacids, and over-the-counter drugs to promote urination.
- Consider conditions with destructive effects on the body as threats to fluid balance. Examples include immobilization, trauma, burns, surgical procedures, and exposure to toxic agents.
- Teach patients to observe for fluid imbalances and to report them promptly. Examples include rapid weight gains and losses; swollen fingers, feet, and ankles; puffy eyelids; muscle weakness; change in skin sensations; and scanty or profuse urine production.
- Help patients and their families understand the significance of maintaining fluid balance and preventing imbalances.
- Be aware that normal physiologic changes associated with aging affect elder patients' ability to maintain fluid balance. Fluid volume deficit is a common fluid and electrolyte disorder in this population. The accompanying Focus on the Older Adult box suggests specific nursing strategies to prevent and correct fluid and electrolyte imbalances.

Table 40-9 lists the risk factors, related assessments, and specific nursing interventions for fluid volume disturbances. Table 40-10 lists the risk factors, related assessments, and specific nursing interventions for electrolyte disturbances.

(text continues on page 1444)

FOCUS ON THE OLDER ADULT

PHYSIOLOGIC CHANGES AND NURSING STRATEGIES FOR FLUID BALANCE PROBLEMS

Physiologic Changes	Nursing Strategies
Altered Sense of Thirst	
• Decreased sense of thirst • Medical conditions, e.g., heart failure or hypertension, requiring medications such as diuretics	• Ensure that oral intake is at least 1,500 mL for 24 hours. • Be aware of schedule for diagnostic tests (and associated dietary and fluid restrictions). • Offer fluids at regular intervals. • Replace fluids as necessary, either orally or IV. • Investigate individual fluid preferences. • Provide assistance or assistive devices for encouraging fluid intake.
Alterations in Renal Functioning	
• Loss of nephrons • Decreased renal blood flow	• Record accurate intake and output. • Note appearance and specific gravity of urine. • Check laboratory values for abnormal levels.

TABLE • 40-9 FLUID VOLUME DISTURBANCES

Risk Factors	Assessments	Nursing Interventions
Fluid Volume Deficit (Hypovolemia)		
GI: Vomiting, diarrhea, suction, fistulas Hemorrhage Excessive sweating Skin trauma, burns, draining wounds Third-space fluid shifts Excessive laxative or diuretic use Polyuria from renal disease or diuretics Hyperglycemia Change in mental status (unable to gain access to fluids, depression, confusion)	Thirst Weight loss over short period Weakness, fatigue, anorexia Dry mucous membranes Poor skin and tongue turgor Sunken eyes Flat neck veins Urine output <30 mL/hr Postural hypotension Weak, rapid pulse ↑Urine specific gravity ↑Hematocrit ↑BUN ↑Serum sodium Altered sensorium	Assess for presence or worsening of FVD. Administer oral fluids if indicated. If patient unable to eat and drink, anticipate TPN or tube feedings to be ordered. Monitor patient's response to fluid intake, either oral or parenteral. Be alert for signs of fluid overload. Provide appropriate skin care.
Fluid Volume Excess (Hypervolemia)		
Compromised regulatory mechanisms: renal failure, CHF, cirrhosis of liver, Cushing's syndrome GI irrigation with hypotonic fluid Excess IV fluids with sodium Corticosteroid therapy Excessive ingestion of sodium-containing substances in diet or sodium-containing medications	Weight gain over short period Peripheral edema (may be pitting) Increased BP Shortness of breath Crackles and wheezes in lungs Full, bounding pulse Neck vein distention Polyuria if renal function is normal Ascites, pleural effusion Pulmonary edema ↓BUN (due to plasma dilution) ↓Hematocrit ↓Serum sodium ↓Urine specific gravity	Assess for presence or worsening of FVE. Encourage adherence to sodium-restricted and fluid-restricted diet, if ordered. Avoid OTC drugs or check with physician or pharmacist about sodium content. Encourage rest periods. Monitor patient's response to diuretics. Teach self-monitoring of weight and intake and output. Attentive skin care. Monitor respiratory status.

GI, gastrointestinal; BUN, blood urea nitrogen; FVD, fluid volume deficit; TPN, total parenteral nutrition; CHF, congestive heart failure; IV, intravenous; BP, blood pressure; FVE, fluid volume excess; OTC, over-the-counter.

TABLE • 40-10   **ELECTROLYTE DISTURBANCES**

Risk Factors	Assessments	Nursing Interventions

Hyponatremia
 	
Loss of sodium, as in:
    Loss of GI fluids
    Use of diuretics
    Adrenal insufficiency
Gains of water, as in:
    Excessive administration of D_5W
    Water intoxication
Disease states associated with
    SIADH (a form of hyponatremia)
Pharmacologic agents that may
    impair water excretion
	Anorexia
	Nausea and vomiting
	Lethargy
	Confusion
	Muscle cramps
	Muscular twitching
	Seizures
	Coma
	Serum Na below 135 mEq/L
	Urine specific gravity <1.010
		Monitor fluid losses and gains.
		Monitor for presence of GI and CNS symptoms.
		Monitor serum Na levels.
		Check urine specific gravity.
		If able to eat, encourage foods and fluids with high sodium content.
		Be aware of sodium content of common IV fluids.
		Avoid giving large water supplements to patients receiving isotonic tube feedings.
		Take seizure precautions when hyponatremia is severe.

Hypernatremia
 	
Water deprivation
Increased sensible and insensible water loss
Ingestion of large amount of salt
Excessive parenteral administration of sodium-containing solutions
Profuse sweating
Diabetes insipidus
	Thirst
	Elevated body temperature
	Tongue dry and swollen, sticky mucous membranes
	Severe hypernatremia
	    Disorientation
	    Hallucinations
	    Lethargy when undisturbed
	    Irritable and hyperactive
	    Focal or grand mal seizures
	    Coma
	Serum Na above 145 mEq/L
	Urine specific gravity >1.015
		Monitor fluid losses and gains.
		Observe for excessive intake of high sodium foods.
		Monitor sodium content of prescriptions and OTC drugs.
		Monitor for changes in behavior such as restlessness, lethargy, and disorientation.
		Look for excessive thirst and elevated body temperature.
		Monitor serum Na levels.
		Check urine specific gravity.
		Give sufficient water with tube feedings to keep serum Na and BUN at normal limits.

Hypokalemia
 	
Diarrhea
Vomiting or gastric suction
Potassium-wasting diuretics
Steroid administration and certain antibiotics
Poor intake as in anorexia nervosa, alcoholism, potassium-free parenteral fluids
Polyuria
	Fatigue
	Anorexia, nausea, and vomiting
	Muscle weakness
	Decreased bowel motility
	Cardiac arrhythmias
	Increased sensitivity to digitalis
	Polyuria, nocturia, dilute urine
	Postural hypotension
	Serum K below 3.5 mEq/L
	ECG changes
	Paresthesias or tender muscles
		Monitor for occurrence of hypokalemia.
		Assess digitalized patients at risk for hypokalemia, which potentiates the action of digitalis
		Prevent hypokalemia by:
		    Encouraging extra K intake if possible
		    Educating about abuse of laxatives and diuretics
		Administer oral K supplements if ordered.
		Be knowledgeable about danger of IV potassium administration.

Hyperkalemia
 	
Decreased potassium excretion:
Oliguric renal failure
Potassium-sparing diuretics
Hypoaldosteronism
High potassium intake, especially in presence of renal insufficiency
Shift of potassium out of cells (acidosis, tissue trauma, malignant cell lysis)
	Vague muscle weakness
	Cardiac arrhythmias
	Paresthesias of face, tongue, feet, and hands
	Flaccid muscle paralysis
	GI symptoms such as nausea, intermittent intestinal colic, or diarrhea may occur
	Serum K >5.0 mEq/L
		Monitor for hyperkalemia, which is life threatening.
		Prevent hyperkalemia by:
		    Following rules for safe administration of K
		    Avoiding giving patients with renal insufficiency K-saving diuretics, K supplements, or salt substitutes
		    Cautioning about foods high in potassium content

Hypocalcemia Surgical hypoparathyroidism Malabsorption Vitamin D deficiency Acute pancreatitis Excessive administration of citrated blood Alkalotic states	Trousseau's and Chvostek's signs Numbness and tingling of fingers and toes Mental changes Seizures Spasm of laryngeal muscles ECG changes Cramps in muscles of extremities Total serum calcium <8.5 mg/dL	Take seizure precautions when hypocalcemia is severe. Monitor condition of airway. Take safety precautions if confusion is present. Educate people at risk for osteoporosis about the need for dietary calcium intake. Discuss calcium-losing aspects of nicotine and alcohol use.

(continued)

TABLE • 40-10 ELECTROLYTE DISTURBANCES *(continued)*

Risk Factors	Assessments	Nursing Interventions
Hypercalcemia Hyperparathyroidism Malignant neoplastic disease Prolonged immobilization Large doses of vitamin D Overuse of calcium supplements Thiazide diuretics	Muscular weakness Tiredness, lethargy Constipation Anorexia, nausea, and vomiting Decreased memory and attention span Polyuria and polydipsia Renal stones Neurotic behavior Cardiac arrest Serum calcium >10.5 mg/dL	Increase mobilization when feasible. Encourage sufficient oral intake. Discourage excessive consumption of milk products. Encourage bulk in the diet. Take safety precautions if confusion is present. Be alert for signs of digitalis toxicity in hypercalcemic patients. Force fluids to prevent formation of renal stones.

Hypomagnesemia
Chronic alcoholism
Intestinal malabsorption
Diarrhea
Nasogastric suction
Drugs
  Thiazide diuretics
  Aminoglycoside antibiotics
  Excessive doses of vitamin D
  Citrate preservative in blood
	Neuromuscular irritability
	  Increased reflexes
	  Coarse tremors
	  Seizures
	Cardiac manifestations
	  Tachyarrhythmias
	  Increased susceptibility to digitalis toxicity
	Mental changes
	  Disorientation
	  Mood changes
	Serum magnesium <1.3 mEq/L
		Assess for magnesium deficit because it predisposes patient to digitalis toxicity.
		Take seizure precautions if necessary.
		Monitor condition of airway because laryngeal stridor can occur.
		Educate patient if abuse of diuretics or laxatives is a problem.
		Educate about intake of foods rich in magnesium.

Hypermagnesemia Renal failure Adrenal insufficiency Excessive magnesium administration during treatment of eclampsia Hemodialysis with hard water or dialysate high in magnesium content	Early sign is serum magnesium level of 3–5 mEq/L Flushing and sense of skin warmth Hypotension Depressed respirations Drowsiness, hypoactive reflexes, and muscular weakness Cardiac abnormalities	If hypermagnesemia is present, be alert for low BP and shallow respirations, lethargy, drowsiness, and coma. Do not give magnesium-containing medications to patient with renal failure or compromised renal function. Be cautious of OTC drugs. Check deep tendon reflexes frequently.
Hypophosphatemia Glucose administration Refeeding after starvation Hyperalimentation Alcohol withdrawal Diabetic ketoacidosis Respiratory alkalosis	Cardiomyopathy Acute respiratory failure Seizures Decreased tissue oxygenation Joint stiffness Serum phosphate <2.5 mg/dL	Be aware that severely hypophosphatemic patients are at greater risk for infection. Administer IV phosphate products cautiously. Introduce hyperalimentation cautiously in patients who are malnourished. Monitor for diarrhea when taking oral supplements. Sudden increase in serum phosphate level can cause hypocalcemia.

Hyperphosphatemia
Renal failure
Chemotherapy
Large intake of milk
Excessive intake of phosphate-containing laxatives (Fleet phosphosoda)
Large vitamin D intake
Hyperthyroidism
	Short-term consequences:
	  Symptoms of tetany, such as tingling of the fingertips and around the mouth, numbness, and muscle spasms
	Long-term consequences:
	  Precipitation of calcium phosphate in nonosseous sites such as the kidneys, joints, arteries, skin, or cornea.
	Serum phosphate >4.5 mg/dL
		Monitor for signs of tetany.
		Be aware that soft tissue calcification can be a long-term complication of chronically elevated serum phosphate levels.
		Instruct patients that use of phosphate-containing laxatives can result in hyperphosphatemia.
		Avoid foods high in phosphorus content.

SIADH, syndrome of inappropriate antidiuretic hormone; ECG, electrocardiographic; CNS, central nervous system.
Data from Smeltzer, S., Bare, B., Hinkle, J., Cheever, K. (2010). *Brunner and Suddarth's textbook of medical-surgical nursing* (12th ed.). Philadelphia: Wolters Kluwer Health/Lippincott Williams & Wilkins; Portable fluids & electrolytes. (2008). Philadelphia: Wolters Kluwer Health/Lippincott Williams & Wilkins; and Porth, C., & Matfin, G. (2009). *Pathophysiology: Concepts of altered health states* (8th ed.). Philadelphia: Wolters Kluwer Health/Lippincott Williams & Wilkins.

Developing a Dietary Plan

Nurses should teach patients about their health conditions and provide information and support to improve health literacy by their patients. Refer to the accompanying Promoting Health Literacy box. Simple dietary changes may help to resolve fluid and electrolyte disturbances. After obtaining a nutritional assessment to identify actual or potential imbalances and food preferences (refer to Chapter 36), initiate teaching based on a nutritional plan that involves both the patient and the person who prepares the patient's meals. Include foods that help to resolve the fluid or electrolyte imbalance and that are acceptable to the patient. For example, for fluid volume deficit, increase foods with high water content (e.g., citrus fruit, melons, celery); for hypokalemia, increase foods with high potassium content (e.g., bananas, citrus fruits, apricots, melons, broccoli, potatoes); and for hypernatremia, avoid foods high in sodium (e.g., processed cheese, lunch meats, canned soups and vegetables, salted snack foods) and eliminate the use of table salt.

When teaching the patient about foods to include or avoid, provide the patient with a written list for reference. Evaluate the patient's understanding of the teaching by having the patient identify foods that can be eaten freely or moderately as well as those to be avoided. Both the patient and person responsible for the patient's food preparation should be able to describe a 24-hour diet plan compatible with the recommended modifications.

Modifying Fluid Intake

Depending on the nature of the fluid or electrolyte imbalance, a patient's fluid intake may need to be increased, decreased, or modified in terms of types of fluids ingested. Nursing responsibilities include:

- Identifying the appropriate fluid modification (e.g., with certain illnesses, the primary care provider may order fluid directives, such as "Restrict fluids to 1,000 mL daily")
- Determining whether the patient understands the rationale for the fluid modification, is motivated to follow the modification, and is capable of adhering to the plan (e.g., a bedridden patient who needs to increase fluid intake cannot do this independently)
- Developing and implementing a plan of care based on the preceding information

The accompanying PICO in Practice box highlights an example of evidence-based decision making regarding nursing intervention for a patient with a fluid imbalance.

INCREASING FLUIDS

Increasing fluids involves an above-average intake of fluids. The usual order reads, "Encourage fluids" and indicates the amount of fluid the patient is to have in each 24-hour period. Typically, the plan of care specifies the amount of fluid to be ingested in 24 hours (for hospitalized patients,

Promoting Health Literacy

IN PATIENTS WITH FLUID OR ELECTROLYTE IMBALANCES

Patient Scenario

Shamala Johnson, 58, had been experiencing complications from diabetes for the previous 10 years. She tells the nurse, "I really thought that I had things under control until lately. I can't believe one more thing has happened." Ms. Johnson was admitted to the hospital with end stage renal failure. "I guess I knew this was coming eventually, but did not expect it so soon!" She initially received dialysis via a temporary dialysis catheter, but had surgery yesterday for an A-V shunt. Her current plan of care includes dietary modifications, including potassium, sodium, protein, and fluid restrictions. The nurse has assisted her with making dietary choices based on the hospital menus, and has arranged a consult with the dietitian. The patient asks, "Do you think I will have to keep this up at home? How will I manage to get the right food? And liquids, can I drink anything? I don't understand this at all!"

Nursing Considerations: Tips for Improving Health Literacy

Confirm her dietary modifications for after discharge. Provide Ms. Johnson with easy to read information about living with renal disease, and managing fluid and electrolyte, as well as protein restrictions. Encourage her to ask her primary care provider as many questions as needed to understand her condition. Explain that there are things she can do to feel in control and follow the suggested regimen. Provide information and resources for support at home. Encourage Ms. Johnson to ask her primary care provider the following three questions:

- What is my main problem?
- What do I need to do?
- Why is it important for me to do this?

What additional measures can you take to help increase health literacy in this patient? What other measures would be helpful for this patient if she did not speak English, could not read, or had other learning deficits?

PICO IN PRACTICE
Asking Clinical Questions

Scenario: You are a staff nurse who works in an emergency department (ED) on the evening shift. One evening, a 3-year-old child is brought to the ED by her mother with complaints of 3 days of diarrhea and vomiting. The child's mother states that several children at her child's daycare center have been sick with a similar "stomach bug" over the course of the past week. The child's mother reports that the child last vomited 8 hours ago when she tried giving her some milk to drink and the child has not had anything to eat or drink since that time. The last episode of diarrhea was this past hour, and the child's mother reports that there may have been some urine mixed with the stool. The child's mucous membranes appear dry and she is lethargic but responds appropriately and lucidly to a variety of stimuli. The mother tells you: "When my oldest child was sick like this a few years ago, I took him here and the doctor gave him an IV (*sic* peripheral intravenous line) and that seemed to perk him right up. I want you to ask the doctor if you can do that for my daughter." You believe the child is only mildly dehydrated based upon your assessment findings and wonder whether oral rehydration should be tried as first-line therapy in treating this child.

- POPULATION: 3-year-old mildly dehydrated children
- INTERVENTION: Oral rehydration
- COMPARISON: IV rehydration
- OUTCOME: Effective rehydration

PICO Question: Is oral rehydration as effective as IV rehydration as a first-line intervention in treating mildly dehydrated 3-year-old children?

Finding: From the National Guidelines Clearinghouse: Cincinnati Children's Hospital Medical Center. (2006). *Evidence-based clinical care guideline for acute gastroenteritis (AGE) in children aged 2 months through 5 years.* Cincinnati, OH: Cincinnati Children's Hospital Medical Center.

This guideline specifies that children aged 2 months through 5 years of age with mild to moderate dehydration be treated with oral rehydration solutions first (i.e., before IV rehydration is tried). A complete protocol for rehydration is included within this guideline.

Level of Evidence: Level I

Recommendation: You recommend to the ED physician that this child be treated first with oral rehydration solutions, following the protocol specified in this guideline. You also recommend that the ED Policy and Procedure Committee develop a protocol for rehydration for mildly and moderately dehydrated young children that is based upon the recommendations found within this guideline.

---

shift totals are helpful [e.g., 7–3, 1,200 mL; 3–11, 900 mL; 11–7, 300 mL]) and the patient's food preferences. Choose or assist with choosing fluids that best provide the calories and electrolytes needed by the patient.

Several techniques are recommended to help the patient take more than average amounts of fluids. Begin by explaining to the patient in understandable terms the rationale for the increased fluids and the specific goal of taking the daily amount of fluid prescribed. This explanation provides the patient with a greater understanding of why he or she needs to increase fluid intake. In addition, this information helps motivate the patient to comply with the treatment. Together with the patient, develop short-term goals for accomplishing the increased fluid intake. For example, the patient will drink a glass of water every hour, a particular beverage by the time a television program is finished, or a pitcher of water by lunch. In general, patients are more likely to reach set goals when they have been involved in setting these goals.

Ensure that a proportionately larger amount of fluid is offered during the early hours of the patient's waking day, rather than large amounts before bedtime. The patient can usually take fluids relatively easily after having few or no fluids during sleeping hours. However, large amounts of fluid at night interferes with the patient's ability to rest and

sleep by being awakened during the night with the need to urinate.

Offering a variety of fluids served at the appropriate temperature is helpful, as is allowing the patient to choose what he or she would like; these measures help the patient comply with the treatment regimen. The likelihood for success also is increased because the patient is more likely to drink more when some liquids are iced and cold and when coffee or tea is hot. Variety also adds interest and makes increasing fluids more palatable. If patients dislike taking fluids (a common problem with children) or have swallowing difficulties, offering a gelatin dessert, flavored frozen water (Popsicles), water ice, or such may meet with more success.

Always have fluids readily available for the patient. Take care to avoid a situation in which patients are unable to secure their own fluids (left with an unfilled water pitcher, an empty glass, a full pitcher out of reach, or a pitcher too heavy to lift). In addition, use attractive, clean, and easy-to-handle cups, glasses, and straws and practices that help to encourage the patient's desire to take fluids.

Patient participation in care promotes autonomy and self-esteem. Therefore, have the patient help keep a record of his or her intake when possible. This often serves as a motivating factor to increase fluid intake. Offer support, understanding, and encouragement in providing nursing care because forcing fluid intake for the person experiencing no thirst can be uncomfortable.

Increasing the fluid intake of patients is among the most common nursing interventions. Use creativity to assist the patient and family to reach desired goals. Having a tea party may be a helpful strategy to use when encouraging a child to increase fluids. When determining the patient's increased fluid intake, be sure to include fluids replaced through nasogastric, gastrostomy, or jejunostomy tubes in the fluid balance summary.

RESTRICTING FLUIDS

Restricting the patient's fluid intake is sometimes necessary. The usual order reads, "Restrict fluids" and indicates the amount of fluid the patient is to have in each 24-hour period.

Several techniques are recommended to help patients restrict their intake of fluids. As with the method for increasing fluids, begin by explaining to the patient in understandable terms the rationale for the fluid restriction and the specified daily amount of fluid prescribed. Then work with the patient to develop short-term outcomes for accomplishing the overall task. Discuss with the patient the time intervals at which fluids will be served. Usually, offering fluids at 1- or 2-hour intervals and between meals is best because food often helps to relieve some feelings of thirst. Provide the fluid in small glasses or cups so that the container appears to contain more fluid than it actually does. Using ice chips also is helpful. Ice chips are about twice the volume of water in its liquid state and help to quench thirst. Remember to include the ice chips as part of the patient's fluid intake. If appropriate, encourage the patient to participate in his or her care by helping to keep a record of intake.

> ➤ *Consider Mr. Park, the patient who received too much IV fluid. As a result of this excess fluid intake and his subsequent development of problems, the nurse would be alert to the possibility that fluid restriction may be ordered. If this occurs, the nurse needs to ensure that Mr. Park understands the reason for the restriction.* ∎

Patients who need to restrict fluid intake often report thirst or dry mouth. Avoid offering patients dry, salty, or sweet foods and fluids because such items tend to increase thirst. Also, attempt to divert the patients' attention from thirst by involving them in activities, and keep fluids not intended for the patient out of sight. Provide understanding, support, and encouragement because limiting fluid intake is uncomfortable for a thirsty person.

Provide oral hygiene at regular intervals so that the patient's mouth remains clean and moist. Lubricate the lips and mucous membranes as indicated. If the patient is capable and cooperative, allow the patient to rinse his or her mouth with water without swallowing the fluid, to avoid exceeding the intake limit. Avoid hard candy and gum, as these actually contribute to drying of the mouth membranes.

Just as with fluid increases, fluid limits should also have shift totals set. This prevents one shift from taking all of the patient's allotted fluid and prepares the patient ahead of time for the fluid limits.

Administering Medications

Patients with fluid, electrolyte, and acid–base imbalances are often prescribed medications as part of the therapeutic regimen. Be knowledgeable about the therapeutic effects of mineral–electrolyte preparations and diuretics, and be alert for adverse effects of other medications, such as steroids and hormone replacements.

MINERAL–ELECTROLYTE PREPARATIONS

Mineral–electrolyte preparations are frequently prescribed to correct electrolyte imbalances. Nursing responsibilities include:

- Accurately administering the medications, following manufacturer's guidelines (e.g., dilute potassium supplements to disguise the unpleasant taste and decrease gastric irritation, monitor ABGs for increased pH after each 50–100 mEq of sodium bicarbonate to avoid overtreatment and metabolic alkalosis)
- Knowing and evaluating the intended therapeutic effect (e.g., with magnesium sulfate, look for decreased restlessness and irritability, decreased muscle tremors, control of convulsions)
- Assessing for adverse effects (e.g., with sodium chloride injection, observe for hypernatremia)
- Knowing the risks associated with administration; for example, IV potassium—IV potassium is never administered via IV bolus, the infusion rate for IV KCl solutions (maximum rate should be 10/mEq/hr) requires careful monitoring. An error can result in sudden hyperkalemia, leading to a fatal cardiac arrhythmia (Smeltzer et al., 2010)
- Assessing for drug interactions (e.g., drugs that increase the effects of minerals and electrolytes include acidifying agents, alkalinizing agents, cation exchange resin, iron salts, potassium salts)
- Teaching patients appropriate self-care behaviors

DIURETICS

Diuretics are drugs that increase renal excretion of water, sodium, and other electrolytes. Although helpful in treating patients with fluid volume excess, they increase the risk for fluid volume deficit and serious electrolyte deficiencies. Careful monitoring (e.g., check urine output and serum electrolytes, particularly serum K^+ level) and education are essential for a patient receiving diuretic therapy.

Administering Intravenous (IV) Therapy

A relatively common form of therapy for handling fluid disturbances is the use of various solutions infused intravenously. The physician or other licensed healthcare professional with prescriptive privileges is responsible for prescribing the kind and amount of solution to be used. The nurse is responsible for initiating, monitoring, and discontinuing the therapy. Refer to the Reflective Practice display at the beginning of the chapter.

TABLE • 40-11   SELECTED IV SOLUTIONS

Solution	Comments
Isotonic Solutions	
5% dextrose in water (D_5W)	Supplies about 170 cal/L and contains 50 g of glucose
	Should not be used in excessive volumes because it does not contain any sodium; thus the fluid dilutes the amount of sodium in the serum. Brain swelling, or *hyponatremic encephalopathy*, can develop rapidly and cause death unless it is promptly recognized and treated.
0.9% NaCl (normal saline)	Not desirable as routine maintenance solution because it provides only Na^+ and Cl^-, which are provided in excessive amounts.
	May be used to expand temporarily the extracellular compartment if circulatory insufficiency is a problem; also used to treat diabetic ketoacidosis.
Lactated Ringer's solution	A roughly isotonic solution that contains multiple electrolytes in about the same concentrations as found in plasma (note that this solution is lacking in Mg^{2+} and PO_4^{3-})
	Used in the treatment of hypovolemia, burns, and fluid lost as bile or diarrhea
	Useful in treating mild metabolic acidosis
Hypotonic Solutions	
0.33% NaCl (⅓-strength normal saline)	A hypotonic solution that provides Na^+, Cl^-, and free water. Na^+ and Cl^- allows kidneys to select and retain needed amounts
	Free water desirable as aid to kidneys in elimination of solutes
0.45% NaCl (½-strength normal saline)	A hypotonic solution that provides Na^+, Cl^-, and free water
	Often used to treat hypernatremia (because this solution contains a small amount of Na^+, it dilutes the plasma sodium while not allowing it to drop too rapidly)
Hypertonic Solutions	
5% dextrose in 0.45% NaCl	A common hypertonic solution used to treat hypovolemia; used to maintain fluid intake
10% dextrose in water ($D_{10}W$)	Supplies 340 cal/L
	Used for peripheral parenteral nutrition (PPN)
5% dextrose in 0.9% NaCl (normal saline)	Replaces nutrients and electrolytes
	Can temporarily be used to treat hypovolemia if plasma expander is not available

Data from *Portable fluids & electrolytes.* (2008). Philadelphia: Wolters Kluwer Health/Lippincott Williams & Wilkins.

As with other therapeutic agents, the nurse must understand the patient's need for IV therapy, the type of solution being used, its desired effect, and untoward reactions that may occur. The contents of selected IV solutions are listed, along with comments about their use, in Table 40-11.

EQUIPMENT

Sterile technique must be observed when accessing a vein to avoid possible catheter-related infection. Disposable infusion tubing and needles are used to help eliminate many possible sources of contamination and to reduce the cost of equipment aftercare.

Equipment varies according to the manufacturer. Be familiar with the equipment used in the facility or home setting. Typically, most solutions for infusions are dispensed in 1-L or 500-mL flexible or rigid plastic containers. Because plastic bags collapse under atmospheric pressure as the solution enters the patient's vein, they do not require a vent for air to enter to replace fluid flowing from the container. Small 50-, 100-, and 250-mL solution bags are available to administer intermittent IV medications (such as antibiotics given by IV piggyback).

Some medications bond with the plastic in IV bags. Therefore, glass bottles are required for certain medications. Glass bottles do not collapse under atmospheric pressure and thus require a vent to allow air to enter the bottle as the fluid leaves the bottle.

IV administration tubing is used to attach the IV container to the patient's venous access. A basic administration set is illustrated in Figure 40-8. Infusion pumps usually require tubing specific for the device. Pump tubing shares many of the same features as tubing used for gravity infusion. Normally an IV administration set includes a spike or piercing pin to access the IV container, a drip chamber for observing fluid drops, a slide clamp to stop fluid flow, a roller clamp to manually regulate the rate of flow, a filter, several injection

FIGURE 40-8. Basic administration tubing for intravenous therapy. *(Photo by B. Proud.)*

ports for administration of medications or additional IV fluids, and a connector at the end of the tubing to connect with the venous access (preferably Luer lock design, threads to screw on). Pump tubing also includes a mechanism that fits into the electronic device to control the infusion rate.

A variety of needles and catheters are commonly used for peripheral IV infusions. IV catheters are plastic tubes that have been mounted on a needle or are threaded through a needle for insertion. Once inserted, the needle is withdrawn, and the flexible catheter remains in the vein. The over-the-needle catheter is easy to insert and stable. Single- or double-winged infusion needles (butterflies) are short-beveled, thin-walled needles with plastic flaps. They are used in pediatric settings and when short-term therapy is expected. Butterfly or scalp vein needles are not flexible, thus are more likely to infiltrate. Other equipment necessary to start an IV infusion is listed in Skill 40-1.

Many devices are available that minimize the potential for injury and promote safety when connecting, accessing, or disposing of IV equipment, including needleless systems and needle-housing systems in which the needle is recessed and protected. Refer to Chapters 27 and 29 for additional information about protective measures and use of IV equipment related to medication administration.

VASCULAR ACCESS DEVICES

Many different options for vascular access devices (IV catheters) are available for delivery of solutions and medications into a vein. The length of time the infusion therapy is needed, the type of medication or product that will be delivered intravenously, and the patient's health status as well as individualized needs determine which option is used. In addition, decisions on insertion site and catheter type should be guided by what will pose the least risk for IV complications (Arbique & Arbique, 2007). The nursing care that is required will depend on the type of device or IV catheter that is utilized. Vascular access devices fall into three main categories: peripheral venous catheters, midline catheters, and central venous access devices (CVADs).

Peripheral Venous Catheters

Over-the-needle catheters, which were previously discussed, are the most common type of peripheral vascular catheter used. When infusion therapy will be brief, a short (<3 inches) peripheral catheter is placed in a peripheral vein. This device is not appropriate for certain therapies—vesicant chemotherapy, drugs that are classified as irritants, or TPN, for example. The insertion site should be rotated at least every 72 to 96 hours for an adult. For a child, the site can remain in place until the IV intervention is completed unless a complication develops (Centers for Disease Control and Prevention [CDC], 2002). The smallest-gauge device is usually selected to minimize trauma to the vein (see Chapter 29 for more discussion on gauges).

Midline Peripheral Catheters

Midline catheters are inserted peripherally, normally just above or below the antecubital fossa into the proximal basilica or cephalic veins. These catheters are longer (>3 inches)

than peripheral venous catheters, and the distal tip dwells in the basilic, cephalic, or brachial vein, at or below the axillary level and distal to the shoulder (Infusion Nurses Society [INS], 2006). These are not considered to be central lines and should not be used to infuse vesicants, hyperosmolar, or irritating solutions. Recommendations for dwell time at a particular insertion site vary from 2 to 6 weeks (Griffiths, 2007; INS, 2006). Follow facility policy for rotation of midline catheter insertion site.

Central Venous Access Devices

Central venous access devices are an integral component of patient care in acute, ambulatory, and subacute care settings, as well as in the home and long-term care facilities. They provide access for a variety of IV fluids, medications, blood products, and TPN solutions and allow a means for hemodynamic monitoring and blood sampling. CVAD are devices where the tip of the catheter terminates in the central venous circulation, usually in the superior vena cava just above the right atrium. All CVADs require radiographic confirmation of position. The patient's diagnosis, the type of care that is required, and other factors (e.g., limited venous access, irritating drugs, patient request, or the need for long-term intermittent infusions) determine the type of CVAD used. Midline catheters, PICC lines, and other central venous devices are not routinely changed in order to reduce the risk of infection. Changing these catheters may pose a greater risk than leaving the catheter in place. However, any central venous catheter may be replaced if suspicion of a catheter-related bloodstream infection exists.

Types of CVADs. Types of CVADs include the following:

- Peripherally inserted central catheters (PICCs)
- Nontunneled percutaneous central venous catheters
- Tunneled central venous catheters
- Implanted ports

PICCs are a type of CVAD, >20 cm depending on patient size, that can be introduced into a peripheral vein (usually the basilic, brachial, or cephalic veins) and advanced so the distal tip dwells in the lower one third of the superior vena cava to the junction of the superior vena cava and the right atrium (INS, 2006) (Fig. 40-9). A specially trained registered nurse or physician can insert this type of catheter. PICC may be inserted in interventional radiology units or, in some institutions, at the bedside. Radiographic verification is always required before use. PICCs may have single or multiple lumens. They are used extensively in the home for IV therapy and have become an increasingly popular venous access device in acute care settings, especially for patients requiring long-term IV therapy (6 weeks to 6 months). PICCs are replaced only as needed, that is, the catheter is no longer patent or the site looks infected.

Indications for use of PICCs include administration of IV antibiotics for an extended period (2–6 weeks), infusion of parenteral nutrition, chemotherapy, continuous narcotic infusions, vesicants, hyperosmolar solutions, blood components, other specific medications (e.g., vasopressors, anticoagulants), and long-term rehydration. Advantages of using a

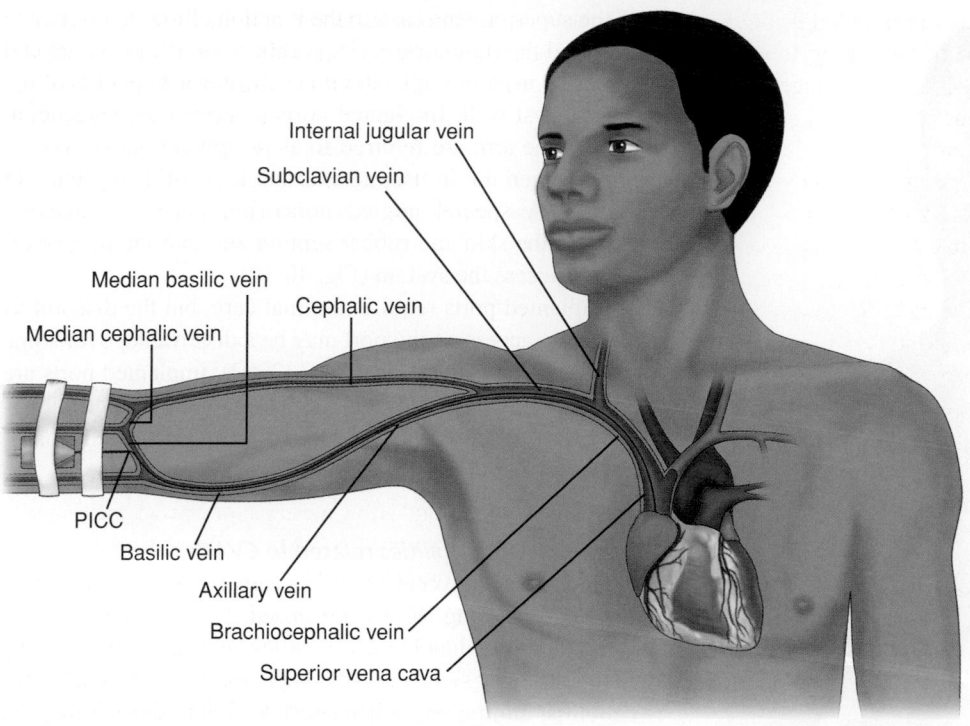

Internal jugular vein

Subclavian vein

Median basilic vein

Cephalic vein

Median cephalic vein

PICC

Basilic vein

Axillary vein

Brachiocephalic vein

Superior vena cava

FIGURE 40-9. Placement of peripherally inserted central catheter (PICC).

PICC include less risk of complications, such as infection and pneumothorax, because the catheter is inserted peripherally (Hammond, 2004). PICCs are also cost effective and provide adequate hemodilution for medications. Guidelines for Nursing Care 40-2 provides information related to nursing care for a patient with a PICC.

Nontunneled percutaneous central venous catheters (Fig. 40-10) have a shorter dwell time (3–10 days). These catheters can have double, triple, or quadruple lumens and are >8 cm, depending on patient size. They are introduced through the skin into the internal jugular, subclavian, or femoral veins and sutured into place. The catheter tip rests in the lower one third

Guidelines for Nursing Care • 40-2

MEASURING FLUID INTAKE AND OUTPUT

Maintenance

Always check agency policy for specific guidelines.

- Use sterile technique when changing dressings (24 hours after insertion and 3 to 7 days thereafter). Also, change dressing if soiled or loose.

- When accessing lumens or injection caps for flushing, drawing blood, or changing the dressing, know that many agencies require nurse and patient to wear a mask.

- Keep external portion of catheter coiled under dressing.

- Change catheter caps every 3 to 7 days based on frequency of access and agency policy. Many agencies have a policy to replace caps once they have been removed (e.g., when blood is drawn).

- Flush using normal saline and heparin (100 u/mL) solution according to agency policy.

- Avoid blood pressure measurement in the involved arm.

- Document:
  Appearance of site
  Length of external part of catheter
  Dates of dressing and cap change
  Flushing frequency and routine
  Any problems

Patient Instruction

- Demonstrate procedures, care, and maintenance of PICC catheter as well as potential complications.

- Provide simple, written instructions for patient/caregiver at home. Instruct concerning reasons to notify nurse or primary care provider.

- Emphasize that there are minimal activity restrictions.

- Instruct to protect insertion site when showering or bathing.

- Advise to wear a Medic-Alert tag if use is long term.

- Avoid strenuous physical activity that may cause displacement of the catheter.

Adapted from: *Best Practices: Evidence-based nursing procedures.* (2007). (2nd ed.). Philadelphia: Wolters Kluwer Health/Lippincott Williams & Wilkins.; and Infusion Nurses Society (INS). (2006). Infusion nursing standards of practice. *Journal of Infusion Nursing, 29*(1S), S1–S92.

FIGURE 40-10. Placement of triple-lumen nontunneled percutaneous central venous catheter.

of the superior vena cava to the junction of the superior vena cava and the right atrium (INS, 2006) in the superior vena cava. Catheters inserted via the femoral vein should have the distal tip dwell in the thoracic inferior vena cava above the level of the diaphragm (INS, 2006). They are mainly used in critical care and emergency settings (Gabriel, 2008a). This type of central venous catheter is associated with a high risk for complications, particularly infection, accounting for most catheter-related bloodstream infections (CDC, 2002). Pneumothorax is another potential complication when the catheter is placed in the subclavian vein.

A *tunneled central venous catheter*, intended for long-term use, is implanted into the internal or external jugular or subclavian vein. The length of this catheter is >8 cm (approximately 90 cm, on average), depending on patient size, and is tunneled in subcutaneous tissue under the skin (usually the midchest area) for 3 to 6 inches to its exit site (Fig. 40-11). The distal tip dwells in the lower one-third of the superior vena cava to the junction of the superior vena cava and the right atrium (INS, 2006). This device is initially sutured into place, but after 7 to 14 days, the sutures are removed. Subcutaneous tissue attaches to a Dacron polyester cuff around the catheter, helping to stabilize the catheter and minimize the risk for infection. Once the exit site is healed, a site dressing is not required. This type of catheter is associated with a lower incidence of infection than is the nontunneled central venous catheter (CDC, 2002).

Another type of long-term CVAD is an *implanted port,* which consists of a subcutaneous injection port attached to a catheter. The distal catheter tip dwells in the lower one third

of the superior vena cava to the junction of the superior vena cava and the right atrium (INS, 2006), and the proximal end or port is usually implanted in a subcutaneous pocket of the upper chest wall. Implanted ports placed in the antecubital area of the arm are referred to as *peripheral access system ports.* When not in use, no external parts of the system are visible. A special angled noncoring needle is inserted through the skin and rubber septum and into the port reservoir to access the system (Fig. 40-12).

Implanted ports require minimal care, but the discomfort related to accessing the port may be a disadvantage for some patients. According to the CDC (2002), implanted ports are associated with the lowest risk for catheter-related bloodstream infections, and patients report improved self-image. Surgery is required for catheter removal.

Nursing Responsibilities related to CVADs. Nursing responsibilities related to central venous catheters include maintaining and changing the sterile dressing, maintaining sterile technique according to facility policy, and carefully assessing for any signs or symptoms of complications, such as phlebitis, cellulitis, infiltration, catheter-related venous thrombosis, and infection or sepsis. Refer to the discussion later in the chapter for more information related to infusion site care. Other nursing interventions include changing the injection caps on the lumens and flushing with a prescribed solution (usually saline and heparin) to prevent clotting and blockage of the lumen, based on facility policy. While caring for patients with CVADs, use the opportunity for health teaching about medical and surgical asepsis and meticulous skin care.

COMPLICATIONS OF IV THERAPY

The patient can be an important source of information regarding the possibility of complications associated with IV therapy. If the patient is uncomfortable, check that the infusion is entering the vein as intended, the flow rate is not too

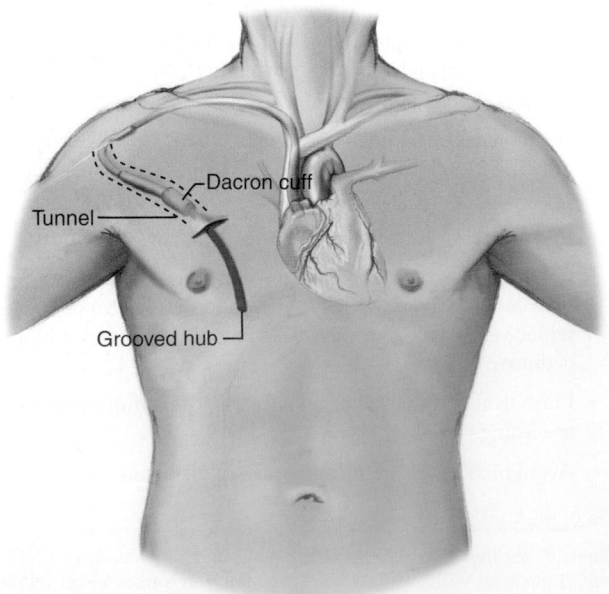

FIGURE 40-11. Placement of tunneled central venous catheter.

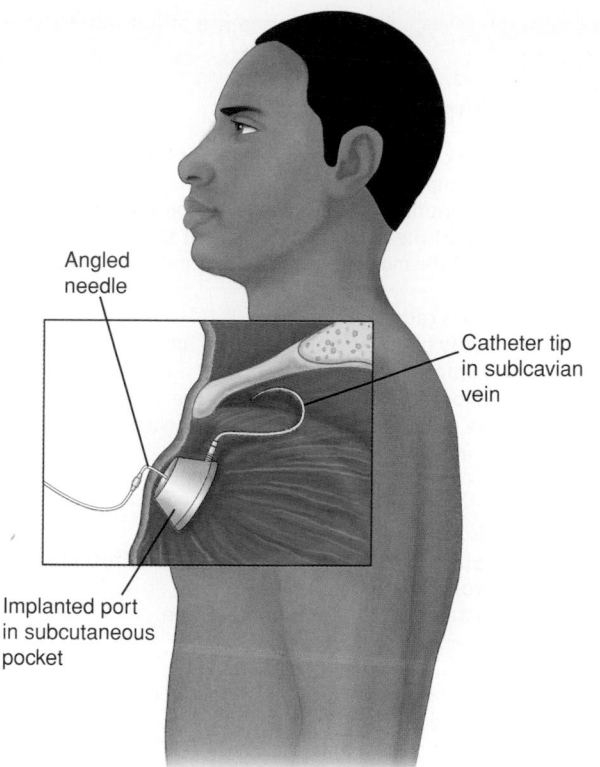

Angled
needle

Catheter tip
in sublcavian
vein

Implanted port
in subcutaneous
pocket

FIGURE 40-12. Placement of an implanted port with the tip in the subclavian vein. Angled needle is inserted through skin and septum into port.

rapid, the patient's position is satisfactory, and the circulatory status of the patient is intact. Anxiety about receiving an infusion can also cause discomfort for the patient.

Local complications, such as infiltration, phlebitis, and thrombophlebitis, occur more frequently than do systemic complications. However, systemic complications (e.g., fluid overload, embolus, sepsis) are more serious and may be life threatening. Catheters are now available that are impregnated with antiseptics and coated with antibiotics, and their use is recommended for patients at high risk for acquiring a catheter-related infection. Consult institutional policy for guidance concerning catheter site care as well as the manufacturer's recommendations and precautions. Table 40-12 defines complications of IV infusions, noting common causes, signs and symptoms, and pertinent nursing considerations. The scales presented in Box 40-1 and Box 40-2 can be used to grade and document infiltration and phlebitis if they occur.

PERIPHERAL VENOUS CATHETER SITE SELECTION

The nurse initiating a peripheral venous access needs to assess for the safest, most appropriate location for each particular patient. The suitability of particular veins for peripheral IV infusions varies with individual circumstances. Selection should be determined after considering the following factors.

Accessibility of a Vein

Keep in mind the following guidelines related to peripheral venous catheters and access sites:

- Determine the most desirable accessible vein. The cephalic vein, accessory cephalic vein, metacarpal, and

---

Box 40-1 INFILTRATION SCALE

Grade and document infiltration according to the most severe presenting indicator.

Grade	Clinical Criteria
0	No symptoms
1	Skin blanched Edema <1 inch in any direction Cool to touch With or without pain
2	Skin blanched Edema 1–6 inches in any direction Cool to touch With or without pain
3	Skin blanched, translucent Gross edema >6 inches in any direction Cool to touch Mild–moderate pain Possible numbness
4	Skin blanched, translucent Skin tight, leaking Skin discolored, bruised, swollen Gross edema >6 inches in any direction Deep pitting tissue edema Circulatory impairment Moderate–severe pain Infiltration of any amount of blood product, irritant or vesicant

(Infusion Nurses Society [INS]. [2006]. Infusion nursing standards of practice. *Journal of Infusion Nursing, 29*(1S), S60).

basilic vein are appropriate sites for infusion (INS, 2006). The superficial veins on the dorsal aspect of the hand can also be used successfully for some people, but can be more painful (I.V. Rounds, 2008). Venipuncture should be initiated at least 2 inches (5 cm) above the crease of the wrist in an adult patient (Masoorli, 2007). Initiate venous access in the distal areas of the upper extremities, as this

---

Box 40-2 PHLEBITIS SCALE

Grade and document phlebitis according to the most severe presenting indicator.

Grade	Clinical Criteria
0	No symptoms
1	Erythema at access site with or without pain
2	Pain at access site with erythema and/or edema
3	Pain at access site with erythema and/or edema Streak formation Palpable venous cord
4	Pain at access site with erythema and/or edema Streak formation Palpable venous cord >1 inch in length Purulent drainage

(Infusion Nurses Society [INS]. [2006]. Infusion nursing standards of practice. *Journal of Infusion Nursing, 29*(1S), p. S59).

TABLE • 40-12   COMPLICATIONS ASSOCIATED WITH INTRAVENOUS INFUSIONS

Complication/Cause	Signs and Symptoms	Nursing Considerations
Infiltration: the escape of fluid into the subcutaneous tissue Dislodged needle Penetrated vessel wall	Swelling, pallor, coldness, or pain around the infusion site; significant decrease in the flow rate	Check the infusion site every hour for signs/symptoms. Discontinue the infusion if symptoms occur. Restart the infusion at a different site. Limit the movement of the extremity with the IV.
Sepsis: microorganisms invade the bloodstream through the catheter insertion site Poor insertion technique Multilumen catheters Long-term catheter insertion Frequent dressing changes	Red and tender insertion site Fever, malaise, other vital sign changes	Assess catheter site daily. Notify physician immediately if any signs of infection. Follow agency protocol for culture of drainage. Use scrupulous aseptic technique when starting an infusion.
Phlebitis: an inflammation of a vein Mechanical trauma from needle or catheter Chemical trauma from solution	Local, acute tenderness; redness, warmth, and slight edema of the vein above the insertion site	Discontinue the infusion immediately. Apply warm, moist compresses to the affected site. Avoid further use of the vein. Restart the infusion in another vein.
Thrombus: a blood clot Tissue trauma from needle or catheter	Symptoms similar to phlebitis IV fluid flow may cease if clot obstructs needle	Stop the infusion immediately. Apply warm compresses as ordered by the primary care provider. Restart the IV at another site. *Do not rub or massage the affected area.*
Speed shock: the body's reaction to a substance that is injected into the circulatory system too rapidly Too rapid a rate of fluid infusion into circulation	Pounding headache, fainting, rapid pulse rate, apprehension, chills, back pains, and dyspnea	If symptoms develop, discontinue the infusion immediately. Report symptoms of speed shock to the primary care provider immediately. Monitor vital signs if symptoms develop. Use the proper IV tubing. Carefully monitor the rate of fluid flow. Check the rate frequently for accuracy. A time tape is useful for this purpose.
Fluid overload: the condition caused when too large a volume of fluid infuses into the circulatory system Too large a volume of fluid infused into circulation	Engorged neck veins, increased blood pressure, and difficulty in breathing (dyspnea)	If symptoms develop, slow the rate of infusion. Notify the primary care provider immediately. Monitor vital signs. Carefully monitor the rate of fluid flow. Check the rate frequently for accuracy.
Air embolus: air in the circulatory system Break in the IV system above the heart level allowing air in the circulatory system as a bolus	Respiratory distress Increased heart rate Cyanosis Decreased blood pressure Change in level of consciousness	Pinch off catheter or secure system to prevent entry of air. Place patient on left side in Trendelenburg position. Call for immediate assistance. Monitor vital signs and pulse oximetry.

allows for future sites proximal to the previous insertion site (INS, 2006). Figure 40-13A illustrates common infusion sites on the arm and hand. Either arm may be used for IV therapy. If the patient is right handed and both arms appear equally usable, usually the left arm is selected to free the right arm for the patient's use.

- Determine accessibility based on the patient's condition. For example, a person with severe burns on both forearms does not have vessels available in these areas.
- Do not use veins in surgical areas. For example, infusions in the arm should not be given on the same side as recent extensive breast surgery because of vascular disturbances in the area, and a patient with a history of axillary node dissection should not have venipuncture in the affected arm. Also, avoid an arm that has a device inserted for dialysis (e.g., fistula or shunt).
- Do not use the antecubital veins if another vein is available. They are not a good choice for infusion because flexion of the patient's arm can displace the IV catheter over time. In addition, by avoiding the antecubital veins for peripheral venous catheters, a PICC line may be inserted at a later time, if needed.

FIGURE 40-13. Peripheral venous access sites. (**A**) Infusion sites on the ventral and dorsal aspects of the lower arm and hand. (**B**) Infusion sites on the scalp of an infant.

• Do not use veins in the leg, unless other sites are inaccessible, because of the danger of stagnation of peripheral circulation and possible serious complications. The cannulation of the lower extremities is associated with risk of embolism and thrombophlebitis (INS, 2006). Some insti-

tutions require a physician's order to insert an IV catheter in an adult patient's lower extremity.

• Additional potential sites for neonates and children include veins of the head, neck, and lower extremities (INS, 2006). Scalp arteries in infants are visible (see Fig. 40-13B). Carefully palpate the site before insertion. If the site is pulsating, do not use.

➤ *Think back to Grace Gilligan, the woman with nausea and vomiting. The nurse would incorporate knowledge of appropriate site selection for adults when determining the location for Grace's venous access.* ∎

Condition of the Vein

The condition of the patient's vein is extremely important. Experience is necessary to acquire skill in palpating a patient's vein to determine its condition. Thin-walled and scarred veins, especially in some older patients, make continued infusion a problem. Attempt only two venipuncture attempts when initiating venous access for a patient. If unsuccessful after two attempts, a colleague with advanced skills, such as a member of the nurse IV team, should attempt to initiate the venous access (Arbique & Arbique, 2007).

➤ *Remember Grace Gilligan, the patient who experienced several unsuccessful IV catheter insertion attempts (Reflective Practice)? The nurse's ability to palpate the patient's veins before attempting venipuncture might have been helpful in determining the best vein to be used. The information provided by palpation also could have indicated that the patient's veins were scarred, thus suggesting the need for a more experienced team member, such as someone from anesthesiology or an IV nurse specialist (as the patient had requested), to perform the procedure.* ∎

Type of Fluid to Be Infused

Keep in mind the following about the type of IV fluid to be infused:

• Select a vein appropriate for the solution. Hypertonic solutions, those containing irritating medications, those administered at a rapid rate, and those with a high viscosity should be given in a large vein to minimize vessel trauma and to facilitate the rate of flow.

• Advise the patient that some medications administered intravenously in a peripheral vein (e.g., potassium chloride and certain antibiotics) may cause irritation and pain; urge the patient to report any discomfort.

Anticipated Duration of Infusion

Consider the anticipated duration of the infusion. Always select a site where restriction in movement is kept to a minimum if this is a consideration. In addition, as stated previously, change peripheral venous catheter sites every 72 to 96 hours, in accordance with facility policy, starting with sites as distal as possible and moving in a proximal direction on the alternate arm.

INITIATION OF AN IV INFUSION

Before the infusion is started, perform a final check of the solution to ensure that it is clear and contains no particles or precipitates. This check is especially important when substances have been added to the solution because some additives create precipitates. Commercially available in-line filters help reduce the risk for contamination by filtering the solution immediately before it enters the patient's vein. Skill 40-1 outlines the procedure for initiating an IV infusion.

Some adults and young children have a fear of needles. In these situations, it may be advisable to use a product that eases the discomfort of venipuncture. Local anesthetic agents include intradermal lidocaine, iontophoresis, low-frequency ultrasonification, pressure-accelerated lidocaine, and topical transdermal agents. The nurse needs to have knowledge of the anesthetic agent used and correct method of administration, based on manufacturer's recommendations and facility policy. The use of a local anesthetic requires monitoring for potential allergic reactions, tissue damage, or inadvertent injection of the drug into the vascular system (INS, 2006). The accompanying Research in Nursing box discusses one type of local anesthetic.

INFUSION REGULATION AND MONITORING

The nurse is responsible for maintaining the proper flow rate while ensuring the comfort and safety of the patient. The primary health care provider prescribes the amount of solu-

tion to be infused within a specified period. The rate is then determined on the basis of the amount of solution to be infused over 1 hour. Maintenance of the flow rate is important because it can directly affect the patient's fluid balance. Too slow a flow may result in a fluid volume deficit because fluid intake is not balancing fluid lost or it may delay the restoration of the balance. Infusing IV fluid too rapidly can overtax the body's capacities to adjust to the increase in the water volume or the electrolytes it contains and may lead to fluid volume excess. Allowing an infusion to get behind schedule and then increasing the rate to catch up might seriously jeopardize the patient's compensatory mechanisms and lead to serious complications.

The use of electronic infusion-control devices (e.g. IV pumps) has become a common, if not required, practice in acute care settings. These devices can be programmed to infuse a certain amount of fluid over a given time, usually milliliters per hour. When using an electronic device, it is not necessary to calculate the drops per minute, as is necessary with a gravity or free-flowing IV. The pump automatically regulates the flow rate at preset limits. An alarm sounds when air is in the tubing, the flow is obstructed, the solution level of the bottle or bag is getting low, or there is increased pressure in the system, such as occurs when an IV infiltrates and fluid flows into the tissues. "Smart pumps," computerized pumps, are beginning to be used in many facilities for IV infusions. Smart pumps also require programming of infusion rates by the nurse, but, in addition, are able to identify dosing limits and practice guidelines to aid in safe administration. They are

---

RESEARCH IN NURSING
Bridging the Gap to Evidence-Based Practice

EPIDERMAL ANESTHETIC FOR VENIPUNCTURE

Needle insertion for venipuncture or intravenous cannulation is painful, frightening, and distressful for children. Topical anesthetics have been used to provide effective local anesthesia for venipuncture. These products require 30 to 90 minutes after application to reach maximum effectiveness. This limits usefulness in acute care situations. Iontophoresis (application of electric current to carry ionized lidocaine through the skin) has also been shown to be an effective analgesic for children undergoing these procedures. It also requires a waiting period, up to 15 minutes, for onset of effect. New systems are being investigated to decrease the wait for onset of effect and provide effective pain relief for venipuncture.

Related Research

Zempsky, W., Bean-Lijewski, J., Kauffman, R., Koh, J., Malviya, S., Rose, J., et al (2008). Needle-free powder lidocaine delivery system provides rapid effective analgesia for venipuncture or cannulation pain in children: randomized, double-blind comparison of venipuncture and venous cannulation pain after fast-onset needle-free powder lidocaine or placebo treatment trial. *Pediatrics, 121*(5), 979–987.

This study's objective was to determine if needle-free powder lidocaine delivery system (a sterile, prefilled, disposable system

that delivers lidocaine powder into the epidermis) produces effective local analgesia within 1 to 3 minutes for venipuncture and peripheral venous cannulation procedures in children. Pediatric patients (3–18 years of age) were randomly assigned to treatment with the needle-free powder lidocaine delivery system (0.5 mg of lidocaine) or a sham placebo system at the antecubital fossa or the back of the hand 1 to 3 minutes before venipuncture or cannulation. All patients rated the administration comfort of the needle-free systems and the pain of the subsequent venous access procedures with the Wong-Baker Faces Pain Rating Scale (from 0 to 5). Patients 8 to 18 years of age also provided self-reports with a visual analog scale, and parents provided observational visual analog scale scores for their child's venous access pain. The authors concluded that the needle-free powder lidocaine delivery system was well tolerated and produced significant analgesia within 1 to 3 minutes.

Relevance for Nursing Practice

Nurses are often responsible for obtaining blood samples from and initiating intravenous access for their patients, including children. Using the most efficient techniques can result in decreased pain and anxiety for both the children and their parents.

For additional research, visit thePoint.

Guidelines for Nursing Care • 40-3

REGULATING IV FLOW RATE

Follow agency's guidelines to determine if infusion should be administered by electronic pump or by gravity.

- Check physician's order for IV solution.
- Check patency of IV line and needle.
- Verify drop factor (number of drops in 1 mL) of the equipment in use.
- Calculate the flow rate:

  EXAMPLE—Administer 1,000 mL D_5W over 10 hours (set delivers 60 gtt/1 mL).

a. Standard formula

$$\text{gtt/min} = \frac{\text{volume (mL)} \times \text{drop factor (gtt/mL)}}{\text{time (in minutes)}}$$

$$\text{gtt/min} = \frac{1,000 \text{ mL} \times 60}{600 \text{ (60 min} \times 10 \text{ h)}}$$

$$= \frac{60,000}{600}$$

$$= 100 \text{ gtt/min}$$

b. Short formula using milliliters per hour

$$\text{gtt/min} = \frac{\text{milliliters per hour} \times \text{drop factor (gtt/mL)}}{\text{time (60 min)}}$$

Find milliliters per hour by dividing 1,000 mL by 10 hours:

$$\frac{1,000}{10} = 100 \text{ mL/hr}$$

$$\text{gtt/min} = \frac{100 \text{ mL} \times 60}{60 \text{ min}}$$

$$= \frac{6,000}{60}$$

$$= 100 \text{ gtt/min}$$

recommended as best practice to avoid unsafe drug therapy (Institute for Safe Medication Practices [ISMP], 2007). Check the infusion every hour or more frequently, if indicated, to determine if the solution is being infused at the proper hourly rate. Skill 40-3 illustrates the use of an infusion pump.

Administration may be achieved by gravity infusion, which requires the nurse to calculate the infusion rate in drops per minute. If using a gravity or free-flowing IV, calculate the drip rate required to achieve the desired infusion rate. A method for determining flow rate is described in the accompanying Guidelines for Nursing Care 40-3. This method requires the nurse to know the amount of solution to be delivered, the total infusion time (in minutes), and the drop factor for the infusion tubing in use. The drop factor, or drops per milliliter of solution, is determined by the size of the opening in the infusion apparatus. It varies among different products from different companies. Most health agencies use the products of a single company. The most common drop factors are macrodrop systems (10, 15, 20 drops per milliliter), a microdrip (60 drops per milliliter), and a blood administration set (10 drops per milliliter). Microdrip or 60 drops per milliliter is used most often when small fluid volumes are administered, such as a rate less than 75 mL per hour. Macrodrop tubing is commonly used for rates greater than 75 mL per hour.

A less commonly used device, a Buretrol, or volume-control device (Fig. 40-14), may be used to reduce the risk for fluid overload or medication overdose. They may also be used to deliver intermittent medications that need to be further diluted and given over a specific time.

A time tape (Fig. 40-15) should be placed on the container of solution to provide a quick reference for the nurse to monitor the rate at which the solution is entering the patient. The tape gives an hourly indication of where the fluid level should be at a given time.

➤ *Consider Jack Soo Park, the patient who received too much IV fluid. When planning Mr. Park's care, the nurse would need to include frequent assessments of the IV infusion to ensure that it is infusing at the proper flow rate. Placing the infusion on an infusion pump would have significantly reduced the potential for an infusion error.* ∎

FIGURE 40-14. Volume-control set.

ABBOTT 1000 mL
UNITED'S Drop Meter

STARTING TIME: _____

Align arrow
with -0- on
Abbott
bottle

____ gtts/min.
____ ml/hr.

| 6 hrs | 8 hrs | 10 hrs | 12 hrs |

50
100
150
200
250
300
350
400
450
500
550
600
650
700
750
800
850
900

DISCONTINUED
TIME   950

NURSE   DATE   RM. NO.   BOTL. NO.

MEDICATION ADDED   SOLUTION   PATIENT

**FOR USE ON
ABBOTT 1000 mL**

UAL DM321

FIGURE 40-15. Sample time tape for IV solution container.

SOLUTION AND TUBING CHANGES

If more than one container of solution is ordered for the patient, attach additional containers using the method determined by the facility. One method for changing the solution and tubing is presented in Skill 40-2.

The frequency of administration set tubing changes varies. Most IV crystalloid fluids of patients with a peripheral or central catheter require tubing to be changed every 72 hours and immediately upon suspected contamination or when the integrity of the product or system has been compromised (INS, 2006). (See the accompanying PICO in Practice box.) However, other fluids, such as TPN solutions, particularly lipid-containing TPN, require tubing changes every 24 hours. It is important to be familiar with the particular policies and procedures of a given facility.

VENOUS ACCESS SITE CARE

Scrupulous care of the infusion site is necessary to help control contamination and to help prevent the introduction of

microorganisms into the bloodstream. Catheter contamination can occur from the following sources:

- Hands of the caregiver
- Skin bacteria that contaminate the catheter during insertion
- Disconnection of the tubing or injection cap from the catheter hub, allowing bacteria to enter the closed system or multiple-lumen catheters

? PICO IN PRACTICE
Asking Clinical Questions

Scenario: You are a staff nurse who works on a surgical step-down unit. Patients who are transferred to your unit from the surgical intensive care unit have intravenous (IV) lines in place. It has long been policy on this unit to routinely change IV tubing every 48 hours. Your hospital has instituted a program that encourages staff to make suggestions that could reduce unnecessary costs. You know that costs would be reduced if IV tubing was changed less frequently. However, you wonder if by doing so, your patients could experience more IV setup-related adverse events such as phlebitis and infections.

- POPULATION: Hospital patients who have had recent surgery
- INTERVENTION: Routine IV tubing change every 48 hours
- COMPARISON: Routine IV tubing change longer than every 48 hours
- OUTCOME: IV setup-related adverse events (e.g., phlebitis and infections)

PICO Question: Among patients who have had recent surgery are routine every 48 hour IV tubing changes associated with lower rates of IV setup-related adverse events, such as phlebitis and infections, than less frequent routine IV tubing changes?

Finding: Joanna Briggs Institute (2008). Management of peripheral intravascular devices. *Best Practice, 12*(5).

Routine replacement of IV tubing no more frequently than every 72 hours is cost-effective and is not associated with a higher rate of adverse events. This recommendation was based upon results from three well-designed and controlled studies.

Strength of Evidence: Level III

Recommendation: You write a proposal that you send to your Nurse Manager and the Nursing Department Policy and Procedure Committee to change the interval for changing IV tubing from 48 hours to 72 hours.

- Poor insertion technique
- Contamination of the catheter hub; inadequate decontamination of hub prior to use
- An IV solution that becomes contaminated when solutions are changed, a medication is added, or the solution is allowed to infuse for too long a period

> *Think back to Grace Gilligan, the woman described in the Reflective Practice display. The numerous attempts at venipuncture increase the patient's risk for possible infection.* ■

Regular dressing changes and tubing replacements are important means of preventing infection. Use of a 2% chlorhexidine-based solution is recommended for skin antisepsis for central venous catheter site care (CDC, 2002; Mimoz et al., 2007). For peripheral catheter site care, chlorhexidine is preferred. However, iodine, povidone-iodine, and 70% alcohol are considered acceptable alternatives (INS, 2006). Transparent semipermeable membrane (TSM) dressings are used most commonly to protect the insertion site. TSM dressings (e.g., Tegaderm or OpSite IV) allow easy inspection of the IV site, permit evaporation of moisture that accumulates under the dressing, and help to secure the catheter. Facility policy generally determines the type of dressing and the intervals for dressing change. The Infusion Nurses Society (INS) recommends TSM IV dressing change at least every 7 days (INS, 2006). Change any dressing that is damp, loosened, or soiled immediately.

Additional manufactured IV securement/stabilization systems are commercially available. These systems are recommended for use on all venous access sites, and particularly central venous access sites, to preserve the integrity of the access device and to prevent catheter migration and loss of access (INS, 2006, p. S44). The use of a stabilization device can also decrease the risk of infiltration, phlebitis, skin damage, occlusion, leaking, and unscheduled restart rates (Smith & Hannum, 2008). These devices include plastic shields and adhesive anchors. Hard plastic shields (Fig. 40-16) that are ventilated and secured with tape are often used in pediatric settings. In addition, they are helpful in minimizing venous access complications with geriatric patients (Smith & Hannum, 2008). Adhesive anchors eliminate the need for tape but are more costly and involve the use of strong adhesives that might make it difficult to change the dressing without dislodging the catheter. Skills 40-3 and 40-4 explain how to monitor an IV site and how to change an IV dressing.

CAPPING A PRIMARY LINE FOR INTERMITTENT USE

When a continuous IV is no longer necessary, the primary IV line can be capped and converted to an intermittent infusion device, commonly referred to as a medication or saline lock, which provides venous access for intermittent or emergency medications. Periodic injection with saline according to facility policy is required to keep the catheter patent. Skill 40-5 describes this technique.

FIGURE 40-16. IV shield in place on hand.

DISCONTINUATION OF THE INFUSION

When the peripheral venous access is no longer required, or when the insertion site shows signs of local complications, the nurse assumes responsibility for discontinuing the access device. After performing hand hygiene, clamp the IV tubing and remove the adhesive strips and sterile dressing. Wear clean gloves because the catheter is withdrawn in line with the vein; do not bend the plastic catheter, which can cause it to break. Apply pressure immediately to the area just above the insertion site until hemostasis is achieved. Apply pressure using a dry sterile gauze pad rather than using an alcohol preparation; alcohol tends to burn and does not stop blood flow from the puncture wound. Apply an occlusive dressing to the site. Document the date and time of removal, the name of the person removing the device, and the assessment of the site.

Nurses or specialized IV team nurses may be responsible for removing a PICC line. Specific protocols must be followed to prevent breakage or fracture of the catheter. Guidelines for removal of a PICC are as follows:

- Wear clean gloves.
- Place the patient in supine position, with the arm straight and the catheter insertion site below heart level (to prevent the risk for an air embolus).
- Remove the dressing carefully while stabilizing the hub of the catheter with one hand.
- Remove the catheter slowly. Grasp the catheter close to the insertion site and slowly ease the catheter out, keeping it parallel to the skin. Continue removing in small increments, using a smooth and gentle motion (*Best Practices,* 2007).
- Apply pressure to the site with a sterile dressing until hemostasis is achieved, and then apply a small sterile dressing to the site.
- Measure the catheter and compare it with the length listed in the chart when it was inserted. This ensures that the entire catheter was removed.
- Document the procedure, catheter length, site assessment, and how the patient tolerated the procedure.

HOME INFUSION

Many patients return to their home from a healthcare facility with IV infusions. Portable infusion pumps and the availability of home care nurses have made this an acceptable alternative. After a patient has been identified as a candidate for home infusion therapy, begin assessment and education to ensure a successful outcome. Candidates for infusion pump IV therapy in the home should meet certain criteria. They should be medically stable, have a full- or part-time caregiver, have access to a telephone, and have a refrigerator available for storage of pre-filled medication cartridges. Patients can receive insulin infusions, pain medication, antibiotic therapy, chemotherapy, or TPN through portable infusion pumps at home.

PICCs are the most common type of catheter used for home care patients. Home care nurses play a crucial role in educating patients concerning successful management of IV catheters and observing for potential complications. The patient and any caregivers must be able to perform necessary skills independently before discharge from the healthcare facility. See Teaching Tips 40-1.

Using Blood and Blood Products

A blood transfusion is the infusion of whole blood or a blood component such as plasma, red blood cells, or platelets into the patient's venous circulation. A blood transfusion is given because of red blood cell loss, such as with a major injury or when the body is not adequately producing cells, such as platelets. Whole blood is used infrequently because the various components can be separated easily and used for replacement therapy. In addition, using whole blood for transfusion can lead to fluid volume overload. The person receiving the blood is the recipient. The person giving the blood is the donor. Steps in administering blood transfusions are described in Skill 40-6.

TYPING AND CROSS-MATCHING

Before a blood product can be given to a patient, it must be determined that the blood of the donor is compatible with that of the patient. If incompatible, clumping and hemolysis of the recipient's blood cells result and death can occur. The laboratory examination to determine a person's blood type is called **typing.** The process of determining compatibility between blood specimens is **cross-matching.**

Blood Types

The four main blood types or groups in the ABO system of blood typing are A, B, AB, and O. Some groups are further broken down into subgroups.

Blood type, an inherited trait, is determined by the type of antigens and antibodies present in the blood. An **antigen** is a substance that causes the formation of antibodies. An **antibody** is a protein substance developed in the body in response to the presence of an antigen that has entered the body. An **agglutinin** is an antibody that causes a clumping of specific antigens. People who have type A blood have an A antigen on their red blood cells, those with type B blood have B antigens on their cells, those in the AB group have both A and B antigens, and people with type O blood have neither A nor B antigens on their red blood cells. People in each blood group have the agglutinins to the red blood cell antigens that they lack. Group A people have the agglutinin for B; group AB people have no agglutinins for A and B, whereas group O people have both A and B agglutinins in their blood serum. If a person with

---

Tips   **TEACHING TIPS • 40-1**

IV THERAPY

Health Topic	Teaching Tip	Why Is This Important?
Sterile technique	• Proper handwashing technique • Dressing changes • Proper technique for infusing medications	The caregiver needs to understand the importance of sterile technique to prevent local systemic infections. If the caregiver is to administer medications, how to access the line in a sterile manner should be discussed by the nurse and then demonstrated by the caregiver.
General information	• Proper technique for using all equipment • Assessing for any indications of an infection or other complications • Obtaining supplies to continue home infusions • Physician orders pertaining to the central line at home • How and why to contact the physician or nurse if questions or problems arise	The caregiver needs to demonstrate how to use any pumps to administer medication. The caregiver should also demonstrate how to flush the central line. The caregiver should understand signs of infection to observe for, as well as any other type of complication associated with a central line. The caregiver needs to know where to obtain supplies and what supplies are needed for care at home. Before discharge, the nurse should ensure that the caregiver understands all physician orders. The caregiver needs to know that resources are available and when it is appropriate to use these resources.

type O blood is transfused with blood from a person with either group A or group B blood, there would be destruction of the recipient's red blood cells because his or her anti-A or anti-B agglutinins would react with the A or B antigens in the donor's red blood cells. This explains why individuals with type AB blood are often called universal recipients (because people in this blood group have no agglutinins for either A or B antigens), and group O people are often called universal donors (because they have neither A nor B antigens).

Rh Factor

The Rh factor is an inherited antigen in human blood. There are five antigens in the Rh system, but the one designated D is of first concern. A person whose blood contains a D antigen is called Rh positive; an Rh-negative person lacks this D antigen. An Rh-negative person must receive blood from another Rh-negative person. If Rh-positive blood is administered to an Rh-negative person, the recipient develops anti-Rh agglutinins. Subsequent transfusion with Rh-positive blood may cause serious reactions with clumping and hemolysis of red blood cells.

SELECTION OF BLOOD DONORS

Blood donors must be selected with care. Not only must the donor's blood be typed accurately, but it is also important to determine that the donor is free of disease. The blood will be tested for human immunodeficiency virus (HIV), hepatitis B and C virus (HBV and HBC), syphilis, West Nile virus, and other viruses that can be transmitted to the recipient.

The donor is examined carefully at the time of donation and receives specific information about eligibility and a confidential method to allow or disallow the distribution of the donated blood. Prospective donors are questioned about their lifestyle and health history, including questions about diseases, past surgeries, tattoos, body piercing, travel, sex, and drug use. Individuals may give blood only if their blood count, temperature, pulse, respiration, blood pressure, and weight are within normal ranges.

Some patients who know in advance that they will need blood can donate their own blood for transfusion (**autologous transfusion**), also called autotransfusion. Autotransfusion eliminates the danger of transmitting cross-infection from donor to recipient and decreases the risk for complications from mismatched blood but requires advance planning (the blood must be donated 5 weeks before the surgery). This practice is growing in popularity. A patient's own blood can also be salvaged during surgery or collected from tubes and drains to allow for autologous transfusions.

BLOOD COMPONENTS

Whole blood is rarely used unless blood loss has been massive. With current technology, whole blood can be easily separated into its components, and patients receive only the blood product they need. For example, a patient may need red blood cells but not the blood plasma and its constituents. Red blood cells in concentrated form, called packed red blood cells, may be used in the following situations:

- Patient with anemia (a reduction in red blood cells or hemoglobin)
- Patient with cardiovascular failure, with a need to increase blood volume and red blood cells while avoiding cardiovascular overload
- Patient with GI bleeding, with a need to maintain adequate hemoglobin levels without increasing blood pressure, which would likely lead to more bleeding

In other situations, only plasma is required, such as when plasma protein or the blood's clotting factor is low. Fresh-frozen plasma is particularly useful in emergencies for immediate restoration of fluid because serum transfusion presents no compatibility problems and time need not be lost seeking donors and matching blood. It is also an excellent blood-volume expander when time is of essence, for example, in a patient who is severely burned and losing plasma rapidly from burn areas. Components of plasma that are used therapeutically include human albumin (used for hypovolemic shock, albuminemia, liver failure), cryoprecipitates (used for bleeding due to hemophilia or disseminated intravascular coagulation), and gamma globulins, the antibody-containing part of plasma (used for gamma globulin deficiencies).

Platelet infusion is indicated for the treatment or prevention of bleeding associated with deficiencies in the number or function of a patient's platelets. The demand for platelets has risen noticeably during the past several decades, and specialized products and preparation methods have been developed to reduce the risk for complications and improve the patient's response to platelet therapy.

INITIATION OF TRANSFUSION

Bar codes on blood products are currently being implemented to identify, track, and assign data to transfusions as an additional safety measure. Blood for transfusion will need to display the usual information such as blood type and Rh factor. In addition, the facility that prepared the blood as well as a code to track the blood back to its donor is required. The procedure for starting a blood transfusion (see Skill 40-6) is basically the same as for an IV solution. If possible, select larger veins because a catheter no smaller than 20 gauge should be used. This size is necessary because of the viscosity of blood. Take and record vital signs just before starting the transfusion and during the beginning of the infusion. Institution policies vary on the frequency of vital signs. If the patient's temperature is 100°F (37.8°C) or higher, notify the primary care provider. Blood that has not been used within 30 minutes after its arrival from the blood bank must be returned, and blood that has been infusing for more than 4 hours must be discontinued to prevent the risk for bacterial contamination. Nurses are also responsible for monitoring the patient for adverse reactions to the blood transfusion. Table 40-13 describes potential transfusion reactions that can be serious.

Administering Total Parenteral Nutrition

Total parenteral nutrition (TPN) is a highly concentrated nutrient solution consisting of dextrose, amino acids, and

TABLE • 40-13 TRANSFUSION REACTIONS

Reaction	Signs and Symptoms	Nursing Activity
Allergic reaction: allergy to transfused blood	Hives, itching Anaphylaxis	• Stop transfusion immediately and keep vein open with normal saline. • Notify primary care provider immediately. • Administer antihistamine parenterally as necessary.
Febrile reaction: fever develops during infusion	Fever and chills Headache Malaise	• Stop transfusion immediately and keep vein open with normal saline. • Notify primary care provider. • Treat symptoms.
Hemolytic transfusion reaction: incompatibility of blood product	Immediate onset Facial flushing Fever, chills Headache Low back pain Shock	• Stop infusion immediately and keep vein open with normal saline. • Notify primary care provider immediately. • Obtain blood samples from site. • Obtain first voided urine. • Treat shock if present. • Send unit, tubing, and filter to lab. • Draw blood sample for serologic testing and send urine specimen to the lab.
Circulatory overload: too much blood administered	Dyspnea Dry cough Pulmonary edema	• Slow or stop infusion. • Monitor vital signs. • Notify primary care provider. • Place in upright position with feet dependent.
Bacterial reaction: bacteria present in blood	Fever Hypertension Dry, flushed skin Abdominal pain	• Stop infusion immediately. • Obtain culture of patient's blood and return blood bag to lab. • Monitor vital signs. • Notify primary care provider. • Administer antibiotics stat.

select electrolytes, vitamins, minerals, and trace elements that must be infused through a central vein because of its hypertonic nature. TPN frequently is given to patients, such as those with severe inflammatory bowel disease, severe pancreatitis, or acquired immunodeficiency syndrome (AIDS), who are unable to meet their nutritional needs through the oral or enteral routes. TPN may be given to a patient before surgery to enhance postoperative recovery. TPN requires careful management for complications such as infection and electrolyte imbalances. Catheter-related infection is a major concern when the patient is receiving TPN infusion. This procedure and related nursing responsibilities are described in Chapter 36.

Evaluating

Ongoing evaluation is integral; throughout nursing care, the nurse must evaluate and readjust his or her plans and interventions. Refer to the accompanying concept map for an illustration of the Nursing Process for Grace Gilligan. Evaluate the effectiveness of the plan of care to promote healthy fluid, electrolyte, and acid–base balance based on the following parameters:

• Are the patient's drinking and eating patterns supplying the needed fluid and electrolytes? Are food and fluid likes and dislikes interfering with the implementation of the care plan? Is the patient having any difficulties with oral fluids, tube feedings, IV therapy, or TPN?

• Is the patient's urine output about equal to the fluid intake? Does the patient void at least once each shift (except when sleeping)? Do urine characteristics (color, odor, specific gravity) indicate healthy functioning of the kidneys and excretion of fluids?

• Are abnormal sources of fluid loss (e.g., vomiting, diarrhea, draining wounds, fistula) responding to treatment? Are these fluid losses effectively being replaced by the designated therapy? Are the signs of fluid volume deficit improving?

• Do the patient's weight and record of fluid intake and output indicate fluid balance?

• Are the signs and symptoms that initially manifested the fluid, electrolyte, or acid–base imbalances absent or improved? Has therapy led to any troublesome new signs or symptoms?

• Is the patient now able to practice self-care behaviors to maintain fluid, electrolyte, and acid–base balance? Can the patient describe appropriate responses to potential future problems?

This evaluation should be ongoing as the plan of care is implemented. As the patient achieves the expected outcomes, these should be noted and reinforced. Before nursing care is terminated, the patient and family should be able to independently promote fluid, electrolyte, and acid–base balance. See the Nursing Plan of Care 40-1 for Jeremiah Stein.

Grace Gilligan, 28 years old, is admitted to the ER with complaints of severe bouts of nausea and vomiting. She has a past medical history of GI problems for which she underwent abdominal surgery several months ago. Her admission assessment reveals that she is awake, alert, and oriented to person, place, and time. Grace complains of dizziness when she sits up suddenly. Assessment reveals poor skin turgor and dry oral mucous membranes. Respirations are even, unlabored at 22 breaths/minute. Lungs are clear. Pulse is 132 beats/minute and weak. BP is 106/52 mm Hg and temperature is 98.9°F. Abdomen is firm, distended, slightly tender with absent bowel sounds. A nasogastric tube was inserted. She reports a 6 pound weight loss over the past 3 days. She has not voided in the past 8 hours. Intravenous therapy is prescribed to restore fluid balance. An X-ray study reveals an intestinal obstruction. She tearfully relates, "I thought my problems were over once I had the surgery."

Priority 1

Deficient Fluid Volume related to nausea and vomiting
Supporting Data:
• Recent abdominal surgery
• Severe bouts of nausea and vomiting
• Nasogastric tube in place
• Abdomen firm, distended without bowel sounds
• X-ray confirmation of bowel obstruction
• Intravenous therapy
• Recent 6 pound weight loss
• Has not voided in past 8 hours
• Dry oral mucous membranes
• C/o orthostatic dizziness
• BP 106/52, pulse 132 beats/minute, respiratory rate 22 breaths/minute

Outcome:
Patient will achieve normal fluid volume, adequate urine output, stable vital signs, good skin turgor, moist mucous membranes, and normal electrolytes.

Nursing Interventions:
• Monitor prescribed intravenous therapy
• Monitor intake and output balance
• Weigh daily
• Vital signs every 4 hours
• Irrigate nasogastric tube every 4 hours with normal saline as prescribed
• Note characteristics and amount of nasogastric drainage
• Perform abdominal assessment
• Provide mouth care every 2 hours
• Assess skin turgor, mucous membranes
• Monitor results of labwork

Evaluation: Intravenous therapy is maintained. Grace voided 250 mL of urine after 4 hours of IV therapy. Vital signs stabilized. Her abdomen remains distended without bowel sounds. A surgical consult was prescribed to evaluate the need for abdominal surgery.

Priority 2

Risk for Imbalanced Nutrition: Less Than Body Requirements related to nausea and vomiting, inability to tolerate oral foods and fluids
Supporting Data:
• Six pound weight loss in 2 days
• NPO with nasogastric tube
• Abdomen distended and firm with absent bowel sounds
• Recent abdominal surgery

Outcome:
Patient will have nutritional needs addressed. Weight will stabilize.

Nursing Interventions:
• Consult dietitian
• Weigh daily
• Perform an abdominal assessment to assist in determining return of bowel function
• Evaluate current weight and compare to ideal body weight
• Prepare to initiate and monitor total parenteral nutrition (TPN)
• Provide frequent mouth care

Evaluation: Grace's abdomen remains distended with absent bowel sounds. She remains NPO and is being evaluated for surgery. Collaborate with dietitian and physician to determine need for TPN.

Priority 3

Anxiety related to change in health status
Supporting Data:
• Severe bouts of nausea and vomiting after recent abdominal surgery
• Uncertainty about health status
• Tearfully states, "I thought my problems were over once I had the surgery."

Outcome:
Patient will report a reduction in anxiety to a manageable level and verbalize feelings surrounding anxiety.

Nursing Interventions:
• Assist patient in identifying support systems and previous coping techniques
• Encourage verbalization of feelings
• Active listening
• Relay accurate information regarding health status, correcting any misperceptions
• Utilize comfort measures such as Therapeutic Touch
• Maintain calm, quiet environment

Evaluation: Grace verbalizes an understanding of rationales for interventions. She is participating in the plan of care and asking questions regarding plan of care.

- - - - - **Relationship**   **Assessment**   **Nursing Diagnosis**   **Outcome Identification**   **Interventions**   **Evaluation**

Concept map illustrating the nursing process for Grace Gilligan.

For Jeremiah Stein

Jeremiah Stein is a 22-year-old man who is a senior in the premed program at a large state university. Although his grades were poor his first year in college, he currently is an honors student and plans to take the MCAT examination in 2 weeks. His overwhelming ambition is to be accepted into a prestigious medical school and to become a psychiatrist. He presents at the campus health clinic with the following assessment findings:

- History of problems with diarrhea since his junior year in high school; self-treatment with kaolin and pectin (Kaopectate) and limiting his food and fluid intake; believes diarrhea is stress related; no medical evaluation to date

- Has had two or three loose bowel movements per day for the past week with urgency and occasional incontinence; believes this is related to anxiety about performance on MCAT and his need for good grades; always thirsty but afraid to drink much; urine output is decreased, and he noted that urine is darker in color and has a stronger odor

Nursing examination: temperature, 99.8°F (37.6°C); pulse, 92 beats/min; respirations, 18 breaths/min; blood pressure, 100/60 mm Hg; skin and mucous membranes are pale and dry; weight is 4 lb less than usual (current weight, 170 lb)

NURSING DIAGNOSIS Deficient Fluid Volume related to prolonged diarrhea and decreased fluid intake secondary to stress management as evidenced by 4-lb weight loss, dry skin and mucous membranes, and report of decreased urine output and concentrated urine

EXPECTED OUTCOME By next week's visit, 3/24/12, the patient will:

- Describe two effective means he has used to cope with stress

Nursing Interventions	Rationale	Evaluative Statement
Explore with the patient (1) what he finds most stressing at present, (2) the control he believes he has over these stressors, and (3) the adequacy of his past and present stress management strategies.	Assisting the patient to eliminate and reduce stress where possible and learn to cope better with unavoidable stress (identify and eliminate causative factors) is critical in controlling stress-related diarrhea.	3/24/12 Outcome not met. Patient reports little progress in coping with stress. With MCATs 1 week away, he feels more tense than ever before. Reports no time to explore stress management techniques.
Assess for other factors contributing to diarrhea and fluid volume deficit.	Diarrhea may have a functional basis.	*Revision:* Goal is appropriate. Encourage visit to counseling center if not before MCATs then as soon as
Teach relation between stress and bouts of diarrhea.	Stress may result in increased intestinal mobility.	possible afterward.
Refer to counseling center on campus for assistance with stress management.	Professional assistance may facilitate identification and management of stressful situation.	*C. Ryan, RN*

EXPECTED OUTCOME By the next week's visit, 3/31/12, the patient will:

- Report that his diarrhea is eliminated or decreased to one or two episodes per day

(continued)

NURSING PLAN OF CARE • 40-1

For Jeremiah Stein (continued)

Nursing Interventions	Rationale	Evaluative Statement
Teach patient to link causative factors with diarrhea and to note anything that brings relief or assists in establishment of usual pattern of defecation.	Being able to make these connections helps patient to assume charge of own condition and to reinforce preventive strategies and successful relief measures.	3/31/12 Outcome met. Patient reports diarrhea decreased to one or two episodes per day.
Make sure patient understands diet: chemically and mechanically nonirritating diet high in calories, protein, and minerals; exclude foods such as cocoa, chocolate, alcohol, cold or carbonated beverages, citrus juices; try frequent, small meals.	Some patients fear eating because it stimulates the gastrocolic reflex and may result in a stool. Eating the proper diet actually reduces bowel irritation and decreases peristalsis.	*Recommendation:* Advise patient that it is important to keep appointment with gastroenterologist because relief may only be temporary. *C. Ryan, RN*
Teach patient proper use of prescribed medications.	Loperamide hydrochloride controls diarrhea, and methylcellulose increases consistency of stool.	

EXPECTED OUTCOME   By next week's visit, 3/31/12, the patient will:

- Demonstrate improved fluid and electrolyte balance as evidenced by (1) maintenance of present weight (170 lb), (2) moist mucous membranes, and (3) report of increased urinary output

Nursing Interventions	Rationale	Evaluative Statement
Explore with patient workable plan for oral replacement of fluids.	Collaboration with patient to determine acceptable sources of fluid intake may allay his fear that fluid intake causes diarrheal episodes.	3/31/12 Outcome partially met. Patient reports diarrhea decreased to once or twice a day. Two days there was no diarrhea. Weight, 169 lb.
Have patient note which calorie- and electrolyte- (sodium and potassium) rich fluids he can tolerate. Increase fluid intake to maintain a normal urine specific gravity.	Increased fluid intake is necessary to compensate for excessive loss in diarrhea and to reestablish fluid balance.	Mucous membranes are moist. Urine output is increased. *C. Ryan, RN*
Instruct patient to weigh himself every other day and to note changes in the volume or appearance of his urine.	All other things being equal, weight loss is a good indicator of continued fluid volume deficit. Other signs include decreased urinary output and high specific gravity.	
Teach patient defining characteristics of electrolyte imbalances associated with prolonged diarrhea—hyponatremia and hypokalemia.	Excreted stool pulls electrolytes with it, especially sodium and potassium.	

(continued)

NURSING PLAN OF CARE · 40-1

For Jeremiah Stein (continued)

SAMPLE DOCUMENTATION	3/31/12, nursing Mr. Stein returned to the clinic reporting that his diarrhea is decreased to one to two episodes per day and that he has an appointment with a gastroenterologist. He believes that modifying his diet, increasing rest periods, and medications (loperamide hydrochloride to control diarrhea and methylcellulose to increase the consistency of stool) were of great help. He still does not know how he can reduce his stress level. Nursing examination revealed temperature, 98.9°F (37.1°C); pulse, 88 beats/min; respirations, 18 breaths/min; blood pressure, 110/60 mm Hg; weight, 169 lb; skin and mucous membranes less dry than on previous visit. States he has not noted much change in urine output but possibly less concentrated. *C. Ryan, RN*

Skill · 40-1 Initiating a Peripheral Venous Access IV Infusion

EQUIPMENT

- IV solution, as prescribed
- Medication administration record (MAR) or computer-generated MAR (CMAR)
- Towel or disposable pad
- Nonallergenic tape
- IV administration set
- Label for infusion set (for next change date)
- Transparent site dressing

- Electronic infusion device (if appropriate)
- Tourniquet
- Time tape and/or label (for IV container)
- Cleansing swabs (chlorhexidine preferred)
- IV securement/stabilization device, as appropriate
- Clean gloves
- Additional PPE, as indicated
- IV pole
- Local anesthetic (if ordered)

- IV catheter (over the needle, Angiocath) or butterfly needle
- Short extension tubing
- End cap for extension tubing
- Alcohol wipes
- Skin protectant wipe (such as SkinPrep)
- Prefilled 2-mL syringe with sterile normal saline for injection

IMPLEMENTATION

ACTION	RATIONALE
1. Verify the IV solution order on the MAR/CMAR with the medical order. Clarify any inconsistencies. Check the patient's chart for allergies. Check for color, leaking, and expiration date. Know techniques for IV insertion, precautions, purpose of the IV administration, and medications if ordered.	This ensures that the correct IV solution and rate of infusion, and/or medication will be administered. This knowledge and skill is essential for safe and accurate IV and medication administration.
2. Gather all equipment and bring to the bedside.	Having equipment available saves time and facilitates accomplishment of procedure.
3. Perform hand hygiene and put on PPE, if indicated.	Hand hygiene and PPE prevent the spread of microorganisms. PPE is required based on transmission precautions.
4. Identify the patient.	Identifying the patient ensures the right patient receives the intervention and helps prevent errors.
5. Close curtains around bed and close door to the room if possible. Explain what you are going to do and why you are going to do it to the patient. Ask the patient about allergies to medications, tape, or skin antiseptics, as appropriate. If considering using a local anesthetic, inquire about allergies for these substances as well.	This ensures the patient's privacy. Explanation relieves anxiety and facilitates cooperation. Possible allergies may exist related to medications, tape, or local anesthetic. Injectable anesthetic can result in allergic reactions and tissue damage.

ACTION

6. If using a local anesthetic, explain the rationale and procedure to the patient. Apply the anesthetic to a few potential insertion sites. Allow sufficient time for the anesthetic to take effect.

Prepare the IV Solution and Administration Set

7. Compare the IV container label with the MAR/CMAR. Remove IV bag from outer wrapper, if indicated. Check expiration dates. Scan bar code on container, if necessary. Compare on patient identification band with the MAR/CMAR. Alternately, label the solution container with the patient's name, solution type, additives, date, and time. Complete a time strip for the infusion and apply to IV container.

8. Maintain aseptic technique when opening sterile packages and IV solution. Remove administration set from package (see Fig. 40-8). Apply label to tubing reflecting the day/date for next set change, per facility guidelines.

9. Close the roller clamp or slide clamp on the IV administration set (Figure 1). Invert the IV solution container and remove the cap on the entry site, taking care to not touch the exposed entry site. Remove the cap from the spike on the administration set. Using a twisting and pushing motion, insert the administration set spike into the entry site of the IV container (Figure 2). Alternately, follow the manufacturer's directions for insertion.

RATIONALE

Explanations provide reassurance and facilitate cooperation of the patient. Local anesthetic decreases the amount of pain felt at the insertion site. Some of the anesthetics take up to an hour to become effective.

Checking label with MAR/CMAR ensures correct IV solution will be administered. Identifying the patient ensures the right patient receives the medications and helps prevent errors. Time strip allows for quick visual reference by the nurse to monitor infusion accuracy.

Asepsis is essential for preventing the spread of microorganisms. Labeling tubing ensures adherence to facility policy regarding administration set changes and reduces risk of spread of microorganisms. In general, IV tubing is changed every 72 to 96 hours.

Clamping the IV tubing prevents air and fluid from entering the IV tubing at this time.

Inverting the container allows easy access to the entry site. Touching the opened entry site on the IV container and/or the spike on the administration set results in contamination and the container/administration set would have to be discarded. Inserting the spike punctures the seal in the IV container and allows access to contents.

FIGURE 1. Closing clamp on administration set.

FIGURE 2. Inserting administration set spike into entry site of IV fluid container.

10. Hang the IV container on the IV pole. Squeeze the drip chamber and fill at least halfway (Figure 3).

11. Open the IV tubing clamp and allow fluid to move through tubing. Follow additional manufacturer's instructions for specific electronic infusion pump, as indicated. **Allow fluid to flow until all air bubbles have disappeared and the entire length of the tubing is primed (filled) with IV solution** (Figure 4). Close clamp. Alternately, some brands of tubing may require removal of cap at end of the IV tubing to allow fluid to flow. Maintain its sterility. After fluid has filled the tubing, recap end of tubing.

Suction causes fluid to move into drip chamber. Fluid prevents air from moving down the tubing.

This technique prepares for IV fluid administration and removes air from tubing. In large amounts, if air is not removed from the tubing, it can act as an embolus. Touching the open end of the tubing results in contamination and the administration set would have to be discarded.

(continued)

Skill · 40-1   Initiating a Peripheral Venous Access IV Infusion   *continued*

ACTION	RATIONALE
12. If an electronic device is to be used, follow manufacturer's instructions for inserting tubing into the device (Figure 5).	This ensures proper use of equipment.

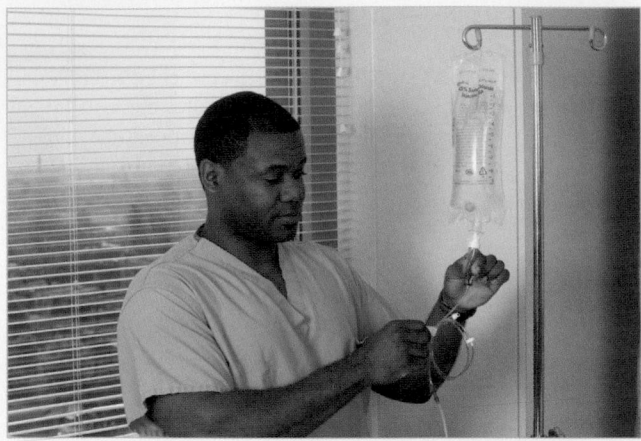

FIGURE 3. Squeezing drip chamber to fill at least halfway.

FIGURE 4. Priming administration set.

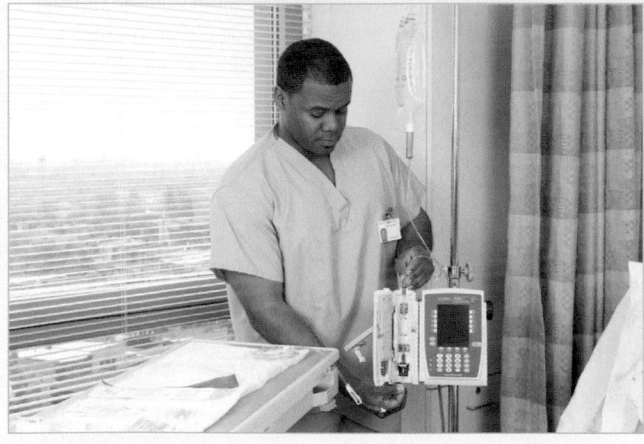

FIGURE 5. Inserting administration set into electronic infusion device.

Initiate Peripheral Venous Access

ACTION	RATIONALE
13. Place patient in low Fowler's position in bed. Place protective towel or pad under patient's arm.	The supine position permits either arm to be used and allows for good body alignment. Towel protects underlying surface from blood contamination.
14. Provide emotional support as needed.	Patient may experience anxiety because he/she may fear needle-stick or IV infusion in general.
15. Open the short extension tubing package. Attach end cap, if not in place. Clean end cap with alcohol wipe. Insert syringe with normal saline into extension tubing. Fill extension tubing with normal saline and apply slide clamp. Remove the syringe and place extension tubing and syringe back on package, within easy reach.	Priming extension tubing removes air from tubing and prevents administration of air when connected to venous access. Having tubing within easy reach facilitates accomplishment of procedure.
16. Select and palpate for an appropriate vein. Refer to guidelines in previous Assessment section.	The use of an appropriate vein decreases discomfort for the patient and reduces the risk for damage to body tissues.
17. If the site is hairy and agency policy permits, clip a 2″ area around the intended site of entry.	Hair can harbor microorganisms and inhibit adhesion of site dressing.

ACTION	RATIONALE
18. Put on gloves.	Gloves prevent contact with blood and body fluids.
19. Apply a tourniquet 3″ to 4″ above the venipuncture site to obstruct venous blood flow and distend the vein (Figure 6). Direct the ends of the tourniquet away from the site of entry. Make sure the radial pulse is still present.	Interrupting the blood flow to the heart causes the vein to distend. Distended veins are easy to see, palpate, and enter. The end of the tourniquet could contaminate the area of injection if directed toward the site of entry. Tourniquet may be applied too tightly so assessment for radial pulse is important. Checking radial pulse ensures arterial supply is not compromised.
20. Instruct the patient to hold the arm lower than the heart.	Lowering the arm below the heart level helps distend the veins by filling them.
21. Ask patient to open and close fist. Observe and palpate for a suitable vein. Try the following techniques if a vein cannot be felt:	Contracting the muscles of the forearm forces blood into the veins, thereby distending them further.
a. Massage the patient's arm from proximal to distal end and gently tap over intended vein.	Massaging and tapping the vein help distend veins by filling them with blood.
b. Remove tourniquet and place warm, moist compresses over intended vein for 10 to 15 minutes.	Warm, moist compresses help dilate veins.
22. **Cleanse site with an antiseptic solution such as chlorhexidine or according to facility policy. Press applicator against the skin and apply chlorhexidine using a back and forth friction scrub for at least 30 seconds. Do not wipe or blot. Allow to dry completely.**	Scrubbing motion and length of time (minimum 30 seconds) is necessary for chlorhexidine to be effective (Infection Control Today [ICT], 2005). Organisms on the skin can be introduced into the tissues or the bloodstream with the needle. Chlorhexidine is the preferred antiseptic solution, but iodine, povidone-iodine, and 70% alcohol are considered acceptable alternatives (INS, 2006).
23. Use the nondominant hand, placed about 1″ or 2″ below entry site, to hold the skin taut against the vein. **Avoid touching the prepared site.** Ask the patient to remain still while you are performing the venipuncture.	Pressure on the vein and surrounding tissues helps prevent movement of the vein as the needle or catheter is being inserted. The needle entry site must remain untouched to prevent contamination from unsterile hands. Patient movement may prevent proper technique for IV insertion.
24. Enter the skin gently, holding the catheter by the hub in your dominant hand, bevel side up, at a 10- to 15-degree angle (Figure 7). Insert the catheter from directly over the vein or from the side of the vein. While following the course of the vein, advance the needle or catheter into the vein. A sensation of "give" can be felt when the needle enters the vein.	This allows needle or catheter to enter vein with minimal trauma and deters passage of the needle through the vein.

FIGURE 6. Applying tourniquet.

FIGURE 7. Stretching skin taut and inserting needle.

(continued)

Skill · 40-1   **Initiating a Peripheral Venous Access IV Infusion**   *continued*

ACTION

RATIONALE

25. When blood returns through the lumen of the needle or the flashback chamber of the catheter, advance either device into the vein until the hub is at the venipuncture site. The exact technique depends on the type of device used.

The tourniquet causes increased venous pressure, resulting in automatic backflow. Placing the access device well into the vein helps to prevent dislodgement.

26. Release the tourniquet. Quickly remove the protective cap from the extension tubing and attach to the catheter or needle. Stabilize the catheter or needle with your nondominant hand.

Bleeding is minimized and the patency of the vein is maintained if the connection is made smoothly between the catheter and tubing.

27. Continue to stabilize the catheter or needle and flush gently with the saline, observing the site for infiltration and leaking.

Infiltration and/or leaking and patient reports of pain and/or discomfort indicate that the insertion into the vein is not successful and should be discontinued.

28. Open the skin protectant wipe. Apply the skin protectant to the site, making sure to cover at minimum the area to be covered with the dressing. Place sterile transparent dressing or catheter securing/stabilization device over venipuncture site. Loop the tubing near the site of entry, and anchor with tape (nonallergenic) close to site.

Skin protectant aids in adhesion of the dressing and decreases the risk for skin trauma when the dressing is removed. Transparent dressing allows easy visualization and protects site. Stabilization/securing devices to preserve the integrity of the access device and to prevent catheter migration and loss of access (INS, 2006, p. S44). Some stabilization devices act as a site dressing also. The weight of the tubing is sufficient to pull it out of the vein if it is not well anchored. Nonallergenic tape is less likely to tear fragile skin.

29. Label the IV dressing with the date, time, site, and type and size of catheter or needle used for the infusion (Figure 8).

Other personnel working with the infusion will know what type of device is being used, the site, and when it was inserted. IV insertion sites are changed every 48 to 72 hours or according to agency policy (Lavery, 2005).

30. Using an antimicrobial swab, cleanse access cap on extension tubing. Remove the end cap from the administration set. Insert the end of the administration set into the end cap (Figure 9). Loop the administration set tubing near the site of entry, and anchor with tape (nonallergenic) close to site. Remove gloves.

Inserting the administration set allows initiation of the fluid infusion. The weight of the tubing is sufficient to pull it out of the vein if it is not well anchored. Nonallergenic tape is less likely to tear fragile skin. Removing gloves properly reduces the risk for infection transmission and contamination of other items.

FIGURE 8. Venous access site with labeled dressing.

FIGURE 9. Inserting administration set into the end cap of venous access device.

31. Open the clamp on the administration set. Set the rate of flow and begin the fluid infusion (Figure 10). Alternately, start the flow of solution by releasing the clamp on the tubing and counting the drops. Adjust until the correct drop rate is achieved. Assess the flow of the solution and function of the infusion device. Inspect the insertion site for signs of infiltration (Figure 11).

Verifying the rate and device settings ensures patient receives correct volume of solution. If catheter or needle slips out of the vein, the solution will accumulate (infiltrate) into the surrounding tissue.

ACTION

FIGURE 10. Initiating IV fluid infusion.

RATIONALE

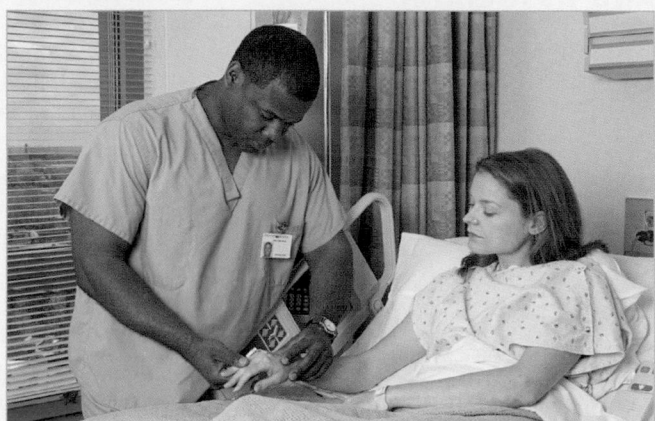

FIGURE 11. Inspecting insertion site.

32. Apply an IV securement/stabilization device if not already in place as part of dressing, as indicated, based on facility policy. Explain to patient the purpose of the device and the importance of safeguarding the site when using the extremity.

These systems are recommended for use on all venous access sites, and particularly central venous access sites, to preserve the integrity of the access device and to prevent catheter migration and loss of access (INS, 2006, p. S44). Some devices act as a site dressing also and may already have been applied.

33. Remove equipment and return patient to a position of comfort. Lower bed, if not in lowest position.

Promotes patient comfort and safety.

34. Remove additional PPE, if used. Perform hand hygiene.

Removing PPE properly reduces the risk for infection transmission and contamination of other items. Hand hygiene prevents transmission of microorganisms.

35. Return to check flow rate and observe IV site for infiltration 30 minutes after starting infusion, and at least hourly thereafter. Ask the patient if he or she is experiencing any pain or discomfort related to the IV infusion.

Continued monitoring is important to maintain correct flow rate. Early detection of problems ensures prompt intervention.

DOCUMENTATION

Guidelines

Document the location where the IV access was placed, as well as the size of the IV catheter or needle, the type of IV solution, and the rate of the IV infusion, as well as the use of a securing or stabilization device. Additionally, document the condition of the site, such as presence of redness, swelling, or drainage. Record the patient's reaction to the procedure and pertinent patient teaching, such as alerting the nurse if the patient experiences any pain from the IV or notices any swelling at the site. If necessary, document the IV fluid solution on the intake and output record.

Sample Documentation

11/02/12 0830 20G IV started in L hand via the dorsal metacarpal vein. Transparent dressing applied. Site without redness, drainage, or edema. $D_5$1/2 NS with 20 mEq KCl begun at 110 mL/hr. Patient instructed to call with any pain or swelling.
—*S. Barnes, RN*

(continued)

Skill · 40-1   Initiating a Peripheral Venous Access IV Infusion   *continued*

UNEXPECTED SITUATIONS AND ASSOCIATED INTERVENTIONS

- *Fluid does not easily flow into the vein:* Reposition the extremity because certain positions that the patient may assume may prevent the IV from infusing properly. If the IV is a free-flowing IV, raise the height of the IV pole. This may promote an increase in IV flow. Attempt to flush the IV with 2–3 mL of saline in a syringe. Check IV connector to ensure that clamp is fully open. If fluid still does not flow easily, or if resistance is met while flushing, the IV may be against a valve and may need to be restarted in a different location.

- *Fluid does not flow easily into the vein, and the skin around the insertion site is edematous and cool to the touch:* IV has infiltrated. Put on gloves and remove catheter. Apply pressure with a sterile gauze pad. Secure gauge with tape over insertion site and restart IV in a new location.

- *A small hematoma is forming at the site while you are inserting the catheter:* The vein is "blowing": a small hole has been made in the vein and blood is leaking out into the tissues. Remove and discard the catheter and choose an alternate insertion site.

- *Fluids are leaking around the insertion site:* Change dressing on IV. If site continues to leak, remove IV to decrease risk of infection and restart it in a new location.

- *IV infusion set becomes disconnected from IV:* Discard IV tubing to prevent infection. Attempt to flush IV with 3 mL of normal saline. If the IV is still patent, the site may still be used, as long as the catheter hub has not been contaminated.

- *IV catheter is partially pulled out of insertion site:* Do not reinsert the catheter. Whether the IV is salvageable depends on how much of the catheter remains in the vein. If this catheter is not removed, monitor it closely for signs of infiltration.

SPECIAL CONSIDERATIONS

General Considerations

- Attempt only two venipuncture attempts when initiating venous access for a patient. If unsuccessful after two attempts, a colleague with advanced skills, such as a member of the nurse IV team, should attempt to initiate the venous access (Arbique & Arbique, 2007).

Infant and Child Considerations

- Hand insertion sites should not be the first choice for children because nerve endings are very close to the surface of the skin, and it is more painful. Once the child can walk, do not use the feet as insertion sites.

- Other potential sites for neonates and children include veins of the head, neck, and lower extremities (INS, 2006). Scalp arteries in infants are visible. Carefully palpate the site before insertion. If the site is pulsating, do not use.

- Do not replace peripheral catheters in children unless clinically indicated (CDC, 2002).

- For neonates, isopropyl alcohol or products containing isopropyl alcohol are not recommended for access site preparation. Povidone-iodine or chlorhexidine solution is recommended but requires complete removal after the preparatory procedure with sterile water or sterile saline to prevent product absorption (INS, 2006, p. S42).

- Chlorhexidine has been associated with contact dermatitis when used for infants weighing less than 1,000 grams. It should be used with caution with this patient population (INS, 2006).

Older Adult Considerations

- Avoid using vigorous friction and too much alcohol at the insertion site. Both can traumatize fragile skin and veins in the elderly.

- To decrease the risk for trauma to the vessel, experienced nurses may omit use of a tourniquet if the patient has prominent but especially fragile veins.

- Catheter stabilization/securing devices should be used routinely with older adults to preserve the integrity of the access device and to prevent catheter migration and loss of access (INS, 2006, p. S44; Smith & Hannum, 2008).

Skill · 40-2   Changing an IV Solution Container and Administration Set

EQUIPMENT

For solution container change:
- IV solution as prescribed
- Medication administration record (MAR) or computer-generated MAR (CMAR)
- Time tape and/or label (for IV container)

For tubing change:
- Administration set
- Label for administration set (for next change date)
- Sterile gauze
- Nonallergenic tape

- IV securement/stabilization device, as appropriate
- Clean gloves
- Additional PPE, as indicated
- Alcohol wipes

IMPLEMENTATION

ACTION	RATIONALE
1. Verify IV solution order on MAR/CMAR with the medical order. Clarify any inconsistencies. Check the patient's chart for allergies. Check for color, leaking, and expiration date. Know the purpose of the IV administration and medications if ordered.	This ensures that the correct IV solution and rate of infusion, and/or medication will be administered. This knowledge and skill is essential for safe and accurate IV and medication administration.
2. Gather all equipment and bring to bedside.	Having equipment available saves time and facilitates accomplishment of procedure.
3. Perform hand hygiene and put on PPE, if indicated.	Hand hygiene and PPE prevent the spread of microorganisms. PPE is required based on transmission precautions.
4. Identify the patient.	Identifying the patient ensures the right patient receives the intervention and helps prevent errors.
5. Close curtains around bed and close door to room if possible. Explain what you are going to do and why you are going to do it to the patient. Ask the patient about allergies to medications or tape, as appropriate.	This ensures the patient's privacy. Explanation relieves anxiety and facilitates cooperation. Possible allergies may exist related to IV solution additive or tape.
6. Compare IV container label with the MAR/CMAR (Figure 1). Remove IV bag from outer wrapper, if indicated. Check expiration dates. Scan bar code on container, if necessary. Compare patient identification band with the MAR/CMAR. Alternately, label solution container with the patient's name, solution type, additives, date, and time. Complete a time strip for the infusion and apply to IV container.	Checking label with MAR/CMAR ensures correct IV solution will be administered. Identifying the patient ensures the right patient receives the medications and helps prevent errors. Time strip allows for quick visual reference by the nurse to monitor infusion accuracy.

FIGURE 1. Comparing IV fluid container label with MAR/CMAR.

| 7. Maintain aseptic technique when opening sterile packages and IV solution. Remove administration set from package. Apply label to tubing reflecting the day/date for next set change, per facility guidelines. | Asepsis is essential for preventing the spread of microorganisms. Labeling tubing ensures adherence to facility policy regarding administration set changes and reduces risk of spread of microorganisms. In general, IV tubing is changed every 72 to 96 hours. |

(continued)

Skill · 40-2 **Changing an IV Solution Container and Administration Set** *continued*

ACTION	**RATIONALE**

To Change IV Solution Container

8. If using an electronic infusion device, pause the device or put on "hold." Close the slide clamp on the administration set closest to the drip chamber. If using gravity infusion, close the roller clamp on the administration set.

The action of the infusion device needs to be paused while the solution container is changed. Closing the clamps prevents the fluid in the drip chamber from emptying and air from entering the tubing during the procedure.

9. Carefully remove the cap on the entry site of the new IV solution container and expose entry site, taking care to not touch the exposed entry site.

Touching the opened entry site on the IV container results in contamination and the container would have to be discarded.

10. Lift empty container off IV pole and invert it. Quickly remove the spike from the old IV container, **being careful not to contaminate it.** Discard old IV container.

Touching the spike on the administration set results in contamination and the tubing would have to be discarded.

11. Using a twisting and pushing motion, insert the administration set spike into the entry site of the IV container. Alternately, follow the manufacturer's directions for insertion. Hang the container on the IV pole.

Inserting spike punctures the seal in the IV container and allows access to contents.

12. Alternately, hang the new IV fluid container on an open hook on the IV pole. Carefully remove the cap on the entry site of the new IV solution container and expose entry site, taking care to not touch the exposed entry site. Lift empty container off IV pole and invert it. Quickly remove the spike from the old IV container, **being careful not to contaminate it (Figure 2).** Discard old IV container. Using a twisting and pushing motion, insert the administration set spike into the entry port of the new IV container as it hangs on the IV pole (Figure 3).

Touching the opened entry site on the IV container or the administration set spike results in contamination and both would have to be discarded. Inserting spike punctures the seal in the IV container and allows access to contents.

FIGURE 2. Removing administration spike from empty IV fluid container.

FIGURE 3. Inserting administration set spike into entry port of new IV fluid container.

13. If using an electronic infusion device, open the slide clamp, check the drip chamber of the administration set, verify the flow rate programmed in the infusion device, and turn the device to "run" or "infuse."

Verifying the rate and device settings ensures patient receives correct volume of solution.

14. If using gravity infusion, slowly open the roller clamp on the administration set and count the drops. Adjust until the correct drop rate is achieved (Figure 4).

Opening clamp regulates flow rate into drip chamber. Verifying the rate ensures patient receives correct volume of solution.

ACTION

FIGURE 4. Reopening the clamp and adjusting the flow rate for a gravity infusion.

To Change IV Solution Container and Administration Set

15. Prepare the IV solution and administration set. Refer to Skill 40-1, Steps 7–11.

16. Hang the IV container on an open hook on the IV pole. Close the clamp on the existing IV administration set. Also, close the clamp on the short extension tubing connected to the IV catheter in the patient's arm.

17. If using an electronic infusion device, remove current administration set from device. Following manufacturer's directions, insert new administration set into infusion device.

18. Put on gloves. Remove the current infusion tubing from the access cap on the short extension IV tubing. Using an antimicrobial swab, cleanse access cap on extension tubing. Remove the end cap from the new administration set. Insert the end of the administration set into the access cap. Loop the administration set tubing near the site of entry, and anchor with tape (nonallergenic) close to site (Figure 5).

FIGURE 5. Making sure clamp is open on new tubing, with short extension tubing taped in place.

RATIONALE

Clamping the existing IV tubing prevents leakage of fluid from the administration set after it is disconnected. Clamping the tubing on the extension set prevents introduction of air into the extension tubing.

Administration set has to be removed in order to insert new tubing into device.

Cleansing the cap or port reduces the risk of contamination. Inserting the administration set allows initiation of the fluid infusion. The weight of the tubing is sufficient to pull it out of the vein if it is not well anchored. Nonallergenic tape is less likely to tear fragile skin.

(continued)

Skill · 40-2   Changing an IV Solution Container and Administration Set   *continued*

ACTION	RATIONALE
19. Open the clamp on the extension tubing. Open the clamp on the administration set.	Opening clamps allows solution to flow to patient.
20. If using an electronic infusion device, open the slide clamp, check the drip chamber of the administration set, verify the flow rate programmed in the infusion device, and turn the device to "run" or "infuse."	Verifying the rate and device settings ensures patient receives correct volume of solution.
21. If using gravity infusion, slowly open the roller clamp on the administration set and count the drops. Adjust until the correct drop rate is achieved.	Opening clamp regulates flow rate into drip chamber. Verifying the rate ensures patient receives correct volume of solution.
22. Remove equipment. Ensure patient's comfort. Remove gloves. Lower bed, if not in lowest position.	Promotes patient comfort and safety. Removing gloves properly reduces the risk for infection transmission and contamination of other items.
23. Remove additional PPE, if used. Perform hand hygiene.	Removing PPE properly reduces the risk for infection transmission and contamination of other items. Hand hygiene prevents transmission of microorganisms.
24. Return to check flow rate and observe IV site for infiltration 30 minutes after starting infusion and at least hourly thereafter. Ask the patient if he or she is experiencing any pain or discomfort related to the IV infusion.	Continued monitoring is important to maintain correct flow rate. Early detection of problems ensures prompt intervention.

DOCUMENTATION

Guidelines

Document the type of IV solution and the rate of infusion such as presence of redness, swelling, or drainage. Record the patient's reaction to the procedure and pertinent patient teaching, such as alerting the nurse if the patient experiences any pain from the IV or notices any swelling at the site. If necessary, document the IV fluid solution on the intake and output record.

Sample Documentation

> 11/3/12 1015 IV fluid changed from $D_5$1/2 NS with 20 mEq KCl/L at 125 mL/hr to $D_5$0.9% NS with 20 mEq KCl/L at 80 mL/hr. IV site intact; no swelling, redness, or drainage noted.
>
> —S. Barnes, RN

UNEXPECTED SITUATIONS AND ASSOCIATED INTERVENTIONS

- *Infusion does not flow or flow rate changes after bag and tubing is changed:* Make sure that the flow clamp is open and the drip chamber is approximately half full. Check the electronic device for proper functioning. Check the IV site for possible problems with the catheter, such as bending of the catheter or position of the patient's extremity, and inspect the IV site for signs and symptoms of complications. Readjust the flow rate.

- *After attaching new IV tubing, you note air bubbles in the tubing:* If the bubbles are above the roller clamp, you can easily remove them by closing the roller clamp, stretching the tubing downward, and tapping the tubing with your finger so the bubbles rise to the drip chamber. If there is a larger amount of air in the tubing, swab the medication port on the tubing below the air with an antimicrobial solution and attach a syringe to the port below the air. Clamp the tubing below the access port. Aspirate the air from the tubing via the syringe. Remember that air bubbles in the tubing can be reduced if the tubing is primed slowly with fluid instead of allowing a wide-open flow of the solution.

Skill · 40-3 Monitoring an IV Site and Infusion

EQUIPMENT
- PPE, as indicated

IMPLEMENTATION

ACTION	RATIONALE
1. Verify IV solution order on MAR/CMAR with the medical order. Clarify any inconsistencies. Check the patient's chart for allergies. Check for color, leaking, and expiration date. Know the purpose of the IV administration and medications if ordered.	This ensures that the correct IV solution and rate of infusion, and/or medication will be administered. This knowledge and skill is essential for safe and accurate IV and medication administration.
2. **Monitor IV infusion every hour or per agency policy. More frequent checks may be necessary if medication is being infused.**	Promotes safe administration of IV fluids and medication.
3. Perform hand hygiene and put on PPE, if indicated.	Hand hygiene and PPE prevent the spread of microorganisms. PPE is required based on transmission precautions.
4. Identify the patient.	Identifying the patient ensures the right patient receives the intervention and helps prevent errors.
5. Close curtains around bed and close door to room if possible. Explain what you are going to do to the patient.	This ensures the patient's privacy. Explanation relieves anxiety and facilitates cooperation.
6. If an electronic infusion device is being used, check settings, alarm, and indicator lights. Check set infusion rate (Figure 1). Note position of fluid in IV container in relation to time tape. Teach patient about the alarm features on the electronic infusion device.	Observation ensures that the infusion control device is functioning and that the alarm is functioning. Lack of knowledge about "alarms" may create anxiety for patient.
7. If IV is infusing via gravity, check the drip chamber and time the drops (Figure 2). (Refer to Guidelines for Nursing Care 40-3 to review calculation of IV flow rates for gravity infusion.)	This ensures that the flow rate is correct. Use a watch with a second hand for counting the drops in regulating a gravity drip IV infusion.

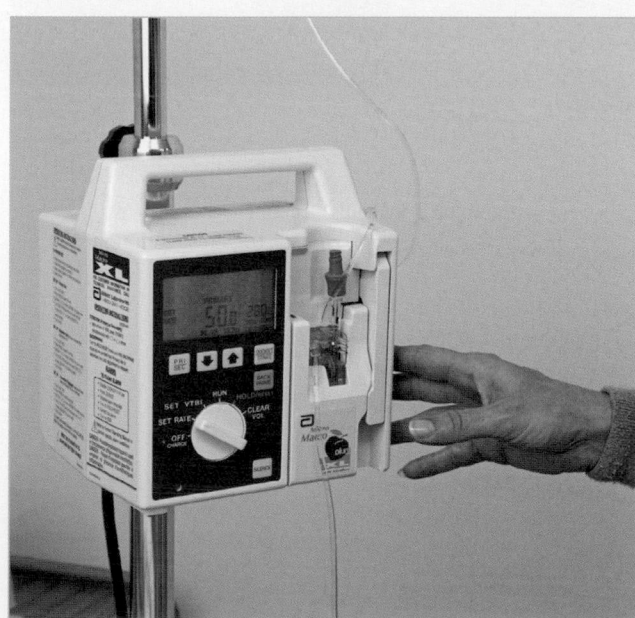

FIGURE 1. Checking the settings of the infusion device.

FIGURE 2. Checking the drip chamber and timing drops.

(continued)

Skill · 40-3 Monitoring an IV Site and Infusion *continued*

ACTION	RATIONALE
8. Check tubing for anything that might interfere with flow (Figure 3). Be sure clamps are in the open position.	Any kink or pressure on tubing may interfere with flow.
9. Observe dressing for leakage of IV solution.	Leakage may occur at the connection of the tubing with the hub of needle or catheter and allow for loss of IV solution.
10. **Inspect the site for swelling, leakage at the site, coolness, or pallor, which may indicate infiltration (Figure 4). Ask if patient is experiencing any pain or discomfort. If any of these symptoms are present, the IV will need to be removed and restarted at another site. Check facility policy for treating infiltration** (Refer to Table 40-12 and Box 40-1.)	Catheter may become dislodged from vein, and IV solution may flow into subcutaneous tissue.

FIGURE 3. Checking the tubing for anything that might interfere with the flow rate.

FIGURE 4. Inspecting IV site.

ACTION	RATIONALE
11. **Inspect site for redness, swelling, and heat. Palpate for induration. Ask if patient is experiencing pain. These findings may indicate phlebitis. Notify primary care provider if phlebitis is suspected. IV will need to be discontinued and restarted at another site. Check facility policy for treatment of phlebitis.** (Refer to Table 40-12 and Box 40-2.)	Chemical irritation or mechanical trauma causes injury to the vein and can lead to phlebitis. Phlebitis is the most common complication related to IV therapy (Lavery, 2005).
12. **Check for local manifestations (redness, pus, warmth, induration, pain) that may indicate an infection is present at the site, or systemic manifestations (chills, fever, tachycardia, hypotension) that may accompany local infection at the site. If signs of infection are present, discontinue the IV and notify the primary care provider.** Be careful not to disconnect IV tubing when putting on patient's hospital gown or assisting the patient with movement.	Poor aseptic technique may allow bacteria to enter the needle or catheter insertion site or tubing connection and may occur with manipulation of equipment.
13. Be alert for additional complications of IV therapy.	
a. **Fluid overload can result in signs of cardiac and/or respiratory failure. Monitor intake and output and vital signs. Assess for edema and auscultate lung sounds. Ask if patient is experiencing any shortness of breath.**	Infusing too much IV solution results in an increased volume of circulating fluid volume. Elderly patients are most at risk for this complication due to possible decrease in cardiac and/or renal functions.

ACTION	RATIONALE
b. Check for bleeding at the site.	Bleeding may be caused by anticoagulant medication. Bleeding at the site is most likely to occur when the IV is discontinued.
14. If possible, instruct patient to call for assistance if any discomfort is noted at site, solution container is nearly empty, flow has changed in any way, or if the electronic pump alarm sounds.	This facilitates cooperation of patient and safe administration of IV solution.

DOCUMENTATION

Guidelines

Document the type of IV solution as well as the infusion rate. Note the insertion site location and site assessment. Document the patient's reaction to the IV therapy as well as absence of subjective reports that he/she is not experiencing any pain or other discomfort, such as coolness or heat associated with the infusion. Additionally, record that the patient is not demonstrating any other IV complications, such as signs or symptoms of fluid overload. Record on the intake and output documents, as needed.

Sample Documentation

11/6/12 1020 IV site right forearm/cephalic vein intact without swelling, redness, or drainage. D_5 0.9% NS with 20 mEq KCL continues to infuse at 110 mL/hr. Patient instructed to call nurse with any swelling or pain.

—S. Barnes, RN

UNEXPECTED SITUATIONS AND ASSOCIATED INTERVENTIONS

- *Patient's lung sounds were previously clear, but now some crackles in the bases are auscultated:* Notify primary care provider immediately. The patient may be exhibiting signs of fluid overload. Be prepared to tell the healthcare provider what the past intake and output totals were, as well as the vital signs and pulse oximetry findings of the patient.

- *IV is not flowing as easily as it previously had been:* Check all clamps on the tubing and check tubing for any kinking. Check that the patient is not lying on the tubing. If the IV is over a joint, reposition the extremity and see if this helps the flow. An arm board may need to be applied. Attempt to flush the IV with 2 to 3 mL of normal saline. If the IV is painful or you meet resistance when attempting to flush, discontinue the IV and restart in another place.

Skill · 40-4 Changing a Peripheral Venous Access Dressing

EQUIPMENT

- Transparent occlusive dressing
- 2% chlorhexidine, povidone-iodine, 70% alcohol
- Adhesive remover (optional)
- Alcohol swabs

- Tape
- Clean gloves
- Towel or disposable pad
- Masks for nurse and patient; sterile gloves (used for catheter with extended

dwell time or if patient is immunocompromised [INS, 2006, p. S57])
- Additional PPE, as indicated

IMPLEMENTATION

ACTION	RATIONALE
1. Determine the need for a dressing change. Check facility policy. Gather all equipment and bring to bedside.	The particular facility's policies determine the type of dressing used and when these dressings are changed. Dressing changes might be required more often, based on nursing assessment and judgment. Immediately change any access site dressing that is damp, loosened, or soiled. Having equipment available saves time and facilitates accomplishment of procedure.

(continued)

Skill · 40-4 Changing a Peripheral Venous Access Dressing *continued*

ACTION	RATIONALE
2. Perform hand hygiene and put on PPE, if indicated.	Hand hygiene and PPE prevent the spread of microorganisms. PPE is required based on transmission precautions.
3. Identify the patient.	Identifying the patient ensures the right patient receives the intervention and helps prevent errors.
4. Close curtains around bed and close door to room if possible. Explain what you are going to do and why you are going to do it to the patient. Ask the patient about allergies to tape and skin antiseptics.	This ensures the patient's privacy. Explanation relieves anxiety and facilitates cooperation. Possible allergies may exist related to tape or antiseptics.
5. Put on mask and place on patient, if indicated. Put on gloves. Place towel or disposable pad under the arm with the venous access. If solution is currently infusing, temporarily stop the infusion. Hold the catheter in place with your nondominant hand and **carefully remove old dressing and/or stabilization/securing device (Figure 1).** Use adhesive remover as necessary. Discard dressing.	Masks should be used for catheter with extended dwell time or if patient is immunocompromised (INS, 2006, p. S57). Gloves prevent contact with blood and body fluids. Pad protects underlying surface. Proper disposal of dressing prevents transmission of microorganisms.

FIGURE 1. Carefully removing old dressing.

6. **Inspect IV site for presence of phlebitis (inflammation), infection, or infiltration.** Discontinue and relocate IV, if noted. (Refer to Table 40-12, Box 40-1, and Box 40-2.)	Inflammation (phlebitis), infection, or infiltration cause trauma to tissues and necessitate removal of the venous access device.
7. **Cleanse site with an antiseptic solution such as chlorhexidine or according to facility policy. Press applicator against the skin and apply chlorhexidine using a back and forth friction scrub for at least 30 seconds. Do not wipe or blot. Allow to dry completely.**	Scrubbing motion and length of time (minimum 30 seconds) is necessary for chlorhexidine to be effective (Infusion Control Today [ICT], 2005). Organisms on the skin can be introduced into the tissues or the bloodstream with the needle. Chlorhexidine is the preferred antiseptic solution, but iodine, povidone-iodine, and 70% alcohol are considered acceptable alternatives (INS, 2006).
8. Open the skin protectant wipe. Apply the skin protectant to the site, making sure to cover at minimum the area to be covered with the dressing (Figure 2). Allow to dry. Place sterile transparent dressing or catheter securing/stabilization device over venipuncture site (Figure 3).	Skin protectant aids in adhesion of the dressing and decreases the risk for skin trauma when the dressing is removed. Transparent dressing allows easy visualization and protects site. Stabilization/securing devices to preserve the integrity of the access device and to prevent catheter migration and loss of access (INS, 2006, p. S44). Some stabilization devices act as a site dressing also.
9. Label dressing with date, time of change, and initials. Loop the tubing near the site of entry, and anchor with tape (nonallergenic) close to site (Figure 4). Resume fluid infusion, if indicated. Check that IV flow is accurate and system is patent (Refer to Skill 40-3).	Labeling helps ensure communication about venous access site dressing change. The weight of the tubing is sufficient to pull it out of the vein if it is not well anchored. Nonallergenic tape is less likely to tear fragile skin.

ACTION

FIGURE 2. Applying skin protectant to site.

RATIONALE

FIGURE 3. Applying transparent dressing to site.

FIGURE 4. Site dressing with label and anchored tubing.

10. Remove equipment. Ensure patient's comfort. Remove gloves. Lower bed, if not in lowest position.	Promotes patient comfort and safety. Removing gloves properly reduces the risk for infection transmission and contamination of other items.
11. Remove additional PPE, if used. Perform hand hygiene.	Removing PPE properly reduces the risk for infection transmission and contamination of other items. Hand hygiene prevents transmission of microorganisms.

DOCUMENTATION

Guidelines

Document the location of the venous access as well as the condition of the site. Include the presence or absence of signs of erythema or redness, swelling, or drainage. Document the clinical criteria for site complications (Refer to Table 40-12, Box 40-1, and Box 40-2). Record the subjective comments of the patient regarding the absence or presence of pain at the site. Record the patient's reaction to the procedure and pertinent patient teaching, such as alerting the nurse if the patient experiences any pain from the IV or notices any swelling at the site.

Sample Documentation

11/15/12 1120 Dressing change to IV site in L hand (dorsal metacarpal) complete. Site without erythema, redness, edema, or drainage. D_5 NS infusing at 75 mL/hr. Patient instructed to call nurse with any pain, swelling, or questions.

—*S. Barnes, RN*

(continued)

Skill · 40-4 Changing a Peripheral Venous Access Dressing *continued*

UNEXPECTED SITUATIONS AND ASSOCIATED INTERVENTIONS	• *Patient complains that IV site feels "funny" and hurts:* Observe venous access site for redness, edema, and warmth. If present, clamp the tubing to stop the IV solution flow, remove the catheter, and apply a gauze dressing. Initiate a new venous access in a different site. Record site assessment and interventions, as well as site for new venous access.

SPECIAL CONSIDERATIONS
Infant and Child Considerations

• For neonates, isopropyl alcohol or products containing isopropyl alcohol are not recommended for access site preparation. Povidone-iodine or chlorhexidine solution is recommended but requires complete removal after the preparatory procedure with sterile water or sterile saline to prevent product absorption (INS, 2006, p. S42).

• Chlorhexidine has been associated with contact dermatitis when used for infants weighing less than 1,000 grams. It should be used with caution with this patient population (INS, 2006).

Skill · 40-5 Capping for Intermittent Use and Flushing a Peripheral Venous Access Device

EQUIPMENT

- End cap device
- Clean gloves
- Additional PPE, as indicated

- 4″ × 4″ gauze pad
- Normal saline flush prepared in a syringe (1–3 mL) according to facility policy

- Antimicrobial wipe
- Tape

IMPLEMENTATION

ACTION	RATIONALE
1. Determine the need for conversion to an intermittent access. Verify medical order. Check facility policy. Gather all equipment and bring to bedside.	Ensures correct intervention for correct patient. Having equipment available saves time and facilitates accomplishment of procedure.
2. Perform hand hygiene and put on PPE, if indicated.	Hand hygiene and PPE prevent the spread of microorganisms. PPE is required based on transmission precautions.
3. Identify the patient.	Identifying the patient ensures the right patient receives the intervention and helps prevent errors.
4. Close curtains around bed and close door to room if possible. Explain what you are going to do and why you are going to do it to the patient. Ask the patient about allergies to tape and skin antiseptics.	This ensures the patient's privacy. Explanation relieves anxiety and facilitates cooperation. Possible allergies may exist related to tape or antiseptics.
5. Assess the IV site. Refer to Skill 40-3.	Complications such as infiltration, phlebitis, or infection necessitate discontinuation of the IV infusion at that site.
6. If using an electronic infusion device, stop the device (Figure 1). Close the roller clamp on the administration set. If using gravity infusion, close the roller clamp on the administration set.	The action of the infusion device needs to be stopped and clamps closed to prevent leaking of fluid when tubing is disconnected.
7. Put on gloves. Close the clamp on the short extension tubing connected to the IV catheter in the patient's arm.	Clamping the tubing on the extension set prevents introduction of air into the extension tubing.
8. Remove the administration set tubing from the extension set. Cleanse the end cap with an antimicrobial swab.	Removing the infusion tubing discontinues the infusion. Cleaning the cap reduces the risk for contamination.
9. Insert the saline flush syringe into the cap on the extension tubing. Pull back on the syringe to aspirate the catheter for positive blood return. If positive, instill the solution over 1 minute or flush the line according to facility policy (Figure 2). Remove syringe and reclamp the extension tubing.	Positive blood return confirms patency prior to administration of medications and solutions (INS, 2006, p. S56). Flushing maintains patency of the IV line. Action of positive pressure end cap is maintained with removal of syringe before clamp is engaged. Clamping prevents air from entering the extension set.

ACTION

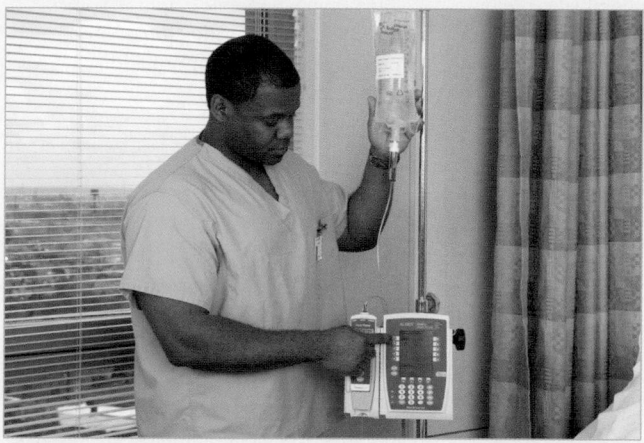

FIGURE 1. Stopping IV fluid infusion.

RATIONALE

FIGURE 2. Flushing venous access device.

10. If necessary, loop the extension tubing near the site of entry, and anchor with tape (nonallergenic) close to site.	The weight of the tubing is sufficient to pull it out of the vein if it is not well anchored. Nonallergenic tape is less likely to tear fragile skin.
11. Remove equipment. Ensure patient's comfort. Remove gloves. Lower bed, if not in lowest position.	Promotes patient comfort and safety. Removing gloves properly reduces the risk for infection transmission and contamination of other items.
12. Remove additional PPE, if used. Perform hand hygiene.	Removing PPE properly reduces the risk for infection transmission and contamination of other items. Hand hygiene prevents transmission of microorganisms.

DOCUMENTATION

Guidelines

Document discontinuation of IV fluid infusion. Record the condition of the venous access site. Document the flushing of the venous access device. This is often done in the MAR. Record the patient's reaction to the procedure and any patient teaching that occurred.

UNEXPECTED SITUATIONS AND ASSOCIATED INTERVENTIONS

- *Peripheral venous access site leaks fluid when flushed:* To prevent infection and other complications, remove from site and restart in another location.
- *IV does not flush easily:* Assess insertion site. Infiltration and/or phlebitis may be present. If present, remove and restart in another location. In addition, the catheter may be blocked or clotted due to a kinked catheter at the insertion site. Aspirate and attempt to flush again. If resistance remains, do not force. Forceful flushing can dislodge a clot at the end of the catheter. Remove and restart in another location. If assessment reveals the catheter has pulled out a short distance, do not reinsert it: it is no longer sterile. Remove and restart in another location.

SPECIAL CONSIDERATIONS

- Some facilities may use end caps for venous access devices that are not positive pressure devices. In this case, flush with the recommended volume of saline, ending with 0.5 mL of solution remaining in syringe. While maintaining pressure on the syringe, clamp the extension tubing. This provides positive pressure, preventing backflow of blood into the catheter, decreasing risk for occlusion.

Skill · 40-6   Administering a Blood Transfusion

EQUIPMENT

- Blood product
- Blood administration set (tubing with in-line filter and Y for saline administration)
- 0.9% normal saline for IV infusion
- IV pole

- Venous access; if peripheral site, preferably initiated with a 20-gauge catheter or larger
- Clean gloves
- Additional PPE, as indicated

- Tape (hypoallergenic)
- Second RN for verification of blood product and patient information

IMPLEMENTATION

ACTION	RATIONALE
1. Verify the medical order for transfusion of blood product. Verify the completion of informed consent documentation in the medical record. Verify any medical order for pretransfusion medication. If ordered, administer medication at least 30 minutes prior to initiating transfusion.	Verification of order ensures patient receives correct intervention. Premedication is sometimes administered to decrease risk for allergic and febrile reactions for patients who have received multiple previous transfusions.
2. Gather all equipment and bring to bedside.	Having equipment available saves time and facilitates accomplishment of procedure.
3. Perform hand hygiene and put on PPE, if indicated.	Hand hygiene and PPE prevent the spread of microorganisms. PPE is required based on transmission precautions.
4. Identify the patient.	Identifying the patient ensures the right patient receives the intervention and helps prevent errors.
5. Close curtains around bed and close door to room if possible. Explain what you are going to do and why you are going to do it to the patient. Ask the patient about previous experience with transfusion and any reactions. Advise patient to report any chills, itching, rash, or unusual symptoms.	This ensures the patient's privacy. Explanation relieves anxiety and facilitates cooperation. Previous reactions may increase risk for reaction to this transfusion. Any reaction to the transfusion necessitates stopping the transfusion immediately and evaluation of the situation.
6. Prime blood administration set with the normal saline IV fluid. Refer to Skill 40-2.	Normal saline is the solution of choice for blood product administration. Solutions with dextrose may lead to clumping of red blood cells and hemolysis.
7. Put on gloves. If patient does not have a venous access in place, initiate peripheral venous access. Refer to Skill 40-1. Connect the administration set to the venous access device via the extension tubing. Refer to Skill 40-1. Infuse the normal saline per facility policy.	Gloves prevent contact with blood and body fluids. Infusion of fluid via venous access maintains patency until blood product is administered. Start an IV before obtaining blood product in case the initiation takes longer than 30 minutes. Blood must be stored at a carefully controlled temperature (4°C) and transfusion must begin within 30 minutes of release from the blood bank.
8. Obtain blood product from blood bank according to agency policy. Scan for bar codes on blood products if required.	Bar codes on blood products are currently being implemented in some agencies to identify, track, and assign data to transfusions as an additional safety measure.
9. Two nurses compare and validate the following information with the medical record, patient identification band, and the label of the blood product: • Medical order for transfusion of blood product • Informed consent • Patient identification number • Patient name • Blood group and type • Expiration date • Inspection of blood product for clots	Most states/agencies require two registered nurses to verify the following information: unit numbers match, ABO group and Rh type are the same, expiration date (after 35 days, red blood cells begin to deteriorate). Blood is never administered to a patient without an identification band. If clots are present, return blood to the blood bank.
10. **Obtain baseline set of vital signs before beginning transfusion.**	Any change in vital signs during the transfusion may indicate a reaction.
11. Put on gloves. If using an electronic infusion device, put the device on "hold." Close the roller clamp closest to the drip chamber on the saline side of the administration set. Close the roller clamp on administration set below the infusion device. Alternately, if using infusing via gravity, close the roller clamp on the administration set.	Gloves prevent contact with blood and body fluids. Stopping the infusion prevents blood from infusing to patient prior to completion of preparations. Closing clamp to saline allow blood product to be infused via electronic infusion device.

ACTION	RATIONALE

12. Close the roller clamp closest to the drip chamber on the blood product side of the administration set. Remove the protective cap from the access port on the blood container. Remove the cap from the access spike on the administration set. Using a pushing and twisting motion, insert the spike into the access port on the blood container, taking care not to contaminate spike. Hang blood container on the IV pole. Open the roller clamp on the blood side of the administration set. Squeeze drip chamber until the in-line filter is saturated (Figure 1). Remove gloves.

Filling the drip chamber prevents air from entering administration set. The filter in the blood administration set removes particulate material formed during storage of blood. If administration set is contaminated, entire set would have to be discarded and replaced.

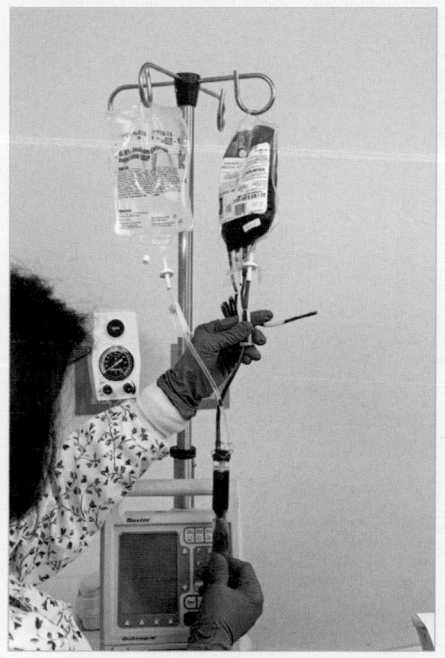

FIGURE 1. Starting transfusion slowly.

13. **Start administration slowly (no more than 25–50 mL for the first 15 minutes). Stay with the patient for the first 5 to 15 minutes of transfusion.** Open the roller clamp on administration set below the infusion device. Set the rate of flow and begin the transfusion. Alternately, start the flow of solution by releasing the clamp on the tubing and counting the drops. Adjust until the correct drop rate is achieved. Assess the flow of the blood and function of the infusion device. Inspect the insertion site for signs of infiltration.

Transfusion reactions typically occur during this period, and a slow rate will minimize the volume of red blood cells infused. Verifying the rate and device settings ensures patient receives correct volume of solution. If catheter or needle slips out of the vein, the blood will accumulate (infiltrate) into the surrounding tissue.

14. Observe patient for flushing, dyspnea, itching, hives or rash, or any unusual comments.

These signs and symptoms may be an early indication of a transfusion reaction.

15. After the observation period (5–15 minutes), increase the infusion rate to the calculated rate to complete the infusion within the prescribed time frame, no greater than 4 hours.

If there have been no adverse effects during this time, the infusion rate is increased. If complications occur, they can be observed and the transfusion can be stopped immediately. Verifying the rate and device settings ensures patient receives correct volume of solution. Transfusion must be completed within 4 hours due to potential for bacterial growth in blood product at room temperature.

(continued)

Skill · 40-6 **Administering a Blood Transfusion** *continued*

ACTION

RATIONALE

16. Reassess vital signs after 15 minutes (Figure 2). Obtain vital signs thereafter according to facility policy and nursing assessment.

Vital signs must be assessed as part of monitoring for possible adverse reaction. Facility policy and nursing judgment will dictate frequency.

FIGURE 2. Assessing vital signs after 15 minutes.

17. Maintain the prescribed flow rate as ordered or as deemed appropriate based on the patient's overall condition, keeping in mind the outer limits for safe administration. Ongoing monitoring is crucial throughout the entire duration of the blood transfusion for early identification of any adverse reactions.

Rate must be carefully controlled, and patient's reaction must be monitored frequently.

18. **During transfusion, assess frequently for transfusion reaction. Stop blood transfusion if you suspect a reaction. Quickly replace the blood tubing with a new administration set primed with normal saline for IV infusion. Initiate an infusion of normal saline for IV at an open rate, usually 40 mL/hour. Obtain vital signs. Notify physician and blood bank.**

If a transfusion reaction is suspected, the blood must be stopped. Do not infuse the normal saline through the blood tubing because you would be allowing more of the blood into the patient's body, which could complicate a reaction. Besides a serious life-threatening blood transfusion reaction, the potential for fluid-volume overload exists in elderly patients and patients with decreased cardiac function.

19. When transfusion is complete, close roller clamp on blood side of the administration set and open the roller clamp on the normal saline side of the administration set. Initiate infusion of normal saline. When all of blood has infused into patient, clamp administration set. Obtain vital signs. Put on gloves. Cap access site or resume previous IV infusion (Refer to Skills 40-1 and 40-5). Dispose of blood-transfusion equipment or return to blood bank according to facility policy.

Saline prevents hemolysis of red blood cells and clears remainder of blood in IV line.

Proper disposal of equipment reduces transmission of microorganisms and potential contact with blood and body fluids.

20. Remove equipment. Ensure patient's comfort. Remove gloves. Lower bed, if not in lowest position.

Promotes patient comfort and safety. Removing gloves properly reduces the risk for infection transmission and contamination of other items.

21. Remove additional PPE, if used. Perform hand hygiene.

Removing PPE properly reduces the risk for infection transmission and contamination of other items. Hand hygiene prevents transmission of microorganisms.

DOCUMENTATION

Guidelines

Document that the patient received the blood transfusion; include the type of blood product. Record the patient's condition throughout the transfusion, including pertinent data, such as vital signs, lung sounds, and the subjective response of the patient to transfusion. Document any complications or reactions, or that the patient received the transfusion without any complications or reactions. Document the assessment of the IV site and any other fluids infused during the procedure. Document transfusion volume and other IV fluid intake on the patient's intake and output record.

Sample Documentation

11/2/12 1100 T 97.6°F P 82 R 14 B/P 116/74. 1 unit of packed blood red cells initiated via left forearm (basilic) 18-gauge venous access without difficulty. Pt states "no discomfort." IV site intact, no swelling, redness, or pain.

—*S. Barnes, RN*

11/2/12 1115 T 97.6°F P 78 R 16 B/P 118/68. 1 unit of packed blood red cells infusing via left forearm (basilic) 18-gauge venous access without difficulty. Pt states "no discomfort." IV site intact, no swelling, redness, or pain.

—*S. Barnes, RN*

11/2/12 1445 T 97.6°F P 82 R 14 B/P 120/74. 1 unit of packed blood red cells completed via left forearm (basilic) 18-gauge venous access without difficulty. Pt denies symptoms of complications. IV site intact, no swelling, redness, or pain.

—*S. Barnes, RN*

UNEXPECTED SITUATIONS AND ASSOCIATED INTERVENTIONS

- *Patient is becoming febrile but is exhibiting no other signs of a transfusion reaction:* Notify primary care provider. The primary care provider may order acetaminophen and an antihistamine for the patient.

- *Patient reports shortness of breath; on auscultation you note crackles bilaterally in the bases:* Compare vital signs to normal vital sounds for this patient. Obtain a pulse oximetry reading. Notify primary care provider. The primary care provider may order a dose of a diuretic or may decrease the rate of the transfusion. Continue to assess the patient for signs and symptoms of fluid overload.

- *Patient is febrile, tachycardic, and complaining of back pain:* Patient is having a transfusion reaction. Stop the transfusion immediately. Obtain new IV tubing with 0.9% sodium chloride. Notify primary care provider and blood bank. Send blood unit, tubing, and filter to the lab. Obtain additional diagnostics tests, such as blood and urine tests, based on facility policy.

SPECIAL CONSIDERATIONS

General Considerations

- If an electronic infusion device is used to maintain the prescribed rate, ensure it is designed for use with blood transfusions prior to initiation of transfusion.

- Never warm blood in a microwave. Use a blood-warming device, if indicated or ordered, especially with rapid transfusions through a CVAD. Rapid administration of cold blood can result in cardiac arrhythmias.

Home Care Considerations

- Home care agencies evaluate patients who are candidates for a blood transfusion at home.

- Home transfusion is not appropriate for patients who are actively bleeding or recently had a reaction to a blood transfusion.

- The nurse transports the blood product to the patient's home in a special cooler. The nurse and the patient's caregiver check the serial number and other identification information together.

● Developing Critical Thinking Skills

1. Assess a healthy individual and a patient whose fluid and electrolyte or acid–base balance is altered using Tables 40-4 and 40-5, which describes parameters to be considered in physical and clinical assessments for fluid, electrolyte, and acid–base balance. Compare and contrast your findings.

2. Review the record of a patient who has been receiving IV fluids over a period of 3 or more days. Note the daily intake and output records, pertinent laboratory values, and clinical behaviors, and make a judgment about the patient's fluid, electrolyte, and acid–base balance. What factors complicate a hospitalized patient's usual ability to remain in balance?

● Practicing for NCLEX

1. Plasma, the liquid constituent of blood, is correctly identified as which of the following?
   a. Interstitial fluid
   b. Intravascular fluid
   c. Intracellular fluid
   d. 40% of total body fluid

2. Potassium functions as which of the following?
   a. The chief electrolyte of extracellular fluid
   b. The most abundant electrolyte in the body
   c. The major cation of intracellular fluid
   d. The chief extracellular anion

3. The movement of the solvent water from an area of lesser solute concentration to an area of greater solute concentration until equilibrium is established is known as:
   a. Osmosis
   b. Diffusion
   c. Active transport
   d. Filtration

4. Which of the following would the nurse use as the most reliable indicator of a patient's fluid balance status?
   a. Intake and output
   b. Skin turgor
   c. Complete blood count
   d. Daily weight

5. Which acid–base imbalance would the nurse suspect after assessing the following arterial blood gas values (pH, 7.30; $PaCO_2$, 36 mm Hg; HCO_3^-, 14 mEq/L)?
   a. Respiratory acidosis
   b. Respiratory alkalosis
   c. Metabolic acidosis
   d. Metabolic alkalosis

6. A patient has been encouraged to increase her fluid intake. Which measure would be most effective for the nurse to implement?

   a. Explaining the mechanisms involved in transporting fluids to and from intracellular compartments
   b. Keeping fluids readily available for the patient
   c. Emphasizing the long-term outcome of increasing fluids when she returns home
   d. Planning to offer most daily fluids in the evening

7. Which of the following would the nurse need to keep in mind when preparing to assist the physician with insertion of a nontunneled percutaneous central venous catheter?
   a. This catheter usually remains in place for 2 to 3 months.
   b. The catheter is introduced via the basilic or cephalic veins in the antecubital space.
   c. Nursing responsibility includes accessing the catheter with an angled needle.
   d. A chest radiograph is required to confirm placement.

8. The nurse alertly assesses the acid–base balance of a patient because she is aware that the patient will be unable to effectively control his carbonic acid supply. This is most likely a patient with bad damage to which of the following?
   a. Kidneys
   b. Lungs
   c. Adrenal glands
   d. Blood vessels

9. The nurse instructs a patient to focus on breathing more slowly as the most effective intervention for which acid–base imbalance?
   a. Respiratory acidosis (carbonic acid excess)
   b. Respiratory alkalosis (carbonic acid deficit)
   c. Metabolic acidosis (base bicarbonate deficit)
   d. Metabolic alkalosis (base bicarbonate excess)

10. Which of the following is the most common etiologic factor related to the nursing diagnosis of Excess Fluid Volume?
    a. Increased need for fluids secondary to fever
    b. Abnormal fluid loss from vomiting
    c. Excessive IV infusion
    d. Decreased fluid intake secondary to depression

11. Which assessment finding would lead the nurse to suspect that a patient's IV has infiltrated?
    a. In the past hour, only 50 mL of fluid has infused.
    b. The insertion site is red, hot, and swollen.
    c. The patient's temperature has risen to 101°F (38.3°C).
    d. The site is pale, cool, swollen, and painful.

12. When developing the teaching plan for a patient at risk for hyperkalemia, which foods would the nurse instruct the patient to avoid?
    a. Carrots and squash
    b. Canned soups and potato chips
    c. Bananas and apricots
    d. Whole-grain cereals and milk

13. Which site would be most appropriate for initiating IV therapy for a patient who has sustained multiple injuries after an automobile accident and has a cast on his right arm?
   a. Left antecubital
   b. Dorsal aspect of either foot
   c. Right hand
   d. Left forearm

14. When implementing the plan of care for a patient receiving IV therapy, which intervention would be most appropriate?
   a. Changing the IV catheter and entry site daily
   b. Changing the tubing every 8 hours
   c. Increasing the rate to catch up if the correct amount has not been infused at the end of the shift
   d. Monitoring the flow rate at least every hour

15. While administering a blood transfusion, when would the nurse assess the patient for a blood transfusion reaction?
   a. 15 minutes after the infusion is started
   b. After the blood is all infused
   c. Every hour
   d. Every 15 minutes

● Answers With Rationale

1. **b.** Intravascular fluid or plasma is extracellular fluid and composes 5% of total body fluid.

2. **c.** Potassium is the major cation of the intracellular fluid. Sodium is the chief electrolyte of extracellular fluid (*a*), calcium is the most abundant electrolyte in the body (*b*), and chloride is the chief extracellular anion (*d*).

3. **a.** Water moves by osmosis. Gases move by diffusion (*b*). Active transport (*c*) is a process that requires energy for the movement of substances through a cell membrane from an area of lesser to higher concentration. Filtration (*d*) is the passage of fluids through a permeable membrane from an area of high pressure to one of low pressure.

4. **d.** Daily weight is the most reliable indicator of a person's fluid balance status. Intake and output (*a*) are not always as accurate and may involve a subjective component. Measurement of skin turgor (*b*) is subjective, and the complete blood count (*c*) does not necessarily reflect fluid balance.

5. **c.** A low pH indicates acidosis. This, coupled with a low bicarbonate, indicates metabolic acidosis. The pH and bicarbonate would be elevated with metabolic alkalosis (*d*). Decreased $PaCO_2$ in conjunction with a low pH indicates respiratory acidosis (*a*); increased $PaCO_2$ in conjunction with an elevated pH indicates respiratory alkalosis (*b*).

6. **b.** Having fluids readily available helps promote intake. Explanation of the fluid transportation mechanisms (*a*)

is inappropriate and does not focus on the immediate problem of increasing fluid intake. Meeting short-term outcomes rather than long-term ones (*c*) provides further reinforcement, and additional fluids should be taken earlier in the day.

7. **d.** A chest radiograph is needed to ensure proper placement for any central venous access device. In addition, nontunneled percutaneous central venous catheters remain in place for 3 to 7 days, are introduced into the subclavian or internal jugular vein, and are never accessed through an angled needle (*c*) (used with an implanted port).

8. **b.** The lungs are the primary controller of the body's carbonic acid supply and thus, if damaged, can affect acid–base balance. The kidneys (*a*) are the primary controller of the body's bicarbonate supply. The adrenal glands (*c*) secrete catecholamines and steroid hormones. The blood vessels (*d*) act only as a transport system.

9. **b.** Breathing more slowly causes accumulation of carbon dioxide to reverse carbonic acid deficit or respiratory alkalosis. Breathing more slowly would further increase a patient's respiratory acidosis (*a*) due to the increased carbon dioxide. Decreasing the respiratory rate would not be effective for a metabolic acid–base balance (*c*).

10. **c.** Excessive IV infusion is the most common factor associated with excess fluid volume. The other alternatives are related to deficient fluid volume.

11. **d.** A decrease in flow rate may indicate an infiltration but is not as significant as the other signs of a pale, cool, swollen, and painful site. Phlebitis is an inflammatory process and results in redness, warmth, and possibly a temperature elevation (*b* and *c*).

12. **c.** Hyperkalemia is an elevated serum potassium level; bananas and apricots are foods high in potassium and should be avoided in this situation. The other foods listed would be allowed. Canned foods and potato chips (*b*) would be avoided if the patient had excess sodium levels.

13. **d.** The left forearm is the best site selection because of the condition of the patient's right arm. The left forearm is preferable to the antecubital space of the left arm (*a*) or the lower extremities (*b*).

14. **d.** The flow rate requires close monitoring, at least every hour. The IV catheter and entry site should be changed every 48 to 72 hours in most circumstances (*a*). The tubing is changed according to agency policy but not at the frequency of every 8 hours (*b*). Increasing the rate may lead to fluid overload (*c*).

15. **d.** The nurse should closely observe a patient for the first 15 minutes and then check the patient thereafter every 15 minutes while he or she is receiving the blood transfusion.

Taylor Suite Resources

The Taylor Suite offers these additional resources to enhance learning and facilitate understanding of this chapter:

- thePoint online resource, http://thepoint.lww.com/Taylor7E
- Student DVD-ROM included with the book
- Study Guide for Taylor's Fundamentals of Nursing
- Skill Checklists for Taylor's Fundamentals of Nursing
- Taylor's Clinical Nursing Skills: *Chapter 15, Fluid, Electrolyte, and Acid–Base Balance*
- Taylor's Video Guide to Clinical Nursing Skills: *Intravenous Therapy and Central Venous Access Devices*

BIBLIOGRAPHY

Advice p.r.n.: Venipuncture. Armed with the facts. (2008). *Nursing, 38(6),* 10.

American Red Cross. Blood eligibility requirements. Available www.redcrossblood.org/donating-blood/eligibility-requirements.

Arbique, J., & Arbique, D. (2007). IV rounds. Reducing the risk of nerve injuries. *Nursing, 37*(11), 20–21.

Best Practices: Evidence-based nursing procedures. (2007). (2nd ed.).Philadelphia: Wolters Kluwer Health/Lippincott Williams & Wilkins.

Bleasdale, S., Trick, W., Gonzalez, I., Lyles, R., Hayden, M., & Weinstein, R. (2007). Effectiveness of chlorhexidine bathing to reduce catheter-associated bloodstream infections in medical intensive care unit patients. *Archives of Internal Medicine, 167*(19), 2073–2079.

Bulechek, G., Butcher, H., & McCloskey Dochterman, J. (Eds.). (2008). *Nursing interventions classification (NIC)* (5th ed.). St. Louis, MO: Mosby Elsevier.

Carpenito-Moyet, L. (2008). *Nursing diagnosis: Application to clinical practice* (12th ed.). Philadelphia: Wolters Kluwer Health/Lippincott Williams & Wilkins.

Centers for Disease Control and Prevention (CDC). (2002). Guidelines for the prevention of intravascular catheter-related infections. *Morbidity and Mortality Weekly Report, 51*(RR10), 1–32. Available at http://www.cdc.gov/mmwr/preview/mmwrhtml/rr5110a1.htm.

Clancy, J., & McVicar, A. (2007a). Intermediate and long-term regulation of acid–base homeostasis. *British Journal of Nursing, 16*(17), 1076–1079.

Clancy, J., & McVicar, A. (2007b). Short-term regulation of acid–base homeostasis of body fluids. *British Journal of Nursing, 16*(16), 1016–1021.

Coggon, J. (2008a). Arterial blood gas analysis 1: Understanding ABG reports. *Nursing Times, 104*(18), 28–29.

Coggon, J. (2008b). Arterial blood gas analysis 2: Compensatory mechanisms. *Nursing Times, 104*(19), 24–25.

David, K. (2007). IV fluids: Do you know what's hanging and why? *RN, 70*(10), 35–40.

Dudek, S. (2006). *Nutrition essentials for nursing practice* (5th ed.). Philadelphia: Lippincott Williams & Wilkins.

Evans, S. (2008). Sticking point. New nurse-led initiatives aim to manage pain for children during venous access procedures. *Advance for Nurses, 10*(1), 27–28.

Fischbach, F., & Dunning, M. (2006). *Common laboratory values and diagnostic tests.* Philadelphia: Lippincott Williams & Wilkins.

Fischbach, F., & Dunning, M. (2009). *A manual of laboratory and diagnostic tests* (8th ed.). Philadelphia: Wolters Kluwer Health/Lippincott Williams & Wilkins.

Fluids & electrolytes: A 2-in-1 reference for nurses. (2006). Philadelphia: Wolters Kluwer Health/Lippincott Williams & Wilkins.

Fluids & electrolytes made incredibly easy. (2008). (4th ed.). Philadelphia: Wolters Kluwer Health/Lippincott Williams & Wilkins.

Gabriel, J. (2008a). Infusion therapy part one: Minimising the risks. *Nursing Standard, 22*(31), 51–56.

Gabriel, J. (2008b). Infusion therapy part two: Prevention and management of complications. *Nursing Standard, 22*(32), 41–48.

Griffiths, V. (2007). Midline catheters: Indications, complications, and maintenance. *Nursing Standard, 22*(11), 48–57.

Hadaway, L. (2006). Technology of flushing vascular access devices. *Journal of Infusion Nursing, 29*(3), 137–145.

Hadaway, L. (2005). Administering parenteral nutrition with other I.V. drugs. *Nursing, 35*(2), 26.

Hammond, T. (2004). Choice and use of peripherally inserted central catheters by nurses. *Professional Nurse, 19*(9), 493–497.

Hankins, J. (2007). I.V. rounds. The role of albumin in fluid balance. *Nursing, 37*(12), 14–15.

Haskal, R. (2007). Current issues for nurse practitioners: Hyponatremia. *Journal of the American Academy of Nurse Practitioners, 19*(11), 563–579.

Holcomb, S. (2008). Third-spacing: When body fluid shifts. *Nursing, 38*(7), 50–53.

Infection Control Today (ICT). (2005). *Chlorbexidine: The prefered skin antiseptic:* Available at www.infectioncontroltoday.com/articles/406/406–52/feat4.htm. Accessed March 9, 2010.

Infusion Nurses Society (INS). (2006). Infusion nursing standards of practice. *Journal of Infusion Nursing, 29*(1S), S1–S92.

Ingram, P. (2006). The safe removal of central venous catheters. *Nursing Standard, 20*(49), 42–46.

Institute for Safe Medication Practices (ISMP). (2007). Smart pumps are not smart on their own. Available at www.ismp.org/Newsletters/acutecare/articles/20070419.asp?ptr=y.

I.V. Rounds. Comparing short peripheral cannula insertion sites. (2008). *Nursing, 38*(5), 60.

Jarvis, C. (2008). *Physical examination & health assessment* (5th ed.). St. Louis: Saunders/Elsevier.

Joanna Briggs Institute. (2008). Best practice. Management of peripheral intravascular devices. *Australian Nursing Journal, 16*(3), 25–28.

The Joint Commission. (2010). *2009 National Patient Safety Goals.* Available at www.jointcommission.org/PatientSafety/NationalPatientSafetyGoals.

Kear, T. (2005). Fluid & electrolyte balance. Nurses' early recognition of imbalances often can prevent complications. *Advance Extra/Advance for Nurses,* Supplement. 27–29.

Konick-McMahan, J. (2008). Calcium imbalances. Hyper- and hypocalcemia can lead to life-threatening events. *Advance for Nurses, 10*(13), 33–35.

Kyle, T. (2008). *Essentials of pediatric nursing.* Philadelphia: Wolters Kluwer/Lippincott Williams & Wilkins.

Lavery, I. (2005). Peripheral intravenous therapy: Key risks and implications for practice. *Nursing Standard, 19*(46), 55–64.

Masoorli, S. (2007). Nerve injuries related to vascular access insertion and assessment. *Journal of Infusion, 30*(6), 346–350.

Migdal, M., Chudzynska-Pomianowska, E., Vause, E., Henry, E., & Lazar, J. (2005). Rapid, needle-free delivery of lidocaine for reducing the pain of venipuncture among pediatric subjects. *Pediatrics, 115*(4), e393–8.

Mimoz, O., Villeminey, S., Ragot, S., Dahyot-Fizelier, C., Laksiri, L., Petitpas, F., et al. (2007). Chlorhexidine-based antiseptic solution vs alcohol-based povidone-iodine for central venous catheter care. *Archives of Internal Medicine, 167*(19), 2066–2072.

Moorhead, S., Johnson, M., Maas, M., & Swanson, E. (Eds.). (2008). *Nursing outcomes classification (NOC)* (4th ed.). St. Louis, MO: Mosby Elsevier.

Morris, W., & Heong Tay, M. (2008). Strategies for preventing peripheral intravenous cannula infection. *British Journal of Nursing, 17*(19) Supplement, S14–S21.

NANDA International. (2009). *Nursing diagnoses: Definitions and classification 2009–2011.* West Sussex, UK: Wiley-Blackwell.

Portable fluids & electrolytes. (2008). Philadelphia: Wolters Kluwer Health/Lippincott Williams & Wilkins.

Porth, C., & Matfin, G. (2009). *Pathophysiology: Concepts of altered health states* (8th ed.). Philadelphia: Wolters Kluwer Health/Lippincott Williams & Wilkins.

Rosenthal, K. (2006). I.V. rounds. Intravenous fluids: The whys and wherefores. *Nursing, 36*(7), 26–27.

Scales, K. (2008). Intravenous therapy: A guide to good practice. *British Journal of Nursing, 17*(19) Supplement, S4–S12.

Scales, K., & Pilsworth, J. (2008). The importance of fluid balance in clinical practice. *Nursing Standard, 22*(47), 50–57.

Smeltzer, S., Bare, B., Hinkle, J., & Cheever, K. (2010). *Brunner & Suddarth's textbook of medical-surgical nursing* (12th ed.). Philadelphia: Wolters Kluwer Health/Lippincott Williams & Wilkins.

Smith, B., & Hannum, F. (2008). Optimizing IV therapy in the elderly. *Advance for Nurses, 10*(18), 27–28.

Sudakin, T. (2006). Supporting nutrition with T.E.N. or T.P.N. *Nursing, 36*(32), 52–55.

Tabloski, P. (2006). *Gerontological nursing.* Upper Saddle River, NJ: Pearson Prentice Hall.

Tsuchida, T., Makimoto, K., Toki, M., Sakai, K., Onaka, E., & Otani, Y. (2007). The effectiveness of a nurse-initiated intervention to reduce catheter-associated bloodstream infections in an urban acute hospital: An intervention study with before and after comparison. *International Journal of Nursing Studies, 44*(8), 1324–1333.

Ulrich, S. P., & Canale, S. W. (2005). *Nursing care planning guides: For adults in acute, extended and home care settings* (6th ed.). St. Louis: Elsevier.

Zempsky, W., Bean-Lijewski, J., Kauffman, R., Koh, J., Malviya, S., Rose, J., et al. (2008). Needle-free powder lidocaine delivery system provided rapid effective analgesia for venipuncture or cannulation pain in children: Randomized, double-blind comparison of venipuncture and venous cannulation pain after fast-onset needle-free powder lidocaine or placebo treatment trial. *Pediatrics, 12*(5), 979–987.

PROMOTING HEALTHY PSYCHOSOCIAL RESPONSES

Every person is a composite of interrelated physiologic, psychosocial, and spiritual dimensions; alterations in one dimension affect the others.

Unit VIII discusses psychosocial considerations in holistic patient care, focusing on sense of self; stress and adaptation; loss, grief, and dying; sensory stimulation; sexuality; and spirituality.

Each individual's sense of self is critical to that person's attitudes toward health and may affect self-care abilities positively or negatively. Additionally, developmental or experiential stressors can motivate or thwart psychosocial growth and self-actualization. Nursing interventions to promote healthy psychosocial responses, including maintaining, strengthening, or changing self-concept, are basic to all aspects of patient care. Because a person's sense of self shapes his or her ability to respond to healthcare interventions, nurses include assessment and intervention to promote a positive sense of self.

Loss, grief, and dying are universal human experiences that most nurses encounter in some form on a daily basis. Effective nurses are competent and willing to assist people struggling with loss, grief, and dying.

Intact and functioning senses are necessary for life, normal growth and development, communication, and pleasurable experiences. Alterations in any of the senses require caring, knowledgeable, and individualized nursing interventions to meet needs, enhance individual independence, and prevent further overload or deprivation.

Sexuality and spirituality are important components of human functioning. These dimensions are an integral part of each person's identity and are critical elements in holistic patient care. Nurses recognize the importance of these areas for optimal health and use their knowledge and skills to assist patients to enhance wellness in these areas.

To facilitate wellness in each of these psychosocial spheres, nurses must develop self-awareness, including knowledge of their own personal attitudes, values, perceptions, and practices, as well as understand how others differ in these characteristics. Nurses, own personal biases, including the ability to accept others who have cultural, spiritual, racial, ethnic, or sexual identity characteristics that differ from their own, affect their ability to plan and provide optimal care. Nursing interventions and therapeutic interpersonal skills are used to elicit concerns, identify needs, implement teaching, make referrals, and demonstrate empathic caring and acceptance.

"The unique function of the nurse is to assist the individual . . . in the performance of those activities contributing to health or its recovery (or to peaceful death) that he would perform unaided if he had the necessary strength, will or knowledge . . . in such a way as to help him gain independence as rapidly as possible."

VIRGINIA HENDERSON (1897–1996) • *the "first lady of nursing," whose career spanned almost 70 years as both author and researcher; her works on nursing principles are research based and have been translated into 25 languages*

41 | Self-Concept

MELISSA MOTSKY

Melissa is a 31-year-old married mother of three children ages 12, 10, and 8 who is a third-year nursing student in academic jeopardy. Melissa cries and calls herself a failure when she speaks to her academic advisor. She sees no way to work herself out of her current predicament.

ANTHONY SANTORINI

Anthony is a middle-aged man with a history of diabetes. He recently underwent a below-the-knee amputation due to complications resulting from poor glucose control. One morning, he states, "I feel like damaged goods. I'm not a whole man anymore."

DELORES SPARKS

Delores is a 72-year-old African American widow, diagnosed with advanced lung cancer 14 months ago. She was living alone in a small apartment until 9 months ago, when she had to move in with her daughter after a lengthy hospital stay because she was no longer capable of living alone, and had a probable prognosis of, at most, 3 months to live. A recent home visit revealed that the patient was increasingly depressed and feeling like a burden to her daughter. She stated, "I'm just an old dish rag, not good for anything anymore."

After completing the chapter, you will be able to accomplish the following:

1. Identify three dimensions of self-concept: self-knowledge, self-expectations, and self-evaluation (self-esteem).

2. Describe major steps in the development of self-concept.

3. Differentiate positive and negative self-concept and high and low self-esteem.

4. Identify six variables that influence self-concept.

5. Use appropriate interview questions and observations to assess a patient's self-concept.

6. Develop nursing diagnoses to identify disturbances in self-concept (body image, self-esteem, role performance, personal identity).

7. Describe nursing strategies that are effective in resolving self-concept problems.

8. Plan, implement, and evaluate nursing care related to select nursing diagnoses for disturbances in self-concept.

KEY TERMS

body image	personal identity
depersonalization	role performance
false self	self-actualization
global self	self-concept
ideal self	self-esteem
identity diffusion	

An individual's self-concept or self-image is crucial to his or her health and well-being throughout life. One's **self-concept,** which is the mental image or picture of self, has the power to either encourage or thwart personal growth. People with deficient self-concept might lack the motivation to learn self-care behaviors in response to illness, injury, and trauma. Nursing efforts aimed at teaching new health behaviors might fail until the patient values himself or herself enough to want to invest energy in self-care. Some patients observing aspects of their negative self-concept that affect their health behaviors might desperately want to make modifications but have no idea how to do so. The experience of illness, diagnostic testing, and treatment can severely threaten the self-concept of a patient. Nurses sensitive to patients' expressions of self-concept can use each nurse–patient interaction to enhance a patient's sense of self and to assist the

patient in resolving self-concept disturbances. (See the accompanying Reflective Practice box for an example.)

There are several variables that contribute to self-concept. For example, as discussed in Chapter 4, as people move through the hierarchy of human needs to higher levels, needs for self-esteem and self-actualization arise. The need for **self-esteem** is the need to feel good about oneself and to believe that others hold one in high regard. The need for **self-actualization** is the need to reach one's potential through full development of one's unique capability. At the other ends of the spectrum are identity diffusion and depersonalization. **Identity diffusion** is the failure to integrate various childhood identifications into a harmonious adult psychosocial identity, which can lead to disruptions in relationships and problems of intimacy. **Depersonalization** is the subjective experience of the partial or total disruption of one's ego and the disintegration and disorganization of one's self-concept (Stuart & Laraia, 2005). See Figure 41-1, which illustrates the continuum of self-concept responses.

OVERVIEW OF SELF-CONCEPT
Dimensions of Self-Concept

As indicated earlier, all of the feelings, beliefs, and values associated with "I" or "me" compose self-concept. Specific components of self-concept include personal identity, body image, self-esteem, and role performance. Crucial to each component are the dimensions of self-concept, which include self-knowledge, self-expectations, and self-evaluation.

People with a positive self-concept usually have greater and more diversified self-knowledge, more realistic perceptions and expectations, and a higher evaluation of themselves or self-esteem, whereas those with negative self-concept tend to exhibit poorer self-knowledge, less realistic perceptions and expectations, and lower self-esteem.

➤ *Consider Anthony Santorini, the patient with a below-the-knee amputation. Analysis of the patient's comments would indicate that the patient is experiencing a negative self-concept. The nurse would need to assess Mr. Santorini more closely to determine his self-knowledge, self-expectations, and self-evaluation for each component of self-concept. This would help the nurse identify possible factors contributing to his status and gain a fuller picture of the patient's current condition.* ∎

Self-Knowledge: "Who Am I?"

Global self is the term used to describe the composite of all the basic facts, qualities, traits, images, and feelings one holds about oneself. These strongly influence a person's ability to manage life events and ensure emotional stability. A person's self-knowledge includes:

• Basic facts (sex, age, race, occupation, cultural background, sexual orientation)

REFLECTIVE PRACTICE

Challenge to Interpersonal Skills

Mrs. Delores Sparks is a 72-year-old widowed African American woman. Before her diagnosis of advanced lung cancer 14 months ago, she lived alone in a small apartment. Nine months ago, following a lengthy hospital stay, she moved in with her daughter when it was determined that she was no longer capable of living alone and probably had, at most, 3 months to live. I was visiting her during my home health nursing experience and growing more and more concerned with her depression. Mrs. Sparks verbalized that she felt like a burden to her daughter, who has three children herself and was currently taking care of a granddaughter born to her eldest, unmarried daughter. Mrs. Sparks was being treated for her depression, but I was concerned about the effects all this was having on her self-concept. She told me she was like "an old dish rag" that wasn't good for anything anymore.

Thinking Outside the Box: Possible Courses of Action

- Try to cheer her up at each visit.
- Ignore her deteriorating self-concept, since focusing on it may only make her feel worse; it is certainly true that she has enough bad stuff going on in her life to make her feel bad.
- Explore sources of positive affirmations of her worth; try to use my professional relationship with her to communicate, "you are a person of worth and I care about you!"

Evaluating a Good Outcome: How Do I Define Success?

- Mrs. Sparks' self-concept improves.
- I learn how to communicate a sense of worth to vulnerable patients.
- I learn how to address problems with self-concept.

Personal Learning: Here's to the Future!

Unfortunately, this situation got worse before it got better. Mrs. Sparks did not always take her meds for depression, and her daughter voiced increasing frustration with her mother's mood. "Mom talks all the time now about how even God doesn't want her. She says that she may have to take her own life since God doesn't seem to be doing it!" The daughter also said that Mrs. Sparks apologized to her constantly for being such a bother. Things didn't start to change until I learned that Mrs. Sparks used to be a very important member of her Baptist church community. She stopped attending services when she got too weak to go out. This was clearly a major loss for her. When I successfully got her minister to visit, he literally turned her life around, providing her with lots of positive reinforcement for how she could use her illness to do God's work. She seemed much more peaceful now. I've also encouraged her to tell me stories about the church work she did in the past and these reminiscences seem to be helpful.

Reflection

How do you think you would respond in a similar situation? Why? What does this tell you about yourself and about the adequacy of your skills for professional practice? Can you think of other ways to respond? What factors may have contributed to the patient's feelings of being a burden to her daughter? Describe the patient's self-concept using the dimensions of self-knowledge, self-expectations, and self-evaluation. What other skills (cognitive, interpersonal, technical, ethical/legal) would you need to respond well in this situation? Do you agree with the criteria to evaluate a successful outcome? Did the nursing student meet the criteria? Please explain your answer.

FIGURE 41-1. Continuum of self-concept responses. (From Stuart, G. W., & Laraia, M.T. [2005]. *Principles and practice of psychiatric nursing* (8th ed., p. 304). St. Louis: Elsevier Mosby. Used with permission.)

- Person's position within social groups
- Qualities or traits that describe typical behaviors, feelings, moods, and other characteristics (generous, hot-headed, ambitious, intelligent, sexy)

Although some labels cannot be changed (e.g., age and race), most are subjective and sensitive to change. Some conditions associated with alterations in self-concept or global self-worth include developmental changes, life crisis, illness, and loss.

> *Think back to Delores Sparks, the older woman with advanced lung cancer who feels like a burden. When assessing the patient's global self-worth, the nurse would need to identify any developmental changes that Mrs. Sparks is experiencing that may be contributing to her current status, such as changes related to her increasing age. In addition, information about role changes, including the inability to care for herself and the need to be dependent due to her illness, in conjunction with the knowledge of her terminal condition and anticipatory grieving related to her death, would be essential for determining her feelings of global self-worth.* ■

Self-Expectations: "Who or What Do I Want to Be?"

Expectations for the self flow from various sources. The **ideal self** constitutes the self one wants to be. These self-expectations develop unconsciously early in childhood and are based on the image of role models such as parents, other caregiving figures, and public figures. These personal expectations might be healthy or unhealthy. Contrast the significance of a child's identifying a television "bad boy" or drug dealer as his hero rather than parents, government leaders, or other professional people. A **false self** might develop in individuals who have the emotional need to respond to the needs and ambitions significant people, such as parents, have for them.

Self-Evaluation: "How Well Do I Like Myself?"

Self-esteem is the evaluative and affective component of the self-concept, sometimes termed self-respect, self-approval, or self-worth. According to Maslow (1954, p. 90), all people "have a need or desire for a stable, firmly based, usually high evaluation of themselves, for self-respect or self-esteem, and for the esteem of others." Accordingly, he identified two subsets of esteem needs: (1) self-esteem needs (strength, achievement, mastery and competence, confidence in the face of the world, independence, freedom) and (2) respect needs or the need for esteem from others (status, dominance, recognition, attention, importance, appreciation). For Maslow, self-esteem comes from two major sources: how competent children think they are in various aspects of life and how much social support they receive from other people. One's

self-esteem, like the various self-images that make up one's self-concept, varies considerably depending on a specific relationship or situation.

Coopersmith (1967) identified the four bases of self-esteem as (1) significance—the way a person feels he or she is loved and approved of by the people important to that person, (2) competence—the way tasks that are considered important are performed, (3) virtue—the attainment of moral–ethical standards, and (4) power—the extent to which a person influences his or her own and others' lives. According to Coopersmith, people with high, medium, and low self-esteem differ in their expectations of the future, in their affective reactions, and in their basic styles of adapting to environmental demands. People with high self-esteem, for example, are accustomed to being well received and successful. They are able to approach people, tasks, and new situations freely, with confidence in their ability to interact and to get along with people and to respond successfully to life's challenges.

Three major self-evaluation feelings or affects found in individuals are: (1) pride, based on a positive self-evaluation; (2) guilt, based on behaviors incongruent with ideal self; and (3) shame, associated with low global self-worth. These affects are learned in early childhood within relationships with significant others and maintained through practice.

Sullivan (1953) proposed the self-representations of "good-me" and "bad-me" based on reflected appraisals of the self, learned in the context of a child's early relationship with significant others, especially parents. The child's feelings of self-esteem and self-worth develop out of his or her perceptions of the parenting figure's feelings, or affects, expressed in caring for the child. Sullivan posited that children perceived their parents' relative anxiety through a process he termed "empathy." Children exposed to higher levels of parental anxiety are at risk for developing lower self-esteem and a greater self-representation of "bad-me." As the child developed further, he or she would begin to behave in ways that confirmed the earlier self-appraisals.

Sullivan and his most important interpreter within nursing, Hildegarde Peplau (1997; 1952), emphasized the fluidity of self-appraisals throughout the life span. They taught that positive interaction at any point in a person's life with new significant others (such as nurses) who are less anxious and more accepting and nurturing than prior figures can have a positive, growth-promoting effect on that person's self-esteem and self-concept.

Bowlby (1969) developed attachment theory, which describes modes by which a young child develops and maintains feelings about the self as well as values and beliefs about the world. Attachment is a process by which the child maintains felt security via an interpersonal bond with close caregivers, most notably parents. Through a learning process based on the child's perception of the caregiver's thoughts and reactions toward him or her, the child forms a sense of self as secure or insecure, calm or anxious, likable or not. Through this process, a child also develops beliefs and feelings about others as well as individual perceptions of situations and events. Depending on how healthy the child's attachment experience is with the early caregiver, the growing child's self-esteem might vary greatly. The child's thoughts and feelings about events might closely match reality or might be distorted and out of touch with reality. Such patterns tend to remain relatively fixed into adulthood.

Formation of Self-Concept

Although self-concept is largely considered to be a social creation that develops as a result of interactions with others (Fig. 41-2), contemporary nursing researchers and others recognize that certain inborn tendencies, such as temperament when interacting with social and interpersonal experiences, are crucial in the formation of self-concept (McClowry, 2003). Psychoanalysts have also emphasized the importance of inborn traits, such as innate aggression, because they affect a child's interpersonal experiences and shape self-concept (Freud, 1961). According to the theoretical formulations stated above, the formation of self-concept includes the following:

1. An infant learns that the physical self is different from the environment. If basic needs are met, warmth and affection are experienced, and the caregivers' anxiety is minimized, then the child begins life with positive feelings about self.

2. The child next internalizes (incorporates into self) other people's attitudes toward self, including attitudes directed toward the child's innate tendencies, such as temperament and aggression. This internalization forms the foundation of self-concept. Parents or other direct caregivers play the most influential role; peers play the second most influential role. Later, the child continues to behave in ways that confirm this early self-concept.

3. The child or adult internalizes the standards of society.

FIGURE 41-2. Interaction between caregivers and the infant are important to the child's development. Feeding, holding, cuddling, and cooing are forms of interaction.

Stages in the development of the self include self-awareness (infancy), self-recognition (18 months), self-definition (3 years), and self-concept (6–7 years). Psychological conditions that foster healthy development of the self in children include:

*   Emotional warmth and acceptance
*   Effective structure and discipline
*   Clearly defined standards and limits, so that children understand what goals, procedures, and conduct are approved
*   Adequately defined roles for both older and younger members of the family
*   Established methods of handling children that produce the desired behavior, discourage misbehavior, and deal with infractions when they occur
*   Encouragement of competence and self-confidence
*   Helping children meet challenges
*   Appropriate role models
*   A stimulating and responsive environment

Formation of self-concept is further described in developmental theories, especially in Erikson's stages of development, Piaget's cognitive developmental stages, and Havighurst's developmental tasks (see Chapters 18 and 19).

Factors Affecting Self-Concept

Almost any life experience can influence a person's self-concept. Key factors include developmental considerations, culture, internal and external resources, history of success and failure, stressors, and illness or trauma.

Developmental Considerations

As a person matures, the criteria that mark the experiences necessary for a positive self-concept change. Although the infant needs a supportive environment in which all human needs are met, the growing child needs the freedom to explore and develop the ability to meet increasing personal needs. Table 41-1 highlights developmental changes affecting self-concept, related implications for nursing, and potential causes of self-concept disturbances.

➤ *Think back to Anthony Santorini, the middle-aged patient with an amputation. For the adult, society emphasizes an intact body, fitness, style, and beauty as important to fulfill role expectations. However, for Mr. Santorini, the amputation is an irreversible body change that affects these areas, ultimately altering his view of how he can function. As a result, he feels that he can no longer function in his role as a man.* ■

Culture

As a child internalizes the values of parents and peers, culture begins to influence a sense of self. If the culture is relatively stable, little tension might be experienced between

TABLE • 41-1 DEVELOPMENTAL CHANGES AFFECTING SELF-CONCEPT

Developmental Period	Changes Affecting Self-Concept	Implications for Nursing	Potential Causes of Disturbances in Self-Concept
Infancy	• No self-concept at birth • Beginning differentiation of self and nonself	• Teach parents the critical importance of providing consistent and affectionate parenting • Assess if the parents have reasonable expectations of the infant: sleeping, eating, other awake behaviors	• Unmet basic human needs • Lack of adequate body and sensory stimulation • Parents' lack of acceptance of the infant's appearance or behavior • Poor match between parent's and child's temperament or needs
Childhood	• An intact body is important to the young child who fears bodily mutilation • During middle childhood, a sense of being trusted and loved, of being competent and trustworthy develops • Differences between self and others are strong	• If invasive procedures are indicated, explain simply to the child what is being done and offer the child support • Assess the parents' ability to provide the type of developmental environment in which the child's self-concepts can evolve positively	• Dysfunctional family • Too much or too little structure • Sensory perceptual impairments
Adolescence	• Development of secondary sex characteristics; rapid body changes • Sense of self is consolidated • Emphasis on sexual identity • Parental influences on self-concept are often rejected; peers become more important; movement is toward development of own identity	• Assess adolescent's self-knowledge and understanding of body changes • Counsel adolescent regarding mature and healthy use of independence he or she craves • Provide anticipatory guidelines regarding hazards to life, health, human functioning	• Inability to accept body • Inability to resolve competing pulls to be both a child and an adult • Unhealthy peer pressure • Identify confusion
Adulthood	• Society places emphasis on intactness of body, fitness, energy, sexuality, style, productivity, sophistication, beauty • Important to meet role expectations well	• Assess how realistic the adult's expectations are and the incentive they provide for growth and development • Assist patient to deal constructively with negative influences in self-image • Preretirement counseling	• Inability to fulfill conflicting role expectations • Failure to accept role responsibility (e.g., parenting responsibilities) • Unreasonable expectations • Irreversible body change related to trauma, illness • Unsatisfying job • Failure to develop new goals to give meaning and purpose to life • Multiple stressors
Later years	• Declining physical and possibly mental abilities • Multiple losses • Increasing dependency • Impending death • Diminished choices/options	• Assess how the older person is adjusting to effects of aging • Counsel regarding meaningful use of time • Explore resources • Assess depression; substance abuse • Recognize and value elders' life experience	• Loss of significant work (retirement); feelings of uselessness • Death of spouse, significant others • Diminished physical attractiveness, strength, overall health • Multiple stressors • Fear of dependency • Change may be more difficult

what culture expects of the child and what the child expects of self. When parents, peers, and the adult world confront the child with different cultural expectations, the sense of self might be confused. For example, an adolescent might realize his or her parents live by the work ethic and believe it is necessary to rise early every day and put in a full day's work.

The adolescent's peer group has few demands placed on it and encourages the adolescent to hang out with the group. The adolescent's vocational aptitudes, meanwhile, are leading him or her to consider a music career in a rock group, which will keep the adolescent out late many nights doing something the parents do not classify as work.

Children of immigrants whose values and practices of their culture of origin vary from the culture of adoption face cultural dissonance. Parents might expect children to behave according to their own cultural norms; peers and society, as well as the adolescent's desire to "belong," create the desire to abandon old cultural beliefs, attitudes, and practices among many of these children. Conflict between parents and children, as well as cultural confusion, might occur.

Internal and External Resources

The personal strengths an individual recognizes, develops, and uses are powerful but subjective determinants of self-concept. For example, one person might use humor as both an effective coping mechanism and a successful interpersonal tool. Another person might use humor to avoid facing conflict and might feel badly about being known as a joker or clown. The degree to which an individual integrates healthy, useful internal resources or personal strengths is associated with how well a person has been able to establish a positive self-concept in the context of nurturing experiences. Self-concept is also associated with the ability to identify and use external resources such as a network of support people (see the accompanying Research in Nursing box), adequate finances, and organizational supports. People who feel more positively about themselves tend to feel connected to others and to society; they can identify and use more external resources. On the other hand, people who feel disconnected and alone tend to perceive and use fewer environmental resources.

> *Remember Delores Sparks, the older adult woman who feels like a burden? The nurse would need to assess the situation more closely to determine what external resources and supports are available for Mrs. Sparks. In the Reflective Practice display, the patient's minister helped to provide one means of support. Subsequently, Mrs. Sparks began to feel better about herself.* ■

History of Success and Failure

People with a history of repeated failure (in school, friendships, work, or marriage) might perceive themselves as failures and actually perpetuate this image by unconsciously encouraging others to treat them this way. They might come to fear success and actually find it easier to fail even though they do not like themselves that way. Thus, failure influences an individual's self-concept negatively (e.g., Sullivan's "bad-me" self-representation), and his or her self-concept instructs the person to continue to fail. On the other hand, a series of successful experiences, especially when experienced in the context of an accepting, nurturing, caring relationship, might condition a person to strive for the next success, and a positive self-concept might be forged that expects success and makes it happen.

> *Think back to Melissa Motsky, the struggling nursing student. Consider how multiple less than satisfactory life*

NURSING RESEARCH
Bridging the Gap to Evidence-Based Practice

PROMOTING POSITIVE SELF-CONCEPT

Social support, positive role function, and satisfaction with healthcare have been demonstrated to have a positive influence on the experience of dealing with illness. As an external resource for patients, nurses can help promote a positive self-concept.

Related Research

Liu, H-E. (2008). Changes of satisfaction with appearance and working status for head and neck tumor patients. *Journal of Clinical Nursing.* 17(14):1930–1938.

This study examines the change of satisfaction with appearance and body image of patients who have undergone head and/or neck tumor surgery. After receiving even micro-reconstructive surgery, patients' views on their body image worsened. This negative feeling carried over to some of the patients' occupations, changing their jobs as a result of the procedure.

Relevance to Nursing Practice

Nurses should incorporate job rehabilitation and body image into the daily care of head and neck cancer patients. Not only is it an essential part of their recuperation process, but it will also aid them in returning to their lives, potentially negating or lessening the negative impact.

For additional research, visit the Point.

Related Research

Hautala, L. A., Junnila, J., Helenius, H., Vaananen, A. M., Liuksila, P. R., Raiha, H., et al. (2008). Towards understanding gender differences in disordered eating among adolescents. *Journal of Clinical Nursing,* 17(13):1803–1813.

This study focuses on the gender differences in disordered eating among adolescents. The article highlights the need to detect disordered eating both in male and female adolescents. Although popular conception tends to view only girls as victims of disordered eating, gender differences in disordered eating are relatively small in adolescence. To enhance the detection of eating disorder symptoms, both girls and boys should be screened for these problems in secondary school.

Relevance to Nursing Practice

Nurses can and should use this information obtained from adolescents' healthcare records to identify those who may need further intervention, including adolescent boys. In this way, disordered eating can be treated at the earliest stage.

experiences may culminate in Ms. Motsky's sense of personal failure such as academics, relationships, role performance in her family and work experience. ■

Crises or Life Stressors

Life stressors or crises (e.g., marriage, divorce, acute or chronic illness, an exam, a new job or job loss, a gray hair, a fire) might call forth a personal response and mobilize an individual's talents, resulting in good feelings about oneself, or it might result in emotional paralysis with diminished self-concept. People vary greatly in their perception of what constitutes a crisis or stressor, as well as the degree to which such experiences might disrupt or diminish self-concept. However, major stressors place anyone at relative risk for maladaptive responses such as withdrawal, isolation, depression, extreme anxiety, substance abuse, or exacerbation of physical illness. How the person perceives the stressor (threat, challenge, defeat) and his or her ability to mobilize personal strengths and other resources are determined largely by that person's self-concept, which, in turn, is influenced by the response the person chooses.

Aguilera (1998) described three factors that determine a person's response to crisis: (1) the person's perception of the event or situation, (2) the person's situational supports (external resources), and (3) the coping mechanisms the person possesses (internal resources.) All of these factors are related to self-concept. The degree of strength an individual has in each area is related to his or her precrisis self-concept. Similarly, each of these conditions can alter self-concept either positively or negatively during or after crisis. Intervention to strengthen any of these three areas can help people better cope with crisis and emerge with enhanced self-concept.

> *Recall Anthony Santorini, the patient who had an amputation. To promote an enhanced self-concept, the nurse would need to assess his perception of the situation and his coping mechanisms to gain further insight into Mr. Santorini's self-concept. In addition, the nurse would need to investigate any support systems available to Mr. Santorini such as family, friends, and community resources that might be helpful in fostering a more positive self-concept.* ■

Aging, Illness, or Trauma

Many people take a healthy body for granted. Society encourages a kind of denial of the eventuality of aging, chronic illness, and the necessity to integrate crisis and change throughout each person's lifetime. Society emphasizes and rewards youth, health, and narrow norms for physical attractiveness while devaluing seniors, those with chronic illness, and those whose appearance does not correspond to movie-star stan-

FIGURE 41-3. An illness or alteration in function may present a crisis situation, which affects the patient's self-concept. Changes may be positive or negative.

dards. Thus, even the suggestion of disease, the sudden impact of illness, trauma, or bodily disfigurement, or signs of the aging process might pose serious threats to the self (Fig. 41-3). People vary greatly in their response to aging, illness, and trauma. This is due to the threats to self-concept and internal beliefs about the self that these conditions may pose. Refer again to the Research in Nursing box.

> *Consider Delores Sparks, the woman described in the Reflective Practice display. Aging, by itself, can influence one's self-concept. However, the patient also is faced with the loss of independence and personal space, reliance on others for daily care, knowledge that she has a terminal illness, and the prospect of death in the near future. All of these factors are contributing to Mrs. Sparks' current status.* ■

THE NURSING PROCESS

Nurses who role model good health behaviors are more effective teachers. Use the Promoting Health Display 41-1 for yourself before using it with others. Before nurses can successfully identify and resolve self-concept disturbances in patients, they must be comfortable with themselves and possess an adequate self-concept (Gustafsson & Willman, 2003; Lin et al., 2004). Box 41-1 provides an additional resource for enhancing your self-concept as a nurse.

PROMOTING HEALTH • 41-1

Self-Concept

Use the assessment checklist to determine how well you are meeting your need for positive self-concept. Then develop a prescription for self-care by choosing appropriate behaviors from the list of suggestions.

Assessment Checklist

❑ almost always   ❑ sometimes   ❑ almost never

❑ ❑ ❑ 1. I have established appropriate expectations and goals for myself.

❑ ❑ ❑ 2. I have effective and satisfying relationships with others.

❑ ❑ ❑ 3. I cope effectively with change and loss.

❑ ❑ ❑ 4. I accept and feel good about myself.

Self-Care Behaviors

1. Accept normal variations in physical appearance and capabilities.
2. Use problem-solving and decision-making strategies to define expectations and set goals.
3. Set priorities and accept that no one person can be all things to all people.
4. Forget past mistakes; carrying around "excess baggage" is unhealthy.
5. Emphasize strengths and abilities in self.
6. Take an active part in group activities in school, work, church, or the community.
7. Volunteer time, talents, or services.
8. Avoid excessive alcohol and drugs.
9. Live life one day at a time.
10. Get help for self-concept disturbances that interfere with healthy social and professional activities.

Box 41-1   ENHANCING SELF-CONCEPT FOR NURSING PROFESSIONALS

Important Goals for Enhancing Self-Concept
- Identify basic unmet human needs, exploring positive means to meet these needs.
- Schedule time every day to meet personal needs.
- Assess the effect of feedback from significant others on self-esteem.
- Describe personal strengths accurately.
- Develop a realistic plan to achieve goals for personal growth and development.

Strategies for Enhancing Self-Concept in Relation to One's Professional Practice
- *Dispel the myth that it is necessary to know all there is to know about nursing to be a good nurse.* At no one point in time does any nurse ever have it all together. Acceptance of the need to learn new theories or new procedures frees you from having to practice defensively (i.e., pretend to be on top of every new development) and is a great stimulus for professional growth and development.
- *Realistically evaluate strengths and weaknesses.* Build a periodic review into your practice and be fair in your self-evaluation. "I think I'm giving better care than ever before and I know my patients are appreciative, but I'm sensing a lot of tension between myself and a couple of the other nurses. . . ."
- *Accentuate the positive.* Many of us have a knack for forgetting the 99 things we did well and focusing on our one error. Errors need to be taken seriously and

evaluated but not to the exclusion of overlooking positive accomplishments.
- *Develop a conscious plan for changing weaknesses into strengths.* Professional growth and development depend on strong motivation to become better at what you do. "Realizing that I never know what to say when a patient receives bad news, I can try to avoid these patients or consciously plan to develop better interpersonal skills." Nurses are tremendous resources for each other. Tapping into each other's strengths is a great way to build self-esteem mutually. "You always seem to know the right thing to say or do with patients. Do you mind if I observe for a while and then 'try on' some of your behaviors?"
- *Work to develop team self-esteem.* A basic interpersonal principle that seems to work well in practice is to offer to others what you want yourself. Because our sense of self is strongly influenced by the feedback we receive from others, positive reinforcement of our strengths and sincere offers to help correct deficiencies are needed by everyone.
- *Actively demonstrate your commitment to nursing and concern about nursing's public image.* To feel good about yourself, you need to be able to experience pride in your profession. Active participation in professional organizations can offer many personal rewards—not the least of which is enthusiasm and pride in being a nurse. Monitoring the media's portrayal of nursing and providing appropriate feedback contributes to individual and corporate nursing self-esteem.

Assessing

The nurse assessing self-concept focuses on the patient's personal identity, body image, self-esteem, and role performance. A general assessment of self-concept should be included in every comprehensive nursing assessment. It is as important to identify and label a patient's positive self-concept as it is to note problems.

> *Remember Melissa Motsky, the mom in academic jeopardy described at the beginning of the chapter? Although she states that "she is a failure," the nurse would need to assess her for any indications of a positive self-concept. For example, the nurse would need to question Ms. Motsky further about her feelings about other key life events and her performance. The nurse would then use this information, building on positive aspects to foster a positive self-concept as Ms. Motsky faces academic challenges.* ∎

Patients experiencing illness or trauma resulting in body disfigurement, altered functioning, or life crises that arrest development and thwart the achievement of life goals are at high risk for problems related to self-concept and should be assessed more carefully. If potential problems surface during the interview, a more thorough assessment should be carried out.

> *Think back to Anthony Santorini, the patient who had an amputation. The patient's statement about being "damaged goods" would lead the nurse to suspect an alteration in self-concept. However, the nurse needs to investigate the patient's comments more closely to determine the underlying reason. Although the loss of his leg may be paramount, the patient's statements may be related to feelings of guilt for not having complied better with his diabetic regimen to reduce his risk of complications. Mr. Santorini may be blaming himself for his current state. Or possibly the patient fears how others will react to him. Once the information is obtained, the nurse can individualize Mr. Santorini's care. If this information is overlooked, the patient may be at higher risk for problems in the future. Thus, a thorough assessment is key.* ∎

The accompanying Focused Assessment Guide highlights elements common to any self-concept assessment and high-risk factors.

It is important when conducting this assessment to realize the limitations of self-reporting. A patient might give what he or she believes are the desired or socially acceptable responses to interview questions. "Why, of course I like myself. I'm a pretty good person. Yes, I have friends." For this reason, the patient's responses must be evaluated in relation to observations made about the patient and what is known about the patient from other sources. When the nursing assessment reveals a clustering of these behaviors, it is important to discuss this finding with the patient. This is especially true when there is a discrepancy between the patient's words and behavior. "You've told me that you feel in control of your situation right now and are committed to the treatment plan, but I notice you're not taking your medications regularly and you did mention that you are drinking more heavily. . . ."

Personal Identity

When assessing self-concept, the information needed first is the patient's description of self. **Personal identity** describes an individual's conscious sense of who he or she is. "How would you describe yourself to others?" Pay special attention to the labels used by the patient and the order in which they appear. A simple exercise consists of asking patients to "Make a list of 10 labels that you believe identify yourself (e.g., gay man, student, Italian American, opera fan, premed major). Put the most important label first, and then list the others in order of decreasing importance. (What if the order were reversed?) To what extent do you think your way of organizing information about yourself affects your behavior?"

It is important to discover whether individuals are comfortable with their perceived identity. Developmental changes, trauma, and cultural and gender dissonance might all place a patient at risk for personal identity disturbances.

Personal Strengths

Many patients focus naturally on their deficiencies; asking pointed questions about personal strengths can help a patient identify positive factors:

> *"What are some of your personal strengths . . . qualities you are proud of . . . things you do well?"*
> *"What special talents or abilities do you have?"*
> *"What has helped you cope in the past when things were tough?"*

> *Consider Delores Sparks, the woman described in the Reflective Practice display. Obtaining information about Mrs. Sparks' personal strengths would be key to planning appropriate interventions to foster a positive self-concept. Assessment revealed that one of the areas important to her was her participation in her church community. The nurse used this information, contacting her minister, to provide support.* ∎

Body Image

Body image is the subjective view a person has about his or her physical appearance. Body image disturbances can be expected with any alteration in bodily appearance, structure, or function.

When a disturbed body image is suspected, carefully interview and observe the patient to identify the nature of the threat to the person's body image (functional significance of

FOCUSED ASSESSMENT GUIDE • 41-1

SELF-CONCEPT

Factors to Assess	High-Risk Factors	Questions and Approaches
Personal identity	• Developmental changes • Trauma • Gender dissonance • Cultural dissonance	How would you describe yourself to others? • Personal characteristics and traits • Strengths • Fears
Body image	• Loss of body part or function • Disfigurement • Developmental changes	Describe your body to me. What do you like most/least about your body? Is there anything about your body that you would like to change?
Self-esteem	• Unhealthy interpersonal relationships • Failure to achieve developmental milestones • Failure to achieve life goals • Failure to live up to personal moral code • Sense of powerlessness	Tell me something about your sense of satisfaction with yourself. Tell me about your relationship with others. Who would you like to be? Who or what has influenced your self-expectations? Are these expectations realistic? • *Significance:* What is your response when you feel unloved or unappreciated by those who are important to you? • *Competence:* How do you feel about your ability to do the things in life that are important to you? • *Virtue:* To what degree are you satisfied with the way you are able to live up to your moral standards? • *Power:* To what extent do you feel able to control what happens to you in life? How does this make you feel?
Role performance	• Loss of valued role • Ambiguous role expectations • Conflicting role expectations • Inability to meet role expectations	Many of us "wear many hats." What roles (wife, mother, student, athlete, nursing aide, dancer) are most important to you? How do you feel about your ability to do all the things your roles demand of you? Are these roles satisfying for you?

the part involved, importance of physical appearance, visibility of the part involved), the meaning the patient attaches to the threat, the adequacy of the patient's coping abilities, response of family members and significant others, and help available to the patient and his or her family.

The patient's response to the deformity or limitation is assessed, including changes in independence–dependence patterns and in socialization and communication.

➤ *Recall Anthony Santorini, the middle-aged man who had an amputation. The patient voiced concerns that he was not "whole" anymore. The nurse would need to assess the underlying factors associated with this feeling. Is the feeling related to the actual loss of a body part, fear of further disfiguration due to continued complications, inability to function independently, or fear of how others will react*

to the loss? Additional inquiry is needed to determine the value Mr. Santorini places on physical appearance and the meaning he attaches to his extremities, such as ability to walk, work, or just get around the house or his environment. The nurse could then work with the patient and assist with adapting to the loss of his leg. Incorporating information about the use of a prosthesis may be helpful as he begins to adapt to his body change. ■

RESPONSE TO DEFORMITY OR LIMITATION

Adaptive and maladaptive responses to deformity or limitation follow:

• *Adaptive responses:* Patient exhibits signs of grief and mourning (shock, disbelief, denial, anger, guilt, acceptance).

• *Maladaptive responses:* Patient continues to deny and to avoid dealing with the deformity or limitation, engages in self-destructive behavior, talks about feelings of worthlessness or insecurity, equates deformity or limitation with whole person, shows a change in ability to estimate relationship of body to environment.

INDEPENDENCE–DEPENDENCE PATTERNS

Adaptive and maladaptive responses to changes in independence–dependence patterns follow:

• *Adaptive responses:* Patient assumes responsibility for care (makes decisions), develops new self-care behaviors, uses available resources, interacts in a mutually supportive way with family.
• *Maladaptive responses:* Patient assigns responsibility for his or her care to others, becomes increasingly dependent or stubbornly refuses necessary help.

Self-Esteem

When a patient has shared perceptions of self, use the opportunity to ask questions about if the patient likes himself or herself, if the patient is pleased with his or her expectations, and the progress the patient is making to realize these expectations. For example, you might state:

> *"Tell me what you like about yourself."*
> *"What would you change about yourself if you could?"*

You can obtain a quick indication of a patient's self-esteem by using a graphic description of self-esteem as the discrepancy between the "real self" (what we think we really are) and the "ideal self" (what we think we would like to be). Have the patient plot two points on a line—real self and ideal self (Fig. 41-4). The greater the discrepancy, the lower the self-esteem; the smaller the discrepancy, the higher the self-esteem.

A person's ideal self may differ dramatically from the current sense of self and positively or negatively influence

High self-esteem

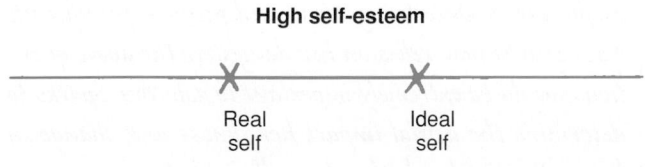

Real   Ideal
self   self

Low self-esteem

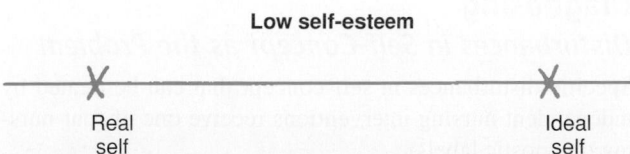

Real   Ideal
self   self

FIGURE 41-4. The patient who perceives his or her real self as relatively close to the ideal self has high self-esteem. The patient who perceives his or her real self as far from the ideal self has low self-esteem.

behavior and personal development. If indicated, question the patient about self-expectations:

> *"You've told me something about who you are and how you view yourself now. Tell me who you would like to be in the future."*
> *"What life goals are important to you?"*
> *"Where do you see yourself 5 years from now? In 10 years?"*
> *"Are these expectations realistic?"*
> *"Are your expectations stemming from who you would like to be or from who you think you should be?"*
> *"Who or what has influenced your self-expectations?"*

This helps assess whether the patient possesses life goals that are positively motivating personal development. Unrealistic expectations need to be identified, and their source needs to be explored with the patient. For example:

> *"You seem to feel that it is necessary to be all things to all people—no matter what this costs you. How might this belief have developed? Is it helpful to you?"*
> *"What I'm hearing is that your performance must always be perfect, that although you allow others to make mistakes, you cannot allow yourself this luxury. Tell me more about this."*
> *"Then, unless you graduate at the top of your class, you will not be satisfied? Why is this so important? Is this type of achievement realistic with your abilities? What will this success both benefit and cost you?"*
> *"You state you have no goals for the future. When you wake up each morning, what gets you out of bed? What keeps you moving?"*

If the need for a more detailed assessment is indicated, you'll next explore the concepts of socialization and communication, significance, competence, virtue, and power.

SOCIALIZATION AND COMMUNICATION

Adaptive and maladaptive responses to socialization and communication follow:

• *Adaptive responses:* Maintains usual social patterns, communicates needs and accepts offers of help, serves as support for others
• *Maladaptive responses:* Isolates himself or herself, exhibits superficial self-confidence, is unable to express needs (becomes hostile, ashamed, frustrated, depressed)

To assess the quantity and quality of the patient's interpersonal relationships, as information in this area identifies the level of social support and relatedness the person has, you might ask:

> *"Tell me about the people in your life."*
> *"Who do you feel is important to you?"*
> *"Is there anyone you feel you can depend on for help if you need it?"*
> *"How do you feel about your relationships?"*

"Tell me about changes you've noticed in your ways of meeting and interacting with others."

"Many people have 'people' problems. Are your relationships causing you any problems right now?"

SIGNIFICANCE

To assess the patient's feelings of significance, you might ask:

"Are there people in your life with whom you share a close relationship?"

"To what extent do you feel loved and approved of by the key people in your life?"

"Does it bother you when you feel unloved or when others fail to appreciate you?"

"In what ways do you let family members and friends know that you like them or are proud of their accomplishments?"

COMPETENCE

To assess the patient's feelings of competence, you might ask:

"What are the things you need to do to feel important?"

"Is anything interfering with your ability to execute these tasks?" ("How does this make you feel?")

"How important to you is it to feel that others value your work?"

VIRTUE

To assess the patient's sense of virtue, you might ask:

"Tell me something about the moral–ethical principles that govern your life."

"How must you live to describe yourself as a 'good' person?"

"How do you feel about your ability to live this way?"

"Describe any difficulties you experience in living up to your moral principles that you would like to discuss."

"In what ways can the nurses help you to live better according to your moral standards?"

POWER

To assess the patient's sense of power, you might ask:

"How important is it to you to 'be in control' of your life (health)?"

"To what extent did you feel 'in control' of your life (health) before this illness (trauma, crisis, and so forth)?"

"To what extent do you feel 'in control' of your life (health) currently?"

"What is it that makes you feel not in control?"

"How might you change this? How can nurses help you to develop and gain more control?"

Role Performance

We all play many roles. Life roles such as our occupation or profession can constitute a major portion of our identity. Our ability to successfully execute societal as well as our own expectations regarding role-specific behaviors, or our **role performance,** is easily compromised by illness and injury. Often, illness or developmental processes such as aging make it necessary to alter or relinquish previous roles. Generally, people experience such alterations as major losses. Thus, all people whose roles are altered or compromised are at risk for disturbances in self-concept. With any patient who has experienced compromised role performance, the following questions are indicated:

"What major roles describe you—son, daughter, spouse, parent, employer or employee, student, club member, and so on?"

"How important is it to you to be good in each of these roles?"

"Tell me how successful you think you are in each of these roles."

"What roles or expectations would you change if you could?"

"How do you feel about the need for changes in your current role?"

"What new skills or behaviors might be necessary to help you resume or modify current roles?"

"What is it like for you to lose a role that's been important to you?"

"How is life going to be different now? What other role options do you have?"

"How can I help you identify other role options or direction?"

> Think back to Delores Sparks, the woman with advanced lung cancer now living with her daughter. The change in living situation and dependence on her daughter for everyday activities has definitely affected the patient's role performance. Once living alone and fairly self-sufficient, Mrs. Sparks now relies on her daughter. The above questions would be extremely important to ask Mrs. Sparks to determine the actual impact her illness and change in living situation has had on her self-concept. ■

Diagnosing
Disturbances in Self-Concept as the Problem

Specific disturbances in self-concept that can be treated by independent nursing interventions receive one of four nursing diagnostic labels:

• *Disturbed Body Image:* The state in which one experiences confusion in the mental picture of one's physical self (NANDA International, 2009)

- *Chronic Low Self-Esteem* or *Situational Low Self-Esteem* or *Risk for Situational Low Self-Esteem:* The state in which an individual experiences or is at risk for experiencing negative self-evaluation about self or capabilities (NANDA International, 2009)
- *Ineffective Role Performance:* The state in which an individual experiences or is at risk for experiencing a disruption in the way he or she perceives his or her role performance (NANDA International, 2009)
- *Disturbed Personal Identity:* The state in which an individual experiences or is at risk for experiencing an inability to distinguish between self and nonself (NANDA International, 2009)

Common etiologies and defining characteristics for these diagnoses are found in the accompanying box, Examples of NANDA Nursing Diagnoses: Disturbances in Self-Concept.

In addition, *Readiness for Enhanced Self-Concept* is a pattern of perceptions and ideas about the self that is sufficient for well-being and can be strengthened (NANDA International, 2009). This is a wellness diagnosis.

Disturbance in Self-Concept as the Etiology

Because disturbances in self-concept have the potential to affect so many other areas of human functioning, they may serve as etiologies for numerous problem statements. Examples of these follow:

- Impaired Adjustment related to change in health status (increasing dependency, need for ongoing medical evaluation and treatment, and so forth)
- Anxiety related to irreversible change in body image (e.g., amputation, mastectomy, burn); delayed development of secondary sex characteristics (body image); discrepancy between real and ideal self (self-esteem); perceived incompetence in important roles; loss of key roles (child or spouse dies, separation, retirement, graduation)
- Ineffective Coping related to inability to identify personal strengths, low self-esteem, "I know I can't manage this"; role conflict
- Anticipatory or Dysfunctional Grieving related to change in body image, loss of key roles
- Ineffective Health Maintenance related to low self-esteem—"Why bother?"
- Hopelessness related to low self-esteem, overwhelming role demands, belief that nothing will change (destiny is controlled externally)
- Deficient Knowledge: How to help children develop High Self-Esteem related to lack of experience with parenting
- Noncompliance (specify) related to low self-esteem
- Altered Parenting related to disturbance in role performance (rejection of parent role)
- Posttrauma Syndrome related to disturbance in personal identity
- Self-Care Deficit related to learned helplessness, low self-esteem—"I can't"

- Disturbed Sensory Perception related to disturbance in personal identity (ability to distinguish between self and nonself)
- Ineffective Sexuality Patterns related to changed body image, disturbance in self-concept
- Impaired Social Interaction or Social Isolation related to low self-esteem, disturbance in personal identity
- Disturbed Thought Processes related to disturbance in personal identity
- Risk for Self-Directed Violence related to disturbance in self-concept, overwhelmed by failure to live according to moral–ethical standards

Important Distinctions

When assessment data point to an alteration in self-concept, the first task is to determine whether the altered self-concept is the problem, the cause of the problem (etiology), or merely a sign that a problem exists (defining characteristics). Self-concept data seem to fit well in all three categories. It is important that an accurate determination be made because this directs the outcomes developed for the patient and related nursing interventions.

➤ *Consider Delores Sparks and the following nursing diagnoses:*

Situational Low Self-Esteem related to perceived failure in role of mother and grandmother manifested by feelings of being a bother and not good for anything anymore. Assessment data point to a disturbance in self-esteem as the priority problem. Nursing energies will be directed to helping the patient evaluate herself positively despite the stress of the illness and loss of independence.

Ineffective Health Maintenance related to decreased self-esteem as manifested by feelings of depression. Here, low self-esteem is contributing to the patient's problem of failing to maintain her health as much as possible by following through with actions, and by voicing thoughts of ending her own life. Nursing energies will be best directed to improving the patient's use of health resources; one of the means used will be to help her to value herself enough to choose healthy behaviors.

Ineffective Coping related to difficulty accepting changes in health status and role resulting from terminal illness as manifested by low self-esteem statements ("I feel like an old dish rag, not good for anything anymore") and thoughts about ending her life ("since God isn't doing it"). Here, low self-esteem statements are the cues that led to the identification of the problem statement. One of the criteria used to evaluate nursing intervention to increase the patient's coping skills will be a reduction in or elimination of low self-esteem statements. ■

Examples of NANDA Nursing Diagnoses

Disturbances in Self-Concept

Nursing Diagnoses	Related Factors	Sample Defining Characteristics
Disturbed Body Image	Irreversible changes in body image such as amputation, mastectomy, hysterectomy, colostomy, scars, burns, disfiguring skin disorder	"Look at me. Nothing can ever be the same again. I feel less whole. When I look in the mirror, all I see is my (stump, missing breast, scar). I know when others look at me they feel repulsed or at the very least pity me."
	Effects of treatment (e.g., braces, casts)	Thirteen-year-old adolescent girl with scoliosis wearing a Milwaukee brace (covers pelvic area and has rods in the front and back that extend up to the chin): "I feel dumb in this thing . . . it's bad enough that my back is crooked but this makes me look like a freak. Besides, it's hot. Must I wear it to school?"
	Difficulty accepting development of secondary sex characteristics or delayed development of same	Fifteen-year-old adolescent boy, sophomore in high school, height 5'1", weight 88 lb: "When am I going to grow up and start looking like the other guys in my class?" No pubic hair; penis, testes, and scrotum are the same size and proportion as in childhood
	Extreme thinness or obesity	Twenty-year-old woman, height 5'7"; weight 200 lb: "I hate my body . . . I've been fat all my life and I'm always on a diet. Why can't I be like everyone else?"
Low Self-Esteem	Feeling unloved or unapproved of by significant others	Twelve-year-old son of parents in the process of getting a divorce: "No matter what I do to make my dad like me he acts like I don't exist. When he's home, he fights with mom, but mostly he's away. I wouldn't even care if he yelled at me so long as he noticed me. I wonder why he doesn't like me?"
	Feelings of incompetence	Forty-two-year-old car salesperson, with company for 18 years: "What's wrong with me? I do my job, I'm also never absent, I have a good sales record, but I keep getting passed over for promotions. I think I'm too old to move to a different company, but I don't want to just sell cars for someone else for the rest of my life!"
	Failure to live according to personal moral ethical code	Thirty-three-year-old single computer programmer: "I should have known I'd get pregnant—I deserve it. I knew I was wrong to go to bed with this guy. Basically, I've tried to live the way I think I should all my life up until now. What if something's wrong with the baby because of my sin?"
	Powerlessness	Sixty-seven-year-old alert widow with degenerative joint disease: "It may be hard for me to move around now, but darn it—there's nothing wrong with my mind. The kids think they are helping me by making all my decisions, but they aren't. I'm not a doddering old lady in a nursing home."

(continued)

Examples of NANDA Nursing Diagnoses

Disturbances in Self-Concept (continued)

Nursing Diagnoses	Related Factors	Sample Defining Characteristics
Ineffective Role Performance	Rejection of role	Twenty-two-year-old mother 2 days after birth of her second son (first son is 15 months old): "I don't know who my husband got to watch our son. I never wanted to be a mother anyway. My husband and I have never had any time for ourselves—and things aren't going to get any better."
	Role conflict Role fatigue Multiple life stressors	Twenty-one-year-old, full-time junior nursing student who failed a major exam; is married and the mother of an 18-month-old daughter; works every other weekend in a hospital as an ECG technician: "I'm trying so hard to get my grades up, but I don't know what else I can do. My husband seems to be losing patience with me more and more and I sometimes feel awful about neglecting my daughter. I'd stop working but we need the money. I want nursing so bad but I'm getting awfully tired."
	Changing personal resources (physical health, mental abilities, motivation)	Fifty-year-old college chemistry teacher begins exhibiting signs of early Alzheimer's disease; forgets where she is and what she is doing; began rambling in class and saying things that made no sense—much to the class's amusement. Later cried and called herself "stupid."
Disturbed Personal Identity	Unresolved crisis	Eighty-eight-year-old man who lost his wife 6 months ago; wife took care of all his needs; sits alone in the house all day: "We always did everything together. I wish I had died first. What shall I do?"
	Declining physical, mental, or sensory abilities	Same 88-year-old man 3 months after admission to long-term care institution, medical diagnosis "rule out depression/dementia"; has become increasingly withdrawn, never initiates conversation; responses to questions are sometimes inappropriate: "What do you mean, what's my name? Who cares? I want to go home to my wife."
	Rejection of membership in minority group	Fifteen-year-old Cambodian girl recently emigrated to the United States with family; in constant conflict with parents as she rejects her family's culture in hopes of fitting in with a peer group: "Sometimes I feel like I no longer know who I am or how I should act. I feel lonely inside and afraid."

Outcome Identification and Planning

Whenever nurses care for patients, nursing interventions need to be supportive of the following patient outcomes. The patient will achieve the following:

- Describe self realistically, identifying both strengths and deficiencies

- Verbalize realistic expectations for self based on who he or she would like to be
- Verbalize that self is liked, or at least "OK"
- Communicate his or her feelings and needs in a way that is comfortable and effective in meeting needs
- Nurture relationships in which needs for love and worth are mutually met (significance)

- Assume role-related responsibilities with confidence (competence)
- Express satisfaction with ability to live according to one's moral–ethical standards (virtue)
- Demonstrate confidence in ability to accomplish what is desired (power)

Sample outcomes for patients with specific disturbances in self-concept follow:

- Describe the relation between self-concept and behavior
- Identify faulty thinking that reinforces a negative self-concept (distortions and denials, faulty categorizing, inappropriate standards)
- Integrate positive self-knowledge into self-concept
- Report feeling better about himself or herself

Implementing

Nursing interventions to assist patients to develop and maintain a positive self-concept might vary tremendously from one patient to another. It is important to be comfortable with your own self-concept before you can address problems in patients. Specific nursing strategies addressed in this section include helping patients identify and use personal strengths, helping at-risk patients maintain a sense of self, enhancing or modifying the self-concept, developing a positive body image, and working with parents and educators to develop self-esteem in children, adolescents, and older adults. These and other nursing interventions are summarized in the accompanying Examples of Nursing Intervention and Nursing Outcome Classifications (NIC/NOC) box.

Helping Patients Identify and Use Personal Strengths

When confronted with a major stressor, many people forget that they have histories of successful coping and numerous personal strengths. Patients at high risk for giving up are those with low self-esteem or multiple stressors perceived as being overwhelming.

Although attributing strength to a patient sounds like something nurses would do naturally, nurses frequently fall into the trap of "doing" for patients (i.e., solving their problems rather than helping them to identify and tap their personal power and strengths). Moreover, patients continually instruct nurses about how they should be perceived, and some patients successfully communicate a manipulative helplessness that encourages the nurse to take charge. An appropriate nursing response in this case is, "I wonder why you want me to speak with your physician about treatment alternatives. I'm sure you would feel much better hearing this information firsthand. If you'd like, I will stay here while you talk with the physician."

Patients experiencing powerlessness might need help to recognize their strengths (Fig. 41-5). Examples of personal strengths that might better equip a person to respond to life's challenges include:

- healthy functioning body
- ability to adjust to/function with chronic bodily malfunction
- cognitive abilities
- positive self-concept
- interpersonal skills
- sense of meaning and purpose in life
- belief system
- social support network
- meaningful work
- hobbies and other interests
- education
- life experience and a past history of effective coping
- good sense of humor
- spirituality
- healthy nutritional state
- ability to make decisions

Examples of Nursing Intervention and Nursing Outcome Classifications (NIC/NOC)
Selected Self-Awareness Enhancement Activities

Nursing Interventions	Nursing Outcomes
• Encourage patient to recognize and discuss thoughts and feelings. • Assist patient to realize that everyone is unique. • Assist patient to realize the impact of illness on self-concept. • Assist patient to change view of self as victim by defining own rights, as appropriate. • Assist patient to be aware of negative self-statements. • Assist patient to identify guilty feelings. • Explore with patient the need to control. • Assist patient to identify positive attributes of self.	• Verbalization of self acceptance • Acceptance of self-limitations • Open communication • Confidence level • Acceptance of compliments from others • Acceptance of constructive criticism • Description of pride in self • Feelings about self-worth

From Bulechek, G. M., Butcher, H. K., & Dochterman, J., (Eds.). (2008). *Nursing interventions classification (NIC),* (5th ed., p. 631). St. Louis: Mosby. A full listing of nursing activities for each nursing intervention can be found in this book.
From Moorhead, S., Johnson, M., Maas, M. L., & Swanson, E. (2008). *Nursing outcomes classification (NOC),* (4th ed., p. 638). St. Louis: Mosby Elsevier.

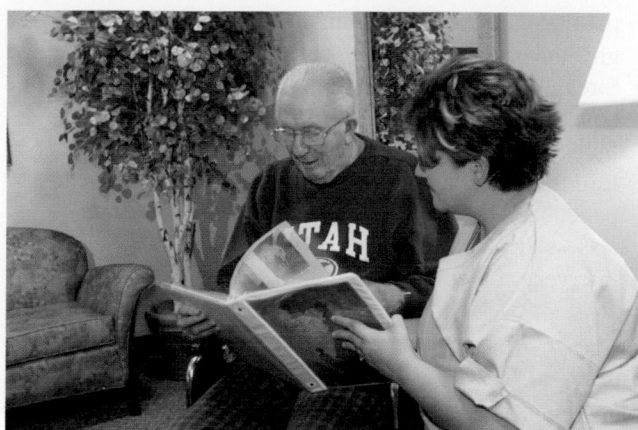

FIGURE 41-5. The nurse helps the patient recognize his self-worth and strengths.

Specific strategies that can be used to help patients identify and use personal strengths include the following:

- Encourage patients to identify their strengths.
- Replace self-negation with positive thinking (see Box 41-2).
- Notice and reinforce patient strengths.
- Encourage patients to will for themselves the strengths they desire and to try them on.
- Help patients cope with necessary dependency resulting from aging or illness.

Box 41-2 **EXPLORING AND DEVELOPING THE POSITIVE**

Example: Twenty-year-old mother, who perceives herself as "a failure in everything I try," states that her husband feels childrearing is the woman's responsibility and she is terrified.

Immediate goal: Assist mother to better understand her feelings of failure by exploring them with her. This paves the way for her to recognize her strengths as a mother.
- Ask her to tell you in detail about her failures.
   "What makes you feel like you are a failure at everything?"
   "What terrifies you about your responsibilities as a mother?"

Long-term goal: Develop confidence in parenting skills, see herself as good mother.
- Explore and reinforce the patient's personal qualities and strengths that will help her to reach her goal.
   "You look like a natural mother when you hold your baby; some women are afraid at the beginning to even hold their infants."
   "That's good that you are talking with your baby. Babies quickly sense how a parent feels about them."
- Teach the patient how to substitute positive self-talk for negative self-talk.
   Negative self-talk (mother during feeding): "She's awfully fussy tonight, I mustn't be doing this right. . . . It was probably dumb luck that she took to breast so well this morning. . . ."
   New positive self-talk: ". . . but she fed so well this morning and the nurse said her weight is good. I wonder what else might be making her fussy . . . maybe she's wet. . . ."

Helping At-Risk Patients Maintain a Sense of Self

People who are acutely ill are often separated not only from their strengths, but also from any real sense of self. This is largely because, as patients in healthcare facilities, they are removed from their personal roles, environments, and belongings, and stripped of their individuality by staff caring for them. One patient, a college president who was recovering from serious complications after surgery for ovarian cancer, shared the following:

> When I first got sick, it didn't matter how people treated me because I knew who I was. As I've grown sicker and weaker, I become whomever people make me. If a nurse walks in here and moves me like meat, I become a slab of meat. My sense of self seems more and more dependent on how people respond to me.

Help patients maintain a sense of self and worth by doing the following:

- Use looks, speech, and judicious touch to communicate worth.
- Acknowledge the patient's status, roles, individuality.
- Speak to the patient respectfully and in a nonpatronizing manner.
- Converse with the patient about his or her life experience.
- Address the patient by preferred name whenever entering the patient's room.
- Offer the patient a simple explanation before initiating any procedure.
- Move the patient's body respectfully if the patient is unable to do this.
- Respect the patient's privacy and sensibilities.
- Acknowledge and allow expression of negative feelings.
- Help the patient to recognize strengths and explore alternatives.

It is important to keep in mind that patients are people first and foremost. A person's illness does not define who that person is. Too often, there is a tendency for all healthcare professionals to focus primarily on a patient's illness, and the whole person is forgotten or ignored, with potential negative consequences for that patient's sense of self, such as lack of motivation to learn or execute important healthcare behaviors. The way nurses care for patients can directly impact self-concept; self-concept, in turn, directly impacts health. This type of caring does not require additional nursing time or energy. It does require from the nurse continual reaffirmation that nursing is a person-centered profession and that nothing is more important at any moment of a nurse's workday than the person being served.

Modifying a Negative Self-Concept

The time is ripe for change when a patient realizes that a negative self-concept is hindering personal development related to healthcare. One option is using a cognitive–behavioral approach to assist the patient in modifying self-concept. The general principle involved here is to help the patient alter his or her perspective of a situation from a more negative view to a more positive view, a process known as "reframing." Once a person can view his or her situation more positively, a wider variety of behavioral options, coping mechanisms, or internal or external supports can be identified and activated. While any person's self-concept is usually firmly entrenched and naturally resists change, you should remain optimistic that change is possible, if even in small increments. Helpful nursing interventions include the following:

- Help the patient identify and describe in detail how he or she thinks and feels about situations related to self-concept (identify the patient's faulty thinking patterns).
- Explore with the patient alternative ways of viewing the same situation (reframe the patient's thinking about the situation).
- Teach the patient to "red flag" faulty thinking behavior as soon as he or she is aware of it. The goal is to replace the negative thinking and self-talk with thinking and self-talk that will develop a more positive self-image.
- Help the patient explore the positive dimensions of himself or herself that he or she wishes to develop, and incorporate this new knowledge into the self-concept.

Developing a Positive Body Image

Interventions for body image disturbances vary according to the nature of the disturbance. Interventions may include any combination of the following:

- Express interest in and acceptance of the patient through verbal and nonverbal expression. Allow the patient to share his or her feelings openly. Sitting quietly by the patient for a few minutes, with a few words such as "How are things?" or "Tell me what's going on with you" communicates to the patient your willingness and readiness to share his or her experience.
- Explore with the patient his or her feelings about altered body image and his or her perceptions about the meaning and consequences of such alteration.
- Support the patient through the various stages of loss, grief, and mourning (shock, disbelief, denial, anger, guilt, acceptance), remembering that there is no one right way to proceed through these stages. Rather, patients may move fluidly in and out of various stages, sometimes returning to earlier stages. Some patients may need to learn that it is okay to cry, to be angry, or to feel depressed.
- Use play therapy with children so that they can describe their feelings and work through their grief using the non-threatening medium of dolls or animals.
- Use self-reflection to gain awareness of your attitudes and feelings toward the patient. Be careful that facial expressions, words, or body positioning do not communicate to the patient disgust, fear, or rejection.
- While communicating support to the patient who is slow to develop and use appropriate self-care behaviors, firmly insist that the patient participate in his or her care to the extent that the patient is able. Whenever possible, provide the patient with honest answers to his or her questions or

put the patient in touch with the appropriate person to give the answers.
- Strengthen the decision-making ability of the patient by honestly exploring alternatives; help the patient to imagine living with the consequences of different courses of action.
- Reinforce the patient's personal strengths and help the patient and family to identify all possible resources.
- Assess the response of the patient's significant others and intervene if they negatively influence the patient.

Developing Self-Esteem in Children and Adolescents

Nurses who work in practice settings where they have access to groups of parents, adult caregivers, or teachers can offer specific guidelines for creating developmental environments that build high self-esteem. Box 41-3 offers five strategies for building self-esteem in children. Because some parents and educators may not have experienced these aids to personal growth themselves, it is beneficial to role-model these behaviors when interacting with children.

Important learning tasks for children include understanding and accepting oneself, feelings, and others; independence; goals and purposeful behavior; mastery, competence, and resourcefulness; emotional maturity; and choices and consequences.

Enhancing Self-Esteem in Older Adults

The many losses associated with aging (e.g., diminished strength and physical health, interpersonal losses, retirement, shrinking income) make older adults especially vulnerable to disturbances in self-concept, particularly chronic low self-esteem. Society's generally negative view of aging compounds the problem. When interacting with older adults, employ the following interventions to enhance and maintain self-esteem in this population:

- Identify one's own attitudes and feelings about aging and elders.
- Address seniors respectfully, communicating that you take their concerns seriously.
- Respect and affirm seniors' intellect, individuality, personal strengths, culture, and spirituality.
- Adjust communication style to accommodate any sensory or cognitive deficits.
- Encourage sharing of life experiences.
- Assist individuals to identify strengths and coping mechanisms to deal with present problems.
- Provide a safe environment for elders to communicate such concerns as interpersonal or physical loss, feelings about illness and death, sexuality, or financial issues.
- Advocate for seniors needing help in attaining services necessary to meet their healthcare needs.
- Explore the personal meaning of dependency for the person, and help seniors adapt both physically and emotionally to any necessary dependency.

The Focus on the Older Adult box describes nursing interventions to promote self-esteem in older adults.

Box 41-3   BUILDING SELF-ESTEEM IN CHILDREN

Strategy One: Looking at the Positive and the Negative

Instruct parents to write an honest description of their child for a stranger. Next, have the parents underline the child's positive and negative qualities.

To reinforce the positive qualities, (1) notice examples of ability in many different circumstances and point this out to the child, (2) find occasion to frequently and honestly praise the child, and (3) give the child an opportunity to show ability frequently.

To address the negative qualities constructively, ask: (1) What need is being expressed by this behavior? (2) Can I see a positive quality being expressed by this behavior? (3) How can I help my child express this quality and meet her needs in a more positive way?

Reexamine the list of negative qualities and ignore those that are a matter of taste, preference, or personal style.

Strategy Two: Listening

The following guidelines can help parents to use listening to communicate to a child, "You are important. What you say matters to me. You matter to me."
1. Make sure that you are ready to listen.
2. Give your child your full attention.
3. Minimize distractions.
4. Be an active listener.
5. Invite your child to talk.

Listen for the point of a child's story ("What is she trying to tell me? Why is this important to him?"). Don't feel that you have to fix things. Listen for and respond to the feelings.

Strategy Three: Using the Language of Self-Esteem

Feedback that enhances self-esteem has three components: (1) a description of the behavior (describe the behavior without judging it), (2) your reaction to the behavior (language that shares something about yourself), and (3) acknowledgement of the child's feelings. For example, "Thanks for playing with your brother tonight [description]. I was wondering how I was going to pay attention to our guests if he got fussy and was really grateful when I noticed that you kept him occupied and happy [reaction]. I know that there were other things you might have enjoyed doing more [acknowledgment]."

To give correction using the language of self-esteem, (1) describe the problematic behavior, (2) state a reason for the behavior change, (3) acknowledge the child's feelings, and (4) offer a clear statement of what is expected.

Attacking communications: "Don't let me ever hear you talk that way to your mother again."

Language of self-esteem: "I overheard you telling your mom that she should 'Get a life and get off your case.' [description]. When you talk like that it just makes people angry or sad, which isn't very helpful [reason for behavior change]. You probably feel like you are being picked on, and we may have some expectations that are different from those of your friends' parents. I hope you know that this is because we love you and want the best for you [acknowledgment]. In the future, try to talk to others with the same respect you'd like others to show you [statement of expectation]."

Avoid using the following destructive language styles, which tear down self-esteem: overgeneralizations ("You *never* come home on time!"), the silent treatment, and vague or violent threats.

Strategy Four: Helping Children Meet Expectations

To help children meet expectations, (1) be sure that your expectations are reasonable and appropriate for your child's age, (2) plan ahead, (3) be clear about your expectations, (4) focus on the positive, (5) provide choices when possible, and (6) provide rewards.

Strategy Five: Promoting a Feeling of Success

To help children have the courage to try new types of experiences, which results from successfully meeting challenges: (1) let a child know what to expect, (2) let your child practice the necessary skills, (3) be patient, and (4) make it safe to fail.

(Material adapted from McKay, M., & Fanning, P. [2000]. *Self-esteem* [3rd ed.]. Oakland, CA: New Harbinger Publications.)

Evaluating

Nurses who are sensitive to the relationship between self-concept and general well-being consistently evaluate the effect the nursing plan of care has on the patient's self-concept.

> *Think of Anthony Santorini, the patient with a history of diabetes who had an amputation due to complications of the disorder. While educating Mr. Santorini about reducing the risk of further complications, the nurse may detect that the patient is feeling extremely guilty about his lack of compliance in the past. "Why should I even try to change any of these things now? I made myself sick, so I may as well live with the punishment." If the plan of care is to be effective, the nurse must first help this patient value himself sufficiently to want to make the necessary changes.* ∎

When the plan of care includes specific interventions to assist patients with disturbances in body image, self-esteem, role performance, and personal identity, listen carefully to the patient's self-report and observe patient behaviors to see if the disturbances are being resolved. Basically, the patient should be able to meet the following outcomes:

- Is comfortable with body image and able to use it effectively to meet human needs
- Is able to describe self positively
- Is able to meet realistic role expectations without undue anxiety and fatigue
- Is capable of interacting appropriately with environment while recognizing self to be a separate and distinct entity

See the accompanying Nursing Plan of Care 41-1 for Ms. Motsky.

FOCUS ON THE OLDER ADULT

PROMOTING SELF-ESTEEM IN OLDER ADULTS

Area of Concern	Nursing Strategies
Personal identity	• When an older person's sense of self is threatened, assist him or her to find meaning in the experience, to regain mastery to the extent that this is possible, and to evaluate realistically the adequacy of his or her coping strategy. • Teach older people to identify and develop a game plan for confronting anxiety-producing situations. • Help to identify and secure intervention for treatable depressions. • Treat causes of self-identity disturbances such as pain, abusive living arrangements, and substance abuse.
Body image	• Notice and affirm positive physiologic characteristics of older adults. • Teach preventive self-care measures that reduce discomforting signs of aging (e.g., exercise, which maintains muscle mass and joint flexibility; proper nutrition; basic hygiene and skin care measures). • Explore new activities (including hobbies) that are within the changing physical capabilities of the older person.
Self-Esteem	• Assist older adults to identify and use personal strengths. • Communicate that you value older people simply for who they are (unconditional affirmation); know and use the name they prefer; ask them questions about their life, interests, or values. • When appropriate, use the expertise of older adults and ask their advice; let them know you value their life experiences. • Engage older people in activities in which they can be successful. • Allow older people to make tough decisions and confront challenging situations when appropriate; teach protective family members the value of older adults confronting situations that invite continued growth. • Empower older people to meet their own needs; provide necessary knowledge, teach new behaviors, instill the belief that they "can manage."
Role performance	• Explore with older people the many roles they have fulfilled throughout their lifetime; invite reminiscences. • Facilitate grieving over valued roles that are no longer able to be performed. • Remedy, whenever possible, factors that prevent older patients from engaging in valued roles. • Explore new roles.

NURSING PLAN OF CARE · 41-1

For Melissa Motsky

PATIENT CARE STUDY

Melissa Motsky is a 31-year-old married woman, mother of three children (aged 12, 10, 8 years), and junior-level nursing student. She works every other weekend as a nurse's aide. She has just received a letter from the nursing division head informing her that she is in academic jeopardy and will fail out of the program unless her grades improve. She presents this to her adviser.

After talking with Ms. Motsky, who calls herself a failure and who cries as she describes her situation at home, her faculty adviser suspects a serious self-esteem problem and helps her to list factors contributing to her current sense of failure and low self-esteem. The following list is generated:

SIGNIFICANCE

− Receives little understanding, affection, approval from husband. "I stay with him because of the kids. I started back to school because I had to get out of the house and want to make something of myself. He doesn't understand this."

+ "The children are very supportive but get impatient when I have to study and can't spend time with them."

− Feels a failure in all the roles that are important to her—wife, mother, and, now, student. "I jeopardized everything to go back to school—if I fail, it's all over for me. There just isn't enough time or energy to do anything well."

+ "They do love me at work, though, which makes me feel like nursing is what I should be doing."

(continued)

NURSING PLAN OF CARE • 41-1

For Melissa Motsky (continued)

VIRTUE

− "I've always believed that hard work pays off and that if you were faithful to your duty you'd be rewarded by the good life—I'm beginning to doubt that. Maybe I'm a fool for trying so hard."

+ "I do still try to live according to my beliefs and feel okay about this. I treat others as I'd like to be treated."

POWER

− "I always believed I could do anything I put my heart and soul into. But I can't seem to change my marriage, and if I fail out of school, that will be the end of all my dreams."

Key indicators of low self-esteem that also surfaced in the interview included overeating (10-lb weight gain during the past year), difficulty sleeping, fatigue, new sensitivity to criticism, and expressions of feeling unloved, alone, and no longer able to manage. Personal strengths included history of "can do" mentality, high motivation to succeed, and past history of success as mother and nurse's aide.

NURSING DIAGNOSIS Situational Low Self-Esteem related to decreased sense of significance, competence, virtue, and power as manifested by expressions of being a failure, powerlessness, fatigue, tears, weight gain, low academic performance (test grades 68, 74)

EXPECTED OUTCOME By this time next month, 11/2/12, the client will demonstrate increased self-esteem by:

- Expressing positive statements about herself

Nursing Interventions	Rationale	Evaluative Statement
Assist patient to rediscover and "own" personal strengths: identify personal qualities and strengths that have pleased her in the past and explore why this has changed; recommend that she make at least one positive statement about herself each morning and evening.	Patients can lose touch with their strengths, especially when multiple stressors seem to create impossible demands.	11/3/12 Outcome partially met. Patient's statements are of the "This is good, *but . . .*" variety. "I think I'm doing better in school but I don't know if it will continue." *Recommendation:* Continue to identify and reinforce personal strengths.

C. Taylor, RN |
| Consistently interact with the patient as if she had the power to weather the crisis successfully (i.e., "will" strength to her). Role-model positive self-concept behaviors. | Once the patient senses that an authority believes in her power and expects her to use it, she may internalize this knowledge and act on it. | |

EXPECTED OUTCOME By this time next month, 11/2/12, the patient will demonstrate increased self-esteem by:

- Reporting ability to receive negative feedback without falling apart

(continued)

NURSING PLAN OF CARE · 41-1

For Melissa Motsky (continued)

Nursing Interventions	Rationale	Evaluative Statement
Explore with patient to what degree she allows the opinions of others to influence her self-concept.	Significance—sense of being loved and approved of by significant others—is a critical component of self-esteem.	11/3/12 Outcome partially met. Patient reports being able to handle everything except putdowns from her husband. *Recommendation:* Explore origin of power she has given to her husband to influence her sense of self and what she wants to do about this.
Teach how the self-concept filters life experiences; thus, if I feel that I am a failure, I may interpret the words and behaviors of others as confirming this, even though that was not their intention.	Principle of self-consistency: once I am down, I may reinforce this by distorting what I feel, hear, and experience.	*C. Taylor, RN*
Explore with the patient ways she can enhance her self-concept independently of others (e.g., take time each day for herself). Encourage patient to draw on personal strengths.	This facilitates internal locus of control versus external. Spending time on self communicates that self is valuable.	
Teach the patient how to analyze feedback constructively and respond appropriately; *cancel negative thinking*. For example, patient receives care plan back with many corrections and the notation, "sloppy work." *Maladaptive response:* "She hates me. See, this proves I'll never be a good nurse. I wasted my time even doing this." *Adaptive response:* "I spent as much time as I had on this . . . now let me see what I did wrong. Maybe I should make an appointment with my instructor so she can show me how to improve."	It is important to break the cycle of negative thinking, which reinforces negative self-concept.	

EXPECTED OUTCOME By this time next month, 11/2/12, the patient will demonstrate increased self-esteem by

• Getting a passing grade on her next quarterly examination

(continued)

NURSING PLAN OF CARE · 41-1

For Melissa Motsky (continued)

Nursing Interventions	Rationale	Evaluative Statement
Explore study skills with patient; recommend study group.	Poor study skills may also be contributing to her low academic performance. A study group will meet both her social and academic needs.	11/3/12 Outcome met. Grade: 82 *C. Taylor, RN*
Discuss importance of how she *perceives* present situation. If present failures are equated with *defeat*, she may be unable to mobilize her resources to succeed; if present failures represent *challenge*, it may call forth her best efforts and result in success.	The meaning given to present stressor can dramatically affect the patient's response to it and condition her for success or failure.	
Discuss importance of breaking cycle of failure leading to another failure.	If this short-term goal is met, it will set the stage for future successes and contribute to the patient's positive self-concept.	

EXPECTED OUTCOME By this time next month, 11/2/12, the patient will demonstrate increased self-esteem by:

- Verbalizing that the way she is living her life is okay

Nursing Interventions	Rationale	Evaluative Statement
Assist patient to examine her moral–ethical standards; explore sources of these standards and whether the patient feels comfortable with them.	Moral–ethical standards may be uncritically internalized and place the patient in conflict.	11/3/12 Outcome met. Patient stated: "I guess I'm living the best way I know how right now. If things are meant to be different, someone is going to have to show me how." *Recommendations:* Reinforce self-acceptance.
Identify unrealistic standards; patient may need "permission" to be human.	Unrealistic standards (perfectionism, conventionality) may constantly undermine the patient's self-esteem.	*C. Taylor, RN*
Refer if appropriate for counseling.	Support groups on campus (counseling centers, ministries) may be able to meet patient's needs.	

EXPECTED OUTCOME By this time next month, 11/2/12, the patient will demonstrate increased self-esteem by:

- Reporting two recent instances when personal power was effective in accomplishing desired goals

(continued)

NURSING PLAN OF CARE · 41-1

For Melissa Motsky (continued)

Nursing Interventions	Rationale	Evaluative Statement
Identify and affirm patient's use of personal power to accomplish goals.	A negative self-concept may deny or distort personal successes; outside intervention may be necessary to bring these to consciousness.	11/3/12 Outcome met . . . with difficulty. Needed considerable prompting to identify successful use of her personal power. Was ready to attribute passing grade to luck rather than her own efforts. *Recommendations:* Have patient make daily record of her use of personal power and results. *C. Taylor, RN*

SAMPLE DOCUMENTATION

10/2/12 Nursing

Melissa Motsky presented today after receiving academic jeopardy letter. She is strongly motivated to complete nursing program successfully and seems to have the ability to do this. Current multiple life stressors—lack of support from husband, need to mother three children (12, 10, 8), part-time nurse's aide job (necessary for financial reasons), and current academic jeopardy (test grades 68, 74) are all contributing to her low self-esteem and overwhelming sense of being a failure. We together developed a care plan that it is hoped will help her to do better academically, as well as begin to feel better about herself. See attached. She will return 11/2/12 at 10 am for follow-up.

C. Taylor, RN

SOAP Format

10/2/12, 12:30 PM, nursing

Academic jeopardy—Melissa Motsky

S: "I jeopardized everything to go back to school—if I fail, it's all over for me." Reports lack of support from husband, grief that she does not have enough time for children, failure of personal work ethic ("hard work pays off"), and sense of powerlessness.

O: Nursing II quarterly exam grades: 68, 74; weight gain of 10 lb during past year; facial and body expressions of fatigue, profuse tears

A: Low Self-Esteem related to decreased sense of significance, competence, virtue, and power

P: See attached plan of care.

C. Taylor, RN

● Developing Critical Thinking Skills

1. The personal strengths an individual recognizes, develops, and uses are powerful but subjective determinants of self-concept. Identify the strengths that have been major determinants of your self-concept (e.g., power, intelligence, physical attractiveness, goodness, humor, "can-do" attitude) and explore how this is helping you to succeed in nursing. Discuss with another student ways that nurses can assist patients to recognize, develop, and use personal strengths to cope better with the stress of injury and illness.

2. Role play with another student your responses to the following patients, and then reverse roles. Reflect on the effects different types of nursing presence and response have on a patient's self-concept. Discuss the nursing responses that would be most helpful to patients at risk for self-concept disturbances.
   • A male patient who was recently passed over for a promotion states, "I can't believe I've got to deal with

this ulcer. It's just one more thing holding me back from succeeding in this business."

- An anorexic teenager tells you that she can't possibly eat the dinner you brought her and states, "I can't do my usual workout in here, and look how fat I'm getting."
- A middle-aged male patient confides, "I need to talk with someone about how it feels to be a woman trapped in a man's body."
- A woman, after mastectomy, refuses to look at the incision site and notes, "If I can't bring myself to look at this, how can I ever expect my husband to want me again?"
- A resident in a nursing home says, "Don't trouble yourself about me. I'm sure you have lots of people to take care of who are more deserving of your time and attention."

● Practicing for NCLEX

1. Robert, aged 19 years, has Down syndrome and is mildly developmentally disabled with an intelligence quotient of 82. He told his nurse, "I'm a good helper. You see I can carry these trays because I'm so strong. But I'm not very smart, so I have just learned to help with the things I know how to do." Robert most likely has which of the following?
   a. Negative self-concept and low self-esteem
   b. Negative self-concept and high self-esteem
   c. Positive self-concept and fairly high self-esteem
   d. Positive self-concept and low self-esteem

2. Joe was asked to make a list of 20 words that describe him. After 15 minutes, Joe listed the following: 25 years old, male, named Joe; then declared he couldn't think of anything else. Joe has demonstrated which of the following?
   a. Lack of self-esteem
   b. Deficient self-knowledge
   c. Unrealistic self-expectation
   d. Inability to evaluate himself

3. Joe was able to list only three facts, traits, or qualities to describe himself. The nurse then asked him to list facts, traits, or qualities that he would like to be descriptive of himself or that he thinks he should have. Joe quickly listed 25, all of which were characteristic of a successful man. When asked if he knew anyone like this, he replied, "My father." This discrepancy between Joe's description of himself as he is and as he would like to be indicates which of the following?
   a. Negative self-concept
   b. Joe's modesty (lack of conceit)
   c. Body image disturbance
   d. Low self-esteem

4. David and his wife decided that she will get a job so that David can go to pharmacy school, as he has wanted to do for some time. Their three teenagers, who were involved in the decision, are also getting jobs to buy their own clothes. David plans to work 12 to 16 hours weekly. He states, "I was always an A student, but I may have to settle for Bs now because I don't want to neglect my family, and I need to work a few hours so that my wife won't have to work overtime." David's self-expectations are:
   a. Realistic and positively motivating his development
   b. Unrealistic and negatively motivating his development
   c. Unrealistic but positively motivating his development
   d. Realistic but negatively motivating his development

5. Which of the following statements made by the parent of a child you are seeing in clinic needs to be followed up with teaching about how to foster healthy development of the self in children?
   a. "I love my child so much I 'hug him to death' every day."
   b. "I think children need challenges, don't you?"
   c. "My husband and I both grew up in very restrictive families. We want our children to be free to do whatever they want."
   d. "My husband and I have different ideas about discipline, but we're talking this out because we know it's important for Johnny that we be consistent."

6. Which intervention would you take first to assist a woman who states that she feels incompetent as the mother of a teenage daughter?
   a. Recommend that she discipline her daughter more strictly and consistently
   b. Make a list of things her husband can do to help her improve
   c. Assist the mother to identify both what she believes is preventing her success and what she can do to improve
   d. Explore with the mother what the daughter can do to improve her behavior

7. Which of the following patients is least likely to develop problems related to self-concept?
   a. A 55-year-old woman television news reporter undergoing a hysterectomy (removal of uterus)
   b. A young clergyperson whose vocal cords are paralyzed after a motorbike accident
   c. A 32-year-old accountant who survives a massive heart attack
   d. A 23-year-old model who just learned that she has breast cancer

For questions 8 to 11, read the patient data below and use the following letters to indicate the diagnosis that data suggest (each response may be used only once):
a. Personal Identity Disturbance
b. Body Image Disturbance
c. Self-Esteem Disturbance
d. Altered Role Performance

8. Juanita Sanchez has been in the United States only 3 months and has recently suffered the loss of her

husband and job. She states that nothing feels familiar . . . "I don't know who I am supposed to be here" and she misses home (Nicaragua) terribly.

9. Jim Boa, a sophomore in high school, has missed a lot of school this year because of leukemia. He said he feels like he is falling behind in everything and misses "hanging out at the mall" with his friends most of all.

10. Kelly Smith, a college freshman away from home for the first time, says, "Why did I have to be born into a family of big bottoms and short fat legs! No one will ever ask me out for a date. Oh, why can't I have long thin legs like everyone else in my class? What a frump I am."

11. Marissa Yule, a 33-year-old businessperson, is now in counseling attempting to deal with a long-repressed history of sexual abuse by her father. "I guess I should feel satisfied with what I've achieved in life, but I'm never content, and nothing I achieve makes me feel good about myself . . . I hate my father for making me feel like I'm no good. This is an awful way to live."

12. Nancy, 36 years old, who was divorced 5 years earlier, entered the emergency department with severe burns and cuts on her face after an auto accident in a car driven by her fiancé of 3 months. Three weeks later, her fiancé has not yet contacted her. Nancy states that he is so busy and she is too tired to have visitors anyway. Nancy frequently lies with her eyes closed and head turned away. These data suggest that:
   a. There is no disturbance in self-concept.
   b. This patient has ego strength and high self-esteem but may have a disturbance of body image.
   c. The area of self-esteem has very low priority at this time and should be ignored until much later.
   d. It is probable that there are disturbances in self-esteem and body image.

13. Which of the nursing interventions below is least likely to assist a severely ill patient with cancer to maintain a positive sense of self?
   a. Making it a point to address the patient by name each time you enter the room
   b. Fatiguing the patient as little as possible by performing all procedures in silence
   c. Continuing to respect the patient's privacy and sensibilities
   d. Offering the patient a simple explanation before moving her in any way

14. Doris, 16 years old, has a nursing diagnosis of Body Image Disturbance related to severe acne. In planning nursing care, an appropriate goal for this nursing diagnosis is "The patient will
   a. make above-B grades in all tests at school."
   b. demonstrate by diet control and skin care increased interest in control of acne."
   c. report that she feels more self-confidence in her music and art, which she enjoys."
   d. express that she is very smart in school."

15. A 4 1/2-year-old boy required stitches for a laceration on the eyebrow. After the doctor held him, visited with him, and explained what was going to be done and that his eye would get better and look just like it did before, the boy placed his hands under his hips as instructed and quietly permitted the procedure. He then expressed pride in himself. Evaluation of the effect of this health-care experience is best expressed in which of the following?
   a. The doctor did an excellent job.
   b. The child's self-esteem was enhanced and fear of bodily mutilation decreased, and the parents were given an excellent role model.
   c. The child was made the center of attention and the situation exaggerated, thus encouraging the child to become self-centered.
   d. These interventions consumed too much physician time to be evaluated positively.

● Answers With Rationale

1. *c.* The data point to Robert having a positive self-concept ("I'm a good helper") and fairly high self-esteem (realizes his strengths and limitations). The statement "But I'm not very smart" is accurate and is not an indication of a negative self-concept.

2. *b.* Joe's inability to list more than three items about himself indicates deficient self-knowledge. There are not enough data provided to determine whether he lacks self-esteem, has unrealistic self-expectations, or is unable to evaluate himself.

3. *d.* Low self-esteem is characterized by great discrepancy between the ideal and real selves. There are no data in this item to suggest that Joe has either a negative self-concept or a body image disturbance. The data do indicate something more serious than modesty.

4. *a.* David's self-expectations are realistic, given his multiple commitments, and seem to be positively motivating his development.

5. *c.* Each option with the exception of *c* correctly addresses some aspect of fostering healthy development in children. Because children need effective structure and development, giving them total freedom to do as they please may actually hinder their development.

6. *c.* The first intervention priority with a mother who feels incompetent to parent a teenage daughter is to assist the mother to identify what is preventing her from being an effective parent and then to explore solutions aimed at improving her parenting skills. The other interventions may prove helpful, but they do not directly address the mother's problem with her feelings of incompetence.

7. *a.* Based simply on the facts given, the 55-year-old news reporter would be least likely to experience body image or role performance disturbance because she is

beyond her childbearing years, and the hysterectomy should not impair her ability to report the news. The young clergyperson's inability to preach (*b*), the 32-year-old's massive myocardial infarction (*c*), and the model's breast resection (*d*) have much greater potential to result in self-concept problems.

8. *a.* An unfamiliar culture, coupled with traumatic life events and loss of husband and job, had resulted in this patient's total loss of her sense of self: "I don't know who I am supposed to be here." Her very sense of identity is at stake, not merely her body image, self-esteem, or role performance.

9. *d.* Important roles for Jim are being a student and a friend. His illness is preventing him from doing either of these well. This self-concept disturbance is basically one that concerns role performance.

10. *b.* Clearly, this patient's concern is with his or her body image.

11. *c.* Marissa's self-concept disturbance is mainly one of devaluing herself and thinking that she is no good. This is a self-esteem disturbance.

12. *d.* The traumatic nature of Nancy's injuries, her fiancé's failure to contact her, and Nancy's response, that is, her withdrawal, all point to potential problems with both body image and self-esteem. It is not true that self-esteem needs are of low priority.

13. *b.* Each option with the exception of *b* should assist the patient to maintain a positive sense of self. Working in silence with the patient may be preferable to idle chatter, but the idea is to address the patient by name, give simple explanations of procedures, and communicate by simple words of caring that he or she is a person of worth.

14. *b.* All of these patient goals may be appropriate for Doris, but the only goal that directly addressed her body image disturbance is *b*.

15. *b.* The physician enhanced the child's self-esteem by teaching him how to participate effectively, decreased his fear of bodily mutilation by telling him that his eyebrow would heal and look normal, and gave the parents an excellent role model.

Taylor Suite Resources

The Taylor Suite offers these additional resources to enhance learning and facilitate understanding of this chapter:

- thePoint online resource, http://thepoint.lww.com/Taylor7E
- Student DVD-ROM included with the book
- Study Guide for Taylor's Fundamentals of Nursing

BIBLIOGRAPHY

Aguilera, D. C. (1998). *Crisis intervention: Theory and methodology* (7th ed.). St. Louis, MO: Mosby.

Bowlby, J. (1969). *Attachment and loss: Vol I: Attachment.* NY: Basic Books.

Bulechek, G. M., Butcher, H. K., & Dochterman, J. (Eds.) (2008). *Nursing interventions classification (NIC)* (5th ed.). St. Louis: Mosby.

Chen, C., Li, C., & Wang, J. (2005). Self-concept: Comparison between school-aged children with congenital heart disease and normal school-aged children. *Journal of Clinical Nursing, 14*(3), 394–402.

Coopersmith, S. (1967). *The antecedents of self-esteem.* San Francisco: Freeman.

Freud, S. (1961). The ego and the id. In J. Strachey (Ed.), *The standard edition of the complete psychological works of Sigmund Freud* (Vol. XIX, pp. 3–63.). London: The Hogarth Press.

George, T. B. (2007). Development of the self-concept of nurse in nursing students. *Research in Nursing and Health, 5*(4), 191–197.

Gustafsson, B., & Willman, A. M. (2003). Nurses' self-relation—becoming theoretically competent: The SAUC model for confirming nursing. *Nursing Science Quarterly, 16*(3), [265], 266–271.

Harter, S. (1999). *The construction of the self.* New York: Guilford.

Knauth, D. G., & Skowron, E. A. (2004). Psychometric evaluation of the differentiation of self inventory for adolescents. *Nursing Research, 53*(3), 163–171.

LeMone, P. (1991). Analysis of a human phenomenon: Self concept. *Nursing Diagnosis, 2*(3), 126–130.

Lin, Y., Shiah, I., Chang, Y., Lai, T., Wang, K., & Chou, K. (2004). Evaluation of an assertiveness training program on nursing and medical students' assertiveness, self-esteem, and interpersonal communication satisfaction. *Nurse Education Today, 24*(8), 656–665.

Maslow, A. (1954.) *Motivation and personality.* New York: Harper and Row.

McClowry, S. G. (2003). *Your child's unique temperament: Insights and strategies for responsive parenting.* Champaign, IL: Research Press.

McKay, M., & Fanning, P. (2000). *Self-esteem* (3rd ed.). Oakland, CA: New Harbinger Publications.

Moorhead, S., Johnson, M., Maas, M. L., & Swanson, E. (2008). *Nursing outcomes classification (NOC)* (4th ed.). St. Louis: Mosby Elsevier.

NANDA International. (2009). *Nursing diagnoses: Definitions & classification, 2009–2011.* West Sussex, UK: Wiley-Blackwell.

Peplau, H. E. (1952). *Interpersonal relations in nursing.* New York: G.P. Putnam & Sons.

Peplau, H. E. (1997). Peplau's theory of interpersonal relations. *Nursing Science Quarterly, 10*(4), 162–167.

Stuart, G. W. & Laraia, M. T. (2005). *Principles and practice of psychiatric nursing,* (8th ed., p. 304). St. Louis: Elsevier Mosby.

Sullivan, H. S. (1953). *The interpersonal theory of psychiatry.* New York: W. W. Norton & Co.

Swinney, J. E. (2002). African Americans with cancer: The relationships among self-esteem, locus of control, and health perception. *Research in Nursing & Health, 25*(5), 371–382.

Wade, T. D., Davidson, S., & O'Dea, J. A. (2003). A preliminary controlled evaluation of a school-based media literacy program and self-esteem program for reducing eating disorder risk factors. *International Journal of Eating Disorders, 33*(4), 371–383.

42 Stress and Adaptation

MEI FU

Mei Fu is a 24-year-old graduate student. She is married, has two small children, and is taking courses toward a degree in physical therapy. Her husband is also a graduate student. Although she lived in China until 3 years ago, she speaks English well. After several months of headaches and diarrhea, Mrs. Fu made an appointment at the student health clinic.

JOAN ROGERRIO

Joan, a middle-aged woman with a history of inflammatory bowel disease, comes to the outpatient clinic with complaints of increasing episodes of diarrhea. She says, "I think my bowel disease is flaring up again." Further assessment reveals she started a new job a month ago after being out of the workforce for the past 15 years. "Since the children are in school most of the day, my husband and I decided it was time for me to go back to work to help out financially," she says.

SARAH KELLER

Sarah, a nursing student, comes to the student health center complaining that she feels sick. She says, "I'm supposed to start my critical care rotation tomorrow and I'm terrified not only of the tubes and machines, but also of my instructor. I had her for my health assessment class and it was really a disaster. I feel sick and I am just shaking all over."

LEARNING OBJECTIVES

After completing the chapter, you will be able to accomplish the following:

1. Summarize the mechanisms involved in maintaining physiologic and psychological homeostasis.

2. Explain the interdependent nature of stressors, stress, and adaptation.

3. Differentiate the physical and emotional responses to stress, including local adaptation syndrome, general adaptation syndrome, mind–body interaction, anxiety, and coping and defense mechanisms.

4. Discuss the effects of short-term and long-term stress on basic human needs, health and illness, and the family.

5. Compare and contrast developmental and situational stress, incorporating the concepts of physiologic and psychosocial stressors.

6. Explain factors that cause stress in the nursing professions.

7. Integrate knowledge of healthy lifestyle, support systems, stress management techniques, and crisis intervention into hospital-based and community-based care.

KEY TERMS

adaptation

anxiety

burnout

caregiver burden

coping mechanisms

crisis

crisis intervention

defense mechanisms

fear

fight-or-flight response

general adaptation syndrome (GAS)

homeostasis

inflammatory response

local adaptation syndrome (LAS)

psychosomatic disorder

reflex pain response

stress

stressor

Stress (a word taken from the term "distress") is a part of life: Everyone feels stress at one time or another. Books and magazines are full of articles about stress, discussing everything from the stressful effects of performing one's job to the positive (or negative) stress of holidays. Television advertisements for over-the-counter remedies promise fast relief from stress headaches and upset stomachs. Stress is blamed for obesity, drug and alcohol use, divorce, and child abuse. Feeling "stressed out" is common, and taking "stress breaks" to do

physical exercise is recommended in many work settings. With stress such a part of everyday life, it is easy to see that an additional health problem, such as an illness or injury, can increase the physical and psychological effects of stress.

The experience of stress and the responses to it are unique to each individual. The process of responding to stress is constant and dynamic and is essential to a person's physical, emotional, and social well-being. Stress is a major component in health and illness. Nurses need to understand the concepts and levels of stress when providing nursing care to patients in all settings. Nurses themselves are subject to stress from the demands of their career, and need to know healthy ways of responding (see the accompanying Reflective Practice display for an example).

BASIC CONCEPTS OF STRESS AND ADAPTATION

The basic concepts of stress and adaptation include stress, stressors, adaptation, and homeostasis.

Stress

Stress is a condition in which the human system responds to changes in its normal balanced state. Stress results from a change in the environment that is perceived as a challenge, a threat, or a danger. The major sources of stress in our society arise from interpersonal relationships and performance demands rather than from actual physical threat (Pender, Murdaugh, & Parsons, 2006). Not only is stress a part of everyday experience, but a person's responses to stress are also necessary to life. Stress affects the whole person in all the human dimensions (physical, emotional, intellectual, social, spiritual), positively or negatively.

> *Think back to Sarah Keller, the nursing student complaining of feeling ill. By her own reports, she was feeling overwhelmed and extremely anxious about her upcoming critical care clinical rotation. The stresses included lack of confidence in manipulating the equipment and machines of the unit and the demands that might be placed on her by the instructor. As a result, she exhibited physiologic responses to these stresses. These stresses could also affect her ability to function intellectually and socially.* ■

The perception of stress and the responses to it are highly individualized, not only from person to person, but also from one time to another in the same person. In addition, each person's perception of and responses to stress are structured by his or her culture, family, genetic inheritance, and life experiences.

Stressors

A **stressor** is anything that is perceived as challenging, threatening, or demanding. Stressors may be internal (e.g., an

REFLECTIVE PRACTICE

Challenge to Technical Competency

I went to the student health center this afternoon because I was feeling sick. Tomorrow I am supposed to begin my critical care rotation. My instructor is the same one that I had for health assessment and that rotation was really a disaster. She has the reputation for being the hardest instructor in the school. She terrifies me. But I'm just as terrified of the tubes and machines that I'm going to be faced with in the critical care unit. Skilled with my hands I am definitely not! I'm not even in the unit and already I am quaking. I tried to switch rotations but no luck. Now, I have to decide what to do tomorrow. I already feel a migraine coming on!

Thinking Outside the Box: Possible Courses of Action

- Call in sick! Obviously, this can't be a long-term strategy.
- Grin and bear it! Just try to do my job and for the most part fade into the woodwork.
- Try to find a preceptor in critical care to whom I can explain my fears and have her/him help me develop the skills (and comfort!) I definitely need.

- Be honest with my instructor about my fears and the stress I am experiencing and ask for HELP!

Evaluating a Good Outcome: How Do I Define Success?

- I develop the skills (and comfort) I need to effectively provide care in a high-tech environment.
- No patient is harmed because of my lack of skill.

- I learn to manage my stress and use it to my advantage.
- I pass this rotation with flying colors!

Personal Learning: Here's to the Future!

After some hard reflection (and the wise counsel of my mother), I decided I was giving my fear of this rotation (and instructor!) way too much power over me! I realized that nursing would continue to put me in new and frightening situations. But escape just couldn't be my "modus operandi." So urging myself to "bite the bullet," I got to the clinical area. Immediately after preconference, I literally grabbed my instructor and told her I had to talk to her before I began giving care. While she'll never be called

"warm and fuzzy," she surprised me by being understanding. Then she spent some extra time orienting me to the unit and helping me develop comfort with a lot of equipment I'd be using that day. I learned an important lesson in confronting fear and not letting it get the best of me. Hopefully, I can remember this the next time "flight" seems more attractive than "fight"!

Sarah Keller, Georgetown University

Reflection

How do you think you would respond in a similar situation? Why? What does this tell you about yourself and about the adequacy of your skills for professional practice? Can you think of other ways to respond? Explain the autonomic nervous system responses the nursing student was experiencing. Describe the defense mechanisms the nursing student used. What other skills (cognitive, interpersonal, technical, ethical/legal) would you need to respond well in this situation? How did the nursing student use task-oriented reactions and attack behavior? What personal factors may have influenced the nursing student's reaction? Propose some strategies that would be appropriate for the nursing student to use to cope with stress. Do you agree with the criteria to evaluate a successful outcome? Did the nursing student meet the criteria? Please explain your response.

---

illness, a hormonal change, or fear) or external (e.g., loud noise or cold temperature). As with stress, the perception and effects of the stressor are highly individualized. Stressors themselves are neither positive nor negative, but they can have positive or negative effects as the person responds to change.

> Consider Joan Rogerrio, the middle-aged woman who is returning to the workforce and experiencing a reoccurrence of her inflammatory bowel disease. The decision to return to work was fostered by the family's financial need, which could be considered a stressor. The stress of returning to work after a 15-year absence

exerted a negative effect, resulting in frequent episodes of diarrhea. ▪

Adaptation

When a person is in a threatening situation, immediate responses occur. Those responses, which are often involuntary, are called coping responses. The change that takes place as a result of the response to a stressor is **adaptation.** Adaptation is, to some degree, an ongoing process as a person strives to maintain balance in his or her internal and external environments (Fig. 42-1). Adaptation also occurs in families and groups. Adaptation is necessary for normal growth and development, the ability to tolerate changing

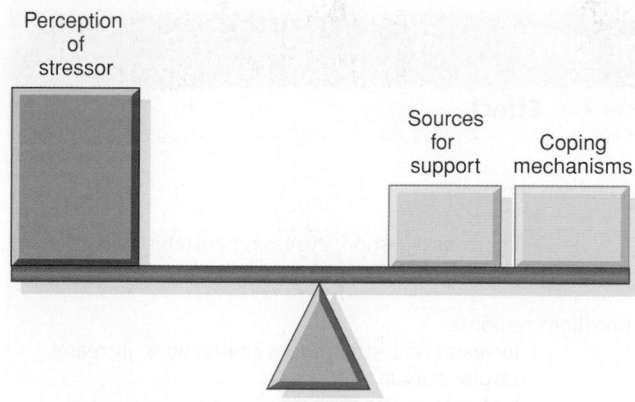

A balance is achieved when the perception of the stressful event is realistic and support and coping mechanisms are adequate

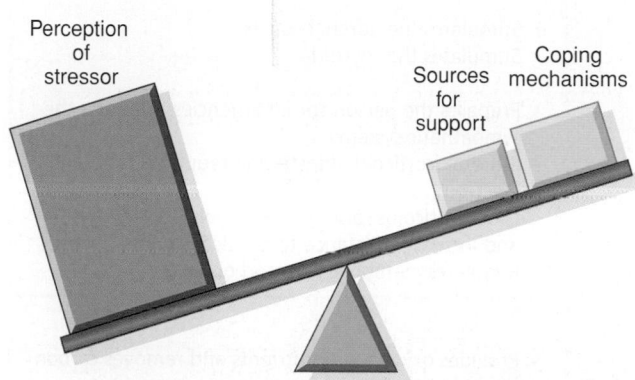

An imbalance can occur if the perception of the event is exaggerated or if sources for support or coping mechanisms are inadequate

FIGURE 42-1. A realistic perception of a stressful event, sources for emotional support, and appropriate coping mechanisms are components of a system of balances during stress.

situations, and the ability to respond to physical and emotional stressors.

Homeostasis

Our bodies are always interacting with a constantly changing environment. The environment includes the external environment, which surrounds our bodies, and the internal environment, which includes the mechanisms that regulate body functions and the fluids that surround body cells. To maintain health, the body's internal environment must remain in a balanced state. Various physiologic mechanisms within the body respond to internal changes to maintain relative constancy in the internal environment, which is called **homeostasis.**

Throughout history, people have believed that health is the result of a balanced state. Some of the most important people in medical history, including Hippocrates (the father of medicine) and Claude Bernard (the father of physiology), believed in and wrote about this balanced state. Originally, the focus was on life processes that occur within the body such as heart rate, blood pressure, and water balance. The concept of homeostasis has been expanded to include both physiologic and psychological balance.

MAINTENANCE OF PHYSIOLOGIC AND PSYCHOLOGICAL HOMEOSTASIS

The effects of physiologic and psychological stress are interrelated, as are the mechanisms that are consciously or unconsciously used to maintain homeostasis in response to stress. For example, the mechanisms described below, including the general adaptation syndrome (GAS) and mind–body interaction, are physiologic responses to either physical or emotional stressors.

Physiologic Homeostasis

The autonomic nervous system and the endocrine system primarily control homeostatic mechanisms. Involved to a lesser degree are the respiratory, cardiovascular, gastrointestinal, and renal systems. These mechanisms are self-regulating, occur without conscious thought, and usually function to correct abnormal conditions. On a simple level, they are like a thermostat regulating a furnace. When the temperature in a house falls below the preset temperature on the thermostat, the thermostat turns on the furnace, which heats the house to the desired temperature and then shuts off.

The regulatory mechanisms of the body are reacting constantly to internal changes to maintain homeostasis and health. The homeostatic mechanisms of the body systems are summarized in Table 42-1. They are important in understanding the consequences of both short-term and long-term stress, which can threaten physiologic homeostasis and result in illness. Box 42-1 provides examples of illnesses known to be associated with stress.

Local Adaptation Syndrome

The **local adaptation syndrome (LAS)** is a localized response of the body to stress. It involves only a specific body part (such as a tissue or organ) instead of the whole body. The stress precipitating the LAS may be traumatic or pathologic.

Box 42-1 EXAMPLES OF PHYSICAL ILLNESSES ASSOCIATED WITH STRESS

Autoimmune disorders
  Graves' disease (hyperthyroidism)
  Rheumatoid arthritis
  Ulcerative colitis
  Psoriasis
  Myasthenia gravis
Cardiovascular disorders
  Hypertension
  Coronary artery disease
Respiratory disorders
  Asthma
Gastrointestinal disorders
  Esophageal reflux
  Constipation
  Diarrhea
  Ulcerative colitis

TABLE • 42-1   HOMEOSTATIC REGULATORS OF THE BODY

System	Action	Effect
Autonomic Nervous		
Parasympathetic—Functions under normal conditions and at rest (Cranial and sacral nerves)		
	• Regulates heart rate	• Slows rate
	• Stimulates secretion of digestive juices and digestive tract smooth muscle	• Improves digestion, increases peristalsis
	• Stimulates insulin secretion	• Increases uptake of glucose by cells
Sympathetic—Functions under stress conditions to bring about the fight-or-flight response		
	• Stimulates heart rate and force	• Increases rate, strengthens contractions, increases cardiac output
	• Dilates skeletal muscle blood vessels	• Increases muscle strength
	• Dilates blood vessels to the brain	• Increases mental alertness
	• Stimulates release of glycogen stores	• Increases blood glucose levels
Endocrine		
Pituitary	• Secretes hormones: Adrenocorticotropic hormone (ACTH) Thyroid-stimulating hormone (TSH)	• Stimulates the adrenal cortex • Stimulates the thyroid
Adrenals	• Medulla produces epinephrine and norepinephrine	• Prepares the person for emergencies; supports the sympathetic system
	• Cortex secretes mineralocorticoids, glucocorticoids, and androgens	• Mineralocorticoid aldosterone regulates fluid and electrolytes • Glucocorticoids raise glucose levels (for energy) and increase resistance to physical stress
Thyroid	• Secretes thyroid hormone and calcitonin	• Regulates metabolic rate and growth
Other		
Cardiovascular	• Serves as transport system and pump	• Provides oxygen and nutrients and removes carbon dioxide and wastes from cells
Renal	• Filters, excretes, and reabsorbs metabolic products and water	• Maintains fluid, electrolyte, and acid–base balance
Respiratory	• Intake and output of oxygen and carbon dioxide	• Necessary for metabolism; helps maintain acid–base balance
Gastrointestinal	• Takes in food and fluids • Eliminates waste products	• Energy sources; maintains fluids and electrolytes

LAS is a primarily homeostatic short-term adaptive response. Although the body has many localized stress responses, the two most common responses that influence nursing care are the reflex pain response and the inflammatory response.

REFLEX PAIN RESPONSE

The **reflex pain response** is a response of the central nervous system to pain. It is rapid and automatic, serving as a protective mechanism to prevent injury. The reflex depends on an intact, functioning neurologic reflex arc and involves both sensory and motor neurons. For example, if you step into a bathtub of dangerously hot water, sensors in your skin detect the heat and immediately send a message to the spinal cord. A message is then sent to a motor nerve, which activates the muscles in your leg to pull back your foot. All of this happens before you consciously realize that the water is too hot to be safe.

INFLAMMATORY RESPONSE

The **inflammatory response** is a local response to injury or infection. It serves to localize and prevent the spread of infection and promote wound healing. When you cut your

finger, for example, you often develop the symptoms of the inflammatory response—pain, swelling, heat, redness, and changes in function. The inflammatory response is discussed in Chapter 32.

General Adaptation Syndrome (GAS)

The **general adaptation syndrome (GAS)** is a biochemical model of stress developed by Hans Selye (1976). The GAS describes the body's general response to stress, a concept essential in all areas of nursing care. The three stages in the GAS are alarm reaction, stage of resistance, and stage of exhaustion (Fig. 42-2). Although the alarm stage is short term (minutes to hours), the length of the resistance and exhaustion stages varies greatly, depending on such variables as the severity and duration of the stressor, the previous health of the person, and the immediacy and effectiveness of healthcare interventions.

The GAS is a physiologic response to stress, but it is important to remember that the response results from either physical or emotional stressors. The stages occur with either physical or psychological damage to the person. Obvious

FIGURE 42-2. The general adaptation syndrome (general response to stress).

alertness. (If you recall the last time you almost had a car crash, you can easily identify these body reactions!) During the second phase of the alarm reaction, countershock, there is a reversal of body changes.

STAGE OF RESISTANCE

Having perceived the threat and mobilized its resources, the body now attempts to adapt to the stressor. Vital signs, hormone levels, and energy production return to normal. If the stress can be managed or confined to a small area (LAS), the body regains homeostasis. If the damage to the body is too great (e.g., with severe injury and bleeding or a major illness such as cancer or a heart attack), the adaptive mechanisms fail.

STAGE OF EXHAUSTION

Exhaustion results when the adaptive mechanisms are exhausted. Without defense against the stressor, the body may either rest and mobilize its defenses to return to normal or reach total exhaustion and die.

Psychological Homeostasis

To maintain mental well-being, humans also must maintain psychological homeostasis. As discussed in Chapter 4, each person needs to feel loved and a sense of belonging, to feel safe and secure, and to have self-esteem. When these needs are not met or a threat to need fulfillment occurs, homeostatic measures in the form of coping or defense mechanisms help return the person to emotional balance.

Everyone frequently encounters physical, psychological, and social changes in their internal and external environments. A person's perception of these changes may be conscious or unconscious. If the person has the necessary resources, adaptation takes place and balance is maintained. If the resources cannot reestablish balance, a state of stress results. The person's responses and the degree of stress depend in part on the nature, intensity, timing, number, and duration of stressors. Adaptation to stress also depends on a person's age, developmental level, past experiences, support systems, and coping mechanisms (see the Focus on the Older Adult box for age-related effects). Adaptive responses include the mind–body interaction, anxiety, and coping/defense mechanisms.

Mind–Body Interaction

Consider the following examples of mind–body interaction:

- Tomorrow, you are scheduled to take a final examination, and you must make a passing score to pass the course and remain in the nursing program. After being awake most of the night, you cannot swallow any food at breakfast, you have a rapid heartbeat, you are filled with feelings of apprehension, and you have diarrhea.
- Since his wife was killed in a car crash, Tom Green has been the sole support of his 4-year-old son, who is developmentally disabled and hyperactive. Tom has been coming to the neighborhood health clinic with increasing frequency over the past 5 months, complaining of weight loss, headaches, and stomach pain.

examples are seen in patients with severe injury or an illness, but GAS is also a factor in mental illness, social isolation, and loss (or lack) of human relationships.

ALARM REACTION

Alarm is initiated when a person perceives a specific stressor and various defense mechanisms are activated. The perception of threat may be conscious or unconscious. The autonomic nervous system initiates the **fight-or-flight response,** preparing the body to either fight off the stressor or to run away from it; however, this is most often not in a literal sense. Hormone levels rise to prepare the body to react. This phase of the alarm reaction, called the shock phase, is characterized by an increase in energy levels, oxygen intake, cardiac output, blood pressure, and mental

FOCUS ON THE OLDER ADULT

SOURCES OF STRESS WITH AGING

Stress, with resultant anxiety, is a risk in the older population. As the number of older adults increases in the population, anxiety is now, and increasingly will be, a significant problem. Not all older patients will experience stress to the point of anxiety, but the following possible causes should always be considered when providing nursing care:

- Invasive or health-related tests or examinations
- Surgical procedures
- Diagnosis of chronic illnesses, including diabetes, cancer, and cardiovascular diseases

- Declining physical and/or mental capabilities
- Retirement
- Loss of spouse and/or significant others
- Increased social isolation
- Chronic pain
- Alcohol abuse
- Loss of independence in living arrangements, driving, and activities of daily living

---

These examples illustrate the relationship between psychological stressors and the physiologic stress response. In the first example, as you begin the test and discover that you know most of the answers, your stress decreases and your symptoms disappear rapidly. Tom's stress, however, is always present and is long term, increasing his risk for developing an illness.

> *Remember Sarah Keller, the nursing student who said she felt she was getting sick from fears about her upcoming clinical rotation in the critical care unit and anticipation of having a strict instructor. As a result of her anticipated fears and lack of confidence, she physiologically responded to the stressors by feeling sick.* ■

What causes this link between psychological stressors and the physiologic stress response? Although the exact cause is not well understood, it is thought that humans react to threats of danger as if they were physiologic threats. A person perceives the threat on an emotional level, and the body prepares itself either to resist the danger or to run away from it (the fight-or-flight response). Box 42-2 lists the physiologic indicators of stress.

Each person reacts in her or his own way. With prolonged stress, some may develop chronic diarrhea while others may develop nausea or heart palpitations. Such illnesses are real and are called **psychosomatic disorders** because the physiologic alterations are thought to be at least partially caused by psychological influences.

Another component of mind–body interaction is the effect of life changes on a person. Researchers have found that the number of changes a person has in his or her life (both positive and negative) is correlated with illness. A life change is defined as an event in a person's life that requires energy for adaptation. When energy is expended to adapt to the event, the person's resistance to illness is lowered. For example, although a holiday celebration with family and friends is considered a positive event in one's life, stressful factors include the time necessary to prepare for the party, worrying about how everyone will get along, and trying to decide how much money to spend.

Anxiety

The most common human response to stress is **anxiety.** Anxiety is a vague, uneasy feeling of discomfort or dread from an often unknown source. It is also a feeling of apprehension caused by anticipating a danger. Anxiety is experienced at some time by all people and can involve one's body, self-perceptions, and social relationships. It is an altering signal that warns of impending danger and enables the individual to take measures to deal with threat (NANDA International, 2009). In contrast, **fear** (a feeling of dread) is a cognitive response to a known threat.

Anxiety is often present before new experiences, such as starting college or beginning a new job, which may be perceived as a threat to one's identity and self-esteem. The four levels of anxiety are mild, moderate, severe, and panic, and each level has different effects. At a mild level, anxiety can have a positive effect—for example, mild anxiety about an upcoming examination can motivate a student to do the required reading and review. Anxiety beyond that level is generally negative and has unpleasant effects. In an attempt to neutralize, deny, or counteract the anxiety, the person develops individual patterns of coping.

Box 42-2   PHYSIOLOGIC INDICATORS OF STRESS

Backache
Constipation or diarrhea
Dilated pupils
Dry mouth
Headache
Increased urination
Increased pulse, blood pressure, and respirations
Nausea
Sleep disturbances
Stiff neck
Increased perspiration
Chest pain
Weight gain or loss
Decreased sex drive

MILD ANXIETY

Mild anxiety is present in day-to-day living. It increases alertness and perceptual fields (e.g., vision and hearing) and motivates learning and growth. Although mild anxiety may interfere with sleep, it also facilitates problem solving. Mild anxiety is often manifested by restlessness and increased questioning.

MODERATE ANXIETY

Moderate anxiety narrows a person's perceptual fields so that the focus is on immediate concerns, with inattention to other communications and details. Moderate anxiety is manifested by a quavering voice, tremors, increased muscle tension, a complaint of "butterflies in the stomach," and slight increases in respirations and pulse.

SEVERE ANXIETY

Severe anxiety creates a very narrow focus on specific details, causing all behavior to be geared toward getting relief. The person has impaired learning ability and is easily distracted. Severe anxiety is characterized by extreme fear of a danger that is not real, by emotional distress that interferes with everyday life, and by avoiding situations that cause anxiety (Murphy, 2008). It is manifested by difficulty verbally communicating, increased motor activity, a fearful facial expression, headache, nausea, dizziness, tachycardia, and hyperventilation.

PANIC

Panic causes the person to lose control and experience dread and terror. The resulting disorganized state is characterized by increased physical activity, distorted perception of events, and loss of rational thought. Panic is manifested by difficulty communicating verbally, agitation, trembling, poor motor control, sensory changes, sweating, tachycardia, hyperventilation, dyspnea, palpitations, a choking sensation, and sensations of chest pain or pressure. The person is unable to learn, concentrates only on the present situation, and often experiences feelings of impending doom. This level of anxiety can lead to exhaustion and death.

Coping Mechanisms

Anxiety often is managed without conscious thought by **coping mechanisms,** which are behaviors used to decrease stress and anxiety. Many coping behaviors are learned, based on one's family, past experiences, and sociocultural influences and expectations. As illustrated in the list that follows, coping behaviors may be positive or negative as they affect health. Typical coping behaviors include the following:

- Crying, laughing, sleeping, cursing
- Physical activity, exercise
- Smoking, drinking
- Lack of eye contact, withdrawal
- Limiting relationships to those with similar values and interests

Moderate, severe, and panic levels of anxiety are greater threats and involve more complex coping mechanisms as the person strives to reduce the stress and anxiety. Coping mechanisms often used at higher levels of anxiety are categorized as task-oriented reactions. Task-oriented reactions involve consciously thinking about the stress situation and then acting to solve problems, resolve conflicts, or satisfy needs. These reactions include attack behavior, withdrawal behavior, and compromise behavior.

Attack behavior occurs when a person attempts to overcome obstacles to satisfy a need; it may be constructive, with assertive problem solving, or destructive, with feelings and actions of aggressive anger and hostility. Withdrawal behavior involves physical withdrawal from the threat, or emotional reactions such as admitting defeat, becoming apathetic, or feeling guilty and isolated. Compromise behavior is usually constructive, often involving the substitution of goals or negotiation to partially fulfill one's needs.

Defense Mechanisms

Other unconscious reactions to stressors, called **defense mechanisms,** often occur. These mechanisms protect one's self-esteem and are useful in mild to moderate anxiety. When extreme, however, they distort reality and create problems with relationships. At that point, the mechanisms become maladaptive instead of adaptive. Common defense mechanisms are summarized in Table 42-2.

EFFECTS OF STRESS

Physiologic and psychological stress affects all of the human dimensions. It strongly influences how one attains basic human needs, it is a factor in health and illness, and it is a component in family reactions to illness. Both long-term stress and crisis situations may seriously affect a person's physical and emotional health.

Stress and Basic Human Needs

Basic human needs, described in Chapter 4, are common to all people. Stress, too, is common to all people. Both the attainment of these needs and the adaptation to stress require energy and motivate behaviors. As a person strives to meet basic human needs at each level, stress can be either a stimulus or a barrier.

How a person meets basic human needs and responds to stress is unique to the individual, depending on his or her sociocultural background, priorities, and past experiences (Box 42-3). In all people, the failure to meet needs results in an imbalance in homeostatic mechanisms and, eventually, illness.

Stress in Health and Illness

The health–illness continuum (described in Chapter 3) is affected by stress. Health and homeostatic balance are at one extreme of the continuum, exhaustion and death are at the other extreme.

TABLE • 42-2 COMMONLY OCCURRING DEFENSE MECHANISMS

Defense Mechanism	Causes	Example
Compensation	A person attempts to overcome a perceived weakness by emphasizing a more desirable trait or overachieving in a more comfortable area.	A student who has difficulty with academics may excel in sports.
Denial	A person refuses to acknowledge the presence of a condition that is disturbing.	Despite finding a lump in her breast, a woman does not seek medical treatment.
Displacement	A person transfers (displaces) an emotional reaction from one object or person to another object or person.	An employee who is angry with a coworker kicks a chair.
Introjection	A person incorporates qualities or values of another person into his or her own ego structure. This mechanism is important in the formation of conscience during childhood.	An older sibling tells his preschool sister not to talk to strangers, expressing his parents' values to his younger sister.
Projection	A person's thoughts or impulses are attributed to someone else.	A person who denies any sexual feelings for a coworker accuses him of sexual harassment.
Rationalization	A person tries to give a logical or socially acceptable explanation for questionable behavior ("behavior justification").	A patient who forgot to keep a healthcare appointment says, "If patients didn't have to wait 3 months to get an appointment, they wouldn't forget them."
Reaction formation	A person develops conscious attitudes and behavior patterns that are opposite to what he or she would really like to do.	A married woman is attracted to her husband's best friend but is constantly rude to him.
Regression	A person returns to an earlier method of behaving.	Children often regress to soiling diapers or demanding a bottle when they are ill.
Repression	A person voluntarily excludes an anxiety-producing event from conscious awareness.	A father may not remember shaking his crying baby.
Sublimation	A person substitutes a socially acceptable goal for one whose normal channel of expression is blocked.	An individual who is aggressive toward others may become a star football player.
Undoing	An act or communication used to negate a previous act or communication	A husband who was physically abusive to his wife may bring her an expensive present the next day.

Stress in a healthy person may promote health and prevent illness. For example, the fear of developing lung cancer may motivate a person to stop smoking, or anxiety about baby care may prompt prospective parents to attend prenatal classes and read childcare books. Stressors in health also facilitate normal growth and development, provide the stimulus for learning constructive adaptive behaviors, stimulate problem-solving abilities, encourage social relationships, and help develop spiritual strength.

The effects of stress on a sick or injured person are, in contrast, usually negative. Stress can cause illness, and illness causes stress. The presence of an illness or a disability demands new coping skills at a time when homeostasis is challenged.

> *Remember Joan Rogerrio, the woman experiencing an exacerbation of her bowel disease. The negative effects of stress exacerbated her illness. As a result, Joan needs to develop new coping skills to deal with the demands of working to minimize the effects of this stressor on her illness.* ■

People who enter healthcare settings as patients are also subjected to situational stressors.

Adaptation to acute and chronic illness or to traumatic injury involves two sets of adaptive tasks:

1. General tasks (as in the case of any situational stress) involve maintaining self-esteem and personal relationships and preparing for an uncertain future.
2. Illness-related tasks include such stressors as losing independence and control, handling pain and disability, and carrying out the prescribed medical regimen.

Box 42-3 EFFECTS OF STRESS ON BASIC HUMAN NEEDS

Physiologic
Change in appetite, activity, or sleep
Change in elimination patterns
Increased pulse, respirations, blood pressure

Safety/Security
Feels threatened or nervous
Uses ineffective coping mechanisms
Is inattentive

Love/Belonging
Is withdrawn and isolated
Blames others for own faults
Demonstrates aggressive behaviors
Becomes overly dependent on others

Self-Esteem
Becomes a workaholic
Exhibits attention-seeking behaviors

Self-Actualization
Refuses to accept reality
Centers on own problems
Demonstrates lack of control

Every situation is different, and each person perceives and reacts to stressors in an individual manner. There is no one "best" way to cope with a given situation. Nursing considerations include the person's major concern, specific illness, sociocultural background, and available resources. For example, an older woman may be anxious about the cost of treatment for her hip fracture, whereas another woman, with the same injury, is seriously worried about the care of her cats while she is in the hospital. As another example, Mary and Jane have both entered the hospital for treatment of breast cancer. Mary is worried about possible disfigurement and death, but she believes that with the help of surgery and chemotherapy, she can overcome the cancer. Jane, on the other hand, comes from a community that has strong fundamental religious beliefs. She believes that the cancer is a punishment from God and refuses treatment, even though she fears death.

Long-Term Stress

Long-term stress is a serious threat to physical and emotional health. As the duration, intensity, or number of stressors increases, a person's ability to adapt is lessened. The failure of adaptive mechanisms is also influenced by a person's state of health and past experiences with stress.

Long-term stress affects physical status, increasing the risk for disease or injury. Recovery and return to normal function are also compromised. High levels of on-going stress are associated with coronary artery disease, hypertension, asthma, rheumatoid arthritis, irritable bowel syndrome, sexual dysfunction, and post-traumatic stress syndrome. It is believed that these diseases are the result of various factors, including the effects of the fight-or-flight response, eating patterns, lifestyle, and coping mechanisms. A person who reacts to stress by overeating, smoking, using alcohol or illegal drugs, or becoming hyperactive puts additional strain on the body. See the Promoting Health Literacy box for tips useful for patients experiencing long-term stress.

Family Stress

The stress that affects an ill person also affects the person's family members or significant others. When the family is viewed as a system, the behavior of the individual is influenced by the family, and any alterations in the individual's behavior in turn affect the family. Stressors for the family include changes in family structure and roles, anger and feelings of helplessness and guilt, loss of control over normal routines, and concern for financial stability. People who were neglected or abused as children are more vulnerable to stress as adults. The family thus is an integral part in the assessment, planning, nursing interventions, and evaluation of actions to promote adaptation to stress.

> *Consider Joan Rogerrio, the woman with an exacerbation of her bowel disease. Her family is already experiencing changes related to her return to work. These changes could be possible stressors for the family. These family stressors are increased by Joan's illness, which may ultimately affect her role performance. Thus, the nurse would need to assess the family situation for the effect of these stressors on the family.* ∎

The family, both as individuals and as a unit, uses many of the same coping and defense mechanisms described previously. Family members may be overly protective, deny the seriousness of the illness, or blame healthcare providers for the patient's condition or behaviors. On the other hand, the family can provide the social support necessary to help the patient manage and adapt to stress. Emotional support from family members allows open expression of feelings and helps meet love and belonging needs. The inclusion of family members in problem solving, teaching and learning activities, and physical care helps both the patient and the family to maintain their self-esteem and feeling of worth. See the Research in Nursing box for a study of nursing interventions that support families experiencing the stress of a critically ill adult.

Caring for a family member at home for long periods can also cause prolonged stress. Called **caregiver burden,** this stress response includes chronic fatigue, sleep problems, and an increased incidence of stress-related illnesses, such as high blood pressure and heart disease.

Prolonged stress can seriously threaten mental health. As coping or defense mechanisms become ineffective, a person may try less effective coping patterns or maladaptive defense mechanisms. As anxiety increases despite these measures, the person may experience difficulties on the job, with personal relationships, and with self-esteem.

Promoting Health Literacy

IN PATIENTS EXPERIENCING LONG-TERM STRESS

Patient Scenario

Eva Weber is a 34-year-old single mother of twin boys. Both boys, now age 6, have had problems with developmental delays and have been diagnosed with attention-deficit disorder. Eva has a job at a dry cleaners but worries constantly that she won't be able to keep it since she has been late frequently because her car is old and breaks down often. Her former husband only pays child support about half the time, often because he has lost his construction job due to chronic alcoholism. When he drinks, he calls her constantly and sometimes comes to her house, beating on the door until she calls the police. She has problems sleeping and has lost 25 pounds, down from 145 to 120 on her 5 foot 9 inch frame. She admits she drinks and smokes too much, but says, "It's the only thing that makes me feel better for a while." Although the nurse practitioner at the local clinic has talked to her about stopping smoking and gaining weight, Eva has not been able to do so.

Nursing Considerations: *Tips for Improving Health Literacy*

Ask Eva to keep a "stress diary," noting when and how often something triggers her stress, how it makes her feel, and listing the things in her life that make her happy.

Teach her how to take one day at a time, encouraging her to believe that she has control over some aspects of her life, but other aspects are uncontrollable. Suggest she ask her primary healthcare provider for some help in stopping smoking in the form of medications and a definite plan for a time to stop. Explain and provide written guidelines for relaxation exercises. Discuss methods of reducing stress other than through alcohol and nicotine, including taking time to relax, talking with a friend, and learning to keep a positive outlook on life. Suggest other activities that are known to reduce stress, such as regular exercise, eating a nutritious diet, learning to say "no," avoiding people who are stressful, being more assertive, and doing something enjoyable each day. Encourage Eva to make an appointment at the clinic and to be prepared to ask her provider the following three questions:

- What is my main problem?
- What do I need to do?
- Why is it important for me to do this?

What additional measures can you take to help maintain health literacy in this patient? What other measures would be helpful for Eva if she did not speak English, could not read, or had other learning deficits?

Crisis

A **crisis** is a disturbance caused by a precipitating event, such as a perceived loss, a threat of loss, or a challenge, that is perceived as a threat to self. Crises may be maturational, situational, or adventitious. Maturational crises occur during developmental events that require role change, such as when a teenager moves into adulthood. Situational crises occur when a life event disrupts a person's psychological equilibrium, such as loss of a job or death of a loved family member. Adventitious crises are accidental and unexpected events, resulting in multiple losses and major environmental changes, such as fires, earthquakes, and floods, that involve not only individuals, but also entire communities.

In a crisis, the person's usual methods of coping are ineffective, resulting in increasingly greater levels of anxiety. This failure produces high levels of anxiety, disorganized behavior, and an inability to function adequately. After the precipitating event, the person's anxiety increases, and phases of the crisis emerge. The anxiety initially activates the person's usual methods of coping. If these are not effective, the person experiences more anxiety because the coping mechanisms are not working. As the crisis continues, the person tries new methods of coping or redefines the threat. This may lead to resolution of the crisis or, if not effective, may result in severe or panic levels of anxiety. The crisis is more likely to be successfully resolved if the person realisti-

cally views the event, if effective coping mechanisms are present, and if situational support systems are available.

FACTORS AFFECTING STRESS AND ADAPTATION

Stress and adaptation are affected by the sources of stress, the types of stressors experienced, and personal factors.

Sources of Stress

Although there are an almost infinite number of sources of stress, they can be categorized into two broad areas—developmental stress and situational stress. Both require adaptive responses.

Developmental Stress

Developmental stress occurs as a person progresses through the normal stages of growth and development from birth to old age (these are described in Chapters 19 and 20). Within each stage, certain tasks must be achieved to resolve the crisis and reduce the stress. Examples associated with developmental stress include the following:

- The infant learning to trust others
- The toddler learning to control elimination
- The school-aged child socializing with peers

RESEARCH IN NURSING
Bridging the Gap to Evidence-Based Practice

SUPPORTING FAMILY MEMBERS OF CRITICALLY ILL ADULTS

The family provides support and comfort for its members during times of stress. However, when a serious illness or injury results in admission of a family member to the critical care unit, both the family and the patient give the responsibility for physical care to members of the healthcare team. Members of the family continue to provide emotional support and to serve as a resource for patient care. The negative effects of the critical care experience on family members include feelings of helplessness and hopelessness as well as feelings of intense emotional distress. Although research has been conducted to identify critical care family needs, little information has been provided about supportive nursing care to meet those needs. The purpose of this study was to detail the process of nursing support for families of critically ill adults from the family members' perspective.

Related Research

Vandall-Walker, V., Jensen, L., & Oberle, K. (2007). Nursing support for family members of critically ill adults. *Qualitative Nursing Research, 17*(9), 1207–1218.

Using the central question "How do family members of the critically ill adult describe and explain nursing support?", a qualitative grounded theory study was conducted. Twenty family members from 14 families were interviewed once or twice in a private area. In addition, staffing patterns, patient assignments, and waiting room configurations were noted. The core category

of the process of nursing support was labeled "Lightening Our Load" and explained the variations in behavior identified in the data from interviews. Participants said that nurses work "was very demanding, there were not enough of them, and they were very busy." The family members believed that nurses had no control over the waiting room or how nurses were assigned, and they all expected nurses to be technically competent. Family members feel supported when nurses engage with and establish a relationship with the family, reassure them and are accountable to them, include them in patient care, and say good-bye when they leave. These supportive nursing interventions help the family "get through" the critical care hospitalization.

Relevance to Nursing Practice

Caring for the critical care patient requires not only an understanding of the patient's family, but also consideration of family members as recipients of nursing support as well. Nurses who work in critical care settings are often very busy and may regard the patient's physical needs as a priority. Family members of critically ill patients may have limited visiting hours and feel they are more hindrance than help. However, taking time to welcome families, to provide information about the care setting, and to demonstrate caring by providing honest answers, listening, and being interested in the patient and family are important interventions in providing family support. In turn, family members who feel supported experience less stress.

For additional research, visit thePoint.

- The adolescent striving for independence
- The middle-aged adult accepting physical signs of aging
- The older adult reflecting on past life experiences with satisfaction

Situational Stress

Situational stress is different from developmental stress. It does not occur in predictable patterns as one progresses through life. Rather, situational stress can occur at any time, although the person's ability to adapt may be strongly influenced by his or her developmental level. Examples of situational stress, which may be either positive or negative, include the following:

- Illness or traumatic injury
- Marriage or divorce
- Loss (belongings, relationships, family member)
- New job
- Role change

> *Recall the three individuals described at the beginning of the chapter. All three are experiencing situational stress, but each is responding differently; Mei is having headaches and diarrhea, Joan is experiencing an exacerbation of her bowel disease, and Sarah is feeling sick and shaky.* ■

Consider pregnancy as an example. A young married couple may be overjoyed at the prospect of becoming parents, whereas an unmarried adolescent may be panic-stricken when she discovers she is pregnant. The situations and the developmental levels of the young couple and the adolescent will have a major effect on the adaptations they will make. A person's physical and psychosocial capacities to cope with the situation depend not only on his or her stage of maturation, but also on the support systems available.

Types of Stressors

Stressors are both physiologic and psychosocial. A physiologic stressor may in turn cause psychosocial stress, and vice versa.

Physiologic Stressors

Physiologic stressors have both a specific effect and a general effect. The specific effect is an alteration of normal body structure and function. The general effect is the stress response. Primary physiologic stressors include chemical agents (drugs, poisons), physical agents (heat, cold, trauma), infectious agents (viruses, bacteria), nutritional imbalances, hypoxia, and genetic or immune disorders.

EXAMPLES OF PSYCHOSOCIAL STRESSORS

- Accidents: cause stress for the victim, the person who caused the accident, and the families of both
- Stressful or traumatic experiences of family members and friends
- Horrors of history, such as Nazi concentration camps, the dropping of the atomic bomb on Hiroshima, and the September 11, 2001 terrorist attacks
- Fear of aggression or mutilation, such as muggings, rape, murder, and terrorism
- Events of history that are brought into our homes through television such as wars, earthquakes, and violence in schools
- Rapid changes in our world and the way we live, including changes in economic and political structures and rapid advances in technology

Psychosocial Stressors

There are an almost infinite variety of psychosocial stressors, which become so much a part of our daily lives that we often overlook them. To illustrate the many types of psychosocial stressors, consider those listed in Box 42-4. Psychosocial stressors include both real and perceived threats. The person's responses are continuous and include individualized coping mechanisms for responding to anxiety, guilt, fear, frustration, and loss. The mechanisms serve to maintain psychological homeostasis.

Personal Factors

A person's adaptation to stress, whether positive or negative, is influenced by a number of personal factors. One's physiologic reserve and genetic inheritance are important in maintaining homeostasis and adapting to stressors. The ability to adapt is decreased in the very young, the very old, and those with altered physical or mental health, who do not have the necessary physiologic reserve to cope with physical changes such as dehydration or fluid excess. Adequate nutrition and sleep are necessary for enzyme function, immune responses, wound healing, and energy production and restoration. Malnutrition, dietary deficits or excess, and sleep deprivation all impair one's ability to adapt to stress. Social factors and life events are also implicated in adaptation to stress, with people who have strong support systems and relationships better able to adapt to stress and remain healthy.

STRESS AND ADAPTATION IN NURSING

Nursing involves activities and interpersonal relationships that are often stressful (Fig. 42-3). Activities identified as highly stressful include the following:

- Assuming responsibilities for which one is not prepared
- Working with unqualified personnel
- Working in an environment in which supervisors and administrators are not supportive

- Caring for a patient during a cardiac arrest or for a patient who is dying
- Experiencing conflict with peers

The stress is even greater for two groups of nurses—new graduates, who must adjust to an environment different from that experienced as students, and nurses who work in settings such as intensive care and emergency care. Patients in hospitals are more acutely ill; this combined with a shortage of nurses and a downsizing in staff has resulted in an increase in patient care assignments and longer working hours or more overtime, also creating stress. Nurses may worry not only about the future of their positions, but also about the safety of their patients. The anxiety is complicated by the expectations of nurses. Even though they may have strong negative feelings and reactions, their role does not include behaviors and verbal expressions that are less than positive and supportive.

Student nurses also experience stress and may have difficulty adapting to the requirements and responsibilities of caring for others. Factors causing stress in student nurses include the following:

- Fear of failing the classroom or clinical laboratory components of each course
- Fear of failing the licensure examination after graduation
- The demands of the nursing program
- Fear of injuring patients
- The need to balance work and study
- The need to meet financial and family responsibilities

➤ *Recall Sarah Keller, the nursing student described in the Reflective Practice display. She was feeling overwhelmed with the responsibilities of caring for patients in a high-tech environment. This feeling was compounded by her concerns about the assigned instructor. Subsequently, Sarah began to feel ill.* ■

FIGURE 42-3. Some nursing specialties can be more stressful than others. To prevent burnout and alleviate personal stress, a nurse may need to work in another area of nursing temporarily or permanently.

Most nurses and student nurses enjoy their education and work and cope with physical and emotional demands effectively. Some, however, become overwhelmed and develop symptoms of stress. The complex of behaviors is called **burnout.** Burnout can be compared with the exhaustion stage of anxiety and is characterized by a wide range of behaviors. Some nurses try to become "supernurses," expecting perfection in themselves and others. Some withdraw and do only minimal work, still others resort to drugs or alcohol. Many nurses who cannot handle the stress leave the profession.

What can graduate and student nurses do to help reduce stress and prevent burnout? The first step in preventing a stress level high enough to cause burnout is to identify and accept the stress. The same stress reduction techniques that are used for patients have positive benefits for nurses as well (see "Encouraging Use of Stress Management Techniques" in the Nursing Process section). Nurses must accept that they have the same needs and are as individual as their patients. By recognizing the early signs of stress and taking steps to reduce it, nurses can continue to be effective and productive as well as satisfied in the profession. (See Focused Critical Thinking Guide 42-1).

FOCUSED CRITICAL THINKING GUIDE • 42-1

Stress and Anxiety

You are a senior nursing student in your community health course. You have been assigned to visit and provide ongoing assessments for Charles Obedide, a 28-year-old man who was involved in a serious motorcycle crash a year ago and is paralyzed from the waist down. Charles initially participated fully in his rehabilitation and has been living independently in an apartment that is wheelchair accessible. However, a month ago, Charles was ill for 2 weeks, lost his job, and broke up with his girlfriend. When you made your last home visit, Charles was restless, had an increased pulse, and did little talking. At this visit, Charles is wearing dirty clothes and has a strong body odor, and there are several empty beer cans on the table in the kitchen. Charles begins to cry, saying, "I am so upset—I can't sleep or eat—I need help." What would you do?

1. Identify Goal of Thinking

Identify the level of anxiety experienced by Charles and begin interventions to help Charles decrease his level of anxiety.

2. Assess Adequacy of Knowledge

Pertinent circumstances: Charles has had numerous losses in the past year, including loss of body function and changes in body image. He has recently lost his job, a major source of economic support and self-concept. He lost his girlfriend, a major source of support. Previously, Charles was clean and well groomed. There was no previous evidence of drinking. His parents live nearby and are supporting and loving.

Prerequisite knowledge: Before you decide what to do in this situation, you need to assess the level of anxiety experienced by Charles. You need to know the typical behaviors of each level and be able to recognize that Charles has severe anxiety. You must recognize that Charles needs interventions to regain equilibrium.

Room for error: Charles requires and has asked for help. You are unsure of your abilities to help him to deal

effectively with his anxiety. You realize that his frustration with the situation could make him angry. You also know that depression and the potential for self-violence are risks unless something is done to reduce his anxiety.

Time constraints: Although you are not certain about how serious his problem is, you understand that Charles needs help in reducing his anxiety soon. There is time for you to ask for guidance from your instructor.

3. Address Potential Problems

There are several potential barriers to critical thinking in this situation. You realize Charles needs help in reducing his level of stress, which in turn causes you anxiety. You are also somewhat frightened about his appearance and behavior. You do not believe your own abilities are developed well enough to help Charles adequately, but at the same time, you do know he needs help.

4. Consult Helpful Resources

Your best source of information is Charles himself. You ask him what you can do to help him. He replies, "Just get someone here to help me." You ask his permission to call his mother and he agrees. His mother says she will be there in 5 minutes. You call your instructor, and she tells you to call the home health agency for further instructions.

5. Critique Judgment/Decision

When his mother arrives, she says she had no idea he was so distressed. She talks to the home health agency staff, who report that they have called Charles's physician and will continue to follow up on needed care and referrals for professional counseling. You believe you made the right decisions: you identified that Charles needed help, you contacted his mother to provide support, you contacted your instructor, and you contacted the home health agency. You also remained calm during the situation, despite your own anxiety.

THE NURSING PROCESS FOR THE PATIENT WITH STRESS AND ANXIETY

Self-awareness of stress and anxiety is essential when caring for patients. Before reading further, use Promoting Health 42-1 to see how well you are meeting your own needs for adaptation and role-modeling healthy behaviors when you are stressed. This tool can also be used with others to develop assessment and teaching skills for healthy responses to stress.

> ➤ *Remember Joan Rogerrio, the woman returning to work after an absence of 15 years. The nurse could use the tool in Promoting Health 42-1 as part of the patient's assessment. Then the nurse could use those items identified as "sometimes" and "almost never" as a basis for teaching Joan measures to adapt and cope with her stressors.* ∎

Assessing

Stress and anxiety are problems that nurses encounter in patients of all ages and in all settings. Stress is assessed through a health assessment, including a nursing history and physical assessment. Risk factors for, or indicators of, stress may be identified through standardized tests or open-ended questions to elicit information. The patient's willingness to share information is affected by the level of stress experienced as well as the coping or defense mechanisms in use.

Nursing History

The nursing history assists the nurse in identifying stressors and how the person perceives and copes with stress. Manifestations of anxiety, as well as questions and leading statements to identify stress and anxiety, are listed in Focused Assessment Guide 42-1.

Physical Assessment

There are no specific guidelines for the physical assessment of stress. Physical indicators of stress, in addition to those listed in the Focused Assessment Guide, may include cardiac dysrhythmias, chest pain, headache, hyperventilation, diarrhea, tense muscles, and skin lesions, such as eczema. These manifestations are the result of the mind–body interaction described earlier.

Diagnosing

Assessment data may reveal stress to be the problem or the etiology of a problem.

Stress as the Problem

The following nursing diagnoses may be made when stress is the cause of the problem:

- Anxiety related to conflicts about values and goals in life, threat to self-concept, threat of death, threat of or change in health status, threat to or change in environment or role, situational/maturational crisis, or unmet needs.

PROMOTING HEALTH • 42-1

Stress and Adaptation

Nurses who design care plans for patients to reduce stress must also examine themselves as a factor in the success of that plan of care. The nurse who wishes to encourage healthy adaptation to stress must demonstrate behaviors that support a healthy lifestyle. Use the assessment checklist to determine how well you are adapting to stress. Then develop a prescription for self-care by choosing the appropriate behaviors from the list of suggestions.

Assessment Checklist

| ❑ almost always | ❑ sometimes | ❑ almost never |

❑ ❑ ❑ 1. I have realistic perceptions of new situations, self, and others.

❑ ❑ ❑ 2. I understand my own personal physical and emotional responses to stress.

❑ ❑ ❑ 3. I anticipate and prepare for change.

❑ ❑ ❑ 4. I have the ability to satisfactorily solve problems and make decisions.

Self-Care Behaviors

1. Accept as positive indicators of growth the changes that come with different parts and stages of life.
2. Maintain an open mind about change—change what you can, and accept what you cannot change.
3. Avoid self-defeating behaviors to cope with stress such as smoking, alcohol, and drugs.
4. Practice methods of stress management that work best for you: relaxation techniques, exercise, hobbies.
5. Set realistic goals.
6. Develop problem-solving strategies for use in stressful situations.
7. Accept help from others.
8. Take life one day at a time.

FOCUSED ASSESSMENT GUIDE • 42-1

ANXIETY

Factors to Assess	Questions and Approaches
Subjective data: Heart palpitations Difficulty breathing Problems with appetite or sleep Feelings of sadness, apprehension, anger, mistrust, helplessness, hopelessness Changes in sexual desire	• "Have you noticed that you sometimes feel your heart beating or have difficulty breathing?" • "Tell me about your appetite and sleep." • "Of the following, which best describes how you are feeling: sad, apprehensive, angry, mistrustful, helpless, hopeless?" • "Tell me about any changes you have noticed in your sexual desire." • "How does your body feel when you are upset?"
Objective data: Dry mouth Increased perspiration Tremors Tachycardia Increased blood pressure Dilated pupils Crying Restlessness Rapid speech Pacing around the room Lack of facial expression	• Note body posture and movements. • Inspect skin and mucous membranes. • Take and record vital signs. • Note general affect.
Ability to verbalize anxiety	• "You have been very quiet today. Has something happened since our last visit?" • "It must be very frightening to be told that you have cancer." • "I notice you seem upset. Would you like to talk about it?" • "What has caused you to feel stressed in the past?" • "What do you do to feel better when you feel anxious?"

• Stress Overload related to single parenthood, inadequate economic resources, and chronic illness.
• Moral Distress related to cultural conflicts, end-of-life decisions, conflicting information about ethical decision making, or treatment decisions.
• Defensive Coping related to loss of job and economic security
• Ineffective Denial related to continued smoking behavior
• Decisional Conflict related to placement of parent in nursing home
• Disabled Family Coping related to lack of knowledge about home care of child on ventilator

Samples of three of these diagnoses are highlighted in the accompanying box, Examples of NANDA Nursing Diagnoses.

Stress as the Etiology

Stress and anxiety may affect many other areas of human functioning. In the following nursing diagnoses, stress and anxiety are involved in the etiologies of other problems:

• Imbalanced Nutrition: Less Than Body Requirements related to inadequate caloric intake while striving to excel in gymnastics
• Caregiver Role Strain related to long-term stress of care for parent with Alzheimer's disease
• Social Isolation related to feelings of worthlessness and apprehension following failure in school
• Spiritual Distress related to inability to accept diagnosis of terminal illness
• Hopelessness related to presence of disabling physical injuries
• Disturbed Sleep Pattern related to anxiety about terminally ill spouse

Outcome Identification and Planning

The nurse plans and implements care to decrease anxiety and facilitate adaptation in the patient with stress. The expected outcomes of the plan must be mutually determined with the patient or family members. Examples of the expected

Examples of NANDA Nursing Diagnoses

Stress and Adaptation

Nursing Diagnoses	Related Factors	Sample Defining Characteristics
Anxiety	Unmet needs, situational/ maturational crises, threat to self-concept, stress, threat to or change in role status, health status, interaction patterns, role function, environment, economic status	Behavioral: • Restlessness, fidgeting, insomnia • "I am so worried about my son getting married." Affective: • Irritable, jittery, focused on self, worried, apprehensive • "I just know I won't be able to do what I have to in this new job." Physiologic: • Tremors, increased pulse and respirations, urinary urgency, perspiration, diarrhea, dry mouth, nausea, respiratory difficulties • "I can't eat or sleep, and my heart feels like it's going to jump out of my chest." Cognitive: • Preoccupation, confusion, decreased attention and concentration, tendency to blame others • "What did you just tell me? I can't seem to remember, and it's all my husband's fault for leaving me."
Ineffective Coping	Inability to appraise stressors, inadequate choices of practical responses, and/or inability to use available resources	• "I know my bad grades are my fault, but I just can't make myself go to class or study." • "I have been so down lately, so I go out and drink a lot and feel better for a while." • "When I get upset, I get in my car and drive down the highway at 90 miles an hour." • "I know I have a lump in my breast, but it's probably nothing."
Ineffective Denial	A conscious or unconscious attempt to disavow the knowledge or meaning of an event to reduce anxiety, but leading to detriment of health	• "I do have a lot of heartburn, but I take something I bought at the store and it feels better." • "I have noticed some bright red blood when I have a bowel movement, but I figure it's just my hemorrhoids."

outcomes of the plan of care may include that the patient will achieve the following:

- Decrease the level of anxiety by verbalizing feelings and using support systems
- Develop effective coping skills through problem-solving skills and anxiety-reducing techniques
- Describe a reduction in anxiety and an increase in comfort

Implementing

Nurses may use a variety of interventions to help patients decrease stress and to facilitate coping. If the patient's anxiety seems too great or the nurse is uncomfortable with the interventions, a referral should be made. Referrals may be made, for example, to a professional counselor, to individuals who have experienced the same type of surgery or health problem, or to the patient's rabbi, minister, or priest.

The nursing interventions discussed in this section include teaching healthy activities of daily living, encouraging use of support systems, and practicing stress management techniques. See the accompanying box, Examples of Nursing Interventions and Nursing Outcomes Classifications (NIC/NOC), for activities and related outcomes for anxiety reduction.

Methods should be selected carefully, based on the person's physical and emotional characteristics, family and social structure, and previously used coping mechanisms

Examples of Nursing Interventions and Nursing Outcomes Classifications (NIC/NOC)

Anxiety Reduction

Nursing Interventions	Nursing Outcomes
• Use a calm, reassuring approach. • Explain all procedures, including sensations likely to be experienced during the procedure. • Stay with the patient to promote safety and reduce fear. • Listen attentively. • Encourage verbalizations of feelings, perceptions, and fears. • Instruct patient on the use of relaxation techniques. • Assess for verbal and nonverbal signs of anxiety.	• Anxiety Level. • Anxiety Self-Control. • Coping. • Information Processing. • Stress Level.

Data from Bulechek, G., Butcher, H., & Dochterman, J. M. (Eds). (2008). *Nursing interventions classification (NIC)* (5th ed.). (p. 138). St. Louis: Mosby Elsevier; and Moorhead, S., Johnson, M., Maas, M., & Swanson, E. (Eds). (2008). *Nursing outcomes classification (NOC)* (4th ed.). (p. 747). St. Louis: Mosby Elsevier. A full listing of interventions and outcomes may be found in these books.

that were successful. Guidelines for Nursing Care 42-1 lists nursing interventions to reduce stress and anxiety for patients as they enter a healthcare setting.

Teaching Healthy Activities of Daily Living

A person's normal lifestyle greatly influences his or her perceptions of and reactions to stressors. For example, a person who is overweight, sedentary, and chronically tired is at increased risk for developing an illness as a result of stress. These factors are also stressors and further increase the risk. Exercise, rest, and good nutrition are important components of stress reduction.

➤ *Think about Sarah Keller's lifestyle as a nursing student. The workload involved with school and the factors associated with stress in nursing students described previously place Sarah at risk for stress. In addition, other factors, such as demands from family members or a need to work part-time, decrease her ability to maintain a healthy lifestyle with exercise, rest, and good nutrition.* ■

EXERCISE

Regular exercise helps maintain physical and emotional health. The benefits of exercise include an improved musculoskeletal system, more effective cardiovascular function, weight control, and relaxation. Exercise improves one's general sense of well-being, relieves tension, and enables coping with day-to-day stressors. General health guidelines recommend that an exercise program consist of 30 to 45 minutes of moderate activity above usual activity on most days of the week. People who are overweight, chronically ill, or older than 35 years of age should have a physical examination before beginning such a program. The type of exercise depends on

Guidelines for Nursing Care • 42-1

REDUCING ANXIETY ON ADMISSION TO A HEALTHCARE FACILITY

1. Assess physical status, sensory status, and cognitive status.
2. Assess cultural/ethnic background, including beliefs about healthcare, dietary restrictions, and language spoken.
3. Assess past experiences with the healthcare system, including medical–surgical treatment for illness or injury.
4. Assess concerns and stressors.
5. Assess amount and type of support systems available.
6. Provide information about the environment:
   a. Ensure all healthcare providers introduce themselves by name and title.
   b. Explain policies and routines.
   c. If the hospital is the setting, provide verbal and written guidelines for use of equipment, telephone, television, meals, and visiting hours.
7. Provide and discuss the patient's rights specific to care in the agency or institution.
8. Mutually determine expected outcomes of the plan of care.
9. Provide information about all diagnostic procedures, surgical procedures, activity, and diet.

what the person enjoys—for example, walking, jogging, bicycling, swimming, or sports such as golf or tennis.

REST AND SLEEP

Rest and sleep help the body maintain homeostasis and restore energy levels. Adequate rest can provide "insulation" against stress, but stress may interfere with one's ability to sleep. Although each person has individual needs, 7 to 8 hours of sleep a day is recommended. Relaxation techniques can be used during both health and illness to facilitate rest and sleep. Hospitalized patients may require additional nursing interventions to relieve pain and promote comfort to get needed rest.

NUTRITION

Nutrition plays an active role in maintaining the body's homeostatic mechanisms and in increasing resistance to stress. (Nutrition is discussed in detail in Chapter 36.) Obesity and malnutrition are major stressors and greatly increase the risk for illness. People of all ages should maintain a normal body weight and should follow these guidelines established by the U.S. Senate Committee on Nutrition and Human Needs:

- Reduce intake of salt, refined sugar, animal fat, and cholesterol.
- Eat more fruit, vegetables, and whole grains.
- Eat less red meat and more fish and poultry.

Encouraging Use of Support Systems

Support systems provide emotional support that helps a person identify and verbalize feelings associated with stress. Other valuable contributions include providing information and services, maintaining positive self-concept, and establishing an avenue for new relationships and social roles. In addition, families and support groups provide an accepting environment, allowing the person to explore problem-solving methods and try out new coping skills. There are support groups for almost every situation; examples are listed in Box 42-5.

Encouraging Use of Stress Management Techniques

Stress creates emotional distress that often produces physical signs and symptoms. One person may have tension headaches,

---

Box 42-5	**EXAMPLES OF SUPPORT GROUPS**

Alcoholics Anonymous
Overeaters Anonymous
Weight Watchers
Parents Without Partners
Reach to Recovery (cancer)
Ostomy clubs
Child abuse support groups
Sudden infant death support groups
Stroke clubs
Assertiveness training groups

---

another becomes irritable, another clenches his fists. Many people take legal or illegal drugs, drink or smoke to excess, or eat compulsively. These behaviors can be modified and adaptive mechanisms strengthened through specific techniques aimed at managing stress. Only a few techniques are included here, but the literature describes many stress reduction methods, including exercise, prayer, art therapy, music therapy, massage, and Therapeutic Touch. Chapter 28 provides further information. Students should learn different methods they can use for themselves and in varied clinical situations.

RELAXATION

Relaxation techniques are useful in many situations, such as childbirth, pain, anxiety, sleeplessness, illness, and anger, and other uses are being discovered. Relaxation promotes a body reaction opposite to that of the fight-or-flight response: respiratory, pulse, and metabolic rates; blood pressure; and energy use are all decreased.

Relaxation can be taught to individuals or groups and is especially helpful because it allows a person to control his or her feelings and behaviors. Various techniques can be used, but most involve rhythmic breathing, reduced muscle tension, and an altered state of consciousness (HEALTHbeat, 2008). Relaxation is discussed as a comfort measure in Chapter 35. Two helpful relaxation activities, to be practiced three or four times at each session, are deep breathing and progressive muscle relaxation (Guidelines for Nursing Care 42-2).

MEDITATION

Meditation has four components: quiet surroundings, a passive attitude, a comfortable position, and a word or mental image on which to focus. A person practicing meditation sits comfortably with closed eyes, relaxes the major muscle groups, and repeats the selected word silently with each exhalation. Alternatively, the person may focus on a pleasant scene and mentally place himself or herself in it while breathing slowly in and out. This exercise should be performed for 20 to 30 minutes twice a day.

> *Sarah Keller, the nursing student, could learn to perform relaxation exercises or practice meditation. Both techniques would be helpful in reducing her stress.* ∎

ANTICIPATORY GUIDANCE

Anticipatory guidance focuses on psychologically preparing a person for an unfamiliar or painful event. Nurses use this technique to teach patients about procedures and the surgical experience. When patients know what to expect, their anxiety is reduced and their coping mechanisms are more effective. For example, before performing a painful procedure (such as ambulating for the first time after surgery), teaching would include information about the pain involved—onset, severity, cause, and methods of relief. With this knowledge, the patient feels less threatened and tolerates the procedure more easily.

A related process is anticipatory socialization, in which people prepare themselves for roles to which they aspire but

Guidelines for Nursing Care • 42-2

RELAXATION ACTIVITIES

Deep Breathing

1. Sit comfortably and place your hands on your stomach. Inhale slowly and deeply, letting your abdomen expand as much as possible. Hold your breath for a few seconds.
2. Exhale slowly through your mouth, blowing through puckered lips. When your abdomen feels empty, begin again with a deep inhalation.

Progressive Muscle Relaxation

1. Tighten your hand into a fist and notice how it feels. Hold the tension for a few seconds.
2. Loosen your grip, relax the muscles in your hand, and let the tension slip away.
3. Continue to tighten–hold–relax each muscle group: hands, arms, shoulders, face, chest, back, abdomen, legs, feet.

---

do not yet occupy. This process may be used, for example, to prepare expectant parents for the role of parenting, thereby enhancing the potential of the child to experience normal growth and development.

GUIDED IMAGERY

In guided imagery, a person creates a mental image, concentrates on the image, and becomes less responsive to stimuli (including pain). The nurse sits by the patient and reads a description of a scene or an experience that the patient has described as happy, pleasant, or peaceful. The patient is then "guided" through the image. For example, using a soothing, soft voice, the nurse might start as follows: "You are floating in your swimming pool. The water is cool and comfortable. Birds are singing in the trees. The roses are perfuming the air." As the patient becomes more and more focused on the scene, the nurse needs only to verbally "paint the picture" at intervals.

BIOFEEDBACK

Biofeedback is a method of gaining mental control of the autonomic nervous system and thus regulating body responses, such as blood pressure, heart rate, and headaches. A measurement device (e.g., skin temperature sensors) is used, and the patient tries to control the readings through relaxation and conscious thought. Over a period of time, the feedback of the change in readings teaches the person to control physiologic functions that normally are considered involuntary responses.

Providing Crisis Intervention

A crisis is a situation that cannot be resolved by usual coping mechanisms. As a result, the person cannot function normally and requires interventions to regain equilibrium. **Crisis intervention** is a five-step problem-solving technique designed to promote a more adaptive outcome, including improved abilities to cope with future crises. The steps are as follows:

1. Identify the problem. This may be more difficult than it appears, as the cause of the crisis is often difficult for the person to identify accurately. Until it is clear, a solution is impossible.
2. List alternatives. All possible solutions to the problem need to be listed. An appropriate solution to a

problem is much more likely if many options are considered.
3. Choose from among alternatives. Each option needs to be carefully considered, using a "what would happen if" approach. The alternative chosen will be highly individualized, based on the person's priorities and values.
4. Implement the plan. The alternative chosen is put into action. The nurse may need to provide support and encouragement so that action is taken.
5. Evaluate the outcome. In this final step, the effectiveness of the plan needs to be carefully considered. If it did not work as well as expected, another alternative should be chosen. If it did work, it has the positive benefit of improving self-confidence and future problem-solving efforts.

The major factor in helping patients adapt to high levels of stress is to identify and plan individually for situations causing the stress. Facilitate recognition of his or her own stress level and specific responses to stress. Encourage adoption of a philosophy of accepting what cannot be changed and changing what cannot be accepted. Emphasize the importance of accepting help from others and giving support to others when needed, as well as being actively involved in problem solving and decision making. Nurses must use therapeutic communication skills in all interactions.

Evaluating

The evaluation of the plan of care is based on the mutually established expected outcomes. It is important to observe both verbal and nonverbal cues when evaluating the usefulness of the plan. In general, the plan is considered to be successful if the patient and family achieve the following:

- Verbalize causes and effects of stress and anxiety
- Identify and use sources of support
- Use problem solving to find solutions to stressors
- Practice healthy lifestyle habits and anxiety-reducing techniques
- Verbalize a decrease in anxiety and an increase in comfort

See the Nursing Plan of Care 42-1.

NURSING PLAN OF CARE · 42-1

For Mei Fu

Remember Mei Fu, the 24-year-old graduate student with a husband and two small children? At her clinic appointment, the nurse conducted a health history and physical assessment of Mrs. Fu and noted the following data:

- Patient is a thin woman who appears her stated age. She is currently in school and expects herself to make the highest grades. She also cares for her two children and her husband. Although her husband encourages her to go to school, he believes it is the wife's responsibility to provide all child and house care. She has had no previous serious illnesses or surgery.
- Patient reports having frequent headaches, rating the pain as a 3 on a scale of 0 (no pain) to 10 (worst possible pain). She also reports having 4 to 6 bowel movements each day, sometimes with abdominal cramping. The diarrhea does not seem to be related to any type of foods eaten. Both the headaches and the diarrhea have been present for the past 2 months. During the interview, the patient appeared restless and talked rapidly. Questions often had to be repeated.
- Physical assessment reveals slight tachycardia, a fine hand tremor, and visible perspiration. Large muscle groups are tense and fists clenched. No tenderness is noted on abdominal palpation. Pupils are equal in size and react to light and accommodation. Nasal mucosa is normal.

NURSING DIAGNOSIS   Anxiety related to stress of achievement in school and care of family as manifested by rapid speech, tachycardia, tremor, tense muscles, headache, and diarrhea.

EXPECTED OUTCOME   By her return appointment in 2 weeks, 10/20/12, Mrs. Fu will:

- Identify sources of and responses to stress

Nursing Interventions	Rationale	Evaluative Statement
Ask Mrs. Fu to keep a diary of hours spent in school-related activities and family care, number and times of headaches, and circumstances that occurred before diarrhea.	Identifying sources of stress and the physical responses to stress is the first step in planning coping strategies to reduce stress.	10/20/12 Outcome met. Mrs. Fu kept a diary as requested. She identified that she does not have any time for herself. Her headaches are worse during the week. She often has diarrhea when papers are due or when her husband and children are demanding of her time. *S. Aird, RN, FNP*

EXPECTED OUTCOME   By her return appointment, 10/20/12, Mrs. Fu will:

- Identify sources of personal strength and support

Nursing Interventions	Rationale	Evaluative Statement
Ask Mrs. Fu to make a list of the people who are important to her and provide her comfort. Ask her to discuss how these people can help her cope with her situation. Ask Mrs. Fu to describe her strengths as a woman, a mother, a wife, and a student.	Identifying support people and areas of personal strength provides the patient with the means to manage stress and enhances self-concept.	10/20/12 Outcome met. Mrs. Fu stated that her family is her greatest source of support, but they are in China and she misses them very much. She does have a very good friend who is also a good listener. She identified her strengths as being a person who cares for others and a good student. She said she is also a good artist, but has not had time for art for months.

S. Aird, RN, FNP

(continued)

NURSING PLAN OF CARE · 42-1

For Mei Fu (continued)

EXPECTED OUTCOME   By her return appointment, 10/20/12, Mrs. Fu will:

- Describe lifestyle changes that include eating a well-balanced diet with three meals a day, walking for 20 to 30 minutes four times a week, and sleeping restfully 7 hours a night

Nursing Interventions	Rationale	Evaluative Statement
Discuss with Mrs. Fu the food pyramid and the importance of eating foods from each group. Also, discuss why she should eat three meals a day.	Adequate nutrition helps maintain the homeostatic mechanisms of the body and increases resistance to stress.	10/20/12 Outcome met. Mrs. Fu was given a copy of the food pyramid, and food preparations were discussed. Although the Fu's have a healthy diet, Mrs. Fu often was too busy to eat more than a few bites. She said that she is making a big effort to eat three times a day.
Discuss with Mrs. Fu the benefits of regular exercise in reducing stress.	Exercise improves well-being, relieves tension, and facilitates coping with daily stressors.	She is walking to school and enjoys the time by herself. She arranged this time by asking her husband to take the children to school.
Discuss with Mrs. Fu the importance of sleep in reducing stress.	Adequate rest and sleep restore energy and facilitate coping with stressors.	She is sleeping better, and averages 7 hours most nights. *S. Aird, RN, FNP*

EXPECTED OUTCOME   By her return appointment, 10/20/12, Mrs. Fu will:

- Practice relaxation for 20 minutes each day

Nursing Interventions	Rationale	Evaluative Statement
Teach and have Mrs. Fu practice progressive muscle relaxation. Suggest that she buy a tape to facilitate the technique (tapes for relaxation are widely available). Recommend that she plan a time when she can be alone and use 20 minutes to complete the technique.	Relaxation promotes a response opposite to the stress response; decreases heart rate, respiratory rate, blood pressure, and metabolic processes.	10/20/12 Outcome met. Mrs. Fu said that at first she had difficulty in finding time to be alone, but she feels so much better after she relaxes that she insists on the time. She did buy a tape and says it helps her very much. *S. Aird, RN, FNP*

EXPECTED OUTCOME   By her return appointment, 10/20/12, Mrs. Fu will:

- Report a decrease in headaches and diarrhea and an increase in her ability to provide self-care to manage stress

(continued)

NURSING PLAN OF CARE · 42-1

For Mei Fu (continued)

Nursing Interventions	Rationale	Evaluative Statement
Assess frequency and severity of headaches and bowel movements. Assess patient's self-report of coping with stressors.	Decreasing stress in daily life often is effective in decreasing physical responses. Self-care of stress is critical in effective management.	10/20/12 Outcome met. Mrs. Fu reports she has noticed fewer headaches in the past week, and the diarrhea is almost gone. Mrs. Fu verbalized the importance of continuing to practice a healthy lifestyle and relaxation. She said she has spent time with her friend and has gotten out her sketchpad. She stated that she believes she can manage her life much better now. *S. Aird, RN, FNP*

SAMPLE DOCUMENTATION

10/06/12, 10 am, nursing

Initial visit to student health center by Mrs. Fu to discuss physical problems of headache and diarrhea. History and physical assessment findings indicated large number of personal stressors, manifested by physical signs and symptoms. Assessment data supported nursing diagnosis: Anxiety related to stress of achievement in school and care of family. Discussion centered on identifying sources of stress, physical responses to stress, sources of support, and personal strength. Teaching strategies included diet, exercise, sleep, and progressive muscle relaxation. Patient's progress will be monitored at next visit on 10/20/12.

S. Aird, RN, FNP

● Developing Critical Thinking Skills

1. Identify the nursing activities and relationships that cause you the most stress. What are your personal warning signs that a situation is becoming stressful? What do you do to decrease your level of stress? Who is most important in helping you do this?

2. List nursing interventions you would use to reduce stress in the following situations:
   • A newly married young woman who found a lump in her breast and is undergoing a breast biopsy
   • The parents of a 2-year-old who are sitting in the surgical waiting room as their child undergoes brain surgery
   • The daughter (and caregiver) of a woman with severe Alzheimer's disease

● Practicing for NCLEX

1. A college student's roommate says she is "so stressed." What happens within the human body as a result of stress?
   a. Becomes increasingly disorganized
   b. Responds to changes in its normal balanced state
   c. Responds to negative changes in its internal environment
   d. Is less likely to respond appropriately to stimuli

2. Which of the following would a nurse identify as an external stressor?
   a. High environmental temperature
   b. Changes in hormone levels
   c. Fear of the dark
   d. Current intestinal infection

3. How does the body maintain the internal environment at a constant state?
   a. Internalization
   b. Adaptation
   c. Cellular integrity
   d. Homeostasis

4. Which of the following individuals would a nurse assess as experiencing developmental stress?
   a. An infant who learns to turn over.
   b. A school-aged child who learns how to add and subtract.
   c. An adolescent who is a "loner."
   d. A young adult who has a variety of friends.

5. The body responds in a variety of ways to stressors. The reflex pain response and the inflammatory response illustrate which of the following responses to stress?
   a. Localized
   b. Negative
   c. Generalized
   d. Positive

6. A nurse is caring for a patient in the shock phase of the GAS. Which response by the patient would be expected?
   a. Decreasing pulse
   b. Increasing sleepiness
   c. Increasing energy levels
   d. Decreasing respirations

7. What term is used to describe a vague feeling of discomfort or dread with an unknown source?
   a. Fear
   b. Concern
   c. Panic
   d. Anxiety

8. Toward the end of the semester, as final examinations near, a student finds himself sleeping more than usual. What best describes his behavior?
   a. Coping mechanism
   b. Defense mechanism
   c. Offense mechanism
   d. Adapting mechanism

9. A patient has just been diagnosed with cancer but responds as though this is impossible. Which of the defense mechanisms is being demonstrated?
   a. Projection
   b. Denial
   c. Displacement
   d. Repression

10. Home care of patients by family members for long periods of time can cause long-term stress and increased risk for illness. What is used to describe this stress response?
    a. Home care chronicity
    b. Patient burnout
    c. Residual stress
    d. Caregiver burden

11. A nurse is teaching a patient a relaxation technique. Which statement demonstrates the need for more teaching?
    a. "I must breathe in and out in rhythm."
    b. "I should take my pulse and expect it to be faster."
    c. "I can expect my muscles to feel less tense."
    d. "I will be more relaxed and less aware."

12. A nurse is teaching a patient about a painful diagnostic procedure. Which type of stress reduction activity would be the most effective?
    a. Progressive muscle relaxation
    b. Meditation
    c. Anticipatory guidance
    d. Biofeedback

13. A nurse teaches problem solving to a college student who is in a crisis situation. What statement best illustrates the student's understanding of the process?
    a. "I need to identify the problem first."
    b. "Listing alternatives is the initial step."
    c. "I will list alternatives after I develop the plan."
    d. "I do not need to evaluate the outcome of my plan."

14. A patient with hypertension is learning to use biofeedback. The nurse understands that which body system is being used with this technique?
    a. Integumentary system
    b. Musculoskeletal system
    c. Autonomic nervous system
    d. Central nervous system

15. A new nursing graduate is considering employment. What setting is considered most stressful for nurses?
    a. Cancer treatment center
    b. Long-term care facility
    c. Operating room
    d. Intensive care unit

● Answers With Rationale

1. *b.* Stress, by definition, causes changes in the normal balanced state.

2. *a.* High environmental temperatures are an external stressor.

3. *d.* To maintain health, the internal environment must remain in balance; this balance is maintained through various physiologic mechanisms as they respond to internal changes.

4. *c.* The adolescent who is a loner is not meeting a major task (being a part of a peer group) for that level of growth and development.

5. *a.* The local adaptation syndrome is a localized response of the body to stress. These responses are homeostatic and short-term; the most common are the reflex pain response and the inflammatory response.

6. *c.* The body perceives a threat and prepares to respond by increasing the activity of the autonomic nervous and endocrine systems. The initial or shock phase is characterized by increased energy levels, oxygen intake, cardiac output, blood pressure, and mental alertness.

7. *d.* Anxiety is a psychological response to an unknown threat.

8. *a.* Mild anxiety is often handled without conscious thought through the use of coping mechanisms, which are behaviors used to decrease stress and anxiety. Sleeping is a coping mechanism.

9. *b.* Denial occurs when a person refuses to acknowledge the presence of a condition that is disturbing.

10. *d.* Reactions of family members to home care for long periods of time, called caregiver burden, include chronic fatigue, sleep disorders, and an increased incidence of stress-related illnesses, such as hypertension and heart disease.

11. *b.* No matter what the technique, relaxation involves rhythmic breathing, a slower pulse, reduced muscle tension, and an altered state of consciousness.

12. *c.* Anticipatory guidance focuses on psychological preparation of the patient for an unfamiliar or painful event. When patients know what to expect, their anxiety is reduced and their coping mechanisms are more effective.

13. *a.* Although identifying the problem may be difficult, a solution to a crisis situation is impossible until the problem is identified.

14. *c.* Biofeedback is a method of gaining control of the autonomic nervous system and regulating body responses to stress such as increased blood pressure, increased heart rate, and headaches.

15. *d.* Patients in intensive care units have complex needs and are at greater risk for death; their care is often stressful.

Taylor Suite Resources

The Taylor Suite offers these additional resources to enhance learning and facilitate understanding of this chapter:

- thePoint online resource, http://thepoint.lww.com/Taylor7E
- Student DVD-ROM included with the book
- Study Guide for Taylor's Fundamentals of Nursing

BIBLIOGRAPHY

The American Institute of Stress. (2008). Stress in the workplace, job stress, occupational stress, job stress questionnaire. Available at http://www.stress.org/topic-workplace.htm?AIS= 16f30694133458211b0edfc3b9ae8d2d

Barclay, L., & Mlurata, P. (2008). Stress management, lifestyle modification help control systolic BP in elderly patients. *Medscape.* Available at http://www.medscape.com/viewarticle/ 572519

Bayat, M., Erdem, E., & Kuzucu, E. (2008). Depression, anxiety, hopelessness, and social support levels of the parents of children with cancer. *Journal of Pediatric Oncology Nursing, 25*(5), 247–253.

Borgatti, J. C. (2008). Stress busters and sanity savers. *American Nurse Today, 3*(2), 38–39.

Bulechek, G., Butcher, H., & Dochterman, J. M. (Eds.). (2008). *Nursing interventions classification (NIC)* (5th ed.). St. Louis: Mosby.

Crane, P., & Clements, P. (2005). Psychological response to disasters: Focus on adolescents. *Journal of Psychosocial Nursing and Mental Health Services, 43*(8), 31–38, 48–49.

Dowd, T., Kolcaba, K., Steiner, R., & Fashinpaur, D. (2007). Comparison of healing touch, coaching, and a combined intervention on comfort and stress in younger college students. *Holistic Nursing Practice, 21*(4), 194–202.

Getting a grip on stress. (2008). *Nursing, 38*(3). 33.

HEALTHbeat. (2008). Reprinted from *Stress management: Techniques for preventing and easing stress.* A special health report from Harvard Medical School. Boston: Harvard Health Publications. Available at www.health.harvard.edu or HEALTHbeat@hms.harvard.edu.

Hyer, K., & Brown, L. (2008). The impact of event scale-revised. *American Journal of Nursing, 108*(11), 60–68.

MayoClinic.com. (2009). *Stress management.* Available at http://www.mayoclinic.com/health/stress-management/ MY00435.

MayoClinic.com. (2008). *Stress management: Understand your sources of stress.* Available at http://www.mayoclinic.com/ health/stress-management/SR00031.

Miller, M. C. (2006). Caregiver stress: When helpers need help. *Harvard Mental Health Letter, 22*(11), 8.

Moorhead, S., Johnson, M., & Maas, M., & Swanson E. (Eds.). (2008). *Nursing outcomes classification (NOC)* (4th ed.). St. Louis: Mosby.

Murphy, K. (2008). Shedding the burden of depression & anxiety. *Nursing, 38*(4), 34–41.

NANDA International. (2009). *Nursing diagnoses: Definitions & classification 2009–20011.* Oxford, UK: Blackwell Wiley.

Pattison, N. (2005). Psychological implications of admission to critical care. *British Journal of Nursing, 14*(13), 708–714.

Pender, N., Murdaugh, C., & Parsons, M. (2006). *Health promotion in nursing practice* (5th ed.). Upper Saddle River, NJ: Prentice Hall.

Porth, C. M., & Matfin, G. (2009). *Pathophysiology: Concepts of altered health states* (8th ed.). Philadelphia: Lippincott Williams & Wilkins.

Research suggests why stress may add pounds. (2007). *Harvard Mental Health Letter, 24*(6), 7.

Seyle, H. (1976). *The stress of life.* New York: McGraw-Hill.

Shindle, M. (2008). Walking the labyrinth: An exercise in self-healing. A stroll through a labyrinth might just reduce your stress, renew your spirit, and spark your creativity. *American Nurse Today, 3*(8), 28–29.

State of the science: Professional partners supporting family caregivers. (2008). *American Journal of Nursing, (September, 2008, Supplement to AJN. Entire issue).*

Tak, S. H. (2006). An insider perspective of daily stress and coping in elders with arthritis. *Orthopaedic Nursing, 25*(2), 127–142.

Vandall-Walker, V., Jensen, L., & Oberle, K. (2007). Nursing support for family members of critically ill adults. *Qualitative Nursing Research, 17*(9), 1207–1218.

Loss, Grief, and Dying

43

YVONNE MALIC

Yvonne, a 20-year-old single woman, has just given birth to a baby, 11 weeks premature. The newborn weighs 2 pounds 2 ounces (1,021 g) and is immediately admitted to the neonatal intensive care unit because of severe respiratory distress. Up until this point, Yvonne had a normal pregnancy and was expecting a healthy baby girl. "I was so happy to be pregnant and I wanted to be a mother so much. But my baby is so tiny! And now the doctors are telling me that she has less than a 50% chance of surviving the next 24 hours."

MANUEL PEREZ

Manuel is a 68-year-old man who moved to a retirement community with his 69-year-old wife 2 months ago. "We were looking forward to traveling and playing lots of golf. But she had this stroke, and now she has permanent brain damage." Mr. Perez is sitting at his wife's bedside, holding her hand, and crying. "The doctors are asking me if I want to continue treatments that are keeping her alive. They mentioned donating her organs. I don't know what to do. We never talked about what we would want."

ANNA MARIA ESPOSITA

The Espositas have been married for 19 years and have two children, Jorge, who is 16, and Marita, who is 13. It has been 2 years since Mrs. Esposita was diagnosed with ovarian cancer, and this period has been difficult for the entire family. At present, she is extremely cachexic (thin) and in the end stage of her illness. She initially tried aggressive treatment, and several chemotherapy regimens failed. During her last hospitalization 2 months ago, a decision was made not to continue treatment, and Mrs. Esposita told her family she wanted to die at home.

LEARNING OBJECTIVES

After completing the chapter, you will be able to accomplish the following:

1. Explain the concepts of loss and grieving, including types of loss and grief reactions.

2. Describe the signs of impending death.

3. Compare and contrast the five emotional stages of dying defined by Kübler-Ross.

4. Identify ethical and legal issues in end-of-life care, including advance directives, physician orders, and euthanasia.

5. Articulate and defend a personal response to a patient's plea, "Please help me die."

6. Explain six factors that affect loss, grief, and dying.

7. Describe physiologic, psychological, and spiritual care of a dying patient and family.

8. Use the nursing process to plan and implement care for dying patients and their families.

9. Outline nursing interventions when providing post-mortem care.

10. Discuss the role of the nurse in caring for the family of a dying patient.

KEY TERMS

active euthanasia	euthanasia
actual loss	grief
advance directive	loss
anticipatory loss	hospice
bereaved	mourning
comfort-measures-only order	palliative care
	perceived loss
death	terminal illness
do-not-resuscitate order	terminal weaning
dysfunctional grief	

There is the potential for loss, grief, and death at any stage of one's life. This is especially true for persons experiencing altered health and for members of their family. A wide variety of losses may occur, including loss of a body part or function, loss of one's ability to care for oneself or to perform valued family or work roles, and death, which may be the most difficult loss of all. Death may be as difficult for healthcare professionals as it is for surviving family members. The goals of nursing include promoting a peaceful death through compassionate palliative care and facilitating coping with disability and death. The nurse is often the person providing support and care when loss or death occurs. To provide effective care, the nurse must have accepted his or her own feelings about death and understand the stages of grieving and dying. (For an example, see the Reflective Practice box.)

CONCEPTS OF LOSS AND GRIEF

The types of loss as well as the varied responses to a loss are important concepts when planning and implementing nursing interventions to facilitate effective coping and adaptation.

Loss

Loss occurs when a valued person, object, or situation is changed or inaccessible so that its value is diminished or removed. There are several types of loss, all of which everyone may experience at some time. **Actual loss** can be recognized by others as well as by the person sustaining the loss, for example, loss of a limb, of a child, of a valued object such as money, and of a job. **Perceived loss,** such as loss of youth, of financial independence, and of a valued environment, is experienced by the person but is intangible to others. Directly related to actual and perceived loss are physical and psychological loss. A person who loses an arm in an automobile crash suffers from both the physical loss of the arm and the psychological loss that may be caused by an altered self-image and the inability to return to his or her occupation. These losses are simultaneously physical, psychological, and actual. A person who is scarred but does not lose a limb may suffer a perceived and psychological loss of self-image.

> Remember Mr. Perez, whose wife has brain damage from a recent stroke. The nurse could use knowledge of the types of losses to help Mr. Perez deal with all the recent changes in his life, including the loss of his wife as a partner. ∎

Other types of loss are maturational loss, situational loss, and anticipatory loss. Maturational loss is experienced as a result of natural developmental processes. As examples, the first child may experience a loss of status when her sibling is born and the parent of a single child may experience a sense of loss when the child begins school. Situational loss is experienced as a result of an unpredictable event, including traumatic injury, disease, death, or national disaster. **Anticipatory loss** occurs when a person displays loss and grief behaviors for a loss that has yet to take place (Fig. 43-1). Anticipatory loss is often seen in the families of patients with serious and life-threatening illnesses and may lessen the effect of the actual loss of a family member.

> Think back to Yvonne Malic, the 20-year-old single mother of the premature neonate described in the beginning of the chapter. The nurse could use knowledge of anticipatory loss to assist Yvonne in coping with the seriousness of her neonate's condition. ∎

REFLECTIVE PRACTICE
Challenge to Ethical and Legal Skills

Anna Maria Giordano was a 49-year-old female attorney who had recently suffered a major cerebral hemorrhage. I came in contact with Ms. Giordano on one of my off-site clinical rotations when I accompanied a social worker for a day at a large medical center. According to most of the nurses and physicians, and the documentation in her chart, her prognosis looked very poor. Due to the fact that she was a lawyer, her advance directives were very clear, appearing to say exactly what she wanted. In essence, her advance directive stated that if she was in a comatose condition and that it appeared as if there was no hope for recovery, she did not want life-sustaining treatment. Although testing did not reveal brain death, almost all the physicians agreed that her condition had little to no hope for improvement. However, one neurosurgeon felt that her condition was improving, with hopes for her recovery; therefore, he had no intention of stopping the life-sustaining treatment. Her family members from Boston had come earlier in the week to discuss treatment options and were given two points of view by two different physicians. Upon hearing the determination of a poor prognosis along with seeing no improvement in the patient's condition over the past few weeks, it was clear from her advance directives that this is not what she wanted.

Thinking Outside the Box: Possible Courses of Action

- Ignore the entire situation: It didn't entirely concern me, since I was only observing as a nursing student for 1 day.
- Talk to the social worker about what I thought was stated in the advance directives, and ask why it wasn't being followed.
- Challenge the doctor as to why he was telling the family that the patient was improving when her assessments for the past 3 weeks had shown no improvement.

Evaluating a Good Outcome: How Do I Define Success?

- The patient is properly diagnosed and her wishes from her advance directives are followed as clearly as they are stated.
- Since the patient is unable to speak, her power of attorney is able to convey what the patient would want.
- The family and the patient's power of attorney are fully informed about the patient's condition so that they can make an educated decision based on what the patient would want.
- My personal and professional integrity are affirmed.

Personal Learning: Here's to the Future!

I chose to talk to the social worker about the patient's advance directives. The social worker was very aware of the situation, explaining that in the past, this neurosurgeon had given other patients' families more optimistic views of the situation, refusing to stop life-sustaining treatment. The social worker explained that she was in the process of bringing this issue to an ethics committee to discuss the situation and hoped that something would be resolved. She also explained that advance directives are often difficult to follow precisely. If the patient is unable to communicate, then the power of attorney takes over, trying his or her best to do what the patient would want. At these times, it can become very subjective. Therefore, following the advance directives is not as simple as one would think it would be.

Although my actions were not extraordinary in this situation, I felt that I learned quite a bit about advance directives, especially trying to honor the patient's and family's wishes. I had learned about advance directives in the past in my previous classes. However, this was the first time I had ever had to deal with them in actual practice. I was able to see how difficult it can be when making such an important decision. I was impressed by the way that the social worker was handling the case; I only hope that I would act in a similar fashion if I were ever faced with a situation like this in the future.

*Kathryn Southerton,
Georgetown University*

Reflection

How do you think you would respond in a similar situation? Why? Are there any factors that might affect your response? If so, explain what these factors are and their possible effect. What do you think might be influencing the neurosurgeon's refusal to end the life-sustaining treatment? How would you respond to this neurosurgeon? In what stage of grief do you think that the neurosurgeon is? The nursing student? The social worker? What does this tell you about yourself and about the adequacy of your skills for professional practice? Can you think of other ways to respond? What other skills (cognitive, interpersonal, technical, ethical/legal) would you need to respond well in this situation? Have you ever been involved in a situation involving an advance directive? If so, were the patient's wishes followed? If not, why not? Do you agree with the criteria used to evaluate a successful outcome? Was professional integrity affirmed? Explain.

FIGURE 43-1. A terminally ill patient's husband begins the grieving process.

Grief

Grief is an internal emotional reaction to loss. It occurs with loss caused by separation, as well as with loss caused by death. For example, many people who divorce experience grief. Loss of a body part, a job, a house, or a pet may cause grief. **Mourning** is the actions and expressions of that grief, including the symbols and ceremonies (including a funeral or final celebration of life) that make up the outward expressions of grief. People who are **bereaved** are in a state of grieving from loss of a loved one.

Grief Reactions

Reactions to grief and dying are similar. The stages of these reactions overlap and vary among individuals (see Factors That Affect Grief and Dying, later in this chapter). One person may skip a reaction stage, whereas another may repeat an earlier stage. Each person is different, and patients and family members may be at different reaction stages. There are several theories of the stages of reactions to grief and death. Two discussed here are by Engel and Kübler-Ross. More important than the actual stages of any given grief reaction is the idea that grief is a process that varies from person to person.

Engel (1964) was among the first to define stages of grief. Engel's six stages are 1) shock and disbelief, 2) developing awareness, 3) restitution, 4) resolving the loss, 5) idealization, and 6) outcome. Shock and disbelief are usually defined as refusal to accept the fact of loss, followed by a stunned or numb response: "No, not me." Developing awareness is characterized by physical and emotional responses such as anger, feeling empty, and crying: "Why me?" Restitution involves the rituals surrounding loss—with death, it includes religious, cultural, or social expressions of mourning, such as funeral services. Resolving the loss involves dealing with the void left by the loss. Idealization is the exaggeration of the good qualities that the person or object had, followed by acceptance of the loss and a lessened need to focus on it. Outcome, the final

resolution of the grief process, includes dealing with loss as a common life occurrence.

Kübler-Ross (1969), a pioneer in the study of grief and death reactions, defined five stages of reaction similar to Engel's. These stages—(1) denial and isolation, (2) anger, (3) bargaining, (4) depression, and (5) acceptance—are discussed later in the chapter.

Dysfunctional Grief

Dysfunctional grief is abnormal or distorted; it may be either unresolved or inhibited. In unresolved grief, a person may have trouble expressing feelings of loss or may deny them; unresolved grief also describes a state of bereavement that extends over a lengthy period. With inhibited grief, a person suppresses feelings of grief and may instead manifest somatic (body) symptoms, such as abdominal pain or heart palpitations.

DYING AND DEATH

Dying may occur suddenly as a result of an accident, injury, or illness or it may occur after a prolonged experience of debilitating disease such as cancer, acquired immunodeficiency syndrome (AIDS), or Alzheimer's disease.

Definitions of Death

The accurate definition of death has proven difficult over time, as technological advances, such as cardiopulmonary resuscitation, have been able to restore lost functions and "bring a person back to life." The Uniform Definition of Death Act (1981) provides a legal definition of **death** as follows: An individual who has sustained either (1) irreversible cessation of all functions of circulatory and respiratory functions, or (2) irreversible cessation of all functions of the entire brain, including the brain stem, is dead. A determination of death must be made in accordance with accepted medical standards.

A Harvard University Medical School committee later added that the nonreversible loss of brain function, accompanied by the more traditional signs, should be the definitive definition of death. These "Harvard criteria" are generally accepted with the understanding that errors in certification of death could occur in conditions that might not permanently suspend life processes, such as from hypothermia (extreme cold), drug or metabolic intoxication, or circulatory shock. In addition, special attention must be paid when a child under the age of 5 is involved. Most protocols require two separate clinical examinations. The medical criteria used to certify a death are:

- cessation of breathing
- no response to deep painful stimuli
- lack of reflexes (such as the gag or corneal reflex) and spontaneous movement

These clinical signs may be further confirmed by an electroencephalogram and/or cerebral blood flow study.

Signs of Impending Death

The clinical signs of impending or approaching death include:

- Difficulty talking or swallowing
- Nausea, flatus, abdominal distention
- Urinary and/or bowel incontinence or constipation
- Loss of movement, sensation, and reflexes
- Decreasing body temperature with cold or clammy skin
- Weak, slow, or irregular pulse
- Decreasing blood pressure
- Noisy, irregular, or Cheyne-Stokes respirations
- Restlessness and/or agitation
- Cooling, mottling, and cyanosis of the extremities and dependent areas

As death nears, the patient may have a decreased level of consciousness or agitated delirium. Although decreased consciousness and agitation are both normal at the end of life, they are very distressing to the patient's family.

Good Death

A good death is one that allows a person to die on his or her own terms, relatively free of pain with dignity. It is free from avoidable distress and suffering for patients, families, and caregivers; in general accord with patients' families wishes; and reasonably consistent with clinical, cultural, and ethical standards (Institute of Medicine, 1997). The definition of a good death varies for each patient, but there are factors important for a good death. These factors include control of symptoms, preparation for death, opportunity to have a sense of completion of one's life, and a good relationship with healthcare professionals. Although the indicators for care that promote a good death listed in Box 43-1were developed by the American Geriatric Society (2007), they apply to persons of all ages. Nurses play a critical role in focusing the healthcare team's attention on meeting the needs of dying persons and their families.

Responses to Dying and Death

People have varying attitudes about death. Increasing numbers are choosing to die at home surrounded by loved ones. Others die alone or in intensive care units surrounded by healthcare professionals and technological equipment. Although each person reacts to the knowledge of impending death or to loss in his or her own way, there are similarities in the psychosocial responses to the situation. Kübler-Ross (1969) studied the emotional responses to death and dying in depth, and nursing and other helping professions have used her findings extensively.

The stages of dying, much like the stages of grief, may overlap, and the duration of any stage may range from as little as a few hours to as long as months. The process varies from person to person. Some people may be in one stage for such a short time that it seems as if they skipped that stage. Sometimes a person returns to a previous stage. According to Kübler-Ross, the five stages of dying, with common reactions, are:

Box 43-1 PROVIDING CARE TO FACILITATE A GOOD DEATH

Although death occurs at any age, the probability of death increases as one grows older. These selected position statements by The American Geriatrics Society Ethics Committee (2007) provide guidance for all healthcare providers in providing excellent care for dying patients of any age.

- The care of the dying patient should be guided by the values and preferences of the individual patient. Independence and dignity are central issues for many dying patients, particularly in the elderly. Maintaining control and not being a burden can also be relevant concerns.
- Palliative care of dying patients is an interdisciplinary undertaking that attends to the needs of both patient and family.
- Care for dying patients should focus on the relief of symptoms, not limited to pain, and should use both pharmacologic and nonpharmacologic means.
- Physicians and other healthcare professionals, at all levels of training, should receive in-depth, insightful, and culturally sensitive instruction in the optimal care of dying patients.
- Adequate funding for research on the optimal care of dying patients is essential to improving end of life care.

---

1. *Denial:* The patient denies the reality of death and may repress what is discussed. The patient may think, "They made a mistake in the diagnosis. Maybe they mixed up my records with someone else's."
2. *Anger:* The patient expresses rage and hostility and adopts a "why me?" attitude: "Why me? I quit smoking and I watched what I ate. Why did this happen to me?"
3. *Bargaining:* The patient tries to barter for more time: "If I can just make it to my son's graduation I'll be satisfied. Just let me live until then." Many patients put their personal affairs in order, make wills, and fulfill last wishes, such as trips, visiting relatives, and so forth. It is important to meet these wishes, if possible, because bargaining helps patients move into later stages of dying.
4. *Depression:* The patient goes through a period of grief before death. The grief is often characterized by crying and not speaking much: "I waited all these years to see my daughter get married. And now I may not be here to see her walk down the aisle. I can't bear the thought of not being there for the wedding— and of not seeing my grandchildren."
5. *Acceptance:* When the stage of acceptance is reached, the patient feels tranquil. The reality of death has been accepted and the patient is prepared to die. The patient may think, "I've tied up all the loose ends: made the will, made arrangements for my daughter to live with her grandparents. Now I can go in peace knowing everyone will be fine."

THE DYING PERSON'S BILL OF RIGHTS

I have the right to be treated as a living human being until I die.

I have the right to maintain a sense of hopefulness, however changing its focus may be.

I have the right to be cared for by those who can maintain a sense of hopefulness, however changing this might be.

I have the right to express my feelings and emotions about my approaching death in my own way.

I have the right to participate in decisions concerning my care.

I have the right to expect continuing medical and nursing attention even though "cure" goals must be changed to "comfort" goals.

I have the right not to die alone.

I have the right to be free from pain.

I have the right to have my questions answered honestly.

I have the right not to be deceived.

I have the right to have help from and for my family in accepting my death.

I have the right to die in peace and dignity.

I have a right to retain my individuality and not be judged for my decisions, which may be contrary to beliefs of others.

I have the right to discuss and enlarge my religious and/or spiritual experiences, whatever these may mean to others.

I have the right to expect that the sanctity of the human body will be respected after death.

I have the right to be cared for by caring, sensitive, knowledgeable people who will attempt to understand my needs and will be able to gain some satisfaction in helping me face my death.

Reprinted with permission from Barbus, A. J. (1975). The dying person's bill of rights. *American Journal of Nursing, 75*(1), 99.

Terminal Illness

In the case of a **terminal illness,** an illness in which death is expected within a limited space of time, the physician is usually responsible for deciding what, when, and how the patient should be told. The nurse, along with members of the clergy and other healthcare professionals, may be involved with these decisions and in discussing the patient's condition with him or her. Most patients want to know their diagnosis and prognosis as soon as possible so that they can begin appropriate planning and take care of business and personal affairs. It is critical for terminally ill patients and their families to have some sense of how the disease is most likely to progress and what this will mean for the patient. All who are involved with the patient's care should know exactly what the patient and the family have been told; members of the patient's healthcare team need to communicate among themselves. *Cultural influences may dictate how much information is desired and which family members are to be informed.*

Effect on the Patient

Many patients realize without being told that they have a terminal illness, picking up this knowledge from nonverbal communication by their families and by healthcare professionals. Patients must be allowed to go through the stages of the grieving process and supported in their decision making. Competent patients have the right to consent to and/or refuse any and all indicated medical treatment—even life-sustaining treatment—and should be made aware of this right. In the past, patients and family members complained about receiving care they did not want and of not being allowed to die. In today's climate of cost-conscious decision making, some patients and family members are complaining that they are being denied costly life-sustaining treatment because of inadequate personal funds or insurance or because they are deemed a poor "investment" of scarce resources. Remember that a patient's wishes should, if possible, be followed. Box 43-2 lists the rights of people who are dying.

Effect on the Family

The family and significant others of terminally ill patients should be encouraged to participate in planning the patient's care. Healthcare personnel should be available to discuss the patient's condition with family members and should offer support and care as the family begins the grieving process (Fig. 43-2). The family may want to make arrangements with the patient for funeral or memorial services, depending on which stage of grief both the patient and the family members are in.

Palliative Care and Hospice

Palliative care means taking care of the whole person—body, mind, and spirit, heart and soul. It views dying as something natural and personal. The goal of palliative care is to give patients with life-threatening illnesses the best quality of life they can have by the aggressive management of symptoms. **Hospice** care is care provided for people with

FIGURE 43-2. The nurse offers support to a patient's grieving spouse.

limited life expectancy, often in the home. While hospice care focuses on the needs of the dying, palliative care is appropriate across the spectrum of disease and illness. Both palliative care and hospice are discussed in Chapter 10.

Ethical and Legal Dimensions

Multiple treatment options and sophisticated life-support technologies may make it difficult to draw the line between promoting life and needlessly prolonging the dying process. In these cases, healthcare decision making is complicated for patients and healthcare professionals alike. Patients have a legally and morally protected right to consent to and refuse medical therapies. Legal foundations for the patient's freedom to choose include the common law right of self-determination and the constitutionally supported right of privacy (discussed in Chapters 6 and 7). Discussions about legalizing physician-assisted suicide and physician-administered lethal injections ("aid in dying") pose new ethical challenges. As patients and families struggle with end-of-life treatment decisions, they are increasingly looking to nurses for information, advice, and support. Nursing care priorities are highlighted in the accompanying Examples of Nursing Diagnoses box. Box 43-3 provides information about related Internet resources for patients and families dealing with grief, loss, and end-of-life concerns.

Advance Directives

Decisions about healthcare are becoming increasingly complex. Patients, family members, and healthcare professionals are voicing frustration as they grapple with complex decisions about prolonging life. Some of the most difficult cases involve patients who are no longer able (competent) to indicate their treatment preferences. Two kinds of written **advance directives** can minimize difficulties by allowing individuals to state in advance what their choices would be for healthcare should certain circumstances develop. Living wills provide specific instructions about the kinds of healthcare that should be provided or foregone in particular situations. A durable power of attorney for healthcare appoints an agent the person trusts to make decisions in the event of subsequent incapacity. A combination directive is illustrated in Figure 43-3. One popular

---

Box 43-3 — END-OF-LIFE WEB RESOURCES

AARP Grief and Loss Programs, http://www.AARP.org/
Aging with Dignity, http://www.agingwithdignity.org/
Dying Well, http://www.dyingwell.org/
GriefNet, http://www.griefnet.org/
Growth House, http://www.growthhouse.org/
Hospice Foundation of America,
    http://www.hospicefoundation.org/
HospiceNet, http://www.hospicenet.org/
National Resource Center on Diversity in End-of-Life Care,
    http://www.ncrd.com/AboutUs.htm
GrievingChild.org, http://www.grievingchildren.org/

---

directive in the United States titled *Five Wishes* (*Aging with Dignity*, 2007) allows individuals to specify:

1. The person I want to make care decisions for me when I can't
2. The kind of medical treatment I want or don't want
3. How comfortable I want to be
4. How I want people to treat me
5. What I want my loved ones to know.

Many means have been suggested to ensure that adult patients have an opportunity to learn about and use advance directives to indicate their wishes about life-prolonging treatment and to appoint surrogate decision makers should they lose decision-making capacity. Nurses play an important role in facilitating this dialogue. In the United States, the Patient Self-Determination Act of 1990 requires all hospitals to inform patients about advance directives. **Because the status of advance directives varies from state to state, it is important for nurses to be familiar with federal and state laws concerning these directives.** Nurses can also be instrumental in developing institutional policies that ensure that patients on admission are encouraged to talk with family, significant others, and healthcare professionals about their treatment preferences.

Do-Not-Resuscitate or No-Code Orders

To prevent the improper use of cardiopulmonary resuscitation, which is designed to prevent unexpected death, some physicians will write do not resuscitate (DNR), or no code, on the chart of a patient if the patient or surrogate has expressed a wish that there be no attempts to resuscitate the patient. A **do-not-resuscitate order** means that no attempts are to be made to resuscitate a patient who stops breathing or whose heart stops beating. However, many physicians are reluctant to write these orders, especially when this issue is a source of conflict between the patient and family or between individual family members.

In some cases, a physician who believes the patient will not benefit from resuscitative measures may indicate verbally to the nurse that only a slow-code (or "show-code") should be called; that is, in the case of cardiopulmonary or respiratory arrest, calling a code and resuscitating the patient are to be delayed until these measures will be ineffectual. Many healthcare institutions have policies forbidding their use. It is likely that a nurse could be charged with negligence in the event of a slow-code and resultant patient death.

The standard of care still obligates healthcare professionals to attempt resuscitation if a patient stops breathing or his or her heart stops (cardiopulmonary arrest) and there is no DNR order to the contrary. For this reason, it is important for nurses to clarify a patient's code status if the probable benefits of resuscitation are negligible or if the nurse has reason to believe a patient would not want to be resuscitated. Many states now allow patients living at home to craft special orders that allow emergency medical technicians called to the home in the event of cardiopulmonary arrest to respect the patient's wishes not to be resuscitated.

(text continues on page 1555)

Examples of NANDA Nursing Diagnoses

Loss and Impending Death

Nursing Diagnoses	Related Factors	Sample Defining Characteristics
Death Anxiety	Newly diagnosed terminal illness	"This can't be happening to me. . . . I know I'm going to die. . . . Why should I try and fight this? Mother fought this same diagnosis and died, why should I hope to be any different?"
Caregiver Role Strain	Hospital discharged dying patient because of inadequate insurance	Spouse has dark circles under eyes, reports unable to sleep through night, decreased appetite, and general lack of energy. "I want to do everything I can for Tony, but I feel so overwhelmed. . . . I don't think anyone prepared me for everything I now find myself needing to do for him. . . . I'm always afraid that I'll hurt him or do something wrong." "I don't want to complain, but I miss being able to go out with my friends. Last week, I didn't even get to church because Tony wasn't feeling well Sunday morning and asked me not to leave. . . . Sometimes I think I'll just go crazy."
Decisional Conflict	Repeat hospitalizations for aspiration pneumonia and new inability to swallow	Family has requested ethics consult because they are split about pending decisions for initiation of artificial nutrition and hydration and advisability of future hospitalizations and continued aggressive treatment; patient has Alzheimer's disease and has been in a nursing home for last 5 years.
Ineffective Coping	Inability to accept death of 42-year-old son who died of a heart attack 2 years ago; failure of coping mechanisms that worked in the past	70-year-old widow who lived alone with son until his death 2 years ago has become a recluse and eats just enough to keep herself alive, seems to exist on gin, cigarettes, and chocolate. "Mothers aren't supposed to outlive their children . . . why didn't God take me first? I just want to die and be with Bernie. . . ."
Ineffective Denial	Inability to believe that she has AIDS and that husband was bisexual	Patient who is just "getting her life back in order" (left abusive husband 1 year ago and is newly happily remarried) learns that she has AIDS. "This can't be happening to me . . . after all I've been through . . . I hear what you are saying but I don't believe you . . . there must be some mistake. . . ." Breaks next appointment and refuses to respond to repeated urgings to seek treatment.
Grieving	Knowledge that fetus is anencephalic	"I don't know how this can be happening to us. . . . We've tried to do everything right. . . . We've waited for this baby for so long. . . . It's hard to believe that our baby won't be normal and that if what the doctors say is true she will only live for a few hours or days at most. . . ."
Complicated Grieving	Inability to accept death of anencephalic infant; no grief resolution	Two years after birth of anencephalic infant who died 3 days after delivery, couple has failed to come to peace with child's death; divorce pending; wife has lost 15 pounds, and her husband complains that she "really let herself go, she quit her job, mopes around the house all day, and isn't interested in anything anymore."
Hopelessness	Inability to accept son's diagnosis of leukemia and favorable prognosis linked to knowledge of death of neighbor's son who had similar diagnosis	"Don't be leading us on. . . . We know what leukemia means, we have neighbors who lost a son to leukemia. . . . It's not true that you can treat this. . . ." Parents refuse to believe favorable prognosis; after hearing diagnosis, they become apathetic and withdrawn. "Marge and Joe tried to do everything to save their son and failed, why should we even try? Nothing else in our lives has worked out."

D.C., Maryland and Virginia

ADVANCE DIRECTIVE

My Durable Power of Attorney for Health Care, Living Will and Other Wishes

I, _____ , write this document as a directive regarding my medical care.

Put the initials of your name by the choices you want.

PART 1. MY DURABLE POWER OF ATTORNEY FOR HEALTH CARE.

_____   I appoint this person to make decisions about my medical care if there ever comes a time when I
            cannot make those decisions myself:

NAME _____ PHONE HOME _____ WORK _____

ADDRESS _____

_____

          If the person above cannot or will not make decisions for me, I appoint this person:

NAME _____ PHONE HOME _____ WORK _____

ADDRESS _____

_____

_____   I have not appointed anyone to make health care decisions for me in this or any other document.

***I want the person I have appointed, my doctors, my family, and others to be guided by the decisions I
have made below:***

PART 2. MY LIVING WILL.

These are my wishes for my future medical care if there ever comes a time when I can't make these decisions
for myself.

A. **These are my wishes if I have a *terminal condition:***
   Life-Sustaining Treatments

   _____   I do not want life-sustaining treatments (including CPR) started. If life-sustaining treatments are
              started, I want them stopped.
   _____   I want life-sustaining treatments that my doctors think are best for me.

   _____   Other wishes: _____

   Artificial Nutrition and Hydration

   _____   I do not want artificial nutrition and hydration started if it would be the main treatment keeping me
              alive. If artificial nutrition and hydration is started, I want it stopped.
   _____   I want artificial nutrition and hydration even if it is the main treatment keeping me alive.

   _____   Other wishes: _____

   Comfort Care

   _____   I want to be kept as comfortable and free of pain as possible, even if such care prolongs my
dying   or shortens my life.

   _____   Other wishes: _____

B. **These are my wishes if I am ever in a *persistent vegetative state:***

   Life-Sustaining Treatments

   _____   I do not want life-sustaining treatments (including CPR) started. If life-sustaining treatments are
              started, I want them stopped.
   _____   I want life-sustaining treatments that my doctors think are best for me.

   _____   Other wishes: _____

FIGURE 43-3. Example of an advance directive (Used with permission of District of Columbia Hospital Association,
Washington, DC.) *(continued)*

Artificial Nutrition and Hydration

_____   I do not want artificial nutrition and hydration started if it would be the main treatment keeping me alive.
If artificial nutrition and hydration is started, I want it stopped.

_____   I want artificial nutrition and hydration even if it is the main treatment keeping me alive.

_____   Other wishes: _____

Comfort Care

_____   I want to be kept as comfortable as possible, even if such care prolongs my dying or shortens my life

_____   Other wishes: _____

C. **Other Direction**

You have the right to be involved in all decisions about your medical care, even those parts not dealing with terminal conditions or persistent vegetative states. If you have wishes not covered in other parts of this document, please indicate them here.

_____

_____

PART 3. OTHER WISHES.

A. **Organ Donation**

_____   I do not wish to donate any of my organs or tissues.
_____   I want to donate all of my organs and tissues.
_____   I only want to donate these organs and tissues: _____

_____   Other wishes: _____

Autopsy

_____   I do not want an autopsy.
_____   I agree to an autopsy if my doctors wish it.

_____   Other wishes: _____

If you wish to say more about any of the above choices, or if you have any other statements to make about your medical care, you may do so on a separate sheet of paper. If you do so, put here the number of pages you are adding: _____

PART 4. SIGNATURES.

You and two witnesses must sign this document for it to be legal.

A. **Your Signature**

By my signature below I show that I understand the purpose and the effect of this document.

SIGNATURE _____ DATE _____

ADDRESS _____

B. **Your Witnesses' Signatures**

I believe the person who has signed this advance directive to be of sound mind, that he/she signed or acknowledged this advance directive in my presence, and that he/she appears not to be acting under pressure, duress, fraud or undue influence. I am not related to the person making this advance directive by blood, marriage or adoption, nor, to the best of my knowledge, am I named in his/her will. I am not the person appointed in this advance directive. I am not a health care provider or an employee of health care provider who is now, or has been in the past, responsible for the care of the person making this advance directive.

Witness #1

SIGNATURE _____ DATE _____

ADDRESS _____

Witness #2

SIGNATURE _____ DATE _____

ADDRESS _____

FIGURE 43-3. (*Continued*)

Comfort Measures Only and Other Special Orders

When a discussion is taking place about resuscitation, it is appropriate to question the use of other life-sustaining interventions, such as the use of dialysis, ventilatory support, artificial nutrition and hydration, blood transfusions, antibiotics and other medications, and surgery. Whereas some patients may want aggressive life-sustaining treatment and such treatment is medically beneficial, other patients may be at a point in their illness at which they choose to terminate all life-sustaining measures and allow the disease to progress naturally to death. There is no moral obligation to initiate or continue the use of life-sustaining treatment that is minimally effective or is a burden. However, laws may place constraints on those who decide to withhold or withdraw life-sustaining treatment for incompetent patients. Nurses should be familiar with pertinent federal and state laws and the policies in their institution or agency concerning the withholding or withdrawing of life-sustaining treatment. Nurses should also be familiar with the forms used to indicate patient preferences about end-of-life care.

Patients may request a **comfort-measures-only order,** which indicates that the goal of treatment is a comfortable, dignified death and that further life-sustaining measures are no longer indicated. A do-not-hospitalize order is being used for patients in nursing homes and other residential settings who have elected not to be hospitalized for further aggressive treatment.

Terminal Weaning

Terminal weaning is the gradual withdrawal of mechanical ventilation from a patient with a terminal illness or an irreversible condition with a poor prognosis. In some cases, competent patients decide that they wish their ventilatory support ended; more often, the surrogate decision makers for an incompetent patient determine that continued ventilatory support is futile. Although it may be expected that a patient will not be able to survive the weaning, death is never a certain outcome, and it is not unusual for a patient to initiate spontaneous respirations once ventilatory support is withdrawn and live for several hours to several days. Competent patients and family members should be prepared for all possibilities. A nurse's role in terminal weaning is to participate in the decision-making process by offering helpful information about the benefits and burdens of continued ventilation and a description of what to expect if terminal weaning is initiated. Supporting the patient's family and managing sedation and analgesia are critical nursing responsibilities. Unfortunately, many agencies and institutions do not have policies for this area. Nurses involved in terminal weaning should consult the literature and be familiar with the latest research.

Active and Passive Euthanasia

Euthanasia literally means "good dying." The two types of euthanasia are active euthanasia and passive euthanasia.

Active euthanasia is taking specific steps to cause a patient's death. *Passive euthanasia* is defined as withdrawing medical treatment with the intention of causing the patient's death. In other words, active euthanasia is **doing something** to end a patient's life, whereas passive euthanasia is **not doing** something to preserve a patient's life. In assisted suicide (which could be considered a form of active euthanasia), the clinician provides the patient with the means to cause his or her own death (e.g., provides a prescription for a lethal dose of barbiturates). In active euthanasia, the clinician acts directly to cause the death of the patient (e.g., administers a lethal dose of medication).

Until recently, most societies maintained that the distinction between "killing" and "allowing to die" was morally relevant. This meant that passive euthanasia, the withholding or withdrawing of medically ineffective or disproportionately burdensome therapies, was morally and legally justified even when this hastened or directly caused a patient's death. On the other hand, making a lethal combination of drugs available to a patient wishing to die (assisted suicide) or administering a lethal injection or carbon monoxide, even when performed with compassionate intent at the request of a patient (active euthanasia), was deemed both immoral and illegal. Some are questioning the validity of this distinction today, and there are efforts to legalize assisted suicide and active euthanasia in numerous countries. In the United States, physician-assisted suicide is legal in Oregon. It is important for nurses to understand the arguments for and against assisted suicide and active euthanasia and to clarify what they believe (Box 43-4).

The American Nurses Association (ANA) (1994) issued position statements stating that assisting in suicide and participating in active euthanasia are in violation of the Code for Nurses, the ethical traditions and goals of the profession, and its covenant with society. Nurses may be confronted by patients who seek assistance in ending their lives. Unless nurses think through this issue carefully, they will be unprepared to respond to the request, "Nurse, please help me die."

Death Certificate

U.S. law requires that a death certificate be prepared for each person who dies. The law specifies what information needs to be supplied. Death certificates are sent to local health departments, which compile many statistics from the information. The mortician assumes responsibility for handling and filing the death certificate with proper authorities. A physician's signature is required on the certificate, as well as that of the pathologist, the coroner, and others in special cases. The nurse's responsibility is to ensure that the physician has signed a death certificate.

Organ Donation

Patients who express a wish to donate functional organs, such as heart, corneas, liver, lungs, and kidneys, can fill out an organ donor consent card (Fig. 43-4). In addition, depending on

---

Box 43-4 **ETHICAL CHALLENGES: THINKING CRITICALLY ABOUT ASSISTED SUICIDE AND ACTIVE EUTHANASIA**

Nurses are often the first to hear a patient's plea, "Please help me die." It is critical for nurses to reflect carefully on what they believe about assisted suicide and active euthanasia and how this influences the responses they make to patients. Assisted suicide is illegal in all states in the United States except Oregon.

- Should the principle of respect for autonomy be expansive enough to embrace respect for, and acquiescence to, a competent patient's request for assistance in dying?
- Does the right to privacy entail a right, in effect, to decide the time and manner of one's death and to gain assistance in implementing that decision?
- Is there such a thing as *rational* suicide?
- If assisted suicide and active euthanasia were to become accepted practices, would this simply represent a logical, defensible extension of the well-established moral basis for refusal of treatment and withholding/withdrawing treatment?

- Are assisted suicide and active euthanasia acts of mercy, morally grounded in the principles of benefiting and not harming patients and expressive of the virtues of compassion and beneficence?
- Is it possible to conceive of situations in which a nurse or a physician has a duty to help a patient die (specifically via active euthanasia/assisted suicide)?
- Is refusal to accede to a patient's request for assisted suicide or active euthanasia a form of abandonment, or are there limits to the duty to respect autonomy, right to privacy, and self-determination?
- Are calls for assisted suicide and active euthanasia emblematic of failure to provide adequate palliative care and to address the suffering of the dying?
- If medicine and nursing possess an "internal" morality, are assisted suicide and active euthanasia consistent with that morality?

---

state law, signing the back of one's driver's license indicates approval of organ donation. The family of a deceased patient also may decide to donate the patient's functional organs. The nurse should be able to review options and provide consent forms to interested patients and their families. Until recently, most organs were retrieved from totally brain-dead patients. New protocols for retrieving organs from non–heart-beating cadavers are raising multiple practice concerns. Comprehensive attention to optimal patient and family care at the time of withdrawal of life-sustaining therapy needs to remain the nurse's priority. The scarcity of organs has resulted in legislation mandating hospitals and other healthcare agencies to notify transplantation programs of potential donors.

> ➤ *Think back to Mr. Perez, who was asking about advance directives and organ donation after his wife had a stroke. The nurse could incorporate knowledge of organ donation to provide appropriate information for Mr. Perez so that he can make the most informed decision possible.* ∎

Signed by the donor and the following two witnesses in the presence of each other:
Signature of Donor   Date of Birth of Donor
Date Signed   City and State
Witness   Witness
This is a legal document under the Uniform Anatomical Gift Act or similar laws in all 50 states
Delaware Valley TRANSPLANT PROGRAM   For further information call **800 KIDNEY-1** 2401 Walnut St., Suite 404 Philadelphia, PA 19103

UNIFORM DONOR CARD

Print or type name of donor

In the hope that I may help others, I hereby make this anatomical gift, if medically acceptable, to take effect upon my death. The words and marks below indicate my desires.

I give: a) _____ any needed organs or parts

b) _____ only the following organs or parts

Specify the organ(s) or parts(s)

for the purpose of transplantation, therapy, medical research or education:

c) _____ my body for anatomical study if needed

Limitations or special wishes, if any

FIGURE 43-4. Example of an organ donor card.

Autopsy

An autopsy is an examination of the organs and tissues of a human body after death. Obtaining consent for autopsy is a legal requirement. The closest surviving family member or members usually have the authority to determine whether an autopsy is performed. Some religious groups prohibit autopsies except for legal purposes.

It is usually the physician's responsibility to obtain permission for an autopsy. Sometimes the patient may grant this permission before death. The nurse can assist by explaining the reasons for an autopsy. Many relatives find comfort when they are told that the knowledge gained from an autopsy may contribute to advances in medical science as well as establish the exact cause of death.

If death is caused by accident, suicide, homicide, or illegal therapeutic practice, the coroner must be notified, according to law. The coroner may decide that an autopsy is advisable and can order that one be performed, even though the patient's family has refused consent. In some cases, a death that occurs within 24 hours of admission to the hospital must be reported to the coroner.

FACTORS THAT AFFECT GRIEF AND DYING

Many factors, including age, family relationships, socioeconomic position, and cultural and religious influences, affect a person's reaction to and expression of grief. Like the stages of grief reaction, these factors vary from person to person.

Developmental Considerations

Children do not understand death on the same level as adults do, but their sense of loss is just as great. Both terminally ill children and their siblings are likely to talk and ask questions about death in an attempt to understand it. Terminally ill children require parental love and support as well as social interaction with other children. Death of a parent or another significant person can retard a child's development or may cause the child to regress developmentally. Children need to go through the same grief reactions as adults to accept such a loss and maintain emotional well-being.

The loss of a parent by a middle-aged adult helps to prepare the adult for the loss of a spouse or significant other and to accept his or her own eventual death. Older people may lose a spouse or friends and relatives their own age. As this happens, they reminisce about life, put their lives and the purpose of living in perspective, and prepare themselves for their own inevitable death.

Family

Family roles have an important effect on a person's reactions to and expressions of grief. For example, the eldest sibling may feel a need to "be strong" and, therefore, may not grieve openly; a person who loses a spouse may display the same type of behavior to "protect the children."

The death of a child is a devastating experience for the family. The family needs time to accept the reality of the situation, opportunities to talk and to be listened to, and the experience of being able to express themselves behaviorally in a nonjudgmental environment. For example, the family of a terminally ill child may express feelings of guilt by wondering if they were responsible for the impending death. A sibling may suppress a guilt feeling for having wished the ill child (or a parent) dead.

Socioeconomic Factors

A bereaved family may suffer more acutely if there is no health or life insurance or pension after the death of the family provider. Such families face not only the loss of a loved one, but also an economic loss that may further disrupt family life. Older people especially may be placed in a difficult position because the death of a spouse may result in the decrease or even elimination of a source of retirement income for the surviving spouse. This reduction in income may lead to loss of home, community, and support systems.

Cultural, Gender, and Religious Influences

Culture influences a person's expression of grief. In many families in the Western culture, grief is a private matter shared only with the family. As such, many people internalize their feelings of grief and may not express their feelings of loss to others. On the other hand, cultural background may necessitate that the patient's and family's public display be emotional and distressed, with loud weeping and moaning.

Although gender roles have become less differentiated in the past few decades, male and female reactions to death may differ. Whereas men are often expected to be stoic and not cry in public, women may be judged as "cold" if they do not grieve publicly. The widow who has a job may not be as emotionally distraught as the woman who needed her husband for financial and other support. Likewise, the widower who has not taken care of the children or the house may view the future more bleakly than the man who has cooked meals and changed diapers. Some ethnic traditions may be ingrained in certain people. For example, the woman may be expected to be weak and need support, whereas the man may be expected to be emotionally supportive. This varies from culture to culture and from person to person.

Faith and religious practices play an important role in the expression of grief and provide comfort and solace to the person experiencing loss. At the same time, others may blame God for their suffering and the death of their loved one and turn away from God. Many people who have put spiritual matters in the background of their lives have found death to be an impetus for a return to earlier practices of religion. The thought of death also invites many to contemplate life's big questions: Is there life after death? Is there a supreme being? And if there is a supreme being where do I stand in relationship to him/her? What is the ultimate source of meaning in my life? See Chapter 46 for a discussion of spiritual care.

Cause of Death

The grief response often depends on the cause of death. Many deaths are sudden and involve shock as well as normal grieving in the survivors. Death from disease may generate several types of responses, including the belief that the death is a punishment (e.g., when AIDS was first diagnosed in homosexuals and drug users), terror and panic (e.g., when people are reminded of the devastation caused by plagues of earlier centuries), and guilt (e.g., when family and friends believe that they could have prevented the death).

Accidental death is often associated with feelings of bad luck. The guilt response can be enormous, especially when children die as the result of an accident. Death while defending a country usually is viewed by most of society as honorable and necessary. Violent deaths occur daily, especially in larger cities. Suicide accounts for a great number of violent deaths; in fact, among teenagers, it has become a major concern. It is also believed that many accidental deaths are actually suicides.

THE NURSE AS ROLE MODEL

Holistic care of the terminally ill patient and family almost always involves some personal emotional investment. It is unrealistic and unfair to expect nurses to handle circumstances surrounding death without feelings. The best policy seems to be taking the time to explore one's own feelings and express them (Promoting Health 43-1).

The nurse who neglects to deal with personal feelings about life, dying, and death is in a questionable position for analyzing and considering the needs of patients facing death. A nurse's own feelings play a major role in determining the care given to a patient with a terminal illness. The following are some questions the nurse should use to help clarify his or her thinking and feelings about dying and death:

- If I could control the events that result in my own death, where would I want to be? What cause of death would I choose? Whom would I want to have present during my terminal illness?
- What fears do I have about death?

- How would I answer these same questions for a patient for whom I have been caring?
- How could I improve the quality of care for a terminally ill patient for whom I am caring?
- If I were a member of the patient's family, what things would I want a nurse to do for me?

The nurse who cares for a patient for an extended period may undergo a grief reaction when the patient dies (Fig. 43-5). Grief after the death of a patient is natural, and the nurse should allow himself or herself to go through the grieving process rather than shut off the grief. The nurse should also address personal health needs.

THE NURSING PROCESS FOR GRIEVING OR DYING PATIENTS AND FAMILIES

The nursing process is a helpful tool when caring for patients who are grieving or dying and their families and significant others.

PROMOTING HEALTH • 43-1

Grieving

If a past or current loss is influencing your everyday functioning, use the assessment checklist to see how well you are responding to the losses in your life. Then develop a prescription for self-care by choosing appropriate behaviors from the list of suggestions.

Assessment Checklist

❑ almost always	❑ sometimes	❑ almost never

❑ ❑ ❑ 1. I can name the personal losses that are currently influencing my state of well-being.

❑ ❑ ❑ 2. I have a plan for coping with these losses that is in place and helping me to cope.

❑ ❑ ❑ 3. I understand the importance of grieving, and I actually set time aside for this self-care measure.

❑ ❑ ❑ 4. I am comfortable with my feelings and am able to give them expression.

❑ ❑ ❑ 5. There is someone who knows and accepts me well enough to allow me to share openly and honestly.

❑ ❑ ❑ 6. I value being a supportive presence for people with life-threatening illnesses.

❑ ❑ ❑ 7. I respond genuinely to the concerns and feelings of dying patients and their families; I am not afraid to cry with patients and to allow my feelings to show.

Self-Care Behaviors

1. Make a list of the losses that are interfering with your present state of well-being. These may include the loss of health, valued role, image/reputation, relationship, material object, job, or person.
2. Determine whether or not you are addressing these losses in a conscious fashion, and identify coping strategies that may be of help.
3. Try implementing a "tried and true" or new coping strategy.
4. Talk about one of these losses with a friend, religious leader, or counselor/therapist. Assess your comfort level in sharing your feelings openly. Ask the person you are sharing with how he or she thinks you are responding.
5. Be honest about any maladaptive coping strategies you may be using to cope such as addictions, apathy ("Who cares?"), withdrawal and passivity, depression, and acting out. Get any help you need to replace these maladaptive coping measures.
6. Reflect upon what your level of comfort in being with people who are dying reveals about your own acceptance of the fact that we will all die.

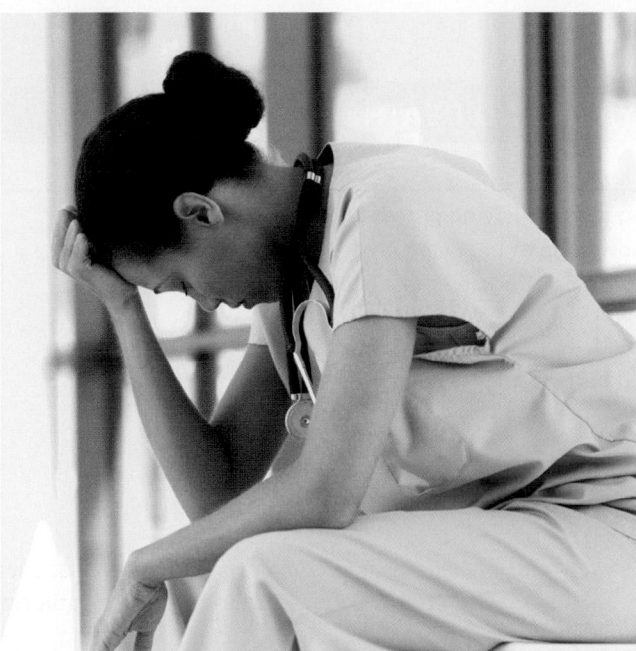

FIGURE 43-5. A nurse grieves the loss of a patient.

Assessing

Focused assessment for those experiencing loss, grief, and dying is directed toward determining the adequacy of the patient's and family's knowledge, perceptions, coping strategies (see Chapter 42), and resources. Pertinent interview questions are highlighted in Focused Assessment Guide 43-1. Physical assessment of both the dying patient and of concerned family, friends, and family caregivers is essential to diagnosing some problems.

Diagnosing

The data the nurse collects about how a patient or the patient's caregivers are responding to an actual or impending loss, or to impending death may support several different nursing diagnoses. Samples of these diagnoses with examples of their defining characteristics are given in the box, Examples of NANDA Nursing Diagnoses, earlier in this chapter.

Response to Loss as the Problem

Nursing diagnoses that specifically address human responses to loss and impending death in the problem statement include Caregiver Role Strain, Decisional Conflict, Ineffective Denial, Ineffective Coping, Grieving or Complicated Grieving, Hopelessness, Ineffective Family Therapeutic Regimen Management, and Powerlessness. Nursing Diagnoses help determine the appropriate care. Box 43-5 provides an overview of the nursing process related to Decisional Conflict.

Response to Loss as the Etiology

Difficulty responding to loss or impending death may also affect other areas of human functioning and result in different diagnoses. Examples of nursing diagnoses for which the experience of loss as the etiology may include:

- Anxiety related to inability to predict how the last stage of illness will play itself out
- Interrupted Family Processes related to stress of caring for dying mother
- Fatigue related to constant demands of caring for dying family member
- Fear related to perceived loss of control and increasing need to be dependent in final stages of illness
- Deficient Knowledge related to lack of experience in caring for dying family member at home
- Situational Low Self-Esteem related to inability to accept need for assistance as disease progresses
- Spiritual Distress related to inability to reconcile diagnosis and pain with belief in a loving God
- Bathing, dressing, or feeding Self-Care Deficits related to decreasing strength as terminal illness progresses

Outcome Identification and Planning

Nursing care should be directed toward the achievement of the following goals or outcomes for grieving and dying patients and their families. The patient or family will:

- Demonstrate freedom to express feelings, needs, fears, and concerns
- Identify and use effective coping strategies
- Accept need for help as appropriate and use available resources
- Make healthcare decisions reflecting personal values and goals; ultimately feel peaceful about role in decision making
- Declare preferences regarding treatment options
- Report sufficient relief of pain to interact meaningfully with family and to attend to everyday concerns
- Experience a dignified and comfortable death
- Resolve grief after a suitable period of mourning and resume meaningful roles and daily activities (family or significant others)

The patient and the family should take an active role in planning for care. Such planning takes the patient's preferences into consideration, facilitates the acceptance of death by the patient and the family, and provides interventions to meet holistic needs.

Implementing

In addition to promoting a comfortable, dignified death, the nurse's aims in caring for dying patients and their families include facilitating coping of the dying person and family and promoting health and preventing illness of the family. The accompanying Focus on the Older Adult display provides indicators for a comfortable, dignified, and peaceful death.

Developing a Trusting Nurse–Patient/Family Relationship

Communication is a lifelong need up to the moment of death and should be maintained at all times with the patient and family. To develop meaningful communication, the nurse must

(text continues on page 1562)

FOCUSED ASSESSMENT GUIDE • 43-1

THE EXPERIENCE OF LOSS, GRIEF, DYING, AND DEATH

Assessment Priorities

- Patient and family's understanding of medical condition, prognosis, and dying process
- Patient and family's attitude toward death and dying and knowledge of the dying process
- Patient's preferences for end-of-life treatment and care: desire to be at home or in a hospital; decisions concerning treatment, resuscitation, advanced life support, organ donation, etc.
- Documented evidence of advance care planning
- Existence of advance directive **(It is critical that the authorized decision maker be known to all members of the healthcare team.)**
- Religious beliefs
- Cultural influences
- Stage of grief and death reaction
- Adequacy of coping behaviors
- Adequacy of resources
- Physiologic needs of the patient, for example, personal hygiene, pain control, nutritional and fluid needs
- Psychological needs of the patient and family, for example, fear of the unknown, pain, separation
- Spiritual needs of the patient and family: need for meaning and purpose, for love and relatedness, for forgiveness, for hope

Factors to Assess	Questions and Approaches
Adequacy of knowledge base	What have you been told about your condition? What do you know about this condition? Please describe what you have been told about your treatment options. Is there anything you don't understand about what your doctor is recommending? What else would you like to know about your present condition and treatment options? Do you know how to contact your doctor and to get the information you need/desire? *Objective is to identify whether or not the knowledge the patient and family possess will allow them to make informed decisions that will serve their best interests.*
Realism of expectations/ perceptions	Have you had any previous experiences with this condition or with the death of someone you love? What are your expectations in this case? How do you see the next few weeks (days) playing out? What are your fears, hopes, concerns, worries? What good do you think might be happening in the midst of all this? *Objective is to discover whether the patient and family have unrealistic expectations or misperceptions about the diagnosis, prognosis, and care options that will interfere with their decision making and coping.*
Adequacy of coping strategies	Dealing with our own dying is a once-in-a-lifetime experience, and sometimes we begin the process feeling totally unprepared. Tell me something about how you think you are coping with all this. How well do you think those around you are coping? How can I help you develop or tap the resources that will help you to cope better? *Objective is to identify whether the patient and the patient's family are using effective coping strategies. If you detect problems, try to identify coping strategies they have used effectively in the past. Also, identify and address destructive habits that have not served them well in the past such as addictions, destructive relationships, passivity, and acting out. Creatively problem solve about new strategies they might try.*
Adequacy of resources	What is helping you to get through this? Do you think the resources available to you are adequate? If the sky was the limit, what help would you wish for? What is interfering with your getting the help you need? What are some of the community resources that might be of help to you? Are you using these? *Objective is to assess the adequacy of the human, financial, spiritual, and psychological resources available to the patient. Questions should be directed to determining what, if anything, is interfering with the patient using whatever resources are available to facilitate coping.*
Physical response	A physical assessment of the patient and the patient's family and caregivers should be performed to detect problems with coping that result in fatigue, decreased energy, decreased self-care (deficient grooming, unplanned weight loss), and other maladaptive responses.

Box 43-5   NURSING PROCESS RELATED TO DECISIONAL CONFLICT

Patients and the surrogate decision makers for incompetent patients frequently feel overwhelmed when they need to make life-and-death decisions about end-of-life care. The NANDA diagnosis for this response follows:

> Decisional Conflict: The state of uncertainty about course of action to be taken when choice among competing actions involves risk, loss, or challenge to values and beliefs (NANDA, 2009, p. 293)

Assessment Priorities

The objective of assessment is to identify individuals and families who are at high risk for decisional conflict and to provide the support they need to make appropriate end-of-life care decisions that advance the patient's interests before problems develop. Potential problems when this need is overlooked include postponement of decision making, which interferes with the patient receiving optimal care; vacillation in decision making, which disturbs continuity of care for the patient; and escalation of conflict concerning decision making, which may result in a standoff between participating parties—the patient, individual family members, and healthcare professionals.

- Detect difficulties with making decisions: fear; insufficient or erroneous information; inadequate support; conflict between religious convictions, personal moral beliefs, and choice one wants to make; and reluctance to assume responsibility for making life-and-death decision.
- Identify what is causing the decision making to be hard for the patient or family and what type of information or support could reverse this.
- Identify potential conflicts between what the patient wants and what his or her family or caregivers believe should be done.
- Observe the patient or his or her surrogate decision makers for physical signs of distress that reflect feeling overwhelmed by the decision that needs to be made: signs of fatigue and general exhaustion, signs of agitation and distress, and signs of growing anger and alienation.
- Read the chart carefully to identify decisions that are pending and note the lack of movement toward a decision or toward resolution of existing conflict.

Expected Outcomes

The morally and legally valid decision maker will achieve the following:

- Describe care options (including the option of nontreatment), listing the advantages and disadvantages of each
- Seek clarification of options, if necessary, and whatever support is needed
- Express fears, concerns, and hopes
- Make an informed and voluntary choice
- Make end-of-life decisions that reflect the patient's values and goals, advancing his or her interests
- Make end-of-life decisions that are consistent with the aims of medicine and nursing

Interventions

Nursing measures revolve around identifying and supporting the morally and legally valid decision maker. The following should be considered:

- Competent patients—those who can (1) understand the information needed to make the decision, (2) reason in accord with a relatively consistent set of values, and (3) communicate a preference—have the right to consent to and to refuse any and all indicated medical treatment.
- Surrogates of previously competent patients are to be guided by what is known about the patient's values and preferences. These surrogates may be designated in an advance directive, or there may be state or province law designating a hierarchy of surrogates, such as spouse, parent, adult child, sibling; the morally valid surrogate is the one who best knows the patient and the patient's preferences.
- Surrogates deciding for a never-competent patient (child or profoundly retarded adult) must be guided by a determination of what is in the patient's best interests by referring to more objective and socially shared values.

The nurse clarifies the goal of treatment (cure, stabilization of functioning, preparation for a comfortable and dignified death) and makes sure that treatment decisions are consistent with this goal. Nursing intervention may be helpful in making sure that everyone is clear about the goal of care and changes in the goal of care as the patient's condition changes. Because some physicians are reluctant to accept preparation for a comfortable, dignified death as an appropriate goal of medicine, some patients have received unwanted care that needlessly prolonged their dying. Conversely, decisions are being made today for financial and other reasons that deprive patients of wanted end-of-life care.

The nurse serves as an advocate for the patient and the family unless what the patient or family wants violates the profession of nursing and nursing's code of ethics or one's own conscience. Interventions include the following:

- Providing whatever information and support the patient or family needs to make an informed and voluntary decision
- Referring the patient or family to sources that can clarify problematic aspects of the decision, such as religious authority, ethicist, legal counsel
- Identifying and addressing coercive influences on decision making, being sensitive to cultural norms; for example, whereas a controlling husband may be violating his wife's freedom to make autonomous choices in one culture, in another, it is customary for the husband (or male elder in the family) to make choices for a woman.

Documentation of end-of-life care preferences of competent, or previously competent, patients is important. This includes a written record of communication, a living will, durable power of attorney for healthcare, and a medical advance directive. These preferences must be communicated to those who are ordering care.

- Mediating sources of conflict
- Referring patient or family to an ethics consult team or ethics committee if conflict cannot be resolved

FOCUS ON THE OLDER ADULT

MEASURING QUALITY OF CARE AT THE END OF LIFE

The American Geriatric Society developed the following statement of principles about quality care at the end of life, but these indicators would seem to work well for persons of all ages:

1. *Physical and emotional symptoms.* Pain, shortness of breath, fatigue, depression, fear, anxiety, nausea, skin breakdown, and other physical and emotional problems often destroy the quality of life at its end. Symptom management is regularly deficient. Care systems should focus on these needs and ensure that people can count on a comfortable and meaningful end of their lives.

2. *Support of function and autonomy.* Even with an inevitable and progressive decline with fatal illness, much can be done to maintain personal dignity and self-respect. Achieving better functional outcomes and greater autonomy should be valued.

3. *Advance care planning.* Often, the experience of patient and family can be improved just by planning ahead for likely problems, so that decisions can reflect the patient's preferences and circumstances rather than responding to crises.

4. *Aggressive care near death—site of death, CPR, and hospitalization.* Although aggressive care is often justified, most patients would prefer to have avoided it when short-term outcome is death. High rates of medical interventions near death should prompt further examination of provider judgment and care system design.

5. *Patient and family satisfaction.* The dying patient's peace of mind and the family's perception of the patient's care and comfort are extremely important. In the long run, we can hope that the time at the end of life will be especially precious, not merely tolerable. We must measure both patient and family satisfaction with these elements: the decision-

making process, the care given, the outcomes achieved, and the extent to which opportunities were provided to complete life in a meaningful way.

6. *Global quality of life.* Often a patient's assessment of overall well-being illuminates successes and shortcomings in care, which are not apparent in more specific measures. Quality of life can be good despite declining physical health, and care systems that achieve this should be valued.

7. *Family burden.* How healthcare is provided affects whether families have serious financial and emotional effects from the costs of care and the challenges of direct caregiving. Current and future pressures on funding healthcare are likely to displace more responsibility for services and payment onto families.

8. *Survival time.* With pressures upon healthcare resources likely to increase, there is new reason to worry that death will be accepted too readily. Purchasers and patients need to know survival times vary across plans and provider systems. In conjunction with information about symptoms, satisfaction, and the other domains listed here, such measures will allow insights into the priorities and trade-offs within each care system.

9. *Provider continuity and skill.* Only with enduring relationships with professional caregivers, can patient and family develop trust, communicate effectively, and develop reliable plans. The providers also must have the relevant skills, including rehabilitation, symptom control, and psychological support. Care systems must demonstrate competent performance on continuity and provider skill.

10. *Bereavement.* Often healthcare stops with the patient's death, but the suffering of the family goes on. Survivors may benefit with relatively modest interventions.

Used with permission, *The American Geriatric Society.*

---

develop a trusting relationship with the patient. The nurse needs to develop listening skills and the ability to recognize both verbal and nonverbal cues given by the patient and family. These skills are discussed in Chapter 21.

Be willing to discuss the patient's fears and doubts openly and to serve as a nonjudgmental listener. However, talking with dying patients is often difficult. The following suggestions by Rancour (personal communication) provide assistance.

- Often, when patients initiate conversations about dying, you may feel unprepared for their questions. They can take you by surprise, and can often lead you to believe that the patient expects a crystal ball response. Remember that the purpose of all such discussions is to keep the lines of communication open with the patient. The idea is to make the subject of dying discussible, and to communicate to the patient that it does not make you afraid to do so. An open-ended statement, such as "Tell me what concerns you the most" provide a means of encouraging communication.

- Some patients may be too fearful to ask physicians such questions. They often approach staff who they perceive as less intimidating or more approachable. The question often comes in the middle of the night, when there are no distractions, when anxiety or pain may keep the patient

awake, when the patient may feel most alone with psycho-spiritual distress. In any case, it is often on the nurse's watch when questions about dying may arise.

- Because of the surprising nature of such questions, you may feel tempted to escape ("I've got to go take that patient's vital signs right now."), or pass the buck ("That sounds like a question for your doctor.") Be vigilant about such impulsive behavior and realize that it only serves your own need to reduce your anxiety, but does nothing to assist the patient with his own. It is well within the scope of your professional practice as a competent nurse to provide counseling and death education, especially when the patient asks you for it or indicates an unmet need for such information and support. *When in doubt, ask a question in response, such as* "What do you feel about that?" *or* "What have you been told already?" This will accomplish several things. First, it will help you to regain your composure. The second point of asking a question is that it will give you more information about what is on the patient's mind so that your intervention can be as specific and responsive to that patient as possible.

- Do not provide false reassurance. It is important to remember that avoiding discussions about death robs the patient of precious time to accomplish goals that produce hope (Box 43-6). People who are dying hope for many

Box 43-6 ENABLING HOPE IN THE TERMINALLY ILL

These guidelines are the product of an interdisciplinary team of those providing care for the terminally ill. They are presented to encourage anyone providing care for the terminally ill to consider the crucial place of hope in their caring and also their own potential to enable such hope.

Hope
Hope is the ingredient in life that enables an individual both to consider a future and to actively bring that future into being. Hope originates in imagination but must become a valued and realistic possibility for that individual in order to energize action. Hope has the capacity to embrace the reality of an individual's suffering without escaping from it (false hope) or being suffocated by it (despair, helplessness, hopelessness).

Hope is unique to each person. During terminal illness, the future being considered will become more focused, yet hope is essential for an individual to transcend despair and complete crucial life tasks.

Enabling Hope
Acknowledging Individual Uniqueness
To enable such hope, the care provider must acknowledge *the uniqueness of the individual* and take seriously the dreams of the terminally ill person within the changing nature of the illness. Steps that can be taken to translate hope into accomplishment must be considered. For this to happen, care providers need to do the following:
- Consider all language used, and appreciate how easily hopes can be disabled by such terms as "hopeless situation" or "nothing more can be done."
- Encounter the individual's feelings at his or her own level; be willing to stay at that individual's level and allow him or her to lead.
- Be willing to take the necessary time to establish rapport with the individual in order that his or her hopes can be shared in a supportive atmosphere. Where appropriate, use physical contact to build trust.
- Realize the changing nature both of the disease and the accompanying hopes. At one point, a hope for a cure may be the necessary activating force for an individual to undergo treatment; at another, a hope to consider one's dying may give the energy to complete crucial life tasks or endure the many losses of terminal illness.

Granting Control
A factor crucial to the nourishing of hope within an individual is that of *control*. An individual must be willing to take the necessary action to achieve what is hoped for. Terminal illness places many restrictions upon an individual and often robs that person of a feeling of being able to control the situation, thus leading to increasing helplessness and hopelessness. To counter this, efforts must be made not only to support an individual in hoping, but also to grant the person control in bringing realistic hopes into being.

To help support an individual's sense of control in order to enable active hoping, care providers need to do the following:
- Provide honest and accessible information regarding the progress of the illness.

- Allow an individual to express and work through many hopes in order to develop those hopes appropriate to him or her in the present context.
- Allow for freedom of choice regarding treatment options to the degree possible within the setting.
- Maximize the present possibilities for achieving hopes while allowing for the changing realities of terminal illness.

Being Aware of One's Own Feelings
Hope is strengthened by those who care for and support a terminally ill individual. Within the context of illness and suffering, hope may be fragile and must be nurtured in relationships with professional caregivers, family, and friends. To enable hope, care providers must be aware of their own hope for that individual.

Care providers need to do the following:
- Recognize their own assumptions regarding that particular individual and how those assumptions may inhibit the enabling of hope for that person.
- Be aware of how their own hope for that individual may differ from the hope being expressed by that person.
- Resist judging expressed hope and be willing to explore such hope further.
- Accept the individual's present suffering. Avoid giving "false hope" that minimizes the reality of the situation ("It can't be that bad," or "Don't worry, everything will be fine") or encouraging despair by focusing only upon the illness ("God can't possibly heal you now. That cancer's all through you!").

Supporting Spirituality
A component of hope is *spirituality*. Supported by faith in God, hope is the capacity to transcend present suffering, to lift one's perspective to future possibilities, and so to enable that individual to accomplish important life tasks. This capacity to transcend is facilitated by one's belief in the presence of God within the changing context of terminal illness.

To enable this spiritual aspect of hope, care providers need to do the following:
- Accept the individual's own spiritual journey and present level of faith (or lack of).
- Be open to expressed hopes that link with religious belief (e.g., "God will cure me" or "I pray that God will take me home soon").
- Allow for spiritual struggle and its resultant emotions (e.g., anger when "the cancer is back and God has failed to cure me!"). Recognize that the level of spiritual struggle during terminal illness may increase to enable the accomplishment of crucial hope for life tasks such as reconciliation and forgiveness.
- Be prepared to accept the reality of death as an aspect of hope. Accept an individual who has shifted hope to how he or she wishes to die, to life after death, to a meeting with deceased loved ones, and so on.
- Enable an individual to have access to whatever means and rites of religion that will encourage his or her hope.

Courtesy of Ted Creen, D.Min., Palliative Care Pastoral Consultant, 865 2nd Ave. West, Owen Sound, Ontario, Canada; 519-376-7886.

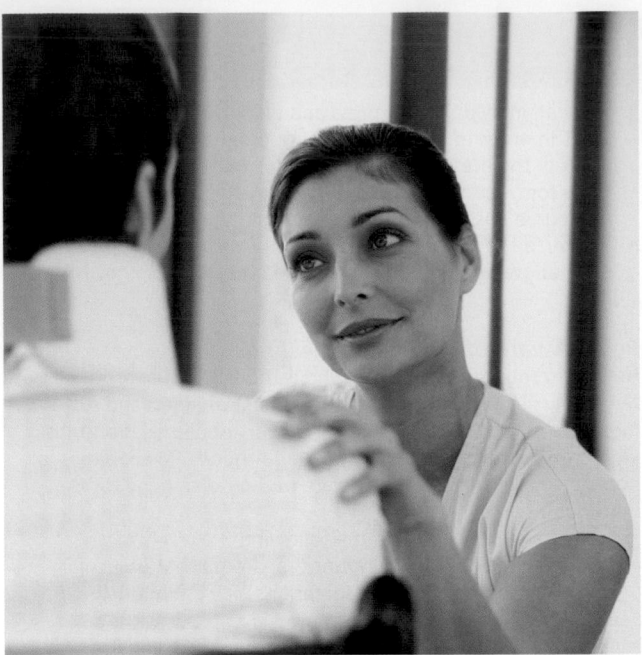

FIGURE 43-6. The nurse displays empathy and compassion.

things even when they cannot hope for a cure, such as hope for freedom from pain, to be surrounded by loved ones, and for the rest of their allotted time to be spent in meaningful pursuits.

A caring nurse feels at ease in crying with the grieving person and sharing experiences with fears, loneliness, and death. This allows the griever the freedom to express his or her deepest concerns. Nonverbal communication is equally important. A smile, holding a hand, and eye-to-eye contact are all meaningful (Fig. 43-6). The warmth behind the gesture and the honest concern of the nurse are what count.

The sense of hearing is believed to be the last sense to leave the body; many patients retain a sense of hearing almost to the moment of death. Demonstrate kindness and thoughtfulness by speaking to the comatose patient and encouraging family members to do likewise. Explain to the patient the nursing care being given and the noises in the unit.

Explaining the Patient's Condition and Treatment

All involved healthcare personnel should know exactly what the patient and family have been told. Telling them different things puts the nurse and other team members at cross-purposes and sets up distrust on the part of the family. Because patients and families often direct questions about the patient's prognosis to the nurse, it is up to the nurse to take the initiative in ensuring that terminology, prognosis, and the description of the progress are consistently presented and explained.

Explain the patient's condition and treatment to both the patient and the family. Patience is required during explanations. The patient and family members may be so over-whelmed by the diagnosis that they do not hear all the information that is shared with them. Question them to learn how much they have retained, then the information they missed can be repeated. Explain care options, as well as the expected outcomes of each option, fully.

Sadly, many healthcare professionals do not embrace "good dying" as a legitimate aim of medical and nursing care. As a result, the dying of many patients is painfully prolonged because no one initiates a patient/family conference to clarify the treatment goals when cure is no longer an option (see Promoting Health Literacy in Caregivers of Terminally Ill Patients). The nurse plays a key role in transitioning the patient and family in preparing for a comfortable and dignified death. Here, the primary focus is palliative, such that the patient and/or family accepts that death is inevitable and now focuses on how to spend the remaining days. For some, this means a referral to hospice or a palliative care program. Nurses play an important role in ensuring that timely prognostic information is given to patients and families so that they can decide how to spend their last days. Some patients want to "die fighting" and will insist upon intensive, life-sustaining treatment until every system fails. Others will choose not to have further treatment and want to spend their last days in a comfortable setting.

Teaching Self-Care and Promoting Self-Esteem

Encourage the patient to retain independence and make decisions as long as possible. Allow the patient to manage personal hygiene practices and self-feeding for as long as possible. After the patient is confined to bed, the creative nurse and family caregivers should attempt to find self-care activities the patient can perform. When physical abilities fail, determining when to take medication, for example, may be all the control the patient can retain.

Having familiar objects in view can help make the patient feel more comfortable and secure. Whether the patient is at home or in a healthcare agency, it is desirable to have the environment reflect personal preferences. This gives the patient some degree of control when health and other activities of daily living have slipped out of the patient's reach. It also supports self-esteem.

In the transition from independence to interdependence and ultimately to dependence, the patient may experience depression and express frustration and grief about "being a burden." It is crucial for professional and nonprofessional caregivers to respond to the dying patient as a person of worth whose life has meaning and value. Chapter 21 discusses practical ways in which nurses can use looks, touch, words, and actions to communicate respect and caring.

Teaching Family Members to Assist in Care

Preparing family members to assist in providing care yields benefits to both the patient and family members. Having loved ones near comforts the patient. The family members, too, are comforted by knowing that they helped comfort the

Promoting Health Literacy

IN CAREGIVERS OF TERMINALLY ILL PATIENTS

Patient Scenario

Marlene Bough is a 47-year-old wife of a 49-year-old man who is nearing the end of his life as a result of widely metastasized thyroid cancer. Mr. Bough was initially diagnosed almost 5 years ago, but treatment is no longer able to control the growth of malignant tumors throughout his body. He has almost constant pain, is unable to walk, and has severe pulmonary and cardiovascular impairments. The doctors have told the couple that there is no more that can be done to prolong Mr. Bough's life and that he has, at the most, less than 6 months to live. Mrs. Bough has taken a family leave from her job as a third-grade teacher so she can care for Mr. Bough at home, even though she is very concerned about being able to care for him and afraid she will cause him further pain.

Nursing Considerations: *Tips for Improving Health Literacy*

Schedule a home care planning meeting for Marlene and others who have indicated a desire to be helpful (daughter, sister-in-law, brother, colleagues at her school) and discuss how each person can help. Include times for family and friends to stay with Mr. Bough so Marlene can have some time away from the care responsibilities. Demonstrate and have Marlene practice moving Mr. Bough in bed, providing

hygiene, and administering pain medications. Discuss the responsibilities of the hospice provider and the goals of palliative care. Provide a written list of phone numbers for healthcare providers, including those that would be available at any time. Encourage Marlene to ask her husband, "What concerns you most?" and then to talk openly about what kind of treatment he wants for his final days. Include the following questions: "Where do you want to die?", "What kind of medical treatment do you want and do not want?", "What do you consider a good death?", "What kind of funeral service do you want?", and "Where do you want to be buried?" Ensure that advanced planning documents are completed. Encourage Marlene to take some time for herself, to recognize the stress of her husband's care, to welcome the help of others, and to use support people and groups after her husband's death. At that time, ask her to be prepared to ask the following three questions of herself and her healthcare provider:

- What is my main problem?
- What do I need to do?
- Why is it important for me to do this?

What additional measures can you take to help maintain health literacy in this woman? What other measures would be helpful for Marlene if she did not speak English, could not read, or had other learning disabilities?

patient. Teach family members how to provide care to the patient. Family members may not want to provide physical care themselves but may want to know what to expect and how they can psychologically aid the patient. Provide assistance in this area by explaining the patient's condition, what treatment the patient is undergoing, and what result the family can expect from the treatment. Knowing the facts may help family members to cope better with impending loss. The accompanying Research in Nursing box highlights factors that affect family caregivers when giving care.

Meeting the Needs of Dying Patients

Nursing interventions to meet the needs of dying patients are discussed below and examples of dying care activities are provided in the accompanying Examples of Nursing Interventions and Nursing Outcomes Classifications (NIC/NOC) box.

ADDRESSING PHYSIOLOGIC NEEDS

Physiologic care of the patient involves meeting physical needs such as personal hygiene, pain control, nutritional and fluid needs, movement, elimination, and respiratory care.

Personal hygiene includes cleanliness of the skin, hair, mouth, nose, and eyes. Frequent baths and linen changes may be necessary. The mouth and nose should be kept free of mucus, and secretions should be wiped from the eyes.

The physician will determine the medication and dosage needed for pain control, but the patient's wishes should be considered. (See Chapter 35 for a further discussion of pain control.) Some patients prefer and are able to control their own medication. If the patient requires nutritional support, he or she should be encouraged to take sips of water or ice chips if still able to swallow. The dying patient may elect to forego artificial nutrition and hydration because the burdens of feeding and hydrating artificially may outweigh the benefits. Problems with elimination include the development of incontinence, constipation, and/or urinary retention. Absorbent pads or a nearby bedpan may be used for patients experiencing incontinence, laxatives or enemas may be used for relieving constipation, and catheterization may be required for urinary retention. Bed linens should be changed often. Periodic movement should also be assisted; regular changes of position help prevent pressure ulcers. Repositioning the conscious patient in semi-Fowler's position can facilitate respirations; positioning the unconscious

RESEARCH IN NURSING
Bridging the Gap to Evidence-Based Practice

HOW FAMILY MEMBERS COPE WITH END-OF-LIFE CARE AT HOME

Patients who are terminally ill often choose to die at home and are supported in this choice by many healthcare providers as a way to enhance the dying experience for the patient and for their family members. This shift to the setting for healthcare as a patient nears end-of-life is contingent upon the availability and readiness of members of the family to assume care of the patient at home. Family caregivers become responsible for providing most of the physical and emotional care of the patient, for managing complex care in the home, and for organizing and coordinating health services on behalf of the dying person. Although research has established that caregiving places considerable burden on family caregivers, little is known about the factors that influence caregiver's ability to cope with providing care at home.

Related Research

Stajduhar, K., Martin, W., Barwidh, D., & Fyles, G. (2008). Factors influencing family caregivers' ability to cope with providing end-of-life cancer care at home. *Cancer Nursing, 31*(1), 77–85.

Using both qualitative and quantitative methodology, this study collected data from family caregivers of home care patients with cancer who were diagnosed with advanced cancer and had a life expectancy of 6 months or less. Data were analyzed and five themes were conceptualized. The themes were (1) the caregiver's approach to life (having a "just do it" positive attitude), (2) the patient's illness experience (caregivers coped best when the patient was "doing well"), (3) the patient's recognition of the caregivers' contribution to their

care (coping was facilitated by patients recognition and appreciation of caregiving efforts), (4) the quality of the relationship between the caregiver and dying person (caregiving was easier when the relationship was based on mutual love and respect), and (5) the caregiver's sense of security (security in the caregiving role was enhanced by having family and friends to listen and provide hands-on help, access to relevant and timely information, and support from the healthcare system when it was needed).

Relevance to Nursing Practice

Although this study focused on patients with terminal cancer, the findings are applicable to family caregivers of all patients who require end-of-life care at home. As the population of older adults increases, so too will the number of people who wish to die at home increase. Nurses must be able to teach the skills of physical care and the importance of maintaining comfort. It is also important for nurses to know how to help family members learn to talk with the patient about dying and what the patient wants to facilitate a good death. The family caregiver must know that other family members and friends support what is being done and that it is often a difficult and lonely responsibility. Nurses can provide emotional support through referrals for hospice care and spiritual support, and by being available to provide information throughout the end-of-life care. Caring for the caregiver of a dying patient is an important nursing role.

For additional research, visit the Point.

Examples of Nursing Interventions and Nursing Outcomes Classifications (NIC/NOC)

Grief Facilitation

Nursing Interventions	Nursing Outcomes
• Assist patient to identify the initial reaction to the loss • Encourage expression of feelings about the loss • Listen to expressions of grief • Make empathetic statements about grief • Encourage identification of greatest fears concerning loss • Support progression through personal grieving stages • Include significant others in discussions and decisions as appropriate • Communicate acceptance of discussing loss • Encourage patient to implement cultural, religious, and social customs associated with the loss • Assist in identifying modifications needed in lifestyle	• Grief resolution • Coping • Family coping • Family resiliency • Psychosocial adjustment: Life change

Bulechek, G., Butcher, H., & Dochterman, J., (Eds.). (2008). *Nursing interventions classification (NIC)* (5th ed., p. 665). St. Louis: C. V. Mosby Inc. A full listing of nursing activities for each nursing intervention can be found in this book.

Moorhead, S., Johnson, M., Maas, M. & Swanson, E. (Eds.) (2008). *Nursing outcomes classification (NOC)* (4th ed., p. 815). St. Louis: C.V. Mosby. A full listing of nursing outcomes for each nursing diagnosis can be found in this book.

patient in a semiprone position allows drainage of saliva and mucus. Oxygen therapy may be necessary for some patients.

ADDRESSING PSYCHOLOGICAL NEEDS

When people speak of their fears of death, responses typically include fear of the unknown, pain, separation, leaving loved ones, loss of dignity, loss of control, and unfinished business. Kübler-Ross believes that there is still another, more overwhelming and more significant fear that often is repressed and unconscious: that of the catastrophic, destructive force that has befallen a person and that the person cannot change. Kübler-Ross points out that terminally ill people communicate this fear of a destructive force but do so largely through symbolic language. A person may use nonverbal language, such as a facial expression, a particular kind of handclasp, or, in the case of children, drawings and manner of play with toys. Verbal communication may also be used symbolically.

A fear of isolation, of having to face death alone, is a primary concern of the dying patient. Support the patient by indicating his or her presence, giving full attention, and showing that he or she cares. Encourage the presence of family members in the room and sharing of reminiscences.

ADDRESSING NEEDS FOR INTIMACY

Terminally ill patients and their sexual partners may feel uncomfortable discussing their needs for intimacy. Partners may wish to be physically intimate with the dying person but are afraid of "hurting" him or her and also afraid that an open expression of sexuality is somehow "inappropriate" when someone is dying. Encourage discussion and suggest ways to be physically intimate that will meet the needs of both partners. A loving foot massage or a tender, cradling body embrace may be exactly what a dying person needs in his or her last moments.

ADDRESSING SPIRITUAL NEEDS

Although not all patients follow specific spiritual or religious beliefs, most require some form of spiritual care. Many terminally ill patients find great comfort in the support they receive from their religious faith. Help in obtaining the services of clergy or pastoral care workers as each situation indicates. Most patients need to feel that their lives have meaning; many feel a need for hope in the face of death. Spiritual needs are discussed more fully in Chapter 46.

Meeting the Needs of the Family

The nurse can provide care for the family facing loss by listening to their concerns. Family members need to verbalize their worries and fears, and nurses and other healthcare personnel can provide support by being nonjudgmental listeners. Likewise, nursing care of the grieving family involves communication and listening. Application of the communication skills discussed in Chapter 21 and earlier in this section aid the nurse in being a nonjudgmental listener. Feedback to the family can be provided by summarizing or

paraphrasing, without questioning the validity of the family's emotions. Be sure that all family members, including children, are able to participate in the grieving process. Family members may need to be reminded to get rest and to eat. Too many visitors may tire the patient; when explanations are offered, most relatives readily understand this.

The reality of death can be made less painful by preparing the family ahead of time. When the process has been explained to the family, they are better prepared to understand the needs of the dying person and how to support him or her.

Explain the steps of the grieving process to all family members ahead of time so that they will recognize the specific stages as they experience them and understand that the process is normal. They will be able to recognize that other members of the family are going through the same stages, perhaps at different times. This preparation allows for better understanding and communication within the family.

Death creates a change in family roles. As one person (the dying person) leaves a role, adjustments must be made within the family to compensate. Each member plays a part in that compensation, and the nurse can help with these adjustments.

Providing Postmortem Care

When a patient dies, the nurse's responsibilities include caring for the patient's body, caring for the family, and discharging specific legal responsibilities. The latter involve ensuring that a death certificate is issued and signed, labeling the body, and reviewing organ donation arrangements, if any.

CARING FOR THE BODY

After the patient has been pronounced dead, the nurse is responsible for preparing the body. The body is placed in normal anatomic position to avoid pooling of blood, soiled dressings are replaced, and tubes are removed. In most cases, it is unnecessary to wash the body; the mortician normally attends to this. Some religions strictly forbid washing of the body, whereas in others a special person must perform it. In cultures in which the family's washing of the deceased's body is considered the last service a family can give a loved one, the family should be given the necessary supplies and left alone in the room with the body. If an autopsy is to be performed, any tubes that were in place should not be removed. In such cases, the nurse should follow the hospital's policy.

The nurse is legally responsible for placing identification tags on either the shroud or garment the body is clothed in and the ankle to ensure that the body can be identified even if it is separated from its shroud. The nurse also places an identification tag on the patient's dentures or other prostheses to ensure that the mortician receives these. The importance of proper and complete identification cannot be overemphasized. The patient's body may be placed in the hospital's morgue refrigerator if mortuary arrangements were not made before the patient's death. If the patient died

Through the Eyes of a Student

We had had several day-shift clinical rotations, but this was our first evening clinical experience. We were unsure as to what the evening would be like. We knew the evening would provide us with a new outlook on nursing, but we were not prepared for what unfolded.

I had been taking care of a patient when another nursing student asked if I would check in on her patient while she had her dinner break. Each of the students knew this patient because we all had the pleasure of caring for him. I was told he was lying in bed watching television and that he had changed his code status to "DNR" (do not resuscitate) just that day. When I went to check on him, I found him lying in bed but not watching television. His eyes were closed as if he were sleeping peacefully. I spoke his name several times without a response. At the same time, I was also checking for a radial pulse. When I couldn't find his pulse, I swiftly walked to find the instructor. Together we went back to him and assessed his condition. There were no radial or carotid pulses. His chest was not rising and the instructor listened to his heart with a stethoscope. There wasn't a heartbeat. I stood there feeling helpless and low spirited. This was a man to whom we had all grown close. His family came to see him and to say a few final words. Tears were shed not only by his family but also by those of us who had cared for him.

Our first evening clinical was an extremely emotional night. We were all quiet as we walked down the hallway to go home. The student who was caring for him that night was stopped by his daughter and two young granddaughters. One granddaughter was wearing his hat and the other was carrying his belt. This man's daughter was broken-hearted by his death, yet needed to know that he wasn't alone when he died. The student told her that I had been the one with him. The daughter seemed relieved to know that he was not by himself when he died.

As I look back on that evening, I'm sad that this man is no longer with us. I did not know him for very long, but he touched me in a way that helped me understand the true meaning of nursing: not only to care for the sick, disabled, or enfeebled, but also to be human and offer support for grieving families.

—*Joyce A. Shearman, Delaware County Community College, Media, Pennsylvania*

of a communicable disease, the body may require special handling to prevent the spread of disease. Requirements for such handling are usually specified by local laws and are contingent on the disease-causing organism, mode of transmission, and other characteristics.

CARING FOR THE FAMILY

After a patient has died, the nurse provides support and care to the patient's family (see Through the Eyes of a Student). In most cases, this involves listening to the family's expressions of grief, loss, and helplessness. Because comforting words are often difficult to find, offer solace and support by being an attentive listener. Family members may need to see the patient's body to accept the death fully; in such cases, arrange for family members to view the body before it is discharged to the mortician.

Sudden death creates unique problems for the family. In the case of sudden injury or illness, the physical needs of the patient are paramount to the healthcare team. This means that family members are not provided as much emotional support or information as they would be if the patient's illness were prolonged, nor are they permitted to exercise as many options regarding the patient's care. The family that loses a member unexpectedly has not had an opportunity to begin the grieving process or to share in grieving with the deceased person. Allow family members to express grief and provide emotional support. Most often, the family is in the emergency department waiting room when death is confirmed. They are stunned, bewildered, and numb. Do not rush them from the waiting room, rather, provide them with a private place to begin their grieving. Acknowledge their shock and listen to their grief. The family needs guidance in making plans and help in making decisions.

It is appropriate for the nurse who was caregiver or who took care of the patient for a prolonged period to attend the funeral. It also is appropriate for the nurse to make a follow-up call to the patient's family after the funeral or memorial service to offer both concern and care for the family's well-being. Follow-up visits are important to give support to the family. If the nurse assesses that the family is not coping well, appropriate referrals should be made. If the patient was cared for by a hospice, the family is offered grief support for up to a year following the death.

CARING FOR OTHER PATIENTS

Because it is not unusual for nurses in institutional settings to provide care to more than one patient at a time, after the death of one patient, the nurse must continue to provide care to the other patients. Other patients are often aware of a death and may need to be consoled; this is particularly true of a patient who has shared a room with the deceased patient. Other patients may have grief reactions and should be supported through the grief process by the nurse. Death of a patient may cause depression in other patients and may make them more aware of their own future deaths.

Evaluating

The plan of nursing care for dying patients is effective if patients meet the outcome of a comfortable, dignified death and family members resolve their grief after a suitable time of mourning and resume meaningful life roles and activities. See Nursing Plan of Care 43-1.

NURSING PLAN OF CARE · 43-1

For Mrs. Esposita and Her Family

Remember Mrs. Esposita, the woman with terminal cancer who is dying at home? The nurse who has been visiting Mrs. Esposita at home asked for assistance from her colleagues in devising a plan of care for Mr. Esposita. Until now, Mrs. Esposita wanted nothing to do with the local hospice because of a reported "bad experience" a neighbor had. Her insurance will not provide for all the home nursing care she needs, and her husband and children have been trying to meet her needs for nursing as well as run the house and meet their own needs. A demanding woman, Mrs. Esposita never seems satisfied with anything anyone does, and the family is looking utterly frustrated, angry, and fatigued. Jorge is coping by "opting out"; he frequently spends the night with friends and doesn't even call home to report on his whereabouts. Marita's grades have fallen, and she has dropped out of cheerleading and other school activities so that she can take care of her mother. Mr. Esposita, who has been silent until now, recently confided that he doesn't know how much longer he can go on this way, and seemed horrified to hear himself say, "I just wish she would die already and get this all over with!" He is very concerned about the changes in his children and feels powerless to change what is happening. For her part, Mrs. Esposita seems oblivious to her family's needs and, even in her weakened state, multiplies pleas for assistance. She seems to be afraid of dying and never wants to be left alone.

NURSING DIAGNOSIS Caregiver Role Strain related to multiple losses and burdens associated with caregiving responsibilities as manifested by self-report, breakdown in family relationships, fatigue, and anger.

EXPECTED OUTCOME By the next home visit on 10/17/2012, Mr. Esposita will:

- Talk openly about his feelings and share his frustrations about his present situation.

Nursing Interventions	Rationale	Evaluative Statement
Plan visits for when there is time for private conversation with Mr. Esposita; initiate conversations by telling him that it is not unusual for family caregivers to feel fatigued, powerless, frustrated, angry, and emotionally distant. Encourage him to talk about what he is feeling: "You seemed surprised at yourself when you said that you wished your wife would 'just die.' This isn't an unusual wish for someone in your situation. . . . Tell me more about what you are feeling now. . . ."	This will normalize what Mr. Esposita is experiencing and communicate that someone cares about him and about what he is experiencing. Simply giving voice to what he is feeling and sharing this with a healthcare professional may help him to accept and address what he takes to be negative and possibly shameful feelings.	10/17/12 Outcome partially met. Mr. Esposita states that he feels better now that he is sharing some of what he's been holding in for such a long time, but he still believes that if he was really a good husband he wouldn't feel this way. Also, states that it is hard for him to find words to express everything that he is feeling. *Revision:* Continue to encourage Mr. Esposita to talk about what he is experiencing and provide a private opportunity for this to happen. *E. McLoughlin, RN*

EXPECTED OUTCOME By 10/17/12, the patient will

- Develop a realistic caregiving plan that matches his ability to care with his wife's need for care and that identifies other resources for his wife's unmet needs.

(continued)

NURSING PLAN OF CARE • 43-1

For Mrs. Esposita and Her Family (continued)

Nursing Interventions	Rationale	Evaluative Statement
Assist Mr. Esposita to identify what his wife's actual needs for care are; how much of this care it is reasonable to expect the family to provide; and other potential caregiving sources.	Mr. Esposita may need "permission" to not meet his wife's unrealistic needs. The nurse's authority may be useful in helping him to believe that he can be a good and faithful husband and still fail to meet her expectations. Identifying other caregiving resources will ensure that Mrs. Esposita's needs will be met.	10/17/12 Outcome not met. To date, Mr. Esposita has been unable to identify any additional caregivers for Mrs. Esposita and continues to feel the need to assume all responsibility for her care when he is home. *Revision:* Bring list of community resources to Mr. Esposita, including church group, and plan with him to contact these sources. Reinforce that it is OK to ask for help.
Explain to Mrs. Esposita that her family may not be able to meet all her needs for care but that every effort will be made to ensure these needs are met by other caregivers.	Even if the nurse's sympathies are with the family, it is critical to communicate to the patient that you are committed to her and intent on doing all in your power to ensure that her needs are met. If the patient's needs are met, it will improve her relationships with her family.	*E. McLoughlin, RN*
Assist Mr. Esposita to identify and use new resources: identify at least one new support person who can sit with Mrs. Esposita and relieve the family of some of this burden; explore the family's reluctance to use hospice and evaluate other community resources. Use appropriate referrals.	The family may be feeling unnecessarily overwhelmed because they have failed to explore the availability of other resources. A gentle push may be needed to make this happen. If a "sitter" can be obtained for several hours in the evening, this would give Mr. Esposita time after work to do something with his children or for himself.	

EXPECTED OUTCOME   By 10/24/12 Mr. Esposita will

- Report feeling more in control and less depressed and angry.

(continued)

NURSING PLAN OF CARE • 43-1

For Mrs. Esposita and Her Family (continued)

Nursing Interventions	Rationale	Evaluative Statement
Lead Mr. Esposita in a discussion that aims to identify everything that is making him feel powerless; then list those factors over which he has no control and those he can influence or change.	This will break the cycle of his thinking that there is nothing at present over which he can exert control. Simply making the list is a first step toward taking action.	10/24/12 Outcome met. Mr. Esposita reports that even though most of his situation remains unchanged, he no longer feels powerless and is less depressed and angry. He expressed gratitude for this intervention and says it has given him new energy. *E. McLoughlin, RN*
Provide opportunities for Mr. Esposita to control decision making over those aspects of his life and his wife's care for which he can exert control. Affirm constructive decision making and ask him how it feels to be "back in control" of at least some aspects of his life. Discuss with Mr. Esposita those factors he can change, and assist him in making decisions.	This is an example of "guided discovery"; you are allowing Mr. Esposita to experience himself as once again in charge and to allow this experience to define his self-image. Reinforcement of his success affirms his self-image of one who is in charge. Types of support that can be given to caregivers include emotional (concern, trust), appraisal (affirms self-worth), informational (useful advice), and instrumental assistance or tangible goods.	

SAMPLE DOCUMENTATION

10/24/12, 12 PM, Nursing

Met with Mr. Esposita this morning and talked about the plan to identify other caregivers who might be able to "sit" with his wife on some evenings in order to give him time to do things for his children and himself. He reported no progress in identifying anyone but also stated that he hadn't really made any efforts to locate someone: "Who would want to help us? Besides, I wouldn't want to inflict my wife and her moods on anyone right now." Explained that there are many individuals and groups who provide exactly this type of assistance and that his wife's moods were not uncommon for someone in her situation. Jointly, made a list of possible caregiver resources, including some family members who had earlier expressed an interest in helping out, the parish nurse service from his church, and finally the local hospice. If the first two sources do not work out, will explore family reluctance to use hospice resources more carefully because this may be their best hope. Will evaluate progress made on 10/24/12.

E. McLoughlin, RN

● Developing Critical Thinking Skills

1. Recall personal losses (death of a family member or friend; loss of a significant relationship, job, or opportunity) and recollect what you were experiencing at the time. Try to remember what your expectations were from those to whom you looked for support, and how your ability to cope was influenced by whether those expectations were met. Remembering that no two people respond to loss in exactly the same way, develop a list of nursing measures to help patients dealing with loss. Compare your list with those of other students and incorporate their ideas.

2. Compare and contrast the care a patient dying of cancer would receive in a critical care unit and at home with hospice care. Identify the advantages and disadvantages of each. Talk with family members and friends about their preferences. Use your analysis to help describe these options to prospective patients.

3. Role-play a situation with a peer in which you counsel a woman with cancer who is told that cure is no longer an option and that she has less than 6 months to live. Reflect on how your experiences, beliefs, and values might affect what you say to patients and how you say it.

● Practicing for NCLEX

1. A woman who is firmly committed to natural childbirth and who has attended each natural childbirth class in preparation for labor and delivery undergoes a cesarean delivery when her fetus displays signs of distress. Inconsolable, she cries and calls herself a failure as a mother. What type of loss is she experiencing? Select all that apply.
   a. Actual
   b. Perceived
   c. Psychological
   d. Anticipatory
   e. Physical

2. What term describes the period of acceptance of loss and grief during which the person learns to deal with loss through actions and expressions of grief?
   a. Anticipatory grieving
   b. Bereavement
   c. Mourning
   d. Stages of death and dying

3. A nurse interviews an 82-year-old resident of a nursing home who says that she has never gotten over the death of her son 20 years ago. She reports that her life fell apart after that and she never again felt like herself or was able to enjoy life. What type of grief is this woman experiencing?
   a. Abbreviated
   b. Anticipatory
   c. Complicated
   d. Inhibited

4. A home health nurse has been visiting a patient with AIDS who says, "I'm no longer afraid of dying. I think I've made my peace with everyone, and I'm actually ready to move on." This reflects his progress to which stage of death and dying?
   a. Acceptance
   b. Anger
   c. Bargaining
   d. Denial

5. A nurse is visiting a patient with AIDS who is dying at home. During the visit, he breaks down and cries and tells the nurse that it is unfair that he should have to die now when he's finally made peace with his family and wants to live. Which response by the nurse would be most appropriate?
   a. "You can't be feeling this way. You know you are going to die."
   b. "It does seem unfair. Tell me more about how you are feeling."
   c. "You'll be all right; who knows how much time any of us has."
   d. "Tell me about your pain. Did it keep you awake last night?"

6. A nurse is caring for a terminally ill patient during the 11 PM to 7 AM shift. The patient says, "I just can't sleep. I keep thinking about what my family will do when I am gone." What response by the nurse would be most appropriate?
   a. "Oh, don't worry about that now. You need to sleep."
   b. "What seems to be concerning you the most?"
   c. "I have talked to your wife and she told me she will be fine."
   d. "I have to go and give medicines now."

7. A patient tells a nurse that he has no one he trusts to make healthcare decisions for him should he become incapacitated. What should the nurse suggest he prepare?
   a. Combination advance medical directive
   b. Durable power of attorney for healthcare
   c. Living will
   d. Proxy for healthcare

8. Which of the following responses by a nurse would best reflect adherence to the position of the American Nurses Association?
   a. A nurse promises a dying patient that he/she will do everything possible to keep the patient comfortable but that he/she cannot administer an injection or overdose to cause the patient's death.
   b. A nurse tells a dying patient who is on a ventilator that under no condition can he be removed from the ventilator because this is active euthanasia and is expressly forbidden by the Code for Nurses.
   c. After exhausting every intervention to keep a dying patient comfortable, the nurse says, "I think you are now at a point where I'm prepared to do what you've been asking me. Let's talk about when and how you want to die."
   d. In response to a patient who asks for assistance in committing suicide, a nurse replies, "I'm personally opposed to assisted suicide, but I'll find you a colleague who can help you."

9. A patient diagnosed with breast cancer who is not in the end stages of her illness has been in the medical intensive care unit for 3 weeks. Her husband tells the nurse caring for the patient that he and his wife often talked about the end of her life and that she was very clear about not wanting aggressive treatment that would merely prolong her dying. The nurse and husband both agree that this seems to be all that therapy is now doing for her. The nurse would suggest that the husband speak to his wife's physician about which type of order?
   a. Comfort-measures-only
   b. Do-not-hospitalize
   c. Do-not-resuscitate
   d. Slow-code-only

10. Which of the following would be least appropriate for a nurse to do when involved in the terminal weaning of a patient?
    a. Participate in the decision-making process by offering the family information about the advantages and disadvantages of continued ventilatory support
    b. Explain to the family what will happen at each phase of the weaning and offer support
    c. Check the orders for sedation and analgesia, making sure that the anticipated death is comfortable and dignified
    d. Tell the family that death will occur almost immediately after the patient is removed from the ventilator

11. All of the following diagnoses may apply to a young couple who gave birth to a premature infant with serious respiratory problems who has been in the neonatal intensive care unit for the last 3 months. The couple has a 22-month-old son at home. Which diagnosis would be most appropriate based on the following assessment data: report of chronic fatigue and decreased energy, guilt about neglecting son at home, shortness of temper with one another, and apprehension about continued ability to go on this way?
    a. Grieving
    b. Ineffective Coping
    c. Caregiver Role Strain
    d. Powerlessness

12. Which of the nursing actions would a nurse correct if he saw a nursing assistant doing it?
    a. Talking to a comatose patient, explaining what is happening at each step along the way when providing his care.
    b. Sitting on the side of the bed of a dying patient holding her hand and crying with her
    c. Listening to the daughter of a dying patient about the demands of care associated with artificially feeding her father.
    d. Telling a dying patient to sit back and relax and that he will wash him because it's easier that way

13. A nurse is providing postmortem care. Which of the following nursing actions violates the standards of caring for the body after a patient has been pronounced dead and is not scheduled for an autopsy?
    a. Maintaining the patient in a comfortable sitting position until the family has arrived to say good-bye
    b. Placing identification tags on both the shroud and the ankle
    c. Removing soiled dressings and tubes
    d. Preparing to transfer the body to the morgue

14. The family of a patient who has just died asks to be alone with the body and asks for supplies to wash the body. The nurse providing care knows that the mortician usually washes the body. Which response would be most appropriate?
    a. Inform the family that there is no need for them to wash the body since the mortician typically does this

    b. Explain that hospital policy forbids their being alone with the deceased patient and that hospital supplies are to be used only by hospital personnel
    c. Give the supplies to the family but maintain a watchful eye to make sure that nothing unusual happens
    d. Provide the requested supplies, checking if this request is linked to their religious or cultural customs and asking if there is anything else you can do to help

15. A 70-year-old woman who has had a number of strokes refuses further life-sustaining interventions, including artificial nutrition and hydration. She is competent, understands the consequences of her actions, is not depressed, and persists in refusing treatment. Her doctor is adamant that she cannot be allowed to die this way, and her daughter agrees. An ethics consult has been initiated. Who would be the appropriate decision maker?
    a. Patient
    b. Daughter
    c. Doctor
    d. Ethics consult team

Answers With Rationale

1. **a, b,** and **c.** The loss experienced by the woman is actual, perceived, and psychological.

2. **c.** Mourning is defined as the period of acceptance of loss and grief during which the person learns to deal with loss.

3. **c.** Dysfunctional grief extends the mourning period for an abnormally long time, characterized by abnormal or distorted expressions of grief.

4. **a.** The patient's statement does reflect the acceptance stage of death and dying defined by Kübler-Ross.

5. **b.** The nurse would want to validate that what the patient is saying has been heard and invite him to share more of his feelings, concerns, and fears.

6. **b.** Using an open-ended question allows the patient to continue talking.

7. **c.** The living will is a document whose precise purpose is to allow individuals to record specific instructions about the type of healthcare they would like to receive in particular end-of-life situations.

8. **a.** The American Nurses Association position statement states that nurse-assisted suicide and participation in active euthanasia violate the Code for Nurses and the ethical traditions of the profession.

9. **a.** Comfort-measures-only order. The wife would want all aggressive treatment to be stopped at this point and all care to be directed to a comfortable, dignified death.

10. **d.** Because there are no guarantees how any patient will respond once removed from a ventilator, and because it is possible for the patient to breathe on his or her own and live for hours, days, and, rarely, even

weeks, the family should definitely not be told that death will occur immediately.

11. *c.* The defining characteristics for the NANDA diagnosis Caregiver Role Strain fit the set of assessment data provided.

12. *d.* Because it is good to encourage dying patients to be as active as possible for as long as possible, it is generally not good practice to perform basic self-care measures the patient can perform simply because it is "easier" to do it this way.

13. *a.* Because the body should be placed in normal anatomic position to avoid pooling of blood, leaving the body in a sitting position is contraindicated.

14. *d.* The family may want to wash the body for personal, religious, or cultural reasons and should be allowed to do so.

15. *a.* Because this patient is competent, she has the right to refuse therapy that she finds to be disproportionately burdensome, even if this hastens her death. Neither her daughter nor her doctor has the authority to assume her decision-making responsibilities unless she asks them to do this. The ethics consult team is not a decision-making body; it can make recommendations but has no authority to order anything.

Taylor Suite Resources

The Taylor Suite offers these additional resources to enhance learning and facilitate understanding of this chapter:

- thePoint online resource, http://thepoint.lww.com/Taylor7E
- Student DVD-ROM included with the book
- Study Guide for Taylor's Fundamentals of Nursing

BIBLIOGRAPHY

Aging with Dignity. (2007). *Five wishes*. Available http://www.agingwithdignity.org/5wishes.html

American Geriatrics Society (AGS) (2007). *Position Statement The care of dying patients*. American Geriatrics Society, Ethics Committee. New York: New York.

American Nurses Association (ANA). (1991). *Position statement on promotion of comfort and relief of pain in dying patients*. Washington, DC: Author.

American Nurses Association (ANA). (1995). *Position statement on assisted suicide*. Washington, DC: Author.

Barclay, L., & Lie, D. (2008). *End-of-life discussions may reduce aggressive care in terminally ill patients*. Medscape. Available at http://cme.medscape.com/viewarticle/581679.

Beckstand, R. L., Callister, L. C., & Kirchoff, K. T. (2006). Providing a "good death": Critical care nurses' suggestions for improving end-of-life care. *American Journal of Critical Care, 15*(1), 38–46.

Bulechek, G., Butcher, H., & Dochterman, J. M. (Eds). (2008). *Nursing interventions classification (NIC)* (5th ed.). St. Louis: Mosby Elsevier.

Emanuel, L., Ferris, F., von Gunten, C., & Von Roenn, J. (2008). *The last hours of living: Practical advice for clinicians*. Medscape. Available at http://cme.medscape.com/viewprogram/5808?src=top10

Engel, G. L. (1964). Grief and grieving. *American Journal of Nursing, 64*(9), 93–98.

Ferrell, B., & Coyle, N. (2008). *The nature of suffering and the goals of nursing*. Cary, NC: Oxford University Press.

Fields, L. (2007). DNR does not mean no care. *Journal of Neuroscience Nursing, 39*(5), 294–296.

Holtslander, L. (2008). Ways of knowing hope: Carper's fundamental patterns as a guide for hope research with bereaved palliative caregivers. *Nursing Outlook, 56*(1), 25–30.

Huggins, M., & Brooks, L. (2007). Discussing end-of-life care with older patients: What are you waiting for? *Geriatrics & Aging, 10*(7), 461–464.

Institute of Medicine. (1997). *Approaching death: Improving care at the end of life*. Washington, DC: National Academy Press.

Johnson, J., & Johnson, M. (2003). *Grief: What it is and what you can do*. Omaha, NE: Centering Corporation.

Kantor, D. (2008). Caring for the dying patient. *American Journal of Nursing, 108*(11), 72CCC–73CCC.

Kübler-Ross, E. (1969). *On death and dying*. New York: Macmillan.

Kübler-Ross, E. (1978). *To live until we say goodbye*. Englewood Cliffs, NJ: Prentice Hall.

Kübler-Ross, E. (1997). *On death and dying: What the dying have to teach doctors, nurses, clergy, and their own families*. New York: Simon & Schuster.

Love, A. W. (2007). Progress in understanding grief, complicated grief, and caring for the bereaved. *Contemporary Nurse, 27*(1), 73–83.

Lowery, S. (2008). Communication between the nurse and family caregiver in end-of-life care: A review of the literature. *Journal of Hospice and Palliative Nursing, 10*(1), 35–45.

Moorhead, S., Johnson, M., Maas, M., & Swanson, E. (Eds). (2008). *Nursing outcomes classification (NOC)* (4th ed.). St. Louis: Mosby Elsevier.

NANDA International. (2009). *Nursing diagnoses: Definitions & classification, 2009–2011*. Oxford, UK: Wiley-Blackwell.

National Consensus Project for Quality Palliative Care. (2008). *Clinical practice guidelines for quality palliative care*. Available at http://www.nationalconsensusproject.org/Guidelines

President's Commission for the Study of Ethical Problems in Medicine and Biomedical and Behavioral Research. (1981). *Defining death*. [Publication No. 81-600150]. Washington, DC: U.S. Government Printing Office.

Rancour, P. (2008). Personal communication.

Rancour, P. (2008). *Tales from the pager chronicles*. Indianapolis, IN: Sigma Theta Tau International.

Stajduhar, K. (2008). Factors influencing family caregivers' ability to cope with providing end-of-life cancer care at home. *Cancer Nursing, 31*(1), 77–85.

Thomas, R., Wilson, D., Justice, C., Birch, S., & Sheps, S. (2008). A literature review of preferences for end-of-life care in developed countries by individuals with different cultural affiliations and ethnicity. *Journal of Hospice and Palliative Nursing, 10*(3). Available at http://www.medscape.com/viewarticle/575049.

Ufema, J. (2007). *Insights on death & dying*. Philadelphia: Lippincott Williams & Wilkins.

Watson, L. A. (2008). Informing critical care patients of a loved one's death. *Critical Care Nurse, 28*(3), 52–64.

Sensory Functioning

44

ORI SOLTES

Ori, a 28-year-old man, is in the intensive care unit after a motor vehicle crash that resulted in multiple internal injuries as well as fractures. He is being monitored continuously and receiving mechanical ventilation. On the 5th day after the crash, he begins to exhibit transient episodes of acute confusion.

DOLORES PIROLLA

Dolores, a 74-year-old woman, comes to the older adult clinic with her 77-year-old husband who was diagnosed with macular degeneration and progressive vision loss. She states, "Now I've noticed he's also having difficulty hearing me. I'm worried because he doesn't want to leave the house and we hardly see any of our friends anymore. We used to go out to the movies or dinner at least once a week. Lately, if we get out once a month, that's a lot!"

MURIEL HAO

Muriel is a 56-year-old woman who had surgery 2 days ago. She denies any complaints of pain or discomfort. She is receiving intravenous therapy via an infusion pump. She states, "Please stop that beeping. It's driving me nuts and I can't rest."

After completing the chapter, you will be able to accomplish the following:

1. Describe the four conditions that must be met in each sensory experience.

2. Explain the role of the reticular activating system in sensory experience.

3. Identify etiologies and perceptual, cognitive, and emotional responses to sensory deprivation and sensory overload.

4. Perform a comprehensive assessment of sensory functioning using appropriate interview questions and physical assessment skills.

5. Develop nursing diagnoses that correctly identify sensory/perceptual alterations that may be treated by independent nursing interventions.

6. Describe specific nursing interventions to prevent sensory alterations, stimulate the senses, promote health literacy, and assist patients with sensory difficulties.

7. Develop, implement, and evaluate a plan of nursing care to help patients safely meet individualized sensory/perceptual outcomes.

KEY TERMS

adaptation	sensoristasis
arousal	sensory deficit
auditory	sensory deprivation
disturbed sensory perception	sensory overload
gustatory	sensory perception
kinesthesia	sensory reception
olfactory	stereognosis
proprioception	stimulus
reticular activating system (RAS)	tactile
	visceral

A person's senses are vital to survival, growth and development, and the experience of bodily pleasure. Nurses encounter many patients who have impaired sensory functioning that places them at risk for injury, disturbed growth and development, and decreased well-being. Moreover, the stress of illness or trauma and the need for diagnosis and treatment may quickly result in sensory deprivation or overload, with serious disturbances in visual, perceptual, cogni-

tive, or emotional functioning (see the accompanying Reflective Practice box for an example). Nurses are in the position to use knowledge of sensory functioning to support positive outcomes for patients. For example, awareness of the intensities and sources of sound, ways to control noise, and the assessment of patients' perceptions of and responses to sound can provide nurses with a basis for therapeutic manipulation of the environment.

THE SENSORY EXPERIENCE
Components and Conditions

The sensory experience consists of two components: reception and perception. **Sensory reception** is the process of receiving data about the external or internal environment through the senses. The senses by which individuals maintain contact with the external environment are vision (visual), hearing (**auditory**), smell (**olfactory**), taste (**gustatory**), and touch (**tactile**). In addition, **stereognosis** is the sense that perceives the solidity of objects and their size, shape, and texture.

Individuals orient themselves internally by the kinesthetic and visceral senses. (**Kinesthesia** refers to awareness of positioning of body parts and body movement; **visceral** pertains to inner organs.) The kinesthetic and visceral senses arise internally from muscles and hollow organs, respectively, and are the body's basic orienting systems. **Proprioception** is the term used to describe the sense, usually at a subconscious level, of the movements and position of the body and especially its limbs, independent of vision. This sense is gained primarily from input from sensory nerve terminals in muscles and tendons and the fibrous capsules of joints combined with input from the vestibular apparatus.

Sensory perception is the conscious process of selecting, organizing, and interpreting data from the senses into meaningful information. Perception is influenced by the intensity, size, change, or representation of stimuli, as well as by past experiences, knowledge, and attitudes.

For a person to receive the necessary data to experience the world, four conditions must be met:

- A **stimulus**—an agent, act, or other influence capable of initiating a response by the nervous system—must be present.
- A receptor or sense organ must receive the stimulus and convert it to a nerve impulse.
- The nerve impulse must be conducted along a nervous pathway from the receptor or sense organ to the brain.
- A particular area in the brain must receive and translate the impulse into a sensation.

> *Think back to Muriel Hao, the 56-year-old woman unable to rest because of the machine's beeping. The nurse would incorporate knowledge of sensory reception and perception to determine that the patient is experiencing a continuous and large amount of auditory stimuli from the beeping of the machine. In addition, the nurse would need*

REFLECTIVE PRACTICE
Challenge to Technical Skills

All throughout nursing school, we are taught theory, and from that theory we are to use critical thinking to determine how to care for a particular patient, focusing on the patient, not the machines surrounding them. "You'll learn that later," they say.

I was assigned to care for Muriel Hao, a 56-year-old woman who had surgery 2 days ago. As I walk into her room, I check to see if she is comfortable and whether she needs anything at that particular point in time. She asks me one favor. "Please stop that beeping. It's driving me nuts and I can't rest." So I look at the machine, dumbfounded, and worried that the patient is going to think I am incompetent because I cannot even work a simple machine. No theory from a classroom is going to teach me how to make the machine stop beeping. To make things worse, every facility has different machines. As nursing students, we go from one facility to another, trying to get accustomed to the equipment and technologies of each one. I assume that things will get easier once I have steady employment in a facility. If that particular facility changes its technologies, I would hope that there would be an in-service on the new technology. But what do I do now, as a nursing student?

Thinking Outside the Box: Possible Courses of Action

- Press the buttons on the machine, and hope that the beeping goes away.
- Seek out someone who does know how to work the machine and have them fix it so I don't do more damage.

- Find someone who knows how to work the machine, have them fix it, and then have them explain to me how to fix it so I can do it next time.

Evaluating a Good Outcome: How Do I Define Success?

- Personal integrity is maintained (if I can't fix it, I feel stupid, and that's an insult to my integrity).
- Professional integrity remains intact (if I can't fix it, I will feel incompetent as a nurse—if I can't even fix a machine, how am I supposed to help a person?).

- The patient expresses relief that the beeping has stopped and she is now able to rest.

Personal Learning: Here's to the Future!

Although this does not seem like a huge or very troublesome problem, every nursing student can probably attest to feeling this way at least once. The first few times it happened to me, I just asked someone to fix it for me, thinking it was a one-time problem. Then I realized that this is something that I was facing over and over again. So I asked someone to show me how to fix the problem if it should occur again. I understood what to do and knew how to do it. Then we switched hospitals and I was confused once again. In today's environment of ever-changing technology, I realized that it is not just the students who feel this way. Nurses, too, have these same feelings. We all learn new things every day, whether it's from a patient, another nurse, a doctor, or a technical specialist. We just need to know that it's okay to ask questions. Moreover, not knowing how to work with a piece of equipment does not mean that you are incompetent with people. Learning in the healthcare field is an ongoing process.

Michele Jordan, Georgetown University

Reflection

How do you think you would respond in a similar situation? Why? What does this tell you about yourself and about the adequacy of your skills for professional practice? Are there any other possible courses of actions that the nursing student should have identified? If so, please explain. What patient needs was the nursing student addressing? What personal needs? Describe the patient's sensory experience, addressing the major components and four conditions necessary to experience the world. Can you think of other ways to respond? What other skills (cognitive, interpersonal, technical, ethical/legal) would you need to respond well in this situation? What measures might have been appropriate for the nursing student to do in preparation for this patient assignment? Do you agree with the criteria to evaluate a successful outcome? Did the nursing student meet the criteria? Please explain why or why not.

to keep in mind other sources of stimuli, such as possible visual stimuli from the lighted numbers on the machine, tactile stimuli from being touched to determine the possible problem associated with the machine, and internal stimuli associated with pain and discomfort from surgery. ■

Arousal Mechanism

To receive stimuli and respond appropriately, the brain must be alert or aroused. The **reticular activating system (RAS),** a poorly defined network that extends from the hypothalamus to the medulla, mediates arousal. The optimal arousal state of the RAS is a general drive state called **sensoristasis.**

Cortical radiations

Special sensory input

Reticular formation

Input from cranial and spinal nerves

FIGURE 44-1. Nerve impulses from all the sensory tracts reach the reticular activating system (RAS), which then selectively allows certain impulses to reach the cerebral cortex and to be perceived.

Nerve impulses from all the sensory tracts reach the RAS, which then selectively allows certain impulses to reach the cerebral cortex and be perceived. The mesencephalic portion of the RAS appears to be the center of the system. Stimulation of this area produces the most pronounced and long-lasting effects on the cerebral cortex (Fig. 44-1). With its many ascending and descending connections to other areas of the brain, the RAS serves to monitor and to regulate incoming sensory stimuli, thus maintaining, enhancing, or inhibiting cortical **arousal.** States of arousal or awareness are described in Box 44-1.

The body quickly adapts to constant stimuli. In addition, the repeated stimulus of a continuing noise, such as city traffic, or a noxious odor eventually goes unnoticed. Therefore, a stimulus must be variable or irregular to evoke a response. This phenomenon is termed **adaptation.** Impulses that are not acted on when received may be used at a later date in response to the same or similar stimuli. The memory process involves the storage of that material. For example, thought and memory are used when a new sensory experience occurs and the individual uses a response based on previous knowledge and experience.

DISTURBED SENSORY PERCEPTION

When a patient is admitted to a health agency, he or she is confronted with stimuli that are different in quality and quantity than that to which he or she is accustomed. For example, a patient confined to bed rest may receive many fewer stimuli, whereas one undergoing multiple diagnostic tests may receive a greater-than-normal level of sensory input. These and other typical experiences are likely to result in disturbed sensory perceptions experienced by the patient. Being sensitive to how visual stimuli, noises, and touch are stimulating the patient, combined with paying attention to the patient's need for privacy and for social interaction, can significantly reduce disturbances in sensory perception.

Severe sensory alterations can occur, especially in certain areas, such as the critical care or intensive care units (termed intensive care unit [ICU] psychosis). Factors contributing to severe sensory alteration include sensory overload, sensory deprivation, sleep deprivation, and cultural care deprivation.

> ➤ *Consider Ori Soltes, the young man in the ICU. The nurse would need to assess Mr. Soltes closely for underlying reasons for his confusion. Although the possible causes are numerous and most likely multiple in nature, the nurse*

Box 44-1 STATES OF AROUSAL/AWARENESS

Conscious States

Delirium	Disorientation, restlessness, confusion, hallucinations, agitation, alternating with other conscious states
Dementia	Difficulties with spatial orientation, memory, language, changes in personality
Confusion	Reduced awareness, easily distracted, easily startled by sensory stimuli, alternates between drowsiness and excitability; resembles minor form of delirium state
Normal consciousness	Aware of self and external environment, well-oriented, responsive
Somnolence	Extreme drowsiness, but will respond normally to stimuli
Minimally conscious states	Part consciousness; sleep–wake cycles present; some motor function, including automatic movements; inconsistently follows commands
Locked-in Syndrome	Full consciousness; sleep–wake cycles present; quadriplegic, auditory and visual function preserved; emotion preserved.

Unconscious States

Asleep	Can be aroused by normal stimuli (light touch, sound, etc.)
Stupor	Can be aroused by extreme and/or repeated stimuli
Coma	Cannot be aroused and does not respond to stimuli (coma states can be further subdivided according to the effect on reflex responses to stimuli) (see Glasgow Coma Scale, Chapter 25)
Vegetative State	Cannot be aroused. Sleep–wake cycles, postures or withdraws to noxious stimuli, occasional nonpurposeful movement, random smiling or grimacing.

would need to address the possibility of sensory deprivation and overload as contributing to the patient's confusion. ■

Box 44-2 provides an overview of sensory deprivation and sensory overload with related nursing interventions.

Sensory Deprivation

Sensory deprivation results when a person experiences decreased sensory input or input that is monotonous, unpatterned, or meaningless. With decreased sensory input, the RAS is no longer able to project a normal level of activation to the brain. As a result, the individual may hallucinate simply to maintain an optimal level of arousal. Factors placing a patient at high risk for sensory deprivation include the following:

- An environment with decreased or monotonous stimuli (such as institutionalized patients or those confined to a small living area at home, on bed rest, or in isolation)
- Impaired ability to receive environmental stimuli (patients with impaired vision or hearing; with bandages or casts that interfere with vision, hearing, or tactile stimulation; or with affective disorders who "close out" the environment)
- Inability to process environmental stimuli (patients with spinal cord injuries or brain damage, those who are confused or disoriented, or are taking prescribed or recreational drugs affecting the central nervous system)

➤ *Remember Dolores Pirolla, the wife of the older man with vision deficits who was developing hearing deficits? The nurse would incorporate knowledge of risk factors for sensory deprivation when developing the patient's plan of care. In this case, Mr. Pirolla's sensory deficits involving vision and now hearing are impacting his ability to receive environmental stimuli. Thus, the nurse would develop a plan of care that addresses measures to ensure that the patient and his wife receive adequate stimulation from the environment.* ■

Sensory deprivation can lead to perceptual, cognitive, and emotional disturbances. *Perceptual responses* result from inaccurate perception of sights, sounds, tastes, smells, and body position, coordination, and equilibrium. These responses can range from mild distortions such as daydreams, to gross distortions such as hallucinations. *Cognitive responses* involve the patient's inability to control the direction of thought content. Typically, attention span and ability to concentrate are decreased. The patient may demonstrate difficulty with memory, problem solving, and task performance. *Emotional responses* typically are manifested by apathy, anxiety, fear, anger, belligerence, panic, or depression. Rapid mood changes also may occur (see Box 44-2 for additional information). In a discussion of the relationships among visual impairment, loss of hearing, and cognitive function in older adults, Wahl and Heyl (2003) found that

cognitive capacity and nonimpaired sensory function were closely related to higher cortical functions.

Sensory Overload

Sensory overload is the condition that results when a person experiences so much sensory stimuli that the brain is unable to either respond meaningfully or ignore the stimuli. The person feels out of control and may exhibit all of the manifestations observed in sensory deprivation. The amount and quality of stimuli necessary to produce overload may differ greatly from one individual to another and is influenced by factors such as age, culture, personality, and lifestyle.

In some patients, especially those coming from a quiet environment with unvarying stimuli, the experience of being hospitalized quickly results in sensory overload. In such patients, the brain is assaulted by the constant presence of strangers who not only demand to be spoken to, but also touch and poke at the body; by the strange sights, odors, sounds, and feels of the unfamiliar environment; by the constant presence of pain or discomfort from dressings, intravenous (IV) lines, drainage tubes, or endotracheal tubes; and by the ever-present worries about the meaning and course of the illness.

Nursing care focuses on reducing distressing stimuli and helping the patient to gain control over the environment (see Box 44-2).

➤ *Now consider Ori Soltes, the young man in the ICU. When assessing Mr. Soltes and his confusion, the nurse would need to be alert for factors that would contribute to sensory overload, such as bright lights, noises from the various monitoring devices, and frequent examinations. In addition, the nurse would need to assess for possible factors contributing to sensory deprivation. For example, the patient is receiving mechanical ventilation. As a result, healthcare team members may limit verbal communication with the patient, thus reducing some auditory stimuli that he would receive. Additionally, the patient is in bed with multiple injuries, also restricting his ability to interact with the environment.* ■

Sensory Deficits

Impaired or absent functioning in one or more senses is termed **sensory deficit.** Examples of sensory deficits include impaired sight and hearing, altered taste, numbness and paralysis that result in altered tactile perception, and impaired kinesthetic sense. These deficits may be reversible or permanent, may occur gradually or all at once, and may be present at birth or evolve later. Awareness of a patient's sensory deficits is necessary to determine whether the patient is able to compensate for the deficit. Illness and hospitalization may threaten a patient's usual adaptive patterns and require new self care abilities. Patients with evolving deficits will require assistance in coping and in learning to compensate skillfully.

➤ *Think again of Dolores Pirolla, the wife of the man with vision and hearing deficits. The nurse would need to assess both the patient and his wife to determine how each is coping. From the description at the beginning of the chapter, Mr. Pirolla appears to be experiencing prob-* *lems coping with the vision changes. As a result, both Mr. and Mrs. Pirolla are beginning to experience social isolation. The nurse would incorporate this information when developing a plan of care for the patient and his wife.* ■

(Box 44-2)   OVERVIEW OF SENSORY DEPRIVATION AND SENSORY OVERLOAD

Sensory Deprivation
Sensory deprivation is insufficient quantity or quality of stimuli; may result from decreased sensory input or monotonous, unpatterned, and unmeaningful input.

Defining Characteristics	Contributing Factors	Patients at Risk
Physical behaviors: drowsiness, excessive yawning	*Decreased environmental stimuli:* institutionalized environment; separation from significant others and usual sources of stimuli; treatments that decrease access to stimuli, such as bed rest or isolation	Institutionalized patients, especially those in long-term care settings
Escape behaviors: eating, exercising, sleeping, running away to escape the deprived environment		Patients with communicable diseases (e.g., AIDS)
		Patients confined to bed
Changes in perception: unusual body sensations; preoccupation with somatic complaints (dry mouth, palpitations, difficulty breathing, nausea); change in body image; illusions and hallucinations	*Impaired ability to receive environmental stimuli:* impaired vision, hearing, taste, smell, touch resulting from treatments such as bandages or body casts that interfere with reception of stimuli, or as a result of depression and other affective disorders	Patients with sensory alterations (e.g., impaired vision or hearing, or patients with eye patches or body casts)
Changes in cognitive behavior: decreased attention span, inability to concentrate, decreased problem solving and task performance		Patients who are depressed
		Patients from a different culture
Changes in affective behavior: crying, increased irritability and annoyance over small matters, confusion, panic, depression	*Inability to process environmental stimuli:* spinal cord injuries, brain damage, confusion, dementia, medications that depress the central nervous system	Patients with a disturbance of the nervous system

Nursing Interventions
Maintain sufficient level of arousal by increasing sensory stimuli from all sensory modalities:
- Instruct the patient in self-stimulation methods: counting, singing, reading, reciting poetry.
- Structure meaningful tangible stimuli into patient's external environment; include a variety of people, ideas, sensations; a pet may provide excellent stimulation.
  - Visual stimulation:
    Colorful sheets, pajamas, robes
    Colorful uniform tops for the nurse
    Face-to-face human contact
    Clocks, calendars, wristwatches
    Pictures, flowers, greeting card
  - Auditory stimulation:
    Call person by name
    Conversation that communicates caring as well as orients patient
    Reading to the patient
    Television, radio, iPod
  - Gustatory and olfactory stimulation:
    Attention to oral hygiene and properly fitting dentures
    Food of different textures, colors, temperatures served attractively
    Smelling food before eating it and recalling pleasurable aromas from the past
    Seasoning foods or having favorite foods brought from home

- Tactile stimulation:
  Backrubs and foot soaks
  Turning and repositioning
  Passive range-of-motion exercises
  Hair brushing, combing, washing
  Hugs
  Touching of arms or shoulders
- Cognitive input:
  Orient patient to environment
  Encourage patient participation in self-care
  Discuss current events or patient's occupation, hobbies, or interests
  Reinforce reality without arguing with a patient who is hallucinating. "No, I don't see a man standing there but the linen hamper may be confusing you."
- Emotional input: Encourage patient to share fears, concerns, and perceptions; reassure patient that illusions and misperceptions do occur with sensory deprivation
- Incorporate culturally assistive, supportive, facilitative acts into nursing care.
- *Caution:* Because it can be difficult to distinguish the behavioral manifestations of sensory deprivation from sensory overload, introduce more stimulation cautiously. If the added stimulation only increases the patient's maladaptive behaviors, consider reducing sensory input because the patient may be experiencing sensory overload.

(continued)

Box 44-2   **OVERVIEW OF SENSORY DEPRIVATION AND SENSORY OVERLOAD** *(continued)*

Sensory Overload
Sensory overload is excessive stimuli over which an individual feels little control; brain is unable meaningfully to respond to or ignore stimuli.

Defining Characteristics	Contributing Factors	Patients at Risk
Similar to those observed in sensory deprivation Elderly patients and patients who have suffered a stroke are more likely to experience a confusion or agitation. Young patients are more likely to seek the comfort of their parents' embrace to block out sensory overload.	*Increased internal stimuli:* pain, pressure and discomfort of intrusive tubes (e.g., intravenous lines [IVs], catheters; endotracheal tubes; nasogastric tubes), worry about state of health or need to make treatment decisions *Increased external stimuli:* unfamiliar healthcare environment, such as lights, noises, sounds, odors, movement, and constant presence of strangers, many of whom touch the body; intrusive procedures such as diagnostic tests and treatments; scratchy linens *Inability perceptually to disregard or selectively ignore some stimuli:* nervous system disturbances, medications such as caffeine that stimulate the central nervous system arousal mechanism	Acutely or chronically ill patients Patients in pain Patient with intrusive monitoring or treatment equipment Hospitalized patients, especially those in critical care settings Patients with disturbances of the nervous system

Nursing Interventions
- Provide a consistent, predictable pattern of stimulation to help the patient develop a sense of control over the environment.
- Offer simple explanations before procedures, tests, and examinations.
- Establish a schedule with the patient for routine care such as eating, bathing, turning, positioning, coughing, and exercising.

- Speak calmly with the patient and move slowly; communicate confidence.
- Explore with the patient what stimuli are most distressing and develop a plan to reduce or eliminate these (e.g., incoming phone calls, visitors); earplugs or pain medication may be indicated. Noise-reducing headphones may be helpful.
- Be careful not to cause sensory deprivation.
- Identify and, wherever possible, eliminate culturally inappropriate stimuli.

(Adapted from Lee, K. A. [1991]. Sensory overload, sensory deprivation, and sleep deprivation. In M. L. Patrick, S. I. Woods, R. F. Craven, J. S. Rokosky, & P. M. Bruno [Eds.], *Medical-surgical nursing* [2nd ed.]. Philadelphia: J. B. Lippincott.)

FACTORS AFFECTING SENSORY STIMULATION

The amount of stimuli different individuals consider optimal appears to vary considerably. Factors influencing the amount and quality of stimuli needed to maintain cortical arousal include developmental considerations, culture, personality and lifestyle, stress and illness, and medication.

Developmental Considerations

Different types of sensory stimulation are needed for growth as sensory receptors, organs, and the nervous system mature. Although the newborn is capable of rudimentary perceptual discrimination at birth, many neural pathways are immature and must be stimulated to develop, become refined, and function adequately. Appropriate stimulation includes soothing, holding, rocking and changes of position (tactile and kinesthetic sensations), singing and being talked to (auditory sensations), and changing patterns of light and shade, such as through the use of mobiles and bright objects (visual sensations). In contrast, the neonatal ICU may be a source of inappropriate sensory stimulation. To facilitate developmentally supportive care, it is recommended that medically fragile infants have limited light and visual and vestibular stimulation to simulate being in the womb.

For children, engaging in developmentally appropriate play will develop muscles and coordination, provide an outlet for surplus physical energy, develop communication skills, provide sources of learning, act as a stimulant to creativity, develop social skills, teach sex roles, provide an outlet for the release of emotional energy, and develop self-insights.

Sensory functioning tends to decline progressively throughout adulthood as the result of aging or chronic illness. The adult may experience the need to compensate for the loss of one type of stimulation by increasing other sources of sensory stimuli. See the accompanying box, Focus on the Older Adult: Sensory Functioning.

FOCUS ON THE OLDER ADULT

SENSORY FUNCTIONING

Age-Related Changes	Nursing Strategies
Decrease in vision	• Ensure the patient is using corrective lenses such as contacts, glasses, and/or magnifiers. • Administer medications that enhance vision, such as medications that lower intraocular pressure in older adult patients with glaucoma. • Provide adequate lighting and clear pathways of clutter to prevent injury. • Provide enlarged print. • Encourage the patient to visit the ophthalmologist annually.
Decrease in hearing	• Ensure the patient is using appropriate and functioning hearing assistive devices. • When communicating with the patient, use a lower tone. • Speak to the patient so that he/she can visualize mouth movements.
Decreased sense of touch	• Protect the patient's skin from temperature extremes. • Assess the extremities for breaks in the skin, blisters, drainage, or open wounds. • Ensure the patient is ambulating with assistive devices.
Sensory deprivation	• Discourage the use of sedatives. • Assess the effect of medications on the patient's central nervous system. • Provide interaction with children and pets. • Encourage the patient to participate in exercise classes and provide activity therapy. • Ensure that institutionalized elderly adults share meals with four individuals per table. • Ensure homebound elderly adults have frequent visits from family and community resources such as Meals on Wheels or church volunteers.
Sensory overload	• Orient the patient to person, place, and time. • Decrease environmental noise. • Encourage patient to participate in nursing care.

Culture

An individual's culture may dictate the amount of sensory stimulation considered normal. For example, the amount of touching a child experiences in a Puerto Rican family may be different from that experienced by a child in a German family. Similarly, male and female roles may be culturally defined; for example, although men are expected to respond to the challenges of out-of-the-home sensory stimuli, the woman who attempts to do so may be scorned if her place is considered to be in the home. Ethnic norms, religious norms, income group norms, and the norms of subgroups within a culture all influence the amount of sensory stimulation sought by an individual and perceived as meaningful.

Moreover, sensory deprivation, sensory overload, and sleep deprivation are all related to or affected by an individual's cultural practices, values, and beliefs. The nurse who is sensitive to the patient's culture attempts to determine what constitutes acceptable levels of stimuli from the patient's viewpoint. For example, in certain cultures, touching is viewed as a natural and welcome custom, whereas other cultures may view it as insulting or offensive. Similarly, patients may find comfort in cultural and religious symbols of care and healing that are absent in a hospital environment. Thus, nurses must be aware of the aspects of the patient's culture to deliver culturally competent care.

Personality and Lifestyle

Apart from a person's culture, different personality types demand different levels of stimulation. One person may thrive on a steady stream of fast-paced changes and excitement, whereas another may feel best when daily routines are rigidly structured and life sends no challenges necessitating changes. Lifestyle choices can dramatically influence the quantity and quality of stimuli received by an individual. The nurse who elects to work in the emergency room of a large city hospital is exposed to vastly different stimuli than the nurse making home visits in a rural setting.

Stress and Illness

Increased sensory stimulation may be sought during periods of low stress simply to maintain cortical arousal. During high-stress periods, multiple stressors may already be overloading the sensory system, and decreased sensory stimulation is desired. Illness, a time of stress, can affect the reception of sensory stimuli and their transmission and perception. Therefore, the stress of physical illness, pain, hospitalization, testing, surgery, or treatment may provide more stimulation than an individual can process and respond to without assistance.

▶ *Think back to Muriel Hao, the woman who had surgery 2 days ago. Most likely, Ms. Hao is experiencing sensory overload from all of the events of the past several days. In addition, the constant beeping of the equipment is adding to this overload.* ■

Medication

Medications that alert or depress the central nervous system may interfere with the perception of sensory stimuli. Certain medications may also contribute to the impairment of sensory functioning by decreasing reception (e.g., captopril, an antihypertensive agent, can cause taste alteration).

THE NURSING PROCESS FOR SENSORY STIMULATION
Assessing

When assessing a patient for disturbed sensory perceptions, interview the patient and examine him or her for sensory deficits and manifestations of sensory deprivation or overload. Be sure to include an assessment of the patient's environment to determine whether it is providing adequate sensory stimulation for healthy development.

Identifying At-Risk Patients

Patients may be at risk for sensory disturbances for different reasons. Often there are *physiological* reasons that place individuals at risk. Aging, for example, is often accompanied by diminished senses. Diseases can also diminish senses. Diabetes-related neuropathies can result in a loss of sensation in limbs rendering the diabetic unable to feel hot objects such as bath water, which can result in burns. Certain drugs affect taste. *Social and environmental* factors likewise place individuals at risk. Humans need appropriate human and environmental stimulation. When either or both are deficient or excessive, problems may result. *Lifestyle* factors may also place individuals at risk such as engaging in work or leisure activities that are potentially harmful to eyes or ears such as exposure to chemicals, flying objects, and loud noises.

Assessment of the Sensory Experience

When assessing a patient's sensory experience, structure the history using the components of the sensory experience—stimulation, reception, and transmission–perception–reaction. See the Focused Assessment Guide 44-1. Because patients may adapt to sensory impairments, it may be helpful to include someone the patient knows well (e.g., spouse or parent) in the assessment to see if that person has noticed behavioral characteristics in the patient that suggest a sensory disturbance (e.g., "I've noticed he turns the television volume much louder than ever before."). Also, recognize that individuals may develop acuity in certain senses to compensate for losses in others. For example, many persons who are blind have acute hearing. It is helpful to begin by asking patients to evaluate their sensory functioning: "How would you rate your vision (hearing, etc.): Excellent, good, fair, poor, or bad?"

The mental status exam is included in assessments of sensory functioning. Chapter 25 provides a detailed description

of how to assess levels of awareness (see also Box 44-1), levels of consciousness, memory, abstract reasoning, and language. The mini-mental status examination (MMSE) is one of the most widely used clinical instruments for quickly detecting cognitive impairment and assessing its severity, as well as for monitoring cognitive changes over time (http://www.minimental.com/).

STIMULATION

Assess whether there have been any recent changes in sensory stimulation, for example, reduction of stimulation from one or more sensory modalities ("Since my husband died, no one touches me anymore. It sounds crazy, but I'm hungry to be touched!") or new or unusual stimulation ("Ever since my granddaughter moved in with me, my house is always noisy. I can't stand the constant noise and her smoking."). Assess whether the type of stimulation present is developmentally appropriate. *High-risk patients* for problems related to stimulation include children in nonstimulating environments, older people, terminally ill patients, patients on bed rest, patients in isolation, and patients requiring intensive nursing in a critical care setting.

RECEPTION

Assess for anything that may interfere with sensory reception and describe any *corrective devices* the patient uses for sensory impairments (eyeglasses, contact lenses, hearing aids). If corrective devices are necessary, assess whether or not the patient is actually using them, has the proper equipment, and understands related care. For example, ask the patient, "When were your eyes last examined," or "Are there batteries for your hearing aid?" The Reception section of the Focused Assessment Guide 44-1 highlights assessment strategies for each sense. Patients at *high risk* for reception problems include people with visual, auditory, or other sensory impairments.

➤ *Consider Dolores Pirolla and her husband who has visual and hearing deficits. The nurse would need to assess the amount and type of stimulation Mr. Pirolla is receiving. In addition, the nurse would need to investigate what measures the couple uses to adapt to the progressive visual changes. Doing so would provide a sound basis on which to build the plan of care. See Box 44-3 for sample documentation of Mr. Pirolla's assessment of sensory functioning.* ■

TRANSMISSION–PERCEPTION–REACTION

Be alert for patients at high risk for transmission–perception–reaction problems, such as the patient who is confused or who has a nervous system impairment. Use everyday interactions as multiple opportunities to assess patients' abilities to transmit, perceive, and react to stimuli.

DEFINING CHARACTERISTICS OF SENSORY DEPRIVATION AND OVERLOAD

Complete the assessment of the patient's sensory functioning by assessing for specific indicators of sensory deprivation

FOCUSED ASSESSMENT GUIDE • 44-1

SENSORY STIMULATION

Factors to Assess	Questions and Approaches
Stimulation	"Does your current environment overly, insufficiently, or appropriately stimulate you?" "Are you bored? Why?" "Are you able to read? Watch television? Knit? Why not?" "Are there other people in your home during the day? Do you spend much time together? How do you spend the time?" "Who visits you while you are in the hospital?" Note reduction in the patterns or meaningfulness of stimulation in each sensory modality, changes in stimulation other than decreases (e.g., new or unusual stimulation), or developmental appropriateness of stimulation.
Reception	"Does anything interfere with the functioning of your senses?" "Describe any corrective devices you use for sensory impairments."
Assess for visual disturbances.	"Please read my name tag (or this page of print)." Note if the patient can correctly identify objects directly in front of the eyes as well as those requiring peripheral vision. Note eye rubbing, squinting, movements indicating faulty vision (bumping into furniture, overreaching or underreaching for objects), changes in the appearance of the eye (cataracts, swelling), and complaints of eye pain, spots, halos, or other visual disturbances.
Assess for auditory disturbances.	"Repeat the words that I will speak softly close to each ear." Note if the patient is able to hear equally well from both ears, distinguish voices, locate the direction of a sound, if the patient needs to face the person speaking and relies on lip reading, if the patient's responses to questions include blank looks, many nods, smiling, or inappropriate responses indicating faulty hearing. Note complaints of ringing or buzzing in ears.
Assess for gustatory (taste) disturbances.	"Close your eyes, stick out your tongue, and tell me if what I place on your tongue is sweet, sour, bitter, or salty." "Have you been experiencing any strange tastes (bitter, metallic) or aftertastes lately?" Note if the patient is able to differentiate sweet, sour, bitter, or salty tastes or reports unusual, persistent taste sensations. Note deficient oral hygiene, ill-fitting dentures, braces, or anything else that might contribute to gustatory disturbances.
Assess for olfactory (smell) disturbances.	"Close your eyes and tell me what you smell." "Have you smelled odors lately that others cannot smell, or have you been especially sensitive to odors?" Note if the patient can correctly identify common odors (coffee, vanilla) or has noticed increased sensitivity to odors.
Assess for tactile (touch) disturbances.	"Close your eyes and tell me when you feel something (brush skin with cotton ball), if what you feel is dull or sharp (use both ends of safety pin), hot or cold (use items from food tray). Now, keep your eyes closed and tell me what I am placing in your hand (coin, cotton ball, paper clip)." Note if the patient can correctly sense touch and distinguish sharp and dull, hot and cold, and different shapes. Note if the patient reports decreased sensation in any part of the body; numbness, pins and needles, tingling; or abnormal sensitivity to pain or touch.
Assess for kinesthetic and visceral disturbances.	Note if the patient withdraws from being touched. "Have you noticed any changes in the way you perceive your body?" "Do you feel any unusual pressure or pain inside your body?" Note if the patient seems unsure of his or her body parts or body position and if he or she experiences new internal sensations (fullness, pressure, pain).

(continued)

FOCUSED ASSESSMENT GUIDE • 44-1

SENSORY STIMULATION *(continued)*

Factors to Assess	Questions and Approaches
Transmission–perception–reaction	"Are you aware of any problems with your nervous system?" "Have you found it difficult to communicate verbally?" Note consciousness, orientation, appropriateness of responses, ability to perform usual self-care activities, ability to follow simple commands, decision-making abilities, pathology affecting central nervous system, or prescribed or recreational drug use that affects the central nervous system.
Behavioral manifestations of sensory deprivation or overload	
Perceptual responses	Mild to gross sensory distortions (illusions, hallucinations)
Cognitive responses	Thought disorganization, slowness of thought, decreased attention/concentration, difficulty with problem solving and task performance
Emotional responses	Rapid mood changes, anxiety, panic

or overload (see Box 44-2 earlier in the chapter). Observe for boredom, inactivity, slowness of thought, daydreaming, increased sleeping, thought disorganization, anxiety, panic, illusions, and hallucinations. Be knowledgeable of the patient's usual state to enhance your ability to identify changes stemming from sensory deprivation or overload.

> *Think back to Muriel Hao, the woman who had surgery 2 days ago. The patient's complaints of inability to rest due to the machine's beeping should alert the nurse to the possibility of sensory overload. Additionally, to confirm the suspicions, the nurse would need to review the patient's medical record to gather more data about the patient's usual state and behavior.* ∎

Physical Assessment

Physical examination skills related to the senses are discussed in Chapter 25. Ear and eye tests, whether performed by a physician or nurse, should be considered when planning care. Problems with the neurologic system indicate the necessity of further assessment of the sensory experience.

Assessment of the Ability to Perform Self-Care

Alterations in sensory functioning may limit an individual's ability to perform everyday activities safely. Exercise empathy by trying to imagine how you would get through a day if you lacked sight, hearing, or other senses. Ideally, this exercise will help in fashioning a plan of care responsive to the needs of patients. Patients with new sensory alterations and their family caregivers will need to be instructed about practical ways to modify their home environment for safety. The Home Safety Council (HSC) is a national nonprofit organization solely dedicated to preventing the home-related injuries that result in nearly 20,000 deaths and 21 million medical visits, on average, each year (http://www.homesafetycouncil.org/). Patients can be referred to this Web site for practical guides and charts. Additionally, it is important to recognize that patients who are out of their home environment will need to be oriented to their

---

Box 44-3 SAMPLE DOCUMENTATION OF A TARGETED ASSESSMENT

Mr. Anthony Pirolla came to the clinic with his wife who reported a new concern about his hearing.

Chief complaint: Difficulty hearing.

Signs and symptoms: According to his wife, Mr. Pirolla frequently fails to answer her questions or answers inappropriately. She also reports that he plays the radio and television louder than before. He complains that people seem to be "mumbling" more than usual—especially in church. Patient denies ringing or buzzing in ears.

Onset/duration: Mr. Pirolla states that he's had difficulty hearing since Christmas (2 months ago)—when the whole family came to visit. Mrs. Pirolla believes he had difficulty starting in the summer.

Predisposing factors: In his youth, Mr. Pirolla worked construction and was frequently around loud equipment. He is 77.

Effect on patient: Patient no longer enjoys going out or being with friends and has become more reclusive.

Self remedies: None.

Intervention: Referred Mr. Pirolla to the clinic's audiologist.

C. Taylor, RN

new surroundings. Patients need to know how to call the nurse, how to use the lights and television, and how to navigate safely to the bathroom. Before leaving a patient's room, do a quick check to ensure that the environment is safe—especially for patients with sensory impairments.

Diagnosing

Disturbed Sensory Perception as the Problem

When assessment data point to sensory disturbances that can be treated independently by nursing interventions, nursing diagnoses are developed and labeled. The North American Nursing Diagnosis Association (2009) recognizes the following diagnostic labels for sensory/perceptual problems:

- **Disturbed Sensory Perception:** A state in which the individual or group experiences or is at risk for a change in the amount, pattern, or interpretation of incoming stimuli. These alterations may be further specified as visual, auditory, gustatory, olfactory, tactile, or kinesthetic. Sensory deprivation, sensory overload, and uncompensated sensory loss may also be used to further specify the disturbed sensory perception and in some cases may be the etiology.
- **Acute Confusion:** The abrupt onset of a cluster of global, transient changes and disturbances in attention, cognition, psychomotor activity level of consciousness, or sleep–wake cycle
- **Chronic Confusion:** An irreversible, long-standing, or progressive deterioration of intellect and personality characterized by decreased ability to interpret environmental stimuli or decreased capacity for intellectual thought processes and manifested by disturbances of memory, orientation, and behavior
- **Impaired Memory:** The state in which an individual experiences the inability to remember or recall bits of information or behavior skills. Impaired memory may be attributed to pathophysiologic or situational causes that are either temporary or permanent.

Common etiologies for disturbed sensory perception include the following:

- Altered environmental stimuli: excessive or insufficient
- Altered sensory reception, transmission, or integration
- Chemical alterations: endogenous (e.g., electrolytes) or exogenous (e.g., drugs)
- Psychological stress

See Examples of NANDA Nursing Diagnoses in which disturbed sensory perception is the problem.

Disturbed Sensory Perception as the Etiology

Because disturbed sensory perceptions affect many other areas of human functioning, they serve as etiologies for multiple problem statements. Examples may include the following:

- Activity Intolerance related to impaired balance and coordination (kinesthetic alteration)

- Anxiety related to paranoia stemming from hearing impairment, sensory deprivation (specify setting), sensory overload
- Impaired Verbal Communication related to difficulty receiving, transmitting, and perceiving sensory stimuli
- Ineffective Coping related to sensory overload (multiple stressors)
- Deficient Diversional Activity related to impaired vision or hearing
- Delayed Growth and Development related to nonstimulating home environment
- Risk for Injury related to decreased or impaired sensation (specify visual, auditory, tactile, kinesthetic)
- Deficient Knowledge about means to Compensate for Sensory Impairment (blindness, deafness, and so forth) related to lack of previous experience with this problem, unavailability of resources
- Deficient Knowledge of providing a Developmentally Stimulating Environment related to lack of experience with children's growth and development
- Impaired Physical Mobility related to impaired balance and coordination (kinesthetic alteration)
- Impaired Parenting associated with failure to Provide Stimuli for Growth related to lack of knowledge, decreased motivation to provide for child's growth and development
- Powerlessness related to inability to interact meaningfully with environment
- Self-Care Deficit: (specify) related to visual impairment, auditory impairment, tactile impairment
- Disturbed Body Image related to kinesthetic impairment (distorted sense of body parts), sensory deprivation
- Low Self-Esteem related to effects of disturbed sensory perception (specify visual, auditory, etc.)
- Ineffective Role Performance related to sensory/perceptual alteration (blindness, deafness, and so forth)
- Disturbed Personal Identity related to sensory deprivation or overload
- Sexual Dysfunction related to decreased sensation
- Impaired Skin Integrity related to absent tactile sensation (injury)
- Disturbed Sleep Pattern related to sensory deprivation or overload
- Impaired Social Interaction related to inability to receive and process interactional stimuli
- Social Isolation related to visual or auditory impairment
- Disturbed Thought Processes (specify illusions, hallucinations, decreased attention or concentration, etc.) related to sensory deprivation or overload

Outcome Identification and Planning

In whatever setting nurses encounter and care for patients, optimal sensory stimulation is a priority. Nursing care focuses on the patient outcomes that follow. The patient will:

- Live in a developmentally stimulating and safe environment
- Exhibit a level of arousal that enables the brain to receive and meaningfully organize patterns of stimulation

Examples of NANDA Nursing Diagnoses

Disturbed Sensory Perception

Nursing Diagnoses	Related Factors	Sample Defining Characteristics
Disturbed Sensory Perception: Sensory Deficit or Excess Visual	Eye patches after surgery	"I never realized before how sight-dependent I am. I don't know what time of day it is now unless I have the radio on or smell food coming in." "It's frightening not to know who is in my room and what they are doing." Patient observed sitting in room with blank facial expression; frequently comments on how bored he or she is and how slowly time is passing; hesitant to move about room without assistance although he or she has been oriented repeatedly
Auditory	Effects of aging	"You're right. I don't always hear what people are saying anymore so I try not to get involved in conversations. If people insist on talking, I just nod and hope I'm giving the right response." Able to hear moderately spoken word close to right ear; cannot hear same from left ear; often startled when someone approaches from left side Sits close to television and radio; loud volume, no history of hearing testing
Gustatory or olfactory	Chemotherapy	"I always seem to have a bitter taste in my mouth now and can't stomach certain foods at all that I used to enjoy, like beef, tomatoes, coffee. . . . I also can't take sweets, and I used to be a real sweets junkie." "Sometimes the very smell of certain foods or even the thought of eating nauseates me." Patient has been receiving vincristine (cancer chemotherapeutic agent) for past 3 months; some nausea and vomiting; history of poor oral hygiene
Tactile	Psychological stress	"I don't know why I feel this way, but I'm hypersensitive to touch. If anyone even brushes against me, I feel burning pain. Even the weight of my clothes against my skin bothers me. I'm trying to move my body as little as possible and keep it protected—but that's obviously impossible when even a breeze assaults me." Patient observed holding the body stiffly looking like he or she does not know what to do with the arms and legs; dressed only in a loose-fitting outfit; reports that he or she sits at home all day afraid to go out
Kinesthetic	Clinitron bed therapy	"I've been in this bed for 2 weeks now and I've lost all sense of my body . . . it's a curious weightless feeling that I have . . . sort of like floating in Jell-O. I'm no longer sure where my body begins and ends, and when I try to lift an arm or leg I feel like I'm in slow motion. I hope I'll be able to walk when I get out of here."

(continued)

Examples of NANDA Nursing Diagnoses

Disturbed Sensory Perception (continued)

Nursing Diagnoses	Related Factors	Sample Defining Characteristics
Disturbed Sensory Perception: Sensory Deprivation	Isolation	"One of the worst things that has happened to me since I found out I had AIDS is that everyone is afraid of me—and no one touches me. I'm so lonely. I've always needed a lot of people around." "Here in the hospital I think I'm going crazy. I can't leave this room. Everyone who comes in looks the same dressed in those yellow gowns. Lately, I've seen some bizarre things that I know can't be real. I look at the clock and it turns into a swirling sun with a sad face that keeps coming closer and closer to me and I'm terrified I'll burn up if it gets too close. That's crazy, isn't it? I'm really losing it now." Disturbed sleep for past 2 weeks; during the day, yawns excessively and catnaps; limited attention span; states he or she is unable to concentrate on anything.
Disturbed Sensory Perception: Sensory Overload	Trauma of rape and aftercare	"When is everyone going to stop touching me? First, he wouldn't stop. Now, everyone here is poking at me, looking at me, asking me hundreds of questions. . . . Why did I have to report this and come to the hospital? Oh, please leave me alone. Get out of here everyone."

- Demonstrate intact functioning of the senses: vision, hearing, taste, smell, touch, and kinesthetic and visceral awareness
- Schedule appropriate health screening exams for sensory functioning
- Maintain orientation to time, place, and person
- Respond appropriately (verbally and nonverbally) to sensory stimuli while executing self-care activities

Patients with impaired sensory functioning require individualized outcomes similar to the following. The patient will:

- Report feeling safe and in control of the environment
- Describe different types of meaningful stimuli present in the environment
- Demonstrate (describe) appropriate self-care behaviors for visual impairment, hearing impairment, or other sensory impairment
- Verbalize acceptance of the sensory deficit

Implementing

The nurse can assist patients to improve sensory functioning by teaching patients and significant others methods for stimulating the senses, teaching patients with intact and impaired senses appropriate self-care behaviors, and interacting therapeutically with patients experiencing sensory impairments. Safety is always a special concern for patients with sensory alterations. Ensure that the patient's environment is as free of danger as possible and assist the patient to develop new self-care behaviors to compensate for sensory impairments. See the accompanying Examples of Nursing Interventions and Nursing Outcomes Classifications (NIC/NOC) for Balance. Safety considerations are discussed in Chapter 26 in more detail. The nursing interventions described here relate to preventing sensory alteration, stimulating the senses, meeting the needs of vision- and hearing-impaired people, communicating with a confused person, and communicating with an unconscious person. Communication guidelines for patients with sensory deficits are also highlighted in Chapter 21.

Preventing Disturbed Sensory Perception and Stimulating the Senses

The most effective means by which sensory alteration can be managed is prevention. The key to prevention is, with the patient's help, to create a functional and meaningful environment while keeping limitations in mind. The creation of such an environment requires careful observation, analysis, and creative planning.

Although numerous nursing measures can be considered in planning care, determining their appropriateness depends on the circumstances. Promote the patient's well-being by offering care that provides rest and comfort (see Chapters 34 and 35). Attempt to control patient discomfort whenever possible.

> *Recall Muriel Hao, the woman who had surgery 2 days ago. The patient verbalizes an inability to rest due to the "beeping of the machine." The initial priority would be to stop the machine from beeping. The nurse would need to*

**Examples of Nursing Interventions and
Nursing Outcomes Classifications (NIC/NOC)**

Exercise Therapy: Balance

Nursing Interventions

- Determine patient's ability to participate in activities requiring balance
- Evaluate sensory functions (e.g., vision, hearing, proprioception)
- Provide opportunity to discuss factors that influence fear of falling
- Provide safe environment for practice of exercises
- Instruct patient on importance of exercise therapy in maintaining and improving balance

Nursing Outcomes

- Balance
- Body Positioning: Self-Initiated
- Coordinated Movement
- Sensory Function: Proprioception

From Bulechek, G. M., Butcher, H. K., & Dochterman, J., (Eds.). (2008). *Nursing interventions classification (NIC)* (5th ed., p. 336). St. Louis: Mosby. A full listing of nursing activities for each nursing intervention can be found in this book.
From Moorhead, S., Johnson, M., Maas, M. L., & Swanson, E. (2008). *Nursing outcomes classification (NOC)* (4th ed., p. 811). St. Louis: Mosby Elsevier.

investigate the underlying problem related to the machine's beeping, such as a low battery or an occlusion. Once the cause is determined, the nurse can then focus on comfort measures. ■

Be aware of the need for sensory aids and prostheses, such as eyeglasses, contact lenses, hearing aids, dentures, canes, and artificial limbs, making them available as needed. Social activities, as shown in Figure 44-2, help to stimulate the senses and mind. Enlist the aid of family members to participate in or encourage these activities. Also encourage physical activity and exercise, which help maintain normal sensory perceptions and decrease the likelihood of sensory alteration (exercises are discussed in Chapter 33).

Provide stimulation for as many senses as possible. Varied sights, sounds, smells, body positions, and textures can be helpful in providing a variety of sensations. For example, music therapy has been found to benefit selected physiologic

variables such as pulse rate, respiratory rate, and mood state in patients receiving mechanical ventilation. Listening to music can ameliorate the stress response and promote non-pharmacologically induced relaxation for the study subjects. See the accompanying Research in Nursing box. All nurses, but especially critical care nurses, can be confident in implementing this nonpharmacologic, independent intervention to promote relaxation without worry of untoward side effects, which are sometimes caused by pharmacologic sedation. Consider cultural factors when stimulating senses and when offering nursing care. This is especially important when caring for patients from cultures different from one's own. (See Chapter 28 for a discussion of common complementary and alternative therapies.)

Teaching About Sensory Experiences

Teaching is a significant nursing responsibility that helps prepare patients for sensory experiences. An informed patient is better able to handle fears, frustration, and confusion. Therefore, explain procedures before performing them or having the patient experience them. Explanations also help prevent the patient from feeling that his or her space and body are being invaded.

Allow individuals experiencing perceptual and thought distortions the opportunity to acknowledge that fact. Discussing such experiences and being reassured that these experiences are normal and usually temporary generally eases anxiety.

▶ *Remember Ori Soltes, the young man in the ICU who becomes confused? The nurse needs to acknowledge the patient's confusion, reorienting him frequently. In addition, the patient's ability to communicate is limited as a result of the ventilator. Therefore, the nurse should provide the patient with alternative means to communicate,*

FIGURE 44-2. The nurse helps the patient find methods for stimulating his or her senses. Family members may participate in sensory activities.

RESEARCH IN NURSING
Bridging the Gap to Evidence-Based Practice

BENEFITS OF SENSORY STIMULATION THROUGH MUSIC THERAPY

By providing patients with sensory stimulation through such activities as music therapy, patients are able to benefit physiologically as well.

Related Research

Stouffer, J. W., Shirk, B. J., & Polomano, R. C. (2007). Practice guidelines for music interventions with hospitalized pediatric patients. *Journal of Pediatric Nursing, 22*(6), 448–456.

Music therapy is an effective complementary approach that can achieve specific therapeutic outcomes in the clinical management of pediatric patients. Growing research on music interventions has generated scientific knowledge about how this modality benefits patients and has formed the basis for effective protocols that can be used in practice. Although it can be challenging to translate research-based protocols into routine clinical care at the bedside, it is essential that music therapy interventions are aligned with evidence-based information and that accepted standards be established by the music therapy discipline to achieve the greatest benefit.

The importance of partnerships between nurses and music therapists is emphasized to enhance the success of music-based treatments. This discussion synthesizes research findings

For additional research, visit the Point.

that can be used to design pediatric practice guidelines in the application of music therapy.

Related Research

Vozzella, S. (2007). Sensory stimulation in dementia care: Why it is important and how to implement it. *Topics in Geriatric Rehabilitation. Function and Cognition, 23*(2), 102–113.

This study focuses on the importance of stimulation and various ways to stimulate a patient suffering from dementia. Patients with dementia need constant stimulation, whether in a hospital setting, or at home. There are multiple ways of providing the necessary stimulation, whether through auditory, visual, olfactory, tactile, taste, and/or kinesthetic activities. Through using sensory exciting techniques, the patient will become much more engaged.

Relevance to Nursing Practice

As a patient's comfort and happiness are important aspects of health, nurses must consider the ways that dementia patients, in particular, can be engaged. Providing an atmosphere where senses can be stimulated is essential.

---

such as paper and pencil or a blackboard to write on so that the patient can make his needs known. The nurse also would need to reinforce explanations about all the equipment and technologies to which the patient is being exposed. Doing so may help to alleviate some of his anxiety. ■

Patients and family members can be guided in sensory self-stimulation, and parents can be aided in stimulation of newborns, infants, and children. Teaching Tips 44-1 gives helpful suggestions for teaching patients about protecting and stimulating sensory function and includes suggestions that the nurse can use in a variety of situations. Table 44-1 provides additional information on stimulating the senses for patients and nurses.

Promoting Health Literacy

Risk factors for inadequate health literacy include advanced age, low educational level, poverty, inability to read, learning disabilities, and lack of English proficiency. Patients with sensory impairments are also at risk for inadequate health literacy because of hearing or visual impairments or confusion and an inability to process or remember what is heard. See the Promoting Health Literacy box. You can also go to www.jointcommission.org in the public policy reports section to find the Joint Commission white paper, "What Did the Doctor Say?": Improving Health Literacy to Protect Patient Safety.

Meeting the Needs of Patients With Reduced Vision

Always check with the physician to discover if a visual problem is temporary, permanent, partial, or complete, and the degree to which the problem is likely to affect the patient's everyday functioning. This information is vital to developing a realistic teaching plan or plan of care.

The first priority is to teach patients self-care behaviors for maintaining vision and preventing blindness. These include:

- Avoid rubbing eyes.
- Avoid eyestrain.
- Avoid damage from ultraviolet rays.
- Protect eyes from foreign bodies.
- Keep eyeglasses clean, protected, and adjusted.
- Avoid nonprescription eyedrops and seek attention for symptoms.
- Avoid cleaning eyes or contact lenses with soiled articles.
- Use caution with aerosol sprays.
- Use caution with ammonia, lye, and so on.
- Visit your physician frequently if you are prone to eye problems.
- Know the danger signals that indicate serious eye problems: persistent eye redness; pain or discomfort, especially after injury; visual disturbances; crossing eyes; growth on or near the eyes; discharge or increased tearing; and pupil irregularities.

TEACHING TIPS • 44-1

SENSORY FUNCTIONING

Health Topic	Teaching Tip	Why Is This Important?
Hearing	• Avoid loud noise that is concentrated at the ear canal, such as with earphones. • Decrease background or loud noises. • Use ear plugs when using loud machinery, including lawn mowers, grass trimmers, or industrial equipment. • Have regular hearing assessments. Children should be assessed in school yearly. • Do not insert objects such as cotton-tipped applicators into the ear. • Avoid cleaning of the ear. • Have ear pain evaluated by a physician or nurse practitioner. • Be aware of the signs and symptoms of hearing loss.	Hearing loss occurring as an individual ages is called **presbycusis.** Presbycusis is the deterioration of nerves and structures within the inner ear. Many occupations result in hearing loss due to increased noise. Thus, the use of ear-protective devices can decrease the development of hearing loss. Instructing the patient on signs and symptoms of hearing loss and interventions to be implemented can help to slow the development of hearing loss.
Vision	• Protect the eye from damage due to ultraviolet rays with sunglasses and tinted windows. • Provide adequate light for working or reading. • Stimulate vision with colors and shapes. • Use large print to assist in readability. • Have an annual eye examination. • Avoid rubbing the eyes. • Use cleaning products or aerosol products safely in a well-ventilated area. • Use eye shields when in contact with harmful or toxic products, such as blood or body fluids or cleaning products. • Avoid nonprescription eyedrops.	The education of the patient to maintain adequate eye function enhances the patient's quality of life. The avoidance of strain on the eye stimulates vision, thus enhancing sensory perception.
Taste (gustatory)	• Practice oral care three times per day to prevent infection and decay. • Visit the dentist biannually for dental cleaning and examination. • Notify the dentist about pain or sensitivity to hot or cold. • Provide nutritional foods that are high in fiber, low in fat and sugar. • Enhance taste with use of spices.	Prevention of mouth disease enhances the taste and enjoyment of foods.
Smell	• Use aromatherapy to reduce stress. • Protect the nose from noxious fumes. • Eliminate disturbing odors with adequate ventilation. • Visit the physician or nurse practitioner when experiencing nasal congestion or diminished sense of smell. • Avoid wearing heavy colognes or perfumes. • Enhance the sense of smell by remembering pleasant odors.	The sense of smell is important in assisting the individual to relax, particularly during times of stress. It is important to evaluate any difficulty with the sense of smell and nasal congestion, since the nose lies in close proximity to the ear and the brain. Thus, the prevention of infection is a primary aspect of care.
Touch	• Protect the skin from extremes in temperature. • Provide various textures in the environment. • Provide touch such as during the bath or massage therapy. • Instruct on all aspects of invasive procedures.	Protecting the skin from temperature changes decreases damage to the skin and underlying tissues. The use of a variety of textures stimulates nerve fibers and tactile sense.
Sensory Overload	• Reduce the number and type of stimuli. • Provide periods of rest. • Provide explanation of sounds and activities within the environment. • Use relaxation techniques to enhance rest.	Sensory overload can be prevented by using these measures. As a result, the patient is able to organize stimuli to decrease anxiety and stress.
Sensory Deprivation	• Provide reading material, audiovisual stimulation, and interactive activities. • Provide stimulation through visitors, phone conversations, and e-mail. • Use Therapeutic Touch. • Encourage the use of assistive devices such as hearing aids and glasses. • Provide a radio and television. • Orient to time, place, and person.	Increasing sensory perception enhances the patient's responses, helping to create a meaningful environment.

TABLE • 44-1	**STIMULATING THE SENSES**	
Sense	**Teaching Patients**	**Nursing Interventions**
Vision	Surround yourself with different colors and with an environment that changes (walk through a mall, sit by a window where you see people come and go). Develop a sensitivity to changes in nature (weather patterns, dawn-to-night cycle, changing seasons, changes in a plant or animal). Use visual devices to keep oriented (watches, calendars, newspaper, television). Use crossword puzzles and games to stimulate mental activities. Create favorite scenes in your mind, paying attention to tiny details.	Wear visually stimulating and comforting colors. Keep meaningful visual stimuli such as photos, greeting cards, toys, or flowers near patient. Position patients with impaired mobility where they can see out a window or watch local traffic on the unit.
Hearing	Decrease or eliminate distressing auditory stimuli (change bedroom, talk with family members about noise of stereos and other such equipment, use earplugs, use headphones to listen to soft music). Develop a sensitivity to different sounds (music, chirping birds, night sounds, different voices). Use the telephone to maintain contact with family and friends. Use television, radio, CDs to keep current and to stimulate mental activities. Recall favorite sounds of the past with the situations in which they were heard.	Speak in a warm and pleasant tone and communicate caring to the patient. Use your voice to orient patient to environment and current situation (e.g., procedure, treatment). Avoid speaking about the patient to others within the patient's hearing. Remember that patients overhearing snatches of conversation outside their room often presume it is about *them!* Decrease extraneous noise (intercom, movement of carts, loud conversations of staff); use carpets and sound-absorbing material whenever possible.
Taste	Experiment with foods of different tastes (seasonings), colors, temperature, and textures; realize that as taste buds age, things will no longer taste the same. Practice thorough oral hygiene and have regular dental examinations. Recall foods that tasted especially good in the past and the events surrounding these tastes (e.g., grandparent baking cookies or homemade bread).	Consult with the dietitian about preparing meals with varied taste sensations; serve meals attractively. Perform routine oral hygiene for patients who are unable to do this for themselves.
Smell	Consciously savor smells that are pleasant; decrease or eliminate noxious odors. Recall pleasant aromas or smells from the past and the events surrounding them (e.g., smell of the ocean as the vacation house was neared, smell of fresh pine in the house at Christmas, the body scent of a loved person or animal).	Keep the patient's room well ventilated, using opportunities when the patient is out of the room to air it out. Remove dressings, drainage, and any equipment with odors from the patient's room as quickly as possible. Encourage patients to focus on pleasant or familiar smells, such as coffee, newspaper, or flowers. Avoid wearing heavy perfumes.
Touch	Consciously surround yourself with different textures and let yourself feel and enjoy them (scratchy afghan; a puppy's moist, wet tongue; soft petal of a flower; smooth silk scarf; mug of hot chocolate). Allow these textures to evoke memories of past tactile experiences (grandchild's hug may bring back memories of hugs from own children, scrap of fabric may recall a prom dress or wedding gown or baby blanket). Recognize the need to be touched and tell someone, "I need a hug today!" Receive tactile stimulation from a pet.	Include different textures in the patient's environment (silky pillow sham from home, soft sheepskin, wooly blanket). Respect the patient's need and desire to be touched or not touched (touch the patient's forearm or shoulder, hug the patient). Use physical care (bath time, foot soaks, hair care, back massages, turning and positioning, passive range of motion) to provide tactile stimulation. Limit intrusive procedures and times when the patient needs to be uncomfortably manipulated.

General Nursing Strategies in the Hospital or Other Residential Care Setting

Encourage the patient to participate in activities that require exploration of the environment (exercise, feeling, tasting, touching, moving, listening).

Use conversation to explore areas of interest to the patient.

Encourage the patient to share feelings.

Familiarize the environment by encouraging the patient to wear own clothes and keep personal items nearby.

Suggest the use of self-stimulation techniques—humming, singing, whistling, reciting, memory review, and problem solving.

Promoting Health Literacy

IN PATIENTS WITH HEARING DEFICITS

Patient Scenario

Mr. Rosato is 84 and until recently had no difficulty hearing. He lives in a nursing home because of complications from several serious diseases: diabetes, congestive heart failure, high blood pressure, degenerative joint disease. His daughter, who visits frequently, informed you, the nurse manager, that he seems to be having increasing difficulty with hearing—although he denies this. She shared that he sometimes answers questions inappropriately or asks folks to speak louder and she noticed that his television volume is always loud. She made an appointment for him with an audiologist but shares that she doesn't know the first thing about hearing disorders.

Nursing Considerations: *Tips for Improving Health Literacy*

Compliment the daughter's keen observation, report that sensory disorders are common among the elderly, and tell her how important the visit with the audiologist is. Give her an information sheet about hearing disorders and tips on finding out more information about the disorder online from a credible source. Encourage her to be prepared to ask the audiologist three questions:

- What is her father's main problem?
- What do they need to do?
- Why is it important for them to do this?

What additional measures can you take to help increase health literacy in this patient/family? What other measures would be helpful if Mr. Rosato and/or his daughter do not speak English, cannot read, or have other learning deficits?

When communicating with patients with reduced vision, follow these guidelines:

- Acknowledge your presence in the patient's room. Identify yourself by name.
- Speak in a normal tone of voice. Remember that the blind person is unable to pick up most nonverbal cues during communication.
- Explain the reason for touching the person before doing so.
- Keep the call light or bell within easy reach of the person and place the bed in the lowest position.
- Orient the person to sounds in the environment.
- Orient the person to the arrangement of the room and its furnishings. Clear pathways for the person and do not rearrange furnishings. Clarify this fact with housekeeping personnel also.
- Assist with ambulation by walking slightly ahead of the person, allowing the person to grasp your arm.
- Stay in the person's field of vision if he or she has partial or reduced peripheral vision.
- Provide diversions using other senses.
- Indicate to the person when the conversation has ended and when you are leaving the room.

Meeting the Needs of Patients With Reduced Hearing

Temporary hearing losses are most often conductive in nature, that is, they are due to a problem with the external or middle ear (wax buildup, foreign-body obstruction, infection). However, sensorineural hearing losses caused by inner ear or central nervous system problems may not be totally correctable. Health teaching to prevent hearing problems includes the following recommendations for patients:

- Avoid excessive noise.
- Avoid inserting sharp objects into ears.
- Avoid excessive cleaning of ears.
- Avoid practices that can cause infection; treat infection early.
- Know the symptoms of hearing loss: asking frequently that statements be repeated, inability to hear at a distance, need to see the person who is talking, leaning forward or turning an ear toward the speaker, answering inappropriately, talking too loudly, inability to carry on a phone conversation, strained facial expression.

When communicating with patients who have hearing deficits or impairments, follow these guidelines:

- Orient the person to your presence before initiating conversation. This may be done by moving so you can be seen or by gently touching the person.
- Decrease background noises (television, radio) if possible before you speak.
- Make sure that hearing aids (if applicable) are working optimally.
- Position yourself so that the light is on your face and the person can see your lips and expressions.
- Talk directly to the person while facing him or her or angle the chair so that your voice reaches the ear that hears best. If the person is able to lip-read, use simple sentences and speak in a quiet, natural manner and pace. Be aware of nonverbal communication.
- Do not chew gum, cover your mouth, or turn away when talking with the person.
- Demonstrate or pantomime ideas you wish to express, as appropriate.

- Use sign language or finger spelling, as appropriate.
- Write any ideas that you cannot convey to the person in another manner.

Aids for individuals with reduced hearing include TDD (telecommunication devices), infrared systems, computers, voice amplifiers, amplified telephones, low-frequency door-bells and telephone ringers, closed-caption TV decoders, flashing alarm clocks, and flashing smoke detectors.

> *Consider Dolores Pirolla, the wife of the patient who has a visual deficit and is now demonstrating signs of a hearing deficit. The nurse would incorporate knowledge of the guidelines (for communicating both with persons with reduced vision and hearing) when developing a teaching plan to assist Mrs. Pirolla in dealing with her husband's condition. In addition, the nurse could enlist the aid of social services to help Mrs. Pirolla in obtaining supportive services for her husband's visual impairment and for obtaining assistive devices for her husband to minimize the effects of the hearing deficit.* ■

Communicating With a Patient Who is Confused

The patient who lacks the mental ability to process environmental stimuli may be aware of this inability and find it frustrating. This patient needs support to make adjustments to this limitation.

> *Most likely, Ori Soltes, the patient in the ICU who becomes confused, is experiencing a high level of frustration. Due to his accident, the patient suddenly is thrust into an environment filled with unfamiliar sights, sounds, and activities, leading to feelings of being overwhelmed physically and emotionally. His level of frustration may be further increased by his inability to speak, secondary to receiving mechanical ventilation.* ■

Other patients may be oblivious of the deficiency. In both instances, always protect the safety of the patient while providing optimal sensory stimulation. Nursing interventions include the following:

- Use frequent face-to-face contact to communicate the social process (use touch when appropriate, walk arm in arm, hug, give a backrub).
- Speak calmly, simply, and directly to the patient and allow sufficient time for the patient to think before responding.
- Orient and reorient the patient to the environment and fill the patient's personal space with as many personal objects as possible.
- Use conversation, watches, clocks, calendar, newspaper, television, radio, and other such devices to orient the patient to time, place, and person.

- Clearly communicate that the patient is expected to perform all self-care activities of which the patient is capable.
- Keep the emphasis on patient strengths rather than on deficiencies and verbally reinforce strengths.
- Offer the patient simple explanations for care, new activities, and so on.
- Vary environmental stimuli gradually while keeping the environment structured enough that the patient feels comfortable and at home.
- Use objects from the patient's past (baseball, picture of a train, photograph) to spark reminiscences and discussions.
- Reinforce reality if the patient is delusional.

A list of selected cognitive stimulation activities may be found in Chapter 21.

Communicating With a Patient Who is Unconscious

The following are recommended guidelines for communicating with a patient who is unconscious:

- Be careful of what is said in the person's presence. Hearing is believed to be the last sense lost; therefore, the person is often likely to hear what is being said, even though there does not appear to be a response.
- Assume the person can hear you. Talk with the person in a normal tone of voice about things you would ordinarily discuss.
- Speak to the person before touching. Remember that touch can be an effective means of communicating with the unconscious person.
- Keep environmental noises at as low a level as possible. This helps the person focus on the communication.

Evaluating

While implementing a plan of nursing care designed to decrease excessive sensory stimuli or increase meaningful stimuli, evaluate the plan's effectiveness by observing for a decrease in the behavioral manifestations of sensory deprivation or overload. It may be concluded that the plan of care is working if a patient who had begun to withdraw and spend most of the day lying in bed with a blank facial expression appears more alert and begins to initiate conversations and to take an interest in personal care. Also evaluate the patient's ability to interact appropriately with the environment while practicing necessary self-care behaviors as well as the patient's need for nursing care versus his or her ability to manage the plan of care independently.

Ideally, the patient and family learn to manipulate the environment to promote optimal sensory stimulation for growth and development. Patients with specific sensory impairments are evaluated for their knowledge of the impairment, acceptance and management of the treatment regimen, and their ability to perform necessary self-care activities. See the accompanying concept map for Ori Soltes and the Nursing Plan of Care 44-1 for Mrs. Philomela Palikias.

Ori Soltes, a 28-year-old man, is in the Intensive Care Unit (ICU) after a motor vehicle crash that resulted in multiple internal injuries as well as fractures. He is being monitored continuously and receiving mechanical ventilation via endotracheal tube. On the fifth day after the crash, he begins to exhibit transient episodes of acute confusion. Bilateral wrist restraints are being utilized to prevent self-extubation. In order to maintain adequate ventilation and control anxiety, intravenous sedation is prescribed as needed. His vital signs are as follows: BP 132/68 mm Hg, pulse 116 beats/minute, respirations 30 breaths/minute.

Priority 1

Nursing Diagnosis: Disturbed Sensory Perception: Sensory Overload related to excessive environmental stimuli.
Supporting Data:
- ICU environment
- Frequent examinations
- Multiple monitoring devices with alarms
- Lighted environment
- Wrist restraints
- Endotracheal intubation and mechanical ventilation
- Intravenous sedation
- BP 132/68 mm Hg, pulse 116 beats/min, respiratory rate 30 breaths/min

Priority 2

Nursing Diagnosis: Acute Confusion related to alteration in sleep–wake cycle.
Supporting Data:
- Transient episodes of confusion
- Frequent examinations
- Excessive environmental stimuli
- Restraints required to prevent self-extubation
- Critically ill with multiple monitoring modalities

Priority 3

Nursing Diagnosis: Impaired Verbal Communication related to endotracheal intubation and mechanical ventilation.
Supporting Data:
- Unable to verbalize needs due to endotracheal intubation
- Wrist restraints
- Multiple contacts with health team members

Outcome:
Patient will experience a reduction in environmental stimuli and normalization of vital signs.

Outcome:
Patient will become oriented to person, place, and time.

Outcome:
Patient will achieve alternate methods of communication.

Nursing Interventions:
- Cluster nursing interventions as tolerated to provide uninterrupted rest periods
- Eliminate nuisance alarms by maintaining appropriate alarm limits
- Dim lights when feasible
- Administer sedation as needed
- Release restraints every hour for 10 minutes while at bedside
- Communicate in soft, calm tones
- Explain all procedures prior to initiating them
- Monitor vital signs for physiologic signs of excessive stimuli
- Consider use of music therapy

Nursing Interventions:
- Reorient to person, place, and time
- Talk to patient prior to initiating touch
- Explain all procedures prior to performing them
- Encourage family to visit, talk, and provide Therapeutic Touch to the patient
- Ask family to bring in familiar objects and pictures
- Provide uninterrupted periods of sleep by clustering care activities
- Use clear, concise, and simple communication

Nursing Interventions:
- Talk directly to patient rather than talking over patient
- Establish an alternative means of communication such as picture board
- Communicate through nonverbal means, such as Therapeutic Touch
- Explain all procedures before starting
- Ascertain patient's areas of interest and talk to patient regarding these topics
- Place call bell within reach at all times

Evaluation: Ori's environment has been managed to reduce stimuli. Sedation has only been required every 4 hours. Vital signs have returned to normal.

Evaluation: Ori continues to exhibit transient periods of confusion, but with decreasing frequency. Continue interventions.

Evaluation: Ori has been unable to use picture board due to his weakened condition. Continue interventions.

- - - - - **Relationship**   **Assessment**   **Nursing Diagnosis**   **Outcome Identification**   **Interventions**   **Evaluation**

Concept map displaying the nursing process for Ori Soltes.

NURSING PLAN OF CARE · 44-1

For Philomela Palikias

Two days ago, Mrs. Philomela Palikias delivered by cesarean birth a 32-week-old, small-for-gestational-age infant girl weighing 3 lb, 8 oz. Because of her size and respiratory distress, the infant was placed in the neonatal intensive care unit (NICU). Postpartal assessments indicate that Mrs. Palikias's physical progress is satisfactory. However, the nurses are concerned about her mental status. Mrs. Palikias arrived in the United States 3 months ago with her husband. Both speak only Greek and neither has family in the United States.

Recorded in the patient's progress notes the evening of her Second postpartal day is the following nursing assessment:

12/4/12, 9 PM, nursing
Patient refused to get out of bed again this evening—demonstrates no interest in seeing baby; to date has not ambulated to NICU. Refusing to learn and participate in self-care activities—expressing breast milk or performing perineal care. Nurses throughout the day reported sudden mood changes—apathy, frustration, panic, and hostility. Unable to find someone who speaks Greek to serve as translator. Husband does not speak English but appears concerned about his wife.

—N. Gable, RN

NURSING DIAGNOSIS   Disturbed Sensory Perception: Mixed Sensory Deprivation and Overload related to unfamiliar hospital environment (different culture) and stress of cesarean birth and infant's prematurity as manifested by patient not demonstrating interest in baby or self-care activities; limited ability to concentrate on new tasks (pericare, expressing breast milk); sudden mood changes—apathy, frustration, panic, hostility

EXPECTED OUTCOME   Before discharge, the patient will:

• Demonstrate increased comfort in the hospital environment (decreased or absent mood swings—apathy, frustration, panic, hostility)

Nursing Interventions	Rationale	Evaluative Statement
Secure assistance of an interpreter and work with the interpreter to do the following:		12/6/12 Outcome met. Patient is quiet but no longer apathetic, fearful, or hostile. Moving about in hospital with more confidence.
• Orient the patient to her surroundings (explaining reasons for equipment, procedures, treatment).	Sensory deprivation results from *meaningless*, unpatterned stimuli; once the patient understands her environment, she can respond to it appropriately.	*N. Gable, RN*
• Reassure the patient that what she is experiencing is normal given her recent stresses (moving to new country, cesarean birth of first child, infant's prematurity).	Patients experiencing strange perceptual, cognitive, and affective responses to sensory deprivation and overload often fear they are going crazy and hesitate to share their feelings.	
• Determine the patient's needs.	The patient herself is best able to voice her needs.	
Have the interpreter teach the nurse several Greek words and make recommendations about how the patient can personalize her environment, such as having her husband provide her with usual food, music, and other familiar items.	Contributing to sensory deprivation is the absence of familiar sounds (native languages, sights, tastes, or scents). Having access to familiar food and the like may reduce sensory deprivation.	

(continued)

NURSING PLAN OF CARE • 44-1

For Philomela Palikias (continued)

Nursing Interventions	Rationale	Evaluative Statement
See if the interpreter can explain usual customs regarding childbirth and aftercare in Greece.	Including culturally familiar childbirth and aftercare customs in the plan of care enhances patient well-being and cooperation in the plan of care.	
Limit the number of nurses and other persons interacting with the patient; attempt to have the same nurse caring for her each shift.	A trusting nurse–patient relationship can develop.	
Schedule care to allow for uninterrupted periods of sleep and rest.	Sleep deprivation contributes to other sensory alterations.	

EXPECTED OUTCOME   Before discharge, the patient will:

- Resume independent self-care activities

Nursing Interventions	Rationale	Evaluative Statement
Use services of interpreter to teach patient importance of ambulating and becoming independent again in self-care measures.	Regaining independence enhances patient's sense of well-being.	12/6/12 Outcome partially met. Patient is ambulating, but she resists pericare and is fearful when expressing breast milk. *Recommendation:* Continue teaching with assistance of interpreter.
Have interpreter write simple directions for follow-up care, times when baby may be visited after patient is discharged, and so on. Share these instructions with the patient's husband.	Cognitive responses to sensory deprivation and overload include decreased attention span and concentration and problem-solving ability. Written instructions and husband's knowledge reinforce the patient's learning.	*N. Gable, RN*
See if husband has bilingual friends or work acquaintances who might be willing to help the patient when she gets home until she has established a comfortable routine of care for the baby and is knowledgeable about community resources.	Careful discharge planning is necessary to ensure that the patient can manage new parenting responsibilities in an unfamiliar country.	

EXPECTED OUTCOME   Before discharge, the patient will:

- Demonstrate interest in her baby by visiting the NICU, holding the baby, expressing her milk, and other such activities.

(continued)

NURSING PLAN OF CARE · 44-1

For Philomela Palikias (continued)

Nursing Interventions	Rationale	Evaluative Statement
Learn and respect cultural norms for new mothering behaviors.	Nursing care that is not culturally sensitive is deficient.	12/6/12 Outcome met. Patient is now visiting baby in the unit on her own.
Assist the patient to ambulate to unit to see the baby; if interpreter is available, have the person explain equipment surrounding the baby and answer the patient's questions about the baby.	The patient may be refusing to visit the unit to protect herself from barrage of frightening stimuli (sensory overload); the goal is for her to become familiar with the unit so she is able to focus on bonding with her daughter.	*N. Gable, RN*

SAMPLE
DOCUMENTATION

Traditional Note Format

12/5/12, 10 AM, nursing

First session with interpreter and patient at 9 AM. Patient's face brightened as soon as she heard someone speak to her in Greek. Basically, patient shared she did not care too much about what was happening to her but she was terrified about the baby and afraid of what everyone was doing to the baby. Directed interpreter to orient patient to her environment, daily routine, and NICU. Patient appeared anxious when she first saw baby but looked content when able to hold her. Schedule teaching session for tomorrow AM when interpreter will come for 1 hour. Patient currently resting comfortably.

N. Gable, RN

SOAP Format

12/5/12, 9 PM, nursing

Sensory/Perceptual Alterations: Mixed Sensory Deprivation and Overload related to unfamiliar hospital environment stress of cesarean birth and infant's prematurity

S: —

O: Cried after husband left this evening; refused postpartal check; turned away from nurses

A: Still feels overwhelmed by newness of all that is happening to her and tries to shut out what she cannot handle

P: Continue to intervene with help of interpreter; focus on helping patient develop more control over her situation; proceed at slow pace; referral to social services for follow-up care.

N. Gable, RN

● Developing Critical Thinking Skills

1. Describe the practical measures you would take to stimulate the senses of the following sensory-impaired patients. Think carefully about the special sensory needs that accompany different conditions.
   - A deaf child
   - A confused older adult
   - An adult man who has just lost his sight
   - A premature infant whose skin is extremely fragile

2. Visit a critical care unit with other students and list all the factors that contribute to sensory overload or deprivation. Try to identify how the critical care culture evolved in ways that are actually harmful to patients. Discuss which of these factors are unavoidable and which could be modified to better meet patient needs.

Identify individualized nursing strategies to minimize sensory overload and deprivation.

Practicing for NCLEX

1. When assessing a patient's sensory experience, which of the following would the nurse identify as the major components?
   a. The kinesthetic and visceral senses
   b. Reception and perception
   c. The intensity, size, change, or representation of stimuli
   d. Vision, hearing, smell, taste, and touch

2. When evaluating a patient's sensory experience, which four conditions would be essential for a person to receive data and experience the world?
   a. A stimulus, a receptor, an intact nerve pathway, and a functioning brain
   b. The visual, auditory, olfactory–gustatory, and tactile senses
   c. The basic orienting systems arising from muscles, joints, hollow organs, and movement
   d. The reticular activating system, variable stimuli, memory, and motivation

3. When planning the care for a patient related to disturbed sensory perception, the nurse would integrate knowledge of which system as responsible for monitoring and regulating incoming sensory stimuli to maintain, enhance, or inhibit cortical arousal?
   a. General adaptation system
   b. Kinesthetic/visceral system
   c. Reticular activating system
   d. Sensory/perceptual system

4. You notice that Mr. Wong, who has cataracts, is sitting closer to the television than usual. The nurse would interpret the etiologic basis of his sensory problem is an alteration in which of the following?
   a. Environmental stimuli
   b. Sensory reception
   c. Nerve impulse conduction
   d. Impulse translation

5. Which of the following would be most important to include in the plan of care for a patient who is 85 years old and has presbycusis?
   a. Obtaining large-print written material
   b. Speaking distinctly using lower frequencies
   c. Decreasing tactile stimulation
   d. Initiating a safety program to prevent falls

6. Peter Almone is in the late stages of AIDS, which is now affecting his brain as well other major organ systems. He confides to you that he feels terribly alone because most of his friends are afraid to visit. The nurse determines that which of the following would be the least likely underlying etiology for his sensory problems?
   a. Stimulation
   b. Reception

   c. Transmission–perception–reaction
   d. Emotional responses

7. Which factor is least likely to place a patient at high risk for sensory deprivation?
   a. An environment with decreased or monotonous stimuli
   b. Impaired ability to receive environmental stimuli
   c. Impaired ability to process environmental stimuli
   d. Impaired ability to respond to environmental stimuli

8. Which patient would the nurse assess as being at greatest risk for sensory deprivation?
   a. An elderly man confined to bed at home after a stroke
   b. An adolescent in an oncology unit working on homework supplied by friends
   c. A woman in labor
   d. A toddler in a playroom awaiting same-day surgery

9. A patient in an intensive care burn unit for 1 week is in pain much of the time and has his face and both arms heavily bandaged. His wife visits every evening for 15 minutes at 6, 7, and 8 PM. A heart monitor beeps for a patient on one side, and another patient moans frequently. Assessment would suggest that that the patient probably is experiencing which of the following?
   a. Sufficient sensory stimulation
   b. Deficient sensory stimulation
   c. Excessive sensory stimulation
   d. Both sensory deprivation and overload

10. Richard's spinal cord was severed, and he is paralyzed from the waist down. When obtaining data about this patient, which component of the sensory experience would be most important to assess?
    a. Transmission of tactile stimuli
    b. Adequate stimulation in the environment
    c. Reception of visual and auditory stimuli
    d. General orientation and ability to follow commands

11. An 11-year-old 6th grader whose grades have dropped has difficulty completing her work on time, frequently rubs her eyes, and squints. Her visual acuity on a Snellen's eye chart was 160/20. Which nursing diagnosis would be most appropriate?
    a. Deficient Knowledge related to visual impairment
    b. Ineffective Role Performance (Student) related to visual impairment
    c. Disturbed Body Image related to visual impairment
    d. Delayed Growth and Development related to visual impairment

12. Of the four items listed below, which nursing intervention would be best to prevent sensory alterations for a man with a severe hearing deficit who reads lips well?
    a. Turn the radio or television volume up very loud and close the door to his room.
    b. Prevent embarrassment and emotional discomfort as much as possible.

c. Provide daily opportunity for him to participate in a social hour with six or eight people.

d. Encourage daily participation in exercise and physical activity.

13. In a boarding home where most patients have slight to moderate visual or hearing impairment and some are periodically confused, which of the following would be the nurse's first priority in caring for sensory concerns?
a. Maintaining safety and preventing sensory deterioration
b. Insisting that every patient participate in as many self-care activities as possible
c. Emphasizing and reinforcing individual patient strengths
d. Encouraging reminiscence and life review in groups

14. The nursing diagnosis for 8-month-old Sally was Disturbed Sensory Perception: Sensory Deprivation related to inadequate parenting. Since that time, both parents have attended parenting classes. However, both parents work while Sally stays with her 86-year-old grandmother, who has reduced vision. The parents provide appropriate stimulation in the evening. At an evaluation conference at age 11 months, Sally lays on the floor sucking her thumb and rocking her body. Her facial expression is dull, and she vocalizes only in a low monotone ("uh-h-h"). Which statement accurately reflects evaluation about the child's sensory deprivation?
a. Her parents lack motivation to provide necessary stimulation.
b. Her grandmother is unable to improve Sally's care.
c. Sally's sensory deprivation is still severe.
d. This is normal behavior for a child of Sally's age.

15. Which nursing interventions would be least appropriate for an elderly woman in a nursing home with a nursing diagnosis of Disturbed Sensory Perception: Chronic Sensory Deprivation related to the effects of aging? She had walked out the door unobserved and was hit by a car.
a. Ignore when the patient is confused or go along to prevent embarrassment.
b. Encourage self-care and independent decisions.
c. Take walks around the grounds and to the garden daily.
d. Provide daily contact with children, community people, and pets.

● Answers With Rationale

1. *b.* Reception and perception are the major components of any sensory experience. All other choices are merely part of the sensory experience.

2. *a.* A stimulus, a receptor, an intact nerve pathway, and a functioning brain are the four conditions necessary for a person to receive data and experience the world.

3. *c.* The reticular activating system maintains, enhances, or inhibits cortical arousal by monitoring and regulating incoming sensory stimuli. The general adaptation system (*a*) is the system responsible for responding to stress. Kinesthetic and visceral (*b*) are senses that arise internally from muscles and hollow organs and are the body's basic orienting systems. Sensory and perceptual systems (*d*) are the two components of the sensory experience.

4. *b.* Cataracts are interfering with the patient's ability to receive visual stimuli—altered sensory reception. The nature of incoming stimuli (*a*), the conduction of nerve impulses (*c*), and the translation of incoming impulses (*d*) in the brain are not a problem here.

5. *b.* Presbycusis is a normal loss of hearing as a result of the aging process. Speaking distinctly in lower frequencies is indicated. The other choices refer to interventions for other sensory problems.

6. *d.* Emotional responses are an effect of sensory deprivation and although may be occurring with this patient, they are not the underlying etiology for his condition. This patient is receiving decreased environmental stimuli (*a*) (e.g., from his friends), is more than likely experiencing problems with reception because of major organ involvement (*b*), and his impaired brain function will impair impulse transmission–perception–reaction (*c*).

7. *d.* An impaired ability to respond to environmental stimuli places a patient at risk for problems other than sensory deprivation. The other options all pertain to components of the sensory experience that, if impaired, may place a patient at high risk for sensory deprivation.

8. *a.* The patient confined to bed rest at home is at risk for greatly reduced environmental stimuli. All of the other patients are in environments where environmental stimuli are at least adequate.

9. *d.* This patient's bandages may result in deficient sensory stimulation (sensory deprivation), and the monitors and other sounds in the intensive care burn unit may cause a sensory overload. All other options are incomplete responses.

10. *a.* Below-the-waist paralysis makes the transmission of tactile stimuli a problem. Although the other options may be assessed, they are indirectly related to his paralysis and of lesser importance at this time.

11. *b.* An important role for an 11-year-old is that of student. Her impaired vision is clearly disturbing her role performance as a student, as evidenced by her lower grades. Although the other options may also represent accurate diagnoses for this patient, they do not flow from the data that were presented.

12. *c.* Although all the options listed are appropriate, providing daily opportunities for this patient to participate in a social hour builds on his strength of being able to

lip-read and provides sufficient sensory stimulation to prevent sensory deprivation resulting from his hearing loss, thereby meeting his needs.

13. *a.* Safety is a basic physiologic need that must be met before higher-level needs, such as love and belonging, self-esteem, and self-actualization, can be met.

14. *c.* Although the data show that the parents have been motivated to improve their parenting skills, it is clear from the data presented that Sally's sensory deprivation is still severe. The data suggest that the grandmother is not improving Sally's care, but there is nothing to suggest that she is unable to do so (*b*) if shown how.

15. *a.* Even if well motivated, ignoring a patient's confusion to prevent embarrassment may be dangerous, as it was in this case in which the appropriate safety precautions were never implemented. The other options are all appropriate for this patient.

Taylor Suite Resources

The Taylor Suite offers these additional resources to enhance learning and facilitate understanding of this chapter:

- thePoint online resource, http://thepoint.lww.com/Taylor7E
- Student DVD-ROM included with the book
- Study Guide for Taylor's Fundamentals of Nursing

BIBLIOGRAPHY

Alfaro-Lefevre, R. (2006). *Applying nursing process: A tool for critical thinking* (6th ed.). Philadelphia: Lippincott Williams & Wilkins.

Aspin, A. (2004). The concept of snoezelen: Sensory stimulation and relaxation for neonates. *Journal of Neonatal Nursing, 10*(2), 47–51.

Baker, C. (2004). Preventing ICU syndrome in children. *Paediatric Nursing, 16*(10), 32–35.

Baker, R., Holloway, J., Holtkamp, C. C. M., Larsson, A., Hartman, L. C., Pearce, R., et al. (2003). Effects of multi-sensory stimulation for people with dementia. *Journal of Advanced Nursing, 43*(5), 465–477.

Bulechek, G. M., Butcher, H. K., & Dochterman, J. (Eds.). (2008). *Nursing interventions classification (NIC)* (5th ed.). St. Louis: Mosby

Cox, H., Burns, I., & Savage, S. (2004). Multisensory environments for leisure: Promoting well-being in nursing home residents with dementia. *Journal of Gerontological Nursing, 30*(2), 37–45.

Crowley, A. A., Bains, R. M., & Pellico, L. H. (2005). In our community. A model preschool vision and hearing screening program: students and faculty serve a community. *American Journal of Nursing, 105*(6), 52–55.

Cutilli, C. C. (2008). Teaching the geriatric patient: Making the most of "cognitive resources" and "gains." Orthopaedic *Nursing, 27*(3), 195–200.

Gerber, C. S. (2005). Understanding and managing coma stimulation: Are we doing everything we can? *Critical Care Nursing Quarterly, 28*(2), 94–110.

Hope, K. W., Easby, R., & Waterman, H. (2004). Finding the person the disease has: The case for multisensory environments. *Journal of Psychiatric and Mental Health Nursing, 11*(5), 554–561.

The Joint Commission. (2007). "What did the doctor say?:" Improving health literacy to protect patient safety. Available at http://www.jointcommission.org/NR/rdonlyres/F53D5057-5349-4391-9DB9-E7F086873D46/0/health_literacy_exec_summary.pdf.

Kloosterman, N. D. (1991). Cultural care: The missing link in severe sensory alteration. *Nursing Science Quarterly, 4*(3), 119–122.

McNicoll, L., Pisani, M. A., Ely, E. W., Gifford, D., & Inouye, S. K. (2005). Detection of delirium in the intensive care unit: Comparison of confusion assessment method for the intensive care unit with confusion assessment method ratings. *Journal of the American Geriatrics Society, 53*(3), 495–500.

Moorhead, S., Johnson, M., Maas, M. L., & Swanson, E. (2008). *Nursing outcomes classification (NOC)* (4th ed.). St. Louis: Mosby Elsevier,

NANDA International. (2009). *Nursing diagnoses: Definitions & classification, 2009–2011.* Oxford, UK: Wiley-Blackwell.

Thoyre, S. M., & Brown, R. L. (2004). Factors contributing to preterm infant engagement during bottle-feeding. *Nursing Research, 53*(5), 304–314.

Tullmann, D. F., Mion, L. C., Fletcher, K., & Foreman, M. D. (2008). Delirium: Prevention, early recognition, and treatment. In E. Capezuti, D. Zwicker, M. Mezey, T. Fulmer, (Eds.). Evidence-based geriatric nursing protocols for best practice (3rd ed.). New York: Springer Publishing Company.

Stouffer, J. W., Shirk, B. J., & Polomano, R. C. (2007). Practice guidelines for music interventions with hospitalized pediatric patients. *Journal of Pediatric Nursing, 22*(6), 448–456.

Valentjin, S. A., van Boxtel, M. P., van Hooren, S. A., Bosma, H., Beckers, H. J., Ponds, R. W., et al. (2005). Change in sensory functioning predicts change in cognitive functioning: Results from a 6-year follow-up in the Maastricht Aging Study. *Journal of the American Geriatrics Society, 53*(3), 374–380.

Wahl, H., & Heyl, V. (2003). Connections between vision, hearing, and cognitive function in old age. *Generations, 27*(6), 39–44.

White-Traut, R. (2004). Providing a nurturing environment for infants in adverse situations: Multisensory strategies for newborn care. *Journal of Midwifery & Women's Health, 49*(4), Suppl. 36–44.

White-Traut, R. C., Nelson, M. N., Silverstri, J. M., Patel, M., Berbaum, M., Gu, G., & Rey, P. M. (2004). Developmental patterns of physiological response to a multisensory intervention in extremely premature and high-risk infants. *JOGNN: Journal of Obstetric, Gynecologic, and Neonatal Nursing, 33*(2), 266–275.

45 Sexuality

LEARNING OBJECTIVES

After completing the chapter, you will be able to accomplish the following:

1. Describe male and female reproductive anatomy and physiology.

2. Describe the sexual response cycle, differentiating male and female responses.

3. Contrast different types of sexual expression.

4. Identify factors that affect an individual's sexuality.

5. Perform a sexual assessment, using suggested interview questions and appropriate physical assessment skills.

6. Describe types of sexual dysfunctions and the assessment priorities for each.

7. Develop nursing diagnoses identifying a problem with sexuality that may be remedied by independent nursing actions.

8. Plan, implement, and evaluate nursing care related to selected nursing diagnoses involving problems of sexuality.

9. Assess how your personal beliefs and values about human sexuality affect your ability to deliver competent, compassionate, and respectful care to patients with sexual problems.

10. Describe effective responses to sexual harassment by patients or colleagues.

KEY TERMS

abstinence	menopause
biologic sex	menstruation
bisexual	orgasm
contraception	premenstrual (tension)
erogenous zones	syndrome
gay	sexual dysfunction
gender identity	sexual harassment
gender role behavior	sexual health
heterosexual	sexual orientation
homosexual	sexuality
impotence	sexually transmitted
intercourse	infections (STIs)
lesbian	transsexual
masturbation	transvestite
menarche	

A critical component of human identity and well-being, **sexuality** is the degree to which a person exhibits and experiences maleness or femaleness physically, emotionally, and mentally. Sexuality is defined not only by a person's genitalia and hormones but also by their attitudes and feelings. It can also be defined as learned behaviors in how a person reacts to his or her own sexuality and by how one behaves in relationships with others. Culture profoundly influences learned behaviors about sexuality. Sexuality is an integral part of a person's identity and is present in one's demeanor through actions, communications, and physical appearance. (See the Reflective Practice box for an example.)

SEXUAL HEALTH

Sexual health may be defined as the integration of the somatic, emotional, intellectual, and social aspects of sexual being, in ways that are positively enriching and that enhance personality, communication, and love. Because our sexuality is so basic to our sense of self, nurses need to value sexuality as a critical element of health and well-being in general and must be skilled in identifying and meeting problems related to sexual self-concept, body image, and sexual identity.

> *Think back to Amy Liu, the woman who reported changes in sexual desire and pain on intercourse. As a result of these changes, she reported not feeling like a woman anymore. The nurse would interpret her statements as reflecting a change in her self-concept and body image secondary to the sexual health issues.* ■

Sexual identity encompasses a person's self-identity, biologic sex, gender identity, gender role behavior or orientation, and sexual orientation or preference. **Biologic sex** is the term used to denote chromosomal sexual development: male (XY) or female (XX), external and internal genitalia, secondary sex characteristics, and hormonal states. **Gender identity** is the inner sense a person has of being male or female, which may be the same as or different from his or her biologic gender. **Gender role behavior** is the behavior a person conveys about being male or female, which, again, may or may not be the same as biologic gender or gender identity (Pillitteri, 2007).

> *Consider Paul Rojas, the homosexual patient with AIDS. The nurse would need to assess his gender identity and gender role behaviors to gain a fuller understanding of his sexual identity and to provide appropriate care.* ■

People experience sexual gratification in many ways, and what is considered normal differs from one individual to another and among cultures. **Sexual orientation** refers to the preferred gender of the partner of an individual. The origins of sexual orientation are unknown, but there are studies claiming a genetic basis. Certainly, some sexual preferences are culturally determined and may be dictated by opportunity.

REFLECTIVE PRACTICE

Challenge to Interpersonal Skills

During my clinical experience in the HIV/infectious disease clinic, I met Paul Rojas, a single young adult homosexual who was diagnosed with AIDS. One day he came to the clinic for infusion therapy, which usually takes several hours.

I was a 20-year-old, single white female with no personal experience with gay or lesbian friends or with individuals who are bisexual, transsexual, or transvestites. I was confused and uncertain about how to respond to him. How should I approach him? What would we talk about during these several hours at the clinic? I was sure my instructor thought this would be a "great learning experience," but what was I supposed to learn? Usually quite self-confident, I was confused, uncomfortable, and uncertain as to how to act.

Thinking Outside the Box: Possible Courses of Action

- Hide my discomfort and simply provide the technical nursing care Paul needs; spend as little time as possible in his room.
- Refuse this assignment because I am unsure I can provide the care Paul needs.
- Talk with my instructor or another experienced nurse whom I respect about my questions and concerns.

- Share with Paul that this is my first experience working with a homosexual patient and ask him what I should know; spend extra time getting to know him and his experiences with other healthcare professionals.

Evaluating a Good Outcome: How Do I Define Success?

- Provide the nursing care he needs in a manner that is respectful.
- Learn from this experience how to be respectful of all patients and to interact in a way that affirms their human dignity.

- Gain knowledge about gender identity and expression through this experience.

Personal Learning: Here's to the Future!

I didn't know how to raise my questions, so I met Paul totally at a loss and did exactly what I didn't want to do: I completed the technical nursing care such as vital signs and intravenous care and then got out of the room as quickly as possible. It wasn't until almost the end of his treatment that he asked me, "You don't feel comfortable with me, do you?" When I answered truthfully that I didn't, all of a sudden wonderful sharing began. When I look back now and think that I almost allowed my fear to prevent me from getting to know Paul and his world, I could kick myself. I hope I always remember to let patients teach me about themselves and their world.

Reflection

How do you think you would respond in a similar situation? Why? What does this tell you about yourself and about the adequacy of your skills for professional practice? Can you think of other ways to respond? Propose possible factors that may have influenced the nursing student's response to the patient. What other skills (cognitive, interpersonal, technical, ethical/legal) would you need to respond well in this situation? With what issues was the nursing student dealing? The patient? Explain how the nursing student's truthful response to the patient's question affected the therapeutic relationship. Do you agree with the criteria to evaluate a successful outcome? Did the nursing student meet the criteria? Please explain your answer.

Common sexual orientations are as follows:

- A **heterosexual** is one who experiences sexual fulfillment with a person of the opposite gender.
- A **homosexual** is one who experiences sexual fulfillment with a person of the same gender. Homosexual males often use the term **gay;** homosexual females use the term **lesbian.** Heterosexuality and homosexuality can be placed at opposite ends of a continuum, with many variations in between.
- A **bisexual** is a person who finds pleasure with both opposite-sex and same-sex partners. Homosexual or heterosexual people may have bisexual relationships at times.
- A **transsexual** is a person of a certain biologic gender who has the feelings of the opposite sex. The person feels trapped within the body of the wrong sex. The reason behind this is unknown, although many factors are believed to be involved. For many transsexuals, the solution is to change their bodies, through surgery and hormone therapy, to match their inner feelings.
- A **transvestite** is an individual who desires to take on the role or wear the clothes of the opposite sex. Most transvestites are heterosexual, and many keep their lifestyle hidden.

PHYSIOLOGY
Female

The female genitalia are represented by external structures, the appearance of which varies slightly among individuals (see Fig. 25-34 in Chapter 25); and internal genitalia, which are located deep within the pelvis of the female.

External Genitalia

MONS PUBIS

The mons pubis is a pad of fatty tissue that lies over the part of the bony pelvis called the symphysis pubis. In the physically mature female, the mons pubis is covered with coarse pubic hair. It contains many nerve endings that make the mons pubis sensitive to touch and pressure.

LABIA MAJORA AND LABIA MINORA

The labia majora consist of two rounded folds of fatty tissue. The outer lips separate downward from the mons pubis and meet again below the vaginal introitus. The labia majora contain a multitude of sebaceous and sweat glands. They respond to touch during sexual activity. The labia minora are the smaller lips located within the labia majora. They are thin and sensitive structures and are pink. When stimulated by touch, the labia minora may turn a darker pink or even red owing to the presence of many blood vessels. The labia minora have no hair and are smooth.

CLITORIS

The clitoris is found above the urinary meatus at the joining of the labia minora, called the clitoral hood. The clitoris is a small, button-like structure similar to the penis in its reaction to stimuli. The clitoris contains erectile tissue, blood vessels, and nerves. It is extremely sensitive.

HYMEN

The opening of the vagina lies between the urinary meatus and the anus. It may contain a structure called the hymen, which is a thick membrane with no apparent function. At one time, the hymen was thought to represent virginity (not having experienced sexual intercourse), but this is erroneous. Remnants, or "tags," of the hymen may be noted at the vaginal introitus in both sexually active and inactive women.

Internal Genitalia

OVARIES

The female body normally contains two ovaries, one on each side. The ovaries closely resemble an almond in size and shape. When a girl is born, each of her ovaries contains some 200,000 to 400,000 follicles. This number steadily decreases until puberty, when 100,000 to 200,000 follicles remain, and the number continues to decline over the reproductive years. The process of ovulation, which begins in the ovaries, is discussed later in the section on menstruation. The ovaries also secrete the hormones estrogen and progesterone.

FALLOPIAN TUBES

The fallopian tubes are slender structures that extend from either side of the uterus and end in a fringed fashion near each ovary. Their function is to transport a mature ovum (female reproductive cell) from an ovary to the uterus. Fertilization of

the ovum by a sperm usually occurs in the tube. The fertilized ovum then travels the rest of the way to the uterus, where it implants. An unfertilized ovum travels the same path but does not implant and is eventually expelled from the body during menses. Because the lumen of each tube is so narrow, it can easily be damaged by the effects of infection and surgery.

UTERUS

The uterus is a pear-shaped organ about 3 inches long located between the urinary bladder and the rectum. Its primary purpose is to house and nurture a pregnancy (the condition of carrying a developing embryo in the uterus). The uterus comprises three layers:

1. The outermost layer, the perimetrium, consists of elastic tissue.
2. The middle layer, the myometrium, is muscular.
3. The innermost layer, the endometrium, comprises tissue that thickens and sloughs off with menses.

The cervix is the structure at the lower portion of the uterus that connects the uterus and the vagina. The cervix is usually closed, but during the birth process, it dilates and thins out extensively to permit the birth of a baby. The cervix is a smooth pink structure that possesses few nerve endings. When touched, the sensation resembles that of touching the end of one's nose.

VAGINA

The vagina is a tubular, hollow organ that lies between the urethra and the rectum. Its size and shape vary among women. The walls of the vagina are composed of rugae, or ribbed tissue. The vagina serves three purposes: it is (1) a receptacle for the penis during sexual intercourse, (2) a birth canal for the passage of a baby, and (3) an exit for menstrual flow from the uterus. During sexual activity, the walls of the vagina secrete, or "sweat," a thin watery material, sometimes in copious amounts. This lubrication is necessary for the comfortable placement and movement of the penis in the vagina.

> ➤ *Recall Amy Liu, the middle-aged woman complaining of pain with intercourse. The nurse would need to determine if she is experiencing a change in vaginal secretions, possibly due to her surgery or other changes, such as the onset of menopause.* ■

Breasts

Although the breasts are not considered part of the internal or external genitalia, they are an important aspect of female physical sexuality. The breasts consist of fatty and glandular tissues and the nipples. Their size and shape vary widely among women. The nipples are pale to deep pink. Caressing of the breasts can be pleasurable during sexual activity, and many women can be brought to orgasm by this action alone.

Menstruation

Menstruation, often referred to as a woman's "period or menses," is a cycle during which the body prepares for the presence of a fertilized ovum. Cycles are about 28 days long but may vary from 21 to 40 days. The first menstrual period, called **menarche,** is experienced at about 12 years of age, but the age of menarche is individual and may occur anywhere between 8 and 17 years of age. **Menopause,** the cessation of a woman's menstrual activity, occurs between the ages of 45 and 55 years. The woman may experience irregular menses over time before menstruation ends.

THE MENSTRUAL CYCLE

The menstrual cycle is controlled by a series of reactions that rely on feedback from the ovaries to the pituitary gland. Actually, two cycles occur simultaneously: one in the ovaries and one in the endometrium of the uterus (Fig. 45-1).

In the ovaries, in a typical 28-day cycle, the phase from day 4 to 14 is called the follicular phase. During this phase,

a number of follicles mature, but only one produces a mature ovum. At the same time, in the uterus, the endometrium is becoming thick and velvety in preparation for receiving a fertilized egg. This phase in the uterus is called the proliferation phase. Ovulation generally occurs on day 14 when the mature ovum ruptures from the follicle and the surface of the ovary and is swept into the fallopian tube. If sperm are present, the ovum is fertilized at this time. Some women can detect ovulation by the presence of a sharp, cramping pain over the ovulating ovary; this pain is called mittelschmerz, or middle pain, because it occurs in the middle of the cycle.

From day 15 to day 28, the phase in the ovaries is called the luteal phase. The leftover empty follicle fills up with a yellow pigment and is then called the corpus luteum, or yellow body. The purpose of the corpus luteum is to produce hormones that encourage a fertilized egg to grow. If fertilization does not occur, the corpus luteum begins to disintegrate. During the luteal phase in the ovaries, the uterus also undergoes changes. This phase is called the secretory phase. The endometrial lining thickens. However, in the absence of a fertilized egg, the corpus luteum dies and the endometrial lining disintegrates.

At day 28, menses, or the menstrual flow, begins as a result of the uterus shedding the useless portion of its endometrium. Menses lasts for 3 to 7 days, the average length of flow being 5 days. The menstrual discharge is a bloody fluid that also contains endometrial debris, mucus, and enzymes. It is odorless until exposed to the air, when the woman may notice a light, fleshy, pungent odor. Deodorized pads and tampons do little to minimize odor and can cause chemical irritation to the vulva and vagina. Good hygiene and regular bathing are much more effective during menses to prevent odor. Normal blood loss averages 30 to 80 mL. Pads and tampons should be changed frequently to prevent odor and irritation from wetness. Women using tampons should read and follow the manufacturer's suggestions to reduce the risk for toxic shock syndrome. Usually, the flow is the heaviest and is bright red on the first day or two of menses, gradually tapering off to light-brown staining. Many women experience some degree of discomfort either premenstrually or during menses.

There is no scientific rationale supporting abstinence from sexual activity during menses. Many women enjoy sex during menses owing to the increase in vascularity in the pelvic region, which heightens enjoyment. Men may also enjoy the warm wetness the menstrual flow provides to the vagina. If flow is heavy, a diaphragm can be used to hold it back during sexual activity, or a towel can be used to protect the bedding. Some women who experience abdominal cramping during menses, or dysmenorrhea, find that sexual activity and orgasm relieve their discomfort.

For women who want to avoid menstruating altogether, in May 2007 the U.S. FDA approved the first oral contraceptive designed to be taken 365 days a year. Women who use the drug don't have regular menstrual periods although they can have breakthrough bleeding (spotting or light bleeding). While there are obvious advantages to not having menstrual periods, women should be counseled that there are no long-term safety

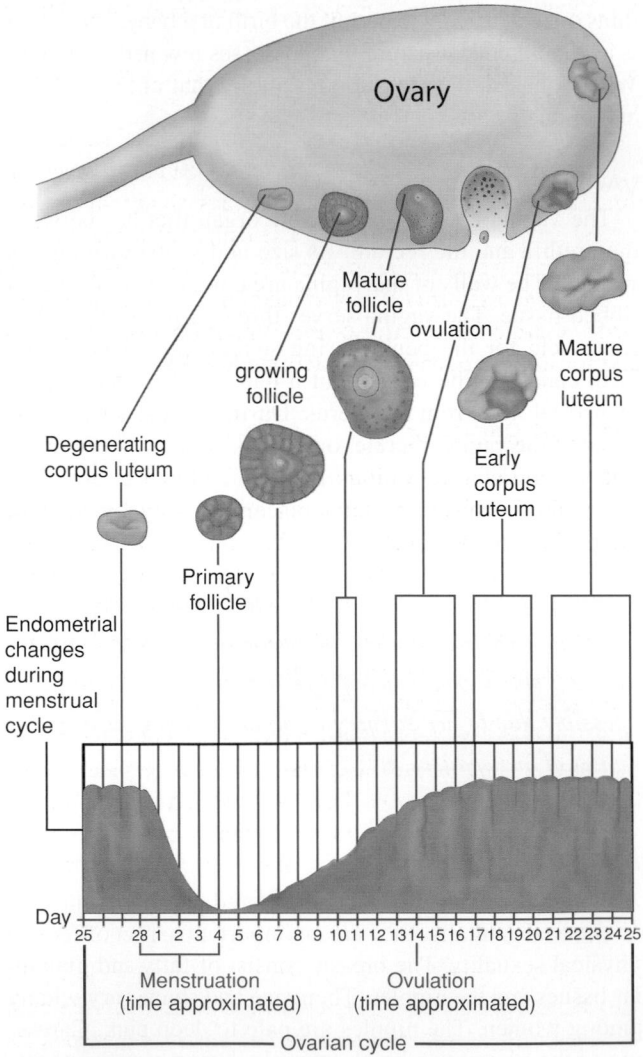

FIGURE 45-1. Schematic representation of one ovarian cycle and the corresponding changes in the endometrium.

data on these drugs. Risks are thought to be similar to those of conventional oral contraceptives: an increased incidence of blood clots, heart attacks and stroke, especially in women who smoke. Positive benefits may include lowering the risk for ovarian cancer and endometrial cancer (Richardson, 2007).

PREMENSTRUAL (TENSION) SYNDROME

Menstrual cycle–related distress, commonly called **premenstrual (tension) syndrome** (PMS), reportedly occurs in 50% to 90% of the female population. PMS is characterized by the appearance of one or more of the following several days before the onset of menstruation: irritability, emotional tension, anxiety, mood changes, headache, breast tenderness, and water retention. Although it is often used to explain unusual behavior (and has been used as a legal defense), its etiology is still uncertain (both physiologic and psychogenic theories have been postulated), as are its effects on women's roles and relationships. Some literature perpetuates a twofold myth: (1) biology and physiology are destiny (many females do and should experience premenstrual distress) and (2) female biology and physiology result in psychiatric disorder, destruction, and violence. Nurses have a great role to play in researching PMS and ensuring that women and the public correctly understand its effects.

Male

Unlike the female genitalia, the male genitalia (illustrated in Fig. 25-35 in Chapter 25) are found primarily outside the body.

External Genitalia

TESTES

The testes, which are about the size of walnuts, feel smooth and are freely movable within the scrotum. Normally, two testes are present. The testes produce sperm and the hormones necessary for the maintenance of male sex characteristics. The primary hormone secreted by the testes is testosterone, which is responsible for a man's deep voice, beard growth, and body hair.

SCROTUM

The scrotum is the loose, bag-like structure that houses the testes. The scrotum hangs between a man's upper thighs. The area around the base of the penis and the scrotum is covered with pubic hair. The looseness of the scrotum is intentional to provide expansion and contraction. When exposed to cool temperatures, the scrotum contracts and draws the testes closer to the body for warmth. In warm temperatures, the scrotum becomes loose and allows the testes to hang farther away from the heat of the body. The testes are sensitive organs and can suffer discomfort, sometimes extreme, if handled roughly or jostled. It is important for men and boys to wear a properly fitted athletic supporter, or jockstrap, when engaged in strenuous physical activity. However, the continuous use of such a support can cause the temperature within the scrotum to rise and the delicate sperm to die because of constant exposure to

high temperatures. Snug-fitting garments such as tight jeans can have the same effect on a man's fertility. The scrotum can be a source of sexual pleasure when lightly stroked, fondled, or caressed during sexual activity.

PENIS

The penis is a tubular structure located above the scrotum. It functions to eliminate urine from the bladder, to ejaculate semen and impregnate a woman, and as a sex organ for sexual pleasure. It consists of the shaft and the glans (head of the penis). In the uncircumcised male, the glans is covered by loose skin (foreskin) that can be retracted. In the circumcised male, the foreskin has been surgically removed, and the glans is exposed. Penis size and shape vary among individuals. Normally, the penis is soft and flaccid and 2.5 to 4 inches long. The dimensions of the penis in no way dictate the man's ability to perform effectively during sexual activity. When an erection occurs, the blood vessels in the shaft of the penis become congested, and the penis becomes hard and erect. The size of the penis during an erection may increase to 5.5 to 7 inches in total length. The penis, particularly the glans, is extremely sensitive to stimulation. Stroking and handling of the shaft of the penis are also pleasurable during sexual activity.

The stimulation that prompts an erection varies. A full bladder on awakening in the morning can cause an erection. Fantasy, memories of a past sexual encounter, and accidental brushing by an attractive stranger can all lead to an erection. An erection in the male does not always signify desire for sexual activity. Exposure of the male patient by the nurse during a bed bath may cause an erection. An erection is a normal physiologic response and not something the man can voluntarily control. The erection ceases if no further stimulation is added. See the accompanying Research in Nursing box.

Internal Genitalia

Tubules from the testes drain into the epididymis, which in turn drains into the vas deferens and ejaculatory ducts. These ducts then drain directly into the urethra. It is believed that the vas deferens acts as a reservoir for sperm between ejaculations.

The seminal vesicles, prostate gland, and Cowper's glands produce a liquid called seminal plasma. The seminal plasma and the sperm collectively make up the semen. The plasma aids in the transport of sperm and also provides energizing nutrients for the sperm. It contains a form of sugar (fructose), mucus, salts, water, base buffers, and coagulators to aid the sperm in their journey. Semen is a thick, creamy white fluid with the consistency of mucus or egg whites.

Breasts

Male breasts contain little real breast tissue, but they still may be stimulated during sexual activity. Although the area of sensitivity is usually limited to the nipple and areola, its stimulation can be as pleasurable an experience for the male as it is for a female.

RESEARCH IN NURSING
Bridging the Gap to Evidence-Based Practice

EFFECT OF NURSE ATTITUDES ON PATIENTS

A nurse's attitudes about sexuality and the human body can directly affect her patient's experiences and self-concept.

Related Research

Zang, Y. B., Chung, L., & Wong, T. (2008). A review of the psychosocial issues for nurses in male genitalia-related care. *Journal of Clinical Nursing, 17*(8), 983–998.

This study examines the response of males to receiving genitalia-related care, and how nurses' attitudes towards performing this procedure may exacerbate the response. Patients who require male genitalia-related care may encounter psychosocial and/or

For additional research, visit thePoint.

sexual dysfunction. Issues surrounding male genitalia-related care for nurses are complicated and may be related to privacy, intimacy, sexuality, dirty work, and emotional discomfort. Age, gender, race, and social class could compound these issues.

Relevance for Nursing Practice

Nurses must be aware of how their negative attitudes or perceptions can affect the response to genitalia-related care. It is the responsibility of nurses to devise strategies of masking their personal view of this procedure, with additional mindfulness as to not cause any additional discomfort for the patient.

Ejaculation

Ejaculation is the expulsion of semen by the rhythmic contractions of the penis. The penis engages in short, jerky movements that produce a spurt of semen with each motion. The period of ejaculation is short, and the penis becomes flaccid after ejaculation. The normal amount of semen per ejaculate is 2 to 6 mL. A fertile man dispels 120 to 160 million sperm per ejaculate. Cowper's glands produce small droplets of fluid during sexual activity that neutralize the acidity of the male urethra and aid in the transport of sperm. This fluid may contain sperm. Therefore, contraceptive measures, if used, must be taken before this fluid can be introduced into the vagina.

Many males, particularly adolescent boys, may experience a phenomenon known as a nocturnal emission, or "wet dream." These ejaculatory episodes occur during sleep without physical stimulation. They are perfectly normal and do not represent any sort of deviation.

SEXUAL RESPONSE CYCLE

The physiologic responses to sexual activity of females and males are more similar than different (Fig. 45-2). Also, body response is essentially the same regardless of the source of stimulation; that is, fantasy, masturbation, and sexual intercourse can all bring about the same body reactions. The sexual response cycle is not limited to the genital organs but is a total-body response that causes many physiologic changes throughout the body. The cycle has four phases: (1) excitement, (2) plateau, (3) orgasm, and (4) resolution; there is a smooth progression from one phase to the next. Although only physiologic responses are discussed here, the emotional and mental involvement of sexual response contributes a great deal to the pleasure and satisfaction of sexual activity.

The human body contains many **erogenous zones,** areas that when stimulated cause sexual arousal and desire. The genitals are an obvious source of sexual pleasure for both men and women, but other areas of the body are also considered erogenous zones. The skin is the largest erogenous

zone. Other areas include the ears, lips, thighs, and breasts. Some people can reach orgasm simply by stimulation of erogenous zones other than the genitals. The most important body organ for sexual arousal and stimulation is the

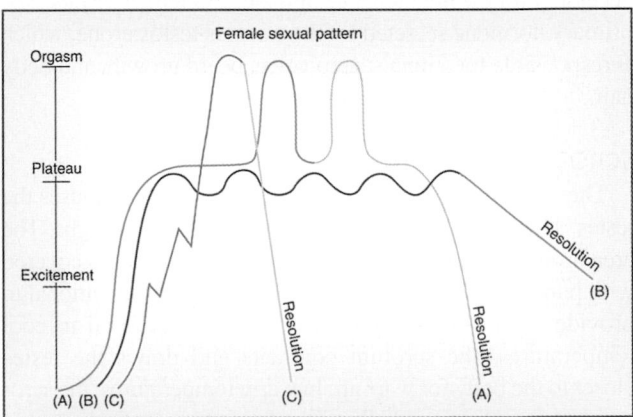

FIGURE 45-2. Male and female sexual response patterns. There are three female patterns shown. (**A**) Steady progression to plateau stage is followed by intense orgasm; subsequent orgasms may occur; resolution is slower. (**B**) Slower progression to plateau stage is followed by minor surges toward orgasm, causing prolonged pleasurable feelings without definitive orgasm; resolution is slowest. (**C**) Rapid progression to plateau stage with some peaks and dips; one intense orgasm follows with rapid resolution. This most closely resembles the male pattern.

brain. It allows individuals freedom to enjoy a sexual experience but also may prevent satisfaction by inhibitions, doubts, and guilt.

Excitement

The excitement phase is initiated by erotic stimulation and arousal. Some of the physiologic changes common in both men and women include an increase in heart rate and blood pressure and the appearance of a pink to red flush to the skin. This sex flush, which is more evident in women than in men, spreads over the face, neck, back, and upper torso. Congestion of the genitals with increased blood flow begins in the excitement phase and causes even more arousal. The length of the excitement phase varies greatly among individuals and even from one experience to another. Women usually enjoy a more prolonged period of stimulation than do men.

During the excitement phase, the woman's breasts swell and the nipples become erect and hard to the touch. Lubrication of the vagina seeps to the outside of the body along the vulvar creases and makes stimulation of the genitals more pleasurable by decreasing friction. The upper two thirds or so of the vagina enlarge and expand. The clitoris enlarges and emerges slightly from the clitoral hood. The labia also enlarge and separate and turn a deep rosy red with arousal.

The first obvious sign of arousal in the man is an erection of the penis caused by increased pelvic congestion of blood. The scrotum noticeably elevates, thickens, and enlarges. The skin of the penis and scrotum turns a deep reddish-purple in response to congestion and arousal. Male nipples may also harden and become erect.

Plateau

The intensity of the plateau phase is greater than that of excitement but not enough to begin orgasm. Desire and arousal continue to build and intensify. This phase varies from a few minutes to 15 to 20 minutes. In the female, the clitoris retracts and disappears under the clitoral hood. It is thought that the clitoris performs in this mysterious way as the body's protection against overstimulation. In the male, secretions from Cowper's glands may appear at the glans of the penis during the plateau phase.

Orgasm

The term **orgasm** defines the climax and sexual explosion of the tension that has been building over the preceding phases. Orgasm lasts only seconds, but it is an extremely intense reaction. Characteristics of the orgasm phase are the involuntary spasmodic contractions of the genital organs. The number of contractions felt by the individual depends on the intensity of the orgasm.

The orgasm phase in the female begins with a heightened feeling of physical pleasure, followed by overwhelming release and involuntary contractions of the genitals. Loss of muscular control can also be seen in spastic contractions and twitching of the arms and legs. The number of contractions can be as few as 4 or as many as 20. Areas of the body that

contract spasmodically are the uterus, anal sphincter, rectum, and urethral sphincter. It is believed that women achieve orgasm in a variety of ways. Although some women can achieve orgasm by penile thrusting in the vagina alone, most women need clitoral stimulation to reach orgasm.

During orgasm in the male, involuntary spasmodic contractions occur in the penis, epididymis, vas deferens, and rectum. The male orgasm is most often accompanied by ejaculation of semen from the urinary meatus of the penis. It is not necessary for ejaculation and orgasm to occur simultaneously; rather, it is a coincidence that the two events usually happen at the same time.

Resolution

The resolution phase is characterized by a return to normal body functioning present before the excitement phase. Feelings of relaxation, fatigue, and fulfillment are common. Some people have a need to be held, fondled, and caressed. Physical demonstrations of affection may initiate the sexual response cycle once again. The woman is physiologically capable of immediate response to sexual stimulation. Because of this, many women can achieve multiple orgasms. The man experiences a period during which he is incapable of sexual response, called the refractory period. The length of the refractory period is individual; it might be a few minutes or even days before the man's body responds readily to continued sexual stimulation.

SEXUAL EXPRESSION

The methods by which people gain satisfaction through sexual stimulation are varied. Touch, smell, sight, sounds, feelings, thoughts, and fantasy can all contribute to sexual fulfillment in any form of expression chosen by individuals. Feelings of love for another person are closely associated with desire.

Forms of sexual stimulation include kissing, hugging, stroking, squeezing, breast stimulation, manual stimulation of the genitals, oral–genital stimulation, and anal stimulation. Sexual stimulation may be physical or psychological. Erotic stimulation through the use of films, magazines, and photographs is common. Fetishism, usually practiced by a male, is sexual arousal with the aid of an inanimate object not generally associated with sexual activity. Items such as shoes, leather, rubber, and women's undergarments might be used.

Masturbation

Masturbation is a technique of sexual expression in which an individual practices self-stimulation. It is a way for a person to learn what he or she prefers during stimulation and what feels good. Men masturbate by holding and stroking the shaft of the penis. Women find manual stimulation of the clitoris enjoyable, although variations of technique are numerous. Many myths and misinformation surround masturbation. The reality is that people masturbate regardless of sex, age, or marital status. People might not masturbate because they feel guilty about it or believe self-stimulation is wrong. Masturbation is not "dirty" and will not lead to blindness or insanity.

Sexual Intercourse

The act of **intercourse** (coitus or copulation) is the insertion of the penis into the partner's vagina, anus, or mouth. It usually begins by stimulation of the senses in some way, followed by a period of activity known as foreplay. "Petting" is part of foreplay; it can involve simple stroking of the breasts, arms, back, and neck without genital involvement or may lead to mutual masturbation and orgasm.

Vaginal Intercourse

The act of placing the penis in the vagina, penile–vaginal intercourse, can be accomplished in various positions. The most common position in Western cultures is the missionary position, in which the woman lies horizontally underneath the man. (This position was named by the Polynesians because it was the preferred position for intercourse used by religious missionaries.) Couples may find other positions to be more stimulating and comfortable. Clitoral stimulation is difficult to achieve in the missionary position. Lying side by side, female on top, and rear entry are some examples of coital positions that enable clitoral stimulation. Sexually inhibited people may believe they need "permission" to engage in alternative sexual positions.

When the penis is pushed into the vagina, the man begins rhythmic thrusting movements of his hips to move the penis back and forth along the vaginal walls. The woman might match her partner's hip movements with movements of her own body. These movements continue until orgasm is attained by one person or both.

Simultaneous orgasms, or both people attaining orgasm at the same moment, are difficult to achieve, and a preoccupation with attaining simultaneous orgasms might disrupt the ultimate intimacy and satisfaction possible during coitus.

The period after coitus is just as significant as the events leading up to it. Caressing, hugging, and kissing deepen the couple's intimacy and should be nurtured, not rushed.

Anal Intercourse

Anal intercourse, the act of inserting the penis into the anus and rectum of a partner, is another form of intercourse. Commonly practiced by gay men, it is also used by heterosexual couples. Once the penis (or any object) is placed in the rectum, it should not be introduced into the vagina without thorough cleansing because many microorganisms present in the rectum can cause vaginal infections. Care should be used to avoid injury to the delicate rectal mucosa, and lubrication is essential for comfort. Condoms are now recommended for both types of intercourse to prevent sexually transmitted infections (STIs).

Oral–Genital Stimulation

Stimulation of the genitals by the mouth and tongue might be used during foreplay or as a way to reach orgasm. Cun-

nilingus is stimulation of the female genitals by licking and sucking the clitoris and surrounding structures. Fellatio is stimulation of the male genitals by licking and sucking the penis and surrounding structures. These techniques may be used by one partner or both simultaneously (*soixante-neuf*). More younger people are using oral–genital stimulation as a replacement for vaginal intercourse to reduce the incidence of pregnancy.

Abstinence

Abstinence is not having sex. It is the most effective form of birth control, preventing pregnancy 100% of the time when practiced consistently. Abstinence also prevents the transmission of STIs 100% of the time when practiced appropriately and consistently. Some STIs spread through oral–genital sex, anal sex, or even intimate skin-to-skin contact without actual penetration (genital warts and herpes can be spread this way). Therefore, only avoiding all types of intimate genital contact can prevent these STIs. Avoiding all types of intimate genital contact—including anal and oral sex—is **complete** abstinence. There are no side effects or health risks related to abstinence.

Alternative Forms of Sexual Expression

Alternate forms of sexual expression include voyeurism, sadism, masochism, sadomasochism, and pedophilia.

- Voyeurism is the achievement of sexual arousal by looking at the body of another. Some voyeurs develop complex means to spy on others that involve violations of privacy.
- Sadism refers to the practice of gaining sexual pleasure while inflicting abuse on another person.
- Masochism refers to gaining sexual pleasure from the humiliation of being abused.
- Sadomasochism is the act of practicing sadism and masochism together. It might involve being tied up, biting, hitting, spanking, whipping, pinching, and other activities.
- Pedophilia is a term used to describe the practice of adults gaining sexual fulfillment by performing sexual acts with children.

FACTORS AFFECTING SEXUALITY

Many factors influence a person's sexuality and produce personal feelings regarding sexuality. The brain, rather than the genitals, plays the most significant role in how people perceive themselves as sexual beings.

Developmental Considerations

The process of human development affects the psychosocial, emotional, and biologic aspects of life, and these in turn affect an individual's sexuality. Sexuality is the only distinguishing trait present at conception. From birth onward, gender, or sex, influences behavior throughout life. Table 45-1 summarizes sexuality throughout the lifespan and the nursing implications for each stage.

TABLE • 45-1	DEVELOPMENTAL ASPECTS OF SEXUALITY THROUGH THE LIFE SPAN	
Stage	**Characteristics**	**Nursing Implications and Teaching Guidelines**
Infancy: Birth to 18 mo	• Needs affection and tactile stimulation • Boys have penile erections, and girls have orgasmic potential • Gradually can differentiate self from others • Obtain pleasure from touching genitals • Dressed according to gender • Toys are gender related	• Avoid early weaning to prevent oral deprivation. • Encourage parents to provide ample physical touch, deprivation of which may cause physical and mental underdevelopment. • Self-manipulation of genitals is normal behavior; avoid denoting this as "bad." • Avoid confusion of sex by consistent use of male or female role reinforcement.
Toddler: Age 1–3 yr	• Establishes control over bowels and bladder • Both sexes enjoy fondling genitals • Able to identify own gender • Develops vocabulary related to anatomy	• Allow toddler to designate his or her readiness to toilet training. Strict measures may lead to compulsive behaviors later. • Punishment of genital fondling may lead to guilt and shame regarding sexual behavior later in life. • Use proper terms for body parts.
Preschooler: Age 4–6 yr	• By age 6, sexuality has been internalized and preference for sexual partners determined • Methods of play and dress are in accordance with gender • Enjoys exploring body parts of self and playmates • Engages in masturbation	• Parents may cause anxiety in the child by intolerance of inconsistency of sex-role behavior. • Negative overreaction by parents of child's masturbating behavior can lead to a belief that the genitals and sex are bad and dirty.
School-aged: Age 6–10 yr	• There is attachment to the parent of the opposite sex • Tendency toward having same-sex friends • Curiosity about sex and sharing of fears • Increasing self-awareness	• Same-sex preference for relationships is not related to heterosexual or homosexual tendencies. • Give child the information desired in a clear, factual form. May look to peers for information that may be incorrect.
Preadolescence: Age 10–13 yr	• Puberty begins for most boys and girls with development of secondary sex characteristics • Menarche takes place • May test behavioral limits	• Information is necessary regarding body changes to alleviate fears. This information should be given to the young person before pubertal changes begin. • Parents need to find a satisfactory middle ground for role setting. Rules that are either too rigid or too lenient can interfere with the development of self-confidence and internal value system. • Treat body image changes with a positive attitude to prevent poor self-image.
Adolescence: Age 13–19 yr	• Begins to develop opposite-sex relationships • Sexual fantasies are common • Masturbation is common • May begin to partake in sexual activity ranging from light to heavy petting to full genital intercourse • Girls concerned with reputations and self-image • Boys preoccupied with competitiveness of sexual activity • Incidence of adolescent pregnancies is increasing	• Parents share their beliefs and moral value systems with their children. • Teenagers may share their feelings with parents. Not taking them seriously may lead to lack of trust and communication gap. • Teens need information regarding contraceptive measures and the potential for contracting sexually transmitted infections.

(continued)

		Nursing Implications and
Stage	**Characteristics**	**Teaching Guidelines**

TABLE • 45-1 DEVELOPMENTAL ASPECTS OF SEXUALITY THROUGH THE LIFE SPAN *(continued)*

Stage	Characteristics	Nursing Implications and Teaching Guidelines
Young adulthood: Age 20–35 yr	• Premarital sex is common • Although many young adults choose cohabitation instead of marriage, most marry and begin families before age 30 yr • Knowledge regarding sexual response and activity increases pleasure of relationship • May experiment with various sexual expressions • Develops own value system and respects values of other people • Many couples share financial responsibilities as well as household tasks	• Encourage communication between partners regarding sexual needs and differences. • Teach use of abstinence and contraceptive measures to prevent unwanted pregnancies. • Counsel against promiscuous behavior to guard against sexually transmitted infections and loss of trust of partner. • Daily communication is necessary to vent stresses and work out difficulties.
Adulthood: Age 35–55 yr	• Bodily changes as a result of menopause • Couples focus on quality rather than quantity of sexual experiences • Divorce is common • Grown children begin their own lives and sexual experiences • Sexual satisfaction may actually increase because of loss of fear of pregnancy	• Both men and women need positive reinforcement of what is good about themselves and their relationships. • Teach parents that empty nest syndrome (feelings of loss caused by children leaving) is common. Accentuate positive aspects of this situation. • Encourage couple to use this period as one of renewal for themselves.
Late adulthood and elderly: Age 55 yr and older	• Orgasms may become shorter and less intense in both men and women • Vaginal secretions decrease, and period of resolution in men lengthens • May feel need to conform to stereotypes regarding the aging process and cease sexual activity • Fear of loss of sexual abilities	• Sexual activity need not be hindered by age. • Teach couples that adaptation to bodily changes is possible with use of comfortable positions for intercourse and increased time for stimulation. • Teach alternatives to coitus, such as caressing, hugging, and stroking, when coitus is impossible because of illness or disability. • Couples who have been consistently sexually active throughout their lives may continue their intimate relationship for as long as they desire.

Culture

The manner in which sexuality is perceived by a society in turn influences the individual. Every culture has its own norms regarding sexual identity and behavior. To some degree, culture dictates the duration of sexual intercourse, methods of sexual stimulation, and sexual positions. In some cultures, women might be expected merely to tolerate sex; in others, the woman's participation is encouraged.

Religion

Some people view organized religion as having a generally negative effect on the expression of sexuality. For example, in many religions, the concept of virginity came to be synonymous with purity, and sex became synonymous with sin. In addition, many forms of sexual expression other than male–female coitus are considered unnatural by some religions. As a result of the rigid regulations and negative connotation of sex dictated by some religious groups, a number of sexual dysfunctions can be related to an individual's resulting guilt and anxiety. Most major religions are reexamining their teachings on sexuality in response to challenges posed by their members. Many have recognized the importance of solid sex education within the realm of the church. There is also a new interest in the spirituality of marriage, and churches are examining their role in supporting the intimate/sexual relationship of married couples.

Ethics

Healthy sexuality depends on freedom from guilt and anxiety. What one person believes is wrong might be perfectly natural and correct to another. Some individuals might feel that certain forms of sexual expression are bizarre and the people who participate in them are perverted. If the sexual expression is performed by consenting adults, is not harmful to them, and is practiced in privacy, it is not considered a deviant behavior. Individuals should personally decide with which aspects of sexual expression they are comfortable. Frequently, all an individual needs to alleviate guilt and consequently enhance sexual satisfaction is permission from a healthcare professional to engage in a different form of expression.

Lifestyle

Modern lifestyles greatly affect sexuality and its expression. Both men and women are exposed to stress, and many are under considerable strain to perform and function in the workplace as well as at home. Stressors might be external, such as job and financial demands, or internal, such as a competitive nature. These varied responsibilities place a time restraint on communication between a couple as well as on the energy level and motivation for sexual satisfaction. Although some couples view sexual activity as a release from the stressors of everyday life, most place nurturing relationships and sexual expression far from the top of the list of "things to do." It is crucial to a relationship's survival that a couple set aside priority time—if not for lovemaking, then for intimate, quiet contact. Lifestyle variables can also influence the sexual expression of adolescent and young adults. Those with "time on their hands" and fewer constructive developmental opportunities (education, sports, community service) are more likely to engage in risky sexual behavior.

Childbearing Considerations

All sorts of questions surround childbearing, and the ability (or lack of ability) to procreate can put great pressure on a sexual relationship: Are we ready to be parents? What does it mean to be a responsible parent—especially in this age when an increasing number of prenatal interventions are available to maximize fetal outcomes (quality control)? Should life partners be chosen only if genetic testing reveals a good match for reproduction? If we choose to be sexually active and not have children, what are the best means to prevent unwanted pregnancies? If we become pregnant and choose not to continue the pregnancy, what are our options? If we desperately want a child and discover one or both parties to be infertile, what are our options? The age of biotechnology promises "designer babies" and raises hard questions for individuals and society. Individuals frequently look to nurses for help in sorting through how they ought to respond to these challenges. Experienced nurses are good at detecting when a fear of pregnancy or inability to conceive is interfering with a couple's normal sexual expression or when a changing developmental stage (e.g., menopause) is interfering with normal sexual expression.

Sexually Transmitted Infections

Sexually transmitted infections (STIs) or diseases (STDs), once called venereal diseases, are infections that are spread primarily through sexual contact. They are among the most common infectious diseases in the United States today. More than 20 STIs have been identified, and they affect more than 13 million men and women in this country each year. A Centers for Disease Control and Prevention (CDC, 2008) study estimates that one in four (26%) young women between the ages of 14 and 19—or 3.2 million teenage girls—is infected with at least one of the most common sexually transmitted diseases: human papillomavirus (HPV), chlamydia, herpes simplex virus, and trichomoniasis. The study also finds that African American teenage girls are the most severely affected. Nearly half of the young African American women (48%) were infected with an STI, compared to 20% of young white or Mexican American women (Forhan, 2008).

Table 45-2 lists common types of STIs and their signs and symptoms. The annual comprehensive cost of STIs in the United States is estimated to be well in excess of $10 billion.

According to the National Institute of Allergy and Infectious Diseases (NIAID), understanding the basic facts about STIs—the ways in which they are spread, their common symptoms, and how they can be treated—is the first step toward prevention. News releases, fact sheets, and other NIAID-related materials are available on the NIAID Web site at http://www.niaid.nih.gov. NIAID recommends understanding at least five key points about all STIs in this country today:

1. STIs affect men and women of all backgrounds and economic levels. They are most prevalent among teenagers and young adults. Nearly two-thirds of all STIs occur in people younger than 25 years of age.
2. The incidence of STIs is rising, in part because in the last few decades, young people have become sexually active earlier yet are marrying later. In addition, divorce is more common. The net result is that sexually active people today are more likely to have multiple sex partners during their lives and are potentially at risk for developing STIs.
3. Most of the time, STIs cause no symptoms, particularly in women. When and if symptoms develop, they may be confused with those of other diseases not transmitted through sexual contact. Even when an STI causes no symptoms, a person who is infected may be able to pass the disease on to a sex partner. That is why many doctors recommend periodic testing or screening for people who have more than one sex partner.
4. Health problems caused by STIs tend to be more severe and more frequent for women than for men, in part because the frequency of asymptomatic infection means that many women do not seek care until serious problems have developed.
   - Some STIs can spread into the uterus (womb) and fallopian tubes to cause pelvic inflammatory disease (PID), which in turn is a major cause of both infertility and ectopic (tubal) pregnancy. The latter can be fatal.
   - STIs in women also may be associated with cervical cancer. One STI, human papillomavirus infection (HPV), causes genital warts and cervical and other genital cancers.
   - STIs can be passed from a mother to her baby before, during, or immediately after birth; some of these infections of the newborn can be cured easily, but others may cause a baby to be permanently disabled or even die.
5. When diagnosed and treated early, many STIs can be treated effectively. Some infections have become resistant to the drugs used to treat them and now require newer types of antibiotics. Experts believe that having STIs other than HIV increases one's risk for becoming infected with the HIV virus (NIAID, 2008).

TABLE • 45-2   **SEXUALLY TRANSMITTED INFECTIONS**

Disease	Characteristics
Acquired immunodeficiency syndrome (AIDS)	• Human immunodeficiency virus (HIV) • Positive ELISA and Western Blot tests • Incidence high in IV drug users and homosexual and bisexual men; increased heterosexual transmission • Fatigue, diarrhea, weight loss, enlarged lymph nodes, fever, anorexia, and night sweats
Cervical intraepithelial neoplasia (CIN) Cervical cancer	• Abnormal Pap smears • Women with multiple sex partners, women who began sexual activity before age 18, and women whose partners have multiple female partners • Asymptomatic • Possible vaginal bleeding or spotting
Chlamydia trachomatis Nongonococcal urethritis (NGU) *Chlamydia*	• The most prevalent STI to date • Intracellular bacteria • Vaginal discharge, burning on urination, urinary frequency, dysuria, and urethral soreness • Many women do not have symptoms.
Cytomegalovirus (CMV)	• A virus in the same family as herpes and Epstein-Barr • May be asymptomatic or may be confused with another disease such as pneumonia, mononucleosis, or hepatitis • Not exclusively sexually transmitted
Nonspecific vaginitis *Gardnerella vaginalis*	• Mixed anaerobic bacteria • Foul-smelling, thin, grayish white vaginal discharge • Male partners do not have symptoms.
Neisseria gonorrhoeae "The clap" or "the drip" Gonorrhea	• Gram-negative bacteria • Both men and women may not have symptoms. • Symptoms in men: purulent penile discharge, dysuria, frequency of urination • Symptoms in women: dysuria, abnormal menses, vaginal discharge, pelvic inflammatory disease • Symptoms of pharyngitis if oral sex was practiced • May be accompanied by chlamydial infection • Detected by gonorrhea culture of cervix or penile discharge from men • Newborns exposed at birth are at risk for blindness and pneumonia. • Untreated gonorrhea can result in infertility, skin rash with lesions, and acute arthritis.
Herpes simplex virus type 1 and 2 "Cold sores" Herpes	• A DNA virus • Lesions develop mostly in oral and genital areas. • Appear as single or multiple painful vesicles, which rupture and form ulcer-like lesions; these form scabs as they heal. • First infections last about 10 to 14 days, whereas subsequent infections are shorter in duration. • Recurrences are usually preceded by prodromal symptoms of tingling and fullness.
Human papillomavirus (HPV) Condylomata acuminate Genital warts Venereal warts	• A DNA virus; vaccine now available. • Pale, soft, papillary lesions found around the internal and external genitalia and perianal and rectal areas of the body; vary in size • Profuse watery vaginal discharge, dyspareunia, intense pruritus, and vulvar irritation • Women with HPV are at risk for cervical cancer. • Male partner may or may not have lesions.
Treponema pallidum Syphilis	• A spirochete detected through serologic blood test (VDRL, RPR, STS) • Three stages to disease if left untreated *Primary:* Single painless genital lesion 10 days to 3 months after exposure *Secondary:* Generalized skin rash, enlarged lymph nodes, fever that may appear 2 to 4 weeks after appearance of primary lesion; may last for several years *Latent:* Usually no clinical symptoms present for as long as 20 years; may continue to involve and damage neurologic and cardiovascular organs; dementia, confusion, paralysis, and paresis may occur.
Trichomoniasis "Trich" *Trichomonas vaginalis*	• Protozoan with flagella • Identified on wet-mount microscopic examination of vaginal discharge • May be identified on Pap smear • Usually asymptomatic in male patients • Foul-smelling vaginal discharge, thin, foamy, and green in color, causes itching of vulva and vagina, burning on urination and dyspareunia; "strawberry" cervix may be seen on speculum examination.

Data from National Institute of Allergy and Infectious Diseases. http://www.niaid.nih.gov/topics/sti/default.htm; and from the Centers for Disease Control and Prevention. http://www.cdc.gov/std/healthcomm/fact_sheets.htm.

Having an STI might affect one's self-concept and keep an individual from becoming intimate for fear of spreading the infection. Some STIs, such as HIV that progresses to acquired immunodeficiency syndrome (AIDS), are deadly because there is no cure.

> *Recall Paul Rojas, the homosexual patient with AIDS. The nurse would need to assess the patient's sexual practices and instruct him about sex practices to prevent the transmission of HIV/AIDS. In addition, the nurse would need to investigate the effect that this STI has had on his sexuality.* ■

Sexual Dysfunction

Sexual dysfunction is a problem that prevents an individual or couple from engaging in or enjoying sexual intercourse and orgasm. Dysfunctions might occur as a result of physiologic malfunctions, conflicts with cultural norms, interpersonal problems, or any combination of these. Anxieties and fears concerning the sexual act are almost always present. Patients with severe sexual dysfunctions require intensive professional therapy from a qualified sex therapist.

Male Primary Sexual Dysfunctions
ERECTILE DYSFUNCTION
Erectile dysfunction, also called **impotence,** is the inability of a man to attain or maintain an erection to such an extent that he cannot have satisfactory intercourse. Common causes of impotence (which may be physiologic or psychological) include various illnesses, treatments for these illnesses, and personal anxieties. New medications have revolutionized treatment for erectile dysfunction.

> *Remember Jefferson Smith, the patient with diabetes and hypertension who is having problems with erections. The nurse would review the pathophysiologic effects of diabetes and hypertension on sexual response and would evaluate his current status, including a review of all medications that he is taking, to determine possible contributory factors.* ■

PREMATURE EJACULATION
Premature ejaculation is a condition in which a man consistently reaches ejaculation or orgasm before or soon after entering the vagina. The result is that his partner usually does not have time to reach sexual satisfaction. Causes of the problem are rarely physical.

RETARDED EJACULATION
Retarded ejaculation, also called ejaculatory incompetence, refers to a man's inability to ejaculate into the vagina, or delayed intravaginal ejaculation. The causes of this problem

are similar to those of impotence. When it occurs after the man has experienced normal ejaculations, the cause is most probably due to interpersonal problems.

Female Primary Sexual Dysfunctions
INHIBITED SEXUAL DESIRE
Inhibited sexual desire consists of an inhibition in sexual arousal so that congestion and vaginal lubrication are absent or minimal. Causative factors may be anxiety, negative emotions, fear, interpersonal problems, or physical factors. Orgasmic dysfunction is defined as the inability of a woman to reach orgasm. The causes are similar to those of inhibited sexual desire.

DYSPAREUNIA
Dyspareunia is painful intercourse. Although it is most often described by women, some men may also suffer from this disorder. The cause is usually physical, although psychological problems such as fear and anxiety can cause pain.

> *Consider Amy Liu, the woman who had a hysterectomy and is experiencing pain on intercourse. The nurse would review the patient's history to determine if the problem is physiologic secondary to changes in the reproductive tract from surgery, or psychological, secondary to the changes in self-concept and feelings of not being a woman.* ■

VAGINISMUS
Vaginismus is a rare condition in which the vaginal opening closes tightly and prevents penile penetration. Vaginismus is due to involuntary spastic contractions of the muscles at and around the vaginal opening and the levator ani muscles. The cause of vaginismus may be physical, psychological, or both.

VULVODYNIA
Vulvodynia, a chronic vulvar discomfort or pain characterized by burning, stinging, irritation, or rawness of the female genitalia that interferes with sexual activity, is particularly problematic because little is known about its cause or treatment.

Other Health Conditions

A healthy body, mind, and emotions are necessary for sexual wellness. A primary sexual dysfunction can affect a person's sexual expression. Similarly, any trauma or stress that interferes with an individual's ability to perform daily functions will also affect the expression of sexuality. Illness is no exception.

Diabetes Mellitus
Diabetes mellitus is a hormonal disease in which an inadequate amount of insulin is secreted by the pancreas. Although almost all hormonal disorders affect sexuality in some way,

diabetes is the most prevalent and well known. Erectile dysfunction, or impotence, is a great concern among diabetic men. Treatment to date depends largely on the degree of erectile ability lost. Some men might be candidates for a penile prosthesis, which was developed in 1973. The prosthesis is surgically implanted below the base of the penis, and inflation of the device produces an erection when sexual activity is desired. Pharmacologic management (e.g., Viagra, Levitra, or Cialis) might also be indicated.

> ➤ *Think back to Jefferson Smith, the patient with diabetes and hypertension. The nurse would explore with Mr. Smith his feelings about the effect of his disorder on his sexual function and sexuality. Additional consultation with other members of the healthcare team would be necessary to determine the most appropriate plan for treatment of Mr. Smith's impotence.* ■

It is not uncommon for diabetic women to experience loss of capacity for orgasm (orgasmic dysfunction). Difficulty experiencing arousal and loss of vaginal lubrication have also been reported. Frequent *Monilia* infections of the vagina are also common and can cause discomfort during coitus.

Cardiovascular Disease

Cardiovascular disease is prevalent in North America, and the sexual response cycle can greatly increase the demands on the heart and other structures. A person with a cardiovascular disease might experience much anxiety over the effect the illness will have on sexuality and sexual functioning.

HYPERTENSION

The most significant difficulty a hypertensive person faces regarding sexuality is that the medication used to control the disease frequently causes a change in sexual functioning. These sexual dysfunctions may be relieved by modifying the dose of the medication or switching to a different medication.

> ➤ *Consider Jefferson Smith, the patient with a history of diabetes and hypertension. The nurse would obtain a complete medication history from the patient to determine if his pharmacologic therapy is the underlying cause of his impotence or if the medication is contributing to a preexisting problem associated with his diabetes. This investigation would provide information about whether an adjustment in medication dosage might minimize or alleviate Mr. Smith's impotence.* ■

MYOCARDIAL INFARCTION (HEART ATTACK)

The primary goal after a myocardial infarction (MI) is to allow the heart ample time to heal. Activities of daily living, including sexual activity, should be resumed gradually, and stressors such as overexertion, alcohol consumption, and emotional upheavals should be avoided. In an uncomplicated MI, sexual activity may begin at about the third week of recovery, beginning with masturbation to partial erection in the male. Generally, this activity is gradually increased until 3 months after the MI, when sexual intercourse may be resumed. A comfortable position that places the least stress on the affected partner should be used.

Diseases of the Joints and Mobility

Joint diseases and disorders affect young and old people. Pain, fatigue, stiffness, and loss of range of motion can accompany any of the dozens of known diseases of the joints. The disease itself does not affect sexual functioning, although the manifestation of it can cause discomfort and anxiety.

Surgery and Body Image

Surgery is performed to remove diseased tissue and repair body organs, and it usually requires an incision with resulting scars. The most devastating kinds of surgery are those used to remove cancerous tissue and surrounding structures. Patients are almost always distressed about a diagnosis of cancer and possible death. After surgery, patients need to adjust to major alterations in their bodies. Changes in body image also affect a person's self-perception as a sexual being.

> ➤ *Remember Amy Liu, the woman who had had a hysterectomy. The uterus, because it is a female reproductive organ, is often associated with childbearing and is a major component of a woman's "femaleness." The nurse would interpret the significance of the uterus to the patient's self-concept and how the surgery to remove it has affected her overall feelings of "femininity" and "femaleness." Using this information, the nurse would then correct any misconceptions that Mrs. Liu may have about this reproductive organ and develop an appropriate teaching plan.* ■

Mastectomy is a surgical procedure to remove a breast and surrounding tissue. After such a surgery, a woman's return to sexual functioning depends on many factors, such as support of her partner, the value placed on the breast by the man or woman, and fear of discomfort during sexual activity.

An ostomy is a surgical opening placed on the outside of the body to allow for the passage of secretions and elimination into a closed drainage bag. Grieving over the loss of the natural means to eliminate waste, such as urine or feces, accompanies learning to live with an obvious artificial device. Many people are anxious as to how this apparatus will affect their sex lives and how accepting their partners will be of it.

Spinal Cord Injuries

Thousands of people are victims of spinal cord injuries each year as a result of various types of accidents. This type of injury almost always results in some degree of permanent disability. Such people face multiple adaptations in their lifestyles, including those related to mobility, bowel and bladder control, sexual functioning, and role expectations. The extent of sexual response that remains after a spinal cord injury depends primarily on the level and extent of the injury. Ejaculation and orgasm are most likely to remain with low spinal injuries. Women are more likely to experience orgasm than men, but they complain more about the lack of physical sensations during the excitement phase than do men. Many people find that other erogenous zones become more easily stimulated after the injury.

Chronic Pain

Many chronic illnesses are accompanied by constant pain, and an individual with persistent pain might not desire any sexual contact. However, the desire for human warmth and contact does not cease because of pain. Altered or modified positions for coitus are sometimes necessary, and discussing these with patients can be an important part of implementing the Nursing Process as discussed later in this chapter.

Mental Illness

Various psychological and physical disorders can cause mental illness. The mind plays a powerful role in sexuality, and any disruption of its functioning will no doubt cause some disturbance in sexual functioning. Even a disorder such as mild depression can affect desire and sexual functioning. Sometimes, it is difficult for the partner of a patient who has developed a mental illness to continue the sexual relationship. People afflicted with Alzheimer's disease can lose the memory of any contact with a partner or spouse. At times, patients with mental illness act out in a sexual manner, such as touching themselves or removing their clothing at inappropriate times and places.

Medications

Some medications have side effects that may affect sexual functioning. These include amyl nitrates, anticonvulsants, antidepressants, antihistamines, antihypertensives, antipsychotics, antispasmodics, barbiturates, and narcotics. Recreational drugs including cocaine, ethyl alcohol, and marijuana are used by some to heighten the sexual experience. These drugs can have serious and even deadly side effects.

THE NURSE AS ROLE MODEL

A nurse's attitudes, biases, and prejudices regarding sexuality are readily transmitted to patients through his or her actions, manner of speech, avoidance of certain circumstances, and types of discussion (see the accompanying Focused Critical Thinking Guide and the Nursing Research box earlier in the chapter). The level of knowledge a nurse has about sexual issues can inhibit or promote discussions of sexual health. The nurse who does not have a sound knowledge base of reproductive anatomy and physiology, sexual response, sexual expression, and other issues surrounding sexuality will be unable to assess, teach, or counsel the patient with sexual concerns.

> ▶ *Recall Paul Rojas, the patient described in the Reflective Practice box. The nurse caring for Mr. Rojas needs to be comfortable with his or her own sexuality to ensure that he or she provides nonjudgmental care. In addition, the nurse needs a solid knowledge foundation about sexual orientation and sexual preference to develop an appropriate, unbiased plan of care that meets Mr. Rojas' needs.* ■

Nursing goals to enhance interactions with patients and to promote individual sexual health are as follows: The nurse will be able to:

- Feel comfortable as a sexual being.
- Develop self-awareness regarding sexual topics.
- Develop communication skills that promote discussion of sexual concerns with patients.
- Identify patients with problems related to sexuality and intervene competently and comfortably to meet these needs.
- Practice responsible sexual expression.

THE NURSING PROCESS FOR THE PATIENT WITH A SEXUAL HEALTH NEED

Nurses who role model good health behaviors are more effective teachers. Use the Promoting Health Display 45-1 for yourself before using it with others.

Assessing
Sexual History

The comprehensive health history should include information regarding a patient's reproductive and sexual health, depending on the circumstances in which the patient is receiving care. As a rule, three general categories of patients should have a sexual history recorded by the nurse:

- Any inpatient or outpatient receiving care for pregnancy, STI, infertility, or contraception
- Any patient experiencing sexual dysfunction
- Any patient whose illness will affect sexual functioning and behavior in any way

Information is best obtained from the patient by beginning with nonthreatening questions and progressing to more sensitive concerns (see the accompanying Focused Assessment Guide). Patients usually have no difficulty answering questions regarding their bodies and general reproductive issues such as, "When did your menstrual periods first begin?"

Explain to patients that this information might be helpful in assisting you in the plan of care and in identifying any sexual problems or concerns. The assessment provides an excellent opportunity to teach by helping the patient confront fears. Four general levels of sexual history are:

Level 1: Sexual history as part of a comprehensive health history—obtained by a nurse

Level 2: Sexual history—obtained by a nurse with education and training in sexuality

FOCUSED CRITICAL THINKING GUIDE • 45-1

Sexuality and Nonjudgmental Nursing Care

A 33-year-old white man with AIDS who is living alone at home asks you, the visiting nurse, about the nurse who was substituting for you during your vacation. "I don't like to complain, but he was overly friendly—if you get what I mean. . . . I wasn't comfortable with the way he was touching me and I'd rather not have help with my bath than have him back here." You have to decide how to respond.

1. Identify Goal of Thinking

Clarify what the patient is saying and make a judgment about the behavior behind his concern so that you can respond appropriately.

2. Assess Adequacy of Knowledge

Pertinent circumstances: You have been visiting the patient for the last 2 months following his discharge from a local hospital because of AIDS-related complications. Apart from his clinical picture, you know very little about the patient, who has always seemed private and reserved during your visits. You "feel sorry" that the patient is as sick as he is at this point in his life, and your instinct is to trust him. You really don't know the colleague who was substituting for you because he is a "new hire."

Prerequisite knowledge: Before you can make a judgment about the patient's concern, you need to know more about what actually happened between him and your colleague. You do not know your colleague well because he is a "new hire" and has only been working in the agency for 3 months. You have heard reports that he is gay. You know that the patient is single but do not know his sexual orientation. You will need to talk with your colleague to get his description of his encounter with the patient. You will also need to know more about what touch means to both the patient and your colleague because culture and individual preference can profoundly influence the meaning different individuals give to touch.

Room for error: Life and death do not hinge on how you respond to this patient. However, the well-being of the patient and your colleague's reputation are at stake, so the matter is grave.

Time constraints: You must make some immediate response to the patient. Because you do not have sufficient information to judge what happened, you should not feel pressured to make a definitive response. The patient's well-being will not be jeopardized if you postpone a complete response until you have investigated the complaint.

3. Address Potential Problems

The most serious obstacles to critical thinking in this situation would be false assumptions you (and the patient) might have about homosexuality in general and male homosexual nurses in particular, and the failure to reason carefully about the situation. Your tendency to "go to bat" for patients and to believe whatever a patient tells you "no mat-

ter what" may result in your unfairly and prematurely judging a colleague.

4. Consult Helpful Resources

Your colleague is the first resource you should consult because you need to hear his side of the event before you can think critically about what happened. When you do meet with him, he thanks you for bringing up the subject because he was similarly disturbed by his encounter with this patient. "I guess I'm a touchy-feely kind of guy and generally find that patients respond well to human touch. In the past, patients have told me how much it means to them to have someone massage their back, stroke a forearm, or greet them with a hug. Touch is certainly a big part of the 'therapeutic package' I give each of my patients. I did sense rather quickly, though, that Jim didn't like to be touched and modified my approach. My sense, from a few comments he made, is that he's probably homophobic [afraid of homosexuals]."

After listening to your colleague, you decide you need to learn more about touch, touch as a therapeutic intervention, and homophobia. You can consult the literature or local experts.

5. Critique Judgment/Decision

Wanting to explore the situation more fully, you responded to the patient initially by saying, "I am sorry that you felt uncomfortable by my colleague's care. I want to talk with him about his sense of what happened and will then discuss this with you when I return on Wednesday." After talking with your colleague, you are reasonably assured that he was not intending, inappropriately, to communicate anything of a sexual nature to the patient. On your return visit to the patient, you inform him about your research and judgment and say, "Touch can mean different things to different people. My sense is that Dave simply wanted to communicate that he cares. If he is going about this in the wrong way, he wants to know what he should be doing differently. We certainly don't want this to be a problem for you or any other patient. Would you like to talk more about this or to file a report?"

You initially think you have three options: (1) to agree at the outset that your colleague has behaved in a sexually inappropriate and unprofessional manner, (2) to investigate the incident and conclude that your colleague was in the wrong, or (3) to investigate the incident and conclude that your colleague was in the right. You chose the third and are relieved when the patient seems to accept your explanation. Two months later, when you receive a similar complaint from another male patient, you are troubled. You realize now that there was a fourth option, and that this is the one you should have taken. Convinced by your colleague's sincerity and good intent, you might nonetheless have informed Dave that you need to communicate this patient's concern to your supervisor so that if future incidents are reported there will be a record of repeat complaints.

PROMOTING HEALTH • 45-1

Sexuality

Use the assessment checklist to determine how well you are meeting your sexuality needs. Then develop a prescription for self-care by choosing appropriate behaviors from the list of suggestions.

Assessment Checklist

almost always	sometimes	almost never

☐ ☐ ☐ 1. I feel positive about my sexual identity.

☐ ☐ ☐ 2. I have satisfying relationships with others.

☐ ☐ ☐ 3. I accept sexual needs as a normal part of life.

☐ ☐ ☐ 4. I am comfortable with physical actions that indicate love and belonging (such as touching and hugging).

Self-Care Behaviors

1. Avoid stereotyping typical gender roles.
2. Learn the biologic aspects of sexual functioning.
3. Ask questions about sexual needs and sexual activity when necessary.
4. Enjoy close relationships with others who love you.
5. Give a hug to someone you love.
6. Accept touch from others as a sign of caring and affection.
7. Practice safer sex (e.g., use contraceptives or condoms, and choose partner carefully).
8. Recognize how age, illness, or disability influences sexual needs and expression.

Level 3: Sexual problem history—obtained by a sex therapist

Level 4: Psychiatric/psychosocial history—obtained by a psychiatric nurse clinician

Each level acquires more specific information from the patient regarding sexual health and also requires the interviewer to have more sophisticated preparation and skills. The professional nurse usually performs a sexual history on level 1.

The nurse sets the tone or atmosphere for the interview. The nurse's attitudes will greatly affect the patient's response to the sexual history, and patients will be more cooperative if they sense the nurse's security and ease during the interview. Privacy is essential for the sexual history; doors should be closed and no interruptions allowed. Sit close to the patient and speak in a quiet, relaxed, objective tone of voice. Use eye contact and open body posture. Explain to the patient that no one will have access to this information unless it is significant to the patient's care.

Obtain reproductive health information first, followed by the sexual health history. The best approach is to begin with general open-ended questions and progress to more specific ones. Try to use the language used by the patient because the patient might be reluctant to admit that he or she does not understand certain terms for fear of appearing ignorant or foolish. For example, the patient might use the term "come" to mean climax or orgasm.

It is useful to begin questions with "many people like" or "many people feel." This gives patients security in knowing they are not alone in how they feel and will encourage them to talk about their problems or concerns. For example, "Many people feel that it's helpful to discuss their concerns about sex with their partner. What do you think about this?"

One helpful structure for obtaining information about sexual problems follows:

- Description of the problem: "How would you describe the problem?"
- Onset and cause of the problem: "What do you think caused the problem, or what was happening when you first noticed it?"
- Past attempts at resolution: "What have you tried in the past to correct the problem?"
- Goals of the patient: "What do you wish to accomplish?"

A narrative form of recording a sexual history is generally used because it allows the interviewer to document the data in many of the patient's own words. If a patient is seeking help for a sexual problem, a more specific format will be used in recording information obtained by a skilled therapist.

A few of the major dysfunctions and assessment priorities are briefly discussed in Table 45-3. See also Focus on the Older Adult.

Physical Assessment

Physical examination of the reproductive or genitourinary system for either male or female patients is necessary under the following circumstances:

- As part of a routine physical examination
- Annual women's healthcare examination, including a Pap smear
- Suspected STI
- Suspected pregnancy
- Workup for infertility

FOCUSED ASSESSMENT GUIDE • 45-1

SEXUALITY

Factors to Assess	Questions and Approaches
Reproductive history	Ask women their date of menarche, date of last menstrual period, duration and length of flow in days, number of pregnancies, living children, miscarriages, abortions, method of birth control. Ask men the number of children they have fathered and method of birth control used. Ask both men and women of childbearing age if they have any concerns about their fertility and determine whether there is any interest in the new reproductive technologies and genetic testing options.
History of sexually transmitted infections	"Do you or a sexual partner have a history of sexually transmitted infections? Many people today have questions about sexually transmitted infections that they are reluctant to express. Do you have any questions? Have you noticed any signs that might indicate a problem?"
History of sexual dysfunction	"Have you ever experienced a problem such as erectile dysfunction, failure to achieve orgasm, or pain during intercourse?"
Sexual self-care behaviors	"Do you perform the breast self-exam (testicular self-exam) on a monthly basis? When was your last gynecologic (urologic) examination (Pap smear, mammogram)? Is there a family history of breast disease, ovarian cancer, testicular cancer, colon cancer? With all the attention on safer sex today and responsible parenting, many people have questions about their sexual self-care behaviors. Do you have any such concerns?" (It is important to ascertain whether patients possess the knowledge, attitudes, and skills necessary to promote their own sexual health and that of others.)
Sexual self-concept	
Sexual identity	"How do you feel about yourself as a man or woman? Is anything changing the way you feel about yourself?"
Sexual body image	"Many people have concerns about their sexual body image. Are you comfortable with your physical maleness or femaleness? Have you experienced any physical changes (e.g., baldness, weight loss or gain, impotence, menopause, mastectomy, hysterectomy, sterilization) that are troubling to you?"
Sexual self-esteem	"We all have certain expectations of ourselves. Are you comfortable with the way you are currently expressing yourself sexually and meeting your sexual needs?"
Sexual role performance	"Has anything interfered with your ability to be a spouse, sexual partner, parent (any other valued sex-related roles)?"
Sexual functioning	"It's not unusual for people with health concerns (name specific medical problem, if appropriate) to have questions related to sexuality and sexual functioning. Do you have any questions or concerns that I can help you with? Has anything (if appropriate, substitute the name of a specific disease, surgery, or medication) changed your ability to function sexually?" (Asking patients if they have questions about resuming their usual sexual activity is an appropriate part of discharge planning for many patients.)

- Unusual lump, discharge, or appearance of the genital organs noticed by the patient
- Request for birth control
- Change in urinary function

The examiner may routinely perform a complete physical examination along with assessment of the reproductive system if the patient has not had contact with the healthcare system within 1 year, or if the assessment findings from a complete examination would be useful in diagnosing an ailment or complaint. See Chapter 25 for a detailed description of how to examine the female and male genitalia.

Initially, ask whether the patient has had this type of examination in the past (if this information is not evident by the patient's records). Depending on the patient's knowledge base, explain the progressive steps of the examination and what the patient may feel during the examination. This will give the patient some feeling of control and security during the examination. The nurse's responsibilities during an examination of the reproductive system are as follows:

- Provide information about the examination.
- Teach the patient.
- Provide support to the patient during the examination.

TABLE • 45-3 SEXUAL DYSFUNCTION AND NURSING ASSESSMENT

Sexual Dysfunction	Assessment Priorities
Male	
Erectile dysfunction (impotence)	• History of diabetes, spinal cord trauma, cardiovascular disease, surgical procedure, alcoholism • Use of certain medications such as antihypertensives, antidepressants, or illicit drugs • Determine degree of mental depression that may be present • Obtain specific information regarding the degree of impotence, length of time of disorder, continuing life factors
Premature ejaculation	• Assess what patient defines as his dysfunction and ability to control ejaculation • Assess any causative relationship factors such as anxiety, guilt, lack of time, and new partner
Retarded ejaculation	• History of neurologic disorders, Parkinson's disease, or use of certain medications • Same assessment priorities as for premature ejaculation
Female	
Inhibited sexual desire	• Use of oral contraceptives or other hormonal therapy, use of alcohol or certain medications • History of sexual abuse, rape or incest, depression, or other sexual dysfunctions • Assess any other contributing or relationship factors
Orgasmic dysfunction	• Assess knowledge level regarding sexual response cycle and anatomy • Assess communication pattern between patient and her partner • Assess usual sexual pattern and behavior between patient and her partner • Assess any other contributing factors
Dyspareunia	• History of diabetes, hormonal imbalance, vaginal infection, endometriosis, urethritis, cervicitis, or rectal lesions • Use of antihistamines, alcohol, tranquilizers, or illicit drugs • Assess patient's ability for vaginal lubrication during sexual act • Assess patient's use of coital positions • Assess use of cosmetic or chemical irritants to genitals, such as deodorant tampons, contraceptive creams or jellies, or condoms • Physical assessment of internal and external genitalia • Assess any other contributing factors
Vaginismus	• Assess knowledge regarding anatomy and sexual response • Assess pattern of sexual activity: how often, level of arousal, orgasm • Assess presence of other sexual dysfunctions • History of sexual abuse, trauma, or rape • Assess patient's feelings regarding her partner • Assess any other causative factors, such as fear of pregnancy, anxiety, guilt • Physical assessment of internal and external genitalia

• Perform the examination or assist the examiner, if appropriate, with any procedures or laboratory studies.

Keeping the patient comfortable and respecting his or her privacy and modesty should be primary nursing considerations. Some female patients might be uncomfortable with male examiners and vice versa for religious, cultural, or other reasons. Sensitivity to these concerns allows the examiner to adapt to these concerns (e.g., to ensure that a female nurse is in the room when a female patient is undergoing a pelvic examination by a male physician).

Diagnosing

Nursing diagnoses written to address problems of sexuality belong to one of two categories:

• *Ineffective Sexuality Patterns:* The state in which an individual experiences or is at risk for a change in sexual health, which results in concern regarding own sexuality.

Sexual health is the integration of somatic, emotional, intellectual, and social aspects of sexual being in ways that are enriching and that enhance personality, communication, and love.

• *Sexual Dysfunction:* The state in which an individual experiences or is at risk for change in sexual function that is viewed as unsatisfying, unrewarding, or inadequate

Related diagnoses include Rape-Trauma Syndrome, Impaired (or Risk for Impaired) Parenting, and Readiness for Enhanced Parenting (NANDA, 2009).

Ineffective Sexuality Patterns or Sexual Dysfunction as the Problem

Before a nursing diagnosis is made regarding a sexual problem, carefully review the assessment data to determine whether the situation can be corrected by independent nursing interventions. Although many problems of sexuality experienced by a

FOCUS ON THE OLDER ADULT

NURSING STRATEGIES TO ADDRESS AGE-RELATED CHANGES IN SEXUALITY AND SEXUAL FUNCTION

Factors that contribute to sexual dysfunction in the older adult are essentially the same as those that affect performance at any age: disease or mutilating surgery of the genitourinary tract, diverse systemic diseases, and emotional disturbances coupled with societal attitudes.

Age-Related Changes	Nursing Strategies
Use of multiple medications	• Educate elderly patients, intimate partners, and family about the sexual side effects of specific medications. Sometimes a change in medication dosage or modification in the treatment regimen can reduce sexual dysfunction.
Dependence on alcohol or marijuana to cope with discomforts of aging, resulting in weakened erection, reduced desire, delayed ejaculation	• Before the patient can decide to stop using alcohol or drugs, he or she must realize the need to change his or her behavior. The nurse can assist in attitude and value clarification about substance use, sexuality, and sexual behavior. Refer the elderly patient to a counselor who can assist with sexual performance problems as well as emotional and dependence problems.
Age-related metabolic disorders such as anemia, diabetes, malnutrition, and fatigue may affect the quality of life and cause impotence.	• Symptoms may be initially discussed with the nurse. The patient may be hesitant to discuss sexual problems openly. Listen carefully. Acknowledge that sexual problems in the elderly are not unusual. Even if the nurse does not know all the answers, active listening on the nurse's part may encourage the patient to visit his or her healthcare provider or a counselor. Encourage elderly patients to have a thorough physical evaluation by a healthcare provider.
Obesity may damage cardiac and vascular integrity and reduce self-esteem, resulting in decreased sexual performance and interest.	• Encourage the patient to seek the advice of his or her healthcare provider and to explore weight reduction and health promotion programs.
Many elderly persons are concerned that sexual activity might increase the risk for illness or even death due to stress on the heart or blood pressure.	• Teach the patient that sexual intercourse and similar forms of sexual expression are not considered dangerous for anyone able to walk around a room and may actually offer physiological benefits.
Radical surgery or dysfunction of the genitourinary tract affects sexual capacity and libido. Extensive surgery due to malignancy may make intercourse difficult or impossible.	• Patients need support and guidance in adjusting to these changes. Provide specific suggestions for how to accommodate to the surgical changes while still maintaining a sexually satisfying relationship. Acknowledge the need for sexual expression in some form or other and provide an open, nonjudgmental response when patients display a need for warmth, close contact, and companionship. Touch is particularly important. An atmosphere of trust between the nurse and the elderly patient is essential.
Loss of a spouse	• Explore alternative forms of sexual expression with patients who are widows and widowers. Encourage them to attend a support group and become active socially. Acknowledge that human sexuality crosses a wide spectrum and that the pattern for each individual is an outcome of his or her development, experiences, and sense of personal identity. The basic pattern is not altered by age or loss of a spouse or loved one. It continues to influence one's capacity for involvement in all life activities.

Murray, R., & Zentner, J. (2000). *Health promotion strategies through the life span.* Upper Saddle River, NJ: Prentice Hall.

patient in a healthcare situation are amenable to nursing action, some require the expertise of other specialties.

> An impotent diabetic patient, such as Jefferson Smith described at the beginning of the chapter, who would benefit from a penile implant, needs medical consultation. A patient with a serious sexual dysfunction or one who practices destructive sexual expression needs intensive therapy

by a clinical psychologist, sex therapist, or counselor. Appropriate referrals by the nurse should follow the identification of such problems. ■

Sexual dysfunction may be specified as erectile failure (impotence), premature ejaculation, retarded ejaculation, inhibited sexual desire, orgasmic dysfunction, vaginismus, or dyspareunia. Common etiologies for sexual dysfunction include effects of medication (specify), effects of alcohol consumption, effects of disease process (specify), history of abuse (specify rape, incest), feelings of depression, guilt, anxiety, fear of rejection, miscommunication with partner, fear of pain, effects of birth control method (specify), lack of knowledge, or effects of surgical procedure (specify).

The nursing diagnosis Ineffective Sexuality Patterns can be further specified by loss of desire (to abstinence), increased desire (to promiscuity), or change in sexual expression. Common etiologies for Ineffective Sexuality Patterns include stress (lifestyle, job, family, finances, marital conflict), isolation from partner, effects of pregnancy (specify), feelings of depression, loss of privacy, loss of communication with partner, relationship change (new partner), effects of disease process (sexual position, frequency, mode of expression), change in body image, change in self-concept, or loss of partner. Some nursing diagnoses concerning sexuality are given in Examples of NANDA Nursing Diagnoses: Sexuality.

Examples of NANDA Nursing Diagnoses

Sexuality

Nursing Diagnoses	Related Factors	Sample Defining Characteristics
Sexual Dysfunction: Erectile Dysfunction	Use of antihypertensive medication	• 45-year-old man with a 3-year history of hypertension • Maintained normotensive on reserpine, 0.25 mg daily • "I have had trouble keeping an erection. My wife and I haven't made love in months. We don't talk about it anymore. I guess that part of my life is over." • Patient appears resigned and saddened.
Sexual Dysfunction: Dyspareunia	Effects of menopausal process	• 54-year-old woman whose last menses was 1 year ago • "Whenever my husband and I make love, my vagina burns and stings." • States decrease in vaginal lubrication during past several months
Altered Sexuality Patterns: Change in Sexual Expression	Loss of privacy due to hospitalization	• 23-year-old man hospitalized for past 6 weeks with injuries resulting from car crash; has been in traction for fractured right femur • "I can't take this place anymore! Everyone barges in here whenever they want to—nobody cares about my feelings—a guy can't even act like a guy around here. I wish I could be alone with my wife for a while with no interruptions."
Altered Sexuality Patterns: Loss of Desire	Change in body image due to body-altering surgery	• Surgery for bowel cancer with construction of permanent colostomy 1 month ago • "I know the colostomy was necessary to save my life, but it is so disgusting. I'll never be able to have a relationship with my husband again. It's a real turn-off to me—just imagine what he'll think—how can I expect him to want to make love to a freak?"
Alteration in Comfort: Pain	Abduction of hips in sexual positioning	• 60-year-old woman with a history of osteoarthritis for 6 years • "The act of intercourse hurts my hips so bad that I'm in pain the whole next day. I don't want to stop having intercourse with my husband, but I'm going to have to if this pain gets worse." • Patient states that the missionary position is the only position used during sex with her husband throughout their 40-year marriage.

Ineffective Sexuality Patterns or Sexual Dysfunction as the Etiology

Changes in sexuality can affect other areas of human functioning. In the following nursing diagnoses, problems of sexuality are the etiology of another problem:

- Impaired Adjustment related to loss of sexual partner, loss of sexual body part
- Anxiety related to fear of pregnancy, loss of sexual functioning or desire, effects of disease process on sexual functioning
- Pain related to sexual position, penile penetration, effects of genital surgery, lack of vaginal lubrication
- Ineffective Coping related to effects of body image on sexual expression, change in sexual partner
- Fear related to pain during sexual intercourse, history of sexual abuse
- Anticipatory Grieving related to loss of sexual functioning, effects of surgical excision of genital body part
- Delayed Growth and Development related to sexual exploitation or abuse, sexual guilt, effects of hormonal imbalance, lack of information about sexuality
- Deficient Knowledge (specify: contraceptive methods, spread of STIs, sexual response, genital anatomy, modes of sexual expression, self-examination, effects of disease or medications) related to misinformation, sexual myths, lack of interest in learning, cognitive limitation
- Disturbed Body Image (specify: surgical excision of genital body part, loss of or gain in body weight) related to fear of rejection
- Impaired Social Interaction related to effects of marital separation or divorce
- Social Isolation related to fear of contracting STI, fear of sexual encounter

Outcome Identification and Planning

Nurses should value sexuality as an important aspect of who the patient is and how the patient is identified as a unique human. Specific patient outcomes to promote sexual health follow. The patient will:

- Define individual sexuality.
- Establish open patterns of communication with significant others.
- Develop self-awareness and body awareness.
- Describe responsible sexual health self-care practices, identifying appropriate resources.
- Practice responsible sexual expression (e.g., by 5/1/12, the patient will use rubber condoms during all sexual encounters).

Specific patient outcomes will depend on the nature of the patient's problem or concern. Expected outcomes should be patient-oriented—that is, something the patient desires to do or has the ability to accomplish. For example, it is not enough to advise a method of birth control; rather, the nurse needs to know which method the patient is motivated and able to use.

Implementing

Establishing a Trusting Nurse–Patient Relationship

It is impossible to address a patient's sexuality if trust has not been developed between you and the patient (see Through the Eyes of a Student). To do so, project an objective, nonthreatening, and nonjudgmental attitude and stress that the information the patient gives will be kept confidential. The nurse who is aware of his or her behavior and verbal and nonverbal cues and anticipates the patient's concerns will help the patient trust the nurse with information of an intimate nature. It is important to establish respect for the patient and empathy before discussing sexual issues. Consider all of the patient's circumstances and

Through the Eyes of a Student

I knew it was going to happen sooner or later. Male nurses are not unheard of in this day and age, but some people just aren't yet ready for us—especially Ethel, a 68-year-old black woman with a deep religious conviction. I concluded this because she called on Jesus for help when I told her that I was her student nurse for the day, and that I would be giving her a bath.

"You're my nurse?" she said. "Help me, Jesus. . . . No, no, you just go on and help somebody else, honey. I've already had my bath," she insisted.

Accordingly, I told her she was mistaken and that I understood her anxiety. Then I proceeded to exaggerate the truth by saying that I had done this before, when really I had given baths before, but not to members of the opposite sex. She thought she was having anxiety!

Next I asked my instructor, Lynn, for help. She quickly assessed the situation and tried to comfort Ethel by vouching for

my professional character and abilities, but still no go. Then I tried appealing to her logic.

"This is a hospital where male doctors examine you all the time. Why is this any different?" I asked. "Because you are not a doctor" was her logical reply.

I felt inadequate. I could not give this woman the care she needed because of my gender. Luckily, in the next bed, Michele was about to give her patient a bath. She offered to give Ethel her bath if I would help her with her patients.

Consequently, Ethel got her bath, and I learned that a nurse has to be flexible as well as willing to ask for and accept help when the patient's quality of care is at stake. This is something I hope to remember throughout my nursing career.

—*Daniel E. Zirolli*
Delaware County Community College, Media, Pennsylvania

Promoting Health Literacy

IN PATIENTS WITH ERECTILE DYSFUNCTION

Patient Scenario

Mr. Jefferson, a middle-aged man, has a history of diabetes and hypertension and is receiving numerous medications as treatment. He tells you, his nurse, that he has been having problems "in the bedroom." He reports difficulty attaining and maintaining an erection. "I probably wouldn't mention this except that I see all those ads for medication for erectile dysfunction—so I guess there's something to help me."

Nursing Considerations: *Tips for Improving Health Literacy*

Tell Mr. Jefferson that erectile dysfunction is a common problem for men with his history and medications—and

that there are several ways to successfully address this problem. Give him an information sheet about erectile dysfunction and tips on finding out more information about the disorder online from a credible source. Encourage him to be prepared to ask his clinician three questions:

- What is my main problem?
- What do I need to do?
- Why is it important to do this?

What additional measures can you take to help increase health literacy in this individual? What other measures would be helpful if Mr. Jefferson does not speak English, cannot read, or has other learning deficits?

---

life experiences and view them using a therapeutic, not a pitying, approach. Only when you are accepted as a trusted, caring person will the patient reveal details of his or her private life, including sexual concerns.

➤ *Review the Reflective Practice display for this chapter. Note how the nursing student initially avoided interpersonal contact with the patient, performing the technical aspects of care but ignoring the patient as a person. Communication and trust did not occur until the patient asked the nursing student about the level of discomfort and the nursing student responded truthfully.* ■

Teaching About Sexuality and Sexual Health

Most nursing interventions pertaining to a patient's sexuality involve teaching to promote sexual health. Major goals of patient teaching are a change in knowledge, a change in patient attitude, or a change in behavior. In some situations, patients need assistance in defining or redefining their sexuality and its importance to their lives. Offering information, dispelling fears, and providing positive reinforcement are some ways to assist patients in increasing their knowledge about their bodies and sexual functioning. Patients might need assistance in modifying behaviors or learning new skills to increase the quality of sexual health and functioning. See the Promoting Health Literacy boxes.

Promoting Health Literacy

IN PATIENTS RECEIVING THE HPV VACCINE

Patient Scenario

Mrs. Smith, mother of 15-year-old Diane Smith, was told by her daughter's high school that all girls must get the HPV vaccine. Mrs. Smith knows that Diane has been dating a boy from school for almost a year, but insists that her daughter "is not sexually active and should not have to get the vaccine." She is primarily concerned that this new vaccine is not safe.

Nursing Considerations: *Tips for Improving Health Literacy*

Tell Mrs. Smith that one in four young women between the ages of 14 and 19 is infected with at least one of the most common STIs, which include the human papillomavirus. Also, many girls between the ages of 11 and 26 get the HPV vaccine. Give both Mrs. Smith and her daughter an

information sheet about the human papillomavirus and the HPV vaccine. Encourage the mother and daughter to be prepared to ask the clinician these questions:

- What problem is the HPV vaccine trying to fix?
- What do I need to know in order to make a good decision about getting the vaccine?
- Why does the school think it is important for all girls to get the vaccine?

What additional measures can you take to help increase health literacy in this mother and daughter? What other measures would be helpful if they do not speak English, cannot read, or have other learning deficits? What other measures could you take if the daughter confides in you that she is sexually active? What additional measure would be necessary if the primary reason for refusing the HPV vaccine was religious?

TABLE • 45-4 SEXUAL MYTHS AND FACTS TO REFUTE THEM

Sexual Dysfunction	Assessment Priorities
Each person is born with a certain amount of sexual drive, which if overdrawn in youth leaves little reserve for later years.	Actually, the correlation between sexual activity and length of time it persists throughout life is just the opposite. The more consistently sexually active a person is, the longer the activity continues into the later years of life.
The need for expressing one's sexuality becomes less important in the latter half of one's life.	Physiologically, sexual desire and ability do not decrease markedly after middle age. The expression of one's sexuality, as an integral part of development, follows the overall pattern of health and physical performance.
Sexual abstinence is necessary in training for sports.	Physiologically, the achievement of orgasm is rarely more demanding than most activities encountered in daily life. The desire for sleep that often follows is most commonly due to factors other than physical exhaustion from sexual activities. There is no scientific evidence that sex "weakens" a person.
Excessive sexual activity can lead to mental illness.	The biologic significance of human sexuality has no greater effect on total development than any other necessary biologic function. There is no scientific basis for believing that one will develop a mental or physical illness with excessive or no sexual activity.
Wet dreams are indicators of sexual disorders.	Erotic dreams that culminate in orgasms are normal common physiologic phenomena in at least 85% of men. They can occur at any age after puberty. Some women also report in clinical studies that their sexual dreams culminate in orgasm. In women, this phenomenon is believed to increase with advancing age.
Because of the anatomic nature of the sex organs, women are passive and men are aggressive.	Physiologic studies disprove this myth by showing the woman to be far from passive. Maximum gratification requires each partner to be both passive and aggressive in participating mutually and cooperatively.
It is unnatural for a woman to have as strong a desire for sex as a man—women should not enjoy sex as much as men.	These myths have been reinforced by a society that has traditionally taught women that they are to suppress sexual desires to gain love, security, and society's respect, based on the assumption that it is the basic nature of women to be submissive, dependent, and subordinate. Physiologic studies indicate that, in some respects, the woman's sex drive is not only as strong but may be even stronger than that of the man.
Women who have multiple orgasms or who readily come to climax are nymphomaniacs or promiscuous.	Physiologic studies at this time suggest that we do not know women's sexual potential; these studies indicate that there is a wide range of intensity and duration of orgasmic experience, and the potential for multiple or frequent orgasms within a brief period is not at all uncommon. Therefore, women normally may have greater orgasmic capacity than men with regard to duration and frequency of orgasm.
There is a difference between vaginal orgasm and clitoral orgasm.	Physiologic misunderstanding has produced the myth of separate clitoral and vaginal orgasms rather than their interrelations. Female orgasm is normally initiated by clitoral stimulation, but because it is a total-body response, there are marked variations in intensity and timing. There is no reason to believe that the female response to the sex act is due to a vaginal rather than a clitoral orgasm.
A mature sexual relationship requires the man and woman to achieve simultaneous orgasm.	Although simultaneous orgasm may be desirable, it is unrealistic. Often, it is possible only under the most ideal circumstances and is not a determinant of sexual achievement or of satisfaction (except to someone who accepts this as dogma).
It is dangerous to have intercourse during menstruation.	Because the source of the menstrual flow is from the uterus rather than the vagina, there is no basis for concern about tissue damage to the vagina. Actually, the desire for sex increases during the menses as a result of increased pelvic vasocongestion. There is no physiologic basis for abstinence during the menses.
The larger penis has greater possibilities for producing orgasm in the woman.	Physiologically, there is practically no relation between the size of a man's penis and his ability to satisfy a woman sexually. Furthermore, there is little correlation between penile size and body size and their relation to sexual potency.
The face-to-face coital position is the proper, moral, and healthy one.	Recent knowledge of human sexual practices dispels this myth with the recognition that there is no normal or single most acceptable sexual position. Whatever position offers the most pleasure and is acceptable to both partners is correct for them. Any variation is normal, healthy, and proper if it satisfies both partners.
The ability to achieve orgasm is an indicator of a person's sexual responsiveness.	Achievement of a satisfactory sexual response is the result of numerous physical, psychological, and cultural influences. Too often, the physical fact of orgasm (or lack of orgasm) is taken to be symbolic of sexual responsiveness and seen out of context of the entire relationship between man and woman.

Part of teaching also includes correcting sexual myths and promoting body awareness. Many people believe things about sex that they have heard from family or friends or as part of their culture that are not true or are not based on scientific data. During the assessment or while providing care, take the opportunity to refute sexual myths and teach factual information (Table 45-4).

Patients might need assistance in becoming familiar with what they believe and feel about their sexual selves. Be helpful in a situation in which a patient has difficulty accepting or developing his or her sexuality by promoting self-confidence and a good self-concept in the patient. When patients feel comfortable about themselves and their sensual feelings, they can begin to focus on how they feel about their sexual functioning and specific sexual expressions.

Getting to know one's physical body is important to healthy sexual development. Every man and woman, sexually active or not, needs to be aware of the appearance of his or her genitalia. Some people, because of their background, feel ashamed and repulsed by their bodies; others feel that touching the body is dirty and might feel guilt and anxiety in stimulating themselves. Patients need assistance in improving body awareness if any of these issues are present. Patients can become accustomed to looking at their bodies by looking at nonthreatening anatomy first and then proceeding to the genitals. This can be done in the shower or with the use of a mirror. Knowing what looks normal can be of great importance so that patients can report the development of an unusual appearance later on.

After patients have developed some degree of comfort in looking at their bodies, they can progress to experiencing touch. Again, patients should progress from nonthreatening parts of the body until the genitals can be touched without stress.

A good exercise for women in developing body awareness is the use of Kegel exercises. These exercises promote good vaginal tone by localizing and strengthening the pubococcygeal muscle. A woman can locate this muscle by stopping a stream of urine midway through urination. Contracting this muscle can be repeated at any time of the day in any circumstance because its performance is undetectable. Some women who practice Kegel exercises have found that their sexual satisfaction is improved.

Promoting Responsible Sexual Expression

Patients need to know how to gain satisfactory sexual experiences while behaving responsibly in their activities. Responsible sexuality encompasses these major areas: the form of sexual expression, the prevention of unwanted pregnancy, the prevention of the spread of STIs, and sex education.

FORM OF SEXUAL EXPRESSION

The form of sexual expression used by patients should not inflict unwanted harm on themselves or others. When sexual expression encroaches on the rights of others, it is neither healthy nor desirable. Sexual acts that violate another's rights are usually considered to be acts of aggression or

hostility rather than stemming from sexual need or desire. Rape, in particular, is motivated by the need to dominate and humiliate the victim.

PREVENTION OF UNWANTED PREGNANCY

Contraception is a process or technique for preventing pregnancy by means of a medication, device, or method that blocks or alters one or more of the processes of reproduction in such a way that sexual union can occur without impregnation. The prevention of unwanted pregnancy must be a conscious decision. Anyone considering the possibility of a sexual encounter who is unprepared for pregnancy should refrain from intercourse or obtain a contraceptive method from a healthcare provider or from the pharmacy; it is too late to think about contraception during sexual intercourse. To practice responsible sexuality, the contraceptive method must be used consistently and according to instructions.

PREVENTION OF STIs

The various STIs are widespread. The only sure way to avoid an STI is to remain a virgin until marriage, to marry a person who is a virgin, and thereafter, never to have sex with anyone else. When this is impractical, there are other practices that can decrease a patient's risk for STIs (see Box 45-1). The American College of Obstetricians and Gynecologists' Committee on Health Care for Underserved Women has published a Committee Opinion on Human Immunodeficiency Virus and Acquired Immunodeficiency Syndrome and Women of Color (2008). In the United States, women of color (primarily African American and Hispanic women) comprise most new cases of HIV and AIDS among women. Most women of color acquire the disease from heterosexual contact, often from a partner who has undisclosed risk factors for HIV infection. A combination of testing, education, and brief behavioral interventions can help reduce the rate of HIV infection and its complications among women of color.

SEX EDUCATION

Sex education is critical to healthy sexual development and safe sexual behaviors. See Examples of Nursing Interventions and Nursing Outcomes Classifications (NIC/NOC): Safe Sex Activities. Information received from peers and friends is almost always inadequate and may be erroneous. Parents should be taught to answer children's questions immediately and accurately.

Considering Contraception

Unintended pregnancy remains a significant women's health issue in the United States as well as a critical social issue. In the United States, 50% of all pregnancies are unplanned; in more than half of them (53%), the couple was using some method of contraception. (This and the statistics that follow about contraceptive methods were obtained from Birth Control: Planned Parenthood Federation of America, Inc., http://www.plannedparenthood.com.) Many unintended pregnancies

Box 45-1 WHAT CAN YOU DO TO PREVENT STIs?

The best way to prevent STIs is to avoid sexual contact with others. If you decide to be sexually active, there are things that you can do to reduce your risk of developing an STI.

- Have a mutually monogamous sexual relationship with an uninfected partner.
- Correctly and consistently use a male condom.
- Use clean needles if injecting intravenous drugs.
- Prevent and control other STIs to decrease susceptibility to HIV infection and to reduce your infectiousness if you are HIV infected.
- Delay having sexual relations as long as possible. The younger people are when having sex for the first time, the more susceptible they become to developing an STI. The risk of acquiring an STI also increases with the number of partners over a lifetime.

Anyone who is sexually active should:

- Have regular checkups for STIs even in the absence of symptoms, and especially if having sex with a new partner. These tests can be done during a routine visit to the doctor's office.
- Learn the common symptoms of STIs. Seek medical help immediately if any suspicious symptoms develop, even if they are mild.
- Avoid having sex during menstruation. HIV-infected women are probably more infectious, and HIV-uninfected women are probably more susceptible to becoming infected during that time.
- Avoid anal intercourse, but if practiced, use a male condom.
- Avoid douching because it removes some of the normal protective bacteria in the vagina and increases the risk of getting some STIs.

Anyone diagnosed as having an STI should:

- Be treated to reduce the risk of transmitting an STI to a sex partner or from mother to baby.
- Discuss with a doctor the possible risk of transmission in breast milk and whether commercial formula should be substituted.
- Notify all recent sex partners and urge them to get a checkup.
- Follow the doctor's orders and complete the full course of medication prescribed. A follow-up test to ensure that the infection has been cured is often an important step in treatment.
- Avoid all sexual activity while being treated for an STI.

Sometimes people are too embarrassed or frightened to ask for help or information. Most STIs are readily treated, and the earlier a person seeks treatment and warns sex partners about the disease, the less likely the disease will do irreparable physical damage, be spread to others, or in the case of a woman, be passed on to a newborn baby.

NIAID is a component of the National Institutes of Health (NIH), which is an agency of the Department of Health and Human Services. NIAID supports basic and applied research to prevent, diagnose, and treat infectious and immune-mediated illnesses, including HIV/AIDS and other sexually transmitted diseases, illness from potential agents of bioterrorism, tuberculosis, malaria, autoimmune disorders, asthma, and allergies. News releases, fact sheets, and other NIAID-related materials are available on the NIAID Web site at http://www.niaid.nih.gov.

Examples of Nursing Interventions and Nursing Outcomes Classifications (NIC/NOC)

Safe Sex Activities

Nursing Interventions	Nursing Outcomes
• Discuss patient's attitudes about various birth control methods.	• Affirms self as a sexual being
• Instruct patient on the use of effective birth control methods, as appropriate.	• Exhibits clear sense of sexual orientation
• Encourage patient to be selective when choosing sexual partners, as appropriate.	• Uses healthy coping behaviors to resolve sexual identity issues
• Stress the importance of knowing the partner's sexual history, as appropriate.	• Reports healthy sexual functioning
• Instruct patient on low-risk sexual practices, such as those that avoid bodily penetration or the exchange of bodily fluids, as appropriate.	• Performs sexually if environment conducive
• Instruct patient on the importance of good hygiene, lubrication, and voiding after intercourse, to decrease susceptibility to infections.	• Performs sexually without coercion of partner
	• Describes risks associated with sexual activity

(From Bulechek, G. M., Butcher, H. K., & Dochterman, J. [Eds.]. [2008]. *Nursing interventions classification [NIC]* [5th ed., p. 735]. St. Louis: Mosby; and Moorhead, S., Johnson, M., Maas, M. L., & Swanson, E. [2008]. *Nursing outcomes classification [NOC]* [4th ed., p. 650–651]. St. Louis: Mosby Elsevier.

result from the use of less effective methods of contraception, such as condoms, spermicide, or barrier methods. The past several years have seen the development of new, easier to use, and more effective methods of contraception. Nurses and nurse practitioners have a responsibility to provide information to women regarding their many contraceptive options.

Patients choose contraception for many reasons and might contact healthcare providers specifically to obtain information about birth control. Some people use contraception for the orderly spacing of pregnancies in a family; others may want to prevent pregnancy from occurring until a family is desired. Some people choose a permanent method to prevent pregnancy from ever occurring. Factors that affect a person's choice of a contraceptive method include age, marital status, desire for future pregnancy, religious beliefs, level of education, cost, and ease of use. Other considerations are the woman's knowledge about available methods, her perceptions of the various methods, and in many cases, her previous experience with contraception.

All contraceptive methods have advantages and disadvantages. Understanding and explaining the available methods thoroughly is a must so that the patient can choose the one that will best meet his or her situation and needs (Box 45-2).

When choosing a contraceptive method, the patient should consider the following:

- How well will it fit into my lifestyle?
- How convenient will it be?
- How effective will it be?
- How safe will it be?
- How affordable will it be?
- How reversible will it be?
- Will it protect against STIs?

METHODS OF CONTRACEPTION
Behavioral

Abstinence is considered a behavioral method of contraception. There are two types of abstinence: continuous and periodic. Choosing abstinence does not mean that a person is sexless. Most people are abstinent at some time in their lives. Abstinence can be a positive way of dealing with sexuality when it represents a well-thought-out decision regarding one's mind, body, spirit, and sexual health.

Continuous abstinence involves not having any sex with a partner at all. It is 100% effective in preventing pregnancy and STIs. However, individuals may find it difficult to abstain for long periods of time. Ending abstinence without being prepared to protect against an unplanned pregnancy or infection might cause additional problems.

Periodic abstinence and fertility awareness methods are two methods of contraception that involve charting a woman's fertility pattern. Periodic abstinence is a method used by some sexually active women to prevent pregnancy. They become familiar with their fertility patterns and abstain from vaginal intercourse on the days they think they could become pregnant. Women who monitor their fertility to prevent pregnancy either abstain from vaginal intercourse for at least one third of each menstrual cycle or use barrier methods during the fertile or "unsafe" period.

Three basic charting methods can be used to predict ovulation in order to plan or prevent pregnancy:

- *Temperature method:* The woman takes her temperature every morning before getting out of bed. Her temperature will rise between 0.4°F and 0.8°F on the day of ovulation and will remain at that level until her next period.
- *Cervical mucus method:* The woman observes the changes in her cervical mucus throughout the first

Box 45-2   KNOWLEDGE DEFICIT: CONTRACEPTIVE METHODS

Assessment Priorities
- Determine past use of contraceptive methods.
- Assess effectiveness and satisfaction with past methods.
- Assess the patient's current knowledge of contraceptive methods.
- Assess frequency of the patient's sexual activity.
- Identify any methods that are unacceptable to the patient.
- Assess motivation of the patient to use certain methods.
- Assess the patient's level of comfort with manipulation of genital body parts.
- Obtain complete patient history and perform a physical examination if indicated.

Expected Outcomes
The patient will achieve the following:
- Choose a contraceptive method that the patient is motivated to use.
- List the adverse effects or danger signs associated with the contraceptive method.
- List the steps needed to use the contraceptive method effectively.
- Use the contraceptive with every act of sexual intercourse.

- Choose a back-up method.
- Report back to the healthcare setting for follow-up as directed.

Nursing Interventions
- Describe in terms at the patient's level of understanding each contraceptive method for which the patient needs information (give objective information in matter-of-fact manner to avoid bias by nurse).
- Describe the effectiveness of each method and side effects or possible complications.
- Instruct the patient in the use of a chosen method, giving step-by-step instructions.
- Advise the patient of the importance of having a back-up method on hand.
- Instruct the patient in the use of the back-up method.
- Have the patient obtain a physical examination if indicated by the chosen contraceptive method (e.g., the pill).
- Instruct the patient to report back in a specified period for follow-up of use of method if indicated (follow-up visits to a healthcare facility are important, particularly if a patient elects to use the pill).

part of the menstrual cycle, until after ovulation. Cervical mucus is normally cloudy, but a few days before ovulation it becomes clear and slippery and can be stretched between the fingers. This indicates the most fertile phase of the cycle. The couple must abstain from vaginal intercourse or use a barrier method during this period to avoid pregnancy.

• *Calendar method:* The woman charts her menstrual cycle on a calendar. The couple must refrain from intercourse or use a barrier method during "unsafe" days.

The best approach to monitoring fertility is to use all three methods; the combination of these methods is called the symptothermal method. Of 100 couples who use any of these methods for 1 year, 20 women will become pregnant with typical use. The failure rate is higher in single women. Using the methods carefully and consistently and avoiding unprotected vaginal intercourse during the fertile phase can give better results.

Coitus interruptus (withdrawal), one of the oldest and most widely used contraceptive methods, is the withdrawal of the penis from the vagina before ejaculation. Pregnancy cannot occur if sperm is kept out of the vagina. Of every 100 women whose partners use withdrawal as a method of contraception, 27 will become pregnant during the first year of typical use. However, pre-ejaculate can contain enough sperm to cause a pregnancy. Pregnancy is also possible if pre-ejaculate or semen is spilled onto the vulva.

Barrier Methods

Barrier methods include the condom, diaphragm, cervical cap, and vaginal sponge used in combination with a spermicidal agent.

Diaphragm. The diaphragm has been used in various forms since ancient times. It is a dome-shaped device made of latex rubber that mechanically prevents semen from coming into contact with the cervix. It is also used to hold a spermicidal jelly in place against the cervix. The diaphragm is placed in the vagina before sexual activity. It fits between the pelvic notch at the front of the vagina to behind the cervix at the back. It should not be detected by either the woman or her partner when correctly situated in the vagina. A diaphragm must be individually fitted during a pelvic examination. The woman needs to be familiar with her body and able to handle her genitals for diaphragm placement and removal. The diaphragm must be worn during each episode of sexual activity and consistently used with a spermicidal agent. Twenty of 100 women who use the diaphragm will become pregnant during the first year of typical use; 6 will become pregnant with perfect use.

Condom. The traditional condom, or "rubber," is used by men, although it is appropriate for a woman to have a condom available for her partner's use. The condom is rolled over the erect penis and collects the semen after ejaculation occurs. If the condom does not have a nipple receptacle end, a small space should be left at the end of the condom to collect sperm (this prevents breakage). Condoms are available over the counter and have had a surge of popularity with the

recent increase in the incidence of HIV/AIDS and other STIs.

A female condom is also available. The female condom is a ringed pouch that unrolls in the vagina. Advantages include the fact that the male does not need to have an erection for the pouch to be used, and it offers significant protection from STIs.

Of 100 women whose partners use condoms, about 14 will become pregnant during the first year of typical use; 2 women will become pregnant with perfect use. The latex condom protects against STIs, including HIV. The latex condom offers better protection against STIs than any other birth control method because it blocks the exchange of body fluids that may be infected.

Cervical Cap. The cervical cap is a thimble-shaped rubber device that is placed over the cervix and may be left there for up to 3 days at a time. Its mechanism of action is similar to that of the diaphragm. Not all women can wear a cervical cap because of individual anatomic differences. There is some evidence to suggest that the cervical cap can cause cervical inflammation and increase the risk for pelvic infection.

Spermicides. Spermicides are used with barrier methods but can also be used alone. Spermicides come in creams, jellies, foams, and suppositories. Although readily available, spermicides are not as effective alone as when combined with another method, such as a diaphragm or a condom.

Vaginal Sponge. The vaginal sponge is a barrier method that contains a spermicide. The sponge acts not only as a barrier between the semen and the cervix but also as a reservoir to hold semen. The vaginal sponge carries some risk of toxic shock syndrome (TSS) and is contraindicated for use in women who have a past history of TSS. Women who use the vaginal sponge must follow package directions carefully and remove the sponge within 24 hours. The vaginal sponge is about as effective as the diaphragm.

Hormonal

Hormonal methods are based on the feedback mechanism of hormones of the menstrual cycle. Synthetic estrogens and progestin chemical compounds are used in the form of a pill, shot, or implant to prevent ovulation.

Oral Contraceptives. The oral contraceptive ("the pill") is the most common contraceptive method and the most popular method for women in their 20s. Most of the harmful side effects and dangers associated with taking the pill are related to the estrogen component. However, most pills currently available contain a small dose of estrogen. The pill has many beneficial noncontraceptive effects. It has been shown to protect women against the development of breast, ovarian, and endometrial cancer. Taken consistently and as prescribed, the pill is almost 100% effective in guarding against pregnancy. However, the cost might be prohibitive to some women. The woman must also be motivated to take a pill every day at the same time. A health history and physical examination by a healthcare provider are necessary to obtain a prescription for oral contraceptives. Some women should not take the pill if they have certain physiologic disorders or diseases. Smoking increases the risks associated with oral contraceptives. Remind women who are taking the pill to take measures to protect themselves from STIs.

Norplant System. The Norplant System is a reversible, 5-year, low-dose progestin-only contraceptive. The system consists of six matchstick-size capsules (made of Silastic tubing) that are placed just under the skin of the woman's upper arm. The average annual pregnancy rate over 5 years is less than 1%. The most common side effect is a change in the menstrual bleeding pattern, including prolonged menstrual bleeding, spotting between menstrual periods, or no bleeding at all.

Implanon. In the Implanon system, a single etonogestrel-containing rod is implanted in the woman through the use of a disposable insertion kit. Removal requires a small incision and takes about 3 minutes. The single-rod system contains 68 mg of etonogestrel in an ethylene vinyl acetate (EVA) copolymer core surrounded by an EVA membrane. The rod releases 67 mcg of etonogestrel daily. This method of contraceptive approaches 100% efficacy. The most common reason for discontinuation is weight gain.

Depo-Provera. Depo-Provera is the brand name of a progestin-only hormonal birth control system. It uses a hormone similar to progesterone, one of the hormones made by a woman's ovaries that regulates the menstrual cycle. It is called depot medroxyprogesterone acetate (DMPA). An injection of DMPA in the buttock or arm can prevent pregnancy for 12 weeks and is 99.7% effective. Protection is immediate if the injection is given on the first day of the woman's period. Irregular bleeding is the most common side effect for women using DMPA. Of every 1,000 women who use Depo-Provera, only 3 will become pregnant during the first year of use.

Transdermal Contraceptive Patch. The transdermal contraceptive patch (Evra) supplies continuous daily circulating levels of ethinyl estradiol (20 mcg) and norelgestromin (150 mcg). The patch is applied weekly on the same day of each week for 3 weeks, followed by a patch-free week. It may be applied to any of four sites: lower abdomen, upper outer arm, buttock, or upper torso (excluding the breast). Women who use the contraceptive patch demonstrate more effective use compared with those using oral contraceptive pills. The patch has been found to have an overall annual probability of pregnancy (method failure plus user failure) of 0.8%. This contraceptive method has the same contraindications as oral contraceptives. The most common side effects include breast symptoms, headache, application site reactions, nausea, upper respiratory tract infection, and dysmenorrhea.

Vaginal Ring. The vaginal ring (NuvaRing) is a soft, flexible, transparent ring made of ethylene vinyl acetate copolymer. It releases approximately 120 mcg of etonogestrel and 15 mcg of ethyl estradiol daily. Each ring is inserted into the vagina and used for one cycle, which consists of 3 weeks of continuous use followed by a ring-free week. Women can insert and remove the ring themselves. It does not need to be fitted, nor does it require particular placement within the vagina. The ring works by inhibiting ovulation in much the same way oral contraceptives do. Used appropriately, the vaginal ring is 99.3% effective in protecting against pregnancy. Benefits of the vaginal ring include ease of use, self-insertion, high degree of effectiveness, and low incidence of negative or adverse effects. The most common side effects include headache, vaginal discharge, vaginitis, vaginal discomfort, foreign body sensation, coital problems, and ring expulsion.

Intrauterine Devices

The intrauterine device (IUD) is an object that is placed by a physician or nurse practitioner within the uterus to prevent implantation of a fertilized ovum. IUDs are small devices made of flexible plastic that provide reversible birth control. IUDs usually prevent fertilization of the egg, but the precise mechanism by which it works is unknown. IUDs seem to affect the way the sperm or egg moves. It may be that substances released by the IUD immobilize sperm. Another possibility is that the IUD prompts the egg to move through the fallopian tube too fast to be fertilized. IUDs that contain copper are more effective for two reasons. The copper affects the behavior of enzymes in the lining of the uterus to prevent implantation and also causes the production of increased amounts of prostaglandin. Only 8 of 1,000 women using copper IUDs will become pregnant with perfect use.

Combination hormonal and IUD contraceptive methods include a T-shaped device with a steroid reservoir around the vertical stem (Mirena). It releases 20 mcg of levonorgestrel daily and provides contraception for up to 5 years. Fertilization is prevented because the device causes changes in cervical mucus and endometrial morphology, inhibition of sperm migration, alteration of sperm–egg binding and ovarian function as well as a foreign body reaction by the uterus. Failure of implantation may occur in some women. Estradiol levels are managed within the usual range of women who are not using contraceptives. Normal function of the ovaries and fertility are restored as quickly after discontinuation as with any IUD. Efficacy approaches 100%. An additional benefit of this contraceptive method is that it controls menorrhagia in pre- and perimenopausal women. Adverse side effects peak at 3 months of use and reduce in frequency after that. The most common side effects include bleeding, depression, headache, acne, and weight changes.

Both types of IUDs have a filament string that serves two purposes. It allows for easier removal by a clinician, and it allows the woman or her clinician to check if the IUD is still in the correct position.

Emergency Contraception

Emergency contraception, often called the "morning after" pill, is designed to reduce the risk of pregnancy after unprotected intercourse. Emergency contraception is provided in two ways:

1. Increased doses of specific oral contraceptive pills. Emergency contraceptive pills can reduce the risk of pregnancy when taken up to 120 hours after unprotected intercourse (ideally within 72 hours).
2. Insertion of a copper IUD within 5 to 7 days after unprotected intercourse.

Sterilization

Sterilization methods should be regarded as permanent and irreversible in both men and women. Although sterilization can sometimes be surgically reversed, the results are not always satisfactory. Sexual desire and ability are unaffected by sterilization.

Sterilization in women is accomplished by surgically severing the fallopian tubes. This procedure, known as tubal ligation, prevents the ovum from traveling down the tube. Tubal ligation is usually performed on an outpatient basis, sometimes under local anesthesia. Postoperative care and recovery time are required after a tubal ligation.

Sterilization in men is accomplished by surgically severing the vas deferens, which prevents sperm from entering the semen. The vasectomy is usually performed in a physician's office under local anesthesia. The man and his partner must use an alternative form of contraception until he has produced two semen analyses with zero sperm. It usually takes about 4 to 6 weeks for all stored sperm to be eliminated from the man's ductal system.

Future Trends

Private industry remains a driving force behind contraceptive research and development. More than 100 experimental contraceptive methods are being studied around the world. The U.S. government contributes to contraceptive research primarily by funding research conducted at the National Institutes of Health.

Almost 40 million women in the United States are at risk for unintended pregnancy. Given that unintended pregnancies are as likely to end in abortion as in birth, there is a clear need to focus on the prevention of unintended pregnancy. Future trends in contraception are likely to be shaped in part by increased awareness of STIs and continuation of the AIDS pandemic. For at-risk women, the emphasis will be on a highly effective primary means of contraception used in conjunction with a barrier method, such as the condom, to prevent STIs.

Female Contraceptives. Most of the contraceptive products that will soon be available for women are refinements of products already available. New barrier methods for women will include enhanced cervical caps and vaginal sponges with microbicides to protect against STIs. New contraceptive pills, patches, and rings for women will use varied combination of hormones. Injectable progestin products might one day protect against pregnancy for up to 90 days. Oral and/or injectable vaccines may one day immunize women against pregnancy. These vaccines might produce antibodies to attack egg or sperm, or the immune system might create antibodies to a crucial type of protein molecule found on the head of sperm. Contraceptive implants designed to remain effective for 2 or 3 years, as well as biodegradable implants with efficacy of up to 18 months, are under development. Computerized fertility monitors that predict ovulation will offer couples who use fertility awareness methods of contraception a much more sophisticated and accurate charting method. Methods for permanent sterilization will expand to include chemical scarring techniques and insertion of fallopian tube chemical plugs and cryosurgery. Temporary sterilization may be effected by the use of silicone plugs.

Unisex Reversible Contraceptives. The concept of unisex reversible contraception is being explored. This method involves a group of drugs called gonadotropin-releasing hormone (GnRH) agonists and can be used to prevent the release of follicle-stimulating hormone (FSH) and luteinizing hormone (LH) from the pituitary gland. The release of FSH and LH triggers ovulation and spermatogenesis. Blocking the release of these hormones will temporarily suppress fertility for women or men. In addition, various contraceptive injections, implants, and vaccines for men are being researched.

Male Contraceptives. Methods of contraception for men continue to be explored. The challenge of developing a reversible method of contraception for men is complicated because men are always producing sperm. Because of this continuous fertility, the opportunities for reversible intervention that are permitted by women's fertility cycles are not available in men. Effective contraceptive methods for men that do not permanently impair fertility have proven elusive, but research continues. Most research has focused on a hormonal approach to decrease spermatogenesis. The major problem is that interference with steroidogenesis might also interfere with the other actions of testosterone such as sexual function, bone and muscle growth, kidney function, and protein anabolism.

Facilitating Coping With Special Sexual Needs

The nurse can help patients cope with sexual concerns generated by diseases and their treatments. Offer anticipatory guidance and information to patients, stressing the importance of open communication with the patient's partner, and also include the partner in teaching.

Start a discussion about possible sexual positions that can reduce pain during coitus. Show the patient drawings of possible sexual positions. Inform the patient that intercourse may be more comfortable if pain medication is taken before beginning sexual activity.

When teaching patients about medications, mention any sexual side effects that may occur to prevent anxiety and depression. Patients should alert the physician if these side effects occur because often the drug dosage can be modified or the drug changed. If patients are unaware of this, they may discontinue the medication on their own rather than sacrifice sexual functioning, if this is an important aspect of life for them.

Healthcare Needs of Lesbian, Gay Male, Bisexual, and Transgender Individuals

The health of lesbian, gay male, bisexual, and transgender (LGBT) individuals requires addressing several issues important to this diverse group. Stigma, as well as a range of other social and cultural factors, affects the health of LGBT people as well as the ability of the healthcare system and

Box 45-3	HEALTH ISSUES FOR THE GAY, LESBIAN, BISEXUAL, AND TRANSGENDER POPULATION

Sexual Behavior
- Hepatitis A and B
- Enteritis
- Human papillomavirus
- Bacterial vaginosis
- Anal cancer
- Other STIs

Cultural Factors
- Body culture: eating disorders
- Socialization through bars: drug, alcohol, and tobacco use
- Nulliparity: breast cancer
- Parenting: insemination questions, mental health concerns
- Gender polarity in dominant culture: conflicts for transgender and intersex persons

Disclosure of Sexual Orientation or Gender Identity
- Psychological adjustment
- Depression

- Anxiety
- Suicide
- Conflicts with family of origin
- Lack of social support
- Physical/economic dislocation

Prejudice and Discrimination
- Provider bias and lack of sensitivity
- Harassment and discrimination in medical encounters, employment, housing, child custody
- Limited access to care or insurance coverage
- "Pathologizing" of gender variant behavior
- Violence against LGBT population

Concealed Sexual Identity
- Reluctance to seek preventive care
- Delayed medical treatment
- Incomplete medical history (e.g., concealed risk, sexually related complications, social factors)

Dean, L., Meyer, I. H., Robinson, K., Sell, R., Sember, R., Silenzio, V., et al. (2000). Lesbian, gay, bisexual, and transgender health: Findings and concerns. *Journal of the Gay and Lesbian Medical Association, 4,* 101–151; Dibble, S., Eliason, M. J., DeJoseph, J. F., & Chinn, P. (2008). Sexual issues in special populations: Lesbian and gay individuals. *Seminars in Oncology Nursing, 24*(2), 127–130.

providers to care for them. LGBT people come from diverse cultural backgrounds, have varied ethnic or racial identity, and differ in terms of education, age, income, and place of residence. Lesbian, gay, and bisexual people are defined by their sexual orientation, and this definition is complex and variable. Sexual behavior, cultural factors, disclosure of sexual orientation and/or gender identity, prejudice and discrimination, as well as concealed sexual identity each present unique health challenges to this population (Box 45-3).

Other issues that affect healthcare delivery to the LGBT population include the following:

- Public health infrastructure: Efforts to research and address the healthcare needs of LGBT persons are hindered by an inadequate infrastructure to support and fund population-specific initiatives.
- Access to quality health services: Financial, structural, personal, and cultural barriers limit access to screening and prevention services and cause delays in receiving care for acute conditions in the LGBT population.
- Health communication: Negative provider attitudes, lack of provider education regarding unique aspects of lesbian and gay health, and exclusion of same-sex partners in care planning seriously hamper therapeutic communication between members of the LGBT population and those who provide care.
- Educational and community-based programs: Some government agencies, professional organizations, and healthcare organizations address health issues of the LGBT population, but this population still relies heavily on self-created community-based programs to address their special healthcare requirements.

Clearly, significant research is needed regarding the unique experience and healthcare needs of the LGBT population, along with increased education for healthcare providers. Issues of prejudice and inequitable service distribution in the healthcare system will need to be addressed to improve the health of this population.

> *Think back to Paul Rojas, the homosexual patient with AIDS. The nurse needs to be acutely aware of the healthcare delivery system in the community to ensure that Mr. Rojas has access to the most appropriate and needed services. In addition, consultation with social services would be helpful for initiating referrals for appropriate services as Mr. Rojas' condition changes.* ∎

Advocating Sexuality Needs of Patients

A hospital experience or institutionalization puts a strain on a person's individuality and sexual self. Illness may diminish feelings of sexual desire, and the desire for sexual interaction can signal a patient's improving health. The nurse should provide anticipatory guidance because many patients may hesitate to make such a request for fear of being ridiculed. Often, a patient merely desires privacy to hold and caress his or her partner. The intimacy of this act often fulfills the patient's feelings of longing to be needed and loved.

There are many ways to advocate for a patient's sexual needs. Some may seem obvious and commonplace, whereas others may require coming to terms with your own sexuality (Box 45-4).

Box 45-4   ADVOCATING FOR PATIENTS' SEXUAL NEEDS

- All patients should be accepted as sexual beings with the right to be treated with dignity and with sensitivity to their feelings.
- All patients have the right to some degree of privacy.
  - Anticipate the patient's desire for privacy by the simple act of drawing a curtain or closing a door.
  - Patients should be given the option of wearing their own sleepwear to promote sexual identity.
- Potentially shaming situations for the patient should be anticipated.
  - Give information regarding what the procedure is and why it needs to be done, and acknowledge that the patient's embarrassment is normal and understandable.
- Healthcare providers should not simply take for granted that patients do not mind intrusive or embarrassing procedures performed on their bodies and private parts.
- Patients have a right to question the physician regarding sexual needs or future sexual functioning.
  - Anticipate these questions for the patient.
  - Ask patients if they have any concerns regarding sexuality that can be answered by the nurse.

- Nurses can interface with the physician to obtain information required by the patient.
- The atmosphere in healthcare settings needs to allow for sexual expression between patients and their partners.
- Confidentiality is a right of every patient.
  - Do not promise confidentiality if that promise cannot be kept.
  - Allow no one access to the patient's personal records who is not directly involved in the patient's care.
  - Allow no information regarding patients to escape into idle conversation.
- All patients should be referred to formally as Mr., Mrs., Miss, or Ms., according to the patient's preference.
- Visitors, including a visiting spouse, should be referred to as people with genders, rather than as "the visitor."
- Patients should be allowed to keep some personal possessions, if it is practical to do so.

Counseling the Patient Regarding Sexuality

Not all patients with sexual concerns need intensive therapy. Some patients benefit greatly from simply having someone listen to their concerns. Voicing their concerns allows patients to put the information into perspective and focus on what the problem is and how to solve it. When counseling patients, do not offer your own advice, because what is right for one person may be wrong for another. Also, offering false reassurances, such as, "It'll be all right," is unproductive. Rather, adopt an objective, empathic, and receptive attitude to facilitate open communication with the patient.

Abortion Counseling

Abortion remains an issue that deeply divides people. Many believe it is a woman's right to choose whether to continue a pregnancy and then to take safe and legal action if a decision is made to terminate. Others believe that from fertilization onward, a human being exists who commands the full respect and protection we afford adult humans, and thus abortion is always wrong. Some would allow abortion only if it is indicated for a woman's health or in cases of rape. It is important to know what you believe, why you believe this, and how your beliefs are likely to influence your ability to counsel women and couples.

Counseling in Cases of Abusive Relationships and/or Rape

It is not uncommon for nurses to encounter children, adolescents, women, and sometimes men who experience sexual abuse and rape in their relationships or families. The Rape, Incest and Abuse National Network (RAINN) reports that:

- **1 out of every 6 American women** have been the victims of an attempted or completed rape in their lifetime (14.8% completed rape; 2.8% attempted rape).
- **17.7 million American women** have been victims of attempted or completed rape.
- **9 of every 10** rape victims were female in 2003.
- While about **80% of all victims are white,** minorities are somewhat more likely to be attacked.
- About **3% of American men**—or **1 in 33**—have experienced an attempted or completed rape in their lifetime.
- 15% of sexual assault and rape victims are **under age 12.**

Victims of sexual assault are 3 times more likely to suffer from depression, 6 times more likely to suffer from posttraumatic stress disorder, 13 times more likely to abuse alcohol, 26 times more likely to abuse drugs, and 4 times more likely to contemplate suicide. Clearly, nurses need to be alert to evidence of sexual abuse while taking the history and conducting physical examinations. Abuse crosses all socioeconomic and ethnic groups. Become familiar with your legal and clinical responsibilities when a victim is identified. The first priority is getting the victim into a safe environment and mobilizing support for the victim and family. Multiple parties may need therapy. Be familiar with local resources and make appropriate referrals. The National Sexual Assault Online Hotline is a free, confidential, secure service that provides live help over the RAINN Web site http://apps.rainn.org/ohl-bridge/.

Evaluating

To evaluate the plan of care, the nurse needs to use information from the patient for most outcomes. The nurse cannot evaluate the patient by observing his or her expression of sexuality, but the nurse can evaluate how the patient is progressing toward sexuality-oriented goals by his or her appearance, self-confidence, and manner. For example, a patient who has expressed feelings of anxiety in the past over a sexual concern should be observably more confident and free of anxiety if the patient outcomes are being met. Ask the patient about progress toward outcomes. Some outcomes need to be "stepping stones," because not all problems are easily resolved with one-time intervention and direction.

When evaluating a patient's progress, it may help to ask: "In what ways have you been able to achieve [orgasm, increased desire, comfortable intercourse, erection]?" "What methods seemed most effective? Which were not?" "What do you think should be the next step?" Determine from this interaction with the patient whether something more needs to be accomplished. It is not enough to assume that because a set of outcomes has been met, the patient is satisfied with the results. See the Nursing Plan of Care 45-1.

SEXUAL HARASSMENT

Harassment is any annoying or distressing comment or conduct that is known or should be known to be unwelcome. **Sexual harassment** is unwelcome behavior that is sexual or gender-based in nature. This type of harassment usually occurs in the context of an asymmetrical relationship where one person has more formal power than the other (e.g., a faculty member over a student) or more informal power (e.g., one peer over another). Sexual harassment can be directed toward individuals of any age, either gender, and any sexual orientation. There are two forms of sexual harassment: "quid pro quo" and environmental harassment (also called a "hostile" environment).

"Quid pro quo" means something given or withheld in exchange for something else. **Quid pro quo harassment** occurs when an individual's employment or well-being is dependent on agreeing to unsolicited and unwelcome sexual demands. This type of harassment is typically initiated by a person in a position of authority who offers either direct or indirect reward or punishment based on the granting of sexual favors. Quid pro quo harassment is a clear abuse of power and is legally, morally, and ethically wrong.

Hostile environment harassment occurs when behaviors of a sexual or gender-based nature create a hostile, intimidating environment and when this type of environment hurts an individual's work performance, classroom performance, or general sense of well-being. In the workplace, for example, the negative behaviors in hostile environment harassment are not directly linked to job-related consequences; instead, the employee's willingness to suffer the experience of the demeaning environment becomes a condition of employment. This type of harassment is not necessarily caused by a person with formal power. Hostile environment is sometimes difficult to define, as it is not always easy to determine when offensive speech or behavior actually turns to true harassment. Coworkers and peers can create a hostile environment for a member of the group through the following:

- Unwelcome sexually oriented and gender-based behaviors
- Sexual bantering
- Sexual jokes
- Offensive pictures and language
- Sexual innuendoes
- Sexual behavior

Effects of Harassment

Harassment can cause feelings of helplessness, worthlessness, and guilt in the victim. This can often lead to less career satisfaction and feelings of loss of control. Anger is a common emotion experienced by those who have been harassed and may lead to requests for transfer, resignation, or withdrawal from the environment where the harassment occurs. In many cases, job performance is affected due to reduced levels of concentration. Loss of job motivation and skill confidence, along with reduced job satisfaction and organizational commitment, are common.

Responding to Harassment in the Nursing Environment

Inappropriate sexual behavior by a patient may cause the nurse to respond with either passive avoidance or aggressive retaliation. An assertive response is recommended that supports the nurse in maintaining his or her self-respect and encourages the patient to accept responsibility for his or her behavior:

1. Be self-aware: Do not deny feelings about being harassed.
2. Confront: Provide feedback to the patient in a nonthreatening way and clearly state what behavior is or is not acceptable.
3. Set limits: Define clear and reasonable consequences that will be enforced if the behavior continues.
4. Enforce the stated limits: Maintain boundaries.
5. Report: Document the incident and submit to supervisor.

Colleagues may also be the source of harassment. The objective of employers should be to create a positive work environment that is characterized by mutually respectful behavior. Many have taken steps to eliminate hostile work environments by educating employees, developing policies against workplace harassment, and outlining guidelines for responding to sexual harassment:

1. If harassed by a coworker, confront the behavior immediately. An assertive statement is sometimes sufficient to stop the behavior.
2. If the harassment continues, document the date and time and describe the behavior.
3. Consult your supervisor.
4. If the harassment still does not stop, file a grievance with administration.
5. Seek legal advice if all previous efforts to stop the behavior have been unsuccessful.

NURSING PLAN OF CARE · 45-1

For Pete Manheim

Pete Manheim is a 13-year-old adolescent boy attending the area health clinic. He is nervous as he explains to the nurse his need for healthcare. He has noticed "sticky white stuff" around his penis and bedclothes on arising some mornings and fears he may be ill. Pete has also expressed concern about his lack of knowledge regarding sexuality. He has heard a lot of stories from his friends but does not feel he can talk to his parents because the subject has never been broached at home. Also, although Pete is a virgin, he is beginning to feel pressured by his friends, who boast of many sexual experiences.

After spending time in conversation with Pete, the nurse gathered the following data:

- Pete is experiencing nocturnal emissions and has little scientific knowledge about their source.

- Pete is anxious because of the stories regarding sex he has heard from his friends.
- There is no communication or dialogue at home with parents about issues of sexuality.
- Pete is having feelings of insecurity and anxiety about his present virginal status, which he feels he should change.
- Peer pressure from friends is also a concern.

The nurse will work together with Pete to develop a plan of care to correct misinformation and relieve his anxiety. Planning will be directed toward correcting myths and supplying Pete with accurate information. Because Pete has a negligible knowledge base on sexuality, the plan of care will allow for ongoing sessions to augment the initial information. The nurse should outline this plan with Pete to be certain it is acceptable to him.

NURSING DIAGNOSIS   Knowledge Deficit: Adolescent Sexuality Concerns related to misinformation and absent family-based sex education as manifested by self-report

EXPECTED OUTCOME   By the end of the teaching session, the patient will:

- Describe the nature of nocturnal emissions

Nursing Interventions	Rationale	Evaluative Statement
Assess patient's present knowledge base on nocturnal emission and the source of his information.	It is necessary to discover what the patient does know and to build on that knowledge.	8/1/12 Outcome met. Patient able to describe the source of nocturnal emissions.
Use terms that the patient has used and language at the level of the patient's understanding.	This facilitates comprehension.	*R. Gordon, RN*
Teach the patient about nocturnal emissions: • Nocturnal emissions, or "wet dreams," are normal in men of all ages, and they are particularly common in the teenage years. They are not the result of disease. • They occur during sleep as the result of erotic dreams. The "white sticky stuff" is the result of ejaculation of semen from the penis. • This is an involuntary action over which the male has no control.	Knowledge decreases anxiety.	

EXPECTED OUTCOME   By the end of the teaching session, the patient will:

- Differentiate sexual myths from sound knowledge

(continued)

NURSING PLAN OF CARE · 45-1

For Pete Manheim *(continued)*

Nursing Interventions	Rationale	Evaluative Statement
Assess what the patient has heard from peers regarding sexual information:	The nurse can then specifically address the myths to which the patient has been exposed.	8/1/12 Outcome met. Patient was able to differentiate between truth in sexual issues and what is myth.
Myth 1: "A large penis is better for sex than a small one." *Truth:* No relation exists between the size of a penis and the man's ability to perform sexually. When a penis becomes erect, it reaches sufficient size to engage in sexual intercourse.	This enables the patient to develop a positive sexual body image based on fact.	*R. Gordon, RN*
Myth 2: "Jerking off causes blindness. It is a dirty habit." *Truth:* Masturbation or self-stimulation is a natural and healthy outlet for sexual urges. Men and women of all ages masturbate. Masturbation can also teach the person what feels good and what does not. Every person has the right to masturbate if he or she wishes to do so.	The patient is given permission to engage in a sexual activity of a masturbatory nature.	
Myth 3: "It looks bad for a guy to be a virgin—everybody's doing it." *Truth:* No one, whether male or female, should feel pressured into sexual activity at any age. Engaging in sexual activity carries with it a great deal of responsibility and concerns of pregnancy and spread of sexually transmitted infections (STIs). No one needs to know of another person's status if the person chooses not to discuss it.	The patient is given permission to abstain from sexual activity and not to feel pressured by friends. Almost 39% of teens have had sex by age 16 years.	

EXPECTED OUTCOME   By the end of the teaching session, the patient will:

- List the positive aspects of abstinence in a sexual relationship

(continued)

NURSING PLAN OF CARE • 45-1

For Pete Manheim (continued)

Nursing Interventions	Rationale	Evaluative Statement
Assess the patient, including previous discussion of sexual myths and knowledge.	Giving the patient all the information necessary allows him to make an informed decision.	8/1/12 Outcome partially met. Patient able to list verbally all positive aspects of abstinence but is still undecided.
Instruct the patient on the positive aspects of abstinence, including the following:		*Revision:* Reinforce to patient that this is a personal decision that he can make for himself with a good knowledge base. Also, he does not have to make a firm decision for or against abstinence immediately. He should take time to think about this information.
• Engagement in any sexual activity should be a personal decision and not the result of pressure from friends.		
• Abstinence will guarantee protection from pregnancy and from most STIs.	Many young people think they are immune to the consequences of their actions. Therefore, it is important to stress that pregnancy and STIs are very probable results of sexual intercourse.	*R. Gordon, RN*
• People can show affection for each other without sexual involvement.	It is difficult to understand and undertake all the implications of a sexual relationship during the teenage years. The patient learns that a successful sexual relationship requires intimacy, love, and sharing; it should not be merely an outlet for sexual feelings.	
• Every person has the right to say no.	The patient has permission to refuse an activity in which he is not sure he wishes to engage.	

EXPECTED OUTCOME   By the end of the teaching session, the patient will:

• Describe the correct use of rubber condoms

Nursing Interventions	Rationale	Evaluative Statement
Assess what the patient knows about rubber condoms and their use.	Since patient is undecided about whether to initiate a sexual relationship in the future, it is prudent to give him information to protect against pregnancy and STIs.	8/1/12 Outcome met. Patient successfully listed the steps in using a condom.
		R. Gordon, RN
Inform the patient that rubber condoms are available over the counter in drug stores. Prices vary according to type and style.	Patient should know where to purchase condoms and the variety available.	

(continued)

NURSING PLAN OF CARE • 45-1

For Pete Manheim (continued)

Nursing Interventions	Rationale	Evaluative Statement
Teach the patient the steps in using rubber condoms:	Patient should know how to use condoms safely.	
• Roll condom onto the penis as soon as it becomes erect.	Protects against sperm from secretions from Cowper's glands	
• If condom does not have a nipple receptacle end, leave a small space at end of condom to collect semen.	Provides a pocket to collect semen and prevents breakage	
• Immediately after ejaculation, remove penis and condom from vagina by holding onto base of condom.	Prevents spillage of semen into the vagina	
• Discard condom.	Condoms are not meant to be reused. A new condom is used for each act of intercourse.	
Advise the patient to use a condom with every act of intercourse. Spermicides used with condom increase effectiveness.	To be as effective as possible, the condom should be used with every act of intercourse. The rubber condom used with spermicide is effective against pregnancy and the spread of STIs. The woman's use of a spermicide foam in the vagina increases effectiveness.	

EXPECTED OUTCOME   By the end of the teaching session, the patient will:

• Express a decrease in anxiety

Nursing Interventions	Rationale	Evaluative Statement
Assess the patient's anxiety level by verbal and nonverbal behavior.	Patient was anxious when he came into clinic. It is important to evaluate level of anxiety before he leaves. If he is still anxious, reassessment should occur because plan of care may have been unsuccessful.	8/1/12 Outcome met. Patient expressed relief that he is normal. Would like to bring a friend to next session. Future teaching sessions to include these topics identified by patient: • STIs, particularly AIDS • Pregnancy—occurrence and prevention • Sexual expression • Further discussion of sexual myths

R. Gordon, RN

(continued)

NURSING PLAN OF CARE · 45-1

For Pete Manheim (continued)

SAMPLE DOCUMENTATION	8/1/12, 11 am, nursing

SAMPLE DOCUMENTATION

8/1/12, 11 am, nursing
Nursing consultation with 13-year-old patient regarding anxiety about cause and source of nocturnal emissions. Patient also expressed concern about sexual myths he has heard from friends. Stated that much peer pressure exists to become sexually active. Patient admits to possessing little knowledge regarding sexual issues. Feels he cannot discuss sexuality with parents because it is not a topic that has been brought up in the past at home. Will conduct initial teaching session with patient to provide information and decrease anxiety about priority concerns. Patient is willing to return to clinic for at least three more teaching sessions to expand knowledge base of sexuality.

R. Gordon, RN

● Developing Critical Thinking Skills

1. Role-play with another student and perform the interview you would use to obtain a sexual history from the following individuals. Think about how you modified the interview in each situation and why. Identify what made you feel uncomfortable as either the nurse or the patient. Discuss how you can best address this discomfort:
   - Mother voices concern that her 9-year-old son is frequently playing with his penis.
   - Adult man appears distressed when he notes that he has suddenly become impotent with his partner of many years.
   - A high school girl says that her mother tells her something is wrong with her because she is attracted only to women.
   - A new resident in a nursing home complains that he misses his privacy and has nowhere to make love.

2. Describe how you would respond to a newly diagnosed HIV-positive woman with multiple partners who tells you that it is none of your business how she acquired the virus or what she plans to do now that she has it. Think carefully about what is at stake in terms of your response.

3. You know a patient is uncomfortable about undergoing a pelvic examination, and you ask the male physician to wait for you before he begins the examination. He tells you he can't wait and doesn't need your assistance. You know the patient wants another woman in the room. How would you respond, and what is at stake? Does it matter if the reason for the patient's request to have you present is simply preference, is linked to a history of abuse, or is related to her cultural or religious beliefs?

● Practicing for NCLEX

1. What is the term for the cessation of a woman's menstrual activity?
   a. Menarche
   b. Premenstrual syndrome
   c. Menopause
   d. Menstrual dysfunction

2. Masturbation is a technique of sexual expression in which an individual practices self-stimulation. Which of the following is another fact related to masturbation?
   a. Only male adolescents masturbate.
   b. There are serious health risks associated with frequent masturbation.
   c. Individuals who masturbate demonstrate sexual dysfunction.
   d. Masturbation is a means of learning what a person prefers sexually.

3. What term describes stimulation of the female genitals by licking and sucking the clitoris and surrounding structures?
   a. Fellatio
   b. Soixante-neuf
   c. Cunnilingus
   d. Masturbation

4. What is the practice of gaining sexual pleasure while inflicting abuse on another person?
   a. Pedophilia
   b. Voyeurism
   c. Sadism
   d. Masochism

5. Which of the following are appropriate recommendations for anyone who is sexually active to prevent STIs?
   a. Have regular checkups for STIs even in the absence of symptoms.

b. Learn the common symptoms of STIs and seek help immediately if any develop—even if the symptom is mild.

c. Avoid having sex during menstruation.

d. Avoid douching.

e. Avoid anal intercourse, but if practiced, use a male condom.

f. All of the above.

6. A patient tells the nurse that she uses a mechanical barrier for birth control. Which of the following methods fits that category?

a. Diaphragm

b. Oral contraceptive pills

c. Depo-Provera

d. Evra patch

7. A 17-year-old college student calls the emergency room and tells the nurse that she was raped by a professor. She wants to come to the ER but only if the nurse can assure her that they will not call her parents. What should be the nurse's first priority?

a. Getting the patient into a safe environment and mobilizing support for her

b. Encouraging the student to disclose the name of the professor so that his predatory behavior will be stopped.

c. Convincing the student to be assessed for pregnancy, STIs, or other complications.

d. Convincing the student to tell her parents so that she can receive their support.

8. Which of the following statements by a patient indicates a need for teaching about contraception?

a. "Depo-Provera is not effective against sexually transmitted infections, but contraceptive protection is immediate if I get the injection on the first day of my period."

b. "The hormonal ring contraceptive, NuvaRing, protects against pregnancy by suppressing ovulation, thickening cervical mucus, and preventing the fertilized egg from implanting in the uterus."

c. "Abstinence may be an effective method of contraception and may be used as a periodic or continuous strategy."

d. "Withdrawal is an effective method of birth control as well as an effective method of reducing the spread of sexually transmitted infections."

9. What term is defined as the integration of somatic, emotional, intellectual, and social aspects of sexual being in ways that are positively enriching and that enhance personality?

a. Gender role behavior

b. Sexual health

c. Gender identity

d. Sexuality

10. What is the term for unwelcome behavior that is sexual or gender-based in nature?

a. Intimidation

b. Sexual harassment

c. Confrontation

d. Altercation

● Answers With Rationale

1. *c.* Menopause, the cessation of a woman's menstrual cycle, occurs between the ages of 45 and 55 years. The woman may experience irregular menses over time before menstruation ends.

2. *d.* It is a means of learning what a person prefers during stimulation and what feels good. Other facts include that people masturbate regardless of sex, age, or marital status. No known health risks are associated with masturbation. Masturbation is not "wrong" or "dirty."

3. *c.* Cunnilingus is stimulation of the female genitals by licking and sucking the clitoris and surrounding structures.

4. *c.* Sadism refers to gaining sexual pleasure while inflicting abuse on another person.

5. *f.* The National Allergy and Infectious Diseases Institute recommends each of the five statements to those who are sexually active to prevent STIs.

6. *a.* The diaphragm is the only barrier method of contraception listed; all the other methods are hormonal.

7. *a.* While the remaining options may be indicated the *first* priority is to ensure the safety of the woman and to get her the support she needs at this moment.

8. *d.* Withdrawal offers no protection against sexually transmitted infections.

9. *b.* Sexual health is the term that best fits the definition.

10. *b.* Sexual harassment may be defined as any unwelcome verbal or physical advance or sexually explicit statement—such as leers, pats, grabs, jokes, requests for dates, and even rape—that interferes with a person's ability to do his or her job by making him or her feel humiliated, intimidated, or uncomfortable.

Taylor Suite Resources

The Taylor Suite offers these additional resources to enhance learning and facilitate understanding of this chapter:

• thePoint online resource, http://thepoint.lww.com/Taylor7E

• Student DVD-ROM included with the book

• Study Guide for Taylor's Fundamentals of Nursing

BIBLIOGRAPHY

Alfaro-Lefevre, R. (2006). *Applying nursing process: A tool for critical thinking* (6th ed.). Philadelphia: Lippincott Williams & Wilkins.

The American College of Obstetricians and Gynecologists' Committee on Health Care for Underserved Women. (2008). *Opinion on Human Immunodeficiency Virus and Acquired Immunodeficiency Syndrome and Women of Color.* Available at http://www.acog.org/departments/dept_notice.cfm?recno=18&bulletin=4634.

Birth control. Planned Parenthood Federation of America, Inc. Available at http://www.plannedparenthood.org/health-topics/birth-control-4211.htm?__utma=1.2117781371.1274739313.1274739313.1274739313.1&__utmb=1.6.10.1274739313&__utmc=1&__utmx=-&__utmz=1.1274739313.1.1.utmcsr=(direct)|utmccn=(direct)|utmcmd=(none)&__utmv=-&__utmk=35684896

Blair, M. (2004). Sexually transmitted diseases: An update. *Urologic Nursing, 24*(6), 467–474.

Bolte, S., & Zebrack, B. (2008). Sexual issues in special populations: Adolescents and young adults. *Seminars in Oncology Nursing, 24*(2), 115–119.

Bradford, J., Ryan, C., Honnold, J., & Rothblum, E. (2001). Expanding the research infrastructure for lesbian health. *American Journal of Public Health, 91*(7), 1029–1032.

Brown, K., Streubert, G. E., & Burgess, A. W. (2004). Effectively detect and manage elder abuse. *Nurse Practitioner: American Journal of Primary Health Care, 29*(8), 22–27, 31–33.

Bulechek, G. M., Butcher, H. K., & Dochterman, J., (Eds.). (2008). *Nursing interventions classification (NIC)* (5th ed.). St. Louis: Mosby.

Carr, R. L., & Gramling, L. F. (2004) Stigma: A health barrier for women with HIV/AIDS. *Journal of the Association of Nurses in AIDS Care, 15*(5), 30–39.

Centers for Disease Control and Prevention. (2008). Fact sheets. http://www.cdc.gov/std/healthcomm/fact_sheets.htm

Champion, J. D., Shain, R. N., & Piper, J. (2004). Minority adolescent women with sexually transmitted diseases and a history of sexual or physical abuse. *Issues in Mental Health Nursing, 25*(3), 293–316.

Cholewinski, J. T., & Burge, J. M. (1990). Sexual harassment of nursing students. *Image The Journal of Nursing Scholarship, 22*(2), 106–110.

Dean, L., Meyer, I., Robinson, K., Sell, R., Sember, R., Silenzio, V., et al. (2000). Lesbian, gay, bisexual, and transgender health: Findings and concerns. *Journal of the Gay and Lesbian Medical Association, 4,* 101–151.

Dibble, S., Eliason, M. J., DeJoseph, J. F., & Chinn, P. (2008). Sexual issues in special populations: Lesbian and gay individuals. *Seminars in Oncology Nursing, 24*(2), 127–130.

Flinck, A., Paavilainen, E., & Astedt-Kurki, P. (2005). Survival of intimate partner violence as experienced by women. *Journal of Clinical Nursing, 14*(3), 383–393.

Forhan, S. E. (2008). Prevalence of sexually transmitted infections and bacterial vaginosis among female adolescents in the United States: Data from the National Health And Nutrition Examination Survey (NHANES) 2003–2004; Presented at the 2008 National STD Prevention Conference On March 13, 2008 In Chicago. Available at http://Cdc.Confex.Com/Cdc/Std2008/Webprogram/Paper14888.Html

Higgins, A., Barker, P., & Begley, C. M. (2008). "Veiling sexualities": a grounded theory of mental health nurses responses to issues of sexuality. *Journal of Advanced Nursing, 62*(3), 307–317

Krebs, L. U. (2008). Sexual assessment in cancer care: Concepts, methods, and strategies for success. *Seminars in Oncology Nursing, 24*(2), 80–90.

Madison, J., & Minichiello, V. (2000). Recognizing and labeling sex-based sexual harassment in the health care workplace. *Journal of Nursing Scholarship, 32*(4), 405–410.

Magnan, M. A., & Norris, D. M. (2008). Nursing students' perceptions of barriers to addressing patient sexuality concerns. *Journal of Nursing Education, 47*(6), 260–268.

Moorhead, S., Johnson, M., Maas, M. L., & Swanson, E. (2008). *Nursing outcomes classification (NOC)* (4th ed.). St. Louis: Mosby Elsevier.

NANDA International. (2009). *Nursing diagnoses: Definitions & classification, 2009–2011.* Oxford, UK: Wiley-Blackwell.

National Institute of Allergy and Infectious Diseases. Sexually Transmitted Sexually Transmitted Infections. Available at http://www.niaid.nih.gov/healthscience/healthtopics/sti/default.htm. Retrieved August 13, 2008.

Pillitteri, A. (2007). *Maternal and child health nursing* (5th ed.). Philadelphia: Lippincott Williams & Wilkins.

Rawlins, S., & Smith, D. (2002). Innovative contraception: New options in hormonal contraception. *American Journal of Nurse Practitioners, 6*(1), 9–28.

Richardson, M. (2007, September). By the way, doctor, is it safe to take a pill that eliminates periods? *Harvard Women's Health Watch*, 8.

Simpson, P. E., & Fothergill, A. (2004). Challenging gender stereotypes in the counselling of adult survivors of childhood sexual abuse. *Journal of Psychiatric and Mental Health Nursing, 11*(5), 589–594.

Smith, W., Beadle, K., & Shuster, E. (2008). The impact of a group psychoeducational appointment on women with sexual dysfunction. *American Journal of Obstetrics & Gynecology, 198*(6), 697.

Sommers, M. S., & Buschur, C. (2004). Injury in women who are raped: What every critical care nurse needs to know. *DCCN: Dimensions of Critical Care Nursing, 23*(2), 62–68.

Zang, Y., Chung, L., & Wong, T. (2008). A review of the psychosocial issues for nurses in male genitalia-related care. *Journal of Clinical Nursing. 17*(8), 983–998.

Spirituality | 46

KEVIN GARGAN

Kevin, a 38-year-old divorced man on a step-down unit after treatment for a myocardial infarction asks the night nurse, "Did you ever give much thought to whether or not there is a God?" Kevin listed his religion as Protestant but says it's been a long time since he went to church or prayed

CHOI MIN LAI

Choi, a member of the Hmong culture from Laos, is refusing to allow physicians to perform a series of surgical repairs to correct severe deformities of his 8-year-old son's feet. "In our culture, the deformity is a sign of spiritual favor and good luck. Because of Kou's condition, a warrior ancestor whose feet were wounded in battle will no longer be spiritually trapped. You see, Kou is special."

MARGOT ZEUNER

Margot, a 75-year-old woman, is taking care of her 80-year-old husband with advanced Alzheimer's disease, who was just discharged from the hospital and requires constant supervision. When visited at home, she says, "I really miss going to church and seeing everyone. They're so supportive. That was the one thing that helped to keep me going."

After completing the chapter, you will be able to accomplish the following:

1. Identify three spiritual needs believed to be common to all people.

2. Describe the influences of spirituality on everyday living, health, and illness.

3. Differentiate life-affirming influences of religious beliefs from life-denying influences.

4. Distinguish the spiritual beliefs and practices of the major religions practiced in the United States.

5. Identify five factors that influence spirituality.

6. Perform a nursing assessment of spiritual health, using appropriate interview questions and observation skills.

7. Develop nursing diagnoses that correctly identify spiritual problems.

8. Describe nursing strategies to promote spiritual health, and state their rationale.

9. Plan, implement, and evaluate nursing care related to select nursing diagnoses involving spiritual problems.

KEY TERMS

agnostic	spiritual distress
atheist	spiritual healing
faith	spiritual health
hope	spirituality
religion	spiritual needs
spiritual beliefs	

Paying attention to the spiritual dimension of health and well-being is integral to holistic care. Patients facing the losses and limits related to injury, disease, and aging begin to evaluate what is important in life and often ask the "big questions": Is there a God or transcendent being? Does life have meaning and purpose? Am I dying? Is there anyone I can trust to be with me during this hard time? Nurses skilled in spiritual care are able to identify and elicit the inner resources that patients and family caregivers have to promote health and healing with sensitivity to these questions. Many nurses who describe themselves as professional healers use the terms "vocation" or "calling" to describe the work of nursing. They claim to be "standing on holy ground" when they create that

hospitable place where patients can expose their vulnerabilities and face their biggest concerns. We learn, with great humility, that sometimes the most important things we do are accomplished simply by being present to those we serve (see Through the Eyes of a Caregiver). A Baptist woman with a life-threatening cancer who had shared the importance of her spirituality with me recently wrote to me:

> *When you made a cross on my forehead with your thumb, it felt unfamiliar—but perfect. Like a blessing with no conditions—no strings. How liberating. Affirming. Loving. And to think you did it with just your thumb. And your heart. Thank you.*

SPIRITUAL DIMENSION

The "spirit" dimension of the person was first recognized in ancient cultures. One individual often played the roles of both priest and physician ministering to the spirit and the body. Over the years, however, medicine and religion evolved separately. Not until the holistic health movement took root was the person once again viewed as an integrated whole of body, mind, and spirit. Healthcare practitioners began again to probe the relationships among physical, psychological, social, and spiritual health. Two models are currently being used to illustrate these relationships (Fig. 46-1). In the integrated approach, the physio-psycho-socio-spiritual model has four equal dimensions, each of which influences the other. In the unifying approach, the spiritual dimension grounds the physiological, psychological, and sociologic dimensions. While it is interesting to interview professional healers about which model is more consistent with their experience, both demand of the nurse greater competence in identifying and meeting spiritual needs than most practicing nurses today display. National guidelines now mandate spiritual care—see the Joint Commission requirements (2008), the National Palliative Care Consensus Project (2004), and Robert Wood Johnson's Promoting Excellence in End of Life Care Program (2003).

According to Shelly and Fish (1988), there are three **spiritual needs** underlying all religious traditions and common to all people:

1. Need for meaning and purpose
2. Need for love and relatedness
3. Need for forgiveness

Although nurses may differ in their beliefs about how involved they should become in meeting patients' spiritual needs, it is impossible to nurse individuals well while ignoring the spiritual dimensions of health. Nurses can assist patients to meet spiritual needs by offering a compassionate presence; assisting in the struggle to find meaning and purpose in the face of suffering, illness, and death; fostering relationships (with a higher being/humans) that nurture the spirit; and facilitating the patient's expression of religious or spiritual beliefs and practices. (For an example, see the Reflective Practice box on page 1647.)

Through the Eyes of a Caregiver

My name is Janine Landry and I love nursing! I especially have a passion for ER Nursing and I'm pleased to be employed in a faith-based community hospital. I don't feel like I have a job, but rather I look at it as an amazing opportunity to meet people from diverse cultures and beliefs. My work has enabled me to learn and grow both professionally and personally. My dream has always been to become a nurse, to have the opportunity to follow my heart and the purpose of my life—that is, to "*make a difference*." I strive to create an environment of hope and healing and to have an impact on the people from the vulnerable population we serve. I would like to recount a true story that encompasses all that I believe in, and live, as a registered nurse.

I'll never forget the day I walked into the Grey Nuns Hospital and noticed the mission statement posted on the wall. It began with "Healing the Body, Enriching the Mind, Nurturing the Soul," and went on to express the hospital's values and beliefs, all of which I truly support. This mission statement helps to guide my decisions and actions I make every day, and in all areas in which I work. As a clinical nurse educator, I have made it my habit to instruct our newly hired staff to locate the mission statement; read, understand, and respect it; and most importantly; to live it!

In Emergency, we often have repeat visitors and one particular gentleman comes to mind. Fred (*not his real name*) was a "high maintenance" kind of guy who always appeared cranky. He had silky white hair, bright blue eyes, wore a constant frown on his face, and often demanded a lot of attention. Fred had a chronic condition, which resulted in him visiting us on a regular basis. At that time, I was working on the floor and I was often assigned to be his nurse. Fred was somewhat gruff when he spoke to people, and he never called me by my given name, Janine. Although I would remind him, he still chose to call me a myriad of other names.

One day while Fred was in the department awaiting admission to the medical unit, I served him his breakfast tray. He snarled and refused to eat it. I looked at him and said "Fred, you're not eating." He grumbled under his breath and said, "No, I don't want to eat this." "Fred, may I remind you that you're at the Grey Nuns Hospital, and did you know that every meal prepared here is made with love . . . and this breakfast was made especially for you?" "Really . . . it was made with love?" "Absolutely!" Not surprisingly, Fred ate all his breakfast, and later on, he ate his entire lunch. When his wife and friends came to visit him, he would tell them how amazed he was to find out that all his meals were made with love. Every time his wife and daughter would come and visit him, I would look at them and wink; this always made them smile and giggle.

A few months later, Fred was an inpatient once again. Guess which nurse was assigned to him? You're right . . . it was me again. While I was busy changing a wound dressing on his leg, a message came over the hospital intercom system. Fred asked, "What's that noise I hear every morning in this hospital?" "Fred, what may be noise to your ears, is known as a prayer or a reflection to others." He said "What do you call it?" "I personally call it Hope!" "Hope?" "Yes, let me explain. Do you like Neapolitan ice cream?" "Yeah!" "What's your favorite flavor?" "I like all the flavors, but I especially enjoy chocolate and my wife and daughter like the vanilla and strawberry flavors. Why do you ask?" "Imagine this; we'll compare Hope to an entire brick of Neapolitan ice cream that has three individual flavors, right?" Fred nodded and agreed. "For some people, in order to have hope, they need to taste that vanilla flavor, which represents *faith*, and depending on what their beliefs are or what they're faced with at that particular moment, having faith may require *courage*;

that would be the strawberry flavor. Most importantly, to have hope, you need *love*—a sense of love for yourself, to be able to receive love and to love others unconditionally, and for some people it also means loving God. So, just think how lucky you are Fred, knowing your favorite flavor is chocolate . . . that's awesome because everyone knows that chocolate and love are both really good for your heart! You can enjoy each flavor individually . . . and that's o.k. . . . or you can swirl the ice cream and mix it all together to make one flavor; a delicious flavor called HOPE!"

Fred really didn't know how to respond. He looked up at me with his big bright blue eyes and a puzzled look on his face. He then asked me "Are you a tree hugger?" I said no! "Would you ever hug a tree?" I thought about it, and I said "you know, for the right reason and at the right time, yes, I guess I would hug a tree, because a tree symbolizes creation, growth, and change." Fred looked up at me and said, "If I was a tree, what type of a tree would I be?" I quickly replied "Oh . . . without a doubt . . . . you would be an ol' crabapple tree!" Fred started to laugh, it was the first time I had ever heard him laugh, and this laughter came from his toes.

A few weeks later as I was walking in the main lobby of the hospital, I heard a familiar gruff voice calling out to me. I turned around, and sure enough it was Fred and his wife. He asked me to close my eyes and to put out my hand. When I opened up my eyes, Fred had placed the shiniest, most perfect red apple in my hand. I was speechless, but realized that we really had no need for words: our eyes spoke volumes. I'll never forget that moment.

A few months later when Fred returned to the ER, I learned that his wife had recently passed away. Fred was depressed and acutely ill; his chronic condition had worsened and the Cardiologist informed me that Fred was dying and that he was made aware of this. I quickly notified his daughter and then went to his bedside to support him, but he shouted "get out, get away from me, and leave me alone!" I respected his wishes by leaving the room; but I intentionally left the curtain slightly open so that I could continue to monitor him from the nursing desk. While I was charting, I sensed that he was watching me, so I looked up and just like the time before, our eyes silently spoke to each other.

Fred was deteriorating quickly, and his daughter hadn't arrived yet. My shift was over but I couldn't imagine leaving him alone, so I went into his room to say goodnight. Although we both knew it wasn't really "goodnight," I asked him if I could come and sit next to him, and he simply raised his finger and nodded his head. I sat next to him, and for the longest time neither one of us said anything. I held his hand and looked into his blue eyes and said, "what do you need?" His response was "this ol' tree needs a hug!" So I held him tightly in my arms for the longest time, and when his daughter arrived, I gently laid him back and said "good bye." Next, when I stood up, the most amazing thing happened: Fred looked up at me, and despite his labored breathing, he whispered, "Thank you . . . Thank you, Janine." This was truly a precious moment for me because it was the first and only time Fred called me by my given name.

Shortly thereafter, he died. I will never forget this experience because when I walked away I was thinking about the time we had spent together, and although there were many challenging times with this gentleman, I realized that I had grown to respect him. He died with dignity, because I knew who he was, I took the time to get to know what was truly at the "core" of this man. In essence, I got to know what was in his heart . . . and he was truly a gift to me!

—Janine Landry

The Spiritual Dimension: Integrated Approach

The Spiritual Dimension: Unifying Approach

FIGURE 46-1. Spiritual dimensions. No consensus exists about the role of the spiritual dimension in health. (**A**) The *integrated approach* views each of the four dimensions as equal and influencing one another. (**B**) The *unifying model* grounds the physiological, psychological, and social dimensions in the spiritual dimension. (Redrawn from Farran, C. J., Fitchett, G., Quiring-Emblen, C. J., & Burk, J. R. [1989]. Development of a model for spiritual assessment and intervention. *Journal of Religion and Health, 28*[3], 185.)

CONCEPTS RELATED TO SPIRITUALITY AND SPIRITUAL HEALTH

Spirituality, faith, religion, and how these elements influence everyday living and health and illness are important concepts to understand when caring for patients. Although some use the words "spirituality," "faith," and "religion" interchangeably, there are distinctions. These and other concepts are explored below.

Spirituality

Spirituality is anything that pertains to a person's relationship with a nonmaterial life force or higher power. Whereas one person describes spirituality in terms of coming to know, love, and serve God, another speaks of transcending the limits of body and experiencing a universal energy.

Elements of spirituality include:

- Spirituality is experienced as a unifying force, life principle, essence of being.
- Spirituality is expressed and experienced in and through connectedness with nature, the earth, the environment, and the cosmos.
- People express and experience spirituality in and through connectedness with other people.
- Spirituality shapes the self-becoming and is reflected in one's being, knowing, and doing.
- Spirituality permeates life; providing purpose, meaning, strength, and guidance; and shaping the journey (Burghardt & Nagai-Jacobson, 1997).

While attempting a concept analysis of spirituality through a review of related literature, nurse scholar Bernice

Golberg identified the following phenomena: meaning, presencing, empathy/compassion, giving hope, love, religion/transcendence, touch and healing. All appeared to be products of relationships, some physical (presencing, touch and healing), and others emotional (meaning, empathy/compassion, hope, love, and religion/transcendence). Golberg collapsed these categories into one and gave spirituality the label "connection" (1998. p. 836).

Faith

Faith generally refers to a confident belief in something for which there is no proof or material evidence. It can involve a person, idea, or thing, and it is usually followed by action related to the ideals or values of that belief. For example, if I have faith in my doctor, parish nurse, or healer, I am more likely to adhere to a prescribed regimen/plan of care and to experience benefits. Similarly, patients who believe in a loving and all-powerful being who knows them and cares for them are often better able to cope with the suffering related to injury and illness. The declaration made by the World Conference of the Religions of Peace in Kyoto, Japan, in 1970 is an excellent example of a confident belief in something for which there is no proof or material evidence. Baha'i, Buddhist, Confucian, Christian, Hindu, Jain, Jew, Muslim, Shintoist, Sikh, and others discovered that the things that unite them were more important than those that divided them. They discovered that they shared:

- A conviction of the fundamental unity of the human family, of the quality and dignity of all human beings
- A sense of the sacredness of the individual person and his conscience

REFLECTIVE PRACTICE

Challenge to Intellectual Skills

During my pediatric rotation, I encountered a Hmong family from Laos whose 8-year-old son, Kou, had horribly deformed feet. It seemed as if the entire healthcare team was united to persuade, cajole, and if necessary force Choi Min Lai, Kou's father, and his mother to authorize a series of surgical repairs. But the parents were adamant in their refusal. In their culture, the deformity was a sign of spiritual favor and good luck. They believed that a warrior ancestor whose own feet were wounded in battle would be released from a form of spiritual entrapment because of their son's condition. This made Kou special in their community. I admired their fierce championing of their beliefs, but my heart ached for Kou because of the difficulties he would face in U.S. society if his feet were not repaired. I didn't know anything about the Hmong culture or their beliefs. As a result, I didn't know which side I should support. I also didn't know much about the legal rights of the parents to refuse a procedure, which although not life saving would clearly benefit their son.

Thinking Outside the Box: Possible Courses of Action

- Remain detached from the conflict and just observe.
- Try to learn more about the family's cultural and religious beliefs to see if this information could be helpful.
- Contact the hospital attorney to find out about the legal rights of the parents to refuse a procedure that while not life saving would clearly benefit their son.

- Use my relationship with the family to try to persuade them to comply.
- Use my knowledge of Kou and his family to try to persuade the healthcare team to respect their wishes.

Evaluating a Good Outcome: How Do I Define Success?

- The healthcare team chooses a course of action that is beneficial to Kou and simultaneously respects the family's religious and cultural beliefs.
- We respect the legal rights of this family.

- My knowledge of the Hmong religion and culture is increased.
- I am faithful to my advocacy obligations.

Personal Learning: Here's To the Future!

Unfortunately, this issue was not resolved during my rotation. In fact, the conflict continued to grow. When I completed my rotation, the hospital was appealing to the court to force the parents to accept surgery. I came to believe that the rights of the parents should be respected. Their cultural community was so strong, and they clearly did not see Kou's condition as a correctable "health problem" but rather a blessing to be enjoyed. While a few other nurses felt the way I did, the physicians and the social worker felt strongly that the parents were wrong. I learned a lot about the Hmong culture, realizing that my practice will continue to surprise me as I encounter patients and families with beliefs and practices very different from mine. As a result of this experience, I hope I will keep an open mind and always be ready to learn.

Reflection

How do you think you would respond in a similar situation? Why? What does this tell you about yourself and about the adequacy of your skills for professional practice? Can you think of other ways to respond? What influence do you imagine the Lai's culture and religion had on their spirituality? How might the spirituality of the physicians influence their actions? The social worker? Other members of the healthcare team? What other skills (cognitive, interpersonal, technical, ethical/legal) would you need to respond well in this situation? Do you agree with the criteria to evaluate a successful outcome? Based on the information provided in Personal Learning, do you think that a successful outcome would be achieved? Why or why not? What would you determine to be a successful outcome?

- A sense of the value of the human community
- A belief that love, compassion, unselfishness, and the force of inner truthfulness and of the spirit have ultimately greater power than hate, enmity, and self-interest
- A sense of obligation to stand on the side of the poor and the oppressed as against the rich and the oppressors
- A profound hope that good will finally prevail

Faith is a term that may also be used to describe a cultural or institutional religion, such as Judaism, Muslim, or Confucianism. An **atheist** is a person who denies the existence of a higher power; an **agnostic** is one who holds that nothing can be known about the existence of a higher power. They deserve respect for what they choose to believe, just as do those who accept a particular religious creed.

Religion

Spirituality and faith may include **religion,** which refers to an organized system of beliefs about a higher power characterized by set forms of worship, spiritual practices, and codes of conduct. Nurses care for people from many different religious traditions. Although it is impossible for nurses to be knowledgeable about all religions, nurses are better able to meet a patient's spiritual needs when they understand his or her religious beliefs and practices. These can directly influence the patient's response to illness and suffering, self-care practices such as diet and hygiene, birth and death rituals, gender roles, spiritual practices, and moral codes. A brief description of the beliefs and health practices of major religious traditions in the United States is provided in Table 46-1. Figure 46-2 depicts the percentages of different religions in the United States.

The *U.S. Religious Landscape Survey* of 35,000 Americans by the Pew Research Center's Forum on Religion & Public Life (2008) finds that most Americans are religious and they have a nondogmatic approach to faith.

- The majority of Americans who are affiliated with a religion do not believe their religion is the only way to salvation. Almost the same number believe that there is more than one true way to interpret the teachings of their religion.
- More than half of Americans rank the importance of religion very highly in their lives, attend religious services regularly, and pray daily.
- A plurality of adults who are affiliated with a religion want their religion to preserve its traditional beliefs and

practices rather than either adjust to new circumstances or adopt modern beliefs and practices.
- Significant minorities across nearly all religious traditions see a conflict between being a devout person and living in a modern society.
- While more than 9 in 10 Americans (92%) believe in the existence of God or a universal spirit, there is considerable variation in the nature and certainty of this belief. Six in ten adults believe that God is a person with whom people can have a relationship; but one in four—including about half of Jews and Hindus—see God as an impersonal force. While roughly 7 in 10 Americans say they are absolutely certain of God's existence, more than 1 in 5 (22%) are less certain in their belief.
- A similar pattern is evident in views of the Bible. Nearly two thirds of the public (63%) take the view that their faith's sacred texts are the word of God. But those who believe Scripture represents the word of God are roughly evenly divided between those who say it should be interpreted literally, word for word (33%), and those who say it should not be taken literally (27%). And more than a quarter of adults—including two thirds of Buddhists (67%) and about half of Jews (53%)—say their faith's sacred texts are written by men and are not the word of God.

Major Religious Traditions in the U.S.	
	Among all adults %
Christian	**78.4**
Protestant	51.3
Evangelical churches	*26.3*
Mainline churches	*18.1*
Hist. black churches	*6.9*
Catholic	23.9
Mormon	1.7
Jehovah's Witness	0.7
Orthodox	0.6
Other Christian	0.3
Other religions	**4.7**
Jewish	1.7
Buddhist	0.7
Muslim*	0.6
Hindu	0.4
Other world religions	<0.3
Other faiths	1.2
Unaffiliated	**16.1**
Don't know/Refused	**0.8**
	100

* From "Muslim Americans: Middle Class and Mostly Mainstream," Pew Research Center, 2007.

Due to rounding, figures may not add to 100 and nested figures may not add to the subtotal indicated.

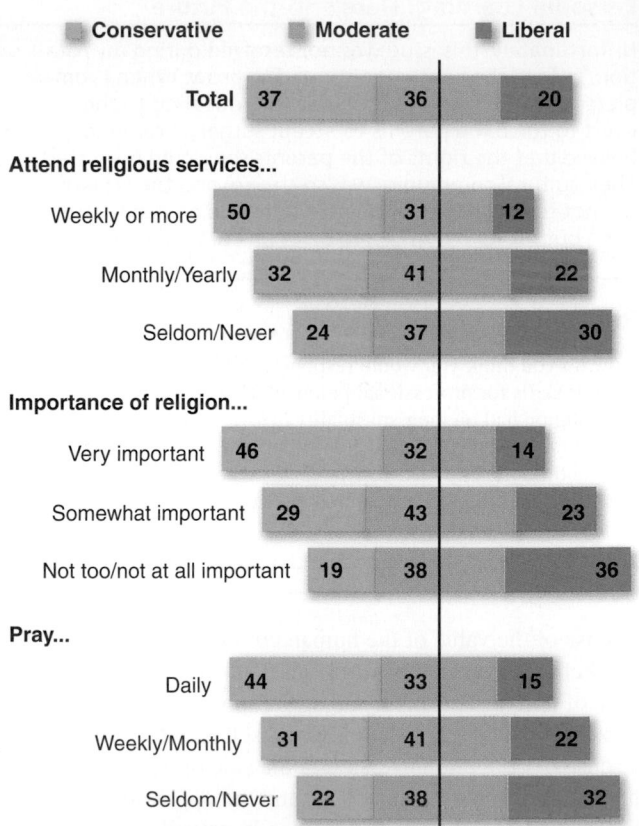

FIGURE 46-2. Based on interviews conducted in English and Spanish with a nationally representative sample of over 35,000 adults, the Pew Research Center's Forum on Religion and Public Life published a landmark survey on religion in the United States. The above graph illustrates the breakdown of U.S. religious practices and political ideology. (Source: U.S. Religious Landscape Survey, Pew Research Center's Forum on Religion & Public Life, http://religions.pewforum.org/. © 2008, Pew Research Center.)

TABLE • 46-1 BELIEFS AND HEALTHCARE PRACTICES OF MAJOR RELIGIOUS TRADITIONS IN THE UNITED STATES

Religion	Beliefs	Select Healthcare Practices
Adventist	Believe in the individual's choice and God's sovereignty. The body is believed to be the temple of the Holy Spirit.	• The taking of all narcotics and stimulants is prohibited because the body is the temple of the Holy Spirit and should be protected. Many groups prohibit meat. • Many regard Saturday as the Sabbath. • Approach to healthcare is holistic.
American Muslim Mission	Accept the Koran as their sacred scripture (see Islam); most stress the importance of cooperation among blacks in business and education to build self-esteem.	• Members are encouraged to obtain healthcare provided by members of the black community. • Major tenets involve prayer rituals, dietary restrictions (prohibitions against pork and alcohol), hygiene (extreme cleanliness), lifestyle modifications, and marital faithfulness.
Baha'i International Community	Believe in a basic harmony between religion and science	• Seek out competent medical care and pray for health • Obligatory prayers, holy days, and the 19-day fast • Permanent sterilization is prohibited, and abortion is discouraged.
Buddhism	Buddha or "the Great Physician" taught the Four Noble Truths to indicate the range of "suffering," its "origin," its "cessation," and the "way" that leads to its cessation. The real cause of human suffering is ignorant craving. The Noble Eightfold Path, which consists of right views, aspirations, speech, conduct, mode of livelihood, effort, mindfulness, and concentration, leads to the cessation of suffering.	• Buddhists do not outwardly proclaim healing through faith. However, spiritual peace and liberation from anxiety attained through the awakening to Buddha's wisdom may be an important factor in expediting healing and the recovery process. • Accepts modern science. The doctrine of avoidance of extremes is applied to the use of drugs, blood, vaccines. • Buddhism does not condone taking lives of any form. • Check with the patient about any special diet restrictions and the observance of holy days.
Christian Scientist	They deny the existence of health crises; sickness and sin are errors of the human mind and can be overcome by altering thoughts, not by using drugs or medicines.	• They will use orthopedic services to set a bone but decline drugs and, in general, other medical or surgical procedures. • They do not allow hypnotism or any form of psychotherapy, which alters the "Divine Mind." • A Christian Science Practitioner may be called to administer spiritual support. • Alcohol and tobacco are not used.
Church of Jesus Christ of Latter Day Saints (Mormons)	Devout adherents believe in divine healing through the "laying on of hands," though many do not prohibit medical therapy. The Church maintains an extensive and well-funded welfare system, including financial support for the sick.	• Disapprove of alcohol, tobacco, and caffeinated beverages • A special undergarment worn by some members should be removed only in an emergency.
Confucianism	Inherent in Confucianism is the appreciation of life and the desire to keep the body from untimely or unnecessary death.	• Appreciate life and desire to keep the body from untimely or unnecessary death • Historically emphasized public health solutions to impending health problems
Daoism (Taoism)	Health is a manifestation of the harmony of the universe, obtained through the proper balancing of internal and external forces. Implicit throughout the Daoist tradition is the tendency to understand salvation in the biomedical sense of health and qualitative improvement and prolongation of human life. The universal principle of the Tao is the mysterious biologic and spiritual life rhythm or order of nature.	• There is a "medicinal" concern for maintaining and prolonging human health and life (sheng). Knowing and living a natural life—following the Tao—is the secret of both health and sagehood. • Long tradition of seeking pragmatic medical techniques, along with its religious techniques of meditation and ritual for establishing a harmony of body and spirit, humanity, and nature (holistic approach)

(continued)

Religion	Beliefs	Select Healthcare Practices
TABLE • 46-1 BELIEFS AND HEALTHCARE PRACTICES OF MAJOR RELIGIOUS TRADITIONS IN THE UNITED STATES *(continued)*		
Hinduism	Doctrine of Transmigration. Moral factors, linked with the all-embracing doctrine of "karma," are believed to be significant in promoting health or causing disease.	• Hindu medicine shows a surprising openness to new ideas, at least in respect to practical treatment. • Many Hindu dietary restrictions conform to individual sect doctrine. • The nurse administering medications should avoid touching patient's lips. • Certain prescribed rites are followed after death; disposal of the body is by cremation.
Jehovah's Witnesses	They oppose the "false teachings" of other sects; opposition often extends to modern science, including medicine.	• Blood transfusions violate God's laws and, therefore, are not allowed. • The courts have not supported the right of Jehovah Witness parents to refuse life-saving treatment for their children. • Use of alcohol and tobacco are discouraged.
Judaism	Formation closely bound with a divine revelation and with commitment to obedience to God's will. The Hebrew Bible is the authority, guide, and inspiration of the many forms of religion of the Jews (currently Reform, Conservative, Orthodox).	• For observant Jews: special needs in the areas of diet, birth rituals, male and female contact, and death • Treatment and procedures should not be scheduled on the Sabbath.
Islam	Allah, one God, who is only one, all seeing, all hearing, all speaking, all knowing, all willing, all powerful Must be able to practice the Five Pillars of Islam May have a fatalistic view of health	• Obligatory prayers, holy days, and fasting (Ramadan), and almsgiving • Koranic law and customs that influence birth, diet (eating pork and drinking alcohol are forbidden), care of women, death and prayer rituals • Some Muslim women are not allowed to make independent decisions; husbands may need to be present when consent is sought.
Native American Religions	Difficult to generalize; notion of cosmic harmony, emphasis on directly experiencing powers and visions and a common view of the cycle of life and death. Death is not the end but the beginning of new life (reincarnation or transcendent hereafter).	• Rituals mark important life changes: birth, puberty, initiation rites, death. • Medicine men and women have specialized spirits from whom they receive the mission to cure. • Common therapeutic measures: sucking, blowing, and drawing out with a feather fan
Protestantism	Worship of the one God revealed to the world through Jesus Christ. Love of neighbor is a central tenet. Other beliefs include sin, redemption, salvation, and a final accounting with God. Care of sick encouraged. God the author and giver of life is also the healer. Most accept modern medical science.	• Religious practices vary according to denomination, may include prayer, faith healing, "laying on of hands," and anointing. • Sacraments: baptism, communion, confirmation
Roman Catholicism	Worship of the one God revealed to the world through Jesus Christ. Love of neighbor is a central tenet. Other beliefs include sin, redemption, salvation, and a final accounting with God. Care of sick encouraged. God the author and giver of life is also the healer. Human life is a gift of God. Many take an antiabortion stance; most accept modern medical science.	• Importance of private devotions and Mass attendance on Sunday • Seven sacraments (importance of baptism, Eucharist, penance, and the anointing of the sick) • Dietary habits • Sexual ethical norms • Only natural means of birth control; abortion, euthanasia, and sterilization are forbidden
Unification Church	God is the living, eternal person who represents universal love and care. God created the world and humans to reflect his nature. The goal of the Unification Church is to unite Christians everywhere as one family under God.	• Most members are still healthy young adults. There is little information available on their interactions with the healthcare team.
Unitarian Universal Association of Churches and Fellowships	Encourage creativity, reason, and living an ethical life. No member is required to adhere to a given creed or set of religious beliefs. The inherent worth and dignity of every person is affirmed.	• Free to accept what they take to be best for their health

The Landscape Survey also reveals that people who are not affiliated with a particular religious tradition do not necessarily lack religious beliefs or practices. In fact, a large portion (41%) of the unaffiliated population says religion is at least somewhat important in their lives, 7 in 10 say they believe in God, and more than a quarter (27%) say they attend religious services at least a few times a year.

Nurses who are unfamiliar with a patient's religion can gain valuable knowledge by discussions with the patient and the patient's family and spiritual adviser.

> *Recall Choi Min Lai, the father of the 8-year-old boy with foot deformities who is refusing surgical repair based on his cultural and religious beliefs. Researching information about the patient's beliefs would be essential in planning this family's care and advocating for the patient and his family.* ∎

It is important to never presume to know what a patient's religious beliefs or practices are upon learning a patient's faith tradition. Many religious groups and individuals work out their own set of beliefs and practices which may or may not be compatible with the tradition at large. Also, you should not interpret the fact that a patient does not belong to an organized religion to mean that the patient has no spiritual needs; a person may be deeply spiritual yet not profess to belong to an organized religion.

Hope

Closely related to spirituality, faith, and religion, **hope** is the ingredient in life responsible for a positive outlook in even life's bleakest moments. It enables an individual both to consider a future and to work to actively bring that future into being. Hope originates in imagination but must become a valued and realistic possibility in order to energize action. Hope has the capacity to embrace the reality of the individual's suffering without escaping from it (false hope) or being suffocated by it (despair, helplessness, hopelessness). Hope is unique to each person. Box 43-6 in Chapter 43 contains a set of suggestions, developed by an interdisciplinary team for enabling hope in the terminally ill, that can apply to any situation in which individuals feel hopeless (Creen, 2002).

Love

Earlier, we noted that people express and experience spirituality in and through connectedness with other people. The popular musical "Les Miserables" put it well in one of its songs, "To love another person is to see the face of God." Love develops from the basic human need to love and be loved, and we cannot be spiritually whole, spiritually healthy, unless this need is met.

Spiritual Health and Healing

Defined most simply, **spiritual health** or well-being is the condition that exists when the universal spiritual needs for meaning and purpose, love and belonging, and forgiveness are met. O'Brien's conceptual model of spiritual well-being in illness (Fig. 46-3) identifies three empirical referents of spiritual well-being: personal faith, spiritual contentment, and religious practice. **Spiritual healing** is the movement toward integration, from brokenness to wholeness.

Spirituality and Everyday Living

Spiritual beliefs and practices are associated with all aspects of a person's life, including health and illness. According to Quinn (2002), the major wisdom traditions address the invisible Spirit—a creative, mysterious, guiding power—by creating principles and practices that:

- Cultivate love of ourselves, our neighbors, of a higher being, and of nature
- Cultivate wisdom that helps us find meaning in life; be in relationships with others; be true to ourselves; live in uncertainty and mystery; deal with suffering, sickness, and death; and honor life's transitions (birth, marriage, death)
- Cultivate awareness of the sacred dimension of life through practices such as worship, prayer, meditation, and singing
- Respect our connectedness as fellow human beings while acknowledging our differences
- Help us be generous in service to others (pp. 13–14)

Religious influences may be life affirming or life denying. Life-affirming influences enhance life, give meaning and purpose to existence, strengthen one's feelings of self-worth, encourage self-actualization, and are health giving and life sustaining. Life-denying influences restrict or enclose life patterns, limit experiences and associations, place burdens of guilt on individuals, encourage feelings of unworthiness, and are generally health denying and life inhibiting.

Spirituality, Health, and Illness

Spiritual beliefs are of special importance to nurses because of the many ways they can influence a patient's level of health and self-care behaviors.

Guide to Daily Living Habits

Certain practices generally associated with healthcare may have religious significance for a patient. For example, many religions have dietary requirements and restrictions. Acceptable birth-control practices are determined by some religious faiths, as are some types of medical treatments (refer back to Table 46-1).

Source of Support

Many people seek support from their religious faith during times of stress. This support is often vital to the acceptance of an illness, especially if the illness brings with it a prolonged period of convalescence or indicates a questionable outcome. Prayer, devotional reading, and other religious practices often do for the person spiritually what protective exercises do for the body physically.

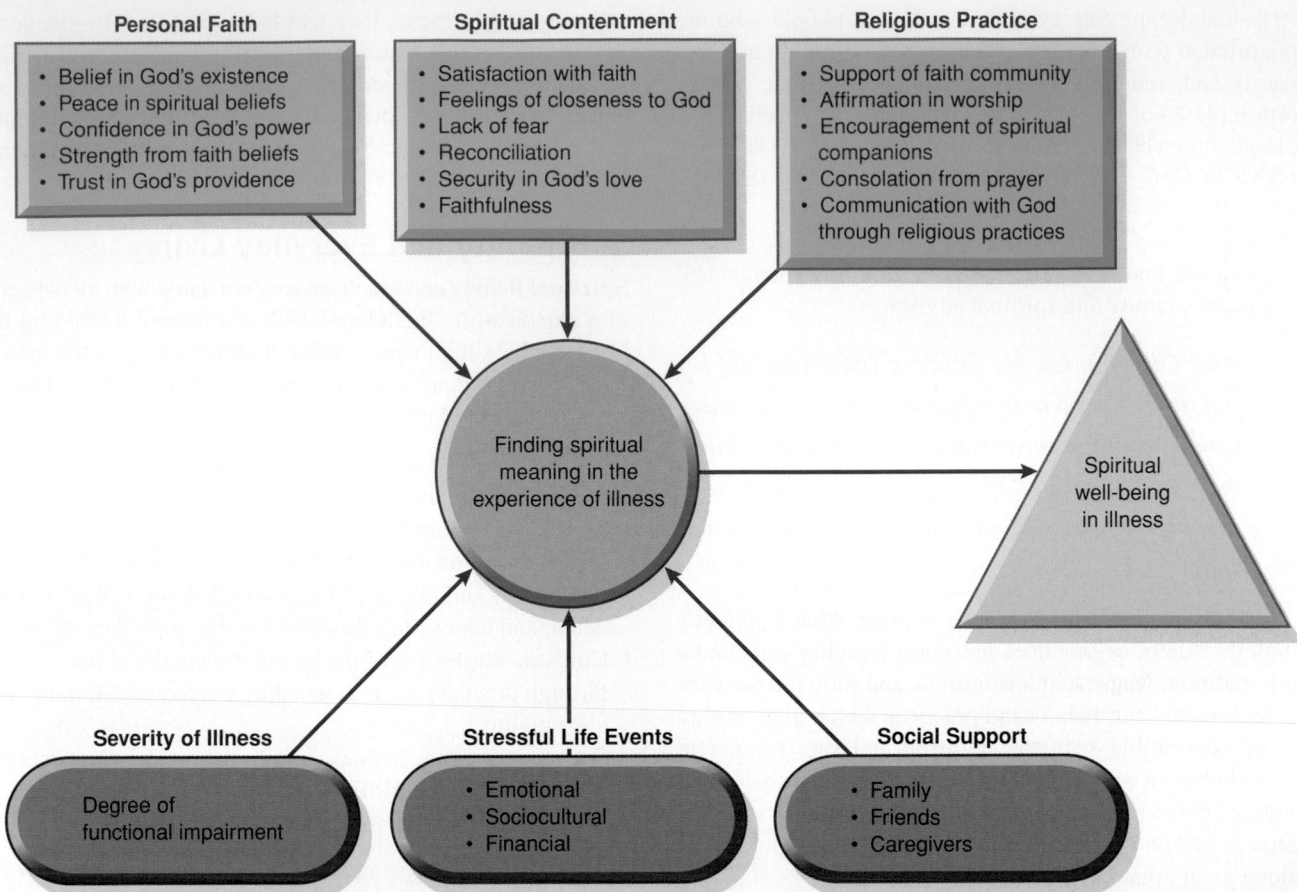

FIGURE 46-3. A conceptual model of spiritual well-being in illness. (Redrawn from O'Brien, M. E. [2003]. *Parish nursing: Healthcare ministry within the church* [p. 109]. Boston: Jones and Bartlett.)

▶ *Think back to Margot Zeuner, the 75-year-old woman caring for her husband with advanced Alzheimer's disease. Assessment reveals that Mrs. Zeuner derived much support from her church group. The nurse, acknowledging the importance of this aspect, could work with Mrs. Zeuner to arrange for assistance at home so that she could attend church activities and continue to receive the support she needs.* ■

Box 46-1 describes how one religion, Buddhism, sees the divine grounding for all human experience, including suffering.

Source of Strength and Healing

The values derived from religious faith cannot be enumerated or evaluated easily. However, the effects attributable to faith are constantly in evidence to healthcare workers. People have been known to endure extreme physical distress because of strong faith. Patients' families have taken on almost unbelievable rehabilitative tasks because they had faith in the eventual positive results of their effort. In the accompanying Through the Eyes of a Patient box, a woman who was faced with life-threatening events describes what

---

Box 46-1 THE CENTER POINT THAT GROUNDS US . . .

. . . I could scarcely make out the large sitting Buddha near the entrance of the house. But what caught my attention was the metal circle with spokes resembling a wheel, hanging over the figure of the Buddha. . . . I asked our host about the wheel. I was told it represented our eternal journey in this life and continuing into the next. Buddha's teachings say that life is suffering. We cannot avoid suffering as we move around the rim of the wheel, which represents perpetual change and the transitory nature of life. But the wheel also symbolizes wholeness or completion because the wheel revolves around the center axis that does not move. That center point represents the presence of the divine. If we remain aware of this center point, we are strengthened for whatever lies ahead.

. . . It is this center point that grounds us in the midst of the many changes in our lives. It is at the center point where we experience the energy and power that turns the wheel. It is at this center point that we connect with the Everywhere Spirit. When we rest in the center point, we find that we have come home again to the place from which we started. But because of the journey, it is as if we had arrived home for the first time. In our journey around the circles of life, we become new persons over and over again.

(From Susan Gregg-Schroeder, *The Journal of Fellowship in Prayer*, April 1999.)

Through the Eyes of a Patient

Seven years ago, I was faced with three life-threatening events in a period of 3 years. Those life-threatening experiences taught me that it is possible to "heal" and to live fully even when we are in the abyss of suffering. I believe everyone would benefit if we redefined "healing." Here are elements I now include in my definition.

Healing is:

- Becoming whole, a life-long journey of becoming fully human, involving the totality of our being: body, mind, emotion, spirit, social, and political context, as well as our relationships with others and with the Divine. Healing does not necessarily mean being happy or getting what we think we want out of life, it means growth, often with pain
- Becoming our authentic self, releasing old unreal self-images, discovering who we really are, not what we think we should be, knowing why we are here and what we really value, restoring our ability to heed our aspirations
- Reconnecting lost aspects of ourselves, paying attention to buried feelings and places inside us that are distressed or sick, enabling us to express our self in fullness, both the light and shadow sides
- Being open to change and new possibilities, responding to problems by changing the picture, being willing to let in more life, to open up to what may have been previously closed or destroyed for us and that which holds promise of giving us new life and fulfillment.
- Facing our fears and refusing to be injured or wounded, changing our belief systems, breaking unnecessary taboos, letting go of what is familiar, and stepping into the unknown
- Accepting that problems, pain, and suffering are part of life and inseparable from us—not a peripheral relationship, not something isolated and avoidable—enabling us to

enter into problems and use suffering, pain, and life-threatening events to enrich our lives.

- Being empowered by the Divine; discovering meaning in our defects, disorders, problems, and disease; experiencing new degrees of creativity and life forces that we might never have imagined before our difficulty; finding that our pains and fears are transformed into relief and confidence.
- Recognizing the value and preciousness of life, knowing that every moment is unique and significant, which usually leads to greater appreciation of the wonder of our minds, bodies, and spirits and of the Divine.
- Having faith and hope—important preconditions for mental and physical health; having a belief in the Divine, the meaning of human life, and the universe; helping us to claim our capacity to create and make something new.
- Finding inner peace, contentment, and tranquility amid the realities of daily life, including its problems, changes, and chaos; experiencing a sense of fullness that makes the burdens of pain or illness lighter.
- Being forgiving of ourselves and others and being forgiven; giving ourselves and others the freedom to let go of rivalry, strife, anger, hatred, fear, and limitations.
- Feeling connected to one another, a sense of interdependence; knowing we are not isolated or autonomous, giving up the illusions of boundaries in life; taking responsibility, acting justly, and accepting that we share our humanity.
- Being loving and loved; loving one's self and wanting to love and serve others, as well as being capable of receiving love; having an ability to trust, a feeling of aliveness, and a sense of greater participation in life.

Used with permission. Carol, J. (2002).
What is healing? Sacred Journey, 53(4), 33–35.

she means by healing, and a caregiver describes a memorable encounter with a burn victim in Through the Eyes of a Caregiver.

Jeff Levin (2001) synthesizes research demonstrating a positive link between health and religion in his seven principles of theosomatic medicine:

1. Religious affiliation and membership benefit health by promoting healthy behavior and lifestyles.
2. Regular religious fellowship benefits health by offering support that buffers the effects of stress and isolation.
3. Participation in worship and prayer benefits health through the physiologic effect of positive emotions.
4. Religious beliefs benefit health by their similarity to health-promoting beliefs and personality styles.
5. Simple faith benefits health by leading to thoughts of hope, optimism, and positive expectations.
6. Mystical experiences benefit health by activating a healing bioenergy or life force or altered state of consciousness.

7. Absent prayer for others is capable of healing by paranormal means or divine intervention (pp. 13–14).

Source of Conflict

Sometimes religious beliefs conflict with prevalent healthcare practices (see Table 46-1). For example, the doctrine of the Jehovah's Witnesses prohibits blood transfusions. In the Islamic religion, humans are regarded as largely helpless in controlling their environment, and illness is accepted as their fate rather than something against which action might be taken. Some Navajos use a lengthy religious ceremony to cure certain diseases, such as tuberculosis. For some people, illness is viewed as punishment for sin and is therefore inevitable.

Such beliefs may require the healthcare worker to modify a treatment plan to accommodate the person's religion. In some instances, acknowledgment of the patient's religious convictions and efforts by health practitioners to accommodate the patient's beliefs can result in quality healthcare without violating the person's religious practices. In other

Through the Eyes of a Caregiver

What's a nice nurse like me doing in a place like this? I belong in Labor and Delivery, with mothers and babies, not in front of our ER trying to help! It is September 11, 2001. Still can't believe what I hear, what I have seen: the World Trade Center buildings, the Pentagon, Pittsburgh. We are at war—oh no! not us! We are the U.S. We don't do homeland war; we are safe.

Oh God! A motorcycle—the driver screaming, "Wounded! Wounded! Pentagon wounded." A hoax? But wait: this is real. No one here to help but me. "How can I help?"

The Pentagon injured—they're coming! His uniform burned but not past recognition. A soldier of the U.S. Army. A U.S. Army officer on a cardboard stretcher, unloaded from the back of an SUV. Time stands still.

"You rode on the sidewalk to get here? The roads were closed?"

His medals still shine.

"I'm here to help you. I will take care of you. Tell me your name."

"I am Brian, and I know you will take care of me. You and God."

Race. Hurry. Run! Doctors, nurses, technicians. Pull, lift. Monitors, IVs, catheters.

"I'm here to help you. I will take care of you."

"I am Brian, and I know you will take care of me. You and God."

His finger is swelling. His ring, it must come off.

"This will hurt, Brian."

"No problem, Ma'am. Just hurry!"

Pull. Pull again. Try harder. Burned skin comes with it. I put it close to my heart. A pocketed wedding ring of a brave man.

I am going to lose it—but his wife will be here soon. Don't lose it. Another soldier.

"Do you know Brian? Take this ring. It's in your pocket now, officer, find his wife."

ET tubes, EKGs, x-rays. Pain, pain, pain.

"You must be Brian's wife. I am so sorry."

How to tell the children? Call his mother? He will be spared. Where was he, the E ring? What did he say to you?

"Before he lost consciousness he told me that God and I were caring for him. He told me he would be OK. He told me he loved you very much. His faith was with him every minute."

Burns, creams, bandages. Lungs OK? Head injury? Critical Care.

I am so angry! This is so wrong, unfair, personal now. I am scared! Whop! whop! whop! The helicopter. Unfrozen air space—for Brian. The Washington Hospital Burn Center.

"I am here to help you. They will take care of you. Good-bye, Brian."

The roads have been closed—tough commute—a whole month! They're reopened today. The Pentagon, a first look. I can see it! Oh, my God, help us! The radio, Q107 News.

"Good news tonight. Word from Washington Hospital Center is that Lt. Colonel Brian . . . has been upgraded from critical condition to stable condition."

Brian, we will never forget. Thank you for letting me take care of you, me and God. You are a hero.

—Judith Rogers, RN
Clinical Educator, Labor and Delivery
Georgetown University

---

situations, an objective explanation of alternative treatments and the predicted consequences of each may help the patient determine acceptable therapy. Whatever the person's decision about healthcare, remember that each person is unique and has a right to pursue his or her own convictions, even though they may differ from those of the healthcare provider.

Healthcare professionals can reduce conflict by attempting to understand how a particular religious culture influences people's thinking about basic questions of biology and ethics. Some of the major questions that religious beliefs, attitudes, and values can affect include (Davis & Zoloth, 1999):

- What is the meaning of suffering?
- How should we regard the physical body and its functions?
- What is the meaning and role of gender differences, sexuality, and reproduction?
- How are we to understand and respond to birth, aging, and death?
- What constitutes the self, and how is selfhood to be assessed?
- How are sin and moral culpability understood? What makes something sinful, and how is sin relieved or absolved?
- What are the tradition's specific bioethical teachings?

> Remember Choi Min Lai, described at the beginning of this chapter. The nurse could use these questions to assess the family's beliefs in greater depth, providing significant data for the healthcare team to incorporate when discussing the possibility of surgery to repair Kou's deformities. Doing so could be helpful in minimizing the conflict between the family and healthcare team. ■

FACTORS AFFECTING SPIRITUALITY

Among the many factors that can influence a person's spirituality, the most important are developmental considerations, family, ethnic background, formal religion, and life events.

Developmental Considerations

Because spirituality has to do with the nonmaterial realm of being, a child must have some capacity for abstract thought before he or she can begin to understand the spiritual self. However, this is not to say that spirituality is meaningless for children. For example, David Heller (1985) interviewed 40 children between 4 and 12 years old who were affiliated with one of four major religions (Judaism, Roman Catholicism, Protestantism, or Hinduism) and discovered that the children had definite perceptions of God. Central themes in all the children's descriptions included the following:

- Notion of a God who works through human intimacy and the interconnectedness of lives
- Belief that God is involved in self-change and growth and transformations that make the world fresh, alive, and meaningful
- Attributing to God tremendous and expansive power and then showing considerable anxiety in the face of this power
- Image of light

As the child matures, life experiences usually influence and mature his or her spiritual beliefs. With advancing years, the tendency to think about life after death prompts some individuals to re-examine and reaffirm their spiritual beliefs. Chapter 18 describes the stages of faith development.

Family

A child's parents play a key role in the development of the child's spirituality. What is important is not so much what parents teach a child about spirituality and religion, but rather what the child learns about spirituality, life, and self from the parents' behavior.

Ethnic Background

Religious traditions differ among ethnic groups. There are clear distinctions between Eastern and Western spiritual traditions as well as among those of individual ethnic groups, such as Native Americans. A person's culture and formal religion have much to do with whether the basic approach to religion is doing something, being someone, or continually striving for harmony.

Formal Religion

Each of the major religious groups discussed earlier in this chapter has several characteristics in common:

- Basis of authority or source of power
- Scripture or sacred word
- An ethical code that defines right and wrong
- A psychology and identity, so that its adherents fit into a group and the world is defined by the religion
- Aspirations or expectations
- Some ideas about what follows death

Life Events

Both positive and negative life experiences can influence spirituality, and they in turn are influenced by the meaning a person's spiritual beliefs attribute to them. For example, if two women who believe in a loving God both lose a child in a car accident, one may bitterly deny God's existence, whereas the other may spend more time in prayer, asking God to help her. Similarly, a chain of successful life experiences (marriage, promotion) may cause one person to assume success and

experience no need for God, whereas for another it occasions deep gratitude and rejoicing.

> *Recall Kevin Gargan who recently experienced a heart attack. It is the experience of his own mortality and the thought that he might have died that now has him questioning whether or not there is a God and if yes, where he stands in relationship to God.* ■

RELIGION AND LAW, ETHICS, AND MEDICINE

Christian Scientists, Jehovah's Witnesses, and members of faith-healing groups are among those challenging the intricate web of rights and responsibilities among individual, society, church, and state. These religious bodies are asking for protection, under the veil of religious freedom, of their right to exercise individual decisions in accordance with scriptural interpretations, even though those decisions may result in the individual's own death or that of a family member, including a child. The most troubling cases are those in which treatable problems, such as bacterial meningitis, diabetes, and bowel obstruction, resulted in the death of minors whose parents chose religious means of healing over traditional medicine. (See Focused Critical Thinking Guide 46-1.) The American Academy of Pediatrics is urging that all child abuse, neglect, and medical neglect statutes be applied without potential or actual exemption for religious beliefs.

Perhaps even more troubling for nurses are situations in which family members insist on care deemed medically futile (i.e., the likelihood of medical benefit is virtually nonexistent) because they believe that God is going to work a miracle. In these cases, simple nursing measures, such as turning or bathing patients, become occasions of pain and torment to both the patient and nurse. Nurses are forced to administer care that they take to be cruel and abusive to patients capable of experiencing pleasure and pain. This nursing care can needlessly prolong a patient's dying. Unfortunately, there are no clear guidelines for drawing the line between promoting life and prolonging the dying process. Although nurses always have the moral right to withdraw from administering care that violates their personal moral code, this does not resolve the problem for the patient. More dialogue is needed on the interaction between religion and law, ethics, and medicine. Ideally, the religious freedom of patients and their families is respected, as is the moral autonomy of caregivers and the integrity of the healing professions. Nurses in these situations should seek the assistance of the ethics committee or ethics consultation service.

> *Consider the situation of Choi Min Lai, the father described at the beginning of this chapter. The nurse is required to respect the family's religious freedom and advocate for them while at the same time acting as a professional member of the healthcare team.* ■

A 16-year-old student approaches you, the school nurse, and confides that she is worried about her brother, who is sick and getting sicker. "My parents are Christian Scientists and have had Christian Science Practitioners in to pray for him, but he seems to be getting worse. I'm afraid he'll die if we don't get him to the hospital." Your first impulse is to visit the student's home to try to see her brother and parents. You immediately remember an article in the paper about the Supreme Court's decision to let stand a Minnesota Court of Appeals ruling upholding an award of $1.5 million to the father of a boy who died in 1989 after his mother, stepfather, and two Christian Scientist Practitioners tried to use prayer to heal his diabetes. Despite their efforts, the boy slipped into a coma and died. What is troubling you is the following comment by Stephen Carter: "By refusing to intervene in *McKown v. Lundman*, the Supreme Court has reinforced a societal message that has grown depressingly common: It is perfectly OK to believe in the power of prayer, so long as one does not believe in it so sincerely that one actually expects it to work—a peculiar fate indeed for our "most inalienable" right" (Carter, S. L. [1996, January 31]. The power of prayer, denied. *The New York Times*, A17). You do believe in the power of prayer and are not sure how you should respond to the student's plea for help for her brother.

1. Identify Goal of Thinking

Clarify 1) what I believe about prayer's power to heal, and 2) what I believe about a parent's right to substitute prayer for modern medicine when a child is seriously ill. Decide how I should respond. What are my professional obligations?

2. Assess Adequacy of Knowledge

Pertinent circumstances: This is the first time I have encountered a family of Christian Scientists. As a school nurse, I am not responsible for my student's brother if he is not in my school and place of employment. That said, I have been asked to help and have the resources to do so.

Prerequisite knowledge: I have no knowledge of what Christian Scientists believe. Moreover, I do not know how the law in our state responds to situations like these. I do not know if any nursing or medical groups have guidelines for situations like these. I immediately get on the Internet to address these deficiencies and also contact my professional nursing organization to see what the law is and if there are any professional organizations that have addressed this issue. I also have to find out how

sick the student's brother is and the probable consequences of his not seeking traditional medical care.

Room for error: The student's brother's very life may depend upon whether or not and how I choose to respond.

Time constraints: Until I learn the exact nature of the boy's medical problems, I cannot know how urgent the need to intervene is.

3. Address Potential Problems

In a situation like this, the most obvious impediments to critical thinking would be (1) the unexamined belief that religion trumps all other considerations ("by golly, this country is founded on respect for religious freedom") and (2) the belief that modern medicine is owed to everyone with a life-threatening illness, no matter what other considerations are present.

4. Consult Helpful Resources

I decide to visit the boy's home with the student and call first to seek the parents' permission. After talking with the parents and seeing the boy, I believe that the boy is in a life-threatening situation because the parents were told that their son has diabetes. I am struck by the love and devotion of both parents and I learn via Internet research that they are doing exactly what their religion prescribes. I later consult with a local Christian Scientist group that confirms this. I learn from my professional nursing organization that there is no consensus about how society should respond in situations like these. Many believe that what these parents are doing is neglect and that if the boy dies, they should be held criminally accountable for manslaughter. Others respect their right to practice their religion. Uncertain of how I should respond, I decide to call Child Protective Services and tell them that I am willing to help if they think my relationship with the daughter would be helpful. I explain to my student what I am doing and tell her to keep me informed and to come back for help if she is not getting the assistance she needs.

5. Critique Judgment/Decision

Child Protective Services did intervene immediately, and the boy was hospitalized and treated against the parents' wishes. While I was happy that the boy's condition was stabilized, I did feel uncomfortable about the disrespect shown to these obviously intelligent, devout, and loving parents. I decided to learn more about how different states are responding to these challenges and to see if nursing can't get involved in some way.

PARISH NURSING

Parish nurse programs are a relatively new movement in faith communities from many denominations. They seek to reclaim the church's role in the ministry of healing and focus again on the impact that spirituality, caring relationships, and a responsibly balanced life can have on health and wellness. Parish nurses and health ministry teams work to reintegrate the healing tradition into the life of faith communities by:

- Interpreting the relationship between faith and health
- Promoting personal responsibility for health and wellness
- Serving as health counselors and educators
- Keeping aware of available resources and making appropriate referrals
- Acting as advocates for people who have health needs but only limited resources
- Recruiting and training volunteers
- Visiting church members
- Initiating caring relationships with the elderly, the chronically ill, and the "worried well."

Parish nurses are not "visiting nurses" or "home health nurses" who provide direct bedside care. The key roles of the parish nurse are health educator, personal health counselor, referral agent, trainer of volunteers, developer of support groups, integrator of faith and health, and health advocate. Nurses who wish to be parish nurses must be registered and compliant with both the state or province practice act and "Scope and Standards of Parish Nursing Practice" (American Nurses Association, 1998).

THE NURSING PROCESS

Nurses who role model good health behaviors are more effective teachers. Use the Promoting Health Display 46-1 for yourself before using it with others. Many nurses approach professional practice as more than a "job" and use the language of "sacred calling" or "vocation" to describe their career choice. Through the Eyes of a Caregiver gives the prayer of one such nurse.

Assessing
Nursing History

Because a person's spirituality and religious beliefs have the potential to influence every aspect of being, an assessment of the patient's spirituality including beliefs and practices, the effect of these beliefs on everyday living, spiritual distress, and spiritual needs should be included in each comprehensive nursing history. There are many guides available to eliciting a spiritual history such as O'Brien (1982), Shelly and Fish (1988), and Puchalski and Romer (2000). One simple guide is Anandarajah and Hight's (2001) HOPE acronym:

H—Sources of hope, meaning, comfort, strength, peace, love, and connection
O—Organized religion
P—Personal spirituality and practice
E—Effects on medical care and end-of-life issue

Additional sample questions are listed in the Focused Assessment Guide 46-1.

If the patient reveals a spiritual problem, use interview questions to determine the specific nature of the problem, its

---

PROMOTING HEALTH • 46-1

Spirituality

Use the assessment checklist to determine how well you are meeting your spirituality needs. Then develop a prescription for self-care by choosing appropriate behaviors from the list of suggestions.

Assessment Checklist

☐ almost always ☐ sometimes ☐ almost never

☐ ☐ ☐ 1. I am comfortable with my spiritual beliefs and values.

☐ ☐ ☐ 2. My beliefs meet my needs for love, belonging, forgiveness, and meaning and purpose.

☐ ☐ ☐ 3. I respect the belief systems of others.

☐ ☐ ☐ 4. I derive sufficient strength from my religious beliefs to meet each day's challenges, especially when confronting pain, suffering, and death.

Self-Care Behaviors

1. Explore personal values and beliefs of self and others.
2. Set aside regular periods to nurture spiritual self.
3. Explore practices that are spiritually supportive.
4. Demonstrate in interaction with others peace, inner strength, warmth, joy, caring, creativity.
5. Respect the belief systems of others.
6. Practice loving relationships with self and others.
7. Seek spiritual assistance to help cope with stress, crisis, or loss.

Through the Eyes of a Caregiver

The Sacred Covenant: A Nurse's Prayer

Gentle God,

You alone are the source of my strength and the center of my life;

Bless my nursing that it may always be guided by the sacred covenant of Your loving care.

Use me as Your instrument in serving the sick;

Use my eyes to look with compassion on those who are broken in body or in spirit;

Use my hands to touch with tenderness those who suffer illness or injury;

Use my lips to speak words of comfort to those who are anxious or afraid.

Dear Lord,

Let me recognize every sickroom as a tabernacle where You dwell; and

Let me not forget, as I care for the ill, that

The ground on which I am standing is holy,

The vocation to which I am called is holy.

Help me to be worthy.

Used with permission. O'Brien, M. E. (2001). The nurse's calling. New York: Paulist Press, p. x.

probable causes, related signs and symptoms, when it began and how often it occurs, how it affects everyday living, the severity of the problem and whether it can be treated independently by nursing or needs to be referred, and how well the patient is coping with the problem.

> *Think back to Kevin Gargan, the man who experienced the heart attack The nurse could use these questions to determine Mr. Gargan's beliefs, thereby developing a plan of care that addresses his current needs. Additionally, this*

FOCUSED ASSESSMENT GUIDE • 46-1

SPIRITUALITY

Factors to Assess	Questions and Approaches
Spiritual beliefs	"Are there particular spiritual or religious beliefs that are important to you? Have these beliefs changed recently? Is your illness challenging these beliefs? Do your religious beliefs in any way dictate a course of action that puts you in conflict with what your physicians are recommending?"
Spiritual practices	"Describe your usual spiritual practices and anything interfering with your ability to perform them. Can I help in any way to secure the aids necessary for these practices (prayer shawl, Bible, crystals, beads, icon)?"
Relation between spiritual beliefs and everyday living	"Describe ways your spiritual beliefs affect everyday living (daily schedule, diet, hygiene, sense of self and the world, relationships). Do you find this influence to be healthy (life affirming) or destructive (life denying)?"
Spiritual deficit or distress	"Are your spiritual beliefs currently causing you any distress?"
Spiritual needs	"In what ways can I and the other nurses help you to meet your spiritual needs?" "Would you like me to contact your spiritual adviser or the hospital's pastoral care minister?"
Need for meaning and purpose	"In what ways do your religious beliefs help or hinder you to understand your current situation and face it with peace and courage?"
Need for love and relatedness	"In what ways do your religious beliefs help or hinder you to meet your need to love and be loved?"
Need for forgiveness	"In what ways do your religious beliefs help or hinder you to feel at peace?"
Significant behavioral observations	Be alert to sudden changes in spiritual practices, mood changes, sudden interest in spiritual matters, and sleep disturbances—all of which may point to unresolved spiritual needs.

assessment would provide valuable information about how the patient is coping with the current situation. ∎

Nursing Observation

Because many patients find it difficult to talk about their spiritual beliefs and problems, also observe the patient's behavior for signs of spiritual distress. A family member or close friend may share significant observations:

- "He's been awfully moody since his heart attack. I can't believe the change in him."
- "I've never seen my father so depressed. He's never in his life been away from the synagogue at Passover. I don't know how to help him."

Significant behavioral observations include sudden changes in spiritual practices (rejection, neglect, fanatical devotion), mood changes (frequent crying, depression, apathy, anger), sudden interest in spiritual matters (reading religious books or watching religious programs on television, visits to clergy), and disturbed sleep. If you observe these behaviors, you should follow up with appropriate interview questions. Often, problems with spiritual distress do not surface until well after a patient's admission history and examination. Effective questions include the following:

- "You've been lying there so quietly. What are you thinking about?"
- "After all you've been through, you must have done a good bit of soul searching. Experiences like these are enough to shake anyone's faith—how is yours holding up?"

Diagnosing

Use each phase of the nursing process when identifying and treating spiritual problems categorized as nursing diagnoses. The NANDA International (2009) diagnoses related specifically to spirituality are:

- Readiness for Enhanced Hope: A pattern of expectations and desires that is sufficient for mobilizing energy on one's own behalf and can be strengthened.
- Hopelessness: Subjective state in which an individual sees limited or no alternatives or personal choices available and is unable to mobilize energy on own behalf.
- Readiness for Enhanced Spiritual Well-being: Ability to experience and integrate meaning and purpose in life through connectedness with self, others, art, music, literature, nature, or a power greater than oneself.
- Impaired Religiosity (or Risk for Impaired Religiosity): Impaired ability to exercise reliance on beliefs and/or participate in rituals of a particular faith tradition.
- Readiness for Enhanced Religiosity: Ability to increase reliance on religious beliefs and/or participate in rituals of a particular faith tradition.
- **Spiritual Distress** (or Risk for Spiritual Distress): Impaired ability to experience and integrate meaning and purpose in life through one's connectedness with self, others, art, music, literature, nature, or a power greater than oneself.

Spiritual distress may be further specified as spiritual pain, alienation, anxiety, guilt, anger, loss, or despair (O'Brien, 1982). Common etiologies for spiritual distress include inability to reconcile current life situations (e.g., illness, death of loved person, divorce) with spiritual beliefs ("God is all-powerful, all-loving, all-wise, and He cares about me") or separation from the religious community or supports. Sample nursing diagnoses of spiritual distress are presented in Examples of NANDA Nursing Diagnoses.

Spiritual distress may affect other areas of human functioning. In the following nursing diagnoses, spiritual distress is the etiology of another problem.

- Impaired Adjustment to Illness related to inability to reconcile illness with spiritual beliefs
- Ineffective Individual Coping related to loss of religion as primary support (feels abandoned by God/higher power)
- Fear related to feeling unprepared for death and afterlife experience
- Dysfunctional Grieving: Despair related to belief that religion is meaningless
- Hopelessness related to belief that no one cares, including God/higher power
- Powerlessness related to feeling victimized by a tyrannical and arbitrary God/higher power
- Self-Esteem Disturbance related to failure to live according to dictates of religion
- Sexual Dysfunction related to values conflict
- Sleep Pattern Disturbance related to spiritual distress
- Risk for Self-Directed Violence related to feeling that life is meaningless

Outcome Identification and Planning
Enhancing Spiritual Health

Show you value spiritual health by being sensitive to the role that spiritual beliefs play in influencing both a person's thoughts about self and the world and his or her interactions with the world. Your interactions with any patient who values spirituality are supportive of the following patient outcomes. The patient will:

- Identify spiritual beliefs that meet needs for meaning and purpose, love and relatedness, and forgiveness.
- Derive from these beliefs strength, hope, and comfort when facing the challenge of illness, injury, or other life crisis.
- Develop spiritual practices that nurture communion with inner self, with God/higher power, and with the world.
- Express satisfaction with the compatibility of spiritual beliefs and everyday living.

Addressing Spiritual Distress

Goals and expected outcomes for patients in spiritual distress need to be individualized and may include a patient achieving some of the following:

- Explore the origin of spiritual beliefs and practices.
- Identify factors in life that challenge spiritual beliefs.

Examples of NANDA Nursing Diagnoses

*Spiritual Distress**

Nursing Diagnoses	Related Factors	Sample Defining Characteristics
Spiritual Pain	Inability to accept death of son	A 46-year-old woman, agnostic, only son died 6 months ago (lung cancer) *"I've often wondered throughout my life if there is a God—thought maybe if I had tried harder I'd have recognized him. Now, I don't care if God exists or not because if he allows this I don't want to know him."* *"My son was my whole life; there's nothing left for me to live for."* Lost 10 lb in 6 months since son died; leaves home only when necessary to purchase food, go to bank, and engage in other routine activities.
Spiritual Alienation	Separated from "faith community"	A 72-year-old Orthodox Jewish man, recently admitted to Protestant nursing home following 3-week hospitalization for stroke *"I guess Yahweh has written me off; first the stroke that killed half my body and then I'm abandoned here where I can't even observe the Sabbath."* *"I want to go home."*
Spiritual Anxiety	Challenged belief and value system	A 37-year-old previously healthy male executive recovering from massive myocardial infarction *"My parents were strict Methodists, but when I left home for college I stopped going to church . . . never gave it much thought . . . there was always something else to do. I started going again but it never meant much."* *"I haven't exactly done anything awful but I've also not been a saint and I find myself wondering if there is a God, what does he think of me."* *"Funny, I guess I thought I'd live forever. I sure never thought about dying and what happens after that."* Often observed lying quietly in bed awake; asked to see minister.
Spiritual Guilt	Failure to live according to religious rules	A 23-year-old, single, Baptist woman being treated for premenstrual syndrome *"I was raised in a strict Baptist home but had to leave . . . I needed more room to be me. I like life here at the university but there's a restlessness in me I can't describe. I've dated several men, one or two I really liked, but I always do something to mess up the relationship. It would kill my mother if she knew I lived with Gary for 3 months."* *"What it really comes down to is my own sense of betraying myself, my family, and my religion. Who am I anyway?"*

(continued)

Examples of NANDA Nursing Diagnoses

*Spiritual Distress** (continued)

Nursing Diagnoses	Related Factors	Sample Defining Characteristics
Spiritual Anger	Inability to accept illness	A 38-year-old homosexual man recently diagnosed with AIDS *"My parents are fundamentalists . . . all I ever heard at home was how much Jesus loves me . . . all the while my mom was beating the daylights out of me. . . . Does He love me? Does He love me so much that He had my parents throw me out when I finally told them I was gay? Does He love me so much that I got AIDS and now no one comes near me?"* Facial features are tight; body held rigidly; speech is sharp, appears angry with God, the world, himself.
Spiritual Loss	Terminal illness; anticipatory grieving; inability to find comfort in religion	A 40-year-old mother of three sons who was diagnosed with ovarian cancer 18 months ago; currently in advanced stage of disease *"I've tried hard to do it all right . . . I read my Bible, prayed every day, went to church each Sunday, loved my husband and kids . . . why is this all happening to me? Why must I lose it all? Where is God now that I need him? Some mornings I wish I could shoot myself and end it all—instead another day drags on. Who can help me?"* Cries frequently, no longer interested in everyday activities of family, no interest in praying, told family not to have pastor call anymore. *"No one can help now."*
Spiritual Despair	Feeling that no one (not even God) cares	A 92-year-old frail widow who lives alone in a two-room apartment; crippled with arthritis; has two married sons she has not seen for years. Says to community nurse who visits every week, *"No one should have to live like this. If it weren't for the neighbor who comes on Saturday with a few groceries and you, I'd be dead. I guess that would be for the best. It's been a long time since I felt like my living or dying would matter to anyone. Because I'm 92 now, I guess even God doesn't want me. Couldn't you do something to put me out of my misery?"*

*NANDA-approved nursing diagnosis label.

- Explore alternatives given these challenges: deny, modify, or reaffirm beliefs; develop new beliefs.
- Identify spiritual supports (e.g., spiritual reading, faith, community).
- Report or demonstrate a decrease in spiritual distress after successful intervention.

Implementing Spiritual Care

A variety of interventions are available to the nurse who wishes to help patients meet their spiritual needs. Like other nursing skills, these interventions need to be practiced before they can be used confidently, competently, and at the right moment. These interventions can be used in the home, hospital, or care center in helping patients meet their spiritual needs. See Examples of NIC/NOC for a list of selected spiritual support activities, and the accompanying Research in Nursing box for nursing roles. Figure 46-4 illustrates an inpatient spiritual care implementation model.

A Word About Ethical and Professional Boundaries

Before exploring spiritual care strategies, remind yourself of the importance of discussing spiritual concerns in a

Examples of Nursing Interventions and Nursing Outcomes Classifications (NIC/NOC)

Selected Spiritual Support Activities

Nursing Interventions	Nursing Outcomes
• Be open to patient's expressions of loneliness and powerlessness • Encourage chapel service attendance, if desired • Encourage use of spiritual resources, if desired • Refer to spiritual advisor of patient's choice • Use values clarification techniques to help patient clarify beliefs and values, as appropriate • Be available to listen to patient's feelings • Express empathy with patient's feelings • Assure patient that a nurse will be available to support patient in times of suffering • Be open to patient's feelings about illness and death	• Quality of faith • Quality of hope • Meaning and purpose in life • Ability to love • Ability to forgive • Ability to worship • Spiritual contentment

(From Bulechek, G. M., Butcher, H. K., & Dochterman, J. [Eds.]. [2008]. *Nursing interventions classification [NIC]* [5th ed., p. 674]. St. Louis, MO: Mosby; and Moorhead, S., Johnson, M., Maas, M. L., & Swanson, E. (2008). *Nursing outcomes classification [NOC]* [4th ed.]. St. Louis: Mosby Elsevier, p. 651.)

respectful manner and as directed by patients. While Figure 46-2, earlier in the chapter, illustrates the importance of religion to many Americans, it is also true that religion means very different things to different individuals. A nurse's offer to pray for a patient may be received gratefully by one and angrily by another who associates prayer with a "last resort" intervention when everything else has failed. The fact that some healthcare professionals confuse spiritual care with proselytizing (trying to convert others to one's own religion) is another source of concern.

NURSING IN RESEARCH
Bridging the Gap to Evidence-Based Practice

ASSESSING SPIRITUAL NEEDS

Research continues to demonstrate the importance of assessing the spiritual needs of patients in order to optimize health outcomes.

Related Research

Mystakidou, K., Tsilika, E. P., Hatzipli, J., Smyrnioti, M., Galanos, A., & Vlahos, L. (2008). Demographic and clinical predictors of *spirituality* in advanced cancer patients: A randomized control study. *Journal of Clinical Nursing, 17*(13): 1779–1785.

This study focuses on the sociodemographic and clinical characteristics of cancer patients, as related to their spiritual beliefs and attitudes. This article displays the factors that allow a more precise estimation of a patient's spiritual beliefs, such as gender, cancer diagnosis, existential/meditative subscale, radiotherapy treatment and external/ritual, and internal/fluid and existential meditative. Addressing patients' spiritual needs is a priority; it affects crucial aspects of psychological functioning. Only after taking into consideration these necessary factors, can an assessment be properly attempted.

Relevance for Nursing Practice

Nurses need to be sensitive to specific patients' demographic and medical characteristics, especially female gender, old age, years of education, performance status, and radiotherapy treatment. Failure to control these factors can lead to a false estimation on patients' spiritual beliefs, and thus degradation of psychological functioning.

Related Research

Lamb, M., Buchanan, D., Godfrey, C., Harrison, Margaret B., & Oakley, P. (2008). The psychosocial spiritual experience of elderly individuals recovering from stroke: A systematic review. *International Journal of Evidence-Based Healthcare, 6*(2), 173–205.

This study examines the spiritual response of adults over 65 after one or more strokes. This article highlights the confusing and terrifying nature of the onset and early period following a stroke, and connectedly, the importance of spiritual connection to the patients' recovery. The period of recovery involves considerable psychological and physical work for elderly individuals to reconstruct their lives. Experiencing a stroke is a life-altering experience for most elderly individuals, involving profound changes in functioning and sense of self.

Relevance for Nursing Practice

In order to better aid older stroke patients, nurses should provide enhanced sensitivity towards spirituality and religion, as an essential conduit to recovery. For those with a spiritual tradition, connectedness to others and spiritual connection is especially important during the time period following the stroke.

For additional research, visit thePoint.

Key

→ Patient process   ---→ Transformative interaction

BCC: Board certified chaplain
Clinicians: Chaplains, physicians, nurses, social workers
Community providers: Community religious leaders, spiritual director, pastoral and community
counselors, faith community nurses, physical therapists, occupational therapists, and others

Physician   Social worker

Nurse   Chaplain

Spiritual screening upon admission to services (nurse, social worker, other)

Patient & family

Spiritual history (physician, nurse, other)

Spiritual assessment (board certified chaplain)

Interdisciplinary team rounds with chaplain as spiritual care expert

Re-evaluate

Community providers; family & friends

Outcomes

Personal and professional preparation

Clinicians and spiritual care providers

Treatment plan

Community providers; family & friends

FIGURE 46-4. Inpatient spiritual care implementation model. (From Puchalski, C., Ferrell, B., Virani, R., Otis-Green, S., Baird, P., Bull, J., et al. [2009]. Improving the quality of spiritual care as a dimension of palliative care: The report of the consensus conference. *Journal of Palliative Medicine, 12*[10], 885–904.)

Puchalski (2006) offers the following hints about professional boundaries:

- Keep the spiritual history patient centered.
- Recognize pastoral care professionals as experts in this field and consult them appropriately.
- Proselytizing is never acceptable in professional settings. Addressing spiritual issues should not be coercive.
- More in-depth spiritual counseling should be under the direction of chaplains and other spiritual leaders.
- Praying with patients should not be initiated by the nurse unless there is no pastoral care available and the patient requests it or in situations where the nurse and patient have a long-standing relationship or share a similar belief system. The nurse can stand in silence as the patient prays in her or his tradition. The nurse can always make a referral to pastoral care for chaplain led prayer (p. 241).

Offering Supportive or Healing Presence

A nurse's gift of supportive presence must underlie all other types of intervention to meet the patient's spiritual needs. The aim of this intervention is to create a hospitable and sacred space ("holy ground") in which patients can share their vulnerabilities without fear. Supportive presence com-

municates value and respect (Fig. 46-5). Chapter 21 presents basic communication skills helpful in establishing this type of presence. Box 46-2 outlines helpful steps for nurses intent on developing the art of healing presence.

The patient who senses that the nurse is sincerely concerned and committed to helping meet human needs is better able to participate in the plan of care. Patients who experience

FIGURE 46-5. The nurse offers supportive presence by holding the patient's hand to show that he or she is sincerely concerned, or simply by being present to communicate value and respect.

Box 46-2   STEPS FOR BEING A HEALING PRESENCE

Inasmuch as it's more art than science, you'll have your own ways of bringing healing presence into your life and the lives of others. Following is a rough order for how you might proceed.

1. Open Yourself
Begin not with the other person but with you. Become present to yourself in a way that is honest, insightful, and accepting. Open to your uniqueness, humanness, prejudices, brokenness, and wholeness. Do this by owning your life story, continually fathoming who you are in a holistic manner, and developing or utilizing a support system to which you hold yourself accountable.

2. Intend to Be a Healing Presence
Aware that healing presence doesn't just occur out of the blue, you intentionally decide to be such a presence with another. Intend to promote healing in its many forms, while being understanding of yourself as you emerge in the day-to-day intricacies of this practice.

3. Prepare a Space for Healing Presence to Take Place
Clear a space to interact with the other or others, assuring as much privacy as possible and creating an atmosphere of calm. Prepare a space also within by placing yourself out of the way and clearing away your personal expectations for what the other should be or do.

4. Honor the One in Your Care
Approach those you accompany as people with dignity and worth. Show your regard for them by honoring their individuality, equality, humanness, separateness, and sacredness. Respect their natural and unique healing capacity.

5. Offer What You Have to Give
Freely and simply make available what you have to offer, realizing it is up to the other or others to accept or not. Offer presence, loving acceptance, empathy, dependability, an unselfish focus on them, your firm belief in them, your willingness to follow their lead, and, as much as anything, hope.

6. Receive the Gifts that Come
Accept with a grateful heart what is yours to receive. This may include living your life more fully as a result of this practice. Other gifts may include uncovering your genuine self, enjoying wonderful relationships, finding personal satisfaction, realizing you have made a difference, receiving your own healing, and exploring some of life's most valuable lessons.

7. Live a Life of Wholeness and Balance
There is more to life than being a healing presence. So, live your days fully, caring for your own needs, setting appropriate boundaries, encouraging your own growth, and nurturing a loving attitude toward life, including the sacred dimension. Affirm and live out the truth of the transforming potential of healing presence. Be grateful for the possibilities.

Used with permission. Miller, J. E., & Cutshall, S. C. (2001). *The art of being a healing presence: A guide for those in caring relationships.* Willogreen Publishing. 10351 Dawsons Creek Blvd, Ste B, Fort Wayne, IN 46825. Phone: 260-490-2222.

respect and affirmation from other humans find it easier to hold spiritual beliefs that meet their needs for meaning and purpose, love and relatedness, and forgiveness.

Facilitating the Practice of Religion

The following are means the nurse can use to help the patient continue normal spiritual practices in the unfamiliar environment of the hospital or care center:

- Familiarize the patient with the religious services and materials available within the institution.
- Respect the patient's need for privacy or quiet during periods of prayer.
- Assist the patient to obtain devotional objects and protect them from loss or damage.
- Arrange for the patient wishing to receive the sacraments to do so.
- Attempt to meet the patient's religious dietary restrictions.
- Arrange for the patient's minister, priest, or rabbi to visit if the patient so wishes.

If the patient has a conflict between spiritual beliefs and the proposed medical therapy, assist the patient in discussing this with the physician. The ill patient in the home may not be able to attend services or meetings to which he or she is accustomed. Aid the patient in finding ways to express his or her spiritual needs.

Nurturing Spirituality

Some patients who experience a need to get in touch with their spiritual self and to nurture their spiritual development look to the nurse for direction. The person who lives life enmeshed in the action and noises of society may feel strangely uncomfortable when illness forces introspection. Be helpful by recommending means to develop a relationship with one's inner world (prayer, reflection, dream analysis, nature walks, enjoying art) and manifest spiritual energy in one's outer world (loving relationships, compassion, forgiveness, joy, service).

Spiritual nurturing for the patient's family caregiver(s) also is important. Recent research findings support the importance and value of caregivers' spirituality, yet as a resource, it is often overlooked. Consider using interventions that enhance a caregiver's ability to take part in church activities to satisfy his or her spiritual needs and to work with church groups to secure helpful services. Using clergy, prayer, forgiveness, and spiritual reading materials as resources for caregivers may also be helpful.

> *Knowledge of the supportive services provided by the church group of Mrs. Zeuner, the 75-year-old woman taking care of her husband with advanced Alzheimer's disease, would be important to include in the plan of care for Mrs. Zeuner and her husband. Supportive services, such as*

respite care, parish nursing, and meals, in addition to the emotional support provided by the group, could be extremely helpful for Mrs. Zeuner in her role as caregiver. ∎

Finally, remember that, as nurses, we cannot give what we don't have. Unless our own spiritual needs are met, we will never be able to be truly present to another. Thus, the art of being a healing presence requires a lifestyle that supports our being a healing presence. It is helpful to reflect on this proverb: *A happy heart is like good medicine. But a broken spirit drains your strength (dries your bones). Proverbs 17:22*

Three ways the nurse can help the patient to nurture his or her own spirituality are by promoting meaning and purpose, promoting love and relatedness, and promoting forgiveness.

PROMOTING MEANING AND PURPOSE

In the book *Man's Search for Meaning*, psychiatrist Victor Frankl, who survived the horrors of the Nazi concentration camps, writes, "Once an individual's search for meaning is successful, it not only renders him happy, but also gives him the capability to cope with suffering" (1985, p. 163). To help patients searching for meaning, explore with the patient what has given his or her life meaning and purpose up to the present, sources of meaning for other people, and possible meanings for the patient's current experience of illness, pain, suffering, or impending death. If desired by the patient, arrange for referral to a spiritual adviser. Explore with the patient spiritual practices from which strength and hope might be derived (e.g., prayer or reading scripture or other spiritual books). You might also want to recommend that the patient read spiritual biographies or Harold Kuschner's book *When Bad Things Happen to Good People* (1983) or Kathleen Brehony's book *After the Darkest Hour: How Suffering Begins the Journey to Wisdom* (2000). Referring the patient to appropriate support groups (e.g., self-help groups for people with stroke, cancer) also is helpful.

PROMOTING LOVE AND RELATEDNESS

First and foremost, always treat the patient with respect, empathy, and genuine caring. It is a good idea to encourage the patient to talk about relationships with others and to identify the origin of negative beliefs about people. Box 46-3 may be a good starting point for reflection on loving kindness.

Encourage conversation about how a patient experiences God or a higher being if that is part of the patient's spiritual beliefs. If appropriate, introduce or reinforce the belief that God is a loving and personal God who is concerned about the patient. Whenever possible, encourage and facilitate visits from the patient's family, friends, and spiritual adviser.

PROMOTING FORGIVENESS

Offer a supportive presence to the patient that demonstrates your acceptance of the patient. Explore with the patient the importance of learning to accept oneself and others, including both strengths and limitations. Explore negative feelings that make it difficult for the patient to seek forgiveness and to believe that he or she is forgiven.

Box 46-3   LOVING KINDNESS MEDITATION

- May you be at peace.
- May your heart remain open.
- May you awaken to the light of your own true nature.
- May you know the power of your higher self.
- May peace of mind be your only goal and forgiveness your only task.
- May you be healed of all pain and hurt.
- May you be a source of healing for others.
- May you know the inner beauty of the person you truly are.
- May you be at peace.

Source unknown.

Explore the patient's self-expectations and assist the patient to determine how realistic these are. Allow the patient to verbalize shame, guilt, and anger, and counsel about the importance of expressing negative emotions in healthy ways. Refer the patient to a spiritual adviser, if appropriate. Offer the patient examples of how not forgiving others can end up hurting only the one who cannot forgive.

Praying With Patients

Patients accustomed to regular periods of prayer but who feel too ill to pray as they would like or who enjoy praying with others may ask the nurse to pray with them or hope that the nurse will suggest this. Because there are many forms of prayer—quiet reflection, silent communion with God or higher power, reading or recitation of formal prayers, silent or loud calling on God or higher power or conversation with God or higher power, lamentations, or reading one's holy book or other religious materials—the nurse can take the lead from the patient by asking, "How would you like us to pray?" The religious background of the patient is considered, along with the type of prayers that have been meaningful in the past. It is also helpful to ask the patient if there is a particular prayer request.

The nurse unaccustomed to praying aloud or in public may find it helpful to have a Bible passage or formal prayer readily available. The prayer may also be a simple expression aloud of the patient's needs and hopes. A sample follows:

Lord God, our Creator and Healer, I entrust Mrs. Smith and her family to your loving care. Bring peace to her mind and health and strength to her body. Be with her [as her treatment begins today, as she goes for surgery, and so on]. We remember all your blessings to us in the past and thank you. We are confident of your help now as we claim your promises.

Prayer should not block communication with the patient. Praying before a patient feels ready to pray may communicate to the patient a lack of interest in the patient's feelings. Because prayer often evokes deep feelings, the nurse should be prepared to spend time with the patient after sharing prayer to respond to these feelings.

Praying for Patients

With research suggesting links between prayer and physical, mental, and spiritual health (Levin, 2001), arguments are being made that healthcare professionals have an obligation to pray for, as well as with, their patients. At the present time, no one is claiming that healthcare professionals are negligent if they fail to pray for patients. This may, however, be an effective intervention strategy. At the very least, nurses ought to be mediators of the spiritual resources patients and their families need.

Counseling Patients Spiritually

The patient who feels that the nurse is sensitive to spiritual needs and comfortable with his or her own spirituality may choose to share spiritual concerns with the nurse rather than with a religious counselor. The nurse who feels competent to counsel the patient may assist the patient to accomplish the following:

- Articulate spiritual beliefs.
- Explore the origin of the patient's spiritual beliefs and practices.
- Identify life factors that challenge the patient's spiritual beliefs (cause spiritual distress).
- Explore alternatives given these challenges: modify lifestyle; deny, modify, or reaffirm beliefs; develop new beliefs.
- Develop spiritual beliefs that meet needs for meaning and purpose, care and relatedness, forgiveness.

To be an effective spiritual counselor, the nurse must be open to different spiritual beliefs and forms of spiritual expression and supportive of the patient's efforts to nurture spiritual growth.

Contacting a Spiritual Counselor

Not every nurse feels comfortable in the role of spiritual counselor. If not, suggest that the patient talk to a pastoral caregiver or spiritual counselor. When a patient expresses a desire to speak to his or her spiritual counselor, help make the appropriate referral or offer to contact the patient's own spiritual adviser. Other options are to contact the healthcare facility's pastoral ministry department or use a referral list of clergy in the local community. If a representative of the patient's own religion is unable to visit within the hospital at a particular time, suggest a visit from a member of the clergy from another faith. The patient, depending on the situation and the immediacy of the need, may welcome such a suggestion.

In a care center setting, you can assist the spiritual counselor by making the counselor feel welcome, answering questions about the patient, directing the counselor to the patient, and ensuring that the patient is ready to receive the counselor. Preparations of the patient's room for the visit may vary, but the following are generally recommended practices:

- The room should be orderly and free of unnecessary equipment and items.
- There should be a seat for the religious counselor at the bedside or near the patient so that both can be comfortable.

- The bedside table should be free of items and covered with a clean, white cover if a sacrament is to be administered.
- The bed curtains should be drawn for privacy if the patient can't be moved to a more private setting.

Some patients and spiritual advisers may value the nurse's participation in prayers, rituals, or the administration of sacraments. When a nursing diagnosis of Spiritual Distress is made, the nurse and the religious counselor often can collaborate on the plan of care and reinforce each other's efforts to assist the patient to meet goals/outcomes. By having good working relations with chaplains and pastoral caregivers, you can quickly direct them to patients most likely to benefit from their visits.

Resolving Conflicts Between Spiritual Beliefs and Treatments

Both the patient and members of the patient's family may experience conflict between a particular spiritual belief or religious law and a proposed medical treatment or health option. The patient may want assistance when conferring with the spiritual adviser about a particular procedure. The nurse's role is to assist the patient in obtaining the information needed to make an informed decision and to support the patient's decision making. Because what the nurse says and the way it is said may powerfully influence the patient's decision, it is important to maintain objectivity. Conflicts that resist resolution may be referred to an ethics committee or consult team (see Chapter 6).

Nursing, Religion, and Conscientious Objection

In recent years, some pharmacists have experienced great media attention by refusing to fill prescriptions for contraceptives. These pharmacists support their refusals by claiming that to fulfill the prescriptions would violate their religious beliefs and convictions. In situations like these, the woman's right to access certain medications is pitted against the pharmacist's right to practice with personal integrity. Nurses can also find themselves in situations where their professional or institutional responsibilities involve participation in activities such as abortion, assisted suicide, and counseling about birth control, which may violate their personal integrity. Thus, it is important for nurses to ensure that they can fulfill the responsibilities of jobs they assume or that they are free to exercise the right of conscientious objection. As legislation addressing these conflicts is in a state of flux, you should be familiar with federal and state guidelines. For example, as this new revision is being written, California is proposing legislation that would forbid healthcare professionals to refuse to care for gay or lesbian patients on the basis of conscientious objection.

Evaluating

The nurse working with a patient and family to achieve specified goals/outcomes to meet spiritual needs can use each patient interaction to evaluate the plan of care. Necessary to the evaluation are sensitivity to what the patient is saying and not saying and observation of the patient when alone as well as when interacting with the family and nurses.

In general, the nurse evaluates the patient's ability to accomplish the following:

- Identify some spiritual belief that gives meaning and purpose to everyday life.
- Move toward a healthy acceptance of the current situation: illness, pain, suffering, impending death.
- Develop mutually caring relationships.
- Reconcile any interpersonal differences causing the patient anguish.
- Verbalize satisfaction with relationship with God/higher being (if this is important).

- Express peaceful acceptance of limitations and failings.
- Express the ability to forgive others and to live in the present.
- Demonstrate an "interior state of peace and joy; freedom from abnormal anxiety, guilt, or a feeling of sinfulness; and a sense of security and direction in the pursuit of one's life goals and activities" (O'Brien, 1982, p. 98).

The nurse helps the patient to determine whether spiritual beliefs are generally life affirming or life denying and whether there is harmony between these beliefs and the patient's everyday life experiences. See Nursing Plan of Care 46-1.

NURSING PLAN OF CARE • 46-1

For Mr. Gargan

Mr. Gargan is a 38-year-old divorced man on a step-down unit after treatment for a myocardial infarction. He owns a small car dealership. His religion is listed as Protestant. Frequently unable to sleep at night, Mr. Gargan often talks with the night nurse and once asked, "Did you ever give much thought to whether or not there is a God?" Sensing much concern behind this question, the nurse asks specific questions to determine whether the patient has spiritual needs that are not being met.

12/26/12, 2 a.m.

Patient again unable to sleep and initiated discussion about God. States that he was raised in a Lutheran home where

everyone went to church on Sunday and tried to live according to God's commandments. Upon leaving home, he stopped going to church (was never a value for his wife) and simply has not given much thought to religion—too busy running his business. Until now, has not experienced any need for God. "But when I think how close I was to dying and that I've no idea what to expect after death—I'm actually scared. Do others feel this way?" Wants to explore religious beliefs—feels lack in his life. Said he would like to talk with hospital minister—will arrange for tomorrow.

E. Nolan, RN

NURSING DIAGNOSIS Spiritual Distress: Anxiety related to concerns about relationship with God as manifested by self-report

EXPECTED OUTCOME Before discharge, the patient will:

- Identify his religious beliefs

Nursing Interventions	Rationale	Evaluative Statement
Assist the patient to (1) identify the spiritual beliefs he had as a child and the origin of these beliefs, (2) evaluate these beliefs in terms of his life experiences, and (3) reaffirm, modify, or reject these beliefs or develop new spiritual beliefs.	Life experiences may challenge religious beliefs that were uncritically held as a child.	12/30/12 Outcome partially met. Patient states he has a much clearer concept of God and no longer fears that God will reject him for ignoring him for so long . . . but believes he also has a lot to learn. *E. Nolan, RN*
Assist the patient to assess whether his newly articulated spiritual beliefs are life affirming or life denying and the degree to which they meet his needs for meaning and purpose, love and relatedness, and forgiveness.	Because spiritual beliefs can exert positive (life-affirming) and negative (life-denying) influences on a person's life, individuals should have some criteria to use when evaluating their beliefs.	
Refer the patient to the hospital minister for assistance with the above.	Patient may value speaking with a minister.	

(continued)

NURSING PLAN OF CARE · 46-1

For Mr. Gargan (continued)

EXPECTED OUTCOME   Before discharge, the patient will:

• Reconcile his life up until the present with God

Nursing Interventions	Rationale	Evaluative Statement
Reassure the patient that many people get involved in day-to-day living to the extent that they forget about God, and that in some religions, people believe that God uses illness and other stressors to invite people to rethink their spiritual beliefs. In these traditions, God is often pictured with open arms waiting to welcome a child home.	Images of a stern and unyielding God ready to strike down transgressors may contribute to a patient's spiritual distress.	12/30/12 Outcome met. "This minister has really helped. I wish I had talked to him a long time ago. I've carried so much guilt about my divorce and some other things—thought God would never forgive me. I feel so much more at peace now." *E. Nolan, RN*
Refer the patient to a spiritual advisor for help in experiencing forgiveness if he mentions guilt feelings.	Guilt often inhibits persons from seeking and experiencing the forgiveness they desire.	
Communicate to the patient the importance of people accepting themselves—with all their strengths and weaknesses.	Many persons have unrealistic self-expectations.	

EXPECTED OUTCOME   Before discharge, the patient will:

• Verbalize that his spiritual beliefs have become a source of strength and peace rather than anxiety

Nursing Interventions	Rationale	Evaluative Statement
Encourage the patient to compare the role of spiritual beliefs in his life before, during, and after hospitalization.	This highlights the positive and negative roles spiritual beliefs can play. It may motivate the patient to continue searching if he values his present experience.	12/30/12 Outcome met. "It's good to be able to feel more peaceful about whatever the future brings. I'm anxious to get out of here because there's a lot I want to do with God's help." *E. Nolan, RN*

EXPECTED OUTCOME   Before discharge, the patient will:

• Increase night sleep to at least 6 undisturbed hours

(continued)

NURSING PLAN OF CARE • 46-1

For Mr. Gargan (continued)

Nursing Interventions	Rationale	Evaluative Statement
Nurse on the 1-to-7 shift checks on patient at beginning of shift to make sure he is comfortable and ready for sleep.	Nursing supervision of the patient at bedtime rules out other factors that may interfere with sleep.	12/30/12 Outcome met. Patient slept last night from midnight to 6 a.m. Will continue to monitor. *E. Nolan, RN*
Use power of suggestion to enhance sleep: *"I'm sure when I check back you'll be sound asleep."*	Suggestion has been shown to enhance the therapeutic effect of other interventions.	
If sleep remains disturbed, try relaxation exercises or guided imagery (see Chapter 42).	As spiritual anxiety decreases, sleep should improve. If sleep does not improve, other contributing factors and interventions will need to be explored.	

SAMPLE DOCUMENTATION	12/27/12 3 p.m., Nursing B. Hanks, Protestant minister, here to see patient at 1 p.m. Afterward, patient said he felt "a whole lot better." Reported minister had assured him that many people in the hospital with a serious illness go through exactly what he is experiencing now—and this thought seemed to decrease much of his anxiety. Minister had reinforced nurse's suggestion that he explore his religious beliefs and he has already jotted down some thoughts. "I knew you fixed bodies in hospitals but didn't know you fix souls, too." Patient looking forward to minister's visit tomorrow. *E. Nolan, RN*

● Developing Critical Thinking Skills

1. Assess your spiritual well-being; that is, to what extent are you able to meet your needs for love and belonging, meaning and purpose, and forgiveness? If confronted with a life-threatening or chronic illness, would you be able to draw on religion or spirituality as a source of strength? Are there any special skills you believe you need to develop to better meet the spiritual needs of your patients? Compare your responses to those of your classmates and explore reasons for the differences you encounter.

2. Poll your classmates and see if they agree strongly, agree, disagree, or disagree strongly with the following statements. Discuss reasons for the differences in your answers and how this is likely to affect your professional practice:
   • Prayer has the power to heal physical, mental, and spiritual illness.
   • Nurses who do not pray for their patients are deficient professional caregivers.
   • Nurses who do not offer to pray with their patients are deficient professional caregivers.

3. How would you respond to a patient who tells you that he isn't very religious but is now wondering if there is a God, and if so, where he stands in relation to God now that his life is in jeopardy? Think about how your personal experience of religion/spirituality colors your response, and determine whether your personal experience of religion/spirituality has prepared you well to respond to these queries.

● Practicing for NCLEX

1. Which of the following statements most correctly differentiates between an agnostic and an atheist?
   a. The terms are used interchangeably, both believing there is no God.
   b. An agnostic denies that humans can know anything about God's existence, whereas an atheist denies God's existence.
   c. They both deny the need for a philosophy of living to guide their life.
   d. No aspect of an atheist's life is influenced by spirituality, whereas an agnostic has spiritual values.

2. A nurse who was raised a strict Roman Catholic stated she couldn't assist patients with their spiritual distress because she recognizes only a "field power" in each individual. She said, "My parents and I hardly talk because I've deserted my faith. Sometimes I feel real isolated from them and also God—if there is a God." Analysis of these data reveals which unmet spiritual need?
   a. Need for meaning and purpose
   b. Need for forgiveness
   c. Need for love and relatedness
   d. Need for strength for everyday living

3. Which statement is true concerning the influence of spirituality and religion on the various aspects of a person's life?
   a. All aspects of life may be influenced by spirituality.
   b. Activities of daily living (eating, bathing, sleeping, dressing) are rarely influenced by religion.
   c. Work and recreation are not influenced by religion.
   d. Whereas physical illness is seldom influenced by religion, mental illness frequently is.

4. A patient whose last name is Goldstein was served on a paper plate a kosher meal ordered from a restaurant because the hospital made no provision for kosher food or dishes. Mr. Goldstein became angry and accused the nurse of insulting him: "I want to eat what everyone else does—and give me decent dishes." Analysis of these data reveals what finding?
   a. The nurse should have ordered kosher dishes also.
   b. The staff must have behaved condescendingly or critically.
   c. Mr. Goldstein is a problem patient and difficult to satisfy.
   d. Mr. Goldstein was stereotyped and not consulted about his dietary preferences.

5. You are least likely to encounter resistance to emergency life-saving surgery for a patient from which of the following families?
   a. Christian Scientist family
   b. Faith Assembly Healer family
   c. Jehovah's Witness family
   d. Orthodox Jewish family

6. When the family desires baptism for an infant, why is it imperative that the nurse provide for baptism to be done?
   a. Baptism frequently postpones or prevents death or suffering.
   b. It is legally required that nurses provide for this care when the family makes this request.
   c. It is a nursing function to assure the salvation of the baby.
   d. Lack of baptism when desired may increase the family's sorrow and suffering.

7. Because the capacity for abstract thought develops as a child grows older, spirituality is understood differently by children of different ages. Which of the following statements is false?
   a. Spirituality and perception of God/higher being is meaningless for the 4- to 5-year-old.
   b. Even young children, 4 to 5 years of age, have definite perceptions of God/higher being and forms of worship.
   c. Children's perceptions of their "spiritual self" mature as they mature.
   d. Children 5 to 11 years of age may show anxiety concerning the power they believe God has.

8. What is the most important source of learning about his or her own spirituality for a child?
   a. His or her church or religious organization
   b. What parents say about God and religion
   c. How parents behave in relationship to one another and their children, to others, and to God
   d. The spiritual adviser for the family

9. Even though a detailed nursing history in which spirituality is assessed is taken on admission, problems with spiritual distress may not surface until days after admission. What is the probable explanation?
   a. Patients usually want to conceal information about spiritual needs
   b. Patients are not concerned about spiritual needs until after their spiritual adviser visits
   c. Family members and close friends often initiate spiritual concerns
   d. Illness increases spiritual concerns, which may be difficult for patients to express in words

10. When a patient needs spiritual counseling, the nurse who is comfortable with his or her own spirituality should do which of the following?
    a. Always call the patient's own spiritual adviser
    b. Consult with the patient about the spiritual adviser with whom he or she wishes to talk
    c. Attempt to counsel the patient and, if unsuccessful, make a referral
    d. Advise the patient and spiritual adviser concerning health options and the correct decision

11. When assessment data point to a spiritual problem that can be treated by independent nursing intervention, it receives which NANDA-approved diagnostic label?
    a. Spiritual Alienation
    b. Spiritual Despair
    c. Spiritual Distress
    d. Spiritual Pain

12. A patient states she feels so isolated from her family and church and even God "in this huge medical center so far from home." An appropriate goal for the patient to relieve her spiritual distress is as follows. The patient will:
    a. Express satisfaction with the compatibility of her spiritual beliefs and everyday living
    b. Identify spiritual beliefs that meet her need for meaning and purpose

c. Express peaceful acceptance of limitations and failings

d. Identify spiritual supports available to her in this medical center

13. A man who is a declared agnostic is extremely depressed after losing his home, his wife, and his children in a fire. His nursing diagnosis is Spiritual Distress: Spiritual Pain related to inability to find meaning and purpose in his current condition. Which of the following is the most important nursing intervention to plan?

a. Ask the patient which spiritual adviser he would like you to call

b. Recommend that the patient read spiritual biographies or religious books

c. Explore with the patient what, in addition to his family, has given his life meaning and purpose in the past

d. Introduce the belief that God is a loving and personal God

14. After having an abortion, the patient told the visiting nurse, "I shouldn't have had that abortion because I'm Catholic, but what else could I do? I'm afraid I'll never get close to my mother or back in the Church again." She then talked with her priest about this feeling of guilt. Which evaluation statement shows a solution to the problem?

a. Patient states, "I wish I had talked with the priest sooner. I now know God has forgiven me, and even my mother understands."

b. Patient has slept from 10 p.m. to 6 a.m. for three consecutive nights without medication.

c. Patient has developed mutually caring relationships with two women and one man.

d. Patient has identified several spiritual beliefs that give purpose to her life.

15. Mr. Brown's teenage daughter had been involved in shoplifting. He expressed much anger toward her and stated he could not face her, let alone discuss this with her: "I just will not tolerate a thief." Which of the following nursing interventions would you take to assist Mr. Brown with his deficit in forgiveness?

a. Assure him that many parents feel the same way.

b. Reassure him that many teenagers go through this kind of rebellion and that it will pass.

c. Assist the patient to identify how unforgiving feelings toward others only hurt the one who cannot forgive.

d. Ask him if he is sure he has spent sufficient time with his daughter.

● Answers With Rationale

1. *b.* An agnostic denies that humans can know anything about God's existence, whereas an atheist denies God's existence. The other options are incorrect.

2. *c.* The data point to an unmet spiritual need to experience love and belonging given her estrangement from her family and God after leaving the church. The other options may represent other needs this nurse has, but the data provided do not support them.

3. *a.* Spirituality can influence all aspects of a person's life, including activities of daily living, work and recreation, and all types of illnesses. The other options are incomplete or false.

4. *d.* On the basis of his name alone, the nurse jumped to the premature and false conclusion that this patient would want a kosher diet.

5. *d.* There is no teaching in the Hebrew scriptures that prohibits emergency life-saving surgery; in fact, most Orthodox Jews would be highly motivated to have the surgery because of the high value attached to preserving life. All of the other groups mentioned might have religious grounds for refusing surgery.

6. *d.* Failure to ensure that an infant baptism is performed when parents desire it may greatly increase the family's sorrow and suffering, and this is an appropriate nursing concern. Whether baptism postpones or prevents death and suffering (answer *a*) is a religious belief that is insufficient to bind all nurses. There is no legal requirement regarding baptism, so answer *b* is false. Although some nurses may believe part of their role is to ensure the salvation of the baby (answer *c*), this function would understandably be rejected by many.

7. *a.* It is false that spirituality and perception of God is meaningless for the 4- to 5-year-old. All the other options are correct.

8. *c.* Children learn most about their own spirituality from how their parents behave in relationship to one another, their children, others, and God/higher being. Less important sources of learning are each of the other options.

9. *d.* Illness may increase spiritual concerns, which many patients find difficult to express. The other options do not correspond to actual experience.

10. *b.* Even when a nurse feels comfortable discussing spiritual concerns, he or she should always check first with patients to determine the spiritual adviser with whom they wish to talk. Calling the patient's own spiritual adviser (answer *a*) may be premature if it is a matter the nurse can handle. Answers *c* and *d* deny patients the right to speak privately with their spiritual adviser from the outset, if this is what they prefer.

11. *c.* The only NANDA-approved nursing diagnosis among the options is Spiritual Distress. The other options may be further specifications of the broader diagnosis Spiritual Distress.

12. *d.* Each of the four options represents appropriate spiritual goals, but identifying spiritual supports available to her in the medical center demonstrates a decreased sense of isolation.

13. *c.* The nursing intervention of exploring with the patient what, in addition to his family, has given his life meaning and purpose in the past is more likely to correct the etiology of his problem, Spiritual Pain, than any of the other nursing interventions listed.

14. *a.* Because this patient's nursing diagnosis is Spiritual Distress: Guilt, an evaluative statement that demonstrates diminished guilt is necessary. Only answer *a* directly deals with guilt.

15. *c.* Because this is the only nursing intervention that directly addresses the patient's unmet spiritual need concerning forgiveness. Answers *a* and *b* may make him feel better initially, but neither addresses his need to forgive. Answer *d* is likely to make him feel guilty.

Taylor Suite Resources

The Taylor Suite offers these additional resources to enhance learning and facilitate understanding of this chapter:

- thePoint online resource, http://thepoint.lww.com/Taylor7E
- Student DVD-ROM included with the book
- Study Guide for Taylor's Fundamentals of Nursing

BIBLIOGRAPHY

Alfaro-Lefevre, R. (2006). *Applying nursing process: A tool for critical thinking* (6th ed.). Philadelphia: Lippincott Williams & Wilkins.

American Nurses Association. (1998). *Scope and standards of parish nursing practice.* Washington, DC: Author.

Anandarajah, G., & Hight, E. (2001). Spirituality and medical practice: Using the HOPE questions as a practical tool for spiritual assessment. *American Family Physician, 63,* 81–89.

Balboni, T., Vanderwerker, L. C., Block, S. D., Paulk, E., Lathan, C. S., Peteet, J. R., & Prigerson, H. G. (2007). Religiousness and spiritual support among advanced cancer patients and associations with end-of-life treatment preferences and quality of life. *Journal of Clinical Oncology, 25*(5), 555–560.

Bephage, G. (2008). Care approaches to spirituality and dementia. *Nursing & Residential Care, 10*(3), 134–137.

Brehony, K. (2000). *After the darkest hour: How suffering begins the journey to wisdom.* New York: Henry Holt and Company.

Bulechek, G. M., Butcher, H. K., & Dochterman, J. (Eds.). (2008). *Nursing interventions classification (NIC)* (5th ed.). St. Louis: Mosby.

Burghardt, M., & Nagai-Jacobson, M. G. (1997). In B. M. Dossey (Ed.), *Core curriculum for holistic nursing.* New York: Aspen Publishers.

Callahan, D., & Campbell, C. S. (Eds.). (1990). Theology, religious traditions, and bioethics: A special supplement. *Hastings Center Report, 20*(6), 18–19.

Carol, J. (2002, August). What is healing? *Sacred Journey, 53*(4), 12–17.

Carson, V. B. (1989). *Spiritual dimensions of nursing practice.* Philadelphia: W. B. Saunders.

Carson, V. B., & Koenig, H. G. (2004). *Spiritual caregiving. Health-care as a ministry.* Chicago: Templeton Foundation Press.

Clarke, E. B., Curtis, J. R., Luce, J. M., Levy, M., Nelson, J., & Solomon, M. Z.; The Robert Wood Johnson Foundation Critical Care End-of-Life Peer Workgroup Members. (2003). Quality indicators for end-of-life care in the intensive care unit. *Critical Care Medicine, 31*(9), 2255–2262

Coles, R. (1990). *The spiritual life of children.* Boston: Houghton Mifflin.

Creen, T. (2002). Enabling hope in the terminally ill. In R. C. Anderson et al. (Eds.). *Palliative care patient and family counseling manual* (2nd ed., pp. 16–17). New York: Aspen Publishers.

Davis, D. S., & Zoloth, L. (1999). *Notes from a narrow ridge: Religion and bioethics.* Hagerstown, MD: University Publishing Group.

Dossey, B. (Ed.). (1989). Spirituality and healing. *Holistic Nursing Practice, 3*(3), entire issue.

Fawcett, T., & Noble, A. (2004). The challenge of spiritual care in a multi-faith society experienced as a Christian nurse. *Journal of Clinical Nursing, 13*(2), 136–142.

Fowler, J. W. (1981). *Stages of faith: The psychology of human development and the quest for meaning.* San Francisco: Harper-Collins.

Frankl, V. (1985). *Man's search for meaning.* New York: Washington Square Press.

Golberg, B. (1998). Connection: An exploration of spirituality in nursing care. *Journal of Advanced Nursing, 27,* 836–842.

Gregg-Schroeder, S. (1999, April). A transforming experience: Circles of Life. *Journal of Fellowship in Prayer,* 23–25.

Hauerwas, S. (1990). *Naming the silences: God, medicine, and the problem of suffering.* Grand Rapids: Erdmans.

Heller, D. (1985). The children's God. *Psychology Today, 19*(12), 22–27.

Hickman, J. S. (2006). *Faith community nursing.* Philadelphia: Lippincott Williams & Wilkins.

Joint Commission Resources (2008). http://www.jcrinc.com/

Kirkham, S. R., Pesut, B., Meyerhoff, H., & Sawatzky, R. (2004). Spiritual caregiving at the juncture of religion, culture, and state. *Canadian Journal of Nursing Research, 36*(4), 148–169.

Koenig, H. G. (2002). *Spirituality in patient care. Why, how, when and what.* Chicago: Templeton Foundation Press.

Koenig, H. G., Lawson, D. M., & McConnell, M. (2005). *Faith in the future. Healthcare, aging and the role of religion.* Chicago: Templeton Foundation Press.

Koss-Chioino, J. D., & Hefner, P. (2006). *Spiritual transformation and healing.* Lanham, MD: Altimira Press.

Kuschner, H. S. (1983). *When bad things happen to good people.* New York: Avon.

Lo, B., Ruston, D., Kates, L. W., Arnold, R. M., Cohen, C. B., Faber-Langendoen, K., et al. (2002). Discussing religious and spiritual issues at the end of life. *JAMA, 287*(6), 749–754.

Levin, J. (2001). God, faith, and health: Exploring the spirituality-healing connection. New York: John Wiley and Sons.

Macrae, J. (1995). Nightingale's spiritual philosophy and its significance for modern nursing. *Image: The Journal of Nursing Scholarship, 27*(1), 8–10.

Miller, J. E., & Cutshall, S. C. (2001). *The art of being a healing presence. A guide for those in caring relationships.* Fort Wayne, IN: Willowgreen Publishing.

Moorhead, S., Johnson, M., Maas, M. L., & Swanson, E. (2008). *Nursing outcomes classification (NOC)* (4th ed.). St. Louis: Mosby Elsevier.

NANDA International. (2009). *Nursing diagnoses: Definitions & classification, 2009–2011.* Oxford, UK: Wiley-Blackwell.

Narayanasamy, A., Clissett, P., Parumal, L., Thompson, D., Annasamy, S., & Edge, R. (2004). Responses to the spiritual needs of older people. *Journal of Advanced Nursing, 48*(1), 6–16.

Narayanasamy, A., & Narayanasamy, M. (2008). The healing power of prayer and its implications for nursing. *British Journal of Nursing, 17*(6), 394–398.

National Consensus Project for Quality Palliative Care (2004). *Clinical practice guide-lines for quality palliative care.* Author. Available at http://www.nationalconsensusproject.org

O'Brien, M. E. (1982). The need for spiritual integrity. In H. Yura & M. Walsh (Eds.), *Human needs and the nursing process* (pp. 81–115). Norwalk, CT: Appleton-Century-Crofts.

O'Brien, M. E. (1999). *Spirituality in nursing.* Boston: Jones and Bartlett.

O'Brien, M. E. (2001). *The nurse's calling.* New York: Paulist Press.

O'Brien, M. E. (2003). *Parish nursing: Healthcare ministry within the church.* Boston: Jones and Bartlett.

O'Brien, M. E. (2007). A Sacred Covenant. The spiritual ministry of healing. Sudbury, MA: Jones and Bartlett.

The Pew Forum on Religion. (2008) The U.S. landmark religion survey. Available at http://religions.pewforum.org/reports#

Puchalski, C., Ferrell, B., Virani, R., Otis-Green, S., Baird, P., Bull, J., et al (2009). Improving the quality of spiritual care as a dimension of palliative care: The report of the consensus conference. *Journal of Palliative Medicine, 12*(10), 885–904.

Puchalski, C., & Romer, A. L. (2000). Taking a spiritual history allows clinicians to understand patients more fully. *Journal of Palliative Medicine, 3*(1), 129–137.

Puchalski, D. M. (2006). A time for listening and caring. Spirituality and the care of the chronically ill and dying. New York: Oxford University Press.

Quinn, A. (2002, August). Spirituality and the family: What religion should I be? *Sacred Journey, 53*(4), 12–17.

Rahner, K. (1971). How to receive a sacrament and mean it. *Theology Digest, 19,* 229.

Ruder, S. (2008). Incorporating spirituality into home care at the end of life. *Home Healthcare Nurse, 26*(3), 158–165.

Shelly, J., & Fish, S. (1988). *Spiritual care: The nurse's role* (3rd ed.). Downer's Grove, IL: InterVarsity Press.

Shapiro, S. L., Brown, K., & Biegel, G. (2007). Self-care for health care professionals: Effects of MBSR on mental wellbeing of counseling psychology students. *Training and Education in Professional Psychology, 1*(2), 105–115.

Sulmasy, D. P. (2006). The rebirth of the clinic: An introduction to spirituality in health care. Washington, DC: Georgetown University Press.

Sweat, M. T. (2005). FAQs in spiritual care. How does spiritual care begin? *Journal of Christian Nursing, 22*(2), 42.

Taylor, E. J. (2007). *What do I say? Talking with patients about spirituality.* Chicago: Templeton Foundation Press.

Taylor, E. J., & Mamier, I. (2005). Spiritual care nursing: What cancer patients and family caregivers want. *Journal of Advanced Nursing, 49*(3), 260–267.

Timmins, F., & Kelly, J. (2008). Spiritual assessment in intensive and cardiac care nursing. *Nursing in Critical Care, 13*(3), 124–131.

Winslow, G. R., & Winslow, B. W. (2003). Examining the ethics of praying with patients. *Holistic Nursing Practice, 17*(4), 170–178.

Equivalents

METRIC UNITS

The metric system, developed by the French, uses the *meter* as the basic unit. The metric system is a decimal system, with prefixes that designate the various multiples or divisibles of 10. The most commonly used prefixes in medicine are:
Milli, which means one one-thousandth (0.001)
Centi, which means one one-hundredth (0.01)
Kilo, which means one thousand (1000)

These prefixes may be affixed to any of the three basic units of measurements, which are

Meter (m), the unit of length
Gram (g), the unit of weight
Liter (L), the unit of volume

Therefore,

1 millimeter (mm) = 0.001 m
1 milligram (mg) = 0.001 g
1 milliliter (mL) = 0.001 L
1 kilometer (km) = 1000 m
1 kilogram (kg) = 1000 g
1 kiloliter (kL) = 1000 L

Length

The meter (a little longer than a yard) and the kilometer (about 0.6 mile) seldom are used in medicine or nursing. The commonly used measure of length is 1 centimeter (cm) = 0.01 m = about 0.4 inch.

Volume

The most frequently used measures of volume are the *liter* and the *milliliter*. Some useful equivalents to know are:

1000 milliliters (mL) = 1 liter (L)
1000 cubic centimeters = 1 liter (L)

Weight

The gram designates the weight of 1 mL of distilled water at 4°C. The most frequently used units of weight are:

1,000,000 micrograms (mcg) = 1 gram (g)
1000 micrograms (mcg) = 1 milligram (mg)

1000 milligrams (mg) = 1 gram (g)
1000 grams (g) = 1 kilogram (kg) = 2.2 pounds (lb)

Metric Units and Their Household Equivalents

Household measurement is inaccurate, with wide variations in the size of teaspoons, teacups, and so forth. The generally accepted household measures are:

60 drops (gtt) = 1 teaspoon (tsp or t)
3 tsp = 1 tablespoon (Tbs or T)
12 Tbs = 1 teacup
16 Tbs = 1 glass (or a standard measuring cup)

APOTHECARY UNITS

In the apothecary system:

The unit of weight is the *grain*.
The unit of volume is the *minim*.

Of the many units of measure in the apothecary system, you should know the following units, abbreviations, and equivalents.

Weight

60 grains (gr) = 1 dram (dr or ʒ)
8 drams (dr or ʒ) = 1 ounce (oz or ℥)

Volume

60 minims (min) = 1 fluid dram (fl dr or f ʒ)
8 fl dr = 1 fluid ounce (fl oz or f ℥)
16 fl oz = 1 pint (pt)
2 pt = 1 quart (qt)
4 qt = 1 gallon (gal)

In the apothecary system, when the symbol or abbreviation is used, the quantity is written in lowercase Roman numerals and follows the symbol. Arabic numerals are used, however, in preference to large Roman numerals. For example:

5 gr = gr v
8 dr = ʒ viii

TABLE • A-1   METRIC AND HOUSEHOLD EQUIVALENTS

Metric Unit	Household Unit
5 mL	1 tsp
15 mL	1 Tbs
180 mL	1 full teacup
240 mL	1 full glass

The quantity one-half may be indicated by the symbol ss.

1½ gr = gr iss
7½ gr = gr viiss

Other fractional parts are expressed as common fractions, for example, gr 1/250, gr 1/10.

When pint, quart, and gallon are written, the quantity is expressed in Arabic numerals, (e.g., 1½ pints or 7½ quarts).

Apothecary Units and Their Household Equivalents

1 drop = 1 minim (m i)
1 tsp = 1 dr (3 i)
1 Tbs = 1/2 oz (ʒ ss)
2 Tbs = 1 oz (ʒ i)
1 teacup = 6 oz (ʒ vi)
1 glass or measuring cup = 8 oz (ʒ viii)
2 measuring cups = 1 pt

TABLE • A-2   MOST COMMONLY USED APPROXIMATE EQUIVALENTS*

Metric	Apothecary	Household
0.06 g	gr i	
0.06 mL	min i	1 drop
1.0 g	gr xv	
1.0 mL	min xv	1/5 tsp
5 mL	(1 dr) 3 i	1 tsp
15 mL	(1/2 oz) ʒ ss	1 Tbs
30 mL	(1 oz) ʒ i	2 Tbs
500 mL	(16 oz) ʒ 16	1 pt
1000 mL	(32 oz) ʒ 32	1 qt

*There are many discrepancies among these approximate equivalents. For example, 30 mL is the accepted equivalent for 1 oz (29.57 mL is the exact equivalent). Such discrepancies are inevitable when two systems are used whose equivalents are not exact. If the discrepancies are within a 10% margin of error, they usually are acceptable in pharmacology.

Normal Adult Laboratory Values*

COMMONLY USED ABBREVIATIONS

kg = kilogram
g = gram
mg = milligram
mcg = microgram
ng = nanogram
mEq = milliequivalent
L = liter
dL = 100 milliliters
mL = milliliter
cu mm (mm^3) = cubic millimeter

nM = nanomolar
mIU = milli-International Unit
pg = picogram
mm = millimeter
mcm = micron or micrometer
mm Hg = millimeters of mercury
mU = milliunit
mcU = microunit
IU = International Unit

*Laboratory values may vary according to techniques used in different laboratories.

TABLE • B-1 HEMATOLOGIC VALUES—REFERENCE RANGES

Determination	Conventional	SI
Coagulation Factors		
Factor I (fibrinogen)	0.15–0.35 g/100 mL	4.0–10.0 mcmol/L
Factor II (prothrombin)	60%–140%	0.60–1.40 mcmol/L
Factor V (accelerator globulin)	60%–140%	0.60–1.40 mcmol/L
Factors VII to X (proconvertin to Stuart factor)	70%–130%	0.70–1.30 mcmol/L
Factor X (Stuart factor)	60%–140%	0.70–1.30 mcmol/L
Factor VIII (antihemophilic globulin)	50%–200%	0.50–2.0 mcmol/L
Factor IX (plasma thromboplastic cofactor)	60%–140%	0.60–1.40 mcmol/L
Factor XI (plasma thromboplastic antecedent)	60%–140%	0.60–1.40 mcmol/L
Factor XII (Hageman factor)	60%–140%	0.60–1.40 mcmol/L
Coagulation Screening Tests		
Bleeding time (Simplate)	2–8 min	180–540 sec
Prothrombin time	9.5–12 sec	Less than 2 sec from control
Partial thromboplastin time (activated)	20–45 sec	25–37 sec
INR	1.0	none
Whole blood clot lysis	No clot lysis in 24 hr	0/day

(continued)

Table • B-1 HEMATOLOGIC VALUES—REFERENCE RANGES *(continued)*		
Determination	**Conventional**	**SI**
Fibrinolytic Studies		
Euglobin lysis	No lysis in 2 hr	0 (in 2 hr)
Thrombin time		Control 15 sec
Complete Blood Count		
Hematocrit	Male: 42%–50% Female: 40%–48%	Male: 0.42–0.52 Female: 0.37–0.48
Hemoglobin	Male: 13–18 g/dL Female: 12–16 g/dL	Male: 8.1–11.2 mmol/L Female: 7.4–9.9 mmol/L
Leukocyte count	5,000–10,000/mm^3	4.3–10.8 × 10^9/L
Erythrocyte count	4.2 million–5.9 million/mm^3	4.2–5.9 × 10^{12}/L
Mean corpuscular volume (MCV)	80–94 mcm^3	80–94 fl
Mean corpuscular hemoglobin (MCH)	27–32 pg	1.7–2.0 fmol
Mean corpuscular hemoglobin concentration (MCHC)	33%–38%	19–22.8 mmol/L
Erythrocyte sedimentation rate (Zeta Centrifuge)	41%–54%	Male: 1–13 mm/h Female: 1–20 mm/h
Erythrocyte Enzymes		
Glucose-6-phosphate dehydrogenase	5–15 U/g Hb	5–15 U/g
Pyruvate kinase	13–17 U/g Hb	13–17 U/g
Ferritin (serum)	Females: 5–100 ng/mL Males: 10–270 ng/mL	
Folic acid, RIA	4–16 ng/mL	
Haptoglobin	50–250 mg/dL	1.0 g–3.0 g/L
Hemoglobin Studies		
Electrophoresis for A$_2$ hemoglobin	1.5%–3.5%	0.015–0.035
Hemoglobin, met- and sulf-	0	0
Serum hemoglobin	2–3 mg/100 mL	1.2–1.9 mcmol/L
Lupus erythematosus (LE) preparation		
Heparin as anticoagulant	0	0
Defibrinated blood	0	0
Muramidase	Serum, 3–7 mcg/mL Urine, 0–2 mcg/mL	3–7 mg/L 0–2 mg/L
Osmotic fragility of erythrocyte	Increased if hemolysis occurs in over 0.5% NaCl; decreased if hemolysis is incomplete in 0.3% NaCl	
Peroxide hemolysis	Less than 10%	<0.10
Platelet count	100,000–400,000/mm^3	150–350 × 10^9/L
Platelet Function Tests		
Clot retraction	50%–100%/2 hr	0.50–1.00/2 hr
Platelet aggregation	Full response to ADP, epinephrine and collagen	1.0
Platelet factor 3	33–57 sec	33–57 sec
Reticulocyte count	0.5%–1.5% red cells	0.005–0.15
Vitamin B$_{12}$	90–280 pg/mL (borderline: 70–90)	66–207 pmol/L (borderline: 52–66)

TABLE • B-2   BLOOD, PLASMA, OR SERUM VALUES—REFERENCE RANGES

Determination	Conventional	SI
Acetoacetate plus acetone	0.3–2.0 mg/dL	3–20 mg/L
Aldolase	1.3–8.2 mU/mL	12–75 nmol sec^{-1}/L
Alpha amino nitrogen	3.0–5.5 mg/100 mL	2.1–3.9 mmol/L
Ammonia	80–110 mcg/100 mL	47–65 mcmol/L
Ascorbic acid	0.4–1.5 mg/100 mL	23–85 mcmol/L
Bilirubin (van den Bergh test)	1 minute: 0.4 mg/100 mL Direct: 0.1–0.2 mg/dL Total: 1.0 mg/100 mL Indirect: 0.1–1.0 mg/dL	Up to 7 mcmol/L Up to 17 mcmol/L
Blood volume	8.5%–9.0% of body weight in kg Toxic level: 17 mEq/L	80–85 mL/kg
Bromsulphalein (BSP)	Less than 5% retention 45 min after 5 mg/kg IV	<0.05 L
Calcium	8.5–10.5 mg/100 mL	2.1–2.5 mmol/L
Carbon dioxide content	24 mEq–32 mEq/L	24–30 mmol/L
Carcinoembryonic antigen (CEA)	0.25 mg/mL	0–2.5 mcg/L
Carotenoids	0.8–4.0 mcg/mL	1.5–7.4 mcmol/L
Ceruloplasmin	27–37 mg/100 mL	1.8–2.4 mcmol/L
Chloride	95–105 mEq/L	100–106 mmol/L
Cholesterol	<200 mg/dL	
Cholinesterase (pseudocholinesterase)	0.5 pH U or more/hr 0.7 pH U or more/hr for packed cells	0.5 arb unit or more
Copper	Total: 100–200 mcg/100 mL	16–31 mcmol/L
Creatine phosphokinase (CPK)	Female: 50–250 mU/mL Male: 50–325 mU/mL	0.08–0.58 mcmol sec^{-1}/L
Creatinine	0.7–1.4 mg/100 mL	60–130 mcmol/L
Ethanol	0.3%–0.4%, marked intoxication; 0.4%–0.5%, alcoholic stupor; 0.5% or over, alcoholic coma	65–87 mmol/L 87–109 mmol/L >109 mmol/L
Glucose	Fasting: 60–100 mg/dL	3.9–5.6 mmol/L
Iron	65–170 mcg/100 mL (higher in males)	9.0–26.9 mcmol/L
Iron-binding capacity	250–410 mcg/100 mL	44.8–73.4 mcmol/L
Lactic acid	0.6–1.8 mEq/L	0.6–1.8 mmol/L
Lactic dehydrogenase isoenzymes	100–225 mU/mL	1.00–2.00 mcmol sec^{-1}/L
Lead	50 mcg/100 mL or less	Up to 2.4 mcmol/L
Lipase	2 U/mL or less	Up to 2 arb units
Lipids, total	400–1,000 mg/dL	3.10–5.69 mmol/L
Magnesium	0.33–2.4 mEq/L	0.8–1.3 mmol/L
5^9 Nucleotidase	0.3–3.2 Bodansky U	30–290 nmol sec^{-1}/L
Osmolality	280–300 mOsm/kg water	285–295 mmol/kg
Oxygen saturation (arterial)	95%–100%	0.96–1.00 L

(continued)

TABLE • B-2   BLOOD, PLASMA, OR SERUM VALUES—REFERENCE RANGES *(continued)*

Determination	Conventional	SI
P_{CO_2}	35–45 mm Hg	4.7–6.0 kPg
pH	7.35–7.45	Same
P_{O_2}	95–100 mm Hg (dependent on age while breathing room air) Above 500 mm Hg while on 100% O_2	10.0–13.3 kPa
Phenylalanine	0–2 mg/100 mL	0–120 mcmol/L
Phosphorus (inorganic)	3.0–4.5 mg/100 mL	1.0–1.5 mmol/L
Potassium	3.8–5.0 mEq/L	3.5–5.0 mmol/L
Primidone (Mysoline)	Therapeutic level, 4–12 mcg/mL	18–55 mcmol/L
Protein, total	6.0–8.0 g/100 mL	60–84 g/L
Albumin	3.5–5.0 g/100 mL	33–50 g/L
Globulin	1.5–3.0 g/100 mL	23–35 g/L
Electrophoresis	% of total protein	% of total protein
Albumin	3.3–5.0 g/dL	0.52–0.68
Globulin		
Alpha$_1$	0.2–0.4 g/dL	0.042–0.072
Alpha$_2$	0.6–1.0 g/dL	0.068–0.12
Beta	0.6–1.2 g/dL	0.093–0.15
Gamma	0.7–1.5 g/dL	0.13–0.23
	0.3–0.7 mg/dL	0–0.11 mmol/L
Sodium	135–145 mEq/L	135–145 mmol/L
Sulfate	0.5–1.5 mg/100 mL	0.05–1.2 mmol/L
Transaminase (SGOT) (aspartate aminotransferase)	7–40 U/mL	0.08–0.32 mcmol sec^{-1}/L
Urea nitrogen (BUN)	10–20 mg/100 mL	2.9–8.9 mmol/L
Uric acid	2.5–8.0 mg/100 mL	0.13–0.42 mmol/L
Vitamin A	50–220 mcg/dL	0.5–2.1 mcmol/L

TABLE • B-3   URINE VALUES—REFERENCE RANGES

Determination	Conventional	SI
Acetone plus acetoacetate (quantitative)	0	0 mg/L
Alpha amino nitrogen	64–199 mg/day; not over 1.5% of total nitrogen	4.6–14.2 mmol/day
Amylase	35–260 U/mL	24–76 arb units
Calcium	150 mg/day or less	3.8 mmol/day or less
Catecholamines	Epinephrine, 10%–40% Norepinephrine, 60%–90%	<55 nmol/day <590 nmol/day
Copper	20–70 mcg/day	0–1.6 mcmol/day
Coproporphyrin	50–300 mcg/day	80–380 nmol/day
Creatine	0–200 mg/24 hr	<0.75 mmol/day
Cystine or cysteine	0	0
Follicle-stimulating hormone		
Follicular phase	5–20 IU/day	Same
Midcycle	15–60 IU/day	
Luteal phase	5–15 IU/day	
Menopausal	50–100 IU/day	
Men	5–25 IU/day	

(continued)

TABLE • B-3   URINE VALUES—REFERENCE RANGES *(continued)*

Determination	Conventional	SI
Hemoglobin and myoglobin	0	
5-Hydroxyindole acetic acid	2–9 mg/day (women lower than men)	10–45 mcmol/day
Phenolsulfonphthalein (PSP)	At least 25% excreted by 15 min; 40% by 30 min; 60% by 120 min	0.25 L
Phosphorus (inorganic)	Varies with intake; average 1 g/day	32 mmol/day
Porphobilinogen	0	0
Protein, quantitative	<150 mg/24 hr	<0.15 g/day

Steroids

17-Ketosteroids (per day)

Age (yr)	Male (mg)	Female (mg)	Male (mcmol/day)	Female (mcmol/day)
10	1–4	1–4	3–14	3–14
20	6–21	4–16	21–73	14–56
30	8–26	4–14	28–90	14–49
50	5–18	3–9	17–62	10–31
70	2–10	1–7	7–35	3–24

Determination	Conventional	SI
17-Hydroxysteroids	3–8 mg/day (women lower than men)	8–22 mcmol/day as hydrocortisone
Sugar		
Quantitative glucose	0	0 mmol/L
Identification of reducing substances		
Fructose	0	0 mmol/L
Pentose	0	0 mmol/L
Titratable acidity	20–40 mEq/day	20–40 mmol/day
Urobilinogen	<0.25 mg/dL	To 1.0 arb unit
Uroporphyrin	Up to 50 mcg in 24 hr	0 nmol/day
Vanilmandelic acid (VMA)	0.7–6.8 mg/24 hr	Up to 45 mcmol/day

TABLE • B-4   CEREBROSPINAL FLUID VALUES—REFERENCE RANGES

Determination	Conventional	SI
Bilirubin	0	0 mcmol/L
Chloride	100–130 mEq/L	
Albumin	15.5–32.0 mg/dL	0.295 g/L 6 2 SD (0.11–0.48)
IgG	0–6.6 mg/dL	0.043 g/L 6 2 SD (0–0.086)
Glucose	50–75 mg/100 mL (30%–50% less than blood)	2.8–4.2 mmol/L
Pressure (initial)	70–180 mm H_2O	70–80 arb units
Protein		
Lumbar	15–45 mg/100 mL	0.15–0.45 g/L
Cisternal	15–25 mg/100 mL	0.15–0.25 g/L
Ventricular	5–15 mg/100 mL	0.05–0.15 g/L

Table • B-5 SPECIAL ENDOCRINE TESTS—REFERENCE RANGES

Determination	Conventional	SI
Steroid Hormones		
Aldosterone	Excretion: 5–19 mcg/24 hr	14–53 nmol/day
Fasting, at rest, 210 mEq sodium diet	Supine: 48 ± 29 pg/mL	133 ± 80 pmol/L
	Upright: (2h) 65 ± 23 pg/mL	180 ± 64 pmol/L
Fasting, at rest, 110 mEq sodium diet	Supine: 107 ± 45 pg/mL	279 ± 125 pmol/L
	Upright: 239 ± 123 pg/mL	663 ± 341 pmol/L
Fasting, at rest, 10 mEq sodium diet	Supine: 175 ± 75 pg/mL	485 ± 208 pmol/L
	Upright: 532 ± 228 pg/mL	1,476 ± 632 pmol/L
Cortisol		
Fasting	8 AM: 5–25 mcg/100 mL	0.14–0.69 mcmol/L
At rest	8 PM: below 10 mcg/100 mL	0–0.28 mcmol/L
20 U ACTH	4-hour ACTH test: 30–45 mcg/100 mL	0.83–1.24 mcmol/L
Dexamethasone at midnight	Overnight suppression test: below 5 mcg/100 mL	<0.14 nmol/L
	Excretion: 20–70 mcg/24 hr	55–193 nmol/day
11-Deoxycortisol	Responsive: over 7.5 mcg/100 mL (after metrapone)	>0.22 mcmol/L
Testosterone	Adult male: 300–1,100 ng/100 mL	10.4–38.1 nmol/L
	Adolescent male: over 100 ng/100 mL	>3.5 nmol/L
	Females: 25–90 ng/100 mL	0.87–3.12 nmol/L
Unbound testosterone	Adult male: 3.06–24.0 ng/100 mL	106–832 pmol/L
	Adult female: 0.09–1.28 ng/100 mL	3.1–44.4 pmol/L
Polypeptide Hormones		
Adrenocorticotrophin (ACTH)	15–70 pg/mL	3.3–15.4 pmol/L
Calcitonin	Undetectable in normals	0
	>100 pg/mL in medullary carcinoma	>29.3 pmol/L
Growth hormone		
Fasting, at rest	Below 5 ng/mL	<233 pmol/L
After exercise	Children: over 10 ng/mL	>465 pmol/L
	Male: below 5 ng/mL	<233 pmol/L
	Female: up to 30 ng/mL	0–1,395 pmol/L
After glucose	Male: below 5 ng/mL	<233 pmol/L
	Female: below 10 mg/mL	0–465 pmol/L
Insulin		
Fasting	6–26 mcU/mL	43–187 pmol/L
During hypoglycemia	Below 20 mcU/mL	<144 pmol/L
After glucose	Up to 150 mcU/mL	0–1,078 pmol/L
Luteinizing hormone	Male: 6–18 mU/mL	6–18 U/L
Preovulatory or postovulatory	Female: 5–22 mU/mL	5–22 U/L
Midcycle peak	30–250 mU/mL	30–250 U/L
Parathyroid hormone	<10 mcl equiv/mL	<10 mL equiv/L
Prolactin	2–15 ng/mL	0.08–6.0 nmol/L
Renin activity		
Normal diet	Supine: 1.1 ± 0.8 ng/mL/hr	0.9 ± 0.6 nmol/L/hr
	Upright: 1.9 ± 1.7 ng/mL/hr	1.5 ± 1.3 nmol/L/hr
Low-sodium diet	Supine: 2.7 ± 1.8 ng/mL/hr	2.1 ± 1.4 nmol/L/hr
	Upright: 6.6 ± 2.5 ng/mL/hr	5.1 ± 1.9 nmol/L/hr
High-sodium diet	Diuretics: 10.0 ± 3.7 ng/mL/hr	7.7 ± 2.9 nmol/L/hr
Thyroid Hormones		
Thyroid-stimulating hormone (TSH)	0.5–3.5 mcU/mL	0.5–3.5 mU/L
Thyroxine-binding globulin capacity	15–25 mcg T_4/100 mL	193–322 mU/L
Total triiodothyronine by radioimmunoassay (T_3)	70–190 ng/100 mL	1.08–2.92 nmol/L
Total thyroxine (T_4) by RIA	4–12 mcg/100 mL	52–154 nmol/L
T_3 resin uptake	25%–35%	0.25–0.35
Free thyroxine index (FT_4I)	1–4 ng/100 mL	12.8–51.2 pmol/L

Glossary

A

Abduction: lateral movement of the body part away from the midline of the body

Absorption: process by which drugs are transferred from the site of entry into the body to the bloodstream

Abstinence: refraining from having sex

Accommodation: (1) ability to adjust the eye to see at various distances; (2) process by which intellectual acts are changed to handle increasingly complex information

Accreditation: process by which an educational program is evaluated and then recognized as having met certain predetermined standards of education

Acid: substance containing a hydrogen ion that can be liberated or released

Acidosis: condition characterized by a proportionate excess of hydrogen ions in the extracellular fluid, in which the pH falls below 7.35

Acquired immunodeficiency syndrome (AIDS): condition in which the body's immune system is rendered ineffective as a result of infection by the retrovirus HIV

Active euthanasia: someone other than the patient commits an action with the intent to end the patient's life, for example, injecting him or her with a lethal dose of a drug

Active exercise: joint movement activated by the person

Active immunity: antibodies against harmful effects of microorganisms or toxins that are self-produced

Active transport: movement of ions or molecules across cell membranes, usually against a pressure gradient and with the expenditure of metabolic energy

Actual loss: loss that can be recognized by others as well as by the person sustaining the loss, such as loss of a limb or a spouse

Actual nursing diagnoses: problems validated by the presence of major defining characteristics and possessing four components: label, definition, defining characteristics, and related factor

Actual problems: health problems that have been validated by the presence of major defining characteristics

Acupuncture: procedure consisting of placing very thin, short, sterile needles at particular acupoints, believed to be centers of nerve and vascular tissue, along a meridian to either increase or decrease the flow of chi along the meridian, restoring the balance of yin and yang, and thereby contributing to healing

Acute illness: rapidly occurring illness that runs its course, allowing the person to return to his or her previous level of functioning

Acute pain: episode of pain that lasts from seconds to less than 6 months

Adaptation: adjustment of living with other living things and environmental conditions

Addiction: a pattern of compulsive use of addictive substances for means other than those prescribed

Addictive: substance to which a person develops a psychological and physiologic dependency

Adduction: movement of a body part toward the midline of the body

Adjuvant: drugs typically used for other purposes, but also used to enhance the effect of opioids by providing additional pain relief

Adolescence: the period of time between childhood and adulthood; a time of rapid physical change, reproductive maturity, and emotional development

Advance directive: written directive that allows people to state in advance what their choices for healthcare would be if certain circumstances should develop

Adventitious breath sounds: abnormal breath sound heard over the lungs

Adverse drug effects: undesirable effects other than the intended therapeutic effect of a drug

Advocacy: protection and support of another's rights

Aerobic bacteria: bacteria that require oxygen to live and grow

Aerobic exercise: exercise that promotes cardiovascular fitness; it increases blood flow, heart rate, and the metabolic demand for oxygen over a period of time

Afebrile: a condition in which the body temperature is not elevated

Affective learning: changes in attitudes, values, and feelings

Ageism: attitudes that stereotype the older adult on the basis of chronologic age

Agency for Healthcare Research and Quality (AHRQ): a group of multidisciplinary experts who use research as well as a broad range of input from professional and consumer organizations and individuals to develop clinical practice guidelines

Agglutinin: an antibody that causes a clumping of specific antigens

Agnostic: person who believes that nothing can be known about the existence of a god

Albuminuria: albumin in the urine; an indication of kidney disease

Alkali: substance that can accept or trap a hydrogen ion; synonym for base

Alkalosis: condition, characterized by a proportionate lack of hydrogen ions in the extracellular fluid concentration, in which the pH exceeds 7.45

Allergic effect: immune system response that occurs when the body interprets the administered drug as a foreign substance and forms antibodies against the drug

Allodynia: characteristic feature of neuropathic pain that occurs after a normally weak or nonpainful stimuli, such as a light touch or a cold drink

Allopathy: (biomedicine), the term generally used to describe "traditional" medical care, dominant for about 100 years, which spearheaded remarkable advances in biotechnology, surgical interventions, pharmaceutical approaches, and diagnostic tools

Alopecia: baldness

Alternative care: general term used to identify various methods of nonhospital healthcare, including residential housing, day-care, respite care, hospice, and extended-care facilities

Alternative modalities: methods not included in the scope of conventional medical care

Alveoli: small air sacs at the end of the terminal bronchioles that are the site of gas exchange

Alzheimer's disease: type of dementia in which discrete patches of brain tissue degenerate; this devastating disease eventually affects all body functions

Ambulatory care: healthcare settings located in areas that are convenient for people to walk into and receive care; may be provided in hospitals, clinics, or centers

Amino acid: basic building blocks used to manufacture protein and the end products of protein digestion

Ampule: glass flask containing a single dose of medication for parenteral administration

Anaerobic bacteria: bacteria that can live without oxygen

Anaerobic exercise: exercise in which the supply of oxygen is less than the demand created by contracting muscles; oxygen debt results

Analgesic drug: pharmaceutical agent used to relieve pain

Anaphylactic reaction/Anaphylaxis: severe reaction occurring immediately after exposure to a drug; characterized by respiratory distress and vascular collapse

Andragogy: the study of teaching adults

Anesthetic: agent that produces states such as loss of consciousness, analgesia, relaxation, and loss of reflexes

Anion: ion that carries a negative electric charge

Ankylosis: fixation or immobilization of a joint

Anorexia: lack or loss of appetite for food

Anorexia nervosa: eating disorder characterized by the denial of appetite and bizarre eating habits

Anoxia: absence of oxygen

Antagonistic effect: combined effect of two or more drugs that produces less than the effect of each drug alone

Anthropometric: measurements of the body and body parts

Antibacterial: agent that kills bacteria or suppresses their growth

Antibody: immunoglobin produced by the body in response to a specific antigen

Anticipatory loss: condition in which a person displays loss and grief behaviors for a loss that has yet to take place

Antigen: foreign material capable of inducing a specific immune response

Antimicrobial: antibacterial agent that kills bacteria or suppresses their growth

Antipyretic: agent that reduces fever

Antiseptic: substance that inhibits the growth of bacteria

Anuria: technically, no urine voided; 24-hour urine output is less than 100 mL

Anus: opening at the end of anal canal

Anxiety: vague sense of impending doom or apprehension precipitated by new and unknown experiences

Apnea: absence of breathing

Applied research (practical research): research designed to directly influence or improve clinical practice

Aromatherapy: the use of essential oils of plants to treat symptoms

Arousal: condition in which the cortical area of the brain receives and responds appropriately to stimuli

Ascites: accumulation of fluid in the peritoneal cavity

Asepsis: absence of disease-producing microorganisms; using methods to prevent infection

Asphyxiation: stoppage of breathing or the lack of air reaching the lungs; synonym for suffocation

Aspiration: misdirection of oropharyngeal secretions or gastric contents into the larynx and lower respiratory tract

Assault: threat or an attempt to make bodily contact with another person without that person's permission

Assertiveness: ability to stand up for oneself and others using open, honest, and direct communication

Assess: to systematically and continuously collect, validate, and communicate patient data

Assimilation: process by which a person interprets information to fit the current level of cognition

Assisted suicide: the act of making a means of suicide (e.g., providing pills or a weapon) available to a patient with knowledge of his or her intention; in assisted suicide, someone makes the means of death available but does not act as the direct agent of death

Atelectasis: incomplete expansion or collapse of a part of the lungs

Atheist: person who denies the existence of a god

Atria: upper chambers of the heart

Atrophy: decrease in the size of a body structure

Attachment: active, affectionate, reciprocal relationship between two persons

Attitude: feeling or emotion, generally including a positive or negative judgment toward people, objects, or ideas

Auditory: pertaining to hearing

Aura: consists of at least seven layers of energy that surround the body and relate to the chakras

Auscultation: listening for sounds within the body

Authoritative knowledge: knowledge that comes from an expert and is accepted as truth based on a perceived level of expertise

Autocratic leadership: leadership style in which the leader assumes complete control over the decisions and activities of the group

Autologous transfusion: occurs when a patient donates his or her own blood for a transfusion

Autonomic bladder: bladder no longer controlled by the brain because of injury or disease; void by reflex only

Autonomy: self-determination; being independent and self-governing

Ayurveda: a science of life that delineates the diet, medicines, and behaviors that are beneficial or harmful for life and considers that balance among people, the environment, and the larger cosmos is integral to human health

B

Bacteria: the most significant and most commonly observed infection-causing agents

Bacteriuria: condition that occurs when bacteria enter the bladder during catheterization, or when organisms migrate up the catheter lumen or the urethra into the bladder; bacteria in the urine

Bandage: piece of gauze or other material used to cover a wound

Basal metabolism: amount of energy required to carry out involuntary activities of the body at rest

Base: substance that can accept or trap a hydrogen ion; synonym for alkali

Base of support: foundation that provides stability for an object

Basic human needs: something essential to the health and survival of humans; common to all people

Basic research (pure research): research designed to generate and refine theory; the findings are often not directly useful in practice

Battery: assault that is carried out

Beliefs: special class of intellectual attitudes based primarily on faith as opposed to fact

Beneficence: principle of doing good

Bereavement: state of grieving or going through the grief process

Bereavement care: continuation of care, usually up to 1 year, for the family after loss of a loved one

Bilateral: pertaining to two sides of the body

Binder: type of bandage, usually designed to fit a large body area

Bioethics: ethics that encompass all those perspectives that seek to understand human nature and behavior, the domain of social science, and the natural world

Biologic sex: term used to denote chromosomal sexual development—male (XY) or female (XX)

Biopsy: removal of a piece of tissue for microscopic examination

Bioterrorism: the deliberate spread of pathogenic organisms into a community to cause widespread illness, fear, and panic

Bisexuality: having sexual feelings for people of both sexes

Blended family: two single-parent families joined together to form a new family unit

Blood pressure: force of blood against arterial walls

Body image: how a person experiences his or her body

Body language: nonverbal communication

Body mass index (BMI): ratio of height to weight

Body mechanics: efficient use of the body as a machine and as a means of locomotion

Body substance isolation (BSI): type of isolation that considers all body substances as potentially infective regardless of a person's diagnosis

Bolus: single injection of a concentrated solution administered intravenously

Bonding: process of initial emotional fusing of the mother and infant that occurs most often in the first few hours after birth and is necessary for later attachment

Bowel incontinence: the inability of the anal sphincter to control the discharge of fecal and gaseous material

Bowel movement: emptying of the intestinal tract; synonym for *defecation*

Bowel training program: program that manipulates factors within a person's control (timing of defecation, exercise, diet) to produce a regular pattern of comfortable defecation without medication or enemas

Bradycardia: slow heart rate

Bradypnea: slow rate of breathing

Breakthrough pain: temporary flare-up of moderate to severe pain that occurs even when the patient is taking around-the-clock medication for persistent pain

Bronchial sounds: those heard over the trachea; high in pitch and intensity, with expiration being longer than inspiration

Bronchodilator: medication that relaxes contractions of smooth muscles of the bronchioles

Bronchoscopy: visual examination of the trachea and bronchi

Bronchovesicular sounds: normal breath sounds heard over the upper anterior chest and intercostal area

Bruit: unusual sound, usually abnormal, heard in auscultation

Buffer: substance that prevents body fluid from becoming overly acid or alkaline

Bulimia: eating disorder characterized by episodes of gorging followed by purging; often occurs in conjunction with anorexia nervosa

Burnout: behaviors exhibited as the result of prolonged occupational stress

C

Calorie: measure of heat, or energy; *kilocalorie,* commonly referred to as a calorie, defined as the amount of heat required to raise 1 kg of water 1°C

Carbohydrate: organic compounds (commonly known as sugars and starches) that are composed of carbon, hydrogen, and oxygen; the most abundant and least expensive source of calories in the diet worldwide

Cardiac output: volume of blood pumped from the left ventricle per minute

Cardinal signs: body temperature, pulse and respiratory rates, and blood pressure; synonym for *vital signs*

Care-based approach: approach to bioethics that directs attention to the specific situations of individual patients viewed within the context of their life narrative

Caregiver burden: stress responses experienced during prolonged periods of home care by family caregivers

Caries: cavities of the teeth

Cartilage: hard nonvascular connective tissue found in the joints as well as in the nose, ear, thorax, trachea, and larynx

Cascade iatrogenesis: downward spiral or sequence of adverse events often triggered by a medical or surgical intervention during the hospitalization of an older adult

Case management: the process of coordinating an individual's healthcare for the purpose of maximizing positive outcomes and containing costs

Cathartic: medication that strongly increases gastrointestinal motility and promotes defecation

Catheter: tube for injecting or removing fluids

Cation: ion that carries a positive electric charge

Center of gravity: point at which the mass of an object is centered

Centers for Disease Control and Prevention (CDC): U.S. government agency whose responsibilities include investigation, identification, prevention, and control of disease

Central venous catheter: venous access device usually introduced into the subclavian or internal jugular veins and passed to the superior vena cava just above the right atrium

Certification: process by which a person who has met certain criteria established by a nongovernmental association is granted recognition

Cerumen: wax in the external ear canals, consisting of a heavy oil and brown pigment

Ceruminal gland: gland found in the external auditory canal that secretes *cerumen*

Chakra: concentrated areas of energy aligned vertically in the body, which relate to each other as well as to specific areas of the body/mind/spirit

Change: process of transforming, altering, or modifying something

Change agent: person who purposefully and systematically implements change

Change-of-shift report: communication method used by nurses who are completing care for a patient to transmit patient information to nurses who are about to assume responsibility for continuing care; may be exchanged verbally in a meeting or audiotaped

Channel: term used in communication theory to denote the medium selected to convey the message; the channel may target any of the receiver's senses

Chart: computerized or paper medical record containing information such as medical orders, assessments, and care; nursing documentation of plan of care, assessments, and interventions; and diagnostic/surgery results

Charting by exception: shorthand method for documenting patient data that is based on well-defined standards of practice; only exceptions to these standards are documented in narrative notes

Cheilosis: ulceration of the lips

Chemical name: precise description of a drug's chemical composition

Chemical terrorism: the deliberate release of a chemical compound that has the potential for harming people's health

Cheyne-Stokes respirations: gradual increase and then gradual decrease in depth of respirations followed by a period of apnea

Child maltreatment: an act or series of acts of commission (abuse) or omission (neglect) by a parent or other caregiver that results in harm, potential for harm, or threat of harm to a child

Chiropractic medicine: science that investigates the relationship between structure (the spine) and function (mainly the nervous system) of the human body to restore and preserve health

Cholesterol: fat-like substance found only in animal tissues; it is important for cell membrane structure, a precursor of steroid hormones, and a constituent of bile; high serum cholesterol levels are a risk factor in the development of atherosclerosis

Chronic illness: irreversible illness that causes permanent physical impairment and requires long-term healthcare

Chronic pain: episode of pain that lasts for 6 months or longer; may be intermittent or continuous

Chyme: semifluid state that food is in when it leaves the stomach

Cilia: microscopic hair-like projections that propel mucus toward the upper airway so that it can be expectorated

Circadian rhythm: rhythm that completes a full cycle every 24 hours; synonym for *diurnal rhythm*

Circumduction: moving the distal part of the limb to trace a complete circle while the proximal end remains fixed

Civil law: rule that regulates relationships among people; synonym for *private law*

Clear liquid diet: diet that contains only foods that are clear liquids at room or body temperature—gelatin, fat-free broth, bouillon, ice pops, clear juices, carbonated beverages, and regular and decaffeinated coffee and tea

Cliché: a stereotyped, trite, or pat answer

Clinical ethics: branch of bioethics concerned with ethical problems that arise within the context of caring for patients

Clinical pathway/critical path/CareMap: case management tools used to communicate the standardized, interdisciplinary plan of care for a particular group of patients; care guidelines and outcomes are specified for each day of the patient's stay

Clubbing: rounding and swelling of nailbeds

Code of ethics: principles that reflect the primary goals, values, and obligations of the profession

Cognition: cerebral functioning; process of perceiving and understanding one's world

Cognitive development: learning that occurs as a result of the internal organization of an event, which forms a mental schema (plan) and serves as a base for further schemata as one grows and develops (Piaget's theory of cognitive development)

Cognitive learning: storing and recalling of new knowledge in the brain

Cognitively skilled: capable of thinking about the nature of things sufficiently to "make sense" of the world and to grasp conceptually what is necessary to achieve valued goals

Coitus: sexual activity in which the penis is placed in the vagina; synonym for *sexual intercourse*

Colic: acute abdominal pain caused by spasmodic contractions of the intestine during the first 3 months of life

Collaborative interventions: interdependent nursing actions performed jointly by nurses and other members of the healthcare team

Collaborative problem: actual or potential health problem that may occur from complications of disease, diagnostic studies, or the treatment regimen; the nurse works together with other members of the healthcare team toward its resolution

Colloid osmotic pressure: pressure exerted by plasma proteins on permeable membranes in the body; synonym for *oncotic pressure*

Colon: section of the large intestine from the cecum to the rectum

Colostomy: an opening into the colon that permits feces to exit through the stoma

Comfort-measures-only order: an order written to indicate that the goal of treatment is a comfortable, dignified death and that further life-sustaining measures are no longer indicated

Common law: law resulting from court decisions that is then followed when other cases involving similar circumstances and facts arise; common law is as binding as civil law

Communication: process of sharing information; process of generating and transmitting meanings

Community: specific population or group of people living in the same geographic area under similar regulations and having common values, interests, and needs

Community-based healthcare: healthcare that is provided to people who live within a defined geographic region or who have common needs; designed to meet the needs of people as they move between and among healthcare settings

Complaint: legal statement of the plaintiff's claim; once filed, it initiates legal proceedings

Complementary/alternative therapies: alternative treatments used with traditional medical interventions

Compliance: act of completing what is expected of one

Comprehensive assessment: health history and complete physical examination, usually conducted when a patient first enters a healthcare setting, provides a baseline for comparing later assessment

Computer-based record: computer-generated patient data collection system that can be distributed among many caregivers in a standardized format, allowing them to compare and uniformly evaluate patient progress easily, or compare the progress of groups of patients with similar diagnoses

Computerized plans of nursing care: plans of patient care developed by computer software programs that enable the nurse to call up screens listing causes, goals, and related nursing interventions for nursing diagnoses and medical diagnoses

Concept: abstract images (ideas) that are formed as impressions from the environment and organized into symbols of reality

Concept mapping: instructional strategy that requires learners to identify, graphically display, and link key concepts

Conceptual framework/model: set of concepts, along with the statements that arrange the concepts into an understandable pattern

Concurrent audit: evaluation of nursing care and patient outcomes conducted while the patient is receiving care; may use direct observation of nursing care, patient interview, and chart review

Concurrent evaluation: the evaluation of nursing care and patient outcomes while the patient is receiving care, conducted by using direct observation of nursing care, patient interviews, and chart review to determine whether the specified evaluative criteria are met

Condom catheter: tube for draining urine; applied externally to the penis and connecting to a collection bag

Confer: to consult with someone to exchange ideas or to seek information, advice, or instructions

Confidentiality: respecting privileged information

Congestion: presence of excessive fluids or secretions in an organ or body tissue

Conscious sedation/analgesia: analgesia used for short-term procedures in which the patient maintains cardiorespiratory function and can respond to verbal commands while the IV administration of sedatives and analgesics raises the pain threshold and produces an altered mood and some degree of amnesia

Constipation: passage of dry, hard, fecal material

Consultation: process in which two or more individuals with varying degrees of experience and expertise deliberate about a problem and its solution

Consumer: the person who uses healthcare services (the patient)

Continuity of care: coordination of services provided to patients before they enter a healthcare setting, during the time they are in the setting, and after they leave the setting

Continuum: graduated scale

Contraception: prevention of conception or pregnancy; also used to describe methods used for birth control

Contractual agreement: pact made between two persons or parties for the achievement of mutually set goals

Contracture: permanently contracted state of a muscle

Convalescent period: stage of an illness that represents recovery from the illness (or surgery)

Coping mechanism: patterns of behavior used to neutralize, deny, or counteract anxiety

Counseling: giving guidance, assisting with problem solving

Crackles: fine crackling sounds made as air moves through wet secretions in the lungs

Credentialing: general term that refers to ways in which professional competence is maintained

Crime: offense against people or property; the act is considered to be against the government, referred to in a lawsuit as "the people," and the accused is prosecuted by the state

Crisis: (1) point at which body temperature drops rapidly to normal; (2) occurs when coping and defense mechanisms are no longer effective, resulting in high levels of anxiety, disorganized behavior, and the inability to function normally

Crisis intervention: five-step problem-solving technique to promote adaptation and improve future coping

Criteria: specified behavior; for example, the measurable criteria in a patient goal specifies how the patient must perform the desired behavior

Critical/collaborative pathway: case management plan that is a detailed, standardized plan of care developed for a patient population with a designated diagnosis or procedure; it includes expected outcomes, a list of interventions to be performed, and the sequence and timing of those interventions

Critical thinking: thought that is disciplined, comprehensive, based on intellectual standards, and, as a result, well-reasoned; a systematic way to form and shape one's thinking that functions purposefully and exactingly

Critical thinking indicators (CTIs): evidence-based descriptions of behaviors that demonstrate the knowledge, characteristics, and skills that promote critical thinking in clinical practice

Cross-matching: act of determining the compatibility of two blood specimens

Cue: significant information that is helpful in making decisions

Cultural assimilation: process that occurs when a minority group, living as part of a dominant group within a culture, loses the cultural characteristics that made it different

Cultural blindness: the process of ignoring differences in people and proceeding as though the differences do not exist

Cultural care deprivation: a lack of culturally assistive, supportive, or facilitative acts in the healthcare setting

Cultural diversity: diverse groups in society, with varying racial classification and national origin, religious affiliation, languages, physical size, gender, sexual orientation, age, disability, socioeconomic status, occupational status, and geographic location

Cultural imposition: tendency of some to impose their beliefs, practices, and values on another culture because they believe that their ideas are superior to those of another person or group

Culturally competent care: care delivered with an awareness of the aspects of the patient's culture

Culture: sum total of human behavior or social characteristics peculiar to a specific group and passed from generation to generation or from one to another within the group

Culture conflict: situation that occurs when people become aware of cultural differences, feel threatened, and respond by ridiculing the beliefs and traditions of others to make themselves feel more secure about their own values

Culture shock: those feelings, usually negative, a person experiences when placed in a different culture

Cumulative effect: condition that occurs when the body cannot metabolize a drug before additional doses are administered

Cutaneous pain: superficial pain usually involving the skin or subcutaneous tissue

Cyanosis: bluish coloring of the skin and mucous membranes

Cystoscopy: direct visual examination of the bladder, ureteral orifices, and urethra with a cystoscope

Cytologic study: study of body cells and fluids

D

Dangling: position in which the person sits on the edge of the bed with legs and feet dangling over the side of the bed

Data: information

Database: all the pertinent patient information that enables a comprehensive and effective plan of care to be designed and implemented

Data cluster: grouping of patient data or cues that points to the existence of a patient health problem

Daycare center: centers that provide care for infants, children, elderly people, and people with special healthcare needs

Death: termination of life

Débridement: cleaning away devitalized tissue and foreign matter from a wound

Decentralized decision-making process: autonomous, accountable professional nursing practice; a characteristic of a democratic leadership style and the heart of a self-governance model of unit organization

Decision making: purposeful, goal-directed effort applied in a systematic way to make a choice among alternatives

Deductive reasoning: cognitive process in which one examines a general idea and then considers specific actions or ideas

Deep vein thrombosis (DVT): formation of a blood clot ("thrombus") in a deep vein

Defamation of character: an intentional tort in which one party makes derogatory remarks about another that diminishes the other party's reputation; slander is oral defamation of character; libel is written defamation of character

Defecation: emptying of the intestinal tract; synonym for *bowel movement*

Defendant: the one being accused of a crime or tort

Defense mechanisms: forms of self-deception; unconscious process the self uses to protect itself from anxiety or threats to self-esteem

Dehiscence: separation of the layers of a surgical wound; may be partial, superficial, or a complete disruption of the surgical wound

Dehydration: decreased water volume in body tissue

Delegation: the transfer of responsibility for the performance of an activity to another individual while retaining accountability for the outcome

Delirium: a temporary state of confusion

Delta sleep: deep sleep, occurring during stage III and especially stage IV in NREM sleep

Dementia: organic impairment of intellectual functioning, gradually leading to interference with social or occupational functioning, memory, and often personality integration

Democratic leadership: leadership style characterized by a sense of equality between the leader and followers

Deontologic: ethical system in which actions are right or wrong independent of the consequences they produce

Dependent action: nursing action carried out at the instruction or order of an authorized healthcare professional other than a nurse; synonym for *physician-initiated* or *physician-prescribed intervention*

Depersonalization: subjective experience of the partial or total disruption of one's ego and the disintegration and disorganization of one's self-concept

Dermis: layer of the skin below the epidermis

Desiccation: dehydration; the process of being rendered free from moisture

Development: increase in the complexity of function and progression to skill advancement

Developmental crisis: predictable patterns of behavior and change occurring throughout the life span

Developmental delay: measure of development that lags behind the normal range for a given age

Developmental task: successful achievement of psychomotor, psychosocial, or cognitive skills at certain periods in life; failure to obtain the developmental task can lead to unhappiness and difficulty with later tasks

Development theory: theory to describe the orderly and predictable process of the growth and development of humans, individualized by social, biologic, and environmental factors

Diagnosis (nursing): analysis of patient data to identify patient strengths and health problems that independent nursing intervention can prevent or resolve

Diagnosis-related groups (DRGs): classification of patients by major medical diagnosis for the purpose of standardizing healthcare costs

Diagnostic error: failure to detect an actual unhealthy behavior

Diarrhea: passage of liquid and unformed stools

Diastolic pressure: least amount of pressure exerted on arterial walls, which occurs when the heart is at rest between ventricular contractions

Dietary Guidelines: recommendations for choosing a healthy diet made by the U.S. Department of Agriculture and the U.S. Department of Health and Human Services

Diffuse pain: pain that covers a large area

Diffusion: tendency of solutes to move freely throughout a solvent from an area of higher concentration to an area of lower concentration until equilibrium is established

Digestion: gastrointestinal system's breakdown process of food into particles small enough to pass into the cells and be used by the cells

Direct transfusion: infusion of blood while it is being taken from the donor

Disaster: an emergency event of greater magnitude that requires the response of people outside the involved community

Discharge planning: systematic process of preparing the patient to leave the healthcare facility and for maintaining continuity of care

Discharge summary: description of where the patient stands in relation to problems identified in the record at discharge; documents any special teaching or counseling the patient received, including referrals

Discipline: specific and unique body of knowledge that uses existing and new knowledge to creatively solve problems and meet human needs within ever-changing boundaries

Disease: pathologic change in the structure or function of the body or mind

Disinfection: process used to destroy microorganisms; destroys all pathogenic organisms except spores

Distribution: movement of drugs by the circulatory system to the site of action

Disturbed sensory perception: a state in which the individual or group experiences or is at risk for a change in the amount, pattern, or interpretation of incoming stimuli

Documentation: written, legal record of all pertinent interventions with the patient—assessments, diagnoses, plans, interventions, and evaluations

Dominant group: group within a culture that has the authority to control the value system and determine the rewards of the system; usually the largest group in a society

Donor: person who donates blood or an organ to be given to another person

Do-not-hospitalize: an order specifying that a patient, usually one who is terminally ill and anticipating death, not be admitted to the hospital in the event of a worsening of condition

Do-not-resuscitate (DNR): an order specifying that there be no attempt to resuscitate a patient in the event of cardiopulmonary arrest

Dosha: the patient's basic condition; understanding dosha is central to Ayurvedic medicine

Dressing: protective covering placed over a wound

Drug: substance that modifies body functions when taken into the living organism; synonym for *medication*

Drug allergy: hypersensitivity caused by previous exposure to a medication; may occur immediately or be delayed; manifestations range from mild to severe

Drug tolerance: tendency of the body to become accustomed to a drug over time; larger doses are required to produce the desired effects

Dry powder inhalers (DPI): types of breath-activated delivery methods for inhaled medications

Dynorphin: the endorphin having the most potent analgesic effect

Dysfunctional grief: abnormal or distorted grief that may be either unresolved or inhibited

Dysphagia: difficulty in swallowing or inability to swallow

Dyspnea: difficult or labored breathing

Dysrhythmia: an abnormal cardiac rhythm

Dyssomnias: sleep disorders characterized by insomnia or excessive sleepiness

Dysuria: difficulty in voiding; may or may not be associated with pain

E

Ecchymosis: collection of blood in subcutaneous tissues that causes a purplish discoloration

Edema: accumulation of fluid in extracellular spaces

Elective surgery: surgery that is recommended but can be omitted or delayed without catastrophe

Electrocardiogram (ECG; EKG): graphic record produced by the electrocardiograph

Electroencephalograph: instrument that measures and records electric impulses of the brain

Electrolyte: substance capable of breaking into ions and developing an electric charge when dissolved in solution

Electromyograph (EMG): instrument that records muscle tone

Electronic medical records (EMR): computer-based records or data that can be distributed among many caregivers in a standardized format

Electrooculogram: recording of the electric current or potential produced by eye movements

Embolism: blocking of an artery by a blood clot or by other foreign matter brought to the site by the blood flow

Embolus: blood clot, foreign body, or air in the circulatory system; plural form is *emboli*

Emergency assessment: rapid focused assessment conducted to determine potentially fatal situations

Emergency surgery: surgery that must be performed immediately to save the person's life or a body organ

Empathy: intellectually identifying with the way another person feels

Endemic: something that occurs with predictability in one specific region or population and can appear in a different geographical location

Endogenous: infection in which the causative organism comes from microbial life the person himself or herself harbors

Endorphins: morphine-like substances released by the body that appear to alter the perception of pain

Endoscopy: direct visualization of hollow organs of the body using an endoscope or flexible, lighted tube

Endotracheal tube: polyvinyl-chloride airway that is inserted through the nose or the mouth into the trachea, using a laryngoscope as a guide

Enema: introduction of solution into the lower bowel

Enkephalins: opioids that are widespread throughout the brain and dorsal horn of the spinal cord and are believed to reduce pain sensation by inhibiting the release of substance P

Enteral nutrition: alternate form of feeding that involves passing a tube into the gastrointestinal tract to allow instillation of the appropriate formula

Entry phase: phase of the home visit in which the nurse develops rapport with the patient and family members, mutually determines outcomes, makes assessments, plans and implements prescribed care, and provides teaching

Enuresis: involuntary urination; most often used to refer to a child who involuntarily urinates during the night

Epidermis: superficial layer of the skin

Epidural analgesia: means of providing pain relief with an opioid injection delivered by way of a catheter inserted in the midlumbar region into the epidural space

Epithelialization: stage of wound healing in which epithelial cells form across the surface of a wound; tissue color ranges from the color of "ground glass" to pink

Erection: condition that results when erectile tissue of the penis fills with blood as a result of stimulation

Erogenous zones: areas of the body that produce sexual desire and arousal when stimulated

Erythema: redness of the skin

Eschar: a thick, leathery scab or dry crust that is necrotic and must be removed for adequate healing to occur

Ethical agency: the ability to behave in an ethical way; to do the ethically right thing because it is the right thing to do

Ethical dilemma: situation that arises when attempted adherence to basic ethical principles results in two conflicting courses of action

Ethical distress: occurrence when the nurse knows the right thing to do but either personal or institutional factors make it difficult to follow the correct course of action

Ethically and legally skilled: capable of conducting one's self in a manner consistent with a personal moral code and professional role responsibilities

Ethics: system dealing with standards of character and behavior related to what is right and wrong

Ethnicity: sense of identification that a cultural group collectively has; the sharing of common and unique cultural and social beliefs and behavior patterns, including language and dialect, religious practices, literature, folklore, music, political interests, food preferences, and employment patterns

Ethnocentrism: belief that one's own ideas, beliefs, and practices are best, superior, or most preferred to those of others

Euphoria: unrealistic sense of well-being

Eupnea: normal respirations

Euthanasia: mercy killing; the deliberate termination of the life of a person

Evaluating: measurement of the extent to which the patient has achieved the goals specified in the plan of care; factors that positively or negatively influence goal achievement are identified, and the plan of care is terminated or revised

Evidence-based practice (EBP): nursing care provided that is supported by sound scientific rationale

Evidence-based practice guideline: guidelines written by a panel of experts that synthesize information from multiple studies and recommend best practices to treat patients with a disease, a symptom, or a disability

Evisceration: protrusion of viscera through an incision

Exacerbation: period in chronic illness when the symptoms of the disease reappear

Excretion: removal of a drug from the body

Exercise: active exertion of muscles involving the contraction and relaxation of muscle groups

Exogenous: infection in which the causative organism is acquired from outside the host

Expected outcome: specific, measurable criteria used to evaluate whether the patient goal has been met

Expectorant: drug that facilitates the removal of respiratory secretions

Expert witness: nurse who explains to the judge and jury what happened based on the patient's record and who offers an opinion as to whether the nursing care met acceptable standards of practice

Expiration: act of breathing out; synonym is *exhalation*

Explicit power: power obtained by virtue of a person's position

Extended-care facility: includes residential care and intermediate or skilled nursing home care

Extended family: nuclear family and other related people

External condom catheter: soft, pliable sheath made of silicone material applied externally to the penis

Extracellular fluid (ECF): fluid outside the cells; includes intravascular and interstitial fluids

Exudate: fluid that accumulates in a wound; may contain serum, cellular debris, bacteria, and white blood cells

F

Fact witness: nurse who has knowledge of the actual incident prompting a legal case; bases testimony on firsthand knowledge of the incident not on assumptions

Failure to thrive (FTT): physical and developmental retardation of infants or children resulting from physical or emotional neglect

Faith: (1) spiritual dimensions of a person's life regardless of religious affiliation; (2) confident belief in something for which there is no proof or material evidence

False self: a sense of self that might develop in individuals who have the emotional need to respond to the needs and ambitions significant people, such as parents, have for them

Family: any group of two or more people who live together and are emotionally involved with each other

Fasting state: abstinence from food and fluids

Fear: a feeling of dread; a cognitive response to a known threat

Febrile: condition in which the body temperature is elevated

Fecal impaction: collection in the rectum of hardened feces that cannot be passed

Fecal incontinence: involuntary or inappropriate passing of stool or flatus

Feces: intestinal waste products

Feedback: verbal and nonverbal evidence that the message is received and understood

Felony: (1) crime punishable by imprisonment in a state or federal penitentiary for more than 1 year; (2) crime of greater offense than a misdemeanor

Feminist ethics: type of ethical approach that aims to critique existing patterns of oppression and domination in society, especially as these affect women and the poor

Fever: elevation above the upper limit of normal body temperature; synonym for *pyrexia*

Fiber: all dietary plant material that is not digestible by gastrointestinal tract, enzymes, and secretions

Fidelity: keeping promises and commitments made to others

Fight-or-flight response: the body prepares itself against threat, to either resist (fight) or evade (flight) the danger

Filtration: passage of a fluid through a permeable membrane whose spaces do not allow certain solutes to pass; passage is from an area of higher pressure to one of lower pressure

Fistula: an abnormal passage from an internal organ to the skin or from one internal organ to another

Flaccidity: decreased muscle tone; synonym for *hypotonicity*

Flatulence: excessive formation of gases in the gastrointestinal tract

Flatus: intestinal gas

Flexibility: ability to use a muscle through its entire range of motion

Flexion: state of being bent

Flow sheets: graphic record of abbreviated aspects of patient's condition (e.g., vital signs, routine aspects of care)

Fluid balance: state in which water and its solutes in the body are in normal proportions and concentrations and are in appropriate body compartments

Fluid imbalance: state in which water and its solutes in the body are in improper proportions and concentrations or are improperly located in body compartments

Fluid volume deficit: deficiency in the amount of both water and electrolytes in extracellular fluid; water and electrolyte proportions remain near normal

Fluid volume excess: excessive retention of water and sodium in extracellular fluid in near-normal proportions

Flushing: red appearance of the skin

Focus charting: a documentation system that replaces the problem list with a focus column that incorporates many aspects of a patient and patient care; the focus may be a patient strength or a problem or need; the narrative portion of focus charting uses the data (D), action (A), response (R) format

Focused assessment: assessment conducted to assess a specific problem; focuses on pertinent history and body regions

Foley catheter: indwelling or retention catheter that remains in place to drain urine

Footdrop: complication resulting from extended plantar flexion

Formal teaching: planned teaching based on learner objectives

Frail-old: term for people over age 75; the fastest-growing segment of the population

Fraud: willful and purposeful misrepresentation that could cause, or has caused, loss or harm to people or property

Fremitus: vibration of the chest wall that can be palpated during the physical examination

Frequency: increased incidence of voiding

Friction: occurs when two surfaces rub against each other; the resulting injury resembles an abrasion and can also damage superficial blood vessels directly under the skin

Friction rub: crackling sounds heard in the chest cavity caused by inflamed pleura rubbing against the chest wall

Full liquid diet: diet that contains milk, plain frozen desserts, pasteurized eggs, cereal gruels, and milk and egg substitutes in addition to clear liquids; contains liquids that can be poured at room temperature

Functional health: level of health defined by one's ability to carry out usual and desired daily activities

Functional incontinence: state in which a person experiences an involuntary, unpredictable passage of urine

Fungi: plant-like organisms (molds and yeasts) that can cause infection

G

Gastrostomy: opening created into the stomach

Gate control theory: theory that explains that excitatory pain stimuli carried by small-diameter nerve fibers can be blocked by inhibiting signals carried by large-diameter nerve fibers

Gay: term used to describe homosexual males

Gender identity: the inner sense a person has of being male or female, which may be the same as or different from biologic gender; synonym is *sexual identity*

Gender role behavior: the behavior a person conveys about being male or female, which may or may not be the same as biologic gender or gender identity

General adaptation syndrome (GAS): biochemical model of stress describing the body's general response to stress

General anesthesia: anesthetic drugs that produce narcosis, relaxation of skeletal muscles, and reduced or absent reflex action

Generic name: name assigned by the manufacturer who first develops a drug; it is often derived from the chemical name

Genomics: the study of the structure and interactions of all genes in the human body, including their interactions with each other as well as the environment.

Gerontologic nursing: nursing specialty concerned with the care of the older adult

Gerontology: study of all aspects of the aging process and their consequences

Gingivitis: inflammation of the gingivae or gums

Global self: term used to describe the composite of all the basic facts, qualities, traits, images, and feelings one holds about oneself

Glossitis: inflammation of the tongue

Glycosuria: presence of sugar in the urine

Goal: an aim or an end

Good Samaritan law: law that holds certain health practitioners blameless when undertaking to aid a person in an emergency

Gram-negative bacteria: bacteria with chemically more complex cell walls that can be decolorized by alcohol

Gram-positive bacteria: bacteria with a thick cell wall that resists decolorization (loss of color) and are stained violet

Granulation tissue: new tissue that is pink/red in color and composed of fibroblasts and small blood vessels that fill an open wound when it starts to heal

Graphic sheet: form used to record specific patient variables

Grief: emotional response to loss. *Dysfunctional grief:* distorted or abnormal grief response, including *inhibited grief* (suppression of grief reaction) and *unresolved grief* (lengthy or denied grief reaction). *Abbreviated grief:* short but genuine grief reaction. *Anticipatory grief:* grief reaction before actual loss

Ground: conducting connection between a source of electricity and the earth

Group dynamics: study of a group's characteristics and ways of functioning

Growth: an increase in body size or changes in body cell structure, function, and complexity

Gurgles: continuous musical sounds that are audible in expiration or inspiration, or both; formerly called *rhonchi*

Gustatory: pertaining to taste

H

Half-life: the amount of time it takes for half a dose of a drug to be eliminated from the body

Halitosis: offensive breath

Healing touch (HT): uses a collection of energy techniques to assess and treat the human energy system, thereby affecting physical, emotional, mental, and spiritual health and healing

Health: state of optimal functioning or well-being

Health-belief model: what people believe to be true about themselves in relation to health

Health literacy: ability to read, understand, and act on health information

Health maintenance organization (HMO): broad term encompassing various healthcare delivery systems that use group practice and provide an incentive to use a prepaid comprehensive healthcare system

Health problem: condition related to health requiring intervention if disease or illness is to be prevented or resolved and coping and wellness are to be promoted

Health promotion: behavior of an individual motivated by a personal desire to increase well-being and health potential

Healthcare-associated infection (HAI): an infection that was not present on admission to the hospital and develops during the course of treatment for other conditions (nosocomial)

Helping relationship: interaction that sets the climate of movement of the participants toward common goals

Hematuria: blood in the urine; if present in large enough quantities, urine may be bright red or reddish brown

Hemolysis: process of freeing a red blood cell of its hemoglobin by destruction of the cell membrane

Hemoptysis: sputum-containing blood

Hemorrhage: excessive blood loss due to the escape of blood from blood vessels

Hemorrhoids: abnormally distended rectal veins

Hemothorax: blood that develops in the pleural space

Heparin lock: intravenous needle or catheter with an injection pad attached at the end

Hesitancy: delay or difficulty in initiating voiding

Heterosexuality: having sexual feelings for a person of the opposite sex

Hierarchy of needs: as defined by Maslow, certain needs are more basic than others; a person strives to at least minimally meet certain needs before attending to others

High-level wellness: functioning to one's maximum potential while maintaining balance and purposeful direction in the environment

HIPAA privacy rule: federal law enacted to ensure that health information is protected while allowing the flow of health information needed to provide and promote high-quality healthcare and to protect the public's health and well-being

Holism: theory and philosophy that focuses on connections and interactions between parts of the whole

Holistic healthcare: healthcare that takes into account the whole person interacting in the environment

Holistic nursing: nursing practice built on a holistic philosophy

Home health agency: agency eligible to receive federal funds that provides home-based care; may be independent, hospital operated, or health department managed

Home healthcare: healthcare services provided in a patient's home

Homeopathy: practice of medicine based on the belief of supporting the body while the symptoms are allowed to "run their course" to stimulate and strengthen the immune system and promote healing

Homeostasis: various physiologic and psychological mechanisms respond to changes in the internal and external environment to maintain a balanced state

Homosexuality: having sexual feelings for a person of the same sex

Hope: ingredient in life responsible for a positive outlook, even in life's bleakest moments

Horizontal violence: anger and aggressive behavior between nurses or nurse-to-nurse hostility

Hospice: a type of end-of-life care for persons who are terminally ill, characterized by the following: (1) patients are kept as free of pain as possible so that they may die comfortably and with dignity; (2) patients receive continuity of care, are not abandoned, and do not lose personal identity; (3) patients retain as much control as possible over decisions regarding their care and are allowed to refuse further life-prolonging technologic interventions; and (4) patients are viewed as individuals with personal fears, thoughts, feelings, values, and hopes

Hospitals: acute-care settings that provide various healthcare services, such as emergency care, in-patient care, surgery, diagnostic tests, and patient education

Host: animal or person on or within which microorganisms live

Hydration: union of a substance with water; term often is used as the opposite of dehydration, in which case it means that there is normal intracellular and extracellular water volume

Hydrometer: instrument used to determine the specific gravity of urine

Hydrostatic pressure: force exerted by a fluid against the container wall

Hypercalcemia: excess of calcium in the extracellular fluid

Hyperkalemia: excess of potassium in the extracellular fluid

Hypermagnesemia: excess of magnesium in the extracellular fluid

Hypernatremia: excess of sodium in the extracellular fluid

Hyperphosphatemia: above-normal serum concentration of inorganic phosphorus

Hyperpyrexia: high fever, above 41°C (105.8°F)

Hypersomnia: condition characterized by excessive sleeping, especially daytime sleeping

Hypertension: blood pressure elevated above the upper limit of normal

Hyperthermia: high body temperature

Hypertonic: having a greater concentration than the solution with which it is being compared

Hyperventilation: condition in which there is more than the normal amount of air entering and leaving lungs

Hypervolemia: excess of plasma

Hypnotic: pharmaceutical agent used to induce sleep

Hypocalcemia: insufficient amount of calcium in the extracellular fluid

Hypokalemia: insufficient amount of potassium in the extracellular fluid

Hypomagnesemia: insufficient amount of magnesium in the extracellular fluid

Hyponatremia: insufficient amount of sodium in the extracellular fluid

Hypophosphatemia: below-normal serum concentration of inorganic phosphorus

Hypoproteinemia: insufficient amount of protein substances in the extracellular fluid

Hypotension: blood pressure below the lower limit of normal

Hypothermia: low body temperature

Hypotonic: having a lesser concentration than the solution with which it is being compared

Hypoventilation: decreased rate or depth of air movement into the lungs

Hypovolemia: deficiency of blood plasma

Hypovolemic shock: shock due to a decrease in blood volume

Hypoxemia: deficient oxygenation of blood

Hypoxia: inadequate amount of oxygen available to the cells

I

Iatrogenic infection: infection that occurs as a result of a treatment or diagnostic procedure

Ideal self: self a person would like to be or thinks he or she should be; includes aspirations, moral ideas, and values

Identity diffusion: failure to integrate various childhood identifications into a harmonious adult psychosocial identity

Idiosyncratic effect: unusual, unexpected response to a drug that may manifest itself by overresponse, underresponse, or response different from the expected outcome

Ileal conduit: urinary diversion in which the ureters are connected to the ileum with a stoma created on the abdominal wall

Ileostomy: opening into the small intestine allows fecal content from the ileum to be eliminated through the stoma

Illness: abnormal process in which any aspect of the person's functioning is altered (in comparison to the previous condition of health)

Imagery: using all five senses to imagine an event or body process unfolding according to a plan

Immunization: process of rendering a person immune or resistant to particular antigenic agents or bacteria

Implement: carry out the plan of care

Implied power: power obtained by force of a person's personality that might enable him or her to have more power to influence others than designated leaders

Impotence: condition in which a man is unable to attain or maintain an erection to such an extent that he cannot have satisfactory sexual intercourse; synonym for *erectile failure*

Incentive spirometer: equipment to help maximize lung inflation

Incident report (variance or occurrence report): tool used by healthcare agencies to document the occurrence of anything out of the ordinary that results in or has the potential to result in harm to a patient, employee, or visitor

Incision: wound made with a sharp, cutting instrument

Incontinence: inability to voluntarily control the discharge of urine or feces

Independent action: (1) nursing action carried out at the instruction or order of a nurse; (2) actions within the legal scope of nursing's independent domain; synonym for *nurse-initiated* or *nurse-prescribed intervention*

Inductive reasoning: cognitive process in which one identifies a specific idea or action and then makes conclusions about general ideas

Indwelling urethral catheter: catheter that remains in place for continuous urine drainage; synonym for *Foley catheter*

Infancy: period from 1 month to 1 year of age

Infection: disease state resulting from pathogens in or on the body

Inference: the judgment reached about a cue

Infiltration: escape of fluid into subcutaneous tissue

Inflammatory response: localized response of the body to injury or infection; protective mechanism that eliminates invading pathogens and allows for tissue repair to occur

Informal teaching: unplanned teaching sessions dealing with the patient's immediate learning needs and concerns

Informed consent: knowledgeable, voluntary permission obtained from a patient to perform a specific test or procedure

Inhalation: (1) act of breathing in; synonym for *inspiration*; (2) administration of a drug in solution via the respiratory tract

Initial assessment: comprehensive nursing assessment resulting in baseline data that enables the nurse to make a judgment about a patient's health status, ability to manage his or her own healthcare, and need for nursing, and to plan individualized, holistic healthcare for the patient

Initial planning: planning that addresses each problem listed in the prioritized nursing diagnoses and identifies appropriate patient goals and the related nursing care

Injection: introduction of medication into the body by a syringe attached to a needle

Inpatient: person who enters a healthcare setting for a stay ranging from 24 hours to many years

Insomnia: difficulty in falling asleep, intermittent sleep, or early awakening from sleep

Inspection: purposeful and systematic observation

Inspiration: act of breathing in; synonym is *inhalation*

Integrative care: care that uses some combination of allopathic and complementary/alternative modalities

Integument: skin

Integumentary system: skin and its appendages (i.e., hair, glands in the skin, and nails)

Intercessory prayer: involves praying for the benefit of another person to the Judeo-Christian God

Intercourse (coitus or copulation): insertion of the penis into the partner's vagina, anus, or mouth

Interdependent action: nursing action performed by the nurse in collaboration with other members of the healthcare team

Intermittent urethral catheter: straight catheter used to drain the bladder for short periods (5–10 minutes)

Intermittent fever: body temperature that alternates between fever and normal or subnormal temperature

Intermittent pulse: normal pulse rhythm broken by periods of irregular rhythm

Internal respiration: exchange of oxygen and carbon dioxide between the circulating blood and the tissue cells

Interpersonal communication: communication that occurs between two or more people with a goal to exchange messages

Interpersonally skilled: capable of establishing and maintaining caring relationships that facilitate the achievement of valued goals while simultaneously affirming the worth of the participants in the relationship

Interstitial fluid: fluid between the cells

Intervention: any action performed to modify an expectation or to enhance outcomes

Interview: planned communication for a specific purpose (e.g., data collection)

Interviewing techniques: communication skills specifically designed to gather and validate information

Intimate partner violence (IPV): domestic violence or battering between two people in a close relationship

Intracellular fluid (ICF): fluid within the cell; synonym for *cellular fluid*

Intractable pain: severe pain that is extremely resistant to relief measures

Intradermal injection: injection placed just below the epidermis

Intramuscular (IM) injection: an injection into deep muscle tissue, usually of the buttock, thigh, or upper arm

Intraoperative phase: period lasting from admission to the operating room area to transfer to the postoperative recovery area after surgery is completed

Intrapersonal communication: communication techniques or self-talk to enhance positive interaction with the patient and family

Intravascular fluid: fluid within the vascular system; synonym for *plasma*

Intravenous (IV) infusion: injection of relatively large quantities of solution into a vein

Intravenous (IV) route: injection of a solution into the vein

Intuitive problem solving: direct understanding of a situation based on a background of experience, knowledge, and skill that makes expert decision making possible

Ion: atom or molecule carrying an electric charge in solution

Irrigation: flushing of a tube, canal, or area with solution

Ischemia: deficiency of blood in a particular area

Isokinetic exercise: exercise involving muscle contractions with resistance varying at a constant rate

Isolation: protective procedure designed to prevent the transmission of specific microorganisms; also called *protective aseptic techniques* and *barrier techniques*

Isometric exercise: exercise in which muscle tension occurs without a significant change in muscle length

Isotonic: having about the same concentration as the solution with which it is being compared

Isotonic exercise: movement in which muscles shorten (contract) and move

J

Jaundice: yellow appearance of the skin

Justice: process that distributes benefits, risks, and costs fairly

K

Kardex care plan: trade name for a care plan documentation system that encompasses (1) prescriptions for nursing care related to activities of daily living; (2) nursing diagnoses and related patient goals and nursing orders; and (3) the nursing care related to diagnostic measures and the medical regimen

Kegel exercises: repetitive contraction and relaxation of the pubococcygeal muscle to improve vaginal tone and urinary continence

Ketosis: an abnormal accumulation of ketone bodies that is frequently associated with acidosis

Kinesthesia: awareness of positioning of body parts and body movement

Korotkoff sounds: series of sounds that correspond to changes in blood flow through an artery as pressure is released

Kussmaul's respiration breathing: an extreme rate and depth of breathing

L

Laissez-faire leadership: leadership style in which the leader relinquishes all power to the group

Language: prescribed way of using words; a means to express thoughts and feelings

Law: rule of conduct established and enforced by the government of a society

Lawsuit: legal action in a court of law

Laxative: drug used to induce emptying of the intestinal tract

Leadership: ability to direct or motivate others toward the achievement of predetermined goals

Learning: increasing one's knowledge; having one's behavior changed in a measurable way as a result of an experience

Learning readiness: patient's willingness to engage in the teaching–learning process (emotional readiness) and experiential readiness to begin the challenge of learning

Lesbian: term for a homosexual female

Liability: legal responsibility for one's acts (and failure to act); includes responsibility for financial restitution of harms resulting from negligent acts

Licensure: to be given a license to practice nursing in a state or province after successfully meeting requirements

Life review/reminiscence: universal phenomenon identified by Butler as a review of one's life through one's recollections

Ligaments: tough fibrous bands that bind joints together and connect bones and cartilage

Line of gravity: vertical line that passes through the center of gravity

Lipid: group name for fatty substances, including fats, oils, waxes, and related compounds

Literacy: ability to read and write

Litigation: process of lawsuit

Living will: advance directive specifying the medical care a person would want or refuse should he or she lack the capacity to consent to or refuse treatment himself or herself

Local adaptation syndrome (LAS): localized response of the body to stress, precipitated by trauma or pathology

Localized symptoms: symptoms that are limited or restricted to a discrete area

Long-term care: facilities for long-term care that provide healthcare and help with activities of daily living for people of any age who are physically or mentally unable to independently care for themselves

Loss: inaccessibility or change in a valued person, object, or situation. *Actual loss:* loss tangible to both the person sustaining the loss and to others. *Perceived loss:* loss tangible only to the person sustaining it. *Physical loss:* loss of life, limb, an object, person, pet, or job. *Psychological loss:* loss that affects a person's self-image. *Anticipatory loss:* loss behaviors displayed before the actual loss occurs

Love and belonging needs: understanding and acceptance of others in giving and receiving love

M

Maceration: softening through liquid; overhydration

Macromineral: mineral that is needed by the body in amount greater than 100 mg/day

Macronutrient: essential nutrient that supplies energy and builds tissue such as carbohydrate, fat, and protein

Macroshock: electric current passing through a relatively large area of a person

Malpractice: act of negligence as applied to a professional person such as a physician, nurse, or dentist

Managed care: an organized, high-quality, cost-effective system of healthcare that influences the selection and use of healthcare services of a population

Management: the act of planning, organizing, directing, and controlling available human resources and financial resources to deliver quality care to patients and families

Masturbation: self-stimulation for sexual satisfaction

Maturational loss: the loss experienced as a result of natural developmental processes

Medicaid: Title XIX (Social Security Act, 1965) to make healthcare available to those people with less than the minimum income who do not qualify for Medicare

Medical asepsis: practices designed to reduce the number and transfer of pathogens; synonym for *clean technique*

Medical diagnosis: statement about a specific disease process using terminology from a well-developed classification system accepted by the medical profession

Medicare: Title XVIII (Social Security Act, 1965) to provide a measure of health coverage to all Social Security recipients

Medication: substance that modifies body functions when taken into the living organisms; synonym for *drug*

Medication record: record documenting all medications administered to the patient, the nurse administering the drugs, and sometimes the reason the drug was administered and its effectiveness

Melatonin: a natural chemical produced at night that decreases wakefulness and promotes sleep

Menarche: initiation of the menstrual cycle

Meniscus: curved surface at the top of a column of liquid in a tube

Menopause: decrease of cyclic hormonal production and cessation of menses in females, usually between ages 45 and 60 years

Menstruation: periodic discharge of bloody secretions through the vagina; usually for 4–5 days each month

Mentorship: relationship in which an experienced person (the mentor) advises and assists a less experienced person

Meridian: part of an intricate structure of 72 energy circuits that nourish and support all cells and organs of the body, through which Qi flows vertically in the body

Message: term used in communication theory to denote the actual physical product of the source or encoder (e.g., a speech, interview, phone conversation, chart)

Metabolic acidosis: proportionate deficiency of bicarbonate ions in the extracellular fluid

Metabolic alkalosis: proportionate excess of bicarbonate ions in the extracellular fluid

Metabolism: (1) chemical changes in the body by which energy is provided; (2) breakdown of a drug to an inactive form; also referred to as *biotransformation*

Metered dose inhaler (MDI): instrument that delivers a controlled dose of medication to narrowed airways with each compression of the canister

Micromineral: mineral or trace element that is needed by the body in an amount less than 100 mg/day

Micronutrient: vitamin or mineral needed in much smaller amount to regulate and control body processes

Microshock: electric current passing through a relatively small area of a person, usually part of the heart

Micturition: process of emptying the bladder; urination; voiding

Middle adult: the adult between the ages of 40 and 60 years; also called *middle adulthood*

Midlife crisis: realization that the halfway point in life has been reached and youthful goals may not have been achieved

Minerals: inorganic elements found in nature

Mini-infusion pump: battery-operated pump for intermittent infusion allowing medication mixed in a syringe to be connected to the primary line and delivered by mechanical pressure applied to the syringe plunger

Minimum data set: a standard established by healthcare institutions that specifies the information that must be collected from every patient

Minority group: group having some physical or cultural characteristic that identifies the people within the group as different from the dominant culture

Misdemeanor: crime of lesser offense than a felony and punishable by fines, imprisonment (usually for less than 1 year), or both

Mixed incontinence: symptoms of urge and stress incontinence are present, although one type may predominate

Moderate sedation/analgesia (conscious or procedural sedation): used for short-term and minimally invasive procedures

Modulation: process by which the sensation of pain is inhibited or modified

Moral development: influence of cultural effects on one's perceptions of justice in interpersonal relationships

Morals: like ethics, concerned with what constitutes right action; more informal and personal than the term *ethics*

Morbidity: frequency that a disease occurs

Mortality: number of deaths

Mourning: period during which a person learns to accept grief

N

Narcolepsy: condition characterized by an uncontrolled desire to sleep

Narrative: descriptive record of the patient's condition; includes patient's response to interventions by health professionals and patient's progress toward goal achievement

Narrative notes: progress notes written by nurses in a source-oriented record

Nasal cannula: disposable, plastic device that delivers oxygen via two protruding prongs for insertion into the nostrils

Nasogastric (NG) tube: tube inserted through the nose and into the stomach

Nasointestinal (NI) tube: tube inserted through the nose and into the upper portion of the small intestine

National Medical Care: healthcare services in Canada, funded by taxes and provided to every Canadian citizen

Naturopathic medicine: a relatively new system of medicine that is not only a system of medicine but also a way of life, with emphasis on patient responsibility, patient education, health maintenance, and disease prevention

Nebulizer: instrument that disperses fine particles of medication into the deeper passages of the respiratory tract where absorption occurs

Necrosis: death of cells and tissue

Negative nitrogen balance: condition resulting in muscle wasting and decreased physical energy for movement and work (e.g., anorexia nervosa and certain cancers)

Negative-pressure wound therapy (NPWT): activity that promotes wound healing and wound closure through the application of uniform negative pressure on the wound bed, reduction in bacteria in the wound, and the removal of excess wound fluid

Negative reinforcement: an ineffective teaching strategy that uses criticism or punishment

Negativism: negative verbalizations and behaviors

Negligence: performing an act that a reasonably prudent person under similar circumstances would not do, or failing to perform an act that a reasonably prudent person under similar circumstances would do

Neonate: period from birth to 28 days of age

Nephrotoxic: capable of causing kidney damage

Neuromodulator: endogenous opioid chemical regulators that appear to have analgesic activity and alter pain perception

Neurons: nerve cells, which conduct impulses from one part of the body to another

Neuropathic pain: pain that results from an injury to or abnormal functioning of peripheral nerves or the central nervous system

Neurotransmitters: substances that either excite or inhibit target nerve cells

Nociceptive pain: pain that is categorized as cutaneous, deep somatic, or visceral in nature

Nociceptors: pain receptors

Nocturia: excessive urination during the night

Nocturnal myoclonus: condition characterized by marked muscle contraction that results in the jerking of one or both legs during sleep

Noise: factors that distort the quality of a message and interfere with the communication process

Noncompliance: nonadherence to a therapeutic recommendation

Nonmaleficence: principle of avoiding evil

Nonproductive cough: forceful expiratory effort without production of mucus; also called a *dry cough*

Nonverbal communication: exchange of information without the use of words

Normal flora: microorganisms that normally inhabit various body sites and are part of the body's natural defense system

Nosocomial: something originating or taking place in the hospital (i.e., infection)

Nosocomial infection: hospital-acquired infection

NPO: nothing by mouth (Latin: *nil per os*)

Non–rapid eye movement sleep (NREM): non–rapid eye movement that characterizes four stages of sleep

Nuclear family: family unit, family of marriage, parenthood, or procreation, and their immediate children

Nuclear terrorism: intentional dispersal of radioactive materials into the environment for the purpose of causing injury and death

Nurse-initiated intervention: independent nursing actions that involve carrying out nurse-prescribed interventions written on the nursing plan of care, as well as any other actions that nurses initiate without the direction or supervision of another healthcare professional and that result from their assessment of patient needs

Nurse practice act: law established to regulate nursing practice

Nursing: profession that focuses on the holistic person receiving healthcare services and provides a unique contribution to the prevention of illness and maintenance of health

Nursing actions: any action performed by a nurse to assist patients to meet health goals: promote wellness, prevent disease or illness, restore health, or facilitate coping with altered functioning

Nursing audit: method of evaluating the outcomes of nursing care or the process by which these outcomes are achieved using a review of patient records

Nursing care conference: formal meeting of nurses to discuss some aspect of patient's care

Nursing care rounds: procedure in which a group of nurses visit patients individually at bedside to gather information that helps to plan and to evaluate nursing care

Nursing diagnosis: actual or potential health problem that an independent nursing intervention can prevent or resolve. *Actual problem* is present. *Possible problem* may be present, but more data are needed to confirm or disconfirm the problem. *Potential problem* may occur; defining characteristics are present as risk factors

Nursing ethics: a subset of bioethics; formal study of ethical issues that arise in the practice of nursing and of the analysis used by nurses to make ethical judgments

Nursing history: assessment of the patient by interview to identify the patient's health status, strengths, health problems, health risks, and need for nursing care

Nursing informatics: specialty that integrates nursing science, computer science, and information science to manage and communicate data, information, and knowledge in nursing practice

Nursing intervention: any treatment, based on clinical judgment and knowledge, that a nurse performs to enhance patient outcomes; there are nurse-initiated, physician-initiated, and collaborative interventions

Nursing Intervention Classification (NIC): first comprehensive, validated list of nursing interventions applicable to all settings that can be used by nurses in multiple specialties and facilitates the work of identifying appropriate interventions

Nursing Outcomes Classification (NOC): developed by the Iowa Outcomes Project and presents the first comprehensive standardized language used to describe the patient outcomes that are responsive to nursing intervention

Nursing order: prescribes the nursing care to be given to assist patient to meet health goals

Nursing plan of care: written guide to direct the efforts of the nursing team as they work with patient to meet health goals; specifies prioritized nursing diagnoses, patient goals, and nursing orders

Nursing process: five-step systematic method for giving patient care; involves assessing, diagnosing, planning, implementing, and evaluating

Nursing research: encompasses both research to improve the care of people in the clinical setting and to study people and the nursing profession, including education, policy development, ethics, and nursing history

Nursing theory: differentiates nursing from other disciplines and activities by serving the purposes of describing, explaining, predicting, and controlling desired outcomes of nursing care practices

Nutrient: specific biochemical substance used by the body for growth, development, activity, reproduction, lactation, health maintenance, and recovery from illness or injury

Nutrition: study of the nutrients and how they are handled by the body, as well as the impact of human behavior and environment on the process of nourishment

O

Obesity: weight greater than 20% above ideal body weight

Objective data: information perceptible to the senses; may be verified by another person

Observation: conscious and deliberate use of the five senses to gather data

Occult blood: blood present in such minute quantities that it cannot be detected with the unassisted eye

Occupational Safety and Health Administration (OSHA): government agency that establishes minimum health and safety standards for workers

Official name: name by which a drug is identified in official publications

Old-old: term used to describe adults over age 75; sometimes referred to as frail-old

Older adult: refers to adults over age of 65

Olfactory: pertaining to smell

Oliguria: scanty or greatly diminished amount of urine voided in a given time; 24-hour urine output is 100 to 400 mL

Oncotic pressure: pressure exerted by plasma proteins on permeable membranes in the body; synonym for *colloid osmotic pressure*

Ongoing partial assessment: assessment that is conducted at regular intervals during care of the patient; concentrates on identified health problems to monitor positive or negative changes and evaluate the effectiveness of interventions

Ongoing planning: planning carried out by any nurse who interacts with the patient to keep the plan up to date, to facilitate the resolution of health problems, to manage risk factors, and to promote function

Opioid: more correct term for narcotic analgesics, since these drugs act by binding to opiate receptor sites in the central nervous system

Opportunist: bacteria that may potentially be harmful

Optional surgery: one not critical to survival or function

Organism: a living being

Organizational communication: process of communication that involves individuals and groups to achieve established goals

Orgasm: apex of sexual activity in which rhythmic contractions of the genital organs and many other physiologic changes occur

Orthopedics: the correction or prevention of disorders of body structures used in locomotion

Orthopnea: type of dyspnea in which breathing is easier when the patient sits or stands

Orthostatic hypotension: temporary fall in blood pressure associated with assuming an upright position; synonym for *postural hypotension*

Osmolarity: concentration of particles in a solution, or a solution's pulling power

Osmosis: passage of a solvent through a semipermeable membrane from an area of lesser concentration to an area of greater concentration until equilibrium is established

Osmotic pressure: drawing power for water or the attraction for water exerted by solute particles

Osteoporosis: condition characterized by loss of calcium from bone tissue

Ostomy: general term referring to an artificial opening; usually used to refer to an opening created for the excretion of body wastes

Outcome: end product of nursing care; patient outcomes are measurable changes in patient behavior or state of health

Outcome and Assessment Information Set (OASIS): assessment instrument representing core items of a comprehensive assessment for adult nonmaternity home care patients and forms the basis for measuring patient outcomes for the purpose of improving the quality of care that is provided

Outcome evaluation: evaluation that focuses on measurable changes in the health status of the patient or the end results of nursing care

Outcome identification: observation of the patient to demonstrate the resolution of the problems identified by the nursing diagnoses and general problem list, along with the time frame for accomplishing these outcomes

Outpatient: person who requires healthcare services but does not need to stay in an institution for those services

Overflow incontinence: involuntary loss of urine associated with overdistention and overflow of the bladder

Overhydration: above-normal amounts of water in extracellular spaces

Ovulation: discharge of ovum from the ovary at about the midpoint of each menstrual cycle

Ovum: female reproductive cell, often called an *egg*

P

Pain: sensation of physical or mental suffering or hurt that usually causes distress or agony to the one experiencing it

Pain threshold: amount of stimulation required before a person experiences the sensation of pain

Pain tolerance: point beyond which a person is no longer willing to endure pain (i.e., pain of greater duration or intensity)

Palliative care: (hospice care), taking care of the whole person—body, mind, spirit, heart and soul—with the goal of giving patients with life-threatening illnesses the best quality of life they can have through the aggressive management of symptoms

Pallor: paleness of the skin

Palpation: method of examining by feeling a part with the fingers or hand

Palpitation: perception of one's own heartbeat

Paracentesis: withdrawal of fluid from a body cavity, usually from the abdominal cavity

Paralysis: absence of strength secondary to nervous impairment

Paralytic ileus: paralysis of intestinal peristalsis

Paraplegia: paralysis of the legs

Parasomnia: patterns of waking behavior that appear during sleep (e.g., sleep walking, sleep talking, nocturnal erections)

Parenteral: outside of intestines or alimentary canal; popularly used to refer to injection routes

Parenteral nutrition: nourishment provided via IV therapy

Paresis: impaired muscle strength or weakness

Paresthesia: numbness and tingling

Partial peripheral nutrition (PPN): nutrition prescribed for patients who require nutrient supplementation through a peripheral vein because they have an inadequate intake of oral feedings

Passive exercise: manual or mechanical means of moving the joints

Paternalism: an action that is based on what a parent would do

Pathogen: disease-producing microorganism

Patient: the person receiving care

Patient care ergonomics: practice of designing equipment and work tasks to conform to the capability of the worker in relation to patient care

Patient-controlled analgesia (PCA): method of controlling pain that involves an infusion pump that holds a vial of an IV analgesic that the patient controls and self-administers in small doses

Patient education: process of influencing the patient's behavior to effect changes in knowledge, attitudes, and skills needed to maintain and improve health

Patient goal: statement describing an expected patient outcome

Patient outcome: expected conclusion to a patient health problem, or in the event of a wellness diagnosis, an expected conclusion to a patient's health expectation

Patient record: a compilation of a patient's health information; the patient record is the only permanent legal document that details the nurse's interactions with the patient

Peak level: highest plasma concentration of a drug

Pedagogy: science of teaching that generally refers to the teaching of children and adolescents

Pediculosis: infestation with lice

Peer review: evaluation at the closest point to the patient and an ongoing tool to use for professional growth

Perceived loss: loss of youth, of financial independence, and of a valued environment experienced by a person, but intangible to others

Perception: conscious process of organizing and interpreting data from the senses into meaningful information

Percussion: act of striking one object against another for the purpose of producing a sound; used to assess the location, shape, size, and density of body tissues

Percutaneous endoscopic gastrostomy tube (PEG): surgically or laparoscopically placed gastrostomy tube

Performance improvement: commitment to healthier patients, quality care, reduced costs, and making a difference; accomplished by discovering a problem, planning a strategy, implementing a change, and assessing the change to see if the goal is met

Perfusion: process by which oxygenated blood passes through body tissues

Periodontitis (periodontal disease): marked inflammation of the gums that also involves degeneration of the dental periosteum (tissues) and bone

Perioperative nursing: wide variety of nursing activities carried out before, during, and after surgery

Perioperative period: three phases of perioperative patient care including the preoperative, intraoperative, and postoperative phases

Peripherally inserted central catheter (PICC): type of venous access device that can be introduced into a peripheral vein and advanced as far as the superior vena cava

Peripheral parenteral nutrition (PPN): prescribed for patients who require nutrient supplementation through a peripheral vein because they have an inadequate intake of oral feedings

Peripheral resistance: restraint to blood flow created by arteriole walls in a partial state of contraction

Peristalsis: involuntary, progressive wave-like movement of the musculature of the gastrointestinal tract

Personal health records (PHRs): information sheets that contain the individual's medical history, including diagnoses, symptoms, and medications

Personal identity: an individual's conscious sense of who he or she is

Personal protective equipment (PPE): gloves, gowns, masks, and protective eye gear designed to minimize or prevent the healthcare worker's exposure to infectious material

Personal space: external environment surrounding a person that is regarded as being part of that person

Petechiae: small, purplish hemorrhagic spots on the skin that do not blanch with applied pressure

pH: expression of hydrogen ion concentration and resulting acidity of a substance

Phagocytosis: engulfing of microorganisms, foreign particles, or other cells by phagocytes

Phantom pain: sensation of pain without demonstrable physiologic or pathologic substance; commonly observed after the amputation of a limb

Pharmacodynamics: process by which drugs alter cell physiology and affect the body

Pharmacokinetics: movement of drug molecules in the body in relation to the drug's absorption, distribution, metabolism, and excretion

Pharmacology: study of actions of chemicals on living organisms

Pharmacotherapeutics: dynamic that achieves the desired therapeutic effect of the drug without causing other undesirable effects

Philosophy: study of wisdom, fundamental knowledge, and the processes we use to develop and construct our perceptions of life

Phlebitis: inflammation of a vein

Phlegm: thick, respiratory secretions

Physical assessment: systematic examination of the patient for objective data to better define the patient's condition and to help the nurse in planning care; usually performed in a head-to-toe format

Physical dependence: phenomenon in which the body physiologically becomes accustomed to an opioid and suffers withdrawal symptoms if the opioid is suddenly removed or the dose is rapidly decreased

Physician-initiated intervention: dependent nursing actions, involving carrying out physician-prescribed orders

Physiologic needs: need for oxygen, food, water, temperature, elimination, sexuality, activity, and rest; these needs have the highest priority and are essential for survival

PIE charting: documentation system that does not develop a separate care plan; the care plan is incorporated into the progress notes in which problems are identified by number, worked up using the problem (P), intervention (I), evaluation (E) format, and evaluated each shift

Piggyback infusion: intermittent IV administration of medications through a primary IV line, with the additive container positioned higher than the primary IV solution

Placebo: Latin word meaning, "I shall please"; an inactive substance that gives satisfaction to the person using it

Plaintiff: person or government bringing a lawsuit against another

Plan: establish patient goals to prevent, reduce, or resolve the problems identified in the nursing diagnoses and determination of related nursing interventions

Planned change: change agent's purposeful, systematic effort to bring about change

Plan of nursing care: written guide that directs the efforts of the nursing team as the nurses work with patients to meet health goals; it specifies nursing diagnoses, outcomes, and associated nursing interventions

Plaque: invisible, destructive, bacterial film that builds up on teeth and eventually leads to the destruction of tooth enamel

Plasma: liquid constituent of blood; synonym for *intravascular fluid*

Pleurae: two-layered membranes; the visceral pleura covers the lungs, and the parietal pleura lines the thoracic cavity

Pleural effusion: fluid in the pleural space

Pleural friction rub: continuous, dry grating sound caused by inflammation of pleural surfaces and loss of lubricating pleural fluid

Pneumonia: inflammation or infection of the lungs

Pneumothorax: air in the pleural space

Podiatrist: one who treats foot disorders; synonym for *chiropodist*

Poison control center: agency that handles poison exposure and provides poison prevention teaching to the general population

Polyp: tumor on a stem that bleeds easily and may become malignant

Polypharmacy: the use of many medications at the same time

Polysomnography: sleep study consisting of an electroencephalographic recording of the stages of sleep and any episodes of apnea, continuous monitoring of arterial oxygen saturation, and an electrocardiographic recording to detect any cardiac dysrhythmias

Polyuria: excessive output of urine (diuresis)

Positive reinforcement: affirmation of the efforts of patients

Possible nursing diagnoses: statements describing a suspected problem for which additional data are needed to confirm or rule out the suspected problem

Possible problems: problems the patient may experience if certain trends in the patient's condition continue unreversed

Postoperative phase: period lasting from admission to the recovery area through recovery and convalescence

Postural hypotension: temporary fall in blood pressure associated with assuming an upright position; synonym for *orthostatic hypotension*

Postvoid residual (PVR): urine that remains in the bladder after the act of micturition; a synonym for *residual urine*

Power: ability to influence others to achieve a desired effect

Preceptorship: process by which an experienced person facilitates an orientee's introduction to new responsibilities through teaching and guidance

Precordium: anterior surface of the chest wall overlying the heart and its related structures

Pre-entry phase: phase of the home visit in which the nurse collects information about the patient's healthcare needs, gathers needed supplies, and evaluates safety factors

Preferred provider organization (PPO): any arrangement whereby patients are channeled to specific organizations as providers of health plans

Premenstrual (tension) syndrome (PMS): menstrual cycle–related distress; occurs a few days before the onset of menstruation

P.R.N. orders: directives commonly written for treatment of symptoms "as needed."

Preoperative phase: period lasting from the decision that surgery is necessary until the patient is transferred to the operating room area

Presbycusis: age-related hearing loss in which there is decreased ability to distinguish higher frequencies

Presbyopia: condition of aging in which decreased elasticity of the eye lens hinders accommodation to close vision

Preschooler: period from ages 3 years to 6 years

Prescription: used by physician to convey medication plans for a patient

Pressure ulcer: any lesion caused by unrelieved pressure that results in damage to underlying tissue

Primary healthcare: essential healthcare based on practical, scientifically sound, and socially acceptable methods and technology, made universally accessible through the community's full participation and at a cost the community can afford

Primary preventive care: care directed toward health promotion and specific protection against illness

Principle-based approach: an approach to bioethics that offers specific action guides

PRN (p.r.n.) order: "as needed" order for medication

Problem-oriented medical record (POR): documentation system organized according to the person's specific health problems; includes database, problem list, plan of care, and progress notes

Process: series of actions, changes, or functions to bring about a result

Process evaluation: evaluation focusing on the nature and sequence of activities carried out by nurses implementing the nursing process

Productive cough: cough that produces respiratory tract secretions (sputum)

Profession: an occupation that meets specific criteria including a well-defined body of specific and unique knowledge, a code of ethics and standards, ongoing research, and autonomy

Professionalism: a way of being/commitment to secure the interests and welfare of those entrusted to one's care

Progress notes: any of a variety of methods of notes that relate how a patient is progressing toward expected outcomes

Proprioception: description of the sense, usually at a subconscious level, of the movements and position of the body and especially its limbs, independent of vision

Protein: vital component of every living cell; composed of carbon, hydrogen, oxygen, and nitrogen

Proteinuria: albumin in the urine; indication of kidney disease

Protocol: written plan that details the nursing activities to be executed in specific situations

Psychogenic pain: pain for which no physical cause can be identified

Psychological loss: loss caused by an altered self-image

Psychomotor learning: acquisition of physical skills

Psychosomatic disorder: physiologic alterations and illness believed to be due to psychological influences

Puberty: period during which primary and secondary sexual characteristics develop and the capability of sexual reproduction is attained

Public health agencies: local, state, provincial, or federal agencies that provide public health services to members of communities

Pulmonary ventilation: movement of air into and out of the lungs

Pulse: wave produced in the wall of an artery with each beat of the heart

Pulse deficit: difference between the apical and radial pulse rates

Pulse oximetry: noninvasive technique that measures the oxygen saturation (SaO_2) of arterial blood

Pulse pressure: difference between systolic and diastolic pressures

Purulent: containing pus

Purulent drainage: comprised of white blood cells, liquefied dead tissue debris, and both dead and live bacteria

Pyorrhea: extensive inflammation of the gums and alveolar tissues; synonym for *periodontitis*

Pyrexia: elevation above the upper limit of normal body temperature; synonym for *fever*

Pyuria: pus in the urine; urine appears cloudy

Q

Qi: represents an invisible flow of energy that circulates through plants, animals, and people, as well as the earth and sky

Qi gong: system of posture, exercise (both gentle and dynamic), breathing techniques, and visualization that regulates the Qi

Qualitative research: method of research conducted to gain insight by discovering meanings

Quality assurance program: ongoing evaluation program designed and implemented to secure the excellence of healthcare; may involve an assessment of structure, process, and outcome standards

Quality improvement: the commitment and approach used to continuously improve every process in every part of an organization, with the intent of meeting and exceeding customer expectations and outcomes (also known as continuous quality improvement [CQI] or total quality management [TQM])

Quantitative research: research involving the concepts of basic and applied research

Quantum leadership: leadership that moves beyond the traditional modes previously experienced by all levels of workers; spawned by the impact of the information age on work and the worker

R

Race: division of human beings based on distinct physical characteristics

Radiography: examination by x-ray film

Range of motion: complete extent of movement of which a joint is normally capable

Rape: sexual violation of a person by someone who uses force, threats, and abuse

Rapid eye movement sleep (REM): stage that constitutes 20% to 25% of a person's nightly sleep; person is difficult to arouse during this stage

Rapport: feeling of mutual trust experienced by people in a satisfactory relationship

Reactive hyperemia: the body's flooding of an area with blood after it has suffered from poor circulation for a period; the occurrence of a blanchable reddening of the skin when pressure is removed

Reality orientation: method of care used to promote awareness of reality in confused or disoriented patients

Receiver (decoder): term used in communication theory that specifies the person or object to which the message is directed

Reception: process of receiving data about the internal or external environment through the senses

Receprocity: process allowing a nurse to apply for and be endorsed as a registered nurse by another state

Recommended dietary allowance (RDA): recommendations for average daily amounts of essential nutrients that healthy population groups should consume over time

Referral: process of sending or guiding someone to another source for assistance

Referral source: a person who recommends home care services and supplies the home healthcare agency with details about the patient's needs

Referred pain: pain in an area removed from that in which stimulation has its origin

Reflex incontinence: emptying of the bladder without the sensation of the need to void

Reflex pain response: automatic response of the central nervous system to the stimulus of pain

Regional anesthesia: anesthetic drug is injected or applied topically to inhibit transmission of sensory stimuli

Regression: behavior that is more characteristic of an earlier age

Rehabilitation: process of restoring a person's highest level of possible wellness and returning that person's ability to live and to work as normally as possible after a disabling illness or injury

Rehabilitation centers: centers specializing in services for patients requiring physical or emotional rehabilitation and for treatment of any type of drug dependency

Reimbursement source: entity that pays for home healthcare services

Relationship: interaction of people over time

Relaxation response: an alert, hypometabolic state of decreased sympathetic nervous system arousal, which can also be viewed as the opposite of Selye's general adaptation syndrome response

Religion: organized system of beliefs about a higher power; often includes set forms of worship, spiritual practices, and codes of conduct

REM: rapid eye movement that characterizes the dream state of sleep

Remission: period in a chronic illness when the disease is present, but the person does not experience symptoms of the disease

Reporting: oral, written, or computer-based communication of patient data with the purpose of informing others

Repression: exclusion of an anxiety-producing event from conscious awareness

Research: process that uses observable and verifiable information (data), collected in a systematic manner, to describe, explain, or predict events

Reservoir: natural habitat for the growth and multiplication of microorganisms

Residual: feeding remaining in the stomach

Residual urine: urine that remains in the bladder after the act of micturition

Respiration: gas exchange between the atmospheric air in the alveoli and blood in the capillaries

Respiratory acidosis: proportionate excess of carbonic acid in the extracellular fluid

Respiratory alkalosis: proportionate deficiency of carbonic acid in the extracellular fluid

Respite care: a type of care provided for caregivers of homebound ill, disabled, or elderly patients

Rest: condition in which the body is in a decreased state of activity, with the consequent feeling of being refreshed

Restless leg syndrome (RLS): a condition in which patients are unable to lie still and report experiencing unpleasant creeping, crawling, or tingling sensations in the legs

Restraint: device used to limit movement or immobilize a client

Retention: inability to void although urine is produced by the kidneys and enters the bladder; excessive storage of urine in the bladder

Retention sutures: sutures used to provide extra support in wounds in obese patients or in wounds with increased risk of dehiscence

Reticular activating system (RAS): network of neurons in the core of the brainstem, with ascending and descending tracts to other areas of the brain that monitor and regulate incoming sensory stimuli and level of arousal

Retrospective audit: evaluation of nursing care and patient outcomes after the patient has been discharged (may use postdischarge questionnaires, patient interviews, or chart review)

Retrospective evaluation: evaluation of nursing care and patient outcomes after the patient has been discharged using postdischarge questionnaires, patient interviews, or chart review to collect data

Review of systems (ROS): physical examination of all body systems in a systematic manner as part of the nursing assessment

Risk factor: something that increases a person's chance for illness or injury

Risk nursing diagnoses: clinical judgments that an individual, family, or community is more vulnerable to develop the problem than others in the same or similar situation

Role performance: ability to successfully execute societal expectations regarding role-specific behaviors

S

Safety and security needs: person's need to be protected from actual or potential harm and to have freedom from fear

Safety event report: documentation describing any injury or potential for injury suffered by a patient in a healthcare agency

Sanguineous: containing or mixed with blood

SBAR: consistent, clear, structured, and easy-to-use method of communication between healthcare personnel; it organizes communication by the categories of: Situation, Background, Assessment, and Recommendations.

Scar: connective tissue that fills a wound area

School-age: period from ages 6 to 12 years

Science: a body of knowledge gained by observing, identifying, describing, investigating, and explaining events and occurrences that are perceived in the world

Scientific knowledge: knowledge arrived at by applying scientific methods

Scientific problem solving: systematic problem-solving process that involves (1) problem identification, (2) data collection, (3) hypothesis formulation, (4) plan of action, (5) hypothesis testing, (6) interpretation of results, and (7) evaluation resulting in conclusion or revision of the study

Scrub nurse: nurse who assists the surgeon during surgery, maintaining surgical asepsis while draping, handling instruments, and handling supplies

Scultetus binder: type of bandage with multiple tails; synonym for *many-tailed binder*

Sebaceous gland: gland found in the skin that secretes an oily substance called sebum

Secondary preventive care: care directed either to health maintenance for patients experiencing health problems or to prevention of complications or disabilities

Self-actualization: reaching of one's potential through full development of one's unique capabilities

Self-actualization needs: highest level on the hierarchy of needs, which include the need for individuals to reach their full potential through development of their unique capabilities

Self-concept: mental image or picture of self; includes body image, subjective self, ideal self, and social self

Self-esteem: person's perception of his or her total being, including self-worth and body image

Self-esteem needs: need to feel good about oneself and to believe others hold one in high regard

Self-governance: employing a decentralized organizational structure for decision making; self-governance at the unit level and respect for, and acknowledgement of, professional autonomy

Semantics: study of the meaning of words

Semen: seminal plasma containing sperm

Semipermeable membrane: selectively permeable membrane that allows water to pass through it but is either impermeable or selectively permeable to solutes

Sensoristasis: arousal state of the reticular activating system; general drive state

Sensory deficit: impaired or absent functioning of one or more senses

Sensory deprivation: condition resulting from decreased sensory input or input that is monotonous, unpatterned, or meaningless

Sensory overload: condition resulting from excessive sensory input to which the brain is unable to meaningfully respond

Sensory/perceptual alteration: disturbance in the body's ability to receive or process data from its internal or external environment

Sensory reception: the process of receiving data about the internal or external environment through the senses

Sentinel event: an unexpected occurrence involving death or serious physical or psychological injury, or the risk thereof

Separation anxiety: condition that occurs when a child is afraid of being sent away from caregivers who are loved and who provide security

Serous: resembling blood serum; clear and watery in appearance

Serous drainage: composed of clear, serous portion of the blood and from serous membranes

Serosanguineous drainage: mixture of serum and red blood cells

Set point: level at which the hypothalamus attempts to maintain body temperature

Sexual dysfunction: condition that prevents a person or couple from engaging in or obtaining satisfaction from sexual activity

Sexual harassment: unwelcome verbal or physical advance or sexually explicit statement (e.g., leers, pats, grabs, jokes, requests for dates, and even rape) that interferes with one's ability to do one's job by making one feel humiliated, intimidated, or uncomfortable

Sexual health: the integration of the somatic, emotional, intellectual, and social aspects of sexual being in ways that are positively enriching and that enhance personality, communication, and love

Sexual orientation: preferred gender of the partner of an individual

Sexuality: degree to which a person exhibits and experiences maleness and femaleness physically, emotionally, and mentally

Sexually transmitted infection (or disease) (STI): disease that spreads from one person to another through intimate sexual contact

Shamanism: a belief that illness originates in the spirit world and usually involves a loss of power; treatment consists of first, restoring the individual's power, and second, treating symptoms

Shearing force: force created when layers of tissue move on one another

Shock: body's reaction to acute peripheral circulatory failure due to an abnormality of circulatory control or to a loss of circulating fluid

Situational crisis: change that results when a person faces an event or situation that causes a disruption in his or her life

Situational leadership: theory of leadership that considers the leader's style, the work group's maturity, and the situation at hand to form a comprehensive approach to management style

Situational loss: experienced as a result of an unpredictable event, including traumatic injury, disease, death, or national disaster

Sitz bath: special type of bath that applies heated water to the pelvic or rectal area

Skin sutures: used to approximate wound tissues and skin; may be silk, synthetic, wire, or metal staples

Skin tests: tests to determine antigen–antibody reaction

Sleep: state of altered consciousness throughout which varying degrees of stimuli preclude wakefulness

Sleep apnea: a condition in which a person experiences the absence of breathing (apnea) or diminished breathing effort (hypopnea) during sleep between snoring intervals

Sleep cycle: passage through the four stages of NREM sleep (I, II, III, IV), then reversal (IV, III, II), and finally, instead of reentering stage I and awakening, entering REM sleep and returning to stage II

Sleep deprivation: a decrease in the amount, consistency, and quality of sleep; results from decreased REM or NREM sleep

Sleep hygiene: nonpharmacologic recommendations like reviewing and changing lifestyles and environment that help an individual get a better night's sleep

Small-group communication: communication that occurs when two or more nurses interact with two or more individuals, allowing the members to achieve a goal through communication

SOAP format: method of charting narrative progress notes; organizes data according to subjective information (S), objective information (O), assessment (A), and plan (P)

Social isolation: sense of aloneness because of decreasing relationships with others, resulting from attitudinal, geographic, financial, or illness-related factors

Social self: way a person believes that others see him or her

Soft diet: regular diet that has been modified to eliminate foods that are hard to digest and to chew, including those that are high in fiber, high in fat, and highly seasoned

Solute: substance dissolved in a solution

Solvent: liquid holding a substance in solution

Somatic pain: pain originating in structures in the body's external wall

Somnambulism: sleepwalking

Sordes: accumulation of mucus and crust formation on the teeth and around the lips

Source (encoder): term used in communication theory to specify the one who prepares and sends a message to the receiver

Source-oriented record: documentation system in which each healthcare group records data on its own separate form

Spasticity: increased muscle tone

Specific gravity: a characteristic of urine that can be determined with manufactured plastic strips or an instrument called a urinometer or hydrometer

Sperm: male reproductive cell; synonym for spermatozoan

Spermicide: chemical agent used to destroy sperm

Sphincter: circular muscle that constricts a passage or closes a natural orifice

Spiritual beliefs: practices associated with all aspects of a person's life, including health and illness that address the invisible "spirit"—a creative, mysterious, guiding power

Spiritual distress: an alteration in spiritual health (e.g., spiritual pain, alienation, anxiety, guilt, anger, loss, despair)

Spiritual healing: movement toward integration, from brokenness to wholeness

Spiritual health: condition that exists when the universal spiritual needs for meaning and purpose, love and belonging, and forgiveness are met

Spirituality: anything that pertains to a person's relationship with a nonmaterial life force or higher power

Spiritual need: lack of anything necessary for spiritual health (e.g., meaning and purpose, love and relatedness, forgiveness)

Spirometer: instrument used to measure lung capacities and volumes; one type is used to encourage deep breathing (incentive spirometry)

Sputum: respiratory secretion expelled by coughing or clearing the throat

Standard: acceptable, expected level of performance established by authority, custom, or consent

Standardized plan of care: prepared plan of care that identifies the nursing diagnoses, patient goals, and related nursing orders common to a specific population (e.g., normal neonates) or problem

Standard Precautions: CDC precautions used in the care of all patients regardless of their diagnosis or possible infection status; this category combines universal and body substance precautions

Standards: rules or guidelines that allow nurses to carry out professional roles, serving as protection for the nurse, the patient, and the institution where healthcare is given

Standards for critical thinking: clear, precise, specific, accurate, relevant, plausible, consistent, logical, deep, broad, complete, significant, adequate (for the purpose), and fair

Standing order: document that details the nursing care to be implemented in specific nursing situations, frequently when a physician is not present; may expand scope of nursing responsibilities

Stat order: single order carried out immediately

Statutory law: law enacted by a legislative body

Stereognosis: the sense that perceives the solidity of objects, their size, shape, and texture

Stereotyping: assigning characteristics to a group of people without considering specific individuality

Sterilization: (1) the process by which all microorganisms, including spores, are destroyed; (2) surgical procedure performed to render a person infertile

Stertorous breathing: noisy respirations

Stimulus: agent, act, or other influence capable of initiating a response by the nervous system

Stoma: artificial opening for waste excretion located on the body surface

Stomatitis: inflammation of the oral mucosa

Stool: excreted feces

Strength (muscle): ability of the muscle to move actively against resistance

Stress: condition in which the human system responds to change in its normal balanced state

Stress incontinence: state in which the person experiences a loss of urine of less than 50 mL that occurs with increased abdominal pressure

Stressor: anything causing a person to experience stress; change in the balanced state

Stridor: harsh, high-pitched sound usually heard on inspiration when upper airways become narrowed

Structure evaluation: (audit) focuses on the environment in which care is provided

Subculture: group of people with different interests or goals than the primary culture

Subcutaneous injection: injection into the subcutaneous tissue that lies between the epidermis and the muscle

Subcutaneous tissue: underlying layer that anchors the skin layers to the underlying tissues of the body

Subjective data (symptoms, covert data): information perceived only by the affected person

Subjective self: how one sees oneself; who one thinks one is

Sublingual: area in the mouth under the tongue

Sudden infant death syndrome (SIDS): sudden death of any infant or young child without demonstrated cause

Sundowning syndrome: describes a phenomenon when a person habitually becomes confused or disoriented with darkness

Suppository: oval- or cone-shaped substance that is inserted into a body cavity and that melts at body temperature

Suprapubic catheter: catheter inserted into the bladder through a small abdominal incision above the pubic area

Surfactant: detergent-like phospholipid that reduces surface tension of the fluid lining the alveoli

Surgical asepsis: practices that render and keep objects and areas free from microorganisms; synonym for *sterile technique*

Susceptibility: degree of resistance of a host to a pathogen

Symptom: abnormality indicative of illness as experienced by the patient; synonym for *subjective data*

Syndrome (nursing diagnoses): cluster of actual or risk nursing diagnoses that are predicted to be present because of a certain event or situation

Synergistic effect: combined effect of two or more drugs is greater than the effect of each drug alone

Systematic reviews: summarized findings from multiple studies of a specific clinical practice question or topic and recommend practice changes and future directions for research; one of the strongest sources of evidence for evidence-based practice

Systemic symptoms: symptoms manifested throughout the entire body

Systolic pressure: highest point of pressure on arterial walls when the ventricles contract

T

Tachycardia: rapid heart rate

Tachypnea: rapid rate of breathing

Tactile: pertaining to touch

Tartar: hard deposit on the teeth near the gum line formed by plaque buildup and dead bacteria

Teaching: planned method or series of methods used to help someone learn

Teaching–learning process: process of patient teaching that encompasses critical steps necessary to provide teaching and to measure learning; the teaching–learning process models the nursing process

Technical competencies: skills that enable a nurse to skillfully manipulate equipment in a manner conducive to achieving a desired goal

Temperament: person's style of approaching people, situations, or events

Temperature: refers to the hotness or coldness of a substance

Tendons: strong, flexible, inelastic fibrous bands that attach muscle to bone

Teratogenic: known to have potential to cause developmental defects in the embryo or fetus

Terminal illness: illness from which there is no reasonable expectation of recovery or cure

Terminal weaning: withdrawal of life-sustaining therapy with the understanding that death may result, generally after a decision is made that the therapy in question is medically futile or disproportionately burdensome

Tertiary preventive care: care directed at helping rehabilitate patients and restore them to a maximum level of functioning after an illness

Theory: statement based on observed facts that explains or characterizes a process, an occurrence, or an event, but cannot be proved directly or absolutely as a fact

Therapeutic range: that concentration of drug in the blood serum that produces the desired effect without causing toxicity

Therapeutic Touch (TT): an alternative therapy that involves using one's hands to consciously direct an energy exchange from the practitioner to the patient to facilitate healing or pain relief

Third-space fluid shift: distributional shift and trapping of body fluids into body spaces such as the pleural, peritoneal, or pericardial, or into the interstitial space (plasma-to-interstitial shift)

Thoracentesis: aspiration of fluid or air from the pleural space

Thrill: abnormal tremor accompanying a vascular or cardiac murmur felt on palpation

Thrombophlebitis: inflammation in a vein associated with thrombus formation

Thrombus: blood clot; plural is *thrombi*

Time-lapsed assessment: an assessment that is scheduled to compare a patient's current status to baseline data obtained earlier

Toddler: period from ages 1 year to 3 years

Tolerance: occurrence of the body's becoming accustomed to an opioid and needing a larger dose each time for pain relief

Tonus: normal, partially steady state of muscle contraction

Topical application: application of a substance directly to a body surface

Tort: wrong committed by a person against another person or his property

Total body water (TBW): total amount of water in the body, expressed as a percentage of body weight. The term *total body fluid* also is used; fluids usually are considered to include water and electrolytes

Total incontinence: continuous and unpredictable loss of urine, resulting form surgery, trauma, or physical malformation

Total parenteral nutrition (TPN): nutritional therapy that bypasses the gastrointestinal tract for patients who are unable to take food orally; meets the patient's nutritional needs by way of nutrient-filled solutions administered intravenously through a central vein

Toxic effects (toxicities): specific groups of symptoms related to drug therapy that carry risk for permanent damage or death

Trace elements: minerals found in the body in quantities less than 5 g and needed in only small amounts (18 mg or less)

Tracheostomy: artificial opening made into the trachea through which a tracheostomy tube is inserted

Tracheostomy tube: curved tube inserted into an artificial opening made in the trachea that comes with varied angles and in multiple sizes

Trade name: drug name selected and trademarked by the company marketing the drug; also called *brand name* or *proprietary name*

Traditional Chinese medicine (TCM): healing system that believes the interaction of people with their environment is most significant in creating health

Traditional family: composed of a husband, wife, and their children, who live together in one house

Traditional knowledge: knowledge passed down from generation to generation

Transcultural nursing: providing nursing care that is planned and implemented in a way that is sensitive to the needs of individuals, families, and groups representing the diverse cultural populations within our society

Transduction: activation of pain receptors

Trans fat: fat that occurs when manufacturers partially hydrogenate liquid oils so that they become more solid and stable; trans fat raises serum cholesterol

Transformational leadership: type of leadership in which the person creates revolutionary change and commits to the personal and professional growth of self and others

Transient incontinence: occurrence which appears suddenly and lasts for 6 months or less and usually is caused by treatable factors, such as confusion secondary to acute illness, infection, and as a result of medical treatment, such as the use of diuretics or intravenous fluid administration

Transmission: conduction of pain sensations from the site of an injury or inflammation along clear and unclear pathways to the spinal cord and then on to higher centers

Transmission-Based Precautions: CDC precautions used in patients known or suspected to be infected with pathogens that can be transmitted by airborne, droplet, or contact routes; used in addition to Standard Precautions

Transsexual: person of a certain biologic gender with the feelings of the opposite sex

Transvestite: individual who desires to take on the role or wear the clothes of the opposite sex

Trauma: injury

Tremor: involuntary muscular movements

Trial: hearing of evidence in a legal case before a judge (and jury) with the intent of reaching a decision or verdict

Trial-and-error problem solving: method of problem solving that involves testing any number of solutions until one is found that works for that particular problem

Triglycerides: predominant form of fat in food and the major storage form of fat in the body; composed of one glyceride molecule and three fatty acids

Trough level: the point when a drug is at its lowest concentration

Turgor: tension of the skin determined by its hydration

Typing: determining a person's blood type

U

Unilateral: affecting or occurring on one side only

Universal Precautions: isolation system that considers blood, body fluids containing blood, semen, and vaginal secretions of all patients as potentially infective

Unlicensed assistive personnel (UAP): individual who is trained to function in an assistive role to the licensed registered nurse in the provision of patient activities as delegated by and under the supervision of the registered professional nurse

Urge incontinence: state in which a person experiences involuntary passage of urine that occurs soon after a strong sense of urgency to void

Urgency: strong desire to void

Urgent surgery: surgery that is not an emergency, but must be done within a reasonably short time frame to preserve health

Urinary diversion: surgical creation of an alternate route for excretion of urine

Urinary incontinence: any involuntary loss of urine

Urinary retention: inability to void although urine is produced by the kidneys and enters the bladder; excessive storage of urine in the bladder

Urination: process of emptying the bladder; micturition; voiding

Utilitarian: action-guiding theory of ethics that states that the rightness or wrongness of an action depends on the consequences of the action

V

Validation: act of confirming or verifying

Valsalva maneuver: forcible exhalation against a closed glottis, resulting in increased intrathoracic pressure

Values: set of beliefs that are meaningful in life and that influence relationships with others

Values clarification: process by which people come to understand their own values and value system

Value system: organization of values ranked along a continuum of importance

Variables: factors in a research study

Variance charting: documentation method in case management that records unexpected events, the cause for the event, actions taken in response to the event, and discharge planning when appropriate

Varicosity: swollen, twisted vein

Vector: nonhuman carriers, such as mosquitoes, ticks, and lice, that transmit organisms from one host to another

Ventilation: exchange of gases

Ventricles: lower chambers of the heart

Veracity: truth telling

Verbal communication: exchange of information using words

Vesicular breath sounds: normal sound of respirations heard on auscultation over peripheral lung areas

Vial: glass bottle with self-sealing stopper through which medication is removed; may be single or multiple dose

Virulence: ability to produce disease

Virus: smallest of all microorganisms; can be seen only by using an electron microscope

Visceral: pertaining to inner organs

Visceral pain: pain originating in the internal organs in the thorax, cranium, or abdomen

Visual: pertaining to sight

Vital signs: body temperature, pulse and respiratory rates, and blood pressure; synonym for *cardinal signs*

Vitamins: organic substances needed by the body in small amounts to help regulate body processes; are susceptible to oxidation and destruction

Voiding: process of emptying the bladder; also called *micturition* or *urination*

Volume-control administration set: intermittent intravenous medication infusion diluted with a small amount of solution

Voluntary agencies: community agencies that are often funded by private donations, grants, or fund-raising and that provide a wide variety of direct services and education

W

Wellness: an active process in which an individual progresses toward the maximum possible potential, regardless of his or her current state of health

Wellness diagnosis: clinical judgment about an individual, family, or community in transition from a specific level of wellness to a higher level of wellness

Wheeze: continuous, high-pitched squeak or musical sound made as air moves through narrowed or partially obstructed airway passages

Whistle-blowing: term generally used to refer to employees who report their employers' violation of the law to appropriate law enforcement agencies outside the employers' facilities

Wound: injury that results in a disruption in the normal continuity of a body tissue

X

X-ray: high-energy electromagnetic wave capable of penetrating solid matter and acting on photographic film; synonym for *roentgen ray*

Y

Yin-yang: energy forces in Chinese teaching that must be in balance for good health; expression of strong emotions results in disharmony and imbalance between these forces

Young adult: adult between the ages of 20 and 40 years

Z

Z-track: Technique used to administer medications intramuscularly that ensures the medication does not leak back along the needle track and into the subcutaneous tissue, reducing pain and discomfort.

Index

Integumentary system
    anatomy of, 917–922
    physiology of, 917–922
Intensive care units (ICUs)
    pressure ulcers in, 930
    use of restraints, 635
Interactions, collaborative, 293
Intercessory prayer, 712
Intercostal muscles, 1351
Interdependent nursing actions, 293
Interdisciplinary care teams, 147–148, 351
Intermediate care facilities, 144
Intermittent positive-pressure breathing (IPPB), 1383
Intermittent urethral catheterization, 1248–1249, 1279–1281, 1280f–1281f
Intermittent urethral catheters, 1246
Internal genitalia, 1607
Internal respiration, 1355
Internal sphincter muscle, 1224
International Classification for Nursing Practice (ICNP®), 194t
International Council of Nurses (ICN), 7
    Code of Ethics for Nurses, 93, 94b
    goals of, 17
    on research, 73
Internet
    end-of-life care resources, 1551
    evidence-based practice resources, 80b
    medical resources on, 718b
    sexual solicitation over, 630
    surfing, 404f
    use by children, 625
Interpersonal skills
    aggressive behaviors, 459–460
    challenges to, 376
    development of, 203–206, 204b
    of nurses, 10–11
Interventions. See also Nursing interventions
    adverse effects, 294–295
    collaborative, 275
    evidence-based practice and, 268
    focused critical thinking guide, 298
    home visits and, 182
    mapping, 298
    modification of, 313
    nurse-initiated, 272–274, 291–292
    physician-initiated, 274–275, 292–293
    selection of, 268
    strategies for, 298
Interviews
    communication techniques, 234b
    motivational, 489–490
    patient variables, 234t
    with patients
        introductory phase, 233
        preparatory phase, 233
        termination, 235
        working phase, 234–235
    skills
        affirming, 489
        open-ended questions, 489
        summarizing, 489
    techniques, 455–456, 456
Intestinal juice, loss of, 1435t
Intestines, peristaltic movements of, 1300f
Intimacy, need for, 1567
Intimacy vs isolation stage (young adulthood), 366, 418
Intimate partner violence (IPV), 631
Intracellular fluid (ICF), 1164, 1416
Intractable pain, 1113
Intradermal injections, 749, 755f, 788–791
Intramuscular injections, 751–755
    administration of, 795–799, 798f
    equipment, 754
    injection sites, 751–754, 753f
        deltoid muscle, 753
        dorsogluteal, 753–754
        needle length, 754t
        vastus lateralis, 753
        ventrogluteal, 752, 752t
    procedure, 754–755, 755b, 755f
Intraoperative phase
    nursing process
        assessing, 836
        diagnosing, 836–387

evaluating, 838
implementing, 838
outcome identification, 387–338
planning, 837–338
of the surgical experience, 820
teaching, 830b
Intrauterine devices (IUDs), 1631
Intravenous injections, 755–757
Intravenous (IV) therapy
    administration set
        changing of, 1471–1474, 1471f–1473f
    bolus administration, 756, 799–802
    complications associated with, 1452t
    complications of, 1450–1451
    discontinuation of, 1457, 1481
    equipment for, 1447–1448
        central venous access devices, 1448
        midline peripheral catheters, 1448
        peripheral venous catheters, 1448
        vascular access devices, 1448
    in fluid disturbances, 1446–1458
    home therapy, 1458
    initiation of, 1454
    intermittent intravenous, 756–757, 806–810, 808f, 809f
    monitoring of, 1454–1456, 1475–1477, 1475f–1476f
    peripheral venous catheter access skill set, 1464–1470
    piggyback delivery systems, 756–757, 802–806
    push administrations, 756, 799–802
    regulation of, 1454–1456
    shield on hand, 1457f
    site monitoring, 1475–1477
    solutions, 756, 1447t, 1456, 1471–1474, 1471f–1473f
    teaching tips, 1458
    tubing changes, 1456
    venous access site care, 1456–1457
    volume-control set, 1455f
Intravenous pyelograms, 1235b
Introjection, as defense mechanism, 1528t
Intuitive problem solving, 196
Intuitive-projective faith, 370
Invasions of privacy, 117–118
Iodine, nutrition summary, 1165tt
IONSYS, 1139
Iowa Outcomes Project, 270
Iron
    nutrition summary, 1165tt
    poisonings, 623t
Iron compounds, 1228
Irradiation injuries, 922f
Irrigation
    continuous closed bladder, 1282–1284, 1283f
    intermittent catheters, 1279–1281
    nasogastric tubes, 1335–1337
Ischemia, pressure ulcers and, 929
Islam, 1650f
Isokinetic exercise, 1012, 1012f
Isolation precautions, 672, 675
Isometric exercise, 1012, 1012f
Isotonic exercise, 1012, 1012f
Isotonic solutions, 1447t
Iyengar, 707

J

Jackson-Pratt drains, 951f, 976–978, 977f
Jaundice, 572, 922
Jehovah's Witnesses, 1650f
Jejunostomy (J) tubes, 744, 1189
Joanna Briggs Institute, 80b
Johnson, Dorothy E., 75t
The Joint Commission (TJC), 445
    abbreviations not used, 331t
    accreditation, 639–640
    on disruptive behaviors in hospitals, 459
    "do not use" list, 735
    on documentation, 191, 324
    emergency preparedness resources, 643t
    on ethics committees, 96
    evaluative programs, 316
    on medication reconciliation, 733, 767

National Patient Safety Goals, 326–329, 639
    on pain management, 1110, 1120, 1138–1139
    patient identification and, 739
    quality initiatives, 318t
    on restraint use, 636
    SBAR Communication, 348
    Sentinel Event Advisory Group, 636
    Sentinel Event Policy, 128, 129
    "Speak Up" initiative, 468
    Web-based resources, 318t
Joints
    ball-and-socket, 1001–1002
    classification of, 1001–1002
    condyloid, 1002
    diseases of, 1616
    exercise, 1036–1037, 1037f
    gliding, 1002
    hinge, 1002
    inspection of, 601
    mobility of, 1008–1009
    palpation of, 601
    pivot, 1002
    saddle, 1002
    structure and function, 1002f, 1018f, 1020
Journal articles, 79t
Judaism, 1650f
Judgment, 201, 310
Justice, principle of, 90, 91t

K

Kaolin and pectin (Kaopectate), 1318
Kapha (relaxed), 705
Kardex card system, 163
Kardex care plans, 277, 342, 343f
Katz Index of Independence, 1019
Kefauver-Harris Amendment, 732
Kegel exercises, 1240, 1627
Keloids, 575t
Keratin, 917
Ketosis, 159
Kidneys. See also Acute renal failure; Chronic renal failure
    anatomy of, 1223
    diseases, 826
    fluid balance and, 1420
    homeostatic mechanisms, 1419t
    physiology of, 1223
KinAir III bed, 890f
Kinesthesia, 1576
Kinesthetic communication, 435, 438b
Kinesthetic sense, 1005
King, Imogene, 74t
Klebsiella sp., 666
Knee
    range of motion, 603f
    reflex testing, 608f
Knee-chest position, 567b
Knowledge
    adequacy of, 199
    deficits, 618, 1636–1640
Kohlberg, Lawrence, 363t, 369–370
Korotkoff sounds, 536, 537t
Kripaula, 707
Kübler-Ross, E., 1548

L

Labels, checking, 738
Labia majora, 1607
Labia minora, 1607
Labor Department, U. S., 131
Laboratory studies, 231, 611t, 659b, 853
Labyrinthine sense, 1005
Lacerations, 922f
Lactating women, 1171
Lactic acid, 1115
Laissez-faire leadership, 499
Language. See also Communication; Vocabularies
    assertiveness skills, 456–457, 457t
    assessment of skills, 606–607
    barriers
        to communication, 458–459
        safety issues, 618